PRINCIPLES AND PRACTICE OF PALLIATIVE CARE AND SUPPORTIVE ONCOLOGY

THIRD EDITION

PRINCIPLES AND PRACTICE OF PALLIATIVE CARE AND SUPPORTIVE ONCOLOGY

THIRD EDITION

Editors

Ann M. Berger, MSN, MD

Pain and Palliative Care
Bethesda, Maryland

John L. Shuster, Jr., MD

Clinical Professor of Psychiatry
The University of Alabama
Research Physician
Tuscaloosa Veterans Affairs Medical Center
Tuscaloosa, Alabama

Jamie H. Von Roenn, MD

Professor of Medicine
Division of Hematology/Oncology
The Feinberg School of Medicine
Robert H. Lurie Comprehensive Cancer Center
Northwestern University
Chicago, Illinois

Lippincott Williams & Wilkins
a Wolters Kluwer business
Philadelphia · Baltimore · New York · London
Buenos Aires · Hong Kong · Sydney · Tokyo

Acquisitions Editor: Jonathan W. Pine, Jr.
Managing Editor: Anne E. Jacobs
Project Manager: Alicia Jackson
Manufacturing Manager: Kathleen Brown
Associate Director of Marketing: Adam Glazer
Design Coordinator and Cover Designer: Stephen Druding
Production Services: Laserwords Private Limited, Chennai, India
Printer: Edwards Brothers

© 2007 by LIPPINCOTT WILLIAMS & WILKINS, a Wolters Kluwer business
530 Walnut Street
Philadelphia, PA 19106 USA
LWW.com

1st edition, © 1998 by Lippincott-Raven Publishers, 2nd edition, © 2002 by Lippincott
Williams & Wilkins

Printed in the USA

Library of Congress Cataloging-in-Publication Data

Principles and practice of palliative care and supportive oncology/
  [edited by] Ann M. Berger, John L. Shuster, Jamie H. Von Roenn.
  —3rd ed.
    p. ; cm.
  Includes bibliographical references and index.
  ISBN-13: 978-07817-9595-1
  ISBN-10: 0-7817-9595-8 (alk. paper)
  1. Cancer—Palliative treatment. 2. Cancer—Complications—Treatment. 3. Cancer pain—Treatment. I. Berger, Ann (Ann M.)
II. Shuster, John L., Jr. III. Von Roenn, Jamie H.
  [DNLM: 1. Neoplasms—therapy. 2. Neoplasms—complications.
3. Pain, Intractable—therapy. 4. Palliative Care. QZ 266 P957
2006]
  RC271.P33P75 2006
  616.99′406—dc22

                          2006018686

10 9 8 7 6 5 4 3 2 1

TO OUR SPOUSES AND CHILDREN, WHOSE LOVE
AND SUPPORT MAKE OUR WORK POSSIBLE

CARL, STEPHEN, REBECCA

SUSAN, MARY GRACE, BEN, MOLLY, JOSEPH

KELVIN, ERIKA, ALEXANDER, KARL

CONTENTS

SECTION I: SYMPTOMS AND SYNDROMES

PART A □ PAIN

PART B □ CONSTITUTIONAL SYMPTOMS

PART C □ GASTROINTESTINAL SYMPTOMS AND SYNDROMES

PART D □ SKIN

PART E □ CARDIOPULMONARY AND VASCULAR SYNDROMES

PART F □ GENITOURINARY SYMPTOMS AND SYNDROMES

PART G □ METABOLIC DISORDERS

PART H □ SELECTED NEUROLOGIC SYMPTOMS AND SYNDROMES

PART I □ SELECTED PSYCHIATRIC SYMPTOMS AND SYNDROMES

SECTION II: ISSUES IN PALLIATIVE CARE

PART A □ DEFINITIONS AND MODELS

PART B □ ASSESSMENT ISSUES

PART C □ THERAPIES WITH PALLIATIVE INTENT

PART D □ OTHER ISSUES IN PALLIATIVE CARE

SECTION III: ETHICAL CONSIDERATIONS IN PALLIATIVE CARE

SECTION IV: SPECIAL INTERVENTIONS IN SUPPORTIVE AND PALLIATIVE CARE

SECTION V: SPECIAL POPULATIONS

SECTION VI: RESEARCH ISSUES IN SUPPORTIVE CARE AND PALLIATIVE CARE

Amy P. Abernethy
Duke University Medical Center
Department of Medicine
Division of Medical Oncology and Transplantation
Durham, North Carolina

Richard J. Ackermann, MD
Professor of Family Medicine
Mercer University School of Medicine
Macon, Georgia

Caroline M. Apovian, MD, FACN, FACP
Associate Professor of Medicine
Boston University School of Medicine
Director, Nutrition and Weight Management Center
Boston Medical Center
Boston, Massachusetts

Robert M. Arnold, MD
Professor of Medicine
Chief, Section of Palliative Care and Medical Ethics
Assistant Director
Institute to Enhance Palliative Care
Director, Institute for Doctor-Patient Communication
Leo H Criep Chair in Patient Care
UPMC Montefiore Hospital
Pittsburgh, Pennsylvania

Noreen M. Aziz, MD, PhD, MPH
Senior Program Director
Bethesda, Maryland

James R. Berenson, MD
Chief of Cancer Research
Associate Director of Research
West Los Angeles VA Medical Center
West Hollywood, California

Ann M. Berger, MSN, MD
Pain and Palliative Care
Bethesda, Maryland

Andrea Bezjak, BMed Sc, MDCM, MSc, FRCPC
The Addie MacNaughton Chair
in Thoracic Radiation Oncology
Associate Professor, Department of Radiation Oncology
University of Toronto
Princess Margaret Hospital
Toronto, Ontario
Canada

Julie A. Biller, MD
Associate Professor of Medicine
Division of Pulmonary/Critical Care Medicine
Medical College of Wisconsin
Milwaukee, Wisconsin

J. Andrew Billings, MD
Palliative Care Services
Massachusetts General Hospital
Boston, Massachusetts

Laura Boxley, BA
Department of Psychology
Loma Linda University
Loma Linda, California

Eduardo Bruera, MD
Professor and Chair
Department of Palliative Care and Rehabilitation Medicine
Unit 8
UT M.D. Anderson Cancer Center
Houston, Texas

Robert A. Burt, JD
The Alexander M. Bickel Professor of Law
Yale Law School, Yale University
New Haven, Connecticut

Lisa C. Campbell
Duke University Medical Center
Department of Psychiatry, Pain Prevention and Treatment
Research Program
Durham, North Carolina

Toby C. Campbell, MD
Clinical Fellow
Department of Medicine
Division of Hematology/Oncology
The Feinberg School of Medicine
Northwestern University
Chicago, Illinois

Jennifer Carlson, RN
Director of Program Integrity
Capital Hospice
Fairfax, Virginia

John A. Carucci, MD, PhD
Chief, Mohs Micrographic and Dermatologic Surgery
Weill Medical College of Cornell University
New York, New York

David Casarett, MD, MA
Center for Health Equity Research and Promotion
Philadelphia VA Medical Center
Assistant Professor, Division of Geriatrics
University of Pennsylvania
Philadelphia, Pennsylvania

Barrie R. Cassileth, MS, PhD
Laurance S. Rockefeller Chair in Integrative Medicine
Chief, Integrated Medicine Service
Department of Medicine
Memorial Sloan-Kettering Cancer Center
New York, New York

Nathan I. Cherny, MBBS, FRACP
Director
Cancer Pain and Palliative Care Service
Department of Oncology
Shaare Zedek Medical Center
Jerusalem, Israel

Andrea Cheville, MD
Director of Cancer Rehabilitation
Assistant Professor
University Penn Health System
Philadelphia, Pennsylvania

Eric M. Chevlen, MD
Director of Oncology
Comprehensive Cancer Care of Meadville
Meadville, Pennsylvania

Nicholas A. Christakis, MD, PhD, MPH
Professor of Medical Sociology
Department of Health Care Policy
Harvard Medical School
Boston, Massachusetts

Daniel Y. Chung, MD
Fellow
Division of Gastroenterology, Hepatology and Nutrition
University of Pittsburgh School of Medicine
Pittsburgh, Pennsylvania

Elizabeth J. Clark, PhD, MPH
Executive Director
National Association of Social Workers
Washington, D.C.

Rebecca A. Clark-Snow, RN, BSN, OCN
Research Coordinator
University of Kansas Medical Center
Kansas City, Kansas

James F. Cleary, MB, BS, FRACP, FAChPM
Associate Professor of Medicine
Director of Palliative Medicine
University of Wisconsin Medical School
Madison, Wisconsin

Jeffrey Crawford, MD
George Barth Geller Professor for Research in Cancer
Chief of Medical Oncology
Department of Medicine
Duke University Medical Center
Durham, North Carolina

Shalini Dalal, MD
Assistant Professor
Department of Palliative Care and Rehabilitation Medicine
Houston, Texas

Davey B. Daniel, MD
Fellow, Hematology/Oncology
Duke University Medical Center
Durham, North Carolina

Gary Deng, MD, PhD
Assistant Attending
Integrative Medicine Service
Memorial Sloan-Kettering Cancer Center
New York, New York

Dorothy B. Doughty, MN, RN, CWOCN, FAAN
Emory University WOC Nursing Education Center
The Emory Clinic
Atlanta, Georgia

Alexandra M. Easson, MD
Department of Surgical Oncology
Princess Margaret Hospital
Toronto, Ontario
Canada

Areej Raed El-Jawahri, BS
Harvard Medical School
Boston, Massachusetts

Linda L. Emanuel, MD, PhD
Buehler Professor of Geriatric Medicine
Director, The Buehler Center on Aging
Principal, The Education on Palliative and End-of-life Care
(EPEC) Project
Northwestern's Feinberg School of Medicine
Chicago, Illinois

Jane M. Fall-Dickson, RN, PhD
Investigator, Laboratory of Symptom Management
Bethesda, Maryland

John T. Farrar, MD, PhD
Senior Scholar
Center for Clinical Epidemiology and Biostatistics
University of Pennsylvania
Philadelphia, Pennsylvania

Betty R. Ferrell, RN, PhD, FAAN
Research Scientist
Department of Nursing Research and Education
City of Hope National Medical Center
Duarte, California

Frank D. Ferris, MD
Medical Director
Palliative Care Standards/Outcome Measures
San Diego Hospice and Palliative Care
San Diego, California

Alan B. Fleischer, Jr., MD
Professor and Chair of Dermatology
Wake Forest University School of Medicine
Winston-Salem, North Carolina

Kenneth D. Friedman, MD
Associate Medical Director
The Blood Center of South East Wisconsin
Milwaukee, Wisconsin

Michael K. Gottlieb, JD, MPH
Yale Law School, Yale University
New Haven, Connecticut

Richard E. Greenberg, MD
Chief, Urologic Oncology
Fox Chase Cancer Center
Clinical Professor of Urology
Temple University School of Medicine
Philadelphia, Pennsylvania

James L. Hallenbeck, MD
Assistant Professor of Medicine
Stanford University School of Medicine
Director, Palliative Care Services
VA Palo Alto HCS
Palo Alto, California

Daniel L. Handel, MD
Pain and Palliative Care Service
Bethesda, Maryland

Bruce P. Himelstein, MD
Palliative Care Program
Children's Hospital of Wisconsin
Milwaukee, Wisconsin

Steven J. Hirshberg, MD
Clinical Assistant Professor of Urology
Temple University School of Medicine
Philadelphia, Pennsylvania

Richard B. Hostetter, MD, FACS
Associate Medical Director and Surgical Oncologist
Center for Cancer Care
Goshen Health System
Goshen, Indiana

Jessica Israel, MD
Division Chief, Palliative Care
Monmouth Medical Center
Drexel University College of Medicine
Long Branch, New Jersey

Juan C. Jimenez, MD
Department of Neurosurgery
Rush University Medical Center
Chicago, Illinois

Albert L. Jochen, MD
Associate Professor of Medicine
Endocrinology, Metabolism
and Clinical Nutrition Medicine
Medical College of Wisconsin
Milwaukee, Wisconsin

Ann Marie Joyce, MD
Gastroenterology Department
Lahey Clinic
Burlington, Massachusetts

Javier R. Kane, MD
Associate Member, Department of Oncology
Director, Palliative and End-of-Life Care
St. Jude Children's Research Hospital
Memphis, Tennessee

Joyson Karakunnel, MD
Bethesda, Maryland

Francis J. Keefe, PhD
Duke University Medical Center
Department of Psychiatry, Pain Prevention
and Treatment Research Program
Durham, North Carolina

Dr. Vaughan Keeley, MA, PhD, MRCGP
Consultant/Head of Service
Palliative Medicine
Derbyshire Royal Infirmary
Nightingale Macmillan Unit
Derby, United Kingdom

Philip S. Kim, MD
Medical Director
St. Francis Pain Center
Wilmington, Delaware

Peter Kirkbride, MB, BS, MRCP, FRCR, FRCPC
Joint National Clinical Lead, Radiotherapy, CSC-'IP'
Clinical Director, Radiation Services
Weston Park Hospital
Sheffield, United Kingdom

Kenneth L. Kirsh, PhD
Assistant Professor of Pharmacy
University of Kentucky
Lexington, Kentucky

Joshua C. Klapow, PhD
Associate Professor
Psychology and Health Care Organization and Policy
Center for Outcomes and Effectiveness Research
and Education
University of Alabama at Birmingham
Birmingham, Alabama

Helena Knotkova, PhD
Department of Pain Medicine and Palliative Care
Beth Israel Medical Center
New York, New York

Michael L. Kochman, MD, FACP
Professor of Medicine
Co-Director Gastroenterology Oncology
Gastroenterology Division
Hospital of the University of Pennsylvania
Philadelphia, Pennsylvania

David A. Kunkle, MD
Resident, Department of Urology
Temple University Hospital
Philadelphia, Pennsylvania

Elizabeth Kvale, MD
Assistant Professor of Medicine
University of Alabama at Birmingham
Birmingham, Alabama

Elizabeth B. Lamont, MD, MS
Assistant Professor of Medicine
Massachusetts General Hospital Cancer Center
and Harvard Medical School
MGH—Institute of Technology Assessment
Boston, Massachusetts

Susan A. Leigh, RN, BSN
Cancer Survivorship Consultant
Tucson, Arizona

Jodi Levinthal, MSW
University of Pennsylvania
Philadelphia, Pennsylvania

Randolph J. Lipchik, MD
Professor of Medicine
Pulmonary and Critical Care Medicine
Medical College of Wisconsin
Milwaukee, Wisconsin

Hannah I. Lipman, MD
Hertzberg Palliative Care Institute
Brookdale Department of Geriatrics and Adult Development
Mount Sinai School of Medicine
New York, New York

Nancy W. Littlefield, RN, BSN, MSHA
Chief Clinical Officer/VP of Operations
Capital Hospice
Fairfax, Virginia

Jerilyn A. Logemann, PhD
Ralph and Jean Sundin Professor
Department of Communication Sciences and Disorders
Professor, Departments of Otolaryngology, Head and Neck
Surgery and Neurology
Robert H. Lurie Comprehensive Cancer Center
of Northwestern University
Evanston, Illinois

W. Scott Long, MD
Connecticut Hospice
Branford, Connecticut;
Assistant Clinical Professor
Yale School of Medicine
New Haven, Connecticut

Russell R. Lonser, MD
Staff Neurosurgeon
Bethesda, Maryland

Charles L. Loprinzi, MD
Professor and Chair
Division of Medical Oncology
The Mayo Clinic
Rochester, Minnesota

Matthew J. Loscalzo, MSW
Associate Clinical Professor of Medicine
Hematology-Oncology
Co-Director Palliative Care
Rebecca and John Moores UCSD Cancer Center
La Jolla, California

Matthew Lublin, MD
Southern California Laparoendoscopic Surgery
Thousand Oaks, California

Fade Mahmoud, MD
Community Hospital Medicine Program
Baystate Medical Center
Tufts University School of Medicine
Springfield, Massachusetts

Andrew Mannes, MD
Department of Anesthesia
Bethesda, Maryland

Mary Jane Massie, MD
Attending Psychiatrist
Department of Psychiatry and Behavioral Sciences
New York, New York

Diane E. Meier, MD
Director, Hertzberg Palliative Care Institute
Catherine Gaisman Professor of Medical Ethics
Mt. Sinai School of Medicine
New York, New York

Sebastiano Mercadante, MD
Director, Anesthesia and Intensive Care Unit
and Pain Relief and Palliative Care Unit
La Maddalena Cancer Center
Scientific Director
Home Care Program
SAMOT
Palermo, Italy

Christine Miaskowski, RN, PhD, FAAN
Professor
Department of Physiological Nursing
University of California
San Francisco, California

Kimberly Miller, MD
Fellow, Department of Psychiatry and Behavioral Sciences
Memorial Sloan-Kettering Cancer Center
New York, New York

Darroch W. O. Moores, MD
Clinical Associate Professor of Surgery
Albany Medical College
Albany Cardiothoracic Surgeons, P.C.
Albany, New York

R. Sean Morrison, MD
Hermann Merkin Professor of Palliative Care
Professor of Geriatrics and Medicine
Vice-Chair for Research
Brookdale Department of Geriatrics and
Adult Development,
Mount Sinai School of Medicine
New York, New York

William A. Mourad, MD
Fellow
Gastroenterology and Nutrition Department
Geisinger Medical Center
Danville, Pennsylvania

J. Cameron Muir, MD
Vice President for Medical Services
Capital Hospice and Capital Palliative Care Consultants
Fairfax, Virginia

Ursula S. Ofman, PsyD
Private Practice
New York, New York

Megan Olden, MA
Department of Psychiatry
Memorial Sloan-Kettering Cancer Center
New York, New York

Kaci Osenga, MD
Clinical Instructor
University of Wisconsin Hospital and Clinics
Madison, Wisconsin

Irene M. O'Shaughnessy, MD, FACP
Associate Professor of Medicine
Associate Chief, Department of Endocrinology, Diabetes and Metabolism
Medical College of Wisconsin
Milwaukee, Wisconsin

Jason E. Owen, PhD, MPH
Assistant Professor
Department of Psychology
Loma Linda University
Loma Linda, California

Judith A. Paice, PhD, RN, FAAN
Director, Cancer Pain Program
Division of Hematology-Oncology
Northwestern University
Feinberg School of Medicine
Chicago, Illinois

Marco Pappagallo, MD
Director, Division of Chronic Pain
Department of Pain Medicine and Palliative Care
Beth Israel Medical Center
Manhattan Campus for the Albert Einstein College of Medicine
New York, New York

Gayatri Palat, MD
Associate Professor
Department of Pain and Palliative Medicine
Amrita Institute of Medical Sciences
Kochi, Kerala, India

Steven D. Passik, PhD
Associate Attending Psychologist
Department of Psychiatry and Behavioral Sciences
Memorial Sloan-Kettering Cancer Center
New York, New York

Domingo G. Perez, MD
Minnesota Oncology Hematology, P.A.
Saint Paul, Minnesota

Eugene Perlov, MD
Hospice Team Physician
VNS Hospice
Brooklyn, New York

Rosemary C. Polomano, PhD, RN, FAAN
Associate Professor of Pain Practice—Clinician Educator
University of Pennsylvania School of Nursing
Philadelphia, Pennsylvania

Russell K. Portenoy, MD
Chairman
Department of Pain Medicine and Palliative Care
Beth Israel Medical Center
New York, New York

Laura S. Porter
Duke University Medical Center
Department of Psychiatry, Pain Prevention and Treatment Research Program
Durham, North Carolina

Thomas J. Prendergast, MD
Assistant Professor of Medicine
Dartmouth Hitchcock Medical Clinic
Lebanon, New Hampshire

Holly G. Prigerson, PhD
Director, Center for Psychooncology and Palliative Care Research
Associate Professor of Psychiatry
Brigham and Women's Hospital
Harvard Medical School
Dana-Farber Cancer Institute
Boston, Massachusetts

Christina M. Puchalski, MD, FACP
Director
The George Washington Institute of Spirituality and Health;
Associate Professor of Medicine
The George Washington University
School of Medicine and Health Sciences
Washington, D.C.

Dianna Quan, MD
Assistant Professor of Neurology
Director, Electromyography Laboratory
University of Colorado Health Sciences Center
Aurora, Colorado

Thomas J. Raife, MD
Associate Professor
Medical Director, DeGowin Blood Center
Section Director
Blood Bank/Transfusion Medicine
Head of Hemapheresis Services
Pathology-C250 General Hospital
Iowa City, Iowa

Barry K. Rayburn, MD
Professor and Head
Section of Advanced Heart Failure, Transplantation and Pulmonary Vascular Disease
Birmingham, Alabama

Christine S. Ritchie, MD, MSPH
Director, Center for Palliative Care
University of Alabama at Birmingham
Birmingham, Alabama

Paul Rousseau, MD
Associate Chief of Staff for Geriatrics and Extended Care
Carl T. Hayden Veterans Administration Medical Center
Phoenix, Arizona

John C. Ruckdeschel, MD, FCCP
Director, President and CEO
Barbara Karmanos Cancer Institute
Detroit, Michigan

Juan Santiago-Palma, MD
Orthopedic Associates of Kankakee, S.C.
Bradley, Illinois

Naheel Sorhill, MD
Division of Hematology/Oncology
Department of Medicine
The UT Health Sciences Center at San Antonio
San Antonio, Texas

David A. Sass, MD
Assistant Professor of Medicine
Director of Hepatology Fellowship Program
Division of Gastroenterology, Hepatology and Nutrition
University of Pittsburgh School of Medicine
Kaufmann Medical Building,
Pittsburgh, Philadelphia

Douglas J. Schwartzentruber, MD, FACS
Medical Director
Center for Cancer Care
Goshen Health System
Goshen, Indiana

Peter A. Selwyn, MD, MPH
Professor and Chairman
Department of Family and Social Medicine
Montefiore Medical Center
Albert Einstein College of Medicine
Bronx, New York

Lauren Shaiova, MD
Memorial Sloan-Kettering Cancer Center
Department of Neurology
Division of Pain and Palliative Care
New York, New York

Christopher Sherwood, RN, CHPCN(c)
Palliative Pain and Symptom Management Coordinator
Brant, Haldimand and Norfolk Counties
Haldimand-Norfolk Community Care Access Centre
Simcoe, Ontario
Canada

John L. Shuster, Jr., MD
Clinical Professor of Psychiatry
The University of Alabama
Research Physician
Tuscaloosa Veterans Affairs Medical Center
Tuscaloosa, Alabama

Rebecca G. Smith, MD, MS
Director of the Musculoskeletal Rehabilitation Program
Department of Physical Medicine and Rehabilitation
Moss Rehab
Elkins Park/Einstein
Elkins Park, Pennsylvania

Michael C. Soulen, MD
VIR Fellowship Program Director
Department of Radiology
University of Pennsylvania Medical Center
Philadelphia, Pennsylvania

Barbara A. Supanich, RSM, MD
Fellow, Palliative Medicine
Clinical Ethicist
Mayo Clinic
Jacksonville, Florida

Christopher D. Still, DO, FACN, FACP
Director, Center for Nutrition and Weight Management
Associate, Department of Gastroenterology and Nutrition
Geisinger Health System
Danville, Pennsylvania

James W. Teener, MD
Director, Neuromuscular Program
Department of Neurology
University of Michigan Health Systems
Ann Arbor, Michigan

Joan M. Teno, MD, MS
Professor of Community Health and Medicine
Brown Medical School
Associate Director
Center for Gerontology and Health Care Research
Providence, Rhode Island

Jay R. Thomas, MD, PhD
Clinical Medical Director
San Diego Hospice and Palliative Care
Associate Clinical Professor of Medicine
University of California, San Diego
San Diego, California

Rodney Tucker, MD
Assistant Professor and Medical Director
UAB Center for Palliative Care
Birmingham, Alabama

James A. Tulsky, MD
Professor of Medicine
Director, Center for Palliative Care
Duke University and VA Medical Centers
Durham, North Carolina

Martha L. Twaddle, MD, FACP, FAAHM
Chief Medical Officer
Midwest Palliative and Hospice Care Center
Evanston, Illinois

Mary L. S. Vachon, RN, PhD
Psychotherapist and Consultant
Professor in the Departments of Psychiatry
and Public Heath Sciences
University of Toronto
Clinical Consultant at Wellspring
Toronto, Ontario
Canada

Mary M. Vargo, MD
Staff Physician—PM and R
Assistant Professor, Case Western Reserve University
Department of Physical Medicine and Rehabilitation
MetroHealth Medical Center
Cleveland, Ohio

Charles F. von Gunten, MD, PhD, FACP
Medical Director, Center for Palliative Studies
San Diego Hospice and Palliative Care
San Diego, California

Jamie H. Von Roenn, MD
Professor of Medicine
Division of Hematology/Oncology
The Feinberg School of Medicine
Robert H. Lurie Comprehensive Cancer Center
of Northwestern University
Chicago, Illinois

Sharon M. Weinstein, MD
Associate Professor of Anesthesiology
Neurology and Oncology
Director, Pain Medicine and Palliative Care
Huntsman Cancer Institute, University of Utah
Salt Lake City, Utah

Mary Wheeler, RN, MSN
Clinical Educator, Institute for Education and Leadership
Capital Hospice
Fairfax, Virginia

Barbara J. Whitlatch, BA
Southern California Cancer Pain Initiative
City of Hope Natl. Med. Center
Duarte, California

Rebecca Wong, MD
Leader, Palliative Radiation Oncology Program
Associate Professor
Department of Radiation Oncology, University of Toronto
Princess Margaret Hospital,
Toronto, Ontario
Canada

Howard Su-Hau Yeh, MD
Hematologist and Medical Oncologist
Berenson Oncology
West Hollywood, California

Christopher B. Yelverton, MD, MBA
Department of Dermatology
Wake Forest University School of Medicine
Medical Center Boulevard
Winston-Salem, North Carolina

James R. Zabora, ScD
Dean, Associate Professor
The Catholic University of America
National Catholic School of Social Services
Washington, D.C.

Wendy C. Ziai, MD, FRCPC
Director, Neurovascular Ultrasound Program
Division of Neurosciences Critical Care
Departments of Neurology, Neurosurgery, Anesthesia
and Critical Care Medicine
Johns Hopkins University School of Medicine
Baltimore, Maryland

I like textbooks. I believe that if they are done well, they play an important role in advancing a field and translating advances into clinical practice, which is often underestimated. They can serve as a foundation stone and a launching pad. They provide comprehensive coverage of the subject matter by allowing a practitioner to get his or her arms around and embrace an entire field. There is a lot of comfort in sitting down and reading a text that gives you the confidence of up-to-date and end-to-end coverage. In that sense they are a foundation stone. Good text books also identify areas where there are gaps in information or our understanding of a field, especially a new one, like palliative care medicine, or the application of information, and can stimulate new research or new applications of existing knowledge. In that sense they serve as a launching pad for the generation of new knowledge.

In fact, when editors plan a book they should look at the content of the book in that way, taking care to provide complete coverage by selecting the appropriate subject matter, and also by editing the content for completeness. They should select authors who work at the cutting edge of their fields, who are able to provide a complete and fresh look at the information offered to the reader. Good textbooks are supplemented by current literature but are not replaced by it, because only a small fraction of current literature in any field alters the way medicine is practiced. The editors of this compendium have done all of that and, by my definition, this book is well done, very well done.

I had the pleasure of being present at the birth of the current textbook as I worked with one of the editors, and had the opportunity to discuss the structure of the first edition with her. From the beginning, this text stretched the definitions and concept of palliative care beyond care for the terminally ill and led the way in visualizing palliation as supporting patients with cancer, and their families, from diagnosis to return to a normal life, or to a more comfortable ending to their life. I have to admit I was one of those physicians concerned with focusing on a separate specialty of palliative care. I was worried that some patients would be lost in the crevice between those who focus on treatment and those who are interested in palliation, as new opportunities arose both in treatment and in supportive care. The more comprehensive view of palliative and supportive care in this text is a strong defense against that happening. The first two editions served as the launching pad for the concept of integrating palliative care into the training and thinking of all cancer specialties. As a result, this book should not be viewed as a text only for health care providers who specialize in palliative care but as a text for all health care providers in the cancer field.

This attitudinal change is apparent in the structure of the current edition. What is also apparent, and dictated the need for a fresh look at the field, is that the tools available to palliate and the resources to support patients and their families have increased substantially. An Institute of Medicine report in 2001 suggested more National Cancer Institute involvement in supporting research in this area, and the National Cancer Institute responded by establishing a group called "Partners in Palliative Care" to share strategies and underline NCI's interest in this area of research. As a result, more grant applications have been received and funded, and major foundations have increased their resources in this area and broadened their definitions of palliation. I can't help but believe that this text, in its first two editions, played a pivotal role in providing a working foundation and the awakening of interest in the field, and is now in a position to consolidate that information in launching this, the third edition, in a refreshingly short period of time.

We find ourselves in an extraordinary time in the history of Oncology. As the famous comic strip character, Pogo, said, "We are faced with insurmountable opportunities". New treatments of a wholly different type are being developed against previously unresponsive tumors, national mortality rates have been falling since 1990 coincident with the application of this new information and, in 2005, for the first time, overall deaths from cancer decreased in the US, despite the increased size and age of the US population. Yet the diagnosis of cancer is still a devastating event in the life of a patient and their families, and it is likely to remain that way for some time to come. Cancer doctors, more than ever, need to be complete physicians, and the information provided in this text will go a long way to ensure that it happens.

Vincent T. DeVita, Jr., MD

Much has changed in the time between the publication of the second and third editions of Principles and Practice of Palliative Care and Supportive Oncology. First of all, two of the textbook's editors are new. There are new chapters covering the topics of Epidemiology and Prognosis in Non-Cancer Diagnoses, Management of Hepatic Disease, Hot Flashes, and Starting a Palliative Care Program. Chapters on topics contained in the second edition have been revised and updated.

Our discipline, Hospice and Palliative Medicine is on the verge of formal recognition as a subspecialty by the American Board of Medical Specialties, with accreditation of fellowship training by the Accreditation Council of Graduate Medical Education. Advances in cancer therapies are making supportive care of cancer patients ever more important and integral to good care and favorable outcomes. The knowledge base continues its steady advance. This is an exciting time in our field.

Still, much has stayed the same with the third edition. We have worked to maintain the focus on practical, clinically applicable information informed by up-to-date reviews of research in palliative care and supportive oncology. We continue to emphasize integrated interdisciplinary care, with a special focus on collaboration with the patient and family to shape care that respects and prioritizes the patient's goals, values, and preferences. For those who practice, teach, or perform research in palliative care and supportive oncology, the unique opportunities to blend scientific knowledge with the primary role of the therapeutic relationship, to witness and be inspired by occasions of genuine healing and growth, and to participate in "doctoring" at its most authentic are the special reward of the work. It is our hope that we have captured the essence of this with the text you hold in your hand.

As always, we wish to thank our contributors, without whose efforts this book would not have been possible. We are grateful that they have so generously shared their gifts in these pages. Thanks also go to the publisher and production staff for their diligent efforts in producing this volume. We are also grateful for the patient forbearance of our families, allowing us the time and offering us the support needed to get the work done. Finally, special thanks are due to Zia Raven, Editorial Assistant, whose tireless effort, professionalism, and gentle clarity of focus simultaneously organized and inspired us.

Ann M. Berger, MSN, MD
John L. Shuster, Jr., MD
Jamie H. Von Roenn, MD

The term supportive oncology refers to those aspects of medical care concerned with the physical, psychosocial, and spiritual issues faced by persons with cancer, their families, their communities, and their health care providers. In this context, supportive oncology describes both those interventions used to support patients who experience adverse effects caused by antineoplastic therapies and those interventions now considered under the broad rubric of palliative care. The term palliative is derived from the Latin pallium: to cloak or cover. At its core, palliative care is concerned with providing the maximum quality of life to the patient-family unit.

In 1990, the World Health Organization (WHO) published a landmark document, Cancer Pain Relief and Palliative Care, which clearly defined the international barriers and needs for improved pain and symptom control in the cancer patient. The WHO definition of palliative care is (1)

> The active total care of patients whose disease is not responsive to curative treatment. Control of pain, of other symptoms, and of psychological, social, and spiritual problems is paramount. The goal of palliative care is achievement of the best quality of life for patients and their families. Many aspects of palliative care are also applicable earlier in the course of the illness in conjunction with anti-cancer treatment.

In 1995, the Canadian Palliative Care Association chose a somewhat broader definition that emphasizes a more expanded role of palliative care (2):

> Palliative care, as a philosophy of care, is the combination of active and compassionate therapies intended to comfort and support individuals and families who are living with a life-threatening illness. During periods of illness and bereavement, palliative care strives to meet physical, psychological, social, and spiritual expectations and needs, while remaining sensitive to personal, cultural, and religious values, beliefs, and practices. Palliative care may be combined with therapies aimed at reducing or curing the illness, or it may be the total focus of care.

In developing this textbook, the editors have brought together those elements of palliative care that are most applicable to the health care professional caring for cancer patients, and have combined this perspective with a detailed description of related therapies used to support patients in active treatment. The editors view these interventions as a necessary and vital aspect of medical care for all cancer patients, from the time of diagnosis until death. Indeed, most patients will have a significant physical symptom requiring treatment at the time of their cancer diagnosis. Even when cancer can be effectively treated and a cure or life prolongation is achieved, there are always physical, psychosocial, or spiritual concerns that must be addressed to maintain function and optimize the quality of life. For patients whose cancer cannot be effectively treated, palliative care must be the dominant mode, and one must focus intensively on the control of distressing symptoms. Planning for the end of life and ensuring that death occurs with a minimum of suffering and in a manner consistent with the values and desires of the patient and family are fundamental elements of this care. Palliative care, as a desired approach to comprehensive cancer care, is appropriate for all health care settings, including the clinic, acute care hospital, long-term care facility, or home hospice.

Palliative care and the broader concept of supportive care involve the collaborative efforts of an interdisciplinary team. This team must include the cancer patient and his or her family, care givers, and involved health care providers. Integral to effective palliative care is the opportunity and support necessary for both care givers and health care providers to work through their own emotions related to the care they are providing.

In organizing this textbook, the editors have recognized the important contributions of medical research and clinical care that have emerged from the disciplines of hospice and palliative medicine; medical, radiation, and surgical oncology; nursing; neurology and neuro-oncology; anesthesiology; psychiatry and psychology; pharmacology; and many others. The text includes chapters focusing on the common physical symptoms experienced by the cancer patient; a review of specific supportive treatment modalities, such as blood products, nutritional support, hydration, palliative chemotherapy, radiotherapy, and surgery; and finally, a review of more specialized topics, including survivorship issues, medical ethics, spiritual care, quality of life, and supportive care in elderly, pediatric, and AIDS patients.

There are many promising new cancer treatments on the horizon. No matter what these new treatments will offer in terms of curing the disease or prolonging life, cancer will remain a devastating illness, not only for the affected patients, but for their families, community, and health care providers. Providing excellent, supportive care will continue to be a goal for all health care providers.

The authors would like to thank our many contributors for their efforts. We are also grateful to our publisher and secretaries, whose oversight and gentle prodding were essential to our success. Finally, we want to express our gratitude to our families and colleagues, who accommodated our needs in bringing the volume to fruition and provided the support we needed throughout the process.

Ann M. Berger, MSN, MD
Russell K. Portenoy, MD
David E. Weissman, MD

References

1. World Health Organization. *Cancer pain relief and palliative care*. Technical Report Series 804. Geneva: World Health Organization, 1990.
2. Canadian Palliative Care Association. *Palliative care: towards a consensus in standardized principles and practice*. Ottawa, Ontario: Canadian Palliative Care Association, 1995.

We would like to thank all of the contributors for their tireless effort. We are also very grateful to Zia Raven, whose oversight, gentle prodding, and years of experience were essential to the success of the book. We would like to thank Jonathan Pine and Anne Jacobs for their efforts in helping us get the book completed. We want to express our gratitude to our families and colleagues for their unstinting support for all of our efforts. Finally, we would like to express appreciation to the patients who continuously teach us, and who are the true heroes.

SYMPTOMS AND SYNDROMES

CHAPTER 1 ■ CANCER PAIN: PRINCIPLES OF ASSESSMENT AND SYNDROMES

NATHAN I. CHERNY

Surveys indicate that pain is experienced by 30–60% of patients with cancer during active therapy and by more than two thirds of those with advanced disease (1). Unrelieved pain is incapacitating and precludes a satisfying quality of life; it interferes with physical functioning and social interaction and is strongly associated with heightened psychological distress. It can provoke or exacerbate existential distress, (2) disturb normal processes of coping and adjustment, and augment a sense of vulnerability, contributing to a preoccupation with the potential for catastrophic outcomes. Persistent pain interferes with the ability to eat, sleep, think, and interact with others and is correlated with fatigue in patients with cancer.

The relationship between pain and psychological well-being is complex and reciprocal; mood disturbance and beliefs about the meaning of pain in relation to illness can exacerbate perceived pain intensity, and the presence of pain is a major determinant of function and mood (3).

The high prevalence of chronic pain among patients with cancer, and the profound psychological and physical burdens engendered by this symptom, oblige all treating clinicians to be skilled in pain management (4). Providing relief from pain in patients with cancer is an ethical imperative, and it is incumbent upon clinicians to maximize the knowledge, skill, and diligence needed to attend to this task.

The undertreatment of cancer pain has many causes, among the most important of which is inadequate assessment (5,6). In a study to evaluate the correlation between patient and clinician evaluation of pain severity, Grossman et al. (6) found that when patients rated their pain as moderate to severe, oncology fellows failed to appreciate the severity of the problem in 73% of cases. In studies of pain relief among patients with cancer in the United States (7) and France (8), the discrepancy between patient and physician evaluation of the severity of the pain problem was a major predictor of inadequate relief.

CANCER PAIN SYNDROMES

A woman with breast cancer who presents with shoulder pain may have any one of a number of pain syndromes including postoperative frozen shoulder, taxol- or bisphosphonate-associated proximal myalgias, radiation or malignant upper brachial plexopathy, metastases in the bony structures of the shoulder, impending fracture of the proximal humerus, C4 radiculopathy associated with epidural encroachment or leptomeningeal metastases, hepatic capsular distension, or

a benign pathology unrelated to the cancer. To arrive at an appropriate therapeutic plan, the treating clinician must be aware of the range of possible causes of the pain, their distinguishing clinical features, and efficient diagnostic strategies to isolate the specific cause as quickly and easily as possible. Lack of awareness of the range of diagnostic possibilities may result in undertreatment.

Cancer pain syndromes are defined by the association of particular pain characteristics and physical signs with specific consequences of the underlying disease or its treatment. Syndromes are associated with distinct etiologies and pathophysiologies and have important prognostic and therapeutic implications. Pain syndromes associated with cancer can be either acute or chronic. Whereas acute pains experienced by patients with cancer are usually related to diagnostic and therapeutic interventions (Table 1.1), chronic pains are most commonly caused by direct tumor infiltration. Adverse consequences of cancer therapy, including surgery, chemotherapy, and radiation therapy, account for 15–25% of chronic cancer pain problems, and a small proportion of the chronic pains experienced by patients with cancer is caused by pathology unrelated to either the cancer or the cancer therapy.

CHRONIC PAIN SYNDROMES

Most chronic cancer-related pains are caused directly by the tumor (Table 1.2). Data from the largest prospective survey of cancer pain syndromes revealed that almost one fourth of the patients experienced two or more pains. Over 90% of the patients had one or more tumor-related pains and 21% had one pain or more caused by cancer therapies. Somatic pains (71%) were more common than neuropathic (39%) or visceral (34%) pains (9). Bone pain and compression of neural structures are the two most common causes of chronic pain (10–14).

Bone Pain

Bone metastases are the most common cause of chronic pain in patients with cancer. Cancers of the lung, breast, and prostate most often metastasize to bone, but any tumor type may be complicated by painful bony lesions. Although bone pain is usually associated with direct tumor invasion of bony structures, >25% of patients with bony metastases are pain free (15), and patients with multiple bony metastases

TABLE 1.1

CANCER-RELATED ACUTE PAIN SYNDROMES

Acute pain associated with diagnostic and therapeutic interventions
Acute pain associated with diagnostic interventions
  Lumbar puncture headache
  Transthoracic needle biopsy
  Arterial or venous blood sampling
  Bone marrow biopsy
  Lumbar puncture
  Colonoscopy
  Myelography
  Percutaneous biopsy
  Thoracocentesis
Acute postoperative pain
Acute pain caused by other therapeutic interventions
  Pleurodesis
  Tumor embolization
  Suprapubic catheterization
  Intercostal catheterization
  Nephrostomy insertion
  Cryosurgery-associated pain and cramping
Acute pain associated with analgesic techniques
  Local anesthetic infiltration pain
  Opioid injection pain
  Opioid headache
  Spinal opioid hyperalgesia syndrome
  Epidural injection pain

Acute pain associated with anticancer therapies
Acute pain associated with chemotherapy infusion techniques
  Intravenous infusion pain
    Venous spasm
    Chemical phlebitis
    Vesicant extravasation
    Anthracycline-associated flare reaction
  Hepatic artery infusion pain
  Intraperitoneal chemotherapy abdominal pain
Acute pain associated with chemotherapy toxicity
  Mucositis
  Corticosteroid-induced perineal discomfort
  Taxol-induced arthralgias

Steroid pseudorheumatism
Painful peripheral neuropathy
Headache
  Intrathecal methotrexate meningitic syndrome
  L-asparaginase–associated dural sinuses thrombosis
  Trans-retinoic acid headache
Diffuse bone pain
  Trans-retinoic acid
  Colony-stimulating factors
5-Fluorouracil–induced anginal chest pain
Palmar–plantar erythrodysesthesia syndrome
Postchemotherapy gynecomastia
Chemotherapy-induced acute digital ischemia
Acute pain associated with hormonal therapy
  Leuteinizing hormone–releasing factor tumor flare in prostate cancer
  Hormone-induced pain flare in breast cancer
Acute pain associated with immunotherapy
  Interferon-induced acute pain
Acute pain associated with growth factors
  Colony-stimulating factor–induced musculoskeletal pains
  Erythropoietin injection pain
Acute pain associated with radiotherapy
  Incident pains associated with positioning
  Oropharyngeal mucositis
  Acute radiation enteritis and proctocolitis
  Early onset brachial plexopathy
  Subacute radiation myelopathy
  Strontium 89–induced pain flare

Acute pain associated with infection
Acute herpetic neuralgia

Acute pain associated with vascular events
Acute thrombosis pain
  Lower-extremity deep venous thrombosis
  Upper-extremity deep venous thrombosis
  Superior vena cava obstruction

typically report pain in only a few sites. The factors that convert a painless lesion to a painful one are unknown.

Pathophysiology

Bone metastases could potentially cause pain by any of multiple mechanisms, including endosteal or periosteal nociceptor activation (by mechanical distortion or release of chemical mediators) or tumor growth into adjacent soft tissues and nerves (16). There have been profound changes in the understanding of the physiology of bone pain. As cancer grows in bone, a wide range of inflammatory mediators is released. The cytokine expression of the tumor cells and their interaction with osteoclasts and osteoblasts determine the nature of the lesion (Fig. 1.1). Osteoclast activity is regulated by a complex set of interactions. Activation of the osteoclast receptor nuclear factor-κB (RANK) leads to the downstream activation of nuclear factor-κB receptor ligand (RANKL), which leads to differentiation, activation, and survival of osteoclasts. Opposing this, the osteoblast-expressed protein

osteoprotegerin (OPG), neutralizes RANKL and prevents the activation of RANK (17). Parathyroid hormone (PTH) is involved in this interaction by upregulating RANKL and by inhibiting OPG gene expression. Recently it has been found that myeloma cells directly express RANKL and indicate that specific blockade of RANKL may be an effective treatment for myeloma bone disease (18). Osteoclastic activity has been shown to be increased by the expression of interleukin-6 and parathyroid hormone–related protein by the tumor (19).

Osteoblastic metastases can be caused by tumor-secreted endothelin-1 (ET-1), insulin-like growth factor, and a variety of other potential osteoblastic factors (20). Among these are the osteogenic factors released by the prostate and other cancer types, called *bone morphogenic proteins* (*BMPs*), which are part of the transforming growth factor (TGF)-β family (21–23). Paradoxically, the stimulation of osteoblasts can increase osteoclast function because osteoblasts are the main regulators of bone-destroying osteoclasts. Therefore, the expression of osteolytic and osteoblastic factors can produce mixed metastases or increased osteolysis.

TABLE 1.2

CANCER-RELATED CHRONIC PAIN SYNDROMES

Tumor-related pain syndromes
Bone pain
 Multifocal or generalized bone pain
  Multiple bony metastases
  Marrow expansion
 Vertebral syndromes
  Atlantoaxial destruction and odontoid fractures
  C7-T1 syndrome
  T12-L1 syndrome
  Sacral syndrome
 Back pain and epidural compression
 Pain syndromes of the bony pelvis and hip
  Hip joint syndrome
 Acrometastases
Arthritides
 Hypertrophic pulmonary osteoarthropathy
 Other polyarthritides
Muscle pain
 Muscle cramps
 Skeletal muscle tumors
Headache and facial pain
 Intracerebral tumor
 Leptomeningeal metastases
 Base of skull metastases
  Orbital syndrome
  Parasellar syndrome
  Middle cranial fossa syndrome
  Jugular foramen syndrome
  Occipital condyle syndrome
  Clivus syndrome
  Sphenoid sinus syndrome
 Painful cranial neuralgias
  Glossopharyngeal neuralgia
  Trigeminal neuralgia
Tumor involvement of the peripheral nervous system
 Tumor-related radiculopathy
  Postherpetic neuralgia
 Cervical plexopathy
 Brachial plexopathy
  Malignant brachial plexopathy
  Idiopathic brachial plexopathy associated with
   Hodgkin's disease
 Malignant lumbosacral plexopathy
 Tumor-related mononeuropathy
 Paraneoplastic painful peripheral neuropathy
  Subacute sensory neuropathy
  Sensorimotor peripheral neuropathy

Pain syndromes of the viscera and miscellaneous
 tumor-related syndromes
 Hepatic distention syndrome
 Midline retroperitoneal syndrome
 Chronic intestinal obstruction
 Peritoneal carcinomatosis
 Malignant perineal pain
  Malignant pelvic floor myalgia
 Adrenal pain syndrome
 Ureteric obstruction
 Ovarian cancer pain
 Lung cancer pain
Paraneoplastic nociceptive pain syndromes
 Tumor-related gynecomastia
 Paraneoplastic pemphigus

Chronic pain syndromes associated with cancer therapy
Postchemotherapy pain syndromes
 Chronic painful peripheral neuropathy
 Avascular necrosis of femoral or humeral head
 Plexopathy associated with intra-arterial infusion
 Raynaud's phenomenon
Chronic pain associated with hormonal therapy
 Gynecomastia with hormonal therapy for prostate
  cancer
Chronic postsurgical pain syndromes
 Postmastectomy pain syndrome
 Postradical neck dissection pain
 Post-thoracotomy pain
 Postoperative frozen shoulder
 Phantom pain syndromes
  Phantom limb pain
  Phantom breast pain
  Phantom anus pain
  Phantom bladder pain
 Stump pain
 Postsurgical pelvic floor myalgia
Chronic postradiation pain syndromes
 Plexopathies
  Radiation-induced brachial and lumbosacral
   plexopathies
  Radiation-induced peripheral nerve tumor
 Chronic radiation myelopathy
 Chronic radiation enteritis and proctitis
 Burning perineum syndrome
 Osteoradionecrosis

The presence of bone metastases stimulates an upregulation of peripheral and central neural processes. Immunocytochemical studies from mouse models indicate alterations in the dorsal horn, including astrocyte hypertrophy and upregulation of dynorphin, that are quite different from those seen in inflammatory and neuropathy pains. In addition, *in vivo* electrophysiology of individual dorsal horn neurons have indicated a profound change and increased excitation within superficial and deep laminae (I and V, respectively). Additionally, there is an increase in the proportion of wide dynamic range (WDR) nerves in lamina I; this is correlated with an increased response to electrical and mechanical stimuli and parallels the development of hyperalgesia and allodynia (24).

Differential Diagnosis

Bone pain due to metastatic tumor needs to be differentiated from less common causes, among which the non-neoplastic causes include osteoporotic fractures (including those associated with multiple myeloma); focal osteonecrosis, which may be idiopathic or related to chemotherapy, corticosteroids (25), or radiotherapy (see subsequent text); and osteomalacia (26).

Multifocal or Generalized Bone Pain

Bone pain may be focal, multifocal, or generalized. Multifocal bone pains are most commonly experienced by patients with

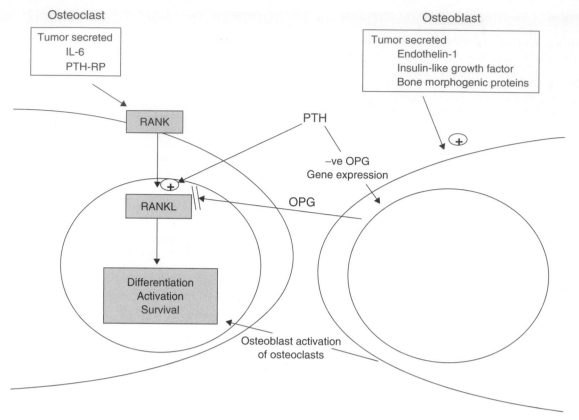

FIGURE 1.1. Tumor interactions with osteoblast and osteoclasts. RANK, osteoclast receptor RANK; RANKL, nuclear factor-κB receptor ligand; OPG, osteoprotegerin; PTH, parathyroid hormone; PTH-RP, parathyroid hormone–related protein; IL-6, interleukin-6.

multiple bony metastases. A generalized pain syndrome is also rarely produced by replacement of bone marrow (27–30). This bone marrow replacement syndrome has been observed in hematogenous malignancies (31–33) and, less commonly, in solid tumors (28). This syndrome can occur in the absence of abnormalities on bone scintigraphy or radiography, increasing the difficulty of diagnosis. Rarely, a paraneoplastic osteomalacia, which is associated with elevated levels of fibroblast growth factor 23 (34), can mimic multiple metastases (35).

Vertebral Syndromes

The vertebrae are the most common sites of bony metastases. More than two thirds of vertebral metastases are located in the thoracic spine; lumbosacral and cervical metastases account for approximately 20% and 10%, respectively (36,37). Multiple-level involvement is common, occurring in >85% of patients (38). The early recognition of pain syndromes due to tumor invasion of vertebral bodies is essential because pain usually precedes the compression of adjacent neural structures, and prompt treatment of the lesion may prevent the subsequent development of neurologic deficits. Several factors often confound accurate diagnosis; referral of pain is common, and the associated symptoms and signs can mimic a variety of other disorders, both malignant (e.g., paraspinal masses) and nonmalignant.

Atlantoaxial destruction and odontoid fracture. Nuchal or occipital pain is the typical presentation of destruction of the atlas or fracture of the odontoid process. Pain often radiates over the posterior aspect of the skull to the vertex and is exacerbated by movement of the neck, particularly flexion (39). Pathologic fracture may result in

secondary subluxation with compression of the spinal cord at the cervicomedullary junction. This complication is usually insidious and may begin with symptoms or signs in one or more extremity. Typically, there is early involvement of the upper extremities and the occasional appearance of so-called pseudo-levels suggestive of more caudal spinal lesions; these deficits can slowly progress to involve the sensory, motor, and autonomic functions (40). Magnetic resonance imaging (MRI) is probably the best method for visualizing this region of the spine (39), but clinical experience suggests that computed tomography (CT) is also sensitive. Plain radiography, tomography, and bone scintigraphy should be viewed as ancillary procedures.

C7-T1 syndrome. Invasion of the C7 or T1 vertebra can result in pain referred to the interscapular region. These lesions may be missed if radiographic evaluation is mistakenly targeted to the painful area caudal to the site of damage. Additionally, visualization of the appropriate region on routine radiographs may be inadequate because of obscuration by overlying bone and mediastinal shadows. Patients with interscapular pain should therefore undergo radiography of both the cervical and the thoracic spine. Bone scintigraphy may assist in targeting additional diagnostic imaging procedures such as CT or MRI that can be useful in assessing the possibility of pain being referred from an extraspinal site, such as the paraspinal gutter.

T12-L1 syndrome. A T12 or L1 vertebral lesion can refer pain to the ipsilateral iliac crest or the sacroiliac joint. Imaging procedures directed at pelvic bones can miss the source of the pain.

Sacral syndrome. Severe focal pain radiating to buttocks, perineum, or posterior thighs may accompany destruction of the sacrum (41). The pain is often exacerbated by sitting or lying down and is relieved by standing or walking (42). The neoplasm can spread laterally to involve muscles that rotate the hip (e.g., the pyriformis muscle). This may produce severe incident pain induced by motion of the hip or a malignant "pyriformis syndrome," characterized by buttock or posterior leg pain that is exacerbated by internal rotation of the hip. Local extension of the tumor mass may also involve the sacral plexus (see subsequent text).

Imaging Investigations of Bone Pain

The two most important imaging modalities for the evaluation of bone pain are plain radiography and nuclear bone scan. In general, CT and MRI are reserved for situations in which the diagnosis cannot be discerned from clinical information and baseline tests in which there are specific diagnostic issues to be resolved that require special techniques.

Plain radiography. Radiography should be the first test ordered to evaluate bone pain and confirm findings of other imaging studies. There are three radiographic patterns of metastatic disease: osteolytic, osteoblastic, and mixed. Osteoblastic areas correspond to the reaction of the host bone to the metastases. This reactive bone forms in a random pattern lacking normal bone structure and often lacking mechanical strength despite its sclerotic, radio-opaque appearance. Lytic lesions with little or no reactive bone formation indicate bone destruction in excess of bone formation. Periosteal thickening or elevation is commonly seen with primary bone neoplasms, rapidly growing tumors, or stress fractures through the underlying bone.

When examining bone radiographs of long bones it is important to evaluate the extent of cortical destruction. The risk of pathologic fracture is high if 50% or more of the cortex is destroyed by the tumor (43–45). Vertebral bodies must be carefully examined for collapse (best viewed on a lateral radiograph) and pedicle erosion (viewed on an anterior/posterior radiograph) because both these findings are associated with enhanced risk of epidural encroachment by tumor.

Bone scan. Technetium bisphosphonate bone scans are valuable in evaluating patients with multifocal pain and in identifying the extent of bony secondaries (46). Three patterns of uptake may indicate bony metastases. The radioisotope most commonly accumulates in the reactive new bone, giving rise to a "hot spot." Less frequently, metastases give rise to cold spots because of the complete absence of reactive bone or poor blood flow (47) or to a pattern of diffuse accumulation of tracer throughout the skeleton (superscan) in the setting of disseminated skeletal disease.

There are several problems associated with bone scans:

1. Bone scans are characterized by high sensitivity and low specificity. Uptake may occur at any skeletal site with an elevated rate of bone turnover in conditions such as trauma (even remote trauma), infection, arthropathy, or even acute osteopenia caused by disuse (46,48–50). Whereas a scan showing multiple lesions strongly suggests metastases, only 50% of solitary foci represents metastases, and in such cases, radiographic correlation is essential.

2. Because bone scans do not evaluate the structural integrity of the bone, positive findings that correspond to painful sites should be further evaluated by plain radiographs, CT scan, or both.

3. There are some situations in which bone scans are notoriously unreliable. Cancers such as melanoma and multiple myeloma may evoke little reactive bone formation, leading to false-negative scans (51–53). In these situations, plain radiography is the preferred initial examination.

Other radionucleotide bone scanning techniques are occasionally used. Single photon emission computed tomography (SPECT) scanning is a bone scanning technique with improved sensitivity and specificity compared to conventional bone scanning (46,54) and conventional positron emission tomography (PET) scanning techniques (55). In patients with diffuse tracer uptake, bone marrow scanning using a tracer linked to antigranulocyte antibody can be helpful in distinguishing a normal scan from a superscan caused by diffuse marrow infiltration (56). Gallium scanning is useful for detecting otherwise undetected bone metastases from lymphomas and soft tissue sarcomas (57).

Computed tomography. CT is a second-tier investigation technique used in the evaluation of bony secondaries. It is effective in evaluating the three-dimensional integrity of bone and to better visualize abnormal lesions identified on bone scan (58). It may be useful in confirming suspicions raised by bone scans and more clearly illustrating the extent of bone destruction. It is particularly helpful in the evaluation of patients with pain in the regions of the pelvic and shoulder girdles and base of the skull who have equivocal or nondiagnostic findings on plain radiography. Spine lesions can also be well visualized by CT using contemporary CT equipment and techniques. The additional yield from MRI is usually very limited.

When confirmation of histologic diagnosis is required, CT-guided biopsy or fine needle aspiration is usually diagnostic (59–61). When the lesion is osteolytic, CT-guided needle biopsy is usually satisfactory (diagnostic accuracy: 80%). When the lesion is osteoblastic or when there is a thick overlying cortical rim, it is extremely difficult to insert a needle and obtain an adequate tissue sample, and such cases may necessitate open surgical biopsy.

Magnetic resonance imaging. MRI is generally reserved for three clinical situations: to arbitrate suspicious lesions that remain ill defined despite plain radiography and CT scan, when bone marrow infiltration is suspected, and in the evaluation of spinal cord compression.

MRI is an excellent method to evaluate bone marrow involvement in diseases such as leukemia, lymphoma, and multiple myeloma that replace the marrow space. Because bone marrow (including hematopoietic or "red" marrow) contains a high percentage of fat, T1-weighted MRI scans generally reveal metastases as focal areas of low signal intensity (62). This approach has also been shown to be very sensitive to solid tumors that metastasize to bone marrow such as breast and lung cancer (63–65).

It is often difficult to distinguish between changes caused by treatment, fracture, and tumor. Indeed, noncontrast MRI cannot reliably distinguish between these changes. In one study the false-positive tumor detection rate was as high as 50% (66). Gadolinium-enhanced bone imaging can be helpful in this situation; tumors commonly demonstrate high or inhomogeneous signal intensity after gadolinium injection, which is not seen in fractures or postoperative changes (67).

Whole body MRI using a moving table has been shown to be an accurate modality for the evaluation of the presence and extent of bony metastases (68,69). Its use in routine practice has not yet been established.

Positron emission tomography ± computed tomography. ^{18}F-Fluoride PET/CT scan has higher sensitivity and specificity than PET scanning alone in detecting bone metastases. This may be a helpful approach in situations in which either CT scan or technetium Tc 99m-methylene diphosphonate bone scintigraphy is inconclusive. In a study, among the 12 patients with bone pain referred for ^{18}F-fluoride PET/CT scan despite negative findings on the Tc 99m-methylene diphosphonate bone scintigraphy, the scan suggested malignant bone involvement in all 4 patients with proved skeletal metastases, a potential benign cause in 4 of 7 patients who had no evidence of metastatic disease, and a soft tissue tumor mass invading a sacral foramen in 1 patient (70).

Back Pain and Epidural Compression

Epidural compression (EC) of the spinal cord or cauda equina is the second most common neurologic complication of cancer, occurring in up to 10% of patients (71). In a large retrospective series, 0.23% of patients with cancer had EC at the presentation of the disease and 2.5% of patients dying of cancer had at least one admission for malignant spinal cord compression (MSCC) in the 5 years preceding their death (72). Breast, lung, and prostate cancers each account for 20–25% of the epidural compression events occurring as complications (72,73). EC is mostly caused by posterior extension of the vertebral body metastasis to the epidural space. Occasionally, EC is caused by tumor extension from the posterior arch of the vertebra or by infiltration of a paravertebral tumor through the intervertebral foramen.

Untreated, EC inevitably leads to neurologic damage. Effective treatment can potentially prevent these complications. The most important determinant of the efficacy of treatment is the degree of neurologic impairment at the time therapy is initiated. Seventy-five percent of patients who begin treatment while they are ambulatory remain so; the efficacy of treatment declines to 30–50% for those who begin treatment while they are markedly paretic and is 10–20% for those who are plegic (74). Despite this, delays in diagnosis are commonplace (75).

Back pain is the initial symptom in almost all patients with EC (71,76), and in 10% it is the only symptom at the time of diagnosis (77). Because pain usually precedes neurologic signs by a prolonged period, it should be viewed as a potential indicator of EC, which can lead to provision of treatment at a time when a favorable response is most likely. Back pain, however, is a nonspecific symptom that can result from bony or paraspinal metastases without epidural encroachment, retroperitoneal or leptomeningeal tumor, epidural lipomatosis due to steroid administration (78), or a large variety of other benign conditions. Because it is infeasible to pursue an extensive evaluation in every patient with cancer who develops back pain, the complaint should impel an evaluation that determines the likelihood of EC and thereby selects patients appropriate for definitive imaging of the epidural space. The selection process is based on symptoms and signs and the results of simple imaging techniques.

Clinical features of epidural extension. Some pain characteristics are particularly suggestive of epidural extension (79). Rapid progression of back pain in a crescendo pattern is an ominous occurrence (80). Radicular pain, which can be constant or lancinating, has similar implications (79). It is usually unilateral in the cervical and lumbosacral regions and bilateral in the thorax, where it is often experienced as a tight, belt-like band across the chest or abdomen (79). The likelihood of EC is also greater when back or radicular pain is exacerbated by recumbency, cough, sneeze, or strain (81). Other types of referred pain are also suggestive of EC, including Lhermitte's sign (82) and central pain due to spinal cord compression, which is usually perceived at some distance below the site of the compression and is typically a poorly localized, nondermatomal dysesthesia (71).

Weakness, sensory loss, autonomic dysfunction, and reflex abnormalities usually occur after a period of progressive pain (79). Weakness may begin segmentally if related to nerve root damage or as a multisegmental or pyramidal distribution if the cauda equina or spinal cord, respectively, is injured. The rate of progression of weakness is variable; in the absence of

treatment, one third of patients will develop paralysis within 7 days of the onset of weakness (83). Patients whose weakness progresses slowly have a better prognosis for neurologic recovery with treatment than those whose weakness progresses rapidly (84,85). Without effective treatment, sensory abnormalities, which may also begin segmentally, may ultimately evolve to a sensory level, with complete loss of all sensory modalities below the site of injury. The upper level of sensory findings may correspond to the location of the epidural tumor or be below it by many segments (79). Ataxia without pain is the initial presentation of EC in 1% of patients; this finding is presumably related to the early involvement of the spinocerebellar tracts (36). Bladder and bowel dysfunction occur late, except in patients with a conus medullaris lesion who may present with acute urinary retention and constipation without preceding motor or sensory symptoms (79).

Other features that may be evident on examination of patients with EC include scoliosis, asymmetrical wasting of paravertebral musculature, and a gibbus (palpable stoop in the spinous processes). Spinal tenderness to percussion, which may be severe, often accompanies the pain.

Imaging modalities. Definitive imaging of the epidural space confirms the existence of EC (and thereby indicates the necessity and urgency of treatment), defines the appropriate radiation portals, and determines the extent of epidural encroachment (which influences prognosis and may alter the therapeutic approach). The options for definitive imaging include MRI, myelography and CT-myelography, or spiral CT without myelographic contrast.

MRI is noninvasive and offers accurate imaging of the vertebrae and intraspinal and paravertebral structures. When available it is generally the preferred mode of evaluation (73). Whenever possible, total spine imaging should be performed because multiple-level involvement is common and other sites may be clinically occult. In a study of 65 patients with cord compression, 32 (49%) showed had multiple-level involvement and of these, 18 (66%) were clinically occult (86). MRI has multiple advantages: metastases can be distinguished from other pathologic processes involving the axial skeleton, epidural and intradural space, and spinal cord. This is particularly true for bacterial abscesses; leptomeningeal carcinomatosis; intradural extramedullary or, rarely, intramedullary metastases or primary tumors; and infectious or inflammatory myelitis.

MRI is relatively contraindicated in patients with severe claustrophobia and certain metallic implants and is absolutely contraindicated for patients with cardiac pacemakers or aneurysm clips. Several other groups who may not be suitable for MRI include very obese patients and those with severe kyphosis or scoliosis.

Previously, myelography was considered the standard examination for imaging the spinal cord (87). In contrast to MRI or CT scan, it is invasive and evaluation may be limited if there is a complete block to the flow of contrast, which precludes the demonstration of the extent of the compressing lesion. It has the advantages of facilitating simultaneous evaluation of the cerebrospinal fluid (CSF) for cytology when leptomeningeal metastases are part of the differential diagnosis.

Postmyelographic CT is a useful tool that provides additional information about the vertebral and paravertebral structures. It can usually define the extent of the cord compression (88) and may help distinguish cord compression caused by displaced bony fragments from soft tissue extension and in the identification of paraspinal tumors with extension through the intervertebral foramina (89).

In addition to immediate patient discomfort, myelography is often complicated by postprocedural side effects that include back pain, headache, vomiting, seizures, and adverse neurobehavioral reactions. The risk of adverse effects is related to the gauge and type of needle used (90), the contrast medium (91), and the anatomy of the EC.

Similar to MRI, CT scanning is noninvasive and provides excellent visualization of the vertebrae, vertebral structural integrity, paravertebral soft tissues, and vertebral foramina. The improved resolution observed with contemporary spiral techniques facilitate clear imaging of the spinal canal contents. Although no comparative data are yet available, in the author's experience, CT scanning of regions identified by either plain radiography or bone scan usually provides excellent visualization of cortical integrity, the intervertebral foramina, and the canal contents. Bone and soft tissue windows are used in a complimentary manner; bone windows allow evaluation of bony integrity and, in particular, cortical breach, while soft tissue windows are used to evaluate the contents of the spinal canal. Using this approach the more expensive and less readily available MRI can be reserved for equivocal cases, when leptomeningeal metastases are suspected, or when total spinal imaging is required.

Algorithm for the investigation of cancer patients with back pain. Given the prevalence and the potentially dire consequences of EC, and the recognition that back pain is a marker of early (and therefore treatable) EC, algorithms have been developed to guide the evaluation of back pain in patients with cancer (Fig. 1.2). The objective of these algorithms is to select a subgroup that should undergo definitive imaging of the epidural space from a large number of patients who develop back pain. Effective treatment of EC before irreversible neurologic compromise occurs is the overriding goal of these approaches.

Pain Syndromes of the Bony Pelvis and Hip

The pelvis and hip are common sites of metastatic involvement. Lesions may involve any of the three anatomic regions of the pelvis (i.e., ischiopubic, iliosacral, or periacetabular region), the hip joint itself, or the proximal femur (92). The weight-bearing function of these structures, which is essential for normal ambulation, contributes to the propensity of the disease at these sites to cause incident pain with ambulation.

Hip joint syndrome. Tumor involvement of the acetabulum or head of the femur typically produces localized hip pain that is aggravated by weight bearing and movement of the hip. The pain may radiate to the knee or medial thigh, and, occasionally, pain is limited to these structures (92,93). Medial extension of an acetabular tumor can involve the lumbosacral plexus as it traverses the pelvic sidewall. Evaluation of this region is best accomplished with CT scan or MRI, both of which can demonstrate the extent of bony destruction and adjacent soft tissue involvement more sensitively than other imaging techniques (94). Important differential diagnoses include avascular necrosis, radicular pain (usually L1), or, occasionally, occult infections (95).

Acrometastases

Acrometastases, metastases in the hands and feet, are rare and often misdiagnosed or overlooked (96). In the feet, the larger bones containing the higher amount of red marrow, such as the os calcis, or talus are usually involved (97,98). Symptoms may be vague and can mimic other conditions, such as osteomyelitis, gouty rheumatoid arthritis, Reiter's syndrome, Paget's disease, osteochondral lesions, and ligamentous sprains.

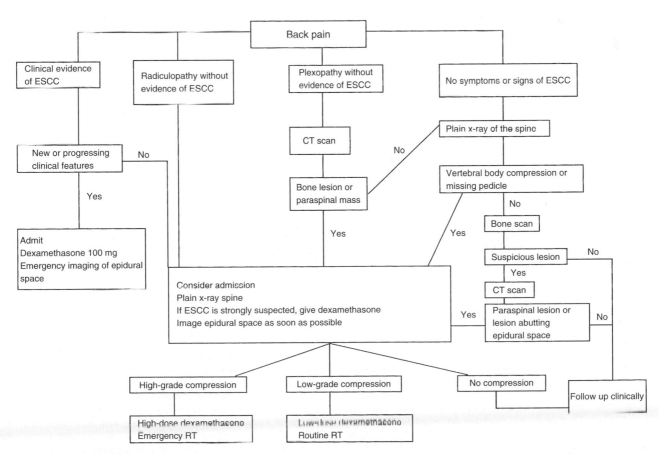

FIGURE 1.2. Algorithm for the management of back pain in a patient with cancer. CT, computed tomography; ESCC, extradural spinal cord compression; RT, radiation therapy.

Arthritides

Hypertrophic Pulmonary Osteoarthropathy

Hypertrophic pulmonary osteoarthropathy (HPOA) is a paraneoplastic syndrome that incorporates clubbing of the fingers, periostitis of long bones, and, occasionally, a rheumatoid-like polyarthritis (99). Periosteitis and arthritis can produce pain, and tenderness and swelling in the knees, wrists, and ankles. The onset of symptoms is usually subacute and may precede the discovery of the underlying neoplasm by several months. It is most commonly associated with non–small cell lung cancer. Less commonly, it mat be associated with benign mesothelioma (100), pulmonary metastases from other sites (101), smooth muscle tumors of the esophagus (102), breast cancer (103), and metastatic nasopharyngeal cancer (104). Effective antitumor therapy is sometimes associated with symptom regression (105). HPOA is diagnosed on the basis of physical findings, radiologic appearance, and radionuclide bone scan (99,106,107).

Other Polyarthritides

Rarely, rheumatoid arthritis, systemic lupus erythematosus, and asymmetric polyarthritis may occur as paraneoplastic phenomena that resolve with effective treatment of the underlying disease (108). A syndrome of palmar plantar fasciitis and polyarthritis characterized by palmar and digital fibromatosis with polyarticular painful capsular contractions, has been associated with ovarian (109), breast (110) and gastric (111) cancers.

Muscle Pain

Muscle Cramps

Persistent muscle cramps in patients with cancer are usually caused by an identifiable neural, muscular, or biochemical abnormality (112). In one series of 50 patients, 22 had peripheral neuropathy, 17 had root or plexus pathology (including 6 with leptomeningeal metastases), 2 had polymyositis, and 1 had hypomagnesemia. In this series, muscle cramps were the presenting symptom of recognizable and previously unsuspected neurologic dysfunction in 64% (27 of 42) of the identified causes (113). Cramps have been reported as an adverse effect of imatinib (114), goserelin (115), and vincristine (116).

Skeletal Muscle Tumors

Soft tissue sarcomas arising from fat, fibrous tissue, or skeletal muscle are the most common tumors involving the skeletal muscles. The skeletal muscle is one of the most unusual sites of metastasis from any malignancy (117,118). The sarcomas occur disproportionately at sites of prior muscle trauma (119). Lesions are usually painless but may present with persistent ache.

Headache and Facial Pain

Headache in the patient with cancer results from traction, inflammation, or infiltration of pain-sensitive structures in the head or neck. Early evaluation with appropriate imaging techniques may identify the lesion and allow prompt treatment, which may reduce pain and prevent the development of neurologic deficits (120).

Intracerebral Tumor

Among 183 patients with new-onset chronic headache as an isolated symptom, investigation revealed underlying intracerebral tumor in 15 cases (121). The prevalence of headache in patients with brain metastases or primary brain tumors is 60–90% (122,123). The headache is presumably produced by traction on pain-sensitive vascular and dural tissues. Patients with multiple metastases and those with posterior fossa metastases are more likely to report this symptom (124). The pain may be focal, overlying the site of the lesion, or generalized. Headache has lateralizing value, especially in patients with supratentorial lesions (125). Posterior fossa lesions often cause a bifrontal headache. The quality of the headache is usually throbbing or steady, and the intensity is usually mild to moderate (125).

Among children, clinical features predictive of underlying tumor include sleep-related headache, headache in the absence of a family history of migraine, vomiting, absence of visual symptoms, headache of <6 months' duration, confusion, and abnormal neurologic examination findings (126).

The headache is often worse in the morning and is exacerbated by stooping, sudden head movement, or Valsalva's maneuvers (cough, sneeze, or strain) (125). In patients with increased intracranial pressure, these maneuvers can also precipitate transient elevations in intracranial pressure called *plateau waves*, which may also be spontaneous and can be associated with short periods of severe headache, nausea, vomiting, photophobia, lethargy, and transient neurologic deficits (127,128). Occasionally, these plateau waves produce life-threatening herniation syndromes (127,128).

Leptomeningeal Metastases

Leptomeningeal metastases, which are characterized by diffuse or multifocal involvement of the subarachnoid space by metastatic tumor, occur in 1–8% of patients with systemic cancer (129). Non-Hodgkin's lymphoma and acute lymphocytic leukemia both demonstrate a predilection for meningeal metastases (129); the incidence is lower for solid tumors alone. Among solid tumors, adenocarcinomas of the breast and small cell lung cancer predominate (130).

Leptomeningeal metastases present with focal or multifocal neurologic symptoms or signs that may involve any level of the neuraxis (129,131,132). More than one third of patients present with evidence of cranial nerve damage, including double vision, hearing loss, facial numbness, and decreased vision (131,132); this is particularly true among patients with underlying hematologic malignancy (132). Less common features include seizures, papilledema, hemiparesis, ataxic gait, and confusion (133). Generalized headache and radicular pain in the low back and buttocks are the most common pains associated with leptomeningeal metastases (132). The headache is variable and may be associated with changes in mental status (e.g., lethargy, confusion, or loss of memory), nausea, vomiting, tinnitus, or nuchal rigidity. Pains that resemble cluster headache (134) or glossopharyngeal neuralgia with syncope (135) have also been reported.

The diagnosis of leptomeningeal metastases is confirmed through analysis of the CSF, which may reveal elevated pressure, elevated protein level, depressed glucose level, and/or lymphocytic pleocytosis. Ninety percent of patients ultimately show positive cytology, but multiple evaluations may be required. After a single lumbar puncture (LP), the false-negative rate may be as high as 55%; this falls to only 10% after three LPs (131,136,137). The sensitivity and specificity of CSF cytology is enhanced by the use of fluorescence *in situ* hybridization (FISH) (138,139) or immunocytochemical techniques (140). Tumor markers, such as lactic dehydrogenase (LDH) isoenzymes (131), carcinoembryonic antigen (141),

β_2-microglobulin (141), and tissue polypeptide antigen (142), may help delineate the diagnosis. Flow cytometry for detection of abnormal deoxyribonucleic acid content may be a useful adjunct to cytologic examination (143).

Gadolinium-enhanced MRI of the neuroaxis can assist in identifying leptomeningeal metastases. When headache is the presenting feature, gadolinium-enhanced MRI examination of the brain is the initial imaging investigation, especially if signs of cranial nerve involvement are present (144,145). If this is nondiagnostic and if the pain distribution indicates spinal involvement, the sensitivity is enhanced by performing an examination of the whole spine. There is evidence that gadolinium-enhanced spinal MRI may be positive in almost 50% of patients without clinical findings related to the spinal region and in 60% of patients with negative CSF cytology (146). Additionally, findings of contrast enhancement of the basilar cisterns, parenchymal metastases, hydrocephalus without a mass lesion, or spinal subarachnoid masses or enhancement may all have therapeutic implications (129).

Untreated leptomeningeal metastases cause progressive neurologic dysfunction at multiple sites, followed by death in 4–6 weeks. Current treatment strategies, which include radiation therapy to the area of symptomatic involvement, corticosteroids, and intraventricular or intrathecal or systemic chemotherapy, are of limited efficacy, and in general, patient outlook remains poor (133,147,148).

Base of Skull Metastases

Base of skull metastases are associated with well-described clinical syndromes (149), which are named according to the site of metastatic involvement: orbital, parasellar, middle fossa, jugular foramen, occipital condyle, clivus, and sphenoid sinus. Cancers of the breast, lung, and prostate are most commonly associated with this complication (149,150), but any tumor type that metastasizes to bone may be responsible. When base of skull metastases are suspected, axial imaging with CT (including bone window settings) is the usual initial procedure (149). MRI is more sensitive for assessing soft tissue extension, and CSF analysis may be needed to exclude leptomeningeal metastases.

Orbital syndrome. Orbital metastases usually present with progressive pain in the retroorbital and supraorbital area of the affected eye. Blurred vision and diplopia may be associated complaints. Signs may include proptosis, chemosis of the involved eye, external ophthalmoparesis, ipsilateral papilledema, and decreased sensation in the ophthalmic division of the trigeminal nerve. Imaging with MRI or CT can delineate the extent of bony damage and orbital infiltration.

Parasellar syndrome. The parasellar syndrome typically presents as unilateral, supraorbital, and frontal headache, which may be associated with diplopia (151). There may be ophthalmoparesis or papilledema, and formal visual field testing may demonstrate hemianopsia or quadrantanopsia.

Middle cranial fossa syndrome. The middle cranial fossa syndrome presents with facial numbness, paresthesias, or pain, which is usually referred to the cheek or jaw (in the distribution of second or third divisions of the trigeminal nerve) (152). The pain is typically described as a dull continual ache but may also be paroxysmal or lancinating. On examination, patients may have hypsthesia in the trigeminal nerve distribution and signs of weakness in the ipsilateral muscles of mastication. Occasionally, patients have other neurologic signs, such as abducens palsy (149,153).

Jugular foramen syndrome. The jugular foramen syndrome usually presents with hoarseness or dysphagia. Pain is usually referred to the ipsilateral ear or mastoid region and may occasionally present as glossopharyngeal neuralgia, with or without syncope (149). Pain may also be referred to the ipsilateral neck or shoulder. Neurologic signs include ipsilateral Horner syndrome, and paresis of the palate, vocal cord, sternocleidomastoid, or trapezius. Ipsilateral paresis of the tongue may also occur if the tumor extends to the region of the hypoglossal canal.

Occipital condyle syndrome. The occipital condyle syndrome presents with unilateral occipital pain that is worsened with neck flexion (154,155). The patient may complain of neck stiffness. Pain intensity is variable but can be severe. Examination may reveal a head tilt, limited movement of the neck, and tenderness to palpation over the occipitonuchal junction. Neurologic findings may include ipsilateral hypoglossal nerve paralysis and sternocleidomastoid weakness.

Clivus syndrome. The clivus syndrome is characterized by vertex headache, which is often exacerbated by neck flexion. Lower cranial nerve (VI–XII) dysfunction follows and may become bilateral (156).

Sphenoid sinus syndrome. A sphenoid sinus metastasis often presents with bifrontal and or retro-orbital pain, which may radiate to the temporal regions (157). There may be associated features of nasal congestion and diplopia. Physical examination is often unremarkable, although unilateral or bilateral sixth nerve paresis can be present.

Painful Cranial Neuralgias

As noted, specific cranial neuralgias can occur from metastases in the base of skull or leptomeninges. They are most commonly observed in patients with prostate and lung cancer (158,159). Invasion of the soft tissues of the head or neck or involvement of sinuses can also eventuate in such lesions. Each of these syndromes has a characteristic presentation. Early diagnosis may allow effective treatment of the underlying lesion before progressive neurologic injury occurs.

Glossopharyngeal neuralgia. Glossopharyngeal neuralgia has been reported in patients with leptomeningeal metastases (135), jugular foramen syndrome (149), or head and neck malignancies (160). This syndrome presents as severe pain in the throat or neck, which may radiate to the ear or mastoid region. Pain may be induced by swallowing. In some patients, pain is associated with sudden orthostasis and syncope (160,161).

Trigeminal neuralgia. Trigeminal pains may be continual, paroxysmal, or lancinating. Pain that mimics classical trigeminal neuralgia can be induced by tumors in the middle or posterior fossa (153,162–164) or by leptomeningeal metastases (134). Sometimes, pain may be caused by perineural spread without evidence of a discrete mass (165). Continual pain in a trigeminal distribution may be an early sign of acoustic neuroma (166). All patients with cancer who develop trigeminal neuralgia should be evaluated for the existence of an underlying neoplasm.

Ear and Eye Pain Syndromes

Otalgia. Otalgia is the sensation of pain in the ear, whereas referred otalgia is pain felt in the ear but originating from a nonotologic source. The rich sensory innervation of the ear derives from four cranial nerves and two cervical nerves that also supply other areas in the head, neck, thorax, and abdomen. Pain referred to the ear may originate in areas far removed from the ear itself. Otalgia may be caused by acoustic neuroma (167) and metastases to the temporal bone or infratemporal fossa (168,169). Referred otalgia is reported among patients with carcinoma of the oropharynx or hypopharynx (170).

Eye pain. Blurring of vision and eye pain are the two most common symptoms of choroidal metastases (171). More commonly, chronic eye pain is related to metastases to the bony orbit, intraorbital structures such as the rectus muscles (172,173), or optic nerve (174).

Uncommon Causes of Headache and Facial Pain

Headache and facial pain in patients with cancer may have many other causes. Unilateral facial pain can be the initial symptom of an ipsilateral lung tumor (175). Presumably, this referred pain is mediated by vagal afferents. Facial squamous cell carcinoma of the skin may present with facial pain due to extensive perineural invasion (176). Patients with Hodgkin's disease may have transient episodes of neurologic dysfunction that has been likened to migraine (177). In some cases this may be a reversible posterior leukoencephalopathy syndrome (RPLS), which is characterized by headache, conscious disturbance, seizure, and cortical visual loss with neuroimaging finding of edema in the posterior regions of the brain (178).

Headache may occur with cerebral infarction or hemorrhage, which may be due to nonbacterial thrombotic endocarditis or disseminated intravascular coagulation. Headache is also the usual presentation of sagittal sinus occlusion, which may be due to tumor infiltration, hypercoagulable state, or treatment with L-asparaginase (179). Headache due to pseudotumor cerebri has also been reported to be the presentation of superior vena caval obstruction in a patient with lung cancer (180). Tumors of the sinonasal tract may present with deep facial or nasal pain (181).

Neuropathic Pains Involving the Peripheral Nervous System

Neuropathic pains involving the peripheral nervous system are common. The syndromes include painful radiculopathy, plexopathy, mononeuropathy, or peripheral neuropathy.

Painful Radiculopathy

Radiculopathy or polyradiculopathy may be caused by any process that compresses, distorts, or inflames nerve roots. Painful radiculopathy is an important presentation of epidural tumor and leptomeningeal metastases (see preceding text).

Postherpetic neuralgia. Postherpetic neuralgia is solely defined by the persistence of pain in the region of a zoster infection. Although some authors use this term if pain persists even after the lesion heals, in most cases a period of weeks to months is required before this label is used; a criterion of pain persisting beyond 2 months after healing of the lesion is recommended (182). One study suggests that postherpetic neuralgia is two to three times more frequent in the cancer population than the general population (183). In patients with postherpetic neuralgia and cancer, changes in the intensity or pattern of pain, or the development of new neurologic deficits, may indicate the possibility of local neoplasm and should be investigated (184).

Cervical Plexopathy

The ventral rami of the upper four cervical spinal nerves join to form the cervical plexus between the deep anterior and lateral muscles of the neck. Cutaneous branches emerge from the posterior border of the sternocleidomastoid. In the cancer population, plexus injury is frequently due to tumor infiltration or treatment (including surgery or radiotherapy) of neoplasms in this region (185). Tumor invasion or compression of the cervical plexus can be caused by direct extension of a primary head and neck malignancy or by neoplastic (metastatic or lymphomatous) involvement of the cervical lymph nodes (185). Pain may be experienced in the preauricular (greater auricular nerve) or postauricular (lesser and greater occipital nerves)

regions or the anterior neck (transverse cutaneous and supraclavicular nerves). Pain may refer to the lateral aspect of the face or head or to the ipsilateral shoulder. The overlap in the pain referral patterns from the face and neck may relate to the close anatomic relationship between the central connections of cervical afferents and the afferents carried in the cranial nerves V, VII, IX, and X in the upper cervical spinal cord. The pain may be aching, burning, or lancinating and is often exacerbated by neck movement or swallowing. Associated features can include ipsilateral Horner syndrome or hemidiaphragmatic paralysis. The diagnosis must be distinguished from EC of the cervical spinal cord and leptomeningeal metastases. MRI or CT scan of the neck and cervical spine is usually required to evaluate the etiology of the pain.

Brachial Plexopathy

The two most common causes of brachial plexopathy in patients with cancer are tumor infiltration and radiation injury. Less common causes of painful brachial plexopathy include trauma during surgery or anesthesia, radiation-induced second neoplasms, acute brachial plexus ischemia, and paraneoplastic brachial neuritis.

Malignant brachial plexopathy. Plexus infiltration by tumor is the most prevalent cause of brachial plexopathy. Malignant brachial plexopathy is most common in patients with lymphoma, lung cancer, or breast cancer. The invading tumor usually arises from adjacent axillary, cervical, and supraclavicular lymph nodes (lymphoma and breast cancer) or from the lung (superior sulcus tumors or so-called Pancoast tumors) (186–188). Pain is nearly universal, occurring in 85% of patients, and often precedes neurologic signs or symptoms by months (187). Lower plexus involvement (C7, C8, and T1 distribution) is typical and is reflected in the pain distribution, which usually involves the elbow, medial forearm, and fourth and fifth fingers. Pain may sometimes localize to the posterior arm or elbow. Severe ache is usually reported, but patients may also experience constant or lancinating dysesthesias along the ulnar aspect of the forearm or hand.

Tumor infiltration of the upper plexus (C5-6 distribution) is less common. This lesion is characterized by pain in the shoulder girdle, lateral arm, and hand. Seventy-five percent of patients presenting with upper plexopathy subsequently develop panplexopathy, and 25% of patients present with panplexopathy (186).

Cross-sectional imaging is essential in all patients with symptoms or signs compatible with plexopathy. Although comparative data on the sensitivity and specificity of MRI and CT scan in evaluating lesions of the brachial plexus is not available, MRI is widely thought to be the best choice for evaluating the anatomy and pathology of the brachial plexus (189,190).

Electrodiagnostic studies may be helpful in patients with suspected plexopathy, particularly when neurologic examination and imaging studies are normal (191). Although not specific for tumor, abnormalities on electromyography (EMG) or somatosensory-evoked potentials may establish the diagnosis of plexopathy and thereby confirm the need for additional evaluation.

Patients with malignant brachial plexopathy are at high risk for epidural extension of the tumor (185,192). Epidural disease can occur as the neoplasm grows medially and invades vertebrae or tracks along nerve roots through the intervertebral foramina. In the latter case, there may be no evidence of bony erosion on imaging studies. The development of Horner syndrome, evidence of panplexopathy, or finding of paraspinal tumor or vertebral damage on CT scan or MRI is highly associated with epidural extension and should lead to definitive imaging of the epidural tumor (185,192).

Radiation-induced brachial plexopathy. Two distinct syndromes of radiation-induced brachial plexopathy have been described: early onset transient plexopathy (see preceding text) and, delayed-onset progressive plexopathy. Delayed-onset progressive plexopathy can occur 6 months to 20 years after a course of radiotherapy that included the plexus in the radiation portal. In contrast to tumor infiltration, pain is a relatively uncommon presenting symptom (18%) and, when present, is usually less severe (186). After supraclavicular node radiotherapy, there is progressively increasing incidence of plexopathy over time, which rises to 56% after 20 years (193). Weakness and sensory changes predominate in the distribution of the upper plexus (C5 and C6 distribution) (194–197). Radiation changes in the skin and lymphedema are commonly associated complications.

On CT scan studies, the typical appearance of radiation fibrosis of the plexus is a diffuse infiltration and loss of tissue planes without a mass lesion (198). There is often associated lymphedema in the arm, which is evident on CT scan, and, occasionally, radiation necrosis of the clavicle or rib or humeral head occurs at the adjacent level (199). Tumor infiltration of the plexus cannot be differentiated from radiation fibrosis by CT scan studies when diffuse infiltration is noted. On MRI, the most common findings observed with radiation fibrosis are thickening and diffuse enhancement of the brachial plexus without a focal mass and/or soft tissue changes with low signal intensity on both T1- and T2-weighted images (190).

Electrodiagnostic studies in patients with radiation fibrosis have been demonstrated to show signs of fibrillation and positive waves associated with denervation. Widespread myokymia is strongly suggestive of radiation-induced plexopathy (200–204). Although a careful history, combined with neurologic findings and the results of tomographic and electrodiagnostic studies, can strongly suggest the diagnosis of radiation-induced injury, repeated assessments over time may be needed to confirm the diagnosis. Rarely, patients require surgical exploration of the plexus to exclude neoplasm and establish the etiology. When caused by radiation, plexopathy is usually progressive (185,205), although some patients plateau for a variable period.

Uncommon causes of brachial plexopathy. Malignant peripheral nerve tumor or a second primary tumor in a previously irradiated site can account for pain recurring late in the course of the patient's illness (206). Pain has been reported to occur as a result of brachial plexus entrapment in a lymphedematous shoulder (196) and as a consequence of acute ischemia many years after axillary radiotherapy (207). An idiopathic brachial plexopathy has also been described in patients with Hodgkin's disease (208).

Lumbosacral Plexopathy

The lumbar plexus, which lies in the paravertebral psoas muscle, is formed primarily by the ventral rami of L1-4. The sacral plexus forms in the sacroiliac notch from the ventral rami of S1-3 and the lumbosacral trunk (L4-5), which courses caudally over the sacral ala to join the plexus (209). Lumbosacral plexopathy may be associated with pain in the lower abdomen, inguinal region, buttock, or leg (210). In the cancer population, lumbosacral plexopathy is usually caused by neoplastic infiltration or compression. Radiation-induced plexopathy also occurs, and occasional patients develop the lesion as a result of surgical trauma, infarction, cytotoxic damage, infection in the pelvis or psoas muscle, abdominal aneurysm, or idiopathic lumbosacral neuritis. Polyradiculopathy from leptomeningeal metastases or epidural metastases can mimic lumbosacral plexopathy.

Malignant lumbosacral plexopathy. The primary tumors most frequently associated with malignant lumbosacral plexopathy include colorectal, cervical, and breast tumors; sarcoma; and lymphoma (188,210). Most tumors involve the plexus by direct extension from the intrapelvic neoplasm; metastases account for only one fourth of the cases. In one study, two thirds of patients developed plexopathy within 3 years of their primary diagnosis and one third presented within one year (210).

Pain is typically the first symptom and is experienced by almost all patients at some point; it is the only symptom in almost 20% of patients. The pain is aching, pressure-like, or stabbing in nature; dysesthesias are relatively uncommon. Most patients develop numbness, paresthesias, or weakness weeks to months after the pain begins. Common signs include leg weakness that involves multiple myotomes, sensory loss that crosses dermatomes, reflex asymmetry, focal tenderness, leg edema, and positive direct or reverse straight leg raising signs.

An upper plexopathy occurs in almost one third of patients with lumbosacral plexopathy (210). This lesion is usually due to direct extension from a low abdominal tumor, most frequently colorectal. Pain may be experienced in the back, lower abdomen, flank or iliac crest, or the anterolateral thigh. Examination may reveal sensory, motor, and reflex changes in a L1-4 distribution. A subgroup of these patients presents with a syndrome characterized by pain and paresthesias limited to the lower abdomen or inguinal region, variable sensory loss, and no motor findings. CT scan may show tumor adjacent to the L1 vertebra (the L1 syndrome) (210) or along the pelvic sidewall, where it presumably damages the ilioinguinal, iliohypogastric, or genitofemoral nerves. Another subgroup has neoplastic involvement of the psoas muscle and presents with a syndrome characterized by upper lumbosacral plexopathy, painful flexion of the ipsilateral hip, and positive psoas muscle stretch test; this has been termed *the malignant psoas syndrome* (211,212). Similarly, pain in the distribution of the femoral nerve has been observed in the setting of recurrent retroperitoneal sarcoma (213), and tumor in the iliac crest can compress the lateral cutaneous nerve of the thigh, producing a pain that mimics meralgia paresthetica (214).

A lower plexopathy occurs in just over 50% of patients with malignant lumbosacral plexopathy (210). This lesion is usually due to direct extension from a pelvic tumor, most frequently rectal cancer, gynecologic tumors, or pelvic sarcoma. Pain may be localized in the buttocks and perineum or referred to the posterolateral thigh and leg. Associated symptoms and signs conform to an L4-S1 distribution. Examination may reveal weakness or sensory changes in the L5 and S1 dermatomes and a depressed ankle jerk. Other findings include leg edema, bladder or bowel dysfunction, sacral or sciatic notch tenderness, and a positive straight leg raising test. A pelvic mass may be palpable.

Sacral plexopathy may occur from direct extension of a sacral lesion or a presacral mass (42). This may present with predominant involvement of the lumbosacral trunk, characterized by numbness over the dorsal medial foot and sole and weakness of knee flexion, ankle dorsiflexion, and inversion. Other patients demonstrate particular involvement of the coccygeal plexus, with prominent sphincter dysfunction and perineal sensory loss. The latter syndrome occurs with low pelvic tumors, such as those arising from the rectum or prostate.

A panplexopathy with involvement of a L1-S3 distribution occurs in almost one fifth of patients with lumbosacral plexopathy (210). Local pain may occur in the lower abdomen, back, buttocks, or perineum. Referred pain can be experienced anywhere in the distribution of the plexus. Leg edema is extremely common. Neurologic deficits may be confluent or patchy within the L1-S3 distribution and a positive straight leg raising test is usually present.

Autonomic dysfunction, particularly anhydrosis and vasodilation, has been associated with plexus and peripheral nerve injuries. Focal autonomic neuropathy, which may suggest the anatomic localization of the lesion (215), has been reported as the presenting symptom of metastatic lumbosacral plexopathy (216).

Cross-sectional imaging, with either CT or MRI, is the preferred diagnostic procedure for the evaluation of lumbosacral plexopathy. Scanning should be done from the level of the L1 vertebral body through the sciatic notch. When using CT scanning techniques, images should include bone and soft tissue windows. Limited data suggests superior sensitivity of MRI over CT scan (217). Definitive imaging of the epidural space adjacent to the plexus should be considered in a patient who has features indicative of a relatively high risk of epidural extension including bilateral symptoms or signs, unexplained incontinence, or a prominent paraspinal mass (192,210).

Radiation-induced lumbosacral plexopathy. Radiation fibrosis of the lumbosacral plexus is a rare complication that may occur from 1 to over 30 years after radiation treatment. The use of intracavitary radium implants for carcinoma of the cervix may be an additional risk factor (218,219). Radiation-induced plexopathy typically presents with progressive weakness and leg swelling; pain is not usually a prominent feature (218,220). Weakness typically begins distally in the L5-S1 segments and is slowly progressive. The symptoms and signs may be bilateral (220). If CT scanning demonstrates a lesion, it is usually a nonspecific diffuse infiltration of the tissues. EMG may show myokymic discharges (220).

Uncommon causes of lumbosacral plexopathy. Lumbosacral plexopathy may occur after intra-arterial cis-platinum infusion (see subsequent text) and embolization techniques. This syndrome has been observed after attempted embolization of a bleeding rectal lesion. Benign conditions that may produce similar findings include hemorrhage or abscess in the iliopsoas muscle (209), abdominal aortic aneurysms, diabetic radiculoplexopathy, vasculitis, and an idiopathic lumbosacral plexitis analogous to acute brachial neuritis (209).

Painful Mononeuropathy

Tumor-Related Mononeuropathy. Tumor-related mononeuropathy usually results from compression or infiltration of a nerve from a tumor arising in an adjacent bony structure. The most common example of this phenomenon is intercostal nerve injury in a patient with rib metastases. Constant burning pain and other dysesthesias in the area of sensory loss are the typical clinical presentation. Other examples include the cranial neuralgias described previously, sciatica associated with tumor invasion of the sciatic notch, and common peroneal nerve palsy associated with primary bone tumors of the proximal fibula and lateral cutaneous nerve of the thigh neuralgia associated with iliac crest tumors.

Other causes of mononeuropathy. Patients with cancer also develop mononeuropathies because of many other causes. Postsurgical syndromes are well described (see subsequent text), and radiation injury of a peripheral nerve occurs occasionally. Rarely, patients with cancer develop nerve entrapment syndromes (such as carpal tunnel syndrome) related to edema or direct compression by tumor (221).

Painful Peripheral Neuropathies

Painful peripheral neuropathies have multiple causes, including nutritional deficiencies, other metabolic derangements (e.g., diabetes and renal dysfunction), neurotoxic effects of chemotherapy, and, rarely, paraneoplastic syndromes.

Paraneoplastic painful peripheral neuropathy. Paraneoplastic painful peripheral neuropathy can be related to injury to the dorsal root ganglion (also known as *subacute sensory neuronopathy* or *ganglionopathy*) or the peripheral nerves (222). These syndromes may be the initial manifestation of an underlying malignancy. Except for the neuropathy associated with myeloma (223,224), their course is usually independent of the primary tumor (222,225).

Subacute sensory neuronopathy is characterized by pain (usually dysesthetic), paresthesias, sensory loss in the extremities, and severe sensory ataxia (226). Although it is usually associated with small cell carcinoma of the lung (227), other tumor types, including breast cancer (228), Hodgkin's disease (229), and varied solid tumors, are rarely associated. Both constant and lancinating dysesthesias occur and typically predate other symptoms. Neuropathic symptoms (e.g., pain, paresthesia, and sensory loss) are asymmetric at onset, with a predilection for the upper limbs. Indeed, in one instance a painful bilateral ulnar neuropathy has been described (230). The pain usually develops before the tumor is evident, and its course is typically independent. Coexisting autonomic, cerebellar, or cerebral abnormalities are common (226). The syndrome, which results from an inflammatory process involving the dorsal root ganglia, may be part of a more diffuse autoimmune disorder that can affect the limbic region, brainstem, and spinal cord (225,226,231). An antineuronal immunoglobulin G antibody ("anti-Hu"), which recognizes a low-molecular-weight protein present in most small cell lung carcinomas, has been associated with this condition (225). Recently, a number of other paraneoplastic antibodies have been identified, including anti-CV2 (232) and anti-Ri (233).

A sensorimotor peripheral neuropathy, which may be painful, has been observed in association with diverse neoplasms, particularly Hodgkin's disease and paraproteinemias (234). The peripheral neuropathies associated with multiple myeloma, Waldenström's macroglobulinemia, small-fiber amyloid neuropathy, and osteosclerotic myeloma are thought to be due to antibodies that cross-react with constituents of the peripheral nerves (234,235). Clinically evident peripheral neuropathy occurs in approximately 15% of patients with multiple myeloma, and electrophysiologic evidence of this lesion can be found in 40% (224). The pathophysiology of the neuropathy is unknown.

Pain Syndromes of the Viscera and Miscellaneous Tumor-Related Syndromes

Pain may be caused by pathology involving the luminal organs of the gastrointestinal or genitourinary tracts, the parenchymal organs, the peritoneum, or the retroperitoneal soft tissues. Obstruction of hollow viscus, including intestine, biliary tract, and ureter, produces visceral nociceptive syndromes that are well described in the surgical literature (236). Pain arising from retroperitoneal and pelvic lesions may involve mixed nociceptive and neuropathic mechanisms if both somatic structures and nerves are involved.

Hepatic Distention Syndrome

Pain-sensitive structures in the region of the liver include the liver capsule, blood vessels, and biliary tract (237). Nociceptive afferents that innervate these structures travel through the celiac plexus, the phrenic nerve, and the lower right intercostal nerves. Extensive intrahepatic metastases, or gross hepatomegaly associated with cholestasis, may produce discomfort in the right subcostal region, and less commonly in the right mid-back or flank (237–240). Referred pain may be experienced in the right neck or shoulder or in the region of the right scapula (238). The pain, usually described as a dull ache, may be exacerbated by movement, pressure in the abdomen, and deep inspiration. Pain is commonly accompanied by symptoms of anorexia and nausea (240). Physical examination may reveal a hard irregular subcostal mass that descends with respiration and is dull to percussion. Other features of hepatic failure may be present. Imaging of the hepatic parenchyma by either ultrasound or CT will usually identify the presence of space-occupying lesions or cholestasis.

Occasional patients who experience chronic pain because of hepatic distension develop an acute intercurrent subcostal pain that may be exacerbated by respiration. Physical examination may demonstrate a palpable or audible rub. These findings suggest the development of an overlying peritonitis, which can develop in response to some acute event, such as a hemorrhage into a metastasis (241).

Midline Retroperitoneal Syndrome

Retroperitoneal pathology involving the upper abdomen may produce pain by injury to deep somatic structures of the posterior abdominal wall, distortion of pain-sensitive connective tissue, vascular and ductal structures, local inflammation, and direct infiltration of the celiac plexus. The most common causes are pancreatic cancer (242–244) and retroperitoneal lymphadenopathy (245–247), particularly celiac lymphadenopathy (248). The reasons for the high frequency of perineural invasion and the presence of pain in pancreatic cancer may be related to the locoregional secretion and activation of growth factor [nerve growth factor (NGF)] and its high-affinity receptor TrkA. These factors are involved in stimulating epithelial cancer cell growth and perineural invasion (249).

In some instances of pancreatic cancer, obstruction of the main pancreatic duct with subsequent ductal hypertension generates pain, which can be relieved by stenting of the pancreatic duct (250).

The pain is experienced in the epigastrium, the low thoracic region of the back, or both locations. It is often diffuse and poorly localized and usually dull and boring in character, exacerbated with recumbency and improved by sitting. The lesion can usually be demonstrated by CT scan, MRI, or ultrasound of the upper abdomen.

Intestinal Obstruction

Abdominal pain is an almost invariable manifestation of intestinal obstruction, which may occur in patients with abdominal or pelvic cancers (251). The factors that contribute to this pain include smooth muscle contractions, mesenteric tension, and mural ischemia. Obstructive symptoms may be due primarily to the tumor or, more likely, due to a combination of mechanical obstruction and other processes, such as autonomic neuropathy and ileus caused by metabolic derangements or drugs. Both continuous and colicky pains occur, which may be referred to the dermatomes represented by the spinal segments supplying the affected viscera. Vomiting, anorexia, and constipation are important associated symptoms.

Peritoneal Carcinomatosis

Peritoneal carcinomatosis occurs most often by the transcelomic spread of abdominal or pelvic tumor; except breast cancer, the hematogenous spread of an extraabdominal neoplasm in this pattern is rare. Carcinomatosis can cause peritoneal inflammation, mesenteric tethering, malignant adhesions, and ascites, all of which can cause pain. Pain and abdominal distension are the most common presenting symptoms. Mesenteric tethering and tension appear to cause a diffuse abdominal or low back pain. Tense malignant ascites can produce diffuse abdominal discomfort and a distinct stretching pain in the anterior abdominal wall. Adhesions

can also cause obstruction of hollow viscus, with intermittent colicky pain (252). CT scanning may demonstrate evidence of ascites, omental infiltration, and peritoneal nodules (253).

Malignant Perineal Pain

Tumors of the colon or rectum, female reproductive tract, and distal genitourinary system are most commonly responsible for perineal pain (254–258). Severe perineal pain after antineoplastic therapy may precede the indications of detectable disease and should be viewed as a potential harbinger of progressive or recurrent cancer (254,255,258). There is evidence to suggest that this phenomenon is caused by microscopic perineural invasion by recurrent disease (259). The pain, which is typically described as constant and aching, is often aggravated by sitting or standing and may be associated with tenesmus or bladder spasms (254).

Tumor invasion of the musculature of the deep pelvis can also result in a syndrome that appears similar to the so-called tension myalgia of the pelvic floor (260). The pain is typically described as a constant ache or heaviness that exacerbates with upright posture. When caused by tumor, the pain may be concurrent with other types of perineal pain. Digital examination of the pelvic floor may reveal local tenderness or palpable tumor.

Adrenal Pain Syndrome

Large adrenal metastases, a common lung cancer, may produce unilateral flank pain and, less commonly, abdominal pain. The pain is of variable severity and can be severe (261). Adrenal metastases can be complicated by hemorrhage, which may cause severe abdominal pain (262).

Ureteric Obstruction

Ureteric obstruction is most frequently caused by tumor compression or infiltration within the true pelvis (263,264). Less commonly, the obstruction can be more proximal, associated with retroperitoneal lymphadenopathy, and an isolated retroperitoneal metastasis, mural metastases, or intraluminal metastases. Cancers of the cervix, ovary, prostate, and rectum are most commonly associated with this complication. Nonmalignant causes, including retroperitoneal fibrosis resulting from radiotherapy or graft versus host disease, are rare (265–267).

Pain may or may not accompany ureteric obstruction. When present, it is typically a dull chronic discomfort in the flank, radiating to the inguinal region or genitalia (268). If pain does not occur, ureteric obstruction may be discovered when hydronephrosis is discerned on abdominal imaging procedures or when renal failure develops. Ureteric obstruction can be complicated by pyelonephritis or pyonephrosis, which often presents with features of sepsis, loin pain, and dysuria. Diagnosis of ureteric obstruction can usually be confirmed by the demonstration of hydronephrosis on renal sonography. The level of obstruction can be identified by pyelography, and CT scanning techniques will usually demonstrate the cause (264).

Ovarian Cancer Pain

Moderate to severe chronic abdominopelvic pain is the most common symptom of ovarian cancer; it is reported by almost two thirds of patients in the 2 weeks' duration before the onset or recurrence of the disease (269). Pain is experienced in the low back or abdomen (270,271). In patients who have been previously treated it is an important symptom of potential recurrence (269).

Lung Cancer Pain

Even in the absence of involvement of the chest wall or parietal pleura, lung tumors can produce a visceral pain syndrome. In a large case series of patients with lung cancer, pain was unilateral in 80% of the cases and bilateral in 20%. Among patients with hilar tumors, the pain was reported to the sternum or the scapula. Upper and lower lobe tumors were referred to the shoulder and the lower chest, respectively (272,273). As previously mentioned, early lung cancers can generate ipsilateral facial pain (175). It is postulated that this pain syndrome is generated by vagal afferent neurons.

Other Uncommon Visceral Pain Syndromes

Sudden-onset severe abdominal or loin pain may be caused by nontraumatic rupture of a visceral tumor. This has been most frequently reported with hepatocellular cancer (274) but also with other liver metastases (275). Kidney rupture due to a renal metastasis from an adenocarcinoma of the colon (276), splenic rupture in acute leukemia (277), rupture of adrenocortical cancers (278), and metastasis-induced perforated appendicitis (279) have been reported. Torsion of pedunculated visceral tumors can produce a cramping abdominal pain (280–282).

Paraneoplastic Nociceptive Pain Syndromes

Tumor-related gynecomastia

Tumors that secrete human chorionic gonadotrophin (HCG), including malignant and benign tumors of the testis (283–285) and, rarely, cancers from other sites (286–288), may be associated with chronic breast tenderness or gynecomastia. Approximately 10% of patients with testis cancer have gynecomastia or breast tenderness at presentation, and the likelihood of gynecomastia is greater with increasing HCG level (289). Breast pain can be the first presentation of an occult tumor (290–292).

Paraneoplastic Pemphigus

Paraneoplastic pemphigus is a rare mucocutaneous disorder associated with non-Hodgkin's lymphoma and chronic lymphocytic leukemia. The condition is characterized by widespread shallow ulcers with hemorrhagic crusting of the lips, conjunctival bullae and, uncommonly, pulmonary lesions. Characteristically, histopathology reveals intraepithelial and subepithelial clefting and immunoprecipitation studies reveal autoantibodies directed against desmoplakins and desmogleins (293,294).

Paraneoplastic Raynaud's Syndrome

Paraneoplastic Raynaud's syndrome is a rare manifestation of solid tumors. It has been reported with lung cancer, ovarian cancer, testicular cancer, and melanoma (295–297).

Chronic Pain Syndromes Associated with Cancer Therapy

Most treatment-related pains are caused by tissue-damaging procedures. These pains are acute, predictable, and self-limited. Chronic treatment-related pain syndromes are associated with either a persistent nociceptive complication of an invasive treatment (such as a postsurgical abscess) or, more commonly, neural injury. In some cases, these syndromes occur long after the therapy is completed, resulting in a difficult differential diagnosis between recurrent disease and a complication of therapy.

Postchemotherapy Pain Syndromes

Chronic painful peripheral neuropathy: toxic peripheral neuropathy. Chemotherapy-induced peripheral neuropathy is a common problem, which is typically manifested by painful paresthesias in the hands and/or feet and signs consistent with an axonopathy, including "stocking-glove" sensory loss, weakness, hyporeflexia, and autonomic dysfunction (298). The pain is usually characterized by continuous burning or lancinating pains, either of which may be increased by contact. The drugs most commonly associated with a peripheral neuropathy are the vinca alkaloids (especially vincristine) (299,300), cis-platinum (301,302), and oxaliplatin (303). Paclitaxel-associated peripheral neuropathy is common but is generally transient and self-limiting (304). Procarbazine, carboplatin, misonidazole, and hexamethylmelamine have also been implicated as causes for this syndrome (305,306). Data from several studies indicate that the risk of neuropathy associated with cis-platinum and oxaliplatin can be diminished by amifostine (307,308), glutathione (309,310), and calcium and magnesium infusion at the time of treatment (311).

Avascular (aseptic) necrosis of femoral or humeral head. Avascular necrosis of the femoral or humeral head may occur either spontaneously or as a complication of intermittent or continuous corticosteroid therapy (312,313) or high-dose chemotherapy with bone marrow transplantation (314). Osteonecrosis may be unilateral or bilateral. Involvement of the femoral head is most common and typically causes pain in the hip, thigh, or knee. Involvement of the humeral head usually presents as pain in the shoulder, upper arm, or elbow. Pain is exacerbated by movement and relieved by rest. There may be local tenderness over the joint, but this is not universal. Pain usually precedes radiologic changes by weeks to months; bone scintigraphy and MRI are sensitive and complementary diagnostic procedures. For the detection of radiographically occult avascular necrosis, radionuclide bone scanning and MRI are both sensitive methods, but MRI is preferred because it has greater sensitivity and specificity than bone scanning (315). Early treatment consists of analgesics, decrease in or discontinuation of steroids, and sometimes surgery. With progressive bone destruction, joint replacement may be necessary.

Plexopathy. Lumbosacral or brachial plexopathy may follow cis-platinum infusion into the iliac artery (316) or axillary artery (317), respectively. Affected patients develop pain, weakness, and paresthesias within 48 hours of the infusion. The mechanism for this syndrome is thought to be small vessel damage and infarction of the plexus or nerve. The prognosis for neurologic recovery is not known.

Raynaud's phenomenon. Among patients with germ cell tumors treated with cisplatin, vinblastine, and bleomycin, persistent Raynaud's phenomenon is observed in 20–30% (318). This effect has also been observed in patients with carcinoma of the head and neck who are treated with a combination of cisplatin, vincristine, and bleomycin (319). Pathophysiologic studies have demonstrated that hyperreactivity in the central sympathetic nervous system results in reduced functioning of the smooth muscle cells in the terminal arterioles (320).

Chronic Pain Associated with Hormonal Therapy

Gynecomastia with hormonal therapy for prostate cancer. Chronic gynecomastia and breast tenderness are common complications of antiandrogen therapies for prostate cancer (321). The incidence of this syndrome depends on the nature of the drugs; it is frequently associated with diethyl stilbestrol (322) and bicalutamide (323), is less common with flutamide (324) and cyproterone (325), and is uncommon among patients receiving luteinizing hormone–releasing hormone (LHRH) agonist therapy (326,327). Gynecomastia in the elderly must be distinguished from primary breast cancer or a secondary cancer in the breast (328,329).

Chronic Postsurgical Pain Syndromes

Surgical incision at virtually any location may result in chronic pain. Although persistent pain is occasionally encountered after nephrectomy, sternotomy, craniotomy, inguinal dissection, and other procedures, these pain syndromes are not well described in the cancer population. In contrast, several syndromes are now clearly recognized as sequelae to specific surgical procedures. The predominant underlying pain mechanism in these syndromes is neuropathic, resulting from injury to peripheral nerves or plexus.

Breast surgery pain syndromes. Chronic pain of variable severity is a common sequel of breast cancer surgery. Although chronic pain has been reported to occur after almost any surgical procedure on the breast (from lumpectomy to radical mastectomy), it is most common after procedures involving axillary dissection (196,330–332). This is a common pain syndrome after axillary lymph node dissection, occurring in 30–70% of patients (330,333–340).

The pain is usually characterized as a constricting and burning discomfort localized to the medial arm, axilla, and anterior chest wall (332,341–344). Pain may begin immediately or as late as many months after surgery. The natural history of this condition appears to be variable, and both subacute and chronic courses are possible (345,346). The onset of pain later than 18 months after surgery is unusual, and a careful evaluation to exclude recurrent chest wall disease is recommended in this setting. On examination, there is often an area of sensory loss within the region of the pain (343). Chronicity of pain is related to the intensity of the immediate postoperative pain (337,347), postoperative complications, and subsequent treatment with chemotherapy and radiotherapy (338). In many cases, pain is chronic and persists over many years (348).

It is most commonly associated with neuropraxia of the intercostobrachial nerve during the process of axillary lymph node dissection (332,343,349). There is marked anatomic variation in the size and distribution of the intercostobrachial nerve, and this may account for some of the variability in the distribution of pain observed in patients with this condition (350). Careful preservation of the nerve at the time of dissection may reduce the prevalence and severity of subsequent pain (351). In some cases pain may be caused by hematoma in the axilla (352).

The risk for, and severity of, pain is correlated positively with the number of lymph nodes removed (353,354) and is inversely correlated with age (336,339,353). There is conflicting data about whether preservation of the intercostobrachial nerve during axillary lymph node dissection can reduce the incidence of this phenomenon (355,356). The incidence is reduced when axillary dissection is avoided either by sentinel node excision without full dissection (357–362) or when nodes are irradiated without dissection (363).

This syndrome must be differentiated from postmastectomy frozen shoulder (364,365), axillary web syndrome (366), and breast cellulitis (367). In some cases of pain after breast surgery, a trigger point can be palpated in the axilla or chest wall.

Postradical neck dissection pain. Chronic neck and shoulder pain after radical neck dissection is common (368). Shoulder pain is most often caused by damage to the spinal accessory nerve (CN XI) (369). In other cases it can result from musculoskeletal imbalance in the shoulder girdle after surgical removal of neck muscles (370). Similar to the droopy shoulder syndrome (371), this syndrome can be complicated by the development of a thoracic outlet syndrome or suprascapular nerve entrapment, with selective weakness and wasting of the supraspinatus and infraspinatus muscles (372). Data from a large survey demonstrated that neck dissections sparing CN XI, and not dissecting level V of the neck when CN XI is spared, are associated with less shoulder and neck pain (373).

Escalating pain in patients who have undergone radical neck dissection may signify recurrent tumor or soft tissue infection. These lesions may be difficult to diagnose in tissues damaged by radiation and surgery. Repeated CT scan or MRI may be needed to exclude tumor recurrence. Empiric treatment with antibiotics should be considered (374,375).

Post-thoracotomy pain. There have been two major studies on post-thoracotomy pain (376,377). In the first study (377), three groups were identified: the largest (63%) had prolonged postoperative pain that abated within 2 months of surgery. Recurrent pain, after resolution of the postoperative pain, was usually due to neoplasm. The second group (16%) experienced pain that persisted after the thoracotomy and then increased in intensity during the follow-up period. Local recurrence of disease and infection was the most common cause of the increasing pain. The final group had a prolonged period of stable or decreasing pain that gradually resolved over a maximum period of 8 months. This pain was not associated with tumor recurrence. Overall, the development of late or increasing post-thoracotomy pain was due to recurrent or persistent tumor in >95% of patients. This finding was corroborated in a more recent study evaluating the records of 238 consecutive patients who underwent thoracotomy, which identified recurrent pain in 20 patients, all of whom were found to have tumor regrowth (376).

Patients with recurrent or increasing post-thoracotomy pain should be carefully evaluated, preferably with a chest CT scan or MRI. Chest radiographs are insufficient to evaluate recurrent chest disease. In some patients, post-thoracotomy pain appears to be caused by a taut muscular band within the scapular region. In such cases, pain may be amenable to trigger point injection of a local anesthetic (378).

Postoperative frozen shoulder. Patients with post-thoracotomy or postmastectomy pain are at risk for the development of a frozen shoulder (330). This lesion may become an independent focus of pain, particularly if complicated by reflex sympathetic dystrophy. Adequate postoperative analgesia and active mobilization of the joint soon after surgery are necessary to prevent these problems.

Phantom pain syndromes. Phantom limb pain is perceived to arise from an amputated limb, as if the limb were still contiguous with the body. Phantom pain is experienced by 60–80% of patients after limb amputation but is severe only in approximately 5–10% of cases (379–381). The incidence of phantom pain is significantly higher in patients with a long duration of preamputation pain and in those with pain on the day before the amputation (382,383). Phantom pain experienced by patients replicates the pain they experienced before the amputation (384). Phantom pain is more prevalent after tumor-related than traumatic amputations, and postoperative chemotherapy is an additional risk factor (381,385). The pain may be continuous or paroxysmal and is often associated with bothersome paresthesias. The phantom limb may assume painful and unusual postures and may gradually telescope and approach the stump. Phantom pain may initially magnify and then slowly fade over time. There is growing evidence that preoperative or postoperative neural blockade reduces the incidence of phantom limb pain during the first year after amputation (386–389).

Some patients have spontaneous partial remission of the pain. The recurrence of pain after such a remission, or the late onset of pain in a previously painless phantom limb, suggests the appearance of a more proximal lesion, including recurrent neoplasm (390).

Phantom pain syndromes have also been described after other surgical procedures. Phantom breast pain after mastectomy, which occurs in 15–30% of patients (337,391–393), also appears to be related to the presence of preoperative pain (392). The pain tends to start in the region of the nipple and then spread to the entire breast. The character of the pain is variable and may be lancinating, continuous, or intermittent (392,393). A phantom rectum pain syndrome occurs in approximately 15% of patients who undergo abdominoperineal resection of the rectum (255,394). Phantom rectal pain may develop either in the early postoperative period or after a latency of months to years. Late-onset pain is almost always associated with tumor recurrence (255,394). Rare cases of phantom bladder pain after cystectomy (395) and phantom eye pain after enucleation (396,397) have also been reported.

Stump pain. Stump pain occurs at the site of the surgical scar several months to years after amputation (398). It is usually the result of the development of neuroma at the site of nerve transection. This pain is characterized by burning or lancinating dysesthesias, which are often exacerbated by movement or pressure and blocked by an injection of a local anesthetic.

Postsurgical pelvic floor myalgia. Surgical trauma to the pelvic floor can cause a residual pelvic floor myalgia, which like the neoplastic syndrome described previously, mimics so-called tension myalgia (260). The risk of disease recurrence associated with this condition is not known, and its natural history has not been defined. In patients who have undergone anorectal resection, this condition must be differentiated from the phantom anus syndrome (see subsequent text).

Chronic Postradiation Pain Syndromes

Chronic pain complicating radiation therapy tends to occur late in the course of a patient's illness. These syndromes must always be differentiated from recurrent tumors.

Radiation-induced brachial and lumbosacral plexopathies. Radiation-induced brachial and lumbosacral plexopathies has been described in the preceding text.

Chronic radiation myelopathy. Chronic radiation myelopathy is a late complication of spinal cord irradiation. The latency of this condition is highly variable but is most commonly 12–14 months. The most common presentation is a partial transverse myelopathy at the cervicothoracic level, sometimes in a Brown-Sequard pattern (399). Sensory symptoms, including pain, typically precede the development of progressive motor and autonomic dysfunction (399). The pain is characterized as a burning dysesthesia localized to the area of spinal cord damage or below. Imaging studies, particularly MRI, are important for the exclusion of epidural metastases and demonstrate the nature and extent of intrinsic cord pathology, which may include atrophy, swelling, or syrinx. On MRI, the signs of radiation myelitis include high-intensity signals on T2-weighted images or gadolinium enhancement of T1-weighted images (400,401). The course of chronic radiation myelopathy is characterized by steady progression over months, followed by a subsequent phase of slow progression or stabilization.

Chronic radiation enteritis and proctitis. Chronic enteritis and proctitis occur as a delayed complication in 2–10% of patients who undergo abdominal or pelvic radiation therapy (402,403). The rectum and rectosigmoid are more commonly involved than the small bowel, a pattern that may relate to the retroperitoneal fixation of the former structures. The latency is variable (3 months–30 years) (402–404). Chronic radiation injury to the rectum can present as proctitis (with bloody diarrhea, tenesmus, and cramping pain),

obstruction due to stricture formation, or fistulae to the bladder or vagina. Small bowel radiation damage typically causes colicky abdominal pain, which can be associated with chronic nausea or malabsorption. Barium studies may demonstrate a narrow tubular bowel segment resembling Crohn's disease or ischemic colitis. Endoscopy and biopsy may be necessary to distinguish suspicious lesions from recurrent cancer (405).

Radiation cystitis. Radiation therapy used in the treatment of tumors of the pelvic organs (i.e., prostate, bladder, colon/rectum, uterus, ovary, and vagina/vulva) may produce a chronic radiation cystitis (406–408). The late sequelae of radiation injury to the bladder can range from minor temporary irritative voiding symptoms and asymptomatic hematuria to more severe complications such as gross hematuria, contracted nonfunctional bladder, persistent incontinence, and fistula formation. The clinical presentation can include frequency, urgency, dysuria, hematuria, incontinence, hydronephrosis, pneumaturia, and fecaluria.

Lymphedema pain. One third of patients with lymphedema as a complication of breast cancer or its treatment experience pain and tightness in the arm (409); pain is a major part of the morbidity among affected patients (410). In some patients, pain is caused by a secondary rotator cuff tendonitis due to internal derangement of tendon fibers resulting from impingement, functional overload, and intrinsic tendinopathy. Conservative treatment with nonsteroidal anti-inflammatory drugs (NSAIDs) and physical therapy (PT) is a safe and effective treatment (411). Some patients develop nerve entrapment syndromes of the carpal tunnels or brachial plexus (196,412). Severe or increasing pain in a lymphedematous arm is strongly suggestive of tumor invasion of the brachial plexus (186,187).

Burning perineum syndrome. Persistent perineal discomfort is an uncommon delayed complication of pelvic radiotherapy. After a latency of 6–18 months, burning pain can develop in the perianal region; the pain may extend anteriorly to involve the vagina or scrotum (413,414). In patients who have had abdominoperineal resection, phantom anus pain and recurrent tumor are major differential diagnoses.

Post–prostate brachytherapy pelvic pain. Patients with prostate cancer who undergo brachytherapy may experience a chronic radiation-related pelvic pain syndrome that is exacerbated by urination or perineal pressure. Data suggests that it may be partly related to higher central prostatic radiation doses (415).

Osteoradionecrosis. Osteoradionecrosis is another late complication of radiotherapy. Bone necrosis, which occurs as a result of endarteritis obliterans, may produce focal pain. Overlying tissue breakdown can occur spontaneously or as a result of trauma, such as dental extraction or denture trauma (416,417). Delayed development of a painful ulcer must be differentiated from tumor recurrence.

Breakthrough Pain

Transitory exacerbations of severe pain over a baseline of moderate pain or less may be described as *breakthrough pain* (418). Breakthrough pains are common in both acute and chronic pain states. These exacerbations may be precipitated by volitional actions of the patient (so-called incident pains), such as movement, micturition, cough, or defecation, or by nonvolitional events, such as bowel distention. Spontaneous fluctuations in pain intensity can also occur without an identifiable precipitant.

Breakthrough pains must be distinguished from exacerbations of pain associated with failure of analgesia. "End-of-dose failure (of analgesia)" is commonly observed as therapeutic levels of the analgesic fall. This phenomenon is observed most commonly when the interval between scheduled doses exceeds the known duration of action of analgesics with short half-life. Because there is substantial interindividual differences in drug metabolism and excretion, some analgesics that may typically have a 4 hour duration of action may be effective for only 2–3 hours in some individuals. Similarly, variability in the duration of analgesic effect is observed with long-acting formulations such as oral morphine or transdermal fentanyl. End-of-dose failure is addressed through either dose or schedule modification.

In a survey by Portenoy and Hagen (418) of 63 patients with cancer having pain who required opioid analgesics, 41 (64%) reported breakthrough pain. Patients had a median of four episodes per day, the duration of which ranged seconds to hours (median/range: 30 minutes/1–240 minutes). Pain characteristics were extremely varied. In 22 patients (43%) they were paroxysmal in onset, with 21 (41%) being both paroxysmal and brief (lancinating pain); the remainder were more gradual. In 15 (29%) patients the pains were related to end-of-dose failure caused by a fixed dose of opioid on a regular schedule. In 28 (55%) patients the pains were precipitated; of these, 22 were caused by an action of the patient (incident pain) and 6 were associated with a nonvolitional precipitant, such as flatulence. The pathophysiology of the pain was believed to be somatic in 33%, visceral in 20%, neuropathic in 27%, and mixed in 20%. Pain was related to the tumor in 82% of cases, the effects of therapy in 14%, and to neither in 4%. Diverse interventions were employed to manage these pains, with variable efficacy. In a study of 194 patients with cancer having pain, Jacobsen et al. (419) reported that 61% reported one or more episodes of breakthrough pain. These episodes were typically paroxysmal (56%), predictable (63%), and precipitated by the patient's actions (67%). They had a mean duration of 20 minutes (range 5 seconds–1.5 hours) and occurred for an average of 10 times per day (range 1–80 times). In a survey of 22 hospice patients by Fine and Busch (420), 86% reported breakthrough pain, with an average of 2.9 episodes per 24-hour period and a mean pain intensity of seven on a ten-point scale. These episodes lasted an average of 52 minutes (range 1–240 minutes). The range of time to relief from breakthrough pains was 5–60 minutes, with a mean of 30 minutes.

Syndromes of Breakthrough Pain

Pain exacerbations represent a heterogeneous phenomenon. The clinical approach to these problems is influenced by the specific underlying mechanism. Therefore, it is useful to define the specific breakthrough pain syndrome.

> Somatic, movement-related pain (volitional and nonvolitional)
> Somatic, nonmovement-related pain
> Neuropathic, movement-related pain
> Neuropathic, nonmovement-related pain
> Visceral pains—volitional
> Visceral pains—nonvolitional

Somatic, movement-related breakthrough pain.

Volitional. Volitional movement is the most common mechanism of breakthrough pain and is most commonly observed when the pain associated with skeletal metastases is exacerbated by movement. This movement is particularly common when the axial skeleton and weight-bearing bones are involved; these episodes are generally predictable. The site of disease involvement influences which volitional movement produces pain. Therefore, the pain associated with vertebral, pelvic, or femoral metastases may be exacerbated by walking. The pain of shoulder girdle or humeral metastases may be exacerbated by reaching or lifting. The pain of rib metastases may be exacerbated by deep breathing. Often,

this sort of breakthrough pain may be prevented or modified by preemptive analgesia, orthotics, bone stabilization, or movement modification.

Nonvolitional. Nonvolitional movements, such as laughing, sneezing, coughing, or myoclonus, may also exacerbate skeletal pain. The spontaneous and nonpredictable nature of these episodes commonly precludes preemptive analgesia, and management must address the possibility of reducing the frequency of the nonvolitional precipitant.

Somatic, nonmovement-related breakthrough pain. Occasionally, somatic structures can spontaneously produce transient exacerbation of pain unrelated to movement. In the setting of cancer pain, this is a relatively uncommon phenomenon. The best recognized syndrome is that of muscle cramps (112,113), which involve a focal transient exacerbation of pain related to a change in muscle tone, but without necessarily involving movement.

Neuropathic, movement-related breakthrough pain. Neuropathic pains are common among patients. Because of the proximity of neural and somatic structures, neuropathic pains are often exacerbated by volitional or nonvolitional movement.

Volitional. Neuropathic pain associated with the compression of neural structures such as the brachial plexus, lumbosacral plexus, spinal cord, and nerve roots are commonly exacerbated by specific volitional activities. Indeed, these associations are often important in the clinical diagnosis. For example, back pain that is exacerbated by lying suggests EC of the cord or nerve roots (79,192,421–423) and headache that is exacerbated by stooping or the Valsalva's maneuver suggests raised intracranial pressure (424).

Nonvolitional. Coughing and sneezing are nonvolitional movements that generate a Valsalva's maneuver (125). Valsalva's maneuvers can precipitate transient elevations in intracranial pressure called *plateau waves*. In patients with cerebral tumors, these plateau waves can be associated with short periods of severe headache, nausea, vomiting, photophobia, lethargy, and transient neurologic deficits (127,128). Occasionally, these plateau waves produce life-threatening herniation syndromes (127,128). Similarly, among patients with spinal cord compression the transient pressure shifts can exacerbate back or radicular pain.

Neuropathic, nonmovement-related breakthrough pain. Transient episodes of spontaneous lancinating or burning pain are a common manifestation of neuropathic pain syndromes. The frequency of pain exacerbations is variable, from many hundred episodes of brief lancinations per day to rare episodes that vary, with weeks to months between the episodes (418). Lancinating neuropathic pains are often of brief duration; this feature has therapeutic implications insofar as responsive analgesia is not likely to take effect until well after the pain has resolved and is therefore not likely to be effective. This sort of pain commonly requires a preventative therapy to diminish the frequency and severity of the episodes (425–428).

Visceral breakthrough pains. Visceral nociceptors respond primarily to mechanical and chemical nociceptive stimuli. Functionally, there is evidence for the existence of three classes of visceral afferents: low-threshold mechanosensitive afferents that respond to distension and contraction, specific chemosensitive afferents, and high-threshold mechanosensitive afferents (429).

Volitional. Initiation of the activity of some visceral organs is influenced by volitional activity; this is true for the upper gastrointestinal tract activity, which is associated with swallowing and digestion, micturition, defecation, and sexual climax (men and women). Indeed, exacerbations of visceral pain may be associated with any one of these activities. Transient visceral pains initiated by volitional activity may benefit from preemptive therapies or specific therapies targeted at the underlying mechanism.

Nonvolitional. Visceral motility is usually spontaneous and is often unrelated to any volitional activity. Spontaneous muscular contractions of hollow organs commonly result in paroxysmal transient pain exacerbations. Pain of this sort is commonly generated by the esophagus, intestines, gallbladder, and urinary bladder. Obstruction or inflammation of any hollow viscus may generate paroxysmal pains associated with spontaneous muscle contraction.

CONCLUSION

Adequate assessment is a necessary precondition for effective pain management. In the cancer population, assessment must recognize the dynamic relationship between the symptom, the illness, and larger concerns related to quality of life. Syndrome identification and inferences about pain pathophysiology are useful elements that may simplify this complex undertaking.

References

1. Goudas LC, Bloch R, Gialeli-Goudas M, et al. The epidemiology of cancer pain. *Cancer Invest* 2005;23(2):182–190.
2. Strang P. Existential consequences of unrelieved cancer pain. *Palliat Med* 1997;11(4):299–305.
3. Zaza C, Baine N. Cancer pain and psychosocial factors. A critical review of the literature. *J Pain Symptom Manage* 2002;24(5):526–542.
4. Emanuel EJ. Pain and symptom control. Patient rights and physician responsibilities. *Hematol Oncol Clin North Am* 1996;10(1):41–56.
5. Von Roenn JH, Cleeland CS, Gonin R, et al. Physician attitudes and practice in cancer pain management. A survey from the Eastern Cooperative Oncology Group. *Ann Intern Med* 1993;119(2):121–126.
6. Grossman SA, Sheidler VR, Swedeen K, et al. Correlation of patient and caregiver ratings of cancer pain. *J Pain Symptom Manage* 1991;6(2):53–57.
7. Cleeland CS, Gonin R, Hatfield AK, et al. Pain and its treatment in outpatients with metastatic cancer. *N Engl J Med* 1994;330(9): 592–596.
8. Larue F, Colleau SM, Brasseur L, et al. Multicentre study of cancer pain and its treatment in France. *Br Med J* 1995;310(6986):1034–1037.
9. Caraceni A, Portenoy RK. An international survey of cancer pain characteristics and syndromes. IASP Task Force on Cancer Pain. International Association for the Study of Pain. *Pain* 1999;82(3):263–274.
10. Foley KM. Pain syndromes in patients with cancer. *Med Clin North Am* 1987;71(2):169–184.
11. Banning A, Sjogren P, Henriksen H. Pain causes in 200 patients referred to a multidisciplinary cancer pain clinic. *Pain* 1991;45(1):45–48.
12. Twycross R, Harcourt J, Bergl S. A survey of pain in patients with advanced cancer. *J Pain Symptom Manage* 1996;12(5):273–282.
13. Daut RL, Cleeland CS. The prevalence and severity of pain in cancer. *Cancer* 1982;50(9):1913–1918.
14. Grond S, Zech D, Diefenbach C, et al. Assessment of cancer pain: a prospective evaluation in 2266 cancer patients referred to a pain service. *Pain* 1996;64(1):107–114.
15. Wagner G. Frequency of pain in patients with cancer. *Recent Results Cancer Res* 1984;89:64–71.
16. Mercadante S. Malignant bone pain: pathophysiology and treatment. *Pain* 1997;69(1–2):1–18.
17. Hofbauer LC, Heufelder AE. Role of receptor activator of nuclear factor-kappaB ligand and osteoprotegerin in bone cell biology. *J Mol Med* 2001;79(5–6):243–253.
18. Heider U, Zavrski I, Jakob C, et al. Expression of receptor activator of NF-kappaB ligand (RANKL) mRNA in human multiple myeloma cells. *J Cancer Res Clin Oncol* 2004;130(8):469–474.
19. Clohisy DR, Perkins SL, Ramnaraine ML. Review of cellular mechanisms of tumor osteolysis. *Clin Orthop Relat Res* 2000;(373):104–114.
20. Guise TA, Kozlow WM, Heras-Herzig A, et al. Molecular mechanisms of breast cancer metastases to bone. *Clin Breast Cancer* 2005;5(Suppl 2):S46–S53.
21. Thomas BG, Hamdy FC. Bone morphogenetic protein-6: potential mediator of osteoblastic metastases in prostate cancer. *Prostate Cancer Prostatic Dis* 2000;3(4):283–285.
22. Yamasaki Y, Nomura T, Mimata H, et al. Involvement of bone morphogenetic protein 2 in ossification of renal cell carcinoma. *J Urol* 2004;172(2):475–476.
23. Yamagishi SI, Suzuki T, Ohkuro H, et al. Ossifying gastric carcinoid tumor containing bone morphogenetic protein, osteopontin and osteonectin. *J Endocrinol Invest* 2004;27(9):870–873.
24. Luger NM, Mach DB, Sevcik MA, et al. Bone cancer pain: from model to mechanism to therapy. *J Pain Symptom Manage* 2005;29(5 Suppl):32–46.
25. Socie G, Cahn JY, Carmelo J, et al. Avascular necrosis of bone after allogeneic bone marrow transplantation: analysis of risk factors for 4388 patients by the Societe Francaise de Greffe de Moelle (SFGM). *Br J Haematol* 1997;97(4):865–870.
26. Shane E, Parisien M, Henderson JE, et al. Tumor-induced osteomalacia: clinical and basic studies. *J Bone Miner Res* 1997;12(9):1502–1511.
27. Jonsson OG, Sartain P, Ducore JM, et al. Bone pain as an initial symptom of childhood acute lymphoblastic leukemia: association with nearly normal hematologic indexes. *J Pediatr* 1990;117(2 Pt 1):233–237.
28. Wong KF, Chan JK, Ma SK. Solid tumour with initial presentation in the bone marrow—a clinicopathologic study of 25 adult cases. *Hematol Oncol* 1993;11(1):35–42.
29. Hesselmann S, Micke O, Schaefer U, et al. Systemic Mast Cell Disease (SMCD) and bone pain. A case treated with radiotherapy. *Strahlenther Onkol* 2002;178(5):275–279.
30. Lin JT, Lachmann E, Nagler W. Low back pain and myalgias in acute and relapsed mast cell leukemia: a case report. *Arch Phys Med Rehabil* 2002;83(6):860–863.
31. Golembe B, Ramsay NK, McKenna R, et al. Localized bone marrow relapse in acute lymphoblastic leukemia. *Med Pediatr Oncol* 1979;6(3): 229–234.
32. Lembersky BC, Ratain MJ, Golomb HM. Skeletal complications in hairy cell leukemia: diagnosis and therapy. *J Clin Oncol* 1988;6(8):1280–1284.
33. Beckers R, Uyttebroeck A, Demaerel P. Acute lymphoblastic leukaemia presenting with low back pain. *Eur J Paediatr Neurol* 2002;6(5): 285–287.
34. Jonsson KB, Zahradnik R, Larsson T, et al. Fibroblast growth factor 23 in oncogenic osteomalacia and X-linked hypophosphatemia. *N Engl J Med* 2003;348(17):1656–1663.
35. Edmister KA, Sundaram M. Oncogenic osteomalacia. *Semin Musculoskelet Radiol* 2002;6(3):191–196.
36. Gilbert RW, Kim JH, Posner JB. Epidural spinal cord compression from metastatic tumor: diagnosis and treatment. *Ann Neurol* 1978;3(1):40–51.
37. Sorensen S, Borgesen SE, Rohde K, et al. Metastatic epidural spinal cord compression. Results of treatment and survival. *Cancer* 1990;65(7):1502–1508.
38. Constans JP, de Divitiis E, Donzelli R, et al. Spinal metastases with neurological manifestations. Review of 600 cases. *J Neurosurg* 1983;59(1):111–118.
39. Bilsky MH, Shannon FJ, Sheppard S, et al. Diagnosis and management of a metastatic tumor in the atlantoaxial spine. *Spine* 2002;27(10):1062–1069.
40. Sundaresan N, Galicich JH, Lane JM, et al. Treatment of odontoid fractures in cancer patients. *J Neurosurg* 1981;54(2):187–192.
41. Nader R, Rhines LD, Mendel E. Metastatic sacral tumors. *Neurosurg Clin N Am* 2004;15(4):453–457.
42. Payer M. Neurological manifestation of sacral tumors. *Neurosurg Focus* 2003;15(2):E1.
43. Hipp JA, Springfield DS, Hayes WC. Predicting pathologic fracture risk in the management of metastatic bone defects. *Clin Orthop* 1995;(312):120–135.
44. Leggon RE, Lindsey RW, Panjabi MM. Strength reduction and the effects of treatment of long bones with diaphyseal defects involving 50% of the cortex. *J Orthop Res* 1988;6(4):540–546.
45. Mirels H. Metastatic disease in long bones. A proposed scoring system for diagnosing impending pathologic fractures. *Clin Orthop* 1989;(249):256–264.
46. Ryan PJ, Fogelman I. The bone scan: where are we now? *Semin Nucl Med* 1995;25(2):76–91.
47. Cahill TR, Oates E. 'Cold lesions' on bone scan. A case of metastatic squamous cell carcinoma of the penis. *Clin Nucl Med* 1991;16(9):633–635.
48. Gaze MN, Neville E, Rooke HW. Bone scan hot spots in a patient with lung cancer: ischaemic necrosis of bone mimicking metastatic carcinoma. *Clin Oncol (R Coll Radiol)* 1991;3(3):177–179.
49. Lee HK, Sung WW, Solodnik P, et al. Bone scan in tumor-induced osteomalacia. *J Nucl Med* 1995;36(2):247–249.
50. Lee S, Coel M, Ko J, et al. Diffuse idiopathic skeletal hyperostosis can resemble metastases on bone scan. *Clin Nucl Med* 1993;18(9):791–792.
51. Munk PL, Poon PY, O'Connell JX, et al. Osteoblastic metastases from breast carcinoma with false-negative bone scan. *Skeletal Radiol* 1997;26(7):434–437.
52. Covelli HD, Zaloznik AJ, Shekitka KM. Evaluation of bone pain in carcinoma of the lung. Role of the localized false-negative scan. *JAMA* 1980;244(23):2625–2627.
53. Schlaeffer F, Mikolich DJ, Mates SM. Technetium Tc 99m diphosphonate bone scan. False-normal findings in elderly patients with hematogenous vertebral osteomyelitis. *Arch Intern Med* 1987;147(11):2024–2026.
54. Han LJ, Au-Yong TK, Tong WC, et al. Comparison of bone single-photon emission tomography and planar imaging in the detection of vertebral metastases in patients with back pain. *Eur J Nucl Med* 1998;25(6):635–638.
55. Uematsu T, Yuen S, Yukisawa S, et al. Comparison of FDG PET and SPECT for detection of bone metastases in breast cancer. *AJR Am J Roentgenol* 2005;184(4):1266–1273.
56. Berna L, Torres G, Carrio I, et al. Antigranulocyte antibody bone marrow scans in cancer patients with metastatic bone superscan appearance. *Clin Nucl Med* 1994;19(2):121–128.

57. Setoain FJ, Pons F, Herranz R, et al. 67 Ga scintigraphy for the evaluation of recurrences and residual masses in patients with lymphoma. *Nucl Med Commun* 1997;18(5):405–411.

58. Pomeranz SJ, Pretorius HT, Ramsingh PS. Bone scintigraphy and multimodality imaging in bone neoplasia: strategies for imaging in the new health care climate. *Semin Nucl Med* 1994;24(3):188–207.

59. Kruyt RH, Oudkerk M, van Sluis D. CT-guided bone biopsy in a cancer center: experience with a new apple corer-shaped device. *J Comput Assist Tomogr* 1998;22(2):276–281.

60. Tikkakoski T, Lahde S, Puranen J, et al. Combined CT-guided biopsy and cytology in diagnosis of bony lesions. *Acta Radiol* 1992;33(3):225–229.

61. Ciray I, Astrom G, Sundstrom C, et al. Assessment of suspected bone metastases. CT with and without clinical information compared to CT-guided bone biopsy. *Acta Radiol* 1997;38(5):890–895.

62. Steiner RM, Mitchell DG, Rao VM, et al. Magnetic resonance imaging of diffuse bone marrow disease. *Radiol Clin North Am* 1993;31(2):383–409.

63. Layer G, Steudel A, Schuller H, et al. Magnetic resonance imaging to detect bone marrow metastases in the initial staging of small cell lung carcinoma and breast carcinoma. *Cancer* 1999;85(4):1004–1009.

64. Hochstenbag MM, Snoep G, Cobben NA, et al. Detection of bone marrow metastases in small cell lung cancer. Comparison of magnetic resonance imaging with standard methods. *Eur J Cancer* 1996;32A(5):779–782.

65. Sanal SM, Flickinger FW, Caudell MJ, et al. Detection of bone marrow involvement in breast cancer with magnetic resonance imaging. *J Clin Oncol* 1994;12(7):1415–1421.

66. Hanna SL, Fletcher BD, Fairclough DL, et al. Magnetic resonance imaging of disseminated bone marrow disease in patients treated for malignancy. *Skeletal Radiol* 1991;20(2):79–84.

67. Cuenod CA, Laredo JD, Chevret S, et al. Acute vertebral collapse due to osteoporosis or malignancy: appearance on unenhanced and gadolinium-enhanced MR images. *Radiology* 1996;199(2):541–549.

68. Lauenstein TC, Freudenberg LS, Goehde SC, et al. Whole-body MRI using a rolling table platform for the detection of bone metastases. *Eur Radiol* 2002;12(8):2091–2099.

69. Engelhard K, Hollenbach HP, Wohlfart K, et al. Comparison of whole-body MRI with automatic moving table technique and bone scintigraphy for screening for bone metastases in patients with breast cancer. *Eur Radiol* 2004;14(1):99–105.

70. Even-Sapir E, Metser U, Flusser G, et al. Assessment of malignant skeletal disease: initial experience with 18F-fluoride PET/CT and comparison between 18F-fluoride PET and 18F-fluoride PET/CT. *J Nucl Med* 2004;15(2):272–278.

71. Posner JB. Back pain and epidural spinal cord compression. *Med Clin North Am* 1987;71(2):185–205.

72. Loblaw DA, Laperriere NJ, Mackillop WJ. A population-based study of malignant spinal cord compression in Ontario. *Clin Oncol (R Coll Radiol)* 2003;15(4):211–217.

73. Loblaw DA, Perry J, Chambers A, et al. Systematic review of the diagnosis and management of malignant extradural spinal cord compression: the Cancer Care Ontario Practice Guidelines Initiative's Neuro-Oncology Disease Site Group. *J Clin Oncol* 2005;23(9):2028–2037.

74. Prasad D, Schiff D. Malignant spinal-cord compression. *Lancet Oncol* 2005;6(1):15–24.

75. Levack P, Graham J, Collie D, et al. Don't wait for a sensory level–listen to the symptoms: a prospective audit of the delays in diagnosis of malignant cord compression. *Clin Oncol (R Coll Radiol)* 2002;14(6):472–480.

76. Ruckdeschel JC. Early detection and treatment of spinal cord compression. *Oncology (Huntingt)* 2005;19(1):81–86. discussion 86, 89–92.

77. Greenberg HS, Kim JH, Posner JB. Epidural spinal cord compression from metastatic tumor: results with a new treatment protocol. *Ann Neurol* 1980;8(4):361–366.

78. Stranjalis G, Jamjoom A, Torrens M. Epidural lipomatosis in steroid-treated patients. *Spine* 1992;17(10):1268.

79. Helweg-Larsen S, Sorensen PS. Symptoms and signs in metastatic spinal cord compression: a study of progression from first symptom until diagnosis in 153 patients. *Eur J Cancer* 1994;30A(3):396–398.

80. Rosenthal MA, Rosen D, Raghavan D, et al. Spinal cord compression in prostate cancer. A 10-year experience. *Br J Urol* 1992;69(5):530–533.

81. Ruff RL, Lanska DJ. Epidural metastases in prospectively evaluated veterans with cancer and back pain. *Cancer* 1989;63(11):2234–2241.

82. Ventafridda V, Caraceni A, Martini C, et al. On the significance of Lhermitte's sign in oncology. *J Neurooncol* 1991;10(2):133–137.

83. Barron KD, Hirano A, Araki S, et al. Experience with metastatic neoplasms involving the spinal cord. *Neurology* 1959;9:91–100.

84. Helweg-Larsen S. Clinical outcome in metastatic spinal cord compression. A prospective study of 153 patients. *Acta Neurol Scand* 1996;94(4):269–275.

85. Helweg-Larsen S, Rasmusson B, Sorensen PS. Recovery of gait after radiotherapy in paralytic patients with metastatic epidural spinal cord compression. *Neurology* 1990;40(8):1234–1236.

86. Heldmann U, Myschetzky PS, Thomsen HS. Frequency of unexpected multifocal metastasis in patients with acute spinal cord compression. Evaluation by low-field MR imaging in cancer patients. *Acta Radiol* 1997;38(3):372–375.

87. Rodichok LD, Ruckdeschel JC, Harper GR, et al. Early detection and treatment of spinal epidural metastases: the role of myelography. *Ann Neurol* 1986;20(6):696–702.

88. Boesen J, Johnsen A, Helweg-Larsen S, et al. Diagnostic value of spinal computer tomography in patients with intraspinal metastases causing complete block on myelography. *Acta Radiol* 1991;32(1):1–2.

89. Helweg-Larsen S, Wagner A, Kjaer L, et al. Comparison of myelography combined with postmyelographic spinal CT and MRI in suspected metastatic disease of the spinal canal. *J Neurooncol* 1992;13(3):231–237.

90. Wilkinson AG, Sellar RJ. The influence of needle size and other factors on the incidence of adverse effects caused by myelography. *Clin Radiol* 1991;44(5):338–341.

91. Killebrew K, Whaley RA, Hayward JN, et al. Complications of metrizamide myelography. *Arch Neurol* 1983;40(2):78–80.

92. Sim FH. Metastatic bone disease of the pelvis and femur. *Instr Course Lect* 1992;41:317–327.

93. Graham DF. Hip pain as a presenting symptom of acetabular metastasis. *Br J Surg* 1976;63(2):147–148.

94. Beatrous TE, Choyke PL, Frank JA. Diagnostic evaluation of cancer patients with pelvic pain: comparison of scintigraphy, CT, and MR imaging [see comments]. *AJR Am J Roentgenol* 1990;155(1):85–88.

95. Mackey JR, Birchall I, MacDonald N. Occult infection as a cause of hip pain in a patient with metastatic breast cancer. *J Pain Symptom Manage* 1995;10(7):569–572.

96. Healey JH, Turnbull AD, Miedema B, et al. Acrometastases. A study of twenty-nine patients with osseous involvement of the hands and feet. *J Bone Joint Surg Am* 1986;68(5):743–746.

97. Freedman DM, Henderson RC. Metastatic breast carcinoma to the os calcis presenting as heel pain. *South Med J* 1995;88(2):232–234.

98. Kouvaris JR, Kouloulias VE, Papacharalampous XN, et al. Isolated talus metastasis from breast carcinoma: a case report and review of the literature. *Onkologie* 2005;28(3):141–143.

99. Martinez-Lavin M. Hypertrophic osteoarthropathy. *Curr Opin Rheumatol* 1997;9(1):83–86.

100. Briselli M, Mark FJ, Dickersin GR. Solitary fibrous tumors of the pleura: eight new cases and review of 360 cases in the literature. *Cancer* 1981;47(11):2678–2689.

101. Davies RA, Darby M, Richards MA. Hypertrophic pulmonary osteoarthropathy in pulmonary metastatic disease. A case report and review of the literature. *Clin Radiol* 1991;43(4):268–271. The above reports in MacintoshPCUNIX TextHTML format.

102. Kaymakcalan H, Sequeira W, Barretta T, et al. Hypertrophic osteoarthropathy with myogenic tumors of the esophagus. *Am J Gastroenterol* 1980;74(1):17–20.

103. Shapiro JS. Breast cancer presenting as periostitis. *Postgrad Med* 1987;82(4):139–140.

104. Daly BD. Thoracic metastases from nasopharyngeal carcinoma presenting as hypertrophic pulmonary osteoarthropathy: scintigraphic and CT findings. *Clin Radiol* 1995;50(8):545–547.

105. Hung GU, Kao CH, Lin WY, et al. Rapid resolution of hypertrophic pulmonary osteoarthropathy after resection of a lung mass caused by xanthogranulomatous inflammation.[In Process Citation]. *Clin Nucl Med* 2000;25(12):1029–1030.

106. Greenfield GB, Schorsch HA, Shkolnik A. The various roentgen appearances of pulmonary hypertrophic osteoarthropathy. *Am J Roentgenol Radium Ther Nucl Med* 1967;101(4):927–931.

107. Sharma OP. Symptoms and signs in pulmonary medicine: old observations and new interpretations. *Dis Mon* 1995;41(9):577–638.

108. Stummvoll GH, Aringer M, Machold KP, et al. Cancer polyarthritis resembling rheumatoid arthritis as a first sign of hidden neoplasms. Report of two cases and review of the literature. *Scand J Rheumatol* 2001;30(1):40–44.

109. Shiel WC Jr, Prete PE, Jason M, et al. Palmar fasciitis and arthritis with ovarian and non-ovarian carcinomas. New syndrome. *Am J Med* 1985;79(5):640–644.

110. Saxman SB, Seitz D. Breast cancer associated with palmar fasciitis and arthritis. *J Clin Oncol* 1997;15(12):3515–3516.

111. Enomoto M, Takemura H, Suzuki M, et al. Palmar fasciitis and polyarthritis associated with gastric carcinoma: complete resolution after total gastrectomy. *Intern Med* 2000;39(9):754–757.

112. Siegal T. Muscle cramps in the cancer patient: causes and treatment. *J Pain Symptom Manage* 1991;6(2):84–91.

113. Steiner I, Siegal T. Muscle cramps in cancer patients. *Cancer* 1989;63(3):574–577.

114. Breccia M, Carmosino I, Russo E, et al. Early and tardive skin adverse events in chronic myeloid leukaemia patients treated with imatinib. *Eur J Haematol* 2005;74(2):121–123.

115. Ernst G, Gericke A, Berg P. Central pain and complex motoric symptoms after goserelin therapy of prostate cancer. *ScientificWorldJournal* 2004;4:969–973.

116. Haim N, Epelbaum R, Ben-Shahar M, et al. Full dose vincristine (without 2-mg dose limit) in the treatment of lymphomas. *Cancer* 1994;73(10):2515–2519.

117. Koike Y, Hatori M, Kokubun S. Skeletal muscle metastasis secondary to cancer—a report of seven cases. *Ups J Med Sci* 2005;110(1):75–83.

118. Di Giorgio A, Sammartino P, Cardini CL, et al. Lung cancer and skeletal muscle metastases. *Ann Thorac Surg* 2004;78(2):709–711.

119. Magee T, Rosenthal H. Skeletal muscle metastases at sites of documented trauma. *AJR Am J Roentgenol* 2002;178(4):985–988.

120. Vecht CJ, Hoff AM, Kansen PJ, et al. Types and causes of pain in cancer of the head and neck. *Cancer* 1992;70(1):178–184.

121. Vazquez-Barquero A, Ibanez FJ, Herrera S, et al. Isolated headache as the presenting clinical manifestation of intracranial tumors: a prospective study [see comments]. *Cephalalgia* 1994;14(4):270–272.

122. El Kamar FG, Posner JB. Brain metastases. *Semin Neurol* 2004;24(4): 347–362.

123. Chidel MA, Suh JH, Barnett GH. Brain metastases: presentation, evaluation, and management. *Cleve Clin J Med* 2000;67(2):120–127.

124. Forsyth PA, Posner JB. Headaches in patients with brain tumors: a study of 111 patients. *Neurology* 1993;43(9):1678–1683.

125. Suwanwela N, Phanthumchinda K, Kaoropthum S. Headache in brain tumor: a cross-sectional study. *Headache* 1994;34(7):435–438.

126. Medina LS, Pinter JD, Zurakowski D, et al. Children with headache: clinical predictors of surgical space-occupying lesions and the role of neuroimaging. *Radiology* 1997;202(3):819–824.

127. Hayashi M, Handa Y, Kobayashi H, et al. Plateau-wave phenomenon (I). Correlation between the appearance of plateau waves and CSF circulation in patients with intracranial hypertension. *Brain* 1991;114(Pt 6):2681–2691.

128. Matsuda M, Yoneda S, Handa H, et al. Cerebral hemodynamic changes during plateau waves in brain-tumor patients. *J Neurosurg* 1979;50(4):483–488.

129. Grossman SA, Krabak MJ. Leptomeningeal carcinomatosis. *Cancer Treat Rev* 1999;25(2):103–119.

130. Jayson GC, Howell A. Carcinomatous meningitis in solid tumours. *Ann Oncol* 1996;7(8):773–786.

131. Wasserstrom WR, Glass JP, Posner JB. Diagnosis and treatment of leptomeningeal metastases from solid tumors: experience with 90 patients. *Cancer* 1982;49(4):759–772.

132. van Oostenbrugge RJ, Twijnstra A. Presenting features and value of diagnostic procedures in leptomeningeal metastases. *Neurology* 1999;53(2):382–385.

133. Balm M, Hammack J. Leptomeningeal carcinomatosis. Presenting features and prognostic factors [see comments]. *Arch Neurol* 1996;53(7): 626–632.

134. DeAngelis LM, Payne R. Lymphomatous meningitis presenting as atypical cluster headache. *Pain* 1987;30(2):211–216.

135. Sozzi G, Marotta P, Piatti L. Vagoglossopharyngeal neuralgia with syncope in the course of carcinomatous meningitis. *Ital J Neurol Sci* 1987;8(3):271–275.

136. Kaplan JG, DeSouza TG, Farkash A, et al. Leptomeningeal metastases: comparison of clinical features and laboratory data of solid tumors, lymphomas and leukemias. *J Neurooncol* 1990;9(3):225–229.

137. Olson ME, Chernik NL, Posner JB. Infiltration of the leptomeninges by systemic cancer. A clinical and pathologic study. *Arch Neurol* 1974;30(2):122–137.

138. van Oostenbrugge RJ, Hopman AH, Arends JW, et al. The value of interphase cytogenetics in cytology for the diagnosis of leptomeningeal metastases. *Neurology* 1998;51(3):906–908.

139. van Oostenbrugge RJ, Hopman AH, Arends JW, et al. Treatment of leptomeningeal metastases evaluated by interphase cytogenetics. *J Clin Oncol* 2000;18(10):2053–2058.

140. Thomas JE, Falls E, Velasco ME, et al. Diagnostic value of immunocytochemistry in leptomeningeal tumor dissemination. *Arch Pathol Lab Med* 2000;124(5):759–761.

141. Twijnstra A, Ongerboer de Visser BW, van Zanten AP. Diagnosis of leptomeningeal metastasis. *Clin Neurol Neurosurg* 1987;89(2): 79–85.

142. Bach F, Soletormos G, Dombernowsky P. Tissue polypeptide antigen activity in cerebrospinal fluid: a marker of central nervous system metastases of breast cancer. *J Natl Cancer Inst* 1991;83(11):779–784.

143. Cibas ES, Malkin MG, Posner JB, et al. Detection of DNA abnormalities by flow cytometry in cells from cerebrospinal fluid. *Am J Clin Pathol* 1987;88(5):570–577.

144. Straathof CS, de Bruin HG, Dippel DW, et al. The diagnostic accuracy of magnetic resonance imaging and cerebrospinal fluid cytology in leptomeningeal metastasis. *J Neurol* 1999;246(9):810–814.

145. Collie DA, Brush JP, Lammie GA, et al. Imaging features of leptomeningeal metastases. *Clin Radiol* 1999;54(11):765–771.

146. Gomori JM, Heching N, Siegal T. Leptomeningeal metastases: evaluation by gadolinium enhanced spinal magnetic resonance imaging. *J Neurooncol* 1998;36(1):55–60.

147. Chamberlain MC. Pediatric leptomeningeal metastases: outcome following combined therapy. *J Child Neurol* 1997;12(1):53–59.

148. Gaumann A, Marx J, Bohl J, et al. Leptomeningeal carcinomatosis and cranial nerve palsy as presenting symptoms of a clinically inapparent gallbladder carcinoma. *Pathol Res Pract* 1999;195(7):495–499.

149. Greenberg HS, Deck MD, Vikram B, et al. Metastasis to the base of the skull: clinical findings in 43 patients. *Neurology* 1981;31(5):530–537.

150. Hawley RJ, Patel A, Lastinger L. Cranial nerve compression from breast cancer metastasis [letter; comment]. *Surg Neurol* 1999;52(4):431–432.

151. Yi HJ, Kim CH, Bak KH, et al. Metastatic tumors in the sellar and parasellar regions: clinical review of four cases. *J Korean Med Sci* 2000;15(3):363–367.

152. Lossos A, Siegal T. Numb chin syndrome in cancer patients: etiology, response to treatment, and prognostic significance [see comments]. *Neurology* 1992;42(6):1181–1184.

153. Bullitt E, Tew JM, Boyd J. Intracranial tumors in patients with facial pain. *J Neurosurg* 1986;64(6):865–871.

154. Moris G, Roig C, Misiego M, et al. The distinctive headache of the occipital condyle syndrome: a report of four cases. *Headache* 1998;38(4): 308–311.

155. Loevner LA, Yousem DM. Overlooked metastatic lesions of the occipital condyle: a missed case treasure trove. *Radiographics* 1997;17(5): 1111–1121.

156. Fink FM, Ausserer B, Schrocksnadel W, et al. Clivus chordoma in a 9-year-old child: case report and review of the literature. *Pediatr Hematol Oncol* 1987;4(2):91–100.

157. Lawson W, Reino AJ. Isolated sphenoid sinus disease: an analysis of 132 cases. *Laryngoscope* 1997;107(12 Pt 1):1590–1595.

158. Gupta SR, Zdonczyk DE, Rubino FA. Cranial neuropathy in systemic malignancy in a VA population [see comments]. *Neurology* 1990;40(6):997–999.

159. McDermott RS, Anderson PR, Greenberg RE, et al. Cranial nerve deficits in patients with metastatic prostate carcinoma: clinical features and treatment outcomes. *Cancer* 2004;101(7):1639–1643.

160. Metheetrairut C, Brown DH. Glossopharyngeal neuralgia and syncope secondary to neck malignancy. *J Otolaryngol* 1993;22(1):18–20.

161. Weinstein RE, Herec D, Friedman JH. Hypotension due to glossopharyngeal neuralgia. *Arch Neurol* 1986;43(1):90–92.

162. Hirota N, Fujimoto T, Takahashi M, et al. Isolated trigeminal nerve metastases from breast cancer: an unusual cause of trigeminal mononeuropathy [In Process Citation]. *Surg Neurol* 1998;49(5):558–561.

163. Barker FG II, Jannetta PJ, Babu RP, et al. Long-term outcome after operation for trigeminal neuralgia in patients with posterior fossa tumors. *J Neurosurg* 1996;84(5):818–825.

164. Cheng TM, Cascino TL, Onofrio BM. Comprehensive study of diagnosis and treatment of trigeminal neuralgia secondary to tumors. *Neurology* 1993;43(11):2298–2302.

165. Boerman RH, Maassen EM, Joosten J, et al. Trigeminal neuropathy secondary to perineural invasion of head and neck carcinomas. *Neurology* 1999;53(1):213–216.

166. Payten RJ. Facial pain as the first symptom in acoustic neuroma. *J Laryngol Otol* 1972;86(5):523–534.

167. Morrison GA, Sterkers JM. Unusual presentations of acoustic tumours. *Clin Otolaryngol* 1996;21(1):80–83.

168. Shapshay SM, Elber E, Strong MS. Occult tumors of the infratemporal fossa: report of seven cases appearing as preauricular facial pain. *Arch Otolaryngol* 1976;102(9):535–538.

169. Hill BA, Kohut RI. Metastatic adenocarcinoma of the temporal bone. *Arch Otolaryngol* 1976;102(9):568–571.

170. Scarbrough TJ, Day TA, Williams TE, et al. Referred otalgia in head and neck cancer: a unifying schema. *Am J Clin Oncol* 2003;26(5):E157–E162.

171. De Potter P. Ocular manifestations of cancer. *Curr Opin Ophthalmol* 1998;9(6):100–104.

172. Weiss R, Grisold W, Jellinger K, et al. Metastasis of solid tumors in extraocular muscles. *Acta Neuropathol (Berl)* 1984;65(2):168–171.

173. Friedman J, Karesh J, Rodrigues M, et al. Thyroid carcinoma metastatic to the medial rectus muscle. *Ophthal Plast Reconstr Surg* 1990;6(2):122–125.

174. Laitt RD, Kumar B, Leatherbarrow B, et al. Cystic optic nerve meningioma presenting with acute proptosis. *Eye* 1996;10(Pt 6):744–746.

175. Sarlani E, Schwartz AH, Greenspan JD, et al. Facial pain as first manifestation of lung cancer: a case of lung cancer-related cluster headache and a review of the literature. *J Orofac Pain* 2003;17(3):262–267.

176. Schroeder TL, Farlane DF, Goldberg LH. Pain as an atypical presentation of squamous cell carcinoma [In Process Citation]. *Dermatol Surg* 1998;24(2):263–266.

177. Dulli DA, Levine RL, Chun RW, et al. Migrainous neurologic dysfunction in Hodgkin's disease [letter]. *Arch Neurol* 1987;44(7):689.

178. Miyazaki Y, Tajima Y, Sudo K, et al. Hodgkin's disease-related central nervous system angiopathy presenting as reversible posterior leukoencephalopathy. *Intern Med* 2004;43(10):1005–1007.

179. Sigsbee B, Deck MD, Posner JB. Nonmetastatic superior sagittal sinus thrombosis complicating systemic cancer. *Neurology* 1979;29(2):139–146.

180. Portenoy RK, Abissi CJ, Robbins JB. Increased intracranial pressure with normal ventricular size due to superior vena cava obstruction [letter]. *Arch Neurol* 1983;40(9):598.

181. Marshall JA, Mahanna GK. Cancer in the differential diagnosis of orofacial pain. *Dent Clin North Am* 1997;41(2):355–365.

182. Portenoy RK, Duma C, Foley KM. Acute herpetic and postherpetic neuralgia: clinical review and current management. *Ann Neurol* 1986;20(6):651–664.

183. Rusthoven JJ, Ahlgren P, Elhakim T, et al. Varicella-zoster infection in adult cancer patients. A population study. *Arch Intern Med* 1988;148(7):1561–1566.

184. Lojeski E, Stevens RA. Postherpetic neuralgia in the cancer patient. *Curr Rev Pain* 2000;4(3):219–226.

185. Jaeckle KA. Nerve plexus metastases. *Neurol Clin* 1991;9(4):857–866.
186. Kori SH, Foley KM, Posner JB. Brachial plexus lesions in patients with cancer: 100 cases. *Neurology* 1981;31(1):45–50.
187. Kori SH. Diagnosis and management of brachial plexus lesions in cancer patients. *Oncology (Huntingt)* 1995;9(8):756–760. discussion 765.
188. Jaeckle KA. Neurological manifestations of neoplastic and radiation-induced plexopathies. *Semin Neurol* 2004;24(4):385–393.
189. van Es HW. MRI of the brachial plexus. *Eur Radiol* 2001;11(2):325–336.
190. Wittenberg KH, Adkins MC. MR imaging of nontraumatic brachial plexopathies: frequency and spectrum of findings. *Radiographics* 2000;20(4):1023–1032.
191. Synek VM. Validity of median nerve somatosensory evoked potentials in the diagnosis of supraclavicular brachial plexus lesions. *Electroencephalogr Clin Neurophysiol* 1986;65(1):27–35.
192. Portenoy RK, Galer BS, Salamon O, et al. Identification of epidural neoplasm. Radiography and bone scintigraphy in the symptomatic and asymptomatic spine. *Cancer* 1989;64(11):2207–2213.
193. Bajrovic A, Rades D, Fehlauer F, et al. Is there a life-long risk of brachial plexopathy after radiotherapy of supraclavicular lymph nodes in breast cancer patients? *Radiother Oncol* 2004;71(3):297–301.
194. Mondrup K, Olsen NK, Pfeiffer P, et al. Clinical and electrodiagnostic findings in breast cancer patients with radiation-induced brachial plexus neuropathy. *Acta Neurol Scand* 1990;81(2):153–158.
195. Olsen NK, Pfeiffer P, Mondrup K, et al. Radiation-induced brachial plexus neuropathy in breast cancer patients. *Acta Oncol* 1990;29(7):885–890.
196. Vecht CJ. Arm pain in the patient with breast cancer. *J Pain Symptom Manage* 1990;5(2):109–117.
197. Schierle C, Winograd JM. Radiation-induced brachial plexopathy: review. Complication without a cure. *J Reconstr Microsurg* 2004;20(2):149–152.
198. Cascino TL, Kori S, Krol G, et al. CT of the brachial plexus in patients with cancer. *Neurology* 1983;33(12):1553–1557.
199. Schulte RW, Adamietz IA, Renner K, et al. Humeral head necrosis following irradiation of breast carcinoma. A case report. *Radiologe* 1989;29(5):252–255.
200. Lederman RJ, Wilbourn AJ. Brachial plexopathy: recurrent cancer or radiation? *Neurology* 1984;34(10):1331–1335.
201. Harper CM Jr, Thomas JE, Cascino TL, et al. Distinction between neoplastic and radiation-induced brachial plexopathy, with emphasis on the role of EMG. *Neurology* 1989;39(4):502–506.
202. Albers JW, Allen AAd, Bastron JA, et al. Limb myokymia. *Muscle Nerve* 1981;4(6):494–504.
203. Flaggman PD, Kelly JJ Jr. Brachial plexus neuropathy. An electrophysiologic evaluation. *Arch Neurol* 1980;37(3):160–164.
204. Roth G, Magistris MR, Le Fort D, et al. Post-radiation branchial plexopathy. Persistent conduction block. Myokymic discharges and cramps. *Rev Neurol (Paris)* 1988;144(3):173–180.
205. Killer HE, Hess K. Natural history of radiation-induced brachial plexopathy compared with surgically treated patients. *J Neurol* 1990;237(4):247–250.
206. Binder DK, Smith JS, Barbaro NM. Primary brachial plexus tumors: imaging, surgical, and pathological findings in 25 patients. *Neurosurg Focus* 2004;16(5):E11.
207. Gerard JM, Franck N, Moussa Z, et al. Acute ischemic brachial plexus neuropathy following radiation therapy. *Neurology* 1989;39(3):450–451.
208. Lachance DH, O Neill BP, Harper CM Jr, et al. Paraneoplastic brachial plexopathy in a patient with Hodgkin's disease. *Mayo Clin Proc* 1991;66(1):97–101.
209. Chad DA, Bradley WG. Lumbosacral plexopathy. *Semin Neurol* 1987;7(1):97–107.
210. Jaeckle KA, Young DF, Foley KM. The natural history of lumbosacral plexopathy in cancer. *Neurology* 1985;35(1):8–15.
211. Stevens MJ, Gonet YM. Malignant psoas syndrome: recognition of an oncologic entity. *Australas Radiol* 1990;34(2):150–154.
212. Agar M, Broadbent A, Chye R. The management of malignant psoas syndrome: case reports and literature review. *J Pain Symptom Manage* 2004;28(3):282–293.
213. Zografos GC, Karakousis CP. Pain in the distribution of the femoral nerve: early evidence of recurrence of a retroperitoneal sarcoma. *Eur J Surg Oncol* 1994;20(6):692–693.
214. Tharion G, Bhattacharji S. Malignant secondary deposit in the iliac crest masquerading as meralgia paresthetica. *Arch Phys Med Rehabil* 1997;78(9):1010–1011.
215. Evans RJ, Watson CPN. Lumbosacral plexopathy in cancer patients. *Neurology* 1985;35:1392–1393.
216. Dalmau J, Graus F, Marco M. 'Hot and dry foot' as initial manifestation of neoplastic lumbosacral plexopathy. *Neurology* 1989;39(6):871–872.
217. Taylor BV, Kimmel DW, Krecke KN, et al. Magnetic resonance imaging in cancer-related lumbosacral plexopathy. *Mayo Clin Proc* 1997;72(9):823–829.
218. Stryker JA, Sommerville K, Perez R, et al. Sacral plexus injury after radiotherapy for carcinoma of cervix. *Cancer* 1990;66(7):1488–1492.
219. Gonzalez-Caballero G, Arroyo-Gonzalez R, Vazquez-Perez AV, et al. Lumbosacral plexopathy 15 years after radiotherapy for carcinoma of the cervix. *Rev Neurol* 2000;30(1):97.
220. Thomas JE, Cascino TL, Earle JD. Differential diagnosis between radiation and tumor plexopathy of the pelvis. *Neurology* 1985;35(1):1–7.
221. Desta K, O'Shaughnessy M, Milling MA. Non-Hodgkin's lymphoma presenting as median nerve compression in the arm. *J Hand Surg [Br]* 1994;19(3):289–291.
222. Grisold W, Drlicek M. Paraneoplastic neuropathy. *Curr Opin Neurol* 1999;12(5):617–625.
223. Rotta FT, Bradley WG. Marked improvement of severe polyneuropathy associated with multifocal osteosclerotic myeloma following surgery, radiation, and chemotherapy. *Muscle Nerve* 1997;20(8):1035–1037.
224. Kissel JT, Mendell JR. Neuropathies associated with monoclonal gammopathies. *Neuromuscul Disord* 1996;6(1):3–18.
225. Dalmau JO, Posner JB. Paraneoplastic syndromes affecting the nervous system. *Semin Oncol* 1997;24(3):318–328.
226. Brady AM. Management of painful paraneoplastic syndromes. *Hematol Oncol Clin North Am* 1996;10(4):801–809.
227. van Oosterhout AG, van de Pol M, ten Velde GP, et al. Neurologic disorders in 203 consecutive patients with small cell lung cancer. Results of a longitudinal study. *Cancer* 1996;77(8):1434–1441.
228. Peterson K, Forsyth PA, Posner JB. Paraneoplastic sensorimotor neuropathy associated with breast cancer. *J Neurooncol* 1994;21(2):159–170.
229. Plante-Bordeneuve V, Baudrimont M, Gorin NC, et al. Subacute sensory neuropathy associated with Hodgkin's disease. *J Neurol Sci* 1994;121(2):155–158.
230. Sharief MK, Robinson SF, Ingram DA, et al. Paraneoplastic painful ulnar neuropathy. *Muscle Nerve* 1999;22(7):952–955.
231. Toepfer M, Schroeder M, Unger JW, et al. Neuromyotonia, myocloni, sensory neuropathy and cerebellar symptoms in a patient with antibodies to neuronal nucleoproteins (anti-Hu- antibodies). *Clin Neurol Neurosurg* 1999;101(3):207–209.
232. Antoine JC, Honnorat J, Camdessanche JP, et al. Paraneoplastic anti-CV2 antibodies react with peripheral nerve and are associated with a mixed axonal and demyelinating peripheral neuropathy. *Ann Neurol* 2001;49(2):214–221.
233. Fasolino M, Sabatini P, Cuomo T, et al. Paraneoplastic subacute sensory neuronopathy associated with anti-ri antibodies. *J Peripher Nerv Syst* 2004;9(2):109.
234. Kelly JJ, Karcher DS. Lymphoma and peripheral neuropathy: a clinical review. *Muscle Nerve* 2005;31(3):301–313.
235. Wicklund MP, Kissel JT. Paraproteinemic Neuropathy. *Curr Treat Options Neurol* 2001;3(2):147–156.
236. Silen W. *Cope's early diagnosis of the acute abdomen*, 16th ed. New York: Oxford; 1983.
237. Coombs DW. Pain due to liver capsular distention. In: Ferrer-Brechner T, ed. *Common problems in pain management*. Chicago: Year Book Medical Publishers, 1990:247–253.
238. Mulholland MW, Debas H, Bonica JJ. Diseases of the liver, biliary system and pancreas. In: Bonica JJ, ed. *The management of pain*. Philadelphia, PA: Lea & Febiger, 1990:1214–1231.
239. De Conno F, Polastri D. Clinical features and symptomatic treatment of liver metastasis in the terminally ill patient. *Ann Ital Chir* 1996;67(6):819–826.
240. Harris JN, Robinson P, Lawrance J, et al. Symptoms of colorectal liver metastases: correlation with CT findings. *Clin Oncol (R Coll Radiol)* 2003;15(2):78–82.
241. La Fianza A, Alberici E, Biasina AM, et al. Spontaneous hemorrhage of a liver metastasis from squamous cell cervical carcinoma: case report and review of the literature. *Tumori* 1999;85(4):290–293.
242. Grahm AL, Andren-Sandberg A. Prospective evaluation of pain in exocrine pancreatic cancer. *Digestion* 1997;58(6):542–549.
243. Kelsen DP, Portenoy R, Thaler H, et al. Pain as a predictor of outcome in patients with operable pancreatic carcinoma. *Surgery* 1997;122(1):53–59.
244. Kelsen DP, Portenoy RK, Thaler HT, et al. Pain and depression in patients with newly diagnosed pancreas cancer. *J Clin Oncol* 1995;13(3):748–755.
245. Sponseller PD. Evaluating the child with back pain. *Am Fam Physician* 1996;54(6):1933–1941.
246. Neer RM, Ferrucci JT, Wang CA, et al. A 77-year-old man with epigastric pain, hypercalcemia, and a retroperitoneal mass. *N Engl J Med* 1981;305(15):874–883.
247. Krane RJ, Perrone TL. A young man with testicular and abdominal pain. *N Engl J Med* 1981;305(6):331–336.
248. Schonenberg P, Bastid C, Guedes J, et al. Percutaneous echography-guided alcohol block of the celiac plexus as treatment of painful syndromes of the upper abdomen: study of 21 cases. *Schweiz Med Wochenschr* 1991;121(15):528–531.
249. Zhu Z, Friess H, diMola FF, et al. Nerve growth factor expression correlates with perineural invasion and pain in human pancreatic cancer. *J Clin Oncol* 1999;17(8):2419.
250. Tham TC, Lichtenstein DR, Vandervoort J, et al. Pancreatic duct stents for "obstructive type" pain in pancreatic malignancy. *Am J Gastroenterol* 2000;95(4):956–960.
251. Ripamonti C. Management of bowel obstruction in advanced cancer. *Curr Opin Oncol* 1994;6(4):351–357.
252. Averbach AM, Sugarbaker PH. Recurrent intraabdominal cancer with intestinal obstruction. *Int Surg* 1995;80(2):141–146.
253. Archer AG, Sugarbaker PH, Jelinek JS. Radiology of peritoneal carcinomatosis. *Cancer Treat Res* 1996;82:263–288.

254. Stillman M. Perineal pain: diagnosis and management, with particular attention to perineal pain of cancer. In: Foley KM, Bonica JJ, Ventafridda V, eds. *Second international congress on cancer pain.* New York: Raven Press, 1990:359–377.
255. Boas RA, Schug SA, Acland RH. Perineal pain after rectal amputation: a 5-year follow-up. *Pain* 1993;52(1):67–70.
256. Miaskowski C. Special needs related to the pain and discomfort of patients with gynecologic cancer. *J Obstet Gynecol Neonatal Nurs* 1996;25(2):181–188.
257. Hagen NA. Sharp, shooting neuropathic pain in the rectum or genitals: pudendal neuralgia. *J Pain Symptom Manage* 1993;8(7):496–501.
258. Rigor BM. Pelvic cancer pain. *J Surg Oncol* 2000;75(4):280–300.
259. Seefeld PH, Bargen JA. The spread of carcinoma of the rectum: invasion of lymphatics, veins and nerves. *Ann Surgery* 1943;118:76–90.
260. Sinaki M, Merritt JL, Stillwell GK. Tension myalgia of the pelvic floor. *Mayo Clin Proc* 1977;52(11):717–722.
261. Berger MS, Cooley ME, Abrahm JL. A pain syndrome associated with large adrenal metastases in patients with lung cancer. *J Pain Symptom Manage* 1995;10(2):161–166.
262. Karanikiotis C, Tentes AA, Markakidis S, et al. Large bilateral adrenal metastases in non-small cell lung cancer. *World J Surg Oncol* 2004;2(1):37.
263. Harrington KJ, Pandha HS, Kelly SA, et al. Palliation of obstructive nephropathy due to malignancy. *Br J Urol* 1995;76(1):101–107.
264. Russo P. Urologic emergencies in the cancer patient. *Semin Oncol* 2000;27(3):284–298.
265. Sklaroff DM, Gnaneswaran P, Sklaroff RB. Postirradiation ureteric stricture. *Gynecol Oncol* 1978;6(6):538–545.
266. Muram D, Oxorn H, Curry RH, et al. Postradiation ureteral obstruction: a reappraisal. *Am J Obstet Gynecol* 1981;139(3):289–293.
267. Goodman M, Dalton JR. Ureteral strictures following radiotherapy: incidence, etiology and treatment guidelines. *J Urol* 1982;128(1):21–24.
268. Little B, Ho KJ, Gawley S, et al. Use of nephrostomy tubes in ureteric obstruction from incurable malignancy. *Int J Clin Pract* 2003;57(3):180–181.
269. Portenoy RK, Kornblith AB, Wong G, et al. Pain in ovarian cancer patients. Prevalence, characteristics, and associated symptoms. *Cancer* 1994;74(3):907–915.
270. Goff BA, Mandel LS, Melancon CH, et al. Frequency of symptoms of ovarian cancer in women presenting to primary care clinics. *JAMA* 2004;291(22):2705–2712.
271. Webb PM, Purdie DM, Grover S, et al. Symptoms and diagnosis of borderline, early and advanced epithelial ovarian cancer. *Gynecol Oncol* 2004;92(1):232–239.
272. Marino C, Zoppi M, Morelli F, et al. Pain in early cancer of the lungs. *Pain* 1986;27(1):57–62.
273. Marangoni C, Lacerenza M, Formaglio F, et al. Sensory disorder of the chest as presenting symptom of lung cancer. *J Neurol Neurosurg Psychiatry* 1993;56(9):1033–1034.
274. Miyamoto M, Sudo T, Kuyama T. Spontaneous rupture of hepatocellular carcinoma: a review of 172 Japanese cases. *Am J Gastroenterol* 1991;86(1):67–71.
275. Marini P, Vilgrain V, Belghiti J. Management of spontaneous rupture of liver tumours. *Dig Surg* 2002;19(2):109–113.
276. Wolff JM, Boeckmann W, Jakse G. Spontaneous kidney rupture due to a metastatic renal tumour. Case report. *Scand J Urol Nephrol* 1994;28(4):415–417.
277. Rajagopal A, Ramasamy R, Martin J, et al. Acute myeloid leukemia presenting as splenic rupture. *J Assoc Physicians India* 2002;50:1435–1437.
278. Stamoulis JS, Antonopoulou Z, Safioleas M. Haemorrhagic shock from the spontaneous rupture of an adrenal cortical carcinoma. A case report. *Acta Chir Belg* 2004;104(2):226–228.
279. Ende DA, Robinson G, Moulton J. Metastasis-induced perforated appendicitis: an acute abdomen of rare aetiology. *Aust N Z J Surg* 1995;65(1):62–63.
280. Reese JA, Blocker SH. Torsion of pedunculated hepatocellular carcinoma. Report of a case in a young woman presenting with abdominal pain. *Mo Med* 1994;91(9):594–595.
281. Andreasen DA, Poulsen J. Intra-abdominal torsion of the testis with seminoma (see comments). *Ugeskr Laeger* 1997;159(14):2103–2104.
282. Abbott J. Pelvic pain: lessons from anatomy and physiology. *J Emerg Med* 1990;8(4):441–447.
283. Daniels IR, Layer GT. Testicular tumours presenting as gynaecomastia. *Eur J Surg Oncol* 2003;29(5):437–439.
284. Duparc C, Boissiere-Veverka G, Lefebvre H, et al. An oestrogen-producing seminoma responsible for gynaecomastia. *Horm Metab Res* 2003;35(5):324–329.
285. Foppiani L, Bernasconi D, Del Monte P, et al. Leydig cell tumour-induced bilateral gynaecomastia in a young man: endocrine abnormalities. *Andrologia* 2005;37(1):36–39.
286. Forst T, Beyer J, Cordes U, et al. Gynaecomastia in a patient with a hCG producing giant cell carcinoma of the lung. Case report. *Exp Clin Endocrinol Diabetes* 1995;103(1):28–32.
287. Wurzel RS, Yamase HT, Nieh PT. Ectopic production of human chorionic gonadotropin by poorly differentiated transitional cell tumors of the urinary tract. *J Urol* 1987;137(3):502–504.
288. Liu G, Rosenfield Darling ML, Chan J, et al. Gynecomastia in a patient with lung cancer. *J Clin Oncol* 1999;17(6):1956.
289. Tseng A Jr, Horning SJ, Freiha FS, et al. Gynecomastia in testicular cancer patients. Prognostic and therapeutic implications. *Cancer* 1985;56(10):2534–2538.
290. Cantwell BM, Richardson PG, Campbell SJ. Gynaecomastia and extragonadal symptoms leading to diagnosis delay of germ cell tumours in young men [see comments]. *Postgrad Med J* 1991;67(789):675–677.
291. Mellor SG, McCutchan JD. Gynaecomastia and occult Leydig cell tumour of the testis. *Br J Urol* 1989;63(4):420–422.
292. Haas GP, Pittaluga S, Gomella L, et al. Clinically occult Leydig cell tumor presenting with gynecomastia. *J Urol* 1989;142(5):1325–1327.
293. Allen CM, Camisa C. Paraneoplastic pemphigus: a review of the literature. *Oral Dis* 2000;6(4):208–214.
294. Camisa C, Helm TN, Liu YC, et al. Paraneoplastic pemphigus: a report of three cases including one long- term survivor. *J Am Acad Dermatol* 1992;27(4):547–553.
295. DeCross AJ, Sahasrabudhe DM. Paraneoplastic Raynaud's phenomenon. *Am J Med* 1992;92(5):571–572.
296. Borenstein A, Seidman DS, Ben-Ari GY. Raynaud's phenomenon as a presenting sign of metastatic melanoma. *Am J Med Sci* 1990;300(1):41–42.
297. Wilmalaratna HS, Sachdev D. Adenocarcinoma of the lung presenting with Raynaud's phenomenon, digital gangrene and multiple infarctions in the internal organs. *Br J Rheumatol* 1987;26(6):473–475.
298. Ocean AJ, Vahdat LT. Chemotherapy-induced peripheral neuropathy: pathogenesis and emerging therapies. *Support Care Cancer* 2004;12(9):619–625.
299. Rosenthal S, Kaufman S. Vincristine neurotoxicity. *Ann Intern Med* 1974;80(6):733–737.
300. Forman A. Peripheral neuropathy in cancer patients: clinical types, etiology, and presentation. Part 2. *Oncology (Huntingt)* 1990;4(2):85–89.
301. Mollman JE, Hogan WM, Glover DJ, et al. Unusual presentation of cis-platinum neuropathy. *Neurology* 1988;38(3):488–490.
302. Siegal T, Haim N. Cisplatin-induced peripheral neuropathy. Frequent off-therapy deterioration, demyelinating syndromes, and muscle cramps. *Cancer* 1990;66(6):1117–1123.
303. Culy CR, Clemett D, Wiseman LR. Oxaliplatin. A review of its pharmacological properties and clinical efficacy in metastatic colorectal cancer and its potential in other malignancies [In Process Citation]. *Drugs* 2000;60(4):895–924.
304. Postma TJ, Vermorken JB, Liefting AJ, et al. Paclitaxel-induced neuropathy. *Ann Oncol* 1995;6(5):489–494.
305. Weiss HD, Walker MD, Wiernik PH. Neurotoxicity of commonly used antineoplastic agents (first of two parts). *N Engl J Med* 1974;291(2):75–81.
306. Weiss HD, Walker MD, Wiernik PH. Neurotoxicity of commonly used antineoplastic agents (second of two parts). *N Engl J Med* 1974;291(3):127–133.
307. Spencer CM, Goa KL. Amifostine. A review of its pharmacodynamic and pharmacokinetic properties, and therapeutic potential as a radioprotector and cytotoxic chemoprotector. *Drugs* 1995;50(6):1001–1031.
308. Penz M, Kornek GV, Raderer M, et al. Subcutaneous administration of amifostine: a promising therapeutic option in patients with oxaliplatin-related peripheral sensitive neuropathy. *Ann Oncol* 2001;12(3):421–422.
309. Cascinu S, Catalano V, Cordella L, et al. Neuroprotective effect of reduced glutathione on oxaliplatin-based chemotherapy in advanced colorectal cancer: a randomized, double-blind, placebo-controlled trial. *J Clin Oncol* 2002;20(16):3478–3483.
310. Cascinu S, Cordella L, Del Ferro E, et al. Neuroprotective effect of reduced glutathione on cisplatin-based chemotherapy in advanced gastric cancer: a randomized double-blind placebo-controlled trial. *J Clin Oncol* 1995;13(1):26–32.
311. Gamelin L, Boisdron-Celle M, Delva R, et al. Prevention of oxaliplatin-related neurotoxicity by calcium and magnesium infusions: a retrospective study of 161 patients receiving oxaliplatin combined with 5-Fluorouracil and leucovorin for advanced colorectal cancer. *Clin Cancer Res* 2004;10(12 Pt 1):4055–4061.
312. Virik K, Karapetis C, Droufakou S, et al. Avascular necrosis of bone: the hidden risk of glucocorticoids used as antiemetics in cancer chemotherapy. *Int J Clin Pract* 2001;55(5):344–345.
313. Cook AM, Dzik-Jurasz AS, Padhani AR, et al. The prevalence of avascular necrosis in patients treated with chemotherapy for testicular tumours. *Br J Cancer* 2001;85(11):1624–1626.
314. Fink JC, Leisenring WM, Sullivan KM, et al. Avascular necrosis following bone marrow transplantation: a case-control study. *Bone* 1998;22(1):67–71.
315. DeSmet AA, Dalinka MK, Alazraki N, et al. Diagnostic imaging of avascular necrosis of the hip. American College of Radiology. ACR appropriateness criteria. *Radiology* 2000;215(Suppl):247–254.
316. Castellanos AM, Glass JP, Yung WK. Regional nerve injury after intra-arterial chemotherapy. *Neurology* 1987;37(5):834–837.
317. Kahn CE Jr, Messersmith RN, Samuels BL. Brachial plexopathy as a complication of intraarterial cisplatin chemotherapy. *Cardiovasc Intervent Radiol* 1989;12(1):47–49.
318. Berger CC, Bokemeyer C, Schneider M, et al. Secondary Raynaud's phenomenon and other late vascular complications following chemotherapy for testicular cancer. *Eur J Cancer* 1995;31A(13–14):2229–2238.
319. Kukla LJ, McGuire WP, Lad T, et al. Acute vascular episodes associated with therapy for carcinomas of the upper aerodigestive

tract with bleomycin, vincristine, and cisplatin. *Cancer Treat Rep* 1982;66(2):369–370.

320. Hansen SW, Olsen N, Rossing N, et al. Vascular toxicity and the mechanism underlying Raynaud's phenomenon in patients treated with cisplatin, vinblastine and bleomycin [see comments]. *Ann Oncol* 1990;1(4):289–292.

321. McLeod DG, Iversen P. Gynecomastia in patients with prostate cancer: a review of treatment options. *Urology* 2000;56(5):713–720.

322. Srinivasan V, Miree J Jr, Lloyd FA. Bilateral mastectomy and irradiation in the prevention of estrogen induced gynecomastia. *J Urol* 1972;107(4):624–625.

323. Soloway MS, Schellhammer PF, Smith JA, et al. Bicalutamide in the treatment of advanced prostatic carcinoma: a phase II multicenter trial. *Urology* 1996;47(1A Suppl):33–37. discussion 48–53.

324. Brogden RN, Chrisp P. Flutamide. A review of its pharmacodynamic and pharmacokinetic properties, and therapeutic use in advanced prostatic cancer. *Drugs Aging* 1991;1(2):104–115.

325. Goldenberg SL, Bruchovsky N. Use of cyproterone acetate in prostate cancer. *Urol Clin North Am* 1991;18(1):111–122.

326. Chrisp P, Goa KL. Goserelin. A review of its pharmacodynamic and pharmacokinetic properties, and clinical use in sex hormone-related conditions. *Drugs* 1991;41(2):254–288.

327. Chrisp P, Sorkin EM. Leuprorelin. A review of its pharmacology and therapeutic use in prostatic disorders. *Drugs Aging* 1991;1(6):487–509.

328. Ramamurthy L, Cooper RA. Metastatic carcinoma to the male breast. *Br J Radiol* 1991;64(759):277–278.

329. Olsson H, Alm P, Kristoffersson U, et al. Hypophyseal tumor and gynecomastia preceding bilateral breast cancer development in a man. *Cancer* 1984;53(9):1974–1977.

330. Maunsell E, Brisson J, Deschenes L. Arm problems and psychological distress after surgery for breast cancer. *Can J Surg* 1993;36(4):315–320.

331. Hladiuk M, Huchcroft S, Temple W, et al. Arm function after axillary dissection for breast cancer: a pilot study to provide parameter estimates. *J Surg Oncol* 1992;50(1):47–52.

332. Vecht CJ, Van de Brand HJ, Wajer OJ. Post-axillary dissection pain in breast cancer due to a lesion of the intercostobrachial nerve. *Pain* 1989;38(2):171–176.

333. Kakuda JT, Stuntz M, Trivedi V, et al. Objective assessment of axillary morbidity in breast cancer treatment. *Am Surg* 1999;65(10):995–998.

334. Keramopoulos A, Tsionou C, Minaretzis D, et al. Arm morbidity following treatment of breast cancer with total axillary dissection: a multivariated approach. *Oncology* 1993;50(6):445–449.

335. Kuehn T, Klauss W, Darsow M, et al. Long-term morbidity following axillary dissection in breast cancer patients–clinical assessment, significance for life quality and the impact of demographic, oncologic and therapeutic factors. *Breast Cancer Res Treat* 2000;64(3):275–286.

336. Warmuth MA, Bowen G, Prosnitz LR, et al. Complications of axillary lymph node dissection for carcinoma of the breast: a report based on a patient survey. *Cancer* 1998;83(7):1362–1368.

337. Tasmuth T, von Smitten K, Kalso E. Pain and other symptoms during the first year after radical and conservative surgery for breast cancer. *Br J Cancer* 1996;74(12):2024–2031.

338. Tasmuth T, von SK, Hietanen P, et al. Pain and other symptoms after different treatment modalities of breast cancer. *Ann Oncol* 1995;6(5):453–459.

339. Smith WC, Bourne D, Squair J, et al. A retrospective cohort study of post mastectomy pain syndrome. *Pain* 1999;83(1):91–95.

340. Carpenter JS, Andrykowski MA, Sloan P, et al. Postmastectomy/postlumpectomy pain in breast cancer survivors. *J Clin Epidemiol* 1998;51(12):1285–1292.

341. Wood KM. Intercostobrachial nerve entrapment syndrome. *South Med J* 1978;71(6):662–663.

342. Paredes JP, Puente JL, Potel J. Variations in sensitivity after sectioning the intercostobrachial nerve. *Am J Surg* 1990;160(5):525–528.

343. van Dam MS, Hennipman A, de Kruif JT, et al. Complications following axillary dissection for breast carcinoma (see comments). *Ned Tijdschr Geneeskd* 1993;137(46):2395–2398.

344. Granek I, Ashikari R, Foley KM. Postmastectomy pain syndrome: clinical and anatomic correlates [Abstract]. *Proc Am Soc Clin Oncol* 1983;3:122.

345. International Association for the Study of Pain: Subcommittee on Taxonomy. Classification of chronic pain. *Pain* 1986;3(suppl):135–138.

346. Ernst MF, Voogd AC, Balder W, et al. Early and late morbidity associated with axillary levels I-III dissection in breast cancer. *J Surg Oncol* 2002;79(3):151–155. discussion 156.

347. Stevens PE, Dibble SL, Miaskowski C. Prevalence, characteristics, and impact of postmastectomy pain syndrome: an investigation of women's experiences. *Pain* 1995;61(1):61–68.

348. Macdonald L, Bruce J, Scott NW, et al. Long-term follow-up of breast cancer survivors with post-mastectomy pain syndrome. *Br J Cancer* 2005;92(2):225–230.

349. Bratschi HU, Haller U. Significance of the intercostobrachial nerve in axillary lymph node excision. *Geburtshilfe Frauenheilhd* 1990;50(9):689–693.

350. Assa J. The intercostobrachial nerve in radical mastectomy. *J Surg Oncol* 1974;6(2):123–126.

351. Torresan RZ, Cabello C, Conde DM, et al. Impact of the preservation of the intercostobrachial nerve in axillary lymphadenectomy due to breast cancer. *Breast J* 2003;9(5):389–392.

352. Blunt C, Schmiedel A. Some cases of severe post-mastectomy pain syndrome may be caused by an axillary haematoma. *Pain* 2004;108(3):294–296.

353. Hack TF, Cohen L, Katz J, et al. Physical and psychological morbidity after axillary lymph node dissection for breast cancer. *J Clin Oncol* 1999;17(1):143–149.

354. Johansson S, Svensson H, Larsson LG, et al. Brachial plexopathy after postoperative radiotherapy of breast cancer patients—a long-term follow-up. *Acta Oncol* 2000;39(3):373–382.

355. Temple WJ, Ketcham AS. Preservation of the intercostobrachial nerve during axillary dissection for breast cancer. *Am J Surg* 1985;150(5):585–588.

356. Salmon RJ, Ansquer Y, Asselain B. Preservation versus section of Intercostal-Brachial Nerve (IBN) in axillary dissection for breast cancer–a prospective randomized trial. *Eur J Surg Oncol* 1998;24(3):158–161.

357. Baron RH, Fey JV, Raboy S, et al. Eighteen sensations after breast cancer surgery: a comparison of sentinel lymph node biopsy and axillary lymph node dissection. *Oncol Nurs Forum* 2002;29(4):651–659.

358. Haid A, Kuehn T, Konstantiniuk P, et al. Shoulder-arm morbidity following axillary dissection and sentinel node only biopsy for breast cancer. *Eur J Surg Oncol* 2002;28(7):705–710.

359. Haid A, Koberle-Wuhrer R, Knauer M, et al. Morbidity of breast cancer patients following complete axillary dissection or sentinel node biopsy only: a comparative evaluation. *Breast Cancer Res Treat* 2002;73(1):31–36.

360. Miguel R, Kuhn AM, Shons AR, et al. The effect of sentinel node selective axillary lymphadenectomy on the incidence of postmastectomy pain syndrome. *Cancer Control* 2001;8(5):427–430.

361. Schrenk P, Rieger R, Shamiyeh A, et al. Morbidity following sentinel lymph node biopsy versus axillary lymph node dissection for patients with breast carcinoma. *Cancer* 2000;88(3):608–614.

362. Swenson KK, Nissen MJ, Ceronsky C, et al. Comparison of side effects between sentinel lymph node and axillary lymph node dissection for breast cancer. *Ann Surg Oncol* 2002;9(8):745–753.

363. Albrecht MR, Zink K, Busch W, et al. Dissection or irradiation of the axilla in postmenopausal patients? Long-term results and long-term effects in 655 patients. *Strahlenther Onkol* 2002;178(9):510–516.

364. Deutsch M, Flickinger JC. Shoulder and arm problems after radiotherapy for primary breast cancer. *Am J Clin Oncol* 2001;24(2):172–176.

365. Johansen J, Overgaard J, Blichert-Toft M, et al. Treatment of morbidity associated with the management of the axilla in breast-conserving therapy. *Acta Oncol* 2000;39(3):349–354.

366. Moskovitz AH, Anderson BO, Yeung RS, et al. Axillary web syndrome after axillary dissection. *Am J Surg* 2001;181(5):434–439.

367. Hughes LL, Styblo TM, Thoms WW, et al. Cellulitis of the breast as a complication of breast-conserving surgery and irradiation. *Am J Clin Oncol* 1997;20(4):338–341.

368. Dijkstra PU, van Wilgen PC, Buijs RP, et al. Incidence of shoulder pain after neck dissection: a clinical explorative study for risk factors. *Head Neck* 2001;23(11):947–953.

369. van Wilgen CP, Dijkstra PU, van der Laan BF, et al. Shoulder complaints after neck dissection; is the spinal accessory nerve involved? *Br J Oral Maxillofac Surg* 2003;41(1):7–11.

370. Talmi YP, Horowitz Z, Pfeffer MR, et al. Pain in the neck after neck dissection. *Otolaryngol Head Neck Surg* 2000;123(3):302–306.

371. Swift TR, Nichols FT. The droopy shoulder syndrome. *Neurology* 1984;34(2):212–215.

372. Brown H, Burns S, Kaiser CW. The spinal accessory nerve plexus, the trapezius muscle, and shoulder stabilization after radical neck cancer surgery. *Ann Surg* 1988;208(5):654–661.

373. Terrell JE, Welsh DE, Bradford CR, et al. Pain, quality of life, and spinal accessory nerve status after neck dissection [In Process Citation]. *Laryngoscope* 2000;110(4):620–626.

374. Bruera E, MacDonald N. Intractable pain in patients with advanced head and neck tumors: a possible role of local infection. *Cancer Treat Rep* 1986;70(5):691–692.

375. Coyle N, Portenoy RK. Infection as a cause of rapidly increasing pain in cancer patients. *J Pain Symptom Manage* 1991;6(4):266–269.

376. Keller SM, Carp NZ, Levy MN, et al. Chronic post thoracotomy pain. *J Cardiovasc Surg (Torino)* 1994;35(6Suppl 1):161–164.

377. Kanner R, Martini N, Foley KM. Nature and incidence of postthoracotomy pain [Abstract]. *Proc Am Soc Clin Oncol* 1982;1:590.

378. Hamada H, Moriwaki K, Shiroyama K, et al. Myofascial pain in patients with postthoracotomy pain syndrome. *Reg Anesth Pain Med* 2000;25(3):302–305.

379. Nikolajsen L, Jensen TS. Phantom limb pain. *Curr Rev Pain* 2000;4(2):166–170.

380. Ehde DM, Czerniecki JM, Smith DG, et al. Chronic phantom sensations, phantom pain, residual limb pain, and other regional pain after lower limb amputation. *Arch Phys Med Rehabil* 2000;81(8):1039–1044.

381. Flor H. Phantom-limb pain: characteristics, causes, and treatment. *Lancet Neurol* 2002;1(3):182–189.

382. Nikolajsen L, Ilkjaer S, Kroner K, et al. The influence of preamputation pain on postamputation stump and phantom pain. *Pain* 1997;72(3):393–405.

383. Weinstein SM. Phantom pain. *Oncology (Huntingt)* 1994;8(5):65–70. discussion 70, 73–74.

384. Katz J, Melzack R. Pain 'memories' in phantom limbs: review and clinical observations. *Pain* 1990;43(3):319–336.

385. Smith J, Thompson JM. Phantom limb pain and chemotherapy in pediatric amputees. *Mayo Clin Proc* 1995;70(4):357–364.

386. Enneking FK, Morey TE. Continuous postoperative infusion of a regional anesthetic after an amputation of the lower extremity. A randomized clinical trial [letter]. *J Bone Joint Surg Am* 1997;79(11):1752–1753.

387. Katz J. Prevention of phantom limb pain by regional anaesthesia. *Lancet* 1997;349(9051):519–520.

388. Nikolajsen L, Ilkjaer S, Christensen JH, et al. Randomised trial of epidural bupivacaine and morphine in prevention of stump and phantom pain in lower-limb amputation [see comments]. *Lancet* 1997;350(9088):1353–1357.

389. Pavy TJ, Doyle DL. Prevention of phantom limb pain by infusion of local anaesthetic into the sciatic nerve [see comments]. *Anaesth Intensive Care* 1996;24(5):599–600.

390. Chang VT, Tunkel RS, Pattillo BA, et al. Increased phantom limb pain as an initial symptom of spinal-neoplasia [published erratum appears in *J Pain Symptom Manage* 1997;14(3):135]. *J Pain Symptom Manage* 1997;13(6):362–364.

391. Kwekkeboom K. Postmastectomy pain syndromes. *Cancer Nurs* 1996; 19(1):37–43.

392. Kroner K, Krebs B, Skov J, et al. Immediate and long-term phantom breast syndrome after mastectomy: incidence, clinical characteristics and relationship to pre-mastectomy breast pain. *Pain* 1989;36(3): 327–334.

393. Rothemund Y, Grusser SM, Liebeskind U, et al. Phantom phenomena in mastectomized patients and their relation to chronic and acute pre-mastectomy pain. *Pain* 2004;107(1–2):140–146.

394. Ovesen P, Kroner K, Ornsholt J, et al. Phantom-related phenomena after rectal amputation: prevalence and clinical characteristics. *Pain* 1991;44(3):289–291.

395. Brena SF, Sammons EE. Phantom urinary bladder pain—case report. *Pain* 1979;7(2):197–201.

396. Nicolodi M, Frezzotti R, Diadori A, et al. Phantom eye: features and prevalence. The predisposing role of headache. *Cephalalgia* 1997;17(4):501–504.

397. Bond JB, Wesley RE. Cluster headache after orbital exenteration. *Ann Ophthalmol* 1987;19(11):438.

398. Davis RW. Phantom sensation, phantom pain, and stump pain. *Arch Phys Med Rehabil* 1993;74(1):79–91.

399. Schultheiss TE, Stephens LC. Invited review: permanent radiation myelopathy. *Br J Radiol* 1992;65(777):737–753.

400. Alfonso ER, De Gregorio MA, Mateo P, et al. Radiation myelopathy in over-irradiated patients: MR imaging findings. *Eur Radiol* 1997;7(3):400–404.

401. Koehler PJ, Verbiest H, Jager J, et al. Delayed radiation myelopathy: serial MR-imaging and pathology. *Clin Neurol Neurosurg* 1996;98(2):197–201.

402. Yeoh EK, Horowitz M. Radiation enteritis. *Surg Gynecol Obstet* 1987;165(4):373–379.

403. Nussbaum ML, Campana TJ, Weese JL. Radiation-induced intestinal injury. *Clin Plast Surg* 1993;20(3):573–580.

404. Tagkalidis PP, Tjandra JJ. Chronic radiation proctitis. *ANZ J Surg* 2001;71(4):230–237.

405. Chi KD, Ehrenpreis ED, Jani AB. Accuracy and reliability of the endoscopic classification of chronic radiation-induced proctopathy using a novel grading method. *J Clin Gastroenterol* 2005;39(1):42–46.

406. Joly F, Brune D, Couette JE, et al. Health-related quality of life and sequelae in patients treated with brachytherapy and external beam irradiation for localized prostate cancer. *Ann Oncol* 1998;9(7):751–757.

407. Pillay PK, Teh M, Chua EJ, et al. Haemorrhagic chronic radiation cystitis–following treatment of pelvic malignancies. *Ann Acad Med Singapore* 1984;13(4):634–638.

408. Perez CA, Grigsby PW, Lockett MA, et al. Radiation therapy morbidity in carcinoma of the uterine cervix: dosimetric and clinical correlation. *Int J Radiat Oncol Biol Phys* 1999;44(4):855–866.

409. Newman ML, Brennan M, Passik S. Lymphedema complicated by pain and psychological distress: a case with complex treatment needs. *J Pain Symptom Manage* 1996;12(6):376–379.

410. McWayne J, Heiney SP. Psychologic and social sequelae of secondary lymphedema. *Cancer* 2005;104(3):457–466.

411. Herrera JE, Stubblefield MD. Rotator cuff tendonitis in lymphedema: a retrospective case series. *Arch Phys Med Rehabil* 2004;85(12):1939–1942.

412. Ganel A, Engel J, Sela M, et al. Nerve entrapments associated with postmastectomy lymphedema. *Cancer* 1979;44(6):2254–2259.

413. Minsky BD, Cohen AM. Minimizing the toxicity of pelvic radiation therapy in rectal cancer. *Oncology (Huntingt)* 1988;2(8):21–25, 28–29.

414. Mannaerts GH, Rutten HJ, Martijn H, et al. Effects on functional outcome after IORT-containing multimodality treatment for locally advanced primary and locally recurrent rectal cancer. *Int J Radiat Oncol Biol Phys* 2002;54(4):1082–1088.

415. Wallner K, Elliott K, Merrick G, et al. Chronic pelvic pain following prostate brachytherapy: a case report. *Brachytherapy* 2004;3(3):153–158.

416. Epstein JB, Rea G, Wong FL, et al. Osteonecrosis: study of the relationship of dental extractions in patients receiving radiotherapy. *Head Neck Surg* 1987;10(1):48–54.

417. Epstein J, van der Meij E, McKenzie M, et al. Postradiation osteonecrosis of the mandible: a long-term follow-up study. *Oral Surg Oral Med Oral Pathol Oral Radiol Endod* 1997;83(6):657–662.

418. Portenoy RK, Hagen NA. Breakthrough pain: definition, prevalence and characteristics. *Pain* 1990;41(3):273–281.

419. Jacobsen P, Kriegstein O, Portenoy R. Breakthrough pain: prevalence and characteristics (Meeting abstract). *Proc Annu Meet Am Soc Clin Oncol* 1994;13:1643.

420. Fine PG, Busch MA. Characterization of breakthrough pain by hospice patients and their caregivers. *J Pain Symptom Manage* 1998;16(3):179–183.

421. Bach F, Larsen BH, Rohde K, et al. Metastatic spinal cord compression. Occurrence, symptoms, clinical presentations and prognosis in 398 patients with spinal cord compression. *Acta Neurochir (Wien)* 1990;107(1–2):37–43.

422. Bernat JL, Greenberg ER, Barrett J. Suspected epidural compression of the spinal cord and cauda equina by metastatic carcinoma. Clinical diagnosis and survival. *Cancer* 1983;51(10):1953–1957.

423. Copeman MC. Presenting symptoms of neoplastic spinal cord compression. *J Surg Oncol* 1988;37(1):24–25.

424. Jaeckle KA. Causes and management of headaches in cancer patients. *Oncology (Huntingt)* 1993;7(4):27–31. discussion 31–32, 34.

425. MacFarlane BV, Wright A, O'Collaghan J, et al. Chronic neuropathic pain and its control by drugs. *Pharmacol Ther* 1997;75(1):1–19.

426. Allen RR. Neuropathic pain in the cancer patient. *Neurol Clin* 1998;16(4):869–888.

427. McQuay HJ, Tramer M, Nye BA, et al. A systematic review of antidepressants in neuropathic pain. *Pain* 1996;68(2–3):217–227.

428. Portenoy RK. Issues in the management of neuropathic pain. In: Basbaum A, Besson J-M, eds. *Towards a new pharmacotherapy of pain.* New York: John Wiley and Sons, 1991:393–416.

429. Janig W. Neurobiology of visceral afferent neurons: neuroanatomy, functions, organ regulations and sensations. *Biol Psychol* 1996;42(1–2):29–51.

CHAPTER 2 ■ DIFFICULT PAIN SYNDROMES: BONE PAIN, VISCERAL PAIN, NEUROPATHIC PAIN

MARCO PAPPAGALLO, LAUREN SHAIOVA, EUGENE PERLOV, AND HELENA KNOTKOVA

Nociception is what occurs physiologically in our bodies during the activation and sensitization of tissue nociceptors, also known as *A-delta* and *C nerve fibers*. Pain corresponds to our awareness of nociception and has been defined as "an unpleasant sensory and emotional experience associated with tissue damage or described in terms of such damage" (1).

In the clinical setting, pain may occur as a response to a noxious event in the tissue, for example, tissue inflammation due to a burn injury, or as a response to an abnormal pathologic process occurring within the nervous system pain pathways. In the first case, the pain signal presumably originates from "healthy" tissue nociceptors activated or sensitized by the local release of algogenic substances (e.g., protons, prostaglandins, bradykinin, adenosine, cytokines, etc.). This type of pain is called *nociceptive*. In the second case, the pain signal is generated ectopically by abnormal peripheral nerve fibers involved in pain transmission and/or by abnormal pain circuits in the central nervous system (CNS); this type of pain has been called *neuropathic*. However, the separation between nociceptive and neuropathic pain states is often blurred. Indeed, as discussed in the subsequent text, neuropathic pain may arise from inflammation (i.e., inflammatory neuropathic pain) (2). Inflammatory and neuropathic mechanisms may be present at the same time or at different times in patients who have been diagnosed with cancer pain syndromes of bone or visceral origin. In fact, cancer pain, whether arising from viscera, bone, or any other somatic structure, is more often than commonly thought the result of a mixture of pain mechanisms. When cancer pain becomes a clinical challenge to treatment, it has been labeled as a difficult pain syndrome.

DIFFICULT PAIN SYNDROMES: PERIPHERAL AND CENTRAL MECHANISMS

The pain signal is transmitted from the peripheral nociceptors, through the dorsal horn of the spinal cord and the thalamus, up to the cortex. In the periphery, nociceptors can be activated by chemical products of tissue damage and inflammation, which include prostanoids, serotonin, bradykinin, cytokines, adenosine, adenosine-5′-triphosphate (ATP), histamine, protons, free radicals, and growth factors. These agents can activate afferent fibers or sensitize them to a range of mechanical, thermal, and chemical stimuli. Notably, a proportion of the afferent fibers that are normally unresponsive to noxious stimuli ("silent" or "sleeping" nociceptors) can be "awakened" by inflammatory chemicals and be stimulated to contribute to pain and hyperalgesia. The products of tissue damage and inflammation interact with receptors located on the A-delta fibers and C fibers to initiate membrane excitability and intracellular transcriptional changes.

Most neuropathic pain conditions develop after partial injuries to the peripheral nervous system (PNS). For example, as observed in animal models of partial nerve injury, both injured and uninjured primary sensory neurons acquire the ability to express genes *de novo* and, therefore, change their phenotype (phenotypic shift). Nerve endings develop sensitivity to a number of factors, such as prostanoids and cytokines [e.g., tumor necrosis factor-α (TNF-α)] (3–6). One example is the upregulation or induction of catecholamine receptors in undamaged nociceptors; in this condition, nociceptors are activated by noradrenaline, and the resulting neuropathic pain has been called *sympathetically maintained pain* (SMP) (7,8). Reversal of the phenotypic shift is associated with the reduction of neuropathic pain (9).

Recent findings suggest that during cancer (and other pathologic inflammatory conditions), a number of diffusible factors might be involved in causing a "neuropathic spin" in the cancer-related pain state. Tissue-related growth factors [e.g., nerve growth factor (NGF)] in combination with specific proinflammatory cytokines (e.g., TNF-α, interleukin-1β (10)) might sensitize nociceptors and generate ectopic and spontaneous activity in tissue nociceptors. In these instances, pain caused by cancer could be classified more properly as inflammatory neuropathic pain. There is considerable hope that the identification of the diffusible factors causing altered gene expression in the dorsal root ganglia (DRG) sensory neurons will direct research to discover more effective treatments. Early and aggressive pain interventions and the use of specific therapies that disengage gene expression might be sufficient to uncouple the phenotypic shift and reverse a difficult pain syndrome into an easy-to-treat condition.

TABLE 2.1

DEVELOPMENT OF PATHOLOGIC PAIN: RELEVANT PERIPHERAL NERVOUS SYSTEM FACTORS

Target—peripheral nervous system mechanisms	Target—activation and cellular effect	Target—clinical importance for	Notes	References
TRPV-1, 2, 3,4 channels	TRPV channels activated by noxious heat, low pH, and capsaicin A subpopulation of primary nociceptive neurons coexpresses TRPV-1 with the ANKTM-1 channels; the ANKTM channels are activated by noxious cold stimulation Nociceptive sensory nerve fibers activation and release of neuropeptides occur	**Inflammatory neuropathic pain**	Activation of TRPV-1 nociceptive neurons leads to the release of neuropeptides, including SP; on endothelial cells, SP binds to the neurokinin-1 receptor and promotes the extravasation of plasma into the interstitial tissue; SP can activate osteoclasts and mast cells; mast cells are known to produce, store, and release NGF (see subsequent text) and proinflammatory cytokines	(11,12)
α-2-Δ subunit of N- and P/Q-type voltage-gated calcium channels	Neuronal membrane voltage changes and nerve fiber activation occur Intracellular calcium influx occurs Nociceptive sensory nerve fiber activation and release of neuropeptides occur	**Inflammatory neuropathic pain**	The gabapentinoids, gabapentin and pregabalin, likely produce their analgesic effect by modulating the activity of the neuronal N- and P/Q-type voltage-gated calcium channels Gabapentinoids bind with high affinity to the α-2-Δ subunit of voltage-gated calcium channels and produce a decrease in intracellular calcium influx Ziconotide, a peptide analgesic derived from the venom of the predatory marine snail *Conus magellaris*, is a neuron-specific (N-type) calcium channel blocker that has recently been approved for intrathecal use	(13–15)
Voltage-gated sodium channels, for example, TTX-R Na (v) 1.8 and TTX-S Na (v) 1.7	Neuronal membrane voltage changes Intracellular sodium influx occurs Nociceptive sensory nerve fiber activation and release of neuropeptides occur	**Inflammatory neuropathic pain**	Chronic inflammation results in an upregulation in the expression of both TTX-S and TTX-R sodium channels Primary nociceptive sensory neurons express multiple voltage-gated sodium channels, of which the TTX-R channel Na (v) 1.8 has been suggested to play a major role in inflammatory pain Observations also suggest that the TTX-S channel Na (v) 1.7 may play a role in pathologic pain; for example, recent studies have shown that the neuropathic pain disorder, known as *familial erythromelalgia*, is a channelopathy caused by mutations in the gene encoding the TTX-S Na (v) 1.7 sodium channel; familial erythromelalgia is an autosomal dominant disease characterized by severe burning pain in distal extremities; the pain is typically relieved by cold temperature or ice pack application to the painful extremities; warm environments and physical exercise aggravate the pain	(16–18)
Proton-gated or ASIC 1, 3 channels	Activated by low pH and by noxious mechanical stimuli Nociceptive sensory nerve fiber activation and release of neuropeptides occur	**Bone pain** **Mechanical pain**	ASICs are amiloride-sensitive channels; the acidic environment created by the osteoclasts during bone resorption activates ASICs; ASICs also appear to play a role in the transduction of mechanical painful stimuli and in the genesis of bone pain	(19)

(continued)

TABLE 2.1

(CONTINUED)

Target–peripheral nervous system mechanisms	Target–activation and cellular effect	Target–clinical importance for	Notes	References
TrkA	Activated by NGF The TrkA–NGF complex is internalized and retrogradely transported to the dorsal root ganglia sensory neuron cell body, where it initiates gene transcription that gives rise to the upregulation of receptors and ion channels (e.g., ASICs), and release of neuropeptides involved in pain transmission	Bone pain Inflammatory neuropathic pain	The sensory innervation of cortical and trabecular bone, as well as bone marrow, is extensive and primarily consists of TrkA-expressing fibers New evidence indicates that NGF plays an important role in cancer bone pain; antibodies directed against NGF are effective against bone pain in animal models of cancer-induced bone pain	(9,20–22)
Purine receptors (P2X3, P2X2/3)	Activated by ATP Nociceptive sensory nerve fiber activation and release of neuropeptides occur	Inflammatory pain Mechanical pain	P2X3 receptors are localized on peripheral sensory afferents; their activation causes nociception and contributes to hyperalgesia and mechanical allodynia ATP may also activate the adenosine receptors (see text)	(23–27)
PAR-2	Activated by mast cell–derived tryptase and other proteinases	Inflammatory neuropathic pain	PAR-2 receptors were recently discovered They are present in primary sensory neurons and are involved in mechanisms of hyperalgesia	(28)
Cannabinoid receptors (CB1, CB2)	Activated by endocannabinoids	Inflammatory neuropathic pain	CB1 receptors are primarily located in the central nervous system and CB2 receptors in the peripheral tissues Recent studies suggest a potential role of cannabinoids not only as anti-inflammatory and antihyperalgesic agents but also in the potentiation of opioid analgesia	(19)
Bradykinin receptors (B1, B2)	Activated by bradykinin	Inflammatory pain	Nociceptive sensory neurons express the bradykinin receptors B1 and B2; expression of B1 receptors is induced by tissue injury, and B1 contributes significantly to inflammatory hyperalgesia	(29)

TRPV, transient receptor potential vanilloid; SP, substance P; ANKTM, ankyrin-like protein with transmembrane domains; NGF, nerve growth factor; TTX-R, tetrodotoxin-resistant; TTX-S, tetrodotoxin-sensitive; ASIC, acid-sensing ion channel; TrkA, tyrosine kinase A; ATP, adenosine-5′-triphosphate; PAR-2, proteinase-activated receptor-2.

Peripheral Mechanisms of Pathologic Pain

In the PNS, several elements of the cellular "machinery" thought to be relevant to the development of pathologic pain have been identified as potential targets for analgesic drugs. These PNS targets are summarized in Table 2.1.

Central Mechanisms of Pathologic Pain

In the CNS, in particular within the spinal cord, a variety of neurobiologic events can occur during the course of ongoing peripheral tissue damage and inflammation (Fig. 2.1) (30). Spinal cord CNS factors known to be relevant to the development of pathologic pain are listed in Table 2.2.

NEUROPATHIC PAIN

Clinical Findings and Diagnosis

The clinical interview of a patient with cancer pain should focus on questions about onset, duration, progression, and nature of complaints suggestive of neurologic deficits (e.g., persistent numbness in a body area, or limb weakness, such as tripping episodes, the progressive inability to open jars, etc.), as well as complaints suggestive of sensory dysfunction (e.g., touch-evoked pain, intermittent abnormal sensations, spontaneous burning, and shooting pains). Notably, patients may report only sensory symptoms and have no neurologic deficits.

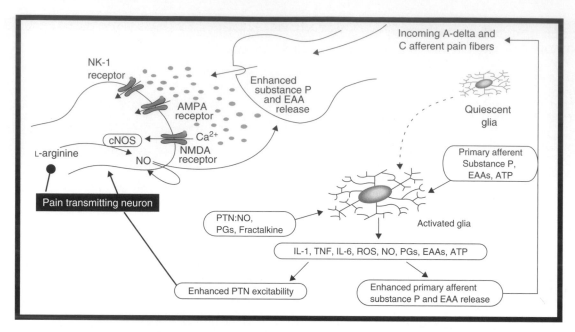

FIGURE 2.1. Central mechanisms of pathologic pain. NK-1, neurokinin-1; AMPA, α-amino-3-hydroxy-5-methyl-4-isoxazole-propionic acid; NMDA, N-methyl-D-aspartate; EAA, excitatory amino acid; ATP, adenosine-5'-triphosphate; cNOS, constitutive nitric oxide synthase; NO, nitric oxide; PTN, pain-transmitting neuron; PGs, prostaglandins; IL, interleukin; TNF, tumor necrosis factor; ROS, reactive oxygen species. (Modified and adapted from Watkins LR, Milligan ED, Maier SF. Glial activation: a driving force for pathologic pain. *Trends Neurosci* 2001;24(8):450–455.)

Patients with neuropathic pain may present with some or all of the following abnormal sensory symptoms and signs:

- *Paresthesias*. Spontaneous, intermittent, painless, abnormal sensations
- *Dysesthesias*. Spontaneous or evoked unpleasant sensations, such as annoying sensations elicited by cold stimuli or pinprick testing
- *Allodynia*. Pain elicited by nonnoxious stimuli (i.e., clothing, air movement, tactile stimuli) when applied to the symptomatic cutaneous area; allodynia may be mechanical (static, e.g., induced by application of a light pressure, or dynamic, e.g., induced by moving a soft brush) or thermal (e.g., induced by a nonpainful cold or warm stimulus)
- *Hyperalgesia*. An exaggerated pain response to a mildly noxious (mechanical or thermal) stimulus applied to the symptomatic area
- *Hyperpathia*. A delayed and explosive pain response to a stimulus applied to the symptomatic area

Allodynia, hyperalgesia, and hyperpathia represent positive abnormal findings, as opposed to the negative findings of the neurologic sensory examination, that is, hypesthesia and anesthesia. Heat hyperalgesia and deep mechanical allodynia (i.e., tenderness on soft tissue palpation) are findings commonly present at the cutaneous epicenter of an inflammatory pain generator, also known as the *zone of primary hyperalgesia*. These findings are indicative of PNS sensitization and are related to a local inflammatory state. On the other hand, the skin surrounding the site of inflammation, also known as the *zone of secondary hyperalgesia*, may present the finding of mechanical allodynia, which can be elicited, for example, by stroking the area with a soft brush. Secondary hyperalgesia is indicative of CNS sensitization. Patients affected by SMP typically complain of cold allodynia/hyperalgesia. This is assessed by providing a cold stimulus, such as placing a cold metallic tuning fork, to the painful region for a few seconds.

Clinical and research tools to assess and measure the intensity and quality of neuropathic pain include the Brief Pain Inventory (BPI) and the Neuropathic Pain Scale (NPS) (41). The BPI is a well-validated instrument that consists of 15 items asking the patient about average pain, worst pain in the past week, whether the patient has received relief from pain treatment, and whether the pain has interfered with daily activities (42). The NPS is a self-report scale for measuring neuropathic pain. It consists of 12 distinct questions, which ask about intensity and quality of the patient's pain. In validation studies, it has been found to have a good predictive power in discriminating between major subgroups of patients with neuropathic pain (42).

Table 2.3 (43) lists the most common neuropathic pain syndromes that have been reported in association with cancer. Neuropathy may result from one or more cancer-related mechanisms (44), for example, compression, mechanical traction, inflammation, or infiltration of nerve trunks or plexi caused by the progression of the primary cancer or by metastatic disease affecting bone or soft tissues. Head and neck cancer and skull-based tumors can cause painful cranial neuropathies by direct nerve compression. Salivary gland cancers may cause painful facial neuropathies. Breast or lung cancer can infiltrate the brachial plexus and cause painful plexitis. Pelvic or retroperitoneal cancer may invade the lumbosacral plexus. If the meninges are affected (meningeal carcinomatosis), the involvement of adjacent roots, spinal nerves, and plexi can occur. Metastatic disease or lymphoma can cause meningeal carcinomatosis and affect multiple spinal roots. Peripheral neuropathies with pain and dysesthesia may also be observed in the presence of lymphomas. Acute inflammatory demyelinating polyneuropathy of the Guillain-Barré syndrome type may occur with lymphomas, particularly Hodgkin's disease.

Antineoplastic therapeutic agents such as cis-platinum, taxoids, and vincristine may cause painful neuropathies. Postradiation plexopathies may arise when >60 Gy (6000 rad)

TABLE 2.2

DEVELOPMENT OF PATHOLOGIC PAIN: RELEVANT CENTRAL NERVOUS SYSTEM FACTORS

Target—central nervous system mechanisms	Target—activation and cellular effect	Target—clinical importance for	Notes	References
NMDA receptors	NK-1 receptors are activated by SP and *NMDA and AMPA* receptors by *EAAs*	Inflammatory neuropathic pain	SP and EAAs can induce central sensitization. NMDA receptors seem to play a relevant role in pain modulation; these receptors are normally inoperative because of the Mg^{2+}-blocking effect; however, in the traditional model of pathologic pain, the intense and/or prolonged "bombardment" of SP and EAAs causes the removal of the Mg^{2+} block from the NMDA receptor and the sensitization of the dorsal horn PTNs	
AMPA receptors	Within the dorsal horn, on incoming nociceptive activity, the small fiber afferents release neuropeptides (*SP,* as well calcitonin gene–related peptide, cholecystokinin, neurokinin A) and *EAAs* (glutamate and aspartate)		The resulting influx of Ca^{2+} causes a series of intracellular changes, including the activation of cNOS, which, in turn, converts L-arginine into NO	
NK-1 receptors	*SP* and *EAAs* cause transient depolarization of the dorsal horn (PTN); EAAs act on several PTN receptors, including NMDA, AMPA, kainate, and the metabotropic receptors			(9,19,31,32)
Microglia Fractalkines Microglia-derived p38 MAP kinase NO, PGs, ATP, and ROS	Increasing evidence suggests that as a consequence of inflammation and/or trauma to peripheral nerves, dorsal horn PTN hyperexcitability is dramatically amplified as a result of spinal cord *microglia activation* It is still unclear what activates the microglia in the spinal cord; however, neuron-to-glia signals exist and include specific substances called *fractalkines*, proteins in the chemokine family, which are expressed on the extracellular surface of spinal neurons and spinal sensory afferents; in specific pathologic states or conditions, fractalkines detach from neurons and bind to activate nearby microglia, the only spinal cells that express fractalkine receptors Several lines of evidence indicate an emerging role of the *microglia-derived p38 MAP kinase* in the development of pathologic pain; in microglia, p38 MAP kinase promotes the synthesis and release of proinflammatory cytokines, including interleukin TNF-α, IL-1β, and IL-6 Microglia activation also leads to an increase in the spinal expression of cyclo-oxygenase and NOS and in the production of *PGs and NO, as well EAAs, ATP, and ROS*	Inflammatory neuropathic pain	Microglia are called the *macrophages* of the central nervous system; when they become activated, in addition to hypertrophy, there is hyperplasia. The tetracycline antibiotic minocycline can specifically inhibit microglial activation. Minocycline prevents the development of hypersensitivity in animal models of neuropathic pain when given before nerve injury; however, minocycline becomes ineffective when administered after the injury Other immunosuppressive or immunomodulatory agents (intrathecal methotrexate and intraperitoneal propentofylline) were tested with the aim of suppressing microglia-derived proinflammatory cytokines It is also known that *in vitro* TNF activates the phosphorylation of p38 MAP kinase (the active form of the kinase); in animal models of neuropathic pain, the TNF antagonist etanercept was found to decrease the hypersensitive pain state in the animal model only when given as a preventive treatment 2 days before the nerve injury; notably, systemic etanercept was shown to affect only the dorsal root ganglia capsaicin-sensitive neuronal p38 MAP kinase and not the spinal microglia p38 MAP kinase	(6,33–40)

NMDA, *N*-methyl-D-aspartate; AMPA, α-amino-3-hydroxy-5-methyl-4-isoxazole-propionic acid; NK-1, neurokinin; SP, substance P; EAAs, excitatory amino acids; PTN, pain-transmitting neuron; MAP, mitogen-activated protein; cNOS, constitutive nitric oxide synthase; NO, nitric oxide; PGs, prostaglandins; ATP, adenosine-5'-triphosphate; ROS, reactive oxygen species; TNF, tumor necrosis factor; IL, interleukin.

TABLE 2.3

CLASSIFICATION OF NEUROPATHIC CANCER PAIN SYNDROMES

Syndromes related to cancer	Clinical examples
Cranial nerve neuralgias	Base of skull or leptomeningeal metastases, head and neck cancers
Mononeuropathy and other neuralgias	Rib metastases with intercostal nerve injury
Radiculopathy	Epidural mass, leptomeningeal metastases
Cervical plexopathy	Head and neck cancer with local extension, cervical lymph node metastases
Brachial plexopathy	Lymph node metastases from breast cancer or lymphoma, direct extension of Pancoast tumor
Lumbosacral plexopathy	Extension of colorectal cancer, cervical cancer, sarcoma, or lymphoma; breast cancer metastases
Paraneoplastic peripheral neuropathy	Small cell lung cancer, antineuronal nuclear antibodies type 1
Central pain	Spinal cord compression
Cachexia	Compression or entrapment neuropathies
Sequela to therapeutic interventions	**Clinical examples**
Hyperalgesia	Extremely high doses of opioids
Postsurgical	Postmastectomy, neck dissection, postthoracotomy
Phantom pain	Postamputation, postmastectomy
Radiation therapy	Myelopathy, plexopathy, neuropathy
Chemotherapy	Neuropathy from cis-platinum, taxoids, vincristine
Parenteral corticosteroids	Perineal burning sensation
Intrathecal methotrexate	Acute meningitic syndrome

Adapted from Martin LA, Hagen NA. Neuropathic pain in cancer patients: mechanisms, syndromes, and clinical controversies. *J Pain Symptom Manage* 1997;14:99–117.

of irradiation are given to the patient. Surgical resection of cancers may result in traumatic injuries to peripheral nerves, with the development of painful neuromas. For example, postthoracotomy pain can be caused by injury to the intercostal nerves, and postmastectomy pain may arise through injury to the intercostobrachial nerve.

Compression or entrapment neuropathies occur in the presence of cachexia; for example, patients with cancer who have lost substantial fat and muscle body weight are prone to develop peroneal neuropathies.

Paraneoplastic autoimmune syndromes due to antineuronal antibodies may present as painful neuropathies. Patients who complain of burning dysesthesias in their feet, hands, and face (in the setting of diagnosed or undiagnosed carcinoma) may have antineuronal nuclear antibodies type 1 (ANNA-1), also known as *anti-Hu*. Most patients who present with sensory neuronopathy and small cell carcinoma of the lung have significantly elevated titers of anti-Hu. All patients with burning dysesthesias of face, hands, and legs and positive titers for anti-Hu should undergo a computed tomography (CT) or magnetic resonance imaging (MRI) of the chest. In fact, small cell carcinoma of the lung may remain undetected by plain chest x-ray. In any case, anti-Hu positivity should prompt a careful search for malignancy, especially for a small cell carcinoma of the lung. Painful dysesthesias develop first in one limb and then progress to involve other limbs, face, scalp, and trunk over weeks or months. In these patients, deep tendon reflexes are reduced or absent and muscle strength is preserved. Patients may be disabled in their ambulation because of the sensory ataxia that is often associated with the painful symptoms.

Therapeutic Interventions for Neuropathic Pain

Management of severe neuropathic pain can be a challenge, and a combination of therapies employing agents from a variety of pharmacologic classes and pain procedures represent the contemporary standard approach (Table 2.4). Treatment includes a wide range of modalities, ranging from opioid and nonopioid analgesics to implantable devices and surgery.

Antiepileptic Drugs

Antiepileptic drugs (AEDs) are becoming the most promising agents for the management of neuropathic pain. The gabapentinoid anticonvulsants gabapentin and pregabalin have both established efficacy in treating neuropathic pain. In May 2002, gabapentin gained U.S. Food and Drug Administration (FDA) approval for the treatment of postherpetic neuralgia (PHN), a state characterized by allodynia and burning pain. However, gabapentin is also known to be effective in treating neuropathic pain from diabetic neuropathy, a state predominantly characterized by spontaneous burning pain (45–47). In December 2004, the gabapentin analog pregabalin gained FDA approval for the treatment of PHN and painful diabetic neuropathy. Gabapentinoids act on neither γ-aminobutyric acid (GABA) receptors nor sodium channels. Recent evidence suggests that gabapentin and pregabalin may modulate the cellular calcium influx into nociceptive neurons by binding to voltage-gated calcium channels, in particular to the α-2-Δ subunit of the channel (48). Trigeminal neuralgia

TABLE 2.4

ANALGESIC ALGORITHM FOR NEUROPATHIC PAIN—STEPS OF INTERVENTION

Pharmacologic Interventions[a]

Moderate to severe pain/functional impairment, with a pain score of >4 on the Brief Pain Inventory:

- Opioid/opioid rotation + gabapentinoids (e.g., gabapentin, pregabalin) + topical therapy for cutaneous allodynia/hyperalgesia[b,c]
- ± Antidepressants (e.g., tricyclic antidepressants, duloxetine, venlafaxine), nongabapentinoid antiepileptic drugs (for intermittent lancinating pain due to cranial neuralgias, consider carbamazepine or oxcarbazepine and/or lamotrigine ± baclofen)
- ± Anti-inflammatory drugs (corticosteroids for acute inflammatory neuropathic pain)
- ± Mexiletine, N methyl-D-aspartate antagonists

Procedure steps

Severe pain/functional impairment, treatment not amenable to conventional drug delivery routes:

- Implantable intrathecal pump or tunneled intraspinal catheter system for neuroaxial analgesia (opioids ± bupivacaine, clonidine, or ziconotide)
- Neurostimulatory procedure by implantable device (spinal cord or motor cortex stimulation)
- Neuroablative procedure (e.g., dorsal root entry zone lesion, midline myelotomy)

[a]On a compassionate basis, according to the patient's clinical condition and pain mechanism, the physician may want to consider an empiric trial of one or more of the emergent topical, oral, or parenteral/intrathecal therapies, as discussed in the text.
[b]In case of sympathetically maintained pain, consider topical clonidine and sympatholytic interventions.
[c]If clinically feasible, trials of topical therapies, for example, lidocaine 5% patch, may be considered for a variety of neuropathic pain states and features.

(a neuropathic condition characterized by brief excruciating lancinating pains) responds extremely well to carbamazepine, while another AED, lamotrigine, has shown some efficacy in treating carbamazepine-resistant trigeminal neuralgia (49). Topiramate has been anecdotally used in the treatment of complex regional pain syndrome (CRPS) type 1 (50). Several new AEDs (e.g., levetiracetam, zonisamide, oxcarbazepine, and tiagabine) have become available for medical use, and some of these, along with topiramate, may have analgesic effect in primary headache and perhaps in neuropathic pain (51,52). Interestingly, in a recent randomized, double-blind, active placebo-controlled, crossover trial, patients with neuropathic pain received lorazepam (active placebo), controlled-release morphine, gabapentin, and a combination of gabapentin and morphine, each treatment given orally for 5 weeks. The study indicated that the best analgesia was obtained from the gabapentin–morphine combination, with each medication given at a lower dose when given as a combination than when given as a single agent (53).

Opioids

Opioids are currently the most potent and effective analgesics used to treat acute and chronic pain, and, as such, they have been prescribed to patients suffering from intractable pain. Morphine, a μ agonist, represents the mainstay for the treatment of moderate to severe nociceptive cancer pain (54). Long

considered to be ineffective for neuropathic pain, opioids have demonstrated efficacy in several recent clinical trials (55–60). A double-blind, placebo-controlled, crossover trial (57) in which 76 patients with PHN received opioids (e.g., controlled-release morphine or methadone), tricyclic antidepressants (TCAs) (e.g., amitriptyline or nortriptyline), and placebo found that both opioids and TCAs provided significantly better pain relief than placebo. Among patients completing the study, most preferred opioids (50%) to TCAs (30%; $p = .02$). The results indicate that opioids are as effective as TCAs in the treatment of PHN.

The analgesic action of the pure opioid agonists (e.g., morphine, methadone, fentanyl, oxycodone, hydromorphone, etc.) is well known and utilized clinically. Among all the analgesic medications currently available, the most powerful and effective drugs are still the agents acting on the μ-, κ-, and Δ-opioid receptors. Opioid receptors are located not only in the CNS (primarily in the dorsal horn) but also peripherally on the nociceptors. Opioids may have a relevant peripheral analgesic effect during painful inflammatory states (61).

The pure opioid agonists are the mainstay for the treatment of severe disabling pain. The treatment of chronic pain may rely on the use of long-acting agents (i.e., methadone, levorphanol) or controlled-release preparations of morphine, fentanyl, and oxycodone. Among the pure opioid agonists, methadone has peculiar properties. It has an intrinsic N-methyl-D-aspartate (NMDA) receptor antagonistic effect, which may add adjuvant analgesic effect in case of neuropathic pain (see subsequent text). Interestingly, recent animal studies suggest that the addition of an extremely low dose of an opioid receptor antagonist (e.g., naltrexone) to morphine in a ratio of 1:1000 may enhance the analgesic efficacy of the opioid agonists (62). Tramadol is an analgesic agent with a weak μ-opioid agonistic effect. Its potency is comparable to that of a codeine–acetaminophen preparation. Notably, in controlled trials, tramadol has shown efficacy in the treatment of neuropathic pain (62–64).

Clinicians should be careful during opioid titration because the requirement for neuropathic pain may be high. The opioid dose should be increased until analgesia is achieved or till side effects become intolerable. Common side effects are constipation, sedation, pruritus, and nausea/vomiting. Rarely, frank confusion may develop. Except for constipation, tolerance occurs for most of the opioid-related side effects (e.g., nausea, vomiting, respiratory depression, and drowsiness). The most feared complication of respiratory depression is rare, especially in patients who are somewhat tolerant to opioids. Unlike anti-inflammatory drugs, opioid agonists have no true "ceiling dose" for analgesia and do not cause direct organ damage. Side effects can often be managed with additional pharmacotherapy, and the clinician may choose to treat the side effects and continue the opioid dose, or "rotate" to another opioid. When converting to another opioid, it is wise to refer to an opioid conversion table or a similar reference and reduce the dose by 50% to avoid incomplete cross-tolerance. Opioid titration and opioid rotation are essential concepts in the management of neuropathic pain. To determine adequate opioid responsiveness, a careful titration of the opioid dose is necessary. However, the development of tolerance to opioid side effects, degree of analgesia, and the development of analgesic tolerance are extremely variable among patients with pain receiving these medications. If severe pain persists or side effects become intolerable during the initial drug trial, trials of different opioids (i.e., opioid rotation) are recommended. Studies indicate that patients on a stable opioid regimen do not report significant impairment in their driving ability, attention, mood, and general cognitive functioning (65).

Antidepressants

Antidepressants also play an important role in the treatment of chronic pain. TCAs, such as amitriptyline, nortriptyline, and desipramine (66), have established efficacy in the treatment of neuropathic pain. They have been used successfully for painful diabetic neuropathy and PHN and provide pain relief in nondepressed patients affected by neuropathic pain. Notably, TCAs such as amitriptyline, doxepin, and imipramine have been found to have potent local anesthetic properties. Amitriptyline appears to be more potent than bupivacaine as a sodium channel blocker (67). TCAs frequently have poorly tolerated adverse effects, including cardiotoxicity, confusion, urinary retention, orthostatic hypotension, nightmares, weight gain, drowsiness, dry mouth, and constipation.

Duloxetine and venlafaxine are both antidepressants that lack the anticholinergic and antihistamine effects of the TCAs (68–70). Duloxetine has recently been approved by the FDA for the treatment of pain secondary to diabetic neuropathy (70,71). Duloxetine and venlafaxine appear to possess an analgesic mechanism of action, with similar TCA-like beneficial properties but fewer side effects. Also, a slow-release preparation of bupropion, an atypical antidepressant, at the dose of 150 mg twice a day, was found to be effective for the treatment of neuropathic pain (72). Selective serotonin reuptake inhibitors (SSRIs), such as paroxetine and fluoxetine, are effective antidepressants but quite ineffective analgesics. While being used for the management of comorbidities such as anxiety, depression, and insomnia, which frequently affect patients with chronic neuropathic pain, SSRIs have not shown the same efficacy as TCAs in the treatment of neuropathic pain (66).

Local Anesthetics

The FDA has approved transdermal lidocaine for the treatment of postherpetic pain (73). In a controlled clinical trial, the transdermal form of 5% lidocaine relieved pain associated with PHN without significant adverse effects (74). There is also early evidence to suggest that the patch provides benefit for other neuropathic pain states (75), including diabetic neuropathy (76), CRPS, postmastectomy pain, and HIV-related neuropathy (77).

Intravenous lidocaine and oral mexiletine have also been utilized in patients with neuropathic pain (78). Mexiletine, an antiarrhythmic local anesthetic, is a sodium channel blocker with analgesic properties for the treatment of neuropathic pain, similar to the properties of some AEDs (e.g., lamotrigine, carbamazepine). Mexiletine is contraindicated in the presence of second- and third-degree atrial–ventricular conduction blocks. Also, the incidence of gastrointestinal side effects (e.g., diarrhea, nausea) is quite high in patients taking mexiletine.

Sodium channel blocking properties are found not only in the traditional local anesthetics, such as bupivacaine and lidocaine, and in the oral antiarrhythmic agent mexiletine but also in several antiepileptic drugs, such as carbamazepine, oxcarbazepine, and lamotrigine, and in the TCAs, such as amitriptyline, doxepin, and imipramine (16,79,80).

Adjuvants and Nonopioid Analgesics for Neuropathic Pain

In addition to the agents discussed in the preceding text, many drugs from a variety of pharmacologic classes can be classified as adjuvant analgesics and used "off label" in the management of patients with chronic intractable pain. In many cases, the mechanisms supporting this analgesic enhancement are still unknown. At present, the evidence that adjuvants and emerging analgesics may possess analgesic properties for the treatment of neuropathic pain has mostly been derived from preliminary clinical investigations and observations.

α₂-Adrenergic Agonists

Drugs acting on the α_2-adrenergic spinal receptors (e.g., clonidine, tizanidine) have been clinically recognized as analgesics (9,81). α_2-Adrenergic agonists are known to have a spinal antinociceptive effect. Controlled trials have shown the effectiveness of intraspinal clonidine for controlling pain (81, 82). Clonidine has been found to potentiate intrathecal opioid analgesia. Moreover, transdermal clonidine has a local antiallodynic effect in patients with SMP (83). Topical clonidine, an α_2-adrenergic agonist, has an analgesic effect in SMP. Clonidine causes local inhibition of noradrenaline release by acting on the adrenergic α_2-autoreceptors of the sympathetic endings (83). Tizanidine is a relatively short-acting, oral α_2-adrenergic agonist with a much lower hypotensive effect than clonidine. Tizanidine has been used for the management of spasticity. However, animal studies and clinical experience indicate the usefulness of tizanidine for a variety of painful states, including neuropathic pain disorders (84–86). The most common side effects of the α_2- adrenergic agonists are somnolence and dizziness (to which tolerance usually develops).

Capsaicin

Capsaicin is the natural substance present in hot chili peppers. Capsaicin activates the recently cloned vanilloid neuronal membrane receptor (87). A single administration of a large dose of capsaicin, after an initial depolarization, appears to produce a prolonged deactivation of capsaicin-sensitive nociceptors. The analgesic effect is dose dependent and may last for several weeks. Capsaicin must be compounded topically at high concentrations (>1%) and administered under local or regional anesthesia (88). Over-the-counter creams must be applied several times a day for many weeks. Controlled studies at low capsaicin concentrations (0.075% or less) have shown mixed results, possibly because of noncompliance.

N-Methyl-D-Aspartate Antagonists

Evidence gleaned from animal experiments shows that NMDA receptors play an important role in the central mechanisms of hyperalgesia and chronic pain (31,32). Dextromethorphan, memantine, and ketamine are NMDA antagonists that may be considered as adjuvants in the management of hyperalgesic neuropathic states poorly responsive to opioid analgesics (70, 89–93). Ketamine and dextromethorphan may be used in conjunction with opioids in the prevention and treatment of analgesic tolerance and the management of allodynia and hyperalgesia. Recent studies indicate that ketamine may have a particular role in the management of cancer pain in those patients who are poorly responsive to opioids. Ketamine as an adjuvant to opioids increase pain relief by 20–30% and allows opioid dose reduction by 25–50% and can be used in both adult and pediatric patients (90,91). Ketamine is able to alter the nociceptive input at the spinal level. Because of the potential neurotoxicity of intrathecal racemic ketamine, the administration of the active compound $S(+)$-ketamine may be a valuable alternative (93). Topical ketamine can provide effective palliation of mucositis pain induced by radiation therapy (92). However, ketamine has a very narrow therapeutic window. Parenteral ketamine can cause intolerable side effects, such as hallucinations and memory impairment. The opioid methadone is a racemic mixture of the isomers D- and L-methadone. D- methadone, although reportedly lacking the opioid agonist effect, has been shown to possess NMDA receptor antagonist activity (94). Methadone's role in the treatment of neuropathic pain (94) may be limited by its long and unpredictable half-life, interindividual variations in pharmacokinetics, and lack of knowledge about appropriate use. Of interest is the possibility that NMDA antagonists may prevent or counteract opioid analgesic tolerance (94,95).

Cannabinoids

Evidence from animal studies and clinical observations indicate that cannabinoids have analgesic properties (94,96,97). Interestingly, the addition of inactive doses of cannabinoids to low doses of μ opioid agonists appears to potentiate opioid antinociception. Moreover, cannabinoids appear to have a predominant antiallodynic/antihyperalgesic effect (94,96–98). The main therapeutic use of cannabinoids in humans is in the prevention of nausea and vomiting caused by chemotherapy. In patients with cancer or acquired immunodeficiency syndrome, Δ-9-*trans*-tetrahydrocannabinol (Δ-9-THC) can be used to increase appetite and treat weight loss.

Several studies have been carried out to assess the therapeutic effectiveness of cannabinoids as analgesics. The major active constituent of cannabis, Δ-9-THC, has been shown to have antinociceptive effects. Δ-9-THC is the most widely studied cannabinoid. Analgesic sites of action have been identified in brain areas, the spinal cord, and the periphery. Cannabinoids appear to have a peripheral anti-inflammatory action and induce antinociception at lower doses than those obtained from effective CNS concentrations. In contrast to the strong preclinical data, good clinical evidence for the efficacy of cannabinoids is lacking. CNS depression seems to be the predominant limiting adverse effect. In chronic neuropathic pain, 1′,1′-dimethylheptyl-Δ8-tetrahydrocannabinol-11-oic acid (CT-3), a THC-11-oic acid analog, at a dose of 40 mg per day, was shown to be more effective than placebo and without major unfavorable side effects. Twenty-one patients with chronic neuropathic pain were randomized in a placebo-controlled, double-blind, crossover trial. Three hours after the administration, the visual analog scale (VAS) values of CT-3 differed significantly from those of the placebo ($p < .02$), whereas, after 8 hours, the differences between the two groups were less marked. Dry mouth and fatigue were the most common CT-3–related side effects ($p < .02$) (96).

Anti-inflammatory and Immunomodulatory Agents

Steroid therapy may be considered for severe inflammatory pain due to cancer-infiltrating structures such as the brachial or lumbosacral plexus, roots, or nerve trunks. Nonsteroidal anti-inflammatory drugs (NSAIDs), for example, cyclo-oxygenase (COX) type-1 and type-2 inhibitors, and acetaminophen have been of little benefit in the treatment of severe neuropathic pain. Several lines of evidence indicate that TNF-α, as well as other proinflammatory interleukins, may play a key role in the mechanism of pathologic intractable pain. Neutralizing antibodies to TNF-α and interleukin-1 receptor may become an important therapeutic approach for severe inflammatory pain resistant to NSAIDs, as well as for other forms of neuropathic inflammatory pain. Thalidomide has been shown to prevent hyperalgesia caused by nerve constriction injury in rats (99,100) and is known to inhibit TNF-α production. TNF-α antagonists or newly developed thalidomide analogs with a better safety profile may play a relevant role in the prevention and treatment of otherwise intractable painful disorders (101). Finally, inhibitors of microglia activation and nuclear factor-κB are being explored, and these lines of research may open new exciting treatment avenues.

Bisphosphonates (e.g., pamidronate, clodronate) have been reported to be efficacious in the treatment of not only bone cancer pain but also CRPS, a neuropathic inflammatory pain syndrome (102,103). The analgesic effect of bisphosphonate is poorly understood. It may be related to the inhibition and apoptosis of activated cells such as osteoclasts and macrophages. This leads to a decreased release of proinflammatory cytokines in the area of the inflammation. In animal models of neuropathic pain (sciatic nerve ligature), bisphosphonates reduced the number of activated macrophages infiltrating the injured nerve, reduced Wallerian nerve fiber degeneration, and decreased experimental hyperalgesia (104).

γ-Aminobutyric Acid Agonists

Baclofen is an analog of the inhibitory neurotransmitter GABA and has a specific action on the GABA-B receptors. It has been used for many years as an effective spasmolytic agent. Baclofen also has shown effectiveness in the treatment of trigeminal neuralgia (61). Clinical experience supports the use of low-dose baclofen to potentiate the antineuralgic effect of carbamazepine in trigeminal neuralgia. Baclofen has also been used intrathecally to relieve intractable spasticity and may have a role as an adjuvant when added to spinal opioids for the treatment of intractable neuropathic pain and spasticity. The most common side effects of baclofen are drowsiness, weakness, hypotension, and confusion. It is important to note that discontinuation of baclofen always requires a slow tapering to avoid the occurrence of seizures and other severe neurologic manifestations.

Benzodiazepines (e.g., alprazolam, lorazepam, diazepam) are GABA-A agonists. Their clinical use in patients with chronic pain is controversial. In a controlled trial, patients with PHN did worse when treated with lorazepam than with placebo or amitriptyline (105). Benzodiazepine-related side effects include depression and disruption of physiologic sleep. In combination with opioids, benzodiazepines cause significant cognitive impairment (65).

Invasive Interventions

Implantable devices, such as intrathecal pumps (IPs), have recently become available for the treatment of neuropathic pain that responds poorly to standard pharmacologic and conservative therapeutic modalities. Among the most commonly utilized implantable devices are spinal cord stimulators (SCSs) and IPs. SCSs have been used successfully in patients with severe limb pain that does not respond to conventional methods. IPs are used to deliver a variety of agents, such as opioids, clonidine, local anesthetics, ziconotide, and baclofen, into the cerebrospinal fluid. Clinical experience and several reports indicate that clonidine and/or local anesthetics administered intrathecally can potentiate opioid analgesia for neuropathic pain (13). Intrathecal morphine is currently the most commonly used analgesic administered by pump. However, before implantation of an intrathecal morphine pump, treatment trials must show that the patient's pain is somewhat responsive to opioids. Combination of intrathecal opioids and bupivacaine enhances the effectiveness of the analgesic regimen and reduces the need for ablative or neurolytic techniques for cancer pain, particularly for visceral and pelvic pain. Pumps can be implanted permanently once trials are successful.

Intraspinally implanted tunneled catheters are also being used for the administration of opioids and/or local anesthetics. Neuraxial analgesia through implanted tunneled catheters can be considered in patients with advanced oncologic disease and pain intractable to standard intervention. Intraspinally implanted tunneled catheters can provide a safe, reliable means of long-term administration of drugs into the epidural space. Utilization of bupivacaine in combination with opioids allows for enhanced pain relief in those patients with pain that is poorly responsive to opioid analgesics. Successful pain management through an intraspinal tunneled catheter system requires a careful education of the patient and caregiver, repeated follow-ups with pain assessment and monitoring of side effects, and close interaction between the patient, caregiver, pharmacist, home care nurse, and physician (106).

Motor cortex stimulation may relieve neuropathic pain. Many publications have corroborated this finding. The mechanism by which stimulation in this area relieves pain is unclear, but long-term results are encouraging. For some specific intractable neuropathic pain disorders, neuroablative procedures might be considered. For example, the dorsal root entry zone (DREZ) lesion has been recommended for the treatment of intractable pain from painful brachial plexopathy. DREZ can also be useful for relieving pain from head and neck cancer. The decision to perform neuroablative surgery should be made only after a thorough comprehensive assessment has been carried out by a multidisciplinary team of pain medicine specialists and after conservative management has failed to produce any improvement in the patient's quality of life. Cordotomy can be an effective treatment for unilateral pelvic and leg pain due to cancer. By sectioning the anterolateral quadrant of the spinal cord, interruption occurs in the spinothalamic tract with subsequent loss of contralateral pain and temperature sensation. The procedure can be done as a percutaneous radiofrequency ablation at C1-2 or through laminectomy. Cordotomy appears to be more effective in addressing intermittent shooting pain than steady burning pain. Unfortunately, the benefit tends to subside with time, and, therefore, its use in treating chronic pain receives little attention. Dorsal root rhizotomies may be beneficial for patients with chest wall pain. It has been hypothesized that malignancies may induce pain through somatic and visceral mechanisms. Midline myelotomy has been advocated as a way of treating visceral pain associated with cancer. Discrete midline myelotomies have also been performed in patients with abdominal/pelvic pain due to cancer, and encouraging results have been reported (107).

BONE PAIN

Metastasis to bone is the most common cause of pain in patients with cancer (108). Bone pain is usually associated with direct tumor invasion of the bone and is often severe and debilitating. Tumors that metastasize to bone most commonly originate in the breast, lung, prostate, thyroid, and kidney. Multiple myeloma causes painful bone lesions. More than two thirds of patients with radiographically detectable lesions will experience bone pain, although many patients experience pain even before skeletal metastases become radiographically apparent.

Immunohistochemical studies have revealed an extensive network of nerve fibers in the vicinity of and within the skeleton, not only in the periosteum but also in the cortical and trabecular bone, as well as in the bone marrow (12). Thinly myelinated and unmyelinated peptidergic sensory fibers, as well as sympathetic fibers, occur throughout the bone marrow, mineralized bone, and periosteum. Although the periosteum is the most densely innervated tissue, when the total volume of each tissue is considered, the bone marrow receives the greatest total number of sensory nerve fibers (109). These sensory fibers express multiple signaling molecules, including neuropeptides and neurotrophins. The presence of receptors for some neuropeptides [e.g., calcitonin gene–related peptide (CGRP) and substance P] on osteoclasts and osteoblasts and the capacity of these receptors to regulate osteoclast formation, and bone formation and resorption have recently been described. Because NGF has been shown to modulate inflammatory neuropathic pain states, in most recent animal models of cancer bone pain, NGF antibody antagonist therapy also has been shown to produce significant reduction in both ongoing and movement-related pain behavior. This treatment was more effective than morphine (21).

It is believed that skeletal lesions result, at least in part, from a disruption of the normal balance between bone formation and bone resorption. In the process, bone nociceptors respond to changes in the bone marrow, as well as cortical, trabecular, and periosteum microenvironments. Inflammatory, immunological, and neuropathic mechanisms develop in the bone in response to the cancer insult, and the patient experiences pain. As osteolysis continues, the bone integrity declines and patients become vulnerable to other complications, including pathologic fractures, nerve compression syndromes, spinal instability, and hypercalcemia.

Although the mechanisms by which these neurochemical pathways cause bone pain are still not completely understood, the prospective for a better understanding of bone pain is thought to be provoking and exciting (110). Moreover, the progress in this field will promote the development of newer and more targeted therapies for pathologic pain.

Clinical Findings and Diagnosis

Pain is commonly the presenting symptom of bone metastases, and the presence of focal pain in a patient with cancer should trigger an investigation. Patients may experience a deep powerful throbbing pain punctuated by sharper intense pain, often triggered by movement (incident or breakthrough pain). On examination, there may also be focal tenderness and swelling at the affected sites. Range of motion is usually severely limited, especially if the joint space is involved. In many patients, normal activities such as deep breathing, coughing, or moving an affected limb can cause intense, often unbearable, pain. Pain may be localized or referred to various sites. Bone pain due to metastases must be differentiated from other bone pain syndromes that are caused by non-neoplastic conditions such as osteoarthritis, osteoporotic fractures, and osteomalacia.

Accurate history and physical examination are the first step in diagnosing bone metastases. Clinicians must remember that pain is generally underassessed. The assessment of pain intensity should rely on the patient's own report of pain. Many different pain scales have been developed, including numeric (0–10) and pictorial scales, among others. The specific pain scale used is less important than using the same scale consistently.

Bone pain may be focal, multifocal, or generalized. Multifocal pain is commonly experienced by patients with multiple sites of bony metastases. Approximately 25% of patients with bone metastases do not complain of pain. Additionally, a patient with multiple sites of osseous metastases may only have a few painful sites (111,112). There is a well-described generalized bone pain syndrome that occurs when there is replacement of bone marrow by tumor. This is observed with myeloproliferative malignancies and less commonly with solid tumors (113).

The vertebral bodies are the most common sites of osseous metastases; more than two thirds of vertebral metastases are found in the thoracic spine because there is a valveless plexus of epidural veins called the *Batson's plexus* in which blood flows rostrally or caudally. This may serve as a route for the metastatic spread of some cancers. The lumbosacral and cervical spine account for approximately 20 and 10% of bone metastases, respectively. Additionally, 85% of patients have multiple-level involvement. Early recognition of pain syndromes of the vertebral bodies is essential because the pain serves as an indicator that compression of adjacent neural structures could be imminent and that neurologic compromise, that is, spinal cord compression, could ensue (114,115). MRI is the best diagnostic tool that can be used, given its best accuracy of extent of disease; clinically, CT can also be diagnostic. Plain films reveal a "moth-eaten" appearance of a bone that has lytic bone metastases. However, plain films and bone scans (scintigraphy) should only be regarded as adjuncts to the former tests.

Occipital pain can indicate the destruction of the atlas or fracture of the odontoid process, and the pain can radiate over the posterior aspect of the skull. This can result in a pathologic fracture and subsequent spinal cord compression at the cervicomedullary junction (116).

Bone metastases at the level of C7-T1 vertebral bodies can cause a pain referral pattern at the infrascapular area, with upper back pain and muscle spasm (117). When T12 or L1 is affected by bone metastases, the referral pattern can often be at the iliac crest or sacroiliac joint; imaging could miss the metastases if it is directed at the pelvis. Sacral syndrome can develop from bone metastases, and referred and/or radiating pain can arise in the buttock, posterior thigh, or perineum (118,119). In addition to this skeletal component, involvement of adjacent structures, such as nerves or muscles, may produce other types of pain. Involvement of adjacent nerve tissue of the peripheral system, such as the lumbar plexus, or central system, such as the spinal cord, can produce not only worrying neurologic deficits but also neuropathic pain syndromes. Many times, epidural disease is the first sign of malignancy in a community setting. Severe back pain is the initial symptom in almost all patients who present with epidural compression. Back pain precedes epidural compression for a prolonged period. Clinically, there is a rapid and crescendo type of pain with epidural disease, and there may or may not be a lancinating quality to the pain or a band-like tightness that wraps around the chest or abdomen. If epidural disease is not diagnosed and treated in a timely manner, paraplegia or quadriplegia may occur. Large lytic metastases present with localized severe pain in the affected bone. The risk of fracture is high; Fidler reported a fracture incidence of 3.7% when 25–50% of the cortex was involved, 61% when the degree of cortical involvement ranged between 50 and 75%, and 79% when >75% of the cortex was involved (119,120). Although any tumor can metastasize to the bone and result in a pathologic fracture, mammary carcinoma is responsible for 50% of such fractures. Multiple myeloma is the second most common cancer to cause pathologic fractures.

In any patient with cancer, the development of an unexplained focal pain should trigger an investigation into the cause, should the goals of care allow it. Clinicians should keep in mind that pain may be referred in numerous patterns, for example, involvement of the hip may refer the pain to the knee or the groin. Plain radiography, CT, MRI, and bone scintigraphy are all measures to image metastatic lesions. In many cases, plain radiography will be adequate in identifying skeletal lesions. MRI is more sensitive at detecting very early skeletal metastases. CT scanning is also more sensitive than plain films and is often used for patients who cannot tolerate or are not candidates for MRI. Bone scintigraphy is more useful when identifying the extent of bone lesions throughout the body.

Therapeutic Interventions for Bone Pain

There are numerous options for the treatment of pain related to bone metastases, including opioid therapy, specific pharmacotherapy, radiotherapy, systemic radionuclide therapy, and surgery (Table 2.5). With the skillful and compassionate use of these measures, even patients with severe pain can expect to achieve adequate relief.

TABLE 2.5

ANALGESIC ALGORITHM FOR BONE PAIN–STEPS OF INTERVENTION

Pharmacologic interventions

Moderate to severe pain/functional impairment, with a pain score of >4 on the on the Brief Pain Inventory:

- Opioid/opioid rotation + i.v. bisphosphonate (e.g., zoledronic acid, pamidronate, ibandronate)
- ± Anti-inflammatory drugs (corticosteroids)
- ± Gabapentinoids, antidepressants, mexiletine, NMDA antagonists

Procedure steps

Severe pain/functional impairment, treatment not amenable to conventional drug delivery routes:

- Implantable intrathecal pump or tunneled intraspinal catheter system for neuroaxial analgesia (opioids ± bupivacaine, clonidine, or ziconotide)
- Radiation or radiopharmaceutical therapy
- Palliative surgery (vertebroplasty, kyphoplasty) for large lytic lesions with risk for fracture
- Neuroablative procedure

NMDA, N-methyl-D-aspartate.

Anti-inflammatory Drugs

Corticosteroids. Steroid therapy may be considered for severe inflammatory pain, especially when bone cancer infiltrates or compresses adjacent nerve tissue structures, such as the brachial or lumbosacral plexi, roots or nerve trunks, or spinal cord. High-dose steroids are used in epidural disease for pain control and for decompression while definitive treatment is planned (121–123).

Nonsteroidal anti-inflammatory drugs. NSAIDs, for example, COX type-1 and type-2 inhibitors, and acetaminophen are commonly used in the treatment of mild to moderate pain evolving from inflammation. NSAIDs share a common mechanism of action, which is the inhibition of COX and, therefore, prostaglandin (PG) production. PGs play important roles in a variety of tissues. For example, PGs, specifically PGE_2 and PGI_2, are responsible for maintaining renal perfusion in patients with compromised kidney function. PGs also act to protect the gastric mucosa and initiate platelet aggregation. Furthermore, PGs function to generate pain by stimulating peripheral sensory neurons during inflammation. The mechanism of action of NSAIDs has been further elucidated by the discovery of two distinct isoforms of COX (COX-1 and COX-2). COX-1 is the constitutive isoform present in, for example, the stomach, kidney, and platelets, and its inhibition is responsible for producing the common side effects of NSAIDs. Conversely, the inducible isoform, COX-2, usually becomes expressed in cells after being activated by proinflammatory cytokines. COX-1 and COX-2 inhibition results in both the adverse and beneficial effects of the NSAIDs. The anti-inflammatory and analgesic effects of the NSAIDs are generally considered equal when comparing agents within the class. However, the frequency with which they produce side effects varies greatly. Caution must be exercised when using NSAIDs in patients with hypertension, impaired renal function, or heart failure. A well-known benefit of the COX-2 inhibitors and acetaminophen is their gastrointestinal safety. However, highly specific COX-2 inhibitors are not void of adverse effects, in particular, the vascular prothrombotic effect. Acetaminophen has a dose-dependent hepatotoxic effect (not to be used at a dose higher than 4 g per day). With the large number of COX inhibitors being available, one must consider the patient's history of response, and the efficacy, safety, and cost-effectiveness of the agent to be prescribed.

Bone Metabolism Modulators

Bisphosphonates. Some of the most important drugs that have emerged in the battle against bone pain are the bisphosphonates, the synthetic analogs of pyrophosphate that bind hydroxyapatite crystals of the bone with a high affinity. They reduce resorption of bone by inhibiting osteoclastic activity and osteolysis. Bisphosphonate therapy has proved highly valuable in the management of numerous bone-related conditions, including hypercalcemia, osteoporosis, multiple myeloma, and Paget's disease. Earlier bisphosphonates, such as etidronate, have been largely replaced by second-generation bisphosphonates, including pamidronate, as well as third-generation bisphosphonates, including zoledronic acid and ibandronate. Multiple studies have demonstrated the efficacy of second- and third-generation bisphosphonates in reducing pain in bone metastases (124–126). Zoledronic acid significantly reduces the overall risk of developing a skeletal-related pathologic event in patients with bone metastasis by an additional 20% in comparison with pamidronate and significantly improves pain and quality of life (127). Ibandronate has been shown to provide significant and sustained relief from metastatic bone pain, improving patient functioning and quality of life. The oral and intravenous formulations of ibandronate appear to have comparable efficacy (128). With a favorable long-term safety profile and the added convenience and flexibility offered by its efficacious oral formulation, ibandronate represents a new therapeutic option for metastatic bone disease management. Recently, a conjugated bisphosphonate, rhenium 186–labeled MAG3-bisphosphonate (^{186}Re-MAG3-HBP), has been developed as a bifunctional radiopharmaceutical (see subsequent text) for the palliation of metastatic bone pain (129). This conjugated form is stable and is expected to be a valuable tool for the palliation of bone pain in the future. However, further research on this drug is necessary.

Calcitonin. Calcitonin may have several pain-related indications in patients who have bone pain, including osseous metastases. The most frequent routes of absorption are intranasal and subcutaneous injection. Calcitonin reduces resorption of bone by inhibiting osteoclastic activity and osteolysis (130).

Radiotherapy

Radiation therapy is a valuable tool in managing pain from bone metastases. Between 60 and 80% of patients with bone metastases will experience a substantial pain reduction after irradiation of the affected area. The procedure itself is relatively quick and unproblematic. The mechanism by which radiation alleviates pain in bone metastases is still unclear; it does not appear to be related directly to tumor shrinkage. Like bisphosphonates, the procedure may be a radiation-mediated effect on osteolysis. Radiotherapy has traditionally been given in many fractions (hyperfractionation) because any single high dose of radiation can cause severe side effects. However, it takes no less than 6 to 9 months after administration of the radiation dose for most of the side effects to manifest. Therefore, patients who are expected to not survive that long should be candidates for hypofractionated palliative radiotherapy. Even a single treatment of 8 Gy (800 rad) is enough for most patients (131). The role of prophylactic radiation to prevent pain from existing metastases is still controversial, and further studies are necessary.

Radiopharmaceuticals

Pain palliation with bone-seeking radiopharmaceuticals has proved to be an effective treatment modality in patients with metastatic bone pain. Bone-seeking radiopharmaceuticals are extremely powerful in treating scattered painful bone metastases for which external beam radiotherapy is impossible because of the large field of irradiation (132,133). Generally, the effectiveness of radioisotopes is satisfactory, but it can be greater when they are combined with chemotherapeutic agents such as cisplatin. The most common and major safety concern related to the adverse effects from radiopharmaceuticals is bone marrow toxicity.

Strontium 89, Samarium 153 (^{89}Sr, ^{153}Sm). The radioisotopes ^{89}Sr and ^{153}Sm have been used for the palliation of pain from metastatic bone cancer. Repeated doses are effective in providing pain relief in many patients, with response rates of between 40 and 95%. Pain relief starts usually 1–4 weeks after the initiation of treatment, continues for up to 18 months, and is associated with a reduction in analgesic use in many patients. Thrombocytopenia and neutropenia are the most common toxic effects, but they are generally mild and reversible. Some studies with ^{89}Sr and ^{153}Sm indicate a reduction of hot spots on bone scans in up to 70% of patients and suggest a possible tumoricidal action (132).

Samarium 153–ethylene diamine tetramethylene phosphonate. ^{153}Sm-ethylene diamine tetramethylene phosphonate (^{153}Sm-EDTPM) is a widely available and extensively tested radiopharmaceutical for systemic therapy in patients with multiple skeletal metastases. Its use is approved for any secondary bone lesion that has been shown to accumulate the traditional marker in bone scans, that is, technetium Tc 99 m-methylene diphosphonate (Tc 99 m-MDP). The short half-life, the relatively low-energy β emissions, and the γ emissions make the ^{153}Sm an attractive radionuclide, allowing therapeutic delivery of short-range electrons at relatively high dose (134).

Rhenium 186-hydroxyethylidene diphosphonate. Rhenium 186-hydroxyethylidene diphosphonate (^{186}Re-HEDP) is a potentially useful radiopharmaceutical agent for the palliation of bone pain, having numerous advantageous characteristics. Bone marrow toxicity is limited and reversible, which makes repetitive treatment safer. Studies using ^{186}Re-HEDP have shown encouraging clinical results of palliative therapy, with an overall response rate of about 70% in painful bone metastases (135). It is effective for fast palliation of painful bone metastases from various tumors, and the effect tends to last longer if patients are treated early in the course of their disease. It is preferred to radiopharmaceuticals with a long half-life in patients who have been pretreated with bone marrow–suppressive chemotherapy.

Surgery

In general, patients with only skeletal metastases have a longer survival than those with visceral metastases. When weighing the risks and benefits of surgery, it is critical to assess the patient's ability to tolerate the procedure. In patients for whom the prognosis is less than a month, surgery is rarely indicated. Patients with cardiopulmonary disease (even unrelated to the cancer) should have a thorough operative assessment. Orthopaedic stabilization of the affected skeletal segment can be helpful for patients with large lytic lesions who are at risk for fracture and can improve the overall quality of life for many patients. However, it should not be used as a substitute for dedicated and effective pain management. Vertebroplasty and kyphoplasty are relatively new techniques that may be efficacious in treating painful vertebral metastasis. These techniques are currently used to treat vertebral compression fractures due to osteoporosis or painful hemangiomas. Vertebroplasty is the injection of bone cement, generally polymethyl methacrylate, into a vertebral body. Kyphoplasty is the placement of a balloon into the vertebral body, followed by an inflation/deflation sequence to create a cavity before the cement injection. These procedures are most often performed in a percutaneous manner on an outpatient or short-stay basis. The risks associated with the procedures are low, but serious complications, such as spinal cord compression, nerve root compression, venous embolism, and pulmonary embolism, including cardiovascular collapse, may occur (136).

VISCERAL PAIN

Visceral pain is common in patients with cancer and becomes evident during cancer infiltration, compression, distention, or stretching of thoracic and/or abdominal viscera. It may be both an early or late manifestation of cancer. Visceral nociceptors are activated by noxious stimuli, including inflammation of the mucosa and omentum and stretching of hollow viscera, as well as organ capsule. Visceral pain is generally diffuse and caused by obstructive syndromes due to tumor involvement of the organ or the organ capsule. Pain can be caused by a primary tumor or metastatic disease to an organ.

Clinical Findings and Diagnosis

Visceral pain may be described as dull, squeezing, colicky, sharp, and deep aching, intermittent or continuous, and can often be perceived as generalized lassitude. Visceral pain is poorly localized and can be accompanied by other symptoms such as nausea, fatigue, and diaphoresis. It may frequently be referred to cutaneous areas overlying or adjacent to the affected structure; referral patterns may vary and actually be distant from the underlying malignancy. The clinician must be knowledgeable about the pain referral patterns to treat the syndrome with precision. An example might be an aching and gnawing right shoulder pain; this may indicate the presence of hepatic metastases or diaphragmatic irritation (137). Pancreatic and endometrial cancer may manifest as back pain. Pain from prostate cancer may appear in the abdomen or lower extremities. Hepatic capsular pain may occur with a primary hepatocellular carcinoma or, more commonly, with liver metastases. The inflammation caused by the disease may result in capsular stretching and produce pain, which is dull and aching in the right subcostal region. Movement may exacerbate the pain; deep breaths cause right diaphragmatic irritation. The treatment for this syndrome is analgesic doses of corticosteroids given in divided dose and opioid analgesics (138,139). Retroperitoneal pain syndrome is most common in pancreatic cancer and retroperitoneal lymphadenopathy. The pain is exacerbated with recumbency and alleviated with forward flexion. The pain is dull, diffuse, and poorly localized. This type of pain should be differentiated from epidural metastasis, and a careful examination and appropriate imaging can confirm the diagnosis. Intestinal obstruction can be the result of gastrointestinal tumor, adhesions, and intra-abdominal or pelvic space-occupying lesions. The pain is characterized as colicky. It is usually associated with nausea and/or vomiting, anorexia, and bloating. Another cause of this syndrome can be an atonic bowel due to ischemia, autonomic denervation, or primary cancer therapies including radiotherapy. Visceral carcinomatosis can cause pain because of multiple mechanisms: peritoneal inflammation, malignant

adhesions, and ascites. Tense ascites produce discomfort from abdominal wall stretching and can also manifest as low back pain. Pelvic and perineal pain can occur in malignancies that arise in the pelvis, including colorectal and genitourinary tumors. The tumor invades the pelvic floor and is frequently both nociceptive and neuropathic pain. Occasionally, patients experience painful spasms in the rectum, bladder, or urethra. The visceral component of this pain syndrome can be marked by tenesmus.

Therapeutic Interventions for Visceral Pain

Treatment includes a wide range of modalities including opioid analgesics (which should be considered for visceral organ pain), steroids, anticholinergics, octreotide (which relieves bowel-obstructive symptoms by decreasing gastric secretions) (140), and adjuvant analgesics given for the neuropathic component.

The pharmacologic treatments for painful spasms are many; the standard treatment may be the anticholinergic medications. Donnatal, which is a combination of atropine, phenobarbital, scopolamine, and hyoscyamine given by mouth three to four times daily, is an old preparation still used for spasms or colicky pain. The anticholinergic medication hyoscyamine has been used as a single agent to treat gastrointestinal spasms at the usual dose of 0.125 mg, one to two tablets every 4 hours as needed. The old antispasmodic combination of chlordiazepoxide, a benzodiazepine, and clidinium, an anticholinergic, (Librax) has also been used to relieve intestinal spasms or cramps.

There are other anticholinergic medications such as propantheline and glycopyrrolate used for much of the same purpose; however, as with all the drugs in this class, the side effects may limit their use excessively. The anticholinergic drugs can be used for bladder spasm due to overactive bladder pathology. Side effects can include mucous membrane dryness, dizziness, and gastrointestinal sluggishness, constipation, and, rarely, obstructive symptoms.

Opioids through IPs or tunneled intraspinal catheter systems, neurolytic blockades, neuroablative procedures, and palliative surgery i.e., bowel resection, percutaneous endoscopic gastrostomy (PEG) tube inserted for the purpose of nutrition, paracentesis, and palliative ostomies, might be an option to relieve the pain associated with the physical obstruction. There are studies under way evaluating the use of peripheral opioid antagonists in the treatment of severe constipation; however, exclusion criteria would include frank obstruction.

Neurolytic Blockade for Visceral Pain

Neurolytic blockade can be efficacious for visceral-related pain in cancer; however, it is usually reserved for patients with a limited prognosis and well-localized pain syndromes. Nerve blocks that are specifically for visceral pain lack durability and have an analgesic benefit of 6 months or less in some cases. Neurolytic blocks are primarily viewed as adjuvant therapy and not as replacing systemic pharmacotherapy for cancer pain. Alcohol and phenol are the most widely used agents (141).

Intrapleural phenol block has been reported to be helpful in managing visceral pain associated with esophageal cancer (142). Certain types of thoracic pain from invasion of the chest wall secondary to a pleural tumor may respond to intercostal neurolytic blocks or paravertebral blockade.

Neurolytic block of the celiac plexus is well described in the literature and has proven efficacy in patients with pancreatic cancer and epigastric and/or back pain. Celiac plexus block has also been used successfully in treating visceral pain from upper abdominal malignancies. In one prospective randomized trial of patients with pancreatic cancer, the pain relief provided by a neurolytic celiac plexus block was equal to that provided by systemic opioids with fewer side effects. (143). Data also support the use of intraoperative neurolytic blockade of the celiac plexus for unresectable pancreatic tumor (144). *Neurolysis of the superior hypogastric plexus* has been used for the treatment of visceral pain from cancer of the lower abdomen and pelvis, including gynecologic, colorectal, and genitourinary malignancies. However, some of these cancers may have a significant retroperitoneal pain component, which may lead to poor results with this type of neurolysis. Reportedly, the procedure seems to carry minimal risks in terms of complications (145). *Neurolysis of the ganglion impar* is used for intractable rectal and perineal pain in patients who often suffer from urgency. The ganglion is located at the sacrococcygeal junction. There are limited published data on this procedure. *Intrathecal neurolytic blockade* might be indicated for patients with advanced or terminal malignancy with intractable, unilateral pain affecting only a few dermatomes (preferably of the thoracic region). The most common complications of intrathecal neurolysis are persistent pain, limb weakness, and urinary and rectal dysfunction.

Epidural neurolytic blockade can be performed by the insertion of a catheter, so that multiple repeated injections can be administered. Epidural neurolysis has been used successfully for unilateral or bilateral pain of thoracic and abdominal visceral origin. It has been described as a safer procedure than intrathecal neurolysis. The duration of analgesia may vary from 1 to 3 months (146).

ANALGESIC ALGORITHMS

The management of severe neuropathic, bone, and visceral cancer pain often represents a difficult treatment challenge. Combination of therapies employing medications from a variety of pharmacologic classes and, at times, procedures corresponds to the contemporary standard approach. Specific agents can be used as treatment trials and courses can be escalated according to the proposed analgesic algorithms for neuropathic, bone, and visceral cancer pain shown in Tables 2.4, 2.5, and 2.6, respectively. The number and variety of options can be confusing and intimidating, even for physicians specializing in the treatment of pain. Dose titration is an important principle to be familiar with when using analgesics, in particular, opioids, AEDs, and antidepressants. Physicians must know how to titrate the dose appropriately while assessing the pain and recognizing and managing drug-related side effects. Patients suffering from difficult cancer pain syndromes need to have treatment plans tailored to their individual problems. As patients become less functional, a more aggressive intervention based on titration and combination therapy will be necessary. The treating physician needs to balance efficacy, safety, and tolerability of several drugs, often used on an "off-label" basis. Moreover, the physician who wishes to utilize the analgesic algorithms should:

1. Know how to assess the quality and features of the pain,
2. Determine the predominant mechanism(s) underlying the difficult cancer pain syndrome,
3. Understand the pharmacology of the analgesics and the indications for the procedures,
4. Recognize and manage side effects of medications and procedure-related adverse events.

TABLE 2.6

ANALGESIC ALGORITHM FOR VISCERAL PAIN—STEPS OF INTERVENTION

Pharmacologic interventions

Moderate to severe pain/functional impairment; with a pain score of >4 on the Brief Pain Inventory:

- Opioid/opioid rotation ± anticholinergic agents
- Corticosteroids, octreotide
- ± Gabapentinoids, antidepressants

Procedure steps

Severe pain/functional impairment, treatment not amenable to conventional drug delivery routes:

- Implantable intrathecal pump or tunneled intraspinal catheter system for neuroaxial analgesia (opioids ± bupivacaine, clonidine, or ziconotide)
- Palliative surgery (if clinically indicated)
- Neurolytic blocks (e.g., celiac plexus, superior hypogastric plexus, ganglion impar, epidural neurolysis)
- Neuroablative procedure

CONCLUSION

Difficult cancer pain syndromes are challenging pain states to treat. Advances are being made in the comprehension of the various mechanisms underlying neuropathic, bone, and visceral pain. If a patient presents with a difficult cancer pain syndrome, a more comprehensive pain assessment and a much more aggressive intervention are going to be needed. Therapeutic interventions can be employed in an escalating regimen to counteract the intensity and the disabling nature of the patient's difficult cancer pain syndrome. Patients suffering from these disorders need to have treatment plans tailored to their individual problems. The employment of agents from a variety of pharmacologic classes represents a contemporary standard approach to pain management. At present, the management of the difficult cancer pain syndrome calls for a balanced combination of therapies that will include analgesic medications, adjuvants, and procedures.

References

1. Merskey H, Bogduk N, eds. Classification of chronic pain, 2nd ed. *IASP task force on taxonomy.* Seattle: IASP Press, 1994:209–214.
2. Pappagallo M. Peripheral neuropathic pain. In: Pappagallo M, ed. *The neurological basis of pain.* New York: McGraw-Hill, 2005:321–341.
3. Allan SM, Tyrrell PJ, Rothwell NJ. Interleukin-1 and neuronal injury. *Nat Rev Immunol* 2005;5:629–640.
4. Empl M, Renaud S, Erne B, et al. TNF-alpha expression in painful and nonpainful neuropathies. *Neurology* 2001;56:1371–1377.
5. Lindenlaub T, Sommer C. Cytokines in sural nerve biopsies from inflammatory and non-inflammatory neuropathies. *Acta Neuropathol (Berl)* 2003;105:593–602.
6. Schafers M, Lee DH, Brors D, et al. Increased sensitivity of injured and adjacent uninjured rat primary sensory neurons to exogenous tumor necrosis factor-alpha after spinal nerve ligation. *J Neurosci* 2003;23:3028–3038.
7. Raja SN, Turnquist JL, Meleka S, et al. Monitoring adequacy of alpha-adrenoceptor blockade following systemic phentolamine administration. *Pain* 1996;64(1).197–204.
8. Ali Z, Raja SN, Wesselmann U, et al. Intradermal injection of norepinephrine evokes pain in patients with sympathetically maintained pain. *Pain* 2000;88:161–168.
9. Scholz J, Woolf CJ. Mechanisms of neuropathic pain. In: Pappagallo M, ed. *The neurological basis of pain.* New York: McGraw-Hill, 2005: 71–94.

10. Schafers M, Brinkhoff J, Neukirchen S, et al. Combined epineurial therapy with neutralizing antibodies to tumor necrosis factor-alpha and interleukin-1 receptor has an additive effect in reducing neuropathic pain in mice. *Neurosci Lett* 2001;310:113–116.

11. Davis JB, Gray J, Gunthorpe MJ, et al. Vanilloid receptor-1 is essential for inflammatory thermal hyperalgesia. *Nature* 2000;405(6783):183–187.

12. Lerner UH. Neuropeptidergic regulation of bone resorption and bone formation. *J Musculoskelet Neuronal Interact* 2002;2:440–447.

13. Katz N. Neuropathic pain in cancer and AIDS. *Clin J Pain* 2000;16:S41–S48.

14. Marais E, Klugbauer N, Hofmann F. Calcium channel alpha(2)delta subunits—structure and gabapentin binding. *Mol Pharmacol* 2001;59:1243–1248.

15. Sutton KG, Martin DJ, Pinnock RD, et al. Gabapentin inhibits high-threshold calcium channel currents in cultured rat dorsal root ganglion neurones. *Br J Pharmacol* 2002;135:257–265.

16. Lai J, Hunter JC, Porreca F. The role of voltage-gated sodium channels in neuropathic pain. *Curr Opin Neurobiol* 2003;13:291–297.

17. Black JA, Liu S, Tanaka M, et al. Changes in the expression of tetrodotoxin-sensitive sodium channels within dorsal root ganglia neurons in inflammatory pain. *Pain* 2004;108(3):237–247.

18. Waxman SG, Dib-Hajj SD. Erythromelalgia: a hereditary pain syndrome enters the molecular era. *Ann Neurol* 2005;57(6):785–788.

19. Knotkova H, Pappagallo M. Pharmacology of pain transmission and modulation. II. Peripheral mechanisms. In: Pappagallo M, ed. *The neurological basis of pain*. New York: McGraw-Hill, 2005:53–60.

20. Mamet J, Lazdunski M, Voilley N. Nerve growth factor drives physiological and inflammatory expressions of acid-sensing ion channel 3 in sensory neurons. *J Biol Chem* 2003;278(49):48907–48913.

21. Sevcik MA, Ghilardi JR, Peters CM, et al. Anti-NGF therapy profoundly reduces bone cancer pain and the accompanying increase in markers of peripheral and central sensitization. *Pain* 2005;115:128–141.

22. Boucher TJ, Okuse K, Bennett DL, et al. Potent analgesic effects of GDNF in neuropathic pain states. *Science* 2000;290(5489):124.

23. Tegeder I, Niederberger E, Schmidt R, et al. Specific inhibition of IkappaB kinase reduces hyperalgesia in inflammatory and neuropathic pain models in rats. *J Neurosci* 2004;24:1637–1645.

24. McGaraughty S, Wismer CT, Zhu CZ, et al. Effects of A-317491, a novel and selective P2X3/P2X2/3 receptor antagonist, on neuropathic, inflammatory and chemogenic nociception following intrathecal and intraplantar administration. *Br J Pharmacol* 2003;140:1381–1388.

25. Pappagallo M, Gaspardone A, Tomai F, et al. Analgesic effect of bamiphylline on pain induced by intradermal injection of adenosine. *Pain* 1993;53:199–204.

26. Sawynok J. Adenosine receptor activation and nociception. *Eur J Pharmacol* 1998;347:1–11.

27. Zhu CZ, Mikusa J, Chu KL, et al. A-134974: a novel adenosine kinase inhibitor, relieves tactile allodynia via spinal sites of action in peripheral nerve injured rats. *Brain Res* 2001;905(1–2):104–110.

28. Vergnolle N, Bunnett NW, Sharkey KA, et al. Proteinase-activated receptor-2 and hyperalgesia: a novel pain pathway. *Nat Med* 2001;7:821–826.

29. Davis AJ, Perkins MN. Induction of B1 receptors *in vivo* in a model of persistent inflammatory mechanical hyperalgesia in the rat. *Neuropharmacology* 1994;33:127–133.

30. Watkins LR, Milligan ED, Maier SF. Glial activation: a driving force for pathological pain. *Trends Neurosci* 2001;24(8):450–455.

31. Bennett G, Deer T, Du PS, et al. Future directions in the management of pain by intraspinal drug delivery. *J Pain Symptom Manage* 2000;20:S44–S50.

32. Bennett GJ. Update on the neurophysiology of pain transmission and modulation: focus on the NMDA-receptor. *J Pain Symptom Manage* 2000;9:S2–S6.

33. DeLeo JA, Tanga FY, Tawfik VL. Neuroimmune activation and neuroinflammation in chronic pain and opioid tolerance/hyperalgesia. *Neuroscientist* 2004;10:40–52.

34. Watkins LR, Maier SF. Glia: a novel drug discovery target for clinical pain. *Nat Rev Drug Discov* 2003;2:973–985.

35. Ledeboer A, Sloane EM, Milligan ED, et al. Minocycline attenuates mechanical allodynia and proinflammatory cytokine expression in rat models of pain facilitation. *Pain* 2005;115:71–83.

36. Milligan ED, Zapata V, Chacur M, et al. Evidence that exogenous and endogenous fractalkine can induce spinal nociceptive facilitation in rats. *Eur J Neurosci* 2004;20:2294–2302.

37. Raghavendra V, Tanga F, DeLeo JA. Inhibition of microglial activation attenuates the development but not existing hypersensitivity in a rat model of neuropathy. *J Pharmacol Exp Ther* 2003;306:624–630.

38. Jin SX, Zhuang ZY, Woolf CJ, et al. P38 mitogen-activated protein kinase is activated after a spinal nerve ligation in spinal cord microglia and dorsal root ganglion neurons and contributes to the generation of neuropathic pain. *J Neurosci* 2003;23:1017–1022.

39. Hashizume H, Rutkowski MD, Weinstein JN, et al. Central administration of methotrexate reduces mechanical allodynia in an animal model of radiculopathy/sciatica. *Pain* 2000;87:159–169.

40. Sweitzer SM, Schubert P, DeLeo JA. Propentofylline, a glial modulating agent, exhibits antiallodynic properties in a rat model of neuropathic pain. *J Pharmacol Exp Ther* 2001;297:1210–1217.

41. Galer BS, Jensen MP. Development and preliminary validation of a pain measure specific to neuropathic pain: the Neuropathic Pain Scale. *Neurology* 1997;48:332–338.

42. Cleeland CS, Ryan KM. Pain assessment: global use of the Brief Pain Inventory. *Ann Acad Med Singapore* 1994;23:129–138.

43. Martin LA, Hagen NA. Neuropathic pain in cancer patients: mechanisms, syndromes, and clinical controversies. *J Pain Symptom Manage* 1997;14:99–117.

44. Amato AA, Collins MP. Neuropathies associated with malignancy. *Semin Neurol* 1998;18:125–144.

45. Backonja M, Beydoun A, Edwards KR, et al. Gabapentin for the symptomatic treatment of painful neuropathy in patients with diabetes mellitus: a randomized controlled trial. *JAMA* 1998;280:1831–1836.

46. Rice AS, Maton S. Gabapentin in postherpetic neuralgia: a randomised, double blind, placebo-controlled study. *Pain* 2001;94:215–224.

47. Rowbotham M, Harden N, Stacey B, et al. Gabapentin for the treatment of postherpetic neuralgia: a randomized controlled trial. *JAMA* 1998;280:1837–1842.

48. Matthews EA, Dickenson AH. Effects of spinally delivered N- and P-type voltage-dependent calcium channel antagonists on dorsal horn neuronal responses in a rat model of neuropathy. *Pain* 2001;92:235–246.

49. Zakrzewska JM, Chaudhry Z, Nurmikko TJ, et al. Lamotrigine (lamictal) in refractory trigeminal neuralgia: results from a double-blind, placebo controlled, crossover trial. *Pain* 1997;73:223–230.

50. Pappagallo M. Preliminary experience with topiramate in the treatment of chronic pain syndromes. *Poster presented at the 17th annual meeting*, San Diego, CA: American Pain Society, 1998.

51. Shi W, Liu H, Zhang Y, et al. Design, synthesis, and preliminary evaluation of gabapentin-pregabalin mutual prodrugs in relieving neuropathic pain. *Arch Pharm (Weinheim)* 2005;338:358–364.

52. Pappagallo M. Newer antiepileptic drugs: possible uses in the treatment of neuropathic pain and migraine. *Clin Ther* 2003;25:2506–2538.

53. Gilron I, Bailey JM, Tu D, et al. Morphine, gabapentin, or their combination for neuropathic pain. *N Engl J Med* 2005;352:1324–1334.

54. Portenoy RK. Opioid therapy for chronic nonmalignant pain: a review of the critical issues. *J Pain Symptom Manage* 1996;11:203–217.

55. Dellemijn PL, Vanneste JA. Randomised double-blind active-placebo-controlled crossover trial of intravenous fentanyl in neuropathic pain. *Lancet* 1997;349:753–758.

56. Gimbel JS, Richards P, Portenoy RK. Controlled-release oxycodone for pain in diabetic neuropathy: a randomized controlled trial. *Neurology* 2003;60:927–934.

57. Raja SN, Haythornthwaite JA, Pappagallo M, et al. Opioids versus antidepressants in postherpetic neuralgia: a randomized, placebo-controlled trial. *Neurology* 2002;59:1015–1021.

58. Rowbotham MC, Twilling L, Davies PS, et al. Oral opioid therapy for chronic peripheral and central neuropathic pain. *N Engl J Med* 2003;348:1223–1232.

59. Suzuki R, Chapman V, Dickenson AH. The effectiveness of spinal and systemic morphine on rat dorsal horn neuronal responses in the spinal nerve ligation model of neuropathic pain. *Pain* 1999;80:215–228.

60. Watson CP, Babul N. Efficacy of oxycodone in neuropathic pain: a randomized trial in postherpetic neuralgia. *Neurology* 1998;50:1837–1841.

61. Pappagallo M. Aggressive pharmacologic treatment of pain. In: Pisetsky DS, Bradley L, eds. *Pain management in the rheumatic diseases. Rheumatic disease clinics of North America*. Philadelphia, PA: WB Saunders, 1999:193.

62. Crain SM, Shen KF. Antagonists of excitatory opioid receptor functions enhance morphine's analgesic potency and attenuate opioid tolerance/dependence liability. *Pain* 2000;84:121–131.

63. Harati Y, Gooch C, Swenson M, et al. Double-blind randomized trial of tramadol for the treatment of the pain of diabetic neuropathy. *Neurology* 1998;50:1842–1846.

64. Sindrup SH, Madsen C, Brosen K, et al. The effect of tramadol in painful polyneuropathy in relation to serum drug and metabolite levels. *Clin Pharmacol Ther* 1999;66:636–641.

65. Haythornthwaite JA, Menefee LA, Quatrano-Piacentini AL, et al. Outcome of chronic opioid therapy for non-cancer pain. *J Pain Symptom Manage* 1998;15:185–194.

66. Max MB, Lynch SA, Muir J, et al. Effects of desipramine, amitriptyline, and fluoxetine on pain in diabetic neuropathy. *N Engl J Med* 1992;326:1250–1256.

67. Sudoh Y, Cahoon EE, Gerner P, et al. Tricyclic antidepressants as long-acting local anesthetics. *Pain* 2003;103:49–55.

68. Grothe DR, Scheckner B, Albano D. Treatment of pain syndromes with venlafaxine. *Pharmacotherapy* 2004;24:621–629.

69. Marchand F, Alloui A, Pelissier T, et al. Evidence for an antihyperalgesic effect of venlafaxine in vincristine induced neuropathy in rat. *Brain Res* 2003;980:117–120.

70. Rowbotham MC, Goli V, Kunz NR, et al. Venlafaxine extended release in the treatment of painful diabetic neuropathy: a double-blind, placebo-controlled study. *Pain* 2004;110:697–706.

71. Goldstein DJ, Lu Y, Detke MJ, et al. Duloxetine vs. placebo in patients with painful diabetic neuropathy. *Pain* 2005;116:109–118.

72. Semenchuk MR, Sherman S, Davis B. Double-blind, randomized trial of bupropion SR for the treatment of neuropathic pain. *Neurology* 2001;57:1583–1588.

73. Galer BS, Rowbotham MC, Perander J, et al. Topical lidocaine patch relieves postherpetic neuralgia more effectively than a vehicle topical patch: results of an enriched enrollment study. *Pain* 1999;80:533–538.

74. Rowbotham MC, Davies PS, Verkempinck C, et al. Lidocaine patch: double-blind controlled study of a new treatment method for post-herpetic neuralgia. *Pain* 1996;65:39–44.

75. Devers A, Galer BS. Topical lidocaine patch relieves a variety of neuropathic pain conditions: an open-label study. *Clin J Pain* 2000;16:205–208.

76. Hart-Gouleau S, Gammaitoni A, Galer B, et al. Open label study of the effectiveness and safety of lidocaine patch 5% (Lidoderm) in patients with painful diabetic neuropathy [abstract]. *Program and abstracts of the IASP 10th world congress of pain.* Seattle, WA: IASP, 2002.

77. Berman SM, Justis JV, HO M, et al. Lidocaine patch 5% (Lidoderm) significantly improves quality of life (QOL) in HIV-associated painful peripheral neuropathy [abstract]. *Program and abstracts of the IASP 10th world congress of pain.* Seattle, WA: IASP, 2002.

78. Wallace MS. Calcium and sodium channel antagonists for the treatment of pain. *Clin J Pain* 2000;16:S80–S85.

79. Hains BC, Klein JP, Saab CY, et al. Upregulation of sodium channel Na(v)1.3 and functional involvement in neuronal hyperexcitability associated with central neuropathic pain after spinal cord injury. *J Neurosci* 2003;23:8881–8892.

80. Roza C, Laird JM, Souslova V, et al. The tetrodotoxin-resistant Na+ channel Na(v)1.8 is essential for the expression of spontaneous activity in damaged sensory axons of mice. *J Physiol* 2003;550:921–926.

81. Khan ZP, Ferguson CN, Jones RM. Alpha-2 and imidazoline receptor agonists. Their pharmacology and therapeutic role. *Anaesthesia* 1999;54:146–165.

82. Eisenach JC, Rauck RL, Buzzanell C, et al. Epidural clonidine analgesia for intractable cancer pain: phase I. *Anesthesiology* 1989;71:647–652.

83. Davis KD, Treede RD, Raja SN, et al. Topical application of clonidine relieves hyperalgesia in patients with sympathetically maintained pain. *Pain* 1991;47:309–317.

84. Fogelholm R, Murros K. Tizanidine in chronic tension-type headache: a placebo controlled double-blind cross-over study. *Headache* 1992;32:509–513.

85. Fromm GH, Aumentado D, Terrence CF. A clinical and experimental investigation of the effects of tizanidine in trigeminal neuralgia. *Pain* 1993;53:265–271.

86. McCarthy RJ, Kroin JS, Lubenow TR, et al. Effect of intrathecal tizanidine on antinociception and blood pressure in the rat. *Pain* 1990;40:333–338.

87. Caterina MJ, Schumacher MA, Tominaga M, et al. The capsaicin receptor: a heat-activated ion channel in the pain pathway. *Nature* 1997;389:816–824.

88. Robbins WR, Staats PS, Levine J, et al. Treatment of intractable pain with topical large-dose capsaicin: preliminary report. *Anesth Analg* 1998;86:579–583.

89. Bell RF, Eccleston C, Kalso E. Ketamine as adjuvant to opioids for cancer pain. A qualitative systematic review. *J Pain Symptom Manage* 2003;26:867–875.

90. Fitzgibbon EJ, Viola R. Parenteral ketamine as an analgesic adjuvant for severe pain: development and retrospective audit of a protocol for a palliative care unit. *J Palliat Med* 2005;8:49–57.

91. Lossignol DA, Obiols-Portis M, Body JJ. Successful use of ketamine for intractable cancer pain. *Support Care Cancer* 2005;13:188–193.

92. Slatkin NE, Rhiner M. Topical ketamine in the treatment of mucositis pain. *Pain Med* 2003;4:298–303.

93. Vranken JH, van der Vegt MH, Kal JE, et al. Treatment of neuropathic cancer pain with continuous intrathecal administration of S +-ketamine. *Acta Anaesthesiol Scand* 2004;48:249–252.

94. Davis AM, Inturrisi CE. d-Methadone blocks morphine tolerance and N-methyl-D-aspartate-induced hyperalgesia. *J Pharmacol Exp Ther* 1999;289:1048–1053.

95. Price DD, Mayer DJ, Mao J, et al. NMDA-receptor antagonists and opioid receptor interactions as related to analgesia and tolerance. *J Pain Symptom Manage* 2000;19:S7–S11.

96. Karst M, Salim K, Burstein S, et al. Analgesic effect of the synthetic cannabinoid CT-3 on chronic neuropathic pain: a randomized controlled trial. *JAMA* 2003;290:1757–1762.

97. Richardson JD. Cannabinoids modulate pain by multiple mechanisms of action. *J Pain* 2000;1(1):2.

98. Richardson JD, Aanonsen L, Hargreaves KM. Antihyperalgesic effects of spinal cannabinoids. *Eur J Pharmacol* 1998;345:145–153.

99. Sommer C, Marziniak M, Myers RR. The effect of thalidomide treatment on vascular pathology and hyperalgesia caused by chronic constriction injury of rat nerve. *Pain* 1998;74:83–91.

100. Ribeiro RA, Vale ML, Ferreira SH, et al. Analgesic effect of thalidomide on inflammatory pain. *Eur J Pharmacol* 2000;391:97–103.

101. George A, Marziniak M, Schafers M, et al. Thalidomide treatment in chronic constrictive neuropathy decreases endoneurial tumor necrosis factor-alpha, increases interleukin-10 and has long-term effects on spinal cord dorsal horn met-enkephalin. *Pain* 2000;88:267–275.

102. Cortet B, Flipo RM, Coquerelle P, et al. Treatment of severe, recalcitrant reflex sympathetic dystrophy: assessment of efficacy and safety of the second generation bisphosphonate pamidronate. *Clin Rheumatol* 1997;16:51–56.

103. Varenna M, Zucchi F, Ghiringhelli D, et al. Intravenous clodronate in the treatment of reflex sympathetic dystrophy syndrome. A randomized, double blind, placebo controlled study. *J Rheumatol* 2000;27:1477–1483.

104. Liu T, van Rooijen N, Tracey DJ. Depletion of macrophages reduces axonal degeneration and hyperalgesia following nerve injury. *Pain* 2000;86:25–32.

105. Max MB, Schafer SC, Culnane M, et al. Amitriptyline, but not lorazepam, relieves postherpetic neuralgia. *Neurology* 1988;38:1427–1432.

106. Mercadante S. Problems of long-term spinal opioid treatment in advanced cancer patients. *Pain* 1999;79(1):1–13.

107. Campbell JN, Sciubba DM. Neurosurgical approaches to the treatment of pain. In: Pappagallo M, ed. *The neurological basis of pain.* New York: McGraw-Hill, 2005:631–639.

108. Banning A, Sjogren P, Henriksen H. Pain causes in 200 patients referred to a multidisciplinary cancer pain clinic. *Pain* 1991;45:45–48.

109. Mach DB, Rogers SD, Sabino MC, et al. Origins of skeletal pain: sensory and sympathetic innervation of the mouse femur. *Neuroscience* 2002;113:155–166.

110. Luger NM, Mach DB, Sevcik MA, et al. Bone cancer pain: from model to mechanism to therapy. *J Pain Symptom Manage* 2005;29:S32–S46.

111. Portenoy RK, Hagen NA. Breakthrough pain: definition, prevalence and characteristics. *Pain* 1990;41:273–281.

112. Kellgren JG. On distribution of pain arising from deep somatic structures with charts of segmental pain areas. *Clin Science* 1939;4:35–46.

113. Jonsson OG, Sartain P, Ducore JM, et al. Bone pain as an initial symptom of childhood acute lymphoblastic leukemia: association with nearly normal hematologic indexes. *J Pediatr* 1990;117:233–237.

114. Constans JP, De Divitiis E, Donzelli R, et al. Spinal metastases with neurological manifestations. Review of 600 cases. *J Neurosurg* 1983;59:111–118.

115. Sorensen S, Borgesen SE, Rohde K, et al. Metastatic epidural spinal cord compression. Results of treatment and survival. *Cancer* 1990;65:1502–1508.

116. Sundaresan N, Galicich JH, Lane JM, et al. Treatment of odontoid fractures in cancer patients. *J Neurosurg* 1981;54:187–192.

117. Stark RJ, Henson RA, Evans SJ. Spinal metastases. A retrospective survey from a general hospital. *Brain* 1982;105:189–213.

118. Portenoy RK, Galer BS, Salamon O, et al. Identification of epidural neoplasm. Radiography and bone scintigraphy in the symptomatic and asymptomatic spine. *Cancer* 1989;64:2207–2213.

119. Ruff RL, Lanska DJ. Epidural metastases in prospectively evaluated veterans with cancer and back pain. *Cancer* 1989;63:2234–2241.

120. Fidler M. Incidence of fracture through metastases in long bones. *Acta Orthop Scand* 1981;52:623–627.

121. Ettinger AB, Portenoy RK. The use of corticosteroids in the treatment of symptoms associated with cancer. *J Pain Symptom Manage* 1988;3:99–103.

122. Vecht CJ, Haaxma-Reiche H, van Putten WL, et al. Initial bolus of conventional versus high-dose dexamethasone in metastatic spinal cord compression. *Neurology* 1989;39:1255–1257.

123. Watanabe S, Bruera E. Corticosteroids as adjuvant analgesics. *J Pain Symptom Manage* 1994;9:442–445.

124. Mystakidou K, Katsouda E, Stathopoulou E, et al. Approaches to managing bone metastases from breast cancer: The role of bisphosphonates. *Cancer Treat Rev* 2005;31:303–311.

125. Smith MR. Osteoclast-targeted therapy for prostate cancer. *Curr Treat Options Oncol* 2004;5:367–375.

126. Wardley A, Davidson N, Barrett-Lee P, et al. Zoledronic acid significantly improves pain scores and quality of life in breast cancer patients with bone metastases: a randomised, crossover study of community vs hospital bisphosphonate administration. *Br J Cancer* 2005;92:1869–1876.

127. Gordon DH. Efficacy and safety of intravenous bisphosphonates for patients with breast cancer metastatic to bone: a review of randomized, double-blind, phase III trials. *Clin Breast Cancer* 2005;6:125–131.

128. Pecherstorfer M. Efficacy and safety of ibandronate in the treatment of neoplastic bone disease. *Expert Opin Pharmacother* 2004;5:2341–2350.

129. Ogawa K, Mukai T, Arano Y, et al. Development of a rhenium-186-labeled MAG3-conjugated bisphosphonate for the palliation of metastatic bone pain based on the concept of bifunctional radiopharmaceuticals. *Bioconjug Chem* 2005;16:751–757.

130. Szanto J, Ady N, Jozsef S. Pain killing with calcitonin nasal spray in patients with malignant tumors. *Oncology* 1992;49:180–182.

131. Hartsell WT, Scott CB, Bruner DW, et al. Randomized trial of short versus long-course radiotherapy for palliation of painful bone metastases. *J Natl Cancer Inst* 2005;97:798–804.

132. Finlay IG, Mason MD, Shelley M. Radioisotopes for the palliation of metastatic bone cancer: a systematic review. *Lancet Oncol* 2005;6:392–400.

133. Nilsson S, Larsen RH, Fossa SD, et al. First clinical experience with alpha-emitting radium-223 in the treatment of skeletal metastases. *Clin Cancer Res* 2005;11:4451–4459.

134. Maini CL, Bergomi S, Romano L, et al. 153Sm-EDTMP for bone pain palliation in skeletal metastases. *Eur J Nucl Med Mol Imaging* 2004;31(Suppl 1):S171–S178.

135. Lam MG, de Klerk JM, van Rijk PP. 186Re-HEDP for metastatic bone pain in breast cancer patients. *Eur J Nucl Med Mol Imaging* 2004;31(Suppl 1):S162–S170.

136. Burton AW, Rhines LD, Mendel E. Vertebroplasty and kyphoplasty: a comprehensive review. *Neurosurg Focus* 2005;18(3):e1.

137. Milne RJ, Foreman RD, Giesler GJ Jr, et al. Convergence of cutaneous and pelvic visceral nociceptive inputs onto primate spinothalamic neurons. *Pain* 1981;11:163–183.

138. Cherny NI. Cancer pain: principles of assessment and syndromes. In: Berger A, Portenoy RK, Weissman D, eds. *Principles and practice of supportive oncology*, 1st ed. Philadelphia, PA: Lippincott Williams & Wilkins, 1998:3–42.

139. Farr WC. The use of corticosteroids for symptom management in terminally ill patients. *Am J Hosp Care* 1990;7:41–46.

140. Ripamonti C, Mercadante S, Groff L, et al. Role of octreotide, scopolamine butylbromide, and hydration in symptom control of patients with inoperable bowel obstruction and nasogastric tubes: a prospective randomized trial. *J Pain Symptom Manage* 2000;19:23–34.

141. Cousins MJ. Techniques for neurolytic neural blockade. In: Cousins MJ, Bridenbaugh PO, eds. *Neural blockade in clinical anesthesia and management of pain*, 3rd ed. Philadelphia, PA: Lippincott Williams & Wilkins, 1998:1007–1061.

142. Lema MJ, Myers DP, Leon-Casasola O, et al. Pleural phenol therapy for the treatment of chronic esophageal cancer pain. *Reg Anesth* 1992;17:166–170.

143. Mercadante S, Nicosia F. Celiac plexus block: a reappraisal. *Reg Anesth Pain Med* 1998;23:37–48.

144. Mercadante S. Celiac plexus block versus analgesics in pancreatic cancer pain. *Pain* 1993;52:187–192.

145. Plancarte R, Leon-Casasola OA, El Helaly M, et al. Neurolytic superior hypogastric plexus block for chronic pelvic pain associated with cancer. *Reg Anesth* 1997;22:562–568.

146. Korevaar WC. Transcatheter thoracic epidural neurolysis using ethyl alcohol. *Anesthesiology* 1988;69:989–993.

CHAPTER 3 ■ OPIOID PHARMACOTHERAPY

JUDITH A. PAICE

Opioids and their derivatives have been used to relieve pain for centuries, and their contribution to relief of suffering is well established. Many of the earliest recorded reports of opioid use are attributed to the Egyptians and extend back many centuries. In the 1600s, Thomas Sydenham promoted the use of laudanum, a mixture of opium, saffron, cinnamon, and cloves in wine (1). Two centuries later, the pharmacist Wilhelm Sertürner extracted morphine from poppy juice, calling this substance morphium after Morpheus, the Greek god of sleep (1). Since that time, many new opioids have been developed, and information about the pharmacodynamics, pharmacokinetics, and pharmacogenomics of these compounds has increased greatly. This understanding has led to improvements in their clinical application, for relief not only of pain but also of dyspnea, cough, and intractable diarrhea. Yet, more than any other agent, opioids generate fear, misunderstanding, and controversy. To address these misconceptions and provide optimal relief, those caring for patients with pain and other symptoms associated with cancer or other life-threatening illnesses must have a strong knowledge base regarding the pharmacology and clinical application of opioids.

PHARMACOLOGY OF OPIOIDS

To fully appreciate the optimal clinical use of opioids, the clinician must understand the pharmacodynamics (the mechanism of opioid analgesia) and the pharmacokinetics (the process by which opioids are absorbed, distributed, metabolized, and excreted) of this class of drugs. The pharmacogenomics of opioids helps explain the variability in response seen in the clinical setting.

Pharmacodynamics

Opioids act through three major types of opioid receptors, including μ (MOR for μ opioid receptor), δ (DOR for δ opioid receptor), and κ (KOR for κ opioid receptor). These receptors are distributed widely throughout the nervous system, including the peripheral nerves, spinal cord, and brain (2). The highest density of opioid receptors include lamina I and II of the dorsal horn of the spinal cord (3). Opioid receptors are also found in the brainstem, including the periaqueductal gray, nucleus raphe magnus, and locus coeruleus, areas known to be involved in the mediation of opioid analgesia (4). More recently, opioid receptors have also been found on immune cells.

Opioid receptors are G protein–coupled, activating a complex cascade of events. These include increased conduction through potassium channels, which hyperpolarizes the sensory neuron. Opioid receptor binding results in diminished conduction through calcium channels, resulting in decreased release of neurotransmitters involved in nociception. Finally, opioid receptor binding leads to inhibition of adenylate cyclase. Together, these actions contribute to the analgesia resulting when an opioid agonist binds to the above receptors.

Pharmacokinetics

As with all other compounds, the absorption, distribution, metabolism, and elimination of an opioid influences the efficacy of the drug. Alterations are of particular concern when caring for patients with advanced malignancy or other life-threatening illness because any of these phases of the opioid may be altered by extensive disease.

Absorption

Absorption is influenced by the lipophilicity of an agent. Morphine and hydromorphone have a partition coefficient (octanol/water) of 1 compared with 115 for methadone and 820 for fentanyl (5). Therefore, fentanyl can cross biologic membranes more avidly when compared with morphine, making it the more appropriate agent for transdermal delivery. The lipophilicity affects the time to maximal serum concentration (C_{max}). The C_{max} for a hydrophilic drug, such as morphine, is approximately 60 minutes after oral administration, 30 minutes after subcutaneous (s.c.) delivery, and 6 minutes or more after intravenous (i.v.) delivery. The half-life of oral morphine is approximately 4 hours. Because steady state is reached in approximately four to five half-lives, it will be reached within approximately 16–20 hours of regular immediate-release oral morphine administration. Little is known about the alterations in absorption of opioids that occur when patients have extensive disease. For example, factors such as shortened transit time may delay the absorption of oral opioids, particularly long-acting or sustained-release compounds.

Distribution

Plasma proteins and lipid solubility of a particular opioid affect the distribution of the drug throughout the vasculature (5). Other mediating factors include body fat stores and total body water. All of these listed above can be significantly altered in older adults or in persons with cachexia and dehydration, the common sequelae of advanced disease.

Metabolism

Most opioids are metabolized through glucuronidation, dealkylation, or other processes, and are then excreted by the kidneys. Although some metabolites produce analgesia (e.g., morphine-3-glucuronide [M3G]), they may also contribute to neurotoxicity (6). Myoclonus has been associated with both M3G and hydromorphone-3-glucuronide (H3G), metabolites that appear to pose a risk for accumulating in patients receiving high doses of opioid for extended periods or in those with renal disease (7). Metabolism is known to be affected by advanced age, liver disease, genetics, and other factors that are prominent in palliative care.

Elimination

Most opioids are excreted renally, with a small percentage eliminated fecally. Experience suggests that patients with renal failure or those receiving dialysis might benefit from the use of agents that are more readily dialyzable, such as fentanyl, as opposed to morphine or codeine (8). However, even in patients who have undergone a successful renal transplantation, the large variability in the kinetics of fentanyl after surgery supports the axiom that all opioid therapy must be individualized (9). Much more research is needed on the interaction between advanced disease and the pharmacokinetics of opioids.

Pharmacogenomics

The field of pharmacogenomics is rapidly growing and much evidence for the variability in response to opioids seen in the clinical setting is related to inborn properties caused by genetic variability (10). The MOR was cloned in 1993 and was called *MOR-1*. More recent work has identified splice variants of the MOR-1 receptor, with different localization of the splice variants within the nervous system (11). The efficacy of morphine varies among the variants, and this may explain, in part, the variability in response to opioids seen in the clinical setting, including efficacy and adverse effects. The translation of this information to the clinical experience includes the practice of opioid rotation when a particular opioid agonist is either ineffective or produces unmanageable adverse effects.

Another clear clinical example of the contribution of pharmacogenomics to the variability in analgesia to opioids is related to codeine. People who are poor metabolizers of the enzyme CYP2D6 derive little analgesic effect from codeine, a prodrug that must be metabolized to morphine to produce analgesia. Approximately 5–10% of whites, 1% of Asians, and 0–20% of African Americans are poor metabolizers (12). Conversely, a recent case report described overdose in a patient taking a small dose of codeine. Analysis revealed him to be an ultrarapid metabolizer of CYP2D6, which theoretically resulted in a rapid, extensive conversion of the drug to morphine (13).

A recent example of the role of pharmacogenomics in cancer pain control is related to the catechol-*O*-methyltransferase (*COMT*) gene, which inactivates dopamine, epinephrine, and norepinephrine in the nervous system. A recent study of 207 white patients with cancer found that polymorphism of the *COMT* gene contributes to variability in response to morphine in pain control (14). A common functional polymorphism (Val158Met) leads to a significant variation in the COMT enzyme activity, with the Met form displaying lower enzymatic activity. Patients with the Val/Val genotype needed more morphine, when compared with the Val/Met and the Met/Met genotype groups. The investigators could not

explain these differences by other factors such as duration of opioid treatment, performance status, time since diagnosis, perceived pain intensity, adverse symptoms, or time until death. Much more research is needed to fully understand the pharmacogenetics of opioids and their implications for those with cancer or other life-threatening illnesses.

CLINICAL APPLICATION

Opioids are a critical component of the armamentarium used to control pain in palliative care. They are indicated in moderate to severe pain, as well as in the management of cough, dyspnea, and severe diarrhea. Because opioids alter pain signal transmission and perception throughout the nervous system, they have an analgesic effect despite the underlying pathophysiology of pain. In fact, despite earlier beliefs, opioids have been shown to be effective in providing relief of neuropathic pain.

Specific Opioids

Opioids are generally categorized as agonists, partial agonists, and mixed agonist–antagonists. Additionally, antagonists to opioids may be used to counteract adverse effects to opioids, although most must be used with significant caution in the palliative care setting.

Agonists

Numerous opioid agonists are available for clinical use. These agents can be subcategorized as alkaloids and synthetic opioids (Table 3.1). Attributes associated with the more commonly used opioids are described in the following text and in Table 3.2.

TABLE 3.1

OPIOIDS BY CLASSIFICATION

Agonists
Alkaloids
  Morphine
  Hydromorphone
  Oxymorphone
  Codeine
  Oxycodone
  Hydrocodone
  Dihydrocodeine
  Heroin
Synthetic opioids
  Phenylpiperidine derivatives—fentanyl, sufentanil, alfentanil, remifentanil, meperidine
  Diphenylheptane derivatives—methadone, propoxyphene
  Morphinan derivatives—levorphanol

Partial agonists
Semisynthetic—buprenorphine

Mixed agonist–antagonists
Semisynthetic alkaloid—nalbuphine
Synthetic benzomorphan derivative—pentazocine
Synthetic morphinan derivative—butorphanol

Antagonists
Naloxone
Naltrexone

TABLE 3.2

PROPERTIES OF COMMONLY USED OPIOIDS

Agent	Routes	Formulations	i.v./s.c.[a] mg	Oral dose mg	Starting dose for adults[b]	Other
Codeine	Oral Parenteral (uncommon)	Codeine sulfate 15, 30, or 60 mg tablets Tylenol No. 2 (15 mg codeine/300 mg acetaminophen) Tylenol No. 3 (30 mg codeine/300 mg acetaminophen) Tylenol No. 4 (60 mg codeine/300 mg acetaminophen) Codeine/guaifenesin liquid (5 mL = 10 mg codeine/100 mg guaifenesin)	130	200	Oral: 30–60 mg	Converted to morphine by CYP2D6; poor metabolizers obtain little pain relief
Fentanyl	Intraspinal i.v. Transdermal Transmucosal	Fentanyl solution for i.v. (Sublimaze) Fentanyl patch (Duragesic, generics) 12.5, 25, 50, 75, or 100 µg/hour Fentanyl oral transmucosal (Actiq) 200, 400, 600, 1200, or 1600 µg units	0.1	NA	NA	Transdermal fentanyl 25 mcg/hour approximately equal to 50 mg oral morphine
Hydrocodone	Oral	Lortab or Vicodin (5 mg hydrocodone/500 mg acetaminophen) Lortab Elixir (15 mL = 7.5 mg hydrocodone/500 mg acetaminophen) Norco (5, 7.5 or 10 mg hydrocodone/325 mg acetaminophen) Hycodan (5 mL = 5 mg hydrocodone/1.5 mg homatropine)	NA	15–30	Oral: 5–10 mg	Role of CYP2D6 unclear
Hydromorphone	Oral Parenteral	Hydromorphone 2, 4, or 8 mg (Dilaudid, generics) Hydromorphone 3 mg suppository	1.5	7.5	Oral: 4–8 mg	Long-acting hydromorphone available outside the United States Toxicity may be due in part to hydromorphone-3-glucuronide

(continued)

TABLE 3.2

(CONTINUED)

Agent	Routes	Formulations	i.v./s.c.[a] mg	Oral dose mg	Starting dose for adults[b]	Other
Levorphanol	Oral Parenteral (uncommon)	Levo-Dromoran 2 mg	2	4	Oral: 2–4 mg	Long half-life; repeated dosing may lead to accumulation. Increased incidence of psychotomimetic effects
Meperidine	Oral Parenteral	Demerol	75–100	300	Not recommended	Not recommended because of toxic metabolite, normeperidine
Methadone	Oral Parenteral	Dolophine and generics (5, 10, 40 mg tablets; 1 mg/mL solution; 10 mg/mL solution)	See text	See text	See text	See text and Tables 3.3 and 3.4
Morphine	Intraspinal Oral Parenteral	Morphine immediate release (15, 30 mg) Morphine sustained release q12h (15, 30, 50, 60, 100, 200 mg) (MS Contin, Kadian, Oramorph, generics) Morphine sustained release q24h (Avinza) (30, 60, 90, 120 mg) Morphine liquid 1 mg/mL, 20 mg/mL Morphine suppository 5, 10, 20, 30 mg	10	30	Oral: 15–30 mg	Avinza and Kadian may be used as sprinkles. Also available in liposomal formulation for epidural administration (DepoDur). Toxicity may be due in part to morphine-3-glucuronide
Oxycodone	Oral	Oxycodone immediate release (5, 15, 30 mg) (OxyIR, Roxicodone, generics) Oxycodone 5 mg/325 mg acetaminophen (Percocet) Oxycodone 5 mg/500 mg acetaminophen (Tylox) Oxycodone sustained release (10, 20, 40, 80 mg) (OxyContin, generics) Oxycodone liquid 5 mg/mL, 20 mg/mL (OxyFast)	NA	20–30	Oral: 5–20 mg	—

[a]Intramuscular injections are not recommended because of variable absorption and pain on injection.
[b]Starting doses are approximations for opioid-naïve adult patients.

Codeine. Codeine is a relatively weak opioid that is more frequently administered in combination with acetaminophen. Codeine is metabolized by glucuronidation primarily to codeine-6-glucuronide, and to a much lesser degree to norcodeine, morphine, M3G, morphine-6-glucuronide, and normorphine (15). As described earlier in the section Pharmacogenomics, codeine is converted to morphine by CYP2D6. The polymorphism seen in this enzyme between various ethnic groups, and between individuals, leads to a significant percentage obtaining reduced analgesia.

Fentanyl. Fentanyl is a highly lipid-soluble opioid (partition coefficient 820) that has been administered parenterally, spinally, transdermally (including an iontophoretically administered patient-controlled device), transmucosally, intranasally, and by a nebulizer for the management of dyspnea (16,17). Dosing units are usually in micrograms because of the potency of this opioid. Questions arise about the efficacy of fentanyl and related compounds, alfentanil, remifentanil, and sufentanil, in the face of extremes in body weight. A recent study of i.v. fentanyl for acute postoperative pain in lean and obese patients found no relationship between plasma levels required for analgesia and total body weight. Therefore, using i.v. dosing on the basis of weight (or milligram per kilogram dosing) in patients with cachexia could lead to underdosing, whereas the same practice in the obese patient could lead to overdose (18). Similar studies are needed to determine the effect of weight on the plasma levels of fentanyl after transdermal delivery, particularly in the often cachectic palliative care patient.

Hydrocodone. Hydrocodone is more potent than codeine and is found only in combination products, primarily acetaminophen, but also ibuprofen. Liquid cough formulations of hydrocodone also contain homatropine. These additives limit the use of hydrocodone in palliative care when higher doses of opioid are required. Hydrocodone is metabolized through demethylation to hydromorphone. Laboratory evidence suggests that CYP2D6 polymorphism may alter the analgesic response to hydrocodone (19).

Hydromorphone. Hydromorphone is a derivative of morphine, with similar properties, and is available as oral tablets, liquids, suppositories, and parenteral formulations (20). Because it is highly soluble and approximately five to ten times more potent than morphine, hydromorphone is used frequently in palliative care when small volumes are needed for s.c. infusions. A long-acting formulation is available outside the United States. Hydromorphone undergoes glucuronidation and the primary metabolite is H3G (15). Recent experience suggests that this metabolite may lead to opioid neurotoxicity, similar to those seen with morphine metabolites, including myoclonus, hyperalgesia, and seizures (7,21,22). This appears to be of particular risk with high doses, prolonged use, or in persons with renal dysfunction (23).

Methadone. Methadone has been gaining renewed popularity in the management of severe, persistent pain. Methadone is a μ & δ agonist and is an antagonist to the N-methyl-D-aspartate (NMDA) receptor, with affinity similar to that of ketamine (24). This antagonism is believed to be of particular benefit in neuropathic pain. A double-blind study in palliative care patients revealed its efficacy in the management of neuropathic pain, although a Cochrane review of existing studies found no obvious clinical effects (25,26). Methadone also blocks the reuptake of serotonin and norepinephrine, another potentially favorable attribute to its use in treating neuropathic pain. The prolonged plasma half-life of methadone (ranging from 15 to 60+ hours) allows for a relatively convenient dosing schedule of every 8 hours. Furthermore, methadone is much less expensive than comparable doses of commercially available continuous-release formulations.

Another advantage of the use of methadone in palliative care is the variety of available routes that can be used, including oral, rectal, s.c., i.v., and epidural (27). Nasal and sublingual administration has been reported to be effective, but preparations are not currently available commercially. The ratio of oral to parenteral methadone is 2:1 and of oral to rectal is 1:1. Subcutaneous methadone infusions may produce local irritation, although using a more dilute solution or changing the needle more frequently can mediate this.

Despite the many advantages, much is unknown about the efficacy of methadone when compared with other agents, the appropriate dosing ratio between methadone and morphine, or the safest and most effective time course for conversion from another opioid to methadone. Despite much anecdotal support for the use of methadone, Bruera et al. conducted a randomized controlled trial in patients with cancer and found no significant difference when compared with morphine (28). Early reports suggested the analgesic ratio of morphine to methadone might be 1:1, yet this appears to be true only for individuals without recent prior exposure to opioids (29). For individuals currently taking another opioid, the dose ratio increases as the dose of oral opioid equivalents increases (30,31). The oral morphine to oral methadone ratio may be 2:1 for patients on <30 mg of oral morphine equivalent daily doses (MEDD) but may be 10:1 or 20:1 for patients on >300 mg oral MEDD (Tables 3.3 and 3.4). An additional complicating factor in the use of methadone is the limited experience in reverse rotation from methadone to another opioid (29,30).

The kinetics of methadone vary greatly between individuals, and causes for the variability include protein binding, CYP3A4 activity, urinary pH, and other factors. Methadone binds avidly to α_1 glycoprotein (AAG), the level of which is increased in advanced cancer, leading to decreasing amounts of unbound methadone and initially delaying the onset of effect. As a result the interindividual variability of the pharmacokinetics of methadone is more pronounced in patients with cancer (24).

Methadone is metabolized primarily by CYP3A4, but also by CYP2D6 and CYP1A2 (24,32,33). Drugs that induce CYP3A4 enzymes accelerate the metabolism of methadone, resulting in reduced serum levels of the drug. Patients report shortened analgesic periods or reduced overall pain relief (34). Drugs that inhibit CYP3A4 enzymes slow methadone metabolism, potentially leading to sedation and respiratory depression. Table 3.5 lists many agents commonly used in palliative care that are CYP3A4 inducers and inhibitors.

TABLE 3.3

METHADONE DOSE RATIOS

Oral morphine equivalent (mg/d)	Dose ratio (morphine: methadone)
<30	2:1
30–99	4:1
100–299	8:1
300–499	12:1
500–999	15:1
>1000	20:1 or greater

These ratios are generally accepted in clinical practice, although these are only as a guide to converting an opioid to methadone. Many factors can increase or decrease serum methadone levels and caution is advised. Frequent assessment of pain and sedation are warranted when converting to methadone or when increasing the dose.

TABLE 3.4

PROTOCOLS FOR THE CONVERSION FROM OTHER OPIOIDS TO METHADONE

Protocol 1–Three- to five-day method
- Calculate an equianalgesic dose of methadone
- Reduce the existing opioid dose by approximately one third and administer one third of the predicted methadone dose (give in three doses or every 8 h); continue to use the existing short-acting opioid for rescue
- On day 2, reduce the existing morphine by another third and increase the methadone dose by one third
- On day 3, discontinue the existing opioid and increase the methadone dose by the remaining third; use a short-acting opioid or methadone for rescue

Protocol 2—Conservative approach
- Start a fixed dose of methadone, 5 or 10 mg, orally q8h for 4–7 d
- Increase the dose by 50% in case of inadequate pain control and continue for another 4–7 d
- Continue increasing the methadone dose by 50% every 4–7 d until pain is relieved
- For rescue, use a short-acting oral opioid every 1 h as needed

Protocol 3—For patients on higher doses of opioids (>600 mg oral morphine equivalents/d)
- Stop the original opioid
- Start methadone at a dose of 5–10 mg orally every 4 h, with rescue doses of 5–10 mg every h allowed as needed
- After 2–3 d, increase the methadone dose by approximately 30% every 4 h
- After 3 d following the switch to methadone, the dose is changed from every 4 h to every 8 h; the rescue doses are administered every 3 h, as needed, at the same single dose as established on days 2 to 3
- The dose can then be increased by up to 30% if further upward titration is required

Protocol 4—For opioid-naïve patients or those on lower doses
- Start methadone at 3–5 mg every 8 h if the patient is opioid naïve or at a dose equivalent to 50% of the daily morphine dose
- Continue for 3 d
- When the patient has pain relief for 6–8 h, change the dose to once daily and allow rescue doses as needed

These are just a few of the many methods for conversion to methadone that have been recommended. Clinicians are advised to carefully assess patients for any signs of sedation; if these appear, reduce or stop the dose of methadone. If at all possible, avoid adding or discontinuing any other medications during conversion or dose escalation, particularly those metabolized by CYP3A4 because these may alter plasma methadone levels.

TABLE 3.5

AGENTS USED IN PALLIATIVE CARE THAT MAY INTERACT WITH METHADONE

Inhibitors of CYP3A4 (may increase serum methadone levels)	Inducers of CYP3A4 (may lower serum methadone levels)
Amiodarone	Carbamazepine
Aprepitant	Dexamethasone
Clarithromycin	Efavirenz
Cimetidine	Ethanol (acute use)
Ciprofloxacin	Isoniazid
Delavirdine	Lopinavir
Diazepam	Nevirapine
Dihydroergotamine	Oxcarbazepine
Diltiazem	Pentobarbital
Disulfiram	Phenobarbital
Erythromycin	Phenytoin
Ethanol (chronic use)	Rifampin
Fluconazole	Risperidone
Fluoxetine	Spironolactone
Haloperidol	St. John's wort
Ketoconazole	Topiramate
Nicardipine	
Norfloxacin	
Omeprazole	
Paroxetine	
Thioridazine	
Venlafaxine	
Verapamil	

Urinary pH can account for a significant amount of the variability seen in methadone plasma levels. Clearance of methadone is greater when the pH is more acidic (<6). As a result, urinary alkalizers, such as sodium bicarbonate, will decrease methadone excretion. Other factors that alter methadone kinetics include drug interactions. In addition to the CYP3A4 interactions listed previously, others have been described. For example, the proton pump inhibitor omeprazole increases gastric pH, increasing the rate of absorption.

Although the extended half-life of methadone allows longer dosing intervals, it also increases the potential of drug accumulation, leading to delayed sedation and respiratory depression. This may occur 2–5 days after initiating the drug or increasing the dose. Another consequence of prolonged or high-dose opioid administration, myoclonus, has been reported with methadone use (35). Finally, controversy exists about the role of methadone in QT-wave interval prolongation (Torsade de pointes). Some question whether this is due to preservatives in the parenteral formulation, although the syndrome has been reported with oral administration of methadone (36). A more recent study of 100 patients taking methadone found that one third had prolonged QT-wave intervals on electrocardiogram, occurring more frequently in men, yet there did not appear to be a risk of serious prolongation (37,38).

Patients currently on methadone as part of a maintenance program for addictive disease will have developed cross-tolerance to the opioids and, as a result, will require higher doses than naïve patients when the drug is used for pain control (39). Prescribing methadone for addictive disease requires a special license in the United States. As a result, prescriptions provided for methadone to manage pain in palliative care should include the statement "for pain."

Morphine. In the past, morphine was considered the "gold standard." We now recognize that because of the wide variability in response, the most appropriate opioid is the agent that works for a particular patient. Morphine is a useful compound for many patients, in that there are a wide range of formulations and routes available for its use. Initial adverse effects are similar to all other opioids, including sedation and nausea that should be anticipated and treated appropriately. These generally resolve within a few days (40). Long-term effects, such as constipation, should be prevented. An active metabolite of morphine, M3G, may contribute to myoclonus, seizures, and hyperalgesia (increasing pain), particularly when clearance is impaired because of renal impairment (6,15,41). In differentiating adverse effects and metabolic effects, the time course of onset should be determined. Adverse effects generally occur soon after the drug has been absorbed, whereas metabolite-induced effects are generally delayed by several days. When adverse effects do not respond to appropriate management, convert to an equianalgesic dose of a different opioid.

Oxycodone. Oxycodone is a synthetic opioid available in a long-acting formulation, as well as immediate-release tablets (alone or with acetaminophen) and liquid. The equianalgesic ratio is approximately 20–30:30 of oral morphine. Metabolites of oxycodone include noroxycodone and oxymorphone. In addition to binding to the MOR, oxycodone binds to the KOR. Side effects appear to be similar to those experienced with morphine; however, one study comparing these two long-acting formulations in persons with advanced cancer found that oxycodone produced less nausea and vomiting (42). Despite significant media attention to oxycodone (OxyContin) and its role in opioid abuse, it does not appear to be inherently "more addicting" than other opioids used in palliative care. Unfortunately, because of this attention several states have restricted the numbers of long-acting or immediate-release tablets that will be distributed to an individual per month.

Tramadol. Tramadol is a synthetic analog of codeine that binds to the MOR and blocks reuptake of serotonin and norepinephrine. As a result of the monoamine action, naloxone will not completely reverse respiratory depression. Furthermore, because of the inhibited reuptake of monoamines, the use of tramadol should be avoided in patients on serotonin selective reuptake inhibitors or tricyclic antidepressants. Tramadol is thought to be approximately one tenth as potent as morphine in patients with cancer (43). Analgesia may be reduced in poor metabolizers of CYP2D6 (43). Individuals on higher doses of tramadol or who have a history of seizures may be at increased risk for seizures. The ceiling dose of tramadol is 400 mg per day.

Other opioids. Meperidine and propoxyphene are not recommended in palliative care or cancer pain management because of the neurotoxic effects of their metabolites, normeperidine and norpropoxyphene, respectively (44). Levorphanol is an analog of morphine that binds to MOR, KOR, and DOR; is an antagonist at NMDA receptors; and is a monoamine reuptake inhibitor. It is not widely used, in part because of limited availability. Oxymorphone is a semisynthetic derivative of morphine that is only commercially available in the United States as a parenteral solution and a rectal suppository. More recently, a long-acting oral formulation has been studied in cancer pain, with positive results (45).

Partial Agonists

Case reports and open label trials suggest that transdermal buprenorphine, a partial agonist, is useful in cancer pain (46). Additionally, a randomized placebo-controlled study in patients with cancer pain revealed an analysis effect of this therapy (47). However, breakthrough medication consisted of sublingual buprenorphine, a product not commercially available in the United States. The interaction of pure and partial opioid agonists may lead to reduced analgesia. Furthermore, studies of buprenorphine suggest there is a ceiling effect for analgesia, limiting the efficacy of this agent in palliative care (48).

Mixed Agonist–Antagonists

Mixed agonist–antagonist opioid analgesics, including butorphanol, nalbuphine, and pentazocine, exhibit a ceiling effect for analgesia, are more likely to cause psychotomimetic effects, and can precipitate the abstinence syndrome if given to a patient physically dependent on a pure opioid agonist (49). As a result, these agents are not recommended in cancer pain management.

Antagonists

Opioid antagonists, such as parenteral naloxone, have been used to reverse acute adverse effects, primarily respiratory depression, caused by opioids. Oral naloxone has been described as being effective in relieving opioid-induced constipation, although one must use bad-tasting solutions intended for parenteral administration (50). Furthermore, higher doses, up to 8–12 mg, can reverse analgesia. New agents, including methylnaltrexone and alvimopan, act peripherally to block opioid receptor binding within the gastrointestinal tract (51,52).

Definitions

Misconceptions about terms such as tolerance, physical dependence, and addiction contribute to inadequate management of pain (Table 3.6). Education of professionals, patients, family members, and the public are needed to overcome the many misconceptions and biases that limit the effective use of this class of analgesics. See Chapter 41 for specific information on substance abuse issues in palliative care.

TABLE 3.6

DEFINITIONS ASSOCIATED WITH OPIOIDS (49,53,54)

Addiction
Addiction is a primary, chronic, neurobiologic disease, with genetic, psychosocial, and environmental factors influencing its development and manifestations. It is characterized by behaviors that include one or more of the following: impaired control over drug use, compulsive use, continued use despite harm, and craving

Physical Dependence
Physical dependence is a state of adaptation that is manifested by a drug class–specific withdrawal syndrome that can be produced by abrupt cessation, rapid dose reduction, decreasing blood level of the drug, and/or administration of an antagonist

Tolerance
Tolerance is a state of adaptation in which exposure to a drug induces changes that result in a diminution of one or more of the drug's effects over time

Pseudoaddiction
Pseudoaddiction is the mistaken assumption of addiction in a patient who is seeking relief from pain

Pseudotolerance
Pseudotolerance is the misconception that the need for increasing doses of drug is due to tolerance rather than disease progression or other factors

Routes of Opioid Administration

Numerous routes of opioid administration are available that are of particular benefit in palliative care. In a study of patients with cancer at 4 weeks, 1 week, and 24 hours before death, the oral route of opioid administration was continued in 62, 43, and 20% of patients, respectively (55). When oral delivery is no longer useful, many alternative routes exist. Sublingual, buccal, rectal, transdermal (including iontophoretic), s.c., intramuscular (i.m.), i.v., pulmonary, nasal, spinal, and peripheral (topical) have all been described. However, the fact that a drug can be administered by a particular route does not imply that it is effective. Lipid solubility and the size of the molecule influence the transport of the opioid across biological membranes, affecting the pharmacokinetics of the agent. The unique clinical challenge of caring for a person unable to swallow because of anatomic abnormalities or loss of consciousness at the end of life leads to the desire to find alternative routes. Yet the attributes of the compound must first be considered.

Oral, Sublingual, Buccal

Numerous options are available when patients are able to swallow tablets or pills, including immediate-release or long-acting tablets, as well as liquids. Morphine's bitter taste may be prohibitive, especially if immediate-release tablets are left in the mouth to dissolve if the patient cannot normally swallow. When patients have dysphagia, several options are available. The 24-hour, long-acting morphine capsule can be broken open and the "sprinkles" placed in applesauce or other soft food. Oral morphine solution can be swallowed or small volumes (0.5–1 mL) of a concentrated solution (e.g., 20 mg per mL) can be placed sublingually or buccally in patients whose voluntary swallowing capabilities are more significantly limited (56). However, buccal and sublingual uptake of morphine is slow and not very predictable because of its hydrophilic chemical nature (57). In fact, most of the analgesic effect of morphine administered in this manner is due to drug trickling down the throat and the resultant absorption through the gastrointestinal tract. Topical morphine mouthwash has been studied to treat chemotherapy-induced oral mucositis and early findings are promising (58).

Enteral, Rectal

If already in place, enteral feeding tubes can be used to access the gut when patients can no longer swallow opioids. The size of the tube should be considered when placing long-acting morphine "sprinkles" to avoid obstruction of the tube. The rectal, stomal, or vaginal route can be used to administer medication when oral delivery is unreasonable. Commercially prepared suppositories, compounded suppositories, or microenemas can be used to deliver the drug into the rectum or stoma. Sustained-release morphine tablets have been used rectally, with resultant delayed time to peak plasma level and approximately 90% of the bioavailability achieved by oral administration (59). Rectal methadone has a bioavailability approximately equal to that of oral methadone (27). Thrombocytopenia or painful lesions preclude the use of these routes. Additionally, delivering medications through these routes can be difficult for family members, especially when the patient is obtunded or unable to assist in turning.

Oral Transmucosal

Oral transmucosal fentanyl citrate (OTFC) is composed of fentanyl on an applicator that patients rub against the oral mucosa for rapid absorption of the drug (60). Clinicians must be aware that, unlike other breakthrough pain drugs, the around-the-clock dose of opioid does not predict the effective dose of OTFC. Pain relief can usually be expected approximately 5 minutes after beginning use (31). Patients should use OTFC over a period of 15 minutes because too rapid use will result in more of the agent being swallowed rather than absorbed transmucosally.

Nasal

Although no pure agonist opioid is commercially available by the nasal route, early studies suggest this may be an alternative. Fentanyl, hydromorphone, and morphine have been investigated (21,61,62).

Parenteral

Parenteral administration includes s.c. and i.v. delivery, routes frequently used in palliative care when other methods are ineffective (40). Intramuscular opioid delivery is inappropriate in the palliative care setting because of the pain associated with this route and the variability in systemic uptake of the drug (49). The i.v. route provides rapid drug delivery but requires vascular access. Subcutaneous boluses have a slower onset and lower peak effect when compared with i.v. boluses, although continuous infusions are equianalgesic (53,63). Subcutaneous infusions may include rates up to 10 mL per hour (although most patients absorb 2–3 mL per hour with least difficulty). Volumes greater than these are poorly absorbed.

Spinal (Epidural/Intrathecal)

Intraspinal routes, including epidural or intrathecal delivery, may allow administration of drugs, such as opioids, local anesthetics, and/or α-adrenergic agonists, in palliative care settings (64). A recent randomized controlled trial demonstrated benefit for patients with cancer who experience pain (65). One must consider the complexity of the equipment used to deliver these medications and the potential caregiver burden. Additionally, not all centers have health care professionals on staff with the specialized knowledge to provide these therapies. Finally, cost is a significant concern related to high-tech procedures.

Intraspinal delivery should be considered when patients experience intolerable adverse effects to opioids and other analgesics, despite aggressive management. Additionally, patients who do not obtain adequate relief from aggressive titration of systemic opioids and other analgesics should be considered for intraspinal drug administration. When systemic opioids are relatively ineffective, this suggests the need for the addition of a local anesthetic, such as bupivacaine, to the infusion. Additionally, pain that is bilateral or midline and is not responsive to systemic analgesics might best be treated with intraspinal drug administration because nerve blocks or other ablative procedures are generally not indicated in these circumstances.

Spinal delivery systems. Percutaneous catheters attached to an external infusion device can be used to deliver medications through the epidural or intrathecal space. Patients with a longer life span would likely benefit from a more permanent catheter that is tunneled to reduce the risk of infection. Dislodgement and infection are the most common complications. Subcutaneous ports, similar to those used to access the venous system, can be implanted and are approved for epidural delivery. Although technically an implanted system, the port must be constantly accessed with a deflected tip needle to allow continuous infusions by an external pump. Implanted pumps are battery driven and programmable, allowing more precise delivery of drug. There is a potential for reduced risk of infection because the pump is entirely implanted. However, they are more expensive and require specially trained staff to refill the device as well as equipment to make programming changes that allow changes in the rate of drug delivery.

Agents administered spinally. Opioids given intraspinally typically include morphine, hydromorphone, fentanyl, remifentanil, and sufentanil. The more lipophilic compounds, such as fentanyl, remifentanil, and sufentanil, are likely to be administered epidurally, whereas more hydrophilic agents, including morphine and hydromorphone, are delivered intrathecally. Adverse effects include those seen with systemic administration of an opioid, with a greater prevalence of pruritus and urinary retention. Local anesthetics are beneficial when treating neuropathic pain, particularly in the pelvis and lower extremities. Clonidine, an α_2-adrenergic agonist, has been shown to be of benefit in providing relief of postoperative, cancer, and labor pain. Hypotension is a potentially dose-limiting adverse effect. The N-specific calcium channel blocker, ziconotide, has been shown to produce analgesia when delivered intrathecally, although the therapeutic window is narrow and adverse effects can be significant.

Topical

Because of the hydrophilic nature of morphine, creams and patches that contain morphine are unlikely to provide analgesia when applied to intact skin. Controversy exists about whether topical morphine or other opioids might be useful in providing pain relief when applied to open areas, such as burns, pressure ulcers, or skin lesions due to venous stasis or sickle cell disease. Several case reports and open-label trials indicate this might be an effective route (66–68). However, a recent randomized controlled trial of topical morphine used to treat painful skin ulcers found no benefit when compared with placebo (69). An analysis of the bioavailability of morphine when delivered to open ulcers found little systemic uptake, a possible explanation for the lack of efficacy (70).

Transdermal

Transdermal fentanyl has been used extensively and a wide range of dosing options (12.5, 25, 50, 75 and 100 µg-per-hour patches) makes this route particularly useful in palliative care (71). Fever, diaphoresis, cachexia, morbid obesity, and ascites may have a significant impact on the absorption, predictability of blood levels, and clinical effects of transdermal fentanyl, although studies are lacking (40). There is some suggestion that transdermal fentanyl may produce less constipation when compared to long-acting morphine, yet the studies demonstrating this effect are small and not sufficiently powered to evaluate this effect (71). A small subset of patients will develop skin irritation because of the adhesive in any patch. Most topical antihistamines have an oil base and would preclude adherence by the patch. Spraying an aqueous steroid inhaler (intended to treat asthma) on the skin and allowing it to dry before applying the patch will often prevent rashes.

A small proportion of patients will experience decreased analgesic effects after only 48 hours of applying a new patch; this should be accommodated by determining whether a higher dose is tolerated with increased duration of the effect or a more frequent (q48h) patch change should be scheduled. As with all long-acting preparations, breakthrough pain medications should be made available to patients using immediate-release opioids.

A new device is being studied that allows patient-controlled analgesia delivered transdermally. The fentanyl-based system allows patients to press the device and administer a very mild electrical current to the skin that allows iontophoretic delivery of a small bolus of fentanyl (72). The system is intended for postoperative or acute pain, although it may one day have a role in providing relief of breakthrough pain in palliative care.

Adverse Effects

The adverse effects associated with opioids are generally well known, although the underlying mechanism for each of these effects might not be fully articulated. More common adverse effects include constipation, cognitive impairment, nausea and vomiting, and sedation. Less common effects include myoclonus, pruritus, and respiratory depression.

Constipation

Patients in palliative care frequently experience constipation, in part because of opioid therapy. Little data exist on the prevalence of opioid-induced constipation or the symptoms that accompany this phenomenon (e.g., bloating, cramping, early satiety, reflux). There is also no evidence-based consensus on the appropriate management of opioid-induced constipation. A prophylactic bowel regimen should be started when commencing opioid analgesic therapy. Bulking or high-fiber agents (e.g., psyllium) are rarely effective and may contribute to worsening constipation, particularly in the patient who cannot take in sufficient amounts of fluid. Oil-based products, such as mineral oil, are not indicated because they prevent the absorption of fat-soluble vitamins and cause incontinence. A daily combination stimulant laxative and softener (e.g., senna and docusate) titrated upward is generally warranted. See Table 3.7 for a list of agents used to prevent and treat opioid-induced constipation. See Chapter 15 for a complete discussion of the management of constipation.

Cognitive Impairment

Anecdotally, patients taking opioids for pain control often report "fuzzy" thinking and an inability to concentrate or perform simple cognitive tasks (such as balancing a checkbook). Few studies have been conducted to explore this phenomenon. A recent double-blind, crossover, controlled trial of patients on sustained-release opioids for pain control examined cognitive performance and memory after administration of oral immediate-release morphine or placebo. There were significant differences in pain reduction, but little effect on sedation. Interestingly, both transient anterograde and retrograde memory impairment and reduced performance on a complex tracking task were observed in those receiving morphine (73). More studies are needed to fully understand the effects of opioids on cognitive functioning.

Nausea and Vomiting

Nausea and vomiting as a result of initial opioid administration are relatively common because of the activation of the chemoreceptor trigger zone in the medulla, vestibular sensitivity, and delayed gastric emptying. Habituation occurs in most cases within several days. Around-the-clock antiemetic therapy can be effective during this period. If persistent, assess for other causes. Table 3.8 provides recommendations for the management of opioid-induced nausea and vomiting. See Chapter 14 for a thorough discussion of the assessment and treatment of persistent nausea and vomiting.

Sedation

Excessive sedation may occur with the initial doses of opioids. If sedation persists, the use of psychostimulants may be beneficial. Starting doses include dextroamphetamine 2.5–5 mg p.o. every morning and midday or methylphenidate 5–10 mg p.o. every morning and 2.5–5 mg midday (74). Adjust both the dose and the timing to prevent nocturnal insomnia and monitor for undesirable psychotomimetic effects (such as agitation, hallucinations, and irritability).

TABLE 3.7

OPIOID-INDUCED CONSTIPATION

PREVENTION

Stimulant laxatives

Senna
Recommended dose: 0.5–2 g
Onset of laxative effect: 6–24 h

Bisacodyl
Recommended dose: 10–30 mg/d oral or one to
  two suppositories

Stool softeners

Docusate sodium
Recommended dose: 100–300 mg/d
Onset to softening: 1–3 d

Combination products include (as well as many generics):
Peri-Colace—Docusate sodium 100 mg and senna 8.6 mg
Senokot-S—Docusate sodium 100 mg and senna 8.6 mg

MANAGEMENT OF PREEXISTING OR INTERMITTENT CONSTIPATION

Category	Agent and dose
Sugars	Lactulose 15–30 mL orally/d
Saline laxative	Magnesium citrate 1–2 bottles/d
	Milk of magnesia 15–60 mL/d
Osmotic laxative	Polyethylene glycol 17–34 g (1–2 heaping teaspoons in 240–480 mL of water)

- If patients are unable to swallow or too weak to assist in evacuation of the stool, laxative suppositories (such as bisacodyl) are indicated
- Glycerin suppositories coat the rectal mucosa, providing some pain relief when stools are painful, and preventing tissue damage
- For patients with neuromuscular dysfunction affecting the bowel (e.g., spinal cord compression), bowel training may be helpful; this includes preventive agents, along with the use of bisacodyl at the same time each day
- Saline-type enemas (e.g., Fleet) may be indicated if suppositories are ineffective

TABLE 3.8

MANAGEMENT OF OPIOID-INDUCED NAUSEA AND VOMITING

- Rule out other causes of nausea and vomiting and treat accordingly
  - A. Other medications (antibiotics, anticonvulsants)
  - B. Tumor (increased intracranial pressure)
  - C. Treatment (radiation to thorax or upper abdomen; chemotherapy)
  - D. Bowel obstruction or constipation
- Treat with centrally acting antiemetics
  - A. Butyrophenones
    - i. Haloperidol 0.5–5 mg every 4–6 h orally or 0.5–2 mg every 3–4 h i.v.; fewer adverse effects at lower doses; as effective as phenothiazines
  - B. Phenothiazines
    - i. Trimethobenzamide 300 mg orally every 6–8 h or 200 mg per rectum every 6–8 h
    - ii. Prochlorperazine 5–25 mg orally every 3–4 h or 25 mg per rectum every 6–8 h; side effects may limit routine use
  - C. Prokinetic agents
    - i. Metoclopramide 5–10 mg orally or i.v. every 6 h
- Consider dexamethasone 4–8 mg every day (although optimal dose is unknown)
- If vestibular component to the nausea is present, add cyclizine 25–50 mg every 8 h orally or 25–50 mg per rectum
- Administer antiemetics on a schedule for the first 2–3 days of opioid therapy, then slowly withdraw to determine whether the patient has developed tolerance to this effect
- If these interventions are inadequate, consider opioid rotation

A recent study conducted in patients with cancer allowed "as-needed" dosing of methylphenidate to manage opioid-induced sedation. Doses up to 20 mg per day did not result in sleep disturbances or agitation, although most subjects took doses in the afternoon and evening (75). Modafinil, a newer agent approved to manage narcolepsy, has been reported to relieve opioid-induced sedation with once daily dosing (76).

Myoclonus

Myoclonic jerking occurs more commonly with high-dose opioid therapy. Opioid rotation may be useful because metabolite accumulation may be implicated, particularly in case of renal dysfunction (6,21,35,41). A lower relative dose of the substituted drug may be possible because of incomplete cross-tolerance. Benzodiazepines, such as clonazepam 0.5–1 mg p.o. q6–8 h, to be increased as needed and tolerated, may be useful in patients who are able to take oral preparations. Lorazepam can be given sublingually if the patient is unable to swallow. Parenteral administration of lorazepam or midazolam may be indicated if symptoms progress. Grand mal seizures associated with high-dose parenteral opioid infusions have been reported, requiring aggressive interventions that include benzodiazepines, barbiturates, and propofol (22). Preservatives in the parenteral opioid solution have been implicated (20). Preservative-free solutions should be used when administering high-dose infusions.

Pruritus

Pruritus is less common with chronic opioid therapy. When pruritus occurs in the palliative care patient, other etiologies also should be explored. Opioid rotation may be indicated because there appears to be variability in the prevalence of pruritus associated with various opioids (53). Antihistamines (such as diphenhydramine) are the most common first-line approach to this opioid-induced symptom when treatment is indicated, although these agents produce sedation and are rarely totally effective. Ondansetron has been reported to be effective in relieving opioid-induced pruritus, but no randomized controlled studies exist. Chapter 20 provides a thorough review of pruritus.

Respiratory Depression

Respiratory depression is greatly feared, although in palliative care, this occurs rarely because most patients are opioid tolerant. Clinicians and family members often fear "giving the last dose" of an opioid. Existing data suggest a lack of correlation between opioid dose, timing of opioid administration, and patient death (77,78).

When respiratory depression [rate <8 per minute and/or hypoxemia (O_2 saturation <90%)] occurs and the cause is clearly associated with opioid use, cautious and slow titration of naloxone should be instituted. Standard doses of naloxone may cause abrupt opioid reversal with pain and autonomic crisis. Dilute one ampule of naloxone (0.4 mg per mL) in 10 mL of injectable saline (final concentration 40 µg per mL) and inject 1 mL every 2 to 3 minutes while closely monitoring the level of consciousness and respiratory rate. Because the duration of effect of naloxone is approximately 30 minutes, the depressant effects of the opioid will recur at 30 minutes and persist until the plasma levels decline (often 4 or more hours) or until the next dose of naloxone is administered (53). If the patient has been on methadone, an infusion of naloxone may be warranted because of the long half-life of this opioid.

Principles of Opioid Use

Effective pain control requires interdisciplinary care that incorporates a thorough assessment, which informs the development of a multimodal treatment plan. Optimally, the plan includes pharmacologic and nonpharmacologic therapies. Because opioids are the mainstay of this treatment plan, clinicians caring for patients must understand basic principles of opioid use that build on the information previously presented in this chapter (Table 3.9).

Prevent and Treat Pain

As much as possible, pain should always be prevented and managed aggressively once it occurs. Prevention includes adequate premedication before invasive procedures and also incorporates patient education to take an immediate-release opioid before a painful activity (e.g., bathing, riding in car).

When in the hospital setting, opioids should be ordered around the clock rather than p.r.n. As-needed dosing of an opioid requires the patient to determine when the pain is sufficiently intense to call the nurse. Furthermore there is great reluctance to "bother" the nurse coupled with a fear of appearing to be "addicted" to the medication. In a recent study conducted on an inpatient medicine unit, around-the-clock dosing provided significantly lower pain intensity with no increased risk of adverse effects (79).

Use Long-Acting and Breakthrough Opioids

Long-acting or sustained-release oral opioid preparations allow convenience and are believed to enhance adherence to the treatment. There are a number of formulations currently available in the United States, including once daily morphine, twice daily morphine, twice daily oxycodone, and transdermal fentanyl. Methadone is often included in this list because it can be given every 8 hours. Selection is based on the patient's ability to obtain relief with a particular opioid; the need for an oral, enteral, or transdermal delivery method; support in the home to adhere to a particular regimen; and preference. When using these sustained-release oral formulations, as well as transdermal fentanyl, several principles should be considered:

1. First, titrate with a short-acting product, such as immediate-release morphine, oxycodone, or hydromorphone; then determine the dose that provides relief during a 24-hour period, and convert this dose to an equivalent sustained-release opioid.
2. Immediate-release opioids should be available for breakthrough pain, with each dose calculated as approximately 5–20% of the 24-hour total sustained-release opioid and administered as frequently as every hour.
3. If the patient consistently requires more than two or three doses of breakthrough medication in a 24-hour period, the total breakthrough dose needed during that time should be added to the sustained-release dose (49).

There is great variability in opioid requirements, such that the dose of the opioid necessary to relieve pain is the correct dose for that individual.

Opioid Rotation

When the treatment of opioid-induced adverse effects is not successful, changing to an alternative opioid, also called *opioid rotation* or *switching*, can be useful. Convert the daily dose of the current opioid, such as morphine, to the equivalent dose of an alternate opioid, such as hydromorphone, using equianalgesic tables as a guide. The 24-hour equianalgesic dose is usually reduced by approximately 20–25% because

TABLE 3.9

PRINCIPLES OF OPIOID ADMINISTRATION IN PALLIATIVE CARE

- Screen for pain frequently; conduct a thorough assessment when the patient reports experiencing pain
- Consider symptoms that frequently occur with pain, including fatigue, depression, and others
- Use opioids as part of a multimodal treatment plan that incorporates nonopioids, adjuvant analgesics, cancer therapies when appropriate, nerve blocks, and other ablative procedures as warranted, as well as nonpharmacologic strategies
- Because pain includes physical, emotional, social, spiritual, and other factors, multidisciplinary care is required
- Prevent pain whenever possible
- Prevent and manage opioid-related adverse effects
- Use sustained-release opioids combined with short-acting opioids for rescue doses
  A. Rescue doses are generally 10–20% of the 24-h sustained-release dose
  B. Rescue doses for parenteral administration are 50–100% of the hourly i.v. or s.c. rate
- Rotate opioids when unmanageable adverse events occur or when relief is inadequate despite aggressive titration
  A. Calculate the appropriate dose using an equianalgesic chart
  B. Reduce the dose by approximately 25–50% to account for cross-tolerance
- Consider patient-related factors when selecting the route of administration
  A. If the patient has dysphagia, choose transdermal or parenteral delivery
  B. Determine whether equipment and cost of parenteral or spinal administration will place a hardship on family caregivers
- Educate patients and families about the most effective strategies for using pharmacologic and nonpharmacologic management
  A. Diaries, flow sheets, and pill boxes will help promote adherence
  B. Knowing how and when to use p.r.n. medications is particularly difficult for many patients and family members; reinforce this information repeatedly
  C. Differentiate p.r.n. medications for pain, nausea and vomiting, and anxiety through color-coding or copying pictures of the pills onto a small poster that explains their use
  D. Consider the patient and family's literacy level when providing any instructional material
- When financial barriers to obtaining opioids exist, explore patient assistance programs
  A. www.needymeds.com
  B. www.togetherrxaccess.com
  C. www.pparx.com
- Never abruptly discontinue an opioid
  A. Gradually reduce the dose by approximately 25–50% to prevent distressing symptoms associated with the abstinence syndrome: agitation, sleeplessness, abdominal cramping, diarrhea, lacrimation, yawning, piloerection

of incomplete cross-tolerance and is titrated as needed (49). Ongoing evaluation of the efficacy of any analgesic regimen is essential, and doses of drug must be titrated on the basis of the patient's self-report of pain.

Multimodal Therapy

For the complicated pain syndromes often seen in advanced disease, opioids alone are rarely sufficient. Adjuvant analgesics, nonsteroidal anti-inflammatory drugs, interventional approaches, along with cognitive–behavioral and physical approaches are warranted (49). See Chapters 4–7 for information on other pharmacologic therapies, nonpharmacologic approaches, and interventional procedures for pain control.

CONCLUSION

For most patients with pain associated with cancer or advanced disease, relief is possible through the use of opioids and other therapies. An understanding of opioid pharmacotherapy is a critical component of pain management in those with cancer or other life-threatening illnesses. The evolving field of pharmacogenomics reinforces and informs the clinical observation that all regimens must be individualized to the patient's needs and responses. One envisions a time when screening to determine the optimal response to a particular opioid will be widely available, preventing the trial and error approach currently required.

Although the science of pain mechanisms and opioid pharmacotherapy is advancing rapidly, myths and misperceptions about addiction persist. In fact, there appears to be an even greater fear of addiction as media attention to celebrity addictive disease increases. To address these misunderstandings, patients, family members, and, often, other clinicians, need extensive education. Pain in people with life-threatening illness is a serious problem in health care that can be addressed only through the combined efforts of scientists, clinicians, regulators, and the public to ensure the availability of opioids to provide relief.

References

1. Zimmerman M. The history of pain concepts and treatment before IASP. In: Mersky H, Loeser J, Dubner R, eds. *The paths of pain 1975–2005*. Seattle: International Association for the Study of Pain, 2005:1–21.
2. Snyder SH, Pasternak GW. Historical review: opioid receptors. *Trends Pharmacol Sci* 2003;24(4):198–205.
3. Yaksh TL, Rudy TA. Analgesia mediated by a direct spinal action of narcotics. *Science* 1976;192(4246):1357–1358.
4. Jensen TS, Yaksh TL. Comparison of antinociceptive action of morphine in the periaqueductal gray, medial and paramedial medulla in rat. *Brain Res* 1986;363(1):99–113.
5. Jackson KC II. Opioid pharmacokinetics. In: Davis M, Glare P, Hardy J, eds. *Opioids in cancer pain*. New York: Oxford University Press, 2005:43–52.
6. Smith MT. Neuroexcitatory effects of morphine and hydromorphone: evidence implicating the 3-glucuronide metabolites. *Clin Exp Pharmacol Physiol* 2000;27(7):524–528.
7. Thwaites D, McCann S, Broderick P. Hydromorphone neuroexcitation. *J Palliat Med* 2004;7(4):545–550.
8. Dean M. Opioids in renal failure and dialysis patients. *J Pain Symptom Manage* 2004;28(5):497–504.
9. Koehntop DE, Rodman JH. Fentanyl pharmacokinetics in patients undergoing renal transplantation. *Pharmacotherapy* 1997;17(4):746–752.
10. Klepstad P, Dale O, Skorpen F, et al. Genetic variability and clinical efficacy of morphine. *Acta Anaesthesiol Scand* 2005;49(7):902–908.

11. Pasternak GW. Molecular biology of opioid analgesia. *J Pain Symptom Manage* 2005;29(5 Suppl):S2–S9.
12. Rogers JF, Nafziger AN, Bertino JS Jr. Pharmacogenetics affects dosing, efficacy, and toxicity of cytochrome P450-metabolized drugs. *Am J Med* 2002;113(9):746–750.
13. Gasche Y, Daali Y, Fathi M, et al. Codeine intoxication associated with ultrarapid CYP2D6 metabolism.[see comment][erratum appears in *N Engl J Med* 2005;352(6):638]. *N Engl J Med* 2004;351(27):2827–2831.
14. Rakvag TT, Klepstad P, Baar C, et al. The Val158Met polymorphism of the human Catechol-O-methyltransferase (COMT) gene may influence morphine requirements in cancer pain patients. *Pain* 2005;116(1–2):73–78.
15. Lotsch J. Opioid metabolites. *J Pain Symptom Manage* 2005;29(5 Suppl):S10–S24.
16. Sathyan G, Jaskowiak J, Evashenk M, et al. Characterisation of the pharmacokinetics of the fentanyl HCl Patient-Controlled Transdermal System (PCTS): effect of current magnitude and multiple-day dosing and comparison with IV fentanyl administration. *Clin Pharmacokinet* 2005;44(Suppl 1):7–15.
17. Mystakidou K, Katsouda E, Tsilika E, et al. Transdermal Therapeutic Fentanyl-System (TTS-F). *In Vivo* 2004;18(5):633–642.
18. Shibutani K, Inchiosa MA Jr, Sawada K, et al. Pharmacokinetic mass of fentanyl for postoperative analgesia in lean and obese patients. *Br J Anaesth* 2005;95(3):377–383.
19. Hutchinson MR, Menelaou A, Foster DJR, et al. CYP2D6 and CYP3A4 involvement in the primary oxidative metabolism of hydrocodone by human liver microsomes. *Br J Clin Pharmacol* 2004;57(3):287–297.
20. Murray A, Hagen NA. Hydromorphone. *J Pain Symptom Manage* 2005;29(5 Suppl):S57–S66.
21. Finn J, Wright J, Fong J, et al. A randomised crossover trial of patient controlled intranasal fentanyl and oral morphine for procedural wound care in adult patients with burns. *Burns* 2004;30(3):262–268.
22. Golf M, Paice JA, Feulner E, et al. Refractory status epilepticus. *J Palliat Med* 2004;7(1):85–88.
23. Lee M, Leng M, Cooper R. Measurements of plasma oxycodone, noroxycodone and oxymorphone levels in a patient with bilateral nephrectomy who is undergoing haemodialysis. *Palliat Med* 2005;19(3):259–260.
24. Benmebarek M, Devaud C, Gex-Fabry M, et al. Effects of grapefruit juice on the pharmacokinetics of the enantiomers of methadone. *Clin Pharmacol Ther* 2004;76(1):55–63.
25. Nicholson AB. Methadone for cancer pain. *Cochrane Database Syst Rev* 2004(2):CD003971, http://gateway.ut.ovid.com/gw2/ovidweb.cgi.
26. Morley JS, Bridson J, Nash TP, et al. Low-dose methadone has an analgesic effect in neuropathic pain: a double-blind randomized controlled crossover trial. *Palliat Med* 2003;17(7):576–587.
27. Dale O, Sheffels P, Kharasch ED. Bioavailabilities of rectal and oral methadone in healthy subjects. *Br J Clin Pharmacol* 2004;58(2):156–162.
28. Bruera E, Palmer JL, Bosnjak S, et al. Methadone versus morphine as a first-line strong opioid for cancer pain: a randomized, double-blind study. *J Clin Oncol* 2004;22(1):185–192.
29. Manfredi PL, Houde RW. Prescribing methadone, a unique analgesic. *J Support Oncol* 2003;1(3):216–220.
30. Moryl N, Santiago-Palma J, Kornick C, et al. Pitfalls of opioid rotation: substituting another opioid for methadone in patients with cancer pain. *Pain* 2002;96(3):325–328.
31. Santiago-Palma J, Khojainova N, Kornick C, et al. Intravenous methadone in the management of chronic cancer pain: safe and effective starting doses when substituting methadone for fentanyl. *Cancer* 2001;92(7):1919–1925.
32. Kharasch ED, Hoffer C, Whittington D, et al. Role of hepatic and intestinal cytochrome P450 3A and 2B6 in the metabolism, disposition, and miotic effects of methadone. *Clin Pharmacol Ther* 2004;76(3):250–269.
33. Wang J-S, DeVane CL. Involvement of CYP3A4, CYP2C8, and CYP2D6 in the metabolism of (R)- and (S)-methadone *in vitro*. *Drug Metab Dispos* 2003;31(6):742–747.
34. Ferrari A, Coccia CPR, Bertolini A, et al. Methadone–metabolism, pharmacokinetics and interactions. *Pharmacol Res* 2004;50(6):551–559.
35. Sarhill N, Davis MP, Walsh D, et al. Methadone-induced myoclonus in advanced cancer. *Am J Hosp Palliat Care* 2001;18(1):51–53.
36. Krantz MJ, Kutinsky IB, Robertson AD, et al. Dose-related effects of methadone on QT prolongation in a series of patients with torsade de pointes. *Pharmacotherapy* 2003;23(6):802–805.
37. Cruciani RA, Sekine R, Homel P, et al. Measurement of QTc in patients receiving chronic methadone therapy. *J Pain Symptom Manage* 2005;29(4):385–391.
38. Reddy S, Fisch M, Bruera E. Oral methadone for cancer pain: no indication of Q-T interval prolongation or torsades de pointes. *J Pain Symptom Manage* 2004;28(4):301–303.
39. Peles E, Schreiber S, Gordon J, et al. Significantly higher methadone dose for Methadone Maintenance Treatment (MMT) patients with chronic pain. *Pain* 2005;113(3):340–346.
40. Hanks GW, Conno F, Cherny N, et al. Morphine and alternative opioids in cancer pain: the EAPC recommendations. *Br J Cancer* 2001;84(5):587–593.
41. Andersen G, Jensen NH, Christrup L, et al. Pain, sedation and morphine metabolism in cancer patients during long-term treatment with sustained-release morphine. *Palliat Med* 2002;16(2):107–114.
42. Lauretti GR, Oliveira GM, Pereira NL. Comparison of sustained-release morphine with sustained-release oxycodone in advanced cancer patients.[see comment]. *Br J Cancer* 2003;89(11):2027–2030.
43. Grond S, Sablotzki A. Clinical pharmacology of tramadol. *Clin Pharmacokinet* 2004;43(13):879–923.
44. Kaiko RF, Foley KM, Grabinski PY, et al. Central nervous system excitatory effects of meperidine in cancer patients. *Ann Neurol* 1983;13(2):180–185.
45. Gabrail NY, Dvergsten C, Ahdieh H. Establishing the dosage equivalency of oxymorphone extended release and oxycodone controlled release in patients with cancer pain: a randomized controlled study. *Curr Med Res Opin* 2004;20(6):911–918.
46. Muriel C, Failde I, Mico JA, et al. Effectiveness and tolerability of the buprenorphine transdermal system in patients with moderate to severe chronic pain: a multicenter, open-label, uncontrolled, prospective, observational clinical study. *Clin Ther* 2005;27(4):451–462.
47. Sittl R, Griessinger N, Likar R. Analgesic efficacy and tolerability of transdermal buprenorphine in patients with inadequately controlled chronic pain related to cancer and other disorders: a multicenter, randomized, double-blind, placebo-controlled trial. *Clin Ther* 2003;25(1):150–168.
48. Johnson RE, Fudala PJ, Payne R. Buprenorphine: considerations for pain management. *J Pain Symptom Manage* 2005;29(3):297–326.
49. Miaskowski C, Cleary J, Burney R, et al. *Guideline for the management of cancer pain in adults and children*. APS Clinical Practice Guidelines Series No. 3. Glenview, IL: American Pain Society, 2005.
50. Meissner W, Schmidt U, Hartmann M, et al. Oral naloxone reverses opioid-associated constipation. *Pain* 2000;84(1):105–109.
51. Yuan C-S. Clinical status of methylnaltrexone, a new agent to prevent and manage opioid-induced side effects. *J Support Oncol* 2004;2(2):111–117. (discussion 119–22).
52. Paulson DM, Kennedy DT, Donovick RA, et al. Alvimopan: an oral, peripherally acting, mu-opioid receptor antagonist for the treatment of opioid-induced bowel dysfunction–a 21-day treatment-randomized clinical trial. *J Pain* 2005;6(3):184–192.
53. Medicine AAoP, Society AP, *Medicine ASoA: definitions related to the use of opioids in the treatment of pain.* 2001.
54. Weissman DE, Haddox JD. Opioid pseudoaddiction–an iatrogenic syndrome. *Pain* 1989;36(3):363–366.
55. Coyle N, Adelhardt J, Foley KM, et al. Character of terminal illness in the advanced cancer patient: pain and other symptoms during the last four weeks of life. [comment] *J Pain Symptom Manage* 1990;5(2):83–93.
56. Zeppetella G. Sublingual fentanyl citrate for cancer-related breakthrough pain: a pilot study. *Palliat Med* 2001;15(4):323–328.
57. Weinberg DS, Inturrisi CE, Reidenberg B, et al. Sublingual absorption of selected opioid analgesics. *Clin Pharmacol Ther* 1988;44(3):335–342.
58. Cerchietti LCA, Navigante AH, Korte MW, et al. Potential utility of the peripheral analgesic properties of morphine in stomatitis-related pain: a pilot study. *Pain* 2003;105(1–2):265–273.
59. Gourlay GK. Sustained relief of chronic pain. Pharmacokinetics of sustained release morphine. *Clin Pharmacokinet* 1998;35(3):173–190.
60. Hanks GW, Nugent M, Higgs CMB, et al. Oral transmucosal fentanyl citrate in the management of breakthrough pain in cancer: an open, multicentre, dose-titration and long-term use study. *Palliat Med* 2004;18(8):698–704.
61. Rudy AC, Coda BA, Archer SM, et al. A multiple-dose phase I study of intranasal hydromorphone hydrochloride in healthy volunteers. *Anesth Analg* 2004;99(5):1379–1386. table of contents.
62. Fitzgibbon D, Morgan D, Dockter D, et al. Initial pharmacokinetic, safety and efficacy evaluation of nasal morphine gluconate for breakthrough pain in cancer patients. *Pain* 2003;106(3):309–315.
63. Nelson KA, Glare PA, Walsh D, et al. A prospective, within-patient, crossover study of continuous intravenous and subcutaneous morphine for chronic cancer pain. *J Pain Symptom Manage* 1997;13(5):262–267.
64. Baker L, Lee M, Regnard C, et al. Evolving spinal analgesia practice in palliative care. *Palliat Med* 2004;18(6):507–515.
65. Coyne PJ, Viswanathan R, Smith TJ. Nebulized fentanyl citrate improves patients' perception of breathing, respiratory rate, and oxygen saturation in dyspnea. *J Pain Symptom Manage* 2002;23(2):157–160.
66. Zeppetella G, Paul J, Ribeiro MDC. Analgesic efficacy of morphine applied topically to painful ulcers. *J Pain Symptom Manage* 2003;25(6):555–558.
67. Ballas SK. Treatment of painful sickle cell leg ulcers with topical opioids. *Blood* 2002;99(3):1096.
68. Long TD, Cathers TA, Twillman R, et al. Morphine-Infused Silver Sulfadiazine (MISS) cream for burn analgesia: a pilot study. *J Burn Care Rehabil* 2001;22(2):118–123.
69. Vernassiere C, Cornet C, Trechot P, et al. Study to determine the efficacy of topical morphine on painful chronic skin ulcers. *J Wound Care* 2005;14(6):289–293.
70. Ribeiro MDC, Joel SP, Zeppetella G. The bioavailability of morphine applied topically to cutaneous ulcers. *J Pain Symptom Manage* 2004;27(5):434–439.
71. Muijsers RB, Wagstaff AJ. Transdermal fentanyl: an updated review of its pharmacological properties and therapeutic efficacy in chronic cancer pain control. *Drugs* 2001;61(15):2289–2307.
72. Sinatra R. The fentanyl HCl Patient-Controlled Transdermal System (PCTS): an alternative to intravenous patient-controlled analgesia in the postoperative setting. *Clin Pharmacokinet* 2005;44(Suppl 1):1–6.

73. Kamboj SK, Tookman A, Jones L, et al. The effects of immediate-release morphine on cognitive functioning in patients receiving chronic opioid therapy in palliative care. *Pain* 2005;117(3):388–395.

74. Rozans M, Dreisbach A, Lertora JJL, et al. Palliative uses of methylphenidate in patients with cancer: a review. *J Clin Oncol* 2002;20(1):335–339.

75. Bruera E, Driver L, Barnes EA, et al. Patient-controlled methylphenidate for the management of fatigue in patients with advanced cancer: a preliminary report. *J Clin Oncol* 2003;21(23):4439–4443.

76. Webster L, Andrews M, Stoddard G. Modafinil treatment of opioid-induced sedation. *Pain Med* 2003;4(2):135–140.

77. Sykes N, Thorns A. The use of opioids and sedatives at the end of life. *Lancet Oncol* 2003;4(5):312–318.

78. Thorns A, Sykes N. Opioid use in last week of life and implications for end-of-life decision-making. *Lancet* 2000;356(9227):398–399.

79. Paice JA, Noskin GA, Vanagunas A, et al. Efficacy and safety of scheduled dosing of opioid analgesics: a quality improvement study. *J Pain* 2005;6(10):639–643.

CHAPTER 4 ■ NONOPIOID AND ADJUVANT ANALGESICS

JAMES F. CLEARY

Analgesic drugs can be divided into three categories: opioids, nonopioids, and coanalgesics. The World Health Organization (WHO) analgesic ladder has clarified the use of these drugs, with opioids being used as step 2 and 3 agents. The term, *nonopioid analgesic*, is applied to acetaminophen and anti-inflammatory agents, drugs that are traditionally WHO step 1 analgesics. The term *coanalgesic* refers to those drugs used for the treatment of pain that have a primary indication other than pain relief (1). These have also been called *adjuvant analgesics* and have been recommended for use throughout the analgesic ladder.

NONOPIOID ANALGESICS

Acetaminophen

Acetaminophen (paracetamol) is a commonly used analgesic that has little clinical anti-inflammatory activity. It is used as initial therapy for mild pain and as a continued medication for cancer pain management in the elderly. Step 2 of the WHO pain ladder has classically included acetaminophen/opioid combination products (Table 4.1). Many clinicians stop acetaminophen once they have moved to step 3 of the WHO ladder. A recent randomized controlled trial (RCT) in patients with cancer has shown that the addition of acetaminophen to opioids used in the treatment of severe pain results in added analgesic effect (2). Safety concerns about the effects of high and continued dosing of acetaminophen on the kidney and liver are well established (3). The current recommendation for maximum dosage of acetaminophen is 4 g per day. As with other analgesic regimens in palliative care, scheduled acetaminophen is usually the most appropriate (Table 4.2).

Nonsteroidal Anti-inflammatory Drugs

Nonsteroidal anti-inflammatory drugs (NSAIDs) are traditional step 1 opioids of the WHO ladder. They are effective in the treatment of mild pain, and have an opioid-sparing effect for moderate to severe pain (4). Many NSAIDs in the United States have both prescription and nonprescription formulations; these are generally equally effective when equivalent doses are given.

NSAIDs are effective through the inhibition of the enzyme cyclo-oxygenase, resulting in the reduction of prostaglandin synthesis. Cyclo-oxygenase has two isoforms: the constitutive variety known as *cyclo-oxygenase-1 (COX-1)* and an inducible variety known as *cyclo-oxygenase-2 (COX-2)*. COX-1 is involved in the normal physiology of the stomach, kidney, and other organs, and platelets. In the stomach, COX-1 participates in the production of prostaglandins that generate the protective barrier of the gastric mucosa and modulates the extent of gastric acid production. COX-2 is found primarily in the brain and kidney, is produced elsewhere in the body in response to pain and inflammation, and is a key element in the inflammatory cascade. The preferential inhibition of COX-2 leads to a relatively improved toxicity profile without loss of anti-inflammatory or analgesic effects. COX-2 inhibitors have a relatively reduced risk of gastrointestinal toxicity and no effect on platelet function. COX-2 inhibitors have continued renal toxicity and a risk of myocardial infarction. It is debatable whether this is a class effect or directly associated with individual drugs.

TABLE 4.1

FORMULATIONS OF OPIOIDS WITH ACETAMINOPHEN

	Acetaminophen dose (mg)	Opioid dose (mg)
Oxycodone	325	2.5, 5, 7.5, 10
	500	5, 7.5
	650	7.5
Hydrocodone	125	2.5
	250	10
	325	5, 7.5, 10
	400	5, 7.5, 10
	500	2.5, 5, 10
	650	7.5, 10
	660	10
	750	7.5, 10
Tramadol	325	37.5
Codeine	125	12
	325	7.5, 15, 30, 60
	650	30
Propoxyphene	325	50, 100
	500	100
	650	100

TABLE 4.2

PRESCRIBING INFORMATION OF COMMON NONOPIOID ANALGESICS

	Usual dose range (24 h)	Usual dose	Frequency
Acetaminophen	2–4 g	325–650 mg	q4h
		650 mg–1 g	q.i.d.
Aspirin	2.4–6 g	600–1500 mg	q.i.d.
Diclofenac	150–200	50, 75 mg	b.i.d.
			t.i.d.
Ibuprofen	1.2–3.2 g	400, 600, 800 mg	q.i.d.
Naproxen	500 mg–1 g	250, 375, 500 mg	b.i.d.
Piroxicam	10–20 mg	10, 20 mg	daily
Sulindac	300–400 mg	150, 200 mg	daily, b.i.d.
Celecoxib	200–400 mg	100, 200 mg	b.i.d.
		200 mg	daily
Valdecoxib	10 mg	10 mg	daily

NSAID gastropathy and nephropathy can be minimized by using these medications carefully in patients with increased risk of gastrointestinal and renal disorders. Good hydration is essential to minimize adverse renal effects. The risk of renal dysfunction is greatest in patients with preexisting renal impairment, heart failure, hepatic dysfunction, hypovolemia, and concomitant therapy with other nephrotoxic drugs such as diuretics, cisplatin, aminoglycosides, and amphotericin B. Older patients with intrinsic renal disease are at increased risk of adverse renal effects from NSAIDs. In addition, the antipyretic and anti-inflammatory effects of NSAIDs may mask the usual signs and symptoms of infection, which may be particularly important in patients with neutropenia.

NSAIDs are effective in the treatment of mild cancer pain and also have an opioid-sparing effect for moderate to severe pain. They may be most useful in the treatment of cancer-related pain when it is associated with inflammation: for example, in patients with pain from bone metastasis. Although, a dose–response relationship exists with both nonselective and COX-2–selective NSAIDs, each individual drug has a maximum therapeutic dose above which there is no additional analgesic effect, but there is an increased risk of toxicity with further dose escalation (ceiling effect). Mercandante et al. (4) confirmed the opioid-sparing nature of NSAIDs. The addition of ketorolac, 60 mg daily, resulted in a significant reduction in opioid dosing. Patients receiving ketorolac had less constipation but more gastric discomfort. This positive effect may be related to the significant potency of ketorolac, which has a limited duration of prescribing (5 days) because of its nephrotoxicity. It is commonly used in both peri- and postoperative analgesia but may be associated with an increased risk of bleeding. A recent Cochrane review of the effects of NSAIDs, alone or combined with opioids, for the treatment of cancer pain showed that NSAIDs had a clear benefit over placebo. There were differences in side effects, while some studies showed improved efficacy of some NSAIDs over others. In terms of the combined therapy of opioids and NSAIDs, there was a statistical advantage for the combination in 9 of 23 studies. Most of the studies were of <7 days' duration, making their applicability to the general cancer population questionable. Most clinicians continue to recommend NSAIDs especially for patients with bone pain. The potential cardiac toxicity of COX-2–selective NSAIDs is not likely to be a factor in the treatment of cancer pain in the palliative care setting, but should be discussed with the patient.

Corticosteroids

Although corticosteroids were not developed for the primary purpose of analgesia, they effectively act with the same mechanism as NSAIDs, decreasing the inflammatory cell response (steroidal anti-inflammatory drugs). In cancer practice, steroids have been used in the treatment of depressed appetite, malignant bowel obstruction, and nausea, and to improve the quality of life generally. Apart from the pain of bowel obstruction, other pain syndromes that are improved with the use of steroids include bone pain, liver capsule pain, and headache from increased intracranial pressure caused by brain metastases. Steroids can reduce the neurologic impact and pain of malignant spinal cord compression, and a response to steroids is in fact a prognostic sign for response to radiotherapy. The reduction of edema around nerves may be an important mechanism in their role in neuropathic pain.

Few studies have formally assessed the effect of corticosteroids on pain; however, studies in hormone-refractory metastatic prostate cancer give some guidance (5). In this study, patients were randomized to receive mitoxantrone and prednisone versus prednisone alone (10 mg daily). Ten of 81 patients (12%) treated with prednisone alone had a reduction in pain compared with 23 of 80 (29%) of those who received mitoxantrone and prednisone. A further seven had no reduction in pain but a >50% reduction in pain medicines. The median duration of pain response, defined as a two-point decrease in pain on a six-point scale without an increase in analgesic medications, was 18 weeks in the prednisone alone arm. Many of these patients had bone disease, suggesting an anti-inflammatory effect of steroids.

Corticosteroids are not without side effects. In the short term, one must be conscious of the potential for fluid retention, hyperglycemia, gastric irritation, and oral candidiasis. When given for a prolonged period, steroids may cause a proximal myopathy immunosuppression leading to opportunistic infections, cushingoid habitus, and some neuropsychiatric syndromes including delirium, especially in the elderly. A mild dysphoria may actually be a positive effect of steroids. Patients administered steroids for more than a few days should be given some form of gastric mucosal protection (e.g., H_2 receptor antagonists, proton pump inhibitors) and an antifungal mouthwash for the prevention of oral thrush. When higher doses are used for more than a few weeks, the addition of prophylaxis for *Pneumocystis* [e.g., trimethoprim/sulfamethoxazole (Bactrim)] may be considered.

COANALGESICS

"Coanalgesics" has become the more common term to describe "adjuvant analgesics," that is, those nonopioid drugs that may have some pain-relieving effects, although pain relief may not be their primary indication in medicine (1). This change in terminology is based on the fact that these agents may be prescribed as first-line therapy for neuropathic pain and not just as adjuvant therapy to opioids. It is more correct to classify these medications on the basis of a drug class and physiologic effect (e.g., "anticonvulsants," "antidepressants," "oral antiarrhythmics," "N-methyl-D-aspartate antagonists," "sympatholytic agents"). Much of the evidence for efficacy and safety of these drugs comes from studies in nonmalignant neuropathic pain rather than malignant pain. However, because the pathophysiologic mechanisms underlying neuropathic pain syndromes are assumed to be similar whether a patient has cancer or not, these agents are used with some success for managing neuropathic pain associated with cancer, but this is not always the case. Given that many patients have mixed etiology of their pain, a clinical trial of these medicines can be undertaken, weighing both the mechanism of the pain and the likely effectiveness and expected side effect profile in individual patients.

Anticonvulsants

Anticonvulsants (Table 4.3) have become commonly used for the treatment of cancer pain, with little evidence of their overall effect (6). In a Cochrane Systematic review, 23 studies were considered for analgesic effectiveness (7). In these studies, which each involved >1000 patients with largely nonmalignant conditions, the primary measure used was the number-needed-to-treat (NNT), allowing better comparison of the effectiveness. NNT is the number of patients required to treat to achieve a >50% reduction in pain intensity in one patient (Table 4.4). Carbamazepine, phenytoin, and gabapentin have been shown to have some analgesic efficacy. A single study with sodium valproate showed no analgesic effect. Newer anticonvulsant medications have also been studied.

Gabapentin has found many uses within medicine, often without clear evidence of effectiveness. Its role in the treatment of cancer-related neuropathic pain has now been confirmed in clinical trials. RCTs with placebo have demonstrated the efficacy and tolerability of gabapentin for the treatment of postherpetic neuralgia (PHN) (8,9) and painful diabetic neuropathy (10). For PHN, the NNT is 3.2 (CI 2.4–5.0), while for diabetic neuropathy the NNT is 3.8 (CI 2.4–8.7) (Table 4.4). Two small open-label studies (11,12) have suggested that gabapentin may be effective in the management of neuropathic pain associated with cancer and cancer treatment. A systemic review showed that these smaller nonrandomized studies supported the randomized controlled studies (13). In a later randomized controlled study, the addition of gabapentin showed an improvement in analgesia in patients already receiving opioids for cancer pain (14). Patients with dysesthesia were more likely to be responsive to gabapentin. The qualities of pain often alleviated by gabapentin, include lancinating, burning, and aching pain, as well as allodynia, confirming the need for a careful and ongoing assessment. In a retrospective review of insurance claim data, the addition of gabapentin to morphine in the treatment of PHN resulted in a reduction in the required morphine dose (15). Gabapentin is well tolerated, with most patients experiencing few intolerable side effects. Treatment is usually started at 100–300 mg per day, with evening dosing often assisting with sleep. The most common side effects are sedation and dizziness with nausea, and confusion, with lower extremity edema occurring infrequently. Although studies and clinical experience have suggested that the effective dosage appears to be in the order of 2700 mg per day, RCTs have not established a clear benefit with dosages >1800 mg per day (administered in three divided doses), but individual dose titration is important. Doses should be reduced in patients with renal insufficiency.

Other anticonvulsants have been and continue to be used in the treatment of neuropathic pain. Carbamazepine is commonly used in the treatment of trigeminal neuralgia. The Cochrane review included three placebo-controlled trials of carbamazepine in patients with trigeminal neuralgia. The review showed an NNT of 2.5 (CI 2.0–3.4) patients to achieve a response in a single patient. Although small controlled trials have demonstrated the efficacy of carbamazepine for painful diabetic neuropathy (NNT = 2.3) (Table 4.4), there is little evidence to support its role in cancer neuropathic pain, with only one study in this population. It may be a difficult drug to use in patients receiving chemotherapy because it is contraindicated in patients with leukocyte counts <4000 per µL or absolute neutrophil count of <1500 per µL. Regular complete blood counts (CBC) are usually recommended, creating considerable burden in the palliative care setting. When studies of the

---

TABLE 4.3

CHARACTERISTICS OF COMMON ANTIEPILEPTICS USED IN THE TREATMENT OF NEUROPATHIC PAIN

	Usual dose	Starting dose	Common side effects
Gabapentin	1800–2700 mg/d (max 3600 mg/d)	300 mg t.i.d. (100 mg at night)	Fatigue, hyperactivity Mood swings
Carbamazepine	500 mg/d	200 mg b.i.d.	Dizziness, ataxia drowsiness, bone marrow suppression
Oxcarbazepine	750 mg/d	300 mg b.i.d.	Fatigue, gastrointestinal, neurologic
Pregabalin	300 mg/d	50 mg t.i.d.	Dizziness, somnolence
Lamotrigine	300 mg/d	50 mg/d	Dizziness, somnolence, skin reactions

TABLE 4.4

NUMBER OF PATIENTS NEEDED TO TREAT (NNT) TO ACHIEVE A 50%
ANALGESIC RESPONSE IN ONE PATIENT

Drug	Condition	Number-needed-to-treat
Gabapentin	Diabetic neuropathy	3.2
	Postherpetic neuralgia	3.8
Carbamazepine	Trigeminal neuralgia	2.5
	Diabetic neuropathy	2.3
Venlafaxine	Diabetic neuropathy	4.5
	Neuropathic pain	5.2
Imipramine	Neuropathic pain	2.7
Capsaicin	Neuropathic pain	5.7
Bisphosphonate	Cancer pain	11 (4 wk)
		7 (12 wk)

different conditions were combined, carbamazepine was found to have increased side effects compared with other anticonvulsants. Oxcarbazepine is a derivative of carbamazepine that has been shown to have analgesic activity in painful diabetic neuropathy (16). Small controlled trials have demonstrated the efficacy of phenytoin for painful diabetic neuropathy (7). Although serum concentrations can be monitored, its poor efficacy and high incidence of intolerable side effects (e.g., confusion, ataxia, nystagmus, nausea) outweighs this potential advantage and has resulted in its minimal clinical use. Loading doses may result in a rapid response to pain, but its nonlinear kinetics makes it a difficult drug to titrate.

Other newer antiseizure medicines have also been studied, with suggestions that they may be useful in the treatment of neuropathic pain. Pregabalin provides effective, safe, and lasting relief from neuropathic pain associated with diabetes (17,18). In 40% of 70 patients receiving pregabalin pain was reduced by more than half compared to 13% of the patients receiving placebo (19). Lamotrigine has been shown to be effective in the treatment of central poststroke pain (20), and in a small randomized study of HIV-associated distal sensory polyneuropathy, the study group of nine patients achieved reduction in average pain but no difference in worst pain when compared to placebo (21). Lamotrigine requires a relatively longer period of dose titration to reduce the likelihood of cutaneous hypersensitivity, which may limit its utility in those with advanced illness.

Antidepressants

A number of tricyclic antidepressant (TCA) drugs, including amitriptyline, nortriptyline, desipramine, doxepin, and imipramine, have well-established analgesic effects independent of their antidepressant effects (22,23). Serotonin and norepinephrine are thought to inhibit pain through interaction with descending pain pathways. Therefore, drugs that inhibit the reuptake of these compounds have been proposed as agents in the treatment of neuropathic pain, with norepinephrine reuptake inhibitors proposed as being more effective than the serotonin reuptake inhibitors (24). The available evidence suggests that antidepressant drugs can relieve both continuous and paroxysmal neuropathic pain. Extensive clinical experience supports their greater utility in continuous pain. Anticonvulsants may be preferred for lancinating or paroxysmal neuropathic pain.

RCTs have demonstrated the efficacy of TCAs for the treatment of postmastectomy pain, PHN, and painful diabetic neuropathy (25) at doses lower than those required for the treatment of depression. In patients with cancer, TCAs are frequently used to treat neuropathic pain associated with surgery, radiation therapy, or chemotherapy, or pain caused by malignant nerve infiltration. Dosing can be started at relatively low doses and titrated slowly upwards. If unsatisfactory side effects are seen, it is prudent to taper these drugs to reduce the risk of withdrawal phenomena such as insomnia and changes in mood. TCAs may worsen conduction abnormalities (e.g., bundle branch block, AV block), so a baseline electrocardiogram (ECG) should be preformed to rule out these conditions, especially in patients who have received anthracycline chemotherapy. Amitriptyline is least tolerated because of its potent anticholinergic effects and is therefore not recommended in patients older than 65. It also has the side effects of sedation and hypotension. Administration of the entire dose of amitriptyline at bedtime promotes sleep and minimizes side effects during daytime.

Many clinicians prefer nortriptyline or desipramine rather than amitriptyline because they cause less sedation and have fewer anticholinergic effects. However desipramine can produce insomnia and should be administered during the day. A comparative crossover study of opioids (e.g., morphine or methadone) versus TCAs (e.g., nortriptyline or desipramine) in the treatment of neuropathic pain showed a trend favoring opioids in terms of pain relief in patients preferring opioids despite some increased side effects (26). Opioids may be a reasonable choice for patients with neuropathic pain rather than chasing the many coanalgesic alternatives.

The newer antidepressants, the selective serotonergic reuptake inhibitors (SSRIs), have produced mixed results in controlled clinical trials. Fluoxetine failed to demonstrate efficacy in a RCT of diabetic neuropathy (27), whereas paroxetine showed efficacy in several small controlled trials (23). Venlafaxine and duloxetine that combine the properties of the TCAs and SSRIs have also been studied.

Venlafaxine is an antidepressant classified as a SSRI and a weak norepinephrine reuptake inhibitor. Venlafaxine extended-release (ER) (75 mg and 150–225 mg) was administered for 6 weeks to patients with painful diabetic neuropathy and compared with placebo (28). The NNT for 50% pain intensity reduction in one patient with venlafaxine ER 150–225 mg was 4.5 at week 6 of therapy, a response suggested by the authors to be equivalent to that of TCAs for neuropathic pain (Table 4.4). The higher dose did not result in a significant percentage reduction from baseline in pain intensity measures. The predominant side effects were nausea and sedation, and seven patients had significant ECG changes. Venlafaxine was compared directly with imipramine in a double-blind placebo-controlled study with a three-way crossover (29). The sum of the individual pain scores during treatment week 4 for the 29 patients was lower with venlafaxine (225 mg, 80% of baseline score; $p = .006$) and imipramine (150 mg, 77%; $p = .001$) than with placebo (100%), with no statistical difference between venlafaxine and imipramine ($p = .44$). NNT to obtain one patient with moderate or better pain relief was 5.2 for venlafaxine and 2.7 for imipramine, questioning the efficacy of venlafaxine when compared with a TCA (Table 4.4). In a placebo-controlled crossover study in a small group of patients with established postmastectomy pain, venlafaxine showed no difference in the primary end point (average daily pain intensity) but there was some improvement in the secondary measures of maximum pain relief and maximum pain intensity (30). The two poor responders had low drug levels, as measured by pharmacokinetics, suggesting that a difference in metabolism may account for the difference in response. The preemptive use of venlafaxine reduced the incidence of postmastectomy pain syndrome (31). Patients administered 2 weeks of venlafaxine, starting the night before surgery, had a greater reduction in chest wall, arm, and axillary pain at 6 months when compared to placebo.

Duloxetine, a balanced and potent dual reuptake inhibitor of serotonin and norepinephrine, was studied in 457 patients with diabetic peripheral neuropathic pain (32). Over a 12-week period, duloxetine 60 and 120 mg per day demonstrated a greater improvement on the 24-hour average pain score when compared with placebo, with the effect starting 1 week after randomization. Duloxetine was also found to have benefits compared with placebo on a number of health-related outcome measures, suggesting that it is worth a trial in patients with neuropathic pain.

Similar to antidepressant effects, there is great variability in the analgesic effects of these different medications within individual patients. The failure of one antidepressant drug does not preclude a trial of others, even within the same subclass.

Local Anesthetic Agents

Local anesthetic agents produce pain relief through the stabilization of neuronal membranes by the inhibition of the ionic fluxes required for the initiation and conduction of impulses. Local anesthetic agents can be administered both topically and systemically.

Topical Local Anesthetic Agents

Topical agents are applied directly on or near the painful body area, where they penetrate the skin, acting locally in the surrounding tissues. Several clinical advantages exist for topical agents over drugs that have a systemic mechanism of action; these include a potential lack of systemic side effects, decreased drug–drug interactions, and a reduced need for dose titration. Topical agents from "compounding pharmacies" should be used cautiously because there may be variability in the concentration and absorption of the active drug.

A local anesthetic topical agent, eutectic mixture of local anesthetics (EMLA), is widely used before the needling of intravascular access devices (33) and does not really have a role in the treatment of neuropathic pain. A lidocaine patch has been approved in the United States for PHN, with the medication applied for 12 hours per day. Blood concentration

of lidocaine on administration of three lidocaine patches was one tenth of the therapeutic concentration required to treat cardiac arrhythmias with intravenous administration (34). Two controlled trials have demonstrated the efficacy, safety, and tolerability of the lidocaine patch in PHN (35,36). Other evidence suggests that the patch is effective for other peripheral neuropathic pain states, such as polyneuropathy, complex regional pain syndrome (CRPS), mononeuropathy, and stump pain (37). Anecdotally, there is some suggestion that it may be useful in the treatment of bone lesions, especially in the vertebrae. A recent meta-analysis of PHN treatment confirms the therapeutic value of topical lidocaine, as well as topical capsaicin (38).

Capsaicin is a naturally occurring compound found in chili peppers. Following prolonged exposure of the vanilloid receptors 1s (VR1s) on nociceptive neurons to capsaicin, there is an influx of calcium into the neurons, resulting in cell death. In a Cochrane review six placebo-controlled trials of 656 patients with neuropathic pain treated for 8 weeks with capsaicin (0.075%), the NNT was 5.7 (39) (Table 4.4). The authors concluded that, although not particularly effective as an analgesic for neuropathic pain, it may be used as an adjunct with other opioids or in patients who are unresponsive or intolerant to other therapies. The application may result in some cutaneous burning at the site of application, and an adequate trial is generally believed to require three to four applications daily for 3–4 weeks.

There is some evidence that topical NSAIDs can be effective for soft tissue pain and perhaps joint pain (40). A trial of a formulation containing diclofenac, ketoprofen, or another NSAID is reasonable when pain is related to chronic soft tissue injury. There is little evidence to suggest any effectiveness in neuropathic pain.

Systemic Local Anesthetic Agents

The systemic administration of local anesthetics may produce analgesia in a variety of pain syndromes and has been an established practice for approximately 40 years (Table 4.5). Kalso et al. found ten studies reporting the use of intravenous lidocaine (41), with the most effective dose being 5 mg per kg infused over 30 minutes. Intravenous lignocaine was effective in four studies in non–cancer-related neuropathic pain, but was without effect in three studies in cancer-related pain. In a more recent systemic review of lignocaine and mexiletine administered systemically, there was clear superiority over placebo but little difference in efficacy or adverse effects when compared with carbamazepine, amantadine, gabapentin, or morphine. Systemic local anesthetics were safe, with no deaths or life-threatening toxicities reported in these trials (42). The use of systemic lidocaine in a hospice setting showed considerable effectiveness in a retrospective chart review (43). Of 89 patients administered parenteral lidocaine initially as a bolus and then as an infusion, 61 were evaluable, with 55 having a major or minor response to pain.

RCTs of mexiletine, the oral analog of lidocaine, have yielded mixed results in the management of neuropathic pain. Positive results were reported in diabetic neuropathy (44,45) and painful mononeuropathy (46), although others failed to report efficacy (47). One criticism of the negative studies is that they failed to allow for necessary dose titration. The most common side effect, nausea, can be reduced by taking mexiletine with food (48). A response to i.v. lidocaine has been shown to be a predictor of a response to oral mexiletine (49). Mexiletine slows cardiac conduction and is contraindicated in patients with second- and third-degree heart block, severe congestive heart failure, and abnormal liver function test results. Other oral agents such as flecainide and tocainide may also be used in a manner similar to that of mexiletine, but the clinical experience is limited.

TABLE 4.5

ADMINISTRATION OF SYSTEMIC PRESERVATIVE-FREE LIDOCAINE
FOR NEUROPATHIC PAIN BY CLINICIANS EXPERIENCED IN TECHNIQUE

Test dose	1–2 mg/kg as slow i.v. push over 3–5 min until side effects or pain relief; patient on telemetry Repeat 15 min × three times until side effects or pain relief Maximum test dose: 300 mg
Continuous infusion	Starting dose: 1 mg/kg/h Titrated according to side effects
Lidocaine side effects	
Mild (at serum levels 3–8 µg/mL)	Numbness and tingling in the fingers and toes Numbness and unusual sensations around the mouth A metallic taste in the mouth Ringing in the ears Lightheadedness and dizziness
Moderate (at serum levels 8–12 µg/mL)	Nausea and vomiting Severe dizziness Decreased hearing Tremors Changes in blood pressure and pulse
Severe (at serum levels >12 µg/mL)	Drowsiness Confusion Muscle twitching Convulsions Loss of consciousness Serious heart problems

N-Methyl-D-Aspartate Antagonists

Preclinical studies during the last decade have established that binding of the excitatory amino acid glutamate to various subunits of the N-methyl-D-aspartate (NMDA) receptor is involved in the mechanisms that may underlie some neuropathic pains and the mechanisms involved in the development of opioid tolerance. In general, clinical experience with NMDA receptor antagonists has been limited. Two studies have reported pain relief with dextromethorphan in patients with diabetic neuropathy but not in those with PHN (50,51). The combination of morphine and dextromethorphan did not result in a significant reduction in morphine dose (52).

Ketamine is an agent most commonly associated with anesthesia and is not familiar to many practicing physicians. A small controlled trial showed the efficacy of ketamine administered as an intravenous infusion in patients with nonmalignant neuropathic pain, but most patients also reported intolerable side effects, such as dissociative experiences (53). A Cochrane review established no clear evidence for the use of ketamine in the cancer pain setting, although only two studies were included (54).

Methadone is suggested to act through NMDA antagonism, as borne out by its prolonged analgesic effect in patients with neuropathic pain (55). Although the racemic mixture DL-methadone is commonly used in clinical practice, D-methadone has been shown to be an antagonist of the NMDA receptor (56).

Memantine, another NMDA antagonist commonly used in the treatment of dementia, has been disappointing in clinical trials of phantom limb pain and other neuropathic pain syndromes such as diabetic neuropathy and PHN (51).

Sympatholytic Agents

It has been suggested that α-Adrenergic agonists such as clonidine have a role in neuropathic pain through interaction with the pain cascade. Two trials reported pain relief in a subpopulation of patients with diabetic neuropathy when treated with transdermal clonidine (57,58). In addition, this α-adrenergic agonist is available for epidural administration in the management of intractable pain. In a controlled trial of patients with cancer pain (59), an infusion of epidural clonidine (30 mcg per hour) was effective in the management of neuropathic pain. Hypotension and bradycardia are possible serious side effects of clonidine, while somnolence and xerostomia are commonly seen.

Bisphosphonates

Bisphosphonates are useful treatments for hypercalcemia and osteoporosis, acting through inhibition of osteoclastic resorption. There is clear evidence that bisphosphonates can delay the onset of painful bone metastases in metastatic cancer from varying primary sites. There is questionable evidence about the role of bisphosphonates in the immediate treatment of pain. In a Cochrane review of 35 randomized studies (3682 subjects), there was some support for the role of bisphosphonates in providing pain relief of bone metastases (60). Any analgesic effect appears to occur over time, with the NNT for an analgesic response of 11 patients at 4 weeks decreasing to 7 at 12 weeks (Table 4.4). The authors concluded that there is insufficient evidence to recommend bisphosphonates for immediate analgesic effect, as first-line therapy, or to define the most effective bisphosphonates or their relative effectiveness for different primary neoplasms. Little new evidence has come to light since this review to change the recommendations. In the palliative treatment of hormone-refractory prostate cancer, the addition of clodronate did not enhance the efficacy of mitoxantrone and prednisone, with responses of 46 and 39%, respectively, in each arm (61). External beam radiotherapy remains a very effective mechanism for the treatment of painful bone metastases (62).

CONCLUSION

With careful attention to the mechanism of the pain, the use of nonopioid analgesics and coanalgesics, both alone and together with opioids, may reduce the amount of opioids required, improving both analgesia and side effects and hence improving quality of life. Continual and frequent reassessment of the severity and character of a patient's pain together with other symptoms is essential to ensure maximal pain control.

References

1. Miaskowski C, Cleary JF, Burney R., et al. *Guideline for the management of cancer pain in adults and children.* Chicago, IL: American Pain Society, 2005.
2. Stockler M, Pillai A, Vardy J. Acetaminophen (paracetamol) improves pain and well-being in people with advanced cancer already receiving a strong opioid regimen: a randomized, double-blind, placebo-controlled cross-over trial. *J Clin Oncol* 2004;22(16):3389–3394.
3. Makin AJ, Williams R. Acetaminophen-induced hepatotoxicity: predisposing factors and treatments. *Adv Intern Med* 1997;42:453–483.
4. Mercadante S, Fulfaro F, Casuccio A. *A randomised controlled study on the use of anti-inflammatory drugs in patients with cancer pain on morphine therapy. Effects on dose-escalation and a pharmacoeconomic analysis. Eur J Cancer* 2002;38(10):1358–1363.
5. Tannock IF, Osoba D, Stockler MR, et al. Chemotherapy with mitoxantrone plus prednisone or prednisone alone for symptomatic hormone-resistant prostate cancer: a Canadian randomized trial with palliative end points. *J Clin Oncol* 1996;14(6):1756–1764.
6. Backonja MM. Use of anticonvulsants for treatment of neuropathic pain. *Neurology* 2002;59(5 Suppl 2):S14–S17.
7. Wiffen P, Collins S Mcquay H, et al. Anticonvulsant drugs for acute and chronic pain (Cochrane review). *Cochrane Database Syst Rev* 2000;(3):CD001133.
8. Rowbotham M, Harden N, Stacey B, et al. Gabapentin for the treatment of postherpetic neuralgia: a randomized controlled trial. *JAMA* 1998;280(21):1837–1842.
9. Rice A, Maton S, Group PNS. Gabapentin in postherpetic neuralgia: a randomised, double blind, placebo controlled study. *Pain* 2001;94:215–224.
10. Backonja M, Beydoun A, Edwards KR. Gabapentin for the symptomatic treatment of painful neuropathy in patients with diabetes mellitus: a randomized controlled trial. *JAMA* 1998;280(21):1831–1836.
11. Caraceni A, Zecca E, Martini C, et al. Gabapentin as an adjuvant to opioid analgesia for neuropathic cancer pain. *J Pain Symptom Manage* 1999;17(6):441–445.
12. Bosnjak S, Jelic S, Susnjar S, et al. Gabapentin for relief of neuropathic pain related to anticancer treatment: a preliminary study. *J Chemother* 2002;14(2):214–219.
13. Mellegers MA, Furlan AD, Mailis A. Gabapentin for neuropathic pain: systematic review of controlled and uncontrolled literature. *Clin J Pain* 2001;17(4):284–295.
14. Caraceni A, Zecca E, Bonezzi C, et al. Gabapentin for neuropathic cancer pain: a randomized controlled trial from the Gabapentin Cancer Pain Study Group. *J Clin Oncol* 2004;22(14):2909–2917.
15. Berger A, Dukes E, McCarberg B, et al. Change in opioid use after the initiation of gabapentin therapy in patients with postherpetic neuralgia. *Clin Ther* 2003;25(11):2809–2821.
16. Beydoun A, Kobetz S, Carrazana E. Efficacy of oxcarbazepine in the treatment of painful diabetic neuropathy. *Clin J Pain* 2004;20(3):174–178.
17. Lesser H, Sharma U, LaMoreaux L, et al. Pregabalin relieves symptoms of painful diabetic neuropathy: a randomized controlled trial. *Neurology* 2004;63:2104–2110.
18. Richter RW, Portenoy R, Sharma U, et al. Relief of painful diabetic peripheral neuropathy with pregabalin: A randomized, placebo-controlled trial. *J Pain* 2005;6:253–260.
19. Rosenstock J, Tuchman M, LaMoreaux L, et al. Pregabalin for the treatment of painful diabetic peripheral neuropathy: a double-blind, placebo-controlled trial. *Pain* 2004;110:628–638.
20. Vestergaard K, Andersen G, Gottrup H, et al. Lamotrigine for central post-stroke pain: a randomized controlled trial. *Neurology* 2001;56:184–190.
21. Simpson DM, Olney R, McArthur JC, et al. A placebo-controlled trial of lamotrigine for painful HIV-associated neuropathy. *Neurology* 2000;54(11):2115–2119.
22. McQuay HJ, Tramer M, Nye BA, et al. A systematic review of antidepressants in neuropathic pain. *Pain* 1996;68(2–3):217–227.
23. Sindrup SH, Jensen TS. Efficacy of pharmacological treatments of neuropathic pain: an update and effect related to mechanism of drug action. *Pain* 1999;83(3):389–400.
24. Mochizucki D. Serotonin and noradrenaline reuptake inhibitors in animal models of pain. *Hum Psychopharmacol* 2004;19(Suppl 1):S15–S19.
25. Max MB, Kishore-Kumar R, Schafer SC, et al. Efficacy of desipramine in painful diabetic neuropathy: a placebo-controlled trial. *Pain* 1991;45(1):3–9; discussion 1–2.
26. Raja SN, Haythornthwaite JA, Pappagallo M, et al. Opioids versus antidepressants in postherpetic neuralgia: a randomized, placebo-controlled trial. *Neurology* 2002;59(7):1015–1021.
27. Max MB, Lynch SA, Muir J, et al. Effects of desipramine, amitriptyline, and fluoxetine on pain in diabetic neuropathy. *N Engl J Med* 1992;326(19):1250–1256.
28. Rowbotham MC, Goli V, Kunz NR, et al. Venlafaxine extended release in the treatment of painful diabetic neuropathy: a double-blind, placebo-controlled study. *Pain* 2004;110(3):697–706.
29. Sindrup SH, Bach FW, Madsen C, et al. Venlafaxine versus imipramine in painful polyneuropathy: a randomized, controlled trial. *Neurology* 2003;60(8):1284–1289.
30. Tasmuth T, Hartel B, Kalso E. Venlafaxine in neuropathic pain following treatment of breast cancer. *Eur J Pain* 2002;6(1):17–24.
31. Reuben SS, Makari-Judson G, Lurie SD. Evaluation of efficacy of the perioperative administration of venlafaxine XR in the prevention of post-mastectomy pain syndrome. *J Pain Symptom Manage* 2004;27(2):133–139.
32. Goldstein DJ, Lu Y, Detke MJ, et al. Duloxetine vs. placebo in patients with painful diabetic neuropathy. *Pain* 2005;116(1–2):109–118.
33. Vaghadia H, al-Ahdal OA, Nevin K. EMLA patch for intravenous cannulation in adult surgical outpatients. *Can J Anaesth* 1997;44(8):798–802.
34. Campbell BJ, Rowbotham M, Davies PS, et al. Systemic absorption of topical lidocaine in normal volunteers, patients with post-herpetic neuralgia, and patients with acute herpes zoster. *J Pharm Sci* 2002;91(5):1343–1350.
35. Rowbotham MC, Davies PS, Verkempinck C, et al. Lidocaine patch: double-blind controlled study of a new treatment method for post-herpetic neuralgia. *Pain* 1996;65(1):39–44.
36. Galer BS, Rowbotham MC, Perander J, et al. Topical lidocaine patch relieves postherpetic neuralgia more effectively than a vehicle topical patch: results of an enriched enrollment study. *Pain* 1999;80(3):533–538.
37. Devers A, Galer BS. Topical lidocaine patch relieves a variety of neuropathic pain conditions: an open-label study. *Clin J Pain* 2000;16(3):205–208.
38. Hempenstall K, Nurmikko TJ, Johnson RW, et al. Analgesic therapy in postherpetic neuralgia: a quantitative systematic review. *PLoS Med* 2005;2(7):e164.
39. Mason L, Moore RA, Derry S, et al. Systematic review of topical capsaicin for the treatment of chronic pain. *BMJ* 2004;328(7446):991.
40. Vaile J, Davis P. Topical NSAIDs for musculoskeletal conditions. A review of the literature. *Drugs* 1998;56:783–799.
41. Kalso E, Tramer MR, McQuay HJ, et al. Systemic local-anaesthetic-type drugs in chronic pain: a systematic review. *Eur J Pain* 1998;2(1):3–14.
42. Challapalli V, Tremont-Lukats I, McNicol E, et al. Systemic administration of local anesthetic agents to relieve neuropathic pain. *Cochrane Database Syst Rev* 2005;(4):CD003345.
43. Thomas J, Kronenberg R, Cox MC, et al. Intravenous lidocaine relieves severe pain: results of an inpatient hospice chart review. *J Palliat Med* 2004;7(5):660–667.
44. Pfeifer MA, Ross DR, Schrage JP, et al. A highly successful and novel model for treatment of chronic painful diabetic peripheral neuropathy. *Diabetes Care* 1993;16(8):1103–1115.
45. Jarvis B, Coukell AJ. Mexiletine. A review of its therapeutic use in painful diabetic neuropathy. *Drugs* 1998;56(4):691–707.
46. Chabal C, Jacobson L, Russell LC, et al. Pain response to perineuromal injection of normal saline, epinephrine, and lidocaine in humans. *Pain* 1992;49(1):9–12.
47. Wallace MS, Magnuson S, Ridgeway B. Efficacy of oral mexiletine for neuropathic pain with allodynia: a double-blind, placebo-controlled, crossover study. *Reg Anesth Pain Med* 2000;25(5):459–467.
48. Sloan P, Basta M, Storey P, et al. Mexiletine as an adjuvant analgesic for the management of neuropathic cancer pain. *Anesth Analg* 1999;89(3):760–761.
49. Galer BS, Harle J, Rowbotham MC. Response to intravenous lidocaine infusion predicts subsequent response to oral mexiletine: a prospective study. *J Pain Symptom Manage* 1996;12(3):161–167.
50. Nelson KA, Park KM, Robinovitz E, et al. High-dose oral dextromethorphan versus placebo in painful diabetic neuropathy and postherpetic neuralgia. *Neurology* 1997;48(5):1212–1218.
51. Sang CN, Booher S, Gilron I, et al. Dextromethorphan and memantine in painful diabetic neuropathy and postherpetic neuralgia: efficacy and dose-response trials. *Anesthesiology* 2002;96(5):1053–1061.

52. Galer BS, Lee D, Ma T, et al. MorphiDex (morphine sulfate/dextromethorphan hydrobromide combination) in the treatment of chronic pain: three multicenter, randomized, double-blind, controlled clinical trials fail to demonstrate enhanced opioid analgesia or reduction in tolerance. *Pain* 2005;115(3):284–295.

53. Oga K, Kojima T, Matsuura M, et al. Effects of low-dose ketamine on neuropathic pain: an electroencephalogram-electrooculogram/behavioral study. *Psychiatry Clin Neurosci* 2002;56(4):355–363.

54. Sang CN. NMDA-receptor antagonists in neuropathic pain: experimental methods to clinical trials. *J Pain Symptom Manage* 2000;19 (1 Suppl):S21–S25.

55. Morley JS, Bridson J, Nash TP, et al. Low-dose methadone has an analgesic effect in neuropathic pain: a double-blind randomized controlled crossover trial. *Palliat Med* 2003;17(7):576–587.

56. Inturrisi CE. Pharmacology of methadone and its isomers. *Minerva Anestesiol* 2005;71(7–8):435–437.

57. Byas-Smith MG, Max MB, Muir J, et al. Transdermal clonidine compared to placebo in painful diabetic neuropathy using a two-stage 'enriched enrollment' design. *Pain* 1995;60(3):267–274.

58. Zeigler D, Lynch SA, Muir J, et al. Transdermal clonidine versus placebo in painful diabetic neuropathy. *Pain* 1992;48(3):403–408.

59. Eisenach JC, DuPen S, Dubois M, et al. The Epidural Clonidine Study Group. Epidural clonidine analgesia for intractable cancer pain. *Pain* 1995;61(3):391–399.

60. Wong R. Wiffen PJ, Bisphosphonates for the relief of pain secondary to bone metastases. *Cochrane Database Syst Rev* 2002;(2):CD002068.

61. Ernst DS, Tannock IF, Winquist EW, et al. Randomized, double-blind, controlled trial of mitoxantrone/prednisone and clodronate versus mitoxantrone/prednisone and placebo in patients with hormone-refractory prostate cancer and pain. *J Clin Oncol* 2003;21(17):3335–3342.

62. McQuay HJ, Collins SL, Carroll D, et al. Radiotherapy for the palliation of painful bone metastases. *Cochrane Database Syst Rev* 2000;(2):CD001793.

CHAPTER 5 ■ NONPHARMACOLOGIC MANAGEMENT OF PAIN

FRANCIS J. KEEFE, AMY P. ABERNETHY, LAURA S. PORTER, AND LISA C. CAMPBELL

Pain is a prevalent and significant problem for persons with cancer. At present, medications are the mainstay of cancer pain management. Despite the fact that medications help many patients with cancer manage pain, there continue to be many patients in whom cancer pain is not effectively managed. Population-based studies demonstrated that in 1969, 66% of patients with cancer complained of pain; in 1987, 72% reported the symptom; and in 1995, 88% reported pain and 66% reported "very distressing" pain (1,2). In response, cancer pain management guidelines have been developed, recommending varying therapeutic building blocks. In 1986, the World Health Organization developed an analgesic ladder to guide the use of pharmacotherapy on the basis of the severity of cancer pain that involved the use of nonopioid and opioid medications with or without adjuvants for escalating severity of pain. Although the validity of the analgesic ladder has been questioned, the basic notion of a guideline-based approach emphasizing medication management has not. More recently, the American Pain Society (APS) developed a cancer pain management guideline that emphasizes pharmacologic strategies and recommends combining these with nonpharmacologic strategies (3).

A wide array of nonpharmacologic interventions is currently being used in the management of cancer pain. A comprehensive review of all of these interventions is not possible in the context of the current chapter. Furthermore, many of these interventions have not been tested in rigorous clinical trials, making a critical analysis of their efficacy difficult, if not impossible.

To illustrate the potential utility of nonpharmacologic interventions for cancer pain, this chapter focuses on a subset of these interventions that are becoming widely used and for which there exists an empirical basis: psychosocial interventions. This chapter is divided into three sections. In the first section, we review the rationale for psychosocial interventions. In the second section, we briefly describe several widely used interventions [psychoeducation, cognitive-behavioral therapy (CBT), hypnosis and imagery, and caregiver-assisted approaches] and critically evaluate their efficacy on the basis of randomized clinical trials. In the final section, we highlight important issues related to the use of psychosocial interventions in cancer pain management.

RATIONALE FOR PSYCHOSOCIAL INTERVENTIONS

Traditionally, cancer pain management has been based on a biomedical model of pain. The chief tenet of this model is that pain is a sensation or symptom due to underlying tissue damage or injury. In cancer, pain can be caused by the tumor itself; tissue damage related to treatments such as surgery, radiation, or chemotherapy; cancer-related infections; immobility; or diagnostic procedures. The biomedical model maintains that pain is most effectively treated by identifying the underlying tissue damage and correcting it.

Clinical observations and research, however, indicate that the traditional biomedical model has limitations. First, the amount of pain that a patient with cancer reports does not correlate well with underlying tissue damage. Some patients with minimal evidence of tissue damage report having excruciating pain, whereas others with considerable tissue damage report little or no pain. Second, even in patients who report the same level of pain, the level of pain-related disability can vary enormously, with some patients becoming much more disabled by their pain than others. Finally, treatments designed to eliminate the underlying cause of cancer pain (e.g., removal of a tumor) often fail to abolish or significantly reduce pain.

Because of these limitations, cancer pain specialists have looked at newer and more complex theories of pain to direct their pain management efforts. Typical of these newer theories is Melzack's neuromatrix theory (4). This theory maintains that pain is a complex and dynamic experience that has sensory, affective, and cognitive dimensions, which are served by underlying somatosensory, limbic, and thalamocortical systems. A key tenet of this theory is that there is a neural network in the brain that integrates multiple inputs to produce pain. The complexity of pain, therefore, reflects the activity of multiple brain inputs (i.e., sensory, cognitive and emotional inputs, and inputs from intrinsic neural inhibitory and stress regulation systems).

The neuromatrix theory has important implications for cancer pain management. First, this theory and the theory it evolved from, Melzack and Wall's gate control theory (5), provide a conceptual rationale for broadening the focus

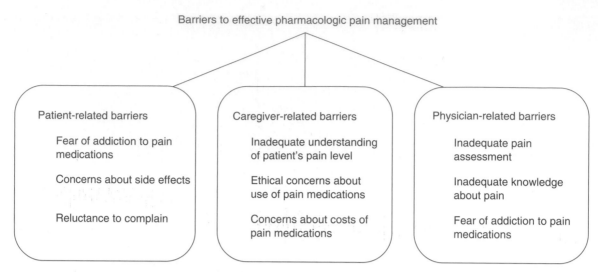

FIGURE 5.1. Barriers to effective pharmacologic pain management.

of assessment efforts to include consideration of cognitive, emotional, social, and cultural factors that can influence cancer pain and disability. Second, by emphasizing the effects of cognition and emotion on pain, this theory has stimulated more widespread use of psychotropic medications (e.g., antidepressants) in cancer pain management. Finally, this theory has highlighted the potential utility of psychosocial interventions in enhancing pain control.

Over the last 20 years, converging lines of evidence have identified important domains of psychosocial factors that can influence the cancer pain experience (6,7). One important domain is made up of the beliefs and attitudes of the patient, caregiver, and physician that function as barriers to effective pharmacologic pain management. Patient-related barriers include concerns about analgesics, fear of addiction, concerns about side effects, fear of the implication of pain, and reluctance to complain (8). Caregiver-related barriers include an unclear role, cost concerns, inadequate understanding of the patient's pain level, and personal ethical concerns about the use of pain medications (9,10). Doctor-related barriers include inadequate pain assessment, inadequate knowledge about pain, fear of tolerance, and fear of addiction (11–13) (Fig. 5.1).

Psychological distress is a second important domain. There is evidence that patients who have high levels of psychological distress experience significantly higher levels of cancer pain than those who report low levels of psychological distress (6). In particular, studies have shown that depression, anxiety, anger, and overall high levels of mood disturbance are linked to the experience of more severe cancer pain (6).

Self-efficacy or the belief that one has a capability to achieve a desired outcome, for example, pain control, is a third important domain. Syrjala and Chapko (14) reported that pretreatment self-efficacy was a significant predictor of the development of pain during bone marrow transplantation therapy. Keefe et al. (15) found that caregivers of patients with cancer who reported high personal self-efficacy with regard to their ability to help their patient partner manage cancer pain at the end of life had much lower levels of caregiver strain and negative mood and increased positive mood, and their patient-partners reported that they were more energetic, spent less time in bed, and had overall higher levels of physical well-being.

Pain catastrophizing, the fourth domain, has been defined as "an individual's tendency to focus on and exaggerate the threat value of painful stimuli and negatively evaluate one's own ability to deal with pain" (16). Of the various forms of pain coping that have been studied, pain catastrophizing has proven to be one of the most consistent predictors of pain and disability (17). In a study of patients with gastrointestinal cancer, we found that patients who engaged in pain catastrophizing reported much higher levels of pain and pain behavior (18).

Social support is a fifth important domain that can influence the pain experience. A review of the literature on social support and cancer pain found that patients who reported high levels of social support experienced much lower levels of pain (6). Indices of social support such as resilience of the social network, level of social activities, and social functioning were all found to be related to decreased pain.

A final important domain that can influence cancer pain is the existential domain. Pain can be a constant reminder of the cancer; persistent or progressive pain a harbinger of advancing disease (19). Hence, progressive pain may imply worsening disease and incite a whirlwind of existential concerns such as "why me?" Conversely, finding meaning in the cancer experience may include reevaluation of the disease and its pain as positive, answering "why me?" by making sense of the disease on a more spiritual or existential level (20). Reappraisal and finding meaning is critical in the coping process. Psychological approaches to pain control can also support the process of finding meaning in and relief from existential suffering.

PSYCHOSOCIAL INTERVENTIONS FOR CANCER PAIN

Evidence that psychological factors can exacerbate pain associated with cancer has heightened interest in the role of psychosocial interventions in cancer pain management. We recently conducted a systematic review and meta-analysis of behavioral therapies for cancer pain management and found that these interventions generally led to improved pain control, with an overall effect size of 0.232 [confidence interval (CI) =0.072–0.392] suggesting that these interventions, as a group, are beneficial as adjuvants in the cancer pain treatment plan (21).

Psychosocial interventions that have been empirically tested can be grouped into four broad categories: cancer pain psychoeducation, CBT, hypnosis and imagery, and caregiver-assisted approaches. An advantage of all of these approaches is that they can be combined with other cancer pain therapies, taking an "adjuvant" role.

PSYCHOEDUCATION

Psychoeducational interventions in pain management were developed in response to the recognition that many patients lack basic knowledge about pain and its management and have misconceptions, particularly about pain medication, that constitute barriers to adequate pain relief. Psychoeducation is probably the most widely used psychosocial intervention in pain management and serves as a natural complement to medical interventions. Several components are commonly included in psychoeducational interventions, such as education about basic principles of pain, instructions for monitoring pain (e.g., keeping a pain diary), guidelines for when to contact health care providers, and recommendations for how to communicate with health care providers about pain. The interventions are typically delivered by nurses who are specially trained for this purpose and are supplemented with videotapes and/or written materials. Interventions can also be tailored to individual patients by including an assessment phase in which the individual learning needs of patients are identified through interviews or questionnaires (22,23).

The effectiveness of psychoeducational interventions has been demonstrated in a number of recent randomized clinical trials. In a series of papers, De Wit et al. (22,24–26) reported on the effectiveness of a tailored Pain Education Program (PEP), which included education about basic principles of pain and pain treatment (given in an oral format supplemented with an audiotape and brochure), instruction in how to report pain in a pain diary, and instruction in simple nonpharmacologic pain management techniques (i.e., cold, heat, relaxation, and massage), as well as encouragement to contact health care providers to talk about the pain experience. The intervention was delivered by a nurse in one 30–60-minute face-to-face session along with two brief (5–15 minute) phone calls during the week after discharge. Results showed that patients who received the PEP intervention had significant increases in pain knowledge and decreases in pain intensity compared to patients who were randomized to standard care. However, pain relief was primarily restricted to the group of patients with better functioning at baseline, indicating that this brief intervention may not be adequate for patients with more complex pain problems.

A randomized controlled trial conducted by Oliver et al. (27) tested the effects of a single-session education and coaching intervention in patients with cancer experiencing at least moderate levels of pain. The intervention was individualized and primarily addressed misconceptions about pain treatment and encouraged communication with health care providers about pain control. Patients receiving this intervention reported significant improvements in average pain severity as compared to controls who received standardized education on controlling cancer pain.

Two studies have tested psychoeducational interventions among hospitalized patients with cancer in Taiwan. The first study (28) randomly assigned patients to receive either a pain education intervention or standard care. Patients in the pain education intervention received a booklet addressing beliefs and concerns about reporting pain and using analgesics that are common among Taiwanese patients with cancer, including fatalism, fear of addiction, the desire to be a "good patient" by not complaining about pain, fear of distracting one's physician from treating the disease, concern that increasing pain signifies disease progression, and concerns about side effects of analgesics. A research assistant spent 30–40 minutes reviewing the content of the booklet with the patient and answering questions. Compared to patients in the control group, patients receiving the pain education intervention demonstrated significant improvements in self-reported barriers to pain management and medication adherence. However, group differences in pain intensity and pain interference were not significant.

The pain education intervention tested in the second study (29) consisted of a booklet that included information on how to prevent or manage side effects of pain medication, an introduction to psychosocial pain interventions, ways to assess and monitor pain intensity, ways to communicate pain problems to health care professionals, and information on common misconceptions about using analgesics. Results indicated that the pain education intervention was effective in reducing pain intensity, negative beliefs about opioids, pain endurance beliefs, and pain catastrophizing, and in increasing a sense of control over pain.

Miaskowski et al. (23) conducted a randomized clinical trial of a self-care intervention in patients with oncologic disorders who had pain from bone metastases. The intervention, PRO-SELF, involved three home visits and three telephone contacts by a nurse and included tailored educational content on pain management and nurse counseling on pain and side effect management, use of a weekly pillbox, and communication with health care providers about unrelieved pain and the need for a change in analgesic prescriptions. Results indicated that patients receiving the intervention had significant reductions in pain intensity and were more likely to have the most appropriate type of analgesic prescription as compared to controls.

A patient- and caregiver-focused cancer pain education strategy was studied in a large randomized controlled trial involving palliative care patients with advanced illness in Australia; >90% of patients had cancer. In this study, the intervention focused on overcoming patient and caregiver barriers to better pain management (e.g., concerns about addiction and side effects, fears that pain implies progressive cancer) in an effort to improve receptiveness to critical information about pain control in the palliative care setting (e.g., round-the-clock dosing, early treatment of constipation, and use of nonpharmacologic interventions). An educational outreach visiting format was used. Patients requiring a caregiver at baseline and randomized to the patient- and caregiver-focused intervention had significantly better performance status than those who did not receive the intervention. This improvement was across their entire time in the palliative care phase of their illness (mean 5 months), a very difficult time in the illness trajectory to modify function. Reports of pain were not significantly improved, and this is still being explored.

A recent study targeting underserved African American and Hispanic patients with cancer found less promising results (30). The intervention used in this study consisted of a culturally specific video and a booklet on pain management. Patients and their family members watched the video, which addressed misconceptions about pain treatment and the importance of reporting pain and insisting on pain relief, and then met with a research nurse who answered questions and emphasized the importance of reporting pain to the health care team. Contrary to expectations, the intervention did not affect pain intensity, pain interference, quality of life, or functional status. The authors speculate that a more intensive education program involving both physicians and patients may be needed for underserved minority patients.

Despite some negative results, the overall pattern of findings suggests that psychoeducational interventions are efficacious in helping patients with cancer manage pain. The interventions that have been tested tend to be brief; although this may be adequate for some patients, others—including medically underserved patients and those with low education and/or complex pain problems—may require more intensive and multifaceted approaches. Specific features of the interventions, including at what point in the illness trajectory they are delivered, where (inpatient vs. outpatient, home vs. clinic), and by whom, have yet to be evaluated.

COGNITIVE-BEHAVIORAL THERAPY

CBT approaches to pain management are based on cognitive and behavioral theories that emphasize the role of thoughts, emotions, and behaviors in influencing pain and pain-related disability. The hallmark of CBT is its insistence that learning to cope with pain is a skill that can be mastered through systematic practice and application. CBT protocols provide patients with training in a variety of coping skills and encourage them to be flexible and creative in the ways they mix and match these skills to deal with challenging pain-related situations. Among the skills commonly taught in CBT are relaxation training, time management/activity pacing, methods for altering overly negative pain-related thoughts, and goal setting. CBT is typically provided by a trained therapist in a series of individual or small group sessions. Multiple sessions are important in that they provide opportunities for learning and mastering the skills. The treatment sessions are interactive and use a combination of instruction, review of home practice, positive reinforcement, guided practice, behavioral rehearsal, and problem solving (Table 5.1).

It is only relatively recently that controlled studies have evaluated CBT for cancer pain. Syrjala et al. conducted one of the first randomized clinical trials (31), in which patients undergoing bone marrow transplantation were randomly assigned to CBT, hypnosis training, attention control, or usual care. The interventions focused on teaching patients to control oral mucositis pain, and were delivered both before and during hospitalization for the transplantation. Whereas patients receiving CBT showed no improvement in their pain, those receiving hypnosis reported a significant reduction in pain. In a subsequent study, Syrjala et al. (32) compared the efficacy of a comprehensive CBT protocol incorporating relaxation training, imagery, distraction, calming self-statements, and goal setting to a CBT protocol that involved only training in relaxation and imagery. Compared to patients assigned to standard care or a therapist support control condition, both CBT protocols produced significant reductions in pain. A limitation of this study was that the sample size was not large enough to detect potential differences between the two CBT protocols.

Dalton et al. (33) tested the effects of CBT in a study of patients with advanced cancer. This study systematically compared a CBT protocol that tailored skills training to patients' pain-coping deficits with a more conventional CBT protocol that provided training in a standard set of pain-coping skills. Results indicated that both CBT protocols were superior to standard care. The tailored CBT protocol was superior to conventional CBT at short-term follow-up (1 month), whereas conventional CBT was superior to tailored CBT at longer-term follow-up (6 months).

In a recent systematic review and meta-analysis of behavioral therapies for cancer pain (21) 7 of the 21 included randomized controlled trials specifically evaluated CBT. Most of the studies examined (five out of the seven) tested CBT protocols that were specifically designed to improve pain control. The CBT interventions were not clearly effective cancer pain adjuvants when compared to the other behavioral therapy subgroups. In general, the studies of CBT interventions were of higher methodological quality than the studies of other behavioral therapies included in the systematic review. CBT was delivered by a PhD-level psychologist in <50% of these cancer pain studies, in contrast to CBT protocols used in the treatment of other persistent pain populations. Interestingly, the participants in these studies had baseline pain levels that were much more variable than those of participants in other studies of behavioral therapy for cancer pain. This variability likely reduced the overall effect size of CBT. It also suggests that, at present, CBT protocols are being used to manage patients with cancer who vary substantially in terms of the pain and pain-related disability. Future studies should test the efficacy of CBT pain management protocols with targeted and more homogeneous populations of patients with cancer (e.g., patients with advanced cancer who have moderate to severe pain).

HYPNOSIS AND IMAGERY

Hypnosis was one of the first psychosocial interventions used in managing cancer pain, with reports of painless breast cancer surgery done under hypnosis dating back to 1829 (34).

TABLE 5.1

COGNITIVE-BEHAVIORAL PAIN MANAGEMENT PROTOCOL

Session	Topics	Pain management goals
1	Rationale for cognitive-behavioral therapy—gate control theory	
2	Progressive relaxation training	
3	Guided imagery	*Diverting attention away from pain*
4	Using focal points	
5	Activity pacing	
6	Pleasant activity scheduling	*Altering activity patterns*
7	Identifying negative thoughts	
8	Challenging negative thoughts to reduce psychological distress	*Reducing negative pain-related emotions*
9	Goal setting	
10	Skills maintenance	*Applying skills in everyday situations and maintaining frequency of skill use*

Source: Adapted from Keefe FJ, Abernethy AP, Campbell LC. Psychological approaches to understanding and treating disease-related pain. *Annu Rev Psychol* 2005;56:601–630.

Over the years, the mechanisms underpinning the effects of hypnosis on pain have evolved and have been the subject of much debate. Opinions about these mechanisms fall into two camps. The traditional camp has argued that through hypnotic induction the hypnotist places an individual in a special state, a hypnotic trance, characterized by focused concentration, suspended peripheral awareness, and increased responsiveness to suggestions of pain relief. The more modern camp, first championed by Barber, has argued that the effects of hypnosis on pain relief are due to high levels of motivation and readiness to accept suggestions from a therapist and the resulting reduction in fear and anxiety that occurs. Research by Barber and others has had a significant influence on the field of clinical hypnosis greatly and has led to a greater emphasis on self-guided hypnosis and the use of hypnosis-like imagery and distraction in awake subjects.

Hypnosis and imagery have a demonstrated role in the management of acute procedural pain in patients with cancer, especially in children. The most compelling study is a randomized trial conducted by Liossi and Hatira (35) on 80 children undergoing lumbar punctures for hematologic malignancies. Children who were either hypnotized ($n = 20$) or provided guided imagery ($n = 20$) before the procedures experienced significantly less pain, anxiety, and behavioral distress than those who were randomized to distraction with play and nonmedical discussions ($n = 20$), or to control ($n = 20$).

Several years earlier, the same group of researchers demonstrated that children undergoing bone marrow biopsy had less pain when hypnotized or exposed to cognitive-behavioral coping skills than when undergoing usual treatment procedure ($n = 30$; 1:1:1 randomization) (36). There was also a trend for hypnosis to be superior to CBT in this study ($p = .20$).

The experiences of adults with acute cancer-related pain are similar to those of children. Women who were given training in hypnosis before breast biopsy reported significantly less postsurgical pain and distress than those randomized to standard care (37). As noted earlier, Syrjala et al. (31) found that the acute mucositis pain associated with bone marrow transplantation could be mitigated with hypnosis; CBT without hypnosis was not as effective. The hypnosis protocol used in this study trained patients in relaxation and patient-directed imagery before the transplantation. Interestingly, the authors later changed the name of their intervention to imagery with relaxation because of patients' negative reaction to the word *hypnosis*.

The role of hypnosis and imagery in chronic malignant pain has also been investigated. In 1983, Spiegel and Bloom randomized 58 women with metastatic breast cancer to weekly group therapy with or without hypnosis (38). The hypnosis component lasted 5–10 minutes per session and focused on teaching patients not to fight the pain and to filter the hurt out by imagining competing sensations in the affected area. In contrast to patients receiving group therapy alone, patients receiving hypnosis plus group therapy reported significant reductions in pain sensation ($p < .02$) and pain suffering ($p < .03$).

In our systematic review and meta-analysis of behavioral therapies for cancer pain (21) we found that the subgroup of studies testing hypnosis and imagery interventions had a larger effect size than the other behavioral interventions studied, with an effect size of 0.419 (CI = 0.059–0.779; $p = .023$). Although this suggests that hypnosis and imagery are more effective than other behavioral therapies for pain control, the large CI indicates that the effects of hypnosis and imagery interventions vary substantially. Although this might be due to differences in setting, it has long been known that there are important individual differences in response to hypnosis and imagery. Some individuals are much more susceptible to pain relief through these interventions than others. To enhance treatment effects, many practitioners screen for hypnotic susceptibility before instituting training in hypnosis or guided imagery.

CAREGIVER-ASSISTED TREATMENTS

Cancer has a profound impact not only on the patient but also on his or her caregivers as well. Caregivers of patients with cancer experience significant levels of psychological distress (39–43) and report particularly high levels of distress when caring for a patient with cancer-related pain (44). Caregivers are often faced with a myriad of tasks and responsibilities including monitoring the patient's symptoms, seeking information relevant to the patient's disease and symptom management, and communicating with health care professionals.

Despite the potential benefits of involving a caregiver in pain management, there have been very few published studies of psychosocial caregiver-assisted pain management interventions in patients with cancer. One study examined the impact of a PEP on family members providing home care to elderly patients with cancer in a quasi-experimental design (45). The program provided patients and their family members with information on pain assessment, pharmacologic interventions, and nonpharmacologic interventions. At the end of the program, family members reported improved psychological functioning and social well-being, and patients reported improvements in pain intensity.

We recently completed a study that tested the effects of a caregiver-guided pain management intervention in patients with cancer pain at end of life (46). In this study, 78 patients with cancer pain who met the criteria for hospice eligibility were randomly assigned to receive either a brief (three session) caregiver-assisted cognitive-behavioral pain management intervention or usual care. The caregiver-assisted intervention integrated educational information about cancer pain with training in three pain-coping skills (relaxation, imagery, and activity pacing) and was delivered by a nurse in the patient's home. Results indicated that patients in the caregiver-assisted intervention tended to report improvements in levels of pain, although this finding was not statistically significant. In addition, caregivers involved in the intervention showed significant improvements in their sense of self-efficacy in helping the patient control pain and other cancer symptoms, and they tended ($p < .06$) to report improvements in their level of caregiver strain. The challenges associated with conducting this type of study in patients and caregivers at the end of life were formidable. Patients and caregivers were often understandably reluctant about committing to a clinical research study at such a stressful time. In addition, at this juncture some patients were experiencing severe pain and had little time or energy to learn and apply coping skills.

Our research team is currently conducting a caregiver-based study focused on symptom management in patients with early stage lung cancer. Unlike patients at the end of life, patients with early stage disease have the opportunity to engage in comprehensive coping skills training and to use these skills over the trajectory of their disease. In this study, patients and their caregivers are randomly assigned to receive either 14 sessions of caregiver-assisted coping skills training or 14 sessions of cancer education. The coping skills intervention trains patients and caregivers in relaxation, pleasant imagery, activity pacing, cognitive restructuring, problem solving, and communication skills. The caregivers, who are primarily spouses, learn the coping skills along with the patients and are taught to coach the patients in the use of these strategies (Table 5.2).

TABLE 5.2

PSYCHOSOCIAL INTERVENTIONS IN CANCER PAIN

Type	Rationale	Components	Effects on pain intensity[a]
Psychoeducation	Many patients lack basic knowledge about pain and its management and/or have misconceptions that constitute barriers to adequate pain relief	Education about basic principles of pain Instructions in monitoring pain and when to contact health care providers Recommendations for how to communicate with health care providers about pain	De Wit et al., 2001a, 2001b, 2001c (+) Oliver et al., 2001 (+) Chang et al., 2001 (−) Lai et al., 2004 (−) Miaskowski et al., 2004 (+) Abernethy et al., 2005 (−) Anderson et al., 2004 (−)
Cognitive-behavioral	This is based on theories that emphasize the role of thoughts, emotions, and behaviors in influencing pain and pain-related disability Learning to cope with pain is a skill that can be mastered through systematic practice and application	Relaxation training Time management/activity pacing Methods for altering overly negative pain-related thoughts Goal setting	Syrjala et al., 1992 (−) Syrjala et al., 1995 (+) Dalton et al., 2004 (+) Liossi and Hatira, 1999 (+)
Hypnosis and imagery	A hypnotic trance is characterized by focused concentration, suspended peripheral awareness, and increased responsivity to suggestions of pain relief High levels of motivation and readiness to accept suggestions lead to pain relief	Hypnotic induction or self-guided hypnosis Imagery	Liossi and Hatira, 2003 (+) Liossi and Hatira, 1999 (+) Montgomery et al., 2002 (+) Syrjala et al., 1992 (+) Spiegel and Bloom, 1993 (+)
Caregiver-assisted	Caregivers report high levels of psychological distress Caregivers are often responsible for helping patients in managing pain	Family members are provided with information and training in pharmacologic and nonpharmacologic interventions	Ferrell et al., 1995 (+) Keefe et al., 2005 (+)

[a]Outcomes are designated positive (+) if the intervention resulted in a decrease in pain intensity, negative (−) if it did not.
This is a selected list of studies. For a comprehensive list see Abernethy AP, Keefe FJ, McCrory DC, et al. *Technology assessment on the use of behavioral therapies for treatment of medical disorders: part 2—impact on management of patients with cancer pain.* Report to the US Agency for Healthcare Research and Quality. Durham, North Carolina: Duke Center for Clinical Health Policy Research, May 5, 2005.

SPECIAL ISSUES AND FUTURE DIRECTIONS

Despite a growing evidence base for psychosocial interventions in managing cancer pain, access to these interventions remains limited. One barrier to access is that health care professionals lack familiarity with these interventions and may view them as being incompatible with pharmacologic approaches to pain management (47). Educational efforts are needed to enhance health care professionals' understanding of psychosocial interventions and how these interventions can serve as adjuvants to pharmacotherapy. Another barrier to access to these interventions is that patients with cancer who need treatment may be too sick or immobile to travel to receive treatment. In the last few years, novel approaches to delivering psychosocial interventions have been investigated (e.g., telephone and Internet). Preliminary research supports the feasibility and efficacy of telephone-based interventions (48). Internet-based approaches to cancer pain management typically take the form of pain education information available on cancer-related Web sites (11). E-mail discussion groups, enhanced with written and video materials about pain, have been shown to reduce pain, disability, and health distress in patients with low back pain (49); however, E-based interventions in pain management have yet to be rigorously evaluated in patients with cancer.

Undertreatment of cancer pain is estimated to occur in 50% of all patients with cancer (50); however, ethnic minority patients with cancer are at even greater risk for undertreatment of their cancer pain (51,52). Culturally sensitive psychosocial interventions may be useful as adjunctive therapies for management of cancer pain and have two primary characteristics. First, they are congruent with the cultural framework and value system of the target group (53). Second, they specifically address interpersonal and intraindividual barriers to adequate pain management among ethnic minority patients with cancer, such as ineffective patient–provider communication during pain assessment and reluctance to take powerful analgesics (e.g., opioids) out of fear of addiction (52). Culturally sensitive pain management interventions are just beginning to be developed and evaluated in ethnic minority patients with cancer. Studies have examined cancer psychoeducation for African American and Hispanic patients with cancer (30) and psychosocial group therapy for Japanese women with breast cancer (54). In our own laboratory, we have examined the efficacy of a partner-assisted coping skills training protocol for pain and other symptom management in African American prostate cancer survivors and their intimate partners. Preliminary findings provide support for the efficacy of the coping skills training intervention for improving symptom-related quality of life in African American prostate cancer survivors (55).

An important issue in the delivery of psychosocial interventions is the optimal dose and intensity of treatment. At present, there is significant variability in the dose/intensity of psychosocial interventions in cancer pain. The dose/intensity ranges from a single, brief episode of pain education (30) to comprehensive pain-coping skills training delivered over weeks and months. Unfortunately, there is no consistent evidence on the best dose/intensity. However, there is growing consensus that one dose does not fit all; rather, interventions need to be tailored to meet the needs of specific populations. In the

TABLE 5.3

STUDIES TESTING EMOTIONAL DISCLOSURE INTERVENTIONS IN PATIENTS WITH CANCER

Study	Population	Treatment conditions	Outcomes
De Moor et al., 2002	Metastatic renal cell carcinoma ($n = 42$)	Expressive writing vs. writing about neutral topic (health behaviors)	Expressive writing led to improvements in vigor and sleep No effect on symptoms of distress, perceived stress, or mood
Stanton et al., 2002	Breast cancer ($n = 60$)	Expressive writing (general) vs. expressive writing (positive feelings only) vs. neutral writing (cancer facts)	Expressive writing (general and positive) led to reduction in medical appointments for cancer-related morbidities Expressive writing (general) led to reduction in physical symptoms Expressive writing (general) led to decreases in psychological distress for women scoring low in cancer-related avoidance, whereas expressive writing (positive) led to decreases in psychological distress for women scoring high in avoidance
Rosenberg et al., 2002	Prostate cancer ($n = 30$)	Expressive writing vs. control	Expressive writing led to improvements in physical symptoms and health care utilization No effects on psychological distress or immunocompetence

area of cancer pain, patient functioning is a primary factor influencing intervention dose and intensity, such that patients experiencing significant fatigue, nausea, and other symptoms require briefer, well-integrated interventions that are efficient in terms of time and cost.

An important future direction is developing and refining novel psychosocial interventions. A psychosocial intervention that could be helpful in managing cancer pain but that has not received systematic attention is emotional disclosure. Emotional disclosure interventions typically consist of having participants write or talk for 15–20 minutes daily for 3–5 days about their deepest thoughts and feelings about stressful experiences. Over the last decade, more than two dozen studies testing variants of this protocol have yielded positive results (56). A recent meta-analysis of the literature on emotional disclosure interventions found that healthy participants who wrote about traumatic topics showed significant improvements in psychological well-being (e.g., affect, adjustment), physical health (e.g., health center visits, self-reported symptoms), physiologic functioning (e.g., immune function), and general functioning (e.g., grade point average, absenteeism) compared to those in a control condition who wrote about neutral topics (57).

Although the effects of an emotional disclosure intervention on cancer pain outcomes have not been tested, several recent studies have examined the effects of this intervention on quality of life outcomes. In one recent preliminary study, de Moor et al. (58) investigated the effect of expressive writing in patients with metastatic renal cell carcinoma. Compared to patients who wrote about a neutral topic (health behaviors), those who wrote about emotional aspects of having cancer experienced significant improvements in a number of outcomes including significant improvements in vigor and sleep, although the small sample size ($n = 21$ in the expressive writing condition) likely precluded the ability of this study to detect many significant effects. In a second recent study, Stanton et al. (59) tested the effects of an emotional disclosure protocol that asked patients with breast cancer to write about their deepest thoughts and feelings about their cancer experience. Results indicated that emotional disclosure led to significant reductions

in physical symptoms and medical appointments for cancer-related morbidities. Emotional disclosure also led to significant reductions in psychological distress, although this effect was apparent only in patients scoring low on cancer avoidance. Finally, in a sample of patients with prostate cancer, emotional disclosure led to improvements in physical symptoms and health care utilization (60). Taken together, these recent studies suggest that in patients with cancer emotional disclosure may have beneficial effects on psychological and physiologic outcomes. Future studies need to examine the effects of emotional disclosure on cancer pain. Along these lines, we are currently conducting a randomized clinical trial testing the efficacy of a new caregiver-assisted emotional disclosure intervention for reducing pain in patients with advanced GI cancer (Table 5.3).

CONCLUSIONS

Nonpharmacologic interventions are of growing interest to persons suffering from cancer pain. Recent theory and research suggests that psychosocial factors can play an important role in the cancer pain experience. Randomized clinical trials suggest that interventions designed to address psychosocial factors can benefit many patients with cancer. Much remains to be learned about psychosocial interventions, including how to reduce barriers to accessing these treatments, optimal dose/timing, and the effectiveness of novel interventions such as emotional disclosure. Nevertheless, the fact that an evidence base has been established for psychosocial interventions for cancer pain management is important and should enhance clinicians' confidence in recommending these nonpharmacologic interventions to their patients.

ACKNOWLEDGMENTS

Preparation of this manuscript was supported by several National Institutes of Health (NIH) Grants (CA91947, CA100734, CA14236, R21 CA8521) and, in part, by funds provided by the Fetzer Institute. Preparation of this chapter was also supported by a Clinical Scientist Career Development Award from the Doris Duke Charitable Foundation.

References

1. Seale C, Cartwright H. *The year before death*. Oxford, UK: Oxford University Press, 1994.
2. Addington-Hall J, McCarthy M. Dying from cancer: results of a national population-based investigation. *Palliat Med* 1995;9:295–305.
3. American Pain Society Cancer Pain Management Guideline Panel. *American pain society guidelines for the management of cancer pain in adults and children*. Glenview, IL: APS, 2004.
4. Melzack R. From the gate to the neuromatrix. *Pain* 1999;6(suppl):121–126.
5. Melzack R, Wall PD. Pain mechanisms: a new theory. *Science* 1965;150: 971–979.
6. Zaza C, Baine N. Cancer pain and psychosocial factors: a critical review of the literature. *J Pain Symptom Manage* 2002;24(5):526–542.
7. Keefe FJ, Abernethy AP, Campbell LC. Psychological approaches to understanding and treating disease-related pain. *Annu Rev Psychol* 2005;56:601–630.
8. Ward SE, Goldberg N, Miller-McCauley V, et al. Patient-related barriers to management of cancer pain. *Pain* 1993;52(3):319–324.
9. Berry PE, Ward SE. Barriers to pain management in hospice: a study of family caregivers. *Hosp J* 1995;10(4):19–33.
10. Ferrell BR. Patient and family caregiver perspectives. *Oncology* 1999;13(5 Suppl 2):15–19.
11. American Cancer Society. *Cancer facts and figures*. 2003. http://www.cancer.org/docroot/STT/stt_0_2003.asp?sitearea=STT&level=1.
12. Mokdad AH, Marks JS, Stroup DF, et al. Actual causes of death in the United States 2000. *JAMA* 2004;291(10):1238–1245.
13. Vuorinen E. Pain as an early symptom in cancer. *Clin J Pain* 1993;9(4): 272–278.
14. Syrjala KL, Chapko ME. Evidence for a biopsychosocial model of cancer treatment–related pain. *Pain* 1995;61(1):69–79.
15. Keefe FJ, Ahles T, Porter L, et al. The self-efficacy of family caregivers for helping cancer patients manage pain at end-of-life. *Pain* 2003;103(1–2): 157–162.
16. Keefe FJ, Lefebvre JC, Egert J, et al. The relationship of gender to pain, pain behavior, and disability in osteoarthritis patients: The role of catastrophizing. *Pain* 2000;87:325–334.
17. Sullivan MJ, Thorn B, Haythornthwaite J, et al. Theoretical perspectives on the relation between catastrophizing and pain. *J Clin Pain* 2001;17:52–64.
18. Keefe FJ, Lipkus I, Lefebvre JC, et al. The social context of gastrointestinal cancer pain: A preliminary study examining the relation of patient pain catastrophizing to patient perceptions of social support and caregiver stress and negative responses. *Pain* 2003;103:151–156.
19. Turk DC. Remember the distinction between malignant and benign pain? Well, forget it. *Clin J Pain* 2002;18(2):75–76.
20. Breitbart W. Spirituality and meaning in supportive care: spirituality-and meaning-centered group psychotherapy interventions in advanced cancer. *Support Care Cancer* 2002;10(4):272–280.
21. Abernethy AP, Keefe FJ, McCrory DC, et al. *Technology assessment on the use of behavioral therapies for treatment of medical disorders: part 2—impact on management of patients with cancer pain. Report to the US Agency for Healthcare Research and Quality*. Durham, North Carolina: Duke Center for Clinical Health Policy Research, May 5, 2005.
22. De Wit R, Van Dam F, Zandbelt L, et al. A pain education program for chronic cancer pain patients: follow-up results from a randomized controlled trial. *Pain* 1997;73(1):55–69.
23. Miaskowski C, Dodd M, West C, et al. Randomized clinical trial of the effectiveness of a self-care intervention to improve cancer pain management. *J Clin Oncol* 2004;22:1713–1720.
24. De Wit R, Van Dam F. From hospital to home care: a randomized controlled trial of a pain education programme for cancer patients with chronic pain. *J Adv Nurs* 2001a;36:742–754.
25. De Wit R, Van Dam F, Loonstra S, et al. Improving the quality of pain treatment by a tailored pain education program for cancer patients in chronic pain. *Eur J Pain* 2001b;5:241–256.
26. De Wit R, van Dam F, Loonstra S, et al. The Amsterdam Pain Management Index Compared to eight frequently used outcome measures to evaluate the adequacy of pain treatment in cancer patients with chronic pain. *Pain* 2001c;91:339–349.
27. Oliver JW, Kravitz RL, Kaplan SH, et al. Individualized patient education and coaching to improve pain control among cancer outpatients. *J Clin Oncol* 2001;19(8):2206–2212.
28. Chang MC, Chang YC, Chiou JF, et al. Overcoming patient-related barriers to cancer pain management for home care patients. A pilot study. *Cancer Nurs* 2002;25(6):470–476.
29. Lai YH, Guo SL, Keefe FJ, et al. Effects of brief pain education on hospitalized cancer patients with moderate to severe pain. *Support Care Cancer* 2004;12:645–652.
30. Anderson KO, Mendoza TR, Payne R, et al. Pain education for underserved minority cancer patients: a randomized controlled trial. *J Clin Oncol* 2004;22:4918–4925.
31. Syrjala KL, Cummings C, Donaldson GW. Hypnosis or cognitive behavioral training for the reduction of pain and nausea during cancer treatment: a controlled clinical trial. *Pain* 1992;48:137–146.
32. Syrjala KL, Donaldson GW, Davis MW, et al. Relaxation and imagery and cognitive-behavioral training reduce pain during cancer treatment: a controlled clinical trial. *Pain* 1995;63:189–198.
33. Dalton J, Keefe FJ, Carlson J, et al. Tailoring cognitive-behavioral treatment for cancer pain. *Pain Manag Nurs* 2004;5:3–18.
34. Barber TX, Spanos NP, Chaves JF. *Hypnosis, imagination, and human potentialities*. New York: Pergamon, 1974.
35. Liossi C, Hatira P. Clinical hypnosis in the alleviation of procedure-related pain in pediatric oncology patients. *Int J Clin Exp Hypn* 2003;51(1): 4–28.
36. Liossi C, Hatira P. Clinical hypnosis versus cognitive behavioral training for pain management with pediatric cancer patients undergoing bone marrow aspirations. *Int J Clin Exp Hypn* 1999;47(2):104–116.
37. Montgomery GH, Weltz CR, Seltz M, et al. Brief presurgery hypnosis reduces distress and pain in excisional breast biopsy patients. *Int J Clin Exp Hypn* 2002;50(1):17–32.
38. Spiegel D, Bloom JR. Group therapy and hypnosis reduce metastatic breast carcinoma pain. *Psychosom Med* 1983;45(4):333–339.
39. Baider L, Kaplan De-Nour A. Adjustment to cancer: Who is the patient—the husband or the wife? *Isr J Med Sci* 1988;24:631–636.
40. Baider L, Perez T, De-Nour AK. Gender and adjustment to chronic disease. A study of couples with colon cancer. *Gen Hosp Psychiatry* 1989;11:1–8.
41. Gotay CC. The experience of cancer during early and advanced stages: the views of patients and their mates. *Soc Sci Med* 1984;18(7):5–13.
42. Haddad P, Pitceathly C, Maguire P. Psychological morbidity in the partners of cancer patients. In: Baider L, Cooper CL, Kaplan De-Nour A, eds. *Cancer and the family*. New York: Wiley, 1996:257–271.
43. Northouse LL, Mood D, Templin T, et al. Couples' patterns of adjustment to colon cancer. *Soc Sci Med* 2000;50:271–284.
44. Miaskowski C, Kragness L, Dibble S, et al. Differences in mood states, health status, and caregiver strain between family caregivers of oncology outpatients with and without cancer-related pain. *J Pain Symptom Manage* 1997;13(3):138–147.
45. Ferrell BR, Grant M, Chan J, et al. The impact of cancer pain education on family caregivers of elderly patients. *Oncol Nurs Forum* 1995;22(8):1211–1218.
46. Keefe FJ, Ahles TA, Sutton L, et al. Partner-guided cancer pain management at end-of-life: a preliminary study. *J Pain Symptom Manage* 2005;29(3):263–272.
47. Zaza C, Sellick SM, William A, et al. Health care professionals' familiarity with nonpharmacological strategies for managing cancer pain. *Psychooncology* 1999;8(2):99–111.
48. Rounds KA, Galinsky MJ, Stevens LS. Linking people with AIDS in rural communities: the telephone group. *Soc Work* 1991;36:13–18.
49. Lorig KR, Lauent DD, Dyo RA, et al. Can a back pain e-mail discussion group improve health status and lower health care cost? *Arch Intern Med* 2002;162:792–796.
50. Cleeland CS, Gonin R, Hatfield AK, et al. Pain and its treatment in outpatients with metastatic cancer. *N Engl J Med* 1994;330(9):592–596.
51. Cleeland CS, Gonin R, Baez L, et al. Pain and treatment of pain in minority patients with cancer: the eastern cooperative oncology group minority outpatient study. *Ann Intern Med* 1997;127:813–816.
52. Anderson KO, Mendoza TR, Valero V, et al. Minority cancer patients and their providers: pain management attitudes and practice. *Cancer* 2000;88:1929–1938.
53. Ard JD, Carter-Edwards L, Svetkey LP. A new model for developing and executing culturally appropriate behavior modification clinical trials for African Americans. *Ethn Dis* 2003;13(2):279–285.
54. Fukui S, Kugaya A, Okamura H, et al. A psychosocial group intervention for Japanese women with primary breast carcinoma. *Cancer* 2000;89:1026–1036.
55. Campbell LC, Keefe FJ, Scipio C, et al. Facilitating research participation and improving quality of life for African American prostate cancer survivors and their intimate partners. A pilot study of telephone-based coping skills training. *Cancer* (in press). 2004;28(5):433–444.
56. Pennebaker JW, Seagal JD. Forming a story: the health benefits of narrative. *J Clin Psycho* 1999;55(10):1243–1254.
57. Smyth JM. Written emotional expression: effect sizes, outcome types, and moderating variables. *J Consult Clin Psychol* 1998;66(1):174–184.
58. de Moor C, Sterner J, Hall M, et al. A pilot study of the effects of expressive writing on psychological and behavioral adjustment in patients enrolled in a phase II trial of vaccine therapy for metastatic renal cell carcinoma. *Health Psychol* 2002;21:615–619.
59. Stanton AL, Danoff-Burg S, Sworowski LA, et al. Randomized, controlled trial of written emotional expression and benefit finding in breast cancer patients. *J Clin Oncol* 2002;20:4160–4168.
60. Rosenberg HJ, Rosenberg SD, Ernstoff MS, et al. Expressive disclosure and health outcomes in a prostate cancer population. *Int J Psychiatry Med* 2002;32(1):37–53.

CHAPTER 6 ■ PHYSIATRIC APPROACHES TO PAIN MANAGEMENT

ANDREA CHEVILLE AND LAUREN SHAIOVA

Rehabilitation has too often remained marginalized in the care of patients with cancer. The perception that rehabilitation only offers meaningful benefit to patients capable of full community and vocational integration with unrestricted life spans is inaccurate and shortsighted. Although physiatry, or physical medicine and rehabilitation, initially emerged as a field dedicated to transforming individuals stricken with anatomically disruptive injuries back to their productive lives, the scope of the field has broadened considerably as medicine has altered the prognoses of many formerly fatal diseases. Integration of rehabilitation services in the care of patients with far-advanced pulmonary and cardiac disease has become standard. Similar services are rarely offered to patients with cancer, even in the early stages of disease.

Physiatric strategies geared toward enhancing pain control can be loosely grouped into three categories:

1. Nonpharmacologic nociceptive modulation
2. Adaptive functional training to allow pain-free mobility and self-care
3. Restoration or preservation of normal biomechanics

These categories are theoretically separate but highly interrelated in practical application. Similar interventions are used to realize the goals of each strategy. It is helpful, however, to consider them individually in developing an integrated plan to control pain, enhance function, and preserve autonomy. The purpose of rehabilitation as outlined in this chapter is to improve the quality of life and survival irrespective of anticipated survival.

FORMULATION OF AN INTEGRATED PAIN MANAGEMENT PROGRAM

Rehabilitative strategies fail in the absence of effective pain control. Adequate pharmacologic analgesia lays a foundation on which physiatry can begin the work of advancing patients from a state of static pain control to that of dynamic pain control. Pain management services allow rehabilitation professionals to effect functional gains and realize therapeutic goals. In turn, information gleaned during attempts to mobilize patients permits refinement of analgesia. Successful pain control is never achieved until the patient moves. For example, formerly mild rest pain related to osseous metastases may become intensely problematic during attempts to transfer and ambulate.

Rehabilitation is an essential component of integrated pain management geared toward symptom control and autonomous function. Ideally, physiatric approaches are seamlessly combined with disease-modifying, pharmacologic, and interventional analgesic strategies. This chapter addresses the three general categories of physiatric interventions (nociceptive modulation, achievement of pain-free function, and restoration of normal biomechanics). Approaches common to each are described, with special attention to the efficacy and limitations in cancer.

NONPHARMACOLOGIC NOCICEPTIVE MODULATION

The capacity of thermal, manual, and electrical modalities to alleviate pain has long been recognized by clinicians. The classical Hippocratic texts outline the use of heat and massage to enhance comfort and reduce the virulence of disease (1). Investigative efforts have revealed the tremendous complexity of the neuroanatomic apparatus subserving nociception. Physiologists are now able to partially explain long-standing clinical observations. This understanding has led to increasing support for the use of manual, thermal, and electrical modalities in conjunction with conventional analgesic therapies.

Massage

Massage is one of the oldest and most widely accepted forms of treatment. Today >75 types of massage are practiced. Some forms are ancient, dating back over thousands of years (2). There has been a considerable increase in the popularity of massage over the last decades. Its use in the treatment of illness ranging from minor myalgias to systemic diseases has become accepted. The physiologic effects of massage have been credited with promoting healing, restoring function, and enhancing physical performance. Specifically, massage is described as assisting with circulation and lymphatic drainage, enhancing the elastic and inelastic properties of connective tissue and muscle, fostering relaxation, counteracting edema, and alleviating muscle pain (3–7). There are many different schools of massage therapy offering a wide variety of approaches for different clinical indications. Those that are most common or relevant to cancer are discussed in subsequent text.

Malignancy was cited as a relative contraindication to massage in the past. The concern stems from the possibility that massage may accelerate dissemination of malignant cells by enhancing the flow of lymph and blood. Several facts illustrate the limitations in this line of reasoning. First, aerobic exercise is a more potent stimulant of blood and lymph flow than massage (8). No association between aerobic exercise and the acceleration of malignant spread has even been suggested. Second, manual lymph drainage, a massage technique specifically designed to enhance the transport capacity of the lymphatic system, is used extensively in the treatment of lymphedema (9). Despite documented acceleration of lymph transport, manual lymph drainage has never been reported to potentiate recurrence or dissemination of cancer cells.

Traditional Swedish Massage

Four basic strokes are used in Swedish massage. These include effleurage, petrissage, friction, and tapotement. Effleurage is a gentle stoking motion that can be applied with varying degrees of force. Superficial stroking has beneficial effects on muscle hypertonicity. It also stimulates the flow of lymph and venous blood. Petrissage is a more vigorous motion that involves kneading muscles and other soft tissue, at times with considerable force. Petrissage is utilized to break up tissue and muscle adhesions. Friction massage involves repetitive circular motions applied with pressure to a small area of tissue. Friction is useful in interrupting muscle hypertonicity. Tapotement involves repetitive alternating movements of the hands. The goal of treatment will determine the rapidity and force of tapotement. Used in concert, the four basic Swedish massage strokes provide tremendous versatility. Each stroke can attenuate most of the pain through counterstimulatory and autonomic effects. Patients with cancer frequently develop muscle pain generators through the adoption of aberrant movement patterns and secondary muscle overuse. Swedish massage can eliminate muscle pain arising from focal hypertonicity, although lasting relief will not be achieved until the causative movement patterns are addressed. Many specialized massage techniques, including those discussed in subsequent text, are refinements of the basic Swedish strokes.

Myofascial Release

Myofascial release techniques are used to restore normal length–tension relationships to muscles and fascia. The capacity of hypertonic muscles to function as pain generators is well established. The potential contribution of contracted fascia to musculoskeletal pain is less appreciated.

Fascia occurs ubiquitously throughout the body's supporting muscles, joints, and viscera. It is densely innervated with nociceptors and can therefore serve as an independent pain generator. Ideally, fascia moves freely in synchrony with the motion of muscles and joints. Many conditions associated with cancer can produce fascial contractures. Examples include radiation fibrosis, immobility, postsurgical scarring, and pain-engendered muscle spasms. Contracted fascia may become painful at rest or with the minimal tension required by routine daily activities. Fascial release techniques are used to release the contracted fascia. Practitioners use vigorous "hands-on" compression and stretching to alter the mobility of affected tissues. Multiple sessions with a skilled practitioner are generally required. Often fascial contractures must be addressed before patients can tolerate therapeutic exercise or aerobic conditioning. Trigger point release involves the strategic application of pressure to discrete foci of increased muscle tone, called *trigger points*. Sustained pressure is applied to a circumscribed, symptomatic area in conjunction with passive range of motion.

Manual Lymphatic Drainage

Manual lymphatic drainage (MLD) or "lymphatic massage" is a highly specialized technique designed to enhance the sequestration and transport of lymph. Specific stroke duration, orientation, pressure, and sequence characterize MLD. This technique stimulates the intrinsic contractility of the lymph vessels, leading to increased interstitial protein sequestration and transport. Through gentle and rhythmic skin distension, congested lymph is directed through the lymphatic system into intact nodal basins. MLD permits shifting of congested lymph to lymphotomes (anatomic regions drained by a specific lymph node bed) with preserved drainage. The massage is very light and superficial, limited to finger/hand pressures of around 30–45 mm Hg. MLD treatments are initiated proximally in lymphostatic regions adjacent to functioning lymphotomes. Lymph is constantly directed toward functional lymph node basins with strategic hand movements. The treatment gradually progresses distally to terminate in the regions farthest removed from intact lymphatics. Cancer treatment is the most frequent cause of lymphedema in developed countries. Progression of disease generally worsens the lymphedema. It may also trigger the onset of lymphedema through nodal infiltration, immobility, and malignant compression of lymph vessels. MLD is safe and can produce surprising levels of analgesia. The latter finding is presumably due to counterstimulatory effects.

Thermal Modalities

This part of the chapter focuses on thermal modalities in the treatment of cancer-related pain. Thermal modalities have been used by physiatrists for many medical conditions associated with disabilities. Thermal modalities commonly employed in rehabilitation medicine include topical heat and cold, hydrotherapy, heat lamps, ultrasound, diathermy, fluidotherapy, and paraffin baths. Each of these is discussed in the following section on modalities used to treat pain in patients with cancer.

Therapeutic Heat

The following discussion is limited to local applications of heat and cold as they pertain to cancer pain management and symptom control. There are three primary modes of heat transfer:

1. Conduction, which includes hot packs and paraffin baths
2. Convection, which includes fluidotherapy, hydrotherapy, and moist air
3. Conversion, which includes radiant heat, laser, microwaves, short waves, and ultrasound

Superficial heating modalities are discussed initially and deep heating modalities subsequently in this section. The integrity of sensation in the area must be tested. Sensory deficits are not an absolute contraindication to the use of heat, but should inform treatment duration and temperature.

Hot packs or hydrocollator packs. Topical heat treatments attempt to warm tissues to between 40 and 45°C. They are primarily used to increase the mobility of a joint or the extensibility of collagen tissue; decrease muscle spasm; assist in the resolution of inflammatory infiltrates, edema, or exudates; increase blood flow; and afford analgesia. Hot packs, also referred to as *hydrocollator* packs (Fig.6.1), are the best-known conductive modality. These packs are available in various sizes and consist of canvas bags filled with silicon dioxide, which absorbs many times its own weight in fluid, acquiring a large heat capacity. Heat is used as a part of cancer therapy and rehabilitation, but certain safeguards must be applied when it is used (10,11). The potential of heat to influence tumor growth is inadequately characterized but should be respected. Heat should not be applied directly to the site of primary tumor or metastases. The advantages of hot packs are many,

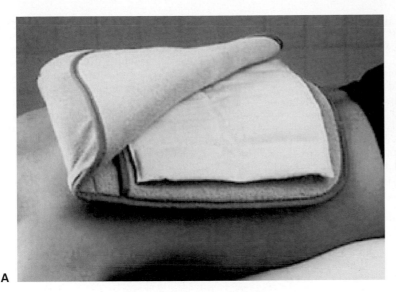
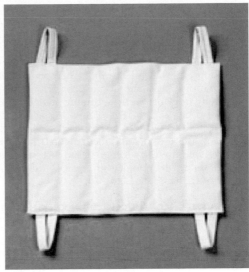

A   B

FIGURE 6.1. Hydrocollator pack shown with (**A**) and without (**B**) cloth cover for skin protection.

including low cost and long life, suitability for use at home and in the hospital, patient satisfaction, and ease of use.

Hydrotherapy. Whirlpool baths and Hubbard tanks are common forms of hydrotherapy. These units, which agitate water, are safe and provide convective heating, massage, and gentle debridement. Treatment goals of hydrotherapy include joint mobilization, debridement, or wound therapy. Temperatures can be adjusted, making this a safe technique for patients with cancer (12,13). Hydrotherapy tanks can be used to immerse the whole body. This is useful in a patient with a large surface area that needs to be treated.

Paraffin baths. The typical paraffin bath is a container filled with a mixture of mineral oil and paraffin maintained at a temperature of 54°C. Although this temperature is somewhat higher than that in water-based therapy, it is tolerated because the mixture has a low heat capacity and an insulating layer of wax builds up on the treated area (14). There are two types of paraffin treatments. One is the dip method, in which a patient repeatedly dips a joint or extremity into the bath, removing the joint between dips to allow the paraffin to solidify. The area is covered or wrapped with plastic for approximately 20 minutes. The paraffin is then stripped off and placed back into the bath.

In the alternate technique the continuous immersion method is used on the affected part of the patient for 20–30 minutes at a time. Heating with this approach ensures a more intense warming of the joint or extremity; this is tolerated because a layer of solid insulating paraffin forms on the skin (15,16). This modality is useful in the treatment of paretic extremities.

Radiant heat/heat lamps. Heat lamps are an inexpensive, versatile, and easy way of warming superficial tissues. Ordinary incandescent light bulbs can produce large amounts of infrared energy, so special infrared sources, such as quartz, are seldom required. Heating rates and temperatures are adjusted by varying the distance between the lamp and the patient (17). This modality may be used in cancer populations when it is advantageous for the skin to stay dry or when heat application without body contact is required. For heating purposes, the portions of the light from yellow to red and the near and far infrared are used. Heat transfer is highest on the skin surface and drops off in deeper tissues.

Ultrasound. Therapeutic ultrasound units produce high-frequency alternating currents of approximately 0.8–1.0 MHz, which are converted by a transducer into acoustic vibrations

(Fig. 6.2) (16). The conversion of the high-frequency alternating voltage into acoustic vibrations is accomplished by the reversal of the piezoelectric effect (18–20) so that deep tissues are heated. This is done by allowing the applicator to produce average ultrasonic intensities of 3–4 W per cm^2. Ultrasound is defined as an acoustic vibration at frequencies too high to be perceived by the human ear. Frequencies <17,000 Hz are called *sound*, whereas those above this level are designated as ultrasound.

Ultrasonic heating occurs at the interface of tissues with different densities. The degree of heat transfer is proportional to the density difference between adjacent tissues. Relatively little heat is absorbed into the subcutaneous fat or musculature. Most energy is converted into heat at the bone surface. This makes ultrasound ideal for pain relief at the bone interface because it does not cause extreme temperature elevation in the superficial tissues. Short-wave and microwave diathermies do not possess the depth of penetration of ultrasound. They have fallen out of practical use in the treatment of pain. These physical modalities may be helpful in the patient with cancer who has pain of muscular or bone origin; however,

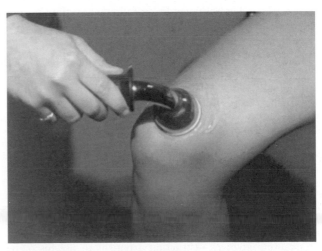

FIGURE 6.2. Therapeutic ultrasound unit being used to alleviate arthritic pain.

heat can increase local blood flow and may be contraindicated in patients with cancer whose pain is at the site of a tumor mass (14,20). This modality may be beneficial and may provide analgesia in an area of local muscle spasm.

Therapeutic Cold. Cold modalities are traditionally used for acute musculoskeletal trauma. Therapeutic cold controls edema and bruising through its vasoconstrictive properties. Its counterstimulatory properties promote analgesia. Therapeutic cold can also be used to reduce muscle spasms (21,22). The depth of penetration of cooling treatments is limited. Although marked decreases in skin and subcutaneous tissue temperatures are possible, cooling of deeper tissue is restricted to a few degrees. It should be avoided in areas of the body that have been previously irradiated (20).

Transcutaneous Electrical Nerve Stimulation

There is no evidence base for the use of transcutaneous electrical nerve stimulation (TENS) in the cancer population. However, TENS is generally well tolerated without serious side effects and a trial can be considered when pharmacologic and/or procedural approaches fail to control pain. TENS has been anecdotally reported to reduce pain associated with cancer-related lymphedema and dermal ulceration.

Non–Transcutaneous Electrical Nerve Stimulation

Indications for electrical stimulation of muscles or other tissues are extremely limited among patients with cancer. If pain is considered myogenic, electrical current may be trialed to reduce muscle strain, spasms, or tightness (14,23).

FUNCTION-ENHANCING THERAPIES

Classically, rehabilitation focuses on reducing the level of disability and handicap associated with a particular impairment. For example, the severe lower extremity motor deficits associated with complete paraplegia can be mitigated through the prescription of an appropriate wheelchair, instruction on independent transfer techniques, and use of assistive devices for performing activities of daily living (ADLs). A similar clinical approach can be extremely effective in reducing the functional morbidity associated with cancer pain. Discrete functional impairments can be identified and alternative means devised for accomplishing affected tasks. The goals behind this clinical approach are twofold: pain is reduced while the patients' functional status is enhanced. Strategies routinely employed toward this end are outlined in the following sections.

Compensatory Strategies

A fundamental rehabilitation approach involves instructing patients in compensatory strategies for mobility and the performance of ADLs. Compensatory strategies assume that a task associated with pain can be accomplished in an alternate, less painful manner. For example, a patient with a pathologic femoral fracture could be taught how to transfer from a seated to a standing position using the arms and unaffected leg for weight bearing. By deconstructing the tasks required for mobility and ADL performance into discrete steps, therapists can determine which step(s) in a task sequence produce pain. This approach allows intact, painless physiologic systems and adaptive equipment to substitute for impaired structures. Therapeutic exercise is often used to supplement this approach. An example involves instructing a patient to use his or her "good" leg and a toe loop to raise a plegic or painful extremity into bed during a sit-to-supine transfer.

Compensatory strategies can be used to minimize tactile stimulation of structures rendered allodynic by malignant involvement of the nervous system. Osseous structures affected by bone metastases can be "deweighted" to various degrees contingent on the risk of fracture and the degree of pain engendered by their use. Patients with cancer and vertebral compression fractures can be taught how to transfer without imposing painful flexion moments on the affected portions of the spine. It is critical to determine the musculoskeletal integrity of the extremities that will be used to relieve painful structures. This is particularly important for patients whose cancers have a predilection for osseous spread.

Adaptive Equipment—Mobility

Many patients require adaptive devices for safety and autonomy while moving about at home or in their communities. Ready access to such devices is essential if patients with advanced cancer are to remain socially integrated within their communities. Too often patients' social spheres collapse with disease progression. Adaptive equipment for mobility ranges in price and complexity from prefabricated single-point canes to motorized wheelchair systems. Handheld assistive devices include canes, crutches, and walkers. A variety of available devices are shown in Figure 6.3. Canes and walkers can be adapted to distribute weight bearing to intact structures to minimize the risk of pathologic fracture. An example is the platform crutch, fourth from the left in Figure 6.3. Broad redistribution of weight is particularly important for patients with extensive osseous disease. Handheld assistive devices can greatly benefit patients with sensory impairments. Tactile feedback transmitted through the device supplements deficits in sensory input. Chemotherapy-induced neuropathy is a common source of sensory impairment.

The use of assistive devices enables deconditioned patients with limited exertional tolerance to participate in aerobic conditioning. Platform rolling walkers reduce the energy required for ambulation. As the patients' stamina improves they are gradually transitioned to fewer and fewer supportive devices.

Adaptive Equipment—Wheelchairs and Scooters

Patients with severe deconditioning, paresis, osseous instability, or other sources of impaired mobility may require a wheelchair. Even when deficits are presumed transient, a wheelchair can sustain community integration and fragile social connections. Wheelchair tolerance and use are enhanced if an appropriate system is provided. There are many variables that can be specified to best serve the requirements and address the deficits of each patient. Armrests, for example, can be detachable to facilitate patient transfers. They are also available in "desk length," enabling patients to maneuver close to desks and tables. Trough armrests can be used for patients requiring greater control of their upper extremities.

Seating systems are elements of wheelchair prescription with tremendous importance. If patients are uncomfortable, wheelchair use will suffer. Use of air cell, gel-filled, custom-molded, and contoured foam cushions improves patient tolerance for sustained sitting and minimizes skin breakdown. Chairs can be equipped with reclining backs, lateral trunk supports, and headrests to optimize patient comfort and stability. Cloth backing should not be used in the seating systems of patients at risk for vertebral compression fractures. Patients tend to slump forward in pronounced kyphosis, thereby increasing compressive forces on the anterior vertebral bodies.

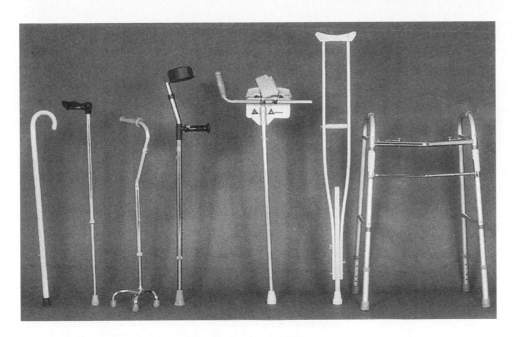

FIGURE 6.3. Common handheld assistive devices to facilitate patient mobility.

Wheelchairs are available in manual and motorized configurations. Patients with sufficient strength to self-propel should be provided with handrims. These are placed slightly lateral to the wheel and are smaller in diameter. Patients with cancer should not be provided with small-diameter handrims. These require greater force per stroke. Knobby projections can be added to the handrims. These "lugs" assist patients with poor grip related to distal arm weakness. If self-propulsion is not feasible, a motorized wheelchair is required. These chairs provide a high degree of independence but are significantly more costly. Add-on power packs can be used to convert manual chairs to motorized power. These best serve individuals for whom a manual chair suffices most of the time.

Many patients with advanced cancer benefit from the use of motorized wheelchairs. Often, the capacity to self-propel is lost as disease progresses. For this reason, anticipatory provision with a motorized chair is generally warranted. Wheelchair control can be adjusted to capitalize on muscle groups with sufficient power to manipulate a joystick or switch. "Sip-and-puff" drive control is available for patients with upper extremity paresis. Voice-controlled units remain experimental. Motorized scooters represent an excellent option for patients who are able to ambulate and transfer independently, but with insufficient endurance for extended ambulation.

Home and automobile adjustments must be considered when prescribing a wheelchair. Commercially purchased ramps are sufficient for many patients, requiring no home modification. If patients do not have access to a vehicle that is able to accommodate a motorized wheelchair or scooter, a collapsible manual chair equipped with an add-on power pack may represent the best option.

Adaptive Equipment—Activities of Daily Living

ADLs refer to the myriad functions required for personal grooming, hygiene, and feeding. Dependence for self-care has been shown to erode the quality of life of chronically ill patients (24,25). Minimizing each patient's requirement for external assistance is rehabilitation's most cherished goal. In self-care this is achieved through the provision of appropriate assistive devices. Scoop dishes or plate guards (Fig. 6.4) can help patients with impaired motor control or those who have the use of only one upper extremity to feed themselves. These devices allow patients to independently position food on their utensils. Nonskid mats, such as Dycem, can be helpful for patients with poor dexterity. Eating utensils can be easily adapted to the needs of each patient. Weight can be added for decreased stability or a bulbous handle can be used for reduced grip strength. A rocker knife (Fig. 6.5) can be used for impaired bilateral coordination. The knife is pushed down into food and rocked back and forth until the food is cut. These devices might reduce pain and improve motor control in patients with cancer who have neurogenic pain and impairments that affect their upper extremities.

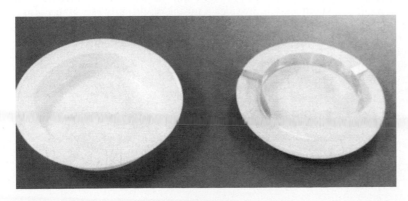

FIGURE 6.4. Scoop dishes to allow independent feeding for patients with impaired motor function.

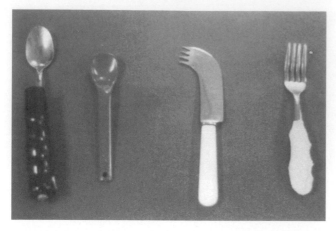

FIGURE 6.5. A rocker knife (third from the left) with other assistive devices for independent feeding.

Many devices are available to assist patients with independent dressing. Use of these devices can significantly reduce the requirement of applying stress on painful structures. When fine motor coordination is poor, fastening can be eased through the use of larger buttons, button aids, zipper pulls, elastic shoelaces, and Velcro. For patients who experience pain when reaching and grasping garments, reachers can retrieve items of clothing. A dressing stick (a long stick with a hook at the end) can help to pull clothing on. Stocking aids and long-handled shoehorns may help in a similar manner. A comparable array of assistive devices can be obtained to facilitate independent grooming.

Assistive devices for dressing and grooming should be explored when patients experience pain while stabilizing the upper trunk or scapular girdle or while abducting the shoulder. Patients with impaired or painful ADL performance should be referred for an occupational therapy evaluation. Most of the devices mentioned in this section can be readily obtained or fabricated by certified occupational therapists.

RESTORATION OF NORMAL BIOMECHANICAL ALIGNMENT

Cancer and its treatment have the capacity to adversely impact normal musculoskeletal physiology and biomechanics. Pain plays an important facilitatory role in the patients' adoption of maladaptive movement patterns. Significant biomechanical adaptations may occur as patients attempt to avoid painful postures or movements. Malignant lesions, particularly osseous metastases, can undermine the essential supporting structures of the musculoskeletal system. Tumors originating in or invading nerves or muscles may cause severe weakness and pain, requiring patients to recruit alternate, unaffected muscles in an effort to preserve their functional status. Patients with lower extremity sarcomas undergoing limb salvage procedures are an excellent example. Substantial portions of the knee and hip extensor muscles may be resected. Continued ambulation requires recruitment of intact muscles and biomechanical adaptations. Nonsurgical anticancer treatments, including radiation therapy and chemotherapy, can also injure nerves and muscles. Ongoing biomechanical alterations are therefore an inescapable consequence of cancer and are experienced by virtually all patients.

Adaptive techniques become essential if patients are to remain mobile. Many biomechanical adaptations are adopted without conscious effort to avoid pain or to compensate for soft tissue contractures or muscle weakness. Unfortunately, the short-term benefit of such maneuvers may ultimately lead to long-term functional decompensation. For example, weight shifting and postural realignment used to relieve pressure from a compromised acetabular joint can eventually produce aberrant gait mechanics with associated pathology of the contralateral hip and bilateral sacroiliac joints. Another common clinical example involves patients with head and neck cancer undergoing surgical neck dissection. These patients frequently develop spinal accessory nerve palsies with resulting weakness of the ipsilateral trapezius muscle. In an effort to continue using their affected upper extremities, patients recruit the remaining intact shoulder girdle muscles in a disorganized and deviant manner. Although this maneuver may initially enhance shoulder abduction and forward flexion, rotator cuff and myofascial pathology eventually develop and may be a source of intense pain.

Three principal rehabilitative strategies permit restoration of normal alignment. Manipulative techniques abruptly return musculoskeletal structures to proper alignment through the controlled application of exogenous force. The therapeutic targets of such maneuvers are axial and appendicular joints. Manipulation is of limited benefit unless therapeutic exercise is concomitantly initiated. Therapeutic exercise, the second essential approach in biomechanical restoration, is frequently the initial and often the sole approach required. Muscles play a critical role in maintaining joint alignment and in modulating the body's many complex biomechanical rhythms (e.g., the gait cycle and scapulothoracic motion required for overhead reaching activities). Therefore, muscle weakness, contracture, and fatigability must be addressed if normal biomechanics are to be lastingly restored. Orthotics comprise the third strategy commonly used to align musculoskeletal structures for pain relief and functional enhancement. If weakness is severe, or if structures have been undermined to an irreparable degree, exogenous support (e.g., orthotics) can substitute and afford biomechanical normalcy. Often, as in the management of vertebral compression fractures, the use of orthotics is integrated with therapeutic exercise. For these patients, the back extensor muscles can be strengthened while axial alignment is maintained through the use of an extension brace. Each of these three strategies (manipulation, exercise, and orthotics) is separately addressed in this section.

Manipulation or Manual Medicine

Manipulation has not been routinely offered to patients with cancer despite the high prevalence of musculoskeletal dysfunction in this population. The overuse of muscle groups through maladaptive movement patterns can lead to spasm, malalignment, disproportionate muscle tone, and chronic pain. Manipulation provides a means of abruptly restoring normal biomechanical patterns and relief from musculoskeletal pain. Functional patterns can then be reinforced through physical therapy. Clearly, the potential of harming patients with cancer having irradiated tissue, bone metastases, and muscle weakness through the inappropriate application of exogenous force must be respected (26).

In the past, "manipulation" has traditionally been equated with high-velocity, thrusting techniques designed to maintain maximal, painless movement of the musculoskeletal system in postural balance (27). In actuality, a broad range of manipulative techniques has been developed. Manual approaches may involve stretching, passive soft tissue release, or strategic muscle contraction to produce counterstrain. The goal of manipulation or manual medicine is to restore optimal body mechanics and improve motion in restricted areas. This is accomplished by treatments that attempt to both restore mechanical function of joints and normalize altered reflex patterns in the muscles that control them (28). Manual medicine techniques are potentially useful for treatment of any musculoskeletal problem associated with a loss of functional range of motion. Pain complaints commonly treated with manual medicine techniques include "sciatica," facet syndromes, mechanical cervical and lumbar pain, and piriformis syndrome.

Mobilization with impulse, or high-velocity, low-amplitude manipulation, is an approach widely equated with manual medicine. This technique is used to restore normal mobility to a discrete, dysfunctional segment (29). Similar effects can be achieved through the *articulatory technique,* which involves the combined use of leverage, patient ventilation, and a fulcrum to mobilize a joint limitation (30). This technique relies on repeated low-velocity, high-amplitude movements. *Muscle energy* is a gentle technique involving active muscle contraction by the patient against resistance supplied by the practitioner (31). Similar to the preceding approaches, the goal of muscle energy is to restore normal excursion to hypomobile segments. Strain and counterstrain is an additional well-tolerated technique designed to restore pain free range of motion. It attempts to place a joint in a position of greatest comfort or ease by reducing exaggerated afferent proprioceptive activity.

Muscle energy techniques (METs) are used to restore normal joint and soft tissue movement through volitional muscle recruitment. METs are an extension of joint mobilization techniques, but rather than applying exogenous force, METs rely on the patients' self-generated force. The practitioner places the patient in a strategic position and asks him or her to push against the practitioner's counterforce to facilitate joint and soft tissue movement. As normal motion is restored, soft tissue and joint restrictions decrease. METs reestablish normal length–tension relationships in the muscle and restore normal accessory joint movement. METs are generally well tolerated by patients. They may be the preferred initial manual technique in patients with cancer.

Manual medicine techniques should be used only in those patients having a reproducible musculoskeletal dysfunction. Each type of treatment technique has its own set of contraindications. Malignancy was considered an absolute contraindication to high-velocity, low-amplitude thrusting maneuvers in the past. However, in experienced hands, symptomatic musculoskeletal structures known to be unaffected by malignancy are candidates for safe manipulation. A cancer diagnosis warrants the initial use of less forceful techniques. Muscle energy, strain, and counterstrain measures should be applied first, in an effort to safely achieve benefit. Caution must be taken in patients with severe osteoarthritis, genetic disorders with hypermobility, and metabolic bone disease.

Patients with mechanical pain or pain that can be reproduced through muscle recruitment in the absence of a local tumor may be candidates for manual techniques. Osteopathic physicians are taught manipulation as an integral part of their medical education. Referral to an osteopathic physician specializing in pain management and manual medicine is an appropriate initial step. Success depends largely on the skill and experience of the treating professional. Therefore, identification of a qualified individual is essential. Many physical therapists are trained in manual medicine. Physical therapy prescriptions should specify the desired treatment and precautions related to each patient's cancer. For assistance in locating a qualified professional, the American Osteopathic Association can be contacted at (800) 621-1773 or http://www.osteopathic.org/.

Therapeutic Exercise

The prescription of exercise as a means of enhancing strength, coordination, stamina, and flexibility is a cornerstone of rehabilitation medicine. The recognition that our muscles and connective tissue respond predictably to imposed demands has produced an elegant body of clinical research. Exercise should be prescribed at a clinically appropriate dose and frequency to optimize benefit and prevent injury. Too often the degree of infirmity found in patients with advanced cancer has resulted in their exclusion from exercise programs. Such patients can benefit significantly from conservative, incremental strengthening and conditioning programs despite their precarious health. This capacity has been demonstrated in other disease states characterized by comparable levels of morbidity (32,33).

When patients are hospitalized and are medically stable, exercise can begin with gentle active and active-assisted twice-daily ranging of the extremities. Brief isometric muscle contractions can be performed in the bed against gravity or with gravity eliminated. Isometric or static contractions are those involving no angular motion of the joint on which the exercising muscle acts. One brief isometric contraction per day was demonstrated to prevent loss of strength in bedridden patients with rheumatoid arthritis (34).

Such an approach does not endanger the patient and minimizes deconditioning. As patients recover, exercise can be performed in a seated position isometrically or isotonically against resistance. An isotonic contraction is dynamic, with the tension on the muscle remaining constant throughout the contraction. More demanding resistive exercise, designed to build strength, can begin with resistance being offered by a Theraband. As patients improve, weighted ankle and wrist cuffs or free weights can be used. Resistive exercise has effectively improved strength in the elderly (35,36) and in patients with acquired immunodeficiency syndrome (37). Clinical investigation with acquired immunodeficiency syndrome and aged patients suggests that the use of anabolic steroids augments the effect of exercise on cachectic muscles (38,39).

Aerobic conditioning differs from resistive exercise in its emphasis on continuous rhythmic contraction of large muscle groups. Jogging and cycling are examples. Conditioning programs have been demonstrated to benefit patients with end-stage chronic obstructive pulmonary disease (40) and end-stage congestive heart failure (41–43). Such programs do not significantly alter the patients' cardiopulmonary status. However, the enhanced aerobic capacity of their muscles permits them to perform daily activities at a lower percentage of their maximal aerobic capacity. Progressive aerobic conditioning is extensively integrated in the standard care for patients with cardiopulmonary disorders, yet it is not routinely provided to patients with cancer. Several investigations have demonstrated significant benefit with respect to fatigue, functional status, pain, and nausea when aerobic conditioning is administered concurrently with the delivery of adjuvant chemotherapy for breast cancer (44), or after high-dose chemotherapy during bone marrow transplantation (45).

Most of the research on exercise in the person with cancer has looked at the effect of aerobic exercise on functional capacity and quality of life. Presently, there is no consensus on an ideal type, frequency, intensity, duration, or mode of exercise. The trend of these studies indicates that there is a good cardiopulmonary response to interval training at 50–70% of the heart rate reserve or while working at an exertion of 11–14 on the 6–20 perceived rate of exertion scale (44,45). The intensity of the exercise program is dependent on baseline fitness levels, intensity of cancer treatment, and stage of cancer. While undergoing treatment, most studies recommend decreasing the intensity to the lower end of the heart rate range. Once active cancer therapy is over, the program should progress toward the higher end of the range. The intensity must also take into account daily laboratory test values and patterns of fatigue associated with treatment. For example, fatigue seems to peak in the period between the middle and end of the radiation cycle, and the program should account for this pattern. Finally, the duration and frequency should closely match the guidelines of the American College of Sports Medicine. It is recommended that patients exercise for a total of 20–30 minutes, three to five times per week. This recommendation must be applied carefully to patients with advanced cancer. Exercise may entail walking slowly for 5–10 minutes. The goal of a conditioning exercise program is to regularly stress the muscular aerobic apparatus to maintain or enhance physical capacity.

Exercise can also be used to enhance coordination, biomechanical balance, and flexibility. Motor learning and muscle recruitment are enhanced by appropriately prescribed exercise. Such neural factors, together with enhanced strength, account for improved biomechanics and coordination. Patients with cancer whose functional decline arises from subtly impaired motor execution are excellent candidates for therapeutic exercise programs.

Orthotics

Orthotics are braces designed to alter articular mechanics when their integrity is compromised by weak muscles, pain, impaired sensation, bone metastases, or disrupted anatomic integrity. Orthotics may be used therapeutically to provide support, restore normal alignment, protect vulnerable structures, address soft tissue contractures, substitute for weak muscles, or maintain joints in positions of least pain. This latter application is particularly relevant for patients with advanced cancer. Many prefabricated orthotics are available "off the shelf." Although prefabricated braces often suffice, patients may require more expensive custom orthoses for optimal benefit. Orthotics can be used to address the pathology in virtually any articular structure. The use of these devices in patients with cancer must be tempered by the overarching

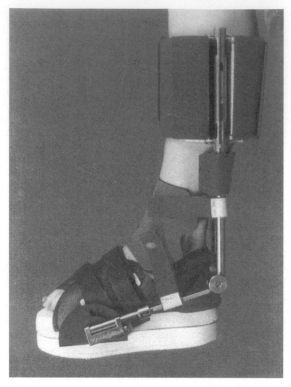

FIGURE 6.7. Dynamic splint (Dynasplint) for gentle stretching of soft tissue contractures.

mandate for patient comfort. For example, a molded body jacket (Fig. 6.6) would provide maximal stability for a patient with diffuse vertebral metastases. However, the discomfort associated with wearing such devices, as well as the difficulty donning and doffing them, makes their use undesirable for many patients with advanced cancer. Similarly, Dynasplint produces orthotics designed to apply steady pressure on the joints to elongate contracted soft tissue (Fig. 6.7).

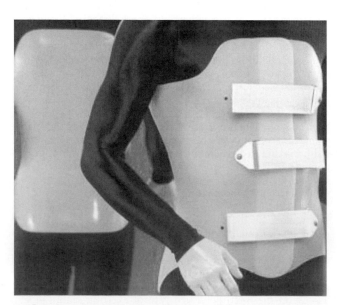

FIGURE 6.6. Custom-molded body jacket. This device is commonly used in patients with cancer who have vertebral metastases. Comfort and ease of donning are important considerations.

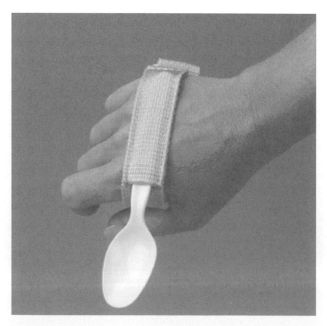

FIGURE 6.8. Universal cuff with plastic spoon inserted into the palmar pocket.

Although many patients with cancer develop soft tissue contractures related to radiation therapy, the cost–benefit ratio of Dynasplint prescription must be carefully weighed before use in patients with advanced cancer.

Orthotics range from highly technical to remarkably simple. A commonly prescribed orthotic is the universal cuff (Fig. 6.8). This simple band encircles the metacarpal heads and has a small pocket into which eating utensils, brushes, pens, and so on, can be inserted. For patients with distal upper extremity weakness related to neural compromise or joint pain, this device can restore the capacity for independent feeding, grooming, and keyboard manipulation. Orthotics of potential benefit to patients with cancer include the sternal–occipital mandibular immobilizer, molded ankle–foot orthotic, and the Jewett brace. The sternal–occipital mandibular immobilizer (Fig. 6.9) deweights cervical vertebrae, thereby alleviating pain and instability in patients with cervical bone metastases. The molded ankle–foot orthotic (Fig. 6.10) is used extensively for patients with impaired ankle dorsiflexion due to tibialis anterior weakness. The Jewett brace (Fig. 6.11) is an anterior hyperextension orthotic designed to reduce compression of the anterior spinal elements. This device may control pain related to the extensive metastatic involvement of the vertebral bodies. By limiting flexion, the device limits progressive vertebral collapse.

Referral to an orthotist or physical medicine and rehabilitation specialist ensures that patients are provided appropriate orthoses. However, many rehabilitation professionals lack experience in dealing with patients with cancer, particularly those with advanced disease. It is important to communicate each patient's prognosis, goals of treatment, financial resources, and

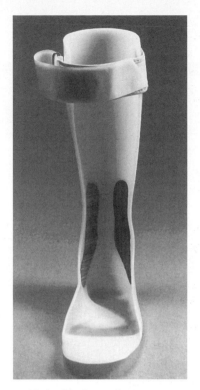

FIGURE 6.10. Molded ankle–foot orthotic.

symptom-control issues to the rehabilitation professional. This increases the likelihood that patients will receive an orthotic suited to their unique requirements (Table 6.1).

Once an orthotic is in use, ongoing scrutiny of dermal integrity becomes a critical dimension of care. Patients with cancer are rendered vulnerable to skin breakdown by a host

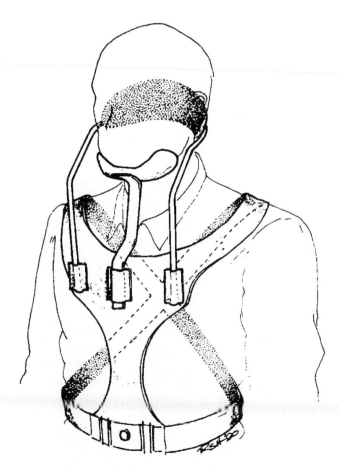

FIGURE 6.9. Sternal–occipital mandibular immobilizer orthosis.

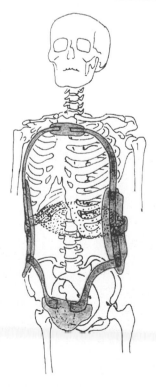

FIGURE 6.11. Jewett hyperextension orthotic.

TABLE 6.1

COMMON ORTHOSES USED FOR SPINAL STABILIZATION IN PATIENTS WITH CANCER

Orthotic	Description	Indication for patients with cancer
	Cervical orthoses	
Collars		
Soft collar	Constructed of soft foam and affording little constriction of neck movement Functions as a reminder to avoid neck movement	Used in the absence of instability for pain and muscle spasm

Rigid collar
  Philadelphia
  Newport
  Miami J
  California Stif-neck immobilizing
  Malibu
	Constructed of firm Plastazote or polyethylene
	Incorporates head through occiput and chin supports
	Offers some control of flexion and extension, but little limitation of rotation or lateral bending
		Indicated during soft tissue healing after cement and pin stabilization

Post appliances
  Two-poster orthosis
  Four-poster orthosis
  Sternal–occipital mandibular immobilizer
	Constructed of an anterior sternal plate, a posterior interscapular plate, and chin and occipital supports connected by rigid anterior and posterior metal struts
	Flexion–extension and rotation are well controlled, but lateral bending is restricted by only 34%
		Indicated during radiation if pain and minor instability are present and after bone grafting with fixation

Halo vest device	Comprised of four posts fixed to a vest and rostrally attached to a graphite ring held in place by pins inserted into the skull Offers optimal, although still incomplete, cervical stabilization in all directions	Useful for significant instability of the cervical spine after stabilization and bone grafting, but rarely indicated in the context of malignancy
Minerva	Total contact device that potentially offers more rotatory and lateral bending motions Extends from head to thorax	Indicated for stabilization during radiation or after surgery when greater control of lateral and rotatory cervical movement is required
	Thoracolumbosacral orthoses	

Corsets
  Lumbosacral
  Thoracolumbosacral
	Constructed of canvas with posterior rigid or semirigid struts
	Laced or Velcro closure
	Off-the-shelf availability is very convenient
	Abdominal constriction may not be tolerated by patients with cancer
		Provides comfort during radiation of a stable spine

Rigid braces
  Thoracolumbosacral orthoses
    Jewett
	Prevents flexion
	No abdominal apron
	Three-point pressure system over the sternum and hypogastrium anteriorly and over the upper lumbar spine posteriorly
	May place excessive hyperextension forces on lumbar vertebrae
		Used to reduce pain and offer support in patients with anterior compression fractures, often when conservative management is indicated

Knight Taylor	Reduces flexion at the thoracolumbar junction Poor restriction of extension and lateral bending Axillary straps must be prohibitively tight for brace to function	Indicated for pain relief in a stable or mildly unstable spine
Body Jacket	Generally fabricated of polypropylene Total contact design distributes pressure over a wide area Challenging to don and doff	Postoperatively after stabilization or for an unstable spine
Lumbosacral orthoses Chairback brace	Designed to control flexion–extension and lateral motion Consists of two paraspinal uprights and two uprights in the midaxillary line	Can provide pain relief for mild instability during or after radiation therapy

of factors, several of which may collude in a given patient. Impaired dermal sensation, lymphedema, compromised nutritional status, immobility, diminished microarterial perfusion, and radiation-induced soft tissue change can render the skin prone to breakdown. Dermal areas with prolonged redness after an orthotic is doffed indicate the need for increased padding, pressure relief, or a return visit to the orthotist.

CONCLUSION

Rehabilitation offers the capacity to enhance pain control while preserving or restoring the capacity of patients with cancer to function independently. Physiatric evaluation can be of particular benefit to patients who experience pain with movement. Ideally, an integrated rehabilitative approach to pain management can be introduced concurrently with disease-modifying, pharmacologic, and interventional analgesic strategies. In the authors' experience, the combined use of modalities (i.e., manual, thermal, and electric) for nociceptive modulation, pragmatic task-oriented therapies for pain-free mobility and ADL performance, and strategies to restore biomechanical alignment optimizes both analgesia and functional autonomy. It is important to note that not all rehabilitation professionals are familiar with the fragility and unique requirements of patients with cancer. For this reason, it is critical that clinicians caring for patients with cancer identify physiatrists; physical, occupational, and speech therapists; masseuses; and orthotists experienced in the care of patients with malignancy.

References

1. Kanemetz HL. History of massage. In: Basmajian JV, ed. *Manipulation, traction, and massage*, 3rd ed. Baltimore, MD: Williams & Wilkins, 1985.
2. Salva SG. *Massage therapy: principles and practice*. Philadelphia, PA: WB Saunders, 1999.
3. Cassar MP. *Handbook of massage therapy*. Oxford, UK: Butterworth–Heinemann, 1999.
4. Goats FC. Massage—the scientific basis of an ancient art: part 2. Physiological and therapeutic effects. *BMJ* 1994;28:153–156.
5. Prentice WE. *Therapeutic modalities for allied health professionals*. New York: McGraw-Hill, 1998.
6. Tappan FM. *Healing massage techniques: a study of Eastern and Western methods*. Reston, VA: Reston Publishing, 1980.
7. Werner R. *A massage therapist's guide to pathology*. Philadelphia, PA: Lippincott Williams & Wilkins, 1998.
8. Hoffman MD, Sheldahl LM, Kraemer WJ. Therapeutic exercise. In: Delisa J, Gans BM, eds. *Rehabilitation medicine principles and practice*, 3rd ed. Philadelphia, PA: Lippincott Williams & Wilkins, 1998:697–743.
9. Kasseroller R. *Compendium of Dr. Vodder's manual lymph drainage*. Heidelberg, Germany: Karl F. Haug Verlag, 1998:697–743.
10. Walsh NE. Pain management for cancer patients. *Cancer rehabilitation symposium, 48th annual assembly of the American Academy of Physical Medicine and Rehabilitation*. Baltimore, MD, 1986.
11. Dietzel F, Kern W. Kann hohes mutter-liches Fieber beim Kind auslosen. *Originalmitteilungen ist ausschlie der Verfasser verantwortlich Naturwissenschaften* 1971;2:24–26.
12. Hayashi S. Der Einfluss der Ultaschallwellen und ultrakurzzwellen auf den maligen. *Tumor J Med Sciences Biophysics Japan* 1940;6:138.
13. Delisa JA, Miller RA, Melnick RR, et al. Rehabilitation of the cancer patient. In: DeVita V, Hellman S, Rosenberg S, eds. *Principles and practice of oncology*, 2nd ed. Philadelphia, PA: JB Lippincott, 1985:2155–2188.
14. Basford JR. Physical agents. In: Delisa JA, ed. *Rehabilitation medicine—principles and practice*, 2nd ed. Philadelphia, PA: JB Lippincott, 1993:404.
15. Borrell RM, Henley EJ, Ho P, et al. Fluidotherapy: evaluation of a new heat modality. *Arch Phys Med Rehabil* 1977;58:69–71.
16. Borrell RM, Parker R, Henley EJ, et al. Comparison of *in vivo* temperatures produced by hydrotherapy, paraffin wax treatment and fluidotherapy. *Phys Ther* 1980;60:1273–1976.
17. Robinson JE. Review of concepts presented related to the physics of heating: emphasis on clinical applications. *Natl Cancer Inst Monogr* 1982;61:531–533.
18. Cameron BM. Experimental acceleration of wound healing. *Am J Orthod* 1961;3:336–343.
19. Child SZ, Vive B, Fridd C, et al. Ultrasonic treatment of tumors-II Moderate hyperthermia. *Ultrasound Med Biol* 1980;6:341–344.
20. Bergmann L. *Der ultraschallund seine anwendung in wissenschaft and technik*. Stuttgart, Germany: S. Hirzel Verlag, 1949.
21. Landon BR. Heat or cold for the relief of low back pain. *Phys Ther* 1967;47:1126–1128.
22. Knight KL. Cryokinetics in rehabilitation of joint spasms. In: *Cryotherapy: theory, technique and physiology*, 1st ed. Chattanooga, TN: Chattanooga Corporation, 1985:55.
23. Melzack R, Wall PD. Pain mechanisms: a new theory. *Science* 1965;150:971.
24. Breitbart W, Rosenfeld B, Pessin H, et al. Depression, hopelessness, and desire for hastened death in terminally ill patients with cancer. *JAMA* 2000;284(22):2907–2911.
25. Natterlund B, Gunnarsson LG, Ahlstrom G. Disability, coping and quality of life in individuals with muscular dystrophy: a prospective study over five years. *Disabil Rehabil* 2000;22(17):776–785.
26. Gerber L, Hicks J, Klaiman M, et al. Rehabilitation of the cancer patient. In DeVita VT, Hellman S, Rosenberg SA, eds. *Cancer: principles & practice of oncology*, 5th ed. Philadelphia, PA: Lippincott-Raven, 1997:2925–2956.
27. Neumann H. *Introduction to manual medicine*. Heidelberg, Germany: Springer-Verlag, 1989.
28. Korr IM. Somatic dysfunction, osteopathic manipulative treatment, and the nervous system: a few facts, some theories, many questions. *J Am Osteopath Assoc* 1986;86:109–114.
29. Heilig D. The thrust technique. *J Am Osteopath Assoc* 1981;81:244–248.
30. Greenman PE. *Principles of manual medicine*. Baltimore, MD: Williams & Wilkins, 1989.
31. Mitchell FL, Moran PS, Pruzzo NA. *An evaluation and treatment manual of osteopathic muscle energy procedures*. Valley Park, MO: Mitchell, Moran, and Pruzzo, 1979.
32. De Lateur BJ, Giaconi RM, Alquist AD. Fatigue and performance data from normal subjects and patients with several neuromuscular and musculoskeletal syndromes: response to training. *Proc AAEE* 1988;6:27–33.
33. Gerber LH, Hicks JE. Exercise in the rheumatic diseases. In: Basmajian JV, ed. *Therapeutic exercise*. Baltimore, MD: Williams & Wilkins, 1990:333–350.
34. Leiberson WT. Brief isometric exercises. In: Basmajian J, ed. *Therapeutic exercise*, 4th ed. Baltimore, MD: Williams & Wilkins, 1984:236–256.
35. Frontera WR, Meredith CN, O'Reilly KP, et al. Strength conditioning in older men: skeletal muscle hypertrophy and improved function. *J Appl Physiol* 1988;64(3):1038–1044.
36. Meredith CN, Frontera WR, O'Reilly KP, et al. Body composition in elderly men: effect of dietary modification during strength training. *Am Geriatr Soc* 1992;40(2):155–162.
37. Nixon S, O'Brien K, Glazier RH, et al. Aerobic exercise interventions for people with HIV/AIDS (Cochrane Review). *Cochrane Database Syst Rev* 2001;1:CD001796.
38. Strawford A, Barbieri T, Van Loan M, et al. Resistance exercise and supraphysiologic androgen therapy in eugonadal men with HIV-related weight loss: a randomized controlled trial. *JAMA* 1999;281(14):1282–1290.
39. Kenny AM, Prestwood KM, Gruman CA, et al. Effects of transdermal testosterone on bone and muscle in older men with low bioavailable testosterone levels. *J Gerontol A Biol Sci Med Sci* 2001;56(5):M266–M272.
40. Celli BR. Pulmonary rehabilitation for patients with advanced lung disease. *Clin Chest Med* 1997;18(3):521–534.
41. Borer JS, Bradni-Pifano S, Puigbo JJ, et al. Rehabilitation of patients with left ventricular dysfunction and heart failure. *Adv Cardiol* 1986;33:160–169.
42. Shabetai R. Beneficial effects of exercise training in compensated heart failure. *Circulation* 1988;78:775–776.
43. Williams RS. Exercise training of patients with left ventricular dysfunction and heart failure. *Cardiovasc Clin* 1985;15:219–231.
44. Winningham ML, Nail L, Barton-Burke M, et al. Fatigue and the cancer experience: the state of the knowledge. *Oncol Nurs Forum* 1994;21:23–36.
45. Dimeo FC, Tilman MH, Bertz H, et al. Aerobic exercise in the rehabilitation of cancer patients after high dose chemotherapy and autologous peripheral stem cell transplantation. *Cancer* 1997;79:1717–1722.

CHAPTER 7 ■ NEUROSURGICAL INTERVENTIONAL APPROACHES TO PAIN

ANDREW MANNES, PHILIP S. KIM, AND RUSSELL R. LONSER

Interventional and neurosurgical procedures can be utilized to supplement pharmacologic and complementary approaches to treat pain (see chapters 3 and 4). Pharmacologic therapies are described elsewhere in this text and includes principles of analgesic management using opioid agents and adjuvant medications. The primary indications for interventional techniques are for patients whose pain is either poorly responsive to systemic analgesic therapies or for those who suffer from intolerable side effects, in whom efforts to manage adverse effects are unsuccessful. Patients can experience severe dose-limiting side effects that prevent optimal titration to therapeutic levels. For example, systemic opioids can produce constipation, nausea, vomiting, or sedation.

Patient's response to analgesic medicinal therapies has been best described in the cancer population. The oral administration of analgesics based on recommendations, including those outlined by the World Health Organization, has provided satisfactory relief to most patients. However, the poorly relieved pain experienced by 5–15% (1–3) of the approximately 500,000 patients who die each year from cancer represents a significant need for additional methods, including interventional and neurosurgical procedures, that can offer symptom relief.

Aside from optimizing pain control while minimizing side effects, interventional pain therapies can also enhance functional abilities and physical and psychological well-being, enhancing the patient's quality of life (4). It has also been reported that better pain management utilizing interventional techniques may result in increased life. Further, reducing patient visits for symptom management could potentially reduce costs (5).

INITIAL EVALUATION

For the interventionalist, it is important to understand the patient's prognosis, associated comorbidities, and patient's and family's expectations. An initial evaluation for interventional pain therapies should ascertain the patient's general medical condition along with the primary disease. A complete history is required, including a general medical, disease-specific (e.g., patients with oncologic disorders need to be thoroughly evaluated for possible local recurrence or new metastases), and pain histories. Specific pain history would include the following: quality of pain, pain intensity, alleviating and exacerbating factors, temporal characteristics, duration, and associated features (e.g., numbness, weakness, vasomotor

changes). Psychosocial evaluation should assess the presence of psychological symptoms (e.g., anxiety, depression), and psychiatric disorders (e.g., major depression, delirium) should be similarly addressed. The nature and meaning of the presenting pain needs to be distinguished from anxiety and suffering affecting all aspects of one's life. The ability to cope and the availability of psychosocial support systems need to be assessed and reinforced with proper health and social professionals. A final assessment should determine the patient's expectation of therapeutic interventional options.

The physical examination includes a general medical examination, with emphasis on neurologic findings. Specific examination of the site of pain and surrounding anatomic regions are important. For example, if a patient has motor and sensory deficits in a particular region, neurolysis techniques become a more acceptable therapeutic option.

Appropriate selection of an intervention is based on therapeutic goals. If the presenting pain is expected to be transient (pain that will be alleviated by primary radiation therapy or chemotherapy, pain that is associated with the treatment of the primary disease, or pain that is) then the intervention should likewise be reversible. However, if the pain is expected to be chronic, a technique that results in more permanent effects is indicated. Life expectancy must be considered when selecting an appropriate intervention. If the patient's life expectancy is short, treatment strategies should strive to minimize the frequency and level of interventions and recovery time and should focus on optimizing a patient's quality of life. A patient with a longer life expectancy may warrant more extensive and expensive interventions (i.e., implantable devices). Certain procedures may not be indicated for patients with longer life expectancy such as neuroablative procedures that are associated with permanent loss of function or a theoretical risk of developing deafferentation pain syndromes.

Therefore, once a definitive diagnosis has been made, a treatment plan should characterize the expected outcome, define contingencies, and plan for reassessment. Longitudinal monitoring of pain and response to interventional therapies is essential and allows implementation of additional options (e.g., complementary therapies, pharmacologic strategies, and behavioral and psychological approaches).

This chapter includes some of the frequently utilized procedures in the palliative care pain population (Table 7.1). Not all indications and contraindications are included and consultation with a pain practitioner should be considered before referring the patient for evaluation and treatment.

TABLE 7.1

COMPARISON OF INTERVENTIONAL PAIN PROCEDURES

	Nerve blocks	Neurolytic procedures	Neurostimulation	Neuraxial infusion
Advantages	Ease of performance Useful for diagnostic and therapeutic relief	Ease of performance Provides long-term relief	Nondestructive Reversible	Nondestructive Reversible
Disadvantages	Provides short-term relief	Risk of associated sensory and motor deficits	Requires costly equipment and surgical implantation	Requires costly equipment and possible surgical implantation Requires pharmaceutical and ancillary support

APPROACHES TO INTERVENTIONS

Pharmacologic management of pain can be viewed as a continuum of indirect and direct drug delivery paradigms (4). Indirect drug delivery (i.e., systemic analgesia) refers to the administration of an analgesic into the bloodstream, which is then transported to the receptor site in neural tissue:

1. By systemic absorption
2. By formulation of depot for sustained and continuous release
3. Through the bloodstream

Direct drug delivery is the administration of an agent to the targeted neural tissue involved in nociception. By delivering directly to the nociceptive pathways, one can achieve a pronounced analgesic effect at a lower dose with fewer side effects. An example of this is comparing equianalgesic morphine doses in the intrathecal, epidural, and intravenous spaces (Table 7.2) (6).

Interventional pain therapies are usually minimally invasive techniques that can be divided into direct drug delivery, neuroablation, neural blockade, and neurostimulation. Direct drug delivery involves the administration of analgesics, usually opioids and local anesthetics, directly into nociceptive pathways. Other potential agents such as α_2-agonists and calcium channel blockers can be administered. Neuroablation refers to direct chemical, thermal, or surgical destruction of nociceptive pathways. Neurostimulation or neuroaugmentation refers to the application of direct electrical stimulation to inhibit nociceptive transmission. Not all pain, however, can be adequately addressed using these techniques. In such cases, one can consider consultation with a neurosurgeon about surgical intervention.

Direct Drug Delivery

Neuraxial direct drug delivery involves accessing the epidural or subarachnoid (intrathecal) space by a needle or the

TABLE 7.2

EQUIANALGESIC MORPHINE CONVERSIONS AMONG ROUTES OF ADMINISTRATION

Oral	Parenteral	Epidural	Subarachnoid
300 mg =	100 mg =	10 mg =	1 mg

placement of a continuous infusion system. In general, neuraxial infusion should be considered when severe pain cannot be controlled with systemic drugs and/or because of dose-limiting toxicities. Neuraxial infusions can also be considered when there is an immediate need for using various nonopioid analgesics. Specifically, local anesthetics can have a profound analgesic effect on many intractable opioid-unresponsive pain conditions. Although it is possible to give local anesthetic systemically, higher local concentrations can be achieved, resulting in profound neural blockade through direct drug delivery.

Neuraxial delivery systems have two components: an intraspinal or epidural catheter and a delivery mode (e.g., bolus dosing, syringe pump, internal port, or internal or external pump). There are basically five types of neuraxial drug delivery systems, and familiarization with these systems allows the clinician to understand the respective advantages and disadvantages of each (7,8).

The simplest, least expensive, and least invasive option, a percutaneous catheter, is typically made of nylon, polyurethane, or polyamide and can be wire reinforced. These catheters are routinely placed in surgical and obstetric patients to manage operative and postoperative pain and are designed for short-term use (<1 week). But a catheter may be maintained for longer periods without problems and may suffice for the duration of the patient's life. If there is a complication, these catheters can be discontinued by removing the dressing and withdrawing the catheter. However, these catheters can cause localized tissue reaction at the site of insertion, can migrate, and are susceptible to accidental displacement.

The next type of drug delivery system uses the same type of catheter as that mentioned in the preceding text, but it is tunneled subcutaneously to decrease the incidence of migration. Placement can be performed in a clinic and requires a small incision with multiple needle insertions. Tunneling the catheter is better suited for the outpatient or the home-bound patient.

Implanted catheters with subcutaneous injection site are technologically more advanced and require a minor surgical procedure, resulting in higher costs (for placement). Sterile preparation and the use of fluoroscopy are essential. These systems can be placed in the epidural or intrathecal space. There are two basic designs: exteriorized or completely internalized injection port. In the first design, the proximal catheter is tunneled from the exit site in the back and exteriorized usually along the midaxillary line. This catheter can include an antimicrobial cuff that reduces both infection and catheter migration. In the second design, the port is supported by bone, usually a rib, so as to facilitate needle insertion. It can be used for intermittent bolus dosing or accessed for continuous infusions.

A totally implanted catheter with implanted reservoir and manual pump is being developed by Medtronics, Inc. (Minneapolis, MN). The Algomed implantable patient-activated device is not yet commercially available. It is composed of an implanted reservoir with a manual pump. This design allows patient-controlled analgesia by pressing the activation valve and pumping chamber, providing a bolus of medication. Because the entire device is implanted, the reservoir is refilled by inserting a needle into a subcutaneous port in the control pad.

A totally implanted catheter with implanted infusion pump is available in two basic designs. The simpler design is a constant fixed infusion pump in which the dose can be adjusted by a clinician changing the concentration (Johnson & Johnson). The second type includes a programmable, peristaltic infusion pump with a drug reservoir, an electronic module, and an antenna allowing reprogramming of drug flow rates (Medtronic Inc., Minneapolis, MN). The clinician controls the pump through an external programmer head (such as a pacemaker) to alter the dose, give single doses, or change the continuous infusion rate.

Recently, Medtronic has received U.S. Food and Drug Administration (FDA) approval for a patient activation device that will allow the patient to receive a medical direct bolus of medication when the device is activated.

Typically, a percutaneous test catheterization of the epidural or intrathecal space would be performed to assess the efficacy and starting doses of medication before implanting a permanent delivery system. There are several approaches to trial the drugs, including bolus dosing, by accessing the intrathecal space with a spinal needle, or by placement of a catheter and continuous infusion—either in the epidural or intrathecal space. Ideally, the method utilized for clinical assessment would best emulate the intended route (e.g., a trial with a continuous intrathecal catheter for evaluating future implantable pump placement). Although the complication rate is low, implantable devices can have problems with catheter failure, infection, seroma, wound dehiscence, and catheter tip fibroma formation (reported with high-concentration morphine) (9). They also require health care provider visits for routine refills and adjustment of dosing.

The selection of the appropriate neuraxial drug(s) and delivery system for an individual patient is based on several considerations (7,10):

1. Patient life expectancy
2. Economics and cost-effectiveness
3. Choice of epidural versus subarachnoid route of administration

Patient life expectancy and duration of need is difficult to predict. The more sophisticated implantable systems are expensive devices that require a trial catheter, adjustments of medications, and a surgical procedure for placement. One study by Bedder et al. suggest that an implanted pump system is a more viable financial alternative compared to other drug delivery systems for a period over 3 months (11). The less sophisticated percutaneous and tunneled catheters are best suited for patients with a limited life expectancy of <1 month. Both epidural and subarachnoid drug delivery can be equally effective. The duration of therapy will usually predict the type of infusion system selected. Catheter obstruction, fibrosis, and loss of analgesic efficacy are well described in long-term epidural drug systems (7). Therefore, intrathecal drug delivery systems are best suited for a protracted duration of therapy (>3 months). A decision-making algorithm for using neuraxial analgesia is shown in Figure 7.1 (12).

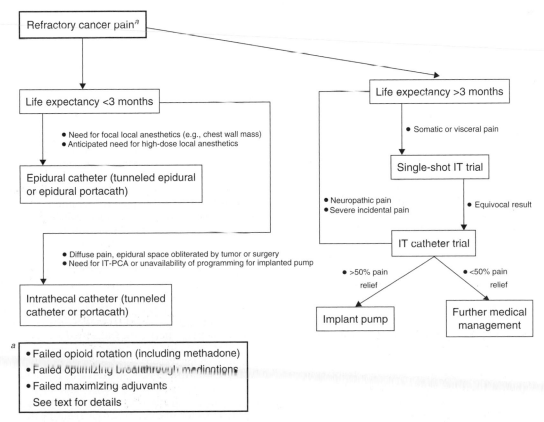

FIGURE 7.1. A decision-making algorithm for patients with refractory cancer-related pain. IT-PCA, intrathecal patient-controlled analgesia.

Multiple pharmacologic preparations have been administered through the neuraxial drug delivery systems. The gold standard is morphine, which is widely used and successful. When intrathecal morphine provides inadequate relief, other opioids, such as hydromorphone, meperidine, methadone, fentanyl, and sufentanil, have been used. As tolerance develops, one might switch opioids and/or use them in combination with coanalgesics, which include local anesthetics (e.g., tetracaine, bupivacaine), α_2- agonists (e.g., clonidine), and GABA B agonists (baclofen). Most recently, ziconotide, a calcium channel blocker that is the synthetic equivalent of a peptide produced by a snail, has been approved for use in intrathecal pumps (13). Drug selection is based on the patient's pain symptoms using clinical strategies which have been developed (e.g., the 2003 Polyanalgesic Consensus Conference) (14). The guidelines and algorithms were developed by an expert panel, evaluating existing literature and algorithms for various intrathecal drugs. The optimal drug dosage, concentration, and issues related to compounding of drugs has been reviewed.

Complications from neuraxial catheter and pump placement may result from anatomic changes, infection, fluid collection, catheter migration, or device failure. Patients with suspected block of the subarachnoid circulation due to tumor extension or subarachnoid hemorrhage/arachnoiditis may have a poor response to the delivery of intrathecal analgesia. Evidence of an obstruction should be sought using magnetic resonance imaging (MRI) or myelography to determine the level of obstruction. Retesting the efficacy of analgesia by placing the injectant proximal to the obstruction may yield improved analgesic response. Migration or fracture of the catheter should be suspected if the patient reports sudden changes in pain relief or if a fluid collection is seen at the insertion site. Percutaneously placed catheters can be bolused with a test dose of a local anesthetic to assess function. Myelography should be performed with implantable catheters or pumps (through a side port) to determine catheter placement and function when displacement or catheter rupture is suspected.

An infection of the site does not always necessitate immediate removal of a catheter. Superficial infections may only require a course of antibiotics. However, persistent or progressive tissue infection or central nervous system (CNS) involvement necessitates immediate removal of the catheter and/or pump.

A growing body of case reports and studies supports the benefits of direct drug (intrathecal) delivery systems. In a study of 202 patients experiencing refractory cancer pain who were randomized to receive either an implantable drug delivery system or comprehensive medical management (15), the patients receiving implantable intrathecal pump had reported successful pain control with a reduction in common drug toxicities such as fatigue and diminished level of consciousness. Overall, there was an improvement in the quality of life measures and survival over the 6 months in the patients receiving implantable intrathecal pump.

Peripheral Nerve/Plexus Drug Delivery

Blockade of peripheral nerves and neural plexi is commonly performed to provide regional anesthesia and analgesia to patients undergoing surgical procedures (15–18). Modified constant infusion systems typically deliver local anesthetics directly to peripheral nerves and neural plexi in patients with inadequate analgesia or intolerable toxicities from systemic medications. Specific localized pain syndromes related to a mononeuropathy, plexopathy, and peripheral neuropathy may benefit from peripheral nerve infusion.

Continuous neural blockade of the brachial plexus is common for postoperative pain. A technique of placing a catheter along the brachial plexus and self-contained infusion system has been described (16,17). A case report describes the successful 2-week management of pain from Pancoast's syndrome with a brachial plexus infusion system using local anesthetics (19). Other potential areas where neural infusion could be performed include the lumbosacral plexus, paravertebral and selected peripheral nerves, and sympathetic chain.

The current self-contained peripheral nerves/plexi infusion system is a modification of neuraxial infusion systems (16–20). The advantages of this system are the simplicity and the minimal invasiveness of the placement of the system. However, the patient can experience a localized tissue reaction or catheter migration and has a risk of infection for implantations of >1 month's duration. Implantable technology must be improved to provide a completely implanted infusion system for long-term continuous nerve/plexi analgesic infusion.

Neural blockade with longer-acting local anesthetics such bupivacaine can provide hours of relief until a more long-term solution can be offered. This window of analgesia can also provide time to titrate systemic medications such as steroids, antidepressants, and anticonvulsants. Many times diagnostic neural blockade will predict the response to neuroablative techniques.

Neuroablation

Neuroablation should be initiated in the following conditions (21):

1. If systemic therapies fail to provide adequate relief and quality of life
2. If neuraxial drug administration fails
3. To accommodate patient preference
4. Early in the natural history of disease (e.g., cancer) in the presence of discrete well-defined pain generators

Contemporary minimally invasive neurolytic techniques can be divided into chemical lysis, cryoneurolysis, and radiofrequency and surgical ablation (22). Chemical neurolysis involves the injection of a destructive chemical such as alcohol or phenol. Historically, other chemicals such as chlorocresol, ammonium salts, and iced and hypertonic saline have been used (22). Ethyl alcohol dehydrates and precipitates neural tissue. Phenol (carbonic acid) denatures neural tissue as well, with an apparently lower incidence of neuritis (22). Radiofrequency neurolysis has numerous advantages compared to chemical neurolysis. Radiofrequency neurolysis involves the placement of insulated needles to localize nociceptive pathways and then pinpoint a heat lesion. The extent of the lesion can be controlled by the size of the probe, duration of application, and the temperature at the tip of the needle. Because a more precise controlled lesion can be performed, radiofrequency lesioning is preferred for cordotomy, rhizotomy, and gangliolysis. The use of pulsed radiofrequency as an alternative to conventional radio frequency ablation (RFA) techniques is being explored. This technique uses a narrow pulsed current, allowing for cooling time, and a lower tissue temperature ($42°C$ in pulsed radiofrequency vs. $80°C$ in RFA) with no histologic signs of tissue damage (23). Several studies have reported reversible antinociceptive effects; therefore, pulsed radiofrequency may be better suited for treating patients with reversible disease or treatment related pain.

Like radiofrequency neurolysis, cryoneurolysis has an advantage in producing a controlled lesion. Cryoneurolysis is produced by disrupting neuronal transmission by allowing rapid expansion of compressed gas, causing the formation of an "ice ball" at the tip of the needle (22). Nerves encompassed in the frozen tissue develop ice crystals that result in degeneration.

However, the architecture of the perineurium and epineurium is not affected, thereby allowing resprouting of the axons without subsequent neuroma formation. The clinical effects are variable and are a function of precise needle tip localization (duration of freezing and lowest temperature achieved). The longevity of the effects needs to be considered when utilizing this technique. If the pain is expected to resolve, the recovery of nerve function would be desirable. However, if the targeted pain is expected to be chronic, relief from symptoms may be short lived. Rarely, peripheral and central nerves can be surgically interrupted. Neurosurgical techniques are included in greater detail in this chapter.

Neurolytic procedures, by definition, often cause irreversible damage to the neurons, but other structures in proximity to the intended site can be damaged because of extension of the therapy or accidental needle migration. Therefore, the resulting effects may include not only the neurons responsible for conveying pain but also lesion neurons that convey touch, proprioception, bladder and bowel control, and motor function. Therefore, these procedures are best performed by trained and experienced practitioners. Although not essential, using local anesthetic blocks is a good trial before implementing an irreversible blockade. It will emulate the level of pain relief that can be provided by the neurolytic procedure while allowing the patient to experience other side effects associated with deafferentation. This includes evaluating the untoward effects such as "numbness" in the affected region that some patients find less desirable than the original pain.

The efferent neuronal pathway can also be a target for interventional therapies. Botulism toxin, a neurotoxin produced by *Clostridium botulinum*, blocks acetylcholine release from nerve terminals, resulting in muscle relaxation. Therapeutic benefit can be achieved by carefully injecting botulinum toxin A into various muscle groups in patients with myofascial pain, migraines, and spastic conditions.

Neurolytic Procedures

Head and neck pain. Peripheral neurolysis can be done at various neural structures throughout the body (22,24,25). The head and neck region is richly innervated, and disease resulting in pain in this region (e.g., cancer) is difficult to manage (22). Pain is often aggravated by simple movements related to coughing, swallowing, talking, and eating. The cranial nerves typically affected by neoplastic growth and surgical and radiation therapy are V, VII, IX, and X. Potential problems exist for the pain interventionalist in understanding anatomic distortion due to cancer and cancer therapies. The avoidance of damage to cranial nerves IX and X is critical for ventilatory and swallowing control.

The cell bodies of the sensory neurons innervating the face, forehead, and upper neck are localized to the trigeminal ganglia (cranial nerve V). The ganglia or branches of the afferent fibers can be selectively targeted by several approaches. Surgical rhizotomies have been supplanted by percutaneous approaches and open surgical microvascular decompression. Radiofrequency thermogangliolysis is the most popularly utilized technique, with >14,000 cases reported in 33 publications (22). Technically similar to chemical neurolysis, a radiofrequency probe is placed along the divisions of the trigeminal ganglion through the foramen ovale and a brief thermal lesion is performed. In one large series, at 2-year follow-up, 28.3% of patients had recurrence of symptoms after one treatment and 8.3% has recurrence after multiple treatments (26). Trigeminal balloon compression is a surgical approach in which a Fogarty balloon catheter is placed and inflated to perform neurolysis, with reported results being similar to those of radiofrequency neurolysis (27). Microvascular decompression is discussed in the section Other Neurosurgical

Procedures. Eye pain can also be conveyed along the fifth cranial nerve. Pain symptoms may arise from localized pathology or may be referred (e.g., migraine), and patient referral to an ophthalmologist is warranted.

Intractable hiccups (singultus) can be treated with phrenic nerve blocks (22). This is done with fluoroscopic guidance to determine whether one hemidiaphragm is predominant in spasm and should be blocked. If the local anesthetic block is successful, a neurolytic phrenic technique can be done surgically or with RFA (28).

Upper and lower extremity. Upper and lower extremity pain can be difficult to treat with interventional neurolytic approaches. The nerves of the brachial and lumbosacral plexi are mainly mixed nerves with motor and sensory components. Difficulties exist in selectively blocking only the sensory components of the nerves and plexi. Subarachnoid and dorsal root neurolysis can be performed with a limited incidence of motor deficits (29). The injection of phenol in the brachial plexus provided four patients with cancer with good to excellent pain relief for 12 weeks (24). Intractable shoulder pain was managed effectively with suprascapular neurolysis using phenol or absolute alcohol (25).

Thorax and abdomen. Thoracic and abdominal wall pain can be treated with multiple intercostal or paravertebral nerve blocks. If adequate relief is obtained, a percutaneous neurolysis can be performed. Subarachnoid neurolysis can also be performed if the dermatome(s) involved in the pain generator can be identified. Doyle reported a series of 46 hospice patients treated with multiple phenol intercostal blocks (30). The patients received a range of total relief from 1–6 weeks (mean: 3 weeks). Peripheral neurolysis of various branches of the lumbosacral plexus (iliohypogastric, ilioinguinal) has been similarly performed for pain in the lower abdomen/pelvic region (31).

Sympathetic Ganglion Neurolytic Blocks

Neuropathic, intra-abdominal, pelvic, and perineal pain can be treated with various sympathetic ganglion neurolytic approaches (32). Unlike the somatic nerves, selective blockade of the sympathetic nervous system will not result in altered motor or sensory function (although other sympathetic mediated function may be lost).

Celiac plexus and splanchnic blocks are among the frequently utilized neurolytic blocks for neuropathic or cancer pain (33–36). Sympathetic blocks are indicated for treating abdominal and referred back pain secondary to abdominal pathology, especially pancreatic cancer. Pancreatic cancer involving the head of the pancreas is more responsive than that of the tail of the pancreas (37). In addition to providing pain relief, celiac plexus blocks can reduce sympathetic tone, leaving unopposed parasympathetic activity, thereby enhancing gastrointestinal motility—a major benefit for patients with cancer requiring systemic opioids. Serious complications involving the kidney, lung, aorta, and vena cava have been minimized with fluoroscopic or computed tomographic (CT) guidance and modification of the original techniques. A randomized study of early intervention of alcohol versus placebo celiac blocks demonstrated statistically significant pain relief and prolonged survival ranging from 3–9 months in alcohol-treated patients (38). A preemptive interventional approach may lead to improved survival rates, but more studies are needed.

An alternative therapy to the celiac axis neurolysis targets the nerves that condense to form the plexus, specifically the greater, lesser, and least splanchnic nerves (derived form the thoracic chain) (39). Neuroablative therapy applied to the splanchnic nerves can achieve the same therapeutic result as celiac plexus neurolysis, although some practitioners think the technique is safer. The lesions must be applied bilaterally, but there is less likelihood for intraperitoneal, bowel, or arterial injections or trauma to these structures.

Interventional pain therapies for intractable perineal pain are predisposed to the potential risk of rectal and urinary incontinence. In cases of preexisting incontinence with surgical diversion, a neurolytic subarachnoid saddle block is simple and effective. Other target structures for pelvic and perineal pain include the superior hypogastric plexus and ganglion impar. The superior hypogastric plexus consists of sympathetic and parasympathetic fibers that innervate the pelvis including the vagina, uterus, cervix, testis, ovaries, and bladder (40). Patients with advanced disease experiencing refractory pain in this region could obtain significant pain relief with a neuroablative procedure.

Sympathetic innervation to the head, neck, and upper extremities can be interrupted with a stellate ganglion block and the lower extremities with a lumbar sympathetic block. An initial injection or series of injections with local anesthetics are useful for diagnosis, and possibly for treatment. A successful injection will reduce the patient's pain symptoms and produce evidence of sympathetic blockade (e.g., temperature chance in affected limb) without somatic motor or sensory loss. If symptom relief is reproducible but transient, a trial using a dorsal column stimulator or a neurodestructive procedure using RFA, chemical neurolysis, or surgical procedure can be considered. Early initiation of treatment after an injury or the appearance of symptoms may elicit a better response than that seen with patients who have experienced chronic symptoms.

Other neurolytic approaches may involve interruption of various CNS pathways. Subarachnoid and epidural neurolysis have been reported in various case reports and series (22,41). The disadvantage is the potential spread of these chemicals on other central structures, leading to potential myelopathies. Painful conditions may require multiple-level neurolysis, greatly compounding the probability of serious complications. The use of implantable pumps has reduced the need for this procedure.

Neurostimulation

Neurostimulation is the application of precisely targeted electrical stimulation on nociceptive pathways. Electric stimulation has a long history in medicine in treating various ailments. Beyond the application of electrodes on the skin such as a transcutaneous electrical nerve stimulation (TENS), electrodes have been applied directly to nociceptive pathways.

Spinal cord stimulation (SCS) uses epidural electrodes placed along the dorsal columns to block nociception (42, 43). The system entails the surgical placement of epidural electrodes, cables, and radiofrequency transmitter or battery. Minimal discomfort is encountered in the placement of the system and in the postoperative period.

The mechanism of SCS is based on the gate control theory (Melzack and Wall) (43). It postulates that stimulating large nerve fibers (A beta fibers) can inhibit or modulate smaller nerve fibers (A delta or C fibers) transmitting nociceptive input, possibly at the dorsal root or horn of the spinal cord. Strategically placed epidural electrodes stimulate the dorsal columns (A beta fibers) to inhibit or modulate nociceptive input (A delta or C fibers). Ongoing research suggests that SCS may inhibit transmission in the spinothalamic tract, activate central inhibitory mechanisms influencing sympathetic efferent neurons, and release various inhibitory neurotransmitters.

SCS can be applied to treat neuropathic pain conditions including arachnoiditis, complex regional pain syndrome (formerly, reflex sympathetic dystrophy), neuropathies, brachial and lumbosacral plexopathies, radiculopathies, deafferentation

syndromes, phantom limb pain, and postherpetic neuralgia (44). Visceral syndromes such as interstitial cystitis, chronic abdominal pain, and chronic pancreatitis have been treated with limited success. SCS for cancer pain is limited to the dynamic nature and progression of neoplasms. SCS may have a role in stable neuropathic cancer pain related to cancer treatments and stable neoplasms.

VERTEBROPLASTY

Vertebroplasty is an image-guided, outpatient procedure, which may be used to treat pain associated with vertebral compression fractures caused by metastatic tumors or osteoporosis. Most vertebroplasties are performed for osteoporotic compression fractures, but patients with cancer pain can experience significant symptom relief with this procedure. Patients with anterior osteolytic lesions that are not amenable to surgical interventions may be candidates for this less invasive intervention. Contraindications for vertebroplasty include >70% vertebral collapse, epidural disease, asymptomatic stable fractures, or infection (45). However, there is growing evidence that these guidelines may not be absolute contraindications (46).

During vertebroplasty, one or two bone biopsy needles are inserted into the collapsed vertebral body through a small incision in the patient's back and acrylic bone cement is injected through the cannula to stabilize the fracture. The procedure typically requires a local anesthetic; conscious sedation is sometimes helpful, depending on the patient's condition and tolerance for medications that can compound hypotension. For many patients, however, vertebroplasty provides immediate (within 72 hours) and lasting relief from pain. Many patients are able to increase their level of activities within only a few days of the procedure.

Clinical studies show increasing success rates and extremely low complication rates. However, risks include infection, an allergic reaction to methacrylates, pulmonary embolism from intravascular injection, and weakness from displacement of fracture or extravasation of the injection into the intrathecal space.

NEUROSURGICAL PROCEDURES FOR PAIN

Despite optimized medical therapy and the use of interventions, some patients will still not achieve a satisfactory level of symptom control and may require neurosurgical procedures for pain relief. Although these procedures can be quite effective in treating specific cancer pain syndromes, careful patient selection is critical to maximize potential benefit. Neurosurgical treatment of medically refractory cancer pain usually involves the interruption of the specific involved pain-sensory pathways. These interventions most often include cordotomy, myelotomy, and other nervous system ablative procedures.

Cordotomy

Cordotomy is used for patients with unilateral medically intractable cancer pain below the level of C5 (17,48). Cordotomy involves lesioning of the anterior spinothalamic tract of the spinal cord that transmits nociceptive impulses from the contralateral half of the body. Interruption of this tract can be performed by an open operation or percutaneously. Because percutaneous cordotomies can be performed under local anesthesia with minimal morbidity, it has become the preferred technique. Percutaneous cordotomies are performed by placing a needle through the neck contralateral to the pain (because the spinothalamic tract fibers have crossed the spinal cord by this point) at the C1-2 level under CT scan guidance (47). Once the placement of the needle tip in the anterior spinothalamic tracts is confirmed, a permanent thermal lesion is made.

Cordotomy can provide excellent pain relief immediately after the procedure in >90% of patients. The effectiveness of this operation diminishes with time, and at 1-year after cordotomy 50–60% of patients will continue to have adequate pain control. Beyond 1 year, 40% of patients will continue to have adequate analgesia. Complications are rare (usually less than 5%) and frequently transient. Complications include ataxia, ipsilateral paresis, bowel/bladder dysfunction, ipsilateral Horner syndrome, sexual dysfunction, respiratory problems (sleep apnea or respiratory failure), and dysesthesias. Because there is a possibility of loss of ipsilateral diaphragmatic function with cordotomy, preoperative pulmonary function studies and dynamic radiographic studies should be performed to assess respiratory and diaphragmatic function. Patients with any pain ipsilateral to cordotomy will often see an exacerbation of this pain (*mirror-image pain*) and may require a second, staged cordotomy on the contralateral side.

Myelotomy

Myelotomy is primarily used for bilateral or midline pain in the lower half of the body. Patients with medically intractable pelvic, lower extremity, visceral, and perineal pain are potential candidates. Classically, myelotomy has been described as incising through the posterior midline of the spinal cord to ventral pia. It is hypothesized that this interrupts the second-order crossing spinothalamic pain fibers and has been designed to create a level of analgesia corresponding to the level and extent of interruption. This procedure is typically performed in the thoracolumbar region, and a number of open and closed techniques have been described (47).

Because of the variability in reported techniques, the region treated for relief from pain, and follow-up, it is difficult to draw definitive conclusions about the effectiveness of this technique. Nevertheless, some studies have shown that myelotomy provides pain relief in 80–90% of patients immediately after the procedure. Similar to other neurosurgical procedures for pain, the effectiveness of this operation diminishes with time, with reports of variable pain relief at distant time points (approximately 25% to 70% of patients with continued adequate relief). Myelotomy is generally well tolerated with a low rate of morbidity. Complications (approximately 10%) include temporary weakness of the lower extremities, transient loss of pain and temperature sensation, bowel/bladder incontinence, and dysesthesias. Reported mortality rates are generally in the range of 1 to 2%.

OTHER NEUROSURGICAL PROCEDURES

Mesencephalotomy

Candidates for mesencephalotomy include patients with cancer pain of the head and neck or cancer pain of the proximal upper extremity, or in those with diaphragmatic paralysis in whom cordotomy may be dangerous. Mesencephalotomy involves stereotactically creating a lesion in the rostral midbrain in structures lying just medial to the lateral spinothalamic tract (49). The results of several small, uncontrolled, retrospective studies suggest that 50–75% of patients may have

significant pain relief, over both the short term (months) to several years (up to 5 years' follow-up in some studies). Lesions at the level of the superior colliculus are more likely to be successful, but also more commonly lead to problems such as difficulty with extraocular movements and binocular vision (up to 10%) than do lesions that are placed slightly lower in the midbrain, at the level of the inferior colliculus.

Hypophysectomy

Candidates for hypophysectomy include patients with severe bone pain as a result of metastatic disease (breast or prostate carcinomas). Although both animal studies and clinical work has shown a connection between the pituitary gland and hypothalamus and pain and pain relief, the exact mechanisms remain poorly understood. Several groups in the 1960s and 1970s reported satisfying results with respect to both pain relief and tumor regression in up to 60% of patients treated with total hypophysectomy through a trans-sphenoidal approach. Other methods of hypophysectomy, such as direct trans-sphenoidal injection of absolute ethanol and Gamma knife radiation, have also been shown to provide moderate or even complete pain relief in most selected patients (50). These results can be difficult to predict, however, and may result from a variety of factors, including endocrine effects due to loss of cortisol, thyroid-stimulating hormone, or growth hormone, or due to stimulation of endorphin pathways; activation of stress-analgesic responses; or even a direct neurolytic effect. The natural consequence of the removal of the pituitary is panhypopituitarism, which carries with it significant morbidity. In addition, the need to perform these procedures under general anesthesia in patients who have been medically compromised potentially has led to waning interest in these approaches, except in carefully selected situations.

Microvascular Decompression

Microvascular decompression, an open neurosurgical approach, is based on the theory that aberrant torturous vessels compress the trigeminal nerve root entry zone at the brainstem, causing pain. By surgically placing an Ivalon or Teflon sponge between the artery and nerve, one can alleviate the facial pain. In one study, 90% of patients had sustained pain relief over 5 years and 46% recurrence of pain in 8.5 years (51).

SUMMARY

Interventional or surgical procedures may dramatically improve a patient's quality of life. Although they provide additional valuable tools when a medicinal or complementary approach fails to provide satisfactory symptom relief, the variability of patient presentation, including progression of disease, results in tremendous unpredictability of the outcome results. Pain may be alleviated in the treated site(s) while other pain elsewhere will not be affected. The distribution of locally administered drug(s) can also be variable, leading to a lessening rather than the complete resolution of the pain symptoms. The duration of the therapeutic effects may be only transient because of incompleteness of the procedure's effects. In rare cases, the intervention may further transiently aggravate or even permanently worsen pain symptoms, or other adverse events may further deteriorate the patient's quality of life. Therefore, the risks and benefits must be carefully weighed. Several texts on interventional pain that provide additional information on the indications, procedure, and risks are included in the references (52,53).

Despite the above cautions, advances in pain interventional techniques continue to improve the therapeutic benefit while reducing the risks. Imaging techniques allow greater visualization and, therefore, facilitate greater ease and precision in needle placement. This provides greater specificity in targeting pain pathways and reduces untoward effects. Further, new therapies that target novel sites are in various stages of clinical development. For example, neurolytic drugs that delete only pain-specific fibers (sparing other afferent and efferent pathways) have demonstrated safety and efficacy in preclinical testing (54).

Finally, more work is needed to validate the use of some of the many current pain interventions. Although interventional techniques are frequently utilized, many therapies have not undergone rigorous blinded controlled studies to determine efficacy. This is by no means an easy task and represents an ethical dilemma because of the necessity of withholding therapies that could increase suffering in this patient group.

References

1. Hanks GW, Justins DM. Cancer pain: management. *Lancet* 1992; 339(8800):1031–1036.
2. Meuser T, Pietruck C, Radbruch L, et al. Symptoms during cancer pain treatment following WHO-guidelines: a longitudinal follow-up study of symptom prevalence, severity and etiology. *Pain* 2001;93(3):247–257.
3. de Leon-Casasola OA. Interventional procedures for cancer pain management: when are they indicated? *Cancer Invest* 2004;22(4):630–642.
4. American Society of Anesthesiologists. Practice guidelines for cancer pain management. A report by the American Society of Anesthesiologists Task Force on Pain Management, Cancer Pain Section. *Anesthesiology* 1996;84(5):1243–1257.
5. Smith TJ, Coyne PJ, Staats PS, et al. An Implantable Drug Delivery System (IDDS) for refractory cancer pain provides sustained pain control, less drug-related toxicity, and possibly better survival compared with Comprehensive Medical Management (CMM). *Ann Oncol* 2005;16(5):825–833.
6. Ferrante FM. Opioids, In: Ferrante FM, ed. *Postoperative pain management.* New York: Churchill Livingstone, 1993:161.
7. Ferrante FM. Neuraxial infusion in the management of cancer pain. *Oncology* 1999;13(5 Suppl 2):30–36.
8. Kim PS. Interventional cancer pain therapies. *Semin Oncol* 2005;32(2):194–199.
9. Yaksh TL, Hassenbusch S, Burchiel K, et al. Inflammatory masses associated with intrathecal drug infusion: a review of preclinical evidence and human data. *Pain Med* 2002;3(4):300–312.
10. Mercadante S. Neuraxial techniques for cancer pain: an opinion about unresolved therapeutic dilemmas. *Reg Anesth Pain Med* 1999;24(1):74–83.
11. Bedder M, Burchiel K, Larson A, et al. Cost analysis of two implantable narcotic delivery systems. *J Pain Symptom Manage* 1991;6:368–373.
12. Burton AW, Rajagopal A, Shah HN, et al. Epidural and intrathecal analgesia is effective in treating refractory cancer pain. *Pain Med* 2004;5(3):239–247.
13. Staats PS, Yearwood T, Charapata SG, et al. Intrathecal ziconotide in the treatment of refractory pain in patients with cancer or AIDS: a randomized controlled trial. *JAMA* 2004;291(1):63–70.
14. Hassenbusch SJ, Portenoy RK, Cousins M, et al. Polyanalgesic consensus conference 2003: an update on the management of pain by intraspinal drug delivery—report of an expert panel. *J Pain Symptom Manage* 2004;27(6):540–563.
15. Ripamanti C, Brunelli C. Randomized clinical trials of an implantable drug delivery system compared with comprehensive medical management for refractory cancer pain: impact of pain drug related toxicity and survival. *J Clin Oncol* 2003;21(14):2801–2802.
16. Ilfeld B, Morey TE, Enneking FK, et al. Continuous infraclavicular brachial plexus block for postoperative pain control at home. *Anesthesiology* 2002;96(6):1297–1304.
17. Ilfeld B, Morey TE, Wright TW, et al. Continuous interscalene brachial plexus block for postoperative pain control at home: a randomized, double-blinded, placebo-controlled study. *Anesth Analg* 2003;96:1089–1095.
18. Klein S, Greengrass RA, Grant SA, et al. Ambulatory surgery for multi-ligament knee reconstruction with continuous dual catheter peripheral nerve blockade. *Can J Anaesth* 2001;48(4):375–378.
19. Swerdlow M. Spinal and peripheral neurolysis for managing Pancoast Syndrome. *Adv Pain Res Ther* 1982;4:135.
20. Ekatodramis G, Borgeat A, Huledal G, et al. Continuous interscalene analgesia with ropivacaine 2 mg/ml after major shoulder surgery. *Anesthesiology* 2003;98(1):143–150.
21. American Society of Anesthesiologists Task Force on Pain Management, C.P.S.. Practice guidelines for cancer pain management. *Anesthesiology* 1996;84(5):1243–1257.
22. Patt R, Cousins M. Techniques for neurolytic neural blockade. In: Cousins M, Bridenbaugh P, eds. *Neural blockade in clinical anesthesia and management of pain.* Philadelphia, PA: Lippincott Williams & Wilkins, 1998:1007–1061.
23. Cohen SP, Foster A. Pulsed radiofrequency as a treatment for groin pain and orchialgia. *Urology* 2003;61(3):645.
24. Patt R, Millard R. A role for peripheral neurolysis in the management of intractable cancer pain. *Pain* 1990;5(suppl):S358.
25. Patt R. Peripheral neurolysis. In: Patt R, ed. *Cancer pain.* Philadelphia, PA: JB Lippincott, 1993:359–376.
26. Meglio M, Cioni B. Percutaneous procedures for trigeminal neuralgia: microcompression versus radiofrequency thermocoagulation. Personal experience. *Pain* 1989;38(9):9–16.
27. Mullan S, Lichtor T. Percutaneous microcompression of the trigeminal ganglion for trigeminal neuralgia. *J Neurosurgery* 1983;59:1007.
28. Twycross R. *Pain relief in advanced cancer.* Edinburgh: Churchill Livingstone, 1994.
29. Swerdlaw M. Subarachnoid and extradural blocks. *Adv Pain Res Ther* 1979;2:325.
30. Doyle D. Nerves blocks in advanced cancer. *Practitioner* 1982;226:539.
31. Mehta M, Ranger I. Persistent abdominal pain. *Anaesthesia* 1971;26:330–333.
32. Leon-Casasola OA. Critical evaluation of chemical neurolysis of the sympathetic axis for cancer pain. *Cancer Control* 2000;7(2):142–148.
33. Black A, Dwyer B. Coeliac plexus block. *Anaesth Intensive Care* 1973;1:315.
34. Chapman CR, Donaldson GW. Issues in designing trials of nonpharmacologic treatments of pain. *Adv Pain Res Ther* 1991;18:699.
35. Filshie J, Golding S, Robbie DS, et al. Unilateral computerized tomography guided coeliac plexus block: a technique for pain relief. *Anaesthesia* 1983;38:498.
36. Gimenex A, Martinez-Noguera A, Donoso L, et al. Percutaneous neurolysis of the celiac plexus via the anterior approach with sonographic guidance. *Am J Radiol* 1993;161:1061.
37. Rykowski JJ, Hilgier M. Efficacy of neurolytic celiac plexus block in varying locations of pancreatic cancer: influence on pain relief. *Anesthesiology* 2000;92(2):347–354.
38. Lillemoe KD, Cameron JL, Kaufman HS, et al. Chemical splanchnicectomy in patients with unresectable pancreatic cancer: a prospective randomized trial.. *Ann Surg* 1993;217:447.
39. de Leon-Casasola OA. Critical evaluation of chemical neurolysis of the sympathetic axis for cancer pain. *Cancer Control* 2000;7(2):142–148.
40. Cariati M, De Martini G, Pretolesi F, et al. CT-guided superior hypogastric plexus block. *J Comput Assist Tomogr* 2002;26(3):428–431.
41. Ferrer-Brechner T. Epidural and intrathecal phenol neurolysis for cancer pain. *Anesthesiol Rev* 1981;8:14.
42. Tasker R. Percutaneous cordotomy: neurosurgical and neuroaugmentative intervention. In: Patt RB, *Cancer pain.* Philadelphia, PA: JB Lippincott, 1993:482.
43. Melzack R, Wall PD. Pain mechanisms: a new theory. *Science* 1965; 150(699):971–979.
44. Tasker R. Neurostimulation and percutaneous neural destructive techniques. In: Cousins M, Bridenbaugh P, eds. *Neural blockade in clinical anesthesia and management of pain.* Philadelphia: Lippincott Williams & Wilkins, 1998:1063–1111.
45. Jensen ME, Kallmes DE. Percutaneous vertebroplasty in the treatment of malignant spine disease. *Cancer J* 2002;8(2):194–206.
46. Hentschel SJ, Burton AW, Fourney DR, et al. Percutaneous vertebroplasty and kyphoplasty performed at a cancer center: refuting proposed contraindications. *J Neurosurg Spine* 2005;2(4):436–440.
47. Kanpolat Y, Akyar S, Caglar S, et al. CT-guided percutaneous selective cordotomy. *Acta Neurochir (Wien)* 1993;123(1–2):92–96.
48. White JC, Sweet WH. Anterolateral cordotomy: open versus closed comparison of end results. In: Bonica J, Liebeskind JC, Albe-Fessard D, eds. *Advances in pain research and therapy.* New York: Raven Press, 1979.
49. Bosch DA. Stereotactic rostral mesencephalotomy in cancer pain and deafferentation pain. A series of 40 cases with follow-up results. *J Neurosurg* 1991;75(5):747–751.
50. Hayashi M, Taira T, Chernov M, et al. Gamma knife surgery for cancer pain-pituitary gland-stalk ablation: a multicenter prospective protocol since 2002. *J Neurosurg* 2002;97(5 Suppl):433–437.
51. Loeser J. Tic couloureux and atypical facial pain. In: Wall P, Melzack R, eds. *Textbook of pain.* Edinburgh: Churchill Livingstone, 1994:688–710.
52. Waldman SD, Winnie AP, eds. *Interventional pain management.* Philadelphia, PA: WB Saunders, 2001.
53. Neural blockade. In: Cousins MJ, Bridenbaugh PO, eds. *Clinical anesthesia and management of pain.* Philadelphia, PA: Lippincott Williams & Wilkins, 1998.
54. Karai L, Brown DC, Mannes AJ, et al. Deletion of vanilloid receptor 1-expressing primary afferent neurons for pain control. *J Clin Invest* 2004;113(9):1344–1352.

CHAPTER 8 ■ ASSESSMENT AND MANAGEMENT OF CANCER-RELATED FATIGUE

CHRISTINE MIASKOWSKI AND RUSSELL K. PORTENOY

Fatigue is a highly prevalent symptom in populations with cancer and is often identified as a major impediment to function and quality of life (QOL) (1–4). It occurs at all stages of illness and is particularly prevalent during periods of active treatment and when the disease becomes advanced. It is now recognized as a serious clinical problem deserving focused strategies for assessment and treatment.

Despite its importance in the clinical setting, there has been limited research on fatigue. The epidemiology is poorly defined and the range of clinical presentations remains anecdotal. The possibility of discrete syndromes linked to specific predisposing factors or potential etiologies, and described by unique phenomenologies and pathophysiologies, has not been explored. Indeed, very few data are available to confirm the importance of any particular etiology, and pathophysiologic mechanisms for cancer-related fatigue are entirely conjectural. Perhaps most important, only a limited number of clinical trials has evaluated putative therapies for fatigue (for reviews, see refs 4–10). Treatment, when it is offered, is based largely on extrapolation of data from other clinical settings and anecdotal experience.

Nonetheless, significant progress has been made during the past decade. A definition of clinical fatigue has been developed and can now be used to define cases for survey research and clinical trials. Epidemiologic studies have begun to characterize fatigue trajectories in varied populations of patients with cancer, including those receiving chemotherapy (CTX) or radiation therapy (RT); those receiving specialist-level palliative care; and those who have survived cancer (for review, see ref 4). The commonalities and differences among these groups may add to an understanding of fatigue etiology or pathophysiology. Finally, clinical guidelines for management based on limited evidence and best practice have been developed, including recently published guidelines by the National Comprehensive Cancer Network (NCCN) (11).

DEFINITION OF FATIGUE

Although the case definition of fatigue as a clinical syndrome is essential for research and the development of rationale treatment guidelines, it has been difficult to define the criteria for diagnosis. Fatigue is a symptom and, as such, is inherently subjective. This subjective phenomenon must be distinguished from the "normal" fatigue common in the population, and the data that would be helpful to make this distinction on the basis of phenomenology, severity, duration, or impact have been lacking.

Recently, a multidisciplinary panel of clinicians and researchers convened by the NCCN revised practice guidelines for cancer-related fatigue. The Fatigue Practice Guidelines Panel defined cancer-related fatigue as "a persistent, subjective sense of tiredness related to cancer or cancer treatment that interferes with usual functioning" (11). An earlier definition, which was accepted as a diagnosis in the *International Classification of Diseases, 10th Revision, Clinical Modification*, states that fatigue is a multidimensional phenomenon that develops over time, diminishing energy, mental capacity, and the psychological condition of patients with cancer (Table 8.1) (11,12).

EPIDEMIOLOGY OF CANCER-RELATED FATIGUE

Studies have begun to explore the prevalence of fatigue in patients receiving cancer treatments or palliative care, as well as in cancer survivors. Most of these studies were performed before the effort to develop consensus concerning case definition and variation in the findings is related, in part, to the application of different criteria for diagnosis. To date, only two studies have evaluated the consensus-derived diagnostic criteria in patients receiving CTX or CTX and RT (13,14). In those studies, the percentage of patients who met the stringent diagnostic criteria for cancer-related fatigue ranged from 17 to 21%.

In other studies, fatigue associated with CTX has been far more variable. Prevalence rates for fatigue have ranged from 4% at the initiation of CTX to 91% at the end of treatment, and fatigue has been shown to vary during the course of treatment (15–18). In one study (16), 43% of the variance in fatigue was ascribed to disease symptoms and 35% to the toxicity of treatment.

Among those undergoing RT, the prevalence of fatigue has ranged from 8 to 92% (for review, see ref 4). This wide range may reflect the varying patient populations, types of RT, and fatigue assessment instruments used in the various studies. In a study of patients with rectal cancer who were receiving concomitant CTX and RT, the prevalence of moderate to severe fatigue rose from 44% at baseline to 59% at the end of treatment (19).

Fatigue prevalence has been high in the few studies that have been performed in populations with advanced cancer.

TABLE 8.1

CRITERIA FOR CANCER-RELATED FATIGUE

The following symptoms have been present everyday or nearly everyday during the same 2-wk period in the past month:

Significant fatigue, diminished energy, or increased need to rest, disproportionate to any recent change in activity level

Plus five (or more) of the following:

Complaints of generalized weakness or limb heaviness

Diminished concentration or attention

Decreased motivation or interest in engaging in usual activities

Insomnia or hypersomnia

Experience of sleep as unrefreshing or nonrestorative

Perceived need to struggle to overcome inactivity

Marked emotional reactivity (e.g., sadness, frustration, or irritability) to feeling fatigued

Difficulty completing daily tasks attributed to feeling fatigued

Perceived problems with short-term memory

Postexertional malaise lasting several hours

The symptoms cause clinically significant distress or impairment in social, occupational, or other important areas of functioning

There is evidence from the history, physical examination, or laboratory findings that the symptoms are the consequence of cancer or cancer-related therapy

The symptoms are not primarily a consequence of comorbid psychiatric disorders such as major depression, somatization disorder, somatoform disorder, or delirium

Adapted from Cella D, Peterman A, Passik S, et al. Progress toward guidelines for the management of fatigue. *Oncology* 1998;12:1–9, with permission.

Donnelly et al. (20), found that 48% of patients reported "clinically important" fatigue. In a prospective study that compared 95 palliative care patients with age- and sex-matched volunteers (21), 75% of the patients had severe fatigue.

Only a limited number of studies have evaluated fatigue levels in cancer survivors (13,22–24). Prevalence rates for fatigue ranged from 17 to 56%. These studies included patients with different cancer diagnoses (e.g., breast cancer, Hodgkin's disease) and evaluated them at different times after treatment (e.g., 2 years to 12 years). These differences may explain the wide range of prevalence rates in these studies.

Recent studies have begun to explore the patterns and correlates of cancer-related fatigue (for review, see ref 4). Most of these studies are descriptive cross-sectional studies that have evaluated relatively small, homogeneous samples of patients. Overall, increased levels of fatigue were found to correlate with decreases in health-related QOL in patients receiving RT (25,26), CTX (27), and in long-term cancer survivors (22).

Several studies have examined the putative biologic correlates of fatigue. Results have generally been unrevealing. In a sample of patients with lung cancer who underwent RT (28), neither weight loss nor prealbumin levels (a marker of impaired nutritional status) correlated with fatigue severity. In another study of patients who underwent autologous bone marrow transplantation for lymphoma (29), no correlation was found between fatigue and serum levels of inflammatory cytokines [i.e., interleukin [IL]-6, tumor necrosis factor (TNF), soluble NF receptor]. In another study (30), no correlation was found between fatigue and mild Leydig cell dysfunction in survivors of various hematologic malignancies. Finally, in a

study of men undergoing RT for prostate cancer (31), fatigue and serum IL-1 levels were found to increase between weeks 1 and 4, but no statistical correlation was found between the measures.

Cancer-related fatigue has been associated with a variety of psychological and demographic variables, other symptoms, and disease and treatment variables (4). Although the results have not been consistent across studies, the strongest correlates of fatigue severity appear to be psychological distress and symptom distress.

In a large case-controlled study of patients with breast cancer (22), the type of adjuvant treatment (i.e., CTX, RT, or both) did not predict fatigue levels, but fatigue was significantly predicted by levels of depression and pain. Another study found that fatigue after adjuvant CTX for breast cancer did not correlate with specific demographic disease or treatment characteristics, but was associated with other symptoms (i.e., poor sleep, menopausal symptoms), the use of catastrophizing as a coping strategy, and the presence of a psychiatric disorder (32). In contrast, prior CTX use was associated with greater fatigue in two other studies (33,34). Several studies have demonstrated a specific relationship between depression and fatigue (27,35–37), and anxiety was a significant predictor of chronic fatigue in a study of Hodgkin's disease survivors (38).

Given the variability in cancer populations and the complexity of fatigue, it is not surprising that studies have identified a range of potential correlates. A variety of patterns would be expected to exist if subtypes of cancer-related fatigue can be identified. More research is needed, however, before the incomplete and conflicting data can be reconciled. Studies must apply consistent case definition and assessment approaches to confirm and expand on the biologic, demographic, disease and treatment, and psychological correlates of fatigue in different groups of cancer patients.

Many parallels exist between cancer and other incurable, progressive diseases, such as acquired immunodeficiency syndrome (AIDS). Several studies have reported prevalence rates for fatigue in patients with AIDS that range from 54 to 65% (39–41). In one study (30), strong associations were found between the occurrence of fatigue and the number of AIDS-related physical symptoms, current treatment for human immunodeficiency virus–related medical disorders, anemia, and pain. In another study (40), women, Hispanics, the disabled, and those with inadequate income or insurance reported higher fatigue intensity scores. Additional research on the prevalence and correlates of fatigue in other chronic medical conditions is also warranted.

PATHOGENESIS OF FATIGUE

The mechanisms that precipitate or sustain fatigue in the cancer population are not known. The diversity of factors that may predispose to fatigue, cause it directly, or influence its expression, combined with the equally complex phenomenology of the symptom, suggest that it is not one disorder with a single mechanism. Rather, it is more likely that the fatigue associated with cancer or other medical illnesses actually represents a final common pathway to which many mechanisms may potentially contribute (3,42,43).

On theoretical grounds, it may be proposed that some fatigue is caused by abnormalities in energy metabolism related to increased need, decreased substrate, or the abnormal production of substances that impair intermediate metabolism or the normal functioning of muscles. Increased need, for example, could be associated with the hypermetabolic state that can accompany tumor growth, infection, fever, or surgery. Decreased substrate may account for the fatigue associated with anemia, hypoxemia of any cause, or poor nutrition.

Based on limited studies of muscle function in cancer patients, it has been suggested that some fatigue could be related to abnormal accumulation of muscle metabolites, such as lactate (44). There is no evidence linking this mechanism to fatigue, however, and if it were to occur, it could still reflect an epiphenomenon related to more fundamental disruption in metabolic activity.

The mechanisms that have been most intensively studied involve the production of cytokines, such as ILs, TNF, and others. There is good evidence that these compounds play a role in the cachexia experienced by some patients with cancer or AIDS (45). The link between cachexia and fatigue observed in the clinical setting, combined with the fatigue that often accompanies the exogenous administration of the biologic response modifiers when used as cancer therapy, suggests that similar mechanisms may be involved in the pathogenesis of at least some types of fatigue (46). However, as noted previously, several studies that have examined the relationship between serum cytokines and fatigue did not find significant correlations. At the present time, there is no direct evidence that any cytokine is causally related to the occurrence of fatigue. Measurement of these and other biochemical factors concurrent with systematic symptom assessment is needed to confirm the relationship.

Other mechanisms for fatigue probably exist as well. Changes in the efficiency of neuromuscular functioning could occur as a direct result of neurologic diseases, such as peripheral neuropathy, and result in fatigue. It is interesting to speculate that the fatigue sometimes reported in association with immobility and lack of exercise may also be due to reduced efficiency of neuromuscular functioning.

Again on theoretical grounds, cancer-related fatigue could also result from a sleep disorder. A sleep disorder could possibly cause disturbed arousal mechanisms or, equally plausible, be an indicator of a disorder of arousal. These disorders could be primary or related to metabolic disturbances or the use of centrally acting drugs. In one study (47), the relationships between daytime inactivity and nighttime restlessness and cancer-related fatigue were evaluated in 72 women who were undergoing the first of three cycles of CTX after surgery for stage I/II breast cancer. Women who were less active during the day and who had more nighttime awakenings consistently reported higher levels of cancer-related fatigue at the midpoints of each CTX cycle. In addition, the number of awakenings had the strongest association with the severity of fatigue. Additional work is warranted to determine the role that sleep disturbance and/or activity intolerance plays in the development of cancer-related fatigue.

Although it would be reasonable to assume that the extent of tumor burden or the presence of metastatic disease would be associated with increased levels of fatigue, several studies have not found significant correlations (21,24,48). However, these studies involved relatively small numbers of patients. Recent work by Stone et al. (49), which compared four groups of patients (i.e., recently diagnosed breast or prostate cancer patients, inoperable small cell lung cancer patients, and a group of patients receiving inpatient palliative care) found that the latter two groups had higher levels of fatigue. A significant correlation was found between increased tumor burden and increased fatigue. In addition, in a study of elderly patients newly diagnosed with different cancers, increased levels of fatigue were found in patients with late stage disease versus early stage disease (50). These findings suggest that tumor burden may in fact be involved in the pathophysiologic mechanisms of cancer-related fatigue.

Finally, it may be useful to postulate a mechanism of fatigue that may be specifically related to an affective disorder. The improvement in fatigue often noted by patients who were successfully treated for a major depression provides some support for this speculation.

Ultimately, it may be possible to assess the fatigue reported by a patient with cancer and infer from this assessment the nature of the underlying mechanism(s). This approach may in turn provide new avenues for therapies targeted to the specific mechanisms involved. A great deal more research is needed before this goal can be attained.

ASSESSMENT OF FATIGUE

Fatigue is a subjective, multidimensional symptom associated with a broad spectrum of physiologic disorders. Detailed characterization of the symptom, combined with an understanding of the most likely etiologic factors, is needed to fashion a therapeutic strategy that aims to minimize or reverse the likely causes and provide whatever symptomatic therapies are practicable.

Assessment of Fatigue Characteristics

The comprehensive assessment of fatigue begins with a detailed description of its phenomenology and the elaboration of hypotheses concerning etiology and pathogenesis. This information is acquired through the history, physical examination, and review of laboratory and imaging studies.

As noted, fatigue is multidimensional. Some of the dimensions that could be used to characterize fatigue are like those that could be applied to any other symptom, such as severity or associated distress. Other dimensions are unique to fatigue (Table 8.1). The quality of the fatigue varies substantially across patients and is one factor that suggests the potential to define meaningful subgroups. Patients may describe fatigue in terms that relate to lack of vitality, muscular weakness, dysphoric mood, somnolence, or impaired cognitive functioning. Commonly, the description will focus on several disturbances. In some cases, this description of fatigue quality will suggest an approach to therapy. For example, a patient who reports diminished energy throughout the day and somnolence in the morning may be describing an untoward reaction to a centrally acting drug taken at night. If such an agent is identified, a treatment strategy could be developed that would first address the morning symptoms by changing the drug regimen and then attempt to manage whatever residual fatigue remained.

The temporal characteristics of the fatigue complaint represent another important dimension. Acute fatigue has a recent onset and is anticipated to end in the near future. Chronic fatigue may be defined as fatigue that persists for a period of weeks and is not anticipated to remit soon. Although there is imprecision in this distinction, it is important in therapeutic decision making. A patient who is perceived to have chronic fatigue typically warrants a more intensive assessment and an approach to management focused on long-term as well as short-term goals.

Other temporal features, such as onset and course, are also clinically relevant. Fluctuation in the levels of fatigue that is linked to a discrete event, such as the administration of an antineoplastic therapy, is strong evidence of causation. Information about factors that exacerbate or relieve fatigue should be specifically queried. Like the course over time, this information may suggest an etiology or pathophysiologic mechanism, or may be therapeutically relevant.

In clinical practice, the assessment of fatigue must always include an evaluation of severity. The clinician should adopt one scale and use it consistently over time. The patient should be given a specific frame of reference when responding. For example, the patient might be asked to indicate the level of

Verbal rating scales

None	Mild	Moderate	Severe	

None	Mild	Moderate	Severe	Very severe

Numeric scale

"On a 0 to 10 scale, where "0" equals no fatigue and "10" equals the worst fatigue imaginable, how severe has fatigue been, on average, during the past week"

Four-point numeric scale (e.g., Common toxicity criteria of the National Cancer Institute)

	0	1	2	3	4
Fatigue (lethargy, malaise, asthenia)	None	Increased fatigue over baseline, but not altering normal activities	Moderate (e.g., decrease in performance status by 1 ECOG level *or* 20% Karnofsky or *Lansky*) or causing difficulty performing some activities	Severe (e.g., decrease in performance status by ≥2 ECOG levels *or* 40% Karnofsky *or Lansky*) loss of ability to perform some activities	Bedridden

Visual analog scale

No fatigue	Worst possible fatigue

FIGURE 8.1. Examples of unidimensional measures of fatigue severity. ECOG, Eastern Cooperative Oncology Group.

fatigue "on average during the past week." The clinician can choose a different frame of reference, if this is desired, as long as the same instructions are given whenever the patient is evaluated.

Instruments for the Assessment of Fatigue

Unidimensional fatigue measurement typically focuses on severity (Fig. 8.1). This assessment can be accomplished using a verbal rating scale (none, mild, moderate, severe), an 11-point numeric rating scale (where 0 equals "no fatigue" and 10 equals "the worst fatigue imaginable"), or a visual analog scale (also called a *linear analog scale assessment*). The linear analog scale is typically a 100-mm line anchored on the ends with opposing descriptors (e.g., "no fatigue" and "worst possible fatigue"). The psychometrics of a linear analog and a numeric scale have been evaluated in a medically ill population (51) and verbal rating scales and numeric scales have been incorporated into many symptom checklists (52–54).

Other types of unidimensional scales have been used to assess fatigue severity. The validated quality of life (QOL) measure created for the European Organization for Research and Treatment of Cancer, the European Organization for Research and Treatment of Cancer QOL Questionnaire C30, has a subscale for fatigue that may be used independently (55). The three items in this subscale (Were you tired? Have you felt weak? Did you need a rest?) are graded on four-point verbal rating scales, and the sum provides the global score. The nine-item Fatigue Severity Scale (56) and the vigor/fatigue subscale of the Profile of Mood States (57) also measure global fatigue severity.

Multidimensional fatigue questionnaires provide information about a range of characteristics other than intensity (58). There are now many validated instruments of this type (Table 8.2) (56,59–67) and these have their major use in research.

There are advantages and disadvantages in selecting a multidimensional assessment instrument. Most important, multidimensional assessment allows analyses that potentially clarify the nature of a fatigue syndrome or the type of response that occurs after an intervention. For example, a multidimensional instrument could help clarify the extent to which an intervention such as epoetin alfa affects fatigue in general, the cognitive component of fatigue, or mood.

There may also be disadvantages. Each questionnaire covers a differing set of domains, and investigators must review a measure carefully before assuming that it addresses the issues relevant to the specific situation. For example, many questionnaires do not assess sleep disturbance, mood disturbance, or cognitive impairment, and some do not evaluate fatigue-associated distress, temporal characteristics (e.g., onset, duration, fluctuation, course), or factors that worsen or relieve the fatigue.

To complement a multidimensional questionnaire, specific items can be developed, or additional validated questionnaires can be added to the questionnaire packet. The use of single

TABLE 8.2	O

MULTIDIMENSIONAL FATIGUE QUESTIONNAIRES

Piper fatigue scale (47)
Lee fatigue scale (48)
Fatigue assessment questionnaire (49)
Functional assessment of cancer therapy—anemia/fatigue (50)
Fatigue symptom inventory (51)
Brief fatigue inventory (52)
Cancer fatigue scale (53)
Schwartz cancer fatigue scale (54)
Multidimensional fatigue inventory (55)

items is simpler, but will not allow for a complete evaluation of the symptom experience and may limit the ability to determine correlations between the various dimensions of fatigue and various demographic and clinical correlates.

Other Fatigue-Related Evaluation

Identification of factors that may be contributing to the fatigue can suggest the use of a specific primary therapy directed to the etiology itself. All patients should undergo a medical and neurologic examination, and an evaluation of psychological status. Most patients should be screened for relevant hematologic or metabolic disturbances. The degree to which this and other types of laboratory or radiographic evaluation are pursued must be decided on a case-by-case basis. An extensive and costly evaluation that may be burdensome to the patient is justified only when the etiology is uncertain and the findings of the evaluation could lead to a change in therapy.

Assessment of Related Constructs

The occurrence of fatigue in the context of a progressive medical illness obligates the clinician to assess the symptom in a broader context. Chronic cancer-related fatigue cannot be addressed clinically without an understanding of the patient's overall QOL, symptom distress, and the goals of care. These constructs constantly inform decision making.

QOL is itself a subjective, multidimensional construct that reflects the overall perception of well-being. The most relevant dimensions that contribute to QOL, or conversely, to the degree of suffering, pertain to physical, psychological, social, and existential or spiritual concerns (66,67). To fully characterize the impact of fatigue, the assessment should attempt to discern the degree to which this symptom contributes to impairment in QOL and, concurrently, identify other factors that may be equally or more important. These factors may include other symptoms, progressive physical decline, independent psychological disorders, social isolation, financial concerns, spiritual distress, or others. This larger assessment allows the development of a therapeutic strategy that should be more likely to yield improved QOL than one focused entirely on a single symptom.

In assessing physical and psychological concerns, it is important to recognize that most cancer patients experience multiple symptoms concurrently (68,69). Studies have generally demonstrated that pain, fatigue, and psychological distress are the most prevalent symptoms across varied cancer populations. The construct of global symptom distress has been useful to characterize overall symptom burden (52–54), and in some situations it is useful to consider symptom distress as the critical issue when assessing QOL. Patients who report fatigue should always be queried about the presence of other symptoms.

The issues encountered in the assessment of fatigue may also be clarified by another construct, the goals of care. At any point during the course of the disease, the patient, the patient's family, and clinicians may emphasize one or more of the major goals in this setting:

1. To cure or prolong life
2. To maintain function
3. To provide comfort

The assessment of the goals of care derives from both the patient's desires and knowledge of the medical realities. Lack of clarity or disagreement about the goals of care can skew the assessment process and undermine the relationship with the patient and family. To avoid these problems, ongoing assessment of the goals of care and communication with the patient and family about these goals must be considered among the most important and challenging aspects of patient care.

MANAGEMENT OF FATIGUE

The comprehensive assessment of the patient with cancer-related fatigue allows the development of a strategy that attempts to ameliorate this symptom while addressing disease management and other palliative needs more broadly. In some cases, therapy for fatigue should be aggressively pursued, whereas in others, interventions for fatigue can be subordinated to other therapeutic imperatives. These priorities should be developed collaboratively with the patient.

An algorithm for the treatment of fatigue has been developed on the basis of the limited existing data and clinical experience (Figs. 8.2A, B) (70). After setting realistic expectations, the fundamentals include decisions about treatment for potential contributing causes and decisions about a variety of symptomatic therapies, both pharmacologic and nonpharmacologic.

Establishing Realistic Expectations

Education of the patient about the nature of fatigue, the options for therapy, and the anticipated results is an essential component of any therapeutic approach to fatigue (See the section Patient Education). In some situations, such as fatigue associated with advanced disease and organ failure, there are limited expectations for reversal of the symptom and this should be explained to the patient as part of a plan to improve adaptation. If there is reason to believe that the fatigue will be transitory, this information alone can sometimes suffice as therapy.

Primary Interventions

Interventions for fatigue can involve primary management of factors that are believed to be causally related, symptomatic interventions, or both. Although the range of factors associated with fatigue (Table 8.3) offers many opportunities for primary interventions, the decision to pursue a specific therapy is often difficult. None of these interventions has been studied as primary treatments for fatigue. There may be many potential factors, and their relative importance is often unclear. In the medically frail, interventions must be undertaken cautiously. The trial-and-error process of manipulating first one and then another contributing factor can be time-consuming and frustrating for the patient. Some of the potential causes for fatigue, such as the use of centrally acting drugs, are extremely prevalent, and it is often difficult to justify efforts to alter these factors when there is risk in doing so and they are so commonly used without the complication of fatigue.

Some primary interventions pose relatively little burden for the patient. The threshold for implementing these interventions is low. For example, all patients who complain of fatigue should undergo review of the drug regimen. Centrally acting drugs that are not essential should be eliminated or reduced. Polypharmacy is extremely common, particularly in the setting of advanced cancer, and there is often a tendency to continue drugs that have questionable benefit due to concerns about worsening symptoms if they are stopped. The experience of fatigue shifts the therapeutic index and clearly justifies a trial of dose reduction, at the least. The drugs that are usually considered in this case include antiemetics, hypnotics or anxiolytics, antihistamines, and analgesics. If pain is controlled

TABLE 8.3

POSSIBLE PREDISPOSING FACTORS OR ETIOLOGIES OF CANCER-RELATED FATIGUE

MEDICAL/PHYSICAL CONDITIONS
- Associated with the underlying disease itself
- Associated with treatment for the disease
  - Chemotherapy
  - Radiotherapy
  - Surgery
  - Biological response modifiers
- Associated with intercurrent systemic disorders
  - Anemia
  - Infection
  - Pulmonary disorders
  - Hepatic failure
  - Heart failure
  - Renal insufficiency
  - Malnutrition
  - Neuromuscular disorders
  - Dehydration or electrolyte disturbances
- Associated with sleep disorders
- Associated with immobility and lack of exercise
- Associated with chronic pain
- Associated with the use of centrally acting drugs (e.g., opioids)

PSYCHOSOCIAL FACTORS
- Associated with anxiety disorders
- Associated with depressive disorders
- Stress-related
- Related to environmental reinforcers

with an opioid, the experience of distressing fatigue often justifies cautious dose reduction (e.g., 25% of the total daily dose) to determine whether fatigue improves without worsening pain.

The threshold for intervening in an effort to reduce physical inactivity, insomnia, some metabolic abnormalities, or depressed mood is also usually low. Suggestions to pursue exercise, if possible, and nonpharmacological therapy for a sleep disorder, are often accepted enthusiastically by patients (See the section Symptomatic Therapy: Nonpharmacological Approaches). Prescription of a hypnotic can be useful but clearly requires careful monitoring. If sleep duration increases but the patient perceives it to be nonrestorative, the desired goal has not been achieved. As might be expected, the use of a centrally acting hypnotic may worsen daytime fatigue in some patients.

Fatigue can be associated with varied metabolic disturbances. Some, such as the derangements associated with renal failure, may not be treatable in the context of the overall disease. Others, such as dehydration, hypercalcemia, hypothyroidism, adrenal insufficiency, or hypoxia, can be managed at little risk. Interventions to improve these disturbances may be warranted in the overall approach to the fatigued patient.

A trial of an antidepressant in a fatigued patient with major depression is strongly indicated. More challenging is the decision to implement antidepressant therapy in the patient who has dysphoric mood but is not anhedonic and lacks other psychological criteria for the diagnosis of major depression. Although there are some risks with this therapy, most clinicians perceive

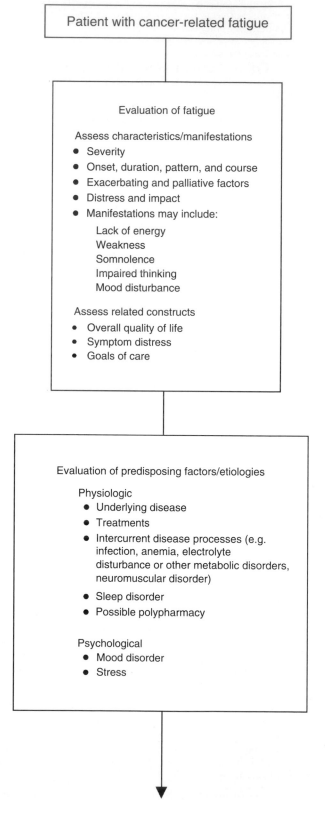

A

FIGURE 8.2 A, B: Algorithm proposed for the treatment of cancer-related fatigue. Hb, hemoglobin. (Adapted from Potency RK, Itri LM. Cancer-related fatigue: guidelines for evaluation and management. *Oncologist* 1999;4:1–10, with permission.)

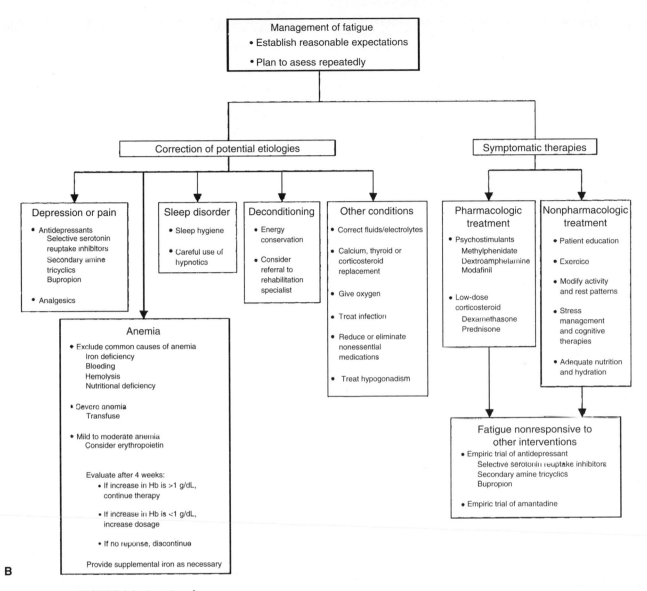

FIGURE 8.2. (*continued*)

that a treatment trial is warranted with any significant degree of depressed mood, particularly if there are other targets for the drug, such as anxiety or pain. In the setting of fatigue, a trial of a relatively less sedating antidepressant, such as one of the selective serotonin or serotonin and norepinephrine reuptake inhibitors, bupropion, or one of the secondary amine tricyclic antidepressants (such as desipramine or nortriptyline) is appropriate. A small open label study suggested that modified-release bupropion reduced fatigue in some patients with cancer (71).

Extensive data indicate that anemia may be a major factor in cancer-related fatigue and the impairment in QOL that it causes (72). Anecdotally, transfusion therapy for severe anemia can promptly reverse fatigue. The introduction of recombinant human erythropoietin (rHuEPO) was a major advance and numerous studies have established that erythropoietin increases hemoglobin and reduces the risk of red blood cell transfusion regardless of baseline hemoglobin level (for review, see refs 8–10). A meta analysis has established the benefits of anemia management with erythropoietin on fatigue and QOL (73) and physicians now commonly treat anemia with the goal of achieving Hb levels adequate to relieve

anemia-related fatigue. Evidence-based guidelines indicate that there is strong evidence for treatment in patients with hemoglobin ≤10, for whom an increase in hemoglobin reduces transfusion risk as well as improves symptoms (74). Treatment of more mild degrees of anemia to improve fatigue and QOL is also supported by data from controlled randomized trials (75), and there is a suggestion that the largest improvement in QOL per gram per deciliter change in hemoglobin actually occurs between 11 g/dL and 12 g/dL.

Symptomatic Therapy

Pharmacologic approaches. There have been few clinical trials of pharmacologic therapies for fatigue associated with medical illness. Clinical experience with psychostimulant drugs has been favorable and a trial of a stimulant to address fatigue is now commonplace. Evidence of effectiveness and clinical experience are most extensive for methylphenidate (76–79). Modafinil has been studied for fatigue related to a variety of chronic disorders other than cancer. Although randomized controlled trials in some disorders have been negative (80,81), other trials have shown benefit (82,83). It is usually well tolerated and its use has grown in the cancer population. Other psychostimulant drugs, including methamphetamine and amphetamine, are occasionally used empirically. Atomoxetine, a nonamphetamine stimulant approved for attention deficit disorder, could be potentially tried for this indication, but use for clinical fatigue of any type has been very limited.

In medically fragile patients, the initial dose of methylphenidate is usually 2.5–5.0 mg once or twice daily. This dose is gradually escalated until favorable effects occur or toxicity supervenes. Most patients require low doses, but effects are clearly dose-dependent, and dose titration should be undertaken in the absence of side effects; doses above 60 mg per day are uncommon but sometimes needed. Effects may wane over time, a change that could reflect tolerance or progression of the underlying cause of the fatigue, and dose escalation may be needed to maintain effects. The risk of toxicity increases with the dose, however, and the ability to regain lost efficacy may be limited.

The starting doses for modafinil is usually 100–200 mg daily. Occasional patients require titration to 2–3 times this dose. Dextroamphetamine and amphetamine are administered in doses that are similar to those of methylphenidate for this indication.

The potential toxicities associated with the psychostimulants include anorexia; insomnia; anxiety, confusion, and other organic brain syndromes; tremor; and tachycardia. These effects can be particularly problematic in the medically ill, who may be predisposed to the same symptoms for other reasons. Relative contraindications include preexisting anorexia, severe insomnia, anxiety, or agitation (particularly if associated with paranoid ideation), and significant heart disease. To ensure safety, dose escalation of the psychostimulants should be undertaken cautiously, and at intervals long enough to evaluate the incipient development of the potential toxicities.

The use of low-dose corticosteroids as a treatment for fatigue has also been supported empirically (84,85). This treatment is usually considered in the population with advanced disease and multiple symptoms. There have been no comparative trials of the different agents in this class. Therapy is usually undertaken with dexamethasone, 1–2 mg twice daily, or prednisone, 5–10 mg twice daily.

Amantadine has been used for the treatment of fatigue due to multiple sclerosis for many years (73). However, a recent systematic review of the use of amantadine for fatigue in multiple sclerosis concluded that whereas amantadine treatment was well tolerated, its efficacy in decreasing fatigue in patients with multiple sclerosis is poorly documented (86). Additional trials are needed to determine the efficacy of this drug in other clinical populations.

As noted previously, a therapeutic trial with an antidepressant drug is clearly appropriate if fatigue is related to a clinical depression. If fatigue is severe, the use of an antidepressant that is relatively less likely to be sedating, such as bupropion or one of the selective serotonin reuptake inhibitors, serotonin and norepinephrine selective reuptake inhibitors or secondary amine tricyclics, would be preferred. Some patients appear to experience increased energy disproportionate to any clear effect on mood during treatment with one of these drugs. In those with refractory severe fatigue and no depression, it may be reasonable to consider a trial of an activating antidepressant as a primary treatment for the fatigue. Bupropion has been used empirically for this purpose, with some favorable observations. Further study of this drug for fatigue is warranted. A randomized trial of paroxetine in a cancer population did not reveal a positive effect on fatigue (87).

Nonpharmacologic approaches. As noted, all patients with distressing fatigue require education to set realistic expectations. This communication is the simplest of the diverse

NONPHARMACOLOGIC INTERVENTIONS TO MANAGE FATIGUE

Patient education
Exercise
Modification of activity and rest patterns
Stress management and cognitive therapies
Adequate nutrition and hydration

nonpharmacologic approaches that can be used to manage this symptom. Although there have been empiric evaluations of these nonpharmacologic therapies, anecdotal experience suggests that several types of interventions may be useful (Table 8.4). Studies are needed to evaluate the effectiveness of these techniques.

Patient preferences must be considered in developing a nonpharmacologic strategy for fatigue. Participation is unlikely unless the patient perceives a substantial chance of benefit and only modest burden. More than one type of nonpharmacologic intervention may be useful depending on the etiology of the fatigue.

Patient education. Patient education that contains both procedural and sensory information has been shown to be effective in reducing pain and improving outcomes (88,89). Inadequate information may lead to needless anxiety. As noted previously, the fatigued patient should receive information about the nature of the symptom, the options for therapy, and the expected outcomes. Many patients assume that the problem reflects worsening of the disease and information about alternative explanations, if any are identified, can be very reassuring. There are large individual differences in patients' preferences for information, and the effort to educate, which is appropriate to the patient's educational level and readiness to learn, should be provided.

As part of the educational process, patients may find it beneficial to keep a diary of their fatigue. The diary may help clinicians and patients discern a pattern to the fatigue and monitor its severity. This information may be useful in developing a management plan that modifies specific activities and incorporates appropriate periods of rest.

Exercise. Of the nonpharmacologic interventions for cancer-related fatigue, exercise has the strongest evidence of a therapeutic benefit (4,6,7). These studies have demonstrated significantly lower levels of fatigue in patients who exercised compared with controls. However, data that would allow the selection of the most appropriate exercise program for patients with various types of cancer or cancer treatments are not available.

Some general principles should be followed when prescribing exercise for a cancer patient. The exercise prescription should be individualized and consider such factors as the patient's age, gender, physical condition, and any intercurrent medical conditions that may affect the individual's ability to exercise. Anecdotally, the type of exercise that appears to be most beneficial in ameliorating fatigue is exercise that involves rhythmic and repetitive movement of large muscle groups. This effect is achieved through walking, cycling, or swimming. An exercise program should be initiated gradually and patients should not exercise to the point of exhaustion. Exercise needs to be done for several days out of the week for beneficial effects to occur.

Contraindications to low-intensity exercise include cardiac abnormalities, recurrent or unexplained pain, onset of nausea with exercise, extreme fatigability, or cyanosis. A referral to an exercise physiologist may be warranted to have a more thorough evaluation and a specific exercise prescription developed for each individual patient.

Modification of activity and rest patterns. The use of a diary to assess fatigue may identify specific activities that are associated with increased levels of fatigue. This information can facilitate a plan to modify, schedule, or pace these activities throughout the day. Brief, scheduled rest periods may help to reduce fatigue. Naps should be allowed only during the day because a period of sleep in the late afternoon or evening may interfere with the patient's ability to sleep at night.

One of the most important interventions in the area of activity and rest pattern modification is an assessment for sleep disturbances and patient education about basic sleep hygiene principles. Again, education about sleep hygiene principles should be tailored to the individual patient. One of the fundamental principles is the establishment of a specific bedtime and wake time. A specific wake time appears to be particularly important in maintaining a normal sleep–wake rhythm. An additional strategy is the establishment of routine procedures before sleep. For example, patients may read a book or watch television before falling asleep (90).

Exercise on a consistent basis tends to improve sleep and promote deeper sleep. If exercise is also used, it should be performed at least 6 hours before bedtime. Intense exercise raises the body temperature for at least 6 hours and it appears preferable for this period to pass before sleep.

Additional sleep hygiene measures include reduced environmental stimuli (e.g., loud noises, light) and the use of diversional activities (e.g., music, massage) to promote sleep. Patients should also be instructed to avoid stimulants (e.g., caffeine, nicotine, steroids, methylphenidate) and central nervous system depressants (e.g., alcohol) before sleep (90).

Stress management and cognitive therapies. Anxiety, difficulties in coping with cancer or its treatment, or sleep disturbances are some of the factors that may contribute to the development of fatigue. These factors may be ameliorated using stress-reduction techniques or cognitive therapies (e.g., relaxation therapy, hypnosis, guided imagery, distraction). Research has demonstrated that distraction (e.g., gardening, listening to music, taking quiet walks) may be effective in reducing the symptom, particularly for patients with fatigue associated with deficits in attention (91,92). A referral to a psychiatrist or a psychologist for counseling and training in stress management techniques or cognitive therapies may be warranted in some patients.

Adequate nutrition and hydration. Cancer and its treatment can interfere with dietary intake. Fatigued individuals may also underestimate the amount of food and fluid they ingest. To aggressively manage fatigue, patients' weight, hydration status, and electrolyte balance should be monitored and maintained to the extent possible. Regular exercise may improve appetite and increase nutritional intake. Referral to a dietitian for dietary planning and suggestions for nutritional supplements may be beneficial if one of the causes of fatigue is inadequate food or fluid intake.

CONCLUSION

Despite the high prevalence and distress associated with fatigue, relatively little is known about its epidemiology, etiologies, and management. No definitive information is available on the types of mechanisms that may produce fatigue in discrete populations. Therefore, the development of mechanism-based interventions is extremely difficult.

With burgeoning interest in palliative care, it is likely that increasing attention will focus on the problem of fatigue. Extensive research is needed before the symptom will be adequately characterized in terms of phenomenology, pathogenesis, and management.

References

1. Vogelzang N, Breitbart W, Cella D, et al. Patient, caregiver, and oncologists perceptions of cancer-related fatigue: results of a tripart assessment survey. *Semin Hematol* 1997;34(Suppl 2):4–12.
2. Curt G, Breitbart W, Cella D, et al. Impact of cancer-related fatigue on the lives of patients: new findings from the fatigue coalition. *Oncologist* 2000;5:355–360.
3. Stasi R, Abriani L, Beccaglia P, et al. Cancer-related fatigue—evolving concepts in evaluation and treatment. *Cancer* 2003;98:1786–1801.
4. Lawrence DP, Kupelnick B, Miller K, et al. Evidence report on the occurrence, assessment, and treatment of fatigue in cancer patients. *J Natl Cancer Inst Monogr* 2004;32:40–50.
5. Ahlberg K, Ekman T, Gaston-Johansson F, et al. Assessment and management of cancer-related fatigue in adults. *Lancet* 2003;362:640–650.
6. Mock V. Evidenced-based treatment for cancer-related fatigue. *J Natl Cancer Inst Monogr* 2004;32:112–118.
7. Stevinson C, Lawlon DA, Fox KR. Exercise interventions for cancer patients: systematic review of controlled clinical trials. *Cancer Causes and Control* 2004;15:1035–1056.
8. Bohlius J, Langensiepen S, Schwarzer G, et al. Erythropoietin for patients with malignant disease. *Cochrane Database Syst Rev* 2004;14(3):210–215.
9. Jones M, Schenkel B, Just J, et al. Epoetin alfa improves quality of life in patients with cancer: results of metaanalysis. *Cancer* 2004;101(8):1720–1732.
10. Djulbegovic B. Erythropoietin use in oncology: a summary of the evidence and practice guidelines comparing efforts of the Cochrane review group and Blue Cross/Blue Shield to set up the ASCO/ASH guidelines. *Best Pract Res Clin Haematol* 2005;18(3):455–466.
11. National Comprehensive Cancer Center Network Practice Guidelines. *Cancer-Related Fatigue Panel 2004.* Guidelines version 1.2004, March. Rockledge, PA: National Comprehensive Cancer Network. (Available at http://www.nccn.org), 2004.
12. Cella D, Peterman A, Passik S, et al. Progress toward guidelines for the management of fatigue. *Oncology* 1998;12:1–9.
13. Cella D, Davis K, Breitbart B, et al. Cancer-related fatigue: prevalence of proposed diagnostic criteria in a United States sample of cancer survivors. *J Clin Oncol* 2001;19:3385–3391.
14. Sadler IJ, Jacobsen PB, Booth-Jones M, et al. Preliminary evaluation of a clinical syndrome approach to assessing cancer-related fatigue. *J Pain Symptom Manage* 2002;23:406–416.
15. Richardson A, Ream EK. Self-care behaviours initiated by chemotherapy patients in response to fatigue. *Int J Nurs Stud* 1997;34:35–43.
16. Hurny C, Bernhard J, Joss R, et al. "Fatigue and malaise" as a quality-of-life indicator in small-cell lung cancer patients. The Swiss Group for clinical cancer research (SAKK). *Support Care Cancer* 1993;1:316–320.
17. Jacobsen PB, Hann DM, Azzarello LM, et al. Fatigue in women receiving adjuvant chemotherapy for breast cancer: characteristics, course, and correlates. *J Pain Symptom Manage* 1999;18:233–242.
18. Gaston-Johansson F, Fall-Dickson JM, Bakos AB, et al. Fatigue, pain, and depression in pre-autotransplant breast cancer patients. *Cancer Pract* 1999;7:240–247.
19. Wang XS, Janjan NA, Guo H, et al. Fatigue during preoperative chemoradiation for resectable rectal cancer. *Cancer* 2001;92:1725–1732.
20. Donnelly S, Walsh D, Rybicki L. The symptoms of advanced cancer: identification of clinical and research priorities by assessment of prevalence and severity. *J Palliat Care* 1995;11:27–32.
21. Stone P, Hardy J, Broadley K, et al. Fatigue in advanced cancer: a prospective controlled cross-sectional study. *Br J Cancer* 1999;79:179–186.
22. Bower JE, Ganz PA, Desmond KA, et al. Fatigue in breast cancer survivors: occurrence, correlates, and impact on quality of life. *J Clin Oncol* 2000;18:743–753.
23. Loge JH, Abrahamsen AF, Ekeberg O, et al. Hodgkin's disease survivors are more fatigued than the general population. *J Clin Oncol* 1999;17:253–261.
24. Okuyama T, Akechi T, Kugaya A, et al. Factors correlated with fatigue in disease-free breast cancer patients: application of the Cancer Fatigue Scale. *Support Care Cancer* 2000;8:215–222.
25. Irvine DM, Vincent L, Graydon JE, et al. Fatigue in women with breast cancer receiving radiation therapy. *Cancer Nurs* 1998;21:127–135.
26. Lovely MP, Miaskowski C, Dodd M. Relationship between fatigue and quality of life in patients with glioblastoma multiformae. *Oncol Nurs Forum* 1999;26:921–925.
27. Redeker NS, Lev EL, Ruggiero J. Insomnia, fatigue, anxiety, depression, and quality of life of cancer patients undergoing hemotherapy. *Sch Inq Nurs Pract* 2000;14:275–290.
28. Beach P, Siebeneck B, Buderer NR, et al. Relationship between fatigue and nutritional status in patients receiving radiation therapy to treat lung cancer. *Oncol Nurs Forum* 2001;28:1027–1031.
29. Knobel H, Loge JH, Nordoy T, et al. High level of fatigue in lymphoma patients treated with high dose therapy. *J Pain Symptom Manage* 2000;19:446–456.

30. Howell SJ, Radford JA, Smets EM, et al. Fatigue, sexual function and mood following treatment for hematological malignancy: the impact of mild Leydig cell dysfunction. *Br J Cancer* 2000;82:789–793.
31. Greenberg DB, Gray JL, Mannix CM, et al. Treatment-related fatigue and serum interleukin-1 levels in patients during external beam irradiation for prostate cancer. *J Pain Symptom Manage* 1993;8:196–200.
32. Broeckel JA, Jacobsen PB, Horton J, et al. Characteristics and correlates of fatigue after adjuvant chemotherapy for breast cancer. *J Clin Oncol* 1998;16:1689–1696.
33. Mast ME. Correlates of fatigue in survivors of breast cancer. *Cancer Nurs* 1998;21:136–142.
34. Woo B, Dibble SL, Piper BF, et al. Differences in fatigue by treatment methods in women with breast cancer. *Oncol Nurs Forum* 1998;2:915–920.
35. Irvine D, Vincent L, Graydon JE, et al. The prevalence and correlates of fatigue in patients receiving chemotherapy and radiotherapy. A comparison of fatigue experienced by health individuals. *Cancer Nurs* 1994;17: 367–378.
36. Akechi T, Kugaya A, Okamura H, et al. Fatigue and its associated factors in ambulatory cancer patients: a preliminary study. *J Pain Symptom Manage* 1999;17:42–48.
37. Hann DM, Garovoy N, Finkelstein B, et al. Fatigue and quality of life in breast cancer patients undergoing autologous stem cell transplantation: a longitudinal comparative study. *J Pain Symptom Manage* 1999;17:311–319.
38. Loge JH, Abrahamsen AF, Ekeberg O, et al. Fatigue and psychiatric morbidity among Hodgkin's disease survivors. *J Pain Symptom Manage* 2000;19:91–99.
39. Breitbart W, McDonald MV, Rosenfeld B, et al. Fatigue in ambulatory AIDS patients. *J Pain Symptom Manage* 1998;15:157–167.
40. Voss JG. Predictors and correlates of fatigue in HIV/AIDS. *J Pain Symptom Manage* 2005;29(2):173–184.
41. Henderson M, Safa F, Easterbrook P, et al. Fatigue among HIV-infected patients in the era of highly active antiretroviral therapy. *HIV Med* 2005;6(5):347–352.
42. Gutstein HB. The biological basis of fatigue. *Cancer* 2001;92:1678–1683.
43. Wagner LI, Cella D. Fatigue and cancer: causes, prevalence, and treatment approaches. *Br J Cancer* 2004;91:822–828.
44. Burt ME, Aoki TT, Gorschboth CM, et al. Peripheral tissue metabolism in cancer-bearing man. *Ann Surg* 1983;198:685–691.
45. Billingsley KG, Alexander HR. The pathophysiology of cachexia in advanced cancer and AIDS. In: Bruera E, Higginson I, eds. *Cachexia-anorexia in cancer patients*. New York: Oxford University Press, 1996:1–22.
46. Neuenschwander H, Bruera E. Asthenia-cachexia. In: Bruera E, Higginson I, eds. *Cachexia-anorexia in cancer patients*. New York: Oxford University Press, 1996:57–75.
47. Berger AM, Farr L. The influence of daytime inactivity and nighttime restlessness on cancer-related fatigue. *Oncol Nurs Forum* 1999;26:1663–1671.
48. Bruera E, Brenneis C, Michaud M, et al. Association between asthenia and nutritional status, lean body mass, anemia, psychological status, and tumor mass in patients with advanced breast cancer. *J Pain Symptom Manage* 1989;4:59–63.
49. Stone P, Richards M, A'Hearn R. A study to investigate the prevalence, severity, and correlates of fatigue among patients with cancer in comparison with a control group of volunteers without cancer. *Ann Oncol* 2000;11:561–567.
50. Given CW, Given B, Azzouz F, et al. Predictors of pain and fatigue in the year following diagnosis among elderly cancer patients. *J Pain Symptom Manage* 2001;21:456–466.
51. Brunier G, Graydon J. A comparison of two methods of measuring fatigue in patients on chronic haemodialysis: visual analogue vs Likert scale. *Int J Nurs Stud* 1996;33:338–348.
52. de Haes JCJM, van Kippenberg FCE, Neijt JP. Measuring psychological and physical distress in cancer patients: structure and application of the Rotterdam Symptom Checklist. *Br J Cancer* 1990;62:1034–1038.
53. McCorkle R, Young K. Development of a symptom distress scale. *Cancer Nurs* 1978;1:373–378.
54. Portenoy RK, Thaler HT, Kornblith AB, et al. The memorial symptom assessment scale: an instrument for the evaluation of symptom prevalence, characteristics, and distress. *Eur J Cancer* 1994;30A:1326–1336.
55. Aaronson NK, Ahmedzai S, Bergman B, et al. The European Organization for Research and Treatment of Cancer QLQ-C30: a quality-of-life instrument for use in international clinical trials in oncology. *J Natl Cancer Inst* 1993;85:376–385.
56. Krupp LB, LaRocca NG, Muir-Nash J, et al. The fatigue severity scale: application to patients with multiple sclerosis and systemic lupus erythematosus. *Arch Neurol* 1989;46:1121–1123.
57. Cella DF, Jacobsen PB, Orav EJ, et al. A brief POMS measure of distress for cancer patients. *J Chronic Dis* 1987;40:939–942.
58. Meek PM, Nail LM, Barsevick A, et al. Psychometric testing of fatigue instruments for use with cancer patients. *Nurs Res* 2000;49(4):181–190.
59. Piper BF, Dibble SL, Dodd MJ, et al. The revised Piper fatigue scale: psychometric evaluation in women in breast cancer. *Oncol Nurs Forum* 1998;25:677–684.
60. Lee KA, Hicks G, Nino-Murcia G. Validity and reliability of a scale to assess fatigue. *Psychiatry Res* 1991;36:291–298.
61. Glaus A. *Fatigue in patients with cancer—analysis and assessment. Recent results in cancer research*. Berlin, Germany: Springer-Verlag, 1996.
62. Yellen SB, Cella DF, Webster MA, et al. Measuring fatigue and other anemia-related symptoms with the Functional Assessment of Cancer Therapy (FACT) measurement system. *J Pain Symptom Manage* 1997;13:63–74.
63. Hann DM, Jacobsen PB, Azzarello LM, et al. Measurement of fatigue in cancer patients: development and validation of the Fatigue Symptom Inventory. *Qual Life Res* 1998;7:301–310.
64. Mendoza TR, Wang XS, Cleeland CS, et al. The rapid assessment of fatigue severity in cancer patients: use of the Brief Fatigue Inventory. *Cancer* 1999;85:1186–1196.
65. Okuyama T, Akechi T, Kugaya A, et al. Development and validation of the cancer fatigue scale: a brief, three-dimensional, self-rating scale for assessment of fatigue in cancer patients. *J Pain Symptom Manage* 2000;19:5–14.
66. Schwartz AL. The Schwartz cancer fatigue scale: testing reliability and validity. *Oncol Nurs Forum* 1998;25:711–717.
67. Smets E, Garssen B, Bonke B, et al. The multidimensional fatigue inventory: psychometric qualities of an instrument to assess fatigue. *J Psychosom Res* 1995;39:315–329.
68. Miaskowski C, Dodd M, Lee K. Symptom clusters: the new frontier in symptom management research. *J Natl Cancer Inst Monogr* 2004;32:17–21.
69. Dodd MJ, Miaskowski C, Paul S. Symptom clusters and their effect on the functional status of patients with cancer. *Oncol Nurs Forum* 2001;28(3):465–470.
70. Portenoy RK, Itri LM. Cancer-related fatigue: guidelines for evaluation and management. *Oncologist* 1999;4:1–10.
71. Cullum JL, Wojciechowski AE, Pelletier G, et al. Bupropion sustained release treatment reduces fatigue in cancer patients. *Can J Psychiatry* 2004;49(2):139–144.
72. Cortesi E, Gascón P, Henry D, et al. Standard of care for cancer-related anemia: improving hemoglobin levels and quality of life. *Oncology* 2005;68(Suppl 1):22–32.
73. Jones M, Schenkel B, Just J, et al. Epoetin alfa improves quality of life in patients with cancer: results of metaanalysis. *Cancer* 2004;101(8):1720–1732.
74. Djulbegovic B. Erythropoietin use in oncology: a summary of the evidence and practice guidelines comparing efforts of the Cochrane Review group and Blue Cross/Blue Shield to set up the ASCO/ASH guidelines. *Best Pract Res Clin Haematol* 2005;18(3):455–466.
75. Chang J, Couture F, Young S, et al. Weekly epoetin alfa maintains hemoglobin, improves quality of life, and reduces transfusion in breast cancer patients receiving chemotherapy. *J Clin Oncol* 2005;23(12):2597–2605.
76. Sarhill N, Walsh D, Nelson KA, et al. Methylphenidate for fatigue in advanced cancer: a prospective open-label pilot study. *Am J Hosp Palliat Care* 2001;18(3):187–192.
77. Schwartz AL, Thompson JA, Masood N. Interferon-induced fatigue in patients with melanoma: a pilot study of exercise and methylphenidate. *Oncol Nurs Forum* 2002;29(7):E85–E90.
78. Bruera E, Driver L, Barnes EA, et al. Patient-controlled methylphenidate for the management of fatigue in patients with advanced cancer: a preliminary report. *J Clin Oncol* 2003;21(23):4439–4443.
79. Hanna A, Sledge G, Mayer ML, et al. A phase II study of methylphenidate for the treatment of fatigue. *Support Care cancer* 2005;14(3):210–215.
80. Stankoff B, Waubant E, Confavreux C, et al. Modafinil for fatigue in MS: a randomized placebo-controlled double-blind study. *Neurology* 2005;64:1139–1143.
81. Sevy S, Rosenthal MH, Alvir J, et al. Double-blind, placebo-controlled study of modafinil for fatigue and cognition in schizophrenia patients treated with psychotropic medications. *J Clin Psychiatry* 2005;66:839–843.
82. Fava M, Thase ME, DeBattista C. A multicenter, placebo-controlled study of modafinil augmentation in partial responders to selective serotonin reuptake inhibitors with persistent fatigue and sleepiness. *J Clin Psychiatry* 2005;66:85–93.
83. Rabkin JG, McElhiney MC, Rabkin R, et al. Modafinil treatment for fatigue in HIV+ patients: a pilot study. *J Clin Psychiatry* 2004;65:1688–1695.
84. Bruera E, Roca E, Cedaro L, et al. Action of oral methylprednisolone in terminal cancer patients: a prospective randomized double-blind study. *Cancer Treat Rep* 1985;69:751–754.
85. Tannock I, Gospodarowicz M, Meakin W, et al. Treatment of metastatic prostatic cancer with low-dose prednisone: evaluation of pain and quality of life as pragmatic indices of response. *J Clin Oncol* 1989;7:590–597.
86. Taus C, Giuliani G, Pucci E, et al. Amantadine for fatigue in multiple sclerosis. *Cochrane Database Syst Rev* 2003;(2):CD002818.
87. Roscoe JA, Morrow GR, Hickok JT, et al. Effect of paroxetine hydrochloride (Paxil) on fatigue and depression in breast cancer patients receiving chemotherapy. *Breast Cancer Res Treat* 2005;89:243–249.
88. Johnson J, Fuller S, Endress MP, et al. Altering patients' responses to surgery: an extension and replication. *Res Nurs Health* 1978;1:111–121.
89. Yates P, Aranda S, Hargraves M, et al. Randomized controlled trial of an educational intervention for managing fatigue in women receiving adjuvant chemotherapy for early-stage breast cancer. *J Clin Oncol* 2005;23(25):6027–6036.
90. Lee K, Cho M, Miaskowski C, et al. Impaired sleep and rhythms in persons with cancer. *Sleep Med Rev* 2004;8(3):189–212.
91. Cimprich B. Attentional fatigue following breast cancer surgery. *Res Nurs Health* 1992;15:199–207.
92. Cimprich B. Developing an intervention to restore attention in cancer patients. *Cancer Nurs* 1993;16:83–92.

CHAPTER 9 ■ FEVER AND SWEATS

KACI OSENGA AND JAMES F. CLEARY

TEMPERATURE AND ASSOCIATED SYMPTOMS

Temperature has long been used in clinical medicine and was included in the cardinal signs of inflammation described as "tumor, rubor, dolor, and fever." The measurement of temperature by a thermometer, in the sublingual, subaxillary or rectal locations, is not a clinical skill practiced regularly by doctors. In most cases, temperature is recorded by other health workers or by patients themselves. Normal body temperature is considered to be 37°C, the average core temperature for an adult population.

Temperature is tightly controlled within a narrow range in each individual. Fever is defined as any elevation in the core body temperature above the normal and results from the upregulation of body temperature. More commonly, a temperature greater that 38°C is considered a clinically significant fever. In oncologic practice and many clinical studies, a significant fever is defined as a single temperature reading greater than 38.5°C or three readings (at least an hour apart) of more than 38°C. The term *fever* (or pyrexia) *of unknown origin*, FUO (PUO), is used commonly and often incorrectly in the daily practice of medicine. An FUO is defined as an illness lasting at least 3 weeks with a fever higher than 38°C on more than one occasion and which lacks a definitive diagnosis after 1 week of evaluation in a hospital (1).

Fever is often accompanied by other symptoms, including sweating and rigors. Sweating, when it accompanies fever, is a cooling response by the body wherein heat is released from the body as it evaporates water on the skin's surface. Rigors and shivering also contribute to temperature control and are rapid muscle spasms designed to increase heat production within the body. For adult humans and most large mammals, shivering is the major means of increased heat production in response to a cold environment. Nonshivering thermogenesis, a process involving heat production in brown adipose tissue, is important in the temperature control of infants.

CONTROL OF TEMPERATURE

It is proposed that core body temperature is controlled by neurologic mechanisms centered at the anterior hypothalamus. The onset of fever in patients results from an elevation of the body's regulated set-point temperature through a resetting of the temperature "gauge" in the hypothalamus (2). This may be caused by various drugs or by endogenous pyrogens. As a result of the reset hypothalamic temperature, the body increases the core body temperature to this new level

(Fig. 9.1) through shivering or nonshivering thermogenesis. The continued presence of pyrogen at the hypothalamus results in the maintenance of this higher temperature. Eventually, either as a result of a decrease in the quantity of pyrogen or the administration of an antipyretic, the hypothalamic temperature is reset to a lower or normal level. The core body temperature is therefore lowered through sweating. This control mechanism may be suppressed in patients administered steroids or anti-inflammatory agents. Older patients may not be able to mount the anticipated febrile response.

The endogenous pyrogens that are responsible for the onset of fever are largely derived from monocytes and macrophages. These cells, as a result of challenge by either endotoxin or infective sources, release tumor necrosis factor (TNF) and interleukin (IL)-1 β. Their production is part of the complex cascade that results in the stimulation of other cytokines, such as iIL-6, IL-8, and changes in prostaglandin metabolism. Serum levels of IL-6 and IL-8 have been found to correlate with core body temperature in patients with febrile neutropenia (3). The ultimate end point of this cascade is the activation of granulocytes, monocytes, and endothelial cells. Although fever appears to be associated with enhanced function of the immune system, it must nonetheless be noted that a direct connection

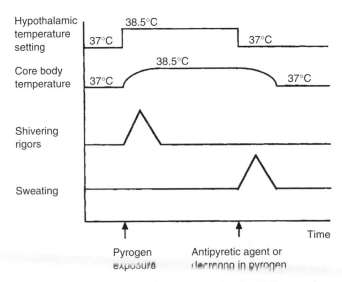

FIGURE 9.1. Physiologic mechanisms associated with fever and accompanying symptoms. (Adapted from Boulant JA. Thermoregulation. In: Mackowiak P, ed. *Fever: basic mechanisms and management.* New York: Raven Press, 1991:1–22, with permission.)

between such phenomena and a beneficial effect of fever on outcome of infections has not been established. Fever, in fact, may be deleterious in the setting of autoimmune disorders or infections (4).

ETIOLOGY OF FEVER IN CANCER PATIENTS

Fever is commonly seen in patients with cancer, both in those with and without infection. The wide range of etiologies of fever in patients with cancer will be considered in relation to the pathophysiology of fever in these patients.

Tumor

Fever associated with tumor is believed to be associated with the release of pyrogens, either directly from a tumor or from tumor stimulation of immunologic mechanisms that cause an elevation in temperature through action on the anterior hypothalamus. The classic association of fever to particular tumor diagnoses relates more to tumors associated with a diagnosis of FUO (Table 9.1). In the combined results of six studies documenting the etiology of FUO, 23% of adults meeting the defined diagnosis were found to have malignancy as the cause (8% of children) (5). In another study of 111 elderly (age >65 years) patients with FUO, 26 had associated malignancy, with 15 patients diagnosed with lymphoma, and 4 with renal cell carcinoma (6). Almost 7000 cancer patients with fever were reviewed by Klastersky et al., and only 47 (0.7%) fit the diagnostic criteria for an FUO (7). Twenty-seven of the 47 had leukemia or lymphoma, with disease rather than infection being the cause of the fever in only 11. Tumor was responsible for fever in seven patients with widespread metastatic carcinomas; in six of these, large liver metastases were present.

Hodgkin's disease has classically been associated with the Pel-Ebstein fever (Fig. 9.2), where a patient experiences 3- to 10-day cycles of fever alternating with periods of normal temperature (8). Although the presence of fever is an important prognostic indicator in patients with Hodgkin's disease, there has been some discussion (9) about the value of Pel-Ebstein fever as a diagnostic tool particularly because the original description of the Pel-Ebstein fever was made in two patients who were subsequently found, on pathologic review, not to have Hodgkin's disease.

Although classical teaching is that fever is associated with particular tumors, fever also occurs in patients with many of the more common cancers (Table 9.2). Forty-one percent of those who underwent autopsy had evidence of infection as an explanation of their fever (10). The incidence of infection among the autopsied patients was 50% for acute leukemia, 75% in patients with lymphoma, and 80% in those with chronic lymphocytic leukemia. Infection was only found in

TABLE 9.1

TUMORS CLASSICALLY ASSOCIATED WITH FEVER

Hodgkin's disease
Lymphoma
Leukemia
Renal cell carcinoma
Myxoma
Osteogenic sarcoma

TABLE 9.2

INCIDENCE OF FEVER WITHOUT EVIDENCE OF INFECTION AT AUTOPSY IN PATIENTS OF DIFFERENT PRIMARY TUMOR TYPES

Primary site	Number of patients observed	Number of patients with fever without associated infection	
		Number	%
Stomach	1498	573	41
Kidney	208	39	19
Colon and rectum	113	75	66
Liver and gallbladder	98	43	44
Uterus	81	19	36
Squamous skin cancer	41	20	49
Esophagus	20	7	35
Breast	48	16	33
Lung	17	8	47
Small bowel	17	1	6
Prostate	11	7	64
Bladder	10	6	60
Bone	10	7	70

From Boggs DR, Frei E. Clinical studies of fever and infection in cancer. *Cancer* 1960;13:1240–1253, with permission.

a third of those with chronic myeloid leukemia, 17% with Hodgkin's disease, and 15% of patients with lung cancer.

Infection (Including Neutropenia)

Although infection and fever can be a common presentation in patients with cancer, it is of particular concern in patients with neutropenia. Neutropenia, defined as a peripheral blood neutrophil count of <500 per µL, results from either increased destruction or decreased production of white blood cells. Decreased production by the bone marrow may result from either disease involving the marrow or from myelosuppression by chemotherapy. The cause of fever is not identified in approximately 60–70% of patients with neutropenia (11). Risk factors for the development of fever in the setting of neutropenia have been identified and include a rapid decrease in the neutrophil count and a protracted neutropenia of <500 cells per µL or >10 days (12). Twenty percent of patients with 1 week of chemotherapy-induced neutropenia develop a fever and the rate of infection increases with lengthening periods of neutropenia. Other factors that may alter the risk of the patient with neutropenia include phagocyte function, the status of the patient's immune system, and alterations in the physical defense barriers of the body (e.g., mucositis).

Fever and neutropenia in patients with cancer are associated with a high risk of medical complications with a death rate ranging from 4 to 12%. Twenty-one percent of patients with febrile neutropenia at the Dana Farber Cancer Center developed serious medical complications (13). The investigators identified four risk groups for patients with febrile neutropenia. Group 1 consisted of inpatients at the time of onset of fever; group 2, outpatients who developed significant comorbidity within 24 hours of presentation; group 3, outpatients with uncontrolled cancer but without serious concurrent comorbidity;

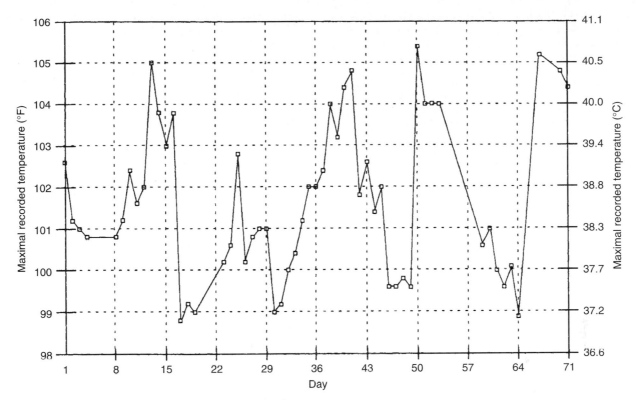

FIGURE 9.2. A 50-year-old man had fever, night sweats, and nonproductive cough for 10 weeks. He took antipyretic medications during the febrile periods. His wife recorded his temperatures, shown in the preceding text, on 56 of the 71 days. Biopsy of a rapidly enlarging cervical lymph node revealed nodular sclerosing Hodgkin's lymphoma. The patient's fevers and other symptoms promptly disappeared after the first cycle of doxorubicin, bleomycin, vinblastine, and dacarbazine. [From Good GR, Dinubile MJ. Images in clinical medicine. Cyclic fever in Hodgkin's disease (Pel-Ebstein fever). *N Engl J Med* 1995;332:436, with permission.]

and group 4, outpatients without serious concurrent comorbidity and whose cancer was well controlled. The model was validated in 444 patients with febrile neutropenia, of whom 36% had a significant comorbidity, 27% had serious medical complications, and 8% died. Group 1 had the greatest risk and group 4 had little risk in relation to medical complications and risk (Table 9.3).

An important component of this study was the identification within 24 hours of onset of fever of those patients at low risk of medical complication. These low-risk patients were

TABLE 9.3

INCIDENCE OF MULTIPLE MEDICAL COMPLICATIONS AND MORTALITY IN PATIENTS WITH FEBRILE NEUTROPENIA AS DEFINED BY RISK[a]

Patient group	Number of patients	Multiple complications (%)	Deaths (%)
Group 1	268	51 (19)	25 (9)
Group 2	43	3 (7)	5 (12)
Group 3	29	3 (10)	4 (14)
Group 4	104	0 (0)	0 (0)
All patients	444	57 (13)	34 (8)

[a]Risk groups are defined in text.
From Talcott JA, Siegel RD, Finberg R, et al. Risk assessment in cancer patients with fever and neutropenia: a prospective, two center validation of a prediction rule. *J Clin Oncol* 1992;10:316–322, with permission.

at risk of developing medical complications (5%) but these were either transient and asymptomatic or were heralded by at least 7 days of medical deterioration and therefore readily detectable by appropriate follow-up. Two additional risk factors—a latency period of <10 days from the time of chemotherapy administration to the onset of fever, and neutropenia and age >40—correlated with the occurrence of more frequent complications. Mucositis was associated with decreased risk of medical complications, suggesting that infection associated with mucositis may be responsive to antibiotics. The identification of a causative organism or positive blood cultures was not associated with increased risk.

In a multinational study, a risk-index score was developed to "stage" those patients with febrile neutropenia (14). Predictive factors included blood pressure, presence of chronic obstructive pulmonary disease or solid tumor, previous fungal infection in patients with hematologic malignancies, outpatient status, status of hydration, and age in relation to 60 years. On the validation set, a Multinational Association for Supportive Care in Cancer risk-index score ≥21 identified low-risk patients with a positive predictive value of 91%, specificity of 68%, and sensitivity of 71%. In a further population, the risk index accurately identified patients at low risk for complications. This risk index may be useful in the selection of patients for studies that test strategies to treat febrile neutropenia.

On the basis of a number of retrospective studies, similar definitions of low risk have been applied to pediatric patients with fever and neutropenia (15). Low risk included evidence of bone marrow recovery in culture-negative patients who were afebrile for at least 24 hours and who had no other reason to continue intravenous antibiotics in the hospital. The control of any localized infection and the patient's ability to return promptly in the event of fever or other complications were also necessary. In a prospective study of 70 patients who met the criteria and who were discharged home with neutropenia, none was readmitted with fever. Seven patients who were inadvertently discharged without evidence of marrow recovery were readmitted with recurrence of fever. Neutropenic children with positive cultures were also assessed to identify risk factors for bacteremia (16). Of the cases of bacteremia, 92.5% occurred in those where cancer was not controlled, were <1 year of age, <10 days past their last chemotherapy, and had no evidence of marrow recovery.

Organisms (Bacteriology)

A basic understanding of the classification and sensitivities of the different organisms is essential to understand the infection in patients with cancer. Over time there have been changes in the underlying organisms associated with febrile neutropenia as evidenced by progressive studies by the European Organization for Research and Treatment of Cancer (EORTC) group (17). Gram-negative organisms were the leading cause of infection in patients with febrile neutropenia, but their incidence has decreased from 71% of identified causative organisms during the 1973–1978 period to 31% during the 1989–1991 period. Infection by one of these gram-negative organisms—*Pseudomonas aeruginosa*—has been a driving force in the selection of antibiotics. However, the incidence of pseudomonas infection has also decreased over the last few years as reflected by an incidence of only 0.1% of febrile neutropenic cases at the National Cancer Institute (18). The incidence of both acute and chronic fungal infections has also increased, with up to 33% of patients with febrile neutropenia not responding to a week of antibiotic therapy, after having a systemic fungal (*Candida* or *Aspergillosis*) infection (19).

The incidence of gram-positive organisms has increased from 29% during the 1973–1978 period to 69% during the 1989–1991 period, requiring a review in treatment regimens used in patients with febrile neutropenia. Some of these gram-positive organisms such as coagulase-negative staphylococci or *Corynebacterium jeikeium*, represent indolent infections that are methicillin resistant and only susceptible to vancomycin, quinupristin-dalfopristin and linezolid. Other gram-positive bacteria such as *Staphylococcus aureus*, viridans streptococci and pneumococci may cause fulminant infections with serious complications and possibly death if not treated promptly. Gram-negative bacilli, especially *P. aeruginosa*, *Escherichia coli* and *Klebsiella* species, remain prominent causes of infection and must be treated with selected antibiotics (20).

Location

Infections can occur throughout the body and need to be sought carefully through history and examination. Collapse, consolidation, and superimposed infection may develop behind an obstructing bronchial tumor. Aspiration pneumonia may occur in those with esophageal tumor either secondary to an obstruction or as a result of a tracheo-esophageal fistula.

The gastrointestinal system is the most common site of indigent organisms causing infection in patients with neutropenia. *Clostridium difficile* infection may present with fever and diarrhea and must be considered in those who are already taking antibiotics. Fungal and viral infections of the esophagus need to be suspected in those with dysphagia and odynophagia. Anaerobic infections may be a factor in severe mucositis or gingivitis and in those patients with perianal discomfort. Spontaneous bacterial peritonitis may be a cause of fever in patients with ascites. A urinary catheter increases the risk of urinary tract infection as does the presence of urinary obstruction, but the presence of asymptomatic bacteriuria

in a patient with non-neutropenic cancer is not usually an indication for antibiotic treatment.

Central nervous system infections can be difficult to diagnose and usually require lumbar puncture to confirm. Infection is the most common complication of Ommaya reservoirs, used to administer intraventricular chemotherapy, and is more likely to occur in those with previous radiotherapy or in whom repeated surgical procedures have been necessary (21). Most infections are due to *Staphylococcus epidermidis* and can usually be successfully treated with antibiotics (22).

Particular attention to sites of recent surgery is essential in assessing infection. Surgical collections may include infected hematomas that develop following surgery. The skin is also a common site of infection that may range from infected decubitus ulcers to herpes zoster infections. The use of percutaneous catheters in oncology has created another portal for the introduction of infection in patients with cancer. Of a total of 322 indwelling devices placed in 274 patients with cancer by a single surgeon, device-related sepsis occurred in 28 of 209 patients (13%) with catheters and 6 of 113 patients (5%) with subcutaneous ports (23). Triple lumen catheters were associated with a higher rate of thrombosis but not of infection. The complications of 1630 venous access devices for long-term use in 1431 consecutive patients with cancer were reviewed (24). Of the catheters inserted, 341 of 788 (43%) had at least one device-related infection compared with 57 of 680 (8%) of the completely implanted ports ($p = .001$). The number of infections per 1000 device days was 2.77 for catheters compared with 0.21 for ports ($p = .001$). The predominant organisms isolated in catheter-related bacteremia were gram-negative bacilli (55%) compared with gram-positive cocci (65.5%) in port-related bacteremia. Patients with solid tumors were less likely to have device-related infectious morbidity compared with patients with hematologic cancers.

Transfusion-Related

Blood products, administered extensively to patients with cancer, may be associated with febrile reactions. The incidence of side effects following the administration of over 100,000 units of red blood cells to more than 25,000 patients with cancer over a 4-year period was retrospectively reviewed (25). Of all transfused units, 0.3% had a transfusion-associated reaction; 51.3% were febrile nonhemolytic, and 36.7% were allergic urticarial reactions. Only 17 hemolytic reactions (4 immediate, 13 delayed) were documented. The incidence of transfusion-related side effects was significantly lower in this study than that reported in the noncancer population. Infection may also be a source of fever in patients receiving blood products. The Canadian Red Cross (26) estimated that the true positive rate of bacterial contamination of platelet concentrate units was between 4.4 and 10.7 per 10,000 units and recommended screening of all such units. The percentage of those patients developing bacteremia or septicemia from infected units was not discussed.

Thrombosis

Trousseau's self diagnosis of gastric cancer on the basis of venous thrombosis is a reminder that patients with cancer are at particular risk of thrombosis. Deep-vein thrombosis may present with fever and, given the uncertainty of clinical diagnosis, investigation may be necessary in the "at risk" patient. Pelvic thrombophlebitis may sometimes occur after pelvic surgery and, if septic, may manifest with either low- or high-grade fever. Pulmonary embolus also needs to be considered in the differential diagnosis of fever in patients with cancer. Of 97 patients with confirmed pulmonary embolus in the Urokinase PE Trial, 17 had associated malignancy (27). Of those with confirmed malignancy, 54% had a fever >37.5°C and 19.6% had a fever >38°C. Forty-one percent of the patients with cancer had associated sweating. Pulmonary infarction, with the primary signs of tachypnea, tachycardia, and fever, may be a presentation of pulmonary thrombi. Other thrombotic syndromes, such as cerebral venous thrombosis, although associated with fever, are not common in the setting of malignancy.

Hemorrhage

Gastrointestinal bleeding may present with fever and should be considered in the differential diagnosis of a patient with low-grade fever and sweats. However, in a major review of fever in patients with cancer (10), serious hemorrhage was followed by fever in a minority of cases; the usual sequence has been that of hemorrhage in an already febrile patient.

Drugs

Drug-associated fever is an ill-defined syndrome in which fever is the predominant manifestation of an adverse drug reaction. It is normally a diagnosis of exclusion (28). The drugs commonly associated with fever are antibiotics, cardiovascular drugs, central nervous system drugs (e.g., phenytoin), cytotoxics, and immune therapy drugs (either as biologic response modifiers or growth factors). Antimicrobial agents were responsible for 46 of 148 drug-related fevers in a review of the experience of two hospitals in Texas and the United Kingdom with a mean lag time from initiation of treatment to onset of fever of 21 days (median, 8 days). For 11 cases of cytotoxic-induced fever, the mean lag time was 6.0 days with a median of 0.5 days. Shaking chills were more common with the administration of cytotoxic-associated fever than with other drugs (29).

Cytotoxics

There is a diverse range of cytotoxic drugs whose administration is associated with fever (Table 9.4). The febrile response to bleomycin was described in the original phase 1 studies (30) and characteristically occurs 3–5 hours after injection. It is more common after intravenous than after intramuscular injection. It is seen in approximately 25% of patients who were administered the drug. The fever becomes less frequent with repeated injections. An anaphylactic reaction manifested by hyperpyrexia, shock, hypotension, urticaria, and wheezing occurs in 1% of patients administered bleomycin (31). Fever following the administration of cisplatin was also reported in early clinical trials (32). Streptozocin administration may result in fever associated with chills, as can cytarabine and etoposide. Fever can occur after the administration of 5-fluorouracil and high-dose methotrexate. Confusion concerning the etiology of a fever arises more commonly in the situation of intensive chemotherapeutic regimens where patients with neutropenia may be administered cytotoxic agents that cause fever. Awareness of the symptoms produced by the different agents assists in discerning the etiology of the fever.

Antibiotics

Antibiotics commonly associated with fever are penicillins, cephalosporins, and amphotericin. Out of 50 patients who were administered at least 100 mg of amphotericin-B over a minimum of 3 days, fever was experienced by 34% and chills by 56%, with rates of 2.6 and 3.5 mean episodes per patient per treatment course, respectively (33). In patients who had received 20 mg or more of amphotericin-B per day for at least 10 consecutive days, shivering occurred first at the test dose, with the percentage of patients who shivered increasing with each successive dose and peaking at the fifth therapeutic dose (34).

Opioids

Intravenous injection of morphine is often associated with sweating and vasodilatation, but not necessarily with fever. Fever may occur as a result of the interaction between meperidine (pethidine) and monoamine oxidase inhibitor, which is to be avoided. Drug withdrawal is associated with a syndrome that includes fever and needs to be suspected in febrile patients with cancer in whom opioids have been suddenly stopped. Withdrawal from benzodiazepines may also be associated with fever.

Biological Therapy

Interferons (IFN) are associated with the development of fever (35). Partially purified IFN administered at low doses intramuscularly induces a fever (38–40°C) within 6 hours that persists for approximately 4–8 hours. More severe side effects are seen with intravenous and intrathecal administration, or in patients older than 65 years. The use of highly purified recombinant DNA IFN induces similar side effects. IFN at doses of 50–120 MU results in a sharp febrile response with severe rigors, peripheral cyanosis, vasoconstriction, nausea and vomiting, severe muscle aches, and headaches. In those patients receiving IFN daily, the febrile response and accompanying symptoms usually decrease in intensity and disappear within 7–10 days. Fever however persists, with intermittent (nondaily) injections resulting in peaks at 6–12 hours, and tends to last longer than the normal 4–8 hours. The administration of other biologic factors is associated with the onset of fever (e.g., TNF). The administration of growth factors is also associated with the onset of fever, although the incidence following granulocyte colony-stimulating factor (G-CSF) is very low. Fever occurs much more commonly following granulocyte macrophage colony-stimulating factor (GM-CSF) administration than following G-CSF administration.

Graft versus Host Disease

Chronic graft versus host disease is very much like a systemic collagen vascular disease and may be associated with infection, with or without the presence of fever. Acute graft versus host disease is associated with fever. Infection is also common.

Radiation-Induced Fever

Patients receiving radiotherapy alone may present with fever a few hours after the initial treatment. Acute radiation

TABLE 9.4

CYTOTOXIC AGENTS ASSOCIATED WITH FEVER AFTER ADMINISTRATION

Bleomycin	Mustine
Cisplatin	Mithramycin
Cytarabine	Streptozocin
Cyclophosphamide	Thiotepa
Etoposide	Vinblastine
5-Fluorouracil	Vincristine
Methotrexate	

pneumonitis may develop 2–3 months after completion of radiation therapy. A high spiking fever may be part of the syndrome that consists of dyspnea and an unproductive cough. Lung biopsy may be necessary to establish the diagnosis.

Other Diseases

Other diseases that may cause fever may coexist in patients with cancer (e.g., systemic lupus erythematosus and rheumatoid arthritis). Careful review of past medical history and current symptoms is essential.

DIAGNOSIS

The classical teaching that history provides 95% of the diagnosis is certainly true when it comes to the symptoms of fever in patients with cancer. Following the physical examination, the use of diagnostic aids is very much dependent on the relevant history. Although two thirds of patients with neutropenia do not have an identifiable cause of the fever, culture of relevant body fluids is still essential. However, routine surveillance cultures in patients with neutropenia, before the development of fever, are not cost productive (36). Although a chest x-ray (CXR) may not be an indicator in symptomatic patients presenting with febrile neutropenia (37), a recent CXR may be an important baseline in a patient without respiratory symptoms or signs but who is likely to have a prolonged period of neutropenia.

The diagnosis of fever due to the cancer itself can be confirmed with the use of naproxen (38). Proponents of "the naproxen test" state that it does not result in a decrease in temperature in patients with infection. Successful treatment of "neoplastic" fever was demonstrated in 21 patients with cancer, with 15 responding to a dose of 250 mg per day, whereas others responded following an increase in the dose of naproxen administered. The true sensitivity and specificity of this test is uncertain, but the authors stress that infectious fever and noninfectious fever due to drug toxicity, allergic reaction, and adrenal insufficiency need to be excluded before considering the diagnosis as "neoplastic fever."

TREATMENT

Primary to any treatment of fever in patients with cancer is the treatment of the underlying cause of fever. Antibiotics should not be used to control fever in patients without neutropenia in the absence of evidence of infection, but nonsteroidal anti-inflammatory drugs may be useful in the treatment of fever associated with infection.

Physical cooling (e.g., through sponging) alone is likely to be uncomfortable for patients with fever and should be reserved for those in a hot and humid environment that may impede evaporative heat loss or for those with defective heat loss mechanisms (39). Sponging, when it is done, should be with tepid water because the use of cold water will induce shivering, which increases patient discomfort and causes an elevation in temperature (40).

Agents that lower body temperature (antipyretics) primarily comprise three groups:

1. Pure antipyretics that do not work in the absence of pyrogen, and do not affect normal temperature at usual therapeutic doses (e.g., acetaminophen)
2. Agents that cause hypothermia in afebrile subjects by directly impairing thermoregulatory function

3. Those that are antipyretic at lower doses and cause hypothermia at higher doses (e.g., chlorpromazine)

Only salicylates, acetaminophen, and ibuprofen have been approved for antipyretic use in the United States, and none of these agents is likely to cause hypothermia in normothermic patients. Aspirin is not recommended for use in children because of the risk of Reye's syndrome, a disease process that results in liver failure (41). Aspirin has been the standard of reference in nearly two thirds of clinical comparisons of antipyretic activity, but only one comparison of aspirin has been performed in patients with cancer (42). Every patient with low-grade fever received doses of aspirin and placebo in random order. No useful conclusions could be drawn, as the mean reduction in temperature for the patients on 600 mg of aspirin was only 0.3°C, a difference that is not statistically significant from that for the patients on placebo.

In children, acetaminophen has a dose–response effect, with doses of 5, 10, and 20 mg per kg bringing about a reduction in temperature of 0.3, 1.6, and 2.5°C, respectively, after 3 hours (39). Aspirin and acetaminophen appear equally effective at approximately 10 mg per kg. Ibuprofen, 0.5 mg per kg, is about as effective as 10 mg per kg of aspirin and 12.5 mg per kg of acetaminophen, and probably lasts longer. Indomethacin has been reported to be more effective than these three compounds in limiting febrile responses to IFN (43) but is not approved for antipyretic use in the United States. Indomethacin (75 mg), naproxen (500 mg), and diclofenac sodium (75 mg) have been found to be equally effective in the management of paraneoplastic fever (44). Steroids may be useful in treating fever, acting in the same manner as nonsteroidal anti-inflammatory drugs. Steroids may be particularly effective in patients who are imminently dying.

Treatment of Infection

The treatment of fever in a non-neutropenic patient with cancer is not in itself a medical emergency. Shock associated with such a patient may well become an emergency. A thorough review of the history and examination and the performance of appropriate tests should guide both the timing and the type of treatment initiated.

The presence of fever in a patient who is immunocompromised is a medical emergency and empirical therapy should be initiated as soon as possible. Patients at risk of neutropenia should be instructed to record their temperature and to report the presence of fever to health care staff. An overall schema for the use of antimicrobial agents in neutropenic patients with unexplained fever is presented in Figure 9.3. Antibiotic recommendations by The Infectious Diseases Society of America (IDSA) Consensus Statement on Febrile Neutropenia (20,45), updated in 2002, should be considered together with more recent studies on the choice of antibiotics in febrile neutropenia. The decision as to the antibiotic regimen to be used rests with each institution and must take into consideration local experience and infection trends.

The initial choice of antibiotic regimens is most commonly an aminoglycoside with an antipseudomonal cephalosporin (cefepime or ceftazidime); an aminoglycoside and antipseudomonal carboxypenicillin or ureidopenicillin (ticarcillin-clavualanic acid or piperacillin-tazobactam); or an aminoglycoside with a carbepenem (imipenem-cilastatin or meropenem) (20). These regimes have been extensively used with similar results and are particularly recommended for those at high risk for *Pseudomonas* infection, including patients with cancer with severe mucositis and those known to be colonized with the organism. Given the nephro- and ototoxicity associated with aminoglycosides and carboxypenicillins, serum

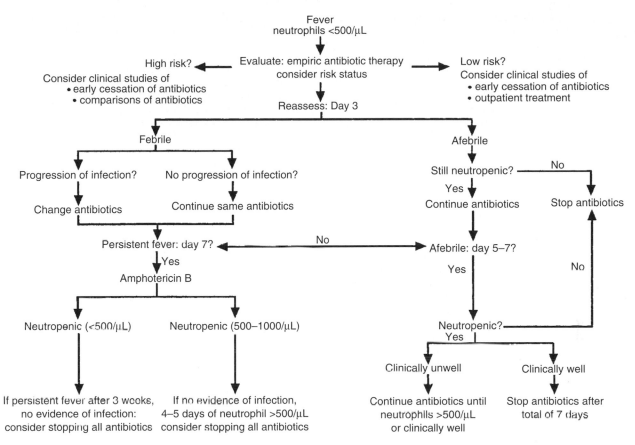

FIGURE 9.3. Clinical approach to the treatment of patients with febrile neutropenia.

concentrations of these drugs should be monitored regularly. The advantages of combination therapy include the possible synergistic effects against some gram-negative bacilli and reduction in the emergence of drug-resistant organisms (20). Although safe, the latter regimens are expensive and may not provide adequate coverage of staphylococcal infections. The addition of vancomycin to any of the regimens mentioned provides additional coverage against staphylococcal infections and, if used initially, results in fewer incidences of treatment failure. Other studies have shown no difference in mortality and morbidity rates in those patients in whom vancomycin was added at a later date.

The use of monotherapy was not strongly supported by the committee (20,45). Although initial results of such therapy were good, modification has been required often enough for combination therapy to be preferred as initial therapy. The panel recommended that monotherapy with a third- or fourth-generation cephalosporin (cefepime or ceftazidime) or a carbepenem (imipenem-cilastatin or meropenem) be considered in patients at low risk of infection (brief period of neutropenia prior to fever and with neutrophil counts between 500 and 1000 per μL) and that these patients be closely monitored (20). A meta-analysis has subsequently been performed on 13 studies that compared ceftazidime monotherapy with different combination therapies (46). No difference was found in treatment failure, and there was no difference in outcome when febrile and bacteremic episodes were considered independently. Similar percentages of modifications for monotherapy and combination therapy were made. In a more recent multicenter, randomized controlled trial involving the treatment of 876 febrile, neutropenic episodes in 696 patients (47), single-agent ceftazidime was found to be safer than piperacillin and tobramycin combined, with similar effectiveness (62.7%

versus. 61.1%; $p > .2$). Infectious mortality was 6% for ceftazidime and 8% for the combination therapy; 38 episodes of superinfection developed in each group. An adverse event occurred in 8% of the episodes treated with ceftazidime, compared with 20% with combination therapy ($p < .001$). It is to be noted that 83% of the patients enrolled in the study had leukemia and had undergone transplantation and they often experienced profound and prolonged neutropenia.

It is essential to continually review a patient's clinical situation and therapy. The consensus panel agreed that by day 3, a patient with neutropenia who was either afebrile or had continuing fever but with no progression of the infective process, could continue on the same antibiotics. Antibiotics should be changed if fever persisted and there was progression of the infective process. Either vancomycin could be added at that stage (if not already in use) or monotherapy in the form of a third-generation cephalosporin could be commenced. If the patient remained both neutropenic and febrile after a week and was unlikely to have white cell recovery in the near future, amphotericin should be added (48). Antianaerobic therapy should be considered in patients with persistent fever and severe oral mucositis, necrotizing gingivitis, or perianal tenderness.

The current duration of antibiotic treatment, where patients with febrile neutropenia have been admitted to hospital for antibiotic treatment until their neutropenia resolved, is based on the results of a 1979 study (49). Early stopping of antibiotics at day 7 in 17 patients with resolved fever but persistent neutropenia resulted in the recurrence of fever in 7 patients, of whom 2 died. The consensus committee considered cessation of antibiotics in patients without fever who were clinically well but with a neutrophil count of <500 per μL. They considered that therapy could be stopped after 7 days provided that the patient was carefully observed, mucous membranes and skin were intact, and no invasive procedure or ablative chemotherapy was imminent, although this was not strongly supported by scientific data.

More recent studies have suggested that in patients at lower risk of complications, outpatient treatment and early stopping of antibiotics may be possible. Thirty patients with febrile neutropenia, identified to have a low complication risk after 48 hours of inpatient intravenous treatment, were continued on the same antibiotics at home until neutropenia resolved (50). Four patients were readmitted with medical complications (hypotension, 3; acute renal failure, 1) and five others were readmitted for observation. Overall costs were similar for those treated at home and for those who were medically eligible for home treatment but were treated in the hospital. The higher-than-expected cost of home treatment related to extended periods of neutropenia in these patients. Attempts have been made to shorten hospital stays by discontinuing intravenous antibiotics in blood culture–negative patients who remained clinically stable and afebrile after 48 hours of treatment (51). In a retrospective review of 134 admissions for neutropenic fever, the median duration of intravenous antibiotics decreased significantly from 7 days before institution of such a policy to 5 days (4–6) and 4 days (3–5) over the next two consecutive 6-month periods. The median duration of hospital stay decreased from 10 days to 7 days (5–8) and 6 days (5–7) over the same periods. The authors concluded that intravenous antibiotics might be discontinued in patients who remained afebrile and clinically stable for 48 hours and who had negative blood cultures, resulting in a shorter duration of hospital stays, with the potential for reduction in hospital costs.

Early stopping of antibiotics together with a selective decontamination regimen (neomycin, polymyxin, amphotericin, and pipemidic acid) was prospectively studied in 52 adult patients with hematologic malignancies and a neutrophil count <500 per μL (52). Patients experienced 77 febrile episodes while receiving the oral antibiotics and further treatment (either broad-spectrum or disease-specific antibodies) was initiated only if clinical signs or microbiologic culture results indicated an infection. Consequently, antibiotics were adjusted according to culture findings or discontinued if evidence of infection was lacking after 72–96 hours. For the 40 episodes without confirmed infection, the median duration of therapy was 3 days (range, 0–13 days) and the survival rate 100%, with 15 receiving no additional antibiotics. For the 37 episodes with confirmed infection, the median duration of therapy was 12 days (range, 1–49 days, p <.0001) and the survival rate 85%. Broad-spectrum therapy was only used for the duration of neutropenia in 18% of the treated episodes, and none of the six deaths could be attributed to the withholding or stopping of broad-spectrum therapy. It was concluded that in patients with febrile neutropenia on this selective decontamination regimen, the standard prolonged administration of broad-spectrum antibiotics was not necessary. The authors recommended that systemic antibiotics be discontinued after 3–5 days if infection is unlikely, that a narrower antibiotic spectrum be chosen according to the clinical situation, and that empirical antifungal treatment be considered after 7 days for this population. Although very promising, the findings of this study need to be confirmed in randomized clinical trials before their widespread implementation.

The place of outpatient treatment of low-risk patients with neutropenia was examined at the M. D. Anderson Cancer Center (53). Oral ciprofloxacin combined with clindamycin was as effective in the control of infection as was the combination of intravenous aztreonam and clindamycin. However, the oral regime was associated with increased renal toxicity that resulted in the early termination of the study. The authors recommended the development of better outpatient antibiotic regimens and urged caution as none of their patients had gram-negative bacteremias or pneumonias, a group that may be difficult to treat. Outpatient treatment was further studied in Pakistan, where 188 low-risk patients with febrile neutropenia were randomized to receive either inpatient or outpatient oral ofloxacin (54). The investigators had previously found oral ofloxacin to be as effective for inpatient care as their standard intravenous regimen (55). The patient group consisted of patients with both solid tumors and leukemias and excluded those in whom the duration of neutropenia was likely to exceed 7 days. Fever control was the same in both groups, with 78% of inpatient and 77% of outpatient fevers resolving without modification of the initial treatment. However, 21% of the outpatients required hospitalization. Mortality was 2% in those assigned inpatient treatment and 4% in outpatients, with one death occurring outside of the hospital.

The oral administration of empirical, broad-spectrum antibiotics in low-risk patients was tested in a randomized, double-blind, placebo-controlled study of patients who had fever and neutropenia during chemotherapy for cancer (56). Hospitalized patients were randomized to receive either oral ciprofloxacin plus amoxicillin-clavulanate or intravenous ceftazidime. Out of 116 episodes in each group, treatment was successful in 71% of episodes in the oral-therapy group and 67% of the intravenous-therapy group. Concerns have been raised as to the selection of patients in this study. However, this approach may be useful, but it should be limited to that subset of patients with low-risk factors who are not otherwise on quinolone prophylaxis and in whom close monitoring and surveillance can be performed. Those with an identifiable cause of infection should be treated with the appropriate antibiotics. The issue of limited treatment in low-risk groups needs to be more clearly defined and addressed in further clinical studies (Fig. 9.3).

In summary, for patients with fever who continue to have neutropenia for a week or more, broad-spectrum antibiotic therapy for the duration of the neutropenia along with empirical antifungal therapy in those who remain febrile is the current consensus. The use of narrow-spectrum agents or abbreviated courses of antibiotics in these patients needs further study, as does their role in patients at low risk of complications.

Vascular access devices often create a treatment dilemma in patients with febrile neutropenia. These may be left in place in most patients, even if bacteremia is detected, and managed with antibiotic and local care (57). Catheters should be removed if they are nonpatent, associated with thrombosis, have evidence of septic emboli, or if there is a subcutaneous tunnel infection. Prompt removal of catheters is also indicated with *Candida* spp. fungemia and bacteremia due to *Bacillus* spp. or a bacteremia that persists for >48 hours after initiation of appropriate antibiotics.

Antiviral medications may be required in patients with neutropenia as well as who are immunocompromised and without neutropenia. However, the empirical use of antiviral drugs in the management of febrile neutropenia in patients without mucosal lesions or evidence of viral disease is not indicated. The recommended dose of acyclovir for the treatment of established herpes infections in the immunocompromised patients ranges from 5 mg per kg q8h i.v. for herpes simplex to 10–12 mg per kg q8h i.v. for herpes zoster.

Although popular throughout the 1970s and 1980s, the use of granulocyte infusions has faded in recent years, despite evidence of efficacy. In a review (58) of the use of granulocyte transfusions, this decline was related to the administration of ineffective doses of granulocytes. The authors recommended that physicians assess the outcome of persistent febrile neutropenia in their own institutions and, if poor, the addition of granulocyte transfusions, at therapeutic doses (2–3 × 10^10 PMN), may be useful along with other changes such as the use of different antibiotics. The use of G-CSF in the collection of white cells was also considered, but it requires more work before it can be used as a standard treatment.

Treatment of Transfusion Reactions

Transfusion reactions can be prevented by the filtration of blood products and also by premedication with an antihistamine. The use of erythropoietin in anemia associated with malignancy may reduce the need for blood transfusions, thereby avoiding both transfusion reactions and a source of infection. The cost of such treatment needs to be considered carefully.

Treatment of Amphotericin-Related Febrile Reaction

For the prevention of amphotericin-related fever and rigors, 12.5–25.0 mg of intravenous meperidine is useful. However, slowing the rate of amphotericin may reduce toxicity. Amphotericin given over 45 minutes was much more toxic in relation to fever and rigors than the same dose given over 4 hours (59). Less meperidine was required for the control of symptoms in the 4-hour infusion arm. In another study, no difference was found between a 45-minute and a 2-hour infusion (60). Other opioids may have the same effect on the treatment of these rigors.

PROPHYLAXIS

Prophylaxis, either in the form of antibiotics or other supportive treatment, may be useful in the prevention of febrile neutropenia.

Growth Factors

Hematologic colony-stimulating factors (CSFs) reduce treatment-associated myelosuppression by shortening the duration of neutropenia and by reducing the nadir of neutrophil counts. However, concern about their appropriate clinical use led to the continued updating of guidelines from the American Society of Clinical Oncology (61). These guidelines, initially released in 1994, have resulted in a small improvement in the use of G-CSF (62). Two indications for the use of G-CSF administration were addressed—primary CSF use in those receiving their initial chemotherapy and secondary use in those who have previously had chemotherapy-induced neutropenia.

To assess a benefit in primary prevention, the incidence of Grade 4 neutropenia following the use of CSF in different randomized treatment protocols was considered. The incidence of neutropenia ranged from 0% in patients with breast cancer receiving the combination of cyclophosphamide, doxorubicin, and 5-fluorouracil to 98% of 102 patients with lung cancer who were administered cyclophosphamide, doxorubicin, and etoposide. G-CSF was found to decrease the incidence of febrile neutropenia significantly where the placebo group had an incidence of neutropenia >40%. However, in these randomized CSF trials, no difference in infectious mortality, response rates, or survival between CSF- and placebo-treated patients was documented. It was recommended that CSFs be used only with those protocols where the incidence of neutropenia was likely to be >40% without their use. Recently, the National Comprehensive Cancer Network has issued guidelines advocating the use of CSFs in patients with a 20% risk of developing febrile neutropenia (63). When less myelotoxic chemotherapy is planned, primary administration of CSFs should be reserved for those patients who are at high risk from neutropenic complications because of host- or disease-related factors. Individual cases should also be considered in patients at higher risk of chemotherapy-induced, infectious complications (e.g., extensive prior chemotherapy). Elderly patients tolerate chemotherapy as well as younger patients do and should not receive CSFs purely on the basis of age. Recently, pegfilgrastim, which is produced by the covalent binding of a 20-kD polyethylene glycol moiety to the N-terminus of filgrastim, has been shown to have a sustained CSF effect (64). Pegylated agents have longer half-lives, superior physical and thermal stability, greater protection from enzymatic degradation, more stable plasma concentrations, and reduced immunogenicity (65). Pegfilgrastim has largely been used in the prevention of chemotherapy-induced neutropenia. A phase II dose-finding study compared single injections of pegfilgrastim (30, 60, or 100 µg per kg) and daily filgrastim (5 µg per kg) in patients with breast cancer treated with four cycles of doxorubicin and docetaxel. Treatment with both drugs began 24 hours following the completion of chemotherapy (66). Results demonstrated that a single dose of pegfilgrastim was as effective in supporting neutrophil counts and as safe as daily filgrastim (67). Similarly, two randomized, double-blind, phase III trials in patients with breast cancer treated with myelosuppressive chemotherapy demonstrated that a single dose of pegfilgrastim provided comparable neutrophil support as an average of 11 daily injections of filgrastim (68). Currently, pegfilgrastim is administered once (6 mg), 24 hours following the completion of chemotherapy prior to the development of neutropenia.

There were few studies concerning the secondary administration of CSFs available to the American Society of Clinical Oncology working group. If a patient has already experienced chemotherapy-induced neutropenia, then CSF can be used if there is proven benefit in maintaining the dose. It is important to remember that there was no difference in infectious mortality, tumor response, or survival for the primary use of CSF. In the absence of a reason to maintain the same dose of chemotherapy, dose reduction should be considered, especially if other toxicities not responsive to CSFs are present. No evidence has been found to support the routine use of CSFs in patients with febrile neutropenia, although those at particularly high risk may have some benefit. Febrile neutropenia may result in delays in chemotherapy or dose reductions. Unfortunately, there is no data on response rate or mortality from large randomized trials. Therefore, there has been no evidence to recommend the use of CSFs to increase chemotherapy dose intensity outside of the clinical trials addressing this issue. CSFs may be useful for mobilizing peripheral blood stem cells, and they have a benefit in reducing the period of neutropenia in autologous and peripheral blood stem cell transplants. However, there was no indication for their use in patients receiving combined chemotherapy and radiotherapy. When used, the group recommended a G-CSF dose of 5 µg/kg/day (GM-CSF, 250 µg/m^2/day), without dose escalation, administered 24–72 hours after chemotherapy until the neutrophil count is >10,000 per µL after the neutrophil nadir. These recommendations are also supported by the European Society of Medical Oncology (ESMO). The ESMO, however, reported that achieving a target absolute neutrophil count of >10,000 per µL was not necessary as long as there was evidence of a sufficient/stable count (69).

The implications, including cost, of the use of G-CSF in the treatment of small cell lung cancer at the University of Indiana were reviewed (70). The overall incidence of neutropenia was 18% in the 137 patients treated with standard chemotherapy and in whom dose reductions were allowed in subsequent courses. The estimated total cost of this treatment was approximated to be $192,000. There would have been more than a sixfold increase in cost ($1,200,000) if primary treatment of all patients with G-CSF had taken place. The cost of the secondary use of G-CSF in those with a previous episode of fever and neutropenia ($272,000) would have been less than twice that of not using growth factors at all. The authors concluded that the routine use of G-CSF in patients with small cell lung cancer treated with standard-dose chemotherapy was expensive and not associated with obvious therapeutic benefits or cost savings. They suggested that careful analysis of the incidence of infectious complications, rather than granulocyte nadir and duration, be performed.

Other Prophylactic Measures

Although total protected environments (involving laminar flow, the oral administration of nonabsorbable antibiotic, and cutaneous decontamination) reduce the incidence of infection, their use proved cumbersome and expensive, and they have largely been abandoned (18), particularly for those patients for whom the duration of neutropenia is likely to be short. Individual components of these regimens, however, continue to be used in many treatment protocols.

Antibiotic Prophylaxis for Patients with Afebrile Neutropenia

There have been mixed results from the oral administration of nonabsorbable drugs such as gentamycin, nystatin, and vancomycin. The consensus panel could make no recommendation as to the use of the drugs but agreed strongly that the use of aminoglycosides in this situation should be avoided (20). In a recent review, the use of nonabsorbable antibiotics without concurrent patient isolation was not recommended because of the unpalatability of the antibiotics, their cost, the emergence of resistant organisms, and the lack of constant efficacy (18).

Prospective, randomized controlled trials have consistently shown that agents such as trimethoprim-sulfamethoxazole (TMP-SMX) and quinolones are more effective and better tolerated for infection prophylaxis. The consensus panel reported two types of oral antibiotics to be considered for chemoprophylaxis. Studies of prophylaxis with TMP-SMX were reviewed in the 1997 report of the IDSA Fever and Neutropenia Panel. These studies revealed that those patients treated with TMP-SMX prophylaxis had significantly fewer infections than those treated with placebo. There were few adverse effects, and bacterial resistance was noted. There is currently no consensus on the routine use of TMP-SMX during periods of neutropenia. There are several disadvantages to using TMP-SMX as chemoprophylaxis—adverse reactions caused by sulfonamide drugs, myelosuppression, development of drug-resistant bacteria, and oral candidiasis. It is important to note that the spectrum of TMP-SMX does not include P. aeruginosa (45).

Similar to TMP-SMX, the oral quinolones have been used extensively for prophylaxis in patients with neutropenia. One difference, however, is that they are ineffective against Pneumocystis carinii and lack activity against gram-positive organisms. A recent survey of 3600 physicians in the United States revealed that 45% use fluorquinolone prophylaxis routinely in patients receiving chemotherapy (71). Norfloxacin,

an oral quinolone, has been found to reduce gram-negative infection when compared with Bactrim, but the possibility of the development of resistance prevented the Consensus group from recommending its routine use. Kern and Kurrle reported 128 patients with neutropenia who were randomized to receive either ofloxacin or TMP-SMX as prophylaxis. They demonstrated that gram-negative bacillary infections occurred significantly less frequently in the ofloxacin group, but there was no difference in the frequency of gram-positive bacterial or fungal infections. The role of prophylactic ciprofloxacin in reducing the incidence of neutropenic fever in 88 consecutive men receiving intensive chemotherapy for germ cell tumors was reviewed. In total, 88 men received 429 courses of chemotherapy and prophylactic ciprofloxacin was prescribed for 168 courses. The incidence of fever in these patients was significantly reduced from 15% (20/131) to 5% (6/109) ($p = .02$) with prophylactic ciprofloxacin. Two patients, one of whom had received prophylactic ciprofloxacin, died of chest infections that were confirmed on postmortem. The results of this nonrandomized, retrospective study suggest that prophylactic ciprofloxacin, 250 mg twice a day, is effective in reducing the incidence of fever complicating neutropenia during chemotherapy for germ cell tumors. To be cost-effective, however, it should be given only to patients with neutropenia (72). Ciprofloxacin (750 mg twice a day) was found to be as safe and effective as TMP-SMX (160 mg per 800 mg twice a day) in the prevention of bacterial infections in 146 bone marrow transplant patients. However, ciprofloxacin was associated with a lower incidence of C. difficile enterocolitis and infections caused by gram-negative bacilli, indicating an advantage due to its use in transplant patients (73). Cullen, et al. in 2005 reported on 1565 patients in a randomized, double-blind, placebo-controlled trial randomized to receive levofloxacin ($n = 781$) or placebo ($n = 784$) for 1 week during the expected neutropenic period following myelosuppressive chemotherapy for solid tumors and lymphoma. The investigators demonstrated that during the first cycle of chemotherapy, 3.5% of patients in the levofloxacin group had at least one febrile episode, as compared with 7.9% in the placebo group ($p < .001$). Similarly, during the entire course of chemotherapy, 10.8% of patients in the levofloxacin group had at least one febrile episode, as compared with 15.2% of patients in the placebo group ($p < .001$). They concluded that among patients receiving chemotherapy for solid tumors or lymphoma, the prophylactic use of levofloxacin reduces the incidence of fever, probable infection, and hospitalization (74). A similar study conducted by Bucaneve, et al. demonstrated the efficacy of prophylactic levofloxacin in preventing febrile episodes in high-risk patients with neutropenia. Although not designed to monitor for levofloxacin-resistant organism, the investigators note a greater number of levofloxacin-resistant gram-negative organisms among patients receiving prophylactic levofloxacin compared to the placebo group (75). Other agents such as penicillin and rifampin have been added to quinolone prophylaxis with some success in preventing febrile, bacteremic episodes in patients with neutropenia.

To summarize, the panel recommended that all patients at risk for P. carinii pneumonitis, regardless of neutropenia, receive prophylaxis with TMP-SMX. Because of the concern regarding antibiotic-resistant bacteria resulting from the overuse of antibiotics, there is no consensus to recommend TMP-SMX or quinolones for routine use for all patients with afebrile neutropenia. The panel reported that the efficacy of prophylaxis with TMP-SMX and quinolones in reducing the number of infectious episodes during neutropenic periods are adequate and would warrant recommendation from the standpoint of efficacy alone. However, concern regarding the emergence of drug-resistant organisms due to extensive antibiotic use, plus the fact that prophylaxis with TMP-SMX or quinolones has not significantly reduced mortality rates prevented the consensus panel from recommending the routine use of this prophylactic therapy (20).

Prophylaxis also extends to antiviral medications. Acyclovir use decreases the incidence of herpetic gingivostomatitis in patients with neutropenia, and the administration of acyclovir decreases the incidence of cytomegalovirus pneumonitis in patients who have undergone bone marrow transplant.

ETHICAL CONSIDERATIONS OF TREATMENT OF INFECTIONS

There is no doubt that if the intention of treatment is to ensure the prolongation of survival, then treatment of the infective episode needs to be initiated. Dilemmas may arise in those patients in whom the intention of treatment is palliation. Antibiotics may make a patient feel more comfortable, but they may also prolong the dying process. A balance between the two should be assessed in each individual patient, including in particular factors such as prognosis and treatment goals.

Even if a patient is nearing death, indications for commencement of antibiotics may include convulsions or mental changes attributed to fever, extreme temperature ($>40°C$), extreme age (very young and very old), and a past history of adverse reaction to fever, marked subjective discomfort pronounced by patient, a prolonged high fever causing significant hypercatabolic state, and a reduced cardiac or pulmonary function to the extent that further tachycardia or tachypnea may be harmful. Further issues pertaining to this will be discussed in other chapters.

References

1. Petersdorf RG, Beeson PB. Fever of unexplained origin: report of 100 cases. *Medicine* 1961;40:1–29.
2. Boulant JA. Thermoregulation. In: Mackowiak P, ed. *Fever: basic mechanisms and management*. New York: Raven Press, 1991:1–22.
3. Engel A, Kern WV, Murdter G, et al. Kinetics and correlation with body temperature of circulating interleukin-6, interleukin-8, tumor necrosis factor alpha and interleukin-1 beta in patients with fever and neutropenia. *Infection* 1994;22:160–164.
4. Ashman RB, Mullbacher A. Host damaging immune responses in virus infections. *Surv Immunol Res* 1984;3:11–15.
5. Greenberg SB, Taber L. Fever of unknown origin. In: Mackowiak P, ed. *Fever: basic mechanisms and management*. New York: Raven Press, 1991:183–195.
6. Esposito AL, Gleckman RA. Fever of unknown origin in the elderly. *J Am Geriatr Soc* 1978;26:498–505.
7. Klastersky J, Weerts D, Hensgens C, et al. Fever of unexplained origin in patients with cancer. *Eur J Cancer* 1973;9:649–656.
8. Good GR, Dinubile MJ. Images in clinical medicine. Cyclic fever in Hodgkin's disease (Pel-Ebstein fever). *N Engl J Med* 1995;332:436.
9. Asher R. *Richard Asher talking sense*. London: Pittman Medical, 1972:21–22.
10. Boggs DR, Frei E. Clinical studies of fever and infection in cancer. *Cancer* 1960;13:1240–1253.
11. Pizzo PA. Evaluation of fever in the patient with cancer. *Eur J Cancer Clin Oncol* 1989;25:S9–16.
12. Bodey GP, Buckley M, Sathe YS, et al. Quantitative relationships between circulating leucocytes and infection in patients with acute leukemia. *Ann Intern Med* 1966;64:328–340.
13. Talcott JA, Siegel RD, Finberg R, et al. Risk assessment in cancer patients with fever and neutropenia: a prospective, two center validation of a prediction rule. *J Clin Oncol* 1992;10:316–322.
14. Klastersky J, Paesmans M, Rubenstein EB, et al. The Multinational Association for Supportive Care in Cancer risk index: a multinational scoring system for identifying low-risk febrile neutropenic cancer patients. *J Clin Oncol* 2000;18(16):3038–3051.
15. Buchanan GR. Approach to treatment of the febrile cancer patient with low-risk neutropenia. *Hematol Oncol Clin North Am* 1993;7:919–935.
16. Pappo AS, Buchanan GR. Predictors of bacteremia in febrile neutropenic children with cancer [Abstract]. *Proc Am Soc Clin Oncol* 1991;10:331.
17. Klastersky J. Therapy of infections. In: Klastersky J, Schimpff SC, Senn HJ, eds. *Handbook of supportive care in cancer*. New York: Marcel Decker Inc, 1994:1–44.
18. Pizzo PA. Management of fever in patients with cancer and treatment-induced neutropenia [see comments]. *N Engl J Med* 1993;328:1323–1332.
19. Pizzo PA, Robichaud KJ, Witebsky FG. Empiric antibiotics and antifungal treatment for cancer patients with prolonged fever and neutropenia. *Am J Med* 1982;72:101–111.
20. Hughes WT, Armstrong D, Bodey GP, et al. 2002 Guidelines for the use of antimicrobial agents in neutropenic patients with cancer. *Clin Infect Dis* 2002;34:730–751.
21. Machado M, Salcman M, Kaplan RS, et al. Expanded role of the cerebrospinal fluid reservoir in neurooncology: indications, causes of revision, and complications. *Neurosurgery* 1985;17:600–603.
22. Siegal T, Pfeffer MR, Steiner I. Antibiotic therapy for infected Ommaya reservoir systems. *Neurosurgery* 1988;22:97–100.
23. Eastridge BJ, Lefor AT. Complications of indwelling venous access devices in cancer patients. *J Clin Oncol* 1995;13:233–238.
24. Groeger JS, Lucas AB, Thaler HT, et al. Infectious morbidity associated with long-term use of venous access devices in patients with cancer [see comments]. *Ann Intern Med* 1993;119:1168–1174.
25. Huh YO, Lichtiger B. Transfusion reactions in patients with cancer. *Am J Clin Pathol* 1987;87:253–257.
26. Blajchman MA. Bacterial contamination of blood products and the value of pretransfusion testing. *Immunol Invest* 1995;24:163–170.
27. Manganelli D, Palla A, Donnamaria V, et al. Clinical features of pulmonary embolus. Doubts and certainties. *Chest* 1995;107:S25–S32.
28. Mackowiak PA. Drug fever. In: Mackowiak PA, ed. *Fever: basic mechanisms and management*. New York: Raven Press, 1991:255–265.
29. Mackowiak PA, LeMaistre CF. Drug fever: a critical appraisal of conventional concepts. An analysis of 51 episodes diagnosed in two Dallas hospitals and 97 episodes reported in the English literature. *Ann Intern Med* 1987;106:728–733.
30. Sonntag RW. Bleomycin (NSC-125066): phase I clinical study. *Cancer Chemo Reports—Part 1* 1972;56:197–205.
31. Ma DD, Isbister JP. Cytotoxic-induced fulminant hyperpyrexia. *Cancer* 1980;45:2249–2251.
32. Ashford RF, McLachlan A, Nelson I, et al. Pyrexia after cisplatin [letter]. *Lancet* 1980;2:691–692.
33. Clements JS Jr, Peacock JE Jr. Amphotericin B revisited: reassessment of toxicity. *Am J Med* 1990; 88:22N–27N
34. Carney-Gersten P, Giuffre M, Levy D. Factors related to amphotericin-B-induced rigors (shivering) [see comments]. *Oncol Nurs Forum* 1991;18:745–750.
35. Quesada JR, Talpaz M, Rios A, et al. Clinical toxicity of interferons in cancer patients: a review. *J Clin Oncol* 1986;4:234–243.
36. Kramer BS, Pizzo PA, Robichaud KJ, et al. Role of serial microbiologic surveillance and clinical evaluation in the management of cancer patients with fever and granulocytopenia. *Am J Med* 1982;72:561–568.
37. Feusner J, Cohen R, O'Leary M, et al. Use of routine chest radiography in the evaluation of fever in neutropenic pediatric oncology patients. *J Clin Oncol* 1988;6:1699–1702.
38. Chang JC, Gross HM. Neoplastic fever responds to the treatment of an adequate dose of naproxen. *J Clin Oncol* 1985;3:552–558.
39. Clark WG. Antipyretics. In: Mackowiak P, ed. *Fever: basic mechanics and management*. New York: Raven Press, 1991:297–340.
40. Steele RW, Tanaka PT, Lara RP, et al. Evaluation of sponging and of oral antipyretic therapy to reduce fever. *J Pediatr* 1970;77:824–829.
41. Pinsky PF, Hurwitz ES, Schonberger LB, et al. Reye's syndrome and aspirin. Evidence for a dose response effect. *JAMA* 1988;260:657–661.
42. Seed JC. A clinical comparison of the antipyretic potency of aspirin and sodium salicylate. *Clin Pharmacol Ther* 1965;6:354–358.
43. Paolozzi F, Zamkoff K, Doyle M, et al. Phase I trial of recombinant interleukin-2 and recombinant beta-interferon in refractory neoplastic diseases. *J Biol Response Mod* 1989;8:122–139.
44. Tsavaris N, Zinelis A, Karabelis A, et al. A randomized trial of the effect of three non-steroid anti-inflammatory agents in ameliorating cancer-induced fever. *J Intern Med* 1990;228:451–455.
45. Hughes WT, Armstrong D, Bodey GP, et al. Guidelines for the use of antimicrobial agents in neutropenic patients with unexplained fever. *J Infect Dis* 1990;161:381–396.
46. Sanders JW, Powe NR, Moore RD. Ceftazidime monotherapy for empiric treatment of febrile neutropenic patients: A meta-analysis. *J Infect Dis* 1991;164:907–916.
47. De Pauw BE, Deresinski SC, Feld R, et al. Ceftazidime compared with piperacillin and tobramycin for the empiric treatment of fever in neutropenic patients with cancer. A multicenter randomized trial. The Intercontinental Antimicrobial Study Group [see comments]. *Ann Intern Med* 1994;120:834–844.
48. Group EIATC. Empiric antifungal therapy in febrile granulocytopenic patients. EORTC International Antimicrobial Therapy Cooperative Group. *Am J Med* 1989;86:668–672.
49. Pizzo PA, Robichaud KJ, Gill FA, et al. Duration of empiric antibiotic therapy in granulocytopenic patients with cancer. *Am J Med* 1979;67:194–200.

50. Talcott JA, Whalen A, Clark J, et al. Home antibiotic therapy for low-risk cancer patients with fever and neutropenia: a pilot study of 30 patients based on a validated prediction rule. *J Clin Oncol* 1994;12:107–114.

51. Tomiak AT, Yau JC, Huan SD, et al. Duration of intravenous antibiotics for patients with neutropenic fever. *Ann Oncol* 1994;5:441–445.

52. de Marie S, van den Broek PJ, Willemze R, et al. Strategy for antibiotic therapy in febrile neutropenic patients on selective antibiotic decontamination. *Eur J Clin Microbiol Infect Dis* 1993;12:897–906.

53. Rubenstein EB, Rolston K, Benjamin RS, et al. Outpatient treatment of febrile episodes in low-risk neutropenic patients with cancer. *Cancer* 1993;71:3640–3646.

54. Malik IA, Khan WA, Karim M, et al. Feasibility of outpatient management of fever in cancer patients with low-risk neutropenia: results of a prospective randomized trial [see comments]. *Am J Med* 1995;98:224–231.

55. Malik IA, Abbas Z, Karim M. Randomised comparison of oral ofloxacin alone with combination of parenteral antibiotics in neutropenic febrile patients. *Lancet* 1992;339:1092–1096.

56. Freifeld A, Marchigiani D, Walsh T, et al. A double-blind comparison of empirical oral and intravenous antibiotic therapy for low-risk febrile patients with neutropenia during cancer chemotherapy. *N Engl J Med* 1999;341(5):305–311.

57. Newman KA, Reed WP, Schimpff SC, et al. Hickman catheters in association with intensive cancer chemotherapy. *Support Care Cancer* 1993;1:92–97.

58. Strauss RG. Granulocyte transfusion therapy. *Hematol Oncol Clin North Am* 1994;8:1159–1166.

59. Ellis ME, al-Hokail AA, Clink HM, et al. Double-blind randomized study of the effect of infusion rates on toxicity of amphotericin B [see comments]. *Antimicrob Agents Chemother* 1992;36:172–179.

60. Cleary JD, Weisdorf D, Fletcher CV. Effect of infusion rate on amphotericin B-associated febrile reactions. *Drug Intell Clin Pharm* 1988;22:769–772.

61. Ozer H, Armitage JO, Bennett CL, et al. American Society of Clinical Oncology. 2000 update of recommendations for the use of hematopoietic colony-stimulating factors: evidence-based, clinical practice guidelines. American Society of Clinical Oncology Growth Factors Expert Panel. *J Clin Oncol* 2000;18(20):3558–3585.

62. Benson AB III, Desch CE, Flynn PJ, et al. American Society of Clinical Oncology. 2000 update of American Society of Clinical Oncology colorectal cancer surveillance guidelines. *J Clin Oncol* 2000;18(20):3586–3588.

63. McNeil C. NCCN Guidelines advocate wider use of colony-stimulating factor. *J Natl Cancer Inst* 2005;97(10):710–711.

64. Biganzoli L, Untch M, Skacel T, et al. Neulasta (Pegfilgrastim): A once-per-cycle option for the management of chemotherapy-induced neutropenia. *Semin Oncol* 2004;31(Suppl 8):27–34.

65. Yowell SL, Blackwell S. Novel effects of with polyethylene glycol modified pharmaceuticals. *Cancer Treat Rev* 2002;28(Suppl A):3–6.

66. Holmes FA, Jones SE, O'Shaughnessy J, et al. Comparable efficiency and safety profiles of once-per-cycle pegfilgrastim and daily filgrastim in chemotherapy-induced neutropenia: a multicenter dose-finding study in women with breast cancer. *Ann Oncol* 2002;13:903–909.

67. Holmes FA, O'Shaughnessy JA, Vukelja S, et al. Blinded, randomized, multicenter study to evaluate single administration pegfilgrastim once per cycle versus daily filgrastim as an adjunct to chemotherapy in patients with high-risk stage II or stage III/IV breast cancer. *J Clin Oncol* 2002;20:727–731.

68. Crawford J. Once-per-cycle pegfilgrastim (Neulasta) for the management of chemotherapy-induced neutropenia. *Semin Oncol* 2003;30(Suppl 13):24–30.

69. Greil R, Jost LM. ESMO recommendations for the application of hematopoietic growth factors. *Ann Oncol* 2005;16(Suppl 1):i80–i82.

70. Nichols CR, Fox EP, Roth BJ, et al. Incidence of neutropenic fever in patients treated with standard-dose combination chemotherapy for small-cell lung cancer and the cost impact of treatment with granulocyte colony-stimulating factor. *J Clin Oncol* 1994;12:1245–1250.

71. Freifeld A, McNabb J, Anderson F, et al. Low-risk patients with fever and neutropenia during chemotherapy: current clinical practice patterns. *J Clin Oncol* 2004 ASCO Ann Meet Proc (Post-Meeting Edition) (14S (July 15 Supplement), 2004;22:8089.

72. Counsell R, Pratt J, Williams MV. Chemotherapy for germ cell tumours: prophylactic ciprofloxacin reduces the incidence of neutropenic fever. *Clin Oncol (R Coll Radiol)* 1994;6:232–236.

73. Lew MA, Kohoe K, Ritz J, et al. Ciprofloxacin versus trimethoprim/sulfamethoxazole for prophylaxis of bacterial infections in bone marrow transplant recipients: a randomized, controlled trial. *J Clin Oncol* 1995;13:239–250.

74. Cullen M, Steven N, Billingham L, et al. Antibacterial Prophylaxis after chemotherapy for solid tumors and lymphomas. *N Engl J Med* 2005;353:988–998.

75. Bucaneve G, Micozzi A, Menichetti F, et al. Levofloxacin to prevent bacterial infection in patients with cancer and neutropenia. *N Engl J Med* 2005;353:977–987.

CHAPTER 10 ■ HOT FLASHES

DOMINGO G. PEREZ AND CHARLES L. LOPRINZI

Nearly three fourth of menopausal women experience hot flashes (1), which are usually described as a sudden and disturbing sensation of intense warmth that starts in the chest and then progresses to the neck and face. Red blotches can appear on the skin, and the increase in skin temperature can lead to profuse sweating. This feeling of intense warmth is often accompanied by palpitations and anxiety. Hot flashes usually last about 4 minutes, but they can last for as little as a few seconds or for 10 minutes or longer. In some women, hot flashes occur every 20 minutes, while in others they occur only once a month. Hot flashes typically start 1 or 2 years before menopause and continue to occur for 1 to 5 years, but in some women they can occur for a longer period of time. Hot flash symptoms can have serious detrimental effects on a woman's work, recreation, sleep, and general perception of quality of life (2).

Hot flashes can be a significant problem for patients with cancer. In many premenopausal women with breast cancer and other gynecologic malignancies, the precipitation of menopause by oophorectomy, chemotherapy, radiotherapy, or hormonal manipulation can lead to the rapid onset of hot flash symptoms that are more frequent and severe than those associated with natural menopause (3). Discontinuation of estrogen replacement therapy in women newly diagnosed with breast or uterine cancer often results in hot flash symptoms. In addition, tamoxifen and the aromatase inhibitors, the most commonly prescribed agents for the treatment of breast cancer, are associated with an increased risk of hot flashes (4). Postmenopausal women with a history of hot flashes are more likely to have hot flashes when exposed to tamoxifen.

Hot flashes are also a common problem in men undergoing androgen deprivation therapy for prostate cancer. Hot flashes have been reported to occur in up to 70% of men after orchiectomy, 80% of men receiving neoadjuvant hormonal therapy before radical prostatectomy, and 70–80% of men receiving long-term androgen deprivation therapy (5–7).

PATHOPHYSIOLOGY OF HOT FLASHES

In humans, perspiration and vasodilatation, the classic mechanisms of heat loss that are activated during hot flashes, are centrally regulated by the thermoregulatory nucleus in the medial preoptic area of the hypothalamus (8). The thermoregulatory nucleus activates perspiration and vasodilatation to keep core body temperature within a tightly regulated range known as the thermoregulatory zone. In menopausal women with hot flashes, the thermoregulatory zone is shifted downward and is narrower than in menopausal women who do not have hot flashes (9). Therefore, in women with hot flashes, small changes in body temperature (as low as 0.01°C) may trigger the mechanisms of heat loss that lead to hot flash symptoms (10).

The dramatic decrease in sexual hormone levels that occurs in menopausal women and in men receiving androgen deprivation therapy is thought to be responsible for lowering and narrowing the thermoregulatory zone. However, sexual hormones have profound effects on multiple neuroendocrine pathways (11) and the exact mechanisms by which they affect the thermoregulatory zone are poorly understood. Therefore, when discussing the pathophysiology of hot flashes and the possible mechanism of action of any of the nonhormonal agents currently in use for the treatment of this problem, only an educated guess can be made.

Since estrogen withdrawal results in decreased central serotonergic activity (12) and some of the newer antidepressants (i.e., venlafaxine and paroxetine) have been shown to relieve hot flashes in placebo-controlled, randomized clinical trials (vide infra), serotonin (5-HT) is thought to play an important role in mediating the thermoregulatory effects of estrogen. In particular, the 5-HT$_{2A}$ receptor has been closely associated with thermoregulation in mammals. Multiple animal and human studies have shown that central expression of the 5-HT$_{2A}$ receptor decreases after estrogen withdrawal and that estrogen treatment reverses this change in estrogen-deficient animals and women (12,13). In addition, tamoxifen has been shown to block the positive effects of estrogen on central 5-HT$_{2A}$ receptor expression in ovariectomized rats (14). Since estrogen withdrawal and tamoxifen treatment result in decreased central expression of 5-HT$_{2A}$ receptors, it is possible that the efficacy of the newer antidepressants against hot flashes is due, at least in part, to their ability to cause a "compensatory" increase in central 5-HT$_{2A}$ signaling (15).

Norepinephrine has also been implicated in the pathophysiology of hot flashes. Estrogen withdrawal leads to increased norepinephrine levels in the hypothalamus (9), which are thought to contribute to the lowering and narrowing of the thermoregulatory zone. In keeping with this theory, several placebo-controlled, randomized clinical trials have shown that clonidine, a centrally acting α_2-adrenergic receptor agonist, is moderately effective in decreasing hot flashes (vide infra).

---

*Portions of this manuscript were adapted with permission from Perez DG, Loprinzi CL. Nonhormonal agents for the treatment of hot flashes. *Compr Ther* 2005;31(2):224–236.

The neuroendocrine pathways that govern thermoregulation in mammals are extraordinarily complex and, as yet, incompletely understood. There is a clear need for further studies to clarify the pathophysiology of hot flashes and to guide the clinical development of more targeted nonhormonal treatments for this problem.

TREATMENT OF HOT FLASHES

Nonpharmacologic Interventions

Multiple nonpharmacologic interventions have been claimed to be of help in alleviating hot flashes. These include the use of fans, air conditioners, cold water, special diets, exercise programs, acupuncture, meditation, relaxation techniques, paced respiration, biofeedback, and so on. However, none of these strategies has been tested in controlled, randomized clinical trials and the placebo effect likely plays a significant role in their apparent efficacy. Indeed, placebo-controlled, randomized clinical trials in women with hot flashes have consistently shown a 20 to 30% reduction in hot flash frequency and severity in women in the placebo group over a 4-week period (*vide infra*). This must be kept in mind when evaluating anecdotal evidence or pilot studies.

Pharmacologic Interventions

Hormonal Therapy

Estrogen. Estrogen reduces hot flashes by 80 to 90% in women with this problem (16). However, there are many situations in which estrogen treatment is contraindicated. For instance, women with a history of coronary artery disease, venous thromboembolism, and uterine cancer should not take estrogen. The use of estrogen in women with a history of breast cancer is controversial. Several prospective and retrospective studies suggest that at least some breast cancer survivors (women with small tumors, negative lymph node status, long disease-free survival, or estrogen receptor–negative tumors) can be safely treated with estrogen replacement (17). However, in the absence of data from large, well-designed randomized clinical trials proving the safety of estrogen treatment in women with a history of breast cancer, most physicians will avoid using estrogen in this patient population. Moreover, the results of the Women's Health Initiative study (18) and other recent studies suggest that long-term estrogen treatment should not be recommended for most women for a variety of reasons.

Progestational agents. Several pilot studies in the 1970s and 1980s suggested that medroxyprogesterone decreased hot flashes. Subsequently, a placebo-controlled, randomized clinical trial of megestrol 40 mg daily in 97 women with history of breast cancer and 66 men receiving androgen deprivation therapy for prostate cancer showed a reduction in hot flashes of 75–80% in the treatment group compared to 20–25% in the placebo group (19). Three years after the completion of the study, one third of the women were still taking megestrol, and this group of women reported having less hot flashes that women who had stopped taking the medication (20). The intramuscular long-acting progestational agent depomedroxyprogesterone acetate (DMPA) has also been shown to be useful for the treatment of hot flashes. In a randomized clinical trial of DMPA versus megestrol acetate, both agents were found to have similar efficacy (21). A placebo-controlled, randomized clinical trial of a progesterone cream in 102 postmenopausal women showed a reduction in hot flashes of 83% in the treatment group compared to 19% in the placebo

group, after 4 weeks of therapy (22). This benefit was still present after 12 months with continued use of the progesterone cream. Adverse effects of progestational agents include vaginal bleeding upon discontinuation of the medication, weight gain, bloating, and thromboembolic phenomena.

Despite the proved efficacy of progestational agents for the treatment of hot flashes, many physicians are wary of using hormonally active agents in patients with a history of breast cancer. Though there is some evidence that progestational agents are active against breast cancer (23), *in vitro* data suggest that they can increase epithelial cell proliferation, a potentially undesirable effect in patients with a history of breast cancer (24). In addition, megestrol was reported to increase the prostate specific antigen (PSA) level in a patient with prostate cancer who was being treated with this agent for hot flashes (25). Given the ongoing debate on this issue, patients need to be counseled before starting a progestational agent if they have a history of breast or prostate cancer.

Nonhormonal Therapy

The reluctance to use hormonally active agents in patients with a history of breast cancer provided the impetus for finding nonhormonal agents that could help alleviate this problem. The following is a brief summary of their clinical development.

Newer antidepressants. In the 1990s, several authors reported reductions in hot flash frequency and severity in postmenopausal women who were taking several of the newer antidepressants for other reasons. Since then, the results of 18 prospective studies of several newer antidepressants for the treatment of hot flashes have been reported. These studies have been reviewed in detail elsewhere (26). Given the reluctance to use estrogen or even a progestational agent in women with a history of breast cancer, many of these studies were done in this patient population, but some studies have been done in noncancer patients and in men with prostate cancer. Self-completed daily hot flash diaries were used to document the frequency and severity of hot flashes. Data on toxicity, quality of life and mood status were commonly obtained. The main efficacy measures used in most studies were the change from baseline in the weekly average number of daily hot flashes and average hot flash score (defined as the number of mild hot flashes plus twice the number of moderate hot flashes plus three times the number of severe hot flashes plus four times the number of very severe hot flashes during that week).

Venlafaxine. Venlafaxine selectively inhibits serotonin, norepinephrine, and dopamine reuptake, in order of decreasing potency. The efficacy of venlafaxine for the treatment of hot flashes was first studied in 1997 in a small pilot study (27). This study included women with a history of breast cancer and men receiving androgen deprivation therapy for prostate cancer. Patients were treated with venlafaxine 12.5 mg twice a day for 4 weeks. Of the 31 patients originally enrolled, 25 completed the study. Eighty-two percent of the patients were women. The average number of daily hot flashes decreased from 6.6 at baseline to 4.3 during the last week of the study. The average hot flash score decreased by 55%. Patients reported significant improvement in fatigue, sweating, and difficulty sleeping, and, at the completion of the study, 64% of the patients chose to continue venlafaxine.

Subsequently, the same investigators conducted a placebo-controlled, double-blind, randomized clinical trial to assess more definitely the efficacy and toxicity of venlafaxine in breast cancer survivors with hot flashes (28). Women were randomized to four treatment arms:

1. Placebo (*n* = 56)
2. Venlafaxine extended release (ER) 37.5 mg daily for 4 weeks (*n* = 56)

3. Venlafaxine ER 37.5 mg daily for 1 week, followed by 75 mg daily for 3 weeks ($n = 55$)
4. Venlafaxine ER 37.5 mg daily for 1 week, followed by 75 mg daily for 1 week, followed by 150 mg daily for 2 weeks ($n = 54$).

Sixty-nine percent of the women were taking tamoxifen. Complete information was available for 191 of the 221 women originally enrolled onto the study. After 4 weeks of treatment, the median frequency of hot flashes decreased 19, 30, 46 and 58% in women in groups 1, 2, 3 and 4, respectively, ($p < .001$ for all groups compared to placebo). Hot flash activity decreased more than 50% in 20, 45, 63 and 55%, respectively. Beck Depression Inventory (BDI) scores improved by a mean of 1.6, 2.4, 4.8 and 3.2 points, respectively. Overall quality of life decreased by 3 points in the placebo group compared to an average increase of 3 points in patients taking venlafaxine ER ($p = .02$). Dry mouth, nausea, constipation, and decreased appetite were significantly more common in patients taking venlafaxine. Venlafaxine ER 150 mg daily was associated with significantly more adverse effects. Efficacy was similar whether tamoxifen was being used or not.

At the completion of the study, treatment was unblinded and women were offered the option of participating in an 8-week, open-label, continuation study (29). Of the 221 women originally enrolled onto the double-blind study, 157 participated in the continuation study. At the time of data analysis, complete information was available for 102 women. Sixty-six percent of women were taking tamoxifen. At the completion of the study, 26 women were taking venlafaxine ER 37.5 mg daily, 35 were taking 75 mg daily, 6 were taking 112.5 mg daily, and 34 were taking 150 mg daily. Among women initially randomized to placebo, the mean hot flash score decreased 62% at the end of the 8-week period. An additional mean reduction in hot flash score of 26% was reported for women originally randomized to venlafaxine 37.5 mg daily. For the 75 mg and 150 mg groups, the 60% reduction in hot flash score achieved in the double-blind study was maintained throughout the continuation phase. Side effects, including mood changes, trouble sleeping, abnormal sweating, and fatigue were reported by fewer women during the continuation phase than during the baseline week.

The long-term efficacy and toxicity of venlafaxine in women with hot flashes was evaluated in two recent randomized clinical trials. In the first trial (30), 80 healthy postmenopausal women with hot flashes were randomized to placebo ($n = 40$) or venlafaxine ER ($n = 40$). Women received venlafaxine 37.5 mg daily for 1 week, followed by 75 mg daily for 11 weeks. Sixty-one women completed the study (32 in the placebo group and 29 in the treatment group). After 12 weeks of treatment, there were no statistically significant differences between the two groups in terms of hot flash frequency and severity. Dryness of the mouth, insomnia, and decreased appetite were significantly more common in the venlafaxine group. However, mental health, and vitality were significantly improved in the venlafaxine group, and 93% of women in this group chose to continue venlafaxine at the conclusion of the study. In the second trial (31), which has been published in abstract form only, 60 healthy postmenopausal women with hot flashes were randomized to placebo ($n = 20$), venlafaxine 37.5 mg daily ($n = 22$) or venlafaxine 75 mg daily ($n = 18$). After 3 weeks of therapy, hot flashes increased by 10% in the placebo group, while they decreased by 65 and 51% in women taking venlafaxine 37.5 mg and 75 mg, respectively. From this point on, all women in the venlafaxine groups (except six women in the 75 mg group who withdrew from the study) received 37.5 mg daily. After 4 months of treatment, hot flashes decreased by 78% in the venlafaxine group compared to 2% in the placebo group. Nausea and dryness of the mouth, the most

frequent side effects, were more common in the venlafaxine groups and were dose related.

The efficacy of venlafaxine for the alleviation of hot flashes in men undergoing androgen deprivation therapy was evaluated in two small studies. In the first study (32), men were treated with venlafaxine 12.5 mg b.i.d. for 4 weeks. Of the 23 men originally enrolled in the study, 16 completed the study and were evaluable. Of these, 10 (63%) had a greater than 50% reduction in their hot flash scores at the end of the study. Median weekly hot flash scores decreased by 54%, and the average incidence of severe and very severe hot flashes decreased from 2.3 per day at baseline to 0.6 per day at the end of the study ($p = .003$). Treatment was well tolerated. In the second study (33), which has been published only in abstract form, the initial dose of venlafaxine was 75 mg daily, but this dose had to be decreased to 37.5 mg daily after one of the first four patients developed grade 2 toxicity. Of the 20 patients originally enrolled, 17 completed the study and were evaluable. After 4 weeks of treatment, the weekly average hot flash score decreased by 58%, and 71% of patients experienced more than a 50% reduction in their hot flash scores. The average weekly frequency of hot flashes decreased from 58.6 at baseline to 29 at the end of the study ($p = .0001$). Overall quality of life ($n = 15$) increased by an average of 1.3 points ($p — .01$). BDI scores ($n = 11$) improved by an average of 3.5 points ($p = .01$). Treatment was well tolerated and 75% of patients expressed their wish to continue venlafaxine. The results of the 75 mg per day arm of this venlafaxine trial is illustrated in Figure 10.1 along with results from several other trials.

Finally, venlafaxine and medroxyprogesterone have been compared in a randomized clinical trial that has been published in abstract form only (34). Women were randomized to venlafaxine 37.5 mg daily for 1 week followed by 75 mg daily ($n — 109$), medroxyprogesterone acetate (MPA) 400 mg IM once ($n = 109$), or MPA 500 mg IM every 2 weeks for three doses ($n = 9$, arm closed prematurely due to slow accrual). Of the 227 women originally randomized, 185 were evaluable. At the end of the study, women in the MPA arm experienced a reduction in median hot flash frequency of 85% compared to 52% in the venlafaxine arm ($p < .0001$), with a reduction in median hot flash score of 88% compared to 57% in the venlafaxine arm ($p < .0001$). Twenty-four percent of women in the MPA arm reported no hot flashes at week 7 compared to 1% of women in the venlafaxine arm ($p < .0001$). Women in the MPA arm had significantly less constipation, abnormal sweating, hot flash distress, sleepiness, and trouble sleeping.

Fluoxetine. Fluoxetine is a serotonin reuptake inhibitor with negligible effects on the noradrenergic system. The efficacy of fluoxetine for the treatment of hot flashes was studied in an 8-week, placebo-controlled, double-blind, crossover clinical trial in women with a history of breast cancer or apprehension regarding the use of estrogen (35). Women were randomized to fluoxetine 20 mg daily or placebo, and, after 4 weeks, patients were crossed over. Of the 81 women originally enrolled onto the study, 66 provided complete data. Fifty-four percent of women were taking tamoxifen. By the end of the first treatment period, hot flash scores decreased by 50% in the fluoxetine group versus 36% in the placebo group, but this difference was not statistically significant. Crossover analysis, however, demonstrated a significantly greater improvement in hot flash score with fluoxetine than with placebo ($p = .02$). In addition, fluoxetine was associated with a greater reduction in the number of daily hot flashes ($p = .01$). There was no statistically significant difference in adverse events. Efficacy was similar whether tamoxifen was being used or not.

The long-term efficacy and toxicity of fluoxetine and citalopram were compared in a placebo-controlled, double-blind,

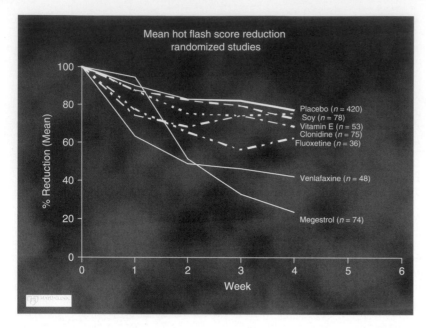

FIGURE 10.1. The figure illustrates data from a series of randomized, placebo-controlled, double-blinded clinical trials conducted by Mayo Clinic/North Central Cancer Treatment Group investigators. Pooled placebo patients (420 subjects) illustrate that a placebo decreases hot flashes by about 25% over a 4-week period of time. In the individual studies, Soy was not significantly better than a placebo (actually doing worse than the placebo in the individual trial), but vitamin E did do a little better. Clonidine was better than the placebo (shown also by other investigators). Fluoxetine fared a bit better than a placebo. Venlafaxine and Megestrol acetate were much better than was a placebo.

randomized clinical trial (36). One hundred fifty healthy postmenopausal women with hot flashes were randomized to placebo (n = 50), fluoxetine (n = 50) or citalopram (n = 50). Women were started on fluoxetine or citalopram 10 mg daily. The dose of both fluoxetine and citalopram was increased to 20 mg after 1 month and to 30 mg after 6 months. Women were treated for a total of 9 months. There were no statistically significant differences among the three groups with respect to hot flashes at any time during the study. Discontinuation rates were 40% in the placebo group, 34% in the fluoxetine group and 34% in the citalopram group. Insomnia improved significantly in the citalopram group compared to the placebo group.

Paroxetine. Paroxetine is a selective serotonin reuptake inhibitor with minimal effects on the reuptake of norepinephrine. The efficacy of paroxetine against hot flashes was initially studied in two small pilot studies in women with a history of breast cancer. In the first study (37), women were treated with paroxetine 10 mg daily for 1 week, followed by paroxetine 20 mg daily for 4 weeks. Of the 30 women originally enrolled, 27 completed the study. After 5 weeks of treatment, the mean hot flash frequency decreased by 67%, while the mean hot flash severity score decreased by 75%. There was a statistically significant improvement in depression, sleep, anxiety, and quality of life scores. Furthermore, 25 (83%) of the women chose to continue paroxetine after the end of study. The most common adverse effect was somnolence, resulting in drug discontinuation in two women and dose reduction in two others. In the second study (38), 13 women were treated with paroxetine 10 mg daily for 3 days, followed by 20 mg daily. After 5 weeks of treatment, 11 women (85%) were still having hot flashes, but the percentage of women still rating their hot flashes as "quite a bit" or "extremely severe" had declined from 100% to 38% (p = .008). The average rating for hot flash severity decreased significantly to the "moderately severe" range (p = .002). In addition, significant improvements were observed in general, emotional and mental fatigue. Rates of clinically significant depressive symptoms decreased and sleep quality improved significantly.

On the basis of these encouraging results, a placebo-controlled, double-blind, randomized clinical trial of paroxetine controlled release (CR) in menopausal women with hot flashes was conducted (39). One hundred sixty-five women were randomized to placebo (n = 56), paroxetine CR 12.5 mg daily (n = 51) or paroxetine CR 25 mg daily (n = 58) for

6 weeks. Among the 139 women who completed the study, the hot flash score had decreased by 62 and 65% in the lower and higher-dose paroxetine groups, respectively, compared to a 38% reduction in the placebo group, after 6 weeks of therapy. The mean daily hot flash frequency decreased from 7.1 to 3.8 in women taking paroxetine CR 12.5 mg, from 6.4 to 3.2 in women taking paroxetine CR 25 mg, and from 6.6 to 4.8 in women taking placebo. Of 104 women with baseline and week 6 data who received paroxetine CR, more than half experienced a 50% or more reduction in hot flash frequency and severity and were considered responders. The response rates were 58% for those receiving 12.5 mg, 63% for those receiving 25 mg, and 43% for those receiving placebo. Although not statistically significant, the odds of being a responder were almost twice greater for women taking paroxetine 12.5 mg than for those taking placebo (OR 1.95, 95% CI 0.86–4.40, p = .1). In contrast, the odds of being a responder were more than 2.5 times greater for women taking paroxetine 25 mg than for those taking placebo (OR 2.56, 95% CI 1.15–5.68, p = .02). The improvement in hot flash symptoms was independent of tamoxifen use. Adverse events were reported by 54% of women taking placebo and by 58% of women taking paroxetine CR.

The efficacy of paroxetine for the treatment of hot flashes in men undergoing androgen deprivation therapy was evaluated in a small pilot study (40). Twenty-six men were treated with extended release paroxetine 12.5 mg daily for 1 week, followed by 25 mg for 1 week, followed by 37.5 mg for 1 week. During the fourth treatment week, depending on hot flash control and adverse effects, patients could either take 37.5 mg or decrease the dose to 25 mg or 12.5 mg. Of the 26 patients originally enrolled, 18 completed the study. In these patients, the median frequency of hot flashes decreased from 6.2 per day at baseline to 2.5 per day at the end of the study. Hot flash scores decreased from 10.6 per day to 3 per day. Treatment was well tolerated.

Citalopram. Citalopram is a potent and specific serotonin reuptake inhibitor. The efficacy of citalopram against hot flashes was evaluated in two small pilot studies. In the first study (41), women with hot flashes and a history of breast cancer or apprehension regarding the use of estrogen were treated with citalopram 10 mg daily for 1 week, followed by 20 mg daily for 3 weeks. Of the 26 women originally enrolled, 15 completed the study and were evaluable. By the end of the study, the mean hot flash frequency had decreased by 58%, and the mean hot flash score by 64%. Women who finished the study also reported decreased, tension, and depression, as well as an improved mood. In the second study (42), 30 women with persistent hot flashes despite treatment with venlafaxine were treated with citalopram 10 mg daily for 1 week followed by 20 mg daily for 3 weeks. Complete hot flash data were available for 22 patients. Mean and median hot flash scores were reduced by 53% ($p < .001$). Mean hot flash frequencies were reduced by 45% ($p < .001$). Nineteen women (65% of women originally enrolled onto the study and 86% of women who completed the study) chose to continue on citalopram. Finally, in the recent placebo-controlled, double-blind, randomized clinical trial of fluoxetine and citalopram noted above (36), neither antidepressant had any significant effects on hot flashes compared to placebo, either in the short- or the long-term.

Sertraline. Sertraline is a very potent and selective serotonin reuptake inhibitor that appears to have little effect on dopamine and norepinephrine metabolism. In a placebo-controlled, double-blind, randomized crossover clinical trial (43) published in abstract form only, 62 women with hot flashes who were taking adjuvant tamoxifen for breast cancer were randomized to sertraline 50 mg daily or placebo. After 6 weeks of therapy, women were crossed over. Of the 62 women randomized, 47 completed the first 6 weeks of the study. After 6 weeks of therapy, 27% of women in the placebo group ($n = 22$) had a 50% reduction in the frequency of hot flashes compared to 36% of women in the treatment group ($n = 25$), but this difference was not statistically significant. After 12 weeks of therapy, women were asked which tablets worked best ($n = 36$) and which of the two 6-week periods was better ($n = 37$). Fifty-six percent of women reported that sertraline worked best, 17% reported that placebo worked best and 28% had no preference. Forty-nine percent of patients preferred the sertraline period, 11% the placebo period, and 41% had no preference.

Mirtazapine. Mirtazapine has antihistaminic, antiserotonergic, and α_2-blocking activity without any significant effect on the synaptic reuptake of catecholamines. In a small pilot study (44), women with hot flashes and a history of breast cancer or apprehension regarding the use of estrogen were treated with mirtazapine 7.5 mg at bedtime during the first week, 15 mg at bedtime during the second week, and 30 mg at bedtime during the third week. During the fourth and last week of the study, women could take either 15 or 30 mg. Of the 27 women originally enrolled, 16 completed the study. The median reduction from baseline in total daily hot flashes and weekly hot flash scores were 53 and 60%, respectively. Patients reported improvements in tension and trouble sleeping. Increased appetite and dry mouth were the most common side effects.

Interactions between Tamoxifen and the Newer Antidepressants. It is important to bear in mind that some of the newer antidepressants have clinically important interactions with other drugs metabolized by the cytochrome (CYP) P-450 system. For instance, paroxetine, a potent CYP2D6 inhibitor, decreases the plasma concentration of endoxifen, a tamoxifen metabolite much more potent than tamoxifen itself. A recent study (45) indicated that, in women with breast cancer taking tamoxifen for adjuvant purposes, the risk of recurrence is higher in women with a less metabolically active CYP2D6 genotype (i.e., in those with lower endoxifen levels) (46). Therefore, it appears prudent to avoid using paroxetine in women who are taking tamoxifen. Venlafaxine is a weak CYP2D6 inhibitor and does not appear to have any significant effects on endoxifen levels (45).

Gabapentin. The exact mechanism of action of the γ-aminobutyric acid analog gabapentin has yet to be determined, but it is widely used in the treatment of a variety of neurologic disorders including neuropathic pain, migraine, and so on. The efficacy of gabapentin for the treatment of hot flashes was first noted serendipitously in a group of six patients at the University of Rochester (47). All six patients reported a 75–100% reduction in hot flashes within 72 hours of starting gabapentin for other reasons. In a subsequent pilot study in 20 women with hot flashes (48), the 16 women who completed the study experienced a 66% reduction in hot flash frequency after 4 weeks of treatment. Similar results were obtained in another pilot study (49). A placebo-controlled, double-blind, randomized clinical trial of gabapentin 900 mg daily in 59 postmenopausal women without a history of breast cancer (50) showed a reduction in hot flash scores of 54% in the treatment group compared to 31% in the placebo group, after 12 weeks of therapy. Side effects included lightheadedness, dizziness, and edema. Subsequently, a placebo-controlled, randomized clinical trial of gabapentin in breast cancer survivors showed similar results (51). A placebo-controlled, randomized clinical trial of gabapentin in men receiving androgen deprivation therapy for prostate cancer is ongoing.

Clonidine. Clonidine is a centrally acting α_2-receptor agonist with antihypertensive properties. The efficacy of transdermal clonidine for the treatment of hot flashes was shown in a placebo-controlled, randomized clinical trial (52). However, the use of the patch was associated with significant side effects (fatigue, dry mouth, and constipation). Another placebo-controlled, randomized clinical trial of clonidine 0.1 mg orally every night in 194 women with history of breast cancer who were taking tamoxifen (53) showed a decrease in hot flashes of 37% in the clonidine group compared to 24% in the placebo group, after 8 weeks of therapy. Patients in the clonidine group had more side effects, especially insomnia (41% in the clonidine group versus 21% in the placebo group). Therefore, although clonidine decreases hot flashes, its limited efficacy and unfavorable toxicity profile greatly limit its use.

Bellargal. Belladonna is a plant extract that has antimuscarinic properties. In combination with phenobarbital and ergotamine (Bellargal), belladonna was used in the 1970s and 1980s for the management of hot flashes. However, available data suggest only a small benefit for Bellargal over placebo. In one placebo-controlled, randomized clinical trial (54), hot flashes decreased by 75% in the Bellargal group compared with 68% in the placebo group after 2 weeks of therapy, but this small difference was lost after 8 weeks. Since safer and more efficacious nonhormonal treatments for hot flashes became available, Bellargal has fallen out of favor.

Vitamin E. There are some data supporting the use of vitamin E for the treatment of hot flashes. A single placebo-controlled, randomized, crossover clinical trial of vitamin E 800 IU daily in 120 women (55) suggested that, on average, women taking vitamin E had one less hot flash per day than women taking placebo. Side effects were similar in the treatment and the placebo groups.

Soy. Soy is a prominent source of phytoestrogens. The North Central Cancer Treatment Group (NCCTG) conducted a placebo-controlled, double-blind, randomized clinical trial of a soy isoflavone preparation (150 mg daily) in 177 women with history of breast cancer (56). This study did not show any significant effect on hot flash frequency or severity. A recent review of all the hot flash trials of soy products concluded that, overall, soy decreased hot flashes 5% more than placebo (57). Given the well-known publication bias, this minimal difference does not bode well for soy as a hot flash remedy. In addition, there is an ongoing debate over whether soy decreases, or increases, the risk of breast cancer.

Black cohosh. The herbal remedy black cohosh (*Cimicifuga racemosa*) has been approved for the treatment of hot flashes in Germany, where several relatively small studies suggested that it relieved hot flashes. However, two recent placebo-controlled, randomized clinical trials did not show any statically significant difference in the frequency or severity of hot flashes between the black cohosh and the placebo groups (58,59).

RECOMMENDATIONS

Based on the available data and the risks and benefits associated with each of the above treatment modalities, the following recommendations can be made.

If a patient has mild symptoms that do not interfere with her or his daily activities, a trial of vitamin E 800 IU would be a reasonable option. This readily available and inexpensive therapy may allow a patient to get the well-known placebo effect and something else. It should be kept in mind, however, that it may take several weeks for this effect to take place.

If a patient has more severe symptoms, it is reasonable to start one of the newer antidepressants or gabapentin. At this time, one agent cannot be recommended over the other as they have not been compared in randomized clinical trials. Such a trial is currently under way. Among the newer antidepressants, venlafaxine and paroxetine seem reasonable first options, with the caveat that paroxetine and other strong CYP2D6 inhibitors should be avoided in women with breast cancer who are taking tamoxifen. Venlafaxine should be started at a dose of 37.5 mg daily. If necessary, this dose can be increased to 75 mg daily. Higher doses do not seem to result in additional benefit and are associated with more toxicity. For paroxetine, a dose of 12.5 mg daily is recommended. Higher doses do not seem to be more effective and are also associated with more toxicity. When using gabapentin, it is reasonable to start with 300 mg at bedtime for 3 days and then titrate the dose up to 300 mg t.i.d. Data from nonrandomized studies suggest that higher doses may be more effective. Finally, based on the results of a recent randomized clinical trial of MPA versus venlafaxine in women with hot flashes (34), a single dose of MPA 400 mg i.m. appears to be a very reasonable option. However, before using MPA, women need to be told that this is a hormonal preparation and that there are no good data regarding its positive or negative effects on breast cancer risk (Figure 10.1).

Although no placebo-controlled, randomized clinical trials of any of the newer antidepressants have been conducted in men with hot flashes undergoing androgen deprivation therapy for prostate cancer, the results of three pilot studies of venlafaxine and paroxetine suggest that these agents are also effective in this patient population. The results of these studies should ideally be confirmed in placebo-controlled, randomized clinical trials, but given their similarity with those obtained with the same agents in women with hot flashes, for which data from placebo-controlled, randomized clinical trials are available, the use of venlafaxine and paroxetine in men with hot flashes seems justified.

References

1. McKinlay SM, Jeffreys M. The menopausal syndrome. *Br J Prev Soc Med* 1974;28:108–115.
2. Daly E, Gray A, Barlow D, et al. Measuring the impact of menopausal symptoms on quality of life. *BMJ* 1993;307:836–840.
3. Carpenter J, Andrykowski MA, Cordova M, et al. Hot flashes in postmenopausal women treated for breast carcinoma. *Cancer* 1998;82:1682–1691.
4. Love RR, Cameron L, Connell BL, et al. Symptoms associated with tamoxifen treatment in postmenopausal women. *Arch Intern Med* 1991;151:1842–1847.
5. Buchholz NP, Mattarelli G, Buchholz MM. Post-orchiectomy hot flushes. *Eur Urol* 1994;26:120–122.
6. Schow DA, Renfer LG, Rozanski TA, et al. Prevalence of hot flushes during and after neoadjuvant hormonal therapy for localized prostate cancer. *South Med J* 1998;91:855–887.
7. Lanfrey P, Mottet N, Dagues F, et al. Hot flashes and hormonal treatment of prostate cancer. *Prog Urol* 1996;6:17–22.
8. Casper RF, Yen SS. Neuroendocrinology of menopausal flushes: an hypothesis of flush mechanism. *Clin Endocrinol (Oxf)* 1985;22:293–312.
9. Freedman RR, Krell W. Reduced thermoregulatory null zone in postmenopausal women with hot flashes. *Am J Obstet Gynecol* 1999;181:66–70.
10. Freedman RR, Norton D, Woodward S, et al. Core body temperature and circadian rhythm of hot flashes in menopausal women. *J Clin Endocrinol Metab* 1995;80:2354–2358.
11. McEwen B. Estrogen actions throughout the brain. *Recent Prog Horm Res* 2002;57:357–384.
12. Bethea CL, Lu NZ, Gundlah C, et al. Diverse actions of ovarian steroids in the serotonin neural system. *Front Neuroendocrinol* 2002;23:41–100.
13. Moses-Kolko EL, Berga SL, Greer PJ, et al. Widespread increases of cortical serotonin type 2A receptor availability after hormone therapy in euthymic postmenopausal women. *Fertil Steril* 2003;80:554–559.
14. Summer BE, Grant KE, Rosie R, et al. Effects of tamoxifen on serotonin transporter and 5-hydroxitryptamine(2A) receptor binding sites and mRNA levels in the brain of ovariectomized rats with or without acute estradiol replacement. *Mol Brain Res* 1999;73:119–128.
15. Sipe K, Leventhal L, Burroughs K, et al. Serotonin 2A receptors modulate tail-skin temperature in two rodent models of estrogen deficiency-related thermoregulatory dysfunction. *Brain Res* 2004;1028:191–202.
16. Notelovitz M, Lenihan JP, McDermott M, et al. Initial 17-beta-estradiol dose for treating vasomotor symptoms. *Obstet Gynecol* 2000;95:726–731.
17. Col NF, Hirota LK, Orr RK, et al. Hormone replacement therapy after breast cancer: a systematic review and quantitative assessment of risk. *J Clin Oncol* 2001;19:2357–2363.
18. Women's Health Initiative Investigators. Risks and benefits of estrogen plus progestin in healthy postmenopausal women: principal results from the Women's Health Initiative randomized controlled trial. *JAMA* 2002;288:321–333.
19. Loprinzi CL, Michalak JC, Quella SK, et al. Megestrol acetate for the prevention of hot flashes. *N Engl J Med* 1994;331:347–352.
20. Quella SK, Loprinzi CL, Sloan JA, et al. Long-term use of megestrol acetate by cancer survivors for the treatment of hot flashes. *Cancer* 1998;82:1784–1788.
21. Bertelli G, Venturini M, Del Mastro L, et al. Intramuscular depot medroxyprogesterone versus oral megestrol for the control of postmenopausal hot flashes in breast cancer patients: a randomized study. *Ann Oncol* 2002;6:88388.
22. Leonetti HB, Longo S, Anasti JN. Transdermal progesterone cream for vasomotor symptoms and postmenopausal bone loss. *Obstet Gynecol* 1999;94:22528.
23. Dixon AR, Jackson L, Chan S, et al. A randomised trial of second-line hormone vs single agent chemotherapy in tamoxifen resistant advanced breast cancer. *Br J Cancer* 1992;66:4024.
24. Hofseth LJ, Raafat AM, Osuch JR, et al. Hormone replacement therapy with oestrogen or estrogen plus medroxyprogesterone acetate is associated with increased epithelial proliferation in the normal postmenopausal breast. *J Clin Endocrinol Metab* 1999;84:445965.
25. Sartor O, Eastham JA. Progressive prostate cancer associated with use of megestrol acetate administered for control of hot flashes. *South Med J* 1999;92:415–416.
26. Perez DG, Loprinzi CL. Newer antidepressants and other non-hormonal agents for the treatment of hot flashes. *Compr Ther* 2005;31(2):224–236.
27. Loprinzi CL, Pisansky TM, Fonseca R, et al. Pilot evaluation of venlafaxine hydrochloride for the therapy of hot flashes in cancer survivors. *J Clin Oncol* 1998;16:2377–2381.
28. Loprinzi CL, Kugler JW, Sloan JA, et al. Venlafaxine in management of hot flashes in survivors of breast cancer: a randomized controlled trial. *Lancet* 2000;356:2059–2063.
29. Barton D, La VB, Loprinzi C, et al. Venlafaxine for the control of hot flashes: results of a longitudinal continuation study. *Oncol Nurs Forum* 2002;29:33–40.
30. Evans ML, Pritts E, Vittinghoff E, et al. Management of postmenopausal hot flushes with venlafaxine hydrochloride: a randomized, controlled trial. *Obstet Gynecol* 2005;105:161–166.
31. Karogelopoulos S, Kampas N, Petrogiannopoulos C, et al. Long-term management of menopausal hot flashes with venlafaxine. *2004 World Congress of Gynecological Endocrinology*, abstract 95. 2004.
32. Quella SK, Loprinzi CL, Sloan J, et al. Pilot evaluation of venlafaxine for the treatment of hot flashes in men undergoing androgen ablation therapy for prostate cancer. *J Urol* 1999;162:98–102.
33. Shafgat A, Titzer ML, Sweeney CJ, et al. A phase II study of venlafaxine for the treatment of hot flashes in men undergoing androgen deprivation for prostate cancer. *2004 Annual Meeting of the American Society of Clinical Oncology*, abstract 8148. 2004.
34. Loprinzi CL. Medroxyprogesterone acetate (MPA) versus venlafaxine for hot flashes: a North Central Cancer Treatment Group Trial. *2005 Annual Meeting of the American Society of Clinical Oncology*, abstract 8014. 2005.
35. Loprinzi CL, Sloan JA, Perez EA, et al. Phase III evaluation of fluoxetine for treatment of hot flashes. *J Clin Oncol* 2002;20:1578–1583.

36. Suvanto-Luukkonen E, Koivunen R, Sundstrom H, et al. Citalopram and fluoxetine in the treatment of postmenopausal symptoms: a prospective, randomized, 9-month, placebo-controlled, double-blind study. *Menopause* 2005;12:18–26.

37. Stearns V, Isaacs C, Rowland J, et al. A pilot trial assessing the efficacy of paroxetine hydrochloride (Paxil) in controlling hot flashes in breast cancer survivors. *Ann Oncol* 2000;11:17–22.

38. Weitzner MA, Moncello J, Jacobsen PB, et al. A pilot trial of paroxetine for the treatment of hot flashes and associated symptoms in women with breast cancer. *J Pain Symptom Manage* 2002;23:337–345.

39. Stearns V, Beebe KL, Iyengar M, et al. Paroxetine controlled release in the treatment of menopausal hot flashes: a randomized controlled trial. *JAMA* 2003;289:2827–2834.

40. Loprinzi CL, Barton DL, Carpenter LA, et al. Pilot evaluation of paroxetine for treating hot flashes in men. *Mayo Clin Proc* 2004;79:1247–1251.

41. Barton DL, Loprinzi CL, Novotny P, et al. Pilot evaluation of citalopram for the relief of hot flashes. *J Support Oncol* 2003;1:47–51.

42. Carpenter LA. Pilot evaluation of citalopram for alleviation of hot flashes in women with inadequate hot flash control with venlafaxine. *2005 Annual Meeting of the American Society of Clinical Oncology*, abstract 8148. 2005.

43. Randomized, placebo-controlled study of sertraline (Zoloft) for the treatment of hot flashes in women with early stage breast cancer taking tamoxifen. *American Society of Oncology annual Meeting 2001*, abstract 1585.

44. Perez DG, Loprinzi CL, Barton DL, et al. Pilot evaluation of mirtazapine for the treatment of hot flashes. *J Support Oncol* 2004;2:50–56.

45. Jin Y, Desta Z Stearns V, et al. CYP2D6 genotype, antidepressant use and tamoxifen metabolism during adjuvant breast cancer treatment. *J Natl Cancer Inst* 2005;97:30–39.

46. Goetz MP, Rae JM, Suman VJ, et al. Pharmacogenomic determinants of outcome with tamoxifen therapy: findings from the randomized North Central Cancer Treatment Group adjuvant breast cancer trial 89–30–52. *2004 San Antonio Breast Cancer Symposium*, abstract 314. 2004.

47. Guttuso TJ Jr. Gabapentin's effects on hot flashes and hypothermia. *Neurology* 2000;54:2161–2163.

48. Loprinzi CL, Barton DL, Sloan JA, et al. Pilot evaluation of gabapentin for treating hot flashes. *Mayo Clin Proc* 2002;77:1159–1163.

49. Thummala AR. Pilot study using gabapentin on tamoxifen-induced hot flashes in women with breast cancer [abstract]. *Program Proc Am Soc Clin Oncol* 2002;21:362a.

50. Guttuso T Jr, Kurlan R, McDermott MP, et al. K Gabapentin's effects on hot flashes in postmenopausal women: a randomized controlled trial. *Obstet Gynecol* 2003;101:337–345.

51. Pandya KJ. A preliminary report of a double blind placebo controlled trial of gabapentin for control of hot flashes in women with breast cancer. A University of Rochester Cancer Center CCOP study. *Proc Am Soc Clin Oncol*. 2004;23:8015.

52. Goldberg RM, Loprinzi CL, O'Fallon JR, et al. Transdermal clonidine for ameliorating tamoxifen-induced hot flashes. *J Clin Oncol* 1994;12:155–158.

53. Pandya KJ, Raubertas RF, Flynn PJ, et al. Oral clonidine in postmenopausal patients with breast cancer experiencing tamoxifen-induced hot flashes: a University of Rochester Cancer Center Community Clinical Oncology Program study. *Ann Intern Med* 2000;132:788–793.

54. Bergmans MG, Merkus JM, Corbey RS, et al. Effect of bellergal retard on climacteric complaints: a double-blind, placebo-controlled study. *Maturitas* 1987;9:227–234.

55. Barton DL, Loprinzi CL, Quella SK, et al. Prospective evaluation of vitamin E for hot flashes in breast cancer survivors. *J Clin Oncol* 1998;16:495–500.

56. Quella SK, Loprinzi CL, Barton DI., et al. Evaluation of soy phytoestrogens for the treatment of hot flashes in breast cancer survivors: a North Central Cancer Treatment Group Trial. *J Clin Oncol* 2000;18:1068–1074.

57. Messina MJ, Loprinzi CL. Soy for breast cancer survivors: a critical review of the literature. *J Nutr* 2001;131(11 suppl):3095S–3108S.

58. Jacobson JS, Troxel AB, Evans J, et al. Randomized trial of black cohosh for the treatment of hot flashes among women with a history of breast cancer. *J Clin Oncol* 2001;19:2739–2745.

59. Pockaj BA, Gallagher J, Loprinzi CL, et al. Phase III double-blinded, randomized trial to evaluate the use of black cohosh in the treatment of hot flashes: a North Central Cancer Treatment Group Study. *2005 American Society of Clinical Oncology Annual Meeting*, abstract 8013. 2005.

CHAPTER 11 ■ ANOREXIA/WEIGHT LOSS

TOBY C. CAMPBELL AND JAMIE H. VON ROENN

Cancer cachexia is a complex metabolic process, due to both host and tumor factors, which results in excess catabolism as well as aberrant fat and carbohydrate metabolism. The syndrome is most commonly seen in patients with advanced cancer and characterized clinically by unintentional weight loss, muscle wasting, anorexia, fatigue, impaired performance status, anemia, and edema (1–4). The incidence of weight loss varies with both the stage and primary tumor site. Tumors of the upper gastrointestinal tract and lung are most frequently associated with weight loss, while it is an uncommon problem for patients with advanced breast cancer (2). Treatment-related symptoms contribute to decreased oral intake but do not cause cachexia. Cachexia is distinguished from starvation (decreased energy intake) by the disproportionate loss of skeletal muscle over adipose tissue and its recognized lack of response to nutritional supplementation (1). The diagnosis of cachexia should be entertained in any patient with involuntary weight loss and muscle wasting.

Multiple clinical investigations have demonstrated the impact of weight loss on prognosis. Involuntary weight loss is associated with decreased overall survival (2,5–7), and decreased response to, and symptomatic benefit from, chemotherapy (8,9). Even in patients with a good performance status, as little as 5% loss in body weight adversely affects prognosis. For many patients, decreasing weight correlates with declines in performance status. The relationship between muscle wasting and mortality has been well documented. Loss of approximately 30% of total body weight or loss of 20% of lean body mass is incompatible with survival (1). In one autopsy series, up to 20% of patients with cancer had no discernible immediate cause of death other than "cachexia" (10).

In this chapter, we will explore the current knowledge of the pathophysiology of the cachexia/anorexia syndrome, discuss its evaluation, and outline pharmacologic and nonpharmacologic treatment options.

PATHOPHYSIOLOGY

Inflammation

The mechanisms underlying cancer-related weight loss are incompletely understood but reflect a complex interplay between symptoms that impact nutritional intake, tumor-related factors, metabolic derangements, and hormone dysregulation. The negative nitrogen balance in patients with cancer cachexia results from an imbalance between protein synthesis (anabolism) and protein degradation (catabolism).

The disproportional loss of muscle mass is mediated, at least in part, by proinflammatory cytokines. Cancer cachexia is associated with a chronic inflammatory response characterized by an increase in acute phase proteins and proinflammatory cytokines (11–13). Elevated levels of proinflammatory cytokines, including interleukin-6 (IL-6), interleukin-1 (IL-1), interferon-γ (IFN-γ), and tumor necrosis factor α (TNF-α) are present in many patients with cancer and their levels seem to correlate with tumor progression. IL-6 levels in newly diagnosed patients with lung cancer are related to the degree of weight loss (14). In patients with pancreatic cancer who have been losing weight, high concentrations of TNF-α and IL-6 in peripheral blood mononuclear cells, increased plasma concentrations of a soluble TNF receptor, and other adhesion molecules have been observed (15). The wasting effect of these proinflammatory cytokines seems to be targeted against the myosin heavy chain of skeletal muscle (16). Similarly, in patients with advanced colon cancer, elevated levels of TNF-α and IL-6 have been associated with anorexia (17). In patients with advanced pancreatic cancer, the presence of an acute phase response is associated with accelerated weight loss, hypermetabolism, anorexia, and shortened survival (15). It has been hypothesized that the increased demand for amino acids for the synthesis of acute phase proteins is met at the expense of skeletal muscle (18). Amidst this cytokine "storm," patients may experience nonspecific signs and symptoms, including depression, anxiety, cognitive impairment, fatigue, and pain (19).

The ubiquitin-proteosome pathway, a regulatory gateway for protein synthesis and degradation in skeletal muscle, may be the final common pathway for cancer-related wasting (20). This pathway, regulated at least in part by proinflammatory cytokines, is downregulated by anticytokine treatment in animal models. The ubiquitin-proteosome proteolytic pathway is responsible for the bulk of basal proteolysis in skeletal muscle and as much as 80% of the muscle degradation in cancer cachexia (21).

Tumor Factors

The excessive catabolism which characterizes cancer cachexia is mediated not only by host factors but also by tumor-derived factors. Proteolysis-inducing factor (PIF) is a tumor-derived glycoprotein which induces protein degradation in skeletal muscle by upregulation of the ubiquitin-proteosome proteolytic system (22). Preliminary data suggests that PIF can be detected in the urine of 80% of patients with unresectable pancreatic cancer (23). The identification of urinary PIF is associated with a greater degree of weight loss compared with those without urinary PIF, 12.5 kg versus 4.5 kg, respectively. Elevated PIF has not been observed in all tumor types in the presence of wasting. The underlying mechanisms of wasting likely vary by tumor type and potentially by other, not yet defined, factors.

Energy Dysregulation

Elevated resting energy expenditure (REE) may contribute to wasting in some patients with cancer. REE has been measured in patients with a variety of cancers with variable results; cancers of the lung and pancreas are most frequently associated with an increase in REE (24). Wasting in the setting of other tumor types is not predictably associated with alterations in REE (24). Hypermetabolism, when present, may occur secondary to tumor growth, increase in the Cori cycle, increase in acute phase protein response, gluconeogenesis, and increased protein turnover.

Dysregulation of the control of energy intake also contributes to the anorexia-cachexia syndrome. There are four neurotransmitters active in the appetite center of the hypothalamus. Neuropeptide Y and Agouti-related peptide (AGRP) are appetite-stimulating neurotransmitters, while opio-melanocortin and the cocaine-amphetamine-related factor (CART) inhibit appetite (25). These neuropeptides regulate the balance between ghrelin, a hormone produced in the stomach that stimulates appetite, and leptin, an anorexigenic hormone produced in fatty tissue (26). Proinflammatory cytokines may stimulate pathologic alterations in the central control of energy intake. Neuropeptide Y–induced feeding is antagonized by IL-1 in rats (27). In addition, IL-1 upregulates central corticotropin-releasing factor, a potent anorexigenic stimulus (28). Proinflammatory cytokines stimulate the expression of leptin and/or mimic the negative feedback from leptin, resulting in long-term inhibition of energy intake (25).

Our understanding of the intracellular mechanisms involved in muscle homeostasis and the impact of host- and tumor-derived factors on cancer cachexia continues to expand. There remain, however, numerous unanswered questions. Although our therapeutic approach once focused entirely on the treatment of nutrition impact symptoms and anorexia, we now recognize the need to consider anabolic as well as anticatabolic interventions.

EVALUATION

The initial evaluation of cancer-associated weight loss includes a detailed history and physical examination to determine the rate and extent of weight loss and to identify treatable, easily reversible causes of weight loss. The evaluation includes a precise measurement of body weight, height, and documentation of premorbid body weight, rate of weight loss, assessment of appetite, review of current medications, and presence of nutrition impact symptoms (dysphagia, nausea, constipation, depression, pain, infection, or altered taste). Both the amount of weight loss and its rate define severity. Weight loss of 2% in 1 week is as significant clinically as weight loss of 5% over 1 month (Table 11.1).

Physical examination is directed at identifying signs of nutrition impact symptoms (e.g., mucositis), skeletal muscle wasting, strength, and mobility. In addition to standard measurements of weight, evaluation of body composition is ideal, as lean body mass is the metabolically active component of body mass. Anthropometric assessments, including midarm circumference using a tape measure and triceps skinfolds using calipers, are useful indicators of change in arm muscle mass. Although anthropomorphic measurements are easy, readily completed, and a potentially useful measure of change, there is

TABLE 11.1

DEFINITION OF SIGNIFICANT WEIGHT LOSS

Time frame	% Weight
1 wk	2
1 mo	5
3 mo	7.5
6 mo	10

variation in results when measurements are taken by different clinicians.

Bioelectric impedance analysis (BIA) is another simple bedside technique to monitor changes in body composition. BIA is based on the differential resistance to a low-intensity electrical current by the fat and lean tissue body compartments. Measured values of reactance and resistance obtained by BIA can be used in regression equations to estimate fat and lean tissue and total body water. The BIA equipment is relatively inexpensive and easy to use. A measurement takes only approximately 10 minutes and involves no discomfort for the patient. Accurate measurements of weight and height and consistent positioning of the electrodes are essential to obtain accurate body composition data with BIA. The BIA technique is most useful for monitoring change.

More accurate measurement techniques for the assessment of body composition include underwater weighing, whole body counting of potassium, nitrogen, and other elements, dual energy x-ray absorptiometry, and estimation of total body water and extracellular water by dilution techniques. These methods are only reasonable considerations in the research setting.

Standardized, validated nutrition assessment tools are available but not routinely utilized. The Patient-Generated Subjective Global Assessment (PG-SGA) of Nutritional Status is a screening tool that can be utilized to identify patients in need of intervention. This tool is accepted as the standard for the nutritional assessment of patients with cancer by the American Dietetic Association. The assessment includes a patient report of weight and weight change, food intake, symptoms, activities, function, and a physician evaluation of the disease and its related nutritional requirements.

Body weight is objective and simple to measure, but it is only one, late manifestation of the cancer cachexia syndrome. Early in the trajectory of disease and/or for research, more objective tools for analysis, including measurement of lean body mass, strength, energy expenditure, and biochemical assays of inflammatory mediators, are important concerns. At the bedside, nutritional interventions must fit a particular patient's goals of care. Dahele and Fearon advocate focus on patient-centered outcomes, such as quality of life, performance status, and activity level (1). Although a patient with end-stage cancer may not gain weight with an appetite stimulant, it may effectively relieve anorexia and allow the social pleasure of eating dinner with family and friends. On the other hand, a patient with a new diagnosis of cancer and wasting might be best served by a combined anticatabolic and anabolic approach. Recommendations for treatment of weight loss and anorexia must be anchored by a discussion of the goals of care.

TREATMENT

The first step in the management of cancer-related weight loss is identification and treatment of nutrition impact symptoms.

TABLE 11.2

NUTRITION IMPACT SYMPTOMS

Mucositis
Nausea/vomiting
Constipation
Early satiety
Severe diarrhea
Bloating/ascites
Anorexia
Xerostomia
Depression
Dementia
Cranial nerve palsies
Dysgeusia
Gastrointestinal obstruction

Table 11.2 lists common, potentially treatable, nutrition impact symptoms. Unfortunately, for most of the patients with involuntary weight loss and muscle wasting, treatment of these symptoms does not reverse the progressive cachexia. The impact of aggressive symptom control on oral intake and, more specifically, wasting may improve sense of well-being but is unlikely to adequately treat the wasting.

Role of Caloric Supplementation

Decreased energy intake and anorexia contribute to weight loss. Intense caloric repletion, at first glance, seems a rational intervention for weight-losing patients with cancer, and many patients and families focus their energies on increasing intake. However, in advanced patients with cancer, the striking difference between starvation, an absolute lack of calories, and cachexia highlights the inadequacy of caloric supplementation as a primary treatment for cachexia (see Table 11.3). In starvation, adaptations lead to decreased energy expenditure, relative preservation of muscle mass, and decreased proportional loss of muscle and visceral mass, with continued caloric restriction. In the setting of cancer cachexia, energy expenditure may remain elevated in spite of inadequate energy intake and continued loss of skeletal muscle mass. The lack of benefit from caloric supplementation for advanced wasting is true whether the calories are delivered enterally or parenterally.

Dietary counseling leads to a limited, short-term (about 4 weeks) increase in caloric intake without significant weight gain, difference in tumor response rate, quality of life, or overall survival for most patients (29). There are, however,

TABLE 11.3

STARVATION VERSUS CACHEXIA

	Starvation	Cachexia
Caloric intake	↓↓	↓
Resting energy expenditure	↓ or ↔	↓↑
Body fat	↓↓	↓
Lean body mass	↓↔	↓↓

↔ Unchanged
↓ Reduced
↓↓ Markedly reduced
↓↑ Increased or reduced

specific clinical situations in which temporary nutritional support provides benefit. Patients with severe mucositis—while undergoing bone marrow transplantation—may benefit from a time-limited course of parenteral nutritional therapy. Weisdorf et al. demonstrated improved overall survival for patients who underwent bone marrow transplant randomized to receive parenteral nutrition support (30).

Nutritional support is a standard supportive therapy for patients with head and neck cancer treated with multimodality therapy. Enteral feeding for patients with head and neck cancer leads to fewer treatment delays in patients undergoing radiation and may improve functional ability several months after completion of therapy (31,32). A favorable impact of nutritional support on treatment toxicity was also noted by the Veteran Affairs Total Parenteral Nutrition Cooperative Group. Three hundred ninety five malnourished patients (65% with cancer) were randomized to receive at least 7 days of total parenteral nutrition or no total parenteral nutrition. A subgroup of patients categorized as severely malnourished, who received nutritional support, had fewer operative complications (e.g., anastomotic leaks and bronchopleural fistulas) (33).

An evaluation of 12 randomized, controlled trials of parenteral nutritional support for patients with cancer concluded that "total parenteral nutrition does not result in improvement in overall survival, in a 30% or greater improvement in short-term survival, or in a 10% or greater improvement in response to chemotherapy" (34). This review led to a consensus statement, published in 1989 by the American College of Physicians (ACP), discouraging the use of parenteral nutrition in patients with cancer receiving active tumor therapy (34).

Exercise

Exercise is an important tool to maintain strength, lean body mass, and body weight. Inactivity exacerbates the metabolic abnormalities characteristic of cancer cachexia and is associated with decreased glucose tolerance and increased plasma insulin levels (18). In the experimental setting, bedrest of an otherwise healthy volunteer for 7 days results in 1 to 4% loss of muscle mass of the back and lower extremities as measured by magnetic resonance imaging (MRI). This underscores the need for patients to remain active.

In patients with HIV-related weight loss and in the frail elderly, exercise has been associated with marked improvement in performance status, muscle mass, and strength (35). In particular, resistance training is a potent anabolic stimulus, resulting in improvement in lean body mass in multiple clinical settings. Endurance training attenuates muscle atrophy associated with tumor growth in animals as well (36). A recent review of exercise in patients with cancer observed improvement in fatigue and/or lean body mass with relatively short duration, overall low-intensity exercise programs (37, 38). It is noteworthy that in none of the studies were patients with cachexia evaluated, in spite of the fact that exercise in the frail elderly and in HIV-infected subjects has resulted in significant improvement in muscle strength.

In HIV-infected subjects with weight loss, a progressive resistance exercise program led to an increase in lean body mass on average of 0.5 kg/week (39), and this increase in muscle mass directly correlated with increased strength. There are little data available in patients with cancer cachexia, but a recommendation for progressive resistance exercise, as tolerated, is an essential component of any nutrition intervention plan.

PHARMACOLOGIC AGENTS

Pharmacologic agents for the treatment of cachexia include orexigenic agents, anabolic agents, and anti-inflammatory/

cytokine modulating interventions. Patients with cancer rank anorexia as one of their most noxious symptoms, and many patients and families request therapy to augment appetite (40). Appetite was the primary target of the earliest pharmacologic interventions for cachexia. Orexigenic agents demonstrated to have a favorable impact on appetite include corticosteroids, progestational agents, and dronabinol.

Corticosteroids

Corticosteroids are potent, anti-inflammatory agents that decrease the production of proinflammatory cytokines, including TNF-α, and inhibit prostaglandin metabolism. Multiple, randomized, placebo-controlled trials demonstrate a short-term improvement in appetite, 4–8 weeks, with steroids without a significant impact on weight (41,42). In general, these trials enrolled patients with very advanced disease who were, as a result, treated with short courses (<3 months) of treatment. In this advanced cancer population, improvement in appetite was associated with a self-reported improvement in sense of well-being. In patients with advanced disease, corticosteroids may also reduce pain and increase energy.

Of the available steroids, dexamethasone is preferred because of its long half-life and minimal mineralocorticoid effects. There is no evidence-based dosing recommendation for steroid therapy in this setting. Precise dosing of dexamethasone is patient-dependent, based on response to therapy, and is generally effective in doses ranging from 2 to 8 mg daily. Recommended doses of prednisone are between 20 and 40 mg daily.

Short-term side effects of corticosteroids include hyperglycemia, insomnia, fluid retention, gastritis, delirium, and immune suppression. Corticosteroids have a catabolic effect (muscle wasting, glucose intolerance, etc.), which underscores the ineffectiveness of these agents for treatment of cachexia.

For patients with limited survival (<8 weeks), corticosteroids may provide palliation of anorexia. For bedridden patients, in particular, corticosteroids may be useful for the treatment of anorexia, as exacerbation of muscle wasting is not a major concern. Corticosteroids may be a particularly good treatment choice for patients who require coanalgesia with an anti-inflammatory agent (e.g., the patient with painful bone metastases).

Progestational Agents

Megestrol acetate and medroxyprogesterone are the most effective appetite stimulants available. The mechanism of action of progestational agents is uncertain. Megestrol acetate may stimulate appetite through inhibition of proinflammatory cytokines (e.g., IL-6, IL-1, TNF-α) or through modulation of calcium channels in the satiety center of the ventromedial hypothalamus (43). Decreased levels of TNF-α and IL-6 have been observed in both animals and in clinical trials of megestrol acetate in patients with cancer cachexia. In one trial in patients with head and neck cancer, treatment with megestrol acetate lowered circulating levels of soluble cytokines (44). Whereas appetite was uniformly increased with megestrol acetate compared with placebo, weight gain, and the degree of weight change varied with the megestrol acetate dose in the patient population studied. The beneficial effects of megestrol acetate on weight and appetite are dose dependent, with greater benefit at higher doses (45). Trials evaluating the impact of megestrol acetate on body composition demonstrate that most of the increased weight is due to an increase in fat mass (45).

The clinical efficacy of progesterones for the improvement of appetite and reversal of weight loss has been demonstrated in more than 15 randomized, placebo-controlled trials (45).

A 2005 Cochrane Review, including 30 trials and more than 4000 patients, concluded that megestrol acetate increases appetite and weight in patients with cancer (46). Because the oral suspension (40 mg per cc) is less expensive and more bioavailable than tablets, it is the preferred formulation (47–49). Treatment is generally started at 400 mg/day and increased by 200 mg/day to a maximum of 800 mg/day over a period of 2–4 weeks based on patient's response or initiated at 800 mg/day with dose reduction dictated by response.

Megestrol acetate is generally well tolerated, though it has some potentially important toxicities. Megestrol acetate interacts with multiple hormone receptors, interfering with normal endocrine function. Castrate levels of testosterone are reached during the first week of treatment (45). Laboratory evidence of adrenal insufficiency is common, though its clinical significance is less clear. In patients on megestrol acetate with acute life-threatening conditions, administration of stress doses of steroids should be considered. The risk of deep vein thrombosis, particularly in patients with advanced cancer, is an important consideration for patients treated with megestrol acetate, though randomized clinical trials have not identified thrombosis as a significant toxicity.

Cannabinoids

Cannabis was used as an appetite stimulant in ancient Ayurvedic and Arabic medicine and has long been purported by marijuana users to increase food intake. In a geriatric population, cannabis increases the desire for food, improves taste, decreases pain, and improves mood (50). Despite the recognition of cannabinoid receptors in the central and peripheral nervous system—CB$_1$ and CB$_2$, respectively—and the presence of endogenous cannabinoids, the mechanism of action of cannabinoids is unclear.

Dronabinol, a synthetic THC (delta-9-tetrahydrocannabinol) derivative, has been used as both an antiemetic (with a potency similar to prochlorperazine) and an appetite stimulant. A randomized, placebo-controlled trial of dronabinol 2.5 mg twice daily in patients with AIDS-related wasting demonstrated a patient-reported improvement in appetite that failed to translate into weight gain. A 6-week, dose-ranging, phase II study of dronabinol in patients with advanced cancer reported improvement in mood and appetite but no increase in weight. Dizziness, euphoria, dysphoria, poor concentration, and somnolence are the most common side effects of dronabinol. Dose reduction may lessen or eliminate the adverse effects.

As both dronabinol and megestrol acetate are approved for the treatment of anorexia, a recent trial compared the efficacy of these agents individually and in combination. The North Central Cancer Treatment Group (NCCTG) randomized 469 patients with advanced cancer to megestrol acetate 800 mg with placebo, dronabinol 2.5 mg twice daily with placebo, or combination therapy. Megestrol acetate proved superior to dronabinol as an orexigenic agent, and combination therapy offered no advantage over megestrol acetate alone (51).

Anabolic Agents

Androgens produce weight gain and increase muscle mass in athletes, the elderly, and in patients with HIV cachexia, yet their utility in patients with cancer cachexia is undefined. Whereas a number of agents (growth hormone, testosterone, nandrolone, oxandrolone) are either approved or currently being evaluated for the treatment of AIDS-related wasting, data regarding their use in cancer-associated cachexia are only available with oxandrolone and nandrolone. Nandrolone has been evaluated in a variety of regimens and doses.

Patients with non–small cell lung cancer randomized to receive standard chemotherapy with nandrolone 200 mg intramuscularly maintained weight and hemoglobin level better than patients on a placebo-treated arm. An increase in arm muscle circumference was observed by anthropometric measurements in those patients treated with nandrolone (52). Similar results have been seen in patients with esophageal cancer treated with nandrolone postesophagectomy. In both trials, however, the duration of therapy was relatively short.

Oxandrolone is a synthetic, oral anabolic agent approved for treatment of weight loss following extensive surgery, chronic infection, or severe trauma and to offset protein catabolism associated with the prolonged administration of steroids. In patients with cancer-related weight loss, a phase II trial of oxandrolone (10 mg orally twice daily) in combination with standardized nutritional recommendations and a progressive resistance exercise program (Therabands) demonstrated an increase in total and lean tissue weight with treatment (53). Improvement in weight and lean body mass correlated with improvements in quality of life scores as well as performance status. Treatment was well tolerated overall, with the only adverse effect being a transient increase in transaminases, which was readily reversible with discontinuation of the drug.

A prospective, randomized trial of oxandrolone in patients with advanced cancers of the upper aerodigestive tract has demonstrated similar findings. Sixty-four patients with advanced aerodigestive tract cancers and documented involuntary weight loss were randomized to oxandrolone 10 mg orally twice daily or placebo (54). Oxandrolone therapy resulted in significant increases in weight and lean body mass as compared to placebo-treated patients. Whereas final study results have not yet been published, the increase in lean body mass associated with oxandrolone and the associated improvement in quality of life measures are of significant interest.

Prokinetic Agents

Early satiety as a result of delayed gastric emptying or gastric stasis occurs in up to 60% of patients with anorexia and cancer-related weight loss (55). Autonomic failure, a recognized complication of advanced cancer, may lead to anorexia, nausea, early satiety, and constipation—all of which contribute to reduced food intake (56). Metoclopramide, a central nervous system dopamine and serotonin antagonist, reduces nausea through both central and peripheral effects and enhances the muscular response of the upper gastrointestinal tract to acetylcholine, stimulating motility, and accelerating gastric emptying without increasing gastric, biliary, or pancreatic secretions. In a small, phase II study in advanced cancer patients with anorexia, metoclopramide 10 mg four times daily improved anorexia in 17 of 20 patients (57). Metoclopramide is typically prescribed at this dose. Sustained-release metoclopramide is superior to the short-acting compound for symptom control in a head-to-head comparison (58). Metoclopramide is generally well tolerated but may cause restlessness, extrapyramidal symptoms, confusion, headache, or insomnia. Diarrhea can be dose-limiting.

Anticatabolic/Metabolic Agents

Cytokine-mediated alterations in host metabolism play an important role in disease-related wasting. Thalidomide inhibits TNF-α production primarily by accelerating the degradation of the TNF-α messenger RNA transcript (59). The anti-TNF-α effects of thalidomide might alter the cytokine triggers of cachexia. In early clinical trials in HIV-infected patients with weight loss, thalidomide has demonstrated appetite stimulation and weight gain (60). To date, only one randomized controlled trial of thalidomide in patients with advanced cancer has been reported. Fifty patients with advanced pancreatic cancer who had lost at least 10% of their preillness weight were randomized to receive thalidomide 200 mg daily or placebo (59). At 4 weeks, patients in the thalidomide arm had significant gains in weight and muscle mass, compared with losses in the placebo-treated group. Over the 24 weeks of treatment, thalidomide was able to attenuate the loss of lean muscle mass and weight in this advanced patient population. Thalidomide deserves further investigation in larger phase III clinical trials (61).

The omega-3-fatty acids, derived from dark fish, decrease cytokine production, inhibit the action of proteolysis-inducing factor, and appear to block ubiquitin-proteosome-induced muscle proteolysis (18,43,59). Eicosapentaenoic acid (EPA) has been evaluated in phase I, II, and III trials that suggest weight stabilization in a subset of patients, but no consistent evidence of increased lean body mass or weight. A phase III study of fish oil in advanced cancer patients did not demonstrate improvement in appetite, nutritional status, or weight in treated patients (62). Furthermore, a significant majority of the patients were not able to swallow the prescribed fish oil capsules, primarily because of excessive burping and dysgeusia. A second phase III clinical trial of the NCCTG randomized 421 patients to receive EPA alone, megestrol acetate alone, or a combination of EPA and megestrol acetate (63). A smaller percentage of patients taking the EPA supplement gained ≥ 10% over their baseline weight compared with those taking megestrol acetate, 6% versus 18%, respectively. Appetite improvement was equivalent across all study arms as assessed by an NCCTG questionnaire, but significantly better in the megestrol acetate-containing arms when assessed by the Functional Assessment of Anorexia/Cachexia Therapy questionnaire. In view of the results of multiple randomized trials, as highlighted above, fish oil derivatives appear ineffective for treatment of cancer cachexia.

CONCLUSION

Anorexia and weight loss remain important concerns for patients and their families. To date, improvement in appetite and/or weight has not led to prolonged survival. A change in survival from cachexia treatment and, ideally, its prevention is unlikely until targeted therapies that address the metabolic alterations and anabolic needs of cachectic patients are available.

Treatment recommendations are based on patient goals. Therapy begins with treatment of readily identified reversible nutrition impact symptoms. For patients with very advanced disease, where the prognosis is measured in weeks to months, corticosteroids are an appropriate choice for short-term appetite stimulation to improve the ability to enjoy meals with family and friends. Megestrol acetate, the most effective orexigenic agent, is recommended for patients with decreased appetite and months of survival. Earlier in the course of disease, there are not yet randomized trial data available on which to base a clear recommendation. Long-term, the goal of therapy is to prevent weight loss, replenish lean tissue, and maintain function. This is likely to require combination therapy with exercise, an anabolic agent, and/or an anticatabolic agent, with or without an appetite stimulant.

References

1. Dahele M, Fearon KCH. Research methodology: cancer cachexia syndrome. *Palliat Med* 2004;18:409–417.

2. DeWys WD, Begg C, Lavin PT, et al. Prognostic effect of weight loss prior to chemotherapy in cancer patients. Eastern Cooperative Oncology Group. *Am J Med* 1980;69:491–497.

3. Cohn SH, Gartenhaus W, Sawitsky A, et al. Compartmental body composition of cancer patients by measurement of total body nitrogen, potassium, and water. *Metabolism* 1981;30:222–229.

4. Staal-van den Brekel AJ, Schols AM, ten Velde GP, et al. Analysis of the energy balance in lung cancer patients. *Cancer Res* 1994;54:6430–6433.

5. Ray P, Quantin X, Grenier J, et al. Predictive factors of tumour response and prognostic factors of survival during lung cancer chemotherapy. *Cancer Detect Prev* 1998;22:293–304.

6. Martins S, Pereira J. Clinical factors and prognosis in non-small cell lung cancer clinical trials. *Am J Clin Oncol* 1999;22:453–457.

7. Kim HL, Han K-R, Zisman A, et al. Cachexia-like symptoms predict a worse prognosis in localized T1 renal cell carcinoma. *J Urol* 2004;171:1810–1813.

8. Ross PJ, Ashley S, Norton A, et al. Do patients with weight loss have a worse outcome when undergoing chemotherapy for lung cancers? *Br J Cancer* 2004;90:1905–1911.

9. Slaviero KA, Clarke SJ, Rivory LP. Inflammatory response: an unrecognized source of variability in the pharmacokinetics and pharmacodynamics of cancer chemotherapy. *Lancet Oncol* 2003;4:224–232.

10. Ambrus JL, Ambrus CM, Mink IB, et al. Causes of death in cancer patients. *J Med* 1975;6:61–64.

11. Argiles JM, Alvarez B, Carbo N. The divergent effects of tumour necrosis factor-alpha on skeletal muscle: implications in wasting. *Eur Cytokine Netw* 2000;11:552–559.

12. Barber MD, Powell JJ, Lynch SF, et al. A polymorphism of the interleukin-1 beta gene influences survival in pancreatic cancer. *Br J Cancer* 2000;83:1443–1447.

13. Wigmore SJ, MacMahon AJ, Sturgeon CM, et al. Acute-phase protein response, survival and tumour recurrence in patients with colorectal cancer. *Br J Surg* 2001;88:255–260.

14. Simons JP, Schols AM, Buurman WA, et al. Weight loss and low body cell mass in males with lung cancer: relationship with systemic inflammation, acute-phase response, resting energy expenditure, and catabolic and anabolic hormones. *Clin Sci* 1999;97:215–223.

15. Fearon KC, Barber MD, Falconer JS, et al. Pancreatic cancer as a model: inflammatory mediators, acute-phase response, and cancer cachexia. *World J Surg* 1999;23:584–588.

16. Lazarus DD, Destree AT, Mazzola LM, et al. A new model of cancer cachexia: contribution of the ubiquitin-proteasome pathway. *Am J Physiol* 1999;227:E332–E341.

17. Rich TA, Innominato P, Mormont MC, et al. Performance status, global quality of life, fatigue, and appetite loss are correlated with serum TGFa and IL-6 in patients with metastatic colorectal cancer (MCC). *J Clin Oncol* 2004;22:8024.

18. Baracos VE. Management of muscle wasting in cancer-associated cachexia: understanding gained from experimental studies. *Cancer* 2001;92:1669–1677.

19. Illman BS, Corringham MD, Robinson D Jr, et al. Are inflammatory cytokines the common link between cancer-associated cachexia and depression? *J Support Oncol* 2005;3:37–47.

20. Tisdale MJ. The ubiquitin-proteasome pathway as a therapeutic target for muscle wasting. *J Support Oncol* 2005;3:209–217.

21. Baracos VE, DeVivo C, Hoyle DH, et al. Activation of the ATP-ubiquitin-proteasome pathway in skeletal muscle of cachectic rats bearing a hepatoma. *Am J Physiol* 1995;268:E996–E1006.

22. Lorite MJ, Cariuk P, Tisdale MJ. Induction of muscle protein degradation by a tumour factor. *Br J Cancer* 1997;76:1035–1040.

23. Wigmore SJ, Todorov PT, Barber MD, et al. Characteristics of patients with pancreatic cancer expressing a novel cancer cachectic factor. *Br J Surg* 2000;87:53–58.

24. Fredrix EWHM, Soeters PB, Wouters EFM, et al. Effect of different tumor types of resting energy expenditure. *Cancer Res* 1991;51:6138–6141.

25. Zigman JM, Elmquist JK. Minireview: from anorexia to obesity—the yin and yang of body weight control. *Endocrinology* 2003;144:3749–3756.

26. Shimizu Y, Nagaya N, Isobe T, et al. Increased plasma ghrelin level in lung cancer cachexia. *Clin Cancer Res* 2003;9:774–778.

27. Theologides A, Ehlert J, Kennedy BJ. The calorie intake of patients with advanced cancer. *Minn Med* 1976;59:526–529.

28. Argiles JM, Moore-Carrasco R, Fuster G, et al. Cancer cachexia: the molecular mechanisms. *Int J Biochem Cell Biol* 2003;35:405–409.

29. Ovesen L, Allingstrup L, Hannibal J, et al. Effect of dietary counseling on food intake, body weight, response rate, survival, and quality of life in cancer patients undergoing chemotherapy: a prospective, randomized study. *J Clin Oncol* 1993;11:2043–2049.

30. Weisdorf SA, Lysne J, Wind D, et al. Positive effect of prophylactic total parenteral nutrition on long-term outcome of bone marrow transplantation. *Transplantation* 1987;43:833–838.

31. Daly JM, Hearne B, Dunai J, et al. Nutritional rehabilitation in patients with advanced head and neck cancer receiving radiation therapy. *Am J Surg* 1984;148:514–520.

32. Nayel J, el-Ghoneimy E, el-Haddad S. Impact of nutritional supplementation on treatment delay and morbidity in patients with head and neck tumors treated with irradiation. *Nutrition* 1992;8:13–18.

33. *N Engl J Med*. Perioperative total parenteral nutrition in surgical patients. *N Engl J Med* 1991;325:525–532.

34. *Ann Intern Med*. Parenteral nutrition in patients receiving cancer chemotherapy. *Ann Intern Med* 1989;110:734–736.

35. Evans WJ, Roubenoff R, Shevitz A. Exercise and the treatment of wasting: aging and human immunodeficiency virus infection. *Semin Oncol* 1998;25:112–122.

36. Deuster PA, Morrison SD, Ahrens RA. Endurance exercise modifies cachexia of tumor growth in rats. *Med Sci Sports Exerc* 1985;17:385–392.

37. Galvao DA, Newton RU. Review of exercise intervention studies in cancer patients. *J Clin Oncol* 2005;23:899–909.

38. Lucia A, Earnest C, Perez M. Cancer-related fatigue: can exercise physiology assist oncologists? *Lancet Oncol* 2003;4:616–625.

39. Strawford A, Barbieri T, Van Loan M, et al. Resistance exercise and supraphysiologic androgen therapy in eugonadal men with HIV-related weight loss: a randomized controlled trial. *JAMA* 1999;281:1282–1290.

40. Walsh D, Donnelly S, Rybicki L. The symptoms of advanced cancer: relationship to age, gender, and performance status of 1,000 patients. *Support Care Cancer* 2000;8:175–179.

41. Schell HW. Adrenal corticosteroids therapy in far-advanced cancer. *Geriatrics* 1972;28:131–141.

42. Moertel CG, Schutt AJ, Reitemeier RJ, et al. Corticosteroid therapy of preterminal gastrointestinal cancer. *Cancer* 1974;33:1606–1609.

43. MacDonald N, Easson AM, Mazurak VC, et al. Understanding and managing cancer cachexia. *J Am Coll Surg* 2003;197:143–161.

44. Mantovani G, Maccio A, Bianchi A, et al. Megestrol acetate in neoplastic anorexia/cachexia: clinical evaluation and comparison with cytokine levels in patients with head and neck carcinoma treated with neoadjuvant chemotherapy. *Int J Clin Lab Res* 1995;25:135–141.

45. Jatoi A, Kumar S, Sloan J, et al. On appetite and its loss. *J Clin Oncol* 2000;18:2930–2932.

46. Berenstein EG, Ortiz Z. Megestrol acetate for the treatment of anorexia-cachexia syndrome. *Cochrane Database Syst Rev* 2005;2:CD004310.

47. Loprinzi CL, Kugler JW, Sloan JA, et al. Randomized comparison of megestrol acetate versus dexamethasone versus fluoxymesterone for the treatment of cancer anorexia/cachexia. *J Clin Oncol* 1999;17:3299–3306.

48. Loprinzi CL, Bernath AM, Schaid DJ, et al. Phase III evaluation of 4 doses of megestrol acetate as therapy for patients with cancer anorexia and/or cachexia. *J Clin Oncol* 1993;11:762–767.

49. Loprinzi CL, Ellison NM, Schaid DJ, et al. Controlled trial of megestrol acetate for the treatment of cancer anorexia and cachexia. *J Natl Cancer Inst* 1990;82:1127–1132.

50. Morley JE. Orexigenic and anabolic agents. *Clin Geriatr Med* 2002;18:853–866.

51. Jatoi A, Windschitl HE, Loprinzi CL, et al. Dronabinol versus megestrol acetate versus both for cancer-associated anorexia: A North Central Cancer Treatment Group study. *Proc Am Soc Clin Oncol* 2001;20:388a.

52. Chlebowski RT, Herrold J, Ali I, et al. Influence of nandrolone decanoate on weight loss in advanced non-small cell lung cancer. *Cancer* 1986;58:183–186.

53. Von Roenn J, Tchekmedyian S, Ottery FD. Oxandrolone increases weight, lean tissue, performance status and quality of life scores in cancer related weight loss [Abstract]. *Support Care Cancer* 2002.

54. Von Roenn JH, Tchekmedyian S, Sheng K-N, et al. Oxandrolone in cancer-related weight loss: improvement in weight, body cell mass, performance status and quality of life [Abst 1450]. *Proc Am Soc Clin Oncol* 2002;21:363a.

55. Curtis EB, Krech R, Walsh TD. Common symptoms in patients with advanced cancer. *J Palliat Care* 1991;7:25–29.

56. Inui A. Cancer anorexia-cachexia syndrome: current issues in research and management. *CA Cancer J Clin* 2002;52:72–91.

57. Nelson KA, Walsh TD. Metoclopramide in anorexia caused by cancer-associated dyspepsia syndrome (CADS). *J Palliat Care* 1993;9:14–18.

58. Bruera ED, MacEachern TJ, Spachynski KA, et al. Comparison of the efficacy, safety, and pharmacokinetics of controlled release and immediate release metoclopramide for the management of chronic nausea in patients with advanced cancer. *Cancer* 1994;74:3204–3211.

59. Stroud M. Thalidomide and cancer cachexia: old problem, new hope? *Gut* 2005;54:447–448.

60. Reyes-Teran G, Sierra-Madero J, Martinez del Cerro V, et al. Effects of thalidomide on HIV associated wasting syndrome: a randomized double blind placebo controlled clinical trial. *AIDS* 1996;10:1501–1507.

61. Gordon JN, Trebble TM, Ellis RD, et al. Thalidomide in the treatment of cancer cachexia: a randomized placebo controlled trial. *Gut* 2005;4:540–555.

62. Jatoi A. Fish oil, lean tissue, and cancer: is there a role for eicosapentaenoic acid in treating the cancer anorexia/weight loss syndrome? *Crit Rev Oncol Hematol* 2005;55:37–43.

63. Jatoi A, Rowland K, Loprinzi CL, et al. An eicosapentaenoic acid supplement versus megestrol acetate versus both for patients with cancer associated wasting: A North Central Cancer Treatment Group and National Cancer Institute of Canada collaborative effort. *J Clin Oncol* 2004;22:2469–2476.

CHAPTER 12 ■ DYSPHAGIA/SPEECH REHABILITATION

JERILYN A. LOGEMANN

The speech-language pathologist is the usual professional to evaluate and treat speech and swallowing disorders at all points in a patient's care whether at the time of their initial diagnosis or in palliative care (1). There are several individuals with speech and swallowing problems who are frequently cared for in palliative care by speech-language pathologists. These include patients who have been treated for head and neck cancer and the patients with degenerative neurologic disease. Patients with degenerative neurologic disease most often are those with Parkinson's disease or with motor neuron disease, particularly amyotrophic lateral sclerosis (ALS). Each of these patient types exhibit different problems in their speech and swallowing and requires a different approach to their speech and swallowing management. There is no single remediation technique that can apply to all patients as the following three patients illustrate. Each of these patient types exhibit different speech, voice, and/or swallowing disorders requiring careful assessment and management.

A 56-year-old patient who had undergone chemoradiation for squamous cell carcinoma of the tongue base was treated for postoperative swallowing disorders but did not improve despite intensive swallowing therapy, practice, and his high motivation. After 6 months of living without oral feeding and dealing with chronic aspiration, the patient requested a total laryngectomy. The patient was counseled that after chemoradiation there were many factors that might make it difficult for him to eat well even after a total laryngectomy, which would, however, eliminate aspiration (2). When asked what he meant by "eating," the patient stated that he wanted to take his nutrition by mouth, understanding that it would be unlikely that he could chew and swallow a steak or even mashed potatoes because of his previous chemoradiation. The chemoradiation made generating adequate pressure to push the food through his mouth a problem, especially through the reconstructed pharyngoesophagus. The patient stated that he understood this but did not want to continue nonoral feeding under any circumstance. He was also counseled about voice loss and alternative speech-rehabilitation methods were discussed. After the counseling, the total laryngectomy was completed at the patient's request and the patient returned to full oral intake without meat or other foods that were difficult to chew and swallow. He was able to take soft foods and liquids of all kinds without any aspiration. To this patient communication was less important than eating, but he received a surgical voice restoration procedure, the tracheoesophageal puncture, and was able to communicate effectively.

The patient developed a recurrence in the pharynx and when in palliative care, continued to be able to speak but needed a diet of thinner and thinner foods, as he was unable to generate adequate pressure to swallow anything thicker. Regular swallow reevaluation by the speech-language pathologist, as the patient's function deteriorated, resulted in continued oral feeding until his death.

Another patient after having had a surgical procedure to remove a squamous cell cancer at the base of his tongue with deltopectoral flap reconstruction was referred by his medical oncologist. The closure pulled his remaining oral tongue backward so that it reduced his ability to articulate speech sounds produced at the front of the mouth with his anterior tongue. He also complained that he had followed his surgeon's suggestion to try to swallow mashed potatoes, but after 6 months of trying, he still could not eat by mouth and had a percutaneous endoscopic gastrostomy. After in-depth assessment of speech and swallowing, he was enrolled in active speech and swallowing therapy to improve range of oral tongue movement for speech and range of motion for the remaining tongue base for swallowing as well as therapy to improve his laryngeal elevation during swallowing, which was impaired from scar tissue. The patient was highly motivated and after 4 months of therapy, returned to oral intake, including mashed potatoes, as well as exhibited much improved articulation and speech understandability. Four years later, the patient developed a new tumor in the supraglottic larynx, which could not be resected and was treated with irradiation for palliation. After 6 months, the patient entered palliative care. His speech understandability further reduced because of decreased tongue mobility and hoarseness. His swallowing safety actually improved because his supraglottic tumor narrowed his airway and eliminated aspiration. He had a tracheostomy. As speech intelligibility worsened, various alternative augmentative communication strategies were introduced to allow the patient to communicate effectively with family, friends, and staff.

A third patient, with motor neuron disease, was losing all speech intelligibility and swallowing was worsening. The speech-language pathologist evaluated the patient for a computerized augmentative communication device and found one appropriate for the patient's function of arms and hands. Swallowing was regularly reevaluated to identify safe food consistencies until the time that nonoral feeding was needed. These three patients illustrate the role of the speech-language pathologist in palliative care.

The speech-language pathologist generally approaches the patient in palliative care in the same way as s/he approaches the patient in rehabilitation, beginning by establishing goals to improve or maintain safe and efficient swallow and understandable speech or communication in patients with significant medical problems such as, terminal squamous cell cancer of the head and neck or neurologic disease.

PROCESS FOR PALLIATIVE CARE BY THE SPEECH-LANGUAGE PATHOLOGIST

Although there is no single "best-swallow technique" or "best choice" of communication procedures or aids for all patients, there is a common process used to define the best swallow or speech/communication techniques for each individual patient. The process includes the following:

1. Counseling to allow the patient and family to understand the nature of the speech and swallowing problems the patient exhibits and the types of help that can be provided to them
2. Regular reevaluation of function to define changes in functional needs
3. Regular interaction/therapy as needed

FACTORS DETERMINING FUNCTIONAL NEEDS IN SWALLOWING AND COMMUNICATION

There are a number of factors that determine the patient's functional needs in palliative care. These include the etiology and nature of the patient's dysfunction(s), the patient's and family's reaction to the idea of therapy/intervention, and the patient's goals for their function. As will be described in further detail later in this chapter, various medical diagnoses and the patient's stage of deterioration result in various speech and swallowing problems that must be managed. In the case of chemoradiation, the patient's exact radiation dose, area radiated, and the type of drugs used must be defined and it must be ascertained whether the chemoradiation was concurrent. For surgical procedures, both the extent and location of the resection, the nature of the surgical reconstruction, and location of recurrence of new tumor play major roles in defining the patient's speech and swallowing abilities. Knowledge of the diagnosis is critical to appropriate speech and swallowing management for patients with neurologic disease. Patients with some diagnoses such as Parkinson's disease benefit from active exercise while others such as those with motor neuron disease will worsen with any active exercise.

Parkinson's Disease

The patient with Parkinson's disease often exhibits worsening speech throughout his/her disease progression, which is usually quite slow and frequently lasts for at least twenty or more years. As the patient begins to have more difficulty being understood, they may benefit from a communication device, which ranges from a communication board, enabling them to point to words or letters to spell words, to a computerized system that can be highly sophisticated. If the patient develops dementia, use of some of these instruments may not be possible.

Motor Neuron Disease

The patient with motor neuron disease, most often ALS, may use oral speech for a period of a year or more and then generally needs some type of more sophisticated communication device. All patients with motor speech disorders require full assessment of their ability to use hand manipulations, typing, and other types of motor movements to control the various devices. There are patients with a diagnosis of ALS who use computerized artificial communication systems for years prior to their death.

Partial Laryngectomy

A partial laryngectomy for cancer of the larynx, either a supraglottic (horizontal partial laryngectomy) or hemilaryngectomy (vertical partial laryngectomy) generally causes some change in voice (hoarseness), as well as potential difficulty in protecting the airway during swallowing (3–5), and sometimes unremitting aspiration. There are a number of rehabilitation procedures involving volitional airway protection for swallowing, which patients can be taught, as well as exercises to improve range of motion of residual structures in the larynx (6–8).

Total Laryngectomy

The patient who receives a total laryngectomy will obviously have no voice source any longer and will need to replace that with either an artificial larynx, esophageal speech, or tracheoesophageal puncture (surgical prosthetic) voice restoration (9–14). The latter procedure has become quite popular, as it restores voice rather quickly and the patient does not need to go through the long process of learning esophageal speech. However, to be a good candidate for a tracheoesophageal puncture, the patient must be willing to maintain a small prosthesis in the puncture site and therefore to do more stomal care. If these patients develop a recurrence of their disease, the prosthesis may need to be removed and they may need to use an artificial larynx.

Total laryngectomy also creates changes in swallowing, requiring the patient to increase the effort and pressure needed to swallow postoperatively (6,15–17). However, after total laryngectomy the patient should be able to eat a full, normal diet. Few patients experience more significant swallowing problems related to a stricture or narrowing in their reconstructed pharyngoesophagus or a flap of "extra" mucosa at the base of the tongue known as a *pseudoepiglottis* (6). With recurrence of disease these problems, particularly cervical esophageal strictures, may recur or worsen.

The involvement of the speech-language pathologist in palliative care is a relatively new development but is increasing with some rapidity. In care of patients who are terminally ill, it is important that a team approach be used involving the speech-language pathologist with the gastroenterologist in management of oropharyngeal (speech-language pathologist) and esophageal (gastroenterologist) disorders. In addition, the interaction of speech-language pathologists with the patient's primary care physician and others can facilitate smooth transitions for the patients as their functions may worsen. The constant goal is always to maintain optimal function for the patient in terms of communication with staff and family as well as best nutritional intake.

High-Dose Chemoradiation

Concomitant high-dose chemotherapy and radiation therapy to the head and neck are often called *organ preservation protocols*. They are designed to preserve the anatomic continuity of the upper aerodigestive tract by curing the patient's disease without the need for surgery and at the same time maintaining function. Recent studies have shown, however, that for some patients, some of the functions of the upper aerodigestive tract are not maintained in these protocols, particularly swallowing ability (18). To date, the particular high-dose chemoradiation protocols that have the greatest swallowing toxicity and the tumor locations where greatest toxicity is seen because of these protocols are just beginning to be defined (19). Currently, it appears that the patient with a hypopharyngeal tumor is at the greatest risk. The swallowing disorders of these individuals often are severe and prolonged, and are sometimes permanent. They include severely restricted laryngeal elevation and often virtually absent pharyngeal wall contraction. Reduced opening of the upper esophageal sphincter is a result of both of these problems. During swallowing, there is little pressure generated on the food to drive it through the pharynx and into the esophagus, leaving most of the food in the pharynx to be aspirated after the swallow. Some patients also develop cervical esophageal strictures, which require repeated dilatation, where possible. Some of these patients require conversion to total laryngectomy in an attempt to eat. However, such a conversion may not result in successful return to full oral intake, because total laryngectomy requires generation of even more pressure to drive the bolus through the reconstructed pharyngoesophagus than does normal swallowing. Because these patients already have diminished ability to generate pressure to drive food through the pharynx and, in this case, the pharyngoesophagus, a total laryngectomy will stop chronic aspiration of the patient's own secretions and of food and liquid but may not enable the patient to get adequate nutrition orally.

These swallowing impairments are thought to result from severe fibrosis, particularly in the muscles of the pharynx, which appear to be quite sensitive to radiotherapy. In some cases, this fibrosis continues to worsen over time so that immediately after the completion of their radiotherapy the patient may be able to continue to eat successfully, but a year or two later may be unable to swallow efficiently and safely. If the larynx is in the field of radiotherapy, changes in voice quality may result, most of which are relatively temporary. Ability to articulate speech sounds is relatively unimpaired compared with swallowing function. With any disease recurrence these problems may worsen significantly and a nonoral feeding may be required.

MANAGEMENT OF TUMORS OF THE HARD AND/OR SOFT PALATE

Generally, the patient who has a tumor of the hard palate, which will be surgically removed, should be seen preoperatively by the maxillofacial prosthodontist and is frequently provided an intraoral obturator prosthesis by the maxillofacial prosthodontist at the time of surgery. In that way, when the patient awakens after surgery, they have a temporary prosthesis in place (20,21). This prosthesis is then redesigned once the patient's healing is complete, at 2 to 4 or more weeks postoperatively. With this temporary prosthesis in place, the patient's speech and swallowing are often relatively intact.

Resection of the soft palate

Surgical removal of part or all of the soft palate often requires another type of intraoral prosthesis, a palatal bulb, which extends posteriorly into the surgical defect. If the palate is only partially resected, fitting the prosthesis can be more difficult than if the entire soft palate is removed. The success of a palatal bulb prosthesis depends upon the ability of the patient's lateral pharyngeal walls to move inward to meet the prosthesis to achieve velopharyngeal closure during speech and swallowing (6,22,23). This can be difficult to design, particularly in patients who also have had or will have radiotherapy to the pharynx. Radiotherapy damages pharyngeal wall motion. There are patients who are never able to wear prosthesis successfully to obturate the velopharyngeal port because they have inadequate pharyngeal wall activity. In these patients, the prosthesis may need to be so large that it blocks the passage to the nose completely and is uncomfortable. If the prosthesis is too small, it allows air to pass through the nose, leaving the patient with nasality during speech and leakage of food up the nose during swallowing. Despite the most experienced prosthodontist and speech-language pathologist's input to the design of palatal bulb prosthesis, there is sometimes no ability to achieve an optimum result. The same difficulties occur with attempts at surgical reconstruction of the soft palate. Generally, prosthetics have been more successful than surgical procedures in these patients.

ORAL CANCER SURGICAL PROCEDURES INVOLVING THE TONGUE

In general, the percent of oral tongue and tongue base that are resected and the nature of the surgical reconstruction used will dictate the extent of the patient's speech and swallowing problems postoperatively (24,25). This is true whether the locus of disease is anterior or posterior. Generally, if the patient undergoes resection of more than 50% of the tongue, significant speech, and swallowing defects will result regardless of the nature of the reconstruction. If disease recurs in the region, the patient's muscle strength in the tongue may be reduced so that they are less intelligible.

ANTERIOR ORAL CAVITY RESECTIONS

Resection of part of the anterior floor of the mouth and tongue generally result in changes in speech understandability and swallowing related to reduced range of motion and shaping of the anterior tongue (26–29). The anterior tongue is used to produce speech sounds such as "t," "d," "s," and "z" as well as to lift and contact the food and bring it laterally to the teeth for chewing. After chewing is complete, the anterior tongue also contributes to forming the food into a bolus or ball prior to the start of the swallow. The anterior tongue initiates the oral stage of swallow by propelling the food backward. All of these functions can be affected by resection of the anterior floor of the mouth and tongue. If the surgical reconstruction after the resection further inhibits tongue motion, then greater functional deficit can be anticipated. Generally, because of the severity of the cosmetic defect, resection of the anterior portion of the mandible is not done or, if resected, the anterior mandible is immediately reconstructed.

The patient who has undergone resection of the anterior oral cavity may exhibit some delay in triggering the pharyngeal swallow because the tongue motion is changed postoperatively and oral tongue motion contributes to the sensory input for triggering the pharyngeal stage of swallowing. These patients need speech and swallowing therapy as soon as possible, after healing. The motor control of the pharyngeal stage of swallowing is not impaired unless muscles of the floor of mouth are cut in the anterior resection. The floor of mouth muscles contribute to lifting and pulling the larynx anteriorly and opening the upper esophageal sphincter during swallowing

(30,31). Generally, the patient with an anterior oral resection has less functional sequela than the patient with a more posterior oral cavity resection as described in the subsequent text (32).

POSTERIOR ORAL CAVITY RESECTIONS

The patient who has undergone a posterior oral cavity resection typically, has both speech and swallowing problems because of the removal of tongue tissue and/or because of the type of reconstruction used. Posterior oral cavity resections usually affect oral aspects of swallowing including chewing and propulsion of the food toward the back of the mouth, triggering of the pharyngeal stage of swallowing, and the efficiency of the motor aspects of the pharyngeal stage of swallow as well (6,32). These patients can return to intelligible speech and full oral intake with a fairly normal diet if they have some degree of remaining tongue mobility (33,34) and have speech and swallowing therapy and an intraoral prosthesis (a palatal augmentation or reshaping device) designed to reshape the hard palate to interact with the function of the remaining tongue. If the tumor recurs in this site, both speech and swallowing may be negatively affected.

Pharyngeal Wall Resection

The patient who has radiotherapy or surgery to the pharyngeal wall for a pharyngeal tumor generally has permanent difficulty generating adequate pressure to propel food efficiently through the pharynx for swallowing posttreatment (6). These individuals can have significant residual food left in the pharynx after the swallow and may aspirate. Postural techniques for swallow may sometimes compensate for pharyngeal resections, which tend to be on one side, whereas radiotherapy generally has bilateral effects. Some of these patients will have dietary restrictions because they have difficulty propelling thicker food through the pharynx, which requires greater pressures.

ASSESSMENT FOR SPEECH AND SWALLOWING

Even patients whose diagnoses fall into the same category as ALS, that is, motor speech disorders, may have very different speech and swallowing disorders requiring very different management. Both are first assessed clinically at bedside to define the disordered aspects of their speech and swallowing ability, largely focusing on oral control. Reliable assessment of the pharynx and larynx at bedside is not possible as neither can be visualized without instrumentation.

The pharyngeal assessment normally uses the modified barium swallow (the videofluorographic study of oropharyngeal swallow) and, if needed, followed by the barium swallow to assess the esophagus. Patients with esophageal disorders should be referred to the gastroenterologist for medication or other assistance. The modified barium swallow should provide the patient and caregivers with a complete description of the abnormalities in their oropharyngeal swallow followed by an assessment of the effectiveness of various treatment

---

TABLE 12.1

POSTURAL TECHNIQUES GENERALLY MOST APPROPRIATE FOR EACH SWALLOW DISORDER AND THE PHYSIOLOGIC/ANATOMIC EFFECT(S) OF THE POSTURE ON PHARYNGEAL DIMENSIONS OR BOLUS FLOW

Disorder observed on fluoroscopy	Posture applied	Physiologic/Anatomic effect of posture
Inefficient oral transit (Reduced posterior propulsion of bolus by tongue)	Chin up	Uses gravity to clear oral cavity
Delay in triggering the pharyngeal swallow (Bolus past ramus of mandible but pharyngeal swallow is not triggered)	Chin down	Widens valleculae to prevent bolus entering airway; and narrows airway entrance
Reduced tongue base retraction (Residue in valleculae)	Chin down	Pushes tongue base backward toward pharyngeal wall
Unilateral laryngeal dysfunction (Aspiration during swallow)	Chin down	Places epiglottis in more posterior, protective position
	Head turned to damaged side	Pushes damaged side toward midline
Reduced laryngeal closure (Aspiration during the swallow)	Head rotated to damaged side and chin down	Increases vocal fold closure by applying extrinsic pressure; narrows laryngeal entrance. Places epiglottis in more protective position.
Reduced pharyngeal contraction (Residue spread throughout pharynx)	Lying down on one side	Eliminates gravitational effect on pharyngeal residue
Unilateral pharyngeal paresis (Residue on one side of pharynx)	Head rotated to damaged side	Eliminates damaged side from bolus path
Cricopharyngeal dysfunction (Residue in pyriform sinuses)	Head rotated	Pulls cricoid cartilage away from posterior pharyngeal wall, reducing resting pressure in cricopharyngeal sphincter

Use of postural techniques are generally the first management procedure evaluated during the radiographic swallow study (modified barium swallow) if a patient regularly gets food or liquid into their airway.

techniques that could be appropriate for the patient and be presented to them during the radiographic study. The treatment techniques therefore can be assessed for their immediate effectiveness (22,35,36). Most recent data (37) indicate that approximately 50% of patients can be immediately helped by the introduction of treatment strategies that have an immediate effect including: postural changes to redirect the flow of food, as shown in Table 12.1, heightening of sensory stimulation to facilitate oral awareness of food and faster triggering of the pharyngeal swallow, and voluntary maneuvers or controls to change selected aspects of the pharyngeal swallow including airway entrance closure, vocal fold closure, tongue base movement to increase pressure on the bolus, and the opening of the upper esophageal sphincter. Each of these is shown in Tables 12.2 and 12.3 and their effects defined. The simplest procedures such as, postural change and sensory enhancement procedures, as well as dietary changes, are often easiest for the patient in palliative care because swallow maneuvers or voluntary controls require greater energy and effort on the patient's part. Patients in palliative care may not have the strength needed to successfully execute these swallowing controls. Changes in diet such as, thickening liquids or adding heightened tastes or avoiding certain foods in terms of consistency may be useful as well, although patients often dislike these interventions. However, the patient with motor neuron disease, for example, may actually spontaneously alter their diet to avoid thicker foods that require greater pressure to be swallowed. These patients may also eliminate foods requiring chewing, as they may not be able to lateralize food to the teeth with the tongue and thereby control chewing. There are many commercially available products from a variety of companies such as Novartis, which produce nectar-thickened liquids, honey-thickened liquids, pureed foods, etc., which are broadly available to patients.

Swallowing assessment for patients with suspected pharyngeal and swallow problems includes a radiographic study of swallowing to define the nature of the patient's swallow physiology and to identify effective strategies to assure safe and efficient oral intake. Often the effects of these strategies can be assessed during the radiographic study (6,32–36). Some

of these therapies such as, postural changes can immediately compensate for the patient's swallowing problem so the patient can continue or restart to eat orally (22,36). Sometimes exercise programs can begin to enable the patient to eventually eat without these compensations but in palliative care patients may be too weak to exercise regularly. Typically, compensatory strategies in the area of swallowing may involve changing head position to alter the direction of the flow of the food through the mouth and pharynx, preswallow sensory stimulation to heighten sensory awareness of the food and swallowing maneuvers designed to improve selected aspects of the swallow physiology, as well as a variety of range of motion exercises (6). The effectiveness of these techniques can be assessed during the radiographic study. Swallowing maneuvers are designed to take voluntary control of selected aspects of the pharyngeal stage of swallow such as, closing the true vocal folds, closing the airway entrance, improving laryngeal elevation and thereby upper sphincter opening into the esophagus and improving the pressure generated on the bolus (6–11,31). Patients are instructed to use these maneuvers or other exercises in practice five to ten times per day for 5 minutes each to improve muscle function. Occasionally such voluntary controls must be used during each swallow to enable oral intake (38).

INTERVENTIONS FOR SPEECH AND SWALLOWING

Clinicians are always in search of a single set of procedures that will improve both speech and swallowing. There are some patients who can successfully use one type of exercise for both speech and swallowing. Because the nature of the speech and swallowing impairment in the oral cancer patient relates in large part to the reduction in range of motion created by either surgical procedures or radiotherapy, use of range of motion exercises often improves both speech and swallowing. Speech production relies on the ability of the tongue to make complete or near complete contacts with the palate at various locations. The degree of contact or approximation and the location of this contact or approximation determines the nature of the sound

TABLE 12.2

BOLUS CONSISTENCIES AND SWALLOW PROBLEMS THEY ARE APPROPRIATE FOR

Food consistencies	Disorders for which these foods are most appropriate
Thin liquids	Delayed pharyngeal swallow
	Reduced tongue base retraction[a]
	Reduced pharyngeal wall contraction[a]
	Reduced laryngeal elevation[a]
	Reduced cricopharyngeal opening
Thickened liquids (nectar and/or honey)	Oral tongue dysfunction[a,b]
	Delayed pharyngeal swallow
Purees and Thick foods	Reduced laryngeal closure at the entrance
	Reduced laryngeal closure throughout the larynx
Foods with texture such as yogurt containing small particles of cookie	Sensory dysfunction, poor recognition of food

[a]All of these disorders affect generation of pressure to drive the bolus through the oral cavity and/or pharynx. Thinner foods (liquids) require less pressure to swallow.
[b]Must be combined with airway protection techniques such as, chin down with head turned posture of a voluntary breath hold when swallowing.
The patient should be tested radiographically with each bolus type to see what food consistency can be most efficiently and safely swallowed.

TABLE 12.3

IMMEDIATE EFFECTS OF TREATMENT

	Treatment effects visible during the x-ray study of swallow			Effects not immediately visible on x-ray
Disorder/(Symptoms)	Posture	Heightened sensory stimulation	Swallow maneuvers	Exercise programs (Ref 22)
Reduced lip closure (food lost from mouth)	Chin up	—	—	Lip resistance exercises
Reduced oral tongue range of motion (reduced tongue vertical or lateral motion)	Chin down, then elevated	—	—	Range of motion exercises
Reduced oral tongue strength (increasing residue as food thickens)	Chin up	—	—	Tongue strength; resistance exercises
Pharyngeal delay (bolus passes trigger point but no pharyngeal swallow)	Chin down	Thermal-tactile stimulation	Supraglottic swallow (breathhold)	—
Reduced velopharyngeal closure (nasal regurgitation)	Chin up	—	—	—
Reduced laryngeal elevation (residue on top of larynx, visibly reduced elevation)	Lie down	—	Mendelsohn maneuver (improves laryngeal lifting)	Shaker exercise (strengthens muscles that lift larynx)
Unilateral pharyngeal wall disorder (residue on damaged side, in pyriform sinus)	Head rotation to damaged side	—	Supraglottic swallow (breathhold)	—
Bilateral pharyngeal wall disorder (residue equal in both pyriform sinuses, on both walls)	Lie down	—	Supraglottic swallow (breathhold)	Tongue holding maneuver (strengthens tongue base movement)
Oral and pharyngeal weakness on the same side (residue in mouth and pharynx on same side)	Lean or tilt to strong side	—	—	Range of motion oral and tongue base exercises
Reduced airway entrance closure (penetration)	Chin down and head turned if damage is asymmetrical	—	Super-supraglottic swallow (breath hold while bearing down)	Effortful breath hold
Reduced laryngeal closure (aspiration during swallow)	Chin down and head turned if damage is asymmetrical	—	Super-supraglottic swallow (breath hold while bearing down	Adduction exercises, effortful breath hold
Reduced tongue base (residue in valleculae)	Chin down		Effortful swallow (squeeze hard during swallow)	Tongue base range of motion exercises (yawn, pull tongue straight back, gargle)
Reduced cricopharyngeal opening (residue in pyriform sinuses, visible reduced width of opening)	Head rotation to weak side of the pharynx		Mendelsohn maneuver (improves laryngeal lifting)	Shaker exercise Mendelsohn maneuver

Be sure to examine the combination of posture and swallow maneuvers where feasible.

produced. Similarly, during swallowing, the tongue must make complete contact with the hard palate sequentially from front to back to propel the food into the pharynx. Gravity alone will not provide an efficient swallow.

For patients with Parkinson's disease, the Lee Silverman Voice Treatment focusing on increasing vocal loudness, has been shown to improve both speech and swallowing (39). Other speech and swallowing interventions are prescribed and conducted as needed for each patient based on their assessment. Throughout the patient's speech and swallowing interventions, the social worker or other psychosocial counselor should be providing the patient with needed psychosocial support.

Voice amplification

As some patients become weaker or for patients with respiratory disease, voice may become extremely soft. For these patients, a voice amplifier may be most helpful. The level of loudness can be set as needed.

Voice replacement

The electrolarynx (a type of artificial larynx) can be useful in patients with a very weak voice or extremely poor respiratory support who cannot exhale hard enough to produce voice but who have the ability to articulate. A handheld artificial larynx placed against their neck can transmit sound into the patient's vocal tract. Articulation can be superimposed over this voice source. The speech-language pathologist must train the patient, family, or staff to hold the instrument in the location on the neck that results in best transmission of the sound and clearest speech.

Augmentative/Alternative Communication Devices

The speech-language pathologist will evaluate the patient's need for and ability to use a communication device and identify the best device for the individual patient. Both a voice amplifier and artificial larynx could be classified as augmentative/alternative devices. The speech-language pathologist then works with the patient to facilitate their learning to use the instrument. The speech-language pathologist also works with the staff in the palliative care facility to help them know best how to help the patient to use the instrument effectively. Instruments can range from a computer keyboard for typing to such a keyboard with a switch that can be controlled by eye blinks or eyebrow movements and thereby choose letters to spell words. A website (http://www.cini.org) (40) provides information about the wide range of devices.

THIRD PARTY REIMBURSEMENT STRATEGIES

Unfortunately, Medicare and other third party payers may not provide adequate funding for palliative services. This means the patient may not be able to receive optimal services for the necessary length of time. Many patients are highly motivated to maintain their function. They are able to follow directions easily, so rehabilitation professionals can provide them with written exercises and videotaped examples of exercise programs and can design other interventions that are as cost effective as possible, for as long as needed by the patient to restore optimal function.

In summary, the key to successful palliative care by speech-language pathologists is to begin and maintain ongoing evaluation and treatment planning in a multidisciplinary format that examines the effectiveness of interventions in light of our knowledge of functional effects of the treatments and nature of each patient's potential functional needs. Speech-language pathologists should be involved from the time the patient in palliative care is identified as exhibiting symptoms of any speech, voice, or swallowing problems.

References

1. Eckman S, Roe J. Speech and language therapists in palliative care: what do we have to offer? *Int J Palliat Nurs* 2005;11(4):179–181.
2. Lazarus CL, Logemann JA, Shi G, et al. Does laryngectomy improve swallowing after chemoradiotherapy? *Arch Otolaryngol Head Neck Surg* 2002;128:54–57.
3. McConnel FMS, Mendelsohn MS, Logemann JA. Manofluorography of deglutition after supraglottic laryngectomy. *Head Neck Surg* 1987;9:142–150.
4. Logemann JA, Gibbons P, Rademaker AW, et al. Mechanisms of recovery of swallow after supraglottic laryngectomy. *J Speech Hear Res* 1994;37:965–974.
5. Rademaker AW, Logemann JA, Pauloski BR, et al. Recovery of postoperative swallowing in patients undergoing partial laryngectomy. *Head Neck* 1993;15:325–334.
6. Logemann JA. *Evaluation and treatment of swallowing disorders*, 2nd ed. Austin, TX: Pro-Ed, 1998.
7. Martin BJW, Logemann JA, Shaker R, et al. Normal laryngeal valving patterns during three breath-hold maneuvers: a pilot investigation. *Dysphagia* 1993;8:11–20.
8. Ohmae Y, Logemann JA, Kaiser P, et al. Effects of two breath-holding maneuvers on oropharyngeal swallow. *Ann Otol Rhinol Laryngol* 1996;105:123–131.
9. Logemann JA. Speech therapy after extensive surgery for post cricoid carcinoma. In: Edels Y, ed. *Vocal rehabilitation after laryngectomy*. London: Croom Helm, 1983.
10. McConnel FMS, Sisson GA, Logemann JA. Three years experience with a hypopharyngeal pseudoglottis for vocal rehabilitation after total laryngectomy. *Trans Am Acad Ophthalmol Otolaryngol* 1976;84:63–67.
11. McConnel F, Sisson G, Logemann JA, et al. Voice rehabilitation after laryngectomy. *Arch Otolaryngol* 1975;101:178–181.
12. Singer M, Blom E. An endoscopic technique for restoration of voice after laryngectomy. *Ann Otol Rhinol Laryngol* 1980;89:529–533.
13. Sisson G, McConnel FMS, Logemann JA. Rehabilitation after laryngectomy with a hypopharyngeal voice prosthesis. *Can J Otolaryngol* 1975;4:588–594.
14. Kearney A. Nontracheoesophageal speech rehabilitation. *Otolaryngol Clin North Am* 2004;37(3):613–625.
15. McConnel FMS, Hester TR, Mendelsohn MS, et al. Manofluorography of deglutition after total laryngopharyngectomy. *Plast Reconstr Surg* 1988;81(3):346–351.
16. McConnel FMS, Mendelsohn MS, Logemann JA. Examination of swallowing after total laryngectomy using manofluorography. *Head Neck Surg* 1986;9:3–12.
17. Pauloski BR, Blom ED, Logemann JA, et al. Functional outcome after surgery for prevention of pharyngospasms in tracheoesophageal speakers. Part II: swallow characteristics. *Laryngoscope* 1995;105:1104–1110.
18. Lazarus CL, Logemann J, Pauloski BR, et al. Swallowing disorders in head and neck cancer patients treated with radiotherapy and adjuvant chemotherapy. *Laryngoscope* 1996;106:1157–1166.
19. Logemann JA, Rademaker AW, Pauloski BR, et al. Site of disease and treatment protocols as correlates of swallowing function in head and neck cancer patients treated with chemoradiation. *Head Neck* 2006;28(1):64–73.
20. Logemann JA. Nursing and allied health interventions in cancer control. In: Mettlin K, ed. *Progress in cancer control*. New York: Alan R. Liss, 1981:101–110.
21. Logemann JA. Speech and swallowing rehabilitation for head and neck tumor patients. In: Myers E, Sten D, eds. *Cancer of the head and neck*, 2nd ed. New York: Churchill Livingstone, 1989:1021–1043.
22. Rasley A, Logemann JA, Kahrilas PJ, et al. Prevention of barium aspiration during videofluoroscopic swallowing studies: value of change in posture. *Am J Roent* 1993;160:1005–1009.
23. Hannon DC, Logemann JA, Hurt M. Physiology of pharynx & larynx. In: Meyerhoff WL, Rice DH, eds. *Otolaryngology-head and neck surgery*. Orlando, FL: WB Saunders, 1992:683–698.
24. McConnel FMS, Logemann JA, Rademaker AW, et al. Surgical variables affecting postoperative swallowing efficiency in oral cancer patients: a pilot study. *Laryngoscope* 1994;104(1):87–90.

25. Pauloski BR, Logemann JA, Colangelo LA, et al. Surgical variables affecting speech in treated oral/oropharyngeal cancer patients. *Laryngoscope* 1998;108:908–916.
26. Pauloski BR, Logemann JA, Rademaker A, et al. Speech and swallowing function after anterior tongue & floor of mouth resection w/distal flap reconstruction. *J Speech Hear Res* 1993;36:267–276.
27. Logemann JA, Bytell DE. Swallowing disorders in three types of head and neck surgical patients. *Cancer* 1979;44:1095–1105.
28. Pauloski BR, Logemann JA, Fox JC, et al. Biomechanical analysis of the pharyngeal swallow in postsurgical patients with anterior tongue and floor of mouth resection and distal flap reconstruction. *J Speech Hear Res* 1995;38:10–123.
29. Logemann J. Articulation management of the oral pharyngeal impaired patient. In: Perkins WH, ed. *Current therapy for communication disorders.* New York: Thieme & Stratton, 1983.
30. Kahrilas PJ, Lin S, Chen J, et al. Oropharyngeal accommodation to swallow volume. *Gastroenterology* 1996;111:297–306.
31. Kahrilas PJ, Logemann JA, Krugler C, et al. Volitional augmentation of upper esophageal sphincter opening during swallowing. *Am J Physiol, Gastrointest Physiol 23* 1991;260:G450–G456.
32. Logemann JA, Pauloski BR, Rademaker AW, et al. Speech and swallow function after tonsil/base of tongue resection w/primary closure. *J Speech Hear Res* 1993;36:918–926.
33. Davis J, Lazarus C, Logemann J, et al. Effect of a maxillary glossectomy prostheses on articulation and swallowing. *J Prosthet Dent* 1987;57(6):715–719.
34. Wheeler R, Logemann J, Rosen MS. A maxillary reshaping prosthesis: its effectiveness in improving the speech & swallowing of postsurgical oral cancer patients. *J Prosthet Dent* 1980;43:491–495.
35. Logemann JA. *A manual for videofluoroscopic evaluation of swallowing,* 2nd ed. Austin, TX: Pro-Ed, 1993.
36. Logemann JA, Rademaker AW, Pauloski BR, et al. Effects of postural change on aspiration in head and neck surgical patients. *Otolaryngol Head Neck Surg* 1994;110:222–227.
37. Martin-Harris B, Logemann JA, McMahon S, et al. Clinical utility of the modified barium swallow. *Dysphagia* 2000;15:136–141.
38. Lazarus C, Logemann JA, Gibbons P. Effects of maneuvers on swallowing function in a dysphagic oral cancer patient. *Head Neck* 1993;15:419–424.
39. El Sharkawi A, Ramig L, Logemann JA, et al. Swallowing and voice effects of Lee Silverman Voice Treatment (LSVT®): a pilot study. *J Neurol Neurosurg Psychiatry* 2002;72:31–36.
40. Communication Independence for the Neurologically Impaired (CINI). *A not-for-profit organization disseminating information about available communication technology people with ALS/MND (Lou Gehrig's Disease).* Website: www.cini.org.

CHAPTER 13 ■ CHEMOTHERAPY-RELATED NAUSEA AND VOMITING

ANN M. BERGER AND REBECCA A. CLARK-SNOW

NATURE OF THE PROBLEM

Currently, there are many efficacious antiemetic regimens for nausea and vomiting produced by chemotherapeutic agents. In a study conducted in 1983, patients with cancer ranked nausea and vomiting as the first and second most severe side effects of chemotherapy, respectively (1). After the emergence of new antiemetic agents and alterations in chemotherapeutic regimens, patients' perceptions of the most severe side effects were modified. In a 1993 study, 155 patients with cancer, receiving chemotherapy, reported that they experienced an average of 20 physical and psychosocial symptoms: nausea was ranked as the most severe symptom and vomiting as the fifth (2). Therefore, nausea is also an important efficacy parameter when evaluating an antiemetic.

Use of these antiemetic agents has decreased the incidence and severity of nausea and vomiting induced by chemotherapy; however, these agents have not totally prevented the problem. Chemotherapy-induced nausea and vomiting (CINV) continue to remain a concern for patients receiving cancer treatment. Grunberg et al. (3) reported that in spite of the use of modern antiemetics, CINV continues to be a problem for a significant number of patients receiving cancer chemotherapy. It was observed that the frequency of CINV, particularly delayed nausea and vomiting, is underestimated by oncology physicians and nurses (3). The incidence and severity of nausea or vomiting in patients receiving chemotherapy vary, depending on the type of chemotherapy given, dose, schedule, combinations of medications, and individual characteristics. The consequences of not controlling the nausea and vomiting induced by cancer treatment may lead to medical complications, a failure of the patient to comply with the cancer therapy and follow-up, and a diminished quality of life.

The supportive care of patients receiving agents with the potential to cause nausea and vomiting remains an important aspect of effective management of the oncology patient. In every treatment situation, the primary goal is prevention of CINV. However, despite an improved understanding of the pathophysiology associated with this phenomenon, the identification of predictive factors, the definition of emetic syndromes, and the development of evidence-based guidelines that incorporate the most effective antiemetic agents and regimens available to prevent and treat chemotherapy-induced emesis, there continue to be patients for whom achieving complete control (no vomiting or nausea) is problematic. To this end, patients' quality of life may be significantly compromised in the event of incomplete control.

PATHOPHYSIOLOGY OF NAUSEA AND VOMITING

The precise mechanisms by which chemotherapy induces nausea and vomiting are unknown; however, it appears probable that different chemotherapeutic agents act at different sites and that some chemotherapeutic agents act at multiple sites. The fact that different chemotherapeutic agents cause nausea and vomiting by different mechanisms, and that one chemotherapeutic agent may induce nausea and vomiting by more than one mechanism, helps clinicians to understand why there is no one antiemetic regimen that is effective all of the time.

Mechanisms by which chemotherapeutic agents cause nausea and vomiting are activation of the chemoreceptor trigger zone (CTZ) either directly or indirectly, peripheral stimulation of the gastrointestinal (GI) tract, vestibular mechanisms, cortical mechanisms, or alterations of taste and smell. For most chemotherapeutic agents, the most common mechanism is thought to be activation of the CTZ.

The CTZ is located in the area postrema of the brain and can be reached by emetogenic chemicals through the cerebrospinal fluid or the blood. The thought is that the mechanisms of interaction between the CTZ and chemotherapy involve the release of various neurotransmitters that activate the vomiting center. Either one or a combination of these transmitters may induce vomiting. Some of the neurotransmitters located in the area postrema of the brain that may be excited and lead to emesis include dopamine, serotonin, histamine, norepinephrine, apomorphine, neurotensin, angiotensin II, vasoactive intestinal polypeptide, gastrin, vasopressin, thyrotropin-releasing hormone, leucine-enkephalin, and substance P (4). Other enzymes surround the CTZ, such as adenosine triphosphatase, monoamine oxidase, cholinesterase, and catecholamines; however, their role in chemotherapy-induced emesis is unknown.

Until the 1990s, the neurotransmitter that appeared to be the most responsible for CINV was dopamine. Many effective antiemetics are dopamine antagonists that may bind specifically to the D_2 receptor. However, there is a high degree of variation in dopamine receptor–binding affinity by these drugs. The action of some drugs that cause nausea and vomiting is affected very little or not at all by dopamine antagonists. It is known that not all the important receptors in the CTZ are dopaminergic, as the effect of dopamine antagonists is not equal to surgical ablation of the CTZ. It has also been noted that the degree of antiemetic activity of high-dose metoclopramide cannot be explained on the basis of dopamine blockade alone.

Histamine receptors are found in abundance in the CTZ; however, H_2 antagonists do not work as antiemetics at all. H_1 antagonists alleviate nausea and vomiting induced by vestibular disorder and motion sickness but not nausea and vomiting induced by chemotherapy (5).

Knowledge that opiate receptors are found in abundance in the CTZ, as well as the facts that narcotics have mixed emetic and antiemetic effects that are blocked by naloxone and that naloxone has emetic properties, have led to the proposal of opiates or enkephalins as an antiemetic. High doses of naloxone augments emesis induced by chemotherapy, and low doses of narcotics may reduce emesis. Studies to date have shown that opiates can prevent chemotherapy-induced emesis in laboratory animals; however, both butorphanol and buprenorphine have not proved to be effective antiemetics in patients who had received chemotherapy previously. One study by Lissoni et al. (6) did demonstrate the synthetic enkephalin analog Fk-33-824 was more effective as an antiemetic in patients who received cisplatin; however, it was ineffective for patients receiving cyclophosphamide or epirubicin.

Edwards et al. found that arginine vasopressin levels rise to a greater extent in patients who vomit when they receive chemotherapy as compared with those who do not vomit (7). It has been suggested that perhaps arginine vasopressin plays a role in nausea more than in the vomiting induced by chemotherapy. Dexamethasone, which is a known effective antiemetic, may work by reducing arginine vasopressin levels. Another mechanism of action of corticosteroids as antiemetics may be related to modulation of prostaglandin release.

Some evidence suggests that although no one neurotransmitter is responsible for all CINV, it appears that 5-hydroxytryptamine (5-HT) (serotonin) receptors are particularly important in the pathophysiology of acute vomiting, whereas others may be more important in the pathophysiology of nausea and delayed emesis. The role of the 5-HT type 3 (5-HT$_3$) receptor in chemotherapy-induced emesis was recognized by examining the mechanism of action of high-dose metoclopramide in decreasing cisplatin-induced emesis. High-dose metoclopramide, unlike other D_2-receptor antagonists, has an exceptionally good capacity to decrease the emesis induced by cisplatin administration. It has been recognized that metoclopramide has pharmacologic effects other than dopamine antagonism. Metoclopramide is a weak antagonist of peripheral 5-HT$_3$ receptors and can stimulate GI motility by increasing acetylcholine release from the cholinergic nerves of the GI tract. To test whether a 5-HT$_3$-receptor blockade would decrease cisplatin-induced emesis, Miner et al. (8) took a substituted benzamide, BRL 24924, which has stimulatory effects on the GI tract and is a 5-HT$_3$-receptor blocker, and demonstrated decreased emesis in ferrets that received cisplatin. This study was repeated with a nonbenzamide selective 5-HT$_3$-receptor blocker MDL 72222, which has no GI-stimulating activity. The study revealed that cisplatin-induced emesis was totally blocked by this compound (8). The same conclusion was reached in another study using a different nonbenzamide, the selective 5-HT$_3$ antagonist ICS 205-930 (9). These studies demonstrated the role of 5-HT$_3$-receptor blockade in chemotherapy-induced emesis.

The precise mechanism of action of the 5-HT$_3$-receptor antagonists is unknown; however, the primary effect appears to be peripheral at the site of the 5-HT$_3$ receptors on the vagal afferent neurons. The GI tract contains approximately 80% of the body's supply of serotonin, and it has been suggested that perhaps chemotherapy administration causes release of serotonin from the enterochromaffin cells of the GI tract, which then stimulates emesis through both the vagus and greater splanchnic nerve, and stimulates the area postrema of the brain. After cisplatin administration, there is an increase in urinary excretion of 5-hydroxyindoleacetic acid, the main metabolite of serotonin, and this increase parallels the number of episodes of emesis (10). Studies have shown that the 5-HT$_3$-receptor antagonists decrease emesis from several chemotherapeutic agents, including cisplatin, cyclophosphamide, and doxorubicin (11,12).

An important mechanism whereby chemotherapy may induce emesis is the peripheral effect that is thought to arise from the pharynx and the upper GI tract. It is most likely that chemotherapy does not directly stimulate the peripheral receptors. Rather, neurotransmitters probably are released as a result of local GI irritation or damage. GI tract serotonin, dopamine, opiate, histamine, and cholinergic receptors are most likely involved in the emesis induced by chemotherapy. The peripheral effects may be abolished by vagotomy, indicating that impulses from the GI tract may reach the vomiting center through the vagus and sympathetic nerves.

In addition to serotonin, substance P has recently been identified as an important neurotransmitter involved in CINV. Positron emission tomography imaging of healthy human brains has demonstrated that substance P/neurokinin-1 (NK1) receptors are located centrally in the brain stem (13). Substance P is believed to exert its effect on the emetic reflex primarily through the central mechanism of binding to the NK1 receptors in the midbrain. NK1 receptor antagonists that cross the blood–brain barrier have been shown to inhibit both acute and delayed emesis by cisplatin in animal models and human studies. Hesketh et al. analyzed data from clinical trials for the time course of cisplatin-induced emesis and demonstrated that serotonin-dependent mechanisms appeared to predominate in the first 8–12 hours post-cisplatin, but thereafter, NK1-dependent mechanisms for emesis appeared to have relatively greater importance (14). Specifically, early acute events responsive to 5-HT$_3$-receptor antagonists are likely to be mediated by peripheral serotonin release, whereas later acute and delayed events responsive to NK1 receptor antagonists are more likely to be medicated by substance P acting centrally at the NK1 receptors (14).

Another mechanism that may be involved in chemotherapy-induced emesis could be the therapy's effect on the vestibular system. It is known that patients who have a history of motion sickness experience a greater severity, frequency, and duration of nausea and vomiting from chemotherapy than patients who do not experience motion sickness. The mechanism by which the vestibular system may lead to chemotherapy-induced emesis is unknown; however, it is postulated that sensory information that is received by the vestibular system is different from information that was expected.

Some investigators believe that taste changes induced by chemotherapy may lead to nausea and vomiting. There are two suggested mechanisms for this. First, taste is thought to inhibit some activities incompatible with eating (e.g., oral pain, gag, nausea, vomiting). Damage to taste such as that produced by some chemotherapy might release that inhibition leading to enhancement of gag, nausea, and vomiting. This is supported by a study showing taste damage in women who have suffered from hyperemesis during pregnancy (15). Second, some chemotherapeutic agents may be tasted. For example, in a study of patients with breast carcinoma who received cyclophosphamide, methotrexate, and 5-fluorouracil, 36% reported a bitter taste in their mouth. One third of the patients thought that the bitter taste caused vomiting (16). The exact mechanism by which taste is changed by chemotherapy is unknown; however, it is thought that while the drugs are in the plasma or saliva, they have a direct effect on the oral mucosa or taste buds. Changes in taste may contribute both to nausea and vomiting as well as to anorexia.

Finally, chemotherapy-induced emesis may be induced by direct or indirect effects on the cerebral cortex. Animal studies have shown that nitrogen mustard partially causes

TABLE 13.1

MECHANISMS OF NAUSEA AND VOMITING AFTER CHEMOTHERAPY

Stimulation of chemoreceptor trigger zone
Peripheral mechanisms
    Damage of gastrointestinal mucosa
    Stimulation of gastrointestinal neurotransmitter receptors
Cortical mechanisms
    Direct cerebral activation
    Indirect (psychogenic) mechanisms
Vestibular mechanisms
Alterations of taste and smell

From Berger AM, Clark-Snow RA. Adverse effects of treatment. In: DeVita VT Jr, Hellman S, Rosenberg SA, eds. *Cancer: principles and practice of oncology*, 6th ed. Philadelphia, PA: Lippincott Williams & Wilkins, 2001, with permission.

emesis through direct stimulation of the cerebral cortex. Studies demonstrate that the risk of nausea and vomiting is increased when a patient's roommate is experiencing nausea and vomiting. It is also known that the amount of sleep had before receiving chemotherapy may influence whether a patient develops chemotherapy-induced emesis. In addition, large differences exist in the severity and incidence of nausea and vomiting from the same chemotherapeutic agents in different countries. These studies indicate that indirect psychological effects can mediate CINV.

Apart from there being more than one mechanism by which each chemotherapeutic agent may induce emesis, chemotherapy induces emesis in a manner different from that of other classic emetic agents. Drugs such as apomorphine, levodopa, digitalis, pilocarpine, nicotine, and morphine cause vomiting almost immediately. Nitrogen mustard may also lead to emesis immediately; however, most chemotherapeutic agents and radiotherapy require a latency period before emesis begins. Also, most chemotherapeutic agents do not induce emesis in a monophasic way, as do the classic emetic agents. Chemotherapeutic agents induce emesis with a delayed onset, and the emesis has multiphasic time courses. When managing chemotherapy-induced emesis, one should realize that there is most likely more than one mechanism involved, suggesting that there is not one antiemetic regimen that works for all patients all of the time.

By 1991, >50% of patients received a serotonin antagonist antiemetic (5-HT$_3$) for symptom control; approximately 90% received similar treatment in 1995, with a statistically significant reduction in posttreatment vomiting. Both physicians and nurses acknowledge an improvement in patients' quality of life and treatment compliance with the use of these agents. However, trends over time have not shown an improvement in the control of nausea. In fact, data confirm that there is a significant increase in the duration of posttreatment nausea and no change in the frequency of posttreatment nausea or anticipatory symptoms (17) (Table 13.1).

PHARMACOGENOMICS OF CHEMOTHERAPY-INDUCED NAUSEA AND VOMITING

The use of genetic profiling to more accurately define the functions and limitations of pharmaceuticals is a relatively recent development of modern biomedicine. The pharmacogenomic approach has proved fruitful in the clinical application of drugs targeted toward CINV (18). Several studies have used a standard approach of sequencing candidate genes associated with known emetic pathways to discover possible associations with the differentiated response among patients to treatment of CINV. Polymorphisms in the serotonin receptor and the cytochrome P (CYP)-450 system are each known to be associated with patient response to therapy.

One group sequenced the gene encoding the 3B subunit of the serotonin (5-HT$_3$) receptor (19). They discovered 13 polymorphisms, of which one, a deletion of AAG, was associated with response to ondansetron and tropisetron. There was also a clear gene dosage effect: homozygosity for the trinucleotide deletion greatly increased postchemotherapeutic emesis over heterozygosity for the same mutation, both in the initial 4 hours after chemotherapy and the following 5–24 hours.

The same group studied gene dosage effects in the CYP-450 enzyme family, particularly the CYP-2D6 enzyme (20). The CYP-450 enzymes metabolize serotonin receptor antagonists, thereby reducing their biological half-life and their value as antiemetic therapeutics. Several alleles of the CYP-2D6 gene decrease the effectiveness of the enzyme versus the wild-type allele. Individuals with three copies of the wild-type allele, which increases serotonin antagonist metabolism, had the greatest number of acute postchemotherapeutic emetic episodes under treatment with ondansetron or tropisetron, whereas individuals with three copies of the inactive variant alleles had fewer emetic episodes. Heterozygosity at the locus produced intermediate effects.

Further studies will focus on other candidate genes in emetic pathways, including the NK1 (substance P) receptor, dopaminergic receptors, and tyrosine hydroxylase. At this time, routine genetic testing of patients receiving emetogenic cancer chemotherapy is not indicated; however, it may prove useful in patients demonstrating unusually impaired response to standard antiemetic therapy. Future testing will more definitively establish the relationship between genotype and antiemetic phenotype and may bring genetic profiling into the realm of standard clinical practice.

EMETIC SYNDROMES

Patients undergoing therapy for the treatment and possible cure of cancer with chemotherapy are often faced with the distressing side effects of nausea and vomiting. The goals of antiemetic therapy are as follows:

1. To achieve complete control in all settings
2. To provide maximum convenience for patients and staff
3. To eliminate potential side effects of the agents
4. To minimize the cost of treatment with antiemetic agents and drug administration

As a result of antiemetic investigations, three major, related emetic syndromes have been identified: acute, delayed, and anticipatory emesis. Traditionally, acute emesis is defined as occurring within the first 24 hours of administration of chemotherapy (usually within 1–2 hours) and is generally most severe during the initial 4–6 hours. Delayed emesis has been arbitrarily defined as occurring 24 or more hours after chemotherapy (range of 16–24 hours), with maximal risk at 48 hours. It is most commonly associated with the administration of cisplatin, carboplatin, cyclophosphamide, and doxorubicin. A study that outlines the natural history of delayed emesis concluded that although the emesis associated with this dilemma is less severe than that which is seen in the acute phase, it still poses significant problems with nutrition, hydration, and possibly a prolonged hospital course (21).

TABLE 13.2

FACTORS ASSOCIATED WITH AN INCREASED INCIDENCE OF ANTICIPATORY NAUSEA AND VOMITING

Severe postchemotherapy side effects
Schedule of chemotherapy
Numerous chemotherapy cycles
Chemotherapeutic agents with high emetogenic potential
Age
History of motion sickness
Anxiety
Depression
Taste and odors

From Berger AM, Clark-Snow RA. Adverse effects of treatment. In: DeVita VT Jr, Hellman S, Rosenberg SA, eds. *Cancer: principles and practice of oncology*, 6th ed. Philadelphia, PA: Lippincott Williams & Wilkins, 2001, with permission.

Initial studies revealed that delayed emesis could be controlled with a regimen of metoclopramide and dexamethasone. Because of the possibility of extrapyramidal side effects such as anxiety, akathisia, restlessness, torticollis, or oculogyric crisis, with metoclopramide, patients should be given a prescription for diphenhydramine to be taken at the first sign of an extrapyramidal symptom. In the younger patient, diphenhydramine should be given prophylactically.

Early trials addressing the treatment of delayed emesis with the single-agent serotonin antagonist ondansetron were discouraging and labeled the serotonin antagonists as having low activity. Two randomized studies, one with ondansetron and one with granisetron, indicated efficacy of the serotonin antagonists for delayed emesis in patients receiving chemotherapy of intermediate emetogenicity (22,23). New antiemetic agents that are beneficial in both the prevention and treatment of delayed emesis have been recently identified and approved for use. These agents are discussed later in the section New Agents.

Preventive therapy is imperative for patients to achieve the best outcome. The risk defined for acute emesis is a good predictor of delayed emesis. Patients who do not receive preventive therapy have a 70–90% incidence of delayed emesis with high-risk agents and a 30–60% risk with moderate-risk agents.

Anticipatory emesis (Table 13.2) is a learned or conditioned response that typically occurs before, during, or after the administration of chemotherapy. In this instance, patients may be responding to a variety of stimuli that in most instances were associated with a prior experience when there was inadequate control of emesis. The corresponding psychological mechanism for anticipatory emesis is unknown and is secondary to the direct administration of the chemotherapy agent itself. Therefore, patients must be given the opportunity to receive the optimal antiemetic regimen with their initial course of chemotherapy to prevent acute and delayed emesis, and, consequently, anticipatory emesis. Treatment for the occurrence of anticipatory emesis may include the use of benzodiazepines in addition to antiemetics before and during chemotherapy. Relaxation techniques, guided visual imagery, desensitization, and hypnosis techniques may also be effective (24–27).

In addition to hypnosis, relaxation, imagery, and desensitization, acupuncture is a nonmedicinal complementary therapy that has been shown to have benefits in chemotherapy-related nausea and vomiting. An initial trial was done with 130 patients who had a history of distressing emesis in prior chemotherapeutic regimens. Emesis was reduced in 97% of the subjects (28). A National Institutes of Health consensus trial concluded that acupuncture was effective in reducing chemotherapy-induced emesis; however, placebo effect was a concern (29). A subsequent trial that addressed the issue of placebo effect was done with women with breast cancer receiving high-dose cyclophosphamide, cisplatin, and carmustine. One hundred four women were randomly assigned to receive no needling, minimal needling at control points with mock electrostimulation, or classic antiemetic electroacupuncture once daily for 5 days. The number of emesis episodes were lower in the first 5 days for those receiving electroacupuncture compared with those receiving minimal needling at control points or no needling ($p < .001$). The effect appeared to be of limited duration in that there were no significant differences during the 9-day follow-up (30). Clearly the data are promising; however, additional research is needed in this area.

CONTROL OF EMESIS AND RISK FACTORS

The methodology used in antiemetic trials has identified useful patient characteristics and prognostic factors that may affect antiemetic control. These indicators become important for tailoring antiemetic regimens as well as designing antiemetic trials. Careful studies have identified patient-related risk factors to include prior experience with chemotherapy, alcohol intake history, age, and gender as influencing patient outcomes.

A patient's prior exposure to chemotherapy very often determines success or failure in controlling emesis with future treatment courses. As mentioned earlier in the section Emetic Syndromes, the administration of the appropriate antiemetic during the initial course of chemotherapy can very often eliminate the development of anticipatory emesis, in addition to decreasing the severity of delayed emesis.

Chronic and heavy alcohol usage, defined as more than 100 g of alcohol or five mixed drinks per day, whether in the past or currently, has been shown to positively affect the control of emesis (31,32). Age as a prognostic factor cannot predict patient response to antiemetic therapy. It is, however, an important factor in determining the potential for the occurrence of acute dystonic reactions. Patients aged 30 years or younger are more prone to experience the acute dystonic reactions associated with the dopamine receptor–blocking agents such as phenothiazines, butyrophenones, and substituted benzamides. These side effects are usually characterized by trismus or torticollis. It is also important to remember that within this population of patients, chemotherapy agents that might necessitate antiemetics are often given over several consecutive days, increasing the possibility of the occurrence of acute dystonic reactions (32). A distinct advantage of the 5-HT$_3$ antiemetic agents is that they do not cause acute dystonic reactions, making them an especially beneficial treatment option for children and younger adults.

It has been difficult to explain the rationale for poorer control of emesis in women receiving treatment for various malignancies. A possible explanation may be that women characteristically receive chemotherapeutic regimens that contain highly emetogenic agents such as cisplatin and cyclophosphamide, usually given in combination, and are less likely than men to have a history of a high alcohol intake.

Other contributing factors that may affect the control of emesis include a heightened level of anxiety during the chemotherapy infusion, being prone to motion sickness, and having had severe emesis during pregnancy (33) (Table 13.3).

TABLE 13.3

FACTORS AFFECTING THE CONTROL AND INCIDENCE OF NAUSEA AND VOMITING AFTER CHEMOTHERAPY

PATIENT-SPECIFIC FACTORS
  Previous emesis experience with chemotherapy
  Alcohol intake
  Age
  Gender
  Anxiety
  Expectation of severe side effects
  Roommate experiencing nausea and vomiting
  Motivation level
  Performance status
  Food intake before chemotherapy
  Amount of sleep before chemotherapy
  Severe emesis during pregnancy
  Motion sickness

TREATMENT-SPECIFIC FACTORS
  Drug
  Dose
  Infusion rate

From Berger AM, Clark-Snow RA. Adverse effects of treatment. In: DeVita VT Jr, Hellman S, Rosenberg SA, eds. *Cancer: principles and practice of oncology*, 6th ed. Philadelphia, PA: Lippincott Williams & Wilkins, 2001, with permission.

ANTIEMETIC AGENTS

Most Active Agents

As outlined earlier in the section Pathophysiology of Nausea and Vomiting, antagonism of the 5-HT$_3$ receptor is an important approach to controlling chemotherapy-induced emesis. Several agents are available that exert their efficacy in this manner. Metoclopramide, previously thought to block emesis by antagonism of a dopamine receptor (D$_2$), probably works primarily through the 5-HT$_3$ pathway at higher doses. This explains why higher doses of metoclopramide are more effective. However, metoclopramide is not selective for the 5-HT$_3$ pathway, and development of highly selective antagonists of the 5-HT$_3$ receptor allowed for good antiemetic effect with a lower side effect profile.

Several selective 5-HT$_3$ antagonists are commercially available in many countries: dolasetron, granisetron, ondansetron, and tropisetron. Other similar agents are available in individual countries or are under investigation. Multiple large, randomized clinical trials have shown no clinically significant difference among these drugs when used appropriately (34–36). Further studies have demonstrated that a single oral dose of a 5-HT$_3$ receptor antagonist before chemotherapy has efficacy equivalent to a multiple-dosing regimen (37–39).

Controversy remains concerning the optimal dose of the serotonin antagonists. It appears that maximal benefit occurs once all relevant receptors are saturated. No matter what the emetic source, if best results are to be achieved, an adequate dose should be given. Higher doses are not advantageous once all receptors have been saturated (40,41). In that these are very safe and well-tolerated agents, it has been difficult to define the best dose for regimens, and different doses have been mandated in different countries. As a general rule, the lowest adequately tested dose should be assumed to be the best dose in all settings.

Although some debate persists concerning the best dose of ondansetron, most trials have indicated that the lower dose (8 mg) is as effective as the higher and far more expensive dose of 32 mg (42,43). The latter dose was superior in only one trial and was troubled by a high inadequate treatment rate, indicating a poorly conducted trial. The lower granisetron dose of 0.01 mg per kg is as effective in all circumstances as four times the dose (44). The same recommendations continue for single-agent or combination use.

The side effect profile of the 5-HT$_3$ antagonists provides an advantage over such effective antiemetics as metoclopramide. Central nervous system effects, extrapyramidal reactions, and sedation are not observed with serotonin antagonists; this is particularly beneficial in younger patients. Common side effects include mild headaches usually not requiring treatment, transient transaminase elevations, and mild constipation with some agents.

As indicated, the antiemetic activity of metoclopramide is likely as a serotonin antagonist, although it has substantial dopamine antagonist action as well. This latter mechanism explains the potential for extrapyramidal reactions. Studies have shown that higher doses are more effective. A dose of 3 mg per kg given every 2 hours for two doses in combination with a corticosteroid has been found to be effective (45).

Corticosteroids are valuable antiemetics. Dexamethasone is the most widely studied of all these agents in oral and parenteral preparations and in most countries is very inexpensive. Although the best dose has not been established, it appears that a single dose of 10–20 mg is adequate. Caution must be used when treating patients with diabetes or others with a poor tolerance for corticosteroids. However, the short recommended course makes these agents very safe and easy to use. In preventing delayed emesis, adequate doses of corticosteroids are viewed as advantageous when combined with metoclopramide.

Efficacy for corticosteroids has been clearly defined for cisplatin-containing regimens as well as other types of chemotherapy with lesser emetic potential. The addition of a corticosteroid to 5-HT$_3$ antagonists significantly improves antiemetic efficacy with each of the agents. This is seen with cisplatin as well as with such drugs as anthracyclines, cyclophosphamide, and carboplatin. Therefore a corticosteroid should be added whenever the emetic source is thought to warrant a serotonin antagonist unless a clearly documented reason for not using a corticosteroid in that patient has been demonstrated.

Antiemetics of Lower Activity

Older agents such as phenothiazines, butyrophenones, and cannabinoids, all have some degree of antiemetic efficacy. In general, this efficacy is substantially lower than that seen with the serotonin antagonists (including high-dose metoclopramide), and the side effects are greater. When given intravenously, phenothiazines appear to be more active than when given by other routes but are associated with hypotension (especially orthostatic), which can be severe. Therefore, these agents are not highly recommended. Oral forms of all three of these agents exhibit only modest activity and are of similarly low efficacy.

Several cannabinoids have been tested in chemotherapy-induced emesis and are of both historical and lay press interest. Semisynthetic agents, such as nabilone and levonantradol; tetrahydrocannabinol (THC) (or 9-THC), the active agent in marijuana; and inhaled marijuana, all appear to be of low and equal efficacy, with frequent autonomic side effects.

These toxicities include dry mouth, hypotension, and dizziness. Dronabinol may be useful as an adjuvant to other antiemetics.

Antianxiety agents, such as the benzodiazepine lorazepam, have little efficacy as single agents in carefully conducted trials. However, they function well against anxiety in the emotionally charged atmosphere of receiving chemotherapy, although they add only a minor antiemetic effect to more active agents. They should be regarded as adjuncts to antiemetics and, in that role, can be useful for many patients. Recommended doses range from 0.5–1.5 mg. It is not clear that there is any advantage in giving these agents parenterally rather than orally when given with the most effective antiemetics. In addition, these drugs may be useful when given to patients with anticipatory emesis, starting 1 or more days before the next chemotherapy dosing. Side effects mainly concern sedation, which can be marked in some patients, especially if the drug is given intravenously.

NEW AGENTS

Although substantial progress has been made in the efforts to prevent and control chemotherapy-induced emesis, it remains a significant problem, especially for patients experiencing delayed emesis and for patients undergoing high-dose chemotherapy and multiple cycles of chemotherapy. Investigators have identified substance P, an 11–amino acid neuropeptide found in the GI tract and central nervous system that has been shown to elicit vomiting in animal models. Substance P exerts its effects by binding to a specific neuroreceptor, NK1. A number of compounds that selectively block the NK1 receptor have been identified (46). These NK1 antagonists demonstrate a wide spectrum of clinical activity and have been possibly implicated in depression, bladder irritability, inflammatory bowel disease, asthma, and functional GI diseases. They also demonstrate a wide spectrum of antiemetic activity against numerous emetic stimuli.

In two, large, randomized, double-blind clinical trials, the combination of aprepitant (Emend), an NK1 antagonist administered with a 5-HT$_3$ antagonist and a corticosteroid, was compared with standard therapy (5-HT$_3$ plus a steroid) and was administered to patients receiving high-dose cisplatin (47–49). Antiemetic activity was evaluated during the acute and delayed phase. In both studies, a statistically significant higher proportion of patients receiving the aprepitant

---

TABLE 13.4

EMETIC POTENTIAL OF CHEMOTHERAPEUTIC AGENTS

Level 1 (<10% frequency)
  Androgens
  Bleomycin
  Busulfan (oral <4 mg/kg/d)
  Chlorambucil
  Cladribine
  Corticosteroids
  Fludarabine
  Hydroxyurea
  Interferon
  Melphalan (oral)
  Mercaptopurine
  Methotrexate (<50 mg/m^2)
  Thioguanine (oral)
  Tretinoin
  Vinblastine
  Vincristine
  Vinorelbine
Level 2 (10–30% frequency)
  Asparaginase
  Cytarabine (<1 g/m^2)
  Docetaxel
  Doxorubicin hydrochloride (<20 mg/m^2)
  Etoposide
  Fluorouracil (<1000 mg/m^2)
  Gemcitabine
  Methotrexate (>50 to <250 mg/m^2)
  Mitomycin
  Paclitaxel
  Teniposide
  Thiotepa
  Topotecan
Level 3 (30–60% frequency)
  Aldesleukin
  Cyclophosphamide (intravenous <750 mg/m^2)

Dactinomycin (<1.5 mg/m^2)
Doxorubicin hydrochloride (20–60 mg/m^2)
Epirubicin hydrochloride (<90 mg/m^2)
Hycamtin
Idarubicin
Ifosfamide
Methenamine (oral)
Methotrexate (250–1000 mg/m^2)
Mitoxantrone (<15 mg/m^2)
Level 4 (60–90% frequency)
  Carboplatin
  Carmustine (<250 mg/m^2)
  Cisplatin (<50 mg/m^2)
  Cyclophosphamide (>750 to <1500 mg/m^2)
  Cytarabine (>1 g/m^2)
  Dactinomycin (>1.5 mg/m^2)
  Doxorubicin hydrochloride (>60 mg/m^2)
  Irinotecan
  Melphalan (intravenous)
  Methotrexate (>1000 mg/m^2)
  Mitoxantrone (15 mg/m^2)
  Procarbazine (oral)
Level 5 (>90% frequency)
  Carmustine (>250 mg/m^2)
  Cisplatin (>50 mg/m^2)
  Cyclophosphamide (>1500 mg/m^2)
  Dacarbazine (>500 mg/m^2)
  Lomustine (60 mg/m^2)
  Mechlorethamine
  Pentostatin
  Streptozocin

Adapted from Hesketh P, Kris M, Grunberg SM, et al. Proposal for classifying the acute emetogenicity of cancer chemotherapy. *J Clin Oncol* 1997;15:103, with permission; and American Society of Health-System Pharmacists. Therapeutic guidelines on the pharmacological management of nausea and vomiting in adult and pediatric patients receiving chemotherapy or radiation therapy or undergoing surgery. *Am J Health Syst Pharm* 1999;56:729, with permission.

regimen had a complete response (no vomiting or rescue therapy) when compared with standard therapy. The most commonly observed side effects with this agent are mild and include fatigue, hiccups, constipation, anorexia, and headache.

Aprepitant is the first NK1 receptor antagonist of this class to be approved for the prevention of acute and delayed nausea and vomiting with initial and repeat courses of highly emetogenic chemotherapy when given in combination with a 5-HT$_3$-receptor antagonist and a corticosteroid as part of a 4-day regimen (49).

Aprepitant has been classified as a moderate CYP3A4 inhibitor, and clinicians have been advised to observe caution in those patients receiving concomitant medicines, including chemotherapy that is primarily metabolized through the CYP-450 isoenzyme (CYP3A4), which may result in a potential drug interaction (49).

Palonosetron (Aloxi) is a potent, new, second-generation 5-HT$_3$ antagonist with strong binding affinity and an extended plasma half-life of approximately 40 hours. It has demonstrated efficacy in preventing CINV associated with initial and repeat courses of moderately and highly emetogenic chemotherapy, as well as delayed nausea and vomiting resulting from initial and repeat courses of moderately emetogenic chemotherapy (50). In three, large, phase III clinical trials (51,52), when compared with currently available 5-HT$_3$-receptor antagonists, palonosetron provided patients with improved control during the acute and delayed phases. The side effects observed were similar in severity and frequency as the comparator agents. The most common side effects related to palonosetron were headache and constipation. This agent is currently the only approved antiemetic for the prevention of acute and delayed CINV for moderately emetogenic chemotherapy (53).

TREATMENT OPTIONS BASED ON EMESIS CATEGORY

To appropriately prevent acute and delayed emesis, regimens for both syndromes should be well thought out and based on the emesis risk of the chemotherapy administered. There are several different professional organizations responsible for the development of antiemetic guidelines, including the American Society of Clinical Oncology, the American Society of Health-System Pharmacists, the Multinational Association for Supportive Care in Cancer, and the National Comprehensive Cancer Network (34–36,54).

The actual risk assigned to each chemotherapy agent has been classified into four categories: high, moderate, low, and minimal. Nearly all patients who receive representative agents such as cisplatin, dacarbazine, and nitrogen mustard from the high-risk group experience emesis if preventive antiemetics are not given. Clinical outcomes are significantly improved with the addition of a corticosteroid such as dexamethasone (35,55) (Tables 13.4 and 13.5).

Therefore, for highly emetogenic chemotherapy a combination of 5-HT$_3$-receptor antagonist plus dexamethasone, plus an NK1 antagonist is recommended (Table 13.6). The new serotonin antagonist palonosetron is recommended for acute and delayed protection for the moderately emetogenic chemotherapeutic regimen (Table 13.7).

Guiding principles for the control of acute emesis include the following (56):

1. Use the lowest fully effective dose.
2. Corticosteroids should be added to the regimen containing 5-HT$_3$ antagonists.
3. Oral antiemetics have equivalent efficacy to the intravenous formulation.

TABLE 13.5

RULES FOR IDENTIFYING THE EMETOGENICITY OF COMBINATION CHEMOTHERAPY

The most highly emetogenic agent in the chemotherapeutic combination must first be identified
Level 1 chemotherapeutic agents do not contribute to the emetogenicity of the regimen
Adding one or more Level 2 chemotherapeutic agents increases the emetogenicity of the combination by one level greater than the most emetogenic agent in the combination
Adding Level 3 and 4 agents increases the emetogenicity of the combination by one level per agent

Adapted from Hesketh P, Kris M, Grunberg SM, et al. Proposal for classifying the acute emetogenicity of cancer chemotherapy. *J Clin Oncol* 1997;15:103, with permission; and American Society of Health-System Pharmacists. Therapeutic guidelines on the pharmacological management of nausea and vomiting in adult and pediatric patients receiving chemotherapy or radiation therapy or undergoing surgery. *Am J Health Syst Pharm* 1999;56:729, with permission.

---

4. There is equivalence among the currently available 5-HT$_3$ antagonists other than palonosetron, which is U.S. Food and Drug Administration (FDA) approved for acute and delayed CINV for moderately emetogenic chemotherapy.
5. NK1 antagonists should be added to the 5-HT$_3$ antagonist and dexamethasone for highly emetogenic chemotherapy and considered for moderately emetogenic chemotherapy.

Patients for whom chemotherapy of low risk of emesis has been ordered, benefit from receiving single-agent therapy such as dexamethasone; however, dopamine antagonists, butyrophenones, and phenothiazines may also be considered. No preventive treatment is recommended for minimally emetic chemotherapy, but clinicians are advised to provide patients with a prescription for an antiemetic to be taken on an as-needed basis (56).

RADIATION-INDUCED NAUSEA AND VOMITING

The etiology of radiation-induced emesis, like chemotherapy-induced emesis, is not completely understood. However, it is clear that it is a complex, multifactorial event. The incidence, severity, and onset of radiation-induced emesis appear to be related to the size of the radiation field, the dose per fraction, and the site of irradiation. Radiation-induced emesis occurs acutely in more than 90% of patients who receive total body irradiation for bone marrow transplantation, within 30–60 minutes in more than 80% of patients who receive single high-dose or large-field hemibody irradiation (>500 cGy), and within 2–3 weeks in approximately 50% of patients who receive conventional fractionated radiotherapy (200 cGy per fraction) to the upper abdomen (57). Radiation-induced emesis also occurs in those patients who receive radiosurgery to the area postrema in excess of 350–400 cGy in a single dose. The emesis usually occurs between 1 and 12 hours after the radiosurgery.

The exact mechanism of radiation-induced emesis remains unclear. However, as with chemotherapy-induced emesis, it is thought that it most likely is due to a peripheral mechanism in the GI tract or a central mechanism involving the CTZ. It has

TABLE 13.6

CHEMOTHERAPY-INDUCED NAUSEA AND VOMITING PREVENTION GUIDELINES FOR HIGHLY (LEVEL 5) EMETOGENIC DRUGS[a]

	DAY 1
NK1 and	Aprepitant 125 mg p.o. q.d.
Steroid	Dexamethasone 12 mg p.o. or i.v. q.d. or methylprednisolone 125 mg i.v. q.d.
and 5-HT$_3$ antagonist	Palonosetron 0.25 mg i.v. q.d. (recommended on day 1; due to long half-life no follow-up dose necessary) or ondansetron 16–24 mg p.o. q.d. or ondansetron 8 mg i.v. (maximum 32 mg) i.v. or granisetron 2 mg p.o. q.d. or 1 mg p.o. b.i.d. or granisetron 0.01 mg/kg (maximum 1 mg) i.v. q.d. or dolasetron 100 mg p.o. q.d. or dolasetron 1.8 mg/kg i.v. q.d. or 100 mg i.v. q.d.
and Benz	Lorazepam 0.5–2 mg p.o., i.v. or s.l. q6h sch
	DAY 2–4
NK1 and	Aprepitant 80 mg p.o. q.d. (Day 2 and Day 3)
steroid	Dexamethasone 8 mg p.o. or i.v. q.d. or methylprednisolone 125 mg i.v. q.d.
or 5-HT$_3$ antagonist	Ondansetron 8 mg p.o. or i.v. q.d. or granisetron 2 mg p.o. q.d. or 1 mg p.o. b.i.d. or granisetron 0.01 mg/kg (maximum 1 mg) i.v. q.d. or dolasetron 100 mg p.o. q.d. or dolasetron 1.8 mg/kg i.v. q.d. or 100 mg i.v. q.d.
and Benz	Lorazepam 0.5–2 mg p.o., i.v. or s.l. q6h sch

[a]■ Order of medication not meant to indicate preference
■ Use lowest efficacious dose
■ Be mindful of potential side effects
■ Day 1 medications are to be given prechemotherapy
■ When fractionated doses of Level 3–5 chemotherapy are given or there is a high risk of delayed CINV, daily dexamethasone, daily 5-HT$_3$ (or a one-time dose of palonosetron for 3-day chemotherapeutic regimen), and daily aprepitant (up to 3–5 days) should be given

been proposed that several substances, including dopamine, catecholamines, and prostaglandins, are released and stimulate afferent visceral fibers, an action that then initiates sensory signals to the CTZ. As a result of both preclinical and clinical studies with serotonin antagonists, it has been suggested that serotonin may be released from enterochromaffin cells of the GI tract and may mediate emesis through mechanisms involving the 5-HT$_3$ receptors, visceral afferent fibers, and the CTZ. This mechanism is most likely involved when radiation is applied to the upper abdomen, hemibody, or total body. Radiosurgery to the area postrema most likely induces emesis from the release of serotonin in the CTZ (58).

Clinical studies in the past using metoclopramide, nabilone (cannabinoid derivative), and chlorpromazine in the treatment of radiation-induced emesis revealed a response of 50–58% (59,60). In a nonplacebo trial with domperidone, a dopamine antagonist, a response of 82% was reported (61). A nonrandomized trial comparing ondansetron with other antiemetics reported response rates of 100% for ondansetron versus 43% for other antiemetics and 19% for no antiemetic treatment for patients who received middle- to upper-hemibody irradiation (57). A randomized study by Priestman et al. (62) of patients who received radiotherapy to the abdomen, pelvis, and thoracolumbar spine reported response rates of 45% for

TABLE 13.7

CHEMOTHERAPY-INDUCED NAUSEA AND VOMITING PREVENTION GUIDELINES FOR MODERATELY (LEVEL 3–4) EMETOGENIC DRUGS[a]

	DAY 1
Steroid	Dexamethasone 12 mg p.o. or i.v. q.d.
	or
	methylprednisolone 125 mg i.v. q.d.
and	
5-HT$_3$ antagonist	Palonosetron 0.25 mg i.v. (preferred on day 1; due to long half-life no follow-up dose necessary)
	or
	ondansetron 16–24 mg p.o.
	or
	ondansetron 8 mg (maximum 32 mg) i.v. q.d.
	or
	granisetron 1–2 mg p.o. or 1 mg p.o. b.i.d.
	or
	granisetron 0.01 mg/kg (maximum 1 mg) i.v. q.d.
	or
	dolasetron 100 mg p.o.
	or
	dolasetron 1.8 mg/kg i.v. or 100 mg i.v. q.d.
and	
Benz	Lorazepam 0.5–2 mg p.o., i.v., or s.l. p.o. q6h sch
and maybe	
NK1	Aprepitant 125 mg p.o. **if** using carboplatin, cyclophosphamide, doxorubicin, epirubicin, ifosfamide, irinotecan, or methotrexate
	DAY 2–4
Steroid	Dexamethasone 8 mg p.o. or i.v. q.d.
	or
	dexamethasone 4 mg p.o. b.i.d.
	or
	methylprednisolone 125 mg i.v. q.d.
or	
5-HT$_3$ antagonist	Ondansetron 8 mg p.o. b.i.d. or 16 mg p.o. q.d.
	or
	ondansetron 8 mg (maximum 32 mg) i.v. q.d.
	or
	granisetron 1–2 mg p.o. q.d. or 1 mg p.o. b.i.d.
	or
	granisetron 0.01 mg/kg (maximum 1 mg) i.v. q.d.
	or
	dolasetron 100 mg p.o. q.d.
	or
	dolasetron 1.8 mg/kg i.v. or 100 mg i.v. q.d.
	or
	metoclopramide 0.5 mg/kg p.o. or i.v. q6h sch ± diphenhydramine 25–50 mg p.o. or i.v. q4–6h p.r.n.
	or
	metoclopramide 20 mg p.o. q6h sch ± diphenhydramine 25–50 mg p.o. or i.v. q4–6h p.r.n.
or	
NK1	Aprepitant 80 mg p.o. (continued on day 2–3 is started day 1) and dexamethasone 8 mg p.o. or i.v. q.d.
±	
Benz	Lorazepam 0.5–2 mg p.o., i.v. or s.l. q6h sch

[a] ■ Order of medication not meant to indicate preference
■ Use lowest efficacious dose
■ Be mindful of potential side effects
■ Day 1 medications are to be given prechemotherapy
■ When fractionated doses of Level 3–5 chemotherapy are given or there is a high risk of delayed CINV, daily dexamethasone, daily 5-HT$_3$ (or a one-time dose of palonosetron for 3-day chemotherapeutic regimen), and daily aprepitant (up to 3–5 days) should be given

metoclopramide versus 97% for ondansetron. A randomized, double-blind, placebo-controlled evaluation revealed oral ondansetron to be an effective therapy for the prevention of emesis induced by total body irradiation (63). Ondansetron has been reported to be effective in radiotherapy-induced emesis in children (64) as well as for patients who receive radiosurgery to the area postrema (58).

Data are available from two double-blind, randomized studies in the use of oral granisetron, 2 mg once daily, in radiation-induced nausea and vomiting. In a study involving patients undergoing fractionated upper-abdominal radiation, patients who received oral granisetron had a significantly longer median time to first emesis than did those who received placebo (35 vs. 9 days, respectively) and a longer median time to first nausea (11 days vs. 1 day, respectively) (65). In another study of patients undergoing total body irradiation, patients treated with oral granisetron had significantly greater control compared with the historical control group over the entire 4-day treatment period (22 vs. 0%, respectively) (66).

Fauser et al. (67) reported on the use of oral dolasetron for the control of emesis during total body irradiation and high-dose cyclophosphamide in patients undergoing allogeneic bone marrow transplantation. Approximately two thirds of the patients who received dolasetron during the irradiation and chemotherapy administration period had two or fewer episodes of vomiting, and nausea was reported as mild. This trial concluded that oral dolasetron was effective and safe for the prevention of nausea and vomiting during total body irradiation.

NAUSEA AND VOMITING SECONDARY TO COMORBID CONDITIONS

A number of comorbid conditions also may lead to nausea and vomiting, although most patients with cancer develop nausea and vomiting as a result of chemotherapy or radiotherapy. Because the mechanism of the nausea and vomiting secondary to comorbid conditions is not usually well understood, it is difficult to know which antiemetics may be helpful. Controlled-release metoclopramide has been shown to be safe and effective in managing chronic nausea in patients with advanced cancer.

IMPROVING ANTIEMETIC CONTROL

The coordination of supportive care of patients with cancer involves the multidisciplinary participation of physicians, nurses, pharmacists, dietitian specialists, and, most important, patients and their families. The last two decades have seen dramatic improvements in the prevention and treatment of the side effects of cancer therapy and symptom management. With the introduction of the serotonin antagonist antiemetics and now with the more recent addition of palonosetron, a more potent second-generation serotonin antagonist, as well as aprepitant, the new NK1 antagonist, clinicians are able to provide patients with state-of-the-art therapy to prevent chemotherapy-induced emesis. This can be accomplished through the development of practical and user-friendly guidelines that incorporate precise treatment principles. Until all patients are able to achieve complete control of nausea and emesis from chemotherapy and other specific cancer treatments, investigations and clinical trials of new agents with new mechanisms of action are necessary.

References

1. Coates A, Abraham S, Kaye SB, et al. On the receiving end. Patients' perceptions of the side-effects of cancer chemotherapy. *Eur J Clin Oncol* 1983;19:203.
2. Griffin AM, Butow PN, Coates AS, et al. On the receiving end: patients' perceptions of the side-effects of cancer chemotherapy. *Ann Oncol* 1996;7:189.
3. Grunberg SM, Hansen M, Deuson R, Mavros P. Incidence and impact of nausea/vomiting with modern antiemetics: perception vs. reality (Abstract). *Proceedings of the American Society Clinical Oncology Meeting.* Orlando, FL, 2002.
4. Young RW. Mechanisms and treatment of radiation-induced nausea and vomiting. In: Davis CJ, Lakke-Bakaar GV, Graham-Smith DG, eds. *Nausea and vomiting: mechanisms and treatment.* Berlin, Germany: Springer-Verlag, 1986:94.
5. Fortner CL, Finley RS, Grove WR. Combination antiemetic therapy in the control of chemotherapy-induced drug emetogenic potential emesis. *Drug Intell Clin Pharm* 1985;19:21. PubMed
6. Lissoni P, Barni S, Crispino S, et al. Synthetic enkephalin analog in the treatment of cancer chemotherapy-induced vomiting. *Cancer Treat Rep* 1987;71:6665.
7. Edwards C, Carmichael J, Bayliss P, et al. Arginine vasopressin—a mediator of chemotherapy-induced emesis? *Br J Cancer* 1989;59:467.
8. Miner WD, Sanger GJ, Turner DH. Comparison of the effect of BRL 24924, metoclopramide and domperidone on cisplatin-induced emesis in the ferret. *Br J Pharmacol* 1986;88:374.
9. Costall B, Domeney AM, Nylor RJ, et al. 5-Hydroxytryptamine M-receptor antagonism to prevent cisplatin-induced emesis. *Neuropharmacology* 1986;25:959.
10. Cubeddu L, Hoffman I, Fuenmayor N, et al. Efficacy of ondansetron (GR 38032F) and the role of serotonin in cisplatin-induced nausea and vomiting. *N Engl J Med* 1990;322:810.
11. Cubeddu L, Hoffman I, Fuenmayor N, et al. Antagonism of serotonin S3 receptors with ondansetron prevents nausea and emesis induced by cyclophosphamide-containing chemotherapy regimens. *J Clin Oncol* 1990;8:1721.
12. Bonneterre J, Chevallier B, Metz R, et al. A randomized double-blind comparison of ondansetron and metoclopramide in the prophylaxis of emesis induced by cyclophosphamide, fluorouracil, and doxorubicin or epirubicin chemotherapy. *J Clin Oncol* 1990;8:1063.
13. Hargreaves R. Imaging substance P receptors (NK1) in the living human brain using positron emission tomography. *J Clin Psychiatry* 2002;63(Suppl 11):18.
14. Hesketh PJ, Van Belle S, Aapro M, et al. Differential involvement of neurotransmitters through the time course of cisplatin-induced emesis as revealed by therapy with specific receptor antagonists. *Eur J Cancer* 2003;39:1074.
15. Sipiora ML, Murtaugh MA, Gregpire MB, et al. Bitter taste perception and severe vomiting during pregnancy. *Physiol Behav* 2000;69:259.
16. Fetting JH, Wilcox PM, Sheidler VR, et al. Tastes associated with parenteral chemotherapy for breast cancer. *Cancer Treat Rep* 1985;69:1249.
17. Roscoe JA, Morrow GR, Hickoj JT, et al. Nausea and vomiting remain a significant clinical problem: trends over time in controlling chemotherapy-induced nausea and vomiting in 1413 patients treated in community clinical practices. *J Pain Manage* 2000;20:113.
18. Hesketh PJ. Understanding the pathobiology of chemotherapy-induced nausea and vomiting. *Oncology* 2004;18(10):9–14.
19. Tremblay PB, Kaiser R, Sezer O, et al. Variations in the 5-hydroxytryptamine type 3B receptor gene as predictors of the efficacy of antiemetic treatment in cancer patients. *J Clin Oncol* 2003;21:2147–2155.
20. Kaiser R, Sezer O, Papies A, et al. Patient-tailored antiemetic treatment with 5-hydroxytryptamine type 3 receptor antagonists according to cytochrome P-450 2D6 genotypes. *J Clin Oncol* 2002;20:2805–2811.
21. Kris MG, Gralla RJ, Clark RA, et al. Incidence, course, and severity of delayed nausea and vomiting following the administration of high-dose cisplatin. *J Clin Oncol* 1985;3:1379.
22. Kaizer L, Warr D, Hoskins P, et al. Effect of schedule and maintenance on the antiemetic efficacy of ondansetron combined with dexamethasone in acute and delayed nausea and emesis in patients receiving moderately emetogenic chemotherapy: a phase III trial by the National Cancer Institute of Canada Clinical Trials Group. *J Clin Oncol* 1994;12:1050.
23. Guillem V, Carrato A, Rifa J, et al. High efficacy of oral granisetron in the total control of cyclophosphamide-induced prolonged emesis (Abstract). *Proc Am Soc Clin Oncol* 1998;17:46a.
24. Morrow GR, Morrell C. Behavioral treatment for the anticipatory nausea and vomiting induced by cancer chemotherapy. *N Engl J Med* 1982;307:1476.
25. Burish TG, Jenkins RA. Effectiveness of biofeedback and relaxation training in reducing the side effects of chemotherapy. *Health Psychol* 1992;11:17.
26. Redd WH, Montgomery GH, DuHamel KN. Behavioral intervention for cancer treatment side effects. *J Natl Cancer Inst* 2001;93:810.
27. Genius ML. The use of hypnosis in helping cancer patients control anxiety, pain and emesis: a review of empirical studies. *Am J Clin Hypn* 1995;37:316.

28. Dundee JW, Ghaly RG, Fitzpatrick NT, et al. Acupuncture prophylaxis of cancer chemotherapy-induced sickness. *J R Soc Med* 1989;82:268.

29. NIH Consensus Conference. Acupuncture. *JAMA* 1998;280:1518.

30. Shen J, Wenger N, Glaspy J, et al. Electroacupuncture for control of myeloablative chemotherapy-induced emesis: a randomized controlled trial. *JAMA* 2000;284:2755.

31. D'Acquisto RW, Tyson LB, Gralla RJ, et al. Antiemetic trials to control delayed vomiting following high-dose cisplatin. *Proc Am Soc Clin Oncol* 1986;5:257.

32. Allen JC, Gralla RJ, Reilly L, et al. Metoclopramide dose-related toxicity and preliminary antiemetic studies in children receiving cancer chemotherapy. *J Clin Oncol* 1985;3:1136.

33. Guillem V, Avanda E, Carrato A, et al. Previous history of emesis during pregnancy and motion sickness as risk factors for chemotherapy-induced emesis (Abstract). *J Clin Oncol* 1999;2280(18):590a.

34. ASHP. Therapeutic guidelines on the pharmacologic management of nausea and vomiting in adult and pediatric patients receiving chemotherapy or radiation therapy or undergoing surgery. *Am J Health Syst Pharm* 1999;56:729.

35. Gralla RJ, Osoba D, Kris MG, et al. Recommendations for the use of antiemetics: evidence-based, clinical practice guidelines. *J Clin Oncol* 1999;17:2971.

36. Antiemesis Practice Guidelines Panel. NCCN antiemetics practice guidelines. NCCN Proceedings. *Oncology* 1997;11:57.

37. Lofters WS, Pater JL, Zee B, et al. Phase III double-blind comparison of dolasetron mesylate and ondansetron and an evaluation of the additive role of dexamethasone in the prevention of acute and delayed nausea and vomiting due to moderately emetogenic chemotherapy. *J Clin Oncol* 1997;15:2966.

38. Audhuy B, Cappelere P, Martin M, et al. A double-blind randomized comparison of the antiemetic efficacy of two intravenous doses of dolasetron mesylate and granisetron in patients receiving high dose cisplatin chemotherapy. *Eur J Cancer* 1996;32A:807.

39. Mantovani G, Maccio A, Bianchi A, et al. Comparison of granisetron, ondansetron and tropisetron in the prophylaxis of acute nausea and vomiting induced by cisplatin for the treatment of head and neck cancer: a randomized controlled trial. *Cancer* 1996;77:941.

40. Kris MG, Gralla RJ, Clark RA, et al. Phase II trials of the serotonin antagonist GR38032F for the control of vomiting caused by cisplatin. *J Natl Cancer Inst* 1989;81:42.

41. Kris MG, Gralla RJ, Clark RA, et al. Dose ranging evaluation of the serotonin antagonist BR-C507/75 (GR38032F) when used as an antiemetic in patients receiving cancer chemotherapy. *J Clin Oncol* 1988;6:659.

42. Seynaeve C, Schuller J, Buser K, et al. Comparison of the anti-emetic efficacy of different doses of ondansetron given as either a continuous infusion or a single IV dose, in acute cisplatin-induced emesis. A multicentre, double-blind, randomized parallel group study. *Br J Cancer* 1992;66:192.

43. Ruff P, Paska W, Goedhals L, et al. Ondansetron compared with granisetron in the prophylaxis of cisplatin-induced emesis: a multicenter double-blind, randomized, parallel group study. *Oncology* 1994;5:113.

44. Navari R, Gandara D, Hesketh P, et al. Comparative clinical trial of granisetron and ondansetron in the prophylaxis of cisplatin-induced emesis. *J Clin Oncol* 1995;13:1242.

45. SKris MG, Gralla RJ, Tyson LB, et al. Improved control of cisplatin-induced emesis with high dose metoclopramide and with combination of metoclopramide, dexamethasone and diphenhydramine. Results of consecutive trials in 255 patients. *Cancer* 1985;55:527.

46. Campos D, Rodrigues Pereira J, Reinhardt R, et al. Prevention of cisplatin-induced emesis by the oral neurokinin-1 antagonist, MK-869, in combination with granisetron and dexamethasone or with dexamethasone alone. *J Clin Oncol* 2002;19:1759.

47. Hesketh PJ, Grunberg SM, Gralla RJ, et al. The oral neurokinin-1 antagonist aprepitant for the prevention of chemotherapy-induced nausea and vomiting: a multinational, randomized, double blind, placebo-controlled trial in patients receiving high-dose cisplatin—the Aprepitant Protocol 052 Study Group. *J Clin Oncol* 2003;21:4112.

48. Poli-Bigelli S, Rodrigues-Pereira J, Carides AD, et al. Addition of the neurokinin 1 receptor antagonist aprepitant to standard antiemetic therapy improved control of chemotherapy-induced nausea and vomiting. Results from a randomized, double-blind, placebo-controlled trial in Latin America. *Cancer* 2003;97:3090.

49. Merck and Co. Inc. *Emend (aprepitant) package insert*. Whitehouse Station, NJ: Merck & Co. Inc, March 2003.

50. Peschel C, Tonini G, Porcile G, et al. Single IV dose of palonosetron, a potent 5-HT3 receptor antagonist demonstrates sustained prevention of nausea and vomiting for 5 days following moderately emetogenic chemotherapy. *Proc Am Soc Clin Oncol* 2003;22:760.

51. Rubenstein EB, Gralla RJ, Eisenberg P, et al. Palonosetron compared with ondansetron or dolasetron for prevention of acute and delayed chemotherapy-induced nausea and vomiting: combined results of two phase II trials. *Proc Am Soc Clin Oncol* 2003;22:729.

52. Labianca R, Van der Vegt SG, Mezger JM, et al. Palonosetron is a safe and well tolerated 5-HT3 receptor antagonist: safety results of a phase III trial. *Proc Am Soc Clin Oncol* 2003;22:753.

53. MGI Pharma Inc. *Aloxi (palonosetron HCl) injection package insert*. Minneapolis: MGI Pharma Inc, July 2003.

54. Antiemetic Subcommittee of the Multinational Association of Supportive Care in Cancer (MASCC). Prevention of chemotherapy and radiotherapy-induced emesis: results of the Perugia Consensus Conference. *Ann Oncol* 1998;9:811.

55. Hesketh PJ, Harvey WH, Harker WG, et al. A randomized, double-blind comparison of intravenous ondansetron alone and in combination with intravenous dexamethasone in the prevention of nausea and vomiting associated with high-dose cisplatin. *J Clin Oncol* 1994;12:596.

56. *Columbia Antiemetic Consensus Conference*, New York, April 2001; Presented at the ASCO-MASCC Joint Session, San Francisco, 14 May 2001.

57. Scarantino CW, Ornitz RD, Hoffman LG, et al. Radiation-induced emesis: effects of ondansetron. *Semin Oncol* 1992;19(Suppl 15):38.

58. Bodis S, Alexander E, Kooy H, et al. The prevention of radiosurgery-induced nausea and vomiting by ondansetron: evidence of a direct effect on the central nervous system chemoreceptor trigger zone. *Surg Neurol* 1994;42:249.

59. Priestman TJ, Priestman SG. An initial evaluation of nabilone in the control of radiotherapy-induced nausea and vomiting. *Clin Radiol* 1984;35:265.

60. Lucraft HH, Palmer MK. Randomized clinical trial of levonantradol and chlorpromazine in the prevention of radiotherapy-induced vomiting. *Radiology* 1982;33:621.

61. Reyntjens A. Domperidone as an anti-emetic: summary of research reports. *Postgrad Med J* 1979;55(Suppl 1):50.

62. Priestman TJ, Roberts JT, Lucraft CH, et al. Results of a randomized double-blind comparative study of ondansetron and metoclopramide in the prevention of nausea and vomiting following high dose upper abdominal irradiation. *Clin Oncol* 1990;2:71.

63. Soitzer TR, Bryson JC, Cirenza E, et al. Randomized double-blind, placebo-controlled evaluation of oral ondansetron in the prevention of nausea and vomiting associated with fractionated total-body irradiation. *J Clin Oncol* 1994;12:2432.

64. Jurgens H, McQuade B. Ondansetron as a prophylaxis for chemotherapy and radiotherapy-induced emesis in children. *Oncology* 1992;49:279.

65. Lanciano R, Sherman DM, Michalski J, et al. The efficacy and safety of once-daily Kytril (granisetron hydrochloride) tablets in the prophylaxis of nausea and emesis following fractionated upper abdominal radiotherapy. *Cancer Invest* 2001;19(8):763–772.

66. Spitzer TR, Friedman C, Bushnell J, et al. Oral granisetron (Kytril) and ondansetron (Zofran) in the prevention of hyperfractionated total body irradiation induced emesis: the results of a double-blind, randomized parallel group study (Abstract). *Blood* 1998;92(Suppl 1):278a.

67. Fauser AA, Russ W, Bischiff M. Oral dolasetron mesylate for the control of emesis during fractionated total-body irradiation and high-dose cyclophosphamide in patients undergoing allogeneic bone marrow transplantation. *Support Care Cancer* 1997;5:219.

CHAPTER 14 ■ CHRONIC NAUSEA AND VOMITING

SHALINI DALAL, GAYATRI PALAT, AND EDUARDO BRUERA

Chronic nausea and vomiting are common symptoms in patients with advanced cancer and when present are associated with great distress, significantly impacting the quality of life of patients who experience them (1,2). The reported prevalence of these symptoms varies, depending on patient characteristics and the assessment methods used for diagnosing chronic nausea and vomiting. Fainsinger et al. reported that 71 of 100 patients in a palliative care unit required treatment for nausea in the last week of life (3). Data from the National Hospice Study showed that nausea and vomiting developed in 62% of patients with terminal cancer prevalence rates of 40% in the last 6 weeks of life in women and younger patients reporting higher rates (4). In a prospective study of 1635 patients with cancer referred to a pain clinic, Grond et al. reported a prevalence of 27% for nausea and 20% for vomiting (5).

There is no standardized definition for chronic nausea. For research purposes it is often defined as nausea lasting for more than 4 weeks. In a population of patients with advanced cancer and short life expectancy this definition excludes many patients. For our purposes the presence of nausea for more than 1 week, in the absence of a well-identified, self-limiting cause (e.g., chemotherapy or radiotherapy) will be termed *chronic*. Chronic nausea has many etiologies, is often multifactorial and requires chronic treatment (3). The various contributing etiologies are presented in Figure 14.1. Unfortunately chronic nausea has not been well studied in the palliative care population and therefore the relative contribution of different causes is not known.

The purpose of this chapter is to review the pathophysiology, causes, assessment, and management of chronic nausea.

PATHOPHYSIOLOGY

The pathophysiology of chronic nausea and vomiting is complex with multiple mechanisms of emesis. A number of neural pathways and neurotransmitters are likely to be involved. Much of what we know about nausea and vomiting today is based on research in patients receiving chemotherapy or radiotherapy and in patients with postoperative nausea and vomiting. Chronic nausea in patients with cancer has not been well studied. In this patient population, research is much more difficult because many factors are present that may contribute to the mechanism of emesis. As a result, research on the mechanisms and management of acute chemotherapy or radiotherapy-induced nausea in which there are fewer contributing factors may not apply to the population of patients

with chronic symptoms. In addition the importance of different mechanisms are likely to vary between individual patients. The various pathways and centers known to be involved in the emetic pathway are illustrated in Figure 14.1 and described in detail in the following text.

Vomiting Center and Central Pattern Generator

Good evidence exists that the various stimuli affecting nausea and vomiting are relayed to the brain in an area described several decades ago as the "vomiting center" (VC) (6).

The VC has long been thought to represent the physiologic control center and is located in the lateral reticular formation of the medulla. This center is not a discrete anatomic site, but rather represents a complex array of interrelated neuronal networks coordinated by a "central pattern generator" (CPG). This site includes the nucleus tractus solitarius (NTS) and the dorsal motor nucleus of the vagus (DMV) (7). The NTS is the site where four major afferent neuronal pathways carrying emetogenic signals converge, as follows:

1. Peripheral pathways (through the vagus and splanchnic nerves) from the gastrointestinal (GI) tract, visceral capsules, and the parietal serosal surfaces
2. Neuronal connections from the chemoreceptor trigger zone (CTZ)
3. Vestibular pathways from labyrinth, in response to vertigo and visuospatial disorientation
4. Cortical pathways from higher cortical centers, in response to sensory stimuli (pain, sight, smell) and psychogenic stimuli (memory, conditioning, fear)

One or more of these pathways may be involved in a patient experiencing nausea or vomiting. Each of these four areas respond to certain types of emetic stimuli modulated by specific neurotransmitters that bind to specific receptors.

The NTS is viscerotopically organized into subnuclei that subserve diverse functions related to swallowing, gastric sensation, laryngeal and pharyngeal sensation, baroreceptor function, and respiration. Depending on the intensity and duration of received signals from these various sources, the NTS processes this information, and accordingly the DMV puts out an appropriate vasomotor efferent response inducing nausea, retching, or vomiting (8). Although nausea, a subjective symptom, has not been well studied, vomiting comprising of retching and expulsion phases has been researched in experimental

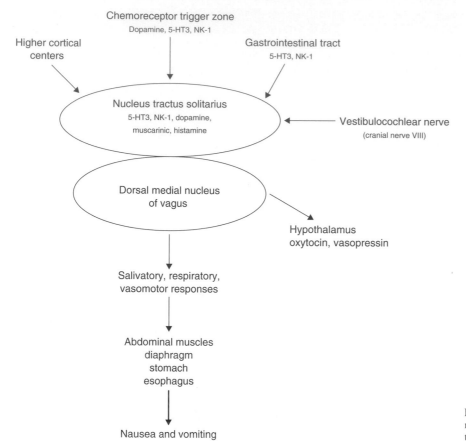

FIGURE 14.1. Emetic pathways and neurotransmitters. 5-HT3, 5-hydroxytryptamine type 3; NK-1, neurokinin-1.

animals. Coordinated combination of events involving neurons controlling the diaphragm, inspiration, blood pressure, heart rate, larynx, pharynx, tongue, esophageal sphincter, and stomach have been found to occur in a sequential manner. Approximately half of the preganglionic motor neurons in the DMV that innervate the lower esophageal sphincter (LES) also innervate the gastric fundus (9). This may have relevance to emesis, as both fundic relaxation and LES relaxation precede emesis. It must be noted that the output neurons that control the muscles involved in emesis are believed to be scattered in the medulla oblongata and therefore there is no discrete site as such. This has supported the concept of the term "central pattern generator" rather than "vomiting center" per se, involving sequential activation of relevant neurons based on the received signals (10). Nausea without vomiting may be due to insufficient stimulation of these neurons. On the other hand, persistent nausea after vomiting may denote persistent stimulation. There is little evidence that antiemetic agents act directly on the CPG.

Vasopressin and oxytocin levels increase in humans experiencing nausea from both illusory self-motion and a number of emetic-producing treatments (11). Changes in neurohypophyseal hormone release from the hypothalamus are relayed from catecholaminergic groups in the ventrolateral medulla and from the NTS (12). These are identified as part of the central pathway by which afferent abdominal vagal stimulation increases plasma vasopressin and arterial pressure. Rise in vasopressin levels may lead to hyponatremia in patients with chronic nausea.

Chemoreceptor Trigger Zone

The CTZ is situated in the area postrema of the medulla. The CTZ is located functionally outside the blood–brain barrier

and therefore samples emetogenic toxins present in cerebrospinal fluid and blood (6). Chemotherapeutic agents, metabolic products (e.g., uremia, hypercalcemia), opioids, and bacterial toxins produce nausea and vomiting by stimulating the CTZ. The CTZ also receives afferent input from peripheral sites (GI tract) through the vagus and splanchnic nerves. The CTZ cannot initiate emesis independently and does so only through stimulation of NTS. A neural pathway connects the two areas.

The predominant neurotransmitters in this area are dopamine (D_2), serotonin 5-hydroxytryptamine type 3 (5-HT3), and neurokinin-1 (NK-1) The involvement of D_2 has been the basis for the use of drugs with antidopaminergic activity such as butyrophenones (haloperidol), phenothiazines, and metoclopramide. 5-HT3 antagonists and NK-1 receptor antagonists are useful for the treatment of chemotherapy- and radiotherapy-induced nausea.

Cortex

The cortex and other areas of the brain, such as the diencephalon and the limbic system, supply afferents to the VC. Raised intracranial pressure, taste, smell, and anxiety can contribute to and stimulate vomiting. The brain cortex is also involved in emesis associated with thoughts, and visual or olfactory stimuli in patients receiving chemotherapy (13).

Vestibulocochlear Nerve

Motion can trigger nausea and vomiting. Opioids can alter the sensitivity of the vestibular center (14) resulting in nausea associated with movement. Motion stimulates receptors in the labyrinth. Impulses are then transmitted to the vestibular nucleus and onto the cerebellum, CTZ, and VC. The frequency of nausea and vomiting is comparatively higher in ambulatory patients as compared to those confined to bed. The predominant neurotransmitters involved at this level are acetylcholine and histamine. Anticholinergics and antihistamines are therefore helpful for treatment.

Gastrointestinal Tract

Stimulation of mechanoreceptors or chemoreceptors in the gut can cause nausea and vomiting. 5-HT3, D_2, acetylcholine, histamine, and substance P (SP) are important neurotransmitters involved in stimulating these receptors. SP binds to NK-1 receptors in the gut (and directly in the vomit center in the brain). GI obstruction, gastric stasis, metastatic disease, bacterial toxins, drugs, chemotherapeutic agents, and irradiation can cause emesis in this way. Abdominal vagal afferents that detect intestinal luminal contents and gastric tone terminate in the NTS (15). In addition, stimulation of the glossopharyngeal or vagus nerves in the pharynx by sputum, candida, or mucosal lesions can cause nausea. Acetylcholine in addition to being a neurotransmitter also increases gut motility and gut secretion.

ETIOLOGY

Chronic nausea in patients with advanced cancer is often multifactorial. Figure 14.2 summarizes the common causes of chronic nausea in this patient population. In many patients the underlying cause or causes are difficult to determine.

Autonomic Failure

In some patients with cancer, chronic nausea is associated with the anorexia cachexia syndrome. In these patients autonomic failure is thought to be the most likely cause of chronic nausea (16). Autonomic failure causes gastroparesis with resulting anorexia, nausea, and early satiety. In addition, other effects on the GI tract include diarrhea and constipation. Autonomic failure also has cardiovascular manifestations such as postural hypotension, syncope, and fixed heart rate.

Autonomic failure was originally described in patients with diabetes mellitus, neurologic disorders, and chronic renal disease (17). It has also been described in patients with advanced cancer. Kris et al. (18) reported delayed gastric emptying in ten patients with cancer who complained of chronic nausea and vomiting. Bruera et al. (19) looked at the incidence of cardiovascular autonomic insufficiency in 43 patients with advanced breast cancer and in 20 healthy controls matched for age and sex. Tests for autonomic failure were performed, and 52% of tests were abnormal in the patient group versus 7% in the control group. Autonomic failure in the group of patients with cancer was more common in those with poor performance status and malnutrition. In another study which included five patients with advanced cancer complaining of unexplained chronic nausea and anorexia, 16 of 23 tests for autonomic function were abnormal, compared to none of 25 tests performed in the control group of five healthy adults (20). None of the five patients had clinical or laboratory evidence of disseminated disease to the abdomen or liver. All had normal endoscopy and barium meals with no evidence of mucosal injury. All five patients had severe gastroparesis (mean emptying time 192 ± 28 minutes) as compared to five controlled (mean emptying time 66 ± 5 minutes) when assessed with a gastric emptying scan. The differences between patients and controls were statistically significant; it was concluded that gastroparesis was the cause of chronic nausea and anorexia in these patients. There have been several other cases reported in the literature of autonomic dysfunction associated with lung and pancreatic cancers (21–23).

The cause of autonomic dysfunction in patients with advanced cancer remains unclear and appears to be multifactorial. Malnutrition itself has been suggested as a cause of autonomic neuropathy (16). Jewish physicians in the Warsaw ghetto during World War II found that their patients who were starving were not able to increase their blood pressure with effort and had a constant tachycardia with no change on standing up (24). Features of autonomic dysfunction have also been described in patients with anorexia nervosa. Studies on animals have suggested that fasting suppresses the activity of the sympathetic nervous system (25). There are isolated case reports suggesting autonomic dysfunction as a paraneoplastic manifestation of advanced cancer (22,26,27). Park et al. (26) reported a patient with bronchial carcinoma who showed postural hypotension and abnormal tests for autonomic dysfunction that disappeared after irradiation of the tumor. In a

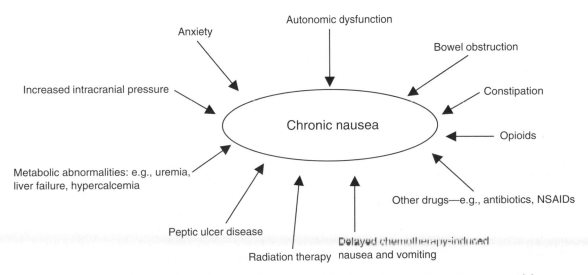

FIGURE 14.2. Causes of chronic nausea in patients with advanced cancer. NSAIDs, nonsteroidal anti-inflammatory drugs.

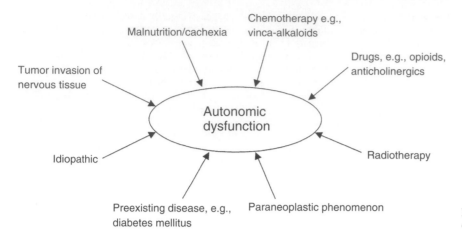

FIGURE 14.3. Possible causes of autonomic dysfunction in patients with advanced cancer.

second report, a patient with small cell carcinoma of the lung developed intestinal obstruction and abnormal tests for autonomic dysfunction. An autopsy demonstrated degeneration of autonomic nerves without tumor involvement in the area. Antineuronal antibodies have been identified in patients with small cell lung carcinoma who demonstrated neurologic signs consistent with autonomic neuropathy (28).

Another possible etiologic factor in autonomic neuropathy in this patient population is direct tumor involvement (29). Cardiovascular autonomic neuropathy has been noted after the administration of chemotherapeutic agents such as vinca alkaloids (30). Drugs such as opioids, anticholinergics, antidepressants, and vasodilators may also have adverse effects on the autonomic nervous system. Many of these drugs are used in the management of cancer-related symptoms. Radiation damage to the autonomic ganglia is also a potential factor. Human immunodeficiency virus (HIV) infection has also been noted to produce autonomic insufficiency (31).

Autonomic dysfunction is a frequent feature in patients with advanced cancer. It should be suspected in patients with unexplained tachycardia, poor performance status, chronic nausea, and malnutrition. Figure 14.3 summarizes the possible causes of autonomic dysfunction in patients with advanced cancer.

Drugs

Opioids are one of the most common causes of chronic nausea in patients with cancer. It is estimated that 6–12% of these patients may experience nausea, with some studies reporting its occurrence as high as 29% (32,33). It may often be difficult to differentiate the cause of opioid-induced nausea due to various comorbidities, conditions, and concomitant drugs, thereby skewing an accurate estimate of its true frequency (34). Patients may often associate nausea with a recent opioid analgesic, creating potential barriers to effective pain management in the form of anticipatory nausea, anxiety, or adherence problems. Opioid analgesia can cause nausea and vomiting in patients after initiation or increase in dose. This usually responds well to antiemetic medication and disappears spontaneously within the first 3 or 4 days of treatment. Some patients, particularly those receiving high doses of opioids, experience chronic and severe nausea (2).

Opioids cause chronic nausea by a number of mechanisms, including stimulation of the CTZ, gastroparesis, constipation, and by increasing sensitivity of the vestibular center. The CTZ being located outside the blood–brain barrier samples emetogenic drugs present in the circulation including opioids, which act on specific nerve cells or opioid receptors. The

presence of opioid receptors in the CTZ in the area postrema is consistent with the observation of morphine and enkephalin-induced vomiting in the dog after local or systemic administration and the abolishment of this response after ablation of the area postrema (35). The CTZ also accepts several medullary neurons, which may be responsible for inhibiting the action potential of these specific nerve cells, thereby keeping the neurons of the CTZ from firing more readily. Neurons originating from the medulla are hypothesized to be enkephalinergic. It is theorized that displacing them by opioids or opioid antagonists may predispose patients to nausea by, in effect, removing inhibitory input into the CTZ. Chronic nausea has been associated with accumulation of active morphine metabolites such as morphine-6-glucuronide. Accumulation of morphine metabolites is more likely with higher doses of opioids but can occur even with lower doses, especially in patients with renal insufficiency (36).

By an unknown mechanism, the vestibular apparatus is directly stimulated by most opioids. This may add to the already decreased threshold for nausea they cause at the CTZ. Distention of the gut, decreased GI emptying time, and constipation may stimulate mechanoreceptors. Stimulation of visceral mechanoreceptors and chemoreceptors is most commonly responsible for nausea and emesis in terminally ill patients receiving opioid drugs. Opioids also decrease GI emptying time, which may cause constipation or fecal impaction. Although not as well defined as the other neuronal inputs, the cortex has direct input into the VC through several types of neuroreceptors. A patient may remember unpleasant feelings of nausea associated with past opioid therapy. When presented with the sight, smell, or even anticipation of taking an opioid again, a strong nausea reflex may result.

Many other drugs can cause nausea. Nonsteroidal anti-inflammatory drugs, antibiotics, and iron supplements can cause nausea irritation of the GI tract. Antibiotics may also cause nausea by a direct effect on the CTZ. Psychoactive medications including tricyclic antidepressants, selective 5-HT3 reuptake inhibitors, and phenothiazines can cause nausea.

Constipation

Constipation is common in patients with advanced cancer. Severe constipation can cause nausea and vomiting, abdominal pain, distension, urinary retention, and cognitive failure (37). There are many factors in patients with advanced cancer that predispose to the development of constipation, including opioid analgesics, immobility, poor oral intake and dehydration, autonomic failure, and other medications. Constipation is often underdiagnosed in this patient population and should be suspected as a cause of nausea in all patients with advanced cancer (38).

Bowel Obstruction

Bowel obstruction is a less common but important cause of nausea and vomiting. It has been reported to occur in 3% of terminally ill patients with cancer, and was found to be present in 15 of 100 consecutive patients admitted to a tertiary palliative care unit (39). Although acute complete bowel obstruction is easy to diagnose, most patients with advanced cancer tend to present with a less clear picture of slow progression from partial to complete bowel obstruction. Some patients have only intermittent obstructive symptoms. These episodes of obstruction may be accompanied by nausea and vomiting.

ASSESSMENT

Because the causes of chronic nausea and vomiting are often multifactorial, the assessment in a given patient should be multidimensional, with awareness that these symptoms are dynamic processes and frequently change in intensity. There are a number of effective systems for assessing the intensity of nausea, such as visual analog scales, numerical scales, and verbal descriptors, but there is no "gold standard" for nausea assessment. As nausea is a subjective symptom, its expression varies from patient to patient and will depend on the individual patient's perception and other factors such as psychosocial issues. From a practical point of view this occasionally leads to a lack of correlation between the observed expression of nausea and the presumed pathophysiology of the underlying condition. It is also important to note that the term *nausea* may mean different things to different individuals and is used by some patients to describe other symptoms, including abdominal discomfort, pain, distension, or early satiety.

Once the intensity of nausea has been assessed, it is important to assess the symptom in the context of other symptoms such as pain, appetite, fatigue, depression, and anxiety. This multidimensional assessment allows formulation of a therapeutic strategy. An example of a validated multidimensional assessment tool is the Edmonton Symptom Assessment System (40,41) The system is based on visual analog scales that assess pain, nausea, anxiety, depression, appetite, shortness of breath, and sense of well-being, among others. Tools such as this can be used to document the intensity of nausea initially, as a baseline assessment, and then on a regular basis, giving the examiner a sense of the therapeutic effect of the management. Such tools allow for a more reproducible assessment from the point of view of research and quality control.

A detailed history and physical examination is essential. It is important to clarify that the patient's expression of nausea does not describe a different symptom such as reflux. Intensity, frequency, exacerbating and relieving factors, onset, and duration of nausea should be documented. If there is coexistent vomiting, the nature of the vomiting should also be documented as the quantity of the vomitus can give a clue to the etiology. Large-volume emesis may indicate gastric outflow obstruction whereas small volume emesis may indicate gastric stasis. The extent to which the emesis interferes with oral intake should be noted, as large and frequent volume vomiting puts the patient at risk of rapid dehydration. A history of syncopal episodes or early satiety should alert the physician of the possibility of autonomic insufficiency.

The etiology of nausea may be related to the underlying cancer diagnosis. It is important to obtain details of tumor involvement and spread, as well as treatment history. In patients with intra-abdominal involvement, nausea with or without vomiting is often seen due to liver metastasis, mechanical obstruction of bowel by tumor, or peritoneal carcinomatosis. The stomach and duodenum can be compressed, causing the "squashed-stomach syndrome." Nausea may be present secondary to primary or metastatic brain involvement by tumor, or leptomeningeal disease. Radiation therapy to the spine or abdomen may be followed by nausea and vomiting.

A detailed medication history is essential. The use of drugs capable of causing nausea, such as opioids, anticholinergics, nonsteroidal anti-inflammatory drugs, and antibiotics, should be specifically noted. Delayed chemotherapy-induced nausea and vomiting (CINV) may be present and refers to symptoms that occur 24 hours after chemotherapy administration and which may last for as many as 6 to 7 days. Cisplatin has an approximate 65-90% likelihood of causing delayed emesis in the absence of antiemetic prophylaxis (42). Patients with HIV may have nausea, which is a side effect of all the drugs of the highly active antiretroviral therapy (HAART) regimen. Patients should be questioned about recent use of steroids because their abrupt inadvertent discontinuation could lead to addisonian crisis presenting with nausea, vomiting, abdominal pain, and hypotension. Emotional experiences, history of anxiety disorder should be explored. Other medical conditions, such as peptic ulcer disease and diabetes, should also be noted. Autonomic failure should be suspected in patients with diabetic neuropathy or chronic renal failure.

Constipation, as already discussed (See the section Constipation), is a common complication in patients with advanced cancer and may cause or aggravate nausea. The frequency of bowel movements; feeling of abdominal distension; rectal soreness; oozing of stool; change in the amount of gases or stool passed recently; laxative use, type, and dose; and date of last bowel movement should be obtained. Unfortunately, clinical impression is likely to be quite unreliable and investigations, such as a plain abdominal x-ray, should be undertaken to help in the diagnosis. The use of a radiologic constipation score may be necessary for adequate diagnosis in some patients, particularly those with cognitive failure. On a plain abdominal x-ray the abdomen is divided into four quadrants. Each quadrant is assessed for constipation: score 0 = no stool; 1 = stool occupying <50% of the lumen; 2 = stool occupying >50% of the lumen; 3 = stool completely occupying the whole lumen of the colon. The total score of all quadrants is calculated and will range from 0 to 12. A score of 7 or greater is suggestive of severe constipation (38).

TABLE 14.1

POSSIBLE FINDINGS ON PHYSICAL EXAMINATION IN PATIENTS WITH CHRONIC NAUSEA AND VOMITING

General inspection
- Cachexia or malnutrition; muscle wasting, decreased skin fold thickness

Abdominal examination
- Bowel obstruction: abdominal distension, increased bowel sounds
- Abdominal masses or ascites
- Constipation: abdominal fullness, including rectal examination

Neurologic examination
- Raised intracranial pressure, papilledema
- Autonomic insufficiency: lying and standing blood pressure, absence of heart rate variation during Valsalva's maneuver

Physical examination may be helpful in identifying possible underlying causes. Table 14.1 summarizes possible findings on physical examination in patients with chronic nausea and vomiting.

Investigations to exclude renal impairment, hepatic failure, and other metabolic abnormalities such as hypercalcemia, hypokalemia, and hyponatremia should be undertaken. A computed tomography scan of the brain may be indicated where brain metastases are suspected. Abdominal x-rays may be useful in assessing nausea. A supine x-ray may indicate the presence of stool and fecal impaction. Erect or decubitus views may show air and fluid levels in the bowel, which is typical of bowel obstruction. Sophisticated investigations, such as gastric emptying scans, are probably not justified for most patients.

MANAGEMENT

Appropriate management of chronic nausea and vomiting depends on a detailed assessment. General supportive measures should be instituted in all patients. In addition specific interventions should be undertaken as appropriate. Due to the lack of well-designed studies there is no convincing data as to the best pharmacologic strategy for treatment of nausea and vomiting and current management is on the basis of expert opinion rather than evidence (43).

Many palliative care specialists are now favoring a mechanistic approach to nausea management, where the initial choice of medication is based on the likely mechanism, and neuropharmacology of the emetic pathway. Response rates of 80–90% have been reported with this approach (44,45). An alternative approach of empiric treatment has been recommended by some, and in studies found to be highly effective (46–49). There have been no head to head comparisons of these approaches.

General Support Measures

General measures should address maintenance of good oral hygiene (poor oral hygiene can contribute to nausea), the creation of a comfortable environment for the patient, regular baths to prevent unpleasant body odors, and attention to diet. Small volumes of food at regular intervals should be considered for patients with early satiety associated with nausea.

Specific Treatment

In patients where an underlying cause or causes have been identified, there should be an attempt to correct these. Metabolic abnormalities should be corrected if possible. In situations where opioid toxicity is suspected, a change of opioids using equianalgesic doses can be expected to improve symptoms of nausea while maintaining pain control (50). Unnecessary medications should be discontinued. Aggressive bowel care, including cleansing enemas and regular laxatives, should be instituted when constipation or stool impaction is suspected. In some cases, such as in patients with brain metastases, symptom control may be attempted with radiation therapy or corticosteroids. If peptic ulcer disease is suspected, appropriate treatment should be instituted.

Pharmacologic Interventions

Many drugs with antiemetic properties are available for the treatment of chronic nausea and vomiting. The various classes of antiemetics and their site of receptor action, if known, are presented in Table 14.2 and further discussed. The choice of an antiemetic should depend not only on the likely etiology of symptoms and the severity of nausea and vomiting,

TABLE 14.2

ESTABLISHED AND EMERGING AGENTS FOR THE TREATMENT OF NAUSEA

Agent	Effects
Dopamine antagonists-central action (e.g., metoclopramide, butyrophenones, phenothiazines)	Block dopamine receptors at chemoreceptor trigger zone.
Dopamine antagonists-peripheral action (e.g., metoclopramide, domperidone)	Promotility effects on gastrointestinal tract.
Antihistamines (e.g., cyclizine, promethazine, dimenhydrinate)	Effects on vomiting center and vestibular apparatus.
Corticosteroids (e.g., dexamethasone)	Reduces raised intracranial pressure. Other antiemetic effects not well understood. Improves sensation of well-being and appetite.
5-HT3 (serotonin) antagonists (e.g., ondansetron, granisetron)	Blocks 5-HT3 receptors in the gut predominantly. Useful in chemotherapy-induced and postoperative vomiting. Metoclopramide at high doses has weak 5-HT3 antagonistic activity.
Progestational agents (e.g., megestrol acetate)	Unknown. Improves appetite, caloric intake, and nutritional variables in cancer cachexia.
Thalidomide	Centrally acting antiemetic effect. Other effects on improving appetite and sensation of well-being.
Cannabinoids	Central effects.
Neurokinin-1 antagonists	Central effects, antagonize substance P.
Octreotide	Reduced gastrointestinal secretions in patients with inoperable bowel obstruction.
Anticholinergic agents (e.g., hyoscine butylbromide, scopolamine)	Reduces gastrointestinal secretions in patients with inoperable bowel obstruction.

5-HT3, 5-hydroxytryptamine type 3.

but also on a drug's potential adverse effects and available routes of administration. Metoclopramide, haloperidol, dexamethasone, hyoscine butylbromide, and cyclizine are the most commonly used antiemetics worldwide (51).

Prokinetic Drugs

The initial pharmacologic management of chronic nausea and vomiting in most patients should involve prokinetic drugs to normalize upper GI motility (2,47,52,53). Metoclopramide hydrochloride is a substituted benzamide used for its prokinetic and antiemetic properties. Cisapride and domperidone are other examples of prokinetic drugs.

Metoclopramide has been established as an effective drug for treating delayed gastric emptying in patients who do not have cancer, in a number of controlled clinical trials (53). Metoclopramide has also been demonstrated to be effective in reversing tumor-associated gastroparesis (18,52) and nausea associated with advanced cancer (2,46,47). Metoclopramide antagonizes D_2 receptors both centrally in the CTZ and peripherally in the GI tract. In addition, it exhibits weak antagonism at the 5-HT3 receptor. It exerts its prokinetic activity through the cholinergic system in the myenteric plexus. Local acetylcholine release, mediated by the serotonin-4 receptors. It stimulates the motility of the upper GI tract without affecting gastric, biliary, or pancreatic secretion and increases gastric peristalsis, leading to accelerated gastric emptying. The resting tone of the gastro-oesophageal sphincter is increased and the pyloric sphincter is relaxed. Duodenal peristalsis is also increased which decreases intestinal transit time. Therefore it appears to play an important role in reversing gastroparesis and bringing about normal peristalsis in the upper GI tract. Anticholinergic medications, including tricyclic antidepressants antagonizes the prokinetic effect. Antiemetic doses are greater than those required for prokinetic effect.

High doses of metoclopramide (1–2 mg per kg given up to five times in 24 hours) may produce 5-HT3 receptor blockade, which may in turn contribute to its antiemetic activity. However these high doses are frequently impractical. Because of its short half-life (3 hours), a continuous infusion of metoclopramide can be effective when intermittent administration fails to control nausea (2). Clinical trials support the view that sustained metoclopramide concentrations are required to suppress nausea and vomiting and possibly other GI symptoms associated with advanced cancer (2,46,47). As a result some patients require frequent administration or continuous infusions for optimal results (54). In one study, 26 cancer patients with a >1-month history of chronic nausea and dyspepsia of advanced cancer were randomized to receive either controlled-release metoclopramide 40 mg 12 hourly or placebo for 4 days (47). Patients were then crossed over to the alternative treatment for another 4 days. On the last day of each treatment phase, nausea was significantly lower in the controlled-release metoclopramide group compared to placebo. Controlled-release metoclopramide was well tolerated and adverse events did not differ between treatments and placebo groups. In another study immediate-release metoclopramide 20 mg 6 hourly was compared to controlled-release metoclopramide 40 mg 12 hourly in patients with advanced cancer and chronic nausea. Nausea scores by day 3 of treatment were significantly lower for patients who received controlled release as compared to immediate-release metoclopramide (46). Metoclopramide occasionally causes acute dystonic reactions. These are more common in younger patients, especially in young women. Motor restlessness (akathisia) may occur in patients receiving high doses of metoclopramide and include feelings of anxiety, agitation, jitteriness, and insomnia. These symptoms may disappear spontaneously or respond to a reduction in dosage.

Domperidone is another drug with antidopaminergic activity. However it does not readily cross the blood–brain barrier and acts primarily on the GI tract. Hence, it is less likely to cause central effects such as extrapyramidal reactions and sedation. Domperidone is not approved for use in the United States and in 2004 the U.S. Food and Drug Administration (FDA) issued a warning against the use of domperidone due to reports of arrhythmias and death with i.v. usage in terminally ill patients with cancer.

Cisapride is a substituted benzamide with prokinetic properties. It stimulates GI motility, probably by increasing the release of acetylcholine in the gut wall at the level of the myenteric plexus, increases the resting tone of the lower oesophageal sphincter, and increases the amplitude of lower oesophageal contractions. Gastric emptying is accelerated and the mouth-to-cecum transit time is reduced. Colonic peristalsis is also increased which decreases colonic transit time. Cisapride apparently lacks antidopaminergic effects (unlike metoclopramide and domperidone). It is reported to be an agonist at serotonin-4 receptors. Cisapride is restricted in this country due to drug–drug interactions resulting in fatal cardiac arrhythmias and is only available by an investigational limited access program for patients meeting strict inclusion criteria. Norcisapride, a less cardiotoxic isomer of cisapride is in early phases of investigation.

Erythromycin has been administered for its prokinetic effects with success in patients with diabetic gastroparesis; however, its efficacy in treatment of nausea is limited due to its adverse GI side effects.

Therefore from a practical standpoint, metoclopramide is the only prokinetic drug available for use, and favored as the drug of first choice for patients with chronic nausea (2). A standard therapeutic ladder for the management of chronic nausea in patients with cancer based on metoclopramide has been developed. Table 14.3 summarizes this regimen. A retrospective assessment of this regimen in 98 terminally ill patients with nausea in a palliative care unit found that most patients without bowel obstruction achieved excellent control of nausea using this regimen. Twenty-five patients (25%) required other antiemetics, 18 because of GI obstruction, three due to extrapyramidal side effects, and four for other reasons.

TABLE 14.3

A METOCLOPRAMIDE-BASED REGIMEN FOR TREATMENT OF CHRONIC NAUSEA

Step 1	Metoclopramide, 10 mg p.o./s.c. q4h + 10 mg p.o./s.c. for rescue
	Poor response after at least 2 d of treatment (consistent complaint of nausea and greater than two extra doses of metoclopramide/d), go to step 2; occasionally patients with severe emesis go to step 3
	Side effects or contraindication (bowel obstruction), go to step 4
Step 2	Metoclopramide (same dose as step 1) + dexamethasone, 10 mg p.o./s.c. b.i.d.
	Poor response after at least 2 d, go to step 3
	Side effects or contraindication, go to step 4
Step 3	Continuous subcutaneous infusion of metoclopramide (60–120 mg/d) + dexamethasone, 10 mg p.o./s.c. b.i.d.
	Poor response, go to step 4
Step 4	Other antiemetics (e.g., haloperidol, dimenhydrinate)

These data suggest that nausea can be controlled in most patients in this population.

Other Centrally Acting Dopamine Antagonists

Phenothiazines (e.g., chlorpromazine) and butyrophenones (e.g., haloperidol) are effective antiemetics. They are D_2 antagonists and act centrally at the CTZ. Other types of receptor activity may also be present, which divides this group into those with a narrow spectrum of activity (such as haloperidol), broader spectrum (chlorpromazine, prochlorperazine, and promethazine), and those with the broadest spectrum of activity (methotrimeprazine). These agents do not increase gastrointestinal motility so are often used in patients presenting with bowel obstruction.

Haloperidol, a narrow spectrum agent, is predominantly a D_2 antagonist with negligible anticholinergic activity. It is therefore less sedating than the others, but has greater extrapyramidal reactions. The oral bioavailability is approximately 65%. It is highly protein bound and is not cleared by the kidney, making it safe in the presence of renal failure. Initial doses range from 0.5–2 mg p.o./i.v./s.c. and can be repeated at 4-hour intervals. In the elderly, doses of 1 mg every 12 hours are usually effective (55). It is an ideal agent in patients with nausea and delirium, and has been successfully combined with 5-HT3 antagonists in cases of intractable nausea (56). When used subcutaneously, it is recommended to keep the concentration of haloperidol below 1.5 mg per mL to avoid precipitation of haloperidol crystals (57).

The broader spectrum agents such as chlorpromazine, prochlorperazine, and promethazine have dopaminergic, cholinergic, and histamine receptor antagonism. Prochlorperazine has low oral absorption (14%) and is usually administered through the rectal or parenteral routes. Side effects include postural tachycardia, dryness of mouth and sedation. Akathisia is common in elderly patients even with low doses. Promethazine has a slightly better oral bioavailability (25%) than prochlorperazine. There is probably little advantage of using this agent over prochlorperazine. Chlorpromazine use for nausea management is limited by its excessive sedation.

Methotrimeprazine, the broadest spectrum agent, has antagonist activity to α-adrenergic, dopaminergic, cholinergic, and histaminic receptors. Although no longer available in the United States, it has been used in other countries in cases of refractory nausea. The drug has a long half-life and can be given once or twice a day. Side effects are similar to other phenothiazines such as dose-dependent orthostatic hypotension and sedation (58).

Olanzapine, an atypical antipsychotic, possesses a unique neurotransmitter binding profile that is similar to methotrimeprazine. Several reports have found olanzapine to be beneficial in nausea management in patients with advanced cancer (59–61). It is also currently undergoing trial for the prevention of chemotherapy-induced nausea and vomiting (62).

Antihistaminics and Anticholinergics

Antihistaminics such as cyclizine, promethazine, and dimenhydrinate are useful antiemetics particularly if a vestibular component to the nausea is identified. Drowsiness is a major side effect.

Antimuscarinic/anticholinergic include tertiary and quaternary ammonium salts. Atropine and scopolamine are tertiary derivatives. These are lipophilic compounds and by crossing the blood–brain barrier may cause excessive sedation and confusion. Glycopyrrolate, on the other hand is a quaternary compound with little central nervous system (CNS) penetration

and is therefore preferred. Anticholinergics have been found to be useful in reducing symptoms of nausea and abdominal colic when associated with mechanical bowel obstruction (63).

Corticosteroids

Corticosteroids have powerful nonspecific antiemetic effects that are not well understood. They may act by modulation of prostaglandin release (64). They can decrease peritumoral edema, therefore reducing intracranial pressure, a known cause of nausea. Corticosteroids are beneficial in combination with other antiemetic agents such as 5-HT3 antagonists or metoclopramide in the prevention and management of acute and delayed chemotherapy-induced emesis (65–67). Corticosteroids are also useful in the management of other symptoms that may coexist with nausea in patients with advanced cancer such as pain, anorexia, and asthenia (68–71).

Serotonin Antagonists

Although the use of serotonin antagonists such as ondansetron, granisetron, and dolasetron in the setting of highly and moderately emetogenic chemotherapy and radiotherapy are well established, there are few published clinical trials on the use of these drugs in managing chronic nausea in patients with advanced cancer. Trials comparing serotonin antagonists and metoclopramide have either had methodologic problems or used inadequate doses of metoclopramide (e.g., 10 mg three times a day). A double-blind randomized placebo-controlled study of 92 patients compared the antiemetic efficacy and safety of ondansetron, placebo, and metoclopramide in the treatment of opioid-induced nausea and emesis in patients with cancer (72). Patients were randomized to receive one of oral ondansetron 24 mg once daily, metoclopramide 10 mg three times daily, or placebo. Study medication was started only if the patient experienced nausea and/or emesis following opioid administration. There was no statistically significant difference between the groups in the proportion achieving complete control of emesis (33% of patients on placebo, 48% on ondansetron, and 52% on metoclopramide) or complete control of nausea (23% of patients on placebo, 17% on ondansetron, and 36% on metoclopramide). The incidence of adverse events was very low and similar in all treatment groups. In another study, single doses of ondansetron 8 mg, 16 mg, or placebo were administered to 520 subjects with pain sufficient to require opioid analgesia (73). Nausea was abated completely in 6.8% of subjects receiving placebo, 14.8% of those receiving ondansetron 8 mg, and 19.4% of those receiving ondansetron 16 mg. Ondansetron 8 mg was not significantly different from placebo; however, the 16-mg dose did show a statistically significant difference ($p = .007$).

There have been some reports of its effectiveness in patients with postoperative nausea and nausea refractory to other treatments (74,75). In one retrospective study seven patients with advanced cancer and nine with late-stage acquired immunodeficiency syndrome (AIDS) were given ondansetron for nausea and vomiting (76,77). All were on at least one other antiemetic, which they continued taking. The addition of ondansetron led to marked improvement in symptom control in 13 of the 16 patients.

Advantages of the serotonin antagonists include less frequent dosing (typically every 8 to 12 hours), availability of an orally dissolving form of ondansetron an option for patients having difficulty with swallowing. Disadvantages include the risk of constipation with long-term use which can be a major disadvantage for a patient with other risk factors such as high-dosage opioid use or decreased gastric motility. Headache is the most common adverse effect. Serotonin antagonists are costly and this may be a significant issue for terminally ill patients with limited resources.

There are reports of serotonin receptor antagonists being more effective than metoclopramide in controlling nausea and vomiting in patients with uremia (78). These agents may also benefit symptoms of pruritus as well which is frequently present in patients with uremia (79). Serotonin and histamine have been reported as possible mediators of uremic pruritus.

Palonosetron is a new 5-HT3 receptor antagonist (second generation) that has antiemetic activity at both central and GI sites. In comparison to the older 5-HT3 receptor antagonists, it has a higher binding affinity to the 5-HT3 receptors, a higher potency, a significantly longer half-life (approximately 40 hours, four to five times longer than that of dolasetron, granisetron, or ondansetron), and an excellent safety profile.

The antidepressant mirtazapine exhibits antagonistic activity at several receptor sites which include 5-α_2 adrenergic, H-1, 5-HT3 and the 5-HT2 receptors. Its antagonistic activity at the 5-HT3 receptor makes it a useful agent in controlling nausea and vomiting. Mirtazapine is anxiolytic by virtue of its antagonism of the 5HT2 receptor, and is strongly sleep inducing. A common side effect of mirtazapine is increased appetite with weight gain when it is used to treat depression. Mirtazapine may be therefore useful as a single agent or an adjunct in the palliative care setting where patients may have nausea associated with depressed mood, anxiety, insomnia, anorexia, and weight loss. Further research on this is warranted.

Progestational Agents

Trials involving progestational agents in the treatment of hormone-responsive tumors found significant body weight gain with or without tumor response (80,81). This prompted studies of these drugs for the treatment of cancer cachexia. Megestrol acetate has been the most widely studied progestational agent in patients with advanced cancer. Several randomized controlled trials have shown that megestrol acetate can improve appetite, caloric intake, and nutritional variables in patients with cancer cachexia (82–87). Simons et al. found improved appetite and possible reduction in nausea and vomiting in patients with advanced-stage, nonhormone-sensitive cancer treated with megestrol acetate (88). Loprinzi et al. in a randomized, placebo-controlled trial of megestrol acetate involving 133 patients, reported a significantly reduced incidence of nausea and vomiting in patients receiving megestrol acetate (83). Reduced nausea has also been reported in other studies of megestrol acetate in cancer cachexia (84,85). Further research is needed to assess the potential role of progestational agents in the treatment of patients with chronic nausea.

Neurokinin-1 Receptor Antagonists

SP is a regulatory neuropeptide belonging to the tachykinin family of peptides. During decades of research there has been much speculation concerning its proposed various physiologic roles including that of emesis. The emetic action of SP has been studied in humans and animal studies. It mediates its action through NK-1 receptors which are abundant in the CTZ, NTS, and the GI tracts (vagal afferents).

SP is co-localized with serotonin in enterochromaffin cells in the GI tract, and SP levels in the peripheral circulation have been reported to be elevated following cisplatin administration in patients (89). SP has been shown in animals to cross the blood–brain barrier, which raises the possibility that SP of peripheral origin may act centrally to induce emesis (90). The specific site of antiemetic action of NK-1 Receptor Antagonists

(RAs) is not known. They may act in the area postrema (91). NK-1 RAs applied to the area postrema have been shown to decrease expulsion and retching episodes induced by morphine and copper sulfate (92). The NK-1 receptor is highly expressed in vagal motor neurons and activation of these receptors in this region potently evokes gastric fundic relaxation (93). Because fundic relaxation is a prodromal event essential for emesis, it is attractive to speculate that these antagonists inhibit fundic relaxation by blocking the NK-1 receptors on preganglionic neurons in the DMV.

In animal studies NK-1 RAs appear to have a broad spectrum of action for diverse causes of emesis (92). In clinical studies, NK-1 RAs have shown efficacy in reducing both acute and delayed CINV when added to other antiemetics (94–96). Aprepitant (Emend) is the first commercially available drug from this new class of agents. Oral aprepitant, in combination with other agents, is indicated for the prevention of acute and delayed chemotherapy-induced nausea and vomiting (CINV) associated with highly emetogenic chemotherapy in adults. NK-1 RAs have also been shown to be beneficial for postoperative nausea and vomiting (97). CNS penetration by the NK-1 RA has been shown to be essential for the prevention of vomiting in the first 4 hours following cisplatin-based chemotherapy, which suggests that the antiemetic effect of NK-1 RAs is mediated centrally, probably in region of the NTS (98).

Aprepitant is generally well tolerated. The most common adverse events in randomized trials were asthenia or fatigue. Other adverse events experienced by aprepitant recipients include anorexia, constipation, diarrhea, nausea (after day 5 of the study) and hiccups.

Aprepitant is eliminated primarily by metabolism of CYP3A4 and is a substrate and moderate inhibitor of CYP3A4. Therefore, potential risk of interaction with drugs metabolized by CYP3A4 may occur. For example A twofold increase in the area under concentration curve (AUC) of dexamethasone, a sensitive substrate of CYP3A4, could be demonstrated when it was combined with aprepitant. Therefore, the dose of dexamethasone should be reduced by approximately 50% when aprepitant is coadministered.

The potential roles of NK-1 RAs in the treatment of chronic nausea and vomiting in advanced cancer is currently unknown.

Thalidomide and Analog

Thalidomide was initially used during the 1950s as a mild anxiolytic, hypnotic, and antiemetic. Its antiemetic effects resulted in its use in the treatment of hyperemesis gravidarum (99), and was found to be effective in the symptomatic therapy of nausea and vomiting caused by malignant, nongastric neoplasms or by the administration of mechlorethamine (100). It was removed from the market after it was found to cause severe teratogenesis when administered to pregnant women. In recent years there has been renewed interest in thalidomide, particularly for use in patients with cancer.

In addition to central antiemetic and sedative effects, thalidomide has complex immunomodulatory, antiinflammatory, anticachectic, and possible antiangiogenic, antidiaphoretic, and analgesic actions (101). It has been shown to downregulate the production of TNF-α and other proinflammatory cytokines, inhibit the transcription factor nuclear factor κB (NFκB), downregulate cyclooxygenase 2, inhibit angiogenesis, and shifts in the ratio of CD4+ lymphocytes (helper T cells) to CD8+ lymphocytes (cytotoxic T cells) (102). The multiplicity of actions may explain the large variety of therapeutic results achieved with the administration of thalidomide. This spectrum of potential effects makes it an interesting drug from a palliative care perspective. Elevation of tumor necrosis factor-α (TNF-α) in the systemic circulation liberated as part of the immune response to antigenic challenge, carcinogenesis, and radiation therapy has been correlated with anorexia, nausea, vomiting, and GI stasis (103). This results from sensory afferent activation of nucleus of the solitary tract (NST) neurons in the medulla by TNF-α producing inhibition of gastric motility (104) Thalidomide can therefore be expected to improve both appetite and chronic nausea and vomiting.

Bruera et al. (105) found that administration of thalidomide 100 mg at night in 37 evaluable patients with advanced cancer and cachexia led to significant improvement in appetite, nausea, and sensation of well-being. Further research is needed to evaluate the effects of thalidomide on chronic nausea.

Lenalidomide

The thalidomide analog and immunomodulatory drug lenalidomide is emerging as a useful treatment for a number of cancers. The FDA recently granted approval for the phase III clinical evaluation of lenalidomide for the treatment of patients with relapsed and refractory multiple myeloma. However, there is a lack of information concerning mechanism of action in these patients and a number of diverse properties, including antiangiogenic activity, have been postulated (106). Its usefulness in chronic nausea and vomiting is not known.

Cannabinoids

δ₉-Tetrahydrocannabinol (THC), the major psychoactive component of marijuana is produced commercially as dronabinol and nabilone for use as antiemetic agents when other agents are not effective. Several studies have demonstrated its efficacy as an antiemetic agent for the treatment of CINV (107–110).

A randomized controlled trial in 139 patients with AIDS cachexia comparing oral dronabinol 2.5 mg twice daily and placebo showed significant improvement in nausea, appetite, and mood but no gain in body weight in those patients taking the drug (111). Side effects, such as somnolence, confusion, and perceptual disturbance, are common. Although there are some case reports in the literature of patient's benefiting with addition of THC to other antiemetic agents in refractory nausea, the effects of cannabinoids in patients with advanced cancer with chronic nausea have not been characterized. In this patient population who frequently have borderline cognitive impairment and are often receiving other medications, such as opioids and other psychoactive drugs, the incidence of side effects is likely to limit their use. The mechanism of action of cannabinoids in emesis control is not clear. THC has been found to inhibit gastric emptying in humans (112). In animal studies THC decreased fundic tone and antral motility by means of cannabinoid (CB1) receptors located in the dorsal ventral columns (113,114). THC-evoked GI stasis and fundic relaxation may be contributory to its antiemetic effects.

Octreotide and Anticholinergic Drugs

In patients with inoperable bowel obstruction, reduction of secretions has been achieved using anticholinergic agents (e.g., hyoscine butylbromide) (115) and octreotide (a somatostatin analogue) (116). Two recent randomized controlled trials have compared anticholinergic agents and octreotide. Mercadante et al. (117), in a study involving 18 patients, found that octreotide treatment produced a significantly reduced number of daily episodes of vomiting and intensity of nausea compared with hyoscine butylbromide. Lower levels of hydration were associated with nausea in both groups. Ripamonti et al. (118) looked at 17 patients who presented with inoperable bowel obstruction and a decompressive nasogastric tube. Patients were randomized to receive either octreotide 0.3 mg or scopolamine butylbromide 60 mg daily for 3 days by subcutaneous infusion. It was possible to remove the nasogastric tube in 13 of the 17 patients. Octreotide significantly reduced the amount of GI secretions at days 2 and 3 as compared to scopolamine butylbromide. Patients who received less parenteral hydration had significantly more nausea and drowsiness. The authors concluded that octreotide should be considered the first-choice drug when a rapid reduction in GI secretions is desired and that parenteral hydration over 500 mL per day may reduce nausea and drowsiness. Further studies are needed to identify the role that hydration plays in the etiology of nausea in this clinical situation.

Surgical Intervention

In patients with nausea or emesis caused by mechanical obstruction, surgical procedures such as percutaneous gastrostomy for gastric outlet obstruction, colostomy, intestinal bypass, or laparotomy for obstruction secondary to tumors or adhesions may be considered for symptom control and improve life expectancy and quality of life. This is provided the patient's general physical condition suggests a life expectancy long enough to result in benefit from surgery. Even when patients appear to be candidates for surgical procedures, these procedures are associated with complications and may not be successful in relieving symptoms (118). In a study, only 56% patients survived 60 days following surgery, and 43% of survivors continued to experience intermittent symptoms of both complete and incomplete bowel obstruction (119,120).

CONCLUSION

Chronic nausea and vomiting are common and distressing symptoms in patients with terminal cancer. These symptoms are likely to be due to several factors, including autonomic failure, opioid analgesics, metabolic abnormalities, constipation, and cachexia. Promotility agents (sometimes in combination with corticosteroids) are in most cases the drug of choice for management of chronic nausea and vomiting. Pharmacologic agents, such as progestational drugs and thalidomide, need further evaluation of their potential beneficial effects in patients with chronic nausea. Despite significant ongoing research into acute chemotherapy-induced and postoperative emesis, research is lacking in chronic nausea. Drugs that have been found to be effective in acute vomiting, such as serotonin and NK-1 RAs, require further evaluation in patients with advanced cancer with chronic nausea.

References

1. Portenoy RK, Thaler HT, Kornblith AB, et al. Symptom prevalence, characteristics and distress in a cancer population. *Qual Life Res* 1994;3:183–189.
2. Bruera E, Seifert L, Watanabe S. Chronic nausea in advanced cancer patients: a retrospective assessment of a metoclopramide-based antiemetic regimen. *J Pain Symptom Manage* 1996;11:147–153.
3. Fainsinger R, Miller MJ, Bruera E, et al. Symptom control during the last week of life on a palliative care unit. *J Palliat Care* 1991;7(1):5–11.
4. Reuben DB, Mor V. Nausea and vomiting in terminal cancer patients. *Arch Intern Med* 1986;146:2021–2023.
5. Grond S, Zech D, Diefenbach C, et al. Prevalence and pattern of symptoms in patients with cancer pain: a prospective evaluation of 1635 cancer patients referred to a pain clinic. *J Pain Symptom Manage* 1994;9:372–382.
6. Borison HL, Wang SC. Physiology and pharmacology of vomiting. *Pharmacol Rev* 1953;5:193–230.
7. Carpenter DO. Neural mechanisms of emesis. *Can J Physiol Pharmacol* 1990;68:230–236.

8. Dienmunsch P, Grelt L. Potential of substance P antagonist as antiemetics. *Drugs* 2000;60:533–546.

9. Hyland NP, Abrahams TP, Fuchs K, et al. Organization and neurochemistry of vagal preganglionic neurons innervating the lower esophageal sphincter in ferrets. *J Comp Neurol* 2001;430:222–234.

10. Lang IM, Sarna SK, Dodds WJ. Pharyngeal, esophageal, and proximal gastric responses associated with vomiting. *Am J Physiol* 1993;265: 963–972.

11. Rowe JW, Shelton RL, Helderman JH, et al. Influence of the emetic reflex on vasopressin release in man. *Kidney* 1979;16:729–735.

12. Gieroba ZJ, Blessing WW. Fos-containing neurons in medulla and pons after unilateral stimulation of the afferent abdominal vagus in conscious rabbits. *Neuroscience* 1994;59:851–858.

13. Morrow GR, Rosenthal SN. Models, mechanisms and management of anticipatory nausea and emesis. *Oncology* 1996;53(Suppl 1):4–7.

14. Gutner LB, Gould WJ, Batterman RC. The effects of potent analgesics upon vestibular function. *J Clin Invest* 1952;31:259–266.

15. Boissonade FM, Sharkey KA, Davison JS. Fos expression in ferret dorsal vagal complex after peripheral emetic stimuli. *Am J Physiol* 1994;266:1118–1126.

16. Henrich WL. Autonomic insufficiency. *Arch Intern Med* 1982;142:339–344.

17. Ewing DJ, Campbell IW, Clarke BF. Assessment of cardiovascular effects in diabetic autonomic neuropathy and prognostic implications. *Ann Intern Med* 1980;92:308–311.

18. Kris MG, Yeh HM, Gralla RJ, et al. Symptomatic gastroparesis in cancer patients. A possible cause of cancer associated anorexia [Abstract]. *Proc Am Soc Clin Oncol* 1985;4:267.

19. Bruera E, Chadwick S, Fox R, et al. Study of cardiovascular autonomic insufficiency in advanced cancer patients. *Cancer Treat Rep* 1986;70:1383–1387.

20. Bruera E, Catz Z, Hooper R, et al. Chronic nausea and anorexia in advanced cancer patients: a possible role for autonomic dysfunction. *J Pain Symptom Manage* 1987;2:19–21.

21. Thomas JP, Shields R. Associated autonomic dysfunction and carcinoma of the pancreas. *BMJ* 1970;4:32.

22. Schuffler MD, Baird HW, Fleming CR, et al. Intestinal pseudo-obstruction as the presenting manifestation of small cell carcinoma of the lung. A paraneoplastic neuropathy of the gastrointestinal tract. *Ann Intern Med* 1983;98:129–134.

23. Gould GA, Ashworth M, Lewis GT. Are cardiovascular reflexes more commonly impaired in patients with bronchial carcinoma? *Thorax* 1986;41:372–375.

24. Apfelbaum-Kowalski E, Pakszwer R, Zarchi J, et al. Pathophysiology of the circulatory system in hunger disease. *Curr Concepts Nutr* 1979;7:125–160.

25. Landsberg L, Young JB. Fasting, feeding and regulation of the sympathetic nervous system. *N Engl J Med* 1978;298:1295–1301.

26. Park DM, Johnson RH, Crean GP, et al. Orthostatic hypotension in bronchial carcinoma. *BMJ* 1972;3:510–511.

27. Mamdani MB, Walsh RL, Rubino FA, et al. Autonomic dysfunction and Eaton Lambert syndrome. *J Auton Nerv Syst* 1985;12:315–320.

28. Anderson NE, Rosenblum MK, Graus F, et al. Autoantibodies in paraneoplastic syndromes associated with small-cell lung cancer. *Neurology* 1988;38:1391–1398.

29. Ingham JM, Bernard EJ. Cardiovascular autonomic insufficiency in a patient with metastatic malignancy. *J Pain Symptom Manage* 1995;10:156–160.

30. Roca E, Bruera E, Politi PM, et al. Vinca alkaloid-induced cardiovascular autonomic neuropathy. *Cancer Treat Rep* 1985;69:149–151.

31. Villa A, Foresti V, Confalonieri F. Autonomic neuropathy and HIV infection [Letter]. *Lancet* 1987;2:915.

32. Aldrete JA. Reduction of nausea and vomiting from epidural opioids by adding droperidol to the infusate in home-bound patients. *J Pain Symptom Manage* 1995;10:544–547.

33. Portenoy RK. Management of common opioid side effects during long-term therapy of cancer pain. *Ann Acad Med Singapore* 1994;23:160–170.

34. Baines MJ. ABC of palliative care. Nausea, vomiting, and intestinal obstruction. *BMJ* 1997;315:1148–1150.

35. Carpenter DO, Briggs DB, Strominger N. Peptide-induced emesis in dogs. *Behav Brain Res* 1984;11:277–281.

36. Hagen NA, Foley KM, Cerbone DJ, et al. Chronic nausea and morphine-6-glucuronide. *J Pain Symptom Manage* 1991;6:125–128.

37. Mancini IL, Bruera E. Constipation in advanced cancer patients. *Support Care Cancer* 1998;6:364.

38. Bruera E, Suarez-Almazor M, Velasco A, et al. The assessment of constipation in terminal cancer patients admitted to a palliative care unit: a retrospective review. *J Pain Symptom Manage* 1994;9:515–519.

39. Fainsinger RL, Spachynski K, Hanson J, et al. Symptom control in terminally ill patients with malignant bowel obstruction (MBO). *J Pain Symptom Manage* 1994;9:12–18.

40. Bruera E, Kuehn N, Miller MJ, et al. The Edmonton Symptom Assessment System (ESAS): a simple method for the assessment of palliative care patients. *J Palliat Care* 1991;7:6–9.

41. Chang VT, Hwang SS, Feuerman M. Validation of the Edmonton Symptom Assessment Scale. *Cancer* 2000;88:2164–2171.

42. Kris MG, Gralla RJ, Clark RA, et al. Incidence, course, and severity of delayed nausea and vomiting following the administration of high-dose cisplatin. *J Clin Oncol* 1985;3:1379–1384.

43. Glare P, Pereira G, Kristjanson LJ, et al. Systematic review of the efficacy of antiemetics in the treatment of nausea in patients with far-advanced cancer. *Support Care Cancer* 2004;12(6):432–440.

44. Bentley A, Boyd K. Use of clinical pictures in the management of nausea and vomiting: a prospective audit. *Palliat Med* 2001;15:247–253.

45. Lichter I. Results of anti-emetic management in terminal illness. *J Palliat Care* 1993;9(2):19–21.

46. Bruera E, MacEachern TJ, Spachynski KA, et al. Comparison of the efficacy, safety and pharmacokinetics of controlled release and immediate release metoclopramide for the management of chronic nausea in patients with advanced cancer. *Cancer* 1994;74:3204–3211.

47. Bruera E, Belzile M, Neumann C, et al. A double blind crossover study of controlled release metoclopramide and placebo for the chronic nausea and dyspepsia of advanced cancer. *J Pain Symptom Manage* 2000;19: 427–431.

48. Mystakidou K, Befon S, Liossi C, et al. Comparison of the efficacy and safety of tropisetron, metoclopramide, and chlorpromazine in the treatment of emesis associated with far advanced cancer. *Cancer* 1998;83:1214–1223.

49. Corli O, Cozzolino A, Battaioto L. Effectiveness of levosulpride versus metoclopramide for nausea and vomiting in advanced cancer patients: a double-blind, randomised, cross-over study. *J Pain Symptom Manage* 2001;22:631–633.

50. de Stoutz ND, Bruera E, Suarez-Almazor M. Opioid rotation for toxicity reduction in terminal cancer patients. *J Pain Symptom Manage* 1995;10:378–384.

51. Dickerson D. The 20 essential drugs in palliative care. *Eur J Palliat Care* 1993;6:130–135.

52. Shivshanker K, Bennett RW Jr, Haynie TP. Tumor associated gastroparesis: correction with metoclopramide. *Am J Surg* 1983;145:221–225.

53. McCallum RW, Ricci DA, Rakatansky H, et al. A multicenter placebo-controlled clinical trial of oral metoclopramide in diabetic gastroparesis. *Diabetes Care* 1983;6:463–467.

54. Bruera E, Brenneis C, Michaud M, et al. Continuous Sc infusion of metoclopramide for treatment of narcotic bowel syndrome [Letter]. *Cancer Treat Rep* 1987;71:1121–1122.

55. Robbins E, Nagel J. Haloperidol parenterally for treatment of vomiting and nausea from gastrointestinal disorders in a group of geriatric patients: double blind, placebo controlled study. *J Am Geriatr Soc* 1975;23:38–41.

56. Cole R, Robinson F, Harvey L, et al. Successful control of intractable nausea and vomiting requiring combined ondansetron and haloperidol in a patient with advanced cancer. *J Pain Symptom Manage* 1994;9:48–50.

57. Storey P, Hill HH, St Louis RH, et al. Subcutaneous infusions for control of cancer symptoms. *J Pain Symptom Manage* 1990;5:33–41.

58. Twycross R, Bankby G, Hallwood P. The use of low dose methotrimeprazine (levopromazine) in the management of nausea and vomiting. *Prog Palliat Care* 1997;5:49–53.

59. Passik SD, Lundberg J, Kirsh KL, et al. A pilot exploration of the antiemetic activity of olanzapine for the relief of nausea in patients with advanced cancer and pain. *J Pain Symptom Manage* 2002;23:526–532.

60. Jackson WC, Tavernier L. Olanzapine for intractable nausea in palliative care patients. *J Palliat Med* 2003;6:251–255.

61. Srivastava M, Brito-Dellan N, Davis MP, et al. Olanzapine as an antiemetic in refractory nausea and vomiting in advanced cancer. *J Pain Symptom Manage* 2003;25:578–582.

62. Navari RM, Einhorn LH, Passik SD, et al. A phase II trial of olanzapine for the prevention of chemotherapy-induced nausea and vomiting: a Hoosier Oncology Group study. *Support Care Cancer* 2005;13:529–534.

63. Davis M. Glycopyrrolate: a useful drug in the palliation of mechanical bowel obstruction. *J Pain Symptom Manage* 1999;18:153–154.

64. Ettinger DS. Preventing chemotherapy induced nausea and vomiting: an update and review of emesis. *Semin Oncol* 1995;22:7.

65. Ioannidis JPA, Hesketh PJ, Lau J. Contribution of dexamethasone to control of chemotherapy-induced nausea and vomiting: a meta-analysis of randomized evidence. *Journal of Clinical Oncology* 2000;18:3409–3422.

66. Bruera ED, Roca E, Cedaro L, et al. Improved control of chemotherapy-induced emesis by the addition of dexamethasone to metoclopramide in patients resistant to metoclopramide. *Cancer Treat Rep* 1983;67:381–383.

67. Antiemetic Subcommittee of the Multinational Association of Supportive Care in Cancer (MASCC). Prevention of chemotherapy- and radiotherapy-induced emesis: results of perugia consensus conference. *Ann Oncol* 1998;9:811–819.

68. Mercadante S. Assessment and management of mechanical bowel obstruction. In: Portenoy RK, Bruera E, eds. *Topics in palliative care*. New York: Oxford University Press, 1997:113–130.

69. Moertel CG, Schutt AJ, Reitemeier RJ, et al. Corticosteroid therapy of preterminal gastrointestinal cancer. *Cancer* 1974;33:1607–1609.

70. Willox JC, Corr J, Shaw J, et al. Prednisolone as an appetite stimulant in patients with cancer. *BMJ* 1984;288:27.

71. Bruera E, Roca E, Cedaro L, et al. Action of oral methylprednisolone in terminal cancer patients: a prospective randomized double-blind study. *Cancer Treat Rep* 1985;69:751–754.

72. Hardy J, Daly S, McQuade B, et al. A double-blind, randomised, parallel group, multinational, multicentre study comparing a single dose of ondansetron 24 mg p.o. with placebo and metoclopramide 10 mg t.d.s. p.o. in the treatment of opioid-induced nausea and emesis in cancer patients. *Support Care Cancer* 2002;10:231–236.

73. Sussman G, Shurman J, Creed MR, et al. Intravenous ondansetron for the control of opioid-induced nausea and vomiting. International S3AA3013 study group. *Clin Ther* 1999;21:1216–1227.

74. Korttila K, Clergue F, Leeser J, et al. Intravenous dolasetron and ondansetron in prevention of post operative nausea and vomiting. A multicenter, double-blind, placebo-controlled study. *Acta Anaesthesiol Scand* 1997;41:914–922.

75. Butcher ME. Global experience with ondansetron and future potential. *Oncology* 1993;50:191–197.

76. Pereira J, Bruera E. Successful management of intractable nausea with ondansetron: a case study. *J Palliat Care* 1996;12:47–50.

77. Currow DC, Coughlan M, Fardell B. Use of ondansetron in palliative medicine. *J Pain Symptom Manage* 1997;13:302–307.

78. Ljutic D, Perkovic D, Rumboldt Z, et al. Comparison of ondansetron with metoclopramide in the symptomatic relief of uremia-induced nausea and vomiting. *Kidney Blood Press Res* 2002;25:61–64.

79. Balaskas EV, Bamihas GI, Karamouzis M, et al. Histamine and serotonin in uremic pruritus: effect of ondansetron in CAPD-pruritic patients. *Nephron* 1998;78:395–402.

80. Tchekmedyian NS, Tait N, Moody M, et al. Appetite stimulation with megestrol acetate in cachectic cancer patients. *Semin Oncol* 1986;13:37–43.

81. Cruz JM, Muss HB, Brockschmidt JK, et al. Weight changes in women with metastatic breast cancer treated with megestrol acetate: a comparison of standard versus high-dose therapy. *Semin Oncol* 1990;17:63–67.

82. Tchekmedyian NS, Hickman M, Siau J, et al. Megestrol acetate in cancer anorexia and weight loss. *Cancer* 1992;69:1268–1274.

83. Loprinzi CL, Ellison NM, Schaid DJ, et al. Controlled trial of megestrol acetate for the treatment of cancer anorexia and cachexia. *J Natl Cancer Inst* 1990;82:1127–1132.

84. Loprinzi CL, Michalak JC, Schaid DJ, et al. Phase III evaluation of four doses of megestrol acetate as therapy for patients with cancer anorexia and/or cachexia. *Semin Oncol* 1993;11:762–767.

85. Beller E, Tattersall M, Lumley T, et al. Improved quality of life with megestrol acetate in patients with endocrine-insensitive advanced cancer: a randomised placebo-controlled trial. Australasian Megestrol Acetate Cooperative Study Group. *Ann Oncol* 1997;8:277–283.

86. Heckmayr M, Gatzemeier U. Treatment of cancer weight loss in patients with advanced lung cancer. *Oncology* 1992;49(Suppl 2):32–34.

87. Bruera E, Macmillan K, Kuehn N, et al. A controlled trial of megestrol acetate on appetite, caloric intake, nutritional status, and other symptoms in patients with advanced cancer. *Cancer* 1990;66:1279–1282.

88. Simons JP, Aaronson NK, Vansteenkiste JF, et al. Effects of medroxyprogesterone acetate on appetite, weight, and quality of life in advanced-stage non-hormone-sensitive cancer: a placebo-controlled multicenter study. *J Clin Oncol* 1996;14:1077–1084.

89. Matsumoto S, Kawasaki Y, Mikami M, et al. Relationship between cancer chemotherapeutic drug-induced emesis and plasma levels of substance P in two patients with small cell lung cancer. *Gan To Kagaku Ryoho* 1999;26:535–538.

90. Freed AL, Audus KL, Lunte SM. Investigation of substance P transport across the blood-brain barrier. *Peptides* 2001;23:157–165.

91. Rudd JA, Ngan MP, Wai MK. Inhibition of emesis by tachykinin NK1 receptor antagonists in Suncus murinus (house musk shrew). *Eur J Pharmacol* 1999;366:243–252.

92. Ariumi H, Saito R, Nago S, et al. The role of tachykinin NK-1 receptors in the area postrema of ferrets in emesis. *Neurosci Lett* 2000;286:123–126.

93. Krowicki ZK, Hornby PJ. Substance P in the dorsal motor nucleus of the vagus evokes gastric motor inhibition via neurokinin 1 receptor in rat. *J Pharmacol Exp Ther* 2000;293:214–221.

94. Navari RM. Reduction of cisplatin-induced emesis by a selective neurokinin 1 receptor antagonist. L-754,030 Antiemetics trials Group. *NEJM* 1999;340:190–195.

95. Hesketh PJ, Grunberg SM, Gralla RJ, et al. The oral neurokinin-1 antagonist aprepitant for the prevention of chemotherapy-induced nausea and vomiting: a multinational, randomized, double-blind, placebo-controlled trial in patients receiving high-dose cisplatin–the Aprepitant Protocol 052 Study Group. *J Clin Oncol* 2003;2:4112–4119.

96. de Wit R, Herrstedt J, Rapoport B, et al. Addition of the oral NK1 antagonist aprepitant to standard antiemetics provides protection against nausea and vomiting during multiple cycles of cisplatin-based chemotherapy. *J Clin Oncol* 2003;21:4105–4111.

97. Diemmusnsh P. Antiemetic activity of the NK-1 receptor antagonist GR 205171 in the treatment of established postoperative nausea and vomiting after major gynaecological surgery. *Br J Anaesth* 1999;82:274–276.

98. Tattersall FD, Rycroft W, Francis B, et al. Tachykinin NK1 receptor antagonists act centrally to inhibit emesis induced by the chemotherapeutic agent cisplatin in ferrets. *Neuropharmacol* 1996;35:1121–1129.

99. Hoffman W, Grospietch G, Kuhn W. Genital malformations in thalidomide-damaged girls. *Geburtshilfe Frauenheilkd* 1976;36:1066–1070.

100. Traldi A, Vaccari GL, Davoli G. Use of the imide of N-phthalylglutamic acid (thalidomide) in the symptomatic therapy of vomiting of many patients with malignant neoplasms or caused by the administration of mechlorethamine HCl. *Cancro* 1965;18:336–341.

101. Peuckmann V, Fisch M, Bruera E. Potential novel uses of thalidomide: focus on palliative care. *Drugs* 2000;60:273–292.

102. Gordon JN, Goggin PM. Thalidomide and its derivatives: emerging from the wilderness. *Postgrad Med J* 2003;79:127–132.

103. Hersch EM, Metch BS, Muggia FM, et al. Phase II studies of recombinant TNF in patients with malignant disease: a summary of the Southwest Oncology Group experience. *J Immunother Emphasis Tumor Immunol* 1991;10:426–431.

104. Emch GS, Hermann GE, Rogers RC. TNF-alpha activates solitary nucleus neurons responsive to gastric distension. *Am J Physiol Gastrointest Liver Physiol* 2000;279:582–586.

105. Bruera E, Neumann CM, Pituskin E, et al. Thalidomide in patients with cachexia due to terminal cancer: preliminary report. *Ann Oncol* 1999;10:857–859.

106. Dredge K, Marriott JB, Macdonald CD, et al. Novel thalidomide analogs display anti-angiogenic activity independently of immunomodulatory effects. *Br J Cancer* 2002;87:1166–1172.

107. Lane M, Vogel CL, Ferguson J, et al. Dronabinol and prochlorperazine on combination for treatment of cancer chemotherapy-induced nausea and vomiting. *J Pain Symptom Manage* 1991;6:352–359.

108. Lucas VS, Laszlo J. Delta 9-Tetrahydrocannabinol for refractory vomiting induced by cancer chemotherapy. *JAMA* 1980;243:1241–1243.

109. Gralla R, Tyson L, Bordin L, et al. Antiemetic therapy: a review of recent studies and a report of a random assignment trial comparing metoclopramide with delta-tetra-hydrocannabinol. *Cancer Treat Rep* 1984;68:163–172.

110. Ungerleider J, Andrysiak T, Fairbanks L, et al. Cannabis and cancer chemotherapy: a comparison of oral delta-THC and prochlorperazine. *Cancer* 1982;50:636–645.

111. Beal JE, Olson R, Laubenstein L, et al. Dronabinol as a treatment for anorexia associated with weight loss in patients with AIDS. *J Pain Symptom Manage* 1995;10:89–97.

112. McCallum RW, Soykan I, Sridhar KR, et al. Delta-9-tetrahydrocannabinol delays the gastric emptying of solid food in humans: a double-blind, randomized study. *Aliment Pharmacol Ther* 1999;13:77–80.

113. Krowicki ZK, Moerschbaecher JM, Winsauer PJ, et al. Delta-9-tetrahydrocannabinol inhibits gastric motility in the rat through cannabinoid CB1 receptors. *Eur J Pharmacol* 1999;371:187–196.

114. Matsuda LA, Bonner TI, Lolait SJ. Localization of cannabinoid receptor mRNA in rat brain. *J Comp Neurol* 1993;327:535–550.

115. Baines M, Oliver DJ, Carter RL. Medical management of intestinal obstruction in patients with advanced malignant disease. A clinical and pathological study. *Lancet* 1985;2:990–993.

116. Mercadante S, Maddaloni S. Octreotide in the management of inoperable gastrointestinal obstruction in terminal cancer patients. *J Pain Symptom Manage* 1992;7:496–498.

117. Mercadante S, Ripamonti C, Casuccio A, et al. Comparison of octreotide and hyoscine butylbromide in controlling gastrointestinal symptoms due to malignant inoperable bowel obstruction. *Support Care Cancer* 2000;8:188–191.

118. Ripamonti C, Mercadante S, Groff L, et al. Role of octreotide, scopolamine butylbromide, and hydration in symptom control of patients with inoperable bowel obstruction and nasogastric tubes: a prospective randomized trial. *J Pain Symptom Manage* 2000;19:23–34.

119. Ripamonti C, Conno FD, Ventafridda V, et al. Management of bowel obstruction in advanced and terminal cancer patients. *Ann Oncol* 1993;4:15–21.

120. Lund B, Hansen M, Lundvall F, et al. Intestinal obstruction in patients with advanced carcinoma of the ovaries treated with combination chemotherapy. *Surg Gynecol Obstet* 1989;169:213–218.

CHAPTER 15 ■ DIARRHEA, MALABSORPTION, AND CONSTIPATION

SEBASTIANO MERCADANTE

DIARRHEA

Diarrhea is a common complication in the cancer population, occurring in 5–10% of patients with advanced disease. Women are more likely to have diarrhea than men after excluding gender-specific cancers (1). Diarrhea is also included among the top ten consequences of adverse drug reactions in hospitalized patients with cancer (2). The consequences of diarrhea can be troublesome, and include loss of water, electrolytes, and albumin, failure to reach nutritional goals, declining immune function, and the risk of bedsores or systemic infection. Diarrhea also brings additional work for the nursing staff or family who have to prevent maceration and bedsores. Moreover, losses of comfort and dignity have to be considered. Severe diarrhea, other than being debilitating, is a costly complication of chemotherapy in colorectal cancer. In patients with colorectal cancer receiving chemotherapy, the median length of hospital stay due to diarrhea was 8 days, translating to a mean cost of $8230 per patient (3).

Although a practical definition is lacking, diarrhea is commonly diagnosed when an abnormal increase in daily stool weight, water content, and frequency, whether or not accompanied by urgency, perianal discomfort, or incontinence, is present as a consequence of incomplete absorption of electrolytes and water from luminal content (4). Common causes among patients with cancer are listed in Table 15.1.

Mechanisms

From the physiopathologic point of view, different mechanisms may produce diarrhea, although it is quite difficult in certain clinical conditions to distinguish among mechanisms that frequently overlap.

Osmotic Diarrhea

The ingestion of a poorly absorbable solute modifies the osmolarity of the luminal content and induces osmotic diarrhea. The proximal small bowel is highly permeable to water; sodium and water influx across the duodenum rapidly adjusts the osmolarity of luminal fluid toward that of plasma, secreting water even after the osmolarity values between luminal contents and plasma are similar. On the contrary, the mucosa of the ileum and colon has a low permeability to sodium and solutes. However, there is an efficient active ion transport mechanism that allows the reabsorption of electrolytes and water even against electrochemical gradients (4).

Carbohydrates and proteins are fermented by colonic bacteria and salvaged as short-chain fatty acids and gases. Anaerobic colonic flora are necessary for the fermentation of fiber into short-chain fatty acids and constitute the bulk of fecal mass.

When large amounts of lactulose, an unabsorbable sugar in the small intestine, are ingested, the protective role of colonic bacteria may be exhausted, resulting in severe diarrhea, proportional to the osmotic force of the malabsorbed saccharide (5). It is characterized by an osmotic gap in stool analysis equivalent to the concentration of the osmotically active agents in fecal fluid that cause diarrhea (4). Similarly, carbohydrate malabsorption may induce osmotic diarrhea, which is characterized by a low stool pH, because of the presence of short-chain fatty acids, a high content of carbohydrates, high stool osmolarity, and flatulence. Moreover, reversible chemotherapy-related hypolactasia and lactose intolerance are not infrequent in patients treated with 5-fluorouracil (5-FU)–based adjuvant chemotherapy for colorectal cancer. Avoidance of lactose during chemotherapy may improve treatment tolerability in these patients (6).

The ingestion of other substances, such as magnesium, sulfate, and poorly absorbed salts may produce osmotic diarrhea. However, there will be a normal pH, unlike in carbohydrate-induced diarrhea. In the perioperative period, massive antibiotic therapy is able to suppress normal colonic metabolism, thereby resulting in diarrhea (5). Osmotic diarrhea commonly subsides as the patient discontinues the poorly absorbable agents.

Secretory Diarrhea

Secretory diarrhea is rarely present as the sole mechanism and is often associated with other mechanisms (5). This kind of diarrhea is associated with an abnormal ion transport in intestinal epithelial cells, with a reduction in absorptive function or increase in the secretion of epithelial cells.

TABLE 15.1

CAUSES OF DIARRHEA IN PATIENTS WITH CANCER

Drugs
Endocrine tumors
Malabsorption
Chemotherapy
Radiotherapy
Concurrent diseases

Unlike in osmotic diarrhea, the anionic gap is small and eating does not markedly increase stool volume. Moreover, diarrhea usually persists despite fasting.

Many factors may affect ion transport in the epithelial cells of the gut. These include bacterial toxins, intraluminal secretagogues (such as bile acids or laxatives) or circulating secretagogues (such as various hormones, drugs, and poisons). Moreover, other medical problems that compromise regulation of intestinal function or reduce absorptive surface area (by disease or resection) can induce secretory diarrhea (7).

Endocrine tumors may cause diarrhea through the release of secretagogue transmitters (8). Diarrhea is a common manifestation of a carcinoid syndrome, occurring in approximately 70% of patients, and seems to be mediated by the release of serotonin and substance P. In the Zollinger-Ellison syndrome, secretory diarrhea is the consequence of gastric hypersecretion caused by a high concentration of circulating gastrin, overwhelming the intestinal absorptive capacity. In a medullary carcinoma of the thyroid, circulating calcitonin is the major mediator of intestinal secretion (4).

Malabsorption due to different mechanisms may equally produce diarrhea (9) (see section on Malabsorption).

Cancer treatment–related diarrhea caused by acute and chemotherapeutic agents such as fluoropyrimidines, paclitaxel, and irinotecan, (3) and graft versus host disease (GVHD) (10) significantly affects morbidity and mortality. Diarrhea is a significant consequence of colorectal chemotherapy, with most patients experiencing grade 3 or 4 diarrhea. Severe diarrhea developed after the first cycle of chemotherapy in 58% of the patients and contributed to a dose reduction, change, or discontinuation of chemotherapy in 9.5, 15.9 and 34.2% of patients, respectively (3). These agents cause acute and chronic damage to the intestinal mucosa, necrosis, and extensive inflammation of the bowel wall. Mucosal and submucosal factors, produced directly or indirectly by the inflamed intestine, stimulate secretion of intestinal fluid and electrolytes. Delayed-onset diarrhea, with an incidence of 20–35% at grade 3–4 level is one of the most important causes of dose-limiting toxicity of irinotecan (11). Similar anatomic changes have been observed in patients with GVHD diarrhea, as well as with radiation enteritis (12). The toxicity grades of these agents seem to depend on individual genotypes (13).

On the other hand, intestinal mucositis also increases the risk of superinfection by opportunistic pathogens such as *Clostridium difficile, Clostridium perfringens, Bacillus cereus, Giardia lamblia, Cryptosporidium, Salmonella, Shigella, Campylobacter,* and *Rotavirus,* particularly in patients who may be neutropenic or immunosuppressed. Bacterial enterotoxins or other infective agents induce secretion probably by a local nervous reflex mediated by enteroendocrine cells or inflammation (4). The incidence of *C. difficile*–induced diarrhea is very high—2.2% in patients receiving standard-dose regimens and 20% in patients receiving high-dose regimens (14).

The use of long-term antibiotics is also associated with diarrhea in patients who recently underwent surgery or are immunocompromised. Agents more frequently causing diarrhea include ampicillin, clindamycin, or cephalosporins, because of the disruption of the normal flora and facilitation of the overgrowth of pathogens. *C. difficile,* an anaerobic organism producing an enteric toxin, induces pseudomembranous enterocolitis, which presents as a severe microbial diarrhea. Other infective agents include *C. perfringens, Staphylococcus aureus, Klebsiella oxytoca,* candida species, and salmonella species (15).

Finally, many drugs may cause diarrhea. Diuretics, caffeine, theophylline, antacids, antibiotics, and poorly absorbable laxative agents and osmotically active solutes, often chronically administered in a palliative care setting, likely produce reflex nervous secretion or directly activate secretory cellular mechanism (4).

Deranged Motility

Defective motility may reduce the contact time between luminal contents and epithelial cells. This commonly occurs in patients with cancer with postsurgical disorders, such as postgastrectomy dumping syndrome, postvagotomy, ileocecal valve resection or neoplastic and chronic diseases, such as malignant carcinoid syndrome, medullary carcinoma of the thyroid, and diabetes. The mechanism by which diabetic neuropathy causes dysmotility is attributed to a sympathetic denervation of the bowel with a prevalence of cholinergic innervation (15). Similarly, procedures such as celiac plexus block produce a sympathetic denervation of the bowel, which may leave a cholinergic innervation unopposed, leading to an increase in intestinal motility and diarrhea, until adaptation mechanisms develop (4).

Spinal cord damage may reduce intestinal mobility favoring bacterial overgrowth, which induces a deconjugation of bile acids in the small bowel and thereby causes diarrhea and steatorrhea. Diarrhea secondary to dysmotility disorders commonly subsides after a 1–2-day fast, determining a small stool volume and an osmolality in the range of 250–300 mOsm.

Assessment

The patient should be questioned in detail about dietary habits, the use of drugs, and previous surgery. Frequency, amounts, and consistency of the stools should be carefully obtained. When the stools are consistently large, light in color, watery or greasy, free of blood, or contain undigested food particles, the underlying disorder is likely to be in the small bowel or the proximal colon. Indeed, small stool diarrhea, in which frequent but small quantities of feces that are dark in color and often contain mucus or blood pass in spite of a sense of urgency, is associated with a disorder of the left colon or rectum (4). Widespread inflammation may simultaneously produce both patterns of diarrhea, confirmed by the passage of nonbloody diarrheal fluid, pus, or exudates. Other useful information includes fecal incontinence, change in stool caliber, rectal bleeding, and small, frequent, but otherwise normal stools.

Timing and spontaneous recovery are also important. Although osmotic diarrhea typically stops or reduces after fasting or stopping the drug previously used, secretory diarrhea persists in spite of fasting. Chemotherapy-induced diarrhea typically occurs 2–14 days after therapy. Radiation colitis is probable in patients who have recently received pelvic radiation for malignancies of the urogenital tract and of the prostate.

A physical examination should precede any further investigation. Signs of anemia, fever, postural hypotension, lymphadenopathy, neuropathy, hepatosplenomegaly, ascites, gaseous abdominal distention or lymphadenopathy, reduced anal sphincter tone, a rectal mass or impaction, and deterioration of nutritional status are of paramount importance in defining the type of diarrhea. Some etiologies may have a typical clinical pattern. For example, carbohydrate malabsorption is typically associated with excessive flatus and mushy stools, whereas intermittent diarrhea and constipation are frequent in diabetic neuropathy, as well as in irritable bowel syndrome or subobstructive disorders. Autonomic neuropathy or anal sphincter dysfunction may be characterized by nocturnal diarrhea and fecal soiling. Alternating diarrhea and constipation suggests fixed colonic obstruction. Fecal impaction may cause apparent diarrhea because only liquids pass a partial obstruction. Symptoms of dumping syndrome after gastric surgery, such as early nausea, abdominal distention, weakness, and diarrhea after a meal followed by hypoglycemia, sweating, dizziness, and tachycardia, are typical. Secretory diarrhea combined with upper gastrointestinal (GI) symptoms caused by refractory peptic ulcer disease is suggestive of a gastrin-secreting tumor. High circulating serotonin levels in carcinoid syndrome cause other effects besides diarrhea, including hypotension, sweating, flushing, palpitation, and wheeziness (4,15). The association of heat intolerance, palpitations, and weight loss suggests possible hyperthyroidism. Intestinal dysmotility or bacterial overgrowth due to diabetes, neoplastic conditions, or postoperative conditions should be suspected, excluding other causes.

Chronic bowel ischemia should be considered in elderly patients with the clinical features of diffuse atherosclerotic disease. Rectal examination and abdominal palpation should be performed to look for fecal masses and to exclude fecal impaction and intestinal obstruction, as well as for perianal fistula or abscess. Rectal involvement is probable in the presence of *tenesmus*, commonly defined as the passing of a little or no stool in spite of a sense of rectal urgency.

Of course, the site of neoplasm and metastases is of paramount importance. An abdominal x-ray will help the diagnosis. The location of the tumor will be verified by computed tomography scan, magnetic resonance imaging, angiography, or laparoscopy.

Laboratory findings should complete the investigation. If feasible, collected diarrhea stool specimen should be submitted for qualitative study. A positive finding in either the stool guaiac or leukocyte test leads to a suspicion of an exudative mechanism, as in radiation colitis, colonic neoplasm, or infective diarrhea. Stool cultures for bacterial, fungal, and viral pathogens, as well as a formal evaluation of the GI tract should complete the initial assessment (12). Gram stain of the stool can diagnose the presence of *Staphylococcus*, *Campylobacter*, or *Candida* infection. Multiple stool cultures should be obtained from patients with secretory diarrhea to rule out microorganisms producing enterotoxins that stimulate intestinal secretion. The presence of a microorganism in the stools is diagnostic.

An anion gap of >50 mmol per L due to a reduction of stool content in sodium and potassium suggests an osmotic diarrhea, whereas lower values (<50 mmol per L) indicate a secretory diarrhea due to active secretion of salts and water.

Treatment

As a general rule, current medication should be revised, considering the use of laxatives, antacids, theophylline preparations, central nervous system drugs, antiarrhythmics, and antibiotics. Dietary advice may be helpful in some circumstances, although difficult to follow by most patients with cancer. A gluten-free diet can reduce abdominal cramping and frequency of bowel movement in the presence of intestinal fermentation with bowel distention. Binders of osmotically active substances (kaolin-pectin) give a thicker consistency to loose stools, producing a viscous, colloidal, absorbent solution, but their antidiarrheal effectiveness is disputable. Apples without the peel are particularly rich in pectin. Other dietary advice include avoiding cold meals, milk, vegetables rich in fibers, fatty meat and fish, coffee, and alcohol.

As diarrhea is associated with the occurrence of dehydration, the patient should be rehydrated, possibly by oral solutions containing glucose, electrolytes, and water. However, clinical signs of dehydration, such as orthostatic hypotension, decreased skin turgor, and a dry mouth, suggest the need for intensive hydration by intravenous route, especially in patients

TABLE 15.2

ETIOLOGY-BASED TREATMENT

Etiology	Treatment
All conditions	Dietary advice, adequate hydration
Radiation-induced diarrhea	Hypofractionated-accelerated radiotherapy and amifostine
	Cholestyramine, aspirin, sucralphate, silicate smectite, steroids
Bacterial overgrowth–related diarrhea	Antibiotics
Antibiotic-associated diarrhea	Discontinuation of antibiotics, start with metronidazole
	Probiotic bacteria
Chemotherapy-induced diarrhea	Alkalization, activated charcoal, loperamide, octreotide
Hormonal gastrointestinal tumors	Octreotide
Diabetic diarrhea	Clonidine

suffering from nausea and vomiting, in whom oral therapy is ineffective (4).

Considering the different mechanisms involved in determining diarrhea in patients with cancer, there are no broadly accepted treatment protocols. Particular strategies have been anecdotally suggested for specific etiologies (Table 15.2). Cholestyramine, aspirin, and sucralfate have been favorably used in radiation-induced diarrhea (16). Silicate smectite has proved a promising drug in the prophylaxis of radiotherapy-induced diarrhea, particularly in patients with a low, irradiated, small bowel volume (17). From recent investigations it seems that the best treatment would be prevention. In gynecologic malignancies, prior operation with low pelvic fields and prior operation with small volume were significantly protective factors for overall diarrhea. Conversely, large volume was a significant factor of overall and moderate to severe diarrhea in patients with large-field operations (18). Hypofractionated and accelerated radiotherapy for prostate cancer were supported with high-dose daily amifostine (1000 mg s.c.) to protect normal tissues against early and late effects, and produced only grade 0–1 cystitis or diarrhea (5/7 grade 0). Amifostine tolerance was excellent (19).

Steroids may exert a positive effect on several conditions associated with diarrhea, including secretory diarrhea, intestinal pseudo-obstruction, radiation-induced enteritis, endocrine tumors due to anti-inflammatory effects, and the capability of reducing the release and effect of inflammation mediators, and promoting salts and water absorption. They are also included in the pharmacologic approach to GVHD-induced diarrhea (12). Budesonide, a topically active steroid, demonstrated a substantial activity in irinotecan and 5-FU–induced diarrhea after failure of loperamide treatment (20).

Antibiotics, such as norfloxacin and amoxicillin-clavulanic acid, are effective in the treatment of bacterial overgrowth–related diarrhea (21). On the contrary, antibiotic-associated diarrhea (pseudomembranous enterocolitis) requires the discontinuation of antibiotics and the starting of either metronidazole or vancomycin (22). Bismuth subsalicylate in doses of 30–60 mL every 30 minutes for eight doses may bring mild symptomatic relief in patients with acute infectious diarrhea with an unknown effect (4). Probiotic bacteria (i.e., live bacteria that survive passage through the GI tract) may have beneficial effects on the host. In a recent review, probiotic bacteria consistently shortened the diarrheal phase of rotavirus infection, although the evidence for other viral or bacterial infections was less strong (23).

Alkalization of the intestinal tract by oral administration of sodium bicarbonate has been reported to be a promising method for preventing delayed diarrhea, a dose-limiting toxicity in patients receiving chemotherapy with irinotecan, without decreasing the blood levels of irinotecan and its active metabolites, thereby improving the tolerability of long-term chemotherapy without reducing the efficacy (24). An oral adsorbent (2 g Kremezin × three times) has been shown to decrease the number of bowel motions, without decreasing the plasma clearance of irinotecan much (25). Activated charcoal, given the evening before the irinotecan dose and then t.i.d. for 48 hours after the dose, reduced irinotecan-induced diarrhea and optimized its dose-intensity, possibly by adsorbing free lumenal SN-38, the irinotecan-active moiety that has a direct effect on mucosal topoisomerase-I (11). Broad-spectrum antibiotics may influence the intestinal toxicity of irinotecan. Although neomycin had no effect on the systemic exposure of irinotecan and its major metabolites, it changed fecal β-glucuronidase activity and decreased fecal concentrations of the pharmacologically active metabolite SN-38. It was associated with an improvement in diarrhea and not with hematologic toxicity, suggesting that bacterial β-glucuronidase plays a crucial role in irinotecan-induced diarrhea without affecting enterocyclic and systemic SN-38 levels (26).

Novel experimental substances may have relevance in this context. RDP58 is an anti-inflammatory agent that inhibits the production of tumor necrosis factor-α, interferon-γ, and interleukin-12. In animals, oral administration of RDP58 significantly decreased the incidence of diarrhea and improved the survival rates of mice treated with toxic doses of irinotecan or 5-FU. RDP58 may have clinical utility in cancer therapy by preventing treatment-associated GI toxicity and potentially increasing the effectiveness of chemotherapy (27).

Clonidine, an α2-agonist, has been reported to be useful in controlling diarrhea in patients with diabetes or in patients with chronic idiopathic secretory diarrhea who presumably present a denervation sympathetic supersensitivity. However, hypotension and sedation may limit the usefulness of clonidine in dehydrated patients or patients with advanced cancer (4).

Opioids have been traditionally used for their antidiarrheal properties owing to the widespread presence of opioid receptors at different peripheral sites, including smooth muscle, myenteric plexus, and spinal cord. It is well known that their activation increases ileocecal tone and decreases small intestine and colon peristalsis (increasing electrolyte and water absorption), also impairing the defecation reflex by inhibiting anorectal sphincteric relaxation and diminishing anorectal sensitivity to distention. As a consequence, the contact time between intestinal mucosa and luminal contents is enhanced by the reduction of colonic propulsive activity, resulting in greater fluid absorption (4). Antidiarrheal effects can be obtained by both oral and parenteral opioids. Among opioids, loperamide is more specific because of the prevalent peripheral effect due to the inability to cross the blood–brain barrier. Loperamide shows the highest antidiarrheal/analgesic ratio among the opioid-like agents and is proved to be the drug of choice because of its few adverse effects. The standard dose of loperamide is 4 mg followed by 2 mg after every unformed stool. The dosage is titrated against the effect and higher doses of 2 mg every 2 hours have been recommended (up to 12 mg per day or more) in conjunction with chemotherapeutic agents associated with a high incidence of diarrhea (28). Loperamide-simethicone combination was significantly more effective than the drugs taken alone in the treatment of acute diarrhea with gas-related abdominal discomfort (29). However, the risk of developing paralytic ileus in the presence of continuous secretion, should be considered as a life-threatening complication. Of interest, opioids may paradoxically cause diarrhea secondary to fecal impaction.

Data from several clinical trials suggest that octreotide may be useful in the symptomatic treatment of diarrhea refractory to other medications (28,30). The mechanism by which octreotide produces these beneficial effects is probably multifactorial, as it suppresses the secretion of many of the gut peptides implicated in the control of secretory and motor activity, and inhibits exocrine secretions from the stomach, pancreas, and small intestine, also facilitating water and electrolyte absorption (31). Octreotide has been found to control diarrhea in several conditions, such as carcinoid tumors, vipoma, gastrinoma, small cell lung cancer, as well as acquired immunodeficiency syndrome–related diarrhea (32). However, hormonal responses to the somatostatin analog do not always parallel clinical responses, probably because of the effects of cosecreted peptides. A dose-response effect of octreotide has been demonstrated. Octreotide seems to be an effective agent in the management of chemotherapy-related diarrhea and refractory GVHD-associated diarrhea (33,34). Doses of 0.3–1.2 mg a day subcutaneously are commonly effective.

Long-acting, biodegradable, microsphere formulation of octreotide for monthly subcutaneous administration (30 mg) has been evaluated for the prophylaxis of diarrhea, speeding the resolution of diarrhea and preventing further episodes during subsequent cycles of chemotherapy (35). A preventive strategy with octreotide LAR as prophylaxis has been proposed for patients with a prior cycle of chemotherapy complicated by persistent diarrhea (36).

MALABSORPTION

An ineffective absorption of breakdown products in the small intestine may occur either because a disorder interferes with the digestion of food or directly with the absorption of nutrients. The digestive and absorptive processes are inextricably linked. The series of events include the reduction of particle size, solubilization of hydrophobic lipids and enzymatic digestion of nutrients to small fragments, absorption of the products of digestion across the intestinal cells, and transport through lymphatics.

Physiopathology of Digestion

The pancreatic secretion of lipase, amylase, and proteases breaks down fat to monoglycerides and fatty acids, carbohydrates to mono- and disaccharides, and proteins to peptides and amino acids. Several processes have been recognized to facilitate the absorption of fat from the aqueous luminal environment. Triglycerides are emulsified together with phospholipids, bile salts, and mono- and diglycerides and dispersed into a variety of phases and particles. Lipid digestion begins in the mouth and in the stomach, active at a low pH, promoting emulsion stability and facilitating the action of pancreatic lipases. Gastric and pyloric motility further promotes emulsification of lipids. This effect is amplified by bile salts and biliary phospholipids, which also influence the absorption of cholesterol and sterol vitamins. Lipolysis to fatty acids and monoglycerides is mediated by pancreatic lipases (4). Protein digestion begins in the stomach. Acid denaturation leads to proteolysis, which is promoted by endopeptidases activated by an acid environment, cleaving the internal bonds of large proteins to form nonabsorbable peptides. Pancreatic peptidases convert proteins and polypeptides into amino acids and oligopeptides. Hormonal and neural stimulation stimulates the release of proenzymes by the pancreas. Enteropeptidases and trypsin activate a cascade of events that promotes the activation of chymotrypsin, elastase, and carboxypeptidase A and B in the duodenum. Digestion of carbohydrates has been described in the section on Osmotic Diarrhea.

The hydrolysis of fat, protein, and carbohydrate by pancreatic enzymes, and the solubilization of fat by bile salts, may be altered by several conditions (4,37). In pancreatic carcinoma or following pancreatic resection, decreased pancreatic enzymes and bicarbonate release may limit the digestion of fat and protein, leading to pancreatic insufficiency. These disorders may also be associated with malabsorption of fat-soluble vitamins. The Zollinger-Ellison syndrome is characterized by an extreme acid hypersecretion, causing a low luminal pH, which inactivates pancreatic enzymes with consequent fat malabsorption. A decrease in intraluminal bile salts due to disruption of the enterohepatic circulation is also seen in patients with Zollinger-Ellison syndrome. Biliary tract obstruction, terminal ileal resection, or cholestatic liver disease results in decreased formation of bile salts or delivery to the duodenum (38). Many postsurgical disorders have been associated with a marked proliferation of intraluminal microorganisms, including an afferent loop of a Billroth II partial gastrectomy, a surgical blind loop with end-to-side anastomosis, or a recirculating loop with side-to-side anastomosis. The final consequence depends on the extension of resection. With limited small bowel resections, malabsorbed bile acids pass into the colon and increase colon motility while decreasing water and electrolyte absorption, resulting in diarrhea. In contrast, after massive small bowel resection, the bile acid pool will decrease because of the loss of intestinal bile salts. This phenomenon is associated with a loss of the absorptive intestinal surface and bacterial overgrowth. These processes will result in steathorrea (47). Bacterial overgrowth causes catabolism of carbohydrates by gram-negative aerobes, deconjugation of bile salts by anaerobes, and the binding of cobalamin by anaerobes. Other than massive resection involving the ileocecal calve, causes of bacterial overgrowth include obstruction or strictures and autonomic neuropathy.

Physiopathology of Absorption

Products of digestion are normally absorbed from the lumen through the enterocyte to appear in the lymphatics or the portal vein. This passage is specific for each digested substance, according to the circumstances. Active transport requires energy to move nutrients against a gradient, whereas passive diffusion allows nutrients to pass according to gradient differentials. Facilitated diffusion is an intermediate mechanism, similar to passive diffusion, but carrier-mediated and subject to competitive inhibition. Endocytosis is a process in which parts of a cell membrane engulf nutrients.

Carbohydrate absorption occurs as monosaccharides, predominantly in the proximal small intestine, although not all the dietary carbohydrate is absorbed. The simple diffusion of monosaccharides across membranes is slow but important in the presence of high luminal concentrations of glucose. When luminal concentrations of glucose are low, specific active transport systems, especially through sodium-coupled transporters, mediate efficient transport of these substances. Monosaccharides may also enter enterocytes by facilitated diffusion. However, the uptake may be limited by enzyme activity, for example, lactase. Xylose is not digested and has a low affinity for carriers. Some of the carbohydrates reach the colon and are fermented by bacteria into short-chain fatty acids

with the production of gases such as hydrogen and methane. Short-chain fatty acids are subsequently absorbed by colonic epithelial cells.

Fat products rapidly diffuse passively into enterocytes, with the rate of transfer depending on the chain length. Fatty acids and monoglycerides are metabolized into triglycerides and assembled with phospholipids and cholesterol esters into chylomicrons. Short- and medium-chain fatty acids have a less complex absorptive mechanism. They may be absorbed intact by passive diffusion or completely hydrolyzed, but they are not re-esterified inside the enterocytes. Lipid absorption is highly efficient; only small amounts of lipids enter the colon. These may be absorbed by the colonic mucosa or undergo bacterial metabolism.

Bile salts are synthesized from cholesterol in the liver, conjugated with amino acids, secreted into the bile, and recycled back to the liver through the portal system. Minimal daily losses are balanced by hepatic synthesis. Passive diffusion and active transport are involved in bile salt transport in the small intestine to limit fecal loss. A certain amount of bile salt in the colonic lumen is essential for normal colonic function. In the colon, bile salts are not absorbed but they stimulate colonic motility and secretion of sodium chloride and water. In contrast, bile salt deficiency may cause constipation (4).

Amino acids are absorbed by enterocytes, oligopeptides are digested by the enterocyte, and brush border by oligo- or dipeptidases. A specific transport mechanism exists for the intracellular transport of amino acids and dipeptides. Protein absorption is efficient and occurs mainly in the jejunum and ileum (39).

Mucosal damage, as observed with radiation enteritis, may impair epithelial cell transport. Other than extensive mucosal damage, lymphatic obstruction and bacterial overgrowth are the principal mechanisms of radiation-induced malabsorption.

A large surgical resection of the small intestine reduces the epithelial surface area available for absorption. The extent and specific level of resection are predictive of severe malabsorption and short-bowel syndrome. Most patients with short-bowel syndrome have either a high jejunostomy with a residual jejunal length <100 cm or a jejunocolic anastomosis. The recovery from massive small bowel resection depends on the adaptive response of the remaining mucosa (39). Resection of >50% of the small intestine still results in significant malabsorption. The inclusion of the distal two thirds of the ileum and ileocecal sphincter in the resected section increases the risk of malabsorption. Preservation of the ileocecal sphincter is important because it may prevent small bowel contamination from colonic flora and may increase the transit time of the intraluminal content.

After intestinal resections, increased amount of bile salts reach the colon, promoting water and electrolyte secretion, unless liver production compensates the losses, as in limited resections. The consequent lack of solubilization of intraluminal fat will worsen the effects of bile salts on the colon mucosa. Enterostomy or intestinal fistulae may also result in a reduced absorption due to the loss of intestinal surface area. A vagotomy may increase the colonic content of bile acids because of an accelerated transit time. Diabetic neuropathy may result in intestinal dysmotility and bacterial overgrowth, and as a consequence, in malabsorption.

Lymphatic transport of chylomicrons and proteins is limited by lymphatic obstruction, leading to dilatation and potential rupture of intestinal lymphatic vessels, causing intestinal leakage of proteins, chylomicrons, and small lymphocytes. Localized ileal tumors, diffuse intestinal lymphomas, metastatic carcinoma, and metastatic carcinoid disease may all lead to lymphatic obstruction, fat malabsorption, and protein-losing enteropathy (4).

Assessment

Patients with malabsorption usually lose weight. If fats are not properly absorbed, the stools are light-colored, soft, bulky, and foul smelling. Documentation of steatorrhea is the cornerstone of the diagnostic evaluation. Malabsorption can cause deficiencies of all nutrients or proteins, fats, vitamins, or minerals selectively. Certain physical signs are frequently associated with specific deficiency states secondary to malabsorption, such as glossitis in folate or vitamin B_{12} deficiency, hyperkeratosis, ecchymoses, and hematuria due to fat-soluble vitamin deficiency (vitamins A and K). Anemia (chronic blood loss or malabsorption of iron, folate, or vitamin B_{12}), leukocytosis with eosinophilia, low serum levels or albumin, iron, cholesterol, and an extension of the prothrombin time are the most common laboratory findings in malabsorption (4). Impaired absorption of calcium and magnesium may induce weakness, paresthesias, and tetany. Osteopenia and bone pain, spontaneous fractures, and vertebral collapse may develop from vitamin D and calcium deficiency. Peripheral neuropathy may occur after gastric resection because of vitamin B_{12} deficiency. Weakness, severe weight loss, and fatigue result from caloric deprivation. In pancreatic carcinoma, floating, bulky, and malodorous stools and increased gas production are often associated with anorexia. Steatorrhea, peripheral lymphocytopenia, hypoalbuminemia, chylous ascites, and peripheral edema are the hallmarks of abnormalities of lymphatic transport. Symptoms of dumping syndrome after gastrectomy include early nausea, abdominal distention, weakness, and diarrhea after a meal, followed by hypoglycemia, sweating, dizziness, and tachycardia.

Other symptoms depend on the disorder that is causing the malabsorption. For example, an obstructed bile duct may cause jaundice; poor blood supply to the intestine may cause abdominal pain.

Malabsorption is suspected when an individual loses weight and has diarrhea and nutritional deficiencies despite eating well, although weight loss alone can have other causes in patients with cancer.

Reviewing current drugs is important in the diagnostic evaluation. Colchicine, neomycin, and clindamycin are the most common drugs causing malabsorption, although the pathophysiologic mechanisms are unknown. Dietary phosphate absorption may be limited by the use of aluminum-containing antacids, resulting in hypophosphatemia and hypercalciuria.

Laboratory tests can help confirm the diagnosis. Tests that directly measure fat in stool samples are the most reliable ones for diagnosing malabsorption of fat. Other laboratory tests can detect malabsorption of other specific substances, such as lactose or vitamin B_{12}. Undigested food fragments may mean that food passes through the intestine too rapidly. Such fragments also can indicate an anatomically abnormal intestinal pathway, such as a direct connection between the stomach and the large intestine that bypasses the small intestine. Small intestinal barium x-rays may define anatomic abnormalities after massive resection. Biochemical examination of the fecal material may give information about the origin of a fistula (pancreatic or enteric). Liver function tests and imaging of the liver or biliary tract may demonstrate parenchymal liver disease as a cause of decreased production of bile salts or a biliary tract obstruction (Table 15.3).

Treatment

After assessing the causes of malabsorption, therapy should be directed to correct the deficiencies, including enzyme replacement, bicarbonate supplements, vitamins, calcium,

---

TABLE 15.3

MALABSORPTION: SIGNS, SYMPTOMS, AND TREATMENT

- Steatorrhea
- Weight loss, weakness, fatigue (caloric deprivation)
- Glossitis (folate or vitamin B_{12} deficiency)
- Hyperkeratosis, ecchymoses, and hematuria (vitamins A and K deficiency)
- Weakness, paresthesias, and tetany (calcium and magnesium deficiencies)
- Early nausea, abdominal distention, weakness, and diarrhea after a meal, followed by hypoglycemia, sweating, dizziness, and tachycardia (after gastric resection)
- Osteopenia and bone pain, spontaneous fractures (vitamin D and calcium deficiencies)
- Chylous ascites—peripheral edema (abnormalities of lymphatic transport)
- Peripheral neuropathy (vitamin B_{12} deficiency)
- Laboratory findings: anemia (iron, folate, or vitamin B_{12} deficiencies) leukocytosis with eosinophilia, peripheral lymphocytopenia, hypoalbuminemia

---

magnesium, and iron. Pancreatic enzyme replacement along with a low-fat, high-protein diet is indicated in the case of malabsorption due to pancreatic insufficiency. The effectiveness of enzyme replacements is variable and, in part, depends on a high enough gastric pH to prevent their degradation in the stomach (40). Large doses of pancreatic extract are required with each meal. Sodium and bicarbonate or anti-H_2 inhibitors and hydrogen-pump inhibitors are mainly added to raise the duodenal pH.

Fat intake should be strictly limited, especially in short-bowel syndrome. Medium-chain triglycerides may be substituted for long-chain triglycerides to improve fat absorption after a small intestinal resection, and they are useful in the presence of lymphatic obstruction because they do not require intestinal lymphatic transport.

For patients with prominent dumping, dietary modification comprising frequent small, dry meals that are high in protein and low in carbohydrates, along with ingestion of substances that prolong the absorption of carbohydrates, such as pectin, may be useful (4).

An aggressive approach should be reserved in the presence of severe malnutrition and dehydration, especially after surgery. Parenteral nutrition is strongly indicated in the immediate postoperative period after massive intestinal resection. The duration of parenteral nutrition is inversely proportional to the length of the remaining intestine. The weaning to oral nutrition depends on several variables including the preoperative nutritional state, the absorptive deficit, and the tolerance to oral intake. Oral feeding should be started as soon as possible, as adaptation of the remaining bowel to resection is facilitated by the early introduction of oral or enteral nutrients. Moreover, intraluminal nutrients stimulate trophic GI hormones regulating mucosal repair. H_2-blocking agents may also favorably influence the rate of adaptation of the remaining intestine after massive resection, possibly by a mucosal trophic effect improving nutrient absorption. Nutrients requiring minimal digestion for absorption should be chosen, such as commercial preparations containing simple sugars, amino acids, or oligopeptides, as well as medium-chain triglycerides. An excessive osmolar load should be avoided to prevent the occurrence of diarrhea. More complex food should be added gradually.

Vitamin B_{12} replacement is necessary after terminal ileal resection. H_2 blockers are used to treat the transient acid hypersecretion after extensive bowel resection or the acid hypersecretion state in patients with gastrinoma (Zollinger-Ellison syndrome) (39). Hydrogen-pump inhibitors produce a greater antisecretory effect than that achieved by H_2-antagonist drugs alone. The use of cholestyramine should be carefully considered. It may be indicated in limited intestinal resections because it binds bile salts and prevents their irritant effects on the colon. However, in short-bowel syndrome after massive intestinal resection, it may reduce the bile salt pool, thereby increasing fat malabsorption. The dose suggested is 4 g three times daily before meals. Aluminum hydroxide exerts similar effects.

Antibiotic-associated malnutrition requires discontinuation of any implicated antimicrobial agents. However, if there is stasis with bacterial overgrowth caused by impaired motility or stricture, such as in radiation enteritis or blind loop syndrome, broad-spectrum antibiotics should be administered. A 10-day course of cephalosporin and metronidazole seems to be effective in suppressing the flora and correcting malabsorption. However, cyclic therapy may be needed (39).

In patients affected by malabsorption due to short-bowel syndrome, it is useful to reduce the intestinal output or the transit time. Loperamide can delay the transit time or reduce secretions (4). Octreotide has been used because of their ability to reduce gastric, pancreatic, and biliary secretions, as well as intestinal transit time (31). Dosages from 0.2–0.6 mg daily have been advocated. It may reduce or shorten the use of parenteral administration in several postoperative conditions, such as enterocutaneous or pancreatic fistulae. Its use in terminally ill patients has been favorably reported (30).

Reversal of a short segment of the bowel or construction of a recirculating loop have been advocated in patients with life-threatening malabsorption and uncontrolled weight loss. However, such operations may have negative consequences, as they can lead to stasis and bacterial overgrowth, further compromising intestinal absorption. More often the benefit is of limited value (4).

CONSTIPATION

Constipation is extremely common in patients with cancer, especially in the advanced stages of disease. The range of prevalence in hospitalized patients receiving cancer treatment varies from 70–10% (41), and is reported by approximately 50% of hospice patients at admission (1,42). Moreover, constipation is considered the first cause of adverse drug reactions in hospitalized patients with cancer (2).

In addition to causing discomfort, constipation affects daily living, nutrition intake, and socialization, therefore compromising quality of life. Untreated constipation may progress to obstipation, which may potentially lead to life-threatening complications associated with bowel obstruction (4).

Pathophysiology

There are many, often concomitant, causes of constipation in patients with cancer (Table 15.4). Constipation may be secondary to systemic diseases or those solely afflicting the GI tract. It may be due directly to a cancer or to secondary effects of the cancer. Furthermore, a great number of substances are known to cause medication-induced constipation, that is, opioid-induced constipation is caused by linkage of the opioid-to-opioid receptors in the bowel and the central nervous system.

TABLE 15.4

CAUSES OF CONSTIPATION IN PATIENTS WITH CANCER

Neurogenic disorders
  Periphery
    Ganglionopathy
    Autonomic neuropathy
  Central nervous system
    Spinal cord lesions
    Parkinson's disease

Metabolic and endocrine diseases
  Diabetes
  Uremia
  Hypokalemia
  Hypothyroidism
  Hypercalcemia
  Pheochromocytoma
  Enteric glucagon excess

Malignancy
  Direct effects
    Cerebral or spinal cord tumors
    Intestinal obstruction
    Hypercalcemia
  Secondary effects
    Inadequate food intake and low-fiber diet
    Poor fluid intake
    Reduced activity
    Previous bowel surgery
    Autonomic neuropathy
    Radiotherapy
    Sedation, low level of consciousness

Drugs
  Opioids
  Nonsteroidal anti-inflammatory drugs
  Anticholinergics
  Anticonvulsants
  Antidepressants
  Diuretics
  Antacids
  Anti-Parkinson drugs
  Antihypertensive agents
  Vinca alkaloids

Constipation is frequently noted in patients with various neurologic disorders. A visceral neuropathy seems to be present in most patients with severe slow-transit constipation. Disturbance in the extrinsic nerve supply to the colon has been found in these patients, along with a lack of inhibitory innervation of colonic circular muscle, and a diminished release of acetylcholine. Patients with advanced cancer frequently complain of GI symptoms, including anorexia, chronic nausea, and early satiety—a symptom complex often associated with physical signs of an autonomic neuropathy. Autonomic neuropathy may also be manifested as severe constipation, including postural hypotension and resting tachycardia. It is a multifactorial syndrome, and malnutrition, decreased activity, diabetes, and drugs, such as vinca alkaloids, opioids, and tricyclic antidepressants, are all possible causative factors (4).

Diabetic dysmotility has traditionally been thought to reflect a generalized autonomic neuropathy. However, secretions of GI hormones may also be important. Decreased amounts of substance P in the rectal mucosa of constipated patients with diabetes has been thought to contribute to the pathogenesis of diabetic constipation.

Peripheral neuropathy is a common complication of cancer chemotherapy. Patients receiving a high cumulative dose of vincristine or cisplatin seem to be at a significantly elevated risk for the development of long-term side effects. These drugs have been shown to cause symptoms of autonomic polyneuropathy with constipation, bladder atony, and hypotension. Whereas many reports describe acute neurologic side effects during therapy, little is known about persistent and late damage to the peripheral nervous system. The long-term neurologic side effects in patients with curable malignancies, such as Hodgkin's disease and testicular cancer, may be particularly troublesome.

Ogilvie's syndrome describes a variety of states with a similar clinical picture due to intrinsic defects in the intestinal smooth muscle, with a massive colonic dilatation in the absence of an obstruction or inflammatory process. Also termed as *pseudo-obstruction*, this syndrome can be categorized into those with myopathic and those with neuropathic features. Several conditions involving the intestinal smooth muscle are associated with colonic pseudo-obstruction, including endocrine and metabolic disorders, neurologic diseases, nonoperative trauma, surgery, nonintestinal inflammatory processes, infections, malignancy, radiation therapy, drugs, and cardiovascular and respiratory diseases. Extensive damage to the submucosal and myenteric nerve plexus associated with lymphoid infiltrate has been observed as a specific disorder, different from other processes that produce intestinal pseudo-obstruction (4).

Long-term denervation abolishes the normal pelvic floor muscle activity. This neurologic impairment may be produced by nerve damage not only following chemotherapy, but also as a consequence of radiotherapy, pelvic surgery, compression, or invasion by neoplastic growth or during prolonged chronic opioid therapy. Loss of the normal rectal muscle tone is also a consequence of prolonged immobility often seen in debilitated patients with cancer. Rectal sensation may be reduced and the rectal capacity to distention may be increased after vincristine treatment or as a consequence of neoplastic involvement of the pelvic sacral nerves. The rectosigmoid junction is a key area in the mechanism of constipation. Rectal outlet obstruction and failure of the puborectalis and anal sphincter muscles to relax are frequent findings in patients with neurologic diseases with intractable constipation. Several mechanisms are possible for constipation by outlet obstruction, including a hyperactive rectosigmoid junction, an increased storage capacity of the rectum, spasticity, and hypertonicity of the anal canal with incoordination of the reflex between rectum and anus. Anismus is a spastic pelvic floor syndrome, recently termed *rectosphincteric dyssynergia*, for its similarity with vesicourethral dyssynergia. Similar extrinsic innervation of the bladder and the rectum has been observed, explaining why patients with severe slow-transit constipation often complain of urologic symptoms.

The integrity of the spinal cord neurons is essential to maintain normal defecation. In patients with spinal cord lesions above the lumbosacral area, incontinence is controlled but defecation is impaired. This is due to the interruption of the cortical pathways, demonstrating the importance of supraspinal control of distal colonic function and defecation. Moreover, colonic response to a meal is reduced. However, appropriate stimuli may be sufficient to result in evacuation. In patients with damage to the cauda equina, transit time is prolonged and the recto–anal inhibitory reflex is weaker, offering little protection against fecal incontinence.

In patients with cancer having Parkinson's disease, constipation is probably caused by the degeneration of the autonomic nervous system, particularly the myenteric plexus. Psychiatric and neurologic diseases are frequently associated with colonic dysmotility (43).

A large variety of metabolic disorders predispose to constipation. Of particular relevance to patients with cancer are dehydration, hypercalcemia, hypokalemia, and uremia. Chronic dehydration can also result in dry stools that are difficult to expel. Many drugs induce constipation.

Many drugs with anticholinergic actions, antiemetics, and diuretics induce constipation. Patients treated with carbamazepine may develop severe constipation that is not dose related but is refractory to the concomitant use of oral laxatives, necessitating drug discontinuation. Selective 5-HT3–receptor antagonists cause constipation. They antagonize the ability of 5-HT to evoke cholinergically mediated contractions of the intestinal longitudinal muscle (44).

One of the most striking pharmacologic features of opioids is their ability to cause constipation. Opioids cause constipation by binding to specific opioid receptors in the enteric and central nervous systems. Opioid receptors have been identified on gut smooth muscle, suggesting that there is a local effect of opioid drugs, although central opioid effects cannot be excluded. Opioids affect the intestines by different mechanisms. Opioids augment the tone and nonpropulsive motility of both the ileum and the colon, thereby increasing transit time. Opioids desiccate the intraluminal content, reducing secretion and increasing intestinal fluid absorption, with an indirect mechanism, possibly by tryptaminergic neurons in the myenteric plexus, resulting in the release of noradrenaline, which antagonize the secretory mechanism of the enterocytes, regulated by α_2-adrenoreceptors. Opioids may also suppress the release of the vasointestinal peptide, an inhibitory neurotransmitter. Vasointestinal peptide is a potent colonic secretagogue and an important inhibitor of smooth muscle contraction. Moreover, the prolonged bowel transit on its own may facilitate the increased intestinal absorption of fluid and electrolytes. Opioid use may lead to fecal impaction, spurious diarrhea, and bowel pseudo-obstruction, causing abdominal pain, nausea and vomiting, and interference with drug administration and absorption (45).

Oral morphine invariably causes constipation when used in repeated doses to treat cancer pain. Although other common unwanted effects, such as sedation, nausea, and vomiting, tend to improve with continued use and often resolve completely, opioid-induced constipation does not get better with repeated administration. It is likely that other factors can contribute to slow intestinal transit, such as immobility, concomitant medications, or disease-related factors. The importance of other factors in the development of constipation is demonstrated by the fact that approximately 50% of hospice patients not on opioids required regular oral laxatives.

Sixty-four percent of patients admitted to a hospice and not receiving opioid analgesia required laxatives, although the doses of laxative required were higher in patients receiving opioids (46). Although there is no correlation between the dose of opioids and the dose of laxatives, an upward titration of laxatives in parallel with increasing doses of morphine has been observed (47). Approximate equivalents of laxatives and typical requirements of opioid therapy have been proposed, but clearly there is large individual patient variation. However, proportionally less laxative is required at a higher opioid dose.

Higher doses of danthron were associated with better physical functioning (but not opioid dose), suggesting that for any given dose of opioid, fitter patients were treated with larger doses of laxatives. Factors other than opioid dose and physical functioning may be more important in contributing to constipation in this group of patients. Less potent opioid drugs, such as codeine, are just as likely to cause constipation as more potent opioids (48).

Postoperative pain relief by both parenteral and intraspinal opioids is often associated with adynamic ileus. Gastric emptying and small bowel transit are inhibited. This is an important consideration for patients with cancer undergoing surgical procedures in which the ileus is likely to be a severe problem. Epidural anesthesia with local anesthetics appears to disrupt GI motility less than systemic opioids (4).

Assessment

A variety of definitions have been used by patients and health care providers—straining, hard stools, the desire but inability to defecate, infrequent stools, and abdominal discomfort. Stool weight and consistency, possible parameters to measure, are unreliable because of the wide range in healthy subjects (4). It is of paramount importance to first establish what the patient means by constipation—if the stools are too small, too hard, too difficult to expel, or too infrequent, or if the patients have a feeling of incomplete evacuation after defecation. Constipation is defined as a decrease in the frequency of the passage of formed stools and characterized by stools that are hard and difficult to pass (41). A frequency of at least three bowel movements per week is viewed as an objective indicator of normality. A careful history should be taken regarding the onset of constipation, bowel habits, and the use of laxatives. Patients who develop progressive constipation in the absence of any clear precipitating cause should be considered for an evaluation that may include determination of electrolytes and renal and hepatic function tests.

Impaction with overflow should be excluded by performing a rectal examination. Therefore, the first step is to completely evacuate the bowel. Multiple oil or saline enemas may be needed. Digital fragmentation is unpleasant, but may permit most of the fecal impactions in the rectum to be diagnosed. A pseudodiarrhea in the presence of impaired anal sphincter function may be discovered. Gentle digital examination of the rectum may reveal a hard mass, a rectal tumor, rectal ulcers, an anal stenosis, anismus, or a lax anal sphincter. Patients with spinal cord lesions may have reduced sensation, but the anal tone is preserved, whereas patients with sacral nerve root infiltration will have a reduced anal tone. The examination of the abdomen may reveal fecal masses in the left iliac fossa. Fecal masses are usually not tender, are relatively mobile, and can be indented with pressure.

An abdominal radiograph may distinguish between constipation and obstruction. Examination after a barium meal may help distinguish between paralytic ileus and mechanical obstruction. Barium studies may help reveal a small intestine motility dysfunction in chronic intestinal pseudo-obstruction. In visceral myopathy, intestinal contractions are infrequent, whereas with a visceral neuropathy, patients tend to have less distension and faster intestinal transit time due to uncoordinated contractions (4).

When constipation is due to ineffective colonic musculature, measurement of colonic transit time may be a useful tool to detect specific areas of the bowel that are not functioning properly. Pieces of radiopaque nasogastric tube are ingested and the progression of markers along the colon is observed by a daily radiograph until total expulsion. This study may demonstrate a delayed transit in the colon, a long storage of feces in the rectum, or a retrograde movement due to a distal spasm (49). A radiologic constipation score has been proposed, assessing the amount of stool in each of the four abdominal quadrants (50).

Treatment

There is a lack of consensus on the definition of constipation and confusion regarding effective methods for prevention and treatment. It could be argued that health care professionals are more intent on monitoring the direct effects rather than the secondary effects of treatment.

The management of constipation should be divided into general interventions and therapeutic measures. An extensive effort should be made to find a specific cause of constipation, and then treatment can be directed at that cause. Etiologic factors, such as physiologic consequences of cancer-associated debility, biochemical abnormalities, including hypercalcemia and hyperkalemia, and drug use, should be identified and reversed wherever possible. An adequate fluid intake is helpful in increasing the stool water content (4).

Fluids, fruit juice, fruit, and bran are all recommended. However, fiber deficiency is unlikely to account for a lower stool weight, and there is no justification for the claim that treatment with bran can return stool output and transit time to normal. In patients with far-advanced cancer, the use of high amounts of fiber is beyond the capacity of most patients. Moreover, dietary fiber seems to have no prophylactic value to prevent constipation in hospitalized patients. Fiber consumption may decrease fluid intake relatively, thereby paradoxically worsening the situation. Since an unfavorable toilet environment, such as lack of privacy or inappropriate posture, may lead to constipation, patients should be provided privacy and appropriate facilities in the hospital setting.

When irreversible causes of constipation cannot be directly treated, symptomatic relief should be provided. Moreover, in spite of prophylaxis, most of these patients will require chronic laxatives, especially in the advanced stage of their disease or when treated with chronic opioid therapy. It is appropriate to begin prophylactic laxative treatment in patients with risk factors for constipation, including the elderly, those who are bedridden, or those requiring drugs known to cause constipation.

A low-rectal impaction should be removed manually. Appropriate sedation and analgesics are usually required to make this procedure comfortable. A more proximal mass can be broken by a sigmoidoscope or by delivering a pulsating stream of water against the stool. The use of enemas and rectal interventions is limited to the acute short-term management of more severe episodes. Therapeutic interventions for the management of constipation are based on the administration of laxatives, either orally or rectally. Laxatives are commonly used in patients with advanced cancer. Sixty-two percent of patients admitted to hospices received laxatives regularly (51). Laxatives will promote active electrolyte secretion, decrease water and electrolyte absorption, increase intraluminal osmolarity, and increase hydrostatic pressure in the gut. Although laxatives can be divided into several groups, no agent acts purely to soften the stool or to stimulate peristalsis. Clinical criteria, responsiveness, acceptability, and the patient's preference should guide the selection of the drug. Table 15.5 outlines different medications that are useful in constipation.

Laxatives

According to their modes of action, they are divided into bulk-forming laxatives, osmotic laxatives, stimulant laxatives, lubricating agents, and others. Bulk-forming laxatives are not recommended for use in palliative care patients, since such patients are normally not able to take in the required amount of fluids.

Patients with advanced cancer are likely to have chronic constipation and will need continuous laxative treatment. No data exist to guide the clinician or patient in the optimal choice of laxatives, as there have been no adequate comparative studies of long-term management of opioid-induced constipation. One of the main limitations of such trials

TABLE 15.5

LAXATIVES USED FOR CONSTIPATION

Class–drugs–doses	Onset	Comments
Lubricant laxatives		
Liquid paraffin 10 mL/d	1–3 d	Paraffin inhalation
Surfactant laxatives		
Docusate 300 mg	1–3 d	Not together with mineral oil
Bulk-forming agents	2–4 d	
Bran (8 g)		If taken with inadequate amount of water can precipitate fecal impaction in intestinal obstruction
Methylcellulosa, ispaghula (4 g)		
Osmotic laxatives	1–2 d	
Lactulose 15 mL b.i.d.		Dose-related cramps, gaseous distention, useful in hepatic encephalopathy
Mannitol		
Sorbitol		
Saline laxatives	1–6 h	
Magnesium salts 2–4 g		Not in renal failure
Sodium salts		
Polyethylene glycol Two sachets daily in water	1–3 d	High volumes of water need to be ingested
Antracenes	6–12 h	Colicky pain
Senna 15 mg		
Dantron 50 mg		Urine pink discoloration
Poliphenolics	6–12 h	Colicky pain
Bisacodyl 10 mg		
Sodium picosulfate 5 mg		
Opioid antagonists		
Naloxone (dose titration)	1–2 h	Possible withdrawal syndrome

is the lack of reliable clinical assessment tools. In a randomized, crossover clinical trial of laxatives in a hospice, lactulose/senna combination produced a significantly greater stool frequency than codanthramer in patients receiving opioids and reduced the usage of rectal measures, although the penalty for this achievement was an increased likelihood of diarrhea (52). In a comparative study conducted with the objective of determining treatment and cost efficiency for senna and lactulose in patients with terminal cancer treated with opioids, no difference was found in defecation-free intervals or in days with defecation between the laxatives (53). In a recent systematic review, the use of docusate for constipation in palliative care has been found to be based on inadequate experimental evidence (54). In a study of healthy volunteers, in which constipation was induced by loperamide, a combination of stimulant and softening laxatives was most likely to maintain normal bowel function at the lowest dose and least adverse effects. Senna was associated with significantly more adverse effects than the other laxatives (55).

Bulk-forming agents are high-fiber foods containing polysaccharides or cellulose derivatives resistant to bacterial breakdown. These agents increase stool bulk and correct its consistency by increasing the mass and the water content of the stool. Evidence of their effect may be observed after 24 hours or more. Their effectiveness and feasibility in the patient with advanced cancer are doubtful, as they require the patients to drink extra fluids to prevent viscous mass formation.

Emollient laxatives are surfactant substances not adsorbed in the gut, acting as a detergent and facilitating the mixture of water and fat. They also promote water and electrolyte

secretion. Stimulant laxatives are the most commonly used drugs to treat constipation. They are represented by the anthraquinone derivatives, such as senna, cascara, and danthron, and the diphenylmethane derivatives, such as bisacodyl and phenolphthalein. This class of drugs acts at the level of the colon and distal ileum by directly stimulating the myenteric plexus. Senna is converted to an active form by colonic bacteria. As a consequence, its site of action is primarily the colon. Danthron and the polyphenolic agents bisacodyl and sodium picosulfate undergo glucuronidation and are secreted in the bile. The enterohepatic circulation may prolong their effect. An increase in myoelectric colonic activity has been observed after the administration of oral senna. Bisacodyl stimulates the mucosal nerve plexus, producing contractions of the entire colon and decreasing water absorption in the small and large intestine. Castor oil is metabolized into ricinoleic acid that has stimulant secretory properties and an effect on glucose absorption. All of these drugs may cause severe cramping. The cathartic action occurs within 1–3 days. Starting doses proposed are 15 mg of senna daily, 50 mg of danthron daily, or 10 mg of bisacodyl daily. Bisacodyl suppositories promote colonic peristalsis with a short onset due to rapid conversion to its active metabolite by the rectal flora. Docusate, alone or in combination with danthron, is most commonly used at doses of 100–300 mg every 8 hours. The effectiveness of docusate has been questioned (4).

Lubricant laxatives are represented by mineral oil. It may be useful in the management of transient acute constipation or fecal impaction, but has little role in the management of chronic constipation. It lubricates the stool surface. Coated feces may pass more easily and the colonic absorption of water is decreased. It may also decrease absorption of fat vitamins. Absorption of small amounts may cause foreign-body reactions in the bowel lymphoid tissue. Liquid paraffin, 10 mL per day, may be given orally or rectally, with an effect noted in 8–24 hours.

Hyperosmotic agents are not broken down or absorbed in the small bowel, drawing fluid into the bowel lumen. Osmotic laxatives are divided into (magnesium) salts, saccharine, alcohols, and macrogols. Lactulose increases fecal weight and frequency but may result in bloating, colic, and flatulence, as well as electrolyte imbalances at high doses. Moreover, it is expensive in comparison to other preparations. The latency of action is 1–2 days. Starting doses are 15–20 mL twice a day. Orally administered macrogol is not metabolized, and pH value and bowel flora remain unchanged. Macrogol hydrates hardened stools, increases stool volume, decreases the duration of colon passage and dilates the bowel wall which then triggers the defecation reflex. Even when given for some time, the effectiveness of macrogol will not decrease (56).

Saline laxatives exert an osmotic effect, increasing the intraluminal volume. They also appear to directly stimulate peristalsis and increase water secretion. The starting dose is 2–4 g daily. Magnesium, sulfate, phosphate, and citrate ions are the ingredients in saline laxatives. Saline laxatives usually produce results in a few hours. Their use may lead to electrolyte imbalances with accumulation of magnesium in patients with renal dysfunction or an excessive load of sodium in patients with hypertension. Moreover, their administration may result in an undesirably strong purgative effect. Administered rectally, they stimulate rectal peristalsis within 15 minutes. Repeated use of a phosphate enema may cause hypocalcemia and hyperphosphatemia or rectal gangrene in patients with hemorrhoids. Glycerin can be used rectally as an osmotic and a lubricant.

Prokinetic drugs. Cisapride is a prokinetic agent that appears to accelerate orocecal transit and stimulate the colon. Cisapride enhances the release of acetylcholine from the myenteric nerve endings. It is devoid of the central antidopaminergic effects that limit the use of metoclopramide. It has been shown to correct impaired propulsion in the small bowel of patients with pseudo-obstruction. Suggested doses are in the range of 2.5–10 mg four times a day. Metoclopramide given by the subcutaneous route, but not by the oral route, seems to be effective in narcotic bowel syndrome. Effects of metoclopramide are mediated by a central and peripheral antidopamine effect and a stimulation of cholinergic receptors (4).

Opioid Antagonists and Opioid Therapy Modification

Opioid-induced constipation can be severe and refractory to therapy with conventional laxatives. Opioid concentration in the enteric nervous system correlates better with opioid-induced, prolonged, intestinal transit time than concentrations in the central nervous system (57) Naloxone is a competitive antagonist of opioid receptors inside and outside the central nervous system and, after systemic administration, it reverses both centrally and peripherally mediated opioid effects. There is now evidence that oral administration of naloxone can reverse opioid-induced constipation, without causing systemic opioid withdrawal in most patients. This route of administration theoretically allows selective blocking of intestinal opioid receptors without blocking the desired opioid effects, as long as hepatic first pass capacity is not exceeded. The low systemic bioavailability due to marked hepatic first-pass metabolism allows for the low plasma levels and high enteric wall concentration. Oral administration of naloxone at a daily dose of approximately 20% of the daily morphine

dose is capable of providing a clinical laxative effect without antagonizing opioid analgesia (58). In another study, the mean dose of naloxone was 17.5 mg per day. Adverse effects of short duration, including yawning, sweating, and shivering, were observed in approximately one third of patients (59). Although oral naloxone doses <2–4 mg or 10% or less of the morphine dose are mostly ineffective, opioid withdrawal may be present. Reversal of analgesia does not seem to be an early symptom of systemic opioid antagonism (60).

In the former reports, the naloxone dose has been based on the preexisting morphine dose and expressed in percentages of daily morphine. However, the reaction to opioid antagonists seems to be proportional to the degree of opioid tolerance rather than to opioid concentration, and the risk of systemic withdrawal may increase if the same percentage relationship is used in patients with high opioid doses. It has been suggested that the initial dose of naloxone should not exceed 5 mg. Dose titration, beginning with a dose of 0.8 mg twice daily and doubling the dose every 2–3 days until favorable effects occur or adverse effects are experienced, independently of the preexisting morphine usage, may be a reasonable approach.

Methylnaltrexone, the first peripheral opioid receptor antagonist and currently under clinical investigation, has the potential to prevent or treat opioid-induced, peripherally mediated side effects, such as constipation, without interfering with analgesia. Methylnaltrexone is an opioid antagonist that cannot penetrate the blood–brain barrier and has been shown to reverse morphine-induced delay of gastric emptying and intestinal transit time after intravenous infusion in volunteers. In a pilot study of subjects receiving chronic methadone therapy, low doses of intravenous methylnaltrexone effectively reversed chronic methadone-induced constipation and delay in gut transit time (61). Future studies are needed in patients with cancer having opioid-associated constipation.

Alvimopan is a potent μ-receptor antagonist without reversing morphine-induced analgesia, because of the minimal systemic absorption (45). In a randomized controlled trial alvimopan in doses of 0.5–1 mg was effective in restoring bowel transit within 8 hours in patients chronically receiving opioids (62)

Constipation may require modification of opioid therapy (63). Opioid switching is a strategy for maintaining or improving analgesic quality directed toward decreasing the effects of previous opiates on the GI tract. Present research indicates that there is a relation between the type of opioid and the degree of constipation, that is, treatment with transdermal fentanyl or methadone tends to cause less constipation compared to morphine or hydromorphone. Among opioids, there may be differences in the analgesia/constipation ratio. Clinical studies have revealed that at doses of oral morphine and transdermal fentanyl that yield equivalent pain relief, constipation differs significantly between the two drugs. Although most of the early studies were not randomized, different methodologies were used, and the analysis was performed while switching patients from oral morphine to transdermal fentanyl, more recent trials are remarkably consistent in that transdermal fentanyl causes less constipation than oral, sustained morphine at the same level of analgesia (4). Differences in pharmacologic profiles, in the affinity to opioid receptor and a higher exposure of opioid-binding receptors in the GI tract following oral administration of morphine compared with transdermal administration of fentanyl, may offer an explanation for the clinically observed variations in the constipation-inducing potentials of equipotent doses of morphine and fentanyl. The lipophilicity profile of fentanyl allows for the ease with which fentanyl penetrates the brain. As less opioid is required to produce a central analgesic effect, less opioid is available in the peripheral circulation to induce constipation. Experimental studies using a castor oil–induced diarrhea model have shown a more favorable analgesia/constipation ratio of subcutaneous fentanyl as compared with oral morphine, although the difference was less pronounced with oral fentanyl. Considerably larger amounts of naloxone were needed to reverse the morphine than the fentanyl-induced antidiarrheal effects (4). Methadone has a high oral bioavailability and a rapid and extensive distribution phase, followed by a slow elimination. The end of the distribution phase is at or below the minimum effective concentration necessary for an effect. This may result in limiting the continuous bathing of intestinal receptors. The high lipophilicity of methadone allows for the maintenance of a low plasma concentration with a relevant clinical effect. Constipation seems to be the symptom that improves most after opioid switching. This could be simply due to different tolerance of different opioids at the level of receptors located in the bowel. Moreover, different reports have shown that methadone therapy may cause less constipation than morphine. In a retrospective analysis, the laxative/opioid dose ratio was lower in patients receiving methadone than in patients on morphine. Moreover, there is a rationale in changing the route of administration. The use of a parenteral administration should also result in a change of the opioid concentration at intestinal receptors. However, in a retrospective study no difference in the doses of laxatives required to maintain regular bowel movements was found between patients receiving oral opioids and those receiving subcutaneous opioids (64).

Therapeutic Strategy

The treatment consists of basic measures and the application of laxatives. Local measures to soften fecal mass are necessary in cases of rectal impaction. The short latency of action of rectal laxatives may be useful to remove hard feces impacted in the rectum. Glycerin suppositories or sorbitol enemas soften the stool by osmosis, also lubricating the rectal wall. Water penetration may be facilitated by a stool softener. Saline enemas cannot be regularly administered and should be used as a last resort if suppositories fail. Any patient requiring an enema should be reevaluated for a possible laxative dose titration.

Practical and economic consideration may influence the choice of drug according to the setting (home, hospital, hospice, or palliative care unit). Although stimulant agents may cause painful colic, softener drugs may be useful in the presence of a hard stool. Peristaltic stimulants are indicated in patients unable to pass soft stool. Senna is the most useful drug in the presence of soft feces in the rectum. All patients commencing opioid analgesia should have a prophylactic laxative unless a contraindication exists, although periodic laxative-free intervals have been advocated for patients with a relatively long prognosis to avoid tolerance.

Laxative dose should usually be titrated according to the response and not according to the dose of opioids. The opioid dose increments do not determine laxative efficacy, indicating that the constipating effect of opioids is not a function of dose. Combination therapy with different mechanisms may be more useful when higher doses of one laxative are required. In patients suspected of having intestinal obstruction, laxatives with a softening action may be tried. However, treatment should be immediately interrupted when transit stops. Patients with colostomies require the same treatment. Before using stimulating agents, an obstruction should be excluded in the absence of feces in a colostomy. Patients with paraplegia often require regular manual evacuation. Glycerin and bisacodyl suppositories should be given to patients with cauda equina syndrome. They may also benefit from the use of cisapride.

Opioid switching may be indicated in cases in which there are serious therapeutic difficulties in maintaining bowel transit.

Opioid switching as well as the use of opioid antagonists should be carefully monitored.

References

1. Komurcu S, Nelson KA, Walsh D, et al. Gastrointestinal symptoms among inpatients with advanced cancer. *Am J Hosp Palliat Care* 2002;19:351–355.
2. Lau PM, Stewart K, Dooley M. The ten most common adverse drug reactions (ADRs) in oncology patients: do they matter to you? *Support Care Cancer* 2004;12:626–633.
3. Dranitsaris G, Maroun J, Shah A. Estimating the cost of illness in colorectal cancer patients who were hospitalized for severe chemotherapy-induced diarrhea. *Can J Gastroenterol* 2005;19:83–87.
4. Mercadante S. Diarrhea, malabsorption, and constipation. In: Berger AM, Portenoy RK, Weissman DE, eds. *Principles and practice of supportive oncology*. Philadelphia, PA: Lippincott–Raven Publishers, 1998:191–206.
5. Clausen MR, Jorgensen J, Mortensen PB. Comparison of diarrhea induced by ingestion of fructooligosaccharide Idolax and disaccharide lactulose: role of osmolarity versus fermentation of malabsorbed carbohydrate. *Dig Dis Sci* 1998;43:2696–2707.
6. Osterlund P, Ruotsalainen T, Peuhkuri K, et al. Lactose intolerance associated with adjuvant 5-fluorouracil-based chemotherapy for colorectal cancer. *Clin Gastroenterol Hepatol* 2004;2:696–703.
7. Schiller LR. Secretory diarrhea. *Curr Gastroenterol Rev* 1999;1:389–397.
8. Jensen RT. Overview of chronic diarrhea caused by functional neuroendocrine neoplasms. *Semin Gastrointest Dis* 1999;10:156–172.
9. Riley SA, Turnberg LA. Maldigestion and malabsorption. In: Sleisinger MH, Fordtran JE, eds. *Gastrointestinal disease*. Philadelphia, PA: WB Saunders, 1993:977–1008.
10. Radu B, Allez M, Gornet JM, et al. Chronic diarrhoea after allogenic bone marrow transplantation. *Gut* 2005;54:161–174.
11. Michael M, Brittain M, Nagai J, et al. Phase II study of activated charcoal to prevent irinotecan-induced diarrhea. *J Clin Oncol* 2004;22:4410–4417.
12. Kornblau S, Benson AB, Catalano R, et al. Management of cancer treatment-related diarrhea. Issues and therapeutic strategies. *J Pain Symptom Manage* 2000;19:118–129.
13. Carlini LE, Meropol NJ, Bever J, et al. UGT1A7 and UGT1A9 polymorphisms predict response and toxicity in colorectal cancer patients treated with capecitabine/irinotecan. *Clin Cancer Res* 2005;11:1226–1236.
14. Hogenauer C, Hammer HF, Krejs GJ, et al. Mechanisms and management of antibiotic-associated diarrhea. *Clin Infect Dis* 1998;27:702–710.
15. Schiller LR. Diarrhea. *Med Clin North Am* 2000;84:1259–1274.
16. Martenson JA, Bollinger JW, Sloan JA, et al. Sucralfate in the prevention of treatment-induced diarrhea in patients receiving pelvic radiation therapy: a North Central Cancer Treatment Group phase III double-blind placebo-controlled trial. *J Clin Oncol* 2000;18:1239–1245.
17. Hombrick J, Frohlich D, Glazel M, et al. Prevention of radiation-induced diarrhea by smectite. Results of a double-blind randomized, placebo-controlled multicenter study. *Strahlenther Onkol* 2000;17:173–179.
18. Huang EY, Hsu HC, Yang KD, et al. Acute diarrhea during pelvic irradiation: is small-bowel volume effect different in gynecologic patients with prior abdomen operation or not? *Gynecol Oncol* 2005;97:118–125.
19. Koukourakis MI, Touloupidis S, Manavis J, et al. Conformal hypofractionated and accelerated radiotherapy with cytoprotection (HypoARC) for high risk prostatic carcinoma: rationale, technique and early experience. *Anticancer Res* 2004;24:3239.
20. Lenfers BH, Loeffler TM, Droege CM, et al. Substantial activity of budesonide in patients with irinotecan (CPT-11) and 5-fluorouracil induced diarrhea and failure of loperamide treatment. *Ann Oncol* 1999;10:1251–1253.
21. Attar A, Flourie B, Ranbaud JC, et al. Antibiotic efficacy in small intestinal bacterial overgrowth-related chronic diarrhea: a crossover, randomized trial. *Gastroenterology* 1999;117:794–797.
22. Gorenek L, Dizer U, Besirbellioglu B, et al. The diagnosis and treatment of *Clostridium difficile* in antibiotic-associated diarrhea. *Hepatogastroenterology* 1999;46:343–348.
23. Saavedra J. Probiotics and infectious diarrhea. *Am J Gastroenterol* 2000;95(Suppl 1):S16–S18.
24. Tamura T, Yasutake K, Nishisaki H, et al. Prevention of irinotecan-induced diarrhea by oral sodium bicarbonate and influence on pharmacokinetics. *Oncologia* 2004;67:327–337.
25. Maeda Y, Ohune T, Nakamura M, et al. Prevention of irinotecan-induced diarrhoea by oral carbonaceous adsorbent (Kremezin) in cancer patients. *Oncol Rep* 2004;12:581–585.
26. Kehrer DF, Sparreboom A, Verweij J, et al. Modulation of irinotecan-induced diarrhea by cotreatment with neomycin in cancer patients. *Clin Cancer Res* 2001;7:1136–1141.
27. Zhao J, Huang L, Belmar N, et al. Oral RDP58 allows CPT-11 dose intensification for enhanced tumor response by decreasing gastrointestinal toxicity. *Clin Cancer Res* 2004;10:2851–2859.
28. Cascinu S, Bichisao E, Amadori D, et al. High-dose loperamide in the treatment of 5-fluorouracil-induced diarrhea in colorectal cancer patients. *Support Care Cancer* 2000;8:65–67.

29. Kaplan MA, Prior MJ, Ash RR, et al. Loperamide-simethicone vs. loperamide alone, simethicone alone, and placebo in the treatment of acute diarrhea with gas-related abdominal discomfort. A randomized controlled trial. *Arch Fam Med* 1999;8:243–248.

30. Mercadante S. Diarrhea in terminally ill patients: pathophysiology and treatment. *J Pain Symptom Manage* 1995;10:298–309.

31. Mercadante S. The role of octreotide in palliative care. *J Pain Symptom Manage* 1994;9:406–411.

32. Cello JP, Grendell JH, Basuk P, et al. Effect of octreotide on refractory AIDS-associated diarrhea: a prospective, multicenter clinical trial. *Ann Intern Med* 1991;115:705–710.

33. Ippoliti C, Champlin R, Bugazia N. Use of octreotide in the symptomatic management of diarrhea induced by graft-versus-host disease in patients with hematologic malignancies. *J Clin Oncol* 1997;15:3350–3354.

34. Wasserman EI, Hidalgo M, Hornedo J, et al. Octreotide (SMS 201-995) for hematopoietic support-dependent high-dose chemotherapy (HSD-HDC)-related diarrhea: dose finding study and evaluation of efficacy. *Bone Marrow Transplant* 1997;20:711–714.

35. Rosenoff SH. Octreotide LAR resolves severe chemotherapy-induced diarrhoea (CID) and allows continuation of full-dose therapy. *Eur J Cancer Care* 2004;13:380–383.

36. Anthony L. New strategies for the prevention and reduction of cancer treatment-induced diarrhea. *Semin Oncol Nurs* 2003;19(Suppl 3):17–21.

37. Westergaard H, Spady DK. The short bowel syndrome. In: Sleisenger MH, Fordtran JS, eds. *Gastrointestinal disease*. Philadelphia, PA: WB Saunders, 1993:1249–1256.

38. Ung KA, Kilander AF, Lindgren A, et al. Impact of bile acid malabsorption on steatorrhoea and symptoms in patients with chronic diarrhoea. *Eur J Gastroenterol Hepatol* 2000;12:541–547.

39. Toskes PP. Malabsorption. In: Wyngaarden JB, Smith LH, Bennett JC, eds. *Cecil textbook of medicine*. Philadelphia, PA: WB Saunders, 1992:667–699.

40. Harewood GC, Murray JA. Approaching the patient with chronic malabsorption syndrome. *Semin Gastrointest Dis* 1999;10:138–144.

41. McMillan S. Assessing and managing opiate-induced constipation in adults with cancer. *Cancer control* 2004;11(Suppl 1):3–9.

42. Sykes NP. Constipation and diarrhoea. In: Doyle D, Hanks GW, MacDonald N, eds. *Oxford textbook of palliative medicine*. New York: Oxford University Press, 1993.299–310.

43. Mercadante S. Nausea and vomiting. In *Palliative care in neurology*, Voltz R, Bernat J, Borasio G, et al. eds, Oxford: Oxford University Press, 2004:210–220.

44. Gershon MD. Review article: serotonin receptors and transporters—roles in normal and abnormal gastrointestinal motility. *Aliment Pharmacol Ther* 2004;20(Suppl 7):3–14.

45. Kurz A, Sessler D. Opioid-induced bowel dysfunction. Pathophysiology and potential new therapies. *Drugs* 2003;63:649–671.

46. Sykes NP. The relationship between opioid use and laxative use in terminally ill cancer patients. *Palliat Med* 1998;12:375–382.

47. Fallon MT, Hanks GW. Morphine, constipation and performance status in advanced cancer patients. *Palliat Med* 1999;13:159–160.

48. Bennett M, Cresswell H. Factors influencing constipation in advanced cancer patients: a prospective study of opioid dose, dantron dose and physical functioning. *Palliat Med* 2003;17:418–422.

49. Sykes N. The treatment of morphine-induced constipation. *Eur J Palliat Care* 1998;5:12–15.

50. Bruera E, Suarez-Almazor M, Velasco A, et al. The assessment of constipation in terminal cancer patients admitted to a palliative care unit: a retrospective review. *J Pain Symptom Manage* 1994;9:515–519.

51. Twycross RG, Harcourt J. The use of laxative at a palliative care center. *Palliat Med* 1991;5:27–33.

52. Sykes NP. A clinical comparison of laxatives in a hospice. *Palliat Med* 1991;5:307–314.

53. Agra Y, Sacristan A, Gonzalez M, et al. Efficacy of senna versus lactulose in terminal cancer patients treated with opioids. *J Pain Symptom Manage* 1998;15:1–7.

54. Hurdon V, Viola R, Schroder C. How useful is docusate in patients at risk for constipation? A systematic review of the evidence in the chronically ill. *J Pain Symptom Manage* 2000;19:130–136.

55. Sykes NP. A volunteer model for the comparison of laxatives in opioid-related constipation. *J Pain Symptom Manage* 1996;11:363–369.

56. Klaschik E, Nauck F, Ostgathe C. Constipation—modern laxative therapy. *Support Care Cancer* 2003;11:679–685.

57. Culpepper-Morgan JA, Inturrisi CE, Portenoy RK, et al. Treatment of opioid-induced constipation with oral naloxone: a pilot study. *Clin Pharmacol Ther* 1992;52:90–95.

58. Sykes NP. An investigation of the ability of oral naloxone to correct opioid-related constipation in patients with advanced cancer. *Palliat Med* 1996;10:135–144.

59. Latasch L, Zimmerman M, Eberhart B, et al. Oral naloxone antagonizes morphine-induced constipation. *Anesthetist* 1997;46:191–194.

60. Meissner W, Schimdt U, Hartmann M, et al. Oral naloxone reverses opioid-associated constipation. *Pain* 2000;84:105–109.

61. Yuan CS, Foss JF, O'Connor M, et al. Effects of intravenous methylnaltrexone on opioid-induced gut motility and transit time changes in subjects receiving chronic methadone therapy: a pilot study. *Pain* 1999;83:631–635.

62. Paulson DM, Kennedy DT, Donovick R, et al. Alvimopan: an oral, peripherally acting, mu-opioid receptor antagonist for the treatment of opioid-induced bowel dysfunction. A 21-day treatment-randomized clinical trial. *J Pain* 2005;6:184–192.

63. Tamayo AC, Diaz-Zuluaga PA. Management of opioid-induced bowel dysfunction in cancer patients. *Support Care Cancer* 2004;12:613–618.

64. Mancini I, Bruera E. Constipation in advanced cancer patients. *Support Care Cancer* 1998;6:356–364.

CHAPTER 16 ■ BOWEL OBSTRUCTION

DOUGLAS J. SCHWARTZENTRUBER, MATTHEW LUBLIN, AND RICHARD B. HOSTETTER

BACKGROUND

Gastrointestinal symptoms in patients with cancer are quite common. These include xerostomia, dysphagia, anorexia, nausea, vomiting, diarrhea, and constipation. These symptoms can be generally improved or ameliorated with a variety of medical interventions (reviewed in (1)). Opioids, chemotherapeutic agents, and tumor can lead to abdominal pain, ileus, constipation, and vomiting that mimic mechanical bowel obstruction. Bowel obstruction may be a primary presentation or a secondary complication of a malignancy. Obstruction can involve either the upper or lower gastrointestinal tract, and the site of obstruction determines the management. Initial management is generally conservative and consists of hydration and nasogastric decompression. The decision to proceed with surgical intervention needs to be individualized to each patient. Palliative management of bowel obstruction is often required in the patient with cancer. Determining the course of palliative therapy can be challenging and one must balance the individual patient's needs and desires with clinically sound judgment. Patients with cancer can be palliated either medically or surgically. Operative treatment of gastrointestinal obstruction accounted for one third of 1022 palliative surgical procedures in a series of 823 patients (2). End-stage patients and patients who are not candidates for surgery should receive effective medical palliation.

INCIDENCE

Upper gastrointestinal obstruction in the US population is more commonly caused by malignancy than ulcer because of the introduction of proton pump inhibitors and H_2 blockers (3). Gastric carcinoma is the most common malignancy causing gastroduodenal obstruction, followed by pancreatic carcinoma (3). Most patients with gastric cancer do not present with obstruction. Patients with pancreatic cancer initially present with upper gastrointestinal obstruction in 6% of the instances (4), but after diagnosis, the incidence of gastroduodenal obstruction increases (5,6). In a review of 350 patients with pancreatic cancer, 25% of patients with unresectable disease developed gastroduodenal obstruction (4).

In contrast to gastroduodenal obstruction, small bowel obstruction in the general population is less commonly the result of malignancy. In a review of 238 patients with a diagnosis of small bowel obstruction, malignancy was the third most common cause of obstruction (7%) after adhesions and hernias, accounting for 88% (7). The incidence of small bowel obstruction is much higher in the cancer population and is generally secondary to metastatic cancers arising from other sites. In a review of 518 patients with ovarian cancer, 127 patients (25%) developed intestinal obstruction (8) that directly correlated with the stage of the disease. In colorectal cancer, 41 of 472 (9%) patients developed small bowel obstruction after primary resection of their cancer (9).

Unlike small bowel obstruction, acute colonic obstruction in the general population is caused by primary malignancy of the colon in most patients. Approximately 15–20% of patients with colon carcinoma present with obstruction (10). In patients presenting with colonic obstruction, 53–78% are due to a primary colorectal carcinoma, whereas only 6–12% are due to extrinsic compression of the colon from metastases (11,12).

ETIOLOGY

In most patients with cancer, symptoms of nausea, vomiting, abdominal pain, and constipation are nonobstructive in origin. Certain chemotherapeutic agents cause ileus, resulting in nausea, vomiting, and constipation. Vincristine is quite notorious for this, and in one series, 46% of patients reported constipation or abdominal pain or both (13). Nonchemotherapeutic agents such as opioids and anticholinergics may also lead to adynamic ileus. Further, patients with malignancy are often bedridden, inactive, malnourished, dehydrated, and have electrolyte imbalances. The common event of postoperative ileus can also be quite protracted in the patient with cancer. These states can lead to bowel dysmotility and the resultant clinical presentation may mimic mechanical bowel obstruction.

When present, mechanical bowel obstruction may involve the upper or lower gastrointestinal tract. The most frequent site of obstruction is the small bowel (14). Gastroduodenal obstruction is rarely benign in nature in the patient with cancer. The obstruction may be secondary to a primary stomach cancer or due to direct extension from the kidney, pancreas, biliary, or colon carcinoma. Ovarian carcinoma can also lead to gastroduodenal obstruction.

In contrast to gastroduodenal obstruction, a significant percentage of small bowel obstructions occurring in the patient with cancer are benign. In the reviewed series, 28% (median) of small bowel obstructions were the result of benign processes such as adhesions from previous oncologic operations (Table 16.1). However, most of the small bowel obstructions (72%) were caused by a recurrence of the intra-abdominal malignancy. Few patients present with primary small bowel tumors as the cause of obstruction (19). A primary

TABLE 16.1

INTESTINAL OBSTRUCTION IN PATIENTS WITH A PREVIOUS DIAGNOSIS OF MALIGNANCY

Author	Patients	Histology	Etiology (%)		Medical treatment (%)		Surgical treatment (%)			
			Benign	Malignant	Success	Recurrence	Success	Recurrence	Morbidity	Mortality
Gallick 1986 (15)	84	All	24	76	12	41	88	33	—	13
Butler 1991 (16)	54	All	32	68	20	45	76	11	49	16
Mäkelä 1991 (14)	85	All	0	100	—	—	55	13	42	22
Tang 1995 (17)	61	All	39	61	29	40	72	33	16	12
Nakane 1996 (18)	85	Gastric	20	80	21	—	48	—	—	6
Woolfson 1997 (19)	75	Nongynecologic	36	64	29	3	76	16	—	22
Edna 1998 (9)	41	Colorectal	51	49	—	—	98	—	—	17
Pothuri 2003 (20)	64	Ovarian	0	100	—	—	71	63	22	6
Median	70		28	72	21	41	74	25	32	15

small bowel tumor (adenocarcinoma, sarcoma, carcinoid, and lymphoma) should be suspected in patients with abdominal pain, weight loss, and occult gastrointestinal bleeding (21). Metastatic small bowel lesions should be considered in patients with the symptoms mentioned in the preceding text and a prior history of cancer of the ovary, colon, stomach, pancreas, breast, or melanoma.

Colorectal, ovarian (gynecologic), and gastric are the most common (nearly 75%) primary tumors in patients with subsequent small bowel obstruction (14–16,18). Less frequent are melanoma, mesothelioma, and a variety of other intra-abdominal and extra-abdominal sites of tumors such as pancreas, breast, or lung. Melanoma is the most common cause of malignant intussusception in the adult population (22). Therefore, small bowel lesions may cause obstruction by their intraluminal occlusion, extraluminal compression, or by intussusception (21).

Colorectal cancer can lead to obstruction of the colon and small bowel obstruction. Primary large bowel obstruction is most commonly caused by colon carcinoma (78% of patients) (12). Noncolonic malignancy (12%) and benign causes (10%) account for the rest. Owing to the increased diameter of the right-sided colon and the fecal consistency, left-sided colon cancer obstructs more readily than right-sided malignancies. Intussusception is an infrequent mechanism of obstruction in these patients (12). Ovarian and prostatic carcinoma may obstruct the colon by peritoneal carcinomatosis or direct extension. Extra-abdominal cancers such as breast cancer metastases may also lead to large bowel obstruction.

Late radiation injury to the bowel may be the source of bowel obstruction (23). The small bowel is the predominant site of obstruction after radiation in approximately 90% of instances.

As mentioned previously, not all bowel obstructions in patients with cancer are mechanical in nature. A patient presenting clinically with obstructive symptoms may have intestinal dysmotility or pseudo-obstruction. The pathophysiology of pseudo-obstruction in the patient with cancer has been attributed to the denervation of the bowel and mesentery by carcinoma, metastatic infiltration of the celiac plexus, and paraneoplastic syndromes (24). Ogilvie's syndrome, as classically described, refers to pseudo-obstruction as a result of extra-abdominal metastatic carcinoma invading the celiac plexus, leading to sympathetic denervation (25). These patients were noted to be free of gastrointestinal involvement by their tumors at exploratory laparotomy despite obstructing symptoms.

DIAGNOSIS

After taking a careful history and performing a physical examination and obtaining blood for studies, patients admitted with obstructive symptoms (such as nausea, vomiting, constipation, cramping abdominal pain, and abdominal distension) should undergo radiographic evaluation of the abdomen (supine and upright) and the chest with plain films. Patients with nondiagnostic plain abdominal films, atypical history and/or physical examination, or protracted courses without resolution of obstructive symptoms are candidates for further radiographic studies.

Many patients with obstructive symptoms may have indeterminate or equivocal plain radiographs, resulting in delayed management. In this patient population, an abdominal computed tomography (CT) scan is invaluable for diagnostic accuracy. In a recent study of 32 patients presenting with clinical suspicion of intestinal obstruction, abdominal CT had a higher sensitivity (93 vs. 77% and specificity (100 vs. 50%) than plain radiographs in diagnosing obstruction (26). Therefore, an abdominal CT scan should be considered for patients with an unclear diagnosis after plain films. Magnetic resonance imaging (MRI) may help distinguish between benign and malignant bowel obstructions (27).

Upper gastrointestinal radiographic contrast studies with small bowel follow through may be useful in further delineating a small bowel obstruction. Barium is generally more useful than water-soluble contrast agents for identifying a distal obstruction because gastrointestinal secretions do not dilute it. If barium remains in the small bowel, it does not become inspissated because the small bowel lacks the water absorptive capacity of the colon. However, a disadvantage of a barium study of the upper bowel is the need to fully cleanse the bowel of this agent before performing any subsequent radiographic studies, and therefore should be used only when the presence of an obstruction in the lower region has been ruled out. Perhaps the greatest utility of the upper gastrointestinal series is in patients with intermittent or partial small bowel obstruction.

For patients with suspected colonic obstruction or both small and large bowel obstruction, a barium enema can be quite useful in determining the presence and location of the large bowel obstruction. In patients with suspected mechanical large bowel obstruction by plain abdominal radiographs, contrast enemas have confirmed the diagnosis in most patients (28). However, as many as one third of patients will have free flow of contrast, ruling out mechanical obstruction and raising the diagnostic possibility of pseudo-obstruction (28). A barium enema should never be attempted if a perforation is suspected and should be terminated promptly if the fluoroscopist detects an obstructing lesion. The colon can absorb water from the barium, which then becomes inspissated above a partially obstructing lesion, making subsequent colonic cleansing very difficult.

Although not widely employed, laparoscopy may be used as a diagnostic tool in patients with suspected small bowel obstruction (29). In one series, 92% of 167 patients were also successfully treated laparoscopically (29).

MANAGEMENT OF MECHANICAL OBSTRUCTION

Overview

An algorithm describing the management of a suspected malignant mechanical bowel obstruction is presented in Figure 16.1. At initial presentation, a history, physical examination, and abdominal plain films should be performed routinely. Patients with obstruction are usually dehydrated and have electrolyte imbalances, owing to persistent vomiting and the inability to tolerate oral liquids. All patients should be aggressively hydrated intravenously and given nothing by mouth. A nasogastric tube should be placed in an attempt to relieve further vomiting and avoid possible aspiration. The electrolyte imbalance should be determined and corrected. Once the patient is

adequately stabilized and hydrated, therapeutic strategies can be entertained.

When upper gastrointestinal obstruction is diagnosed, the etiology is generally secondary to a malignancy. If the patient is able to tolerate an operation, a resection and anastomosis or a gastroduodenal bypass should be performed. Less invasive procedures such as stenting or permanent tube decompression can be offered. In the largest reported series of patients undergoing surgical palliation (operative or endoscopic) for upper gastrointestinal obstruction ($n = 151$), 79% had symptom resolution (2). If the patient is not a candidate for surgery, pharmacologic palliation should be administered.

In the setting of small bowel obstruction, patients with a previously resected malignancy or abdominal surgery may be managed with a trial of conservative therapy. Often the obstruction will resolve as edema and inflammation of the distended bowel subside. If the obstruction resolves, no further treatment is warranted. If the obstruction persists for >3–7 days, patients able to tolerate an operation should undergo an exploratory laparotomy with the intention of reestablishing gastrointestinal continuity. The procedure may involve enterolysis for benign obstruction, resection, bypass, or a diverting ostomy for recurrent cancer. In one of the largest reported series of patients undergoing surgical palliation for small and large bowel obstruction ($n = 97$), 89% had resolution of symptoms (2). Patients with small bowel obstruction who are not candidates for surgery are best managed pharmacologically.

In contrast to small bowel obstruction, mechanical colonic obstruction does not usually resolve with conservative therapy

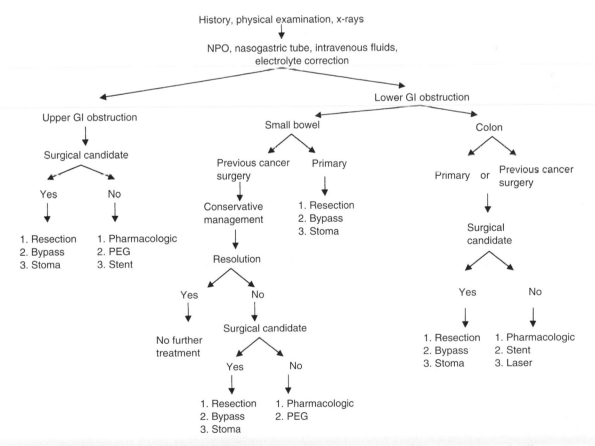

FIGURE 16.1. Management algorithm for malignant bowel obstruction. NPO, nothing by mouth; GI, gastrointestinal; PEG, percutaneous endoscopic gastrostomy.

as this is rarely due to edema or inflammation. If the patient is able to tolerate surgery, a resection should be attempted when feasible. Patients with a large tumor burden can be managed either by bypass or stoma creation. Patients unable to tolerate a major surgical procedure can be managed by less invasive endoscopic ablative therapy, dilatation and stenting, or permanent tube decompression. These smaller procedures can be frequently done at the bedside or under local anesthesia.

Malignant bowel obstruction secondary to peritoneal carcinomatosis has a poor prognosis. Surgical palliation is less effective in patients with ascites, and consequently, nonoperative palliation is advocated in this subset (30,31).

Initial Management

In the absence of fever, leukocytosis, or peritonitis, patients with obstructive symptoms deserve a trial of conservative therapy. Patients need to be monitored with serial physical examinations (preferably by the same clinician) and with daily abdominal radiographs. In the patient with cancer, nasogastric decompression, intravenous hydration, and electrolyte replenishment results in spontaneous resolution of small bowel obstructions in 21% of patients (Table 16.1) in a mean of 3–7 days (15,16). Approximately 40% of patients will need to be readmitted for conservative or surgical management of recurrent obstruction (Table 16.1). Bowel strangulation and gangrene are rare in these circumstances, occurring in 0–5% (15,17), with the exception of one series in which it occurred in 24% of patients (16).

The choice of nasogastric tube or long intestinal tube (i.e., Miller-Abbott, Cantor, Baker) for decompression is individualized by the physician. Both tubes have been reported to have similar success in treating small bowel obstruction. A randomized study failed to identify the superiority of one tube over the other (32). The most common practice is to use the nasogastric tube because of its ease of placement and effectiveness in decompressing the upper gastrointestinal tract. It is more difficult to get long tubes into position (i.e., pass beyond the duodenum), but they can be effective in decompressing the more distal bowel. They may help delineate a site of obstruction through their failure to pass beyond the obstructed point or serve as a port for the instillation of radiographic contrast agents. Long tubes may also provide useful landmarks intraoperatively when faced with carcinomatosis and dense adhesions, locating a suitable segment of small bowel for bypass.

If, during the course of conservative therapy, the patient deteriorates or fails to improve after a clinically acceptable length of therapy, surgical therapy should be considered.

Surgical Management

Gastroduodenal Obstruction

When patients present with gastroduodenal obstruction, the goal is to reestablish gastrointestinal continuity and palliate the symptoms of obstruction. The surgical procedure should be performed with curative intent.

Ten to 20% of patients with pancreatic cancer, not undergoing a resection at initial surgery, eventually require a gastrojejunostomy for palliation of gastric outlet obstruction (6,33). Hence, prophylactic gastrojejunostomy at the time of initial exploration has been advised for patients with unresectable obstruction (5,6,34). Effective palliation is not always achieved. Delayed gastric emptying may occur leading to significant postoperative morbidity (5). Recently, laparoscopic gastroenterostomy has been introduced for the treatment of gastroduodenal obstruction. The procedure can be performed safely with minimal operation times. Good palliation of nausea and vomiting can be expected (35).

Small Intestine Obstruction

As many as one third of patients with cancer undergoing surgery for small bowel obstruction with a previous diagnosis of cancer may have adhesions or a benign cause of obstruction (Table 16.1). In this setting, operative success in resolving their symptoms is usually high. Still, most of the obstructions in patients with a previous diagnosis of cancer are tumor related (median 72%). Three fourths of patients (median 74%) can be surgically relieved of their symptoms. A variety of surgical procedures has been reported to relieve the small bowel obstruction (Table 16.2). Bypass was the procedure most commonly performed, followed by resection, and then stoma creation. Recurrent obstruction after successful surgical relief of symptoms occurs in 25% of patients (Table 16.1). Operative morbidity (median 32%) and mortality (median 15%) are high and reflect the generally comorbid nature of this patient population.

Treatment options are similar for a small bowel obstruction caused by a primary small bowel tumor or an extra-abdominal carcinoma with a metastasis to the small bowel. Patients should be managed by resection with primary anastomosis,

TABLE 16.2

SURGICAL PROCEDURES TO RELIEVE OBSTRUCTION IN PATIENTS WITH CANCER

Author	Surgical procedures	Bypass	Stoma	Resection	Enterolysis	Others
Gallick 1986 (15)	56[a]	16	10	18	12	0
Butler 1991 (16)	45[a]	12	0	19	7	7
Makela 1991 (14)	85	25	25	25	0	10
Tang 1995 (17)	61[a]	29	15	3	14	0
Nakane 1996 (18)	50	14	12	5	10	9
Edna 1998 (9)	41	7	1	16	16	1
Pothuri 2003 (20)	94[a]	33	21	18	0	22
Total	432	136	84	104	59	49

[a]More than one procedure in some patients.

when appropriate, or by bypass, if resection is not warranted or possible.

Primary resection and anastomosis has been advocated in patients with postradiation small bowel obstruction (23). Despite careful selection of patients, anastomotic leak occurred in 11% and was the most common complication.

Colon Obstruction

The surgical management of right-sided and transverse colonic obstruction secondary to a primary colonic malignancy is similar to small bowel obstruction. Right hemicolectomy for obstructive right-colon lesions or extended right hemicolectomy for transverse colon lesions followed by primary anastomosis is generally considered safe in emergent conditions without preoperative bowel preparation (12,36). Obstructive carcinoma of the splenic flexure can be managed by extended right hemicolectomy and immediate anastomosis (36) although including these lesions in a left colon resection is also a valid option. The best approach is one that is individualized for the patient and comfortable to the surgeon.

Owing to improved antibiotics, anesthesia, and operative techniques, the surgical management of obstructive left colon and sigmoid lesions is evolving from the traditional three-stage procedure to a two-stage procedure, and more recently a single-stage procedure (36,37). The presence of peritoneal soiling or inflammation, the condition of the bowel, the stability of the patient, and ultimately the judgment and expertise of the surgeon will dictate the approach used. All three methods have a role that depends on the clinical setting. The three-stage procedure for lesions distal to the splenic flexure involves creation of a proximal (transverse colon) decompressing colostomy, elective resection of the lesion in the mechanically cleansed bowel and primary anastomosis, and closure of the colostomy.

Presently a two-stage procedure is the more common approach and consists of primary resection with the creation of a proximal end colostomy and Hartman pouch or mucous fistula. The second stage reestablishes bowel continuity. Retrospective data as well as a randomized study (38) support the use of a two-stage as opposed to a three-stage approach.

The most recent trend in treating obstructive left colon lesions has been a single-step segmental resection and primary anastomosis in select patients (39,40). Currently, one-stage procedures for obstructing left colon lesions are not advocated in the presence of fecal peritonitis, a large contiguous pelvic abscess, or debilitated patient (37). To accomplish a one-stage procedure in highly select patients and to have a low incidence of anastomotic leak, a variety of approaches that allow mechanical bowel cleaning have been advocated. Preoperative techniques include endoscopic laser relief of obstruction (41) and stenting (42). Intraoperatively, colonic irrigation has been advocated by a variety of groups (10,39,40). The technique consists of proximal (cecal) infusion of saline and distal (above the obstruction) collection of luminal contents in a closed system. Following resection and mechanical cleansing, a primary anastomosis is performed. One small randomized trial compared intraoperative colonic irrigation to manual decompression of the colon and concluded that both methods were equally safe during one-stage procedures (43).

The most aggressive approach of subtotal/total colectomy and ileocolonic/ileorectal anastomosis obviates the need for mechanical bowel cleansing in one-stage procedures (44). Subtotal colectomy can decrease the operative time and complexity associated with colonic irrigation. Any synchronous tumors are also removed. A prospective randomized multi-center trial compared subtotal colectomy to segmental resection following intraoperative irrigation (45). Mortality and complication rates did not differ significantly between the two groups. However, patients undergoing subtotal colectomy reported increased frequency of bowel movement and increased visits to their general practitioner for bowel problems.

Curative resection for malignant colonic obstruction is not possible in all patients. Patients with unresectable disease, either primary, recurrent, or from carcinomatosis may be palliated by bypass or stoma. For high-risk patients, a proximal diverting colostomy is a viable alternative (46). Loop colostomies (independent of location) are generally easier to create and close than divided colostomies, and can be totally diverting.

Medical Management

Pharmacologic

Pharmacologic palliation is most often administered to patients with end-stage cancer. The goal is to decrease symptoms associated with bowel obstruction. Therefore, pharmacologic therapy should attempt to decrease abdominal pain, alleviate nausea and vomiting, reduce gastrointestinal secretions, and, at times, increase bowel motility. Hyoscine butylbromide and opioids (morphine) are agents frequently used to control colicky abdominal pain (47–50) (Table 16.3). Loperamide has also been used to relieve intestinal colic (49).

Emesis is controlled by different classes of pharmacologic agents. Metoclopramide, dimenhydrinate, and haloperidol have all been administered subcutaneously to alleviate nausea and vomiting (47–49). Generally, metoclopramide has been reserved for patients with partial bowel obstruction, as symptoms may be exacerbated if the obstruction is complete. Prochlorperazine (given rectally) and dexamethasone (given intravenously) have also been used to treat nausea and vomiting (48,49) (Table 16.3).

For prophylaxis against crampy abdominal pain and nausea/vomiting, pharmacologic agents that decrease gastrointestinal secretions have been employed. Hyoscine butylbromide, scopolamine, and octreotide have all been used subcutaneously to decrease gastrointestinal secretions successfully and minimize symptoms of obstruction (48,51,52,54). In two separate randomized trials, octreotide was superior to hyoscine butylbromide in alleviating symptoms of malignant bowel obstruction in nonoperable patients (51,52).

Corticosteroids may have palliative effects because they are able to reduce the edema surrounding tumors and points of obstruction. By reducing edema, steroids may lessen the extrinsic or intrinsic compression of the bowel lumen and relieve symptoms. A meta-analysis studying the use of corticosteroids and bowel obstruction could only indicate a trend toward the resolution of bowel obstruction at a daily dose range of 6–16 mg intravenously (55).

The general strategy of combining multiple agents with different activities has been widely accepted for the pharmacologic management of bowel obstruction. However, the large list of agents reported suggests that no single approach has emerged as the standard. A practical approach has been the use of an antisecretory agent such as octreotide, a corticosteroid such as dexamethasone to reduce bowel wall edema and intraluminal secretions, and a prokinetic agent such as metaclopramide in the absence of complete bowel obstruction. A recent report of the combination of propulsive agents (metoclopramide 60 mg per day and amidotrizoato 50 mL bolus, a radiocontrast media) and antisecretory agents (octreotide 0.3 mg per day and dexamethasone 12 mg daily) demonstrated reversal of malignant bowel obstruction in 14 of 15 patients (53). In this study, patients were hydrated and metabolic alterations were corrected. The authors noted that no patient had exacerbation of colic with the use of

TABLE 16.3

PALLIATIVE PHARMACOLOGIC THERAPY

Drug	Class	Dosage	Route	Reference
COLICKY PAIN DRUG				
Hyoscine butylbromide	Anticholinergic	40–80 mg/d	s.c.	(48,51,52)
		0.8–2 mg/d	s.c.	(49)
Morphine	Opioid	2.5 mg/h, increasing by 2.5 mg/h until relief is achieved	s.c.	(50)
		0.5 mg/kg/h increasing by 0.5 mg/kg until relief is achieved	s.c./i.v.	(47)
Loperamide	Antidiarrheal	2 mg/q.i.d.	Oral	(49)
NAUSEA AND VOMITING				
Metoclopramide	Neuroleptic	60–120 mg/d	s.c.	(48,53)
Dimenhydrinate	Antihistamine	50–100 mg p.r.n.	s.c.	(48)
Haloperidol	Neuroleptic	5–10 mg/d	s.c.	(47,49)
Prochlorperazine	Neuroleptic	25 mg/q8h	p.r.	(49)
Dexamethasone	Corticosteroid	8–60 mg/d	i.v.	(48,53)
Scopolamine	Antimuscarinic	40–120 mg/d	s.c.	(54)
Octreotide	Somatostatin analog	0.2–0.9 mg/d	s.c.	(51–54)

the prokinetic agents and attributed these findings to the concomitant use of antisecretory agents.

Optimal pharmacologic management may permit the hydration of some terminally ill patients without the need for intravenous support. But when the oral intake of fluids is contraindicated, the intravenous route may be used. Home care with intravenous hydration and pharmacologic support has been successful in some series (56). However, intravenous access is often difficult in these patients. Hypodermoclysis is an option for hydration in terminally ill patients with cancer. One liter of fluid can be administered subcutaneous per day in a safe and effective manner (57).

Percutaneous Gastrostomy

When pharmacologic management fails to control symptoms in patients who do not have surgical options, percutaneous endoscopic gastrostomy (PEG) for decompression may be an effective procedure to relieve symptoms of obstruction. PEG placement offers an alternative to nasogastric tube decompression and surgical gastrostomy when treating malignant upper gastrointestinal or small bowel obstructions. The PEG tube allows patients to resume oral intake and avoid nasogastric discomfort. In patients with gynecologic malignancies, palliation has been obtained successfully in most patients after PEG placement (58,59). In one study of patients with mostly nongynecologic malignancies, 22 of 24 patients with advanced disease were able to tolerate liquids by mouth after PEG placement and 20 were discharged to home care (60). Complications from PEG placement occurred in <20% of patients (58,59). Further, most patients could return home or to a hospice setting to continue palliative care.

Local Ablation

Another palliative procedure that is less invasive than surgery for the relief of malignant bowel obstructions is local ablation with endoscopic laser therapy or by other means. The laser has been used most frequently in select patients for left-sided colonic obstruction (41,61). The neodymium-yttrium aluminum garnett (Nd-YAG) laser is the most commonly used laser for palliation of symptoms. In a series of 117 patients treated with laser therapy for distal colonic obstruction, 89%

of patients were successfully treated by initial endoscopic laser therapy. A mean number of seven sessions over a period of 7 months was needed to achieve long-term palliation in 65% of patients (61). Laser therapy has also been used concomitantly with metallic stents for distal colonic obstruction (62). After initial treatment of the obstruction with laser therapy, a metallic stent is inserted to increase colonic patency and decrease repeated laser treatments. It is best not to treat patients with obstruction and significant pelvic invasion by endoscopic laser therapy as pain persists after treatment (61). Simple electrocautery and snare piecemeal removal and wire-guided dilatation can be used with relative safety for short-term palliation.

Stenting

Endoscopic metallic stenting is increasingly used for the management of obstructive lesions that are reachable by endoscopes, which include upper and lower intestinal tract and some small bowel lesions. Although stenting for upper gastrointestinal obstruction is always palliative in nature, stenting for colorectal obstruction may be used as a bridge to definitive surgical treatment and palliation.

Most stents are placed under direct endoscopic visualization, and sometimes with radiologic guidance. The site of obstruction is visualized directly or under fluoroscopy with an injection of radiographic contrast. Next, a guidewire is placed across the stricture with either endoscopic or fluoroscopic guidance, or both. The self-expandable metal stent is then threaded over the guide wire, across the obstruction, and released into position. Once the stent is in place, the endoscope can be further advanced to look for other lesions. Repeat contrast injection is sometimes used to verify position, rule out perforation, and look for additional points of obstruction.

Endoscopically or fluoroscopically placed metallic stents have been used selectively for the treatment of gastroduodenal obstructions caused by pancreatic, gastric, and bile duct cancers and by lymphoma. Upper gastrointestinal stents have been placed in the esophagus, stomach, and duodenum, and across previous surgical anastomoses. Technical success in stent placement is >90% in most series and 80–90% of patients experience clinical improvement and are able to tolerate an oral solid or liquid diet (63,64). Complications related to the placement of the stents are uncommon. However, some stents will migrate and obstruct over time. Duration of stent patency is difficult to determine in this patient population as many patients expire before stent occlusion. It should be noted that stents are placed in a highly select patient population and high success rates may be due to the retrospective analyses. Still, the stenting of malignant upper gastrointestinal obstructions remains an attractive, simple procedure to relieve vomiting and the inability to eat in select patients. In a retrospective review of patients with duodenal obstruction, enhanced quality of life was noted in patients undergoing stenting as compared to those undergoing surgical gastrojejunostomy (65). It is to be noted that after duodenal stent placement, the biliary tree is usually inaccessible endoscopically. Consequently, patients with known or impending biliary obstruction should have a biliary stent placed before duodenal stent placement (63).

Stenting is more commonly performed for the resolution of malignant colorectal obstruction than for upper gastrointestinal obstructions. In colorectal obstruction, metallic wall stents may be employed either for the palliation of obstruction in end-stage patients or as a bridge to further definitive surgical management. The use of preoperative stenting allows nonsurgical decompression of the colon and avoids an emergent colostomy. Decompression allows adequate bowel preparation and preoperative optimization. Further, metallic stents have been used after initial laser treatment to maintain colorectal patency (62). In a collective review of 1198 patients with stents for malignant colorectal obstruction, the median technical success rate was 94% with a clinical success rate of 91% (12). Stenting served as a bridge to surgery in 72% of patients. Major complications related to stent placement included perforation in 4%, stent migration in 12%, reobstruction in 7% and mortality in 0.6% of patients (42). Other side effects included bleeding and tenesmus (if the stent is placed too distally in the rectum) (63). In one randomized trial of 30 patients with inoperable left colon cancer, stent placement was compared to stoma creation, and survival was equivalent in both groups (66). The authors claimed a psychological benefit in patients receiving stents because they did not need colostomies.

MANAGEMENT OF NONMECHANICAL OBSTRUCTION

Patients with malignancy may present with nonmechanical colonic obstruction during their course of disease. Colonic pseudo-obstruction has been managed both pharmacologically and by colonoscopic decompression. A mechanical obstruction must be excluded before the initiation of pharmacologic management. Neostigmine has been used effectively to relieve colonic pseudo-obstruction in the nonmalignant setting (67). Further study is warranted to assess the efficiency of neostigmine in pseudo-obstruction associated with malignancy. Most patients with colonic pseudo-obstruction can be conservatively managed initially with a trial of bed rest, intravenous fluids, avoidance of opioids, and pharmacologic therapy. When symptoms worsen or the risk of complication increases, colonoscopic decompression is warranted. Perforation from cecal dilatation is the most severe complication of colonic pseudo-obstruction. Cecostomy was used in the past to prevent this complication. Successful decompression is now performed with colonoscopy. Most (68%) patients are effectively relieved of pseudo-obstruction by colonoscopy (68). If colonoscopy fails, either a right hemicolectomy or cecostomy should be performed for definitive management.

PREVENTION

If one could prevent bowel obstruction, this would be far better than trying to accurately diagnose and treat the condition. Careful attention to fluid and electrolytes to prevent nonmechanical events, and strict adherence to a bowel program when on chronic opioids can obviate most inpatient events of bowel obstruction.

The judicious use of prophylactic surgery to either bypass impending areas of obstruction or create stomas when the progression of cancer would likely obstruct the bowel may be beneficial to the patient. In the presence of extensive disease in the pelvis due to colonic or ovarian carcinoma, a prophylactic stoma is often considered despite the lack of obstructive symptoms at the time. Ten to 20% of patients with pancreatic cancer not undergoing a resection at initial surgery eventually require a gastrojejunostomy for palliation of gastric outlet obstruction (6,33). Hence, prophylactic gastrojejunostomy at the time of initial exploration has been advised for unresectable patients (5,6,34).

CONCLUSION

Bowel obstruction in the patient with cancer continues to be a significant problem. Many effective therapies are now available. The appropriate diagnosis and assessment of comorbidities are critical to the successful resolution of obstruction. Bowel obstruction is managed initially with intravenous hydration, nasogastric tube placement, avoidance of opioids, and correction of electrolyte abnormalities. When possible, mechanical gastroduodenal and colonic obstruction should be treated surgically. Patients with small bowel obstruction should receive a trial of conservative therapy, which often leads to the resolution of symptoms. The decision to proceed with surgical intervention in small bowel obstruction ultimately needs to be individualized to each patient.

Palliative management of bowel obstruction, either medical or surgical, is often required in the patient with cancer. Medical palliation by administration of a variety of pharmacologic agents can control symptoms of nausea, vomiting, pain, and distension in patients who are not candidates for surgery. Minimally invasive surgical procedures, such as PEG, local ablative therapy, and stenting may palliate symptoms without the need for further pharmacologic support.

References

1. Cherny NI. Taking care of the terminally ill cancer patient: management of gastrointestinal symptoms in patients with advanced cancer. *Ann Oncol* 2004;15(Suppl 4):iv205–iv213.
2. Miner TJ, Brennan MF, Jaques DP. A prospective, symptom related, outcomes analysis of 1022 palliative procedures for advanced cancer. *Ann Surg* 2004;240:719–726.
3. Shone DN, Nikoomanesh P, Smith-Meek MM, et al. Malignancy is the most common cause of gastric outlet obstruction in the era of H2 blockers. *Am J Gastroenterol* 1995;90:1769–1770.
4. Andersson A, Bergdahl L. Carcinoma of the pancreas. *Am Surg* 1976;42:173–177.
5. Jacobs PP, van der Sluis RF, Wobbes T. Role of gastroenterostomy in the palliative surgical treatment of pancreatic cancer. *J Surg Oncol* 1989;42:145–149.
6. Singh SM, Longmire WP, Reber HA. Surgical palliation for pancreatic cancer. The UCLA experience. *Ann Surg* 1990;212:132–139.
7. Stewardson RH, Bombeck CT, Nyhus LM. Critical operative management of small bowel obstruction. *Ann Surg* 1978;187:189–193.
8. Tunca JC, Buchler DA, Mack EA, et al. The management of ovarian-cancer-caused bowel obstruction. *Gynecol Oncol* 1981;12:186–192.
9. Edna TH, Bjerkeset T. Small bowel obstruction in patients previously operated on for colorectal cancer. *Eur J Surg* 1998;164:587–592.

10. Lee YM, Law WL, Chu KW, et al. Emergency surgery for obstructing colorectal cancers: a comparison between right-sided and left-sided lesions. *J Am Coll Surg* 2001;192:719–725.

11. Greenlee HB, Pienkos EJ, Vanderbilt PC, et al. Proceedings: acute large bowel obstruction. Comparison of county, veterans administration, and community hospital populations. *Arch Surg* 1974;108:470–476.

12. Buechter KJ, Boustany C, Gaillouette R, et al. Surgical management of the acutely obstructed colon. A review of 127 cases. *Am J Surg* 1988;156:163–168.

13. Sandler SG, Tobin W, Hendernson ES. Vincristine-induced neuropathy. A clinical study of fifty leukemic patients. *Neurology* 1969;19:367–374.

14. Makela J, Kiviniemi H, Laitinen S, et al. Surgical management of intestinal obstruction after treatment for cancer. *Eur J Surg* 1991;157:73–76.

15. Gallick HL, Weaver DW, Sachs RJ, et al. Intestinal obstruction in cancer patients. An assessment of risk factors and outcome. *Am Surg* 1986;52:434–437.

16. Butler JA, Cameron BL, Morrow M, et al. Small bowel obstruction in patients with a prior history of cancer. *Am J Surg* 1991;162:624–628.

17. Tang E, Davis J, Silberman H. Bowel obstruction in cancer patients. *Arch Surg* 1995;130:832–836.

18. Nakane Y, Okumura S, Akehira K, et al. Management of intestinal obstruction after gastrectomy for carcinoma. *Br J Surg* 1996;83:113.

19. Woolfson RG, Jennings K, Whalen GF. Management of bowel obstruction in patients with abdominal cancer. *Arch Surg* 1997;132:1093–1097.

20. Pothuri B, Vaidya A, Aghajanian C, et al. Palliative surgery for bowel obstruction in recurrent ovarian cancer:an updated series. *Gynecol Oncol* 2003;89:306–313.

21. Brophy C, Cahow CE. Primary small bowel malignant tumors. Unrecognized until emergent laparotomy. *Am Surg* 1989;55:408–412.

22. Liaw CC, Wang CS, Ng KK, et al. Enteric intussusception due to metastatic intestinal tumors. *J Formos Med Assoc* 1997;96:125–128.

23. Muttillo IA, Elias D, Bolognese A, et al. Surgical treatment of severe late radiation injury to the bowel: a retrospective analysis of 83 cases. *Hepatogastroenterology* 2002;49:1023–1026.

24. Lautenbach E, Lichtenstein GR. Retroperitoneal leiomyosarcoma and gastroparesis: a new association and review of tumor-associated intestinal pseudo-obstruction. *Am J Gastroenterol* 1995;90:1338–1341.

25. Ogilvie H. Large intestine colic due to sympathetic deprivation. A new clinical syndrome. *Br Med J* 1948;2:671–673.

26. Suri S, Gupta S, Sudhakar PJ, et al. Comparative evaluation of plain films, ultrasound and CT in the diagnosis of intestinal obstruction. *Acta Radiol* 1999;40:422–428.

27. Low RN, Chen SC, Barone R. Distinguishing benign from malignant bowel obstruction in patients with malignancy: findings at MR imaging. *Radiology* 2003;228:157–165.

28. Stewart J, Finan PJ, Courtney DF, et al. Does a water soluble contrast enema assist in the management of acute large bowel obstruction : a prospective study of 117 cases. *Br J Surg* 1984;71:799–801.

29. Franklin ME Jr, Gonzalez JJ Jr, Miter DB, et al. Laparoscopic diagnosis and treatment of intestinal obstruction. *Surg Endosc* 2004;18:26–30.

30. Blair SL, Chu DZ, Schwarz RE. Outcome of palliative operations for malignant bowel obstruction in patients with peritoneal carcinomatosis from nongynecological cancer. *Ann Surg Oncol* 2001;8:632–637.

31. Higashi H, Shida H, Ban K, et al. Factors affecting successful palliative surgery for malignant bowel obstruction due to peritoneal dissemination from colorectal cancer. *Jpn J Clin Oncol* 2003;33:357–359.

32. Fleshner PR, Siegman MG, Slater GI, et al. A prospective, randomized trial of short versus long tubes in adhesive small-bowel obstruction. *Am J Surg* 1995;170:366–337.

33. Sarr MG, Cameron JL. Surgical palliation of unresectable carcinoma of the pancreas. *World J Surg* 1984;8:906–918.

34. Sohn TA, Lillemoe KD, Cameron JL, et al. Surgical palliation of unresectable periampullary adenocarcinoma in the 1990s. *J Am Coll Surg* 1999;188:658–666.

35. Nagy A, Brosseuk D, Hemming A, et al. Laparoscopic gastroenterostomy for duodenal obstruction. *Am J Surg* 1995;169:539–542.

36. Matheson NA. Management of obstructed and perforated large bowel carcinoma. *Baillieres Clin Gastroenterol* 1989;3:671–697.

37. Murray JJ. Nonelective colon resection. Alternatives to multistage resections. *Surg Clin North Am* 1991;71:1187–1194.

38. Kronborg O. Acute obstruction from tumour in the left colon without spread. A randomized trial of emergency colostomy versus resection. *Int J Colorect Dis* 1995;10:1–5.

39. Koruth NM, Krukowshi ZH, Youngson GG, et al. Intra-operative colonic irrigation in the management of left-sided large bowel emergencies. *Br J Surg* 1985;72:708–711.

40. Deen KI, Madoff RD, Goldberg SM, et al. Surgical management of left colon obstruction: the University of Minnesota experience. *J Am Coll Surg* 1998;187:573–576.

41. Eckhauser ML, Mansour EG. Endoscopic laser therapy for obstructing and/or bleeding colorectal carcinoma. *Am Surg* 1992;58:358–363.

42. Sebastian S, Johnston S, Geoghegan T, et al. Pooled analysis of the efficacy and safety of self-expanding metal stenting in malignant colorectal obstruction. *Am J Gastroenterol* 2004;99:2051–2057.

43. Lim JF, Tang CL, Seow-Choen F, et al. Prospective, randomized trial comparing intraoperative colonic irrigation with manual decompression only for obstructed left-sided colorectal cancer. *Dis Colon Rectum* 2005;48:205–209.

44. Arnaud J-P, Bergamaschi R. Emergency subtotal/total colectomy with anastomosis for acutely obstructed carcinoma of the left colon. *Dis Colon Rectum* 1994;37:685–688.

45. SCOTIA Study Group. Single-stage treatment for malignant left-sided colonic obstruction: a prospective randomized clinical trial comparing subtotal colectomy with segmental resection following intraoperative irrigation. The SCOTIA Study Group. Subtotal colectomy versus On-table irrigation and anastomosis. *Br J Surg* 1995;82:1622–1627.

46. Gutman M, Kaplan O, Skornick Y, et al. Proximal colostomy: still an effective emergency measure in obstructing carcinoma of the large bowel. *J Surg Oncol* 1989;41:210–212.

47. Ventafridda V, Ripamonti C, Caraceni A, et al. The management of inoperable gastrointestinal obstruction in terminal cancer patients. *Tumori* 1990;76:389–393.

48. Fainsinger RL, Spachynski K, Hanson J, et al. Symptom control in terminally ill patients with malignant bowel obstruction (MBO). *J Pain Symptom Manage* 1994;9:12–18.

49. Baines M, Oliver DJ, Carter RL. Medical management of intestinal obstruction in patients with advanced malignant disease. *Lancet* 1985;2:990–993.

50. Isbister WH, Elder P, Symons L. Non-operative management of malignant intestinal obstruction. *J R Coll Surg Edinb* 1990;35:369–372.

51. Mercadante S, Ripamonti C, Casuccio A, et al. Comparison of octreotide and hyoscine butylbromide in controlling gastrointestinal symptoms due to malignant inoperable bowel obstruction. *Support Care Cancer* 2000;8:188–191.

52. Mystakidou K, Tsilika E, Kalaidopoulou O, et al. Comparison of octreotide administration vs conservative treatment in the management of inoperable bowel obstruction in patients with far advanced cancer: a randomized, double- blind, controlled clinical trial. *Anticancer Res* 2002;22:1187–1192.

53. Mercadante S, Ferrera P, Villari P, et al. Aggressive pharmacological treatment for reversing malignant bowel obstruction. *J Pain Symptom Manage* 2004;28:412–416.

54. Ripamonti C, Mercadante S, Groff L, et al. Role of octreotide, scopolamine butylbromide, and hydration in symptom control of patients with inoperable bowel obstruction and nasogastric tubes: a prospective randomized trial. *J Pain Symptom Manage* 2000;19:23–34.

55. Feuer DJ, Broadley KE. Systematic review and meta-analysis of corti-costeroids for the resolution of malignant bowel obstruction in advanced gynaecological and gastrointestinal cancers. Systematic review steering committee. *Ann Oncol* 1999;10:1035–1041.

56. Gemlo B, Rayner AA, Lewis B, et al. Home support of patients with end-stage malignant bowel obstruction using hydration and venting gastrostomy. *Am J Surg* 1986;152:100–104.

57. Fainsinger RL, MacEachern T, Miller MJ, et al. The use of hypodermoclysis for rehydration in terminally ill cancer patients. *J Pain Symptom Manage* 1994;9:298–302.

58. Campagnutta E, Cannizzaro R, Gallo A, et al. Palliative treatment of upper intestinal obstruction by gynecological malignancy: the usefulness of percutaneous endoscopic gastrostomy. *Gynecol Oncol* 1996;62:103–105.

59. Pothuri B, Montemarano M, Gerardi M, et al. Percutaneous endoscopic gastrostomy tube placement in patients with malignant bowel obstruction due to ovarian carcinoma. *Gynecol Oncol* 2005;96:330–334.

60. Scheidbach H, Horbach T, Groitl H, et al. Percutaneous endoscopic gastrostomy/jejunostomy (PEG/PEJ) for decompression in the upper gastrointestinal tract. Initial experience with palliative treatment of gastrointestinal obstruction in terminally ill patients with advanced carcinomas. *Surg Endosc* 1999;13:1103–1105.

61. Gevers AM, Macken E, Hiele M, et al. Endoscopic laser therapy for palliation of patients with distal colorectal carcinoma: analysis of factors influencing long-term outcome. *Gastrointest Endosc* 2000;51:580–585.

62. Dohmoto M, Hunerbein M, Schlag PM. Application of rectal stents for palliation of obstructing rectosigmoid cancer. *Surg Endosc* 1997;11:758–761.

63. Baron TH, Harewood GC. Enteral self-expandable stents. *Gastrointest Endosc* 2003;58:421–433.

64. Mergener K, Kozarek RA. Stenting of the gastrointestinal tract. *Dig Dis* 2002;20:173–181.

65. Maetani I, Tada T, Ukita T, et al. Comparison of duodenal stent placement with surgical gastrojejunostomy for palliation in patients with duodenal obstructions caused by pancreaticobiliary malignancies. *Endoscopy* 2004;36:73–78.

66. Xinopoulos D, Dimitroulopoulos D, Theodosopoulos T, et al. Stenting or stoma creation for patients with inoperable malignant colonic obstructions? Results of a study and cost-effectiveness analysis. *Surg Endosc* 2004;18:421–426.

67. Trevisani GT, Hyman NH, Church JM. Neostigmine: safe and effective treatment for acute colonic pseudo-obstruction. *Dis Colon Rectum* 2000;43:599–603.

68. Bode WE, Beart RW Jr, Spencer RJ, et al. Colonoscopic decompression for acute pseudo-obstruction of the colon (Ogilvie's syndrome). Report of 22 cases and review of the literature. *Am J Surg* 1984;147:243–245.

CHAPTER 17 ■ DIAGNOSIS AND MANAGEMENT OF ASCITES

JAY R. THOMAS AND CHARLES F. VON GUNTEN

EPIDEMIOLOGY

Ascites, the accumulation of fluid in the abdomen, is common in patients with certain types of end-stage cancer. Its formation may be a direct result of a malignant process or secondary to unrelated comorbidity. Because the pathophysiology of fluid collection varies, treatment strategies differ. Clinical distinction between the causes of ascites is therefore imperative.

Of all patients with ascites, approximately 80% have cirrhosis (1). Other causes of nonmalignant ascites are accounted for as follows: heart failure, 3%; tuberculosis, 2%; nephrogenic ascites related to hemodialysis, 1%; pancreatic disease, 1%; and miscellaneous entities such as hepatic vein thrombosis (Budd-Chiari syndrome), pericardial disease, and nephrotic syndrome account for approximately 2% (1). Only 10% of patients who have ascites have malignancy as the primary cause (1). In these patients, epithelial malignancies, particularly ovarian, endometrial, breast, colon, gastric, and pancreatic carcinomas, cause over 80% of malignant ascites. The remaining 20% is due to malignancies of unknown origin (2). In one study, Runyon has shown that 53.3% of malignant ascites is associated with peritoneal carcinomatosis, 13.3% is associated with massive liver metastases, 13.3% is associated with peritoneal carcinomatosis and massive liver metastases, 13.3% is associated with hepatocellular carcinoma with portal hypertension, and 6.7% is associated with chylous ascites (3).

In general, the presence of ascites portends a poor prognosis, regardless of the cause. Patients with nonmalignant ascites related to cirrhosis have a survival rate of approximately 50% at 2 years (1). The mean survival in patients with malignant ascites is generally <4 months (4). However, with ascites due to a malignancy that is relatively sensitive to chemotherapy, such as newly diagnosed ovarian cancer or lymphoma, the mean survival may improve significantly (4).

PATHOPHYSIOLOGY

Nonmalignant Ascites

The mechanisms that lead to the development of ascites are many, and controversy exists regarding which factors are most important. The most common cause of nonmalignant ascites is cirrhosis of the liver. In cirrhotic ascites, abnormal sodium retention is mediated by various hormonal and neural mechanisms, similar to those responsible for excess fluid retention in congestive heart failure. A hemodynamic state exists where total blood volume and cardiac output are increased and systemic vascular resistance is low. Studies have implicated nitric oxide as one potential mediator of this arterial vasodilation (5). In response, the vasoconstrictors of the renin–angiotensin–aldosterone system and the sympathetic nervous system are activated. Although atrial natriuretic peptide levels are increased, there is reduced renal responsiveness (6). In addition, arginine vasopressin, a potent vasoconstrictor, is activated in a manner independent of the osmotic state (7). The net result is an increase in total body sodium and water. In conjunction with cirrhosis, which has caused increased hepatic venous and lymphatic resistance, severe portal hypertension ensues. The increase in hepatic venous sinusoidal and portal pressures causes the excess fluid volume to localize to the peritoneal cavity secondary to fluid transudation from the splanchnic capillary bed. Ascites accumulation is also exacerbated by diminished intravascular oncotic pressure, resulting from hypoalbuminemia caused by decreased synthetic capacity of the cirrhotic liver.

Malignant Ascites

Malignant ascites arises through different pathophysiologic mechanisms. First, in peritoneal carcinomatosis, neovascularization and subsequent "leak" from vessels is thought to play a prime role in ascites development. Researchers have identified a vascular growth and permeability factor that increases fluid leak from peritoneal vasculature; vascular endothelial growth factor (VEGF) is a prime candidate for this activity (8). Compared with cirrhotic ascites, high levels of VEGF are present in malignant ascites from gastric, colon, and ovarian cancers (9). In animal models, inhibiting the tyrosine kinase activity of VEGF receptors reduced ascites formation (10). Matrix metalloproteinases (MMP) also appear to be involved in this process. Breaking down the extracellular matrix is an important step in neovascularization and metastatic spread. In animal models, MMP inhibitors significantly reduced malignant ascites (11). Portal pressures may be raised by direct tumor invasion of the liver with resultant hepatic venous obstruction. The resultant portal hypertension leads to transudation of fluid across the splanchnic bed into the abdominal cavity as in cirrhotic ascites. A final mechanism of ascites formation is due to lymphatic obstruction, commonly caused by lymphoma, resulting in chylous ascites.

DIAGNOSIS

History

Patients with ascites commonly notice an increase in abdominal girth, a sensation of fullness or bloating, and early satiety. Other useful features of the history include recent weight gain or ankle swelling. Patients may describe vague, generalized abdominal discomfort or a feeling of heaviness with ambulation. They may also note indigestion, nausea, and vomiting due to delayed gastric emptying, esophageal reflux symptoms due to increased intra-abdominal pressure, or protrusion of the umbilicus.

Physical Examination

Physical examination for ascites includes inspection for bulging flanks, percussion for flank dullness, a test for shifting dullness, and a test for a fluid wave. Jugular venous distension should also be assessed, as it may indicate a potentially reversible cardiac cause of ascites.

The abdominal flanks bulge when significant ascites is present because of the weight of abdominal free fluid. The examiner should look for bulging flanks when the patient is supine. The distinction between excess adipose tissue and ascites may be made by percussing the flanks to assess for dullness (Fig. 17.1). To detect flank dullness in the supine patient, approximately 1500 mL of fluid must be present (12).

If dullness to percussion is found, examination for shifting dullness is a useful maneuver. The flank is tapped, and a mark is made on the skin at the location where the tone changes. The patient is then turned partially toward the side that has been percussed. If the location of the dullness shifts upward toward the umbilicus, it is further evidence of intra-abdominal ascites (Fig. 17.2).

The elicitation of a fluid wave may also help to confirm the diagnosis. The test is performed by having an assistant place the medial edges of both hands firmly down the midline of the abdomen to block transmission of a wave through subcutaneous fat. The examiner places his/her hands on the flanks and then taps one flank sharply while simultaneously using the fingertips of the opposite hand to feel for an impulse

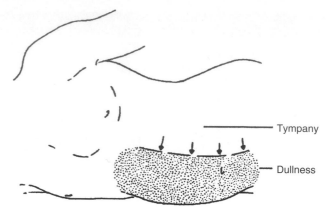

FIGURE 17.2. Tympany and dullness.

transmitted through the ascites to the other flank. This test is 90% specific, but only 62% sensitive (13).

Several additional aspects of the physical examination may also be helpful. The liver may be ballotable if it is enlarged and ascites is present. If ascites is severe, the examiner may discern umbilical, abdominal, or inguinal hernias; scrotal or lower extremity edema; or abdominal wall venous engorgement. The umbilicus may be flattened or slightly protuberant. Two additional maneuvers that have been described for the physical diagnosis of ascites, the puddle sign and auscultatory percussion, are not recommended (13).

Several diagnostic tests may be useful, particularly if the physical examination is equivocal. A plain radiograph of the abdomen may demonstrate a hazy or ground-glass pattern. Ultrasonography or computed tomography scan of the abdomen can readily identify as little as 100 mL of free fluid. These latter tests are most helpful in making the diagnosis when there is a relatively small amount of fluid, or when loculation is present.

Laboratory Abnormalities

A diagnostic paracentesis of 10–20 mL of fluid is useful to confirm the presence of ascites. More importantly, it is essential to help determine its cause. Identifying the cause has profound implications on the treatment to be attempted.

To perform paracentesis, one of two locations is chosen. The first is a midline location 2 cm inferior to the umbilicus. This location is over the linea alba, which is typically avascular. The second is a location 2 cm superior and medial to the anterior iliac spine and lateral to the edge of the rectus sheath, avoiding entry into the inferior epigastric artery. Ultrasonography may be performed if the fluid is difficult to obtain, loculation is suspected, or surgical scarring is present. Previous surgery in the area of the procedure increases the possibility of the bowel being adherent to the abdominal wall.

After careful cleansing and local anesthetizing, a 2-inch, 20-gauge angiocatheter is attached to a 20-mL syringe. To minimize the risk of leaking fluid after the procedure, the Z technique is performed. The skin is displaced 2 cm relative to the deep fascia. The needle is slowly advanced while a small amount of negative pressure is intermittently applied through the syringe until ascitic fluid is obtained. The intermittent pressure helps to avoid trapping omentum or bowel against the needle tip. After the necessary amount of fluid has been obtained, the needle is withdrawn. The fascial planes overlap to prevent fluid leakage, a common complication with a more direct approach.

The color of the fluid should be noted. A white milky fluid is characteristic of chylous ascites. Bloody fluid is almost always

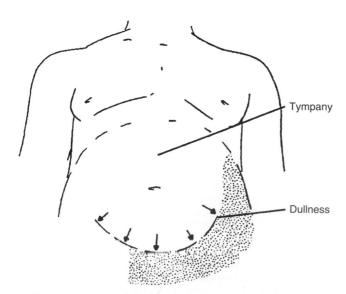

FIGURE 17.1. Shifting dullness.

malignant in origin, although it may be due to abdominal tuberculosis. Initial bloody fluid that clears is more likely related to the trauma of the procedure.

The fluid should undergo cytologic analysis, determination of cell counts with a differential, and determination of albumin and total protein concentrations. A Gram's stain with culture can be performed if infection is suspected, but it has a low sensitivity. Inoculation of ascites directly into blood culture bottles increases the sensitivity of detecting infection up to 85% (14). The cell count, particularly the absolute neutrophil count, is useful in the presumptive diagnosis of bacterial peritonitis. If the neutrophil count is >250 cells per mL, bacterial peritonitis is presumed and empiric antibiotics should be started.

Cytology is the most specific test to demonstrate that the ascites is due to malignancy. Cytology is approximately 97% sensitive with peritoneal carcinomatosis (3), but is not helpful in the detection of other types of malignant ascites such as massive hepatic metastasis or lymphomatous obstruction of lymph vessels. Therefore, the absence of malignant cells does not exclude malignancy as a cause.

In the past, the total protein concentration has been used to classify ascites into the broad categories of exudate (total protein >25 g per L) or transudate (total protein <25 g per L). However, this classification system has limitations and sometimes fails to lead to optimal treatment. It has been superseded by the serum-ascites albumin gradient (SAAG). It is defined as the serum albumin concentration minus the ascitic fluid albumin concentration. The SAAG directly correlates with portal pressure (15). Patients with an SAAG of 1.1 g per dL or more have ascites that is due in part to increased portal pressures, with an accuracy of 97%. Patients with an SAAG less than 1.1 g per dL do not have portal hypertension, with an accuracy of 97% (16).

The superiority of the SAAG to the exudate/transudate characterization is shown by two examples. Cardiac ascites is associated with portal hypertension and would be expected to be transudative; however, the total protein levels in cardiac ascites are often exudative (16,17). In this example, although total protein is not useful for primary categorization, it may be useful to identify some forms of ascites. Furthermore, ascites associated with spontaneous bacterial peritonitis (SBP) would be expected to be exudative consistent with an infection. However, SBP almost exclusively develops in low protein content ascites associated with portal hypertension, and total protein levels are typically in the transudative range (16).

MANAGEMENT

Overall goals for patient care should be considered before specific choices are made for managing ascites. The prognosis, expected response to management of the underlying conditions, and preferences for treatment should be established with the patient and family before any treatment plan is instituted. Each ascites treatment modality has associated burdens and benefits that deserve to be considered and discussed.

Whether ascites has a low or high SAAG is critical in determining the overall management plan. Ascites due to portal hypertension *is* in equilibrium with total body fluid. The most common cause of nonmalignant ascites, cirrhosis, falls within this category. Efforts to restrict salt and to affect fluid balance with diuretics are often successful. Malignant ascites may or may not be responsive to these efforts, depending on their cause. In peritoneal carcinomatosis, the SAAG is low, there is no portal hypertension, and the ascites *is not* in equilibrium with total body fluid (18). Consequently, salt and fluid restriction and diuretics may be of little use. Their injudicious use may result in intravascular volume depletion, diminished renal perfusion, azotemia, hypotension,

and fatigue (2). However, there are high SAAG forms of malignant ascites that are responsive to salt restriction and diuretics. For example, in cases of massive hepatic metastasis, portal hypertension is present, and salt restriction and diuretics are indicated (18). One exception to this rule is nephrotic syndrome in which the SAAG is low but the ascites is diuretic responsive (19). The total protein is also low (<25 g per L) in nephrotic syndrome and is therefore helpful in identifying this form of ascites. See Table 17.1 and Figure 17.3 for a summary.

Interventions for ascites management in the supportive or palliative care setting should be generally reserved for patients who are symptomatic. The following ascites-related symptoms may spur intervention:

- Dyspnea
- Fatigue
- Anorexia or early satiety
- Nausea/vomiting
- Pain
- Diminished exercise tolerance

Dietary Management

The dietary management of ascites with a high SAAG begins with sodium restriction. Patients with cirrhosis may excrete as little as 5–10 mEq of sodium per day in their urine. Limiting sodium intake to 88 mmol or 2 g per day (equivalent to 5 g of sodium chloride per day) is an attainable goal for a motivated patient but does make food less palatable. Considering the patient's goals of care, it may be better to liberalize the sodium intake and control ascites through other methods.

Patients are also prone to develop dilutional hyponatremia. The management of this condition has typically been fluid restriction to 1 L per day. In the patient with advanced disease, when treatment goals are purely palliative, fluid restriction is usually intolerably burdensome. Judicious medical management may be less burdensome. For patients with cirrhotic ascites, serum sodium levels as low as 120 mmol per L are well tolerated and rarely dictate intervention (1).

Pharmacologic Management

For most patients, the pharmacologic management of ascites is palliative. That is, the goal of therapy is to minimize symptoms and optimize quality of life without the expectation that the underlying cause can be reversed.

Systemic chemotherapy may be an effective management strategy for patients with malignant ascites due to a responsive cancer (e.g., lymphoma, breast, or ovarian cancer). In addition to systemic chemotherapy, intraperitoneal chemotherapy is an option. In theory, intraperitoneal chemotherapy can deliver high doses to peritoneal sites with minimal systemic side effects. In practice, intraperitoneal chemotherapy is often limited by uneven distribution and poor tissue penetration. Hyperthermic intracavitary chemotherapy after surgical debulking may overcome some of these limitations and enhance the cytotoxicity of chemotherapy (20,21). Biologically active agents have also been used intraperitoneally to treat malignant ascites. Early clinical trials have used interferon (IFN)-α, IFN-β, IFN-γ, tumor necrosis factor, interleukin-2, anti-VEGF antibodies, anti-VEGF receptor antibodies, VEGF receptor tyrosine kinase inhibitors, and metalloproteinase inhibitors. To date, no phase III clinical trials have been performed. Overall, the efficacy and role of intraperitoneal chemotherapeutic and biologic agents in both curative and palliative care remains to be determined.

Diuretic therapy could be useful for patients whose ascites has a high SAAG, as opposed to low SAAG ascites that is

TABLE 17.1

CAUSES OF ASCITES AND DIURETIC RESPONSIVENESS

Cause of ascites	Serum-ascites albumin gradient	Typical diuretic response
Cirrhosis	High ($\geq$1.1 g/dL)	Yes
Alcoholic hepatitis	High ($\geq$1.1 g/dL)	Yes
Cardiac ascites	High ($\geq$1.1 g/dL)	Yes
Fulminant hepatic failure	High ($\geq$1.1 g/dL)	Yes
Budd-Chiari syndrome	High ($\geq$1.1 g/dL)	Yes
Portal vein thrombosis	High ($\geq$1.1 g/dL)	Yes
Veno-occlusive disease	High ($\geq$1.1 g/dL)	Yes
Acute fatty liver of pregnancy	High ($\geq$1.1 g/dL)	Yes
Myxedema	High ($\geq$1.1 g/dL)	Yes
Tuberculosis (without cirrhosis)	Low ($\leq$1.1 g/dL)	No
Pancreatic ascites (without cirrhosis)	Low ($\leq$1.1 g/dL)	No
Biliary ascites (without cirrhosis)	Low ($\leq$1.1 g/dL)	No
Nephrotic syndrome	Low ($\leq$1.1 g/dL)	Yes
Serositis from connective tissue disease	Low ($\leq$1.1 g/dL)	No
Bowel obstruction/Infarction	Low ($\leq$1.1 g/dL)	No
Mixed ascites (i.e., cirrhosis plus infection or cancer)	High ($\geq$1.1 g/dL)	Yes
Peritoneal carcinomatosis	Low ($\leq$1.1 g/dL)	No
Massive hepatic metastasis	High ($\geq$1.1 g/dL)	Yes

typically diuretic unresponsive. As with any drug therapy in the supportive care setting, the patient's symptoms should first be ascertained and the benefit versus the burden of therapy considered. The goal of diuretic therapy is to reduce extravascular fluid accumulation. Diuretic therapy should be directed to achieve a slow and gradual diuresis that does not exceed the capacity for mobilization of ascitic fluid. In the patient with ascites and edema, edema acts as a fluid reservoir to buffer the effects of a rapid contraction of plasma volume. Approximately 1 L per day (net) can safely be diuresed. In patients with ascites but without edema, diuresis may be achieved at the expense of the intravascular volume, leading to symptomatic orthostatic hypotension. In these patients, a more modest goal is to achieve net diuresis of 500 mL per day. Diuretics should not be administered with the goal to render the patient free of edema and ascites. Rather, only enough fluid should be mobilized to promote the patient's comfort. Overly aggressive diuretic therapy for ascites in a patient with high SAAG ascites has been associated with the hepatorenal syndrome and death (22).

In patients with high SAAG ascites for whom diuretics may be helpful, the renin–angiotensin–aldosterone system is activated. Therefore, the initial diuretic of choice for management is one that acts at the distal nephron to block the effect

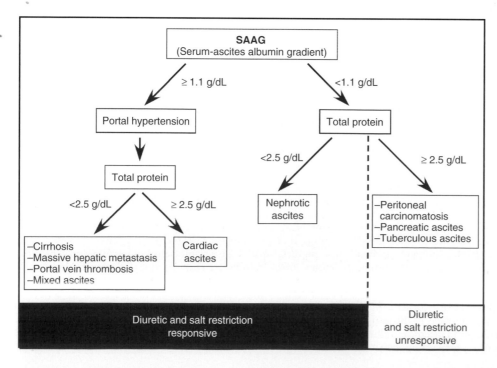

FIGURE 17.3. Predicted responsiveness to salt restriction and diuretics.

TABLE 17.2

DIURETICS

Diuretic	Major site of action	Dosage range	Comments
Spironolactone	Distal tubule	100–400 mg/d	Long half-life, gynecomastia
Amiloride hydrochloride	Distal tubule	10–40 mg/d	—
Triamterene	Distal tubule	100–300 mg/d	—
Furosemide	Loop of Henle	40–160 mg/d	—
Ethacrynic acid	Loop of Henle	50–200 mg/d	Can be used for sulfa allergy

of increased aldosterone activity (23,24). Spironolactone, an aldosterone receptor antagonist, is first-line therapy. Dosing begins at 100 mg per day and can be titrated up to effect or a maximum of 400 mg per day (Table 17.2). Given spironolactone's long half-life, daily dosing is sufficient. Spironolactone may cause painful gynecomastia (25). Amiloride hydrochloride, 10 mg per day, is an alternative. It acts faster and does not cause gynecomastia. It can be titrated up to a dose of 40 mg per day. Because these diuretics are relatively potassium sparing, patients should be advised not to use salt substitutes, as these are usually preparations of potassium chloride. If patients have a suboptimal response despite maximal use of the distal diuretics, a loop diuretic may be added, beginning at low doses (e.g., furosemide, 40 mg orally daily). There is evidence to support the combined use of a distal tubule diuretic and a loop diuretic at the beginning of therapy (24). This combination may effect a more rapid diuresis while maintaining potassium homeostasis. A ratio of 100 mg of spironolactone to 40 mg of furosemide is recommended as a starting point (1). The ratio can be adjusted to maintain normokalemia. The dosages can be increased in parallel until the goals of therapy have been attained, up to a maximum of spironolactone, 400 mg per day, and furosemide, 160 mg per day, or until therapy is limited by side effects (1). If there is no response to this level of therapy, the ascites is considered refractory to diuretic therapy if the following are true: salt intake is appropriately limited, and nonsteroidal anti-inflammatory medications, which can affect glomerular filtration, are not being used.

Aquaretics comprise a new class of agents that can enhance water excretion. There are two types that are in the early stages of clinical evaluation in cirrhotic ascites—κ opioid agonists and vasopressin receptor antagonists. In advanced cirrhosis, hyponatremia and hypo-osmolality are in part due to elevated vasopressin levels that are independent of osmolality. Although the mechanism of action is not clear, κ opioid agonists can increase free water excretion and raise the plasma sodium concentration (26). Renal V2 vasopressin receptors mediate the insertion of water channels in renal tubules rendering them permeable to water. A specific V2 receptor antagonist has been effective in promoting water excretion and correcting hyponatremia (27). The clinical utility of these agents remains to be established.

In the patient who has limited mobility, urinary tract outflow symptoms such as hesitancy and frequency, poor appetite, and poor oral intake, or who has difficulties related to polypharmacy, diuretic therapy may be excessively burdensome. Injudicious diuretic therapy can result in incontinence (with attendant self-esteem and skin care issues), sleep deprivation from frequent urination, fatigue from hyponatremia or hypokalemia, and falls from postural hypotension.

Spontaneous Bacterial Peritonitis Prophylaxis

Patients with cirrhotic ascites with low protein content are at increased risk of SBP (28). This increased risk may be due to decreased opsonin levels in the ascites (29). Patients with SBP may be asymptomatic or may note fever, abdominal pain, nausea/vomiting, or changes in mental status. Studies have indicated that antibiotic prophylaxis (Table 17.3) is effective in preventing SBP. Norfloxacin, 400 mg per day, ciprofloxacin, 750 mg per week, or one trimethoprim and sulfamethoxazole (Septra DS) per day, Monday through Friday, as primary prophylaxis significantly decrease the risk of developing SBP (30–32). A meta-analysis of SBP prophylaxis studies also supports decreased infection rates and improved survival (33). Liver transplant protocols call for the routine use of SBP prophylaxis (34). Prophylaxis raises the concern of drug-resistant organisms. The long-term clinical significance remains unknown, but after 6 months on once-a-week ciprofloxacin there was no evidence of resistance (31). The use of prophylaxis in an individual case is dependent on the overall treatment goals and the disease context.

INVASIVE INTERVENTIONS

Therapeutic Paracentesis

Large-volume therapeutic paracentesis (≥ 5 L) of high SAAG ascites with concurrent colloid infusion is a simple procedure and is associated with minimal morbidity or mortality (35,36). The symptom response is much faster than when diuretics are used alone. In the patient with refractory ascites it may be the only therapeutic modality that is effective. In fact, total paracentesis (mean, 10.7 L) associated with colloid

TABLE 17.3

SPONTANEOUS BACTERIAL PERITONITIS ANTIBIOTIC PROPHYLAXIS

Antibiotic	Dosing regimen
Norfloxacin	400 mg p.o. q.d.
Ciprofloxacin	750 mg p.o. q.wk.
Trimethoprim–sulfamethoxazole DS	One tablet p.o. Monday through Friday

infusion has been shown to be safe (37). If the ascites is in equilibrium with the systemic circulation, as is the case with portal hypertension, there is a risk of hemodynamic compromise. Colloid plasma volume expansion (e.g., 6–8 g of albumin per L of ascites removed) has been used to avoid this complication, but its use remains controversial. Ginès et al. (36) performed large-volume paracentesis with and without albumin. They demonstrated that without albumin, they could measure increases in blood urea nitrogen, plasma renin, and aldosterone, and decreases in plasma sodium, which were avoided by the infusion of intravenous albumin. Although most patients with paracentesis-induced circulatory dysfunction were asymptomatic, increased renin levels are predictive of worse outcome (38). Although no controlled trials have been done to demonstrate that albumin can prevent this morbidity, it seems prudent to use albumin pending more definitive evidence-based guidelines. Although albumin is expensive, it is not known to cause harm. There are no reports of hepatorenal syndrome associated with paracentesis for low SAAG malignant ascites.

Surgical Procedures

Liver transplantation offers cure for a subset of patients with cirrhosis (34) and a subset of patients with small hepatocellular carcinoma (39).

Other surgical techniques offer palliation. Peritoneovenous shunts have been reported for the management of malignant and nonmalignant ascites. They are placed surgically during a 30- to 60-minute procedure while the patient is under local anesthesia. Their purpose is to drain ascites from the peritoneal space through a one-way valve into the thoracic venous system. Unfortunately, the rate of complications is high, including shunt occlusion, heart failure due to fluid overload, infection, and disseminated intravascular coagulation. Stanley et al. (40) and Gines et al. (41) studied serial paracentesis compared with peritoneovenous shunts in patients with cirrhosis. There was no improvement in survival and a high rate of complications with the peritoneovenous shunts was reported. Similarly, Gough and Balderson (42) compared peritoneovenous shunts with nonoperative management in patients with malignant ascites. They found no difference in survival or quality of life. Therefore, although there may be specific cases in which peritoneovenous shunting is advantageous in either nonmalignant or malignant ascites, serial paracentesis remains the first-line therapy.

Externally draining, implanted abdominal catheters may be beneficial for select patients who require repeated large-volume paracentesis for comfort and whose prognosis warrants a surgical procedure. The catheter is surgically placed in the peritoneal cavity with an external drain, which can be accessed intermittently by physicians, nurses, or even trained family members (43). The catheters may be untunneled (e.g., pigtail catheter) or tunneled (e.g., Pleurx catheter). Theoretically, tunneled catheters may lower infection risk, but there are no comparative studies. Furthermore, there are no large, formal comparative trials of implanted catheters versus serial paracentesis in patients with cirrhotic or malignant ascites. A study of 17 patients with an implanted catheter and abdominal carcinoma was complicated by two cases of cellulitis, one case of peritonitis, and eight cases of asymptomatic culture-positive ascites (44). Rosenberg et al. published their experience with Pleurx catheters versus serial paracentesis for malignant ascites and concluded these techniques were equally efficacious and safe (45). However, with no definitive guidance from the literature, use of implanted catheters must be individualized.

The transjugular intrahepatic portosystemic shunt (TIPS) is a procedure performed by interventional radiologists that creates a side-to-side shunt that effectively relieves portal hypertension. The role of TIPS in patients with cirrhosis and refractory ascites remains controversial, potentially due to studies on differing populations. Rossle et al. showed that in comparison to serial large-volume paracentesis, TIPS led to a higher rate of ascites resolution and improved survival without transplantation (46). However, Sanyal et al. found that although TIPS improved ascites control versus paracentesis, there was no improvement in quality of life or survival (47). Given the rate of shunt complications and trend of increased frequency of worse encephalopathy, these authors recommend against TIPS as first-line therapy. TIPS has also been employed in a few cases of malignant ascites associated with portal hypertension. In two cases of malignant portal and hepatic vein occlusion, TIPS improved ascites and quality of life (48). The decision to pursue any of the invasive surgical procedures mentioned in the preceding text is dependent on the patient's goals and the disease context, and must be individualized.

References

1. Runyon B. Current concepts: care of patients with ascites. *N Engl J Med* 1994;330(5):337–342.
2. Sharma S, Walsh D. Management of symptomatic malignant ascites with diuretics: two case reports and a review of the literature. *J Pain Symptom Manage* 1995;10(3):237–242.
3. Runyon B, Hoefs J, Morgan T. Ascitic fluid analysis in malignancy related ascites. *Hepatology* 1988;8:1104–1109.
4. Garrison R, Kaelin L, Galloway R, et al. Malignant ascites: clinical and experimental observations. *Ann Surg* 1986;203:644–649.
5. Martin P, Gines P, Schrier RW. Nitric oxide as a mediator of hemodynamic abnormalities and sodium and water retention in cirrhosis. *N Engl J Med* 1998;339(8):533–541.
6. Gines P, Jimenez W, Arroyo V, et al. Atrial natriuretic factor in cirrhosis with ascites; plasma levels, cardiac release and splanchnic extraction. *Hepatology* 1988;8(3):636–642.
7. Bichet D, Szatalowicz V, Chaimovitz C, et al. Role of vasopressin in abnormal water excretion in cirrhotic patients. *Ann Intern Med* 1982;96:413–417.
8. Senger DR, Galli SJ, Dvorak AM, et al. Tumor cells secrete a vascular permeability factor that promotes accumulation of ascites fluid. *Science* 1983;219:983–985.
9. Zebrowski BK, Liu W, Ramirez K, et al. Markedly elevated levels of vascular endothelial growth factor in malignant ascites. *Ann Surg Oncol* 1999;6(4):373–378.
10. Xu L, Yoneda J, Herrera C, et al. Inhibition of malignant ascites and growth of human ovarian carcinoma by oral administration of a potent inhibitor of the vascular endothelial growth factor receptor tyrosine kinases. *Int J Oncol* 2000;16(3):445–454.
11. Watson SA, Morris TM, Robinson G, et al. Inhibition of organ invasion by the matrix metalloproteinase inhibitor batimastat (BB-94) in two human colon carcinoma metastasis models. *Cancer Res* 1995;55(16):3629–3633.
12. Cattau EL Jr, Benjamin SB, Knuff TE, et al. The accuracy of the physical exam in the diagnosis of suspected ascites. *JAMA* 1982;247(8):1164–1166.
13. Williams JW Jr, Simel DI. Does this patient have ascites? How to divine fluid in the abdomen. *JAMA* 1992;267(19):2645–2648.
14. Runyon BA, Antillon MR, Akriviadis EA, et al. Bedside inoculation of blood culture bottles with ascitic fluid is superior to delayed inoculation in the detection of spontaneous bacterial peritonitis. *J Clin Microbiol* 1990;28:2811–2812.
15. Hoefs JC. Serum protein concentration and portal pressure determine the ascitic fluid protein concentration in patients with chronic liver disease. *J Lab Clin Med* 1983;102:260–273.
16. Runyon BA, Montano AA, Akriviadis EA, et al. The serum-ascites albumin gradient is superior to the exudate-transudate concept in the differential diagnosis of ascites. *Ann Intern Med* 1992;117:215–220.
17. Runyon BA. Cardiac ascites: a characterization. *J Clin Gastroenterol* 1988;10(4):410–412.
18. Pockros PJ, Esrason KT, Nguyen C, et al. Mobilization of malignant ascites with diuretics is dependent on ascitic fluid characteristics. *Gastroenterology* 1992;103(4):1302–1306.
19. Ackerman Z. Ascites in nephrotic syndrome: incidence, patients' characteristics, and complications. *J Clin Gastroenterol* 1996;22:31–34.
20. Loggie BW, Perini M, Fleming RA, et al. Treatment and prevention of malignant ascites associated with disseminated intraperitoneal malignancies by aggressive combined-modality therapy. *Am Surg* 1997;63(2):137–143.

21. Shen P, Hawksworth J, Lovato J, et al. Cytoreductive surgery and intraperitoneal hyperthermic chemotherapy with mitomycin C for peritoneal carcinomatosis from nonappendiceal colorectal carcinoma. *Ann Surg Oncol* 2004;11(2):178–186.

22. Roberts LR, Kamath PS. Ascites and hepatorenal syndrome: pathophysiology and management. *Mayo Clin Proc* 1996;71(9):874–881.

23. Pérez-Ayuso RM, Arroyo V, Planas R, et al. Randomized comparative study of efficacy of furosemide versus spironolactone in nonazotemic cirrhosis with ascites: relationship between the diuretic response and the activity of the renin-aldosterone system. *Gastroenterology* 1983;84:961–968.

24. Fogel MR, Sawhney VK, Neal EA, et al. Diuresis in the ascitic patient: a randomized controlled trial of three regimens. *J Clin Gastroenterol* 1981;3(Suppl 1):73–80.

25. Mantero F, Lucarelli G. Aldosterone antagonists in hypertension and heart failure. *Ann Endocrinol* 2000;61(1):52–60.

26. Gadano A, Moreau R, Pessione F, et al. Aquaretic effects of niravoline, a kappa-opioid agonist, in patients with cirrhosis. *J Hepatol* 2000;32(1):38–42.

27. Wong F, Blei AT, Blendis LM, et al. A vasopressin receptor antagonist (VPA-985) improves serum sodium concentration in patients with hyponatremia: a multicenter, randomized, placebo-controlled trial. *Hepatology* 2003;37(1):182–191.

28. Runyon BA. Low-protein concentration ascitic fluid is predisposed to spontaneous bacterial peritonitis. *Gastroenterology* 1986;91(6):1343–1346.

29. Runyon BA. Patients with deficient ascitic fluid opsonic activity are predisposed to spontaneous bacterial peritonitis. *Hepatology* 1988;8(3):632–635.

30. Grangé JD, Roulot D, Pelletier G, et al. Norfloxacin primary prophylaxis of bacterial infections in cirrhotic patients with ascites: a double-blind randomized trial. *J Hepatol* 1998;29(3):430–436.

31. Rolachon A, Cordier L, Bacq Y, et al. Ciprofloxacin and long-term prevention of spontaneous bacterial peritonitis: results of a prospective controlled trial. *Hepatology* 1995;22:1171–1174.

32. Singh N, Gayowski T, Yu VL, et al. Trimethoprim-sulfamethoxazole for the prevention of spontaneous bacterial peritonitis in cirrhosis: a randomized trial. *Ann Intern Med* 1995;122(8):595–598.

33. Soares-Weiser K, Brezis M, Paul M, et al. Antibiotic prophylaxis of bacterial infections in cirrhotic inpatients: a meta-analysis of randomized controlled trials. *Scand J Gastroenterol* 2003;38(2):193–200.

34. Saab S, Han SH, Martin P. Liver transplantation: selection, listing criteria, and preoperative management. *Clin Liver Dis* 2000;4(3):513–532.

35. Ginés P, Arroyo V, Quintero E, et al. Comparison of paracentesis and diuretics in the treatment of cirrhotics with tense ascites: results of a randomized study. *Gastroenterology* 1987;93(2):234–241.

36. Ginés P, Titó L, Arroyo V, et al. Randomized comparative study of therapeutic paracentesis with and without intravenous albumin in cirrhosis. *Gastroenterology* 1988;94(6):1493–1502.

37. Titó L, Ginès P, Arroyo V, et al. Total paracentesis associated with intravenous albumin management of patients with cirrhosis and ascites. *Gastroenterology* 1990;98(1):146–151.

38. Gines A, Fernandez-Esparrach G, Monescillo A, et al. Randomized trial comparing albumin, dextran 70, and polygeline in cirrhotic patients with ascites treated by paracentesis. *Gastroenterology* 1996;111(4):1002–1010.

39. Llovet JM, Bruix J, Fuster J, et al. Liver transplantation for small hepatocellular carcinoma: the tumor-node-metastasis classification does not have prognostic power. *Hepatology* 1998;27(6):1572–1577.

40. Stanley MM, Ochi S, Lee KK, et al. Peritoneovenous shunting as compared with medical treatment in patients with alcoholic cirrhosis and massive ascites: Veterans Administration Cooperative Study on treatment of alcoholic cirrhosis with ascites. *N Engl J Med* 1989;321(24):1632–1638.

41. Gines P, Arroyo V, Vargas B, et al. Paracentesis with intravenous infusion of albumin as compared with peritoneovenous shunting in cirrhosis with refractory ascites. *N Engl J Med* 1991;325:829–835.

42. Gough IR, Balderson GA. Malignant ascites: a comparison of peritoneovenous shunting and nonoperative management. *Cancer* 1993;71(7):2377–2382.

43. Murphy M, Rossi M. Managing ascites via the Tenckhoff catheter. *Med Surg Nurs* 1995;4:468–471.

44. Belfort MA, Stevens PJ, DeHaek K, et al. A new approach to the management of malignant ascites; a permanently implanted abdominal drain. *Eur J Surg Oncol* 1990;16(1):47–53.

45. Rosenberg S, Courtney A, Omary RA, et al. Comparison of percutaneous management techniques for recurrent malignant ascites. *J Vasc Interv Radiol* 2004;15(10):1129–1131.

46. Rössle M, Ochs A, Gülberg V, et al. A comparison of paracentesis and transjugular intrahepatic portosystemic shunting in patients with ascites. *N Engl J Med* 2000;342(23):1701–1707.

47. Sanyal AJ, Genning C, Reddy KR, et al. The North American Study for the Treatment of Refractory Ascites. *Gastroenterology* 2003;124(3):634–641.

48. Burger JA, Ochs A, Wirth K, et al. The transjugular stent implantation for the treatment of malignant portal and hepatic vein obstruction in cancer patients. *Ann Oncol* 1997;8(2):200–202.

CHAPTER 18 ■ HICCUPS AND OTHER GASTROINTESTINAL SYMPTOMS

NABEEL SARHILL AND FADE MAHMOUD

Gastrointestinal (GI) symptoms are commonly seen in patients with cancer, regardless of the disease site. These symptoms are experienced during the course of the illness or as a result of therapy. However, it should be remembered that many GI problems seen in patients with cancer are also seen in those without cancer. In fact, some GI symptoms are very common, and although they cause distress, they rarely represent life-threatening pathology. This presents a problem, as patients and physicians face the concern that every new symptom is related to the cancer. This chapter focuses primarily on GI symptoms as they relate to cancer and its treatment, but the reader is reminded that most GI symptoms are not directly due to the cancer.

HICCUPS

Definition/Incidence

Hiccup is a spasmodic, involuntary contraction of the inspiratory (external) intercostal muscles and the diaphragm associated with a strong, sudden inspiration, and abrupt glottic closure. The inspiratory effort does not result in lung volume changes and there are minimal ventilatory effects. Hiccups can be classified by their duration; acute (up to 48 hours), persistent or protracted (longer than 48 hours) and intractable (>1 month) (1).

Pathophysiology/Etiology

Hiccup is a primitive reflex that contains three parts. The afferent portion consists of branches of the vagus nerve, the phrenic nerve, and the sympathetic chain from T6–12. The hiccup center is located in the spinal cord between C3 and C5. The efferent limb is primarily the phrenic nerve with involvement of the efferents to the glottis and accessory muscles of respiration (1).

In addition to the neural pathways, numerous anatomic structures are involved in the mechanism of hiccup (epiglottis, larynx, hyoid muscles, superior constrictor of the pharynx, esophagus, stomach, diaphragm, and exterior intercostal, sternocleidomastoid, anterior serratus, and scalene muscles). Given this extensive list, it is not surprising that hiccup has been associated with many conditions affecting the central nervous system (CNS), thorax, mediastinum, and abdominal viscera; although a cause-and-effect relationship has not always been clear. One report listed over 100 causes, the most common being an overdistended stomach (2). Some cancer-related causes of persistent and intractable hiccup are listed in Table 18.1.

Treatment/Management

Management is usually aimed at inhibiting or interrupting the irritated reflex arc. Nonpharmacologic therapies (3) include

TABLE 18.1

CAUSES OF HICCUPS IN THE PATIENT WITH CANCER[a]

Uremia
Alcohol
Hyponatremia, hypokalemia, hypocalcemia
Fever
Diaphragmatic irritation (diaphragmatic tumors, pericarditis)
Pleuritis
Esophageal obstruction
Pericarditis
Hepatomegaly
Subphrenic abscess
Esophageal cancer
Mediastinal tumors
Herpes zoster
Lung cancer
Gastric distension
Gastric cancer
Pancreatic cancer
Intra-abdominal abscess
Bowel obstruction
Gastrointestinal hemorrhage
Short-acting barbiturates
Dexamethasone
Diazepam, chlordiazepoxide
Infections (meningitis)
Grief reaction
Psychosis

[a]A comprehensive list of the causes of hiccups can be found in Launois S, Bizec JL, Whitelaw WA, et al. Hiccup in adults: an overview. *Eur Respir J* 1993;6:563–575.

the Valsalva's maneuver (expiring forcefully against a closed glottis), ocular compression, carotid sinus massage, traction on the tongue, ice water gargles, noxious odors or tastes, breath holding, rebreathing into a paper bag, gagging, drinking from a glass while holding a pencil between the teeth or while bending over head down, taking as many sips of fluid as rapidly as possible without breathing, ingesting granulated sugar, biting a lemon wedge, or inducing emesis. Physical changes that may help stop hiccups include pulling the knees to chest, leaning forward to compress the chest, tapping over the fifth cervical vertebra, or applying ice over the phrenic nerve. Although these measures have not been subjected to controlled clinical trials, most are worth a try. However, many are not practical for these patients, who may be too debilitated to tolerate even simple maneuvers (e.g., holding breath).

Gastric distension being the most common cause of hiccups in patients with cancer, initial treatment should be aimed at relieving the distension and increasing gastric emptying. The insertion of a nasogastric tube may provide quick relief while drug therapy is being provided. Many drugs have been used to treat hiccups (Table 18.2). The literature is based largely on case reports and no definitive clinical evidence is available

TABLE 18.2

COMMONLY USED DRUGS IN THE TREATMENT OF HICCUPS

Drug	Dose	Side effects
Metoclopramide	10 mg p.o. or i.v. three to four times daily	Extrapyramidal symptoms[a]
Chlorpromazine	25–50 mg i.v. three to four times daily, infused slowly 25–50 mg p.o. three times daily	Sedation, hypotension, extrapyramidal symptoms
Haloperidol	1–5 mg p.o. three times daily or s.c. q12h	Sedation, extrapyramidal symptoms
Baclofen	10–20 mg p.o. three times daily	Sedation, confusion; less commonly, nausea and fatigue
Nifedipine	10 mg p.o. three times daily	Hypotension, use with caution in patients with coronary artery disease
Amitriptyline	10 mg p.o. three times daily	Cardiac arrhythmias, blurred vision, urinary retention, dry mouth, constipation, and dizziness
Carbamazepine	200 mg three times daily	Dizziness, drowsiness, nausea or vomiting, low red and white blood cell counts
Diphenylhydantoin	200 mg i.v. once and then 100 mg p.o. four times daily	Enlarged gums, unsteadiness, confusion, lymphadenopathy; fever, muscle pain, skin rash or itching, slurred speech, sore throat, and nervousness or irritability
Valproic acid	15 mg/kg p.o. daily in one to three divided doses	Dizziness, drowsiness, nervousness, upset stomach, vomiting, diarrhea, tremor, sore throat, and drug-induced hepatitis
Gabapentin	300 mg p.o. three times daily	Drowsiness, headache, fatigue, blurred vision, tremor, anxiety, skin rash, itching, fever, flu-like symptoms, seizures
Ketamine (Ketalar)	0.4 mg/kg (one fifth of the usual anesthetic dose) i.v.; supplemental dose of one third to half initial dose may be given for maintenance	Resuscitative equipment should be immediately available during administration of medication
Lidocaine	1 mg/kg i.v. loading dose followed by an infusion of 2 mg/min i.v.	May increase risk of adverse central nervous system and cardiac effects in elderly; high plasma concentrations can cause seizures, heart block, and atrioventricular conduction abnormalities
Ephedrine	25 mg i.m. q6h	Headache, restless, anxiety, tremor, weakness, dizziness, confusion, delirium, hallucinations, palpitations, sweating, nausea or vomiting, and urinary retention Serious side effects include severe hypertension that may lead to cerebral hemorrhage or cardiac ischemia
Methylphenidate (Ritalin)	5 mg p.o. daily or divided b.i.d.; not to exceed 60 mg/d	Insomnia, anorexia, irritability, nervousness, upset stomach, headaches, dry mouth, blurry vision, nausea, hypersensitivity, palpitations, and cardiac arrhythmias
Other therapies	Behavioral conditioning (including other members of the family unit) Hypnosis Acupuncture Phrenic nerve or diaphragmatic pacing	

[a]More common in younger women.

Liu FC, Chen CA, Yang SS, et al. Acupuncture therapy rapidly terminates intractable hiccups complicating acute myocardial infarction. *South Med J* 2005;98(3):385–387; Schiff E, River Y, Oliven A, et al. Acupuncture therapy for persistent hiccups. *Am J Med Sci* 2002;323(3):166–168.

to define the standard treatment. The drugs most commonly used are chlorpromazine (25–50 mg through i.v., orally, or rectally three to four times a day) (4), haloperidol (1–5 mg orally three times daily or subcutaneously every 12 hours) (5), nifedipine (10 mg p.o. three times daily) (6), metoclopramide (10 mg p.o. or i.v. every 6 hours) (7), and baclofen (10–20 mg p.o. three times a day) (8). Chlorpromazine is less attractive in patients with cancer due to side effects of hypotension and sedation. Moreover, Baclofen should be given with caution to the elderly due to frequent side effects of sedation, insomnia, dizziness, weakness, ataxia, and confusion (8). Haloperidol may be a better choice for those taking opioids. If hiccups persist, amitriptyline (10 mg three times a day) (9), carbamazepine (200 mg three times a day) (10), diphenylhydantoin (200 mg i.v. and then 100 mg p.o. four times a day) (11), or valproic acid (15 mg/kg/day in divided doses) (12) can be administered. Gabapentin (300 mg p.o. three times daily) has shown efficacy in treating hiccups among patients with cancer. The mechanism of action is probably related to the increase of endogenous γ-aminobutyric acid (GABA) release which plays a role in the modulation of the excitability of the diaphragm and the other inspiratory muscles (13,14).

Efficacy has been claimed for a variety of drugs that have a peripheral action such as atropine, edrophonium, procainamide, and quinidine. Methylphenidate (10 mg p.o. daily) is reported to be effective in the treatment of hiccups (15).

Various invasive methods have been tried. Gastric aspiration may be useful if overdistension of the stomach is the cause of hiccups. The insertion of a nasogastric tube may also serve a purpose by stimulating the pharynx or causing gagging. High-pressure oxygen inhalation has been tried. Percutaneous stimulation of the phrenic nerve has also been reported. A surgical approach consists of an attack on the phrenic nerve (by a crush technique), usually first attempted on the left. Regardless of treatment, in most cases, hiccups stop because of, or in spite of, therapeutic measures (16,17).

It is important to remember that hiccups in cancer may be extremely distressing and affect the quality of life by interfering with food intake, causing insomnia, or exacerbating pain and other symptoms. For this reason, it may be advisable to pursue diagnosis and treatment more aggressively than in the general population (18).

DYSPEPSIA

Definition/Incidence

Dyspepsia consists of episodic or persistent symptoms that include abdominal pain or discomfort, postprandial fullness, abdominal bloating, belching, early satiety, anorexia, nausea, vomiting, heartburn, and regurgitation. There is considerable overlap between this constellation of symptoms and those of gastroesophageal reflux disease (GERD), biliary tract disease, irritable bowel syndrome, and chronic pancreatitis. This condition is reported in approximately 25% of the population each year, but most do not seek medical care (19,20).

Pathophysiology/Etiology

Results of upper GI endoscopy in 3667 general medical patients with dyspepsia were as follows: normal (34%), gastroesophageal reflux (24%), inflammation (20%), ulcer (20%), and cancer (2%) (19). Dyspepsia is divided into two categories: organic dyspepsia and functional dyspepsia. Patients in the first group have anatomical abnormalities (e.g., peptic ulcer disease, GERD, gastric, or esophageal cancer). Patients in the

second category have symptoms for which no focal lesion can be found (Table 18.3). Recent studies have shown potential associations between specific pathophysiologic disturbances and functional dyspeptic symptoms. Delayed gastric emptying reported in approximately 30% of patients with functional dyspepsia is associated with postprandial fullness, nausea, and vomiting. Impaired gastric accommodation present in 40% of patients with functional dyspepsia is found to be associated with early satiety. Hypersensitivity to gastric distension is observed in 37% of patients with functional dyspepsia and is associated with postprandial pain, belching, and weight loss. Psychosocial factors have also been identified as pathophysiologic mechanisms (21,22).

Dysmotility-like dyspepsia, or gastroparesis, is commonly seen in patients with cancer due to autonomic nervous system dysfunction, use of anticholinergic drugs, or opioids. It is associated with symptoms of bloating, abdominal distension, flatulence, and prominent nausea. Patients with this condition tend to have premature satiety with resultant epigastric heaviness or fullness even after the consumption of small meals (23). The diagnosis of paraneoplastic dyspepsia requires a high index of clinical suspicion. A panel of serologic tests for paraneoplastic autoantibodies, scintigraphic gastric emptying, and esophageal manometry are useful as first-line screening tests. Nuclear scintigraphy is considered the gold standard for diagnosing and quantifying delayed gastric emptying. Seropositivity for type 1 antineuronal nuclear antibody, Purkinje cell cytoplasmic antibody, or N type calcium channel-binding antibodies has been detected in patients with paraneoplastic gastroparesis but its diagnostic value is under investigation (24).

Recent studies have linked gastroparesis to disruption of the interstitial cell of Cajal (ICC). These are fibroblast like cells, which have been identified in the gut by electron microscopy and by immunohistochemistry for Kit protein. Generating electrical slow waves, the ICC are intercalated between the intramural neurons and the effector smooth muscular cells to form a gastroenteric pacemaker system. It has been recently found that loss of the ICC causes dysmotility-like symptoms *in vivo*. A loss of these cells has been detected in patients with paraneoplastic gastroparesis (25).

Other causes of cancer-induced dyspepsia include gastric cancer or lymphoma, gastritis secondary to radiotherapy/chemotherapy, gastric compression secondary to intra-abdominal tumor, hepatomegaly, splenomegaly, ascites, or gastric outlet obstruction due to tumor. Medications that have been associated with dyspepsia include acarbose, alcohol, alendronate, codeine, iron, metformin, nonsteroidal anti-inflammatory drugs, erythromycin, potassium, corticosteroids, and theophylline. Dosage reduction or discontinuation of the offending agent may relieve dyspepsia.

Management/Treatment

The management of organic dyspepsia should be directed at the cause. Treatment may be based on previous history (e.g., obstructing lesion responding to primary tumor treatment) or recent endoscopy findings. In functional dyspepsia, treatment should be based on symptoms (Table 18.3). Nutrition support in gastroparesis begins with encouraging smaller volume, low-fat, low-fiber meals and, if necessary, liquid caloric supplements. Metoclopramide is now the prokinetic drug of choice (26). Controlled-release metoclopramide (20–80 mg q12h) is effective in ameliorating symptoms of the cancer-induced dyspepsia such as nausea, vomiting, loss of appetite, and bloating (27).

Moreover, subcutaneous administration of metoclopramide is an important method, allowing for continued guaranteed

TABLE 18.3

CLASSIFICATION OF NONULCER DYSPEPSIA BY SYMPTOM—TYPE AND THEIR TREATMENTS

Classification	Symptoms	Treatment
Reflux-like	Heartburn, regurgitation without esophagitis	Antacid, H_2 blocker, proton pump inhibitor
Ulcer-like	Epigastric pain relieved by food and antacids, relapse and remission, without ulcer	As above
Dysmotility-like	Abdominal bloating, distension, early satiety, nausea, vomiting	Prokinetic agent, antiflatulence agent
Nonspecific	Symptoms do not fall into one of the three categories in the preceding text	Start simple: antacid, antiflatulence agent (simethicone)

absorption. Low-dosage erythromycin also has a prokinetic role, either alone or in combination with metoclopramide. Domperidone, a centrally acting antiemetic and prokinetic, is not available in US markets. Antiemetics should be used for nausea, which is a very severe debilitating symptom. There should be a low threshold for placing a jejunal feeding tube either by laparoscopy or mini-laparotomy. Parenteral nutrition should be used only briefly during hospitalization and not encouraged or sustained in an outpatient. Most excitingly, the era of gastric electrical stimulation has arrived for patients not responding to standard medical therapy. The dramatic decrease in nausea and vomiting, as well as a sustained evidence of improved quality of life, gastric emptying, nutritional status, and decreased hospitalizations by this device are documented by long-term follow-up of more than a year (28). Gastric pacemaker has been studied in patients with diabetes-induced gastroparesis but not in cancer. Further research is needed in patients with cancer-induced gastroparesis (29,30).

HEARTBURN

Definition/Incidence

Heartburn is the most common GI complaint in the western population; 33–44% of the population complain of heartburn at least monthly and 7–13% may have it daily (31). Heartburn is a retrosternal burning sensation that usually radiates proximally from the xiphoid process to the neck. It is caused by reflux of the gastric content into the esophagus. GERD occurs when the amount of gastric content that refluxes into the esophagus exceeds the normal limit, causing symptoms with or without esophagitis. Although there is no clear evidence that GERD is more common in those with cancer, certain conditions in this population may increase their risk, such as intra-abdominal lesions, which increase pressure on the stomach. In addition to the typical symptoms (heartburn, regurgitation, dysphagia), abnormal reflux can cause atypical symptoms such as coughing, chest pain, and wheezing and also damage to the lungs (pneumonia, asthma, idiopathic pulmonary fibrosis), vocal cords (laryngitis, cancer), ear (otitis media), and teeth (enamel decay). Approximately 50% of patients with reflux develop esophagitis, which is classified on the basis of severity.

Pathophysiology/Etiology

The most important pathophysiologic factor in GERD is frequent transient relaxation of the lower esophageal sphincter (LES). Other factors include anatomic disruption of the LES as in hiatal hernia, transient increase in intra-abdominal pressure, abnormal esophageal peristalsis with impaired clearance of acid, and gastroparesis.

A number of foods, drugs, and neurohumoral factors reduce basal LES pressure, making patients prone to gastroesophageal reflux and heartburn (Table 18.4). Avoiding these foods and medications often constitutes the initial treatment of GERD. Some common agents that increase LES pressure include a protein meal, bethanechol, metoclopramide, and α-adrenergic agonists.

Heartburn is most frequently noted within 1 hour of eating, particularly after the largest meal of the day. Wine drinkers may have heartburn after hearty consumption of red wine but not after white wine. Lying down, especially after a late meal, causes heartburn within 1–2 hours; in contrast to peptic ulcer disease, heartburn does not awaken the person in the early morning. Heartburn may be accompanied by regurgitation, a bitter acidic fluid in the mouth that is common at night or when the patient bends over. The regurgitated material comes from the stomach and is yellow or green, suggesting the presence of bile. It is important to distinguish regurgitation from vomiting. The absence of nausea, retching, and abdominal contractions suggests regurgitation rather than vomiting. Furthermore, the regurgitation of bland material is atypical for acid reflux disease and suggests the presence of an esophageal motility disorder (i.e., achalasia) or delayed gastric emptying.

Many disorders cause epigastric or substernal pain similar to heartburn, making it important to determine the cause in each patient. Causes include collagen-vascular disorders, scleroderma, mixed connective tissue disorders, raised intra-abdominal pressure, gastroparesis, nasogastric tube, prolonged recumbent position, persistent vomiting, pregnancy, hypothyroidism, Zollinger-Ellison syndrome, medications, and some surgical procedures (e.g., myotomy, esophagogastrectomy).

Treatment/Management

Treatment is a stepwise approach. The goal is to control symptoms, to heal esophagitis, and to prevent recurrent esophagitis or complications. The treatment is based on lifestyle modification and control of gastric acid secretion. Lifestyle modification includes losing weight, avoiding precipitating factors such as chocolate, spicy food, alcohol, citrus juice, and tomato-based products. Ask the patient to eat several small meals during the day and avoid large ones, and elevate the head of the bed. Antacids are effective in mild symptoms if given after each meal and at bedtime. More aggressive therapy includes H_2 receptor blockers, sucralfate, or omeprazole. Metoclopramide works very well in GERD among patients with cancer who commonly have gastroparesis. It increases the LES

TABLE 18.4

AGGRAVATING FACTORS FOR HEARTBURN

Low LES pressure	Direct mucosal irritant	Increased intra-abdominal pressure	Others
Certain foods	Certain foods	Bending over	Supine position
Fats	Citrus products	Lifting	Lying on right side
Sugars	Tomato-based products	Straining at stool	Red wine
Chocolate	Spicy foods	Exercise	Emotions
Onions	Coffee		
Coffee	Medications		
Alcohol	Aspirin		
Cigarettes	Nonsteroidal anti-inflammatory drug		
Medications	Tetracycline		
Progesterone	Quinidine sulfate		
Theophylline	Potassium chloride tablets		
Anticholinergic agents	Iron salts		
Adrenergic agonists			
Adrenergic antagonists			
Diazepam			
Estrogens			
Mint, anise, dill			
Benzodiazepines			
Meperidine hydrochloride			
Nitrates			
Calcium channel blockers			

LES, lower esophageal sphincter.

pressure and enhances gastric emptying. Long-term therapy is usually necessary. Approximately 80% of patients have a recurrent but nonprogressive GERD that is controlled with medications. In 20% of patients the disease is progressive and severe complications may occur, such as strictures or Barrett's esophagus. Laparoscopic fundoplication or other palliative procedures should be considered and discussed with patients having cancer. Over the past decade, a new noninvasive endoscopic technique, called *Enteryx*, has been developed to treat GERD (32). This procedure involves the injection of a compound called *ethylene polyvinyl alcohol* into the LES, just within the stomach. The injection is done with guidance from real-time x-ray. The compound is in liquid form outside the body, but when it comes into contact with the tissues inside the body, it turns into an expanding, spongy material. The procedure may cause a sore throat or chest pain. Although this treatment resulted in highly significant improvement at 6 and 12 months, longer follow-up is needed to better assess the duration of efficacy of these positive effects.

EARLY SATIETY

Definition/Incidence

Early satiety is the desire to eat combined with an inability to consume more than an unusually small amount of food. This is in contrast to anorexia, in which there is a reduced desire to eat. Early satiety should be distinguished not only from anorexia, but also from nausea, bloating, postprandial filling, pyrosis, food aversion, and dyspepsia. However, all of these symptoms may be due to the same physiologic abnormality—delayed gastric emptying. Patients generally do not report this symptom unless questioned. The incidence of cancer-related early satiety

varies from 13–62% depending on the study and population being evaluated (33–35).

Pathophysiology/Etiology

Satiety results from overlapping stimuli from the CNS and GI tract affecting food intake. The nutrients ingested and peptide hormones (insulin, glucagon, norepinephrine-stimulating α_2-adrenergic receptors in the medial hypothalamus), along with serotonin and dopaminergic-α-adrenergic receptors in the lateral hypothalamus, all affect satiety. Cholecystokinin may have primary effects on satiety. Exogenous administration of peptides like cholecystokinin and bombesin affect satiety both centrally and peripherally and inhibit feeding activity in animals.

Early satiety may be due to tumor encroachment on the GI tract, inappropriate satiety signals from oropharyngeal receptors, hyperglycemia, or gastric muscle atrophy. Another important cause appears to be reduced upper GI motility due to autonomic nervous system dysfunction, possibly a paraneoplastic syndrome (36). Tumor type and previous chemotherapy treatment have not been shown to affect the incidence of early satiety in cancer. However, patients with taste aversions appear to have a higher incidence of early satiety than those without (37).

Treatment/Management

It is important to determine if early satiety is the reported symptom. If bloating, pyrosis, anorexia, or nausea not due to gastric status is present, it should be treated appropriately. If there is pressure on the stomach ("squashed stomach"), it should be reduced if possible, although in many cases it is not. Problems such as ascites may be amenable to paracentesis, which can provide temporary relief. Those with gastroduodenal ulcers should be treated with appropriate therapy (H_2 blocker, proton pump inhibitor, antibiotic). In patients with cicatrization at the pyloric outlet, balloon dilatation may afford relief for variable periods.

Patients with early satiety should be instructed to eat frequent, small meals, with the bulk of their daily intake consumed early, as gastric stasis increases as the day progresses. They should also be instructed to eat sitting up and avoid liquids at mealtimes, as liquids promote gastric distension and a sense of fullness. Prokinetic agents (e.g., metoclopramide, domperidone) may be of particular use. The rationale for prokinetic agent use in early satiety is based on the assumption that the symptom(s) is due to delayed gastric emptying. Metoclopramide is the drug of choice in the United States (26). It is a dopamine antagonist that increases LES pressure and enhances gastric antral contractility. It is generally well-tolerated orally, but extrapyramidal reactions, which appear to be more common in young women, do occur; insomnia (often noted to be "jumpy legs" on further questioning) and sedation have also been reported. Metoclopramide, 10 mg three times daily orally, is effective treatment for many and enhances food intake. The central effects of metoclopramide may have a direct effect on anorexia to improve appetite in addition to the peripheral effects on gastric contractility. The other prokinetic agents, cisapride and domperidone, are not available in the United States. Cisapride has been removed from the market due to drug interactions causing cardiac abnormalities. Domperidone, also a dopamine antagonist, does not cross the blood–brain barrier, hence its side effect profile is superior to metoclopramide; unfortunately, it has not yet been approved

in the United States. Erythromycin is another prokinetic agent but is less useful in cancer-related gastroparesis as it causes gastric dumping, which is useful in acute gastric stasis (e.g., diabetic gastroparesis). Treatments for early satiety, dyspepsia, and heartburn are listed in Table 18.5.

GASTROINTESTINAL HEMORRHAGE

Definition/Incidence

GI bleeding may originate at any site from the mouth to the anus. It can be occult or overt, with varying degrees of severity. A careful history and physical examination often suggests the site as well as the cause of the bleeding. Although controversial, most agree that 20% loss of circulating volume produces hemodynamic changes and >30% produces shock with organ damage. In the debilitated patient with cancer, the ability to tolerate a GI hemorrhage is compromised and these signs and symptoms may occur with far less blood loss.

The overall incidence of acute upper GI hemorrhage is 100 hospitalizations per 100,000 adults per year (38). In a study of over 15 million people, there was an overall mortality rate of 14% (39). However, in patients younger than 60 years of age without malignancy or organ failure, the mortality was only 0.6%. In 800 admissions to a palliative home care program, the incidence of GI bleeding was 2.3%; those with liver cancer or hepatic metastases were at higher risk (40).

TABLE 18.5

TREATMENT OF DYSPEPSIA, HEARTBURN, AND EARLY SATIETY

Dyspepsia	1. Antacids (aluminum hydroxide, magnesium hydroxide, and simethicone): 10–20 mL or 2–4 tablets p.o. four to six times daily between meals and at bedtime 2. Treat *Helicobacter pylori* 3. Treat peptic ulcer disease with proton pump inhibitors 4. Prokinetic drug: Metoclopramide: 10 mg p.o. or i.v. three to four times daily Controlled-release metoclopramide: 20–80 mg p.o. q12h Domperidone: 10–20 mg p.o. three to four times daily, 15–30 min before meals (not available in the United States) Cisapride: 5–20 mg p.o. four times daily at least 15 min before meals and at bedtime (not available in the United States) Erythromycin: 30–50 mg/kg p.o. daily in two to four divided doses; maximum 2 g daily
Early satiety	1. Eat frequent, small meals, with the bulk of their daily intake consumed early 2. Eat sitting up and avoid liquids at mealtimes 3. Prokinetic drug (e.g., metoclopramide, domperidone, erythromycin) (see preceding text for doses)
Heartburn	1. Lifestyle modification: Weight loss Avoid chocolate, spicy food, alcohol, citrus juice, and tomato-based products Eat several small meals during the day Elevate the head of the bed 2. Antacids (aluminum hydroxide, magnesium hydroxide, and simethicone): 10–20 mL or 2–4 tablets p.o. four to six times daily between meals and at bedtime 3. H_2 receptor antagonist: Cimetidine 300 mg p.o. four times daily or 800 mg p.o. at bedtime or 400 mg p.o. twice daily for up to 8 wk i.m., i.v.: 300 mg every 6 h Ranitidine 150 mg twice daily, or 300 mg once daily at bedtime 4. Proton pump inhibitors: Omeprazole 20 mg p.o. daily

Pathophysiology/Etiology

GI bleeding can be multifactorial, and one should not assume that a tumor is the source of bleeding. In a general population of 2225 patients, duodenal ulcer (24%), gastric erosions (23%), and gastric ulcer (21%) accounted for most of the upper GI bleeding (41). In cancer, gastritis (36%), peptic or stress ulceration (26%), and tumor necrosis (23%) are the most common causes. *Candida* esophagitis, particularly during chemotherapy administration, Mallory-Weiss mucosal tears with significant bleeding in the setting of thrombocytopenia (42), and inflammatory conditions (e.g., radiation therapy) are less common (43). In the general population, 43% of lower GI bleeding is due to diverticulosis (44). Massive lower GI bleeding can be a late complication of the high-dose radiation therapy used for treatment of GI, gynecologic, or genitourinary cancer.

Other causes of bleeding in patients with cancer include thrombocytopenia and coagulopathies secondary to the disease or the treatment. Aggressive chemotherapy may cause stress-related ulceration of the mucosa or suppress bone marrow production. The incidence of GI perforation after chemotherapy is 10%; most of who are patients with lymphoma. GI lymphomas are more common sources of tumor bleeding than other intra-abdominal malignancies. Bleeding is the presenting symptom in 15–28% of patients, but only 3–4% have perforation (45). Hemorrhage has been reported in 27% of those receiving chemotherapy for unresected lymphoma. Resection before treatment may reduce the bleeding and perforation by 50%. Cytosine arabinoside can cause bowel necrosis, and hepatic arterial infusion of fluorodeoxyuridine may cause upper GI toxicity, resulting in gastritis and peptic ulcers. The initiation of chemotherapy has been reported to trigger or accelerate disseminated intravascular coagulation in lymphoma, presumably due to release of thromboplastin-like or other clot-promoting agents (45).

Medications may be responsible for GI bleeding. Drugs usually implicated are corticosteroids, nonsteroidal anti-inflammatory drugs, and aspirin (46). Cephalosporins, streptomycin, isoniazid, penicillin, β-lactam, and amphotericin B may cause bleeding due to clotting factor inhibitors or impairing of platelet function.

Upper Gastrointestinal Bleeding—Diagnostic Evaluation

Hematemesis is the vomiting of blood, either bright red or dark, with a "coffee grounds" appearance. Melena is foul smelling stool with a coal black, sticky, tar-like appearance. Hematemesis and melena indicate that the bleeding may be from the nasopharynx, esophagus, stomach, duodenum, or, rarely, the proximal jejunum. Endoscopy is used to evaluate upper GI bleeding. Hemodynamically unstable patients should undergo emergent endoscopy, as they may benefit from both diagnosis and therapy (e.g., ligation for variceal bleeding).

Lower Gastrointestinal Bleeding—Diagnostic Evaluation

Hematochezia is the passage of red blood from the anus. Blood from the distal colon, rectum, or anus is fresh and usually bright red, whereas blood from the proximal colon is likely to be darker. Bleeding from the cecum or ascending colon may appear black but is not as shiny or tar-like as in melena. Early colonoscopy for the detection of lower lesions may be the first diagnostic step (47). However, when the bleeding is significant it is often difficult to identify the source. A technetium-99–labeled red cell scan may identify the general location of bleeding; however, results are variable. If the source remains unknown, the next step is typically angiography. It can detect the bleeding site as well as allow treatment with intra-arterial infusion of vasopressin or embolization (48).

Treatment/Management

General

It is important to understand the status of the primary disease, the expected survival, and the potential for cure in patients with GI hemorrhage. If the long-term survival rate is poor, patients should not be subjected to unnecessary tests and procedures in their final days. The goal is to determine the source of the hemorrhage, stop the bleeding, and prevent recurrence. Start with a quick assessment of the hemodynamic status including vital signs and postural blood pressure. A sudden increase in pulse or postural hypotension may be the first indication of bleeding. The hematocrit should follow; however, it may take hours to equilibrate. Packed red blood cells should be transfused until the hematocrit is >25%. A coagulopathy should initially be corrected with four units of fresh frozen plasma; thrombocytopenia below 50,000 per mm^3 requires platelet transfusions.

Upper Gastrointestinal Bleeding Treatment

To prevent stress ulceration and recurrent bleeding several medications are now available, although there is no evidence of their benefit in the immediate posttreatment period (Table 18.6) (49). Endotracheal intubation to prevent aspiration may be necessary in massive upper GI bleeding. Supportive measures with antacids, H_2 receptor blockers, and blood products control the bleeding in 60% of patients with gastritis or ulceration. Endoscopic control using BICAP, yttrium-aluminum-garnet (YAG) laser, and other modalities may provide temporary control of bleeding ulceration or tumors. If medical management fails, surgery should be considered. The decision to operate should also be based on the patient's potential quality of life and disease prognosis, as surgery is associated with high morbidity and mortality (50).

Variceal bleeding may be treated with endoscopic sclerotherapy or variceal ligation. Medical management is less

---

TABLE 18.6

DRUGS USED TO PREVENT RECURRENT UPPER GASTROINTESTINAL BLEEDING

Drug	Dose
Antacid	Two tablespoons high-potency liquid, after meals (heartburn)
H_2 blocker	Ranitidine hydrochloride 150 mg p.o. twice daily
	Famotidine, 40 mg, at bedtime
	Nizatidine, 150 mg, at bedtime (duodenal)/150 mg p.o. b.i.d. (gastric ulcer)
Proton pump inhibitor	Omeprazole, 20 mg p.o. daily
Sucralfate	1 g twice daily
Prokinetic	Metoclopramide, 5–15 mg p.o. four times daily

effective, but octreotide acetate, a long-acting synthetic analog of somatostatin (50–100-µg i.v. bolus followed by an infusion at 25–50 µg per hour) may reduce portal hypertension in acute variceal hemorrhage. Balloon tamponade may temporize bleeding until more definitive therapy is begun. However, it is associated with a high rate of complications and mortality. Splenorenal and portosystemic shunts control variceal bleeding in a very select group of patients (51).

Lower Gastrointestinal Bleeding—Treatment

For lower GI bleeding, colonoscopy, radionuclide imaging, or mesenteric angiography may be required to identify the source. However, it may be difficult to determine the source due to significant bleeding when performing colonoscopy. If the bleeding rate is >1 mL per minute, selective mesenteric arteriography is the best procedure to localize the source. When it is not possible to localize the source, subtotal colectomy should be performed. In poor-risk patients, therapy with selective infusion of vasopressin or embolization of the bleeding vessel can be performed, but there is a risk of bowel infarction (52).

The Dying Patient

GI hemorrhage may be a terminal event in advanced cancer, and the family and professional team should be prepared as this can be a very distressing time. Bleeding may occur very rapidly, and the patient will die immediately of asphyxiation (upper GI bleed) or a precipitous drop in blood pressure resulting in cardiac arrest due to massive lower GI bleed. GI hemorrhage prevented a peaceful death in 2% of patients in a study of 200 hospice patients (53). The key to successful symptom management in the final days, particularly in the home, is preparation. It is important to have a plan to control these symptoms. Neuroleptics are the drugs of choice to sedate patients who have catastrophic bleeds (e.g., chlorpromazine, 25 mg i.v. slow push or 50 mg p.r. can be given). Benzodiazepines may increase anxiety (54), and unless the patient is having pain, opioids should not be given, as they may cause restlessness, diaphoresis, and hallucinations (55). It is helpful to have dark sheets and towels available to camouflage the bleeding. Although symptoms can be managed well in most, poor preparation precludes a comfortable death.

BILIARY OBSTRUCTION

Definition/Incidence

Biliary obstruction is the blockage of the flow of bile resulting in increased pressure in the biliary system. Malignant obstruction can occur anywhere in the biliary tree, but it most often affects the extrahepatic biliary tree or liver hilum. Its incidence in malignant disease varies depending on the etiology and stage of disease. Extrahepatic biliary obstruction is common in carcinoma of the head of the pancreas. Less common tumors are in the ampulla, bile duct, gall bladder, or liver. Cholangiocarcinoma, metastatic tumor, or enlarged lymphatic nodes are other causes of biliary obstruction (56).

Pathophysiology/Etiology

Normally, the hepatocyte secretes bile. Blocking the flow raises pressure in the biliary system rendering the hepatocyte unable to secrete more. The pressure needed to stop secretion is 300 mm of H_2O, but there is evidence of cholestasis with lesser pressure. A neural or hormonal mechanism may be responsible for cholestasis before the necessary biliary pressure is reached.

Treatment/Management

Patients usually present in the advanced stage of the disease and surgical resection is rarely possible. Patients with symptomatic biliary obstruction should be evaluated for some type of biliary bypass procedure (57). Although survival is often limited, the symptoms, particularly pruritus, are quite distressing and less amenable to other treatments. Open surgical procedures have not been shown to prolong survival and are associated with greater morbidity and mortality than endoscopically placed stents (58). Unless the patient is moribund, a stenting procedure should be considered, as it may offer dramatic relief.

Stent placement with biliary drainage results in decreased serum bilirubin, and symptoms of pruritus usually resolve within 24–48 hours. The duration of palliation afforded by stenting depends on the underlying disease and the type of stent used to relieve the obstruction (59).

There are two types of endoscopically placed stents: self-expanding metallic stents (SEMS) and plastic stents. The major drawback of plastic stents is occlusion with bacterial biofilm. This results in occlusion and recurrence of jaundice and requires one or more stent changes in 30–60% of patients. In randomized trials comparing plastic stents to SEMS in malignant bile duct occlusion, SEMS provided longer patency rates but had no survival advantage. In a three-arm study comparing plastic stent left in place until dysfunction occurred versus plastic stent routinely changed every 3 months versus SEMS, an initial success rate of 97% was obtained. The plastic stent not routinely changed had the poorest complication-free survival rate. The SEMS were the most cost-effective when life expectancy was >6 months (60,61).

The method to control symptoms associated with biliary obstruction depends on the performance status of the patient, tumor type, and local professional expertise. It is important to remember that patients may appear gravely ill due to infection and obstruction, yet may improve dramatically with antibiotics and a procedure to relieve the obstruction.

HEPATIC FAILURE

Definition/Incidence

Hepatic failure is the severe inability of the liver to function normally, as evidenced by jaundice and abnormal plasma levels of ammonia, bilirubin, alkaline phosphatase, glutamic oxaloacetic transaminase, lactic dehydrogenase, and reversal of the albumin/globulin ratio. It quickly leads to failure of other organs. The hallmark of acute hepatic failure is hepatic encephalopathy and coagulopathy (62).

Pathophysiology/Etiology

Most hepatic failure, regardless of cause, results from massive coagulative necrosis of hepatocytes. Viral hepatitis accounts for approximately 70%, and drug ingestion (primarily acetaminophen) accounts for most of the remaining 30%. Malignant causes are associated with metastatic gastric carcinoma, carcinoid, breast cancer, small cell lung cancer, melanoma, leukemia, and lymphoma. Hepatic failure may be the presenting sign of malignancy in some cases (63). Sinusoidal obstruction with subsequent ischemia has been reported in metastatic liver disease. Occlusion of hepatic venous outflow may occur in the setting of intensive chemotherapy or bone marrow transplantation or recrudescence of hepatitis B virus after treatment.

Clinical Manifestations

Regardless of the cause, hepatic failure begins with nausea and malaise. It proceeds to accumulation of ammonia as a result of diminished urea formation, hepatic encephalopathy, cerebral edema, prolonged prothrombin time, rapidly rising bilirubin, metabolic changes, GI bleeding, sepsis, respiratory failure, renal failure, and cardiovascular collapse (64).

Hepatic Encephalopathy

Hepatic encephalopathy is a complex neuropsychiatric syndrome characterized by cognitive changes, fluctuating neurologic signs, and electroencephalographic changes. In severe cases, irreversible coma and death occur (65). It results from severe hepatocellular dysfunction or intrahepatic and extrahepatic shunting of portal venous blood into the systemic circulation bypassing the liver. Toxic substances are not detoxified by the liver; this leads to metabolic abnormalities in the CNS. Most patients have elevated blood ammonia levels (66). Cognitive changes are due to excessive concentrations of GABA. The role of endogenous benzodiazepine agonists is unclear but may contribute to hepatic encephalopathy. A partial response has been observed in some after administration of a benzodiazepine antagonist (flumazenil) (67). The most common predisposing factor is GI bleeding, which leads to an increase in ammonia production. Hypokalemic alkalosis, hypoxia, CNS-depressing drugs (e.g., barbiturates, benzodiazepines), and acute infection may also trigger hepatic encephalopathy (68).

Reversal of the sleep/wake cycle is among the earliest signs of encephalopathy. Mood disturbances, confusion, alterations in personality, deterioration in self-care and handwriting, and daytime somnolence are also seen. The diagnosis of hepatic encephalopathy is usually one of exclusion (69). There are no diagnostic liver function test abnormalities, although an elevated serum ammonia level is highly suggestive of the diagnosis (69). It is sometimes difficult to distinguish hepatic encephalopathy from other forms of delirium.

Portal Hypertension

Tumor burden may compress the hepatic blood vessels; this can result in portal hypertension, which causes collateral vessels in the esophagus and the stomach to become enlarged and tortuous (varices). Bleeding of the varices is likely because the liver is unable to synthesize vitamin K and clotting factors. Procedures to reduce the pressure include a portalsystemic shunt, and β-adrenergic blockade (e.g., propranolol hydrochloride), if not contraindicated (70).

Spontaneous Bacterial Peritonitis

Spontaneous bacterial peritonitis occurs with ascites without an obvious primary source of infection. The ascitic fluid has low concentrations of opsonic proteins, which normally provide protection against bacteria. Paracentesis reveals cloudy fluid with a white cell count >500 cells per μL (>250 polymorphonuclear leukocytes). Common isolates are *Escherichia coli* and pneumococci and, to a lesser extent, anaerobes. Empirical therapy with i.v. cefotaxime sodium (2 g every 8 hours for at least 5 days) and an aminoglycoside should be initiated if clinically appropriate (69).

TABLE 18.7

ADVERSE PROGNOSTIC INDICATORS IN HEPATIC FAILURE

Indicator	Value
Age	<10 y, >40 y
Cause	Idiosyncratic drug reaction, halothane, non-A, non-B hepatitis
Jaundice	>7 d before onset of encephalopathy
Bilirubin	>300 μ mol/L (18 mg/dL)
Prothrombin time	>100 s
Factor V level	<20%
Clinical status	Respiratory failure Rapid reduction in liver size Coma

Hepatorenal Syndrome

Hepatorenal syndrome is a disorder characterized by worsening azotemia, oliguria, hyponatremia, low urinary sodium, and hypotension, with structurally intact kidneys. It is diagnosed only in the absence of identifiable causes of renal dysfunction. Treatment is usually ineffective. Some patients with hypotension and decreased plasma volume may respond to volume expansion, but care must be taken to rehydrate slowly to avoid variceal bleeding (71).

Treatment/Management

Whenever possible, the inciting agent should be treated or eliminated. There is little role for liver transplant in the patient with cancer. For most, treatment of the underlying disease provides the best method to reverse the process of hepatic failure. It may be useful to review adverse prognostic indicators in hepatic encephalopathy (Table 18.7) before embarking on intensive, supportive therapy in those who survive.

Stenting biliary obstructions may provide relief from jaundice and pruritus. Paracentesis helps control symptomatic ascites. Neuropsychiatric symptoms are distressing and should be controlled with appropriate medications. Flumazenil, a short-acting benzodiazepine antagonist, may have a role in the management of hepatic encephalopathy (65). Reducing oral protein intake in advanced cancer is rarely necessary. Administering lactulose, a nonabsorbable laxative sugar, may help. The initial dose is 30–50 mL every hour until diarrhea occurs; thereafter the dose is adjusted (15–30 mL three times daily) so that the patient has two to four soft stools daily (69).

In the terminal state, it may be appropriate to allow a deteriorating level of consciousness to progress and to forgo treatment. The neuropsychiatric symptoms are controlled with neuroleptics (if hallucinating, chlorpromazine 50–200 mg every 2–3 hours) or with diazepam (if agitated). The goal is to relieve distress without concern for the adverse effect of major tranquilizers on the mental status.

TENESMUS

Definition/Incidence

Tenesmus is a painful spasm of the anal sphincter with a sensation of the urgent need to defecate, with involuntary straining, but with little bowel movement if any. Patients complain of an abnormally frequent desire to defecate and a sensation that evacuation is incomplete. Rectal pain is not commonly caused by organic lesions, which more frequently result in tenesmus. It is a distressing, difficult to control problem. In the patient with cancer it occurs most commonly in cancer of the rectum or after pelvic radiation.

Pathophysiology/Etiology

Tenesmus is thought to be a motility disorder of the rectum, with decreased compliance and high-amplitude pressure waves in the rectal wall. This results in an increased sensitivity to distension of the rectum. Rectal causes of tenesmus include impacted feces, carcinoma, rectal prolapse, rectal polyps, adenoma, hemorrhoids, fissure, proctitis, foreign body, abscess, and hemorrhoids. Infectious causes include *Shigella*, *Campylobacter*, and *Clostridium difficile*.

In the patient with rectal cancer, tenesmus is usually an ominous sign, indicating circumferential growth or ulceration involving the sphincter muscle. Tenesmus typically occurs in the morning on waking and subsides as the day progresses. Accompanying perineal or buttock pain suggests involvement of the sacral nerve plexus. Patients presenting with this symptom complex are unlikely to be candidates for sphincter-saving procedures. Tenesmus can also be caused by damage from radiation therapy (acute and late effect) for rectal cancer or other pelvic structures (e.g., cervix, prostate, bladder, testes).

Treatment/Management

Treatment is based on the cause and is variably effective. Infectious causes should be treated with appropriate antibiotics. Radiation-induced tenesmus is a difficult problem. Symptoms usually resolve spontaneously within 2–6 months (72). Tenesmus and rectal bleeding have been treated with oral sulfasalazine combined with steroid enemas or sucralfate enemas (2 g in 20 mL of tap water) (73).

Curative intent pelvic exenteration effectively controlled pain and tenesmus in 89% and palliative intent in 67% of patients with rectal cancer (74). However, this is a procedure associated with significant morbidity and should not be performed for the sole purpose of controlling pain. Radiotherapy may also provide symptomatic relief, but again, the primary purpose is to control the disease; and it may be most useful in those who have not received chemotherapy (75). Metal expandable stents have been used successfully and are associated with little morbidity but may migrate (76). Lumbar sympathectomy produced complete relief of tenesmus in 10 of 12 patients with cancers in the pelvic region. Duration of relief was 3 days to 7 months (mean, 53 days). In this small series, the only complication was transient hypotension responding to intravenous fluids (77); however, mild, reversible bruising, and stiffness at the needle insertion site often occur. Up to 20% of patients have limb pain, which develops after a 10- to 14-day latent period and spontaneously resolves after a few weeks. Major neurologic deficits are uncommon when lumbar sympathectomy is performed by experienced pain practitioners, making it one of the most important treatment modes currently available.

A general treatment plan should include a laxative and stool softener unless diarrhea is the prominent symptom, in which case an obstructing lesion should be ruled out. Care should be taken when prescribing roughage in those with previous radiation, as the bowel/rectal wall can be traumatized. Dexamethasone (4–16 mg daily) may provide some relief through its anti-inflammatory actions. The calcium channel antagonist nifedipine (10–20 mg two to three times daily) may help to relieve spasms. Epidural opioids and local anesthetics may also be helpful. Systemic opioids should be tried but are less effective, as in other forms of neuropathic pain. Traditional neuropathic pain treatment such as tricyclic antidepressants (e.g., amitriptyline hydrochloride) should be used with caution, as one of the main side effects is constipation.

CONCLUSIONS

GI symptoms are so common in the general, healthy population, that it may be more difficult to evaluate them in those with cancer. Common symptoms may be disease-related or a comorbidity unrelated to the cancer. Both may represent potentially life-threatening problems, and yet the decision to treat may not be clear if based on management guidelines for the general population. Decisions regarding treatment must be evaluated with an understanding of the goals of therapy, potential quality of life, and life expectancy. Consultation with GI specialists and ongoing communication with the patient and family, help to provide the framework in which to make these often difficult decisions.

References

1. Askenasy JJM. About the mechanism of hiccup. *Eur Neurol* 1992;32:159–163.
2. Lewis JH. Hiccups: causes and cures. *J Clin Gastroenterol* 1985;7:539–552.
3. Launois S, Bizec JL, Whitelaw WA, et al. Hiccup in adults: an overview. *Eur Respir J* 1993;6:563–575.
4. Friedgood CE, Ripstein CB. Chlorpromazine (Thorazine) in the treatment of intractable hiccups. *JAMA* 1955;157:309–310.
5. Ives TJ, Flemming MF, Weart CW, et al. Treatment of intractable hiccup with intramuscular haloperidol. *Am J Psychiatry* 1985;142:1368–1369.
6. Lipps DC, Jabbari B, Mitchel MH, et al. Nifedipine for intractable hiccups. *Neurology* 1990;40:531–532.
7. Madanagopolan N. Metoclopramide in hiccup. *Curr Med Res Opin* 1975;3:371–374.
8. Walker P, Watanabe S, Bruera E. Baclofen, a treatment for chronic hiccup. *J Pain Symptom Manage* 1998;16:125–132.
9. Parvin R, Milo R, Klein C, et al. Amitriptyline for intractable hiccup. *Am J Gastroenterol* 1988;63:1007–1008.
10. McFarling DA, Susac JO. Carbamazepine for hiccoughs. *JAMA* 1974;230:962.
11. Petroski D, Patel AN. Diphenylhydantoin for intractable hiccups. *Lancet* 1974;1:739.
12. Jacobson PL, Messenheimer JA, Farmer TW. Treatment of intractable hiccups with valproic acid. *Neurology* 1981;31:1458–1460.
13. Porzio G, Aielli F, Narducci F, et al. Hiccup in patients with advanced cancer successfully treated with gabapentin: report of three cases. *N Z Med J* 2003;116(1182):U605.
14. Hernandez JL, Pajaron M, Garcia-Regata O, et al. Gabapentin for intractable hiccup. *Am J Med* 2004;117(4):279–281.
15. Marechal R, Berghmans T, Sculier P. Successful treatment of intractable hiccup with methylphenidate in a lung cancer patient. *Support Care Cancer* 2003;11(2):126.
16. Aravot DJ, Wright G, Rees A, et al. Non-invasive phrenic nerve stimulation for intractable hiccups. *Lancet* 1989;2:1047.
17. Salem MR. Treatment of hiccups by pharyngeal stimulation in anesthetized and conscious subjects. *JAMA* 1967;202:126–130.
18. Smith HS, Busracamwongs A. Management of hiccups in the palliative care population. *Am J Hosp Palliat Care* 2003;20(2):149–154.
19. Heading RC. Definitions of dyspepsia. *Scand J Gastroenterol* 1991;26(Suppl 182):1–6.
20. Ofman JJ, Etchason J, Fullerton S, et al. Management strategies for Helicobacter pyloriseropositive patients with dyspepsia: clinical and economic consequences. *Ann Intern Med* 1997;126:280–291.
21. Tack J, Lee KJ. Pathophysiology and treatment of functional dyspepsia. *J Clin Gastroenterol* 2005;39(5 Suppl):S211–S216.
22. Fisher RS, Parkman HP. Management of nonulcer dyspepsia. *N Engl J Med* 1998;339:1376–1381.
23. Talley NJ. Nonulcer dyspepsia: current approaches to diagnosis and management. *Am Fam Physician* 1993;47:1407–1416.
24. Lee HR, Lennon VA, Camilleri M, et al. Paraneoplastic gastrointestinal motor dysfunction: clinical and laboratory characteristics. *Am J Gastroenterol* 2001;96(2):373–379.

25. Pardi DS, Miller SM, Miller DL, et al. Paraneoplastic dysmotility: loss of interstitial cells of Cajal. *Am J Gastroenterol* 2002;97(7):1828–1833.
26. Nelson KA, Walsh TD. The use of metoclopramide in anorexia due to the cancer–associated dyspepsia syndrome (CADS). *J Palliat Care* 1993;9:14–18.
27. Wilson J, Plourde JY, Marshall D, et al. Long-term safety and clinical effectiveness of controlled-release metoclopramide in cancer-associated dyspepsia syndrome: a multicenter evaluation. *J Palliat Care* 2002;18(2):84–91.
28. McCallum RW, George SJ. Gastric dysmotility and gastroparesis. *Curr Treat Options Gastroenterol* 2001;4(2):179–191.
29. Forster J, Sarosiek I, Delcore R, et al. Gastric pacing is a new surgical treatment for gastroparesis. *Am J Surg* 2001;182(6):676–681.
30. Abell T, Lou J, Tabbaa M, et al. Gastric electrical stimulation for gastroparesis improves nutritional parameters at short, intermediate, and long-term follow-up. *JPEN J Parenter Enteral Nutr* 2003;27(4):277–281.
31. Nebel OT, Fornes MF, Castell DO. Symptomatic gastroesophageal reflux: incidence and precipitating factors. *Dig Dis Sci* 1976;21:953–964.
32. Johnson DA, Ganz R, Aisenberg J, et al. Endoscopic implantation of Enteryx for treatment of GERD: 12-month results of a prospective, multicenter trial. *Am J Gastroenterol* 2003;98(9):1921–1930.
33. Donnelly S, Walsh D. The symptom of advanced cancer. *Semin Oncol* 1995;22(2 Suppl 3):67–72.
34. Dunlop GM. A study of the relative frequency and importance of gastrointestinal symptoms, and weakness in patients with far advanced cancer. *Palliat Med* 1989;4:37–43.
35. Armes PJ, Plant HJ, Allbright A, et al. A study to investigate the incidence of early satiety in patients with advanced cancer. *Br J Cancer* 1992;65:481–484.
36. Nelson KA, Walsh DT, Sheehan FG, et al. Assessment of upper gastrointestinal motility in the cancer–associated dyspepsia syndrome. *J Palliat Care* 1993;9(1):27–31.
37. Neilson SS, Theologides A, Vickers ZM. Influence of food odors on food aversions and preferences in patients with cancer. *Am J Clin Nutr* 1980;33:2253–2261.
38. Longstreth GF. Epidemiology for hospitalization for acute upper gastrointestinal hemorrhage: a population based study. *Am J Gastroenterol* 1995;90:206–210.
39. Rockall TA, Logan RFA, Devlin HB, et al. Incidence of and mortality from acute upper gastrointestinal haemorrhage in the United Kingdom. *BMJ* 1995;311:222.
40. Mercadante S, Baressi L, Casuccio A, et al. Gastrointestinal bleeding in advanced cancer patients. *J Pain Symptom Manage* 2000;19:160–162.
41. Silverstein FE, Gilbert DA, Tedesco FJ. The national ASGE survey on upper gastrointestinal bleeding. *Gastrointest Endosc* 1981;27:73.
42. Spencer GD, Hackman RC, McDonald GB, et al. A prospective study of unexplained nausea and vomiting after marrow transplantation. *Transplantation* 1986;42:602–607.
43. Kemeny MM, Brennan MF. The surgical complications of chemotherapy in the cancer patient. *Curr Probl Surg* 1987;24:613–675.
44. Boley SJ, DiBiase A, Brandt LJ, et al. Lower intestinal bleeding in the elderly. *Am J Surg* 1979;137:57.
45. Weingrad DN, Decosse JJ, Sherlock P, et al. Primary gastrointestinal lymphoma. *Cancer* 1982;49:1258–1265.
46. Gabriel SE, Jaakkimaenen L, Bombardier C. Risk for serious gastrointestinal complications related to the use of nonsteroidal anti-inflammatory drugs: a meta-analysis. *Ann Intern Med* 1991;115:787–797.
47. Jensen DM, Machicado GA. Diagnosis and treatment of severe hematochezia. The role of urgent colonoscopy after purge. *Gastroenterology* 1988;95:1569–1574.
48. Nusbaum M, Baum S. Radiographic demonstration of unknown sites of gastrointestinal bleeding. *Surg Forum* 1963;14:374–375.
49. Lind T, Aadland E, Eriksson S, et al. Beneficial effects of I.V. omeprazole in patients with peptic ulcer bleeding. *Gastroenterology* 1995;108:A150.
50. Cotlon RB, Rosenberg MT, Waldram RPL, et al. Early endoscopy of esophagus, stomach, and duodenal bulb in patients with hematemesis and melena. *BMJ* 1973;2:505–509.
51. Graham D, Smith JL. The course of patients after variceal hemorrhage. *Gastroenterology* 1981;80:800–809.
52. Jensen DM. Current management of severe lower gastrointestinal tract bleeding. *Gastrointest Endosc* 1995;41:171–173.
53. Lichter I, Hunt E. The last 48 hours of life. *J Palliat Care* 1990;6:7–15.
54. Breitbart W, Marotta R, Platt M, et al. A double-blind trial of haloperidol, chlorpromazine, and lorazepam in the treatment of delirium in hospitalized AIDS patients. *Am J Psychiatry* 1996;153:231–237.
55. Crain SM, Shen F. Opioids can evoke direct receptor-mediated excitatory effects in sensory neurons. *Trends Pharmacol Sci* 1990;11:77–81.
56. Stellato TA, Zollinger RM, Shuck JM. Metastatic malignant biliary obstruction. *Am Surg* 1989;157:381–385.
57. Bear HD, Turner MA, Parker GA, et al. Treatment of biliary obstruction caused by metastatic cancer. *Am J Surg* 1989;157:381–385.
58. Smith AC, Dowsett JF, Russell RCG, et al. Randomized trial of endoscopic stenting versus surgical bypass in malignant low bile duct obstruction. *Lancet* 1994;334:1655–1660.
59. Earnshaw JJ, Hayter JP, Teasdale C, et al. Should endoscopic stenting be the initial treatment of malignant biliary obstruction? *Ann R Coll Surg Engl* 1992;74:338–341.
60. Wagner HJ, Knyrim K, Vakil N, et al. Polyethylene endoprostheses versus metal stents in the palliative treatment of malignant hilar obstruction. A prospective and randomized trial. *Endoscopy* 1993;25:213–218.
61. Schmassmann A, von Gunten E, Knuchel J, et al. Wall stents versus plastic stents in malignant biliary obstruction: effects of stent patency of the first and second stent on patient compliance and survival. *Am J Gastroenterol* 1996;91:654–659.
62. O'Grady JG, Schalm SW, Williams R. Acute liver failure: redefining the syndromes. *Lancet* 1993;342:273–275.
63. McGuire BM, Cherwitz DL, Rabe KM, et al. Small cell carcinoma of the lung manifesting as acute hepatic failure. *Mayo Clin Proc* 1997;72:133–139.
64. Fingerote RJ. Fulminant hepatic failure. *Am J Gastroenterol* 1993;88:1000–1010.
65. Butterworth RF. Pathogenesis and treatment of portal-systemic encephalopathy: an update. *Dig Dis Sci* 1992;37:321–340.
66. Lockwood AH. Hepatic encephalopathy. *Neurol Clin* 2002;20:241–246.
67. Howard CD, Seifert CF. Flumazenil in the treatment of hepatic encephalopathy. *Ann Pharmacother* 1993;27:46–48.
68. Hoyumpa AM, Desmond PV, Avant GR, et al. Clinical conference: hepatic encephalopathy. *Gastroenterology* 1979;78:184.
69. Hoofnagle JH, Carithers RL, Shapiro C, et al. Fulminant hepatic failure: summary of a workshop. *Hepatology* 1995;21:240.
70. D'Amico G, Pagliaco L, Bosch J. The treatment of portal hypertension: a meta-analysis review. *Hepatology* 1995;22:332–354.
71. Wilkinson SP, Portmann B, Hurst D, et al. Pathogenesis of renal failure in cirrhosis and fulminant hepatic failure. *Postgrad Med J* 1975;51:503.
72. Sedwick DM, Howard GC, Ferguson A. Pathogenesis of acute radiation injury to the rectum. A prospective study in patients. *Int J Colorectal Dis* 1994;9:23–30.
73. Regnard CFB. Control of bleeding in advanced cancer. *Lancet* 1991;337:974.
74. Yeung RS, Moffat FL, Falk RE. Pelvic exenteration for recurrent and extensive primary colorectal adenocarcinoma. *Cancer* 1993;72:1853–1858.
75. Midgley R, Kerr D. Colorectal cancer. *Lancet* 1999;353:391–399.
76. Rey JF, Romanczyk T, Graff M. Metal stents for palliation of rectal carcinoma: a preliminary report on 12 patients. *Endoscopy* 1995;27:501–504.
77. Bristow A, Foster JMG. Lumbar sympathectomy in the management of rectal tenesmoid pain. *Ann R Coll Surg Engl* 1988;70:38–39.

CHAPTER 19 ■ ORAL MANIFESTATIONS AND COMPLICATIONS OF CANCER THERAPY

JANE M. FALL-DICKSON AND ANN M. BERGER

ORAL COMPLICATIONS

The effectiveness of standard cancer treatments targeted at improving cure rates, extending survival, or providing palliative treatment, and novel cancer therapies tested in the clinical trial setting, is tempered by patient morbidity manifested as side effects. Nonhematologic side effects have become the primary-dose and treatment-limiting clinical challenges due to the standard use of growth factors. Oral complications are clinically significant side effects and include chemotherapy- and radiation therapy-related stomatitis and chronic graft versus host disease (cGVHD)-related oral manifestations, associated oropharyngeal pain, xerostomia, and oral infection (1). Patient outcomes from these oral complications range from symptoms such as severe oral pain to life threatening medical emergencies such as sepsis. Pathogenic theories of prevention, assessment, and management strategies for these oral complications are presented.

Stomatitis

Chemotherapy-Related Stomatitis

Stomatitis occurs in approximately 40% of chemotherapy patients (2), with about 50% of these patients experiencing severe painful lesions requiring cancer treatment modification and or parenteral analgesia (3). Patients undergoing bone marrow transplantation (BMT) experience incidence rates of stomatitis >60%, and have higher incidence rates for ulcerative stomatitis of up to 78% (4). Oral infection may not only increase the severity of stomatitis, but also has a four times greater relative risk of septicemia due to pathogen entry through damaged mucosal barriers. In the peripheral blood stem cell transplantation (PBSCT) setting, stomatitis typically develops 5 to 7 days post high-dose chemotherapy administration with severe stomatitis usually preceding the white blood cell (WBC) nadir by 2 to 3 days.

Stomatitis clinically presents with asymptomatic erythema. Solitary, white, elevated, desquamative, slightly painful patches may progress to large, contiguous, pseudomembranous, painful lesions. Nonkeratinized mucosa is most affected, including the labial, buccal, and soft palate mucosa, the floor of the mouth, and the ventral surface of the tongue. Typical oral histology of chemotherapy-related stomatitis

includes epithelial hyperplasia, collagen and glandular degeneration, epithelial dysplasia, atrophy, edema of the rete pegs, and vascular changes. The loss of basement membrane epithelial cells exposes the underlying connective tissue stroma and its associated innervation, contributing to increasing oropharyngeal pain levels.

Radiation Therapy–Related Stomatitis

Radiation therapy targeted at the oropharyngeal area almost always causes stomatitis, with severity related to type of ionizing radiation, volume of irradiated tissue, daily and cumulative dose, and duration of radiotherapy. Stomatitis remains a dose- and rate-limiting toxicity in the population receiving irradiation for cancer of the head and neck, and also with hyperfractionated radiotherapy and chemotherapy designed to improve survival time. Radiation therapy interacts directly with DNA leading to chromosomal and cellular mitotic apparatus damage. Total doses of 1600 to 2200 cGy, administered at 200 cGy per day usually leads to atrophic changes in the oral epithelium, and doses >6000 cGy may cause permanent salivary gland changes (5). Pseudomembranes and ulcerations develop in parallel with increase in severity of stomatitis. Although decalcification or hypocalcification of teeth may result from direct dental irradiation, radiation therapy–related dental effects depend mainly on salivary changes that occur from irradiated glands. The addition of total body irradiation to the PBSCT treatment leads to an increased risk of severe stomatitis related to both direct mucosal damage and xerostomia.

Radiation-induced dental effects primarily depend on salivary changes and occur when the glands are included in the field of treatment, rather than on direct irradiation of the teeth themselves. Direct irradiation of teeth may alter the organic or inorganic components in some manner, making them more susceptible to decalcification or hypocalcification. Although there have been no clinical studies to support the possibility that radiation therapy directly affects the pupal chamber, many teeth in the direct irradiated field could be desensitized and therefore, early caries involving the nerve might be asymptomatic. Therefore, meticulous mouth or oral care includes daily fluoride application.

Pathogenesis of Stomatitis

Stomatitis is an inflammation of the mucous membranes of the oral cavity and oropharynx characterized by tissue erythema, edema, and atrophy, often progressing to ulceration (6). The pathogenesis of cancer treatment–related stomatitis remains to be completely elucidated. Mucosal epithelial stem cells that are located in the deep squamous epithelium superior to the basement membrane are subjected to trauma by routine actions such as chewing, swallowing, and digestion. Cancer therapy affects rapidly dividing cells, and therefore the oral basal epithelium cell turnover rate of 7 to 14 days places them at risk for chemotherapy targeting. Sonis (3) proposed a hypothetical model for the pathogenesis of stomatitis and healing that includes four interdependent phases: inflammatory/vascular, epithelial, ulcerative, and healing. Each phase results from cytokine-mediated actions and the direct effect of chemotherapy or radiation therapy on the epithelium which is also influenced by the patient's bone marrow status and oral bacterial flora. Sonis (7) has expanded upon this model recently and has proposed a five-phase biological model of stomatitis that includes dynamic interactions that promote initiation, message generation, signaling and amplification, ulceration, and healing.

The relatively acute inflammatory/vascular phase occurs shortly after chemotherapy or radiation therapy administration (3). Cytokines released from epithelial tissue include tumor necrosis factor-α (TNF-α) that is related to tissue damage, and interleukin-1 (IL-1) both of which incite the inflammatory response and increase subepithelial vascularity that may lead to increased local chemotherapy levels. The epithelial phase demonstrates reduced epithelial renewal and atrophy, and typically begins 4 to 5 days after chemotherapy administration. The cell cycle S-phase specific agents are the most efficient contributors to this phase and include methotrexate, 5-fluorouracil (5-FU), and cytarabine.

The ulcerative/bacterial phase, which begins approximately 1 week postchemotherapy administration with maximum neutropenia, is the most biologically complex stage (3). This phase is probably not chemotherapy agent class specific. During this most symptomatic phase, patients often experience acute oropharyngeal pain leading to dysphagia, decreased oral intake, and difficulty in speaking. Bacterial colonization of mucosal ulceration occurs, and gram-negative organisms release endotoxins that induce the release of IL-1 and TNF-α and production of nitric oxide which may increase local mucosal injury. Radiation therapy and chemotherapy are likely to amplify and prolong this cytokine release, thus exacerbating tissue response. Genetic expression of cytokines and enzymes critical in tissue damage may be modified by transcription factors (3). Healing of oral lesions in the nonmyelosuppressed patient occurs within 2 to 3 weeks through renewed epithelial proliferation and differentiation in parallel with WBC recovery, reestablishment of normal local microbial flora, and decrease in oropharyngeal pain.

Risk Factors

Risk factors for chemotherapy-related stomatitis are complex and conflicting study results are seen (Table 19.1). Younger patients are considered to be at increased risk for stomatitis, and women have been reported to have more severe stomatitis with greater frequency than men. However, Driezen (8) reported no age or gender risk for stomatitis development. In general, children are three times more likely than adults to develop stomatitis due to their higher fraction of proliferating basal cells. Although both alcohol and tobacco may impair salivary function, it has been suggested that tobacco is associated with a decreased incidence of chemotherapy-induced stomatitis (3). One recent study involving 332 outpatients receiving chemotherapy revealed no significant differences in stomatitis incidence between patients who wore dental appliances, had a history of

TABLE 19.1

PATIENT-RELATED AND TREATMENT RELATED-STOMATITIS RISK FACTORS

PATIENT-RELATED

Age >65 and <20 years
Gender
Poor oral health and hygiene
Periodontal diseases
Microbial flora
Chronic low-grade mouth infections
Salivary gland secretory dysfunction
Herpes simplex viral infection
Inborn inability to metabolize chemotherapeutic agent
   effectively
Poor nutritional status
Exposure to oral stressors such as alcohol and smoking
Ill-fitting dental prostheses

TREATMENT-RELATED

Radiation therapy: dose, schedule
Chemotherapy: drug, dose, schedule
Myelosuppression
Neutropenia
Immunosuppression
Reduced secretory protein Immunoglobin A
Oral care during treatment
Infections of bacterial, viral, and fungal origin
Use of antidepressants, opiates, antihypertensives,
   antihistamines, diuretics, and sedatives
Impairment of renal and/or hepatic function
Protein or calorie malnutrition, and dehydration
Xerostomia

IgA, protein Immunoglobin A.
Reference (9,10)
Adapted from Berger AM, Kilroy TJ. Oral Complications. In: DeVita VT Jr, Hellman S, Rosenberg SA, eds. *Cancer: principles and practice of oncology,* 7th ed. Philadelphia, PA: Lippincott Williams & Wilkins, 2004.

oral lesions and a history of smoking and patients who did not, as well as those patients who practiced different oral hygiene regimens (9). Also, drug metabolism affects the incidence and severity of stomatitis in patients who are unable to adequately metabolize or excrete certain chemotherapeutic agents.

Although the full spectrum of treatment-related risk factors for stomatitis remains to be defined, reported risk factors include continuous infusion therapy for breast and colon cancer (5-FU and leucovorin), administration of selected anthracyclines, alkylating agents, taxanes, vinca alkaloids, antimetabolites, antitumor antibiotics, myeloablative conditioning regimens for PBSCT or BMT, and radiation therapy to the head and neck. Drugs that can result in xerostomia include antidepressants, opiates, antihypertensives, antihistamines, diuretics, and sedatives. In general, there are many complicated risk factors for the development of chemotherapy-induced stomatitis, and a lack of stratification criteria and clear definition of risk factors for patients entering clinical trials may contribute to conflicting study results (10).

Radiation Therapy–Related Complications

Long-term effects of head and neck radiation therapy include soft tissue fibrosis, obliterative endarteritis, trismus, non- or slow healing mucosal ulcerations, and slow healing of dental extraction sites. These changes become more substantial over time. Radiation-related fibrotic changes in the muscles of mastication and/or the temporal mandibular joint can develop till 1 year posttreatment. Oral candidiasis is a common acute and long-term oral sequela of head and neck radiation therapy. These candida lesions, which frequently present as angular cheilitis, may appear white and movable, chronic hyperplastic (nonremovable), or chronic erythematous (diffuse patchy erythema).

Osteoradionecrosis (ORN) is a relatively uncommon clinical entity related to hypocellularity, hypovascularity, and tissue ischemia. Higher incidences are seen when total doses to the bone exceed 65 Gy (11). Although ORN may be spontaneous, the etiology is usually trauma such as dental extraction, and may lead to serious conditions such as pathologic fracture, infection of surrounding soft tissues, and severe pain. Most studies have reported ORN after tooth extractions that were not allowed adequate extraction site healing time of 10 to 14 days before start of radiation therapy. The risk of ORN does not diminish over time, and it may even increase following radiation therapy. See below.

Chronic Graft versus Host Disease Oral Manifestations

Patients with cancer who have undergone allogeneic PBSCT frequently develop GVHD, which is an alloimmune condition derived from an immune attack mediated by donor T-cells recognizing antigens expressed on normal tissues. This condition occurs following allogeneic PBSCT due to disparities in minor histocompatibility antigens between donor and recipient, inherited independently of HLA genes (12). Acute GVHD occurs within the first 100 days postallogeneic PBSCT, and cGVHD begins as early as 70 days or as late as 15 months postallogeneic transplant. Mitchell (13) presents a comprehensive overview of treatment strategies for GVHD.

Oral involvement occurs in approximately 80% of patients who experience extensive cGVHD and is a major contributing factor to patient morbidity seen in the allogeneic PBSCT setting (14). Patients may also present with limited disease involving only the oral cavity. Oral cGVHD clinically presents with tissue atrophy and erythema, lichenoid changes (hyperkeratotic striae, patches, plaques, and papules) and pseudomembranous ulcerations seen typically on buccal and labial mucosa and the lateral tongue, angular stomatitis, and xerostomia (14). Patients' decreased oral intake related to oropharyngeal pain may lead to serious problems of weight loss and malnutrition. Oral infections in this population may lead to serious, life-threatening systemic infections (15).

Osteonecrosis

Osteonecrosis of the jaw bone has been associated with the use of bisphosphonate therapy, which is used to treat patients with hypercalcemia related to malignancy, bone metastasis, and metabolic bone diseases (16). Ruggiero, Mehrotra, Rosenberg et al. (17) performed a retrospective chart review of 63 patients with a diagnosis of refractory osteomyelitis and a history of chronic bisphosphonate therapy. A subsample of 56 patients had received intravenous bisphosphonates for at least 1 year and 7 patients were receiving chronic oral bisphosphonate therapy. Lesions were presented with either a nonhealing extraction socket or an exposed jawbone. Both of these conditions were refractory to conservative debridement and antibiotic therapy. Most of these patients required surgical procedures to remove the involved bone. In view of the current trend of increasing and widespread use of chronic bisphosphonate therapy, the authors stated that the associated risk of osteonecrosis of the jaw should alert practitioners to monitor this previously unrecognized potential complication. An early diagnosis might prevent or reduce the morbidity resulting from advanced destructive lesions of the jaw bone.

STRATEGIES FOR PREVENTION AND TREATMENT OF ORAL COMPLICATIONS

Pretherapy Dental Evaluation and Intervention

Oral/dental stabilization before chemotherapy and radiation therapy is critical in avoiding potential serious sequelae. Pretreatment oral/dental stabilization requires close collaboration between an experienced dental team and informed patients to provide adequate cleaning, eliminate sites of oral infection and trauma, and encourage appropriate oral hygiene (18). There exist many private practice or health care institution–specific policies and preventive approaches for oral care for chemotherapy and radiation therapy patients.

Patients scheduled for chemotherapy and/or head and neck radiation therapy should receive dental screening at least 2 weeks before therapy starts. This schedule allows for proper healing of any extraction sites, recovery of soft tissue manipulations, and restoration of teeth necessary to promote optimal mucosal health before, during, and following cancer treatment. Oral hygiene is one of the most important screening areas for all patients regardless of cancer treatment modality. Plaque and gingival hemorrhage on dental pocket probing are clinical signs that necessitate development of the oral/dental treatment plan (e.g., preradiation extractions). These procedures reduce the incidence of oral complications by eliminating bacteria that could lead to local oral infections or sepsis. The dental team must know the patient's total WBC count, absolute granulocyte count, and platelet count following chemotherapy or in preparation for intense chemotherapy or peripheral blood stem cell transplant, especially if the patient requires dental extractions, oral biopsies, or periodontal surgery.

The initial dental appointment includes examination of the patient's dentition for carious lesions and defective restorations, which are sources of potential irritation of the oral mucosa and necessitate replacement. The periodontium, as well as pulp vitality must be evaluated. Periodontal status is a major consideration and thorough screening includes measurement of pocket depth and assessment of furcation involvement. Denture fit assessment is important to avoid ill-fitting dentures that may cause irritation of irradiated tissue and potential ulceration to underlying bone (19). Trismus is anticipated if the temporal mandibular joints and other muscles of mastication are included in the radiation field. Therefore, maximum mouth opening should be recorded before radiation therapy at baseline to compare the interarch distance at various time points postradiation therapy to evaluate the degree of trismus. Comprehensive evaluation also includes assessment of the oral mucosa and the alveolar process to prepare for possible future prosthetic intervention, and also to assess ulcerations, fibromas, irritation, hyperplasia, bony spicules, and tori.

A panoramic radiograph combined with intraoral radiographs as needed is necessary to detect periodontal disease, periapical infections, cyst, third molar pathology, unerupted or partially erupted teeth, and residual root tips. Significant oral/dental problems to address before cancer treatment include poor oral hygiene, periapical pathology, third molar pathology, periodontal disease, defective restorations, dental caries, orthodontic appliances, ill-fitting prostheses, and other potential sources of infection. Also recommended before cancer treatment is root planing, scaling, and prophylaxis, excluding visible tumor located at the site of anticipated dental manipulation, to reduce the bacteria load that could lead to local infection and sepsis. Acyclovir should be considered prophylactically in patients who are seropositive and at high risk for HSV infection reactivation, including BMT patients or those with prolonged myelosuppression. Mucosal lesions with fungal, viral, or bacterial infection require treatment to avoid the risk of systemic infection.

Decisions by the dental team regarding extraction before radiation therapy are based on radiation exposure, type, portal field, fractionation and total dosage, tumor prognosis and expediency of cancer control, and very importantly, the patient's motivation to adhere to the preventive regimen. Teeth with acute and symptomatic periodontal problems should be extracted with careful follow-up examination of these sites before head and neck radiation therapy. The patient is at risk for ORN following tooth extractions that do not allow 10 to 14 days of healing before radiation therapy. Dental appliances fabricated during the pretreatment time period include fluoride carriers and radiation protective mouthguards. Surgical resection of any anatomic oral or pharyngeal structure including soft palate, tongue, hard palate, mandible, or combination will compromise oral function. Sequelae of many resections can be alleviated by intervention with maxillofacial prosthetics that are designed to restore function and cosmesis, with some limitations.

Dental extractions following radiation therapy require collaborations between dental and radiation oncology team members to minimize the risk of ORN. A low incidence of ORN is seen when preradiation therapy dental consultation and appropriate treatment (e.g., extractions) are rendered (20–22). Follow-up and recall of the head and neck cancer patient for dental preventive maintenance and treatment are essential to prevent or attenuate negative sequelae in the oral cavity. Generally, any teeth with acute and symptomatic periodontal problems should be extracted before head and neck radiation therapy. The decision to extract asymptomatic teeth before the commencement of radiation therapy is related to several important factors including radiation exposure, type, portal field, fractionization and total dosage, in addition to tumor prognosis, and expediency of control of the cancer (23). Lack of patient motivation regarding appropriate oral hygiene practices should lead to a decision to extract questionable teeth before radiation therapy.

Teeth that are class II or III mobility without use as abutment teeth for prosthetic retention should also be considered for preradiation extraction therapy. Extractions of residual root tips and impacted teeth should be performed atraumatically with regard to tissue handling. Alveolectomy and primary wound closure are considered to eliminate sharp ridges and bone spicules that could project to the overlying soft tissues. This is particularly important for prosthetic consideration because negligible bone remodeling is predicted after radiation therapy.

Nonvital teeth located in the portal fields that do not have periapical radiolucency and are asymptomatic should be treated endodontically. Endodontics with possible retrograde filings are preferred because of increased ORN risk in the portal fields. Teeth with small amounts of periapical granulomas without periodontal involvement but important for oral function or rehabilitation, should be treated with apicoectomies.

Allowing adequate time for healing of extraction sites before radiation therapy is essential. Healing times of 14 to 21 days are generally considered safe and should be the rule.

Antibiotics are not routinely recommended because there is no evidence that they influence healing in the absence of infection. Careful examination of extraction sites must be performed before radiation therapy commences. Communication between the dentist, patient, and radiation therapist is pivotal for healthy maintenance of the oral cavity. Patients are susceptible to dental caries (decay) at the cervical areas of all teeth after radiation therapy to the head and neck region and need to be instructed about effective daily plaque removal through use of floss, a soft toothbrush, and fluoridated toothpaste at least three to four times a day. Daily compliancy of fluoride for the patient's life is more important than the modality of fluoride application.

Patient and family education and counseling within the context of patient motivation are necessary to promote successful preventive strategies. Communication between and among the dentist, dental hygienist, medical oncologist and/or radiation therapist, oncology nurse, and patient is critical for the successful outcome of oral health following cancer treatment. Patients often receive their cancer treatment in the ambulatory setting and are therefore responsible for their oral care at home. Therefore, specific written instructions are needed regarding appropriate use of oral care agents and instruments for effective daily plaque removal, use of prescribed fluoride treatments, and reportable oral observations and symptoms. Numerous educational materials exist including the comprehensive patient education packet "Oral Health, Cancer Care, and You: Fitting the Pieces Together" (www.nohic.nidcr.nih.gov/campaign/titlepg.htm) that is available through the National Oral Health Information Clearinghouse (24).

Assessment of the Oral Mucosa

Consistent and frequent oral cavity assessment is needed to assess clinical signs before, during, and after the treatment time course, and requires the use of an adequately intense white light to visualize all soft and hard tissues and dentition. Assessment and treatment of oral complications is often performed by medical and nursing staff when the patient is hospitalized, which requires an appropriate knowledge base of clinical signs and symptoms of oral complications and predicted negative sequelae. No standard grading system for severity of oral complications of cancer treatment exists. Numerous available oral complications grading tools are based on two or more clinical parameters combined with functional status, such as eating ability. One commonly used tool is the National Cancer Institute Common Terminology Criteria for Adverse Events v3.0 that includes both descriptive terminology and a severity grading scale for each reportable adverse event (25). Other frequently used oral mucosal assessment tools are discussed in the subsequent text.

Oral Assessment Guide

The Oral Assessment Guide (OAG) (26) is a concise clinical tool to record oral cavity changes related to cancer therapy using eight assessment categories (voice, swallowing, lips, tongue, saliva, mucous membranes, gingiva, and teeth/dentures), each rated on three levels of descriptors: 1 = normal findings; 2 = mild alterations; and 3 = definitely compromised. The overall oral assessment score is the summation of the subscale score with a possible range of 8 to 24. Content-related validity, construct validity, clinical utility, and a high, trained nurse–nurse interrater reliability (r = .912) have been reported (26). The OAG has been used frequently to assess the efficacy of oral care protocols, to compare methods designed to determine the nature and prevalence of stomatitis, and to describe the incidence and severity of stomatitis in (PBSCT) patients.

Oral Mucositis Rating Scale

The Oral Mucositis Rating Scale (OMRS) was developed as "...a research tool for the comprehensive measurement of a broad range of oral tissue changes associated with cancer therapy" (27). The OMRS was originally tested in 60 patients who were 180 to 500 days post PBSCT, to examine the relationship between oral abnormalities and cGVHD (28). Findings demonstrated that oral manifestations and related sequelae most strongly associated with cGVHD included atrophy and erythema, lichenoid lesions located on the buccal and labial mucosa, and oral pain.

The item pool consists of 91 items covering 13 areas of the mouth that are assessed for several types of changes in seven anatomic areas: lips; labial and buccal mucosa; tongue; floor of mouth; palate; and attached gingiva. Each site is divided into upper and lower (lips and labial mucosa), right and left (buccal mucosa), dorsal, ventral, and lateral (tongue), and hard and soft (palate). Descriptive categories are atrophy, pseudomembrane, erythema, hyperkeratosis, lichenoid, ulceration, and edema. Erythema, atrophy, hyperkeratosis, lichenoid, and edema are scored using scales of 0 to 3 (0 = normal/no change, 1 = mild change, 2 = moderate change, and 3 = severe change). Ulceration and pseudomembrane are rated by estimated surface area involved (0 = none, 1 = >0 but ≤1 cm^2, 2 = >1 cm^2 but ≤2 cm^2, and 3 = >2 cm^2). The total possible score is the sum of all item scores with a possible range of 0 to 273. The OMRS has shown clinical and research utility (28).

Oral Mucositis Index

The Oral Mucositis Index (OMI) was developed from the finalized OMRS. A downsized 20-item version of the OMI (OMI-20) was developed and validated through a consensus panel of BMT oral complications specialists in the United States (29). The OMI-20 consists of nine items measuring erythema, nine items measuring ulceration, one atrophy item, and one edema item; all scored from 0 = none to 3 = severe, summed for a possible range of 0 to 60. The two sets of nine items measuring erythema and ulceration may be summed to produce subscale scores ranging from 0 to 27. The OMI-20 has demonstrated internal consistency, test–retest, and inter-rater reliability through evaluation in a sample of 133 adult PBSCT/BMT patients (29).

Oral Mucositis Assessment Scale

The Oral Mucositis Assessment Scale (OMAS) was developed as a scoring system for evaluating the anatomic extent and severity of stomatitis in clinical research studies by a team of oral medicine specialists, dentists, dental hygienists, oncologists, and oncology nurses from the United States, Canada, and Europe (30,31). Oral cavity regions assessed are lip (upper and lower), cheek (right and left), right and lateral tongue, left ventral and lateral tongue, floor of mouth, soft palate/fauces, and hard palate (30). Erythema is rated on a scale 0 to 2 (0 = none, 1 = not severe, and 2 = severe) and ulceration/pseudomembrane is a combined category rated on scores based on estimated surface area involved (0 = no lesion, 1 = <1 cm^2, 2 = 1 to 3 cm^2, and 3 = >3 cm^2) and summed giving a possible score range of 0 to 45 (30,31). Validity and reliability have been demonstrated for the OMAS through clinical research studies (31).

World Health Organization Index

The World Health Organization (WHO) Index gives an overall rating of stomatitis and has frequently been used as a general comparison index to other oral assessment scales (6,32). The WHO Index is scaled as follows: grade 0 = no change; grade 1 = soreness, erythema; grade 2 = erythema, ulcers, can eat solids; and grade 3 = ulcers, requires liquid diet only; and grade 4 = alimentation not possible. Limitations of this instrument are the lack of reliability and validity data, and also the tool's inability to capture the variety of oral changes that are observed with cancer treatment (6).

Assessment of Stomatitis-Related Oral Pain

Oral pain related to cancer treatment is multidimensional. Although this oral pain is often challenging to manage, this is critical to accomplish to avoid suffering and psychological distress (15). Effective oral pain management is promoted through constant communication between and among patient, physician, nurse, and caregiver. Numerous valid and reliable pain intensity assessment tools exist. However, to adequately capture this oral pain experience, it is necessary to use a more comprehensive pain assessment tool such as the painometer (33) whose components include sensory and affective dimensions.

Treatment Strategies

The optimal treatment strategies for oral complications and related sequelae are unknown. Treatment strategies for stomatitis and related oropharyngeal pain are mainly empirical and need testing in the randomized controlled clinical trial setting (Table 19.2). Zlotolow and Berger (34) presented a comprehensive review of clinical research focusing on treatment strategies for oral complications of cancer strategies. Conflicting study results may be attributed to inappropriate design issues, use of limited oral assessment instruments that do not capture variations in oral cavity changes, and incorrect timing and dose of interventions. The only standard forms of care are pretreatment oral/dental stabilization, saline mouthwashes, and oropharyngeal pain management (35). The outcome of any oral care practice standard should be a clean, moist oral cavity that is trauma free, and conducive to healing. Meticulous oral hygiene must be maintained before, during, and following the cancer treatment process.

The need for standardized treatment for stomatitis was appreciated by the Mucositis Study Section of the Multinational Association of Supportive Care in Cancer and the International Society for Oral Oncology through their formulation of the "Clinical Practice Guidelines for the Prevention and Treatment of Cancer Therapy-Induced Oral and Gastrointestinal Mucositis" (36). These guidelines are based on a comprehensive review of more than 8000 English language publications (1966–2001). The publications regarding alimentary tract mucositis were scored using criteria that rated the studies for level of evidence and quality of research design (37).

A standardized approach for the prevention and treatment of chemotherapy- and radiotherapy-induced stomatitis is essential, although the efficacy and safety of most of the regimens have not been established through clinical trials. The prophylactic measures usually used for the prevention of stomatitis include chlorhexidine gluconate (Peridex), saline rinses, sodium bicarbonate rinses, acyclovir, amphotericin B, and ice. Regimens commonly used for the treatment of stomatitis and related pain include a local anesthetic such as lidocaine or dyclonine hydrochloride, magnesium-based antacids (Maalox, Mylanta), diphenhydramine hydrochloride (Benadryl), nystatin, or sucralfate. These agents are used either alone or in different combinations in a mouthwash formulation. Other agents used less commonly include kaolin-pectin (Kaopectate),

TABLE 19.2

FORMULARY OF COMMON TREATMENTS FOR ORAL COMPLICATIONS

	DIRECTIONS FOR USE
PREVENTION OF STOMATITIS	
Chlorhexidine gluconate 0.12% oral rinse	Rinse mouth twice daily for 30 s. Do not swallow.
NaHCO3[a] powder: 3 tbsp or 11.6 g	Combine all ingredients. Rinse mouth two to four times daily. Do not swallow.
NaCl[b] powder: 3 tbsp or 11.6 g	
Distilled water: 1 gallon	
Povidone iodine 0.5% oral rinse	Rinse mouth two to four times daily. Do not swallow.
TREATMENT OF STOMATITIS-ASSOCIATED PAIN	
Carafate suspension, 1 g	Rinse mouth with suspension four times daily. Do not swallow.
Diphenhydramine (Benadryl) 12.5 mg/5 mL; kaolin and pectin (Kaopectate)	Combine equal amounts of each. Rinse mouth with 10 to 15 mL four to six times daily. Do not swallow.
Diphenhydramine (Benadryl) 12.5 mg/5 mL: 30 mL; Maalox 30 mL; Nystatin 100,000 units/mL: 30 mL	Combine all ingredients. Rinse mouth with 15 mL four to six times per day. Do not swallow.
Diphenhydramine (Benadryl), 12.5 mg/5 mL: 30 mL; Viscous lidocaine (Xylocaine) 2%: 30 mL; Maalox: 30 mL	Combine all ingredients. Rinse mouth with 15 mL four to six times per day. Do not swallow.
Diphenhydramine (Benadryl), 12.5 mg/5 mL: 30 mL; tetracycline 125 mg/5 mL suspension 60 mL; nystatin oral suspension, 100,000 units/mL 45 mL; viscous lidocaine (Xylocaine) 2%: 30 mL; hydrocortisone suspension, 10 mg/5 mL: 30 mL; sterile water for irrigation 45 mL	Combine all ingredients. Rinse mouth with 15 mL four to six times per day. Do not swallow.
Gelclair	Follow manufacturer's (Sinclair Pharma Ltd., Surrey, England, United Kingdom) instructions for mixing contents of a single-dose Gelclair packet with 40 mL or 3 tbsp of water. Stir mixture and use at once as a mouth rinse for at least 1 min, gargle, and spit out. Use at least three times per day.
Opioids	May use oral or parenteral opioids, such as patient-controlled analgesia. If oral analgesics are selected, use tablets. Do not use elixir, which has alcohol and will exacerbate stomatitis.
Viscous lidocaine (Xylocaine) 2% solution	Rinse mouth with 10 to 15 mL q2 to 3 h. Do not swallow.
Dyclonine hydrochloride 0.5% or 1% solution	Rinse mouth with 10 to 15 mL q2 to 3 h. Do not swallow.
XEROSTOMIA	
Xerolube, salivary substitute	Rinse mouth four to six times per day.
Salivart synthetic saliva spray	Spray mouth four to six times per day.
Biotene chewing gum	Use as needed.
Pilocarpine	5 mg p.o. three times a day.
Amifostine (Ethyol)	Use 200 mg/m^2 daily as a 3-min intravenous infusion 15 to 30 min before radiation therapy. Hydrate adequately, monitor blood pressure, and administer antiemetics.

Many of the medications listed have been used alone or in combination to treat stomatitis.
[a]NaCl = sodium chloride.
[b]NaHCO3 = sodium bicarbonate.
Adapted from Berger AM, Kilroy TJ. Oral complications. In: DeVita VT Jr, Hellman S, Rosenberg SA, eds. *Cancer: principles and practice of oncology*, 7th ed. Philadelphia, PA: Lippincott Williams & Wilkins, 2004.

allopurinol, vitamin E, beta-carotene, chamomile (Kamillosan) liquid, aspirin, antiprostaglandins, prostaglandins, MGI 209 (marketed as Oratect Gel), silver nitrate, and antibiotics. Oral and sometimes parenteral opioids are used to relieve stomatitis-related pain.

Direct Cytoprotectants

Sucralfate. Sucralfate, which is an aluminum salt of a sulfated disaccharide, has shown efficacy in the treatment of gastrointestinal (GI) ulceration, and has also been tested as a mouthwash for the prevention and treatment of stomatitis. Sucralfate creates a protective barrier at the ulcer site through the formation of an ionic bond to proteins. Additional evidence suggests an increase in the local production of prostaglandin E$_2$ (PGE$_2$) leading to an increase in mucosal blood flow, mucus production, mitotic activity, and surface migration of cells.

Study results with sulcrafate are conflicting. In 1984 and 1985, Ferraro and Mattern (38,39) reported encouraging results for the use of sucralfate for chemotherapy-induced stomatitis. Solomon (40) reported, from a sample of 19 patients receiving chemotherapy, a 55% objective response rate, defined as decrease in one grade on the Cancer and Leukemia Group B (CALGB) oral toxicity rating scale. Pfeiffer et al. (41) found a significant reduction in edema, erythema, erosion, and ulceration in 23 of 40 patients who could be evaluated, who received cisplatin and continuous infusion 5-FU, administered with or without bleomycin. Although not statistically significant, patient preference favored sucralfate. It was noted that 10 patients did not complete the study because swishing the sucralfate or placebo aggravated chemotherapy-induced nausea. The authors suggested that, to help overcome this problem, the solution should have a neutral taste and should not be swallowed. Results from a similarly designed study in a sample of patients receiving remission–induction chemotherapy for acute nonlymphocytic leukemia did not demonstrate sulcrafate efficacy for stomatitis (42). Additional results from this study showed that chronic administration of the sucralfate suspension had no effect on the incidence of GI bleeding and ulceration. However, some patients did report pain relief (42). A phase III study was conducted by the North Central Cancer Treatment Group (NCCTG) to compare sucralfate suspension versus placebo for 5-FU-related stomatitis. Results demonstrated that in the 50 patients who experienced stomatitis, not only did the sucralfate suspension provide no beneficial reduction in 5-FU-induced stomatitis severity or duration, but also that the sucralfate group had considerable additional GI toxicity (43). Additionally, no efficacy was demonstrated for a sucralfate mouthwash for prevention and treatment of 5-FU induced stomatitis in a randomized controlled clinical trial with 81 patients with colorectal cancer, who received either sucralfate suspension or placebo four times daily during their first cycle of chemotherapy with 5-FU and leucovorin (44).

Sucralfate has also been tested in the head and neck radiation therapy population. A prospective double-blind study compared the effectiveness of sucralfate suspension to a formulation of diphenhydramine hydrochloride syrup plus kaolin-pectin on radiotherapy-induced stomatitis. Data regarding pain, helpfulness of mouth rinses, weight change, and interruption of therapy were collected daily, and stomatitis grade was collected weekly. Results showed no statistically significant differences between the two groups. Results from a retrospective comparison with the preceding two groups that used a sample of 15 patients who had not used daily oral rinses, suggested that the use of a daily rinse with a mouth-coating agent may result in less pain, may reduce weight loss, and may help to prevent interruption of radiotherapy related to severe stomatitis (45).

In a study designed to compare outcomes in 21 patients who received standard oral care with 24 patients who received sucralfate suspension four times daily, the sucralfate group showed a significant difference in mucosal edema, pain, dysphagia, and weight loss (46). Results from a pilot study done by Pfeiffer et al. (47) using a sequential sample of patients who received radiotherapy to the head and neck and received sucralfate at the onset of stomatitis showed that most of the patients had decreased pain after sucralfate use. Conversely, a double-blind placebo-controlled study with sucralfate in 33 patients who received radiation therapy to the head and neck demonstrated no statistically significant differences in stomatitis (48). However, the sucralfate group did experience less oral pain and also required a later start of topical and systemic analgesics throughout radiation (48). Dodd, Miaskowski, Greenspan (49) used a pilot randomized controlled clinical trial to evaluate the efficacy of a micronized sucralfate mouth wash compared with a salt and soda mouthwash in 30 patients receiving radiation therapy. All patients also used the PRO-SELF: Mouth Aware Program (PSMA), which is a systematic oral hygiene program. Results demonstrated no significant difference in efficacy between the two groups.

Gelclair. Gelclair (Sinclair Pharmaceuticals, Surrey, England, United Kingdom) is a concentrated, bioadherent gel that has received U.S. Food and Drug Administration (FDA) approval as a 510(k) medical device indicated for the management of stomatitis-related oral pain. Gelclair adheres to the oral surface to create a protective barrier for irritated tissue and sensitized nociceptors. Two open-label, prospective trials evaluated the safety and efficacy of Gelclair in patients with oral inflammatory or ulcerative lesions. Innocenti (50) reported a 92% decrease in oral pain from baseline 5 to 7 hours after Gelclair administration in patients experiencing stomatitis, severe diffuse oral aphthous lesions, and post–oral surgery pain. More than half of these patients reported that the maximum effect of Gelclair lasted longer than 3 hours, and 87% of patients reported overall improvements from baseline for pain with swallowing food, liquids, and saliva following 1 week of treatment (50). From a clinical study that administered Gelclair to patients with stomatitis three times daily before meals as a 2 to 3 minute swish and spit for 3 to 10 days, DeCordi (51) reported significant improvements from baseline for pain, stomatitis severity, and function (51). There were no adverse effects reported during either trial, and patients reported that the taste, smell, texture, and ease of use of Gelclair were acceptable.

Prostaglandins, antiprostaglandins, and nonsteroidal agents. Prostaglandins are a family of naturally occurring eicosanoids, some of which have demonstrated cytoprotective activity. Topical Dinoprostone was administered in a nonblinded study four times daily to 10 patients who were receiving 5-FU and mitomycin with concomitant radiation therapy for oral carcinomas (52). The control group used 14 patients who were receiving identical treatment. Results showed that in 8 of the 10 patients who could be evaluated and who received Dinoprostone, no patient developed severe stomatitis as compared with 6 episodes in the control group. A second pilot study that was conducted with 15 patients who received radiation therapy to the head and neck demonstrated that an inflammatory reaction was detected in only 5 patients in the vicinity of their tumor when treated with topically applied PGE_2, and that no patients developed bullous or desquamating inflammatory lesions (53). A double-blind, placebo-controlled study of PGE_2 in 60 patients undergoing BMT revealed no significant differences in the incidence, severity, or duration of stomatitis. It was noted that the incidence of herpes simplex virus was higher in those on the PGE_2 arm, and that among those patients who developed herpes simplex virus, there was an increase in stomatitis severity (54).

Benzydamine is a nonsteroidal anti-inflammatory drug with reported analgesic, anesthetic, anti-inflammatory, and antimicrobial properties. Epstein and Stevenson-Moore (55) reported in a double-blind, placebo-controlled trial, that benzydamine produced statistically significant relief of pain from radiation-induced stomatitis. Positive responses to benzydamine have been reported in at least two other studies (56,57). Epstein and Stevenson-Moore (55) reported not only a trend toward reduction in pain, but also a statistically significant reduction in both the total area and the size of ulceration. Another study demonstrated that oral indomethacin, an antiprostaglandin, reduced severity of and delayed onset of radiation therapy–related stomatitis (58).

Corticosteroids. No placebo-controlled studies testing the efficacy of corticosteroids for chemotherapy-induced stomatitis have been reported, although two reports have presented pilot work conducted with patients who received radiation therapy. Abdelaal (59) reported the use of a betamethasone and water mouthwash in five patients receiving radiotherapy, whose mucosa remained virtually ulcer free and who did not report any pain. The proposed mechanism of action of the steroid mouthwash was inhibition of leukotriene and prostaglandin production. Another pilot study compared 21 patients receiving radiotherapy, who used an oral rinse consisting of hydrocortisone in combination with nystatin, tetracycline, and diphenhydramine hydrochloride, with patients using a placebo rinse. Although only 12 of the 21 patients could be evaluated by the end of the radiation therapy cycles, there was a statistically significant difference in stomatitis severity as well as a trend toward pain reduction. No patients in the treatment group needed to interrupt the radiation therapy regime, as compared with three patients in the control group (60).

Vitamins and other antioxidants. Vitamin E has been tested in chemotherapy-induced stomatitis because it can stabilize cellular membranes and may improve herpetic gingivitis, possibly through antioxidant activity. Wadleigh et al. (61) demonstrated the efficacy of vitamin E in 18 chemotherapy patients who were randomized to receive topical vitamin E or placebo. Statistically significant results showed that in the vitamin E group, six of nine patients had complete stomatitis resolution within 4 days of initiating therapy, as compared with the placebo group, in which only one of nine had stomatitis resolution during the 5-day study period (61).

Other antioxidants that have been tested for efficacy with stomatitis include vitamin C and glutathione. Azelastine hydrochloride has shown efficacy in the treatment of aphthous ulcers in Behçet's disease. Osaki et al. (62) reported findings from a study with a sample of 63 patients with head and neck cancer who were treated with chemoradiation. Twenty-six patients received regimen 1 (vitamins C and E and glutathione) and 37 patients received regimen 2 (regimen 1 plus azelastine). Study findings showed that in the azelastine group, 21 patients remained at grade 1 or 2 stomatitis, 6 patients had grade 3 stomatitis, and 10 patients had grade 4 stomatitis. In comparison with these findings, in the control group, grade 3 or 4 stomatitis was observed in over half of the subjects. Azelastine suppressed neutrophil respiratory burst both *in vivo* and *in vitro*, and also showed cytokine release suppression from lymphocytes. The study results led the authors to conclude that azelastine, which suppresses reactive oxygen production and stabilizes cell membranes, may be useful to prevent chemoradiation-induced stomatitis (62).

Beta-carotene, which is a vitamin A precursor with known effects on cellular differentiation and has been used for radiation therapy-related stomatitis, also produces regression of oral leukoplakia lesions (63). Mills (64) reported on the use of beta-carotene in treatment-induced stomatitis. Ten patients receiving radiation interspersed with two cycles of chemotherapy were given beta-carotene 250 mg per day for the first 3 weeks of therapy, and then 75 mg per day for the last 5 weeks of therapy. The control group consisted of 10 patients with oral cancer who were receiving identical treatment, but without the beta-carotene. At the end of treatment, there was a statistically significant difference in grade 3 to 4 mucositis in the beta-carotene group; there was no difference in grades 1 and 2 mucositis (64).

Silver nitrate. Silver nitrate, which is a caustic agent, has been tested for radiation therapy–induced stomatitis. Also, because silver nitrate stimulates cell division when applied to normal mucosa, it has potential as a preventive agent for chemotherapy-induced stomatitis. Maciejewski et al. (65) described the use of silver nitrate for patients receiving radiation therapy. Silver nitrate 2% was applied to the left side of the oral mucosa three times daily for 5 days before and during the first 2 days of radiation therapy in 16 patients who received treatment to bilateral opposing fields. The right side of the oral mucosa served as the control. Significantly less severe stomatitis with shorter duration was seen in the silver nitrate group (65). However, a second trial failed to confirm these results (66), indicating that silver nitrate needs further evaluation for chemotherapy-induced stomatitis.

Cryotherapy. Cryotherapy, which is administered in the form of ice chips and flavored ice pops, has been used to prevent stomatitis. Efficacy of cryotherapy for the reduction of 5-FU-induced stomatitis severity was demonstrated from a NCCTG and Mayo Clinic–sponsored controlled randomized trial (67). A subsequent study, with a sample of 178 patients who could be evaluated and who were randomized to receive 30 minutes versus 60 minutes of oral cryotherapy, reported similar degrees of stomatitis in both groups (68). The study recommended the use of 30 minutes of oral cryotherapy preintensitve bolus 5-FU–based chemotherapy. An additional study conducted by the NCCTG and the Mayo Clinic confirmed that oral cryotherapy can reduce 5-FU-induced stomatitis (69). Cryotherapy used to induce vasoconstriction should be considered for patients receiving 5-FU or melphalan when these agents are administered over short infusion times.

Laser. The efficacy of laser treatment for oral lesion and pain control was studied initially in an animal model. One study used four groups of animals with a mucosal lesion, three of which received impulse laser exposure from 60 to 600 pulses, and one of which was untreated (70). Only the group that received 600 pulsed exposures demonstrated more rapid resolution of the mucosal lesion (14 versus 21 to 25 days). A preliminary study was conducted in a sample of 36 patients with diverse cancers and chemotherapy regimens; 16 patients were treated with laser and 20 patients served as controls (71). Results showed reduced stomatitis duration from a mean of 19.3 days in the control arm to 8.1 days in the treatment arm (71). The efficacy of low-energy He/Ne laser (LEL) was studied in a sample of 30 patients through a randomized controlled clinical trial (72). LEL was reported to reduce the severity and duration of stomatitis in this population (72). Laser efficacy for stomatitis needs further testing in the randomized controlled clinical trial setting.

Miscellaneous agents. A descriptive study reported in a sample of 98 patients with diverse malignancies who were treated with either chemotherapy or radiation therapy that Kamillosan liquid taken before and after the onset of stomatitis helped to prevent and decrease the duration of stomatitis (73). The NCCTG conducted a placebo-controlled trial in which patients were randomized to receive chamomile or placebo in addition to an established oral cryotherapy regimen (74). Results from this study demonstrated that the chamomile mouthwash did not reduce 5-FU–associated stomatitis (74).

A phase III study of topical AES-14, which is a novel drug system designed to concentrate delivery of L-glutamine to oral mucosa for ulceration treatment, was conducted with 121 patients at risk for stomatitis (75). Subjects were randomized to either AES-14 or placebo and received protocol treatment from day 1 of chemotherapy up to 2 weeks following the last chemotherapy dose or stomatitis resolution. Results suggested a potential 20% reduction of moderate to severe stomatitis in the AES-14 group, and a 10% increase in grade 0 stomatitis. Oshitani et al. (76) conducted a study regarding the use of topical sodium alginate, which is an agent that has been shown to promote healing of radiation therapy–induced mucositis in esophageal and gastric mucosa. Thirty-nine subjects, who were experiencing stomatitis, were randomized to receive either sodium alginate or placebo. The subjects who received sodium alginate had a reduction in both mucosal erosions and pain (76). Other topical agents used clinically for treatment-induced stomatitis include Kaopectate, diphenhydramine hydrochloride (Benadryl), saline, sodium bicarbonate, and gentian violet. These agents now need to be tested in the clinical trial setting.

Indirect Cytoprotectants

Hematopoietic growth factors. Hematologic growth factors are currently the standard treatment for patients who are treated with high-dose chemotherapy because they have demonstrated well-established efficacy to decrease the duration of chemotherapy-induced neutropenia. Effects of various growth factors such as granulocyte-macrophage colony-stimulating factor (GM-CSF), granulocyte-colony-stimulating factor (G-CSF), epidermal growth factor (EGF), and transforming growth factor (TGF), as well as cytokines such as interleukin 11 (IL-11) in the development and severity of stomatitis have been evaluated in the animal cheek pouch model using Syrian Golden hamsters. Results from these studies have shown increased severity of mucosal damage in animals receiving 5-FU and EGF (77), and in those animals who received TGF-β after chemotherapy, outcomes of decreased incidence, severity, and duration of stomatitis, decreased weight loss, and increased survival were reported (78). *In vitro* studies have demonstrated that EGF is present in saliva, and has the ability to affect growth, cell and migration, and repair mechanisms (59). The development of increased oral toxicity or mucosal repair may be dependent on the timing of EGF administration in relation to chemotherapy (79). Sonis et al. (80) administered EGF or placebo to hamsters in four different treatment schedule settings, and reported that although EGF delayed the stomatitis onset, it showed no beneficial effects regarding stomatitis duration or severity. CSF has been tested as a treatment for stomatitis in numerous studies. Gabrilove et al. (81) reported from a sample of 27 patients with bladder cancer, who received escalating doses of G-CSF during treatment with methotrexate, vinblastine, doxorubicin, and cisplatin. The patients received G-CSF only during the first of two cycles of chemotherapy. Although significantly less stomatitis was seen during the first cycle with G-CSF, a limitation of this study is that positive results may be biased because of possible cumulative chemotherapeutic toxicity with resultant increase in stomatitis severity. Conversely, Bronchud et al. (82) reported from a study of 17 patients with breast or ovarian carcinoma treated with escalating doses of doxorubicin with G-CSF, that G-CSF did not prevent severe stomatitis. A third study was conducted comparing clinical outcomes in a sample of 55 adult patients who received chemotherapy for non-Hodgkin's lymphoma and G-CSF with clinical outcomes in 39 patients who received chemotherapy alone. In those patients who did not receive G-CSF, neutropenia was the primary cause of treatment delay, as compared to stomatitis as the main cause of treatment delay in those patients who received G-CSF (83).

GM-CSF has demonstrated conflicting results in patients receiving diverse cancer treatment modalities. Saarilahlti (84) reported a trend for less severe stomatitis in the GM-CSF group from a randomized controlled clinical trial comparing GM-CSF mouthwashes with sucralfate mouthwashes in a sample of 40 postoperative radiation therapy patients. Conversely, prophylactic use of GM-CSF mouthwash in a randomized trial using a sample of 90 patients undergoing high-dose chemotherapy and autologous PBSCT did not show a reduction of frequency and duration of severe stomatitis (85). The use of CSFs in the treatment of stomatitis remains investigational.

TGF-β3 inhibits epithelial cell growth, and has been studied in the animal model. Sonis et al. (69) conducted a study using Syrian hamsters that demonstrated that topical application of TGF-β3 resulted in a decrease in chemotherapy-related stomatitis severity and duration. Foncuberta et al. (86) reported from two phase II randomized controlled clinical trials evaluating TGF-β3 that TGF-β3 was not effective in the prevention or alleviation of chemotherapy-related stomatitis. The trials used a mouthwash formulation of 10 mL (25 μg per mL) or placebo formulation administered four times daily (or twice daily) in samples of patients with lymphomas or solid tumors. However, IL-1 and IL-11 have demonstrated a cytoprotective effect (87,88)

Keratinocyte growth factors. Recently, palifermin, which is a recombinant human keratinocyte growth factor, has shown efficacy in the reduction of oral mucosal injury induced by cytotoxic therapy (89). Speilberger, Stiff, Bensinger et al. (89) reported from a double-blind study that compared the effect of palifermin with a placebo for the development of stomatitis in 212 subjects with hematologic cancers. Palifermin or placebo was administered intravenously for 3 consecutive days immediately before initiating conditioning therapy using fractionated total body radiation plus high-dose chemotherapy. As compared with placebo, the palifermin group experienced significant reductions in grade 4 stomatitis, soreness of the mouth and throat, use of opioid analgesics, and the incidence of total parenteral nutrition use.

Antimicrobials. Antimicrobials have included systemic antimicrobials, such as antibiotics, antivirals (acyclovir, valcyclovir, ganciclovir), and the antifungal agent, fluconazole. Donnelly, Bellm, Epstein et al. (90) evaluated the evidence regarding the role of infection in the pathophysiology of stomatitis through a comprehensive review of 31 prospective randomized trials. Conclusions from the review indicated that there was no clear pattern of patient type, cancer treatment, or type of antimicrobial agent used, and also that there is a lack of consistent stomatitis assessment.

Oral candidiasis is a common acute and chronic oral sequela of head and neck radiation therapy. These lesions may present as removable (whitish) chronic or hyperplastic (nonremovable), and chronic erythematous (diffused as patchy erythema), and frequently appear as angular cheilitis (first signs or symptoms). Treatment approaches for oral candidiases include mycostatin (troches), nystatin (liquid or ointment), or clotrimazole. Pseudomembranous candidiasis is successfully treated topically. Chronic candidiases usually require much longer treatment and it may be necessary to use oral ketoconazole, fluconazole, or intravenous amphotericin B.

Conflicting reports have been published regarding the use of chlorhexidine mouthwash both for alleviating stomatitis and reducing oral colonization by gram-positive, gram-negative, and Candida species in patients receiving chemotherapy, radiation therapy, or BMT. Most of the studies have not demonstrated the efficacy of chlorhexixdine mouthwash in stomatitis reduction in patients receiving intensive chemotherapy (91). Dodd, Larson, Dibble et al. (92) tested the efficacy of the PSMA program when combined with randomization to one of two mouthwashes (0.12% chlorhexidine or sterile water) for the prevention of chemotherapy-related stomatitis in 222 patients. Although chlorhexidine was found to be no more effective than water regarding stomatitis incidence, days to onset, and severity, the PSMA program appeared to reduce stomatitis incidence (92). Weisdorf et al. (93) and Epstein et al. (94) reported results from studies designed to evaluate the efficacy of chlorhexidine mouth rinse and chlorhexidine and nystatin mouth rinses, respectively, and reported a reduction in oral colonization by Candida species and oral candidiasis. Acyclovir prophylaxis is the currently accepted treatment for HSV and cytomegalovirus (CMV) seropositive BMT patients. A randomized controlled clinical trial conducted in BMT patients compared fluconazole to placebo and reported that fluconazole prevented systemic fungal infections (7% fluconazole vs. 18% placebo) and significantly reduced the incidence of mucosal infection and oropharyngeal colonization by *Candida albicans* (95).

Sutherland and Browman (96) reviewed 59 studies assessing prophylaxis of radiation therapy–induced stomatitis in head and neck cancer patients and reported that interventions chosen on the basis of the biological etiology of stomatitis are effective. A study by Spijkervet et al. (97) evaluated the efficacy of lozenges containing polymyxin E_2 2 mg, tobramycin 1.8 mg, and amphotericin B, 10 mg (PTA) taken four times daily for the oropharyngeal flora related to stomatitis. These researchers compared 15 patients receiving radiation therapy using PTA and two other groups of 15 patients each, one of which was using 0.1% chlorhexidine and the other placebo. Results showed that the selectively decontaminated group had significantly reduced severity and extent of stomatitis as compared with the chlorhexidine and placebo groups. Conversely, Stokman and colleagues (98) analyzed the effects of selective oral flora elimination on radiation-related stomatitis in a randomized controlled clinical trial in 65 patients with head and neck tumors with randomization to either a lozenge of polymyxin E2 1 g, tobramycin 1.8 mg, and amphotericin B 13 mg or placebo. Results showed that selective oral flora elimination in head and neck radiated patients did not prevent the development of severe stomatitis.

IB-367, which is a broad-spectrum antimicrobial peptide found in porcine leukocytes, was tested in a hamster model (99). The results indicated that stomatitis scores were significantly lower in hamsters given topical IB-367, as compared with those animals which received the placebo. Although further study is needed, IB-367 might improve clinical outcomes in patients at risk for the stomatitis development (99). A Nystatin suspension has been studied in the prophylaxis of candidiasis in leukemia and BMT patients. Most of the publications do not support the use of nystatin (94,100–106).

Pharmacologic Modulation

Allopurinol mouthwash has been evaluated for the prevention and treatment of 5-FU–related stomatitis because allopurinol inhibits the enzyme orotidylate decarboxylase and formation of the metabolites of fluorodeoxyuridine monophosphate (FdUMP) and fluorouridine (FUrd) (107). Clark and Selvin (108) demonstrated in a pilot study that an allopurinol mouthwash substantially decreased the incidence and severity of stomatitis in six patients who had received bolus 5-FU. Another pilot study conducted with a sample of 16 patients receiving 5-day 5-FU infusions and using allopurinol mouthwashes four to six times daily also reported that the allopurinol alleviated stomatitis in all patients (109). These positive results have led to allopurinol becoming routine practice in many institutions. However, it is important to note that no protective effect of allopurinol against 5-FU–induced stomatitis was seen in a randomized, double-blind clinical trial conducted by the NCCTG and the Mayo Clinic (110). The study sample consisted of 75 patients who were assigned to either allopurinol mouthwash or placebo during their first 5-day course of 5-FU administered with or without leucovorin (110).

Uridine has been reported to protect host tissues selectively from 5-FU's toxic effects, and importantly without loss of antitumor effect. A study of the efficacy of uridine with regard to stomatitis was conducted in a sample of 29 patients with advanced malignancies who received N-phosphoracetyl-disodium l-aspartic acid (PALA) and methotrexate, each at doses of 250 mg per m^2, and followed at 24 hours by increasing doses of 5-FU (600 to 750 mg per m^2), with both a leucovorin rescue and a uridine rescue for a 72-hour infusion (111). Use of uridine allowed dose escalation of 5-FU to 750 mg per m^2, and a decrease in all 5-FU–related toxicities except stomatitis, and that was the only significant chemotherapy-induced toxicity (111).

The effectiveness of propantheline, which is an anticholinergic agent that causes xerostomia, versus placebo to reduce stomatitis related to etoposide was tested in a pilot study involving 12 patients (112). The hypothesis of the study was that the mucosal toxicity might be related to salivary excretion of etoposide after systemic administration. Results showed a decrease in stomatitis incidence and severity in the propantheline group (112).

Leucovorin calcium has been used in combination with methotrexate to help decrease stomatitis. In a pilot study involving 19 patients with non–small cell lung carcinoma who received edatrexate, less stomatitis was observed than was predicted (113). Decreased stomatitis was observed when reduced folates were given systemically following methotrexate administration (114). However, administration of leucovorin calcium-hyaluronidase mouthwashes in a small crossover study did not reduce the severity of stomatitis induced by high-dose methotrexate (115). Glutamine administration in

animal studies has been shown to lead to a reduction in both morbidity and mortality in the chemotherapy setting, including methotrexate. Glutamine has been reported to preserve the morphologic structure of the GI tract and also to reduce the incidence of bacteremia (116,117). A randomized trial was conducted in 28 patients with GI cancers who received 5-FU and folinic acid, and either 16 g glutamine daily for 8 days or placebo. The authors stated that perhaps both the dose and duration of exposure to the glutamine were insufficient to lead to a decrease in stomatitis (118).

Exercises for Radiation Therapy–Induced Complications

Radiation therapy–induced fibrosis of the masticatory muscles and/or the temporal mandibular joint may be prevented or attenuated through early exercises with trismus appliances post-therapy. Fibrosis of the masticatory muscles may occur up to 1 year postradiation and therefore, jaw-opening exercises should start after oral mucosal healing, and continue for more than 1 year following radiation therapy. Effective exercises in reducing trismus include the use of tongue depressors taped together 10 to 15 times a day for 10-minute sets.

Anti-inflammatory Agents for Oral cGVHD

Almost all patients with extensive cGVHD require systemic immunosuppressive therapy. Therefore, there is a critical need for adjuvant therapies that are both efficacious and avoid the long-term consequences of the corticosteroid therapies. In general, advances in the treatment of cGVHD have been modest. No standard therapy exists for cGVHD that fails to respond to initial therapy or recurs. Patients with symptomatic disease that is limited to the oral cavity have been found to benefit from topical steroids such as dexamethasone (Decadron) elixir (0.5 mg per 5 mL). Decadron elixir has shown efficacy when used as a mouth rinse (10 mL) for 2 to 3 minutes at least four times per day (15). Topical steroids such as Lidex (Syntex, Palo Alto, CA) have also been tried. If local steroids alone are not adequate to control oral disease, then cyclosporine mouth rinses may be tried (15). Even isolated stomatitis may necessitate the use of systemic immunosuppressive therapy. Intraoral psoralen plus ultraviolet A irradiation (PUVA) may be required depending on the patient's condition (15). Clobetasol (Temovate) 0.05%, which is a topical high potency steroid, has been administered three times a day for 2 to 3 weeks depending on the severity of the ulcerative oral cGVHD to decrease inflammation and oral pain. However, these treatments need evaluation in a randomized controlled clinical trial setting.

Treatment Strategies for Osteonecrosis

Traditional treatment of ORN has included antibiotics and surgical debridement and curettage. However, these treatments are not always successful. Recent literature supports the use of hyperbaric oxygen to boost tissue oxygenation in damaged irradiated wounds for anticipated difficult extractions and for patients with radiographic interpretation of trabecular bony pattern avascularity and telangiectasia that covers mucous membranes or gingiva (119). Use of hyperbaric oxygen as an adjunctive treatment needs further evaluation in the randomized controlled clinical trial setting.

Osteonecrosis of the jaw related to bisphosphonate therapy may be refractory to conservative debridement and antibiotic therapy. Patients with this condition may require surgical procedures to remove the involved bone. Practitioners should monitor patients who are receiving bisphosphonate therapy because an early diagnosis may prevent or reduce the morbidity resulting from advanced destructive lesions of the jaw bone

(17). Complete prevention of this complication is not possible. However pretherapy dental care reduces the incidence, and nonsurgical dental procedures are able to prevent new cases (120).

SYMPTOM MANAGEMENT

Oropharyngeal Pain

Stomatitis is the principal etiology of most pain experienced during the 3-week post-BMT period. This pain is often described as the most unforgettable ordeal of BMT. Stomatitis-related oropharyngeal pain is a multidimensional entity. The sensory dimension of stomatitis-related pain has been described with general mucosal inflammation and breakdown as ranging from mild discomfort to severe and debilitating pain requiring opioids for pain management (27). Immunocompromised patients who have developed cancer and are also HIV positive develop larger, more painful lesions than those experienced by noncancer patients. Oral pain associated with cGVHD has been described as severe with reported symptoms of burning, irritation, dryness, and loss of taste. In contrast to the often long lasting oral pain accompanying oral cGVHD, stomatitis-related oral pain in the chemotherapy setting is of usually less than 3 months' duration. The affective dimension of the oral stomatitis pain experience is seen through the effect on the patient's psychological well-being. Alterations in communication, decreased oral intake, and medication usage are viewed as part of the behavioral dimension. The cognitive dimension of pain refers to how this pain influences the patient's thought processes, self-perception, stated pain relief, and the personal meaning of the pain (121). The sociocultural dimension encompasses demographic characteristics, personal, family and work roles, cultural backgrounds, and caregiver perspectives (121). Gender differences have been reported for pain, for example, female subjects in a pilot study testing capsaicin efficacy for stomatitis related pain reported a higher level of pain (122).

Anesthetic Cocktails

Although anesthetic cocktails, composed of agents such as viscous lidocaine (Xylocaine) or dyclonine hydrochloride have been used with some success, these agents provide only temporary pain relief. Also, these agents may alter taste perception that may decrease oral intake. Anesthetic agents provide only temporary pain relief, and alter taste perception that may decrease oral intake. Other analgesics and mucosal coating agents used for pain control include kaolin-pectin, diphenhydramine, Orabase, and Oratect Gel. A prospective, double-blinded study involving 18 patients was designed to compare the efficacy of viscous lidocaine with cocaine 1%, dyclonine hydrochloride 1%, kaolin-pectin solution, diphenhydramine, and saline solution versus placebo for oral pain (123). Dyclonine hydrochloride 1% provided the greatest pain relief, and dyclonine hydrochloride with viscous lidocaine and cocaine 1% provided the longest duration of pain relief (124).

Hospital-based pharmacies commonly formulate and dispense topical mixtures containing an analgesic, an anti-inflammatory agent, and a coating agent for use as an oral comfort measure for patients undergoing cancer treatment. A large clinical research center uses a topical formulation that contains lidocaine viscous 2% (40 mL), diphenhydramine 12.5 mg per 5 mL (40 mL), and Maalox 10 mg (40 mL) and prescribes its use every 3 to 4 hours as needed. Testing these various topical formulations through randomized controlled clinical trials is needed to promote evidence-based practice regarding these treatment recommendations.

Opioids

Severe stomatitis-related oropharyngeal pain may interfere with hydration and nutritional intake and affect quality of life. Management of this severe oropharyngeal pain may require the use of opioids, often administered at high doses by patient-controlled analgesia pumps. Other routes of administration are oral, transmucosal, and parenteral. Topical opioids (morphine 0.08% gel, prepared with taste supplements) were reported in treating stomatitis-related oral pain in a terminally ill patient (125). The efficacy of oral transmucosal fentanyl citrate (Actiq) was compared with morphine sulfate immediate release in a randomized controlled clinical trial for the treatment of breakthrough cancer pain in 134 adult ambulatory cancer patients (126). Study results showed that oral transmucosal fentanyl was more effective than morphine sulfate immediate release in treating breakthrough pain. The efficacy of topical morphine for stomatitis-related pain was evaluated in a sample of 26 patients following chemoradiation for head and neck cancer (127). Subjects were randomized to morphine mouthwash (1 mL 2% morphine solution) or magic mouthwash (equal parts of lodocaine, diphenhydramine, and magnesium aluminum hydroxide). Patients in the morphine group had both significantly shorter duration and lower intensity of oral pain than the magic mouthwash group. Many oncology treatments are now administered in the ambulatory setting necessitating increased use of both patient self-care activities and involvement of patient caregivers in patient pain management plans. Swisher, Scheidler, and Kennedy (128) described a stomatitis pain management algorithm to promote symptom management for the BMT patient who is transitioning from inpatient to ambulatory care. A key component of this successful program was the availability of a multidisciplinary team who could respond to the patients' self-report of oral pain.

When stomatitis-related oral pain is severe and interferes with nutritional intake and quality of life, it is appropriate to use any of the previously cited treatments, as well as oral, transmucosal, or if necessary, parenteral narcotics. Although many of the agents previously mentioned may have some value in palliating the pain, very few controlled clinical trials have established their efficacy. At present, no standard treatment has been defined for the prevention or treatment of stomatitis-related oral pain, and therefore it is essential to continue studies of the treatments already available and to develop any promising new approaches.

Capsaicin

Capsaicin, which is the active ingredient in chili peppers, has been used for diverse pain syndromes, and may have efficacy for cancer treatment–related stomatitis (122). Several studies have presented the efficacy of locally applied capsaicin in a cream vehicle for neuropathic pain syndromes including postherpetic neuralgia and diabetic neuropathy, postmastectomy pain, stump pain, trigeminal neuralgia, reflex sympathetic dystrophy, and Guillain-Barré syndrome. Topical capsaicin is useful as an analgesic for the pain associated with rheumatoid arthritis and osteoarthritis. Intranasal capsaicin spray has shown efficacy for the treatment of pain related to cluster headaches. Capsaicin was tested in a phase I study with chemotherapy and radiation therapy patients (122). The capsaicin was delivered in a taffy candy vehicle (cayenne pepper candy), which the subjects were instructed to let dissolve in their mouths without chewing. After the candy had dissolved, the burn produced by the candy was allowed to fade. The patients rated their pain before and after eating the candy. Partial and temporary pain reduction was reported in 11 patients with stomatitis (122). The patients rated their pain before and after eating the candy. The reduction in pain was statistically very significant. Clinical significance needs to be examined in future research.

Xerostomia

Xerostomia is a major negative sequela for patients who receive radiation therapy to the head and neck. The severity of xerostomia is dependent on the radiation dosage, location, and volume of exposed salivary glands. However, significant xerostomia has not been shown as a sequela in patients treated with chemotherapy alone. The degree of xerostomia is usually reported subjectively by both patients and clinicians, and can affect oral comfort, fit of prostheses, speech, and swallowing. This decrease in quantity and quality of saliva can be devastating to the dentition through the formation of caries. Many of the enzymes (mucin) found in patients who experience xerostomia contribute to the growth of caries-producing organisms. Oral hygiene regimens that include the use of water/saline and daily fluoride application along with brushing teeth at least three times daily may reduce colonization and proliferation of oral pathogens.

Sialogogues have been investigated as stimulants for residual salivary parenchyma (pilocarpine, 5 and 10 mg doses) and subjective improvement has been reported in some patients. Extreme caution with the use of pilocarpine is warranted because of reported side effects of glaucoma and cardiac problems. A randomized controlled trial tested the efficacy of amifostine in a sample of 315 patients with head and neck cancer. The subjects received standard fractionated radiation with or without amifostine (Ethyol), administered at 200 mg per m^2 as a 3-minute IV infusion 15 to 30 minutes before each fraction of radiation (129). Patient eligibility criteria included that the radiation field encompassed at least 75% of both parotid glands. The Radiation Therapy Oncology Group acute and late morbidity score and criteria were used to rate the severity of xerostomia. The incidence of grade 2 or higher acute xerostomia (90 days from the start of radiotherapy) and late xerostomia (9 to 12 months after radiotherapy) was significantly reduced in patients receiving Ethyol. Whole saliva collection 1 year following radiation therapy showed that in the Ethyol group, more subjects produced 0.1 g of saliva (72 versus 49%), and that the median saliva production was greater (0.26 g versus 0.1 g). Stimulated saliva collections showed no difference between the treatment groups. Supporting these improvements in saliva production were the patient's reports of oral dryness (129). Artificial saliva, which usually uses carboxymethylcellulose as a base, has not demonstrated increased oral cavity comfort. Patients have reported subjective improvement in comfort levels through the frequent use of sugarless gum and hard candy. The patient should be encouraged to stop or reduce the use of tobacco and alcohol.

FUTURE RESEARCH DIRECTIONS

Two underlying principles of oral complications in cancer treatment research are that the human model is the most appropriate for clinical research, and that the etiology, progression, and resolution of stomatitis have a multifactorial nature (130). The importance of the transgeneic and gene-targeted murine model to elucidate mechanisms of mucosal injury is also appreciated (130). Synergizing the expertise of clinical researchers and basic scientists promotes formulation of novel hypotheses regarding the contributions of inflammation, sustained cytokine dysregulation, tissue injury and repair mechanisms to the pathogenesis of oral complications.

Evaluation of the efficacy and mechanisms of systemic and topical pharmacologic agents for prevention and treatment of oral complications through experimental designs is needed, and should include pediatric, geriatric, and diverse ethnic populations. Exploration of the optimal dose and timing of interventions for stomatitis and related oropharyngeal pain is needed. Clinically meaningful outcomes for the evaluation of new stomatitis treatments include oropharyngeal pain, need for opioid analgesics, inability to eat soft food, diminished quality of life, and functional status, increased length of hospital stay, and inability to take medication orally (131). Continued psychometric testing of oral cavity assessment tools is also needed. Exploration of the interrelationships among the multiple dimensions of stomatitis-related oral pain at rest and with movement may increase our understanding of this complex phenomenon. Combining quantitative and qualitative research designs to study the complex symptomatology related to oral complications may yield rich results. Outcomes of these research directions include application of the best evidence at the individual patient care level.

CONCLUSION

Oral complications of cancer treatment remain biologically complex and often challenging to treat, and lead to a cascade of negative sequelae. Vital outcomes of oncology treatments that are designed to examine the effect of dose-intensive treatments on clinical and survival outcomes may be compromised when dose reduction or treatment cessation is necessary because of treatment-related oral complications. Although there exist numerous recommendations for prevention and treatment of oral complications and related negative sequelae, there remains a critical need to evaluate these interventions in the randomized controlled clinical trial setting using valid and reliable stomatitis assessment tools to advance the science of oral mucosal toxicities and thereby improve patient care. This clinical research work requires a multidisciplinary team dedicated to both testing innovative treatment approaches, and implementing appropriate findings through evidence-based practice.

References

1. National Institutes of Health Consensus Development Panel. Consensus statement: oral complications of cancer therapies. *Natl Cancer Inst Monogr* 1989;9:3–8.
2. Sonis ST. Oral complications of cancer therapy. In: DeVita VT, Hellman S, Rosenberg SA, eds. *Cancer: principles and practice of oncology*, 4th ed. Philadelphia, PA: JB Lippincott Co, 1993:2389.
3. Sonis ST. Mucositis as a biological process: a new hypothesis for the development of chemotherapy-induced stomatoxicity. *Oral Oncol* 1998;34:39–43.
4. Woo S-B, Sonis ST, Monopoli MM, et al. A longitudinal study of oral ulcerative mucositis in bone marrow transplant recipients. *Cancer* 1993;72:1612–1617.
5. Shih A, Miaskowshi C, Dodd MJ, et al. Mechanisms for radiation-induced oral mucositis and the consequences. *Cancer Nurs* 2003;26:222–229.
6. Hyland SA. Assessing the oral cavity. In: Frank-Stromborg M, Olsen SJ, eds. *Instruments for clinical health-care research*, London: Jones and Bartlett Publishers International, 1997:519–527.
7. Sonis ST. The pathobiology of mucositis. *Nat Rev Cancer* 2004;4:277–284.
8. Driezen S. Description and incidence of oral complications. *Natl Cancer Inst Monogr* 1990;9:11–15.
9. Dodd MJ, Miaskowski C, Shiba GH, et al. Risk factors for chemotherapy-induced oral mucositis: dental appliances, oral hygiene, previous oral lesion, and a history of smoking. *Cancer Invest* 1999;17(4):278.
10. Barasch A, Peterson DE. Risk factors for ulcerative mucositis in cancer patients: unanswered questions. *Oral Oncol* 2003;39:91–100.

11. Vissink A, Jansma J, Spijkervet FKL, et al. Oral sequelae of head and neck radiotherapy. *Crit Rev Oral Biol Med* 2003;14:199–212.

12. Lazarus HM, Vogelsang GB, Rowe JM. Prevention and treatment of acute graft-versus-host disease: the old and the new. A report from the Eastern Cooperative Oncology Group (ECOG). *Bone Marrow Transplant* 1997;19:577–600.

13. Mitchell SA. Graft versus host disease. In: Ezzone S, ed. *Peripheral blood stem cell transplantation: recommendations for nursing education and practice.* Pittsburgh, PA: Oncology Nursing Society, 2004:85–131.

14. Lloid ME. Oral medicine concerns of the BMT patient. In: Buchsel PC, Whedon MB, eds. *Bone marrow transplantation administrative and clinical strategies*, Boston, MA: Jones and Bartlett Publishers, 1995:257–281.

15. Vogelsang GB. How I treat chronic graft-versus-host-disease. *Blood* 2001;97:1196–1201.

16. Merigo E, Manfredi M, Meleti M, et al. Jaw bone necrosis without previous dental extractions associated with the use of bisphosphonates (pamidronate and zoledronate): a four-case report. *J Oral Pathol Med* 2005;34:613–617.

17. Ruggiero SL, Mehrotra B, Rosenberg TJ, et al. Osteonecrosis of the jaws associated with the use of bisphosphonates: a review of 63 cases. *J Oral Maxillofac Surg* 2004;62:527–534.

18. Berger AM, Kilroy TJ. Oral complications. In: DeVita VT, Hellman S, Rosenberg SA, eds. *Cancer: principles and practice of oncology*, 6th ed. Philadelphia, PA: Lippincott-Raven, 1997:2714–2725.

19. Beumer J. Radiation therapy of the oral cavity, sequelae and management. Part I. *Head Neck Surg* 1979;1:303–306.

20. Beumer J, Curtis T, Morris LR. Radiation complications in edentulous patients. *J Prosthet Dent* 1976;36:193.

21. Schweiger JW. Oral complications following radiation therapy: a five year retrospective report. *J Prosthet Dent* 1987;58:78–82.

22. Beumer J, Harrison R, Sanders B, et al. Pre-radiation dental extractions and the incidence of bone necrosis. *Head Neck Surg* 1983;5:514–521.

23. Beumer J, Zlotow I, Curtis T. Rehabilitation. In: Silverman S, ed. *Oral Cancer*, New York: American Cancer Society, 1990.

24. US Department of Health and Human Services. *Oral health, cancer care, and you: fitting the pieces together.* Bethesda, MD: US Department of Health and Human Services, National Institutes of Health, National Institute of Dental and Craniofacial Research, 2002.

25. Cancer Therapy Evaluation Program. *Common terminology criteria for adverse events*, Version 3.0, DCTD, NCI, NIH, DHHS, Bethesda, MD: June 10, 2003.

26. Eilers J, Berger AM, Petersen MC. Development, testing, and application of the oral assessment guide. *Oncol Nurs Forum* 1988;15:325–330.

27. Schubert MM, Williams BE, Lloid ME, et al. Clinical scale for the rating of oral mucosal changes associated with bone marrow transplantation. Development of an oral mucositis index. *Cancer* 1992;69:2469–2477.

28. Schubert MM, Sullivan KM, Morton TH, et al. Oral manifestations of chronic graft-versus-host disease. *Arch Intern Med* 1984;144:1591–1595.

29. McGuire DB, Peterson DE, Muller S, et al. The 20 item oral mucositis index: reliability and validity in bone marrow and stem cell transplant patients. *Cancer Invest* 2002;20:893–903.

30. Sonis ST, Eilers JP, Epstein JB, et al. Mucositis Study Group. Validation of a new scoring system for the assessment of clinical trial research of oral mucositis induced by radiation or chemotherapy. *Cancer* 1999;85:2103–2113.

31. Sonis ST, Oster G, Fuchs H, et al. Oral mucositis and the clinical and economic outcomes of hematopoietic stem-cell transplantation. *J Clin Oncol* 2001;19:2201–2205.

32. World Health Organization. *WHO handbook for reporting results of cancer treatment*, (offset publication No. 48). Geneva: World Health Organization, 1979:15–22.

33. Gaston-Johansson F. Measurement of pain: the psychometric properties of the Pain-O-Meter, a simple, inexpensive pain assessment tool that could change health care practices. *J Pain Symptom Manage* 1996;12:172–181.

34. Zlotolow IM, Berger AM. Oral manifestations of cancer therapy. In: Berger AM, Portnoy RK, Weissman DE, eds. *Principles and practice of palliative care and supportive oncology*. Philadelphia, PA: Lippincott Williams & Wilkins, 2002:282–294.

35. Biron P, Sebban C, Gourmet R, et al. Research controversies in management of oral mucositis. *Support Care Cancer* 2000;8:68–71.

36. Rubenstein EB, Peterson DE, Schubert M, et al. Clinical practice guidelines for the prevention and treatment of cancer therapy-induced oral and gastrointestinal mucositis. *Cancer* 2004;100:2026–2046.

37. Somerfield M, Padberg J, Pfister D, et al. ASCO clinical practice guidelines: process, progress, pitfalls, and prospects. *Classic Pap Curr Comments* 2000;4:881–886.

38. Ferraro JM, Mattern J. Sucralfate suspension for stomatitis [Letter]. *Drug Intell Clin Pharmacol* 1984;18:153.

39. Ferraro JM, Mattern J. Sucralfate suspension for mouth ulcers [Letter]. *Drug Intell Clin Pharmacol* 1985;19:480.

40. Solomon MA. Oral sucralfate suspension for mucositis. *N Engl J Med* 1986;315:459.

41. Pfeiffer P, Madsen EL, Hansen O, et al. Effect of prophylactic sucralfate suspension on stomatitis induced by cancer chemotherapy. A randomized, double-blind cross-over study. *Acta Oncol* 1990;29:171.

42. Shenep JL, Kalwihsky D, Hudson PR, et al. Oral sucralfate in chemotherapy-induced mucositis. *J Pediatr* 1988;113:753.

43. Loprinzi CL, Ghosh C, Camoriani J, et al. Phase III controlled evaluation of sucralfate to alleviate stomatitis in patients receiving fluorouracil-based chemotherapy. *J Clin Oncol* 1997;15:1235.

44. Nottage M, McLachlan S-A, Brittain M-A, et al. Sucralfate mouthwash for prevention and treatment of 5-FU-induced mucositis: a randomized, placebo-controlled trial. *Support Care Cancer* 2003;11:41–47.

45. Barker G, Loftus L, Cuddy P, et al. The effects of sucralfate suspension and diphenhydramine syrup plus kaolin-pectin on radiotherapy-induced mucositis. *Oral Surg Oral Med Oral Pathol* 1991;71:288.

46. Scherlacher A, Beaufort-Spontin E. Radiotherapy of head-neck neoplasms: prevention of inflammation of the mucosa by sucralfate treatment. *HNO* 1990;38:24.

47. Pfeiffer P, Hansen O, Madsen EL, et al. A prospective pilot study on the effect of sucralfate mouth-swishing in reducing stomatitis during radiotherapy of the oral cavity. *Acta Oncol* 1990;29:471.

48. Epstein JB, Wong FLW. The efficacy of sucralfate suspension in the prevention of oral mucositis due to radiation therapy. *Int J Radiat Oncol Biol Phys* 1994;28:693.

49. Dodd MJ, Miaskowski C, Greenspan D. Radiation-induced mucositis: a randomized clinical trial of micronized sucralfate versus salt & soda mouthwashes. *Cancer Invest* 2003;21:21–33.

50. Innocenti M, Moscatelli G, Lopez S. Efficacy of Gelclair in reducing pain in palliative care patients with oal lesions. Preliminary findings from an open pilot study. *J Pain Symptom Manage* 2001;24:456–457.

51. DeCordi D, D'Andrea P, Giorguitti E: potentially an efficacious treatment for chemotherapy-induced mucositis [Abstract]. *Italian Anti-tumor league III congress of professional oncology nurses*, Conegliano, Italy, October 10–12, 2001.

52. Porteder H, Rausch E, Kment G, et al. Local prostaglandin E2 in patients with oral malignancies undergoing chemo and radiotherapy. *J Craniomaxillofac Surg* 1988;16:371.

53. Matejka M, Nell A, Kment G, et al. Local benefit of prostaglandin E2 in radiochemotherapy-induced oral mucositis. *Br J Oral Maxillofac Surg* 1990;28:89.

54. Labor B, Mrsic M, Pavleric A, et al. Prostaglandin E2 for prophylaxis of oral mucositis following BMT. *Bone Marrow Transplant* 1993;11:379.

55. Epstein JB, Stevenson-Moore P. Benzydamine hydrochloride in prevention and management of pain in mucositis associated with radiation therapy. *Oral Surg Oral Med Oral Pathol* 1986;62:145.

56. Epstein JB, Stevenson-Moore P, Jackson S, et al. Prevention of oral mucositis in radiation therapy: a controlled study with benzydamine hydrochloride rinse. *Int J Radiat Oncol Biol Phys* 1989;16:1571.

57. Lever SA, Dupuis LL, Chan SL. Comparative evaluation of benzydamine oral rinse in children with antineoplastic-induced stomatitis. *Drug Intell Clin Pharmacol* 1987;21:359.

58. Pillsbury HC, Webster WP, Rosenman J. Prostaglandin inhibitor and radiotherapy in advanced head and neck cancer. *Arch Otolaryngol Head Neck Surg* 1986;112:552.

59. Abdelaal AS, Barker DS, Fergusson MM. Treatment for irradiation-induced mucositis. *Lancet* 1987;1:97.

60. Rothwell BR, Spektor WS. Palliation of radiation-related mucositis. *Spec Care Dentist* 1990;10:21.

61. Wadleigh RG, Redman RS, Graham Ml, et al. Vitamin E in the treatment of chemo-induced mucositis. *Am J Med* 1992;92:481–484.

62. Osaki T, Ueta E, Yoneda K, et al. Prophylaxis of oral mucositis associated with chemoradiotherapy for oral carcinoma by Azelastine hydrochloride (azelastine) with other antioxidants. *Head Neck* 1994;16:331–339.

63. Garewal HS, Meyskens F. Retinoids and carcinoids in the prevention of oral cancer. A critical appraisal. *Cancer Epidemiol Biomarkers Prev* 1992;1:155.

64. Mills EE. The modifying effect of beta-carotene on radiation and chemotherapy induced oral mucositis. *Br J Cancer* 1988;57:416.

65. Maciejewski B, Zajusz A, Pilecki B, et al. Acute mucositis in the stimulated oral mucosa of patients during radiotherapy for head and neck cancer. *Radiother Oncol* 1991;22:7.

66. Dorr W, Jacubek A, Kummermehr J, et al. Effects of stimulated repopulation on oral mucositis during conventional radiotherapy. *Radiother Oncol* 1995;37:100.

67. Mahoud DJ, Dose AM, Loprinzi CL, et al. Inhibition of fluorouracil-induced stomatitis by oral cryotherapy. *J Clin Oncol* 1991;9:449.

68. Rocke LK, Loprinzi CL, Lee JK, et al. A randomized clinical trial of two different durations of oral cryotherapy for prevention of 5-FU-related stomatitis. *Cancer* 1993;72(7):2234–2238.

69. Cascinu S, Fedeli A, Fedeli SL, et al. Oral cooling (cryotherapy), an effective treatment for the prevention of 5-FU-induced stomatitis. *Oral Oncol Eur J Cancer* 1994;30(4):234.

70. Bugai LP, Saprykina VA, Vakhtin VI, et al. The effect of light from a low intensity impulse laser on the processes of experimental inflammation and regeneration in the oral mucosa. *Stomatologiia* 1991;2:6.

71. Pourreau-Schneider N, Soudry M, Franquin JC, et al. Soft-laser therapy for iatrogenic mucositis in cancer patients receiving high-dose fluorouracil: a preliminary report. *J Natl Cancer Inst* 1992;84:358.

72. Bensadoun RJ, Ciais G, Schubert MM, et al. Low-energy He/Ne laser in the prevention of radiation-induced mucositis. A multicenter phase III randomized study in patients with head and neck cancer. *Support Care Cancer* 1999;7:244–252.

73. Carl W, Emrich LS. Management of oral mucositis during local radiation and systemic chemotherapy. A study of 98 patients. *J Prosthet Dent* 1991;66:361.

74. Fidler P, Loprinzi CL, O'Fallon JR, et al. Prospective evaluation of a chamomile mouthwash for prevention of 5-FU-induced oral mucositis. *Cancer* 1996;77:522.

75. Peterson D, Petit G. Phase III study: AES-14 in chemotherapy patients at risk for mucositis. *Proc Am Soc Clin Oncol* 2003;22:725.

76. Oshitani T, Okada K, Kushima T, et al. Clinical evaluation of sodium alginate on oral mucositis associated with radiotherapy. *Nippon Gan Chiryo Gakkai Shi* 1990;25(6):1129.

77. Spijkervet FKL, Saene HKF, Panders AK, et al. Effect of chlorhexidine rinsing on the oropharyngeal ecology in patients with head and neck cancer who have irradiation mucositis. *Oral Surg Oral Med Oral Pathol* 1989;67:154.

78. Foote RL, Loprinzi CL, Frank AR, et al. Randomized trial of a chlorhexidine mouthwash for alleviation of radiation-induced mucositis. *J Clin Oncol* 1994;12:2630.

79. Sonis ST, Costa JW Jr, Evitts SM, et al. Effect of epidermal growth factor on ulcerative mucositis in hamsters that receive cancer chemotherapy. *Oral Surg Oral Med Oral Pathol* 1992:74:749.

80. Sonis ST, Tracey C, Shklar G, et al. An animal model for mucositis induced by cancer chemotherapy. *Oral Surg Oral Med Oral Pathol* 1990;69:437.

81. Gabrilove JL, Jakubowski A, Scher H, et al. Effect of granulocyte colony-stimulating factor on neutropenia and associated morbidity due to chemotherapy for transitional-cell carcinoma of the urothelium. *N Engl J Med* 1988;318:1414.

82. Bronchud MH, Howell A, Crowther D, et al. The use of granulocyte colony-stimulating factor to increase the intensity of treatment with doxorubicin in patients with advanced breast and ovarian cancer. *Br J Cancer* 1989;60:121.

83. Pettengell R, Gurney H, Radford JA, et al. Granulocyte colony-stimulating factor to prevent dose-limiting neutropenia in non-Hodgkin's lymphoma: a randomized controlled trial. *Blood* 1992;80:1430.

84. Saarilahti K, Kajanti M, Joensuu T. Comparison of granulocyte-macrophage colony-stimulating factor and sucralfate mouthwashes in the prevention of radiation-induced mucositis: a double-blind prospective randomized phase III study. *Int J Radiat Oncol Biol Phys* 2002;2:479–485.

85. Dazzi C, Cariello A, Giovanis P, et al. Prophylaxis with GM-CSF mouthwashes does not reduce frequency and duration of severe oral mucositis in patients with solid tumors undergoing high-dose chemotherapy with autologous peripheral blood stem cell transplantation rescue: a double blind, randomized, placebo-controlled study. *Ann Oncol* 2003;14:559–563.

86. Foncuberta MC, Cagnoni CH, Brandts R, et al. Topical transforming growth factor-β3 in the prevention or alleviation of chemotherapy-induced oral mucositis in patients with lymphomas or solid tumors. *J Immunother* 2001;24:384–388.

87. Zaghloul MS, Dorie MJ, Kallman RF, et al. Interleukin 1 increases thymidine labeling index of normal tissue of mice, not the tumor. *Int J Radiat Oncol Biol Phys* 1994;29:805.

88. Sonis S, Edwards L, Lucey C. The biological basis for the attenuation of mucositis: the example of interleukin-11. *Leukemia* 1999;13:831.

89. Spielberger R, Stiff P, Bensinger W, et al. Palifermin for oral mucositis after intensive therapy for hematologic cancers. *N Engl J Med* 2004;351:2590–2598.

90. Donnelly JP, Bellm LA, Epstein JB, et al. Antimicrobial therapy to prevent or treat oral mucositis. *Lancet Infect Dis* 2003;3:405–412.

91. Wahlin BY. Effects of chlorhexidine mouth rinse on oral health in patients with acute leukemia. *Oral Surg Oral Med Oral Pathol* 1989;68:279.

92. Dodd MJ, Larson PL, Dibble SL, et al. Randomized clinical trial of chlorhexidine versus placebo for prevention of oral mucositis in patients receiving chemotherapy. *Oncol Nurs Forum* 1996;23:921–927.

93. Weisdorf DJ, Bostrom B, Raether D, et al. Oropharyngeal mucositis complicating bone marrow transplantation: prognostic factors and the effect of chlorhexidine mouth rinse. *Bone Marrow Transplant* 1989;4:89.

94. Epstein JB, Vickais L, Spinelli J, et al. Efficacy of chlorhexidine and nystatin rinses in prevention of oral complications in leukemia and bone marrow transplantation. *Oral Surg Oral Med Oral Pathol* 1992;73:682.

95. Slavin MA, Osborne B, Adams R, et al. Efficacy and safety of fluconazole prophylaxis for fungal infections after marrow transplantation- a prospective, randomized, double-blind study. *J Infect Dis* 1995;171:1545–1552.

96. Sutherland SE, Browman GP. Prophylaxis of oral mucositis in irradiated head-and-neck cancer patients: a proposed classification scheme of interventions and meta-analysis of randomized controlled trials. *Int J Radiat Oncol Phys* 2001;1:917–930.

97. Spijkervet FK, Saene HK, van Saene JJ, et al. Effect of selective elimination of the oral flora on mucositis in irradiated head and neck cancer patients. *J Surg Oncol* 1991;46:167.

98. Stokman MA, Spijkervet FKL, Burlage FR, et al. Oral mucositis and selective elimination of oral flora in head and neck cancer patients receiving radiotherapy: a double-blind randomized clinical trial. *Br J Cancer* 2003;88:1012–1016.

99. Loury DJ, Embree JR, Steinberg DA. Effect of local application of the antimicrobial peptide IB-367 on the incidence and severity of oral mucositis in hamsters. *Oral Surg Oral Med Oral Pathol* 1999;87:544.

100. Barrett AP. A long-term prospective clinical study of oral complications during conventional chemotherapy for acute leukemia. *Oral Surg Oral Med Oral Pathol* 1987;63:313.

101. DeGregorio MW, Lee WMF, Linker CA, et al. Fungal infections in patients with acute leukemia. *Am J Med* 1982;73:543.

102. Bender JF, Schimpff SC, Young VM, et al. A comparative trial of tobramycin vs gentamicin in combination with vancomycin and nystatin for alimentary tract suppression in leukemic patients. *Eur J Cancer* 1979;15:35.

103. Barrett AP. Evaluation of nystatin in prevention and elimination of oropharyngeal Candida in immunosuppressed patients. *Oral Surg Oral Med Oral Pathol* 1984;58:148.

104. William C, Whitehouse JMA, Lister TA, et al. Oral anticandidal prophylaxis in patients undergoing chemotherapy for acute leukemia. *Med Pediatr Oncol* 1977;3:275.

105. Carpentieri V, Haggard ME, Lockhart LH, et al. Clinical experience in prevention of candidiasis by nystatin in children with acute lymphocytic leukemia. *J Pediatr* 1978;92:593.

106. Hann IM, Prentice HG, Corringham R, et al. Ketoconazole versus nystatin plus amphotericin B for fungal prophylaxis in severely immunocompromised patients. *Lancet* 1982;1:826.

107. Schwartz PM, Dunigan JM, Marsh JC, et al. Allopurinol modification of the toxicity and antitumor activity of 5-FU. *Cancer Res* 1980;40:1885.

108. Clark PI, Selvin ML. Allopurinol mouthwash and 5-FU-induced oral toxicity. *Eur J Surg Oncol* 1985;11:267.

109. Tsararis N, Caragliuris P, Kosmidus P. Reduction of oral toxicity of 5-FU by allopurinol mouthwashes. *Eur J Surg Oncol* 1998;14:405.

110. Loprinzi CI, Cianflone SG, Dose ASM, et al. A controlled evaluation of an allopurinol mouthwash as prophylaxis against 5-fluorouracil induced stomatitis. *Cancer* 1990;65:1879.

111. Seiter K, Kemeny N, Martin D, et al. Uridine allows dose escalation of 5-FU when given with N-phosphonacetyl-l-aspartate, methotrexate, and leucovorin. *Cancer* 1993;71(5):1875.

112. Ahmed T, Engelking C, Szalyga J, et al. Propantheline prevention of mucositis from etoposide. *Bone Marrow Transplant* 1993;12:131.

113. Lee JS, Murphy WK, Shirinian MH, et al. Alleviation by leucovorin of the dose-limiting toxicity of edatrexate: potential for improved therapeutic efficacy. *Cancer Chemother Pharmacol* 1991;28:199.

114. Ackland SP, Schilsky RL. High-dose methotrexate: a critical reappraisal. *J Clin Oncol* 1987;5:2017.

115. Oliff A, Bleyer WA, Poplack DG. Methotrexate-induced oral mucositis and salivary methotrexate concentrations. *Cancer Chemother Pharmacol* 1979;2:225.

116. Fox AD, Kripke SA, Depaula JA, et al. Effect of a glutamine supplemented enteral diet on methotrexate-induced enterocolitis. *JPEN J Parenter Enteral Nutr* 1988;12:325.

117. O'Dwyer ST, Scott T, Smith RJ, et al. 5-FU toxicity on small intestinal mucosa but not white blood cells is decreased by glutamine [abst]. *Clin Res* 1987;35:367A.

118. Jebb SA, Osborne RJ, Maughan TS, et al. 5-FU and folinic acid-induced mucositis: no effect of oral glutamine supplementation. *Br J Cancer* 1994;70:132.

119. Marx RE, Johnson RP, Kline SN. Prevention of osteoradionecrosis: a randomized prospective clinical trial of hyperbaric oxygen versus penicillin. *J Am Dent Assoc* 1985;111:49–54.

120. Marx RE, Sawatari Y, Fortin M, et al. Bisphosphonate-induced exposed bone (osteonecrosis/osteopetrosis) of the jaws: risk factors, recognition, prevention, and treatment. *J Oral Maxillofac Surg* 2005;63:1567–1575.

121. National Institute of Nursing Research (NINR). *The nature of pain. A conceptual perspective. A report of the NINR priority expert panel on symptom management. Acute pain.* Bethesda, MD: US Department of Health and Human Services, 1994:23–42.

122. Berger A, Henderson M, Nadoolman W, et al. Oral capsaicin provides temporary relief for oral mucositis pain secondary to chemotherapy/radiation therapy. *J Pain Symptom Manage* 1995;10:243–248.

123. Dodd MJ, Miaskowski C, Shiba GH, et al. Risk factors for chemotherapy-induced oral mucositis: dental appliances, oral hygiene, previous oral lesion, and a history of smoking. *Cancer Invest* 1999;17:278–284.

124. Carnal SB, Blakeslee DB, Oswald SG, et al. Treatment of radiation- and chemotherapy-induced stomatitis. *Otolaryngol Head Neck Surg* 1990;102:326.

125. Krajnik M, Zylicz Z, Finlay I, et al. Potential uses of topical opioids in palliative care report of 6 cases. *Pain* 1999;80:121.

126. Coluzzi PH, Schwartzberg L, Conroy JD, et al. Breakthrough cancer pain: a randomized trial comparing oral transmucosal fentanyl (OTFC) and morphine sulfate immediate release (MSIR). *Pain* 2001;91:123–130.

127. Cerchietti LC, Navigante AH, Bonomi MR, et al. Effect of topical morphine for mucositis-associated pain following concomitant chemoradiotherapy for head and neck cancer. *Cancer* 2002;95:2230–2236.

128. Swisher ME, Scheidler VR, Kennedy MJ. A mucositis pain management algorithm: a creative strategy to enhance the transition to ambulatory care. *Oncol Nurs Forum* 1998.

129. Brizel DM, Wasserman TH, Strnad V, et al. Final report of a phase III randomized trial of amifostine as a radioprotectant in head and neck cancer [abstract]. *41st annual meeting of the American Society for Therapeutic Radiology and Oncology*, Texas, 1999.

130. Peterson DE, Sonis S. Executive summary. *J Natl Cancer Inst Monogr* 2001;29:3–5.

131. Bellum LA, Durnell L, Epstein JB, et al. Defining clinically meaningful outcomes in the evaluation of new treatments for oral mucositis: oral mucositis patients provider advisory board. *Cancer Invest* 2002;20:793–800.

CHAPTER 20 ■ PRURITUS

ALAN B. FLEISCHER JR. AND CHRISTOPHER B. YELVERTON

Like the sensation of pain, pruritus (itching) can diminish the quality of life in patients with cancer. Because of the distress pruritus may cause, the cancer clinician should be aware of its importance and its management. Pruritus in patients with cancer may be attributable to a primary skin disease, a coexisting medical condition, a medication, or the cancer itself. Indeed, to quote Krajnik and Zylicz, "There is no one cure for all pruritic symptoms. Better understanding of mechanisms of pruritus may help develop better treatments" (1). A number of notable articles, chapters, and texts on itch have been published by leading authorities (1–13). This chapter focuses on pruritus in patients with cancer and reviews its etiology, diagnosis, and management. Readers should bear in mind that patients with cancer can be affected by the same pruritic conditions that those without cancer may acquire, in addition to cancer and cancer treatment–associated conditions.

PRURITUS SENSATIONS

In simplest terms, *pruritus* is the sensation that provokes scratching. Like the sensation of pain, objective analysis cannot easily confirm the presence or severity of pruritus. Nevertheless, patients are generally thought to be reliable in their assessment of pruritus severity. Scratch marks (*excoriations*), skin thickening (*lichenification*), and visible cutaneous disease support patients' subjective complaints.

To complicate the issue, some patients with typically itchy diseases, such as scabies, deny that they itch. These patients may complain of burning, stinging, tingling, tickling, or a crawling sensation. These symptoms are closely related to pruritus, have similar pathogenic mechanisms, and are treated identically. Bernhard (14) summarized this notion by stating, "one man's itch is another man's tickle... and one man's stinging itch is another man's pain." For most people, itch is readily distinguished from pain, and many patients with severe pruritus would be happy to have pain instead (15).

Pruritus is a distinct, complex sensation that may be considered a primary sensory modality (10). The cutaneous itch response is carried by unique sensory C-fibers (15). Although itch fibers are histologically indistinguishable from pain receptors, they may be distinguished electrophysiologically. These unmyelinated fibers carry sensations to the spinothalamic tract where they are relayed to the thalamus and subthalamus. Experimental injection of histamine into the skin induces itch or pain. This histamine-induced pruritus may be suppressed by systemic antihistamine administration (16).

Because many patients with pruritus show no signs of histamine release (e.g., cutaneous wheal and flare), it is likely that other compounds (e.g., cytokines and neuropeptides) cause most pruritus. Furthermore, the failure of many pruritic conditions to improve with nonsedating antihistamines suggests that histamine is a minor pruritus mediator (17,18). Studies have revealed that pruritus may be caused by opiates, serotonin, and other neuropeptides, prostaglandins, kinins, proteases, and physical stimuli (10). Each of these agents may induce pruritus primarily or act through secondary mediators.

The sensation of pruritus also may arise within the central nervous system. Systemic opioids are known to induce pruritus, and the opioid-antagonists, including naloxone hydrochloride, naltrexone hydrochloride, and nalmefine hydrochloride, decrease the pruritus of cholestatic and other liver disease (19–22). Exogenous opioids administered in small quantities to spinal levels in spinal anesthesia relieve pain and can stimulate itching (23). Plasma from patients with cholestatic itching causes facial scratching when introduced into the medullary dorsal horn of monkeys; this scratching is abolished by administering the opioid receptor antagonist naloxone hydrochloride (24). Although opioids may promote histamine release by mast cells (e.g., exacerbating urticarial itch), opioid peptides generally do not cause any release of histamine when injected alone.

Other central nervous system pruritic phenomena include cerebrovascular accident pruritus (25) and phantom limb or phantom breast pruritus (i.e., pruritus in an amputated extremity or removed breast) (26,27). Therefore, it is clear that pruritus is often not histamine induced and may not arise in the skin.

DERMATOLOGIC DISEASES AND PRURITUS

Many skin diseases may contribute to the sensation of pruritus. Dry skin, or *xerosis*, is commonly seen in patients with cancer who have generalized wasting or have undergone chemotherapy or radiation therapy. Xerosis makes the skin more susceptible to irritation from environmental assault (28).

Many other diseases may present with pruritus, including scabies, atopic dermatitis, dermatitis herpetiformis, bullous pemphigoid, miliaria, pediculosis, and urticaria (29). These cutaneous diseases are often readily diagnosed by careful clinical examination. Signs of dermatologic diseases may be remarkably subtle or nonspecific in any given patient, particularly in the immunocompromised host. There is no substitute for an excellent physical examination of the skin surface (30–36).

PRURITUS AND MALIGNANCY

Pruritus may be associated with virtually any malignancy (Table 20.1) (5,37–52). Some neoplasms, particularly hematologic malignancies, are more frequently associated with pruritus. Primary polycythemia, for example, has a pruritus prevalence of 30 to 50%, and Hodgkin's disease has a prevalence of 15%. Cutaneous T-cell lymphoma, peripheral T-cell lymphoma, and other cutaneous lymphomas are notoriously pruritic. Generally, the etiology of the pruritus in these patients is thought to be related to a poorly understood paraneoplastic

TABLE 20.1

SYSTEMIC CONDITIONS REPORTED TO BE ASSOCIATED WITH GENERALIZED PRURITUS

Organ systems and etiologies	Example
Autoimmune	Sjögren's syndrome
	Progressive systemic sclerosis
	Lupus erythematosus
	Sicca syndrome
Endocrine	Hyperthyroidism
	Hypothyroidism
	Parathyroid disease
Central nervous system	Cerebrovascular accident
	Delusions of parasitosis
	Depression
	Multiple sclerosis
	Neurodermatitis
	Psychosis
	Syrinx
	Brain tumor
Hematopoietic	Paraproteinemia
	Iron deficiency anemia
	Mastocytosis
Liver	Primary biliary cirrhosis
	Extrahepatic biliary obstruction
	Hepatitis
Malignancy	Breast carcinoma
	Carcinoid syndrome
	Cutaneous T-cell lymphoma
	Gastrointestinal tract cancers: tongue, stomach, and colon
	Hodgkin's disease
	Insulinoma
	Leukemia
	Lung cancer
	Multiple myeloma
	Non-Hodgkin's lymphoma
	Polycythemia vera
	Prostatic carcinoma
	Thyroid carcinoma
	Uterine carcinoma
Iatrogenic	Drug ingestion
	Drug-induced cholestasis
	Injection site reaction
Infectious	Human immunodeficiency virus
	Parasitic diseases
	Scabies
	Syphilis
Renal	Chronic renal insufficiency and renal failure
	Dialysis dermatosis

phenomenon. Pruritus may be a presenting symptom in both solid and hematologic cancers (53,54). Gobbi et al. (48) reported that severe pruritus in Hodgkin's disease predicts a poor prognosis. Pruritus may also be a sign of malignant physical obstruction of the biliary system from either a primary or metastatic tumor (50).

PRURITUS AND NONMALIGNANT INTERNAL DISEASES

Patients with cancer are not exempt from having concurrent medical conditions. There is no question that other internal diseases may be associated with pruritus (Table 20.1). Pruritus has been reported to herald the onset of thyroid disease (55), renal insufficiency (56), liver disease (57), iron deficiency (58), diabetes mellitus (59), paraproteinemia (60), Sjögren's syndrome (61), and other conditions. Patients with cancer can independently develop other medical conditions, or the cancer itself may cause a systemic condition, such as biliary obstruction, that may cause pruritus. Mechanisms of pruritus induction in most of these diseases are poorly understood. It has been postulated that renal disease may induce a metastatic calcification, hyperphosphatemia, xerosis, mast cell proliferation, and other changes that might be associated with pruritus.

CANCER THERAPY

Pruritus may be the result of a chemotherapy reaction, radiation therapy, or medications used for symptom management. Pruritus has been reported as an adverse reaction to chemotherapeutic agents, including those listed in Table 20.2 (62–68). Adverse effects of some chemotherapeutic agents may include anemia and other metabolic disturbances, which could also lead to pruritus. New combinations of chemotherapeutic agents in ever increasing dosage regimens will undoubtedly be associated with increased cutaneous toxicity. Pruritus caused by opioids, particularly injectible opioids, used for pain control is also possible. Additionally, pruritus may be caused by other chemicals that may be used in the preparation of medications and medication administration tools (69).

Acute radiodermatitis may cause erythema and pruritus. Additionally, chronic radiodermatitis can be associated with severe xerosis, skin thinning, and ease of irritation. Total body electron beam radiation may make the entire skin surface dry and pruritic.

All clinicians managing patients with cancer are familiar with the typical morbilliform drug rash from antibiotics and other supportive agents. Similar to this eruption is the engraftment phenomenon in bone marrow transplant recipients; however, many pruritogenic drugs do not induce any rash. As stated, opiates may induce pruritus through central nervous mechanisms. Others, such as estrogens or ketoconazole, may precipitate cholestasis and therefore induce pruritus. It is noteworthy that placebo agents may induce pruritus in as many as 5% of the people treated. More than 100 medications are reported to cause pruritus without a rash (63). Careful review of the medication history and simplification of the drug regimen is essential.

NEUROPSYCHIATRIC DISEASE AND PRURITUS

Calnan and O'Neill (70) found that in most patients with a chief complaint of generalized pruritus, the itch began at a

TABLE 20.2

ANTITUMOR AGENTS ASSOCIATED WITH PRURITUS

Interferon-α
Bacille Calmette-Guérin
Bleomycin sulfate
Carboplatin
Carmustine
Chlorambucil
Cisplatin
Cyclophosphamide
Cytosine arabinoside and daunomycin
Daunomycin
Docetaxel
Doxorubicin
Gemcitabine hydrochloride
Hydroxyurea
Imatinib
Interleukin-2 with levamisole hydrochloride or interferon-α
L-Asparaginase
Mechlorethamine hydrochloride
Megestrol acetate
Methotrexate
Mitomycin
Oxaliplatin
Paclitaxel
Procarbazine hydrochloride

time of emotional stress. Edwards et al. (71) later reported that a high level of psychological stress enhances a person's ability to perceive intense itch stimuli. In patients with cancer, psychological stress, depression, anxiety, and organic brain diseases undoubtedly contribute to cutaneous diseases (72–74). Recognition of neuropsychiatric disease may lead to better control.

EVALUATION OF THE PRURITIC PATIENT

Obtaining a focused history, a directed review of symptoms, and a focused clinical examination may lead to a clinical diagnosis. The physician should first probe for likely pharmaceutical agents that could exacerbate pruritus. A temporal history of therapeutic agent initiation within 2 weeks of the onset of pruritus may be helpful. Other historic points of value include an abnormal or excessive bathing history, others in the family or household with similar problems, and symptoms of neuropsychiatric disease. Complete dermatologic clinical examination quickly excludes urticaria, scabies, and a host of other dermatologic diagnoses.

Some patients with long-standing, generalized pruritus may require further evaluation. For practicing dermatologic clinicians, further investigation may be warranted. This evaluation should include a careful history, physical examination, and appropriate, limited, screening laboratory tests. Extensive, undirected evaluation of these patients rarely leads to a specific attributable cause (75).

There is no single list, nor are there specific guidelines for tests that must be performed in any individual patient. Scabies preparations, fungal examinations, and skin biopsies may be needed to diagnose specific dermatologic diseases.

TREATMENT

Treating pruritus in the patient with cancer can take many forms. In general, the primary approaches to management should involve removal of the cause of itch, if possible, in conjunction with control of symptoms. Although there are some specific issues to consider in this population, most of the management is similar to other forms of itch. It is important to devote adequate time to a given therapy to obtain optimum results. Unfortunately, there are very few guidelines regarding the appropriate duration of therapy in chronic pruritus.

Topical Treatment

Ideally, particularly in localized itch, the physician would choose the single topical medication that corrects the underlying condition. Although this scenario occasionally occurs (e.g., permethrin for scabies infestation), symptomatic treatment is less specific. Therefore, the clinician must use all diagnostic skills to provide the patient with reasonable relief. Table 20.3 presents the advantages and disadvantages of different topical agents.

One of the most important aspects of skin therapy that must be addressed is hydration and lubrication of the skin surface (28,76). A simple but sometimes effective therapeutic approach is to apply emollients (lotions, creams, and ointments) on the dry skin twice daily. Emollients with camphor and menthol (e.g., Sarna lotion), phenol, pramoxine (Sarna Sensitive, PrameGel, Pramosone, or Aveeno anti-itch lotion) or benzocaine (Lanacane) may provide relief. Camphor, phenol, menthol, pramoxine, and benzocaine have local anesthetic effects (12).

Age-old remedies such as cool compresses (application of a wet washcloth for 20 minutes) and shake lotions (calamine) may prove highly efficacious. Cooling the skin may provide remarkable pruritus relief. Oatmeal baths (Aveeno) or baths in therapeutic salts may also provide short-term symptomatic relief. Wet wraps may also be indicated for generalized pruritus.

Topical corticosteroids may be useful adjunctive agents for pruritus control. When used properly, they should be prescribed in amounts necessary to cover the affected skin. Table 20.4 provides prescribing quantity information. Although any topical corticosteroid may be useful in a given patient, for widespread pruritus, hydrocortisone (1% or 2.5%) or triamcinolone (0.1%) preparations are generally effective. Because of the relatively thin skin of some cancer patients, long-term use of halogenated corticosteroids should be approached with great caution. Overuse of corticosteroids in unsupervised or overzealous patients is a common cause of dermatological iatrogenic disease (77). Even when topical corticosteroids are required, the use of emollients remains indicated (78,79).

Topical tacrolimus (Protopic) 0.1% ointment is also an effective anti-inflammatory product for itching. It may cause some short-term burning and stinging on topical application, but can be used for long periods of time on any skin site without risk of atrophy (80,81). Although success has been demonstrated with only atopic dermatitis, it is likely to be effective for a broad range of diseases that involve cutaneous inflammation. Pimecrolimus (Elidel) cream is also safe and effective for long-term use, but is less effective than tacrolimus. Like tacrolimus, pimecrolimus causes no long-term atrophy, and neither agent suppresses systemic immune function.

Capsaicin cream (Zostrix) is of limited help in select patients with a wide range of inflammatory and noninflammatory dermatoses (82–84). Topical capsaicin should be applied three times daily and may be used indefinitely. Its application requires careful patient instruction, as it often initially produces

TABLE 20.3

ADVANTAGES AND DISADVANTAGES OF TOPICAL AGENTS

Topical agent	Examples	Advantages	Disadvantages
Emollients and moisturizers	Petrolatum moisturizing lotions	Inexpensive, reduces irritant dermatitis	May be too greasy, insufficient in inflammatory diseases
Corticosteroids	Hydrocortisone Desonide Triamcinolone Fluocinonide Clobetasol	Effective for inflammatory dermatoses, mainstay of topical therapy	May cause atrophy, sensitivity, adrenal suppression
Topical calcineurin inhibitors	Tacrolimus Pimecrolimus	Effective for inflammatory dermatoses, no atrophy	May cause itch or burn on application
Anesthetics	Camphor Pramoxine Benzocaine Prilocaine (EMLA) Menthol	Excellent pruritus relief, no atrophy or adrenal suppression	Potentially sensitizing and short-transient activity
Antihistamines	Diphenhydramine hydrochloride Doxepin hydrochloride	Modest relief, no atrophy or adrenal suppression	Potentially sedating and sensitizing
Cooling agents	Calamine Alcohol	May be soothing and cooling	Calamine leaves visible film Alcohol dries the skin
Miscellaneous	Coal tar	Coal tar is anti-inflammatory	Tar is not elegant and stains
	Capsaicin	Capsaicin works differently than other agents	Capsaicin often burns

EMLA, eutectic mixture of local anesthetics.

significant burning or stinging sensations or superficial burns. In many cases, after 1 or more weeks, the burning sensation diminishes and relief from pruritus follows. Capsaicin is not appropriate for generalized pruritus because of its significant expense and irritation potential.

Other agents have modest topical efficacy in relieving pruritus. The eutectic mixture of local anesthetics (EMLA) lidocaine and prilocaine has been demonstrated to be helpful in experimentally induced pruritus (85) and may prove useful in recalcitrant pruritic conditions. However, it is likely to offer no additional advantages over other anesthetics mentioned. Topical doxepin hydrochloride (Zonalon), an antidepressant and antihistamine, is a noncorticosteroid pruritus medication

with modest demonstrated efficacy (86). Topical doxepin hydrochloride may cause sedation and is particularly likely to cause allergic contact dermatitis. Clinicians should be aware that all topical agents, including emollients, corticosteroids, antihistamines, and anesthetics, have sensitizing potential and may induce allergic contact dermatitis.

Systemic Treatment

In patients with pruritus that interferes with sleep or pruritus that may have a significant neuropsychiatric component, oral antipruritic agents may prove important in symptomatic relief

TABLE 20.4

AMOUNTS OF TOPICAL AGENT PRESCRIBING INFORMATION

Location	One application (g)	Twice daily for 1 wk[a]	Twice daily for 1 mo[a]
Hands, scalp, genitalia, or face	2	30 g (1 oz)	120 g (4 oz)
Upper extremity or one side of trunk	3	45 g (1.5 oz)	180 g (6 oz)
One lower extremity	4	60 g (2 oz)	240 g (8 oz)
Entire body	30–60	540 g (1 lb)	2700 g (5 lb)

[a]Although the twice-daily dosing of topical agents is appropriate for many patients, clinicians employ these agents from daily to four times daily.

TABLE 20.5

SYSTEMIC OR PHYSICAL MODALITY PRURITUS TREATMENTS FOR SPECIFIC CONDITIONS

Disease	Drug or modality	Dosage range	Reference
Renal insufficiency or failure	Ultraviolet B phototherapy	N/A	(56,87,88)
	Activated charcoal	50 g every 4 h	(89)
Hepatic cholestasis	Rifampin	300 mg b.i.d	(90,91)
	Ondansetron	8 mg t.i.d	(91,92)
	Cholestyramine	4–6 g t.i.d with meals	(90)
	Nalmefene	2–10 mg b.i.d	(21,22)
	Naltrexone	25–50 mg daily	
Inflammatory skin diseases	Prednisone	5–60 mg daily	(7–10,12,13)
	Phototherapy	N/A	(87,88,93)
	Thalidomide	100–300 mg daily	(94)
Urticaria	Antihistamines		(13,95)
	Cetirizine	10–20 mg daily	
	Chlorpheniramine	4–12 mg q8–12 h	
	Desloratadine	50–10 mg daily	
	Diphenhydramine	25–50 mg q6–8 h	
	Fexofenadine	60–180 mg daily	
	Hydroxizine	10–100 mg q6h	
	Loratadine	10–20 mg daily	
Neurogenic Itch	Doxepin	10–150 mg qhs	(96)
	Paroxetine	10–50 mg daily	(97)
	Gabapentin	300–1500 mg daily	
Polycythemia	Aspirin	81–325 mg daily	(49)

N/A, not available.

(Table 20.5). Antihistamines, such as hydroxyzine (Atarax) and diphenhydramine hydrochloride (Benadryl), are not only occasionally antipruritic but also have important central nervous system effects. In a review of the pharmacologic control of pruritus nearly two decades ago, Winkelmann (95) stated that the most effective antihistamines have central nervous system effects. Moreover, ensuring adequate sedation can be important now that there is good evidence that pruritus disturbs normal sleep (98). However, some patients, especially the elderly, may have increased sensitivity to antihistamines, and memory impairment or impaired psychomotor function may result from their administration (3,4). Cetirizine hydrochloride (Zyrtec) is an antihistamine that is less sedating than hydroxyzine, but more sedating than the typically nonsedating antihistamines (e.g., desloratadine and fexofenadine hydrochloride).

In conditions other than urticaria, the nonsedating antihistamines may only have marginal therapeutic effect. There are conflicting data on the antipruritic efficacy of terfenadine and acrivastine in atopic dermatitis (18,99). Although they may be useful agents in the treatment of urticaria, nonsedating antihistamines have limited application in nonurticarial conditions. Moreover, the role of histamine in itch mediation in patients with cancer is even more questionable. Burtin et al. (100) found a decreased skin response to histamine injection in patients with cancer. They postulated that the presence of a tumor mimics the effects of general administration of histamine H$_1$ antagonists on the skin response to histamine.

Doxepin hydrochloride, a tricyclic antidepressant with antihistamine activity (96), may be an effective agent for the treatment of refractory pruritus, but in vivo has similar efficacy in suppressing histamine to hydroxyzine.

Systemic corticosteroids for pruritus are often highly effective, but their use can present certain difficulties. All oncologic practitioners are aware that chronic pathologic states, including hypertension, diabetes, fluid retention, and osteoporosis, may all be exacerbated by intramuscular or oral corticosteroids. Systemic corticosteroids are particularly effective for brief periods for morbilliform drug eruptions and allergic or irritant contact dermatitis. Further prolonged use may induce adverse sequelae.

A variety of other systemic agents have been used with some effect in specific disease states (Table 20.5). Activated charcoal (89), naloxone hydrochloride (19,20), naltrexone hydrochloride (22), and cholestyramine (90), for instance, have been demonstrated to be effective in the treatment of pruritus of biliary cirrhosis. Rifampin may be effective in the treatment of pruritus of primary biliary cirrhosis (90,91). Aspirin occasionally exacerbates pruritus but has been reported to be helpful in the treatment of pruritus associated with polycythemia rubra vera (49). Interferon-α has been used with some success in intractable pruritic conditions, especially polycythemia vera (51,52), but its cost and side effects demand careful consideration. Another confounding factor is that 30% of patients receiving Interferon-α, in one published melanoma study, experienced pruritus thought to be associated with the treatment (101). Although purely anecdotal, our experience with thalidomide, a teratogenic anti-inflammatory agent, suggests that this agent is also extremely useful for intractable pruritus if skin inflammation is present (94).

The serotonin agents paroxetine hydrochloride (97) and ondansetron (92) have shown some effect with intractable pruritus, but their mechanism of action is unclear. Although these findings are preliminary, the reported efficacy with this class of pharmacologic agents represents one of the most important recent advances in pruritus. These agents may have a role to play in the pruritus of liver disease and a wide variety of other conditions.

The reader should always bear in mind that if a patient obtains relief with any given medication, the medication cannot always take credit. In a classic study, Epstein and Pinski (102) found that placebo therapy provides pruritus relief with a surprisingly high success rate.

Physical Treatment Modalities

Ultraviolet A (UVA), ultraviolet B (UVB), and psoralen photochemotherapy have been successfully employed in a wide range of pruritic disorders, from atopic dermatitis to renal disease (56,87,93). Because of its high degree of efficacy, UVB is the treatment of choice for uremic pruritus, including our own. We administer UVB, combination UVA-UVB, and psoralen photochemotherapy treatments for pruritus. UV doses are usually administered three times weekly and UV doses are progressively increased until erythema is attained, then the therapy is individually adjusted to accommodate the patients' photosensitivity (88). To attain symptomatic relief, 20 to 30 treatments may be necessary; occasionally, weekly maintenance therapy is continued. As with all other therapies, patients are known to fail phototherapy.

Transcutaneous electrical nerve stimulation (TENS) is another modality that has been described to offer some relief to patients suffering from generalized itch associated with hematologic malignancies (103).

CONCLUSIONS

Pruritus in patients with cancer is common and provides a diagnostic and therapeutic challenge for the physician. Evaluation may be limited to obtaining an excellent history and physical examination. Alternatively, an exhaustive search for systemic disease may occasionally be indicated. The physician should address the therapeutic intervention to correct the underlying cutaneous disease. Systemic antipruritics are often beneficial and well tolerated but have well-known side effects. Above all, diagnosis and therapy should be individualized for the patient.

References

1. Krajnik M, Zylicz Z. Understanding pruritus in systemic disease. *J Pain Symptom Manage* 2001;21:151–168.
2. Lober CW. Pruritus and malignancy. *Clin Dermatol* 1993;11:125–128.
3. Higgins EM, du Vivier AW. Cutaneous manifestations of malignant disease. *Br J Hosp Med* 1992;48:552–554.
4. De Conno F, Ventafridda V, Saita I. Skin problems in advanced and terminal cancer patients. *J Pain Symptom Manage* 1991;6:247–256.
5. Rosenberg FW. Cutaneous manifestations of internal malignancy. *Cutis* 1977;20:227–234.
6. Campbell J. Management of pruritus in the cancer patient. *Oncol Nurs Forum* 1981;8:40–41.
7. Bernhard JD. Clinical aspects of pruritus. In: Fitzpatrick TB, Eisen AZ, Wolff K, et al., eds. *Dermatology in general medicine*, 3rd ed. New York: McGraw-Hill, 1987:78–90.
8. Weisshaar E, Kucenic MJ, Fleischer AB Jr. Pruritus, a review. *Acta Derm Venereol* 2003;83(Suppl 212):5–31.
9. Winkelmann RK. Pruritus. *Semin Dermatol* 1988;7:233–235.
10. Denman ST. A review of pruritus. *J Am Acad Dermatol* 1986;14:375–392.
11. Dangel RB. Pruritus and cancer. *Oncol Nurs Forum* 1986;13.17–21.
12. Gatti S, Serri F. *Pruritus in clinical medicine*. New York: McGraw-Hill, 1991.
13. Fleischer AB Jr. *The management of itching diseases*. New York: Parthenon Publishers, 2000.
14. Bernhard JD. Itches, pains, and other strange sensations. *Curr Chall in Dermatol* 1991:1–10.
15. Schmelz M, Schmidt R, Bickel A, et al. Specific C-receptors for itch in human skin. *J Neurosci* 1997;17:8003–8008.
16. Arnold AJ, Simpson JG, Jones HE, et al. Suppression of histamine-induced pruritus by hydroxyzine and various neuroleptics. *J Am Acad Dermatol* 1979;1:509–512.
17. Krause L, Shuster S. Mechanism of action of antipruritic drugs. *BMJ* 1983;287:1199–1200.
18. Berth-Jones J, Graham-Brown RAC. Failure of terfenadine in relieving the pruritus of atopic dermatitis. *Br J Dermatol* 1989;121:635–637.
19. Bernstein JE, Swift RM, Soltani K, et al. Antipruritic effect of the opiate antagonist, naloxone hydrochloride. *J Invest Dermatol* 1982;78:82–83.
20. Bernstein JE, Swift R. Relief of intractable pruritus with naloxone. *Arch Dermatol* 1979;115:1366–1367.
21. Bergasa NV, Alling DW, Talbot TL, et al. Oral nalmefene therapy reduces scratching activity due to the pruritus of cholestasis: a controlled study. *J Am Acad Dermatol* 1999;41:431–434.
22. Terra SG, Tsunoda SM. Opioid antagonists in the treatment of pruritus from cholestatic liver disease. *Ann Pharmacother* 1998;32:1228–1230.
23. Fischer HB, Scott PV. Spinal opiate analgesia and facial pruritus. *Anaesthesia* 1982;37:777–778.
24. Bergasa NV, Thomas DA, Vergalla J, et al. Plasma from patients with the pruritus of cholestasis induces opioid receptor–mediated scratching in monkeys. *Life Sci* 1993;53:1253–1257.
25. King CA, Huff FJ, Jorizzo JL. Unilateral neurogenic pruritus: paroxysmal itching associated with central nervous system lesions. *Ann Intern Med* 1982;97:222–223.
26. Bernhard JD. Phantom itch, pseudophantom itch, and senile pruritus. *Int J Dermatol* 1992;33:856–857.
27. Lierman LM. Phantom breast experiences after mastectomy. *Oncol Nurs Forum* 1988;15:41–44.
28. Hunnuksela A, Kinnunen T. Moisturizers prevent irritant dermatitis. *Acta Derm Venereol* 1992;72:42–44.
29. Gilchrest BA. *Skin and aging processes*. Boca Raton, FL: CRC Press, 1984.
30. Beare JM. Generalized pruritus: a study of 43 cases. *Clin Exp Dermatol* 1976;1:343–352.
31. Botero F. Pruritus as a manifestation of systemic disorders. *Cutis* 1978;21:873–880.
32. Gilchrest BA. Pruritus: pathogenesis, therapy and significance in systemic disease states. *Arch Intern Med* 1982;142:101–105.
33. Camp R. Generalized pruritus and its management. *Clin Exp Dermatol* 1982;7:557–563.
34. Kantor GR, Lookingbill DP. Generalized pruritus and systemic disease. *J Am Acad Dermatol* 1983;9:375–382.
35. Champion RH. Generalized pruritus. *BMJ* 1984;289:751–773.
36. Kantor GR. Evaluation and treatment of generalized pruritus. *Cleve Clin J Med* 1990;57:521–526.
37. Cormia FE. Pruritus, an uncommon but important symptom of systemic carcinoma. *Arch Dermatol* 1965;92:36–39.
38. Erskine JG, Rowan RM, Alexander JO, et al. Pruritus as a manifestation of myelomatosis. *BMJ* 1977;1:687–688.
39. Mengel CE. Cutaneous manifestations of the malignant carcinoid syndrome: severe pruritus and orange blotches. *Ann Intern Med* 1963;58:989–993.
40. Beeaff DE. Pruritus as a sign of systemic disease, report of metastatic small cell carcinoma. *Ariz Med* 1980;37:831–833.
41. Thomas S, Harrington CT. Intractable pruritus as the presenting symptom of carcinoma of the bronchus: a case report and review of the literature. *Clin Exp Dermatol* 1983;8:459–461.
42. Shoenfeld Y, Weinburger A, Ben-Bassat M, et al. Generalized pruritus in metastatic adenocarcinoma of the stomach. *Dermatology* 1977;155:122–124.
43. Degos R, Civatte J, Blanchet P, et al. Prurit, seule manifestation pendant 5 ans d'une maladie de Hodgkin. *Ann Med Interne (Paris)* 1973;124:235–238.
44. Alexander LL. Pruritus and Hodgkin's disease. *JAMA* 1979;241:2598–2599.
45. Bluefarb SM. *Cutaneous manifestations of malignant lymphomas*. Springfield, IL: Charles C Thomas Publisher, 1959.
46. Stock H. Cutaneous paraneoplastic syndromes. *Med Klin* 1976;71:356–372.
47. Curth HO. A spectrum of organ systems that respond to the presence of cancer: how and why the skin reacts. *Ann N Y Acad Sci* 1974;230:435–442.
48. Gobbi PG, Attardo-Parrinello G, Lattanzio G, et al. Severe pruritus should be a B-symptom in Hodgkin's disease. *Cancer* 1983;51:1934–1936.
49. Fjellner B, Hägermark O. Pruritus in polycythemia: treatment with aspirin and possibility of platelet involvement. *Acta Derm Venereol* 1979;61:505–512.
50. Ballinger AB, McHugh M, Catnach SM, et al. Symptom relief and quality of life after stenting for malignant bile duct obstruction. *Gut* 1994;35.467–470.
51. de Wolf JT, Hendriks DW, Egger RC, et al. Alpha-interferon for intractable pruritus in polycythemia rubra vera. *Lancet* 1991;337:241.
52. Flecknoe-Brown S. Relief of itch associated with myeloproliferative disease by alpha interferon. *Aust N Z J Med* 1991;21:81.
53. Johnson RE, Kanigsberg ND, Jimenez CL. Localized pruritus: a presenting symptom of a spinal cord tumor in a child with features of neurofibromatosis. *J Am Acad Dermatol* 2000;43(5 Pt 2):958–961.
54. King NK, Siriwardana HP, Coyne JD, et al. Intractable pruritus associated with insulinoma in the absence of multiple endocrine neoplasia: a novel paraneoplastic phenomenon. *Scand J Gastroenterol* 2003;38(6):678–680.
55. Barnes HM, Sarkany I, Calnan CD. Pruritus and thyrotoxicosis. *Trans St. Johns Hosp Dermatol Soc* 1974;60:59–62.
56. Gilchrest BA, Rowe JW, Brown RS, et al. Ultraviolet phototherapy of uremic pruritus with ultraviolet light therapy: long term results and possible mechanisms of action. *Ann Intern Med* 1979;91:17–21.
57. Sherlock S, Scheyer PJ. The presentation and diagnosis of 100 patients with primary biliary cirrhosis. *N Engl J Med* 1973;289:674–678.

58. Lewiecki EM, Rahman F. Pruritus: a manifestation of iron deficiency. *JAMA* 1976;236:2319–2320.
59. Stawiski MA, Vorhees JJ. Cutaneous signs of diabetes mellitus. *Cutis* 1976;18:415–421.
60. Zelicovici Z, Lahav M, Cahane P, et al. Pruritus as a possible early sign of paraproteinemia. *Isr J Med Sci* 1969;5:1079–1081.
61. Feuerman EJ. Sjögren's syndrome presenting as recalcitrant generalized pruritus. *Dermatologica* 1968;137:74–86.
62. Breathnach SM, Hinter H. *Adverse reactions and the skin.* Oxford, UK: Blackwell Science, 1992:281–304.
63. Bork C. *Cutaneous side effects of drugs.* Philadelphia, PA: WB Saunders, 1988.
64. Call TG, Creagan ET, Frytak S, et al. Phase I trial of combined recombinant interleukin-2 with levamisole in patients with advanced malignant disease. *Am J Clin Oncol* 1994;17:344–347.
65. Hortobagyi GN, Richman SP, Dandridge K, et al. Immunotherapy with BCG administered by scarification: standardization of reactions and management of side effects. *Cancer* 1978;42:2293–2303.
66. Ogilvie GK, Richardson RC, Curtis CR, et al. Acute and short-term toxicoses associated with the administration of doxorubicin to dogs with malignant tumors. *J Am Vet Med Assoc* 1989;195:1584–1587.
67. Valeyrie L, Bastuji-Garin S, Revuz J, et al. Adverse cutaneous reactions to imatinib (STI571) in Philadelphia chromosome-positive leukemias: a prospective study of 54 patients. *J Am Acad Dermatol* 2003;48(2):201–206.
68. Bhargava P, Gammon D, McCormick MJ. Hypersensitivity and idiosyncratic reactions to oxaliplatin. *Cancer* 2004;100(1):211–212.
69. Georgieva J, Steinhoff M, Orfanos CE, et al. Ethylene-oxide-induced pruritus associated with extracorporeal photochemotherapy. *Transfusion* 2004;44(10):1532–1533.
70. Calnan CD, O'Neill D. Itching in tension states. *Br J Dermatol* 1952;64:274–280.
71. Edwards AE, Shellow WV, Wright ET, et al. Pruritic skin disease, psychological stress, and the itch sensation. *Arch Dermatol* 1976;112:339–343.
72. Musaph H. Psychodynamics in itching states. *Int J Psychoanal* 1968;49:336–340.
73. Whitlock FA. Pruritus generalized and localised. In: Whitlock FA, ed. *Psychophysiological aspects of skin disease.* London: WB Saunders, 1976:110–129.
74. Sheehan-Dare RA, Henderson MJ, Cotterill JA. Anxiety and depression in patients with chronic urticaria and generalized pruritus. *Br J Dermatol* 1990;123:769–774.
75. Fleischer AB Jr. Pruritus in the elderly: management by senior dermatologists. *J Am Acad Dermatol* 1993;28:603–609.
76. Ghiadially R, Halkier-Sorensen L, Elias PM. Effects of petrolatum on stratum corneum structure and function. *J Am Acad Dermatol* 1992;26:387–396.
77. Fransway AF, Winkelmann RK. Treatment of pruritus. *Semin Dermatol* 1988;7:310–325.
78. Watsky KL, Freije L, Leneveu MC, et al. Water-in-oil emollients as steroid sparing adjunctive therapy in the treatment of psoriasis. *Cutis* 1992;50:383–386.
79. Ronayne C, Bray G, Robertson G. The use of aqueous cream to relieve pruritus in patients with liver disease. *Br J Nurs* 1993;2:527–528.
80. Fleischer AB Jr. Treatment of atopic dermatitis: role of tacrolimus ointment as a topical noncorticosteroidal therapy. *J Allergy Clin Immunol* 1999;104:126–130.
81. Kang S, Lucky AW, Pariser D, et al. Long-term safety and efficacy of tacrolimus ointment for the treatment of atopic dermatitis in children. *J Am Acad Dermatol* 2001;44(Suppl 1):S58–S64.
82. Breneman DL, Cardone JS, Blumsack RF, et al. Topical capsaicin for hemodialysis-related pruritus. *J Am Acad Dermatol* 1992;26:91–94.
83. Leibsohn E. Treatment of notalgia paresthetica with capsaicin. *Cutis* 1992;49:335–336.
84. Fusco GM, Giacovazzo M. Peppers and pain: the promise of capsaicin. *Drugs* 1997;53(6):909–914.
85. Shuttleworth D, Hill S, Marks R, et al. Relief of experimentally induced pruritus with a novel mixture of local anesthetic agents. *Br J Dermatol* 1988;119:535–540.
86. Drake L, Breneman D, Greene S, et al. Effects of topical doxepin 5% cream on pruritic eczema. *J Invest Dermatol* 1992;98:605.
87. Morison WL, Parrish J, Fitzpartick TB. Oral psoralen photochemotherapy of atopic eczema. *Br J Dermatol* 1978;98(1):25–30.
88. Zanolli MD, Feldman SR, Clark AR, et al. *Phototherapy and psoriasis treatment protocols.* New York: Parthenon Publishers, 2000.
89. Pederson JA, Matter BJ, Czerwinski AW, et al. Relief of idiopathic generalized pruritus in dialysis patients treated with activated oral charcoal. *Ann Intern Med* 1980;93:446–448.
90. Ghent CN, Carruthers SG. Treatment of pruritus in primary biliary cirrhosis with rifampin. Results of a double-blind, crossover, randomized trial. *Gastroenterology* 1988;94:488–493.
91. Bergasa NV. The pruritus of cholestasis. *Semin Dermatol* 1995;14:302–312.
92. Muller C, Pongratz S, Pidlich J, et al. Treatment of pruritus in chronic liver disease with the 5-hydroxytryptamine receptor type 3 antagonist ondansetron: a randomized, placebo-controlled, double-blind cross-over trial. *Eur J Gastroenterol Hepatol* 1998;10:865–870.
93. Jekler J, Larko O. UVA solarium versus UVB phototherapy of atopic dermatitis: a paired–comparison study. *Br J Dermatol* 1991;125:569–572.
94. Calabrese L, Fleischer AB. Thalidomide: current and potential clinical applications. *Am J Med* 2000;108(6):487–495.
95. Winkelmann RK. Pharmacologic control of pruritus. *Med Clin North Am* 1982;66:1119–1133.
96. Richelson B. Tricyclic antidepressants block H1 receptors of mouse neuroblastoma cells. *Nature* 1978;274:176–177.
97. Zylicz Z, Smits C, Krajnik M. Paroxetine for pruritus in advanced cancer. *J Pain Symptom Manage* 1998;16:121–124.
98. Aoki T, Kushimoto H, Hishikawa Y, et al. Nocturnal scratching and its relationship to the disturbed sleep of itchy subjects. *Clin Exp Dermatol* 1991;16:268–272.
99. Doherty V, Sylvester DGH, Kennedy CTC, et al. Treatment of atopic eczema with antihistamines with a low sedative profile. *BMJ* 1989;298:96.
100. Burtin C, Noirot C, Giroux C, et al. Decreased skin response to intradermal histamine in cancer patients. *J Allergy Clin Immunol* 1986;78:83–89.
101. Guillot B, Blazquez L, Bessis D, et al. A prospective study of cutaneous adverse events induced by low-dose alpha-interferon treatment for malignant melanoma. *Dermatology* 2004;208(1):49–54.
102. Epstein E, Pinski JB. A blind study. *Arch Dermatol* 1964;89:548–549.
103. Tinegate H, McLelland J. Transcutaneous electrical nerve stimulation may improve pruritus associated with haematological disorders. *Clin Lab Haematol* 2002;24(6):389–390.

CHAPTER 21 ■ TREATMENT OF TUMOR-RELATED SKIN DISORDERS

JOHN A. CARUCCI

As the number of patients diagnosed with cancer continues to rise, a concomitant increase in tumor-related skin disorders (TRSDs) can be expected. Management of these conditions, which can be challenging, is essential to the patient's overall sense of comfort and well-being. In some cases, diagnosis of TRSDs may permit early detection of occult malignancy. In this chapter, tumor-associated skin conditions are divided into two groups:

1. Generalized eruptions associated with internal malignancy
2. Cancer-related genodermatoses.

These disorders are reviewed with respect to commonly associated malignancies (Table 21.1). Emphasis is placed on the more common examples of these uncommon conditions and potential management strategies are discussed.

GENERALIZED ERUPTIONS ASSOCIATED WITH INTERNAL MALIGNANCY

Pruritus

Pruritus, or itch, is often nonspecific. It is one of the most common complaints in the elderly patient and is most commonly secondary to xerosis (dry skin, Figure 21.1B) (1). However, intractable pruritus accompanied by severe excoriations may be an indicator of internal malignancy (1). This type of pruritus is most commonly encountered in Hodgkin's lymphoma but may be observed with any internal malignancy (2). There are often no true primary lesions on examination but secondary changes including excoriations and subsequent lichenification and pigmentary alterations can be significant (Figure 21.1A). Pruritus has been reported in up to 25% of patients with Hodgkin's disease and may be an indicator of less favorable prognosis when associated with fever or weight loss (2). Pruritus of Hodgkin's disease is described as intense and burning and usually begins on a localized area.

Pruritus may also be a sign of cholestatic liver disease, renal disease, human immunodeficiency virus (HIV) disease, thyrotoxicosis, or diabetes (1). Infestation with scabies must also be considered in the differential diagnosis.

In contrast to the nonmalignant associations of localized pruritus, adenocarcinoma and squamous cell carcinoma (SCC)

of the brain (3,4), breast (5), colon (6), pancreas (7), and stomach (8) have been associated with generalized pruritus. Unilateral paroxysmal facial pruritus was reported as a presenting sign in two children with brain stem glioma (4). In both cases, pruritus resolved after radiation therapy was given for the glioma.

Intractable pruritus is best evaluated by a dermatologist, who can distinguish primary pruritus from pruritus secondary to some other cutaneous condition. Workup should include a thorough history and physical examination including baseline evaluation of complete blood count (CBC), liver function tests (LFTs), and chest x-ray. Skin biopsy of primary lesions, if present, may determine the cause of the pruritus.

TABLE 21.1

TUMOR-ASSOCIATED SKIN DISORDERS

Tumor-associated disorder	Commonly associated cancer
Pruritus	Hodgkin's lymphoma
Leser-Trelat	Gastric adenocarcinoma
Erythema gyratum repens	Lung cancer
Hypertrichosis lanuginosa acquisita	Lung cancer
Necrolytic migratory erythema	Glucagonoma
Paraneoplastic pemphigus	Non-Hodgkin's lymphoma
	Chronic lymphocytic leukemia
Bazex syndrome	Aerodigestive tract carcinoma
Acanthosis nigricans	Gastric adenocarcinoma
Dermatomyositis	Ovarian carcinoma
Sweet's syndrome	Leukemia
	Colorectal carcinoma
Muir-Torre syndrome	Colorectal carcinoma
Cowden syndrome	Breast carcinoma
	Thyroid carcinoma
Multiple endocrine neoplasia	Pheochromocytoma
	Thyroid carcinoma
Peutz-Jeghers syndrome	Colonic adenoma

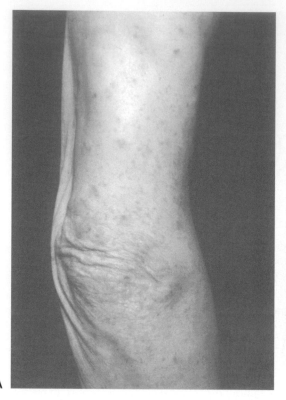
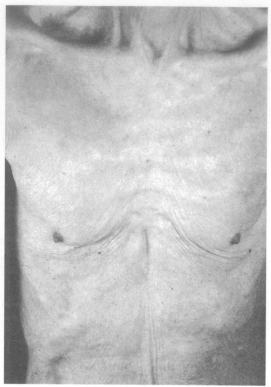

FIGURE 21.1. A: Pruritus in Hodgkin's Disease. **B:** Pruritus associated with xerosis (NYU Skin and Cancer slide collection).

In addition, age-appropriate and symptom-directed cancer screening should be updated. Treatment options include oral antihistamines (especially sedating antihistamines), topical corticosteroids, and ultraviolet light therapy. Zylicz et al. have reported successful treatment of pruritus associated with cholestasis in disseminated cancer using buprenorphine with low-dose naloxone (9).

Sign of Leser-Trelat

The sign of Leser-Trelat is the sudden appearance of numerous seborrheic keratoses in association with internal malignancy. It has been most commonly associated with gastric carcinoma (10). The sign has been attributed separately to Edmund Leser and Ulysse Trelat (11,12). Interestingly, this represents a misnomer because both individuals were actually observing cherry hemangiomas. In fact, it was Hollander who first emphasized the association between internal cancer and seborrheic keratoses in 1900 (13). Little is known about the pathogenesis of Leser-Trelat; however, some investigators point toward increases in tumor-derived growth factors (14).

Seborrheic keratoses are benign lesions and are best described as waxy, hyperpigmented papules or plaques (Figure 21.2). They appear to be "stuck on" and look as though they might be easily peeled away from the surface of the skin. They are extremely common in older individuals and represent no danger to patients. The differential diagnosis may include benign, premalignant, and malignant lesions including lentigines, nevi, actinic keratoses, atypical nevi, pigmented Bowen's disease, and melanoma. Diagnosis can be confirmed by simple skin biopsy performed by a dermatologist. Leser-Trelat is characterized by the sudden eruption of multiple seborrheic keratoses and most commonly affects the back and

chest, although the extremities, groin, and even the face may be affected (12). It must be emphasized that although seborrheic keratoses are common, the sudden appearance of numerous lesions or their appearance before the third decade is not common and should prompt further investigation. Vielhauer et al. have reported the diagnosis of occult renal cell carcinoma in a patient with Leser-Trelat (10). Curative nephrectomy was performed as a result of early diagnosis.

Further investigation in patients with Leser-Trelat should include a complete history and physical examination accompanied by routine blood studies including CBC, LFTs, chest x-ray, mammogram and pap smear for women, and prostate-specific antigen (PSA) for men. Endoscopic evaluation of the colon should also be considered, as should any symptom-directed diagnostic studies.

The presence of seborrheic keratoses itself is not dangerous to the patient and reassurance of this is necessary. If desired, they may be removed by curettage under local anesthesia with little risk of scarring. Other treatment methods include cryosurgery with liquid nitrogen and chemical cauterization with topical application of 70% trichloroacetic acid.

Erythema Gyratum Repens

Erythema gyratum repens is part of the group of gyrate erythemas (15). These are reactive, inflammatory dermatoses that share morphologic characteristics and have been described as "figurate," "polycyclic," and "serpiginous" in appearance (16). None of the gyrate erythemas has the characteristic appearance of erythema gyratum repens.

Erythema gyratum repens was first described by Gamel in 1952, who reported it in association with breast carcinoma (17). Since that time, the overwhelming instances of cases have been associated with internal malignancy (18).

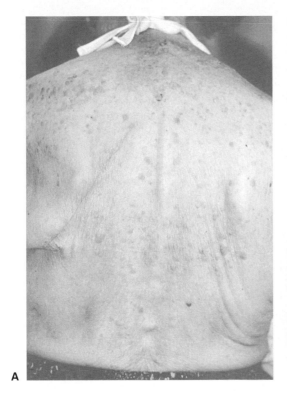
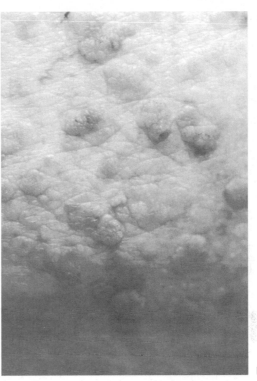

FIGURE 21.2. A: Leser-Trelat associated with lung cancer—note pneumonectomy scar. **B:** Close-up view of seborrheic keratoses in Leser Trelat (Yale Dermatology Residents' slide collection).

On clinical examination, serpiginous, erythematous bands that take on a "wood grain" or "zebra-like" appearance (Figure 21.3) are seen. There is usually scaling associated with the lesions and there are often multiple bands. Lesions may be indurated and are likely to migrate over the course of hours. There may be associated pruritus. Unlike the characteristic clinical picture, histopathologic findings are nonspecific and may include hyperkeratosis, acanthosis, spongiosis, and a superficial perivascular lymphohistiocytic infiltrate (15).

On suspicion of erythema gyratum repens, dermatologic consultation is required for confirmation. Because of the likelihood of association with internal malignancy, screening for internal malignancy should be performed. Standard screening laboratory and imaging studies should be performed with special attention toward ruling out cancer of the lung (18,19). Although most commonly associated with lung cancer (20), erythema gyratum has been reported with breast and renal cancer (21) and, in rare cases, in the absence of malignancy (22). It is especially important to repeat screening tests periodically because the eruption may precede the onset of malignancy (23).

The most effective treatment is removal of the underlying tumor (19). Skin manifestations have resolved after removal of localized tumors or may persist until death in the face of widespread disease. Associated pruritus and inflammation may be relieved with oral antihistamines in combination with midpotency topical corticosteroids.

Hypertrichosis Lanuginosa Acquisita

Hypertrichosis lanuginosa acquisita, also referred to as malignant down, is characterized by the growth of fine, nonpigmented hair that occurs primarily on the face (23). It is most commonly associated with small cell and non–small cell carcinoma of the lung (24) and colorectal cancer (25) and has been reported with carcinomas of the kidney (26) and pancreas (27) and in metastatic melanoma (28). It has been associated with other conditions including shock, thyrotoxicosis, and porphyria and ingestion of drugs including cyclosporine,

FIGURE 21.3. Erythema gyratum repens in a patient with lung cancer (NYU Skin and Cancer slide collection).

streptomycin, phenytoin, spironolactone, diazoxide, minoxidil, interferon, and corticosteroids (23).

The most effective treatment for malignant down is that it successfully treats the underlying tumor. Management of cosmesis may be attempted through electrolysis, depilatories, or shaving. Because the hairs are not pigmented, treatment with hair removal laser would likely be unsuccessful because lasers target melanin in the hair follicle. Treatment with eflornithine HCl cream (13.9%) applied to the affected area twice daily may be successful. This agent inhibits ornithine decarboxylase, a key hair cycle enzyme, and may result in noticeably diminished hair growth (29). The presence of hypertrichosis lanuginosa implies poor prognosis and a survival time of <2 years in most patients (23).

Necrolytic Migratory Erythema

Necrolytic migratory erythema refers to cutaneous manifestations of the glucagonoma syndrome caused by a tumor of the pancreatic islet α-cells (30). The eruption begins as an erythematous patch involving the groin that spreads to the buttocks, perineum, thighs, and extremities (Figure 21.4).

The erythematous areas eventually undergo scaling and blister formation. Erosions occur subsequent to rupture of blisters and healing with induration and pigmentary change follows over the course of several weeks. This may follow a relapsing and remitting course and may be associated with stomatitis. The differential diagnosis includes intertrigo, superficial candidiasis, bullous drug eruption, and pemphigus (30). Histologic findings include dyskeratotic epidermal cells with superficial epidermal necrosis (Figure 21.4D) (30). The diagnostic features include elevated plasma glucagon levels. Dermatologic consultation should be sought to confirm the diagnosis as well as to rule out other skin disorders that may mimic necrolytic migratory erythema. As with other paraneoplastic syndromes, effective tumor therapy results in improvement of cutaneous symptoms (31). Unfortunately, patients with necrolytic migratory erythema may have metastatic disease at presentation. There have been reports of successful treatment using the

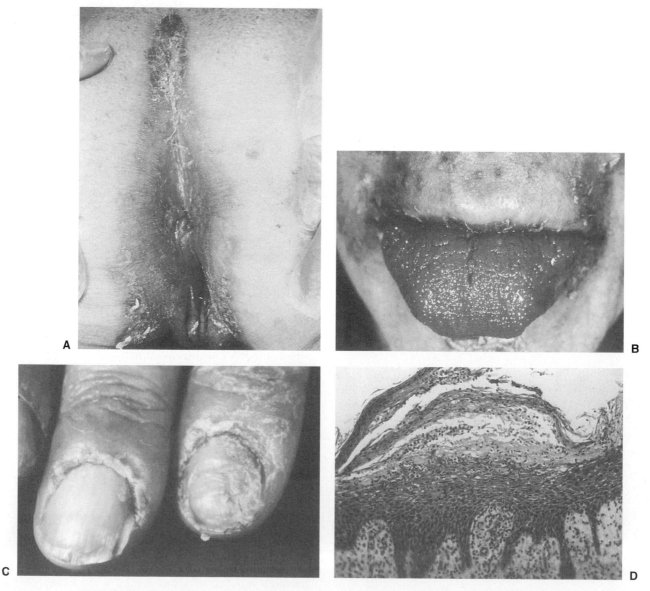

FIGURE 21.4. Necrolytic migratory erythema in the glucagonoma syndrome. **A:** Perianal blistering. **B:** Stomatitis **C:** Characteristic periungual involvement. **D:** Histologic findings include superficial epidermal necrosis and dyskeratotic cells (NYU Skin and Cancer slide collection).

somatostatin analog octreotide. Jockenhovel et al. reported temporary resolution of cutaneous symptoms with octreotide but noted that the drug had no effect on tumor growth (32). Resolution may be noted as early as 1 week after beginning therapy but resistance can develop. Shepherd et al. reported successful treatment of cutaneous symptoms with intravenous amino acids (33). While waiting for response, denuded areas should be gently cleansed twice daily, covered with a bland emollient, and dressed with a nonstick bandage. Appropriate monitoring for secondary infection is indicated and is especially important in the hospitalized patient. Interestingly, one of the originally described patients was recently reported as a long-term survivor 24 years after diagnosis (34). Necrolytic migratory erythema has recently been reported in a patient with myelodysplastic syndrome without glucagonoma or evidence of pancreatic disease (35).

Paraneoplastic Pemphigus

Pemphigus is an immunologically mediated blistering disorder of the skin (36). The three main subtypes, based on target antigens, include pemphigus vulgaris, pemphigus foliaceus (including fogo selvagem, an endemic form), and paraneoplastic pemphigus (PNP). PNP is characterized by severe stomatitis, oral ulcers, and skin lesions with variable morphology (37–39). It is characteristically associated with hematologic malignancies, especially non-Hodgkin's lymphoma and chronic lymphocytic leukemia (38). It has also been associated with spindle cell sarcoma, Waldenstrom's macroglobulinemia, thymoma (malignant and benign), Castleman's tumor and pancreatic carcinoma (39). The pathogenesis centers on production of autoantibodies that attack components of the hemidesmosome and desmosome that function to link the epidermal cells to their basement membrane and to one another (38). Weakening of this scaffolding system renders the epidermal cells more susceptible to shearing forces, resulting in formation of blisters. The blisters rupture and result in erosive stomatitis, oral ulcers, and cutaneous erosions. In PNP there may be autoantibodies that recognize desmoglein 3, desmoglein 1, plakin proteins, and the hemidesmosomal BP230 (BPAg1) antigen (40).

On physical examination, erosive stomatitis and ulceration of the oral mucosa (38,39) are found. There may be associated polymorphous skin lesions (Figure 21.5). The oral lesions are typically painful and interfere with eating. Skin biopsy will reveal varied findings (38,39). Perilesional biopsy will reveal suprabasilar acantholysis of oral epithelium or skin

epidermis. Necrotic keratinocytes along with a scant lymphocytic infiltrate may be observed. Direct immunofluorescence studies may demonstrate deposition of immunoglobulin (Ig)G and C3 on epidermal surfaces and variably along the basement membrane (41). Indirect immunofluorescence studies will show the presence of antibodies that recognize antigens on monkey esophagus as well as transitional epithelium from rat bladder (41). Immunoprecipitation studies will demonstrate the presence of autoantibodies to desmogleins 1 and 3, desmoplakins, or BPAg1. Owing to the complex nature of the disease and its diagnosis, the consideration of PNP demands consultation with a dermatologist.

Treatment can be difficult. Topical therapy is for the most part unrewarding; however, some patients may experience relief with the application of high-potency steroid gels to affected oral mucosa on a twice-daily basis. Viscous lidocaine, in general, is of little value, with most patients complaining of burning rather than experiencing relief. Resolution of ulcers has been obtained with administration of cyclosporine (5 mg per kg) in two to three divided daily doses (38). Cyclosporine, a potent immunosuppressive drug, is not without risk of significant side effects, including hypertension and renal compromise, and should only be administered by physicians who are familiar with its use and its side effects profile. Williams et al. have reported successful treatment of skin and oral lesions in a patient with PNP using mycophenolate mofetil (42). Mycophenolate mofetil is also a potent immunosuppressive agent with potential side effects that include bone marrow suppression. Other options include high-dose cyclophosphamide without stem cell rescue and monoclonal antibody to CD20 (Rituximab) (43).

Bazex Syndrome

Bazex syndrome or acrokeratosis paraneoplastica refers to a cutaneous syndrome of psoriasiform lesions on the ears, fingers, and toes, with associated nail changes that occur in the context of an internal malignancy (Figure 21.6) (44). Bazex et al. initially described this in association with carcinoma

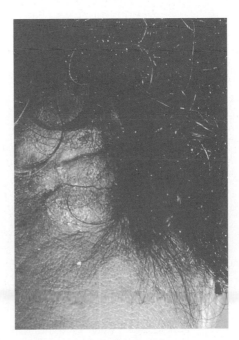

FIGURE 21.6. Bazex syndrome. Psoriasiform dermatitis (Yale Dermatology Residents' slide collection).

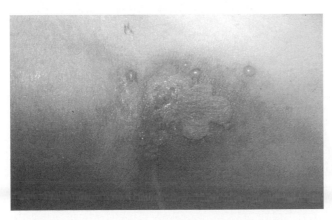

FIGURE 21.5. Paraneoplastic pemphigus. Although paraneoplastic pemphigus commonly affects the oral mucosa, other areas may present with superficial blisters as seen in this patient (NYU Skin and Cancer slide collection).

of the piriform sinus (45). Subsequent reports have described associations primarily with cancers of the aerodigestive tract and carcinomas metastatic to lymph nodes. In addition, Bazex has been reported with colon (46), bladder (47), and neuroendocrine cancer (48) and primary cutaneous SCC (49).

The syndrome may evolve through three stages (44). In the initial stage, there is vesicle formation with thickening of the periungual skin, subungual hyperkeratosis, and nail dystrophy. Erythematous scaled plaques develop on the ears, fingers, and toes. The lesions characteristically affect the dorsal aspects of the digits and the helices of the ears. This stage can last anywhere between 2 and 12 months. The second stage ensues if the tumor remains undiagnosed and untreated and is characterized by progression of skin lesions that are usually refractory to local therapy. With progression, violaceous color changes are noted on the palms and soles. If the tumor remains unrecognized, the third stage of Bazex is characterized by spread of skin lesions to the trunk, extremities, and scalp.

Histopathologic analysis may reveal foci epidermal cytoplasmic eosinophilia and vacuolization of keratinocytes with pyknosis of their nuclei. A perivascular mixed cell infiltrate may be present in the superficial dermis (44). In one report of Bazex syndrome associated with SCC of the tonsil, direct immunofluorescence studies showed deposition of IgA, IgM, IgG, and C3 on the basement membrane (50). The authors stated that this supported an immunologically mediated pathogenic mechanism.

Treatment of the tumor can result in resolution of cutaneous symptoms (51). This was illustrated in a recent report of Bazex on a primary cutaneous SCC of the lower extremity (49). In this case, cutaneous manifestations of Bazex syndrome resolved after excision of the skin cancer.

Acanthosis Nigricans

Acanthosis nigricans can be associated with internal cancers, particularly gastric adenocarcinoma, as well as endocrinopathies resulting in hyperinsulinemia and insulin resistance (52). The pathogenesis may lie in the similarity of insulin and insulin-like growth factor. Binding of insulin-like growth factor receptors by insulin or by tumor-derived growth factors may result in cellular growth and subsequent development of characteristic clinical findings.

On physical examination, velvet-like, hyperpigmented plaques are seen on the neck, axilla, inframammary folds, and groin (Figure 21.7) (53). There may be mucosal thickening as well (54). Microscopic examination shows hyperkeratosis and papillomatosis without epidermal hyperplasia or excess melanin deposition.

Acanthosis nigricans is most frequently associated with adenocarcinoma of the stomach (55) but may be associated with almost any internal cancer. Recently, the coexistence of acanthosis nigricans and Leser-Trelat was reported in a patient with advanced gastric adenocarcinoma (14). In this case, appearance of both conditions preceded other manifestations of the malignancy by 6 months. Treatment is difficult even with successful treatment of the underlying cancer.

Dermatomyositis

Dermatomyositis is characterized by proximal muscle weakness in conjunction with characteristic cutaneous findings and may occur in adults in association with any internal cancer (56). The proximal muscle weakness manifests with inability to perform daily activities such as combing hair, putting

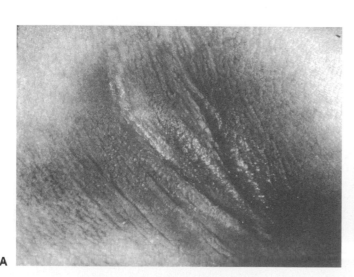
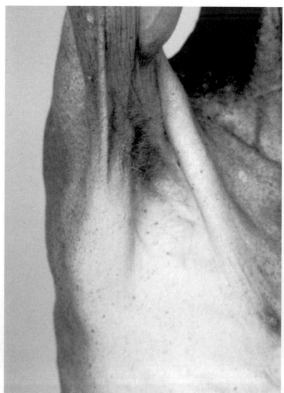

FIGURE 21.7. Acanthosis nigricans. **A:** Acanthosis nigricans is characterized by velvety, hyperpigmented plaques involving intertriginous areas (Yale Dermatology Residents' slide collection). **B:** Acanthosis nigricans in a patient with gastric carcinoma (NYU Skin and Cancer slide collection).

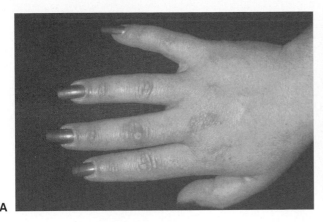
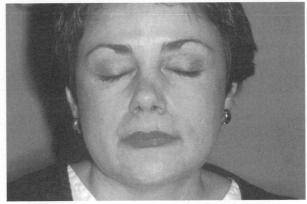

FIGURE 21.8. Dermatomyositis. **A:** Gottron's papule. **B:** Characteristic heliotrope rash (Yale Dermatology Residents' slide collection).

on or removing a shirt or a coat, and rising from a seated position. Cutaneous findings usually involve the periorbital area, chest, back, and fingers.

Cutaneous examination frequently reveals a heliotrope rash, Gottron's papules, and poikiloderma in a shawl-like distribution (Figure 21.8) (56). The heliotrope rash is characterized by an erythematous dermatitis involving the periorbital areas of the face. Gottron's papules are characteristic raised lesions present on the extensor aspects of the fingers. The shawl sign refers to poikiloderma (blotchy erythema with telangiectasias, atrophy, and hypopigmentation) involving the upper chest, shoulders, and upper back.

Skin biopsy is remarkable for superficial and deep perivascular infiltrate and there may be basement membrane thickening as in lupus (56). Laboratory values of creatine phosphokinase (CPK) and aldolase are elevated in dermatomyositis. Anti-jo-1 antibody and antinuclear antibodies may be present (56). The combination of the characteristic cutaneous findings, proximal muscle weakness, and elevated CPK and aldolase values are the diagnostic features.

Dermatomyositis may be associated with any malignancy, particularly ovarian cancer (56). This is supported by the findings of Cherin et al. (57), who reported ovarian cancer in 21% of their female patients over age 40 with dermatomyositis. This represents a significant increase over the percentage of ovarian carcinoma in the general population (~1%). Dermatomyositis has been reported with B cell lymphoma (58), thymoma (59),

colon cancer (60) and metastatic melanoma (61). It should be clear that patients with dermatomyositis must be evaluated for the presence of an internal malignancy with special attention to gynecologic cancers.

Sweet's Syndrome

Acute febrile neutrophilic dermatosis was first described by Robert Sweet (62,63). It is characterized by a combination of acute onset of fever, anemia, neutrophilia, and characteristic skin lesions (23,64,65). Skin lesions can be described as erythematous plaques and blisters that involve the face, neck, chest, and extremities (Figure 21.9). Involvement of the eyes, joints, and oral mucosa as well as involvement of the lung, liver, kidney, and central nervous system has been described (65).

Sweet's syndrome occurs in the context of hematopoietic tumors, especially leukemia, and has been reported with solid malignant tumors (66). It has also been reported with chronic inflammatory disorders (67) and, in rare cases, with pregnancy (68). In one review of 249 cases, it was reported that Sweet's syndrome was associated with hematologic malignancies in 40% of cases and with solid tumors in 7% of cases (64). In a study of cases of Sweet's syndrome associated with solid tumors (66), the most commonly associated malignancies were genitourinary carcinomas (37%), breast carcinomas (23%), and cancers of the gastrointestinal tract (17%).

Sweet's syndrome responds rapidly to oral corticosteroid therapy (67). Other treatments including potassium iodide, colchicine, dapsone, clofazimine, and cyclosporine have been reported (65,67,69).

CANCER-RELATED GENODERMATOSES

Muir-Torre Syndrome

The Muir-Torre syndrome (MTS) was first described by Muir et al. in 1967 (70), and by Torre in 1968 (71), who noted the association of sebaceous adenomas of the skin and internal cancers. The internal cancers were most commonly low-grade colorectal carcinomas. MTS is transmitted in an autosomal dominant manner (72). The skin lesions most often associated with MTS are sebaceous adenomas, sebaceous epitheliomas, sebaceous carcinomas, and keratoacanthoma (KA) (72).

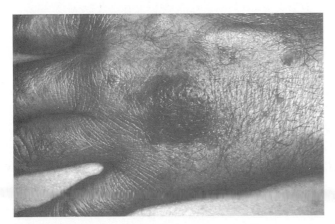

FIGURE 21.9. Sweet's syndrome. An indurated plaque in a patient with Sweet's syndrome in acute myelogenous leukemia (NYU Skin and Cancer slide collection).

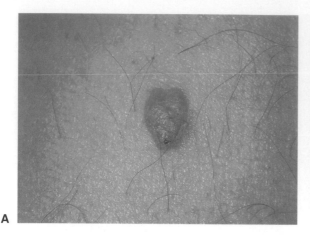

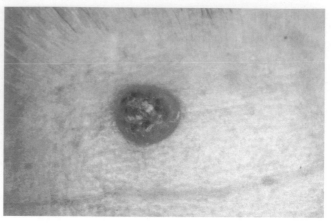

A   B

FIGURE 21.10. Muir-Torre Syndrome. **A:** Sebaceous carcinomas as shown here are seen in Muir-Torre Syndrome (Photo by John Carucci). **B:** Keratoacanthomas may be associated with Muir-Torre syndrome.

On physical examination, sebaceous adenomas appear as flesh- to yellow-colored papules, usually measuring <5 mm. They are commonly located on the face but can occur anywhere. Sebaceous epitheliomas can take on a cystic appearance whereas sebaceous carcinomas typically appear as a papule on the eyelid and can be overlooked in the early stages. Sebaceous carcinomas are common on the eyelid but may appear as cystic lesions on the extremities (Figure 21.10). KAs are a subtype of SCC and usually occur as a rapidly growing nodule with a keratinaceous central core.

The treatment of choice for sebaceous carcinoma and KA-like SCC on the face is Mohs' micrographic surgery (MMS) (73). MMS offers the highest rate of cure and the advantage of tissue conservation due to superior margin control. Sebaceous epitheliomas can be excised with clear margins whereas sebaceous adenomas can be removed by tangential (shave) excision. Incomplete removal is likely to result in local recurrence. Management must proceed beyond treatment of the primary skin lesions. MTS is associated with colorectal, genitourinary, and hematologic malignancies and appropriate cancer screening must be performed on patients and their family members because of the autosomal dominant mode of inheritance (72).

Cowden Syndrome

Cowden syndrome is also known as *multiple hamartoma syndrome* and is characterized by facial and oral lesions when associated with cancers of the breast and thyroid (74). Multiple hamartoma syndrome is inherited in an autosomal dominant manner, and although only approximately 100 cases have been reported so far, it may be more common than originally thought (75). The usual age of presentation is between 20 and 40 years and the primary mucocutaneous manifestations include facial trichilemmomas and oral papillomas (75). Cowden syndrome is believed to be due to mutations in the *PTEN* gene (76).

Trichilemmomas appear as tan to yellow verrucous papules on the center of the face (Figure 21.11). Oral papillomas give a cobblestone appearance to the tongue and oral mucosa (74). There may be associated acral keratotic papules on the hands and wrists and translucent punctate keratoses on the palms and soles.

When Cowden syndrome is suspected, dermatologic consultation is required for confirmation. Appropriate cancer screening should be performed for breast and thyroid carcinomas (77). Trichilemmomas are benign lesions; however,

trichilemmomal carcinoma has been reported in Cowden syndrome (78). Treatment may be attempted by laser ablation, dermabrasion, or shave excision.

Multiple Endocrine Neoplasia

Multiple endocrine neoplasia (MEN IIb) is also known as the *multiple mucosal neuroma syndrome* (79). It is inherited in an autosomal dominant manner because of a mutation on chromosome 10q11.2 but can occur sporadically in up to 50% of cases (79). Patients usually present early and it is to be noted that the appearance of mucosal lesions may precede development of internal cancers by 10 years. It is thought to be due to a mutation in the RET proto-oncogene, which may affect neural crest development (80).

Mucocutaneous signs include neuromas on the tongue, lips, and oral mucosa. These appear as papules or nodules and may involve the palatal, nasal, and laryngeal mucosa (79). Patients with MEN IIb exhibit a marfanoid habitus. Associated internal cancers include pheochromocytoma and medullary carcinoma of the thyroid. Gastrointestinal neuromas may lead to diarrhea, constipation, and megacolon.

If MEN is suspected, consultation with a dermatologist and geneticist is indicated. Patients and family members need to be evaluated for internal malignancies and workup should include urine catecholamine level, thyroid scan, thyroid function

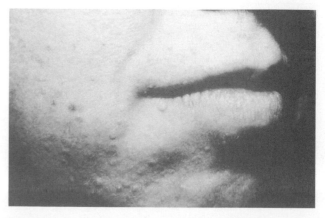

FIGURE 21.11. Cowden syndrome. Perioral trichilemmomas are characteristic in Cowden syndrome (Yale Dermatology Residents' slide collection).

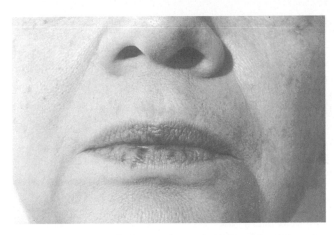

FIGURE 21.12. Peutz-Jeghers syndrome. Labial lentigines in a patient with Peutz-Jeghers syndrome (Yale Dermatology Residents' slide collection).

tests, and computed tomography (CT) scan of the abdomen. Treatment of neuromas by excision often results in recurrence.

Peutz-Jeghers Syndrome

Peutz-Jeghers syndrome (PJS) or periorificial lentiginosis is characterized by perioral skin lesions in association with colonic polyps that have malignant potential (81,82). It can be inherited in an autosomal dominant manner or may occur sporadically (81,82). The pigmented lesions appear around the mouth during the first few years of life and precede the development of colonic polyps by at least 10 years in most cases (81). PJS is associated with loss of heterozygosity or somatic mutations at the lkb1 locus, suggesting that serine/threonine kinase LKB1 acts as a tumor suppressor (83).

The cutaneous lesions are pigmented macules usually measuring between 2 and 5 mm (Figure 21.12) (81). They are uniformly brown to black in color, symmetrical, and occur in the perioral area, buccal mucosa, palms, soles, and digits.

When PJS is suspected, consultation with a dermatologist and a gastroenterologist is required. PJS is associated with hamartomas of the colon, which have the potential to develop into adenocarcinoma. There is also increased risk of ovarian, breast, and pancreatic carcinoma. Therefore, adequate periodic screening is essential for patients with PJS.

Lentigines can be treated successfully with the Q-switched ruby laser (693 nm) (84).

CONCLUSIONS

Tumor-associated skin disorders may appear in many forms with varying degrees of severity. In select cases, prompt diagnosis and effective management can lead to early detection of cancer and alter prognosis. It is therefore essential that any suspected case be evaluated by a dermatologist.

References

1. Duncan WC, Fenske NA. Cutaneous signs of internal disease in the elderly. *Geriatrics* 1990;45(8):24–30.
2. Cavalli F. Rare syndromes in Hodgkin's disease. *Ann Oncol* 1998;9(Suppl 5):S109–S113.
3. Adreev VC, Petkov I. Skin manifestations associated with tumours of the brain. *Br J Dermatol* 1975;92(6):675–678.
4. Summers CG, MacDonald JT. Paroxysmal facial itch: a presenting sign of childhood brainstem glioma. *J Child Neurol* 1988;3(3):189–192.
5. Twycross RG. Pruritus and pain in en cuirass breast cancer. *Lancet* 1981;2(8248):696.
6. Katz SK, Gordon KB, Roenigk HH. The cutaneous manifestations of gastrointestinal disease. *Prim Care* 1996;23(3):455–476.
7. Warren KW, Braasch JW, Thum CW. Diagnosis and surgical treatment of carcinoma of the pancreas. *Curr Probl Surg* 1968;3:3–70.
8. Shoenfeld Y, Weiberger A, Ben-Bassat M, et al. Generalized pruritus in metastatic adenocarcinoma of the stomach. *Dermatologica* 1977;155(2):122–124.
9. Zylicz Z, Stork N, Krajnik M. Severe pruritus of cholestasis in disseminated cancer: developing a rational treatment strategy. A case report. *J Pain Symptom Manage* 2005;29(1):100–103.
10. Vielhauer V, Herzinger T, Korting HC. The sign of Leser-Trelat: a paraneoplastic cutaneous syndrome that facilitates early diagnosis of occult cancer. *Eur J Med Res* 2000;5(12):512–516.
11. Leser E. Ueber ein die krebskranheit beim Menschen haufig begleitendes, noch wenig gekanntes symptom. *Munch Med Wochenschr* 1901;51:2035–2036.
12. Schwartz RA. Sign of Leser-Trelat. *J Am Acad Dermatol* 1996;35(1):88–95.
13. Hollander E. Beitrage zur fruhdiagnose des darmcarcinomas (hereditatsverhaltnisse und hautveranderungen). *Dtsch Med Wochenschr* 1900;26:483–485.
14. Yeh MS, Plunkett TA, Harper PG, et al. Coexistence of acanthosis nigricans and the sign of Leser-Trelat in a patient with gastric adenocarcinoma: a case report and literature review. *J Am Acad Dermatol* 2000;42:357–362.
15. White J. Gyrate erythema. *Dermatol Clin* 1985;3:129–139.
16. Kurzrock R, Cohen PR. Erythema gyratum repens. *JAMA* 1995;273(7):594.
17. Gammel JA. Erythema gyratum repens; skin manifestations in patient with carcinoma of breast. *AMA Arch Derm Syphilol* 1952;66(4):494–505.
18. Boyd AS, Neldner KH. Erythema gyratum repens without underlying disease. *J Am Acad Dermatol* 1993;28(1):132.
19. Boyd AS, Neldner KH, Menter A. Erythema gyratum repens: a paraneoplastic eruption. *J Am Acad Dermatol* 1992;26(5 Pt 1):757–762.
20. Olsen TG, Milroy SK, Jones-Olsen S. Erythema gyratum repens with associated squamous cell carcinoma of the lung. *Cutis* 1984;34(4):351–353, 355.
21. Kwatra A, McDonald RE, Corriere JN Jr. Erythema gyratum repens in association with renal cell carcinoma. *J Urol* 1998;159(6):2077.
22. Kawakami T, Saito R. Erythema gyratum repens unassociated with underlying malignancy. *J Dermatol* 1995;22(8):587–589.
23. Kurzrock R, Cohen PR. Cutaneous paraneoplastic syndromes in solid tumors. *Am J Med* 1995;99(6):662–671.
24. Knowling MA, Meakin JW, Hradsky NS, et al. Hypertrichosis lanuginosa acquisita associated with adenocarcinoma of the lung. *Can Med Assoc J* 1982;126(11):1308–1310.
25. Brinkmann J, Breier B, Goos M. Hypertrichosis lanuginosa acquisita in ulcerative colitis with colon cancer. *Hautarzt* 1992;43(11):714–716.
26. Duncan LE, Hemming JD. Renal cell carcinoma of the kidney and hypertrichosis lanuginosa acquisita. *Br J Urol* 1994;74(5):678–679.
27. McLean DI, Macaulay JC. Hypertrichosis lanuginosa acquisita associated with pancreatic carcinoma. *Br J Dermatol* 1977;96(3):313–316.
28. Begany A, Nagy Vezekenyi K. Hypertrichosis lanuginosa acquisita. *Acta Derm Venereol* 1992;72(1):18–19.
29. Hickman JG, Huber F, Palmisano M. Human dermal safety studies with eflornithine HCl 13.9% cream (Vaniqa), a novel treatment for excessive facial hair. *Curr Med Res Opin* 2001;16(4):235–244.
30. Shyr YM, Su CH, Lee CH, et al. Glucagonoma syndrome: a case report. *Zhonghua Yi Xue Za Zhi (Taipei)* 1999;62(9):639–643.
31. Thorisdottir K, Camisa C, Tomecki KJ, et al. Necrolytic migratory erythema: a report of three cases. *J Am Acad Dermatol* 1994;30(2 Pt 2):324–329.
32. Jockenhovel F, Lederbogen S, Olbricht T, et al. The long-acting somatostatin analogue octreotide alleviates symptoms by reducing posttranslational conversion of prepro-glucagon to glucagon in a patient with malignant glucagonoma, but does not prevent tumor growth. *Clin Investig* 1994;72(2):127–133.
33. Shepherd ME, Raimer SS, Tyring SK, et al. Treatment of necrolytic migratory erythema in glucagonoma syndrome. *J Am Acad Dermatol* 1991;25(5 Pt 2):925–928.
34. Nightingale KJ, Davies MG, Kingsnorth AN. Glucagonoma syndrome: survival 24 years following diagnosis. *Dig Surg* 1999;16(1):68–71.
35. Technau K, Renkl A, Norgauer J, et al. Necrolytic migratory erythema with myelodysplastic syndrome without glucagonoma. *Eur J Dermatol* 2005;15(2):110–112.
36. Camisa C, Warner M. Treatment of pemphigus. *Dermatol Nurs* 1998;10(2):115–118, 123–131.
37. Allen CM, Camisa C. Paraneoplastic pemphigus: a review of the literature. *Oral Dis* 2000;6(4):208–214.
38. Anhalt GJ. Paraneoplastic pemphigus. *Adv Dermatol* 1997;12:77–96, discussion 97.
39. Sklavounou A, Laskaris G. Paraneoplastic pemphigus: a review. *Oral Oncol* 1998;34(6):437–440.
40. Anhalt GJ. Making sense of antigens and antibodies in pemphigus. *J Am Acad Dermatol* 1999;40(5 Pt 1):763–766.

41. Morrison LH. When to request immunofluorescence: practical hints. *Semin Cutan Med Surg* 1999;18(1):36–42.

42. Williams JV, Marks JG Jr, Billingsley EM. Use of mycophenolate mofetil in the treatment of paraneoplastic pemphigus. *Br J Dermatol* 2000;142(3):506–508.

43. Wade MS, Black MM. Paraneoplastic pemphigus: a brief update. *Australas J Dermatol* 2005;46(1):1–8; quiz 9–10.

44. Bolognia JL. Bazex syndrome: acrokeratosis paraneoplastica. *Semin Dermatol* 1995;14(2):84–89.

45. Bazex A, Salvador R, Dupre A. Syndrome para-neoplastique a type d'hyperatose des extremites. Guerison apres le traitement de l'epithelioma larynge. *Bull Soc Fr Dermatol Syphiligr* 1965;72:182.

46. Hsu YS, Lien GS, Lai HH, et al. Acrokeratosis paraneoplastica (Bazex syndrome) with adenocarcinoma of the colon: report of a case and review of the literature. *J Gastroenterol* 2000;35(6):460–464.

47. Arregui MA, Raton JA, Landa N, et al. Bazex's syndrome (acrokeratosis paraneoplastica)–first case report of association with a bladder carcinoma. *Clin Exp Dermatol* 1993;18(5):445–448.

48. Halpern SM, O'Donnell LJ, Makunura CN. Acrokeratosis paraneoplastica of Bazex in association with a metastatic neuroendocrine tumour. *J R Soc Med* 1995;88(6):353P–354P.

49. Hara M, Hunayama M, Aiba S, et al. Acrokeratosis paraneoplastica (Bazex syndrome) associated with primary cutaneous squamous cell carcinoma of the lower leg, vitiligo and alopecia areata. *Br J Dermatol* 1995;133(1):121–124.

50. Pecora AL, Landsman L, Imgrund SP, et al. Acrokeratosis paraneoplastica (Bazex' syndrome). Report of a case and review of the literature. *Arch Dermatol* 1983;119(10):820–826.

51. Wareing MJ, Vaughan-Jones SA, McGibbon DH. Acrokeratosis paraneoplastica: Bazex syndrome. *J Laryngol Otol* 1996;110(9):899–900.

52. Kihiczak NI, Leevy CB, Krysicki MM, et al. Cutaneous signs of selected systemic diseases. *J Med* 1999;30(1–2):3–12.

53. Matsuoka LY, Wortsman J, Goldman J. Acanthosis nigricans. *Clin Dermatol* 1993;11(1):21–25.

54. Ramirez-Amador V, Esquivel-Pedraza L, Caballero-Mendoza E, et al. Oral manifestations as a hallmark of malignant acanthosis nigricans. *J Oral Pathol Med* 1999;28(6):278–281.

55. Fukushima H, Fukushima M, Mizokami M, et al. Case report of an advanced gastric cancer associated with diffused protruded lesions at the angles of the mouth, oral cavity and esophagus. *Kurume Med J* 1991;38(2):123–127.

56. Callen JP. Dermatomyositis. *Lancet* 2000;355(9197):53–57.

57. Cherin P, Piette JC, Herson S, et al. Dermatomyositis and ovarian cancer: a report of 7 cases and literature review. *J Rheumatol* 1993;20(11):1897–1899.

58. Anzai S, Katagiri K, Sato T, et al. Dermatomyositis associated with primary intramuscular B cell lymphoma. *J Dermatol* 1997;24(10):649–653.

59. Nagasawa K. Thymoma-associated dermatomyositis and polymyositis. *Intern Med* 1999;38(2):81–82.

60. Nyui S, Osanai H, Ohba S, et al. Relapse of colon cancer followed by polymyositis: report of a case and review of the literature. *Surg Today* 1997;27(6):559–562.

61. Shorr AF, Yacavone M, Seguin S, et al. Dermatomyositis and malignant melanoma. *Am J Med Sci* 1997;313(4):249–251.

62. Sweet R. Further observations on acute febrile neutrophilic dermatosis. *Br J Dermatol* 1968;80:800–805.

63. Sweet R. Acute febrile neutrophilic dermatosis–1978. *Br J Dermatol* 1979;100:93–99.

64. Burrall B. Sweet's syndrome (acute febrile neutrophilic dermatosis). *Dermatol Online J* 1999;5(1):8.

65. Chan HL, Lee YS, Kuo TT. Sweet's syndrome: clinicopathologic study of eleven cases. *Int J Dermatol* 1994;33(6):425–432.

66. Cohen PR, Holder WR, Tucker SB, et al. Sweet syndrome in patients with solid tumors. *Cancer* 1993;72(9):2723–2731.

67. Cohen PR, Kurzrock R. Sweet's syndrome: a neutrophilic dermatosis classically associated with acute onset and fever. *Clin Dermatol* 2000;18(3):265–282.

68. Satra K, Zalka A, Cohen PR, et al. Sweet's syndrome and pregnancy. *J Am Acad Dermatol* 1994;30(2 Pt 2):297–300.

69. von den Driesch P. Sweet's syndrome (acute febrile neutrophilic dermatosis). *J Am Acad Dermatol* 1994;31(4):535–556; quiz 557–560.

70. Muir E, Bell A, Barlow K. Multiple primary carcinomata of the colon, duodenum, and larynx associated with kerato-acanthomata of the face. *Br J Surg* 1967;54:191–195.

71. Torre D. Multiple sebaceous tumors. *Arch Dermatol* 1968;98:549–551.

72. Schwartz R, Torre D. The Muir-Torre syndrome: a 25-year retrospective. *J Am Acad Dermatol* 1995;33:90–104.

73. Leslie DF, Greenway HT. Mohs micrographic surgery for skin cancer. *Australas J Dermatol* 1991;32(3):159–164.

74. Mallory SB. Cowden syndrome (multiple hamartoma syndrome). *Dermatol Clin* 1995;13(1):27–31.

75. Longy M, Lacombe D. Cowden disease. Report of a family and review. *Ann Genet* 1996;39(1):35–42.

76. Celebi JT, Ping XL, Zhang H, et al. Germline PTEN mutations in three families with Cowden syndrome. *Exp Dermatol* 2000;9(2):152–156.

77. Kacem M, Zili J, Zakhama A, et al. Multinodular goiter and parotid carcinoma: a new case of Cowden's disease. *Ann Endocrinol (Paris)* 2000;61(2):159–163.

78. O'Hare AM, Cooper PH, Parlette HL III. Trichilemmomal carcinoma in a patient with Cowden's disease (multiple hamartoma syndrome). *J Am Acad Dermatol* 1997;36(6 Pt 1):1021–1023.

79. Holloway KB, Flowers FP. Multiple endocrine neoplasia 2B (MEN 2B)/MEN 3. *Dermatol Clin* 1995;13(1):99–103.

80. Goodfellow PJ, Wells SA Jr. RET gene and its implications for cancer. *J Natl Cancer Inst* 1995;87(20):1515–1523.

81. McGarrity TJ, Kulin HE, Zaino RJ. Peutz-Jeghers syndrome. *Am J Gastroenterol* 2000;95(3):596–604.

82. Miyaki M. Peutz-Jeghers syndrome. *Nippon Rinsho* 2000;58(7):1400–1404.

83. Marignani PA. LKB1, the multitasking tumour suppressor kinase. *J Clin Pathol* 2005;58(1):15–19.

84. Kato S, Takeyama J, Tanita Y, et al. Ruby laser therapy for labial lentigines in Peutz-Jeghers syndrome. *Eur J Pediatr* 1998;157(8):622–624.

CHAPTER 22 ■ MANAGEMENT OF PRESSURE ULCERS AND FUNGATING WOUNDS

FRANK D. FERRIS

Skin is one of the vital human organs. It has a highly developed physiology and several essential functions in the regulation of homeostasis and immunity.

Provides protection. Skin surrounds virtually our entire bodies. It is the outer layer of the structures that hold us intact and give shape to our bodies. It also provides protection and a cushion when objects hit our bodies.

Senses environment. Skin is highly innervated. It helps sense the environment and avoid injury. When skin is "wounded" and becomes inflamed or infected, the resulting inflammatory response can sensitize nociceptors, lead to recruitment of additional neurons, and increase neuronal firing of each involved neuron. Patients frequently experience increasing pain associated with the wound and the inflamed structures, that is, hyperalgesia and allodynia (1). Although opioid receptors are not present in normal skin, within minutes to hours of inflammation, they may appear in peripheral sensory nerves (2).

Maintains fluid balance. Skin has a highly developed system of pores that help to control fluid balance. The pores open and close to regulate evaporation and transcutaneous perspiration.

Controls body temperature. Skin also participates in the regulation of body temperature by releasing fluids on the surface as perspiration or sweat to evaporate and cool down the body.

Controls infection. Intact skin presents a physical barrier to infections and immunologic barrier to infections. When skin is "wounded," this barrier is broken and bacteria and other infective agents can colonize or infect the wound and the surrounding tissues and sometimes lead to systemic infections or even sepsis. Wound infections can secrete pathogens that inhibit epithelial cell mitosis and delay granulation and wound healing.

Creates body image. Skin is the most visible organ. Its presence creates a bodily image of who we are. Disfigurement due to wounds may have profound consequences on an individual's body image and the way others respond to her/him. If it is bad enough, the patient may want to withdraw, family members and friends may not want to look at the patient, and health care workers may not want to provide care. At a time when the patient may need more support than ever, she/he may be abandoned by family members and caregivers.

Creates body smells. Skin secretes a number of fluids and substance that have associated smells. Over time, many people develop attractions to each other based on familiar scents. If those scents change or become overwhelmed by odors from putrefying tissues or infections, the effect may be repulsive and lead to isolation and abandonment.

There are multiple potential events that can damage skin integrity and/or function acutely or chronically. For patients with advanced cancer, particularly the elderly, pressure and fungating tumor masses are the most common causes of chronic wounds to the skin and the tissues that lie below it, that is, subcutaneous fat, muscles, bone, tendons, nerves, blood vessels, and so on.

When patients with cancer experience chronic wounds, not only do they suffer from the underlying cancer and their wounds, but their whole being is affected by the multiple physical, psychological, social, spiritual, practical, loss and end-of-life issues that are frequently associated with wounds. To be effective, care of such patients must be consistent with their goals of care and treatment priorities, and manage the whole "wounded" person, not just the "hole" (3,4).

PRESSURE ULCERS

Pressure or decubitus ulcers are encountered frequently in patients with cancer, particularly those who are debilitated by their illness or by treatment (5,6).

The microarterioles that supply blood to the skin run through the subcutaneous fat. In the face of mild pressure, the fat normally cushions and redistributes the pressure. However, when the pressure increases above the capillary filling pressure, the microarterioles close for as long as the pressure is present and the oxygen tension falls in the downstream tissues. Normal skin can withstand 30–60 minutes of poor perfusion but not longer. When the pressure and hypoxia are sustained, ischemia and necrosis can develop relatively rapidly (7,8).

In both general hospital and long-term care, pressure ulcers occur in up to 28% of patients (9). One study of 980 home hospice patients found that 10% of patients developed ulcers during the study period (10).

Pressure points, for example, sacrum, heels, and elbows, are at particular risk for the development of ischemia and pressure ulcers. Thin patients with cachexia who lack subcutaneous fat are even more susceptible. When they are weak, fatigued, and unable to move around by themselves, the risk of developing one or more pressure ulcers is very high. Shear, friction, prolonged presence of moisture associated with incontinence, age-related changes in skin, and poor nutrition further compound the risk (11).

Pressure ulcers most often develop at body sites were the pressure is highest. In supine patients, 60% of pressure ulcers occur in the sacrum, and the greater trochanter and heel account for a further 15%. In patients who are constantly sitting, the ischial tuberosities are more susceptible (4).

MALIGNANT ULCERS

Malignant wounds occur in up to 10% of patients with advanced or metastatic cancer, usually in the last 6 months of life (12). They can evolve from a primary tumor of skin or an invasive underlying mass, a recurrence along a surgical suture line, or a metastasis. They can be both erosive ulcers and/or expanding nodules. If many nodules confluence, the result can be a cauliflower-like wound. They are most commonly associated with cancers that start in the breast, particularly when they reoccur locally (50% or more). Other common sites include the head and neck (up to 30%) and axilla or groin (approximately 5%) (13–15).

Although a tumor initially stimulates neovascularization, a rapidly growing tumor can outstrip its available blood supply and necrose centrally. When the process involves the skin, it frequently becomes friable and produces significant exudate; becomes malodorous as the tissue putrefies and/or becomes infected with anaerobes; and frequently bleeds.

ASSESSMENT

In any patient with cancer who has developed a wound, or is at risk of developing one, start with a comprehensive assessment of the patient's illness context, risk of developing a pressure ulcer, wound, surrounding skin, blood supply, frequently associated issues, for example, pain, odor, or "woundedness."

Illness Context

Assess the context of the patient's illness, including her/his cancer type, stage, and prognosis; functional status, for

TABLE 22.1

CONTEXT ASSESSMENT

Issue	Examples
Cancer type, stage, prognosis	Stage IV breast cancer with metastases to liver, lungs, bone; prognosis 1–2 mo
Comorbidities	Rheumatoid arthritis
	Autoimmune disorders, for example, systemic lupus, vasculitis
Functional status, for example, KPS or PPS	KPS or PPS = 50%
Nutritional/fluid status	Appetite, for example, anorectic
	Degree of cachexia, for example, 20-lb weight loss, albumin 2.1 g/dL
	Mild dehydration with orthostatic hypotension and 1+ pitting ankle edema
Cognitive status	Alert, oriented ×3, normal mini-mental status
Decision-making capacity	Has capacity
Medications that could delay healing	Steroids
	Nonsteroidal anti-inflammatory drugs
	Immunosuppressive medications
Goals of care	Maintain function
	Minimize symptoms
	Interact clearly with family and friends

KPS, Karnofsky; PPS, palliative performance status.

example, Karnofsky (KPS) or Palliative Performance Status (PPS); nutritional, fluid, and cognitive status; decision-making capacity; and goals of care (Table 22.1).

Pressure Ulcer Risk

The risk of developing a pressure ulcer increases as cancer advances, particularly when patients are debilitated (16).

TABLE 22.2

BRADEN PRESSURE ULCER RISK ASSESSMENT

					Score
Sensory perception	Completely limited	Very limited	Slightly limited	No impairment	
Moisture	Constantly moist	Very moist	Occasionally moist	Rarely moist	
Activity	Bedfast	Chairfast	Walks occasionally	Walks frequently	
Mobility	Completely immobile	Very limited	Slightly limited	Walks frequently	
Nutrition	Very poor	Probably inadequate	Adequate	Excellent	
Friction, shear	Problem	Potential problem	No apparent problem		
>16 = not at risk of developing pressure ulcers; 15–16 = low risk; 13–14 = moderate risk; ≤12 high risk.				Total score:	

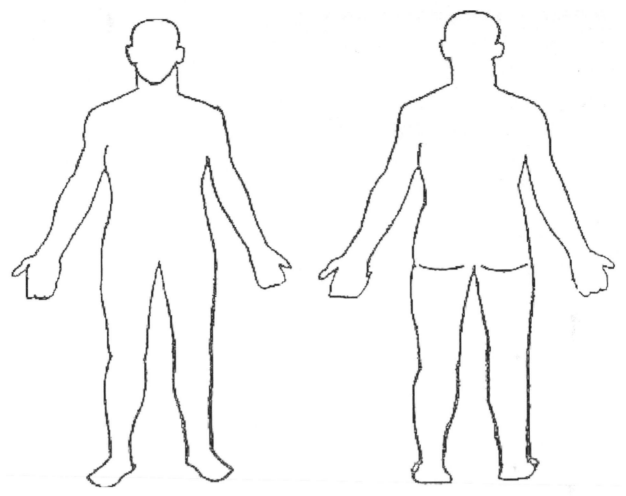

FIGURE 22.1. Wound location. Mark the location of each wound on the body diagrams. Label sites as A, B, C, D.

Periodically assess every patient's risk using either a Braden (17) (http://www.bradenscale.com/) or a Norton (18) risk assessment tool (http://www.ncbi.nlm.nih.gov/books/bv.fcgi?rid=hstat2.table.4948). Both tools examine the most significant risk factors for developing a pressure ulcer including sensory perception, moisture, activity, mobility, nutrition, and friction/shear (Table 22.2, a simplification of the Braden Pressure Ulcer Risk Assessment tool—for complete details, refer to the original tool).

Once a wound develops, assess the following:

1. **The wound,** including the type (etiology), location (Figure 22.1), duration, description of the structure and base/surface, dimensions (best to document with a labeled photograph or diagram (Figure 22.2), exudate, and bleeding (Table 22.3). Observe old dressings for strikethrough (i.e., drainage on the outside of an old dressing) and then remove the dressing slowly, starting from the edges. If dressings adhere to the wound surface, moisten them with normal saline or water to reduce adherence and facilitate removal. If you can anticipate that there will be pain or if there is any pain during the removal process, before continuing start on preemptive anesthesia/analgesia until the patient is comfortable (discussed later in this chapter).
2. **The surrounding skin,** including contamination, maceration, signs of infection, and edema (Table 22.4).
3. **The blood supply,** particularly in lower extremity wounds (Table 22.5).

4. **The frequently associated issues,** for example, odor, pain, "woundedness," anxiety, and depression (Table 22.6).

STAGING

Pressure Ulcers

To help determine the management plan, the National Pressure Ulcer Advisory Panel/Agency for Health Care Policy and Research (NPUAP/AHCPR) developed a system that is widely used to stage pressure ulcers (19).

- *Stage I.* The heralding lesion of skin ulceration is non-blanchable erythema of intact skin when compared with another region of the body. In darker skin, the erythema may appear as persistent blue or purplish discoloration.
- *Stage II.* Partial-thickness skin loss involving epidermis, dermis, or both. The ulcer is superficial and looks like an abrasion, a shallow crater, or a blister.
- *Stage III.* Full-thickness skin loss involving subcutaneous tissue. The ulcer may extend down to, but not through, the underlying fascia. The ulcer looks like a deep crater, with or without undermining of adjacent tissue (i.e., skin that overhangs wound edges).
- *Stage IV.* The ulcer is deep enough to include necrosis and damage to underlying muscle, bone, and/or other supporting structures such as the tendon or joint capsule.

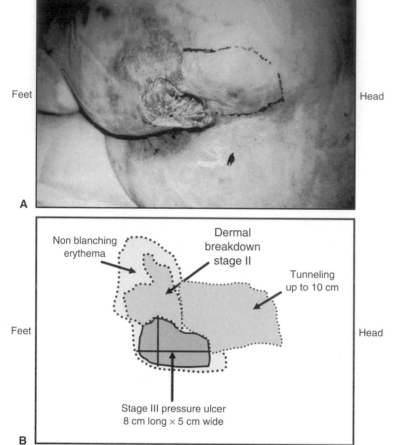

Feet   Head

Feet   Head

FIGURE 22.2. Description of a sacral pressure ulcer. Photograph or trace the circumference of the wound and any damage to surrounding skin onto a transparency or plastic page protector, including areas of tracking or tunneling (indicating measurements, usually in centimeters). Use plastic wrap next to the skin to avoid bacterial or body fluid contamination.

Undermining of adjacent skin and sinus tracts or fistula may also be present.

■ *Stage X.* Unstageable, depth unknown

Malignant Wounds

There is no specific staging system for malignant wounds.

MANAGEMENT

If patients who are at risk of developing a pressure ulcer, or those who are in the process of developing one, are caught early and appropriate prevention and treatment initiated, progression can be arrested and significant morbidity preempted.

Interdisciplinary

Wound care always involves an interdisciplinary team that includes a nurse and physician at a minimum, and may include an enterostomal therapist who is an expert in wound care, a pharmacist, a social worker, a chaplain, a physiotherapist, a dietitian, and so on, especially when the patient's issues are more complex.

Establish Goals of Care

To develop an effective plan of care, start with effective communication with the patient or her/his surrogate decision maker about the context of the patient's illness, the patient's personal goals of care, and possible therapeutic options including their benefits and risks of harm and burden. Carefully guide a decision-making and treatment-planning process that involves the patient, her/his family, and caregivers.

For patients with pressure ulcers, if the blood supply to the surrounding tissues is adequate (i.e., Dorsalis pedis and/or posterior tibial pulses are palpable or ankle brachial index (ABI) >0.5 or toe arterial pressure >40 mm Hg), it may be possible to heal the wound. For many patients with advanced cancer and a short prognosis, it is unrealistic to strive to heal a pressure ulcer. For such patients, it is much more appropriate to focus on stabilizing the wound, relieving interface pressure to prevent further progression, and managing associated symptoms.

For patients with malignant wounds, if it is not possible to treat the underlying cancer, it will not be possible to heal a malignant wound.

PRESSURE ULCERS—WHEN THE GOAL IS TO HEAL

When the goal is to heal a pressure ulcer, management involves conventional wound care strategies (20).

1. Start by reducing the interface pressure.
2. Then prepare the wound bed. Cleanse, debride when there is necrotic tissue or slough with preemptive anaesthesia/analgesia, and control infection and bleeding (21–24).

TABLE 22.3

WOUND ASSESSMENT

	Examples
Type of wound (etiology)	Pressure, malignant cavitating or fungating, chemotherapy extravasation, radiation reaction, diabetic, neurotrophic, arterial, venous, acute surgical, acute trauma
Location	Precise location, ideally placing the wound on a body diagram (Figure 22.1)
Duration	How long the patient has had it
Description of pressure ulcer	Nonblanching erythema of dermis, no breakdown or disruption of epidermis
	Dermal breakdown
	Cavity with breakdown extending to subcutaneous fat, muscle, bone
Description of malignant fungating wound	Nodular, cauliflower, cavitating
	Percent necrosis
Base/surface	Color, for example, black if eschar, red if granulation tissue, or yellow if fibrous tissue or slough
	Friability, for example, tissue breaking down on contact
	Exposed structures, for example, tendon, nerve, major blood vessel
Dimensions (Figure 22.1)	Greatest vertical (head to toe) and horizontal dimensions at right angles
	Greatest depth of open wound using a probe, or height of a raised fungating wound
	Depth of any tracks (e.g., overhanging skin) or tunnels that extend underneath the skin through soft tissue and either dead end (e.g., sinus tracts) or open onto the skin in another location (e.g., fistula)
Exudate	Color, for example, serous, sanguineous, serosanguineous
	Purulence
	Volume, for example, none, mild, moderate, copious
Bleeding	Oozing or frank bleeding
Strikethrough, that is, drainage on the outside of an old dressing	Color, for example, serous, sanguinous, serosanguineous
	Purulence
	Volume, for example, spotting, soaked

3. Once the wound bed has been prepared, dress the wound to promote moist interactive wound healing. If there is a risk of significant shearing, tearing, or regular contamination with exudate, urine or stool that could cause maceration, protect surrounding skin.
4. Pack all dead spaces to keep them open and draining.
5. Layer dressings.
6. Finally, manage all associated issues, including pain, odors, and the patient's "woundedness."

Reduce Interface Pressure

Continuous pressure, particularly over bony prominences, increases the risk of ischemia, skin breakdown, and pain (11). Pressure ulcers can develop within hours if the patient is not moved and circulation remains compromised.

Pressure at an interface is the force per unit area that acts perpendicularly between the body and the support surface. This parameter is affected by the stiffness of the support surface, the composition of the body tissue, and the geometry of the body being supported (16).

TABLE 22.4

SURROUNDING SKIN ASSESSMENT

Contamination	Urine, stool
Maceration due to excess moisture	White hyperkeratosis
	Wet surface
Signs of infection	Erythema, warmth, tenderness
Edema	Type, for example, pitting, nonpitting
	Volume, for example, mild, moderate, severe

- Pressure reduction is a therapeutic strategy to reduce the interface pressure, not necessarily below capillary-closing pressure.
- Pressure relief is a therapeutic strategy to reduce the interface pressure below capillary-closing pressure (25,26).

In patients with advanced cancer, particularly those who are debilitated, and patients with wounds, implement as many strategies to reduce, if not relieve, the interface pressure as much as possible, including repositioning, turning, massaging, supporting, protecting, and avoiding rolling and bunching of bedsheets and dressings.

Position

To minimize sacral pressure in patients who are bedridden, keep the head of the bed as low as possible, ideally at <30 degrees. Raise it only for short periods of social interaction or use foam wedges to support the patient. Avoid resting one limb on another. Use a pillow or another cushioning support to keep legs apart. Protect bony prominences with hydrocolloid dressings.

Turn

When a patient is unable to move by herself/himself, turn the patient from side to side every 1 to 1.5 hour. In addition to reducing pressure, this helps to relieve joint position fatigue in immobilized patients. Use a careful "log-roll" technique to distribute forces evenly across the patient's body and minimize pain on movement. Use a draw sheet to reduce shearing forces that could lead to skin tears. If turning is painful, turn the patient less frequently and/or place the patient on a pressure-reducing surface, for example, air mattress or airbed. As patients approach death, the need for turning lessens as the risk of skin breakdown becomes less important.

TABLE 22.5

BLOOD SUPPLY ASSESSMENT OF EXTREMITIES

Dorsalis pedis or posterior tibial pulses	If palpable, systolic pressure is ≈ 80 mm Hg or greater and perfusion is adequate to facilitate healing.		
Doppler ABI = ankle systolic pressure/brachial systolic pressure (27) (e.g., 80 mm Hg/100 mm Hg = 0.8)	**ABI** >0.8 >0.6 >0.4 <0.4	**Toe arterial pressure** 55 mm Hg >40 mm Hg >20 mm Hg <20 mm Hg	**Risk of not healing** Low Moderate (adequate perfusion) High (inadequate perfusion) Severe
Transcutaneous partial oxygen saturation	>30% indicates adequate perfusion		
Toe arterial pressures (photoplethysmography)	>40 mm Hg indicates adequate perfusion		

ABI, ankle brachial index.

Massage

Massage intermittently to stimulate circulation, shift edema, spread out moisturizing lotions, and provide comfort. This is particularly helpful in dependent areas subject to increased pressure, before and after turning. Avoid massaging skin that is erythematous or broken down.

Support

Therapeutic support surfaces that reduce or relieve pressure include specialty mattresses/beds, chairs, wheelchairs, and positioning devices.

Foam Pads

Simple foam pads are often ineffective. If they are used, they may need to be layered so that they are at least 6–8 inches thick. If the pressure has been reduced adequately, when a hand is placed under a pad at the lowest point of the patient's body, for example, under buttocks, there will be at least 1 inch of noncompressed foam between the hand and the patient.

Three groups of mattresses/beds have demonstrated efficacy:

- *Group 1*. Air or water mattress overlays reduce pressure. If employed early enough in any patient who is

bed-bound, has limited mobility, or is cachectic, they will help prevent pressure ulcers.
- *Group 2*. Low-air-loss beds are used for any patient who is at high risk of developing a pressure ulcer, or for a patient who has developed an ulcer already and the goal is to prevent worsening and/or promote healing.
- *Group 3*. Air-fluidized beds are reserved for patients who need pressure relief. However, patients frequently describe them as overly confining (even "coffin-like"). They are also very expensive.

Cushions

For chairs and wheelchairs, there are a number of pressure-reducing cushions. For chairfast patients who need to use a chair or a wheelchair for a prolonged time, it may be more effective to have them assessed professionally for customized pressure-reducing cushions. Never use round cushions commonly called *donuts*. They redistribute pressure without relieving it.

Protect

Protect thin, fragile skin from friction, moisture, and shear to minimize the risk of skin tears. This is particularly important in cachectic patients who have lost the elasticity and resilience effect previously provided by their collagen and subcutaneous fat. Thin films will reduce shearing forces. Hydrocolloid dressings will add a cushioning effect.

Caution

Be sure that bedsheets do not wrinkle and dressings do not ripple under the patient, as both will produce new pressure points that could lead to ulceration if sustained, particularly in patients with cachexia.

Cleanse

Prepare the wound bed by cleansing and rinsing away exudate, slough, and debris. Although it may be acceptable to use relatively cytotoxic fluids to clean intact skin, for example, hydrogen peroxide, povidone iodine, or sodium hypochlorite, avoid using them in the wound. Although they decrease bacterial burden, they will be cytotoxic to granulation tissue and delay healing (28).

When choosing a wound cleanser, a useful rule of thumb is: "don't put anything into the wound that you wouldn't put into your eye." Unpreserved normal (physiologic) saline or

TABLE 22.6

ASSOCIATED ISSUES

Odor	Fruity or foul smelling
	Just under dressing or throughout the room
Pain (describe for each major site)	Location
	Type, for example, nociceptive, neuropathic, mixed
	Temporal profile, for example, constant, breakthrough, intermittent acute
	Severity, for example, 3/10 on a visual analog scale
	Effect of medications (benefit and adverse effects, e.g., drowsiness, nausea, constipation)
Anxiety	See Chapter 40
Depression	See Chapter 40
"Woundness"	Psychological state
	Body image
	Fear

sterile water are the preferred wound cleansers. Although both can be purchased commercially, saline can also be prepared on the stove-top at home. Mix two teaspoons (10 mL) salt in four cups (1 qt or L) water; boil on the stove 3–20 minutes; cool to room temperature; do not store more than 24 hours. Alternately, use a commercially available wound cleanser with as little cytotoxicity as possible.

Cleanse the wound gently to avoid flushing away migrating epithelial cells or damaging normal tissues using one of the following four techniques:

1. Soak or compress the wound with a saline-moistened gauze.
2. Gently pour the cleanser over the wound.
3. Irrigate the wound with a piston or bulb syringe that delivers 5–8 pounds per square inch (PSI) pressure or, to remove slough or eschar, irrigate with an 18–20 gauge Angiocath on a 30–60 mL syringe held 4–6 inches from the wound, which delivers 5–15 PSI pressure.
4. Use a commercial spray wound cleanser with a predetermined PSI pressure. If there is any pain, stop cleansing, start on preemptive anaesthesia/analgesia until the patient is comfortable, and then continue cleansing.

Maintain good hygiene on surrounding skin using unpreserved normal saline or sterile water, or with a more cytotoxic fluid or commercially available skin cleanser.

Debride

Necrotic tissue (eschar or slough) and contaminated and foreign material can delay wound healing and harbor infections. Optimal wound healing will not occur until these are removed. If there is significant necrotic tissue or slough, and the blood supply to the surround tissue is adequate for healing to occur, that is, ABI >0.5, after cleansing the wound to remove debris, debride as much of the necrotic and contaminated tissue as possible and expose dead spaces. Where possible, debride down to a bleeding base. This converts a chronic wound into an acute wound and decreases surface bacterial burden.

Choose from the available debridement techniques, for example, surgical/sharp, autolytic, enzymatic/chemical, mechanical, or larval, on the basis of a thorough assessment of wound and the goals of care for the patient (Table 22.7). If there is associated gangrene, delay debridement until a line of demarcation between healthy and necrotic tissue develops. Avoid blood vessels, nerves, tendons, or other underlying structures. If using surgical or mechanical debridement, instigate preemptive anaesthesia/analgesia beforehand.

Control Infection

All wounds are colonized by bacteria, fungi, and other infective agents, but this does not mean they are infected. *Staphylococcus epidermis* and *Corynebacterium* are the most common colonizers of wounds. *Proteus, Klebsiella, Pseudomonas,* and *Candida* commonly infect wounds, particularly when there is recurring contamination with urine or feces or immunocompromise.

If present in sufficient quantities, the wound and the surrounding tissue may become infected. Healing can be delayed significantly. Purulent exudates, pain and/or foul odors may be the first signs of local infection. If the odor is fruity and the wound has a greenish tinge, the wound is likely infected with pseudomonal organisms. If the odor is foul/putrid, it is likely infected with anaerobic bacteria.

If the goal is to heal the wound, establishing when a wound has become infected to the point that the bacterial burden impacts healing can be difficult. A careful swab technique to obtain meaningful samples is most important to gain useful cultures. First, cleanse the wound with normal saline or water and remove all debris. Then swab healthy-appearing granulation tissue in a zigzag pattern, gently rotating the tip of the swab. If the wound is dry, premoisten the tip of the swab with a little culture media. If, after culturing swab samples, the cause remains elusive, consider culturing a biopsy from the wound bed.

If the infection is superficial, cleanse the wound with saline or water and apply a topical antibiotic with each change of dressing (Table 22.8) (33). If there is infection in the surrounding tissues, or if wound healing is delayed, add a systemic antibiotic until the infection is cleared. If there is obvious candidal growth or a lot of crusting, mix a topical antifungal, for example, ketoconazole, with the topical antibiotic or alternate them. If the ulcer probes to bone, suspect osteomyelitis and consider 4–6 weeks of systemic antibiotics.

Honey and yogurt may also be very effective topical antibacterials, even when they are diluted (34). Use only honey that has been irradiated to ensure that it is free of clostridium spores.

Control Bleeding

Bleeding is much more of a problem in malignant wounds than in pressure ulcers. If dressings adhere to the wound surface, moisten the dressing with normal saline or water to reduce adherence and facilitate removal. If uncontrolled bleeding occurs in a pressure ulcer, management strategies are the same as those for malignant wounds (see section on "Malignant Wounds").

Dress the Wound and Surrounding Tissue

This section aims to present the principles and suggest a strategy for dressing chronic wounds, not recommend specific dressings. Any reference to commercial products is only to illustrate a point, not to recommend particular products. Contact manufacturers for detailed information about their products and how to use them.

If healing is the goal of pressure ulcer management, the epithelial cells and fibroblasts that must proliferate to form granulation tissue and fill in the wound require a moist environment that is rich in oxygen and the nutrients necessary to sustain their replication and migration. At the same time, the environment must protect the wound, control excessive exudate, and minimize exposure to infective microorganisms that can inhibit healing. By contrast, a dry environment is conducive to necrosis and eschar, and not to healing.

There are seven classes of dressing: foams, alginates, hydrogels, hydrocolloids, films, gauze, and nonstick dressings (Table 22.9). They are distinguished by their absorbency, wear time, and occlusiveness. Within each class, specific products also vary by size, user friendliness, cost/accessibility, adhesive used, and impact on the wound margin and surrounding skin. As studies of different types of moist wound dressings showed no difference in pressure ulcer healing outcomes, use clinical judgment to select a type of dressing most appropriate for a given wound (35,36).

To hold dressings in place, there are a wide range of tapes and stocking products that use varying adhesives and may result in different hypersensitivity reactions.

Dressing Strategy

If healing is the goal, use a dressing strategy that enables the following:

1. *Keep the wound bed continuously moist.* A dry wound needs to have moisture given to it through a hypotonic gel (donates water). If there is excessive wet exudates, a

TABLE 22.7

DEBRIDEMENT TECHNIQUES

Technique	Mechanism	Precautions	Comments
Surgical/sharp	Use of curved scissors, curette, or scalpel.	Make sure there is adequate blood supply for healing to occur: ABI >0.5 Toe pressure >40 mm Hg Transcutaneous oxygen saturation >30%.	Fastest, most effective technique for large areas of necrosis, a high degree of contamination or frank infection. Requires a skilled clinician. Manage procedural pain with preemptive anaesthesia (e.g., topical lidocaine cream or spray, EMLA).
Autolytic	Use of moist interactive dressings (e.g., hydrogels, hydrocolloids, alginates, films) to liquefy necrotic tissue.	Remove as much loose debris as possible when changing dressings (usually q24–48 h initially).	Gentlest technique. Results should be seen within 72 h. Occlusive dressings facilitate autolysis by maintaining a moist environment. Monitor for overhydration and infection.
Enzymic/chemical	Use of collagenase or papain to digest damaged collagen, but not newly formed granulation tissue.	Bacterial infection and bacteremia can occur. Detergents, bleach, hexachlorophene, and heavy metals (e.g., silver, mercury) may inactivate enzymes.	Faster than autolytic debridement (29). To facilitate the process, score eschar without causing bleeding. Do not use on normal or granulation tissue. Enzymes do not facilitate the granulation and re-epithelialization phases of wound care. They may damage normal tissues.
Mechanical	Use of gentle irrigation to remove necrotic tissue. Use an 18–20 gauge Angiocath on a 30–60 mL syringe to keep pressure under 15 PSI.	Excessive force may flush away migrating epithelial cells or damage normal tissue.	Saline wet-to-dry gauze dressings, irrigation, and whirlpool therapy are alternate mechanical debriding techniques. The latter is not recommended as it may cause pain or bleeding and damage normal or granulation tissue that sticks to the dry gauze when the dressing is removed.
Larval	Use of larvae to consume necrotic tissue (30–32).	Use larvae cultured for this purpose. Enclose them within the wound. Monitor their activity closely. Remove them when the debridement is complete.	Relatively rapid technique to debride large volumes of necrotic tissue. May be offensive to patients, families, or staff.

ABI, ankle brachial index; EMLA, eutectic mixture of long-acting anaesthetics; PSI, pounds per square inch.

hypertonic gel, alginate, or foam will remove fluids from the wound.

2. *Control exudate.* This should be done without desiccating the wound bed. Wound exudates can be substantial, especially from stage IV pressure ulcers and malignant wounds. When there are copious exudates, consider uncontrolled edema or increased bacterial burden or infection as possible causes (37).
   Both foams and alginates can absorb fluids that are many times heavier and effectively remove copious exudates from the environment of the wound. By wicking the exudate away from the wound and surrounding skin, the risk of infection and maceration is minimized. By containing the fluid within the dressing, it will not drip onto clothes and bedsheets and it will be more cosmetically pleasing for everyone. Change dressings once strikethrough is present, that is, leakage through to the outside of the dressing.

3. *Keep surrounding skin dry.* In addition to cleansing surrounding skin, zinc oxide or barrier creams or sprays may help protect the skin from prolonged contact or contamination with fluids, for example, exudates, urine, or feces. Some sprays may also increase adherence of adjacent dressing. When the risk is expected to be ongoing, thin film or hydrocolloid dressings placed around the wound with a cutout for the wound dressings can provide further protection (38).

4. *Eliminate dead space.* Loosely fill all cavities with nonadherent dressing materials, for example, alginates or hydrogel-soak gauze.

5. *Consider caregiver time, skill, and burden.* Wound care can be burdensome. Do not create a plan that is not physically or financially possible for the patient and caregivers to adhere to.

6. *Monitor dressings applied near the anus.* Dressings close to the anus/perineum tend to move and bunch up under the tremendous friction and shearing forces in the sacral area.

7. *Dress in layers.* As no single dressing will meet all these criteria, use a layered approach for dressing a wound.

TABLE 22.8

COMMON TOPICAL ANTIBACTERIAL AGENTS

Agent	Staphylococcus aureus	MRSA	Streptococcus	Pseudomonas	Anaerobes	Comments
Cadexomer iodine dressing	√	√	√	√	√	Microspheres of starch cross-linked with ether bridges and iodine Absorbs up to seven times its weight in moisture Slowly releases iodine for antibacterial action without being cytotoxic to epithelial cells Caution with thyroid disease, iodine allergy
Ionized silver dressings	√	√	√	√	√	Slowly releases silver Decreases surface friability Must be used with sterile water, not saline (which precipitates the silver as inactive silver chloride)
Fusidic acid cream/ointment	√	—	√	—	—	Lanolin in ointment base may act as a sensitizer
Gentamicin cream/ointment	√	—	√	√	—	—
Metronidazole gel/cream	—	—	—	—	√	Good penetration and wound deodorizer
Polymyxin B sulfate—Bacitracin zinc	√	√	√	√	√	Broad spectrum; low cost
Polymyxin B sulfate–Bacitracin zinc—neomycin	√	√	√	√	√	Neomycin is a potent sensitizer; may cross-sensitize to other aminoglycosides
Silver sulfadiazine	√	—	√	√	—	Do not use in sulfa-sensitive individuals

MRSA, methicillin-resistant *Staphylococcus aureus*; √, use.

The primary or first layer goes next to the surface of the wound. It can include a hydrogel, an antibiotic, and/or thromboplastin. Subsequent layers rest one on top of the other. Finally, the top or outer layer typically holds the dressing in place and serves as the "aesthetic" covering. There is no minimum or maximum number of layers. Build the best possible combination for the patient's situation on the basis of your clinical judgment.

Although dressing changes may be initially needed once or even twice daily to control infections and remove copious exudate, as the exudate and infection settle and the wound stabilizes, the frequency of dressing changes may be reduced (even to once or twice per week).

Examples

The dressing of stages I–IV pressure ulcers varies considerably. The following examples illustrate the range of strategies that are possible:

Stage I and II Pressure Ulcers. Dry stage I and II pressure ulcers are typically dressed with a transparent film placed directly on the surface of the wound to protect it from contact or irritation. It forms a semiocclusive barrier to the environment. A film dressing is typically changed every 3–5 days (39). Exercise caution when removing it. A strong adhesive can easily lead to tearing of fragile skin. If you are having difficulties removing the dressing, use an adhesive remover to facilitate the process.

When there is limited exudate, a hydrocolloid placed directly on the wound will more effectively absorb the exudate. It forms an occlusive barrier and a moist internal environment to facilitate autolysis and healing. If there is mild necrosis, use a two-layered approach:

1. *Primary dressing (next to the wound).* Apply hydrogel to stimulate autolysis.
2. *Second dressing.* Place a hydrocolloid to form an occlusive barrier and facilitate autolysis and healing.

Hydrocolloid dressings are typically changed every 3–7 days or sooner if leakage occurs. Exercise caution when removing them. Their strong adhesive can easily lead to tearing of fragile skin. If you are having difficulties removing the dressing, use an adhesive remover to facilitate the process.

Stage III and IV Pressure Ulcers. Stage III and IV pressure ulcers are often much more complex to dress, depending on their configuration and the involvement of surrounding tissues. As an example, for a newly diagnosed dry stage IV pressure ulcer with tunneling that is infected, has a foul odor, and

TABLE 22.9

DRESSINGS

Class	Absorbency	Wear time	Types	Comments
1. Foams	4+/4	24 h–7 d	Mesh sponges	Ideal for copious exudate May macerate surrounding skin. Either protect the surrounding skin with petrolatum or zinc oxide ointment, or cut the foam to the inside dimensions of the wound and wick the exudate to secondary dressings.
2. Alginates	3+/4	12–48 or more hours	Sheets, ribbons, or ropes	Seaweed derivative Hemostatic Rope wicks vertically—ideal for packing tracks and tunnels Convert to gel on contact with fluid; can wash off in the shower.
3. Hydrogels	Variable, depending on the tonicity of the gel	24–72 h	Several different bases used in different products, for example, hydrocolloid, propylene glycol, sodium chloride	Facilitate autolytic debridement Use to hydrate
4. Hydrocolloids	Minimal 1–2+/4	24–48 h for debridement 3–7 d for protection	Millimeter thick pads consisting of a membrane or other backing with a hydrophilic layer (e.g., gelatin, pectin) and a hydrophobic layer (e.g., carboxymethylcellulose) Gelatin layer liquefies on contact with fluids, minimizing trauma on removal Usually self-adhesive	Facilitate autolytic debridement Protect bony prominences and areas of potential skin breakdown Occlusive barrier for fluids (e.g., urine, feces) and for showering and swimming Occasional allergies to adhesives Must avoid leakage channels, which can introduce bacteria, and rippling, which can result in new pressure points
5. Transparent films/membranes	None	Up to 7 d	Both adhesive and nonadhesive films	Protect fragile skin from shearing and tearing Permit visualization Oxygen permeable Facilitate re-epithelialization Avoid leakage channels, which can introduce bacteria Barrier for showering and swimming
6. Gauze	Variable 1–2+/4	Variable, depending on strikethrough Up to 7 d	Pads, tapes, nets	Ideal outer dressings Hold dressing in place Cosmetic
7. Nonstick	None	Up to 7 d	Petroleum-coated pads, inert pads, inert mesh	Facilitate nonadherence

is somewhat friable and oozing blood, use a four-layered approach:

1. *Primary layer (next to the wound)*. Isotonic hydrogel with an antimicrobial against anaerobes, for example, metronidazole.
2. *Second layer*. Alginate for its bacteriostatic properties, ease of conforming to the structure of the wound and tendency to turn to gel on contact with fluids, thereby minimizing trauma to the wound surface and washing off easily.
3. *Third layer*. Cotton gauze or an abdominal pad to contain and protect the underlying dressing.
4. *Fourth (outer) layer*. Tape to hold the outer dressing layer in place.

For a particularly friable, bleeding wound, the layering might start with an inert nonadherent mesh dressing placed on the surface of the wound to protect the surface from trauma during repeated dressing changes.

Adjuvant Therapies

In addition to standard wound preparation and dressing strategies, for more challenging wounds, there are a number of adjunctive therapies that could help stimulate the granulation process, for example, vacuum-assisted closure (VAC) therapy (see http://www.kci1.com/35.asp.), warm-up therapy, and electro stimulation. You can read more about these therapies online, or in Krasner's Chronic Wound Care III textbook (4).

PRESSURE ULCERS—WHEN THE GOAL IS TO STABILIZE

When the goal is not to heal a pressure ulcer, the plan of care is based on the assessment of the wound and the surrounding tissues.

Assess and stage the pressure ulcer as discussed earlier.

Management

Reduce Interface Pressure

Always reduce the interface pressure using the techniques described earlier. This will minimize the risk of further progression of the existing pressure ulcers, and reduce the risk that new ulcers will develop.

Cleanse, Debride, Dress

Dry Wounds. If the wound is covered with a dry eschar and there is no sign of pain, odor, or infection in the wound, the eschar or the surrounding tissues, leave the wound alone. The dry eschar may be the most effective barrier against infections. Cleansing or debriding will only soften and ultimately remove the eschar, exposing the underlying tissues to an increased risk of infection and creating the need for routine dressing changes. To reduce bacterial burden, intermittently paint the eschar and the surrounding tissues with an aseptic iodine solution and let it air-dry. While it is contraindicated for healing wounds, the cytotoxicity of iodine can minimize the risk of infection and the need for a more complex wound management strategy (22).

If the wound needs to be covered to protect it, or for aesthetic reasons, cover it with a nonstick, nonocclusive dressing.

Wet Wound. If the wound is open, wet, or infected in the wound bed or surrounding tissues, pursue a conservative wound management strategy to stabilize the wound, control infection, exudate, odors and bleeding, and maintain the best possible body image.

MALIGNANT WOUNDS

The management of malignant wounds is basically the same as for advanced pressure ulcers (12–15,40,41).

For some patients, antineoplastic treatments may offer significant palliation of the symptoms associated with a malignant wound. Radiation therapy may decrease bleeding, pain, and exudate. Chemotherapy or hormonal therapy may even promote wound healing in patients with responsive disease.

Assessment, Staging

Use the same assessment tool (Table 22.1). There is no specific staging system for malignant wounds.

Management

Establish Goals of Care

Ensure that everyone is clear about the goals of care. If there exists chemotherapy or radiation therapy that could treat the underlying cancer and cause it to shrink or disappear, it may be possible to heal the malignant wound. Otherwise, if there is no effective therapy for the underlying disease, there will be no possibility for the wound to heal. Focus goals on stabilizing the wound, controlling infection, exudate, odors and bleeding, and maintaining the best possible body image.

Reduce Interface Pressure

To minimize the risk of developing or extending any pressure ulcers, particularly in cachectic, debilitated patients with cancer who are chairfast or bedridden, reduce the interface pressure as much as possible by repositioning, turning, massaging, supporting on pressure-reducing surfaces, protecting, and avoiding rolling and bunching of bedsheets and dressings as outlined earlier.

Cleanse

To remove necrotic debris and exudate, flush gently with normal saline or water at low pressures, as underlying necrotic tissue may be friable and bleed easily. Avoid cytotoxic wound cleansers.

Maintain good hygiene on surrounding skin using unpreserved normal saline or sterile water, or with a more cytotoxic fluid or commercially available skin cleanser.

Debride

Debride using autolysis or a very gentle surgical/sharp technique. Cautiously remove as much of the putrefying necrotic tissue that may be infected as possible, particularly if there is an associated foul odor. Use caution when approaching the tumor surface that may be friable, painful, and bleed easily, particularly if there is a lot of neovascularization close to the surface.

Control Infection

Most frequently, anaerobes infect the necrotic tissues and slough associated with a malignant wound and produce a foul/putrid odor and a purulent exudate. If the infection is superficial, cleanse the wound with normal saline or water, debride cautiously, and apply a topical antibiotic with each dressing change (Table 22.8) (33). Metronidazole and silver sulfadiazine are the preferred antimicrobials to control anaerobic infections in tumors. They will usually control superficial infections within 5–7 days. If the infection is deep into the tumor, or invades surrounding tissues, add systemic metronidazole 250–500 mg p.o. or i.v. q8h until the infection clears. Caution patients not to drink alcohol while receiving metronidazole. If there is obvious candidal growth or a lot of crusting, mix a topical antifungal, for example, ketoconazole, with the topical antibiotic or alternate them.

Control Bleeding

Bleeding is a common problem in malignant wounds. As tumors outgrow their blood supply, their surfaces become friable, coagulation is frequently impaired, and they become predisposed to oozing from microvascular fragmentation or frank bleeding if a small or large blood vessel is involved.

Dressings may adhere to the wound and tear the surface when the dressing is removed. For this reason, saline wet-to-dry gauze dressings are contraindicated in the management of malignant wounds. If dressings adhere to the wound surface, moisten them with normal saline or water to reduce adherence and facilitate removal. Remove each dressing slowly, starting from the edges. If you can anticipate that there will be pain, or if there is any pain during the removal process, before continuing start on preemptive anaesthesia/analgesia until the patient is comfortable (discussed later in this chapter).

When wound surfaces are particularly friable, apply an inert, nonstick, nonabsorbent synthetic polymer mesh, for example, Mepitel, as the first dressing layer. This does not need to be removed, and other dressings can be changed routinely with much less risk of tissue disruption and bleeding.

If oozing is significant, during each dressing change apply 5–10 mL of low-dose topical thromboplastin as a spray across the wound surface to stimulate coagulation (the 100 or 1,000 units per mL solution is as effective as higher-concentration solutions, and is less expensive). A 0.5–1% silver nitrate solution may be equally effective. Antifibrinolytics, such as topical aminocaproic acid, are occasionally used, although their role is not clear because fibrinolysis is not a major mechanism in wound bleeding.

Alginate dressings are hemostatic and can be left in place as the primary dressing layer for several days. They turn to jelly on absorbing fluids from the wound and are easily washed off, even in the shower, with minimal trauma to the wound surface. Hemostatic surgical sponges may be equally effective.

A short course of high dose per fraction palliative radiation therapy (typically 250–800 cGy/fraction/day) will sclerose most vessels and stop bleeding from a malignant wound in just a few days (42).

For frank bleeding, try silver nitrate sticks, electrocautery, and/or apply gentle pressure for 10–15 minutes. Interventional radiology may be able to stop bleeding from a larger blood vessel by sclerosing it.

In all situations where bleeding is a significant risk, discuss the situation with the patient, family, and caregivers and decide on how and in what setting everyone will cope with a major catastrophic bleed. If bleeding occurs uncontrollably, dark towels lessen the sight of blood and reduce anxiety of the family, caregiver, and staff. If the patient is aware and distressed by the protracted bleeding, sedation with a rapid-acting benzodiazepine (e.g., midazolam or lorazepam) may be warranted.

Dress the Wound and Surrounding Tissues

Follow the same dressing principles outlined in the preceding text for pressure ulcers. Layer the dressings in a manner similar to the approach used for a stage III or IV pressure ulcers.

1. Keep the malignant wound continuously moist. Do not let a necrotic wound surface dry out. It will be much more susceptible to cracking, bleeding, and infection with anaerobes and candida.
2. Control exudate in a manner similar to pressure ulcers. When there are copious exudates (e.g., malignant fistulae from the GI tract), stomal appliances or suction devices such as VAC therapy may be needed to cope with the volume (see http://www.kci1.com/35.asp).
3. Keep surrounding skin dry in a manner similar to pressure ulcers.
4. Eliminate dead space by filling it with nonadherent dressing materials.
5. Consider caregiver time, skill and burden. Care for a malignant wound with copious exudate or bleeding can be burdensome and psychologically difficult, particularly when the wound is in the head and neck area. Health care professionals (HCPs) and family caregivers will need a lot of skill building and support to ensure that they adhere to the plan of care effectively.
6. Monitor dressings applied near the anus. They tend to move and bunch up under the tremendous friction and shearing forces in the sacral area.
7. Dress in layers. Use the same layered technique as for advanced pressure ulcers. Hydrogels and alginates are ideal for friable malignant wounds as they liquefy as they absorb fluids, and can be washed off easily, even in the shower. Alginates are also hemostatic and conform easily to the many crevices and contours of a malignant

wound. Other nonstick dressing, for example, Telfa, will protect and minimize the trauma to a dry malignant wound when the dressing is changed. Ensure that the outer layer is fashioned to optimize the aesthetics for the patient and the family.

ASSOCIATED ISSUES

Odor

Odor emanating from wounds is caused by putrefying tissue and/or infection. When the odor is fruity and there is a green tinge on the wound surface, it is likely emanating from a pseudomonas infection. When the odor is foul/putrid, it is caused by an anaerobic infection in necrotic tissue.

Foul odor can be very distressing to the patient, family, and caregivers. It can lead to embarrassment, depression, and social isolation (43).

Odor management includes the following:

1. *Debride putrefying tissues.* Cleanse the wound carefully to remove any purulent exudate and then debride as much of the necrotic tissue as possible. Treat odorous dressings as biologically contaminated waste. Place them in a plastic puncture-resistant bag and close it securely. Double bag the waste and place in a tightly sealed trash container for pickup and disposal.
2. *Control infection.* If "healing" is not the goal of wound care, cytotoxic cleansers can be used to kill bacteria. Iodine will help keep the wound clean, although some patients find it irritating and painful. For pseudomonas, 0.0025% acetic acid may help inhibit the organism's growth in addition to a topical and/or systemic antibiotic (Table 22.8).

   If there is superficial anaerobic infection, topical treatment with metronidazole or silver sulfadiazine may be sufficient. If there is a deeper tissue infection, add systemic metronidazole 250–500 mg p.o./i.v. q8h until the infection resolves.
3. *Modify the environment.* There are multiple environmental changes that will help patients and families cope with foul odors, including the following:
   a. *Ventilate adequately.* Open windows to allow fresh air into the environment. Run a fan on a low speed so that it circulates air around the room without chilling the patient
   b. *Absorb odors.* Place inexpensive kitty liter or activated charcoal in a flat container with a large surface area under the patient's bed. As long as the air in the room is circulating freely, odors will diminish rapidly. Alternately, burn a flame, for example, a candle, to combust the chemicals causing the odor.
      For particularly odorous wounds, place an occlusive dressing that contains charcoal or a disposable diaper over the wound to contain the odor.
   c. *Alternate odors.* Introduce an alternate odor that is tolerable to the patient and family, for example, aromatherapy, coffee, vanilla, or vinegar. Avoid commercial fragrances and perfumes as many are not tolerated by patients with advanced cancer.

Pain

Pressure ulcers and malignant wounds are often painful unless the patient is paraplegic or has an altered sensorium (44–47). The pain can be constant with or without breakthrough pain, or acute. Constant pain can be the result of a local tissue reaction, underlying cancer, infection, the products of inflammation or increased pressure at a bony prominence. Intermittent acute pain occurs with specific procedures, for example, debridement. Cyclic acute pain occurs with recurring dressing changes (48–50).

To appropriately treat wound-related pain, it is important to know if the pain is nociceptive in origin, that is, the result of normal nociception and nerve function, neuropathic in origin, that is, the result of abnormal nerve function, or mixed.

Pain management follows standard pain management principles:

1. *Treat the underlying cause.* Where possible treat the cancer, control infections, heal the wound, and/or move the patient to a pressure-reducing or relieving surface.
2. *For constant pain.* Provide oral analgesics around the clock. If pain is nociceptive in origin, particularly if it is associated with inflammation, it will likely respond to a nonsteroidal anti-inflammatory drug (NSAID) and/or an opioid analgesic dosed once every half-life. If the pain is neuropathic in origin, a tricyclic analgesic or an anticonvulsant may be needed as an effective coanalgesic.

   For breakthrough pain, provide 10% of the total 24-hour oral dose of opioid every 1 hour as needed.

   Early evidence suggests that topical opioids mixed into a hydrogel, for example, morphine 0.1–0.5%, and placed against the wound surface in the primary dressing layer may reduce constant wound pain (51,52).

   Please note that if "healing" is the goal of wound care, NSAIDs may interfere with angiogenesis and delay wound healing (53).
3. *For both intermittent and cyclic acute pain.* Provide preemptive anaesthesia and/or analgesia. Ensure that the pharmacokinetics of the medication closely follow the temporal profile of the pain.

During debridement, acute intermittent pain will likely last only as long as the procedure. If there is an eschar to debride, score it, then apply EMLA (eutectic mixture of long-acting anaesthetics) "like icing on a cake" 30–60 minutes before the procedure, and cover it with an occlusive film. If there is slough and debris to be removed, apply a 2–4% lidocaine solution to the open wound. If there is likely to be pain at the periphery of the wound, inject s.c. lidocaine (± epinephrine to minimize bleeding) into the surrounding tissues and leave it for 5–10 minutes before commencing debridement.

Similarly, during dressing changes, acute cyclic pain will likely last only as long as the procedure (54,55). As the edges of the dressing are being slowly removed, moisten the wound and the dressing with a 2–4% solution of lidocaine. Allow enough time for the patient to be comfortable.

Careful selection of dressings to minimize tissue adherence, for example, hydrogels, alginates, and nonstick dressings, will minimize pain during dressing changes. If pain persists, consider reducing the frequency of dressing changes.

If local anaesthesia is insufficient, try a very short acting opioid, for example, systemic fentanyl or inhaled nitrous oxide (56).

SUMMARY

Chronic wounds are relatively common in patients with advanced cancer. After doing a comprehensive, whole person assessment, consider what the goals of care and treatment plan for the wound will be in light of the context of the patient's underlying cancer (and other comorbidities). Always use therapies that aim to reduce the risk of developing pressure ulcers. Once a pressure ulcer develops, if the goal is to heal it, follow the conventional wound healing strategies outlined in the text. If the goal is to stabilize, but not heal either a pressure ulcer or a malignant wound, the management will depend on whether the wound is dry or wet. Leave dry, noninfected wounds alone. For wet wounds, use relatively conservative wound cleansing, debridement, and dressing strategies to control infection and odor and minimize bleeding and pain.

Patients living with chronic wounds are inevitably "wounded" far beyond their physical wound. They live from day to day knowing that someone will be putting her/his hands into their body for daily dressing changes. Exudates, bleeding, and odors are embarrassing and distressing. Emotions frequently run high. Anxiety and depression are common, particularly in the face of multiple unexpected losses. Changes in intimacy, relationships, and finances can be dramatic and even lead to social isolation. Questions of meaning, value, purpose in life, "why me," and so on, all surface. To successfully manage these patients, interdisciplinary care must focus on the whole "wounded" person, not just the "hole."

All URLs were last accessed February 19, 2006

References

1. Pain Terminology. International Association for the Study of Pain. Available at http://www.iasp-pain.org/terms-p.html.
2. Hassan AH, Ableitner A, Stein C, et al. Inflammation of the rat paw enhances axonal transport of opioid receptors in the sciatic nerve and increases their density in the inflamed tissue. *Neuroscience* 1993;55(1):185–195. PMID: 7688879.
3. Alvarez OM, Meehan M, Ennis W, et al. Chronic Wounds: Palliative Management for the Frail Population. *Wounds* 2002;14(Suppl 8). See http://woundsresearch.com/wnds/frailsup.cfm.
4. Krasner DL, Rodeheaver GT, Sibbald RG, eds. *Chronic wound care: a clinical source book for healthcare professionals.* 3rd ed. Wayne, PA: HMP Communications, 2001.
5. Walker P. *Update on pressure ulcers. Principles & practice of supportive oncology updates,* Vol. 3 No. 6, 2nd ed. New York : Lippincott Williams & Wilkins, 2000:1–11.
6. Brem H, Lyder C. Protocol for the successful treatment of pressure ulcers. *Am J Surg* 2004;188(1A Suppl):9–17. Review.
7. Leigh I, Bennett G. Pressure ulcers: prevalence, etiology, and treatment modalities, a review. *Am J Surg* 1994;167:25S–30S.
8. Eachempati SR, Hydo LJ, Barie PS. Factors influencing the development of decubitus ulcers in critically ill surgical patients. *Crit Care Med* 2001;29(9):1678–1682.
9. Cuddigan J, Berlowitz DR, Ayello EA. Pressure ulcers in America: prevalence, incidence and implications for the future: an executive summary of the National Pressure Ulcer Advisory Panel Monograph. *Adv Skin Wound Care* 2001;14:208–215.
10. Reifsnyder J, Magee H. Development of pressure ulcers in patients receiving home hospice care. *Wounds* 2005;17:74–79.
11. Walker P. The pathophysiology and management of pressure ulcers. In: Portenoy RK, Bruera E, eds. *Topics in palliative care,* Vol. 3. New York, NY: Oxford University Press, 1998:253–270.
12. Haisfield-Wolfe ME, Rund C. Malignant cutaneous wounds: a management protocol. *Ostomy Wound Manage* 1997;43:56–66.
13. Naylor W. Malignant wounds: aetiology and principles of management. *Nurs Stand* 2002;16:45–56.
14. Collier M. The assessment of patients with malignant fungating wounds—A holistic approach: Part 1. *Nurs Times* 1997;93(44):1–4.
15. Wilkes L, White K, Smeal T, et al. Malignant wound management: what dressings do nurses use? *J Wound Care* 2002;10:65–69.
16. Agency for Health Care Policy and Research. *Pressure ulcers in adults Prediction and prevention, clinical guideline no. 3.* Rockville, MD: AHCPR, 1992. See http://www.ncbi.nlm.nih.gov/books/bv.fcgi?rid=hstat2.chapter.4409.
17. Bergstrom N, Braden BJ, Laguzza A, et al. The Braden scale for predicting pressure ulcer sore risk. *Nurs Res* 1987;36:205–210.
18. Norton D, McLaren R, Exton-Smith AN. *An investigation of geriatric nursing problems in hospitals.* London, UK: National Corporation for the Care of Old People, 1962.
19. Agency for Health Care Policy and Research. *Treatment of Pressure Ulcers, Clinical Guideline No. 15.* Rockville, MD: AHCPR, 1994 See http://www.ncbi.nlm.nih.gov/books/bv.fcgi?rid=hstat2.chapter.5124. See also NPUAP at http://www.npuap.org/.
20. Carson S. Basics of wound healing and treatment. Wound Healer. See http://www.woundhealer.com/wound_healing_at_its_best.htm.
21. Walker P. Management of pressure ulcers. *Oncology (Williston Park)* 2001;15(11):1499–1508, 1511

22. Sibbald RG, Williamson D, Orsted HL, et al. Preparing the wound bed–debridement, bacterial balance, and moisture balance. *Ostomy Wound Manage* 2000;46(11):14–22, 24–28, 30–35.

23. Krasner DL. How to prepare the wound bed. *Ostomy Wound Manage* 2001;47(4):59–61.

24. Vowden K, Vowden P. Wound bed preparation. World Wide Wounds, March 2002. See http://www.worldwidewounds.com/2002/april/Vowden/Wound-Bed-Preparation.html.

25. Bergstrom N, Bennett MA, Carlson CE, et al. *Pressure ulcer treatment. Clinical practice guideline. Quick reference guide for clinicians, no. 15.* Rockville, MD: U.S. Department of Health and Human Services, Public Health Service, Agency for Health Care Policy and Research, AHCPR Pub. No. 95–0653, December 1994.

26. Maklebust J, Sieggreen M. *Pressure ulcers: guidelines for prevention and nursing management,* 2nd ed. Springhouse, PA: Springhouse Corporation, 1996.

27. Sykes MT, Godsey JB. Vascular evaluation of the diabetic foot. *Clin Podiatr Med Surg* 1998;15(1):49–83.

28. Rodeheaver GT. Wound cleansing, wound irrigation, wound disinfection. In: Krasner DL, Rodeheaver GT, Sibbald RG, eds. *Chronic wound care: a clinical source book for healthcare professionals,* 3rd ed. Wayne, PA: HMP Communications, 2001:369–383.

29. Boxer AM, Gottesman N, Bernstein H, et al. Debridement of dermal ulcers and decubiti with collagenase. *Geriatrics* 1968;24:75–86.

30. Thomas S, Andrews A, Jones M, et al. Maggots are useful in treating infected or necrotic wounds. *BMJ* 1999;318(7186):807–808.

31. Jones M. Larval therapy. *Nurs Stand* 2000;14:47–51.

32. Bonn D. Maggot therapy: an alternative for wound infection. *Lancet* 2000;356(9236):1174.

33. Spann CT, Tutrone WD, Weinberg JM, et al. Topical antibacterial agents for wound care: a primer. *Dermatol Surg* 2003;29(6):620–626.

34. Molan PC. Re-introducing honey in the management of wounds and ulcers - theory and practice. *Ostomy Wound Manage* 2002;48(11):28–40.

35. Ovington LG. Dressings and adjunctive therapies: AHCPR guidelines revisited. *Ostomy Wound Manage* 1999;45(Suppl 1A):94S–106S.

36. Ovington L, Peirce B. Wound dressings: form, function feasibility and facts. In: Krasner DL, Rodeheaver GT, Sibbald RG, eds. *Chronic wound care: a clinical sourcebook for healthcare professionals,* 3rd ed. Wayne, PA: HMP Communications, 2001;311–319.

37. Cutting KF. Wound exudate: composition and functions. *Br J Community Nurs* 2003;8(9 Suppl):4–9.

38. White RJ, Cutting KF. Interventions to avoid maceration of the skin and wound bed. *Br J Nurs* 2003;12(20):1186–1201.

39. Wooten MK. Long-term care in geriatrics: management of chronic wounds in the elderly. *Clin Fam Pract* 2001;3.

40. Barton P, Parslow N. Maligant wounds: holistic assessment and management. In: Krasner DL, Rodeheaver GT, Sibbald RG, eds. *Chronic wound care: a clinical sourcebook for healthcare professionals,* 3rd ed. Wayne, PA: HMP Communications, 2001;699–710.

41. Grocott P. The palliative management of fungating malignant wounds. *J Wound Care* 2000;9(1):4–9.

42. Ferris FD, Bezjak A, Rosenthal SG. The palliative uses of radiation therapy in surgical oncology patients. *Surg Oncol Clin N Am* 2001;10(1):185–201.

43. Piggin C. Malodorous fungating wounds: uncertain concepts underlying the management of social isolation. *Int J Palliat Nurs* 2003;9(5):216–221.

44. Krasner D. Using a gentler hand: reflections on patients with pressure ulcers who experience pain. *Ostomy Wound Manage* 1996;42(3):20–22.

45. Reddy M, Keast D, Fowler E, et al. Pain in pressure ulcers. *Ostomy Wound Manage* 2003;49(4 Suppl):30–35.

46. Popescu A, Salcido RS. Wound pain: a challenge for the patient and the wound care specialist. *Adv Skin Wound Care* 2004;17(1):14–20.

47. Naylor W. Assessment and management of pain in fungating wounds. *Br J Nurs* 2001;10(22 Suppl):S33–S36.

48. Moffatt C, Briggs M, Hollinworth H, et al. *Pain at wound dressing changes. EWMA position document.* London, UK: Medical Education Partnership, See http://www.tendra.com/index.asp?id=1321&lang=2.

49. Reddy M, Kohr R, Queen D, et al. Practical treatment of wound pain and trauma: a patient-centered approach. An overview. *Ostomy Wound Manage* 2003;49(4 Suppl):2–15.

50. Krasner D. The chronic wound pain experience: a conceptual model. *Ostomy Wound Manage* 1995;41(3):20–25.

51. Twillman RK, Long TD, Cathers TA, et al. Treatment of painful skin ulcers with topical opioids. *J Pain Symptom Manage* 1999;17(4):288–292.

52. Zeppetella G, Paul J, Ribeiro MD. Analgesic efficacy of morphine applied topically to painful ulcers. *J Pain Symptom Manage* 2003;25(6):555–558.

53. Jones MK, Wang H, Peskar BM, et al. Inhibition of angiogenesis by nonsteroidal anti-inflammatory drugs: insight into mechanisms and implications for cancer growth and ulcer healing. *Nat Med* 1999;5(12):1418–1423.

54. Briggs M, Ferris FD, Glynn C, et al. World Union of Wound Healing Societies EXPERT WORKING GROUP. Assessing pain at wound dressing-related procedures. *Nurs Times* 2004 100(41):56–57. See also http://www.tendra.com/index.asp?id=13153&lang=2.

55. Kammerlander G, Eberlein T. Nurses' views about pain and trauma at dressing changes: a central European perspective. *J Wound Care* 2002;11(2):76–79.

56. Parlow JL, Milne B, Tod DA, et al. Self-administered nitrous oxide for the management of incident pain in terminally ill patients: a blinded case series. *Palliat Med* 2005;19(1):3–8.

CHAPTER 23 ■ LYMPHEDEMA

VAUGHAN KEELEY

For patients with cancer, lymphedema can occur as an aftermath of treatment or it can be a feature of advanced disease. Lymphedema of the arm is a fairly common sequel to treatment for breast cancer, and leg edema may be present in patients with advanced pelvic cancers.

The approaches to management of these two groups may be different. In the former, "supportive" treatment would aim to minimize the edema and enable the patient, with successfully treated cancer, to live as normally as possible with the problem. In the latter, a "palliative" approach would aim to alleviate symptoms as much as possible while ensuring that any burden of treatment would be outweighed by the benefits. Edema in patients with advanced cancer may be only one of a number of problems that is experienced, and would therefore need to be considered in this context.

PATHOPHYSIOLOGY

Lymphedema is defined as the accumulation of a relatively protein-rich fluid in the interstitial space of tissues due to a low output failure of the lymphatic system, that is, lymph transport is reduced (1).

Lymphedema is usually classified into "primary", which defines a group of lymphedemas arising from a congenital abnormality of the development of the lymphatic system, and "secondary", in which extrinsic factors cause damage to the lymphatics. Lymphedema associated with cancer and its treatment is therefore secondary lymphedema.

However, the formation of edema in patients with advanced cancer is usually more complex than this. It is helpful, therefore, to consider the mechanisms of edema formation. Edema is the accumulation of excessive fluid in the interstitial space and results from an imbalance between the formation and drainage of interstitial fluid.

The Formation of Interstitial Fluid

Fluid enters the interstitial space by capillary filtration. The amount of filtrate is determined by the "Starling" forces acting across the capillary wall. These are the hydrostatic pressure gradient, which tends to push fluid from the capillary into the interstitial space, and the colloid osmotic pressure gradient due to plasma proteins that are retained in the capillary which tends to draw water from the interstitial space into the capillary. The volume of filtrate will also be determined by the permeability of the capillary wall (Fig. 23.1).

In the past it was felt that this process occurred largely in the arterial end of the capillary and a degree of reabsorption occurred at the venous end of the capillary. However, current thinking suggests that once fluid reaches the interstitial space its route of exit is through the lymphatic capillary, that is, lymphatic drainage (2). Therefore, edema occurs whenever capillary filtration exceeds lymphatic drainage.

Table 23.1 shows the changes in capillary filtration and lymphatic drainage in a variety of chronic edemas.

In venous edema, for example in chronic venous insufficiency of the leg, capillary filtration is raised because of increased hydrostatic pressure in the capillaries, but this results in increased lymphatic drainage due to the spare capacity of the lymphatic system to transport fluid. When this capacity is exceeded, then edema occurs (high output failure of the lymphatics). The edema in this situation is believed to be of lower protein content than in true lymphoedema described in the preceding text (1). If high output failure of the lymphatic system persists, then there is a gradual deterioration in lymphatic transport capacity and an element of true lymphedema occurs. This situation is often called *edema of mixed etiology*, that is, mixed venous and lymphatic.

In patients with reduced mobility, for example, those with chronic conditions, which means that they spend a lot of time sitting in a chair, the so-called dependency edema can occur. This is, again, a mixture of lymphatic and venous edema. Poor mobility means that the usual muscle pump that aids both venous and lymphatic drainage is impaired, and therefore capillary filtration is increased and lymphatic drainage reduced.

In patients with hypoalbuminemia the colloid osmotic pressure in the plasma is reduced, and therefore capillary filtration is increased, and edema can occur if lymphatic drainage is unable to cope with this.

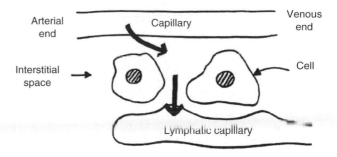

FIGURE 23.1. Diagram to illustrate tissue fluid formation.

TABLE 23.1

CHRONIC EDEMAS

Type	Pathology	Capillary filtration	Lymphatic drainage
Primary lymphedema	Lymphatic hypoplasia	Normal	↓
Secondary lymphedema	Lymphatic drainage	Probably normal	↓
Venous edema	High output failure	↑↑	↑
Lymphovenous edema	Reduced venous and lymphatic drainage	↑↑	↓
Advanced cancer	Lymphatic obstruction, venous obstruction, hypoalbuminemia immobility	↑↑	↓

Post-cancer Treatment Edema

It has long been assumed that axillary lymphadenectomy carried out as part of the surgical treatment for breast cancer has led to lymphedema of the arm in some women because of simple damage to the lymphatics. In addition, those women who have had radiotherapy to the axilla have also been believed to develop lymphedema because of damage to the lymphatics caused by the radiotherapy treatment. However, in recent years, it has become clear that this is perhaps too simplistic a view of the etiology of the edema. Studies have shown that in many women there are also changes in venous (3) and arterial (4) flow in the affected arm. In some women there may also be an underlying predisposition to developing lymphedema (5). Finally, the distribution of the edema, for example, sometimes sparing the hand, sometimes affecting only the hand, and so on, does not necessarily fit with a simple model (6).

Similar mechanisms may contribute to the formation of edema in people who have had groin lymph node dissections for the treatment of tumors such as melanomas of the leg.

Edema in Advanced Cancer

In patients with advanced cancer, the edema is usually of complex etiology (Tables 23.1 and 23.2). A patient may have lymphatic obstruction due to metastatic disease in the lymph nodes or due to previous treatment. There may be extrinsic venous compression causing venous hypertension or even venous thrombosis. In advanced disease, hypoalbuminemia is common, and finally, in association with the cachexia of advanced disease, weakness and immobility may result. These factors will lead to increased capillary filtration and reduced lymphatic drainage. This situation is often seen in patients with advanced pelvic malignancies (Table 23.2).

Chronic Edema

It is likely that very few edemas seen in patients treated for cancer are pure lymphedemas. Indeed, it may be better to use the term "chronic edema." This is defined as :

"A broad term used to describe edema which has been present for more than 3 months and involves 1 or more of the following areas: limb/s, hands/feet, upper body (breast, chest, shoulder, back), lower body (buttocks, abdomen), genital (scrotum, penis, vulva), head, neck, or face. Edema which develops because of a failure in the lymphatic system is referred to as lymphedema, but chronic edema may have a more complex underlying etiology" (7).

Nevertheless the term *lymphedema* tends to be used clinically and in current publications.

INCIDENCE

The literature is not clear about the precise incidence of lymphedema following treatment for cancer (8). Difficulties arise because of a lack of agreement about the definition of the degree of swelling that constitutes lymphedema, and the different ways in which measurements are made.

Cancer treatment–related lymphedema is most commonly seen in patients who have been treated for breast cancer, gynecologic cancers, urologic cancers, those who have had groin dissections for treatment for malignant melanoma, and those who have been treated for head and neck cancer.

TABLE 23.2

CAUSES OF EDEMA IN ADVANCED CANCER

General
- Cardiac failure (which may be secondary to or exacerbated by anemia)
- Hypoalbuminemia
- Late stage chronic renal failure
- Drugs:
  Salt and water retention, e.g., nonsteroidal Anti-inflammatory drugs and corticosteroids
  Vasodilation, e.g., nifedipine
- Malignant ascites

Local
- Lymphatic obstruction/damage
  Surgery/radiotherapy
  Metastatic tumor in lymph nodes or skin lymphatics
  Recurrent infections
- Venous obstruction
  e.g., deep vein thrombosis, superior vena caval obstruction, inferior vena caval obstruction, extrinsic venous compression by tumor, thrombophlebitis migrans
- Lymphovenous edema
  due to immobility and dependency or localized weakness due to neurologic deficit

Breast Cancer–related Lymphedema

Breast cancer–related lymphedema is the type that has been studied most, but even in this group there remain a number of uncertainties about the true incidence and etiology (8). The prevalence of edema in women who have received conventional treatment for breast cancer is reported to be around 25–28% (9), although in some reports the figure is as low as 6% (10). This "conventional" treatment usually involves axillary node sampling in which it is intended to remove a sample of four nodes for staging purposes. Removal of the tumor itself is usually by mastectomy or wide local excision together with postoperative radiotherapy in some instances. It has been argued that with the use of sentinel node biopsy, the incidence of lymphedema may be reduced to approximately 3% (11).

Some of the variations in the results reported may relate to different lengths of follow-up as well as measurement techniques. There is a well-recognized pattern of delay in the onset of swelling which may occur several years after the primary treatment, even in the absence of recurrence of cancer.

The literature is also not consistent in terms of the risk factors identified for the development of lymphedema following treatment of breast cancer, but some of the common factors that emerge include (8) the following:

- Radiotherapy
- The extent of axillary node dissection
- Combined axillary surgery and radiotherapy
- Obesity
- Surgical wound infection
- Tumor stage
- Extent of surgery

Attempts have therefore been made to reduce the incidence of breast cancer–related edema by modifications of surgical and radiotherapy techniques. The following factors should help with this (12):

- Wide local excision rather than mastectomy
- Sentinel node biopsy rather than axillary node sampling
- Avoidance of axillary radiotherapy following axillary node clearance
- Modification of radiotherapy techniques
- Avoidance of arm infections and inflammation

Because of the often-delayed appearance of lymphedema following treatment, it will take some time to determine whether any of these changes will bring about the desired reduction in incidence.

Gynecologic Cancer

The prevalence of lower limb lymphedema after treatment for gynecologic cancers depends upon the type of cancer and surgery carried out. Nevertheless, one study has shown an overall prevalence of 18% in women treated for all gynecologic cancers (13). In 16% of these women the edema developed between 1–5 years following treatment. The prevalence was 47% in women treated for vulval cancer with lymphadenectomy and radiotherapy. However, other studies of vulval cancer have shown a range of between 9% (14) and 70% (15).

Urologic Cancers

There is very little evidence in the literature concerning the incidence of lymphedema of the legs and genitalia following treatment for urologic cancers. The incidence does seem to vary according to the type and location of a tumor and may be up to 50% in advanced stages of penile cancer or following its treatment (16).

Groin Dissection

Again, the literature shows a varied incidence. In one study of groin dissection for malignant melanoma, soft tissue sarcoma, and squamous cell carcinoma, the overall incidence of mild to moderate lymphedema was 21% (17). Sentinel node biopsy in the management of melanomas of the leg has been advocated to reduce the incidence of post-treatment lymphedema.

Other studies have shown the incidence of measurable lymphedema after groin dissection to be >80% after 5 years (18).

Head and Neck Cancer

Lymphedema of the face and submental region can occur following treatment for head and neck cancer. This treatment may involve bilateral lymph node dissections of the neck and postoperative radiotherapy, but there is little evidence in the literature to show how common the problem is.

Incidence of Edema in Advanced Cancer

Edema is a common problem in advanced cancer although, as described in the preceding text, its etiology can be complex. In one study it was shown that edema occurred in approximately one third of patients with advanced disease and was associated with a poor prognosis (19).

CLINICAL FEATURES

Lymphedema Due to Cancer Treatments

Symptoms and Signs

Lymphedema is often described as a firm nonpitting edema. However, in the early stages of its development, the swelling may be soft and pit easily on pressure. As the condition progresses, the edema becomes firmer because of the development of fibrosis and fatty tissue within the subcutaneous space.

The development of typical skin changes in lymphedema also takes a variable amount of time and seems to be more prominent in leg edema than in arm edema.

These changes include the following:

- An increase in skin thickness
- Hyperkeratosis: a buildup of horny scale on the skin surface
- A deepening of skin creases, especially round the ankle and base of toes (Figure 23.2)
- A warty appearance to the skin as hyperkeratosis worsens
- Lymphangiectasia: small blisters due to dilated lymph vessels. These may burst and cause significant leakage (lymphorrhoea). These are said to occur particularly following radiotherapy, which causes fibrosis and obstruction of the deep collecting lymphatics.
- Papillomatosis: with papules consisting of dilated skin lymphatics surrounded by rigid fibrous tissue which may give a "cobblestone" appearance to areas of skin, particularly on the legs

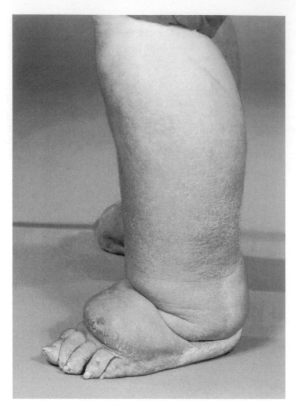

FIGURE 23.2. Lymphedema of the leg.

The physical sign, Stemmer's sign, is the inability to pick up a fold of skin at the base of the second toe and its presence is said to be diagnostic of lymphedema (20).

Pain may be a feature of lymphedema. In one study of various types of lymphedema, 57% of patients reported pain, while 32% described "tightness." Patients with active cancer were more likely to report both tightness and pain (21). Four types of pain were described: tissue pressure, muscle stretch, neurologic, and inflammation. Neurologic pain tended to occur in patients with advanced cancer. When lymphedema first appears, particularly if the swelling develops quickly, pain may occur which subsequently subsides.

In the early stages of the development of lymphedema, limb function and mobility may be normal, but as swelling develops, particularly around the joints, mobility is reduced and this may in turn exacerbate the swelling due to the reduced action of the muscle pump on lymphatic drainage. As a result, the limb can become increasingly heavy and cause further pain and discomfort at the shoulder or hip in the case of arm and leg edema, respectively.

Lymphedema after Breast Cancer Treatment

Patients may often develop symptoms before any objective evidence of lymphedema (22). These symptoms may include a feeling of fullness, tightness, or heaviness of the arm, shoulder, or chest, and an altered mobility of the shoulder. Associated with arm swelling, there may be truncal edema and an asymmetric increase in the subcutaneous fatty tissues.

Some patients may develop symptoms shortly after the initial treatment, and it may be that these are transient changes that will resolve. However, it is not clear whether these will predispose to subsequent development of more persistent lymphedema (22).

In women who have had treatment for breast cancer and who develop edema of the arm, it is important to consider whether there may be recurrence of the breast cancer or whether the edema has developed because of an acute deep vein thrombosis (DVT).

Psychosocial Aspects

Lymphedema, especially following cancer treatment, can be associated with a significant psychological morbidity (23). These may relate to issues of altered body image, disability, and the fear of cancer recurrence. The development of arm swelling can be particularly distressing for women who have had to cope with surgery, radiotherapy and chemotherapy for breast cancer, and their consequences. To have undergone all these treatments and then be left with persistent arm edema as a constant reminder of previous breast cancer can be traumatic.

Complications

The most common complications of lymphedema are as follows:

- Cellulitis
- Lymphorrhoea
- DVT
- New malignancies, especially lymphangiosarcoma

Cellulitis

In lymphedematous limbs there is an altered local immune response (24). This leads to a predisposition to developing infections and new malignancies in the affected area. The most important infection is cellulitis, which can not only be very unpleasant for the sufferer but may also lead to further damage to the lymphatic system and worsening edema, particularly if the cellulitis is recurrent.

Cellulitis in lymphedema is generally believed to be due to infection by beta hemolytic streptococci, although sometimes other bacteria such as staphylococci may be involved.

The usual clinical picture is the development of a flu-like illness with fever, muscular aches, and sometimes headache and vomiting. This is followed by the appearance of red inflamed painful tender areas in the skin of the lymphedematous limb. The skin changes can be very variable ranging from the whole limb being extremely inflamed to a relatively mild patchy rash.

Proving bacterial infection in all cases is difficult. This has led to the idea that some of these episodes are not necessarily infective, and the term *acute inflammatory episodes* or *secondary acute inflammation* has been derived (25) to describe them.

Sometimes it is clear that bacterial infection has entered the tissues through cuts, broken skin, and ruptured lymphangiectasia or papillomas. In the feet the skin between the toes may be cracked because of tinea pedis infections, to which people with lymphedema are predisposed.

A particular feature of lymphedema is the predisposition to recurrent episodes of cellulitis, which may not only be unpleasant in themselves, but may lead to worsening edema.

Lymphorrhoea

This is the leakage of lymph through the skin at sites of laceration or ruptured cutaneous lymph blisters (lymphangiectasia).

This can be particularly distressing if it affects the legs, as large volumes of fluid can leak out. There is an associated increased risk of infection.

Deep Vein Thrombosis

Patients with lymphedema are at risk from DVT in the affected limb, particularly if the limb is very edematous and immobile or if there is an associated abnormality of venous flow because of treatment for malignancy. A DVT can occur even when a patient is wearing a compression garment as treatment for their lymphedema.

Malignancy

Although rare, malignancies can arise in the skin of affected limbs. The most important of these is the lymphangiosarcoma (26). The term *Stewart-Treves syndrome* is used to describe its occurrence in postmastectomy lymphedema. In this situation, the incidence is <0.45% and the mean time from the surgery to onset is approximately 10 years.

Lymphangiosarcoma presents as single or multiple bluishred nodules in the skin, which spread rapidly locally often forming satellite lesions that may become confluent and ulcerate. Unfortunately, the prognosis is poor with a median survival of <3 years.

Edema of Advanced Cancer

Symptoms and Signs

The general symptoms and signs of edema in advanced cancer may be similar to those described in the previous section. However, as the etiology is often more complex, the clinical picture may also vary (Table 23.2). Pure lymphedema is probably unusual in advanced disease, and if it does occur, because of the short prognosis there is not usually time for the more chronic skin changes to develop. Therefore, edema in advanced cancer is often very soft and pitting. The skin can look stretched and shiny rather than thickened as in chronic lymphedema.

Pain is more likely to be a problem in patients with advanced cancer, particularly neuropathic pain resulting from nerve compression or destruction by tumor. This is often severe with tingling, burning, or stabbing features and altered sensation in the area of the pain. Light touch might be more painful than deep pressure (touch-evoked allodynia).

Patients may also be more prone to infections due to poor skin condition (often fragile, thin, and dry), skin tumors, ulceration and reduced resistance to infection because of treatment, or as a feature of advanced disease.

Ulceration of the skin is generally uncommon in lymphedema in comparison with venous disease, but can occur in patients with edema in advanced malignancy. There can be significant associated lymphorrhoea that can cause distress to patients. Superimposed infection by anaerobic bacteria can lead to unpleasant malodorous discharge and increased pain.

Immobility may be worse in patients with advanced malignancy because of generalized weakness or local nerve injury caused by tumor, such as brachial plexus infiltration in breast cancer.

The psychosocial aspects of edema in these situations are often greater, with patients having to cope with progressive disease and impending death, as well as the problems of lymphedema described in the preceding text.

Specific Situations

Locally Advanced Breast Cancer

In locally advanced breast cancer, a particularly severe and intractable type of edema can develop. In this situation the deep lymphatic drainage of the arm may have already been damaged by surgery and radiotherapy, but this can be worsened by the recurrence of disease in axillary lymph nodes and the development of metastatic disease in the skin of the upper arm and chest wall with infiltration of the skin lymphatics. The arm can become extremely swollen. The problem may be exacerbated by brachial plexopathy resulting in immobility of the arm and DVT because of extrinsic venous compression by tumor. In the latter, distended collateral veins may be seen around the shoulder.

The arm can become very heavy, swollen, painful, and dysfunctional. Blisters are common and breakdown of the skin may lead to ulceration and persistent lymphorrhea. The hand and fingers may swell to such an extent as to give the appearance of "a boxing glove" (Figure 23.3).

Advanced Pelvic Malignant Disease

Patients with advanced cancers of the uterus, ovary, prostate, bladder, or rectum may have gross edema of the legs and trunk, often of mixed etiology as follows:

- Lymphatic obstruction from metastatic disease in lymph nodes
- Extrinsic venous compression
- Inferior vena caval obstruction (IVCO)
- DVT
- Hypoalbuminemia
- Fluid-retaining drugs
- Ascites

Ascites

Malignant ascites is common in advanced ovarian, colorectal, gastric, pancreatic, and uterine cancers and is associated with a poor prognosis (median survival 2–3 months) (27). Leg edema is often associated with ascites.

Hypoalbuminemia

Hypoalbuminemia is common in advanced cancer because of the cachexia-anorexia syndrome, which causes a reduction in

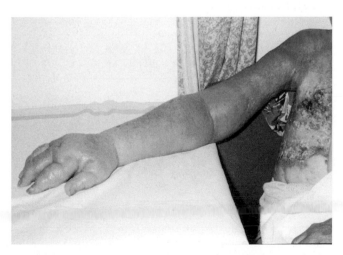

FIGURE 23.3. Lymphedema of the arm in locally advanced breast cancer.

hepatic protein synthesis (28). Hypoalbuminemia may cause edema on its own, but is usually seen in the context of other factors as described in the preceding text.

Superior Vena Caval Obstruction

Superior vena caval obstruction (SVCO) is usually seen in patients with extrinsic compression of the vena cava by metastases in the upper mediastinal lymph nodes. It is particularly common in lung cancer. The features may develop very quickly perhaps because of secondary venous thrombosis. The most common presenting symptoms are as follows:

- Dyspnea
- Neck and facial swelling
- Trunk and arm swelling
- A sensation of choking
- A feeling of fullness in the head
- Headache

On examination, the following may be present:

- Thoracic vein distension
- Neck vein distension
- Facial edema
- Tachypnea
- Facial plethora
- Cyanosis
- Arm edema

The condition can be very distressing for patients and, if untreated, may lead to death.

Inferior Vena Caval Obstruction

Inferior vena caval obstruction usually occurs because of extrinsic compression by retroperitoneal lymphadenopathy or hepatomegaly due to metastatic disease. Patients develop edema of the legs, abdomen, and genitalia, and if the obstruction is above the level of the hepatic veins, ascites may occur as well. Dilated collateral veins are often seen on the abdominal wall.

Complications

Although the complications of edema in advanced cancer may be similar to those of lymphedema described in the preceding text, patients with advanced disease are more prone to venous thrombosis due to the increased coagulability of their blood. They are also more prone to lymphorrhea and infections, but the short prognosis means that the development of lymphangiosarcomas is not an issue.

DIFFERENTIAL DIAGNOSIS AND INVESTIGATIONS

In patients with cancer treatment–related lymphedema, the diagnosis is usually based on the clinical history and examination. However, the possibility of DVT or recurrence of malignant disease does need to be borne in mind.

In patients with advanced malignancy, elucidating potentially reversible contributory factors is an important part of the management of edema (Table 23.2).

Investigations

Specific investigations may include the following:

- Computed tomography scan/magnetic resonance imaging/ultrasound scan to look for recurrent disease
- Full blood count to look for anemia
- Echocardiogram/chest x-ray/brain natriuretic peptide/electrocardiogram to look for evidence of heart failure
- Serum albumin to detect hypoalbuminemia
- Plasma urea and creatinine to look for evidence of renal failure

Deep Vein Thrombosis

In the United Kingdom current diagnostic practice for DVT relies on the use of an algorithm based on signs and symptoms (Well's Score (29)—see Table 23.3) together with d-dimer levels in the blood and an ultrasound examination of the leg to assess deep vein blood flow. Unfortunately, in patients with advanced malignancy the level of d-dimers may be elevated anyway, so this element of the assessment may not be particularly helpful.

A "Well's score" of 2 or higher indicates that the probability of DVT is "likely"; a score of <2 indicates the probability of DVT is "unlikely." In patients with symptoms in both legs, the more symptomatic leg is used.

DVT can be ruled out in a patient who is scored in the "unlikely" category and who has a negative d-dimer test (29). In those with positive d-dimers, a Well's score in the "likely" category, further investigation with ultrasound imaging of the leg is recommended.

Lymphoscintigraphy

Lymphoscintigraphy is a specific examination for lymphedema. Using a subcutaneous injection of a radioactively labeled macromolecule, for example, ^{99m}Tc-labeled protein or colloid. This is taken up by the lymphatics, which can then be detected using an external gamma camera. Although this is a useful technique in the assessment of patients with lymphedema in general, its place in patients who have cancer-related lymphedema is limited. However, practice does vary

TABLE 23.3

"WELL'S SCORE"

Clinical Model for predicting the pretest probability of deep vein thrombosis Clinical characteristic	Score
Active cancer (patient receiving treatment for cancer within the previous 6 months or currently receiving palliative treatment)	1
Paralysis, paresis, or recent plaster immobilization of the lower extremities	1
Recently bedridden for 3 d or more, or major surgery within the previous 12 wk requiring general or regional anesthesia	1
Localized tenderness along the distribution of the deep venous system	1
Entire leg swollen	1
Calf swelling at least 3 cm larger than that on the asymptomatic side (measured 10 cm below tibial tuberosity)	1
Pitting edema confined to the symptomatic leg	1
Collateral superficial veins (nonvaricose)	1
Previously documented deep vein thrombosis	1
Alternative diagnosis at least as likely as deep vein thrombosis	−2

around the world. In the United Kingdom lymphoscintigraphy is rarely done in this situation, as it is felt it is unlikely to affect management, and the diagnosis is usually clear on clinical grounds. However, in other countries isotope lymphoscintigraphy is more commonly performed (30).

MANAGEMENT

Recommendations to Patients Regarding Prevention of Lymphedema

Although there is little evidence to support recommendations for the prevention of the development of lymphedema in those at risk following cancer surgery, for example, axillary lymphadenectomy, it seems reasonable for patients to take sensible precautions to minimize the risk of infection or overload of the lymphatics that may cause further damage to lymph vessels and precipitate overt edema (31). Examples of these are given in Tables 23.4 and 23.5.

Management of Treatment-Related Edema

The mainstay of cancer treatment–related edema is a combination of physical treatments which together are known as *decongestive lymphatic therapy* (DLT) (32). Other terminology is used to describe similar combinations of treatment, for example, complex decongestive therapy (CDT).

The treatment comprises four elements:

- Compression
- Skin care
- Exercise
- Massage: simple lymphatic drainage (SLD) or manual lymphatic drainage (MLD)

Compression is carried out either in the form of a specific multilayer lymphedema bandage (MLLB) or elastic compression garments.

Skin care typically involves the use of a moisturizing cream such as aqueous cream, but also looks at ways of protecting the skin such as avoiding cuts and abrasions, avoiding sun burn, avoiding venipuncture, intravenous infusions, and treating

TABLE 23.4

RECOMMENDATIONS TO PREVENT LYMPHEDEMA AFTER BREAST CANCER TREATMENT

- Avoid injuries including cuts and abrasions, for example, wear gloves when gardening
- Use a thimble when sewing
- Use an oven glove when cooking
- Take care when ironing
- Avoid tight clothing including tight bra straps
- Avoid irritating cosmetics/soaps
- Avoid sunburn
- Avoid extreme sports
- Avoid heavy lifting, e.g., carrying heavy shopping
- Avoid insect bites/cat scratches
- Use an electric razor for shaving
- Avoid obesity
- Avoid injections or venipuncture in the "at risk" arm
- Avoid blood pressure measurement in the "at risk" arm
- Seek medical advice if "at risk" arm becomes inflamed or swollen

TABLE 23.5

RECOMMENDATIONS TO PATIENTS AT RISK OF DEVELOPING LEG LYMPHEDEMA

- Avoid standing for several hours
- Maintain skin hygiene especially feet
- Avoid tight shoes, socks, other clothing
- Avoid walking barefoot outdoors
- Avoid irritating cosmetics or soaps
- Avoid injections in the "at risk" limb
- Avoid insect bites/cat scratches/cuts/injuries
- Treat fungal infections, for example, tinea pedis, early
- Avoid sunburn
- Avoid surgery, for example, for varicose veins, if possible
- Avoid obesity
- Use an electric razor for shaving
- Seek medical advice if "at risk" leg becomes inflamed or swollen

conditions such as eczema. It is often also recommended to avoid having blood pressure measured in the lymphedematous arm. The aim of these recommendations is to improve the skin condition and reduce the likelihood of infections.

Exercise in compression garments encourages lymphatic drainage but some patients may require specific physiotherapy/exercises to improve function if joints have become stiff.

MLD is a type of gentle skin massage applied by trained therapists, which is designed to improve lymph drainage. SLD is based on the principles of MLD, but is carried out by the patient themselves or by a carer.

MLD is said to stimulate contraction of the lymph collectors and enhance protein resorption. The massage technique is designed to improve drainage from congested areas. It includes breathing exercises to improve thoracic duct drainage and gentle superficial massage working distal to proximal, for example, commencing on the trunk, then the proximal part of the limb, and then the distal area, to encourage proximal flow. There are a number of different "schools" of MLD, for example, Vodder, Leduc, Földi and Casley Smith. Although slightly different techniques are employed, the basic principles are shared by all schools (33).

For patients with moderate to severe edema, an intensive phase of treatment over a period of approximately 2 weeks involving compression bandaging (with or without MLD) to reduce the swelling and improve the shape of the limb is carried out. Patients who have associated truncal edema usually require MLD together with compression bandaging. This intensive phase of treatment is followed by the application of compression garments, that is, an elastic stocking or arm sleeve, which is then worn daily indefinitely.

Some patients require repeated courses of bandaging treatment over a period of time. Other patients with more mild edema may be managed with skin care and compression garments alone.

Patients with "mid-line" edema, that is, truncal, breast, genital, or head and neck edema, are best treated with MLD and SLD as these are not areas to which compression garments can be easily applied. Specialist garments for these areas, however, are available and may be helpful in some situations.

Evidence for Effectiveness of Treatments

There is little robust evidence in the literature to validate the individual components of these treatment regimes. Nevertheless, the combination of physical treatments has been shown to produce a sustained improvement in limb volume and a reduction in the incidence of episodes of cellulitis (34). This important study looked at the response to a two-phase treatment program in 299 patients with arm or leg lymphedema. The first phase of treatment consisted of MLD, multilayer bandaging, exercises, and skin care for an average of 15.7 days. This was followed by a second phase of wearing a daytime elastic compression garment, nighttime "wrapping", and exercises. Limb volume measurements were taken at regular intervals and the occurrences of cellulitis recorded. Lymphedema reduction averaged 59% in arm edema and 68% in leg edema. With an average follow-up of 9 months, this improvement was maintained in compliant patients at 90% of the initial reduction. There was also a reduction in the incidence of infection from 1.1 episodes per patient per year before treatment to 0.65 episodes per patient per year following treatment. It should be noted that this study involved patients who had non-cancer-related edema as well as those who had been treated for cancer.

A small number of studies have looked at the effectiveness of individual components of treatment. For example:

- Multilayer bandaging as initial phase of treatment for moderate or severe unilateral lymphedema (≥20% of excess volume compared with normal limb), followed by hosiery achieved greater and more sustained limb volume reduction than hosiery alone (35).
- MLD produced a small added reduction in volume when used with bandaging (36) (mean reduction = 27 mL) or when compared with SLD (37) (mean volume difference = 39 mL). However, it is not clear whether these small changes are of clinical significance.

Other treatments that have been used include pneumatic compression pumps. A variety of these devises is available, ranging from single-chambered sleeves providing intermittent compression to a limb, to multichambered devices (e.g., 5–10 chambers) that produce an intermittent sequential (peristaltic) compression massaging fluid from the distal to the proximal part of the limb (38).

However, there seems to be no major advantage in the use of these pumps and they probably do not have a place in routine practice (39). Nevertheless, in some situations, in which there is firm swelling that is difficult to control, they may have a role as part of a multimodal treatment package.

Surgical treatment of cancer-related lymphedema is again not commonly carried out, although there are some advocates for specific techniques in difficult circumstances. Liposuction has been used in women with breast-cancer–related lymphedema. However, although the reduction in limb volume is good with this technique, patients continue to have to wear compression hosiery and carry out massage techniques following surgery (40).

Drug treatments for lymphedema are generally disappointing. Diuretics seem to have no role in the treatment of pure lymphedema, although they can be helpful if fluid retention is present as well.

Some advocate the use of benzopyrones such as oxerutins or coumarin. However, their evidence for effectiveness is inconsistent in the literature, and coumarin has significant hepatotoxicity (41,42).

Treatment of Infection

Local fungal infections such as tinea pedis are treated with topical antifungals such as Miconazole cream. Fungal nail infections are more difficult to eradicate and may require treatment with oral Terbinafine.

TABLE 23.6

ORAL ANTIBIOTICS FOR THE TREATMENT OF CELLULITIS

1. Amoxycillin 500 mg t.i.d. for at least 14 days.
2. Flucloxacillin 500 mg q.i.d. if evidence of staphylococcal infections, e.g., folliculitis
3. Clindamycin 300 mg q.i.d. to be substituted for the Amoxycillin if there is a poor response to oral antibiotics after 48 h. This is recommended for patients who are allergic to penicillin as the first-line treatment.

Treatment of cellulitis is aimed at group A Streptococci, and depending upon the severity of the problem, may be managed at home with oral antibiotics, but may require admission to hospital for intravenous therapy (Table 23.6).

Bed rest and elevation of the lymphedematous limb is part of the management. Compression garments are not worn until the infection has settled.

If intravenous antibiotics are required, then a regime such as Amoxycillin 2 g t.i.d. intravenously, plus Gentamicin 5 mg per kg intravenously, given in a single daily dose for no more than 7 days may be followed. If there is no response after 48 hours to this management, then Clindamycin 1.5 g q.i.d., i.v. could be substituted. Once the patient's condition begins to improve, a switch can be made to oral antibiotics.

In patients who develop recurrent cellulitis, that is, who have two or more attacks of cellulitis per year, prophylactic antibiotics should be considered if reduction in limb volume by treatment and improvement of skin condition has failed to reduce the incidence of infection. A suggested antibiotic regime is phenoxymethylpenicillin 500 mg daily. The duration of prophylaxis is dependent on individual circumstances, but may need to be life-long in patients in whom attempts to withdraw it have resulted in recurrence of cellulitis.

Management in Patients with Advanced Cancer

The general principles of management are as for patients with lymphedema caused by cancer treatment, but they may have to be modified in the light of circumstances. In view of the complex etiology it is helpful to identify potentially reversible factors as described in the preceding text and treat these accordingly, for example, blood transfusion for anemia.

When uncontrolled tumor is the main cause of the edema, this is unlikely to respond very well to treatment and an emphasis should be based on enhancing the patient's quality of life, respecting their choices and priorities and providing psychological support to the patient and the family. It is important that any burden of treatment should not exceed the benefit gained (43).

Skin Care

Skin care remains important in advanced disease, and the avoidance of trauma is particularly relevant. The shearing forces when putting on and taking off a compression garment may cause damage to the skin and a light support bandage may be more appropriate in these circumstances. Where there is skin breakdown, nonadherent dressings may have to be applied. Occasionally, hemostatic dressings may be needed to control bleeding (e.g., calcium alginate), or topical epinephrine solution 1 in 1000 (1 mg in 1 mL) used when dressings are changed.

Fungating Lesions

Fungating lesions, for example on the chest wall or upper arm, in locally advanced breast cancer may become malodorous because of superadded anaerobic bacterial infection. Topical metronidazole 0.8% gel daily or oral metronidazole 400 mg b.i.d. for 2 weeks is often helpful (44). Topical metronidazole is relatively free from adverse effects but sometimes it is difficult to apply the gel to deeper crevices, and in some situations in which there is profuse discharge the gel is flushed away or diluted, thereby making it less effective. In these circumstances oral metronidazole may be helpful.

Support and Positioning

In very ill patients, support and positioning of swollen limbs using pillows, and so on, may relieve discomfort. It is important to try to avoid the use of an arm sling for people with arm edema, as this may cause pooling of fluid of the elbow and stiffness of the elbow joint (45). However, in some patients with severe arm edema and weakness from brachial plexopathy, a sling that can take the weight away from the shoulders and distribute it across the back may help with comfort and improve steadiness on movement (e.g., Polysling).

Exercise

Exercises need to be adjusted to the patients' abilities and condition. Passive movements may be helpful to reduce stiffness and discomfort, but more active exercise regimes are usually inappropriate.

Massage

The presence of active cancer is often considered to be a contraindication to massage techniques such as MLD and SLD. It is argued that stimulation of lymph flow around the site of a tumor may lead to metastasis (46). There is no evidence either way to support or refute this in the literature, but in the presence of advanced metastatic disease the potential benefits of massage, particularly for truncal edema, outweigh any risk of inducing further metastatic spread. It is important that the patient makes an informed choice in this situation.

Compression

The aim of management in advanced cancer is often to relieve discomfort rather than to aggressively try to reduce limb volume. The skin may be too fragile to tolerate significant compression and therefore modifications of bandaging techniques to provide support from light bandages or from low compression garments are often needed. Shaped Tubigrip is a useful alternative to compression garments. In all circumstances the skin condition needs to be checked regularly, particularly if there is impaired skin sensation, to confirm that the bandage or garment is not causing additional problems (47).

Lymphorrhoea is helped by bandaging. A sterile pad or gauze is used to absorb the lymph and the gentle pressure applied by bandage often stops lymphorrhoea in 24–48 hours (47). Sometimes, however, the bandage may need changing several times a day initially because of the rapid leakage of lymph.

In certain circumstances compression bandaging may increase the amount of fluid leakage. For example, in patients with fungating breast tumors in the axilla or chest wall, the application of a bandage to the ipsilateral swollen arm may result in an increased discharge from the lesion. This is believed to be due to the increased flow of lymph through "open" lymphatics near the skin surface.

Compression bandaging, particularly of the legs, should be avoided in patients with acute heart failure, which may be contributing to their edema in advanced disease, and also in those with acute DVT. Because of the multifactorial nature of the edema, those with bilateral leg swelling, genital, and truncal edema often do not tolerate compression bandaging of the legs. This may be ineffective, or simply push fluid onto the abdominal wall and genital areas making the edema there worse.

Appliances to Aid Mobility and Function

Various aids that may help with walking, dressing, use of swollen hands and arms, and so on, may be provided by an occupational therapist.

Drug Treatments

Corticosteroids. Systemic corticosteroids are often used for a variety of symptoms in advanced cancer. They work by reducing inflammation and peritumour edema and thereby can relieve pressure on neighboring structures such as lymphatics, veins, and nerves. They can therefore have a role in reducing pain and swelling.

Dexamethasone is commonly used as a starting dose of 8–16 mg daily. This is usually given as a trial for 1 week to determine whether it is effective. If the drug is ineffective, it is discontinued at this stage. If it is effective, then the dose is gradually reduced until the lowest level that relieves the symptoms is reached. This usually takes a period of weeks, over which time adverse effects such as fluid retention, gastrointestinal disturbance, weight gain, proximal myopathy, diabetes, and psychosis may develop. Should these occur, the balance of benefit versus the side effects of the drugs should be reviewed with the patient and a decision made whether to continue or gradually withdraw the treatment.

Diuretics

Diuretics may be helpful in the management of edema of advanced cancer if fluid retention, for example, due to drugs, or heart failure is present. Furosemide is commonly used and the dose adjusted according to effect.

Analgesics

Pain associated with edema in advanced cancer may respond to opioid analgesics, but if neuropathic pain is present other approaches such as the use of amitriptyline or one of the anticonvulsant drugs such as gabapentin may be helpful. (see chapter 2)

Treatment of Specific Potentially Reversible Factors

Potentially reversible factors should be treated in the light of a patient's general condition. Aggressive invasive treatment may not be appropriate in patients with a very short prognosis. A detailed description of all the treatment regimes is beyond the scope of this chapter, but a brief summary is given in Table 23.7.

The management of DVT with anticoagulants in patients with advanced cancer is not easy (49). The presence of existing bleeding from tumors such as fungating breast lesions would represent a contraindication. Although patients with advanced cancer are more prone to thrombosis, they are also more prone to hemorrhage if anticoagulated with warfarin. Drug interactions between warfarin and other medications that the person may be taking are common. Furthermore, patients who are anticoagulated to a "routine" level with warfarin, that is, INR = 2–2.5, may still develop further thromboembolic events. Anticoagulation to a higher level is sometimes used but has an associated increased risk of bleeding. Low-molecular-weight heparins, for example, enoxaparin may be a more

TABLE 23.7

TREATMENT OF POTENTIALLY REVERSIBLE FACTORS IN ADVANCED CANCER

Condition	Treatment
Anemia	Blood transfusion
Heart failure	Diuretics, digoxin, angiotensin-converting enzyme inhibitors
Fluid-retaining drugs	Withdraw if possible or use diuretics
Hypoalbuminemia	Treatment generally unrewarding
Malignant ascites	Paracentesis
	Diuretic therapy, for example, with spironolactone with or without furosemide
	Anticancer therapy, for example, in ovarian cancer
Superior vena caval obstruction	Metal stent (48)
	High-dose corticosteroids plus radiotherapy
	Chemotherapy
Inferior vena caval obstruction	Corticosteroids
	Metal stent
Deep vein thrombosis	Anticoagulation with low-molecular-weight heparin or warfarin

appropriate alternative, but are more expensive and require daily subcutaneous injections. The likely risks and benefits of anticoagulation should be considered and an informed decision made with the patient.

CONCLUSIONS

The management of cancer treatment–related lymphedema is not curative, but can help control the significant symptoms experienced by patients. The situation in patients with edema in advanced cancer is different and the treatment is more "palliative" in nature.

It is important to assess patients in the light of the above and decide, with the patients, the most appropriate treatment for. In all situations, the balance of benefit versus burden should be weighed up.

References

1. Consensus Document of the International Society of Lymphology Executive Committee. The diagnosis and treatment of peripheral lymphedema. *Lymphology* 1995;28:113–117.
2. Levick J, McHale N. The physiology of lymph production and propulsion. In: Browse N, Burnand K, Mortimer P, eds. *Diseases of the lymphatics*. London: Arnold, 2003:44–64.
3. Svensson WE, Mortimer PS, Tohno E, et al. Colour Doppler demonstrates venous flow abnormalities in breast cancer patients with chronic arm swelling. *Eur J Cancer* 1994;30:657–660.
4. Svensson WE, Mortimer PS, Tohno E, et al. Increased arterial inflow demonstrated by Doppler ultrasound in arm swelling following breast cancer treatment. *Cancer* 1994;30:661–664.
5. Mortimer PS, Bates DO, Brassington HD, et al. The prevalence of arm oedema following treatment for breast cancer. *Q J Med* 1996;89:377–380.
6. Modi S, Stanton AWB, Mellor RH, et al. Region of distribution of epifascial swelling and epifascial lymph drainage rate constance in breast cancer-related lymphoedema. *Lymphat Res Biol* 2005;3:3–15.
7. Moffat CJ, Franks PJ, Doherty DC, et al. Lymphoedema: an underestimated health problem. *Q J Med* 2003;96:731–738.
8. Williams AF, Franks PJ, Moffat CJ. Lymphoedema: estimating the size of the problem. *Palliat Med* 2005;19:300–313.
9. Logan V. Incidence and prevalence of lymphoedema: a literature review. *J Clin Nurs* 1995;4:213–219.
10. Petrek JA, Heelan MC. Incidence of breast carcinoma-related lymphoedema. *Cancer* 1998;83:2776–2781.
11. Sener SF, Winchester DJ, Martz CH, et al. Lymphoedema after sentinel lymphadenectomy for breast carcinoma. *Cancer* 2001;92:748–752.
12. Meek AG. Breast radiotherapy and lymphoedema. *Cancer* 1998;83:2788–2797.
13. Ryan M, Stainton MC, Slaytor EK, et al. Aetiology and prevalence of lower limb lymphoedema following treatment for gynaecological cancer. *Aust N Z J Obstet Gynaecol* 2003;43:148–151.
14. Van der Velden J, Ansink A. Primary groin irradiation vs primary groin surgery for early vulval cancer (Cochrane Review). In: *The cochrane library*. No. 3, Chichester UK: John Wiley and Sons, 2004.
15. Stehman FB, Bundy BN, Thomas G, et al. Groin dissection versus groin radiation in carcinoma of the vulva: a gynaecologic oncology group study. *Int J Radiat Oncol, Biol Phys* 1992;24:389–396.
16. Okeke AA, Bates DO, Gillatt DO. Lymphoedema in urological cancers. *Eur Urol* 2004;45:18–25.
17. Karakousis CP, Heisler MA, Moore RH. Lymphoedema after groin dissection. *Am J Surg* 1983;145:205–208.
18. Papachristou D, Fortner JT. Comparison of lymphoedema following incontinuity and discontinuity groin dissection. *Ann Surg* 1997;185:13–16.
19. Morita T, Tsunoda J, Inone S, et al. The palliative prognostic index: a scoring system for survival prediction of terminally ill cancer patients. *Support Care Cancer* 1999;7:128–133.
20. Stemmer R. Ein klinisches Zeichen zur Früh-und differential-diagnose des Lymphödems. *VASA* 1976;5:261–262.
21. Badger CM, Mortimer PS, Regnard CFB, et al. Pain in the chronically swollen limb. *Prog Lymphol* 1998;11:243–246.
22. Rockson SG, Miller LT, Senie R, et al. Diagnosis and management of lymphoedema. *Cancer* 1998;83:2882–2885.
23. Tobin MB, Lacey HJ, Meyer L, et al. Psychological morbidity of breast cancer-related arm swelling. *Cancer* 1993;72:3248–3252.
24. Mallon E, Powell S, Mortimer P, et al. Evidence of altered cell mediated immunity in post-mastectomy lymphoedema. *Br J Dermatol* 1997;137:928–933.
25. Casley-Smith JR, Földi M, Ryan TJ, et al. Summary of the 10th international congress of Lymphology working group discussions and recommendations. *Lymphology* 1985;18:175–180.
26. Mulvenna PM, Gillham L, Regnard CFB. Lymphangiosarcomata - experience in a lymphoedema clinic. *Palliat Med* 1995;9:55–59.
27. DeSimone GG. Treatment of malignant ascites. *Prog Palliat Care* 1999;7:10–16.
28. Strasser F Hanks G, Cherny N. et al. The pathophysiology of anorexia/cachexia syndrome. In: Doyle D, et al., eds. *Oxford textbook of palliative medicine*, 3rd ed. Oxford, UK: Oxford University Press, 2004:520–533.
29. Wells PS, Anderson DR, Rodger M, et al. Evaluation of D-dimer in the diagnosis of suspected deep-vein thrombosis. *N Engl J Med* 2003;349:1227–1235.
30. Bourgeois P. Critical analysis of the literature on lymphoscintigraphic investigations of limb oedemas. *Eur J Lymphology* 1997;6:1–9.
31. Földi E, Földi M. Lymphostatic diseases. In: Földi M, Földi E, Kubik S. *Textbook of Lymphology*. Chap 5. Munich, Germany: Urban & Fischer, 2003:275–279.
32. British Lymphology Society Clinical Definitions. 2001. BLS website: www.lymphoedema.org/bls
33. Jenns K. Management Strategies. In: Twycross R, Jenns K, Todd J. *Lymphoedema*. Chap 7. Oxford, UK: Radcliffe Medical Press, 2000:108.
34. Ko DSC, Lerner R, Klose G, et al. Effective treatment of lymphoedema of the extremities. *Arch Surg* 1998;133:452–458.
35. Badger CMA, Peacock JL, Mortimer PS. A randomised controlled parallel group clinical trial comparing multilayer bandaging followed by hosiery versus hosiery alone in the treatment of patients with lymphoedema of the limb. *Cancer* 2000;88:283–287.
36. Johansson K, Albertsson M, Ingvar C, et al. Effects of compression bandaging with or without manual lymphatic drainage treatment in patients with postoperative arm lymphoedema. *Lymphology* 1999;32:103–110.
37. Williams AF, Vadgama A, Franks P, et al. A randomised controlled crossover study of manual lymphatic drainage therapy in women with breast cancer-related lymphoedema. *Eur J Cancer Care* 2002;11:254–261.
38. Bray T, Barnett J. Pneumatic compression therapy. In: Twycross R, Jenns K, Todd J. *Lymphoedema*. Chap 4. Oxford, UK: Radcliffe Medical Press, 2000:236–243.
39. Dini D, Del Mastro L, Gozza A, et al. The role of pneumatic compression in the treatment of post-mastectomy lymphoedema. A randomised phase III study. *Ann Oncol* 1998;9:187–190.
40. Brorson H, Svensson H. Liposuction combined with controlled compression therapy reduces arm lymphoedema more effectively than controlled compression therapy alone. *Plast Reconstr Surg* 1998;102:1058–1067.

41. Casley-Smith JR, Morgan RG, Piller NB. Treatment of lymphoedema of the arms and legs with 5,6 benzo-(alpha)-pyrone. *N Engl J Med* 1993;329:1158–1163.

42. Loprinzi CL, Kugler JW, Sloan JA, et al. Lack of effect of coumarin in women with lymphoedema after treatment for breast cancer. *N Engl J Med* 1999;340:346–350.

43. British Lymphology Society. 2001. Chronic oedema: population of needs. BLS website: www.lymphoedema.org/bls

44. Newman V, Allwood M, Oakes RA. The use of Metronidazole gel to control the smell of malodorous lesions. *Palliat Med* 1989;3:303–305.

45. Badger C. Lymphoedema: management of patients with advanced cancer. *Prof Nurse* 1987;2:100–102.

46. Wittlinger H, Wittlinger G. Absolute contraindications. In: *Textbook of Dr Vodder's manual lymph drainage Vol 1 basic course*, 5th ed, Brussels: Haug International, 1995:74.

47. Mortimer PS, Badger C, Hanks G, et al. Lymphoedema. In: Doyle D, et al., ed. *Oxford textbook of palliative medicine*, 3rd ed. Oxford, UK: Oxford University Press, 2004:640–647.

48. NICE Guidance. Stent placement for vena caval obstruction. *Interventional procedure guidance 79*. London: National Institute for Clinical Excellence, 2004.

49. Johnson MJ, Sherry K. How do palliative physicians manage venous thromboembolism. *Palliat Med* 1997;11:46–48.

CHAPTER 24 ■ PRINCIPLES OF FISTULA AND STOMA MANAGEMENT

DOROTHY B. DOUGHTY

A significant number of patients with solid tumors involving the abdominal organs have surgically created stomas or spontaneously occurring fistulas. Palliative care for these patients must provide effective containment of the effluent and odor, protection of the adjacent skin, and maintenance of fecal and urinary elimination. This chapter addresses the specific needs of patients with stomas or fistulas involving the intestinal or urinary tract.

FISTULA MANAGEMENT

Fistulas are abnormal openings between two internal organs or between an internal organ and the skin. Most fistulas arise from the gastrointestinal (GI) tract and are caused by delayed healing and anastomotic breakdown after a surgical procedure; fistulas may also occur as a result of direct tumor invasion or as a complication of radiation therapy (1–4). Fistula is always a devastating development, and despite significant progress in the management of complications such as sepsis and malnutrition, fistulas continue to be associated with significant morbidity and mortality. For patients with cancer, fistula development may be even more devastating; the addition of a fistula may overwhelm the patient's defenses, both physically and psychologically. Statistics indicate higher mortality rates among this patient population—for example, a retrospective review of patients treated at the National Institutes of Health Clinical Center from 1980 through 1994 revealed a 42% fistula-related mortality rate among patients with cancer who had enterocutaneous fistulas (2). In addition to the issues related to the fistula itself, the development of a fistula may delay or prevent treatment for the underlying malignancy, and malignant involvement of the fistulous tract may prevent closure, even with surgical intervention (2,4). Effective fistula management is therefore a critical component of effective palliative care.

Classification Systems

Fistulas are commonly classified according to the organs involved, point of drainage, or volume of output (1,4). Fistulas are named according to the organs involved and the pathway followed by the effluent (Table 24.1). Fistulas may also be classified as internal or external. Internal fistulas involve an abnormal communication between two internal organs (e.g., enteroenteric or enterocolic fistulas). These fistulas may be silent in that they produce no obvious pathology, but

they can greatly affect the patient's nutritional status by bypassing absorptive segments of the small bowel (4). External fistulas are those communicating with the skin or with organs that drain onto the skin, such as the vagina. These fistulas produce obvious symptoms and present major challenges in management (4). The third mechanism for classifying fistulas is by volume of output. Fistulas producing more than 500 mL of output per day have been labeled *high-output fistulas*, and those producing 200–500 mL per day are generally classified as *low-* or *moderate-output fistulas* (1,4,5). As might be expected, high-output fistulas are associated with greater risk of sepsis, malnutrition, and death than fistulas with low or moderate output (2).

Phases of Fistula Management

Effective fistula management can be divided into several distinct phases: stabilization, investigation, conservative therapy, and definitive management (1,4).

Stabilization

Initial goals in fistula management include normalization of fluid and electrolyte balance, establishment of nutritional support, and elimination of sepsis (1,4–6). Specific fluid and electrolyte needs depend on the type and volume of fistula output; for example, small bowel fistulas usually produce high volumes of effluent containing potassium, sodium, magnesium, phosphate, and zinc (1,4). The patient with a high-output fistula requires close monitoring of fluid—electrolyte balance, with replacement titrated in response to type and volume of

TABLE 24.1

TERMINOLOGY FOR COMMON FISTULAS

Origin	Termination	Name
Small bowel	Skin	Enterocutaneous
Colon	Skin	Colocutaneous
Bladder	Skin	Vesicocutaneous
Small bowel	Vagina	Enterovaginal
Colon	Vagina	Colovaginal
Bladder	Vagina	Vesicovaginal
Rectum	Vagina	Rectovaginal

output and on the basis of laboratory indices. Fluid and electrolyte anomalies remain a significant problem in the management of these patients, and effective management can significantly reduce morbidity (1,4,5,7).

Malnutrition is another major problem associated with GI fistulas, especially high-output fistulas; therefore, prompt initiation of nutritional support is an essential element of care. (5) Patients with small bowel fistulas usually require total parenteral nutrition (TPN), though low-volume enteral intake is frequently advocated to prevent atrophy of the villi; in contrast, patients with colonic fistulas can frequently be managed with oral or enteral nutrition (4,6). Any nutritional support program must include ongoing monitoring of the patient's weight and prealbumin; in addition, the patient receiving enteral or oral nutrition must be monitored for any significant increase in fistula output. While aggressive nutritional support is generally contraindicated in the setting of palliative care, failure to provide such support can produce a catabolic state that causes rapid deterioration in the patient's overall condition. Therefore, decisions regarding nutritional support for the patient with cancer who has a high-output fistula must be made within the context of the overall treatment plan and management goals (1,4).

Fistula development is often associated with intra-abdominal abscess formation, and sepsis is the most common complication of enterocutaneous fistulas. Therefore, initial management includes prompt management of any intra-abdominal infectious process (i.e., drainage of all abscesses and initiation of appropriate antibiotic therapy) (1,4).

Investigation

The second goal in fistula management is to identify the origin of the fistulous tract and any anatomic conditions that would prevent spontaneous closure of the fistula, such as distal obstruction, development of an epithelial-lined tract between the skin and the fistula opening (i.e., pseudostoma formation), complete disruption of bowel continuity, persistent abscess, or tumor involvement of the fistulous tract (1,4,6). Studies commonly involved in the investigative phase of fistula management include fistulograms and radiographic studies of the small bowel (to identify the origin of the fistula) and computed tomography scans (to determine the presence of tumor involvement or persistent abscess) (4,6).

Conservative Management

If there are no anatomic factors that would prevent spontaneous closure of the fistula tract, initial management usually involves medical measures to promote closure as opposed to surgical intervention. This approach is based on studies indicating that a significant proportion of fistulas close spontaneously (if there is no inhibiting pathology) and on the fact that surgical closure is frequently ineffective until the underlying factors contributing to fistula development have been corrected (1,4). Even among patients with cancer, spontaneous closure of fistula tracts is possible: Chamberlain reported a spontaneous closure rate of 33% for enterocutaneous fistulas (2).

Conservative management includes continued attention to fluid and electrolyte balance, nutritional repletion, and control of infection. In addition, measures are instituted to reduce the volume of effluent and collapse the fistula tract. The goal is to ensure sufficient intake of nutrients to support the healing process while minimizing the volume of drainage. Specific measures to reduce fistula output and collapse the fistula tract include limitation (or elimination) of oral intake, administration of octreotide acetate, and implementation of negative pressure wound therapy (NPWT) (1,4,6,8).

NPO status. Elimination or significant restriction of oral intake can markedly reduce fistula output; however, such

restrictions can have a significant and negative impact on quality of life and should therefore be implemented only if fistula closure represents a primary treatment objective (7). If oral intake *is* significantly restricted, it may be beneficial to administer H_2 receptor antagonists to prevent stress ulceration and reduce gastric secretions (4).

Octreotide acetate. Octreotide acetate is a synthetic somatostatin analog that reduces the volume of intestinal secretions and prolongs GI transit time. The data on octreotide acetate's impact on fistula volume and fistula closure are inconclusive; however, in general, octreotide acetate has been shown to reduce the volume of fistula output and in some studies has appeared to significantly reduce the time frame for spontaneous closure. To date, there is no evidence that octreotide acetate actually increases the number or percentage of fistulas closing spontaneously, so the clinician must weigh the potential benefit against the expense of the therapy (3,4,9,10).

Negative pressure wound therapy (NPWT). NPWT was initially developed to manage exudate and promote granulation within chronic wounds; it has recently been approved for use with enteric fistulas and represents a major advance in conservative fistula management. The system with the strongest data related to closure of enteric fistulas is the VAC (vacuum-assisted closure) system of KCI (Kinetic Concepts, Inc., San Antonio, Texas). This therapy involves placement of a contact layer dressing and a porous foam dressing into the wound bed (but not the fistula tract), followed by application of a transparent adhesive drape to seal the entire wound; a small opening is then created in the drape and a suction device (TRAC Pad) is placed over the opening and connected to a portable negative pressure unit. (See Table 24.2 for the recommended procedure.) Therapy is begun at 150 mm Hg continuous negative pressure, and is titrated to the point required to collapse the fistula tract (as evidenced by cessation of fistula drainage), but not beyond −200 mm Hg. Therapy should be continued for at least 3 weeks following the collapse of the fistula tract to assure adequate healing. The therapy is expensive (>\$100.00 per day); therefore, failure to collapse the fistula

---

TABLE 24.2

APPLICATION OF NEGATIVE PRESSURE WOUND THERAPY (VACUUM-ASSISTED CLOSURE) TO PROMOTE FISTULA CLOSURE

1. Ensure appropriateness of therapy (appropriate only for enteric fistulas with potential for spontaneous closure).
2. Apply contact layer such as Adaptic (Johnson and Johnson) or Mepitel (Molnlycke) to wound bed and cover with VersaFoam (white foam). Note that VersaFoam should be cut slightly smaller than the diameter of the wound (to allow for wound contraction).
3. Apply adhesive drape to cover entire wound and 2–4 in. of surrounding skin.
4. Cut a small opening into the drape over the area of the fistula and apply the TRAC Pad over the opening.
5. Initiate suction at −150 mm Hg and observe for fistula drainage. If fistula drainage persists 30 min after initiation of suction, advance to −175 mm Hg and observe for fistula drainage. If fistula drainage persists after 30 min of −175 mm Hg suction, advance to −200 mm Hg. Do not advance beyond −200 mm Hg. If fistula drainage persists after 4 d of suction at −200 mm Hg, discontinue therapy.
6. If negative suction effectively collapses the fistula tract (as evidenced by cessation of fistula drainage), continue therapy for at least 3 wk to permit healing.

tract despite maximum negative pressure for a period of 4 days is generally considered a contraindication to continuation.

Definitive Therapy

When it is recognized that spontaneous closure is unlikely or impossible, a decision must be made regarding further management. The two options are palliative management (with no expectation of closure) and surgical intervention. The increasing availability of laparoscopic procedures makes surgical intervention a feasible option even for patients receiving palliative care (11,12). The optimal surgical approach involves resection of the fistulous tract with end-to-end anastomosis (4–6). If the involved segment of bowel cannot be isolated because of dense adhesions, it may be necessary to perform a bypass procedure, or, occasionally, to divert the fecal stream proximal to the fistula (1,4). If the fistulous tract is embedded in tumor and a radical resection is not feasible, the fistula tract may be defunctionalized by dividing the involved bowel segment proximal and distal to the fistula with a stapling device and performing an end-to-end anastomosis between the proximal and distal limbs of the normal bowel (6). Fistula drainage is therefore reduced to the small volume of mucous and intestinal secretions produced by the isolated segment of bowel containing the fistula (13). There are also reports of a successful "extra-abdominal" approach to fistula closure in a small series of patients with dense adhesions or irradiated tissue (14). Finally, the infusion of fibrin glue into low-output fistula tracts to significantly reduce the time to closure has been reported; however, this approach is not appropriate in high-output fistulas (15).

Palliative Fistula Management

In the patient with advanced malignancy, neither spontaneous closure nor surgical correction of the fistula may be achievable or practical. In this case, therapy is directed toward maintenance of patient comfort through containment of drainage and odor, protection of the perifistular skin, continued attention to fluid—electrolyte balance, nutritional support, and control of sepsis (1,5–7).

A major component of effective fistula management is containment of the effluent and odor and protection of the surrounding skin; these aspects of care have a profound impact on the patient's quality of life (7). Today, fistulas are treated as spontaneously occurring stomas, and ostomy pouches and products are used to protect the skin while containing the drainage and odor (5,6). In addition to promoting the patient's psychological and physical comfort, an effective pouching system permits quantification of output, which is critical for accurate replacement of fluid losses (1,4).

Guidelines for Pouching

Many products and techniques for containing drainage and odor and protecting the perifistular skin are now available. Selection is determined by the type and volume of drainage, the contours of the surrounding tissue, and the integrity of the perifistular skin (1). Additional factors to be considered include the cost and availability of products, the technical difficulty of the procedures compared to the caregiver's cognitive abilities and technical skills, and the availability of professional assistance, such as wound, ostomy, continence also known as enterostomal therapy, or ET nurses and home care nurses (6).

Products for skin protection. The volume and characteristics of the effluent dictate the level of skin protection required. Drainage that contains proteolytic enzymes or is highly alkaline or acidic can produce rapid and severe skin breakdown (especially if the fistula is also high output).

Therefore, gastric, pancreatic, and small bowel fistulas require aggressive protection of all perifistular skin and effective containment of the drainage, if at all possible (1). In contrast, drainage from the colon is usually low volume and nonenzymatic; severe skin breakdown is unlikely, and containment is needed more for odor control than for skin protection. Products available for skin protection include plasticizing skin sealants, pectin-based pastes and wafers, and moisture barrier ointments. The indications and guidelines for use of each of these products are outlined in Table 24.3.

Pouching principles. As noted, effective containment of drainage and odor is best accomplished through successful application of an adherent pouching system, similar to the systems used to contain ostomy output. Successful pouch application requires adherence to the following principles: the pouching system selected should be compatible with the type of drainage; the pouching system must be applied to a dry skin surface; and the surface of the pouching system must "match" the perifistular skin contours (1).

In selecting a system that is compatible with the type of drainage, the clinician should assess the effluent for fluidity and odor. Output that is very fluid and relatively nonodorous can be effectively managed with pouches designed for urinary stomas. These systems are odor-resistant (but not completely odor-proof) and equipped with narrow drainage spouts that cannot accommodate thick effluents. Output that is thick or malodorous should be managed with either fecal pouches or wound drainage systems. These systems are odor-proof and are equipped with tapered openings that permit thick or solid drainage.

The clinician must assure a dry pouching surface to obtain a good seal between the pouch and the skin. Denuded and weeping perifistular skin is common because of the damaging nature of the drainage, and is best treated with a procedure known as *crusting*. A pectin-based powder [Stomahesive Powder by ConvaTec (Princeton, NJ) or Premium Powder by Hollister (Libertyville, IL)] is sprinkled onto the wet skin to absorb the drainage and create a "gummy" surface; the powder is then "sealed" to the skin by blotting over the powder with a moist gloved finger or an alcohol-free skin sealant [e.g., No-Sting Skin-Prep by Smith and Nephew (Largo, FL), or Cavilon No Sting by 3-M (Minneapolis, MN)] (1).

The contours of the pouching system are matched to the patient's skin surface by carefully evaluating the perifistular skin with the patient in both the supine and sitting positions, and then selecting a pouch that is compatible with those contours. If the perifistular contours are fairly smooth, almost any system can be used. However, the patient with deep creases in the perifistular skin usually requires an all-flexible pouching system that will "bend and mold." If the fistula is in a "valley" and the perifistular contours are concave, a convex pouching system is advantageous. It is frequently necessary to use "filler" products (pectin paste, barrier strips, or moldable barrier rings) to fill small defects and create a smoother pouching surface (1).

Pouching procedures. Most fistulas can be managed with a standard pouching procedure using either an ostomy pouch or a wound drainage pouch. The standard pouching procedure is outlined in Table 24.4.

In patients with very irregular abdominal contours or a large associated wound, the standard pouching procedure is frequently ineffective. One pouching procedure that is frequently effective when standard pouching fails is the trough procedure; however, it is important to note that this technique is appropriate only for fistulas located in open wounds. The basic concept is as follows:

1. The perifistular skin is protected with skin barrier paste and overlapping strips of a solid skin barrier (such as Stomahesive).

TABLE 24.3

OSTOMY PRODUCTS AND MANUFACTURERS

Company	Contact information	Product line
Coloplast	Marietta, GA 800-533-0464 www.us.coloplast.com	1-piece and 2-piece pouches, fecal and urinary (flat, flexible, and varying levels of convexity) Skin protective products
ConvaTec	Princeton, NJ 800-325-8005 www.convatec.com	1-piece and 2-piece pouches, fecal and urinary (flat, flexible, and shallow convexity) Skin protective products
Hollister	Libertyville, IL 800-323-4060 www.hollister.com	1-piece and 2-piece pouches, fecal and urinary (flat, flexible, and shallow convexity + convex rings) Skin protective products
Marlen	Bedford, OH 216-292-7060 www.marlenmfg.com	1-piece pouches, fecal and urinary; 2-piece adhesive systems fecal only (flat, flexible, and varying levels of convexity) Skin protective products
NuHope	Pacoima, CA 800-899-5017 www.nuhope.com	1-piece pouches, fecal and urinary (flat, flexible, and varying levels of convexity) Customized pouches, belts and binders, skin protection

2. A large opening is created in a strip of transparent adhesive dressing (such as OpSite by Smith and Nephew, Largo, Florida), a drainable pouch is placed over this opening, and the strip of adhesive dressing and attached pouch are then applied to the inferior aspect of the wound.

3. Additional overlapping strips of a transparent adhesive dressing are used to cover the entire wound and the skin around the wound (1).

The wound therefore becomes a trough, with drainage funneled to the bottom of the wound, where it is collected. Suction can be added to this system for very high-output fistulas. The trough procedure is outlined in Table 24.5 and illustrated in Figure 24.1.

An alternative to the trough procedure for bedbound patients is the closed suction method of management. With this approach, the perifistular skin is again protected with overlapping strips of a skin barrier and skin barrier paste; the wound bed is then lined with a layer of damp fluffed gauze, suction catheters are placed over the gauze inferior to the fistulous opening(s), and damp fluffed gauze dressings are used to cover the suction catheters. Transparent adhesive dressings are then used to completely cover the wound and adjacent skin, and the suction catheters are connected to wall suction.

If all pouching procedures fail, or if the caregiver is unable to manage a pouching system, the focus becomes skin protection and odor control. Skin protection can be provided in one of two

TABLE 24.4

STANDARD POUCHING PROCEDURE

Select an appropriate pouch on the basis of the type of drainage and abdominal contours.
Size the pouch opening appropriately:
  For fistulas or skin-level stomas, size the opening to clear the fistula/stoma margins by 1/4–1/2 in.; this helps to prevent tunneling of the drainage under the barrier and pouch.
  For protruding stomas, size the opening 1/8 in. larger than the stoma.
Treat any skin damage with skin barrier powder ("seal" with damp finger or skin sealant).
Use pectin paste to fill any surface defects and "caulk" around the stoma or fistula opening (a wet finger facilitates paste application). Press pouch into place and use gentle pressure to ensure adherence.
Change pouch every 5–7 d and as needed (for leakage).

TABLE 24.5

TROUGH PROCEDURE FOR FISTULA MANAGEMENT

Treat any damaged skin with skin barrier powder ("seal" with damp finger or skin sealant).
Cut skin barrier strips and apply overlapping strips along periphery of wound. Use pectin paste to caulk the junctions between strips and protect any exposed skin. Note that the strip placed along the inferior aspect of the wound should be a solid U-shaped strip with no overlapping junctions, to prevent leakage.
Select transparent adhesive dressing strips that are approximately 4 in. longer than the widest point of the wound; this assures a 2-in. overlap onto intact skin on each side of the wound bed.
Modify one strip of transparent adhesive dressing as follows:
  With paper backing still in place, cut an opening in the dressing wide enough to encompass the inferior aspect of the wound (if wound diameter is 1 1/2 in. at the inferior aspect, the opening should be cut at least 1 3/4 in. in diameter).
  Select a one-piece ostomy pouch or wound pouch and cut an opening in the pouch that matches the opening in the adhesive dressing.
  Peel paper backing off the pouch and stick the pouch to the nonadhesive surface of the transparent adhesive dressing strip.
Peel paper backing off transparent adhesive dressing strip with pouch attached and apply to the inferior aspect of the wound.
Apply remaining strips of transparent adhesive dressing in overlapping fashion to cover the remaining area of the wound.

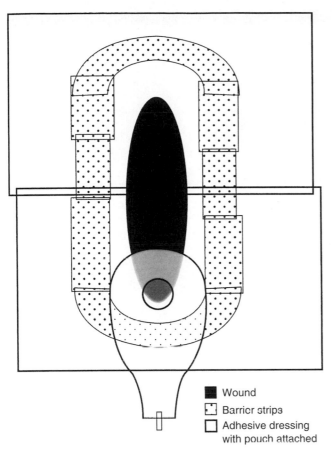

Wound

Barrier strips

Adhesive dressing
with pouch attached

FIGURE 24.1. Illustration of trough procedure for fistula management.

ways: either by placing overlapping strips of skin barrier along the wound edge or by applying a thick layer of a zinc-oxide-based moisture barrier along the wound edges. Absorptive dressings are then used to absorb the effluent; these dressings are best secured with a nonadherent system (e.g., burn netting), which facilitates frequent dressing changes. Odor control can be provided by charcoal cover dressings or by oral deodorants (e.g., chlorophyllin copper complex 100 mg once or twice daily or bismuth subgallate 325–650 mg three times daily). See Table 24.6 for odor-control options.

Vaginal Fistulas

One type of fistula that cannot be managed by pouching is the vaginal fistula. Patients with rectovaginal fistulas may be managed most effectively by maintaining stool in formed state the stool formed to minimize fecal contamination of the vagina. Frequently, patients with vesicovaginal fistulas can be managed effectively by placement of an indwelling urethral catheter to decompress the bladder. Patients with enterovaginal fistulas and patients with combined vesicovaginal fistulas, however, require containment to prevent significant perineal skin breakdown. An effective approach for these patients is outlined in Table 24.7.

Resources

Any patient with a significant fistula can benefit from referral to a Wound, Ostomy, Continence/ET nurse specialist. These nurses specialize in the management of patients with complex wounds and stomas. Information regarding availability of these specialists can be obtained from the national office of the

Wound Ostomy Continence Nursing Society (888-224-9626) or from their Web site (www.wocn.org).

STOMA MANAGEMENT

Urinary or fecal stomas may be created in conjunction with surgical removal of the bladder or rectum due to a malignant tumor or they may be performed for palliative management of advanced disease producing colorectal or ureteral obstruction (16,17). Therefore, palliative care for patients with GI or genitourinary malignancies frequently requires attention to stoma management and maintenance of GI/genitourinary function.

Management of Fecal Diversions

Descending/Sigmoid Colostomy

A descending or sigmoid colostomy is constructed when the rectum or sigmoid colon is removed or bypassed (17–19). The output from a descending/sigmoid colostomy is typically formed stool, and elimination patterns are similar to preoperative bowel patterns for the individual patient. These patients usually have two options for management. One option is to wear an odor-proof pouch and allow evacuation to occur spontaneously. The other option is to regulate bowel elimination through routine colostomy irrigations (20). The patient is taught to instill 500–1500 mL of lukewarm tap water into the stoma through a cone-tip irrigator that prevents bowel perforation as well as backflow of water (18,21–23). The distention of the bowel stimulates peristalsis, which usually causes evacuation of the left colon within 30–60 minutes. Evacuation of this bowel segment typically produces approximately 24–48 stool-free hours. Repeated administration of the same stimulus over time tends to "regulate" bowel emptying so that the potential for fecal spillage between irrigations is reduced. The patient who manages his colostomy with routine irrigation usually can wear a simple stoma cover or a stoma cap between irrigations; the stoma cap provides for absorption of mucus and also deodorizes and vents flatus (18–20,24).

Management issues for the patient with a descending or sigmoid colostomy include measures to control odor, reduce gas, and prevent or manage diarrhea and constipation (20,21,24). Routine measures to control odor include maintenance of an intact pouch seal and a clean drainage "spout"; the pouch material is odor-proof, so odor occurs only if there is a break in the seal or if fecal material is left on the drainage spout. Additional odor-control measures include the use of pouch deodorants (or the addition of 1 teaspoon of mouthwash into the pouch each time it is emptied) or administration of oral deodorants (as outlined in Table 24.6) (21,22). The primary "gas-reduction" strategy is limitation of gas-producing foods, such as broccoli, cabbage, onions, and beans (20–22); additional measures include use of over-the-counter agents such as Beano and Gas-X. Diarrhea can occur as a result of a viral illness or in response to some chemotherapeutic agents, and is managed similar to diarrhea in the patient with an intact rectum and anus. The patient is counseled to remain on a low-fat, low-roughage diet; to increase fluid intake; and to take over-the-counter antidiarrheal medications if desired (20–22). The patient who manages with routine irrigation is instructed to omit irrigations until bowel function and stool consistency return to normal. Constipation is much more common than diarrhea in the patient with advanced malignancy and a descending/sigmoid colostomy; this is due to the antiperistaltic effects of reduced fiber intake, reduced activity, and increased use of analgesics,

TABLE 24.6

OPTIONS FOR ODOR CONTROL

Product type/Examples	Mechanism of action	Indications/Guidelines for use	Companies and locations/ Contact information

Odor-absorbing dressings
    Odor Absorbing
        Dressing (Hollister)
    Carboflex Odor
        Control Dressing
        (ConvaTec)
	Dressing is impregnated with charcoal; when used as cover dressing, odor molecule forced through charcoal for odor elimination	Indicated for odor control with fistulas being managed with dressings as opposed to pouch
		Use as cover dressing; secure on all 4 sides with tape
			Hollister (Libertyville, IL) (800-323-4060)
			ConvaTec (Princeton, NJ) (800-325-8005)

Pouch deodorants
    M9 Deodorizing Drops
        (Hollister) or Adapt
        Deodorizing Lubricant
        (Hollister)
    OAD (Coloplast)
    Commercial
        mouthwash
	Reduce or neutralize odors in pouches to minimize odor when pouch is opened for drainage or replacement	Fecal stomas
		Malodorous wounds or fistulas being managed with pouching
			Add recommended amount to pouch each time pouch is emptied *or* saturate cotton ball with deodorizer and add to pouch each time pouch is emptied

Room deodorants
    REFRESH (Cymed)
    Hex-On (Coloplast)
	Reduce or neutralize odors in air; for use when pouch is emptied or changed	Spray into air just before opening pouch	Cymed (Berkeley, CA) (800-582-0707)
			Coloplast (Marietta, GA) (800-533-0464)

Internal deodorizers
    Devrom (Bismuth
        Subgallate),
        Parthenon Co.
    Derifil (chlorophyllin
        copper complex),
        Rystan
	Significantly reduce or eliminate fecal odor when taken orally on routine basis	Fecal stomas and fistulas
		Follow guidelines for dosage and administration; available over the counter
			Parthenon Co. (Salt Lake City, UT) (800-453-8898)
			Rystan (Little Falls, NJ) (973-256-3737)

a triad common in the setting of advanced disease. Acute constipation can be alleviated by the administration of laxative agents (e.g., bisacodyl, milk of magnesia, or polyethylene glycol preparations) or cleansing irrigations. Constipation should also trigger adjustments in the patient's management program: key elements in an effective program include assurance of adequate fiber and fluid intake (i.e., 28–30 g fiber per day

TABLE 24.7

VAGINAL FISTULA MANAGEMENT

Perform a vaginal examination to determine the size of the vaginal vault [use a topical anesthetic such as viscous lidocaine (Xylocaine) if patient has significant tenderness].

Obtain a soft rubber nipple shield or baby nipple (depending on size of vault) and a mushroom catheter.

Cut a small hole in the tip of the nipple or nipple shield; thread the catheter through so that the mushroom tip is resting within the nipple or shield. Secure the catheter to the nipple or shield with waterproof tape.

Fold the nipple shield down around the catheter, lubricate the nipple shield generously with a water-soluble lubricant, and gently push it into the vagina until the entire shield is in the vault; gently pull back on the catheter until the nipple shield is seated at the vaginal orifice.

Connect open end to bedside drainage unit.

and 30 cc fluid/kg body weight/day). If the patient is unable or unwilling to ingest adequate amounts of dietary fiber, he or she should be counseled to begin a bulk laxative (e.g., Metamucil, Citrucel, Konsyl, Benefiber) at the recommended dose or a bran mixture (1 cup miller's bran plus 1 cup applesauce plus one-fourth cup prune juice) at an initial dose of 2 tablespoons per day. The patient is instructed to increase the daily dose by 1 tablespoon each week until normal bowel patterns are reestablished. The patient must be cautioned regarding the critical importance of sufficient fluid intake and the risk of bowel obstruction if bulking agents are consumed without adequate fluids (25,26). If the patient is unable to maintain adequate fluid intake, bulking agents should be discontinued and the patient should be instructed to drink 2 glasses of prune juice daily; if this is insufficient or if the patient is unable to tolerate this, he or she should be placed on a softener/stimulant combination, such as Peri-colace (docusate and casanthranol) (25).

Transverse Colostomy

A transverse colostomy may be performed to provide fecal diversion in the patient with distal obstruction. Fecal output from the transverse colon is generally mushy in consistency, and the patient typically experiences output after meals and at other unpredictable times (20,21,24). Unlike the descending/sigmoid colostomy, a transverse colostomy cannot be regulated by routine irrigation because of continuous peristalsis in the ascending colon. Therefore, these patients must wear an odor-proof pouch for collection of the stool. Management issues for these patients include odor and gas control and management of diarrhea (as discussed in the section Descending/Sigmoid Colostomy) (21). Constipation usually does not occur because the stool in the transverse colon is quite soft and peristalsis in the ascending colon is fairly continuous; if constipation *should* occur, the management options would be the same as those discussed in the preceding section (Descending/Sigmoid Colostomy).

Ileostomy (or Ascending Colostomy)

An ileostomy is most frequently done when the entire colon and rectum are removed for disease processes such as familial polyposis, multiple colonic tumors, or inflammatory bowel disease (18,19). Cecostomies and ascending colostomies are not usually performed but are occasionally required to relieve acute obstruction of the distal ascending or proximal transverse colon (19). Output from these stomas is a thick liquid that contains proteolytic enzymes, which are extremely damaging to the skin (18,21). Management must therefore include continuous pouching with a well-fitting pouch and meticulous skin care to prevent contact between the peristomal skin and feces.

Ascending colostomy. Management issues for the patient who has undergone an ascending colostomy include skin protection, maintenance of fluid—electrolyte balance, and modifications in medication (20,21,24). The patient is taught to carefully size the pouch so that it fits closely around the stoma and protect any exposed skin with pectin-based paste. Patients are also taught to maintain a daily fluid intake of approximately 2 L and aggressively replace fluids and electrolytes during periods of increased loss (e.g., diarrhea or heavy perspiration); a practical recommendation is to drink a glass of replacement fluid (such as vegetable juice, broth, or a sports drink) each time the pouch is emptied. The patient is taught to recognize signs and symptoms of fluid-electrolyte imbalance and report such symptoms promptly to the physician (18,21). Modifications in medication include avoidance of time-released and enteric-coated medications because these forms are likely to be incompletely and unpredictably absorbed as a result of reduced bowel length and transit time (21).

Ileostomy. The issues of skin protection, fluid–electrolyte balance, and modification in medication are equally critical to the patient who has undergone an ileostomy. In addition, such a patient must be taught how to modify his or her diet to prevent food blockage (18–21,27). Food blockage is a complication unique to such a patient; it occurs when a bolus of fibrous undigested food obstructs the lumen of the bowel at the point where the bowel is brought through the fascia-muscle layer (a point of potential narrowing). Patients who have undergone ileostomies are taught to add foods high in insoluble fiber (raw fruits and vegetables, coconut, popcorn, nuts, etc.) to their diets one at a time and in small amounts, to chew thoroughly, and to maintain adequate fluid intake. They are also taught to recognize and report signs of partial or complete blockage: high-volume malodorous liquid output or no output, coupled with abdominal cramping, distention, and possibly nausea and vomiting (18,20–22). Food blockage is managed by ileostomy lavage performed by the physician or ostomy nurse specialist. A catheter is inserted into the stoma until the blockage is reached and 30–50 mL of warm saline is instilled. The catheter is then removed to allow for returns, and the procedure is repeated until the blockage is removed (18,20–22).

Continent Fecal Diversions

Most continent fecal diversions are performed for nonmalignant conditions affecting the colon, such as familial polyposis and ulcerative colitis (18,28). These patients, however, are not immune to other malignancies that may progress to an advanced state, and their care must include management of the continent diversion.

Continent ileostomy. A continent ileostomy (also known as *Koch Pouch* or *Barnett Continent Ileal Reservoir*) differs from a standard ileostomy in that an internal reservoir is constructed between the proximal bowel and the abdominal stoma. The diversion is made continent by intussuscepting the segment of bowel between the reservoir and the abdominal stoma, therefore creating a one-way valve (18,19,22,28–30). The patient drains the reservoir by intubating the stoma with a large-bore catheter approximately three to four times daily. If the stool is too thick to drain readily, the patient is taught to instill tepid water through the catheter into the reservoir to fluidize the stool (27,28). Management issues include avoidance of foods with peels (because the peels tend to obstruct the drainage catheter) and modifications in medication. In addition to avoiding enteric-coated and time-released medications, these patients must avoid wax-matrix medications because the wax shells do not dissolve and cannot be drained through the catheter. Patients are also instructed to flush the reservoir until clear one or two times daily to prevent pouchitis, an inflammation of the reservoir thought to be caused by bacterial overgrowth (22,28).

Ileal-anal reservoir. An ileal-anal reservoir is performed in conjunction with a colectomy and proctectomy. The sphincter mechanism is preserved. A reservoir is then created from the distal small bowel, and anastomosed to the anal canal (28,30,31). The patient's own sphincter therefore serves as the continence mechanism. The patient who has had an ileal-anal reservoir has mushy stools with residual enzymes; therefore, meticulous skin care is essential at all times and is even more critical during episodes of diarrhea (28,29,32). Such a patient is also at risk for pouchitis, an inflammation of the reservoir characterized by burning, itching, bleeding, and fecal urgency; treatment typically involves clear liquids and antibiotics (e.g., ciprofloxacin and metronidazole), or soluble fiber and probiotics such as VSL-3 (28,31–34).

Management of Retained Nonfunctional Distal Bowel Segment

Patients who have had a loop or double-barrel colostomy and patients with a Hartmann's pouch have a variable length of distal bowel that is nonfunctional. This segment continues to produce mucus, and some patients require periodic low-volume rectal enemas to eliminate inspissated mucus (35). The retained segment may also become inflamed, a condition known as diversion colitis, and characterized by the production of large volumes of mucus; management involves rectal irrigations to eliminate retained mucus, antibiotics, and topical steroids.

A common question among health care professionals is the appropriateness of rectal administration of medications through a "bypassed" rectal segment. Although this segment is no longer in continuity with the bowel, it is still vascularized; this means that medications administered rectally will be at least partially absorbed systemically. Therefore, it is appropriate to administer drugs such as antiemetics rectally, since these drugs are given for their systemic effects; it would of course *not* be appropriate to administer a glycerine suppository rectally for treatment of constipation involving the proximal bowel.

Management of Urinary Diversions

Urinary diversions are required for patients with pelvic malignancies requiring removal of the bladder and for patients with ureteral obstruction that cannot be managed with internally placed ureteral stents. The standard diversion for many years was the intestinal conduit, but the current trend is toward construction of continent diversions or orthotopic neobladders anastomosed to the urethra (16,36).

Intestinal Conduits

Ileal conduits and other intestinal conduits normally produce clear urine with strands of mucus (because a bowel segment is used as the conduit for urinary drainage). Because there is no reservoir for urine collection, urine drainage is almost continuous, and patients must wear a pouch to contain the output (16,21,37). The most important management issues are prevention and recognition of urinary tract infections. Patients are taught to maintain adequate fluid intake and recognize and promptly report signs of infection. Confirmation of urinary tract infection and organism identification are usually accomplished by obtaining a catheterized specimen for culture and sensitivity; these data provide the basis for organism-specific treatment (21).

Ureterostomy

Ureterostomies are rarely constructed because of the numerous associated complications (e.g., ineffective drainage, stenosis, and pouching problems). However, these diversions are occasionally required when it is not feasible to construct an ileal conduit. Output from a ureterostomy is clear urine without mucus, and management is the same as for patients with intestinal conduits. In addition, these patients need to be monitored for evidence of stenosis (i.e., reduced output, flank pain, and chronic urinary tract infections). Stomal dilatation or stoma revision may be required for management (21,38).

Continent Urinary Diversions

The trend in urinary diversions is construction of continent reservoirs. A variety of surgical procedures exist, but all of these involve construction of a low-pressure reservoir; an antireflux mechanism between the reservoir and the ureters; and a continent, catheterizable channel between the reservoir and the abdominal surface (28,36,37). The two most commonly performed are the Koch Urostomy and variations of the ileocecal reservoir (e.g., Indiana Reservoir, Florida Pouch, and Miami Pouch) (16,28,39). Normal output is clear urine with strands of mucus; long-term management involves intermittent intubation and irrigation of the reservoir (with water or saline) to remove the mucus and prevent pouchitis (28). Adequate fluid intake and close adherence to the catheterization schedule help to prevent urinary tract infections (28). These patients typically need only an absorptive pad over the stoma, and significant leakage is uncommon. Patients who develop significant leakage are usually managed by using two-piece pouching systems. This provides for containment of the urinary leakage while maintaining ready access to the stoma for routine catheterizations. (Routine catheterization must be continued to prevent urinary retention and resultant infection.)

Orthotopic Neobladder to Urethra

The newest approach to urinary tract reconstruction after cystectomy is construction of a neobladder with anastomosis to the retained urethral sphincter mechanism. This procedure is limited to patients whose malignancy can be resected adequately without compromising the sphincter (16,40). Because the neobladder is usually a noncontractile reservoir constructed from detubularized bowel, effective emptying depends on effective relaxation of the voluntary sphincter in combination with abdominal muscle contraction to increase the pressure in the reservoir (16,40). Patients must be monitored for urinary retention, and patients who are unable to empty the reservoir completely are taught to augment voluntary voids with clean, intermittent catheterization to prevent urinary stasis and resulting infection (16,40). Another common problem is some degree of urinary leakage, particularly at night (when the voluntary pelvic floor muscles are partially relaxed). Depending on the severity of the leakage, absorbent products may be required for containment (40).

Pouching: Products and Principles

As outlined in the section Fistula Management, the key principles in stoma management include containment of the drainage and odor and protection of the peristomal skin. The degree of skin protection required is dictated by the characteristics of the output. Drainage that is proteolytic or highly acidic or alkaline requires meticulous protection of all peristomal skin, whereas nonenzymatic drainage with a pH that is essentially neutral primarily requires protection against pooling of drainage and subsequent maceration (21). Therefore, ileostomies and ascending colostomies require aggressive skin protection, whereas descending/sigmoid colostomies and urinary diversions primarily require protection against prolonged contact between the drainage and the skin.

Products available for protection of peristomal skin include skin sealants, skin barriers, and pectin-based paste. The use of these products is outlined in Table 24.3. As mentioned earlier, pouching systems are available for both urinary and fecal drainage. Pouching systems are also available as both one-piece and two-piece systems. Typically, one-piece systems are constructed with a barrier ring and tape border to which the pouch is welded, and are available in both precut and cut-to-fit varieties. Two-piece pouches typically consist of an adhesive barrier wafer with an attached flange or an adhesive "landing zone" to which the patient attaches a separate pouch (21,22,24). Application guidelines are the same as those for fistula pouch application (Table 24.4).

Management of Peristomal Complications

Common peristomal complications include epithelial denudation, monilial rash, and allergic reactions to ostomy products. Prompt recognition and appropriate intervention usually result in complete resolution of the problem.

Denudation

Superficial skin loss in the peristomal area is usually caused by a poorly fitting or incorrectly sized pouch that allows contact between the effluent and the peristomal skin. The area of damage typically extends from the stoma along the path taken by the effluent; the area is usually red, raw, and painful (38,41,42). The most important intervention is correction of the underlying problem (i.e., modification of the pouching system). Actual treatment of the denuded areas involves application of a pectin-based powder [e.g., Stomahesive by ConvaTec (Princeton, NJ) or Premium by Hollister (Libertyville, IL)] to the denuded areas; the powder can then be "sealed" by blotting with a moist finger or an alcohol-free skin sealant [e.g., Cavilon No Sting by 3M (Minneapolis, MN) or No-Sting Skin-Prep by Smith and Nephew (Largo, FL)]. Severely denuded areas may require several layers of powder and sealant to provide a thick protective layer. The correctly sized pouching system can then be applied over the treated surface (38).

Monilial Rash

Peristomal yeast rashes can occur as a result of antibiotic administration with resulting overgrowth of yeast organisms in the bowel, or as a result of constant moisture resulting from a leaking pouch or heavy perspiration under the plastic pouch material. The rash has a maculopapular appearance with distinct border (satellite) lesions and is commonly pruritic. Usually it responds promptly to nystatin powder that is dusted onto the peristomal surface and then blotted with a skin sealant or moist finger to create a dry or sticky pouching surface (21,22,38,42).

Allergy

Any product used to protect the peristomal skin or to contain the output can be an allergen. Allergic contact dermatitis is typically characterized by an area of erythema that corresponds to the skin surface exposed to the allergen. The patient typically describes the area as pruritic and tender, and vesicles may be noted in severe reactions (22,38,42). The first step in management is to identify and eliminate the allergen, which can be a challenge when the patient is using a variety of products on the involved skin. Usually the distribution of the reaction helps to identify the offender, although patch testing may be required when the identity of the allergen is unclear (21,38,42). Until the specific allergen is identified and the peristomal skin has normalized, product use should be minimized; for example, use of paste, powder, and sealants should be eliminated if possible, and the patient should be managed with a solid barrier and pouch (such as a two-piece pouching system with a barrier wafer to which the pouch is attached). Patients with severe blistering or pruritus may require topical or systemic antihistamines or corticosteroids in addition to the measures already identified (41). If topical products are used, sprays or vanishing gels should be selected because creams and ointments interfere with pouch adhesion (21,22).

Management of Stomal Complications

Although stomal complications are uncommon, they can interfere with normal ostomy function or with effective containment of the output. Therefore, the clinician needs to be knowledgeable regarding their management.

Peristomal Hernia

Peristomal hernia involves herniation of the bowel through the muscle defect created by the stoma and into the subcutaneous tissue (18,22,38). The hernia usually reduces spontaneously when the patient is in a reclining position and intra-abdominal pressure is reduced. Problems created by peristomal hernias include the potential for strangulation and bowel obstruction, which is uncommon, and difficulty in maintaining an effective pouch seal, which is more common (38,41–43). In the patient with advanced cancer, surgical intervention is usually reserved for emergency situations involving strangulation and obstruction (43). Conservative management commonly includes use of a hernia belt, which is an abdominal binder with a cutout that accommodates the stoma and pouch (38,41,42). The belt is applied while the patient is recumbent and the hernia is reduced, and the resistance provided by the belt helps maintain reduction of the herniated loop of the bowel. Patients who have had colostomy and who manage their stomas with routine irrigation must be cautioned to irrigate only with a cone-tip irrigator (because a catheter could cause perforation of the herniated loop) and instill the irrigation fluid in the recumbent or semirecumbent position (so that the hernia is reduced) (38).

Stenosis

Narrowing of the stoma to a point that interferes with normal function can occur at either the skin level or the fascia level. Stenosis at the skin level may be evidenced by visible narrowing of the stomal lumen, but stenosis at fascia level can be detected only by digital examination. Signs of stenosis include reduced output, cramping pain, abdominal distention (with fecal diversions), and flank pain or infection (with urinary diversions). Stenosis that interferes with normal function requires surgical revision, either local excision of the stenotic area or open laparotomy (22,38,42).

Retraction

Early retraction of the stoma to a plane below skin level can occur postoperatively as a result of tension on the bowel or mesentery or because of breakdown of the mucocutaneous suture line. Late retraction can be caused by ascites or intraperitoneal tumor growth causing abdominal distention or tension on the mesentery. Retraction can also be caused by excessive postoperative weight gain (41). Management involves modification of the pouching system to accommodate the change in peristomal contours; typically, a convex pouching system is required (38,42).

Prolapse

Factors contributing to stomal prolapse include increased intra-abdominal pressure, loop stoma construction, location of the stoma outside the rectus muscle, and formation of an excessively large aperture in the abdominal wall (44). Prolapse is usually quite disturbing for patients; however, prolapse does not represent a surgical emergency unless there is evidence of incarceration and stomal ischemia (41,44). Sometimes a prolapsed stoma can be reduced—the patient is placed in a recumbent position to reduce intra-abdominal pressure, and manual reduction is attempted (45). (If the stoma is very edematous, a hypertonic substance, such as sugar or salt, may be applied topically to reduce the edema before reduction is attempted.) Once the prolapse is reduced, a hernia belt with prolapse overbelt (or a simple abdominal binder) can be used to prevent recurrence. If this approach fails, surgical intervention may be required (22,38,41,42).

Bleeding

Slight stomal bleeding during pouch changes is common because of the vascularity of the stoma. However, significant or spontaneous bleeding is not normal and requires investigation and intervention. Bleeding from the stoma itself can usually be managed by direct pressure, application of ice, or silver nitrate cauterization (38). Bleeding originating from the bowel requires further workup, with intervention determined by the causative factors and the patient's overall status (38).

Specific Issues for Oncology Patients

Some specific ostomy-related issues are relevant only to patients with cancer. These issues include management of a stoma in the radiation field, management of stomatitis, and the impact of advancing disease on self-care and management.

Stoma in Radiation Field

The goal in management of a stoma in the radiation field is to prevent peristomal skin damage (46). If the radiation oncologist wishes to have the pouch removed for each treatment, the patient should be switched to a nonadhesive pouching system [e.g., Hollister one-piece Karaya (Libertyville,

IL) ring pouches with belt attachment or Cook (Wound Ostomy Continence, Spencer, IN) nonadhesive pouches] (47). If the radiation oncologist elects to leave the pouch in place during treatments, the pouching system should be modified to eliminate any metallic agents that could cause scatter of the radiation beam at skin level (e.g., tapes containing zinc oxide) (47). Pectin-based barriers, plastic pouches, and porous paper tape are all safe for peristomal use. Any peristomal damage that does occur can usually be managed by applying a hydrocolloid wafer dressing [e.g., DuoDerm by ConvaTec (Princeton, NJ)] to the peristomal skin under the pouch.

Management of Stomatitis

Stomatitis, a common side effect of both radiation therapy and chemotherapy, is manifested as stomal edema, vasocongestion, and possibly ulceration. The goals of treatment are to prevent secondary infection, trauma and bleeding. Patients who have had colostomy and who manage their stomas with routine irrigation are instructed to omit irrigation during courses of pelvic radiation and during any episodes of stomatitis caused by chemotherapy (47). Patients are also counseled to avoid vigorous cleansing of the stoma and, if the stoma is friable, may be advised to add small amounts of mineral oil to lubricate the inside of the pouch (once radiation is complete). Patients with continent diversions may need to use smaller catheters, additional lubricant, and extreme caution in intubating the reservoir. Patients who develop stomatitis secondary to chemotherapy usually require treatment with antifungal agents (48) because the entire length of the alimentary canal is likely to be affected.

Impact of Advancing Disease on Self-Care and Management

In a patient who has undergone ostomy, one of the most significant issues with advanced disease is self-care and management. It is frequently necessary to modify the patient's management regimen or to teach a family member to change the pouch or intubate the stoma as the patient becomes less able to manage his or her own care. The patient who has undergone colostomy and has managed with irrigation and who is no longer able to perform this procedure needs to be placed on a drainable pouching system. As noted earlier in this chapter, constipation is a common problem for such a patient with advanced cancer, but usually it can be managed with bulk and stimulant laxatives, stool softeners, and irrigations as needed (49). Removal of impacted stool can usually be accomplished by administration of a 1:1 solution of milk and molasses given as an irrigation.

The patient with a continent urinary diversion (or orthotopic neobladder) may be managed by insertion of an indwelling catheter into the reservoir if such a procedure is more feasible for the caregiver than intermittent intubation. The caregiver should be instructed to give irrigations once or twice daily to eliminate retained mucous.

The home health or hospice nurse can be extremely valuable in assisting the patient and family to modify their care routines in the most effective and manageable way.

SUMMARY

Effective management of fistulas and stomas requires containment of drainage and odor as well as protection of the surrounding skin. These aspects of care have a significant impact on the quality of life for patients with advanced disease.

References

1. Rolstad B, Bryant R. Management of drain sites and fistulas. In: Bryant R, ed. *Acute and chronic wounds: nursing management,* 2nd ed. St. Louis, MO: Mosby, 2000: 317–342.
2. Chamberlain R, Kaufman H, Danforth D. Enterocutaneous fistula in cancer patients: etiology, management, outcome, and impact on further treatment. *Am Surg* 1998;64: 1204–1211.
3. Jensen R. Peptide therapy: recent advances in the use of somatostatin and other peptide receptor agonists and antagonists. In: Lewis J, Dubois A, eds. *Current clinical topics in gastrointestinal pharmacology.* Malden, MA: Blackwell Science, 1997: 144–223.
4. Berry S, Fisher J. Biliary and gastrointestinal fistulas. In: Zinner M, Schwartz S, Ellis H, eds. *Maingot's abdominal operations,* Vol. 1, 10th ed. Stamford, CT: Appleton & Lange, 1997: 581–628.
5. Haffejee A. Surgical management of high output enterocutaneous fistulas: a 24-year experience. *Curr Opin Clin Nutr Metab Care* 2004;7(3): 309–316.
6. Erwin-Toth P, Hocevar B, Landis-Erdman J. Fistula management. In: Colwell J, Goldberg M, Carmel J, eds. *Fecal and urinary diversions: management principles.* St. Louis, MO: Mosby, 2004: 381–391.
7. Oneschuk D, Bruera E. Successful management of multiple enterocutaneous fistulas in a patient with metastatic colon cancer. *J Pain Symptom Manage* 1997;14: 121–124.
8. Kinetic Concepts Incorporated. *V.A.C.® Therapy™ clinical guidelines.* San Antonio, TX: KCI Licensing, Inc, 2004.
9. Sancho J, Costanzo J, Nubiola P, et al Randomized double-blind placebo-controlled trial of early octreotide in patients with postoperative enterocutaneous fistula. *Br J Surg* 1995;82: 638–641.
10. Ayache S, Wadleigh R. Treatment of a malignant enterocutaneous fistula with octreotide acetate. *Cancer Invest* 1999;17: 320–321.
11. Regan J, Salky B. Laparoscopic treatment of enteric fistulas. *Surg Endosc* 2004;18: 252–254.
12. Hunerbein M. Endoscopic and surgical palliation of gastrointestinal tumors. *Support Care Cancer* 2004;12(3): 155–160.
13. Xografos G, Peros G, Androulakis G. Palliative surgical treatment in enterocutaneous fistula. *J Surg Oncol* 1997;66: 138.
14. Kearney R, Payne W, Rosemurgy A. Extra-abdominal closure of enterocutaneous fistula. *Am Surg* 1997;63: 406–410.
15. Hwang T, Chen M. Randomized trial of fibrin tissue glue for low-output enterocutaneous fistula. *Br J Surg* 1996;83: 112.
16. Tomaselli N, McGinnis D. Urinary diversions: Surgical interventions. In: Colwell J, Goldberg M, Carmel J, eds. *Fecal and urinary diversions: management principles.* St. Louis, MO: Mosby, 2004: 184–204.
17. Vasilevsky C, Gordon P. Gastrointestinal cancers: surgical management. In: Colwell J, Goldberg M, Carmel J, eds. *Fecal and urinary diversions: management principles.* St. Louis, MO: Mosby, 2004: 126–135.
18. Kodner I. Intestinal stomas. In: Zinner M, Schwartz S, Ellis H, eds. *Maingot's abdominal operations,* Vol. 1, 10th ed. Stamford, CT: Appleton & Lange, 1997: 427–460.
19. Fazio W, Erwin-Toth P. Stomal and pouch function and care. In: Haubrich W, Schaffner F, Berk J, eds. *Gastroenterology,* 5th ed. Philadelphia, PA: WB Saunders, 1995: 1547–1560.
20. Carmel J, Goldberg M. Preoperative and postoperative management. In: Colwell J, Goldberg M, Carmel J, eds. *Fecal and urinary diversions: management principles,* St. Louis, MO: Mosby, 2004: 207–239.
21. Erwin-Toth P, Doughty D. Principles and procedures of stomal management. In: Hampton B, Bryant R, eds. *Ostomies and continent diversions: nursing management.* St. Louis, MO: Mosby, 1992: 29–103.
22. Harford F, Harford D. Intestinal stomas. In: Beck D. ed. *Handbook of colorectal surgery.* St. Louis, MO: Quality Medical Publishers, 1997: 105–128.
23. Roberts D. The pursuit of colostomy continence. *J Wound Ostomy Continence Nurs* 1997;24: 92–97.
24. Colwell J. Principles of stoma management. In: Colwell J, Goldberg M, Carmel J, eds. *Fecal and urinary diversions: management principles.* St. Louis, MO: Mosby, 2004: 240–262.
25. Jensen L. Assessment and management of patients with bowel dysfunction or fecal incontinence. In: Doughty D, ed. *Urinary and fecal incontinence: nursing management,* 2nd ed. St. Louis, MO: Mosby, 2000: 353–384.
26. Fleshman J. Functional colorectal disorders. In: Beck D, ed. *Handbook of colo-rectal surgery.* St. Louis, MO: Quality Medical Publishers, 1997: 198–216.
27. Kelly K. Approach to patient with ileostomy and ileal pouch ileostomy. In: Yamada T, ed. *Textbook of gastroenterology,* 2nd ed. Philadelphia, PA: JB Lippincott Co, 1995: 880–892.
28. Rolstad B, Hoyman K. Continent diversions and reservoirs. In: Hampton B, Bryant R, eds. *Ostomies and continent diversions: nursing management.* St. Louis, MO: Mosby, 1992: 129–162.
29. Hull T, Erwin-Toth P. The pelvic pouch procedure and continent ostomies: overview and controversies. *J Wound Ostomy Continence Nurs* 1996;23: 156–165.
30. Doughty D. History of stoma creation and surgical advances. In: Colwell J, Goldberg M, Carmel J, eds. *Fecal and urinary diversions: management principles.* St. Louis, MO: Mosby, 2004: 3–17.

31. Cohen Z. What are the continuing challenges and issues related to restorative proctocolectomy? In: Boulos P, Wexner S, eds. *Current challenges in colorectal surgery.* Philadelphia, PA: WB Saunders, 2000: 129–143.

32. Hull T. Ileoanal procedures: acute and long-term management issues. *J Wound Ostomy Continence Nurs* 1999;26: 201–206.

33. Gray M, Colwell J. Evidence-based report card from the Center for Clinical Investigation: pouchitis part 2: treatment options and their effectiveness. *J Wound Ostomy Continence Nurs* 2002;29(4): 174–179.

34. Crentsil V, Hanauer S. Inflammatory bowel disease: Medical management. In: Colwell J, Goldberg M, Carmel J, eds. *Fecal and urinary diversions: management principles.* St. Louis, MO: Mosby, 2004: 63–79.

35. Lavery I, Erwin-Toth P. Stoma therapy. In: Mackeigan J, Cataldo P, eds. *Intestinal stomas: principles, techniques, and management.* St. Louis, MO: Quality Medical Publishers, 1993: 60–84.

36. Hald D, Ahlering T, Razor B. The pathogenesis and management of urothelial malignancies. *J Wound Ostomy Continence Nurs* 1996;23: 144–149.

37. Dalton D. Methods of urinary diversion. In: Mackeigan J, Cataldo P, eds. *Intestinal stomas: principles, techniques, and management.* St. Louis, MO: Quality Medical Publishers, 1993: 198–227.

38. Hampton B. Peristomal and stomal complications. In: Hampton B, Bryant R, eds. *Ostomies and continent diversions: nursing management.* St. Louis, MO: Mosby, 1992: 105–128.

39. Gowing-Farhat C. The florida pouch. *Urol Nurs* 1994;14: 1–5.

40. Krupski T, Theodorescu D. Orthotopic neobladder following cystectomy: indications, management, and outcomes. *J Wound Ostomy Continence Nurs* 2001;28: 37–46.

41. Colwell J, Goldberg M, Carmel J. The state of the standard diversion. *J Wound Ostomy Continence Nurs* 2001;28: 6–17.

42. Colwell J. Stomal and peristomal complications. In: Colwell J, Goldberg M, Carmel J, eds. *Fecal and urinary diversions: management principles.* St. Louis, MO: Mosby, 2004: 308–325.

43. Rubin M, Bailey R. Parastomal hernias. In: Mackeigan J, Cataldo P, eds. *Intestinal stomas: principles, techniques, and management.* St. Louis, MO: Quality Medical Publishers, 1993: 245–267.

44. Nogueras J, Wexner S. Stoma prolapse. In: Mackeigan J, Cataldo P, eds. *Intestinal stomas: principles, techniques, and management.* St. Louis, MO: Quality Medical Publishers, 1993: 268–277.

45. Myers J, Rothenberger D. Sugar in the reduction of incarcerated prolapsed bowel: report of two cases. *Dis Colon Rectum* 1991;5: 416–418.

46. Floruta C, Berschorner J, Hull T. Gastrointestinal cancers: medical management. In: Colwell J, Goldberg M, Carmel J, eds. *Fecal and urinary diversions: management principles.* St. Louis, MO: Mosby, 2004: 102–125.

47. Ratliff C. Principles of cancer therapy. In: Hampton B, Bryant R, eds. *Ostomies and continent diversions: nursing management.* St. Louis, MO: Mosby, 1992: 163–194.

48. Goodman M, Ladd L, Purl S. Integumentary and mucous membrane alterations. In: Groenwald S, Frogge M, Goodman Y, et al., eds. *Cancer nursing: principles and practice,* 3rd ed. Boston, MA: Jones & Bartlett, 1993: 737–748.

49. McGuire D, Sheidler V. Pain. In: Groenwald S, Frogge M, Goodman M, et al., eds. *Cancer nursing: principles and practice,* 3rd ed. Boston, MA: Jones & Bartlett, 1993: 530–533.

CHAPTER 25 ■ MANAGEMENT OF DYSPNEA

SHALINI DALAL, GAYATRI PALAT, AND EDUARDO BRUERA

Dyspnea has been defined as an uncomfortable awareness of breathing (1). Although everybody has experienced the sensation and has an intuitive understanding of this symptom, there is no universal agreement as to its definition. Dyspnea is a subjective sensation and cannot be defined by the physical abnormalities that accompany such an unpleasant subjective experience. For the purpose of this chapter, dyspnea is defined as an unpleasant sensation of difficult, labored breathing.

Dyspnea is a frequent and devastating symptom in patients with advanced cancer (2) and has been reported to occur in 21–79% of patients (3). A quality of life and survival prediction study in terminal cancer has shown that health care professionals should focus on physical health-related quality of life indicators, such as nausea and emesis, dyspnea, and weakness, to gather prognostic clues in patients with terminal cancer (4). There is evidence that good symptom control, even by experienced palliative care teams, is achieved less frequently for dyspnea than for other symptoms such as pain or nausea (5). In addition, limited research, and education are available on the adequate assessment and management of dyspnea in cancer patients.

The aim of this chapter is to review the pathophysiology, prevalence, assessment, and treatment of dyspnea in patients with cancer. Discussion of areas where future research should focus is also included.

PATHOPHYSIOLOGY

Dyspnea is frequently associated with abnormalities in the mechanisms that regulate normal breathing. However, the actual expression of dyspnea by a patient results from a complex interaction between the abnormalities in breathing and the perception of those abnormalities in the central nervous system. The origins of dyspnea in different clinical settings can be traced to specific abnormalities. These are discussed in the following paragraphs.

Regulation of Breathing

Figure 25.1 summarizes the regulation of normal breathing. Respiration is integrated as a system with three main components, as discussed in the following sections.

Respiratory Center

The respiratory center is located in the medulla. Its neurons receive information from both central and peripheral chemoreceptors and peripheral mechanoreceptors. It also receives information from the cerebral cortex, which regulates voluntary breathing such as occurs during speaking and singing. Efferent neurons stimulate the diaphragm, the intercostal muscles, and the accessory muscles (6).

Receptors

The levels of oxygen and carbon dioxide in the blood stimulate chemoreceptors located centrally and peripherally. These chemoreceptors are capable of stimulating the respiratory center and increasing respiratory rate (7). Although strong debate continues on this subject, recent evidence suggests that chemoreceptors are probably also able to stimulate the brain cortex directly and cause dyspnea (7). An alternative explanation for the dyspnea caused by increases in PCO_2 and decreases in PO_2 is that chemoreceptors stimulate the respiratory center; increasing the respiratory effort, which stimulates mechanoreceptors capable of stimulating the brain cortex, resulting in the sensation of dyspnea. The mechanoreceptors are located primarily in the respiratory muscles and the lung. These receptors respond to either irritants or, more commonly, pulmonary stretch, including vascular congestion (6).

Respiratory Muscles

The respiratory muscles promote gas exchange. Changes in the PO_2 and PCO_2 are detected by the chemoreceptors. Changes in the tension within the abdominal wall and the lung are detected by the mechanoreceptors. This information is fed back to the respiratory center. Sensory receptors are found inside the respiratory muscles, including the intercostal, sternomastoid, and diaphragm. The balance between the contractual activity and stimulation of the sensory receptors is of great importance in the type of input provided to the respiratory center and the cortex.

Although the three aforementioned factors are the main elements in the regulation of breathing, the actual sensation of dyspnea is a result of cortical stimulation. The sensation of dyspnea has been related to the activation of mechanoreceptors in the respiratory muscles and lung (8). Elegant research has shown that both in normal volunteers and patients, with different stimuli capable of stimulating mechanoreceptors are able to produce dyspnea even in the absence of increased respiratory activity (6). In addition, two other possible mechanisms of dyspnea have been proposed. On one hand, the previously discussed role of chemoreceptor stimulation, on the other hand, some authors have proposed a role for the respiratory center as a potential cause of dyspnea by direct ascending cortical stimulation (7,9).

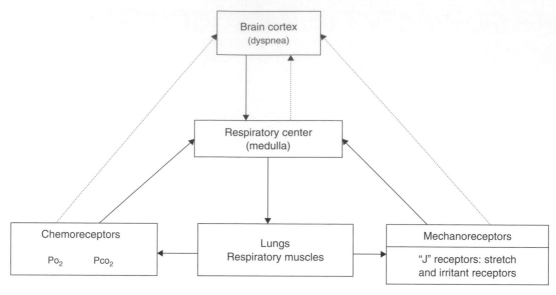

FIGURE 25.1. Regulation of normal breathing. PO_2, partial pressure of oxygen; PCO_2, partial pressure of carbon dioxide.

Production of Dyspnea

Dyspnea is produced by physical and biochemical abnormalities (Fig. 25.2). The perception is then modulated by anxiety, depression, or administration of opioids. Somatization and cultural factors further influence a patient's expression of dyspnea.

A number of researchers have found great variability in the expression of dyspnea among patients with similar levels of functional abnormalities. Among patients with asthma, approximately 15% did not report dyspnea despite severe airflow obstruction (forced expiratory volume in 1 second (FEV_1) of <15% of the predicted) (10). Similarly, among patients with chronic obstructive pulmonary disease (COPD), the complaint of dyspnea was not well correlated with abnormalities in the pulmonary function tests (11). Among these patients who were defined as having disproportionate dyspnea (complaint

of dyspnea in the presence of a mean FEV_1 of 1.8 L), almost all patients were considered to have a psychiatric diagnosis (mostly anxiety and depression) (11). Anxiety has been shown to be an independent correlate of the intensity of dyspnea in patients with cancer (12). This association is not entirely clear as anxiety may contribute to dyspnea but may also arise from its presence.

These studies suggest that some patients have modulators that either amplify or decrease the intensity of the symptom that is perceived at the cortical level. Patients receiving drugs such as opioids for pain can perceive significantly less dyspnea (2).

Finally, the expression of a certain symptom may be influenced by cultural factors, the belief about the mechanism for the symptom, and other factors such as somatization (13). Because neither the production nor the perception of dyspnea can be measured at present, the entire assessment is based on the patient's expression. This issue is discussed in the following section.

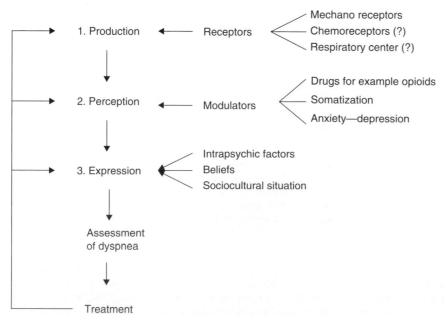

FIGURE 25.2. Stages in the production of dyspnea. ?, hypothesized/suspected but not absolutely clear.

Clinical Situations Associated with Dyspnea

Dyspnea can result from three main pathophysiologic abnormalities (6):

1. An increase in respiratory effort to overcome a certain load (e.g., obstructive or restrictive lung disease, pleural effusion)
2. An increase in the proportion of respiratory muscle required to maintain a normal workload (e.g., neuromuscular weakness, cancer cachexia)
3. An increase in ventilatory requirements (hypoxemia, hypercapnia, metabolic acidosis, anemia, etc.)

In many patients with cancer, different proportions of the three abnormalities may coexist, thereby making the pathophysiologic interpretation of the intensity of dyspnea more complex.

Role of Respiratory Muscles

During recent years a number of authors have found that respiratory muscle weakness has an important role in the dyspnea associated with a number of chronic conditions. Palange et al. (14) found that malnutrition significantly affected the muscle aerobic capacity and exercise tolerance in patients with COPD. They suggested that high wasted ventilation might be responsible for the weight loss. Diaphragmatic fatigue has been associated with dyspnea in patients with COPD (15). In chronically malnourished patients without pulmonary disease, malnutrition reduces respiratory muscle strength and maximal voluntary ventilation. Therefore, malnutrition might impair the respiratory muscle capacity to handle increased ventilatory loads in cardiopulmonary disease (16). In normal volunteers, the sensation of dyspnea has been correlated with respiratory muscle fatigue (17).

A study of patients with cancer determined that the maximal inspiratory pressure, a reliable functional test of the strength of the diaphragm and other respiratory muscles, is severely impaired in patients with cancer and dyspnea (18). Maximal inspiratory pressure has subsequently been found to be an independent correlate of the intensity of dyspnea in a subgroup of patients with advanced cancer and with moderate to severe dyspnea (12).

PREVALENCE OF DYSPNEA

The large variation in reported prevalence of dyspnea (21–79%) is a result of the different natures of patient populations reported by different authors and the lack of a general consensus on the assessment methods for identifying and quantifying the presence and intensity of dyspnea.

Higginson and McCarthy (5) conducted a prospective study in 86 consecutive patients with advanced cancer referred to a Community Palliative Care Service. Eighteen patients (21%) reported dyspnea as their main symptom before death. The symptom assessment scores for patients with dyspnea showed no change overtime, as compared with a significant decrease in the intensity of pain reported by this same patient population. In the National Hospice Study, Reuben et al. (19) reported a high prevalence of dyspnea, with 70% of 1754 patients experiencing this symptom sometime during the last 6 weeks of life. 27.5% of patients reported dyspnea to be present all the time and more than 28% of patients rated the severity of their symptoms as moderate or worse during the self-report assessment. Although 33% of patients had a diagnosis of primary or metastatic lung cancer, 24% of patients with dyspnea did not have any known lung or heart disease or evidence of pleural effusion. Grond et al. (20) reported a

prevalence of dyspnea of 24% among 1635 patients with cancer referred to a pain clinic. Donnelly et al. (21) found dyspnea in 28% of 1000 patients referred for consultation to a palliative care service. Of those patients who reported dyspnea, 63% rated this symptom as moderate or severe.

Twycross and Lack (22) found a prevalence of 51% of dyspnea in 6677 patients admitted to a palliative care program. Muers (23) found breathlessness to be a presenting complaint for 60% of 289 patients with non–small cell lung cancer, half of whom described their shortness of breath as moderate or severe.

A number of authors have reported dyspnea in a significant percentage of patients with advanced cancer without intrathoracic malignancy. The National Hospice Study (19) found a frequency of 24% in patients with no known lung or heart disease. Cachexia occurs in more than 80% of patients with advanced cancer (24). In addition, asthenia, and electrophysiological abnormalities in muscle function are detected in a large proportion of patients with advanced cancer. A recent study of 222 patients with chronic congestive heart failure found that dyspnea was the exercise-limiting symptom in 160 and generalized fatigue in 62 patients. No significant differences were found between any of the cardiovascular parameters of these two groups. The authors concluded that both symptoms are "two sides of the same coin," and that they express the same underlying pathophysiologic process (25). It is possible that in some patients with advanced cancer, dyspnea may be one clinical expression of the syndrome of overwhelming cachexia and asthenia that is highly prevalent in the comprehensive assessment of these patients, including frequent pulmonary function tests.

In summary, dyspnea appears to be a common symptom in patients with advanced cancer. It is reported more commonly in patients during the last weeks of life. Although it is more common among patients with lung cancer or pulmonary metastases, it is also frequent in patients with no demonstrable tumor involvement in the lung. Most patients who develop dyspnea tend to rate this symptom as one of their main problems.

Smoke is considered the major cause of lung cancer although other factors may be involved in its pathogenesis. In developing countries, wood, and other solid fuels (26) are used for cooking and heating. Exposure to biomass smoke has been associated with respiratory diseases such as chronic bronchitis, emphysema, and asthma (27).

Although the causes of dyspnea in cancer are more varied than the causes of dyspnea in COPD, many are similar, thereby providing the justification for recommending the best practice from COPD research to be used in lung cancer. Figure 25.3 summarizes the common causes of dyspnea in patients with cancer.

Less common causes of dyspnea in patients with cancer include atelectasis, phrenic nerve palsy, tracheal obstruction, carcinomatous infiltration of the chest wall, abdominal distention, pneumothorax, and metabolic acidosis. The pathophysiology of dyspnea in most patients with cancer is complex. For example, a given patient may have an increase in respiratory effort necessary to overcome the presence of a large pleural effusion, in addition to an increase in the proportion of respiratory muscle required for breathing because of cachexia and increased ventilatory requirement resulting from severe anemia.

ASSESSMENT

Although most patients with cancer develop dyspnea as a progressive complication over days or weeks, some patients present with sudden onset of dyspnea as an acute medical

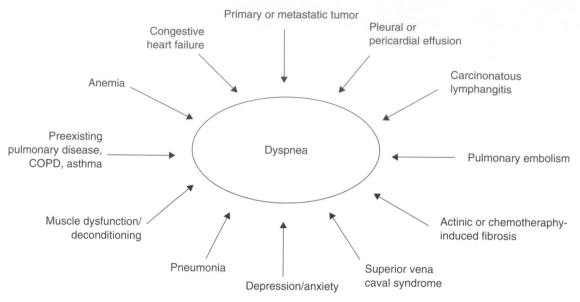

FIGURE 25.3. Common cause of dyspnea in patients with advanced cancer. COPD, chronic obstructive pulmonary disease.

emergency. The management of the latter group always should be considered a medical emergency.

History

The cause of dyspnea can be determined in most patients by taking an adequate history and performing a physical examination. The intensity of dyspnea should be assessed using a validated system. In addition, descriptors of dyspnea may provide a clue as to the pathophysiologic basis of dyspnea.

Intensity of Dyspnea

Because dyspnea is a subjective symptom with multiple potential etiologies, objective findings such as tachypnea or oxygenation saturation levels may not adequately reflect the distress experienced by patients with dyspnea. The presence and intensity of dyspnea should be assessed using validated assessment tools with numerical, verbal analogue, or visual analog scales (28,29). The intensity of dyspnea is included in some of the available supportive care tools, such as the Support Team Assessment Schedule (3) and the Edmonton Symptom Assessment System (29). Quality of life questionnaires, including the European Organisation for Research and Treatment in Cancer Quality-of-Life Core Questionnaire, have provided for a more detailed assessment of the intensity of dyspnea in certain modules (e.g., lung cancer) (30).

In addition, some specific dyspnea questionnaires such as the chronic respiratory questionnaire (CRQ) and the Medical Research Council Scale have been found to be useful in patients with COPD (31,32), and with dyspnea from a variety of respiratory and cardiovascular origins, respectively (33,34). The Borg Category Scale (35) was developed for rating perceived dyspnea during exercise.

One of the main problems associated with assessment of dyspnea is the variable intensity of this symptom according to the level of activity and during different times of the day. In patients with respiratory and cardiovascular diseases, one approach to this problem has been the performance of dyspnea-causing activities (such as progressive exercising on a treadmill or bicycle) to assess pharmacologic and nonpharmacologic interventions (36). However, most patients with cancer are

too ill to participate in these tests. One potentially less invasive approach to dyspnea assessment is breath-holding (37,38) and reading (39) to measure the limiting effects of breathlessness. Immediately after breath-holding, there is a period when no particular respiratory sensation is experienced (20–30 seconds in healthy subjects). This is followed by a second period in which there is progressive discomfort until breaking point. It has been found that training plays an important role in prolongation of total breath-holding time, but has little effect on the period of no respiratory sensation. In addition, the period of no respiratory sensation in patients with COPD is apparently shortened and measurement of this period can be useful in the study of the genesis of dyspnea (38). Breath-holding has not been prospectively validated for use as an assessment tool in cancer dyspnea.

A study (39) looked at a simple test involving reading of numbers in 30 patients with cancer and 30 controls. Patients read fewer numbers, and fewer numbers per breath than controls. Twelve of the 30 patients were unable to complete all five readings in all three tests due to tiredness. The test was found to have good repeatability, both within and between days, and was sensitive to improvement seen following drainage of pleural effusions in 13 patients.

In summary, a large number of scales are available for assessment of the intensity of dyspnea. They range from simple analog and numerical scales to more complex scales, including multiple items. Many of these scales have been adequately validated and are highly reproducible.

Descriptors of Dyspnea

In the case of pain, specific descriptors are associated with specific pathophysiologic syndromes (40). For example, a burning, or numb sensation has traditionally been associated with neuropathic pain. In many cases, the descriptor alone is enough to make a diagnosis and suggest the need for specific drug therapy. Simon et al. (41) attempted to associate specific descriptors with specific pathophysiology in 53 patients with dyspnea caused by a number of known causes. Patients were asked to choose descriptions of their sensation of breathlessness from a dyspnea questionnaire listing 19 descriptors. Cluster analysis then was used to identify natural groupings among those descriptors. Although descriptors, such as "rapid" or "heavy," were associated with exercise, "tight" was frequently associated with asthma, and "suffocating" was frequently associated with congestive heart failure. Mahler et al. (42) used a questionnaire with 15 items that described qualities of breathlessness in 218 patients who sought medical care for breathlessness. The authors concluded that patients with different cardiorespiratory conditions experience distinct qualities of breathlessness and that using a questionnaire containing descriptors of dyspnea might help to establish a specific diagnosis. However, a recent study has suggested that different ethnic groups use different words to describe breathlessness in the presence of air-flow obstruction (43). This requires further clarification. In addition, more research is needed to better characterize the quality of dyspnea associated with specific clinical conditions.

Physical Examination and Investigations

A general physical examination with focus on the cardiac and respiratory systems is essential. A chest radiograph, digital oximetry, and simple blood tests can help in determining its cause. Pulmonary function tests can be particularly useful in the assessment of obstructive and restrictive pulmonary disorders as well as neuromuscular weakness. These tests can be performed repeatedly at the bedside and are useful in assessing the response to different therapies, in particular bronchodilators. The measurement of maximal inspiratory pressure may also be useful in patients with cancer (12).

Multidimensional Assessment

Although some researchers have described a good correlation between the abnormality of pulmonary function tests and the intensity of subjective dyspnea (35), others found this correlation to be extremely poor. In some cases, the authors suggested that the lack of correlation between objective and subjective findings might be due to underlying psychiatric disorders (11).

Figure 25.2 shows the different stages in the production of dyspnea. These are common to other symptoms, such as pain. Neither the production nor perception of dyspnea can be measured. Expression of the intensity of dyspnea can be influenced by a number of factors described in the figure and should not be interpreted as a direct representation of the intensity of production of dyspnea at the level of mechanoreceptors or chemoreceptors.

The complex nature of dyspnea in many patients with cancer means that assessment of dyspnea in isolation is inappropriate and may result in overtreatment or inappropriate treatment of a patient's expression of dyspnea. Multidimensional assessment of dyspnea using tools that look at dyspnea in the context of other physical and psychologic symptoms allows for determination of the part played by other factors such as pain, anxiety, depression, and somatization in the expression of dyspnea. The Edmonton Symptom Assessment System is an example of a validated multidimensional assessment tool (29,44). Identification of the various factors influencing the expression of dyspnea in a given patient allows for the implementation of a multidimensional therapeutic approach for that patient.

TREATMENT

Treatment of dyspnea should focus on a patient's expression of dyspnea rather than his or her apparent level of dyspnea as judged by tachypnea and use of accessory muscles of respiration, or the level of oxygen in the blood. It is not unusual for patients to have marked tachypnea and not report difficulty in breathing or conversely to report severe dyspnea in the absence of tachypnea.

Treatment approaches include therapies aimed at modifying a specific pathophysiologic cause and therapies aimed to provide general symptom control.

Treatments of Specific Pathophysiologic Causes

In patients in whom a specific cause of dyspnea is suspected, appropriate treatment of the potential underlying cause should be initiated. Treatment modalities include radiation therapy, often accompanied by high-dose corticosteroids for superior vena cava syndrome, and chemotherapy for some patients with pleural effusions or carcinomatous lymphangitis. High-dose corticosteroids may also be useful for patients with the latter. Drainage of pleural or pericardial infusions can give rapid relief. Other procedures, such as pleurodesis or creation of a pericardial window, may be necessary when effusions are recurrent.

Reversible airway obstruction is a common cause of dyspnea in patients with cancer who have a history of heavy smoking (45). In these patients optimum treatment of airway obstruction using bronchodilators, corticosteroids, and, if necessary, antibiotics for infective exacerbation of symptoms should considered. In addition, infections including pneumonia are responsible for the deaths of almost half the patients who die of advanced cancer (46). Dyspnea associated with pneumonia can be effectively treated with appropriate antibiotics.

In addition to the aforementioned causes, patients may present with severe anemia, massive ascites, an acute exacerbation of chronic asthma, or acute panic attacks as part of a chronic panic disorder. The latter is characterized by hyperventilation. Occasionally, metabolic acidosis associated with acute renal failure or lactic acidosis can result in hyperventilation. All these diagnoses should be considered during assessment of a patient with dyspnea and advanced cancer because specific therapy may result in rapid symptom relief.

Symptomatic Treatment

Symptomatic management of dyspnea is based on three main elements: oxygen therapy, drug therapy, and general measures of support and counseling. Evidence for the role of these three therapeutic approaches are discussed in subsequent paragraphs. For the purpose of this review, a Medline search of the literature on dyspnea published between 1966 and 2000 was conducted. All studies relating to the symptomatic therapy of dyspnea were reviewed. Studies were classified according to their methodology in three levels of evidence (45).

Oxygen

Long-term oxygen therapy has beneficial effects on the outcome of patients with COPD (47,48). However, the symptomatic effects of this therapy are less clear. Some studies suggest that oxygen has no symptomatic effects in cancer dyspnea (49,50). In addition, the evidence for a beneficial effect of oxygen in patients with congestive heart failure is also controversial.

Table 25.1 summarizes studies that have addressed the use of oxygen for symptom relief in a number of conditions. Only studies with level 1 evidence (randomized controlled trials) are discussed in this chapter. In the case of COPD, most studies suggest that there is a significant symptomatic improvement at

TABLE 25.1

SYMPTOMATIC EFFECT OF OXYGEN THERAPY

Author (reference)	No. of patients	Dose O_2	Disease	Findings	Level of evidence[a]
Bruera et al. (51)	14	O_2 5 L/min or air	Ca[b]	+	I
Bruera et al. (52)	1	O_2 5 L/min or air	Ca[b]	+	I (N of 1)
Booth et al. (53)	38	O_2 4 L/min or air	Ca[c]	both +	I
Swinburn et al. (54)	10/12	O_2 28% 4 L/min or air	ILD/COPD	+/+	I
Liss and Grant (55)	8	O_2 28% or air	COPD	−	I
Davidson et al. (56)	17	4 L/min or air	COPD	+	I
Woodcock et al. (57)	10	O_2 28% 4 L/min or air	COPD	+	I
Dean et al. (58)	12	O_2 40% or air	COPD	+	I
Moore et al. (59)	12	O_2 30%, 50% or air	CHF	+	I
Restrick et al. (60)	12	O_2 2 L/min or air	CHF	−	I

CHF, congestive heart failure; COPD, chronic obstructive pulmonary disease; ILD, interstitial lung disease; +, effective; −, not effective.
[a]Level of evidence, I, randomized controlled trial.
[b]Cancer hypoxemia.
[c]Only six patients had hypoxemia.

rest and during exercise as a result of the administration of supplemental oxygen (54,56–58). However, Liss and Grant (55) found that the administration of 0, 2, or 4 L per minute of oxygen to patients with COPD was not superior to administration of air on resting dyspnea. Oxygen has been found to improve functional capacity in patients with COPD (61,62).

In a systematic review of contemporary management of COPD, domiciliary oxygen therapy is the only intervention that has been demonstrated to prolong survival, but only in patients with resting hypoxia (63). These authors also found a significant increase in breathlessness after nasal anesthesia with lidocaine. The authors suggested that the reduction in breathlessness caused by nasal oxygen is a placebo effect caused by wearing the nasal cannula and is unrelated to gas flow or the increase of arterial oxygen tension. In the case of congestive heart failure, one study found that supplemental oxygen could improve subjective scores for fatigue and breathlessness during steady-state exercise (59). Another study, however, found no significant benefit from supplemental oxygen on the symptomatic scores of patients subjected to regular walking (60).

Although the balance of evidence suggests that oxygen does have symptomatic effects in COPD and also probably in congestive heart failure, patients with dyspnea due to cancer most frequently have restrictive respiratory failure that might not respond to oxygen in the same way. There are three randomized controlled trials in which patients with cancer dyspnea were randomized in a crossover design to 5 L (51,52) or 4 L per minute of oxygen (53). In the first two studies, all patients were hypoxemic on room air. In these patients, oxygen had a significant beneficial effect. In the third study, only 6 of 38 evaluable patients were hypoxemic; both oxygen and air were significantly superior to baseline (53). Swinburn et al. (54) studied the role of oxygen in a group of 10 patients with interstitial lung disease in addition to their main sample of 12 patients with COPD. Results in interstitial lung disease patients were as beneficial as those observed in the COPD group. It is possible that oxygen supplementation could improve function in patients with cancer dyspnea but not many studies have been conducted.

A Danish study aimed to evaluate the effect of noncontinuous oxygen therapy (NCOT) on pulmonary symptoms and sleep quality, and to determine whether patients with a subjective beneficial effect differed from those without effect in terms of patients' characteristics, utilization of oxygen, hospitalization, and survival (64) 254 patients were prescribed oxygen <12 hour daily or to use as needed. Of these patients, 142 (55.9%) answered a questionnaire on hours spent with oxygen and symptomatic effect of oxygen treatment. While on oxygen, 76.3% of the patients reported improved dyspnea score (0–10) more than 0.5 points, 78.3% had improved quality of life, 59.5% improved sleep, 48.5% increased physical activity, 49.3% felt less tired and 40.0% reported improved thinking. Fifty-seven (43.2%) patients reported both improved dyspnea and physical activity whereas seven (5.3%) patients reported that oxygen had no effect on dyspnea but a beneficial effect on physical activity. Only 11 (7.7%) patients reported no subjective improvement on oxygen. Thus, NCOT improved symptoms and well-being in the majority of patients during daily activity, with most pronounced effects on dyspnea, sleep and quality of life. This effect was not significantly associated with number of hours spent with oxygen, underlying disease, hospitalization or survival. Very few patients sensed improved physical activity without relief in breathlessness.

The symptomatic benefits of oxygen in patients with cancer who have nonhypoxic dyspnea are not well defined. In a double-blind, randomized crossover trial study (65), patients with advanced cancer who had no severe hypoxemia (i.e., had an O_2 saturation level of 90%) at rest, oxygen, or air (5 L per min) was administered through nasal cannula during a 6-minute walk test. The outcome measures were dyspnea at 3 and 6 minutes, fatigue at 6 minutes and distance walked. In 33 evaluable patients (31 with lung cancer), no significant differences between treatment groups were observed in dyspnea, fatigue, or distance walked at 3 minutes and at 6 minutes. Therefore the routine use of supplemental oxygen for dyspnea during exercise cannot be recommended.

The main objective of oxygen therapy in patients with advanced cancer is symptomatic relief rather than the prevention of long-term complications; therefore, intermittent use can be acceptable and less psychologically burdensome in patients who present with intermittent exacerbations of dyspnea.

In summary, although more research is needed, there is some compelling evidence for the use of oxygen for symptomatic relief for patients with cancer-related dyspnea. In particular, patients who are hypoxemic on room air are quite likely to benefit from this approach. It is possible that oxygen would be effective in relieving dyspnea at concentrations higher than those required to maintain optimal saturation

TABLE 25.2

N OF 1 STUDY FOR ASSESSMENT OF EFFECT OF
SUPPLEMENTAL OXYGEN ON DYSPNEA

Measurements
  O₂ saturation—pulse oximetry
  Visual analog scale scores of dyspnea: baseline and
    during blinded treatment with oxygen and air
  Patient and investigator selected treatment of choice
  Patient rated differences between the two treatments
Procedure
  1. Baseline 5 min—no treatment
  2. Patient and investigator blinded to treatments,
     either 5 L/min of 100% oxygen or air through face
     mask for 5 min
  3. Followed directly by 5 min of alternate treatment
  4. Repeat steps 1–3 six times

of hemoglobin. Anecdotal experience in patients with cancer and with congestive heart failure suggest that oxygen might give significant symptomatic relief to patients who are not hypoxemic. This hypothesis should be tested in prospective clinical trials.

When there are doubts about the effectiveness of oxygen for symptomatic relief in a given patient, an "N of 1" study can be conducted (52). The method used by the investigators in this study is summarized in Table 25.2. By performing multiple, double-blind crossovers between oxygen and air, it is possible to determine with great accuracy, in <1 hour, whether a specific patient does or does not benefit from the supplemental oxygen.

Pharmacologic Interventions

A number of drugs have been suggested to affect the intensity of dyspnea in patients with cancer and other chronic conditions.

Opioids. Although the exact mode of action of opioids in dyspnea management is unknown, several mechanisms of action, both peripheral, and central in origin, have been postulated. The possible mechanisms of action of opioids include depression of opioid receptors found in the lungs, spinal cord, and central respiratory centers, decrease in anxiety associated with dyspnea, and reduction in the central perception of dyspnea. Opioids may diminish the ventilatory responses to hypoxia and hypercapnia and improve cardiovascular function. Opioids cause venodilation of pulmonary vessels, thereby reducing preload to the heart.

Table 25.3 summarizes studies on the use of opioids in the treatment of dyspnea associated with a number of nonmalignant conditions (66–77). Most of the studies using opioids in varying doses and routes of administration in dyspneic noncancer patients with COPD and interstitial lung diseases but no cancer found opioids to be beneficial in the management of dyspnea. The most recent study by Abernethy et al. (66), randomized patients (n = 42), most of whom had COPD (88%) to 4 days of 20 mg oral morphine with sustained release followed by 4 days of identically formulated placebo, or vice versa. No wash-out period between the 4 day treatment periods was employed, although the authors acknowledge some carryover effect in patients receiving morphine first in sequence. Patients reported significantly less dyspnea according to a visual analog scale and improved sleep when using active treatment. The study concluded that sustained-release morphine was useful in relieving refractory dyspnea with reassuring data concerning adverse effects other than troublesome constipation. Although limited by the small

number of patients, duration of study, and reliance on visual analog scales, this and other studies provide reassurance that opioids have benefits in relieving intractable dyspnea. Large scale studies to investigate the optimum dose, route of opioids and to identify which patients benefit most, while also evaluating adverse effects are warranted. Caution should be exercised in opioid naive patients with COPD because of the risk of respiratory depression and hypercapnia.

Table 25.4 summarizes studies of systemic opioids in the treatment of cancer-related dyspnea. In the case of cancer-related dyspnea, all the published studies have agreed on the beneficial effect of systemic opioids for cancer dyspnea (78–83). However, the optimal type, dose, and modality of administration of opioids have not yet been determined. Cohen et al. (82) treated eight patients with cancer dyspnea with continuous intravenous morphine. Significant symptomatic relief was observed, but the authors found that in this population of patients with no previous exposure to morphine, the continuous intravenous infusion resulted in a significant increase in the levels of PCO₂. Bruera et al. (78,81) conducted two trials using intermittent subcutaneous morphine for the relief of cancer dyspnea. In the second study (81), intermittent doses of up to 2.5 times the regular opioid dose resulted in no significant change in the end-tidal CO₂ level. Most of these patients had already been chronically exposed to opioids and therefore had developed tolerance to their respiratory depressant effects. Mazzocato et al. (79), in a double-blind, crossover trial, looked at the effect of morphine 5 mg in seven opioid-naive elderly patients with cancer and 3.5 mg in addition to their regular dose in two patients already on 7.5 mg oral morphine every 4 hours. They found a significant improvement in dyspnea following treatment with morphine as compared with placebo with no significant changes in oxygen saturation.

Allard et al. (80) looked at the effect of two different doses of opioids on dyspnea in patients receiving regular opioid therapy. Fifteen patient pairs were given supplemental doses of 25% or 50% of the equivalent 4-hourly dose. The findings suggested that 25% of the patient's usual 4-hourly dose was sufficient to reduce dyspnea intensity and tachypnea for 4 hours.

One of the main methodological problems in the design of clinical trials of opioids in cancer dyspnea is the changing intensity of dyspnea both spontaneously and as a result of definite maneuvers. For these reasons, some groups advocate the use of intermittent opioids, as needed, when dyspnea occurs or for the anticipation of dyspnea associated with specific maneuvers.

Nebulized Opioids. During recent years, a number of authors reported symptomatic relief when patients with dyspnea are administered different types and doses of nebulized opioids (summarized in Table 25.5) (84–95). The possibility that opioids might affect receptors in the lung is exciting because of recent evidence suggesting that morphine does have an analgesic effect peripherally (96) and also because a small dose of nebulized morphine might be devoid of systemic opioid side effects.

Pharmacokinetic studies suggest that the systemic bioavailability of nebulized morphine is extremely poor (97). Therefore, the effects reported in most studies would have to be of a local nature. This is further supported by the lack of reports of side effects usually observed when morphine is administered systemically, such as sedation and nausea.

Most studies of patients with COPD but no cancer did not show any benefit with nebulized opioids for dyspnea management. (86,90–95) In patients with cancer, although there was one uncontrolled study which reported beneficial results in dyspnea (87), a subsequent controlled trial showed no symptomatic benefit for nebulized morphine compared

TABLE 25.3

USE OF OPIOIDS IN DYSPNEA ASSOCIATED WITH NONMALIGNANT CONDITIONS

Author (reference)	No. of patients	Opioid	Disease	Study	Level of evidence[a]	Effect on dyspnea	Assessment
Abernethy et al. (66)	42	Sustained-release morphine (20 mg twice daily) or placebo	COPD	8 d	I	+	VAS
Poole et al. (67)	16	Sustained-release morphine (20 mg twice daily) or placebo	COPD	6 wk	I	−	CRQ (36) Categorical scale
Browning et al. (68)	7	Hydrocodone (20 mg/m²/d oral) or placebo	COPD	Acute	I	+	VAS
Woodcock et al. (69)	12	Dihydrocodeine (1 mg/kg oral)	COPD	Acute	I	+	VAS
Johnson et al. (70)	18	Dihydrocodeine (15 mg three times/d) or placebo	COPD	3 wk	I	+	VAS
Robin and Burke (71)	1	Hydromorphone suppositories (3 mg three to four times/d)	COPD	Acute	I (N of 1)	+	Categorical scale
Eiser et al. (72)	4	Diamorphine (2.5, 5.0, or 7.5 mg 6 hourly oral) or placebo	COPD	2 wk	I	−	VAS
Rice et al. (73)	11	Codeine (30 mg four times/d) or promethazine (25 mg four times/d)	COPD	1 mo	I	+	VAS
Light et al. (74)	13	Morphine (0.8 mg/kg oral) or placebo	COPD	Acute	I	+	Borg scale
Sackner (75)	17,8	Hydrocodone (5 mg oral)	COPD	Acute	III	+	Not reported
Chua et al. (76)	12	Dihydrocodeine p.o., dose 1 mg/kg or placebo	CHF	Acute	I	+	Borg scale
Woodcock et al. (77)	16	Dihydrocodeine p.o., dose 30/60 mg three times/d	COPD				

COPD, chronic obstructive pulmonary disease; CHF, chronic heart failure; CRQ, chronic respiratory questionnaire; VAS, visual analog scale; +, effective; −, not effective.
[a]Level of evidence, I, randomized controlled trial; III, retrospective study.

with placebo (86). In a recently published study Bruera et al. (84) compared the effects of nebulized versus subcutaneous morphine on the intensity of dyspnea in 11 cancer patients. On the first day patients were randomized to receive either subcutaneous morphine plus nebulized placebo or nebulized morphine plus subcutaneous placebo. On the second day patients were crossed over. There was no significant difference in dyspnea intensity between nebulized and subcutaneous morphine at 60 minutes. Unfortunately, due to limited sample size, there was insufficient power to rule out a significant difference between both routes of administration. Larger randomized controlled trials in patients with both continuous dyspnea and early stages of dyspnea were recommended. In another crossover study, Grimbert et al. (85) compared nebulized morphine to nebulized normal saline in 12 patients with lung cancer suffering from dyspnea despite conventional treatments. For two periods of 48 hours (separated by a 24-hour wash-out period) patients received 4 mL of morphine sulfate and 4 mL of normal saline 4 hourly

by a jet nebulizer. The aerosols of normal saline and morphine produced the same improvements in the dyspnea scores independently of the mass nebulized. Furthermore the nebulizations did not produce any significant change in respiratory rate or oxygen saturation. The fact that both aerosols lead to a similar improvement in dyspnea scores suggests that humidification of the airways rather than a pharmacologic action may be beneficial in the treatment of dyspnea in terminally ill patients.

For patients unable or unwilling to take an oral agent or for those who have had intolerable adverse effects after systemic administration, the use of nebulized opioids may be advantageous. A variety of opioids have been administered through inhalation for dyspnea. Morphine sulfate 2.5–10 mg, hydromorphone hydrochloride 0.25–1 mg, and fentanyl citrate 25 μg are the most commonly used doses in the United States. The disadvantages of nebulized opioids include increased costs related to equipment, need for using preservative-free drug and complicated method of delivery.

TABLE 25.4

SYSTEMIC OPIOIDS IN THE TREATMENT OF CANCER-RELATED DYSPNEA

Author (reference)	No. of patients	Opioid drug	Disease	Study	Level of evidence[a]	Assessment	Findings
Bruera et al. (78)	10	Morphine s.c., 50% higher than regular scheduled dose	Advanced cancer	Acute	I	VAS	+
Mazzocato et al. (79)	9	Morphine s.c., 5 mg if opioid naive or half daily oral dose	Advanced cancer	Acute	I	VAS and Borg scale	+
Allard et al. (80)	33	Morphine 25% or 50% of 4 hourly opioid dose by same route	Advanced cancer	Acute	I	VAS	+/+
Bruera et al. (81)	20	Morphine s.c., 5 mg bolus or 2.5 times the regular dose	Advanced cancer	Acute	III	VAS	+
Cohen et al. (82)	8	Morphine i.v. bolus, mean dose 5.6 mg/h	Advanced cancer	Acute	III	Categorical scale	+
Ventafridda et al. (83)	5	Morphine s.c., 10 mg Chlorpromazine s.c., 25 mg	Advanced cancer	Acute	III	VAS	+

VAS, visual analog scale; +, effective; +/+, very effective.
[a]Level of evidence, I, randomized controlled trial; III, retrospective study.

In a systematic review Jennings et al examined the use of opioids in patients with advanced disease for management of dyspnea (98). Eighteen studies met the inclusion criteria. Nine trials involving the use of oral or parenteral opioids (67, 69,70,72,74,76–78) and nine trials which studied the use of nebulized opioids. (86–89,91–95) This review found a highly statistically significant effect for oral and parenteral opioids in the management of dyspnea between the opioid and placebo treatment periods. This review did not find a statistically significant effect for nebulized opioids in the management of dyspnea. In the at-rest studies there was some improvement in dyspnea after nebulized morphine, but this was not significantly different from that seen after nebulized saline. However, nebulized normal saline may not be a true placebo as it has a variety of nonspecific actions in patients with dyspnea, including stimulation of facial nerve endings and liquefaction of tenacious secretions (99–101).

Benzodiazepines. Benzodiazepines are commonly used in the management of cancer-related dyspnea. Table 25.6 summarizes studies in which benzodiazepines and other psychotropic drugs were used for the management of dyspnea associated with both exercise and COPD (102–106). Four of the five studies found no significant difference between benzodiazepines and placebo. Mitchell-Heggs et al. (106) studied four patients with COPD in a controlled, single arm, blinded study comparing diazepam and placebo. The authors reported a sustained benefit for three of four patients after diazepam.

In some patients, benzodiazepines may be used when dyspnea is considered to be a somatic manifestation of a panic disorder or when patients have severe anxiety. There is no evidence to support the routine use of benzodiazepines in the management of dyspnea

Corticosteroids. Steroids are useful for managing dyspnea in patients with cancer who have carcinomatous lymphangitis, radiation associated pneumonitis, superior vena caval syndrome or an inflammatory component to their dyspnea (as in asthma). They are highly effective in treating bronchospasm associated with both asthma and COPD (107). Bronchiolitis obliterans organizing pneumonia (BOOP) syndrome after adjuvant radiation therapy for breast cancer has been recently recognized, and treatment with corticosteroids results in rapid improvement (108). On the other hand, evidence exists that corticosteroids induce negative functional and pathologic alterations in several muscle groups (109). It has been suggested that the effects are more pronounced on the diaphragm than on other muscles. These findings might be important because of the frequent presence of cachexia and muscle weakness in patients with advanced cancer. A double-blind placebo-controlled randomized trial indicated that anabolic steroids may counteract the deleterious effects of systemic corticosteroids. Nandrolone treatment restored respiratory muscle function and exercise capacity in patients with moderate to severe COPD patients undergoing pulmonary rehabilitation (110).

Past trials of inhaled corticosteroids have measured the effect on progression of COPD and FEV_1 decline rather than clinical outcomes. A recent meta-analysis (111) suggested that inhaled corticosteroid trials of patients with a mean FEV_1 of <2 L (or <70% of predicted) almost uniformly demonstrated a benefit of inhaled corticosteroids on exacerbations. Long-acting β_2 agonists and tiotropium had similar efficacy and reduced exacerbation rates by 20–25%. Combining a long-acting β_2 agonist with an inhaled corticosteroid resulted in an exacerbation reduction of 30%.

Bronchodilators. Both nebulized and orally administered bronchodilators are useful in the management of bronchospasm associated with both asthma and COPD (107). A large proportion of the patients with cancer-related dyspnea have a history of smoking or COPD. Congleton and Muers (112) demonstrated that almost half of 57 consecutive patients with lung cancer treated by their group had evidence of air-flow obstruction. A strong association was found between

TABLE 25.5

USE OF NEBULIZED OPIOIDS IN DYSPNEA

Author (reference)	No. of patients	Drug	Disease	Level of evidence[a]	Findings	Assessment
Bruera et al. (84)	11	Morphine or Subcutaneous morphine	Cancer	I	Both routes similarly effective	
Grimbert et al. (85)	12	Mophine or normal saline placebo	Lung cancer	I	Same for both	
Davis et al. (86)	79	Morphine (5–50 mg) or placebo	Cancer	I	−	VAS and modified Borg scale
Davis et al. (87)	18	Morphine (12.5 mg) or M-6-glucuronide (4 mg) or placebo	COPD	I	− + −	Objective measurement
Young et al. (88)	11	Morphine (5 mg/5 mL over 12 min) or placebo	COPD	I	+	Patient asked about limiting symptoms
Beauford et al. (89)	8	Morphine (1, 4, or 10 mg) or placebo	COPD	I	−	VAS and objective measurement
Farncombe et al. (90)	54	34 pts morphine 1–30 mg/4 h	Cancer	III	34 patients +12 stopped after 1 and 2 doses	Not described
		17 pts hydromorphone 1–20 mg/4 h 2 pts codeine 15–60 mg/4 h 1 pt anileridine 25–50 mg/4 h	COPD		8 conflicting reports on charts	
Noseda et al. (91)	12	Morphine, dose 10, 20 mg	COPD	I	−	VAS for dyspnea
Masood et al. (92)	12	Morphine (10, 25 mg) or placebo	COPD	I	−	VAS
Leung et al. (93)	9	Morphine, dose 5 mg	COPD/ILD	I	−	VAS
Jankelson et al. (94)	16	Morphine (20, 40 mg) or placebo	COPD	I	−	VAS
Harris-Eze et al. (95)	6	Morphine (2.5, 5 mg) or placebo	COPD/ILD	I	−	VAS

COPD, chronic obstructive pulmonary disease; ILD, interstitial lung disease
VAS, visual analog scale; +, effective; −, not effective.
[a]Level of evidence, I, randomized controlled trial; III, retrospective study.

air-flow obstruction and dyspnea. Of the 17 patients who accepted the offer of a trial of bronchodilator therapy (a combination of nebulized adrenergic and anticholinergic agents four times a day), most experienced significant symptomatic improvement.

Previous studies suggested that dyspnea in some patients with nonreversible obstructive airway disease could improve following the administration of theophylline (113). Aminophylline, theophylline, and caffeine all improve diaphragmatic contractility both in normal volunteers (113–115) and in patients with COPD (116). Because of the frequent presence of asthenia and generalized muscle weakness with or without cachexia, some patients with cancer might benefit from the effect of xanthines on respiratory muscle contractility.

Other Drugs. Nebulized furosemide has been found to be protective against the bronchospasm induced by exercise in patients with asthma (117). It has also been shown to have bronchodilator effect in acute asthma (118,119). There are reports of its use for the treatment of dyspnea in a palliative care setting (120).

Several studies suggested that alcohol might be able to decrease the intensity of dyspnea in patients with COPD (69, 120). Although there is some consistent evidence for a symptomatic benefit for alcohol, the side effects associated with both acute and chronic administration, in addition to the potentially dangerous interaction with other drugs, suggests that alcohol may be an impractical option.

A number of drugs, such as indomethacin (121) and medroxyprogesterone acetate (122), are being studied as a potential treatment for dyspnea, but the evidence for a role of these and other agents is very limited, and they could not be recommended for clinical use.

General Support Measures

A number of measures can be implemented for the support of the patient and the family. Most of these measures can be implemented in the acute-care hospital setting, continuing-care hospitals, and at home.

TABLE 25.6

EFFECT OF BENZODIAZEPINES AND OTHER PSYCHOTROPIC DRUGS ON DYSPNEA

Author (reference)	No. of patients	Psychotropic drug	Condition	Study	Level of evidence[a]	Effect of dyspnea
Stark et al. (102)	6	Diazepam (10 mg daily)	Exercise	Acute	I	−
		Promethazine (25 mg daily)				−
O'Neill et al. (103)	12	Promethazine (25 mg daily) and placebo	Exercise	Acute	I	−
	6	Mebhydrolin (50 mg daily) or placebo (histamine antagonist)	Exercise			−
	6	Chlorpromazine (25 mg) or placebo				+
Woodcock et al. (104)	15	Diazepam (25 mg daily)	COPD	2 wk	I	−
		Promethazine (125 mg)				+
Mann et al. (105)	24	Alprazolam (0.5 mg b.i.d.) or placebo	COPD	3 wk	I	−
Mitchell-Heggs et al. (106)	4	Diazepam (25 mg)	COPD	Acute	I	+

COPD, chronic obstructive pulmonary disease; +, effective; −, not effective.
[a]Level of evidence, I, randomized controlled trial.

Activity Level. Dyspnea is a variable symptom. Most of the aggravating factors are related to muscle effort associated with different physical activities. It is important to educate patients and families so that they can recognize the type of maneuvers associated with episodes of increased dyspnea. Once these maneuvers are recognized, the two most effective approaches are anticipatory symptomatic relief and avoidance of effort. Anticipatory relief can include the administration of doses of drugs for symptomatic relief before the dyspnea-causing maneuver, and psychologic support techniques such as relaxation or imagery. Avoidance of effort involves assisting the patient to the maximum with the maneuver to minimize the muscle effort and the consequent development of dyspnea. This includes the use of different devices to assist the patient with transportation to and from the bathroom and for mobilization. It is important for patients and families to understand that they can remain quite active whereas not necessarily making muscle efforts. With the use of wheelchairs and portable oxygen it is possible for patients to return to the community.

On the other hand, there is substantial recent evidence that exercise programs and pulmonary rehabilitation in patients with COPD improve dyspnea and exercise tolerance (123–127). It is postulated that skeletal muscle dysfunction is an important contributor to exercise intolerance and dyspnea in patients with COPD (126). The dysfunction is probably related to several factors, many of which also exist in patients with advanced cancer patients, such as deconditioning secondary to immobility, malnutrition, and the use of corticosteroids. In addition inflammatory factors, such as interleukins and tumor necrosis factor, contribute to muscle wasting associated with cachexia in cancer patients. The respiratory exercises include controlled breathing, diaphragmatic, and pursed-lip breathing. Postural drainage has, in most parts of the world, been replaced by airway clearance regimens that include forced expiratory maneuvers or technique of breathing at different airflow and lung volume. Percussions and external or internal vibrations are seldom justified in adults.

A meta-analysis to determine the effectiveness of rehabilitation in patients with COPD shows that rehabilitation groups undergoing at least lower extremity training did significantly better than control groups on walking test and shortness of breath (128). Trials that included patients with severe COPD showed that rehabilitation groups did significantly better than control groups only when the rehabilitation programs were 6 months or longer. Trials that included mild/moderate patients with COPD showed that rehabilitation groups did significantly better than control groups with both short- and long-term rehabilitation programs.

Pulmonary rehabilitation programs must be comprehensive and flexible to address each patient's need and include smoking cessation, optimal medical treatment, nutritional intervention, psychosocial support, and health education. The maintenance of benefits after pulmonary rehabilitation is possible with minimal maintenance of activity (129).

Ventilatory support. In patients with severe neuromuscular disorders, positive pressure ventilation provides significant relief for respiratory muscle fatigue. Techniques include continuous positive airway pressure ventilation or intermittent positive pressure ventilation (IPPV) through face or nasal masks. Continuous positive airway pressure ventilation has been shown to reduce inspiratory muscle effort and improve sleep in patients with both COPD and congestive heart failure, and to reduce dyspnea and fatigue in the latter group (130, 131). By providing respiratory muscle relief, these techniques can decrease the sensation of breathlessness at rest and during exercise. The recognition of progressive muscle weakness in patients with cancer and the correlation between maximal inspiratory pressure and dyspnea indicate that some patients in whom respiratory muscle weakness can be demonstrated could possibly benefit from positive pressure ventilation. Specialized personnel, such as a chest physician or a trained chest therapist in an inpatient setting, should initiate these techniques.

Noninvasive ventilation (NIV) provided through a standard face mask by BiPAP, was found to be an effective ventilation support for 18 patients with cancer with "life-support techniques limitation" admitted for an acute respiratory distress, in terms of intensive care unit (ICU) and hospital discharges (132).

Ventilation and End-of-Life-Care. In recent times the simple principles of beneficence and nonmaleficence have been augmented and sometimes challenged by a rising awareness of patient/consumer rights, and the public expectation of greater involvement in medical, social, and scientific affairs which affect them. In a publicly funded healthcare system in which rationing (explicit or otherwise) is inevitable, the additional concepts of utility and distributive justice can easily come into conflict with the individual's right to autonomy.

Burden of mechanical ventilation. Studies on patients with COPD receiving mechanical ventilation have shown that the burden of ICU care for the individual is substantial. Pochard et al. have shown that over and above medical complications and their consequences, in 43 patients receiving IPPV, 88% were depressed, 58% felt unable to communicate, 37% experienced an acute fear of dying, 30% felt intolerable pain, and 21% feared they had been abandoned (133). Even after discharge it is probable that some physical and psychologic effects will never be eliminated. A UK study reported a 1-year mortality rate of 59% following mechanical ventilation in COPD and 53% of survivors were more dependent on carers, were housebound, and having worse exercise tolerance and poorer quality of life than before ICU admission (134).

When there is a doubt about reversibility or when there is not enough time for its assessment, a patient with advanced malignancy may get interventions that are unwarranted and often positively detrimental to quality of life. In such events, based on available evidence, it can be recommended that NIV be resorted to rather than more invasive endotracheal intubation and ventilation.

The use of NIV is associated with a marked reduction in the need for endotracheal intubation, a decrease in complication rate, a reduced duration of hospital stay and a substantial reduction in hospital mortality (135,136). One important factor in success seems to be the early delivery of NIV during the course of respiratory failure (137). NIV allows many of the complications associated with mechanical ventilation to be avoided, especially the occurrence of nosocomial infections. It is important that, at the time of initiation of NIV, a decision is made as to whether progression to intubation and IPPV is appropriate if NIV is unsuccessful.

Nevertheless, it needs to be emphasized that education of the patient and family as well as rehabilitation at home to enable essential activity, supported by adequate drug therapy is the effective measure in dyspnea of advanced malignancy. Ventilatory support can only be a stopgap measure to tide over a potentially reversible event in the course of illness.

Support of the Patient and Family. Explanation of dyspnea and addressing the fears of the patient and family is of great importance. Dyspnea can elicit major psychologic reactions in the patient and the family, both of whom may fear that the patient may "choke to death." It is important to anticipate the possibility of a crisis of respiratory failure. Symptomatic drugs should be made available together with instructions for administration. Telephone numbers of individuals to be contacted should also be made available. Even if patients do not require oxygen at a given time, it is important that oxygen be available immediately if a respiratory crisis occurs.

Because dyspnea is frequently associated with tachypnea and the use of accessory respiratory muscles, patients may appear to be significantly dyspneic even when they are in good symptomatic control. As mentioned previously it is important for the relatives and members of the staff to remember to assess dyspnea only by asking patients how short of breath they feel rather than by estimating their dyspnea from the degree of tachypnea and use of accessory muscles. The goal should be symptomatic therapeutic intervention of the patient's expression of dyspnea rather than relief of the objective variables that accompany this symptom.

Future Research

Many aspects of dyspnea in patients with cancer have not been adequately researched. These include areas of assessment and management. The use of simple noninvasive assessment methods, including reading (serial numbers or a paragraph in loud voice) and breath-holding, should be researched in greater detail. The potential role of descriptors of dyspnea to indicate underlying clinical conditions causing dyspnea should receive closer attention. Areas of treatment, including the roles of nebulized loop diuretics and various opioids, in addition to the effects of xanthines on respiratory muscle contractility, should be addressed by investigators. The effects of exercise training on dyspnea in patients with advanced cancer and the role of positive pressure ventilation in those with demonstrated respiratory muscle weakness should also be investigated.

References

1. Baines M. Control of other symptoms. In: CM Saunders, ed. *The management of terminal disease.* Chicago: Yearbook, 1978.
2. Ahmedzai S. Palliation of respiratory symptoms. In: Doyle D, Hanks GWC, MacDonald N, eds. *Oxford textbook of palliative medicine.* Oxford, England: Oxford University Press, 1993:349–378.
3. Ripamonti C. Management of dyspnea in advanced cancer patients. *Support Care Cancer* 1999;7:233–243.
4. Vigano A, Donaldson N, Higginson IJ, et al. Quality of life and survival prediction in terminal cancer patients: a multicenter study. *Cancer* 2004;101:1090–1098.
5. Higginson I, McCarthy M. Measuring symptoms in terminal cancer: are pain and dyspnoea controlled? *J R Soc Med* 1989;82:264–267.
6. Tobin MJ. Dyspnea: pathophysiologic basis, clinical presentations and management. *Arch Intern Med* 1990;150:1604–1613.
7. Castele RJ, Connors AF, Altose MD. Effects of changes in CO_2 partial pressure on the sensation of respiratory drive. *J Appl Physiol* 1985;59:1747–1757.
8. Manning HL, Schwartzstein RM. Mechanisms of disease: pathophysiology of dyspnea. *N Engl J Med* 1995;333:1547–1553.
9. Altose MA. Dyspnea. In: DH Simmons, ed. *Current pulmonology,* Vol. 7. Chicago: Year Book Medical Publishers, 1986:199–226.
10. Rubinfeld AR, Pain MCF. Perception of asthma. *Lancet* 1976;1:882–884.
11. Burns BH, Howell JBL. Disproportionately severe breathlessness in chronic bronchitis. *QJM* 1969;151:277–294.
12. Bruera E, Schmitz B, Pither J, et al. The frequency and correlates of dyspnea in patients with advanced cancer. *J Pain Symptom Manage* 2000;19:357–362.
13. Fainsinger R, Bruera E. Case report: assessment of total pain. *Perspect Pain Manage* 1991;13–14.
14. Palange P, Forte S, Felli A, et al. Nutritional state and exercise tolerance in patients with COPD. *Chest* 1995;107:1206–1212.
15. Kongragunta VR, Druz WS, Sharp JT. Dyspnea and diaphragmatic fatigue in patients with chronic obstructive pulmonary disease. *Am Rev Respir Dis* 1988;137:662–667.
16. Arora NS, Rochester DF. Respiratory muscle strength and maximal voluntary ventilation in undernourished patients. *Am Rev Respir Dis* 1982;126:5–8.
17. Ward ME, Eidelman D, Stubbing DG, et al. Respiratory sensation and pattern of respiratory muscle activation during diaphragm fatigue. *J Appl Physiol* 1988;65:2181–2189.
18. Dudgeon DJ, Lertzman M. Dyspnea in the advanced cancer patient. *J Pain Symptom Manage* 1998;16:212–219.
19. Reuben DB, Mor V. Dyspnea in terminally ill cancer patients. *Chest* 1986;89:234–236.
20. Grond S, Zech D, Diefenbach C, et al. Prevalence and pattern of symptoms in patients with cancer pain: a prospective evaluation of 1635 cancer patients referred to a pain clinic. *J Pain Symptom Manage* 1994;9:372–382.
21. Donnelly S, Walsh D. The symptoms of advanced cancer: identification of clinical and research priorities by assessment of prevalence and severity. *J Palliat Care* 1995;11:27–32.
22. Twycross RG, Lack SA. *Control of alimentary symptoms in far advanced cancer,* Edinburgh, Scotland: Churchill Livingstone, 1986.
23. Muers MF. Palliation of symptoms in non-small cell lung cancer: a study by the Yorkshire Regional Cancer Organization Thoraxic Group. *Thorax* 1993;48:339–343.
24. Bruera E. Clinical management of cachexia and anorexia in patients with advanced cancer. *Oncology* 1992;49(Suppl 2):35–42.
25. Clark AL, Sparrow JL, Coats AJS. Muscle fatigue and dyspnoea in chronic heart failure: two sides of the same coin? *Eur Heart J* 1995;16:49–52.
26. Hecht SS. Tobacco carcinogenesis and lung cancer. *J Natl Cancer Inst* 1999;91:1194–1210.
27. Montano M, Becerril C, Ruiz V, et al. Matrix metalloproteinases activity in COPD associated with wood smoke. *Chest* 2004;125:466–472.
28. Mador MJ, Kufel TJ. Reproducibility of visual analogue scale measurements of dyspnea in patients with chronic obstructive pulmonary disease. *Am Rev Respir Dis* 1992;146:82–87.
29. Bruera E, Kuehn N, Miller MJ, et al. The edmonton symptom assessment system (ESAS): a simple method for the assessment of palliative care patients. *J Palliat Care* 1991;7:6–9.

30. Bergman B, Aarouson NK, Ahmedzai S, et al. The EORTC QLQ-LC13: a modular supplement to the EORTC core quality of life questionnaire (QLQ-C30) for use in lung cancer clinical trials. EORTC Study Group on Quality of Life. *Eur J Cancer* 1994;30A:635–642.

31. Guyatt GH, Townsend M, Keller J, et al. Measuring functional status in chronic lung disease: conclusions from a randomized control trial. *Respir Med* 1991;85(Suppl B):17–21.

32. Wijkstra PJ, TenVergert EM, Van Altena R, et al. Reliability and validity of the chronic respiratory questionnaire. *Thorax* 1994;49:465–467.

33. Medical Research Council *Committee on research into chronic bronchitis: instruction for use of the questionnaire on respiratory symptoms.* Devon, England: W.J. Holman, 1966.

34. Mahler DA, Rosiello RA, Harver A, et al. Comparison of clinical dyspnea ratings and psychophysical measurements of respiratory sensation in obstructive airway disease. *Am Rev Respir Dis* 1987;135:1229–1233.

35. Mador MJ, Rodis A, Magalang UJ. Reproducibility of Borg scale measurements of dyspnea during exercise in patients with COPD. *Chest* 1995;107:1590–1597.

36. Morgan A. Simple exercise testing. *Respir Med* 1989;83:383–387.

37. Taskar V, Clayton N, Atkins M, et al. Breath-holding time in normal subjects, snorers, and sleep apnea patients. *Chest* 1995;107:959–962.

38. Nishino T, Sugimori K, Ishikawa T. Changes in the period of no respiratory sensation and total breath-holding time in successive breath-holding trials. *Clin Sci (Colch)* 1996;91:755–761.

39. Wilcock A, Crosby V, Clarke D, et al. Reading numbers aloud: a measure of the limiting effect of breathlessness in patients with cancer. *Thorax* 1999;54:1099–1103.

40. Foley K. The treatment of cancer pain. *N Engl J Med* 1985;313:84–95.

41. Simon PM, Schwartzstein RM, Weiss JW, et al. Distinguishable types of dyspnea in patients with shortness of breath. *Am Rev Respir Dis* 1990;142:1009–1014.

42. Mahler DA, Harver A, Lentine T, et al. Descriptors of breathlessness in cardiorespiratory diseases. *Am J Respir Crit Care Med* 1996;154:1357–1363.

43. Hardie GE, Janson S, Gold WM, et al. Ethnic differences: word descriptors used by African-American and white asthma patients during induced bronchoconstriction. *Chest* 2000;117:935–943.

44. Chang VT, Hwang SS, Feuerman M. Validation of the edmonton symptom assessment scale. *Cancer* 2000;88:2164–2171.

45. Cook DJ, Guyatt GH, Laupacis A, et al. Rules of evidence and clinical recommendations on the use of antithrombotic agents. *Chest* 1992;102:305S–311S.

46. Pizzo PA, Meyers J, Freifeld AG, et al. Infections in the cancer patient. In: DeVita VT, Hellman S, Rosenberg SA, eds. *Cancer, principles and practice of oncology,* Vol. 2, 4th ed. Philadelphia, PA: JB Lippincott Co, 1993:2292–2337.

47. Anthonisen NR. Long-term oxygen therapy. *Ann Intern Med* 1983;99:519–527.

48. Nocturnal Oxygen Therapy Trial Group. Continuous or nocturnal oxygen therapy in hypoxemic chronic obstructive lung disease. *Ann Intern Med* 1980;93:391–398.

49. Billings JA. The management of common symptoms. In: Billings JA, ed. *Out-patient management of advanced cancer,* Vol. 41. Philadelphia, PA: JB Lippincott Co, 1985:80–87.

50. Twycross RG, Lack SA. *Therapeutics in terminal cancer,* 2nd ed. Edinburgh, Scotland: Churchill Livingstone, 1990:129–132.

51. Bruera E, de Stoutz N, Velasco-Leiva A, et al. The effects of oxygen on the intensity of dyspnea in hypoxemic terminal cancer patients. *Lancet* 1993;342:13–14.

52. Bruera E, Schoeller T, MacEachern T. Symptomatic benefit of supplemental oxygen in hypoxemic patients with terminal cancer: the use of the N of 1 randomized controlled trial. *J Pain Symptom Manage* 1992;7:365–368.

53. Booth S, Kelly MJ, Cox NP, et al. Does oxygen help dyspnea in patients with cancer? *Am J Respir Crit Care Med* 1996;153:1515–1518.

54. Swinburn CR, Mould H, Stone TN, et al. Symptomatic benefit of supplemental oxygen in hypoxemic patients with chronic lung disease. *Am Rev Respir Dis* 1991;143:913–915.

55. Liss HP, Grant BJB. The effect of nasal flow on breathlessness in patients with chronic obstructive pulmonary disease. *Am Rev Respir Dis* 1988;137:1285–1288.

56. Davidson AC, Leach R, George RJD, et al. Supplemental oxygen and exercise ability in chronic obstructive airways disease. *Thorax* 1988;43:965–971.

57. Woodcock AAS, Gross ER, Geddes DM. Oxygen relieves breathlessness in pink puffers. *Lancet* 1981;1:907–909.

58. Dean NC, Brown JK, Himelman RB, et al. Oxygen may improve dyspnea and endurance in patients with chronic obstructive pulmonary disease and only mild hypoxemia. *Am Rev Respir Dis* 1992;146:941–945.

59. Moore DP, Weston AR, Hughes JMB, et al. Effects of increased inspired oxygen concentrations on exercise performance in chronic heart failure. *Lancet* 1992;339:850–853.

60. Restrick LJ, Davies SW, Noone L, et al. Ambulatory oxygen in chronic heart failure. *Lancet* 1992;334:1192–1193.

61. Davidson AC, Leach R, George RJ, et al. Supplemental oxygen and exercise ability in chronic obstructive airways disease. *Thorax* 1988;43:965–971.

62. MacIntyre NR. Oxygen therapy and exercise response in lung disease. *Respir Care* 2000;45:194–200.

63. Sin DD, McAlister FA, Man SF, et al. Contemporary management of chronic obstructive pulmonary disease: scientific review. *JAMA* 2003;290:2301–2312.

64. Ringbaek TJ, Viskum K, Lange P. Non-continuous home oxygen therapy: utilization, symptomatic effect and prognosis, data from a national register on home oxygen therapy. *Respir Med* 2001;95:980–985.

65. Bruera E, Sweeney C, Willey J, et al. A randomized controlled trial of supplemental oxygen versus air in cancer patients with dyspnea. *Palliat Med* 2003;17:659–663.

66. Abernethy AP, Currow DC, Frith P, et al. Randomised, double blind, placebo controlled crossover trial of sustained release morphine for the management of refractory dyspnoea. *BMJ* 2003;237:523–528.

67. Poole PJ, Veale AG, Black PN. The effect of sustained-release morphine on breathlessness and quality of life in severe chronic pulmonary disease. *Am J Respir Crit Care Med* 1998;157:1877–1880.

68. Browning I, D Alonzo GE, Tobin MJ. Effect of hydrocodone on dyspnea, respiratory drive and exercise performance in adult patients with cystic fibrosis (abstract). *Am Rev Respir Dis* 1988;137:305.

69. Woodcock AA, Gross ER, Gellert A, et al. Effects of dihydrocodeine, alcohol, and caffeine on breathlessness and exercise tolerance in patients with chronic obstructive lung disease and normal blood gases. *N Engl J Med* 1981;305:1611–1616.

70. Johnson MA, Woodcock AA, Geddes DM. Dihydrocodeine for breathlessness in pink puffers. *BMJ* 1983;286:675–677.

71. Robin ED, Burke CM. Risk-benefit analysis in chest medicine. Single-patient randomization clinical trial. Opiates for intractable dyspnea. *Chest* 1986;90:889–892.

72. Eiser N, Denman WT, West C, et al. Oral diamorphine: lack of effect on dyspnoea and exercise tolerance in the pink puffer syndrome. *Eur Respir J* 1991;4:926–931.

73. Rice KL, Kronenberg RS, Hedemark LL, et al. Effects of chronic administration of codeine and promethazine on breathlessness and exercise tolerance in patients with chronic airflow obstruction. *Br J Dis Chest* 1987;81:287–292.

74. Light RW, Muro JR, Sato RI, et al. Effects of oral morphine on breathlessness and exercise tolerance in patients with chronic obstructive pulmonary disease. *Am Rev Respir Dis* 1989;139:126–133.

75. Sackner MA. Effects of hydrocodone bitartrate on breathing pattern of patients with chronic obstructive pulmonary disease and restrictive lung disease. *Mt Sinai J Med* 1984;51:222–226.

76. Chua TP, Harrington D, Ponikowski P, et al. Effects of dihydrocodeine on chemosensitivity and exercise tolerance in patients with chronic heart failure. *Am Coll Cardiol* 1997;29:147–152.

77. Woodcock AA, Johnson MA, Geddes DM. Breathlessness, alcohol and opiates. *N Engl J Med* 1982;306:1363–1364.

78. Bruera E, MacEachern T, Ripamonti C, et al. Subcutaneous morphine for dyspnea in cancer patients. *Ann Intern Med* 1993;119:906–907.

79. Mazzocato C, Buclin T, Rapin CH. The effects of morphine on dyspnea and ventilatory function in elderly patients with advanced cancer: a randomized double-blind controlled trial. *Ann Oncol* 1999;10:1511–1514.

80. Allard P, Lamontagne C, Bernard P, et al. How effective are supplementary doses of opioids for dyspnea in terminally ill cancer patients? A randomized continuous sequential clinical trial. *J Pain Symptom Manage* 1999;17:256–265.

81. Bruera E, Macmillan K, Pither J, et al. The effects of morphine on the dyspnea of terminal cancer patients. *J Pain Symptom Manage* 1990;5:341–344.

82. Cohen MH, Anderson A, Krasnow SH, et al. Continuous intravenous infusion of morphine for severe dyspnea. *South Med J* 1991;84:229–234.

83. Ventafridda V, Spoldi E, De Conno F. Control of dyspnea in advanced cancer patients [Letter]. *Chest* 1990;98:1544–1545.

84. Bruera E, Sala R, Spruyt O, et al. Nebulized versus subcutaneous morphine for patients with cancer dyspnea. *J Pain Symptom Manage* 2005;29:613–618.

85. Grimbert D, Lubin O, De Monte M, et al. Dyspnea and morphine aerosols in the palliative care of lung cancer. *Rev Mal Respir* 2004;21:1091–1097.

86. Davis CL, Penn K, A'Hern R, et al. Single dose randomized controlled trial of nebulized morphine in patients with cancer related breathlessness (Abstract). *Palliat Med* 1996;10:64.

87. Davis CL, Hodder C, Love S, et al. Effect of nebulized morphine and morphine-6-glucuronide on exercise endurance in patients with chronic obstructive pulmonary disease. *Thorax* 1994;49:393.

88. Young IH, Daviskas E, Keena VA. Effect of low dose nebulised morphine on exercise endurance in patients with chronic lung disease. *Thorax* 1989;44:387–390.

89. Beauford W, Saylor TT, Stansbury DW, et al. Effects of nebulized morphine sulfate on the exercise tolerance on the ventilatory limited COPD patient. *Chest* 1993;104:175–178.

90. Farncombe M, Chater S, Gillin A. The use of nebulized opioids for breathlessness: a chart review. *Palliat Med* 1994;8:306–312.

91. Noseda A, Carpiaux JP, Markstein C, et al. Disabling dyspnoea in patients with advanced disease: lack of effect of nebulized morphine. *Eur Respir J* 1997;10:1079–1083.

92. Masood AR, Reed JW, Thomas SH. Lack of effect of inhaled morphine on exercise-induced breathlessness in chronic obstructive pulmonary disease. *Thorax* 1996;50:529–534.

93. Leung R, Hill P, Burdon J. Effect of inhaled morphine on the development of breathlessness during exercise in patients with chronic lung disease. *Thorax* 1996;51:596–600.

94. Jankelson D, Hosseini K, Mather LE, et al. Lack of effect of high doses of inhaled morphine on exercise endurance in chronic obstructive pulmonary disease. *Eur Respir J* 1997;10:2270–2274.

95. Harris-Eze A, Sridhar G, Clemens RE, et al. Low-dose nebulized morphine does not improve exercise in interstitial lung disease. *Am J Respir Crit Care Med* 1995;152:1940–1945.

96. Stein C. The control of pain in peripheral tissue by opioids. *N Engl J Med* 1995;332(25):1685–1690.

97. Davis CL, Lam W, Butcher M, et al. Low systemic bioavailability of nebulized morphine: potential therapeutic role for the relief of dyspnea (Abstract). *Proc Annu Meet Am Soc Clin Oncol* 1992;11:A359.

98. Jennings AL, Davies AN, Higgins JP, et al. A systematic review of the use of opioids in the management of dyspnoea. *Thorax* 2002;57:939–944.

99. Davis C. The role of nebulised drugs in palliating respiratory symptoms of malignant disease. *Eur J Palliat Care* 1995;2:9–15.

100. Schwartzstein RM, Lahive K, Pope A, et al. Cold facial stimulation reduces breathlessness induced in normal subjects. *Am Rev Respir Dis* 1987;136:58–61.

101. Sutton PP, Gemmell HG, Innes N, et al. Use of nebulised saline and nebulised terbutaline as an adjunct to chest physiotherapy. *Thorax* 1988;43:57–60.

102. Stark RD, Gambles SA, Lewis JA. Methods to assess breathlessness in healthy subjects: a critical evaluation and application to analyze the acute effects of diazepam and promethazine on breathlessness induced by exercise or by exposure to raised levels of carbon dioxide. *Clin Sci (Colch)* 1981;61:429–439.

103. Neill PA, Morton PB, Stark RD. Chlorpromazine—a specific effect on breathlessness? *Br J Clin Pharmacol* 1985;19:793–797.

104. Woodcock AA, Gross ER, Geddes DM. Drug treatment of breathlessness: contrasting effects of diazepam and promethazine in pink puffers. *BMJ* 1981;283:343–346.

105. Mann GCW, Sproule BJ. Effect of alprazolam on exercise and dyspnea in patients with chronic obstructive pulmonary disease. *Chest* 1986;90:832–836.

106. Mitchell-Heggs P, Murphy K, Minty K, et al. Diazepam in the treatment of dyspnoea in the pink puffer syndrome. *QJM* 1980;New Series 49(193):9–20.

107. Frew AJ, Holgate ST. Clinical pharmacology of asthma. Implications for treatment. *Drugs* 1993;46:847–862.

108. Miwa S, Morita S, Suda T. The incidence and clinical characteristics of bronchiolitis obliterans organizing pneumonia syndrome after radiation therapy for breast cancer. *Sarcoidosis Vasc Diffuse Lung Dis* 2004;21:212–218.

109. Ferguson GT, Irvin CG, Cherniak RM. Effect of corticosteroids on respiratory muscle histopathology. *Am Rev Respir Dis* 1990;142:1047–1052.

110. Creutzberg E, Wouters E, Mostert R, et al. A role for anabolic steroids in the rehabilitation of patients with COPD? *Chest* 2003;124:1733–1742.

111. Sin D, McAlister F, Man SFP, et al. Contemporary management of chronic obstructive pulmonary disease. *JAMA* 2003;290:2301–2312.

112. Congleton J, Muers MF. The incidence of airflow obstruction in bronchial carcinoma, its relation to breathlessness, and response to bronchodilator therapy. *Respir Med* 1995;89:291–296.

113. Mahler DA, Matthay RA, Snyuder PE, et al. Sustained-release theophylline reduced dyspnea in nonreversible obstructive airway disease. *Am Rev Respir Dis* 1985;131:22–25.

114. Aubier M, De Troyer A, Sampson M, et al. Aminophylline improves diaphragmatic contractility. *N Engl J Med* 1981;305:249–254.

115. Wittmann TA, Kelsen SG. The effect of caffeine on diaphragmatic muscle force in normal hamsters. *Am Rev Respir Dis* 1982;126:499–504.

116. Murciano D, Aubier M, Lecocguic Y, et al. Effects of theophylline on diaphragmatic strength and fatigue in patients with chronic obstructive pulmonary disease. *N Engl J Med* 1984;311:349–353.

117. Bianco S, Vaghi A, Robuschi M, et al. Prevention of exercise-induced bronchoconstriction by inhaled furosemide. *Lancet* 1988;2:252–255.

118. Pendino JC, Nannini LJ, Chapman KR, et al. Effect of inhaled furosemide in acute asthma. *J Asthma* 1998;35:89–93.

119. Tanigaki T, Kondo T, Hayashi Y, et al. Rapid response to inhaled furosemide in severe acute asthma with hypercapnia. *Respiration* 1997;64:108–110.

120. Stone P, Kurowska A, Tookman A. Nebulized furosemide for dyspnoea [Letter]. *Palliat Med* 1994;8:258.

121. Neill PA, Stretton TB, Stark RD, et al. The effect of indomethacin on breathlessness in patients with diffuse parenchymal disease of the lung. *Br J Dis Chest* 1986;80:72–79.

122. Al-Damluji S. The effect of ventilatory stimulation with medroxyprogesterone on exercise performance and the sensation of dyspnoea in hypercapnic chronic bronchitis. *Br J Dis Chest* 1986;80:273–279.

123. Hernandez MT, Rubio TM, Ruiz FO, et al. Results of a home-based training program for patients with COPD. *Chest* 2000;118:106–114.

124. Berry MJ, Rejeski WJ, Adair NE, et al. Exercise rehabilitation and chronic obstructive pulmonary disease stage. *Am J Respir Crit Care Med* 1999;160:1248–1253.

125. Ramirez-Venegas A, Ward JL, Olmstead EM, et al. Effect of exercise training on dyspnea measures in patients with chronic obstructive pulmonary disease. *J Cardiopulm Rehabil* 1997;17:103–109.

126. Casaburi R. Skeletal muscle function in COPD. *Chest* 2000;117:267S–271S.

127. Lacasse Y, Wrong E, Guyatt GH, et al. Meta-analysis of respiratory rehabilitation in chronic obstructive pulmonary disease. *Lancet* 1996;348:1115–1119.

128. Salman GH, Mosier MC, Beasley BW, et al. Rehabilitation for patients with chronic obstructive pulmonary disease, meta-analysis of randomized controlled trials. *J Gen Intern Med* 2003;18(3):213–222.

129. Opdekamp C, Sergysels R. Respiratory physiotherapy in lung diseases. *Rev Med Brux* 2003;24:231–235.

130. Petrof BJ, Kimoff RJ, Levy RD, et al. Nasal continuous positive airway pressure facilitates respiratory muscle function during sleep in severe chronic obstructive pulmonary disease. *Am Rev Respir Dis* 1991;143:928–935.

131. Granton JT, Naughton MT, Benard DC, et al. CPAP improves inspiratory muscle strength in patients with heart failure and central sleep apnea. *Am J Respir Crit Care Med* 1996;153:277–282.

132. Meert AP, Berghmans T, Hardy M, et al. Non-invasive ventilation for cancer patients with life-support techniques limitation. *Support Care Cancer* 2006;14(2):167–171.

133. Pochard F, Lanore JJ, Bellivire F, et al. Subjective psychological status of severely ill patients discharged from mechanical ventilation. *Clin Intensive Care* 1995;6:57–61.

134. Hill AT, Hopkinson RB, Stableforth DE. Ventilation in a Birmingham intensive care unit 1993–1995: outcome for patients with chronic obstructive pulmonary disease. *Respir Med* 1999;92:156–161.

135. Brochard L, Mancebo J, Wysocki M, et al. Noninvasive ventilation for acute exacerbations of chronic pulmonary disease. *N Engl J Med* 1995;333:817–822.

136. Plant PK, Owen JL, Elliott MW. Early use of noninvasive ventilation for acute exacerbations of chronic obstructive pulmonary disease on general respiratory wards: a multicentre randomized controlled trial. *Lancet* 2000;355:1931–1935.

137. Nava S, Ambrosino N, Clini E, et al. Non-invasive mechanical ventilation in the weaning of patients with respiratory failure due to chronic obstructive pulmonary disease. A randomized controlled trial. *Ann Intern Med* 1998;128:721–728.

CHAPTER 26 ■ HEMOPTYSIS

RANDOLPH J. LIPCHIK

Hemoptysis, the coughing or expectoration of blood that originates in the lung, can be an alarming symptom for both patient and physician. It can range from blood-tinged or streaked sputum to *massive hemoptysis*, the latter defined as blood loss of 400–600 mL per day. Massive hemoptysis occurs in fewer than 5% of cases but carries a mortality rate of up to 85% if surgical intervention is not feasible (1,2). The management of hemoptysis, therefore, requires careful consideration of the cause, severity of the process, and functional status of the patient. Management may be more aggressive and invasive early in the course of a malignancy, whereas this could be inappropriate or dangerous for a patient in the terminal stages of an illness.

PATHOGENESIS

The lung is perfused by two distinct circulations that must be considered when determining the source and planned treatment of hemoptysis. The pulmonary circulation delivers blood under low pressure from the right ventricle to the alveolar capillaries for exchange of oxygen and carbon dioxide. The bronchial circulation, which is approximately 1–2% of the cardiac output, arises from the systemic circulation and provides nutrient flow to the lung parenchyma. A detailed review of the anatomy and physiology of the bronchial circulation has been published (3) and is beyond the scope of this chapter. In brief, two or more arteries arise from the aorta or upper intercostal arteries, enter the lung, and eventually form a plexus, which accompanies the branching airways with small, penetrating arteries, forming another plexus that supplies the bronchial mucosa down to the terminal bronchioles. Farther on, they anastomose with both precapillary pulmonary arterioles and pulmonary veins. Bronchial venous return is more complex: Veins from the proximal airways return blood to the right atrium through the azygous, homozygous, or intercostal veins, whereas the intrapulmonary bronchial venous blood returns through the pulmonary veins to the left ventricle. The latter occurs because of anastomoses between bronchial and pulmonary veins and carries the bulk of bronchial venous return. Although the bronchial circulation is nonessential in the normal adult lung, in the setting of chronic inflammation, neoplasm, or repair after lung injury, bronchial blood flow increases because of increases in both the size and number of vessels. Elevations of pulmonary vascular pressure can affect the bronchial circulation because of the many anastomoses between the dual circulations. In general, hemoptysis occurs because of disruption of the high-pressure bronchial vessels, which become abnormally enlarged and exposed within diseased airways.

ETIOLOGY

This discussion concentrates on the malignant causes of hemoptysis, but awareness of other causes is important because many patients have underlying conditions that may become active problems during treatment of a malignant disease. The differential diagnosis for a patient presenting with hemoptysis is extensive (Table 26.1). Some conditions that are more likely to be associated with massive hemoptysis are shown in Table 26.2. In past years, tuberculosis, bronchiectasis, and lung abscess were the most common causes of massive hemoptysis. The incidence of the latter two has declined in industrialized nations, but tuberculosis remains a significant problem worldwide. Experience with tuberculosis has helped us to understand the pathophysiology of massive hemoptysis. Up to 7% of deaths from tuberculosis have been attributed to massive hemoptysis; autopsy examinations have revealed ruptured pulmonary artery aneurysms. Rasmussen has described localized ruptures of aneurysmal portions of pulmonary arteries passing through thick-walled cavities of chronic tuberculosis, the so-called "Rasmussen's aneurysms." Rupture occurs secondary to the infection or the associated inflammatory response (4). Healed calcified mediastinal lymph nodes from prior tuberculosis can erode into the bronchial mucosa, also causing significant bleeding. Tuberculosis distorts lung architecture, causing bronchiectasis with resulting hypertrophy and proliferation of bronchial vessels. Infection or inflammation in these diseased portions of the airway can cause rupture of vessels; the result is massive bleeding caused by the high systemic arterial pressure.

Nonmalignant Conditions

Patients with preexisting cavitary lung disease resulting from mycobacterial infections, sarcoidosis, bullous emphysema, lung abscess, lung infarction, and fibrocavitary disease secondary to rheumatoid disease are at risk for mycetoma formation, most often due to *Aspergillus*. This noninvasive infection results in a thick-walled cavity with vascular granulation tissue and inflammatory cells, the former the result of proliferation of the bronchial circulation. Bleeding is a result of vascular injury from fungal endotoxin, proteolytic activity, or a type 3 hypersensitivity reaction (5). Bacterial superinfection also can promote hemoptysis in the setting.

Deep venous thrombosis and the subsequent thromboembolic disease are common in hospitalized patients, especially those with underlying risk factors. The presence of a malignancy is a major risk factor, and the onset of hemoptysis

TABLE 26.1

CAUSES OF HEMOPTYSIS

Pulmonary	Vascular
Bronchitis	Pulmonary hypertension
Bronchiectasis	Arteriovenous malformation
Pulmonary embolism	Aortic aneurysm
Cystic fibrosis	Traumatic
Infectious	Blunt/penetrating chest injury
Lung abscess	Ruptured bronchus
Mycetoma	Systemic disease
Necrotizing pneumonia	Goodpasture's syndrome
Viral	Vasculitis
Fungal	Systemic lupus erythematosus
Parasitic	Drugs/toxins
Septic embolism	Aspirin
Cardiac	Anticoagulation
Mitral stenosis	Penicillamine
Congestive heart failure	Solvents
Neoplastic	Crack cocaine
Bronchogenic carcinoma	Miscellaneous
Bronchial adenoma	Foreign body
Endobronchial hamartoma	Endometriosis
Metastatic disease	Broncholithiasis
Tracheal tumors	Cryptogenic hemoptysis
Hematologic	Iatrogenic
Coagulopathy	Lung biopsy
Platelet dysfunction	Pulmonary artery catheterization
Thrombocytopenia	Lymphangiography
Disseminated intravascular coagulation	Transtracheal aspirate

Modified from Cahill BC, Ingbar DH. Massive hemoptysis: assessment and management. *Clin Chest Med* 1994;15:147. with permission.

warrants consideration of the possibility of pulmonary embolism and subsequent infarction. With current standard anticoagulation therapy, pulmonary embolism is a treatable condition with a 2.5% mortality rate. In a prospective study of the clinical course of pulmonary embolism, almost 24% of patients died within 1 year of diagnosis. Many cases, approximately 35%, had some form of cancer (6). A less-well-appreciated and studied source of pulmonary embolism is upper extremity thrombosis resulting from indwelling venous catheters. In some series, the incidence of central line thromboembolism has been as high as 12% (7). Although most commonly seen in the pediatric population, there have been reports of inhaled foreign bodies in adults that, if unrecognized, have caused hemoptysis (8).

TABLE 26.2

CAUSES OF MASSIVE HEMOPTYSIS

Pulmonary tuberculosis
Bronchiectasis
Lung abscess
Mycetoma
Bronchogenic carcinoma
Pulmonary carcinoid
Pulmonary arteriovenous fistula
Pulmonary vasculitis
Broncholithiasis

Malignant Conditions

In a retrospective review of 877 cases of lung cancer, Miller and McGregor reported a 19.3% overall incidence of hemoptysis, with non-life-threatening hemoptysis occurring equally among histologic types (9). Twenty-nine cases (3.3%) were massive and terminal events, due almost exclusively to proximal, cavitary squamous cell carcinomas. In only 6 of these 29 cases was there no antecedent nonlethal bleeding. The cause of this sudden catastrophic bleeding was tumor hemorrhage or invasion of a pulmonary artery or vein. In another series, Panos et al. (10) also found an association between cavitary squamous cell tumors and fatal hemoptysis. Metastatic endobronchial disease (carcinoma of breast, colon, kidney, and melanoma) is more likely to cause nonfatal hemoptysis rather than a terminal bleeding event. The incidence of hemoptysis in patients with bronchial carcinoid tumors approaches 50%, resulting from mucosal ulceration or airway inflammation disrupting the bronchial arteries supplying these tumors. The high incidence of symptomatic bleeding is not surprising, as 85% of carcinoids arise in the proximal airway and are often very vascular (11). Malignant tracheal tumors are uncommon; when present, they usually result in obstructive symptoms. Hemoptysis does occur from these tumors, but less frequently than with bronchogenic carcinoma (12). A Danish series of pulmonary hamartoma cases found that only 39% of patients were symptomatic but nearly one fourth of those patients noted hemoptysis (13).

Patients with a hematologic malignancy may develop hemoptysis for many reasons, including thrombocytopenia, coagulation abnormalities, and infections. In one series, fatal hemoptysis was associated strongly with the autopsy findings of vascular invasion, thrombosis, and hemorrhagic infarction secondary to invasive fungal disease (14). Idiopathic alveolar hemorrhage is a rare cause of fatal hemoptysis, accounting for only 2–3% of leukemia deaths, but it also is associated with nonfatal hemoptysis. This is hypothesized to be attributable to the combination of thrombocytopenia and diffuse alveolar damage, the latter a result of chemotherapy, radiotherapy, sepsis, viral infection, or a combination of any of these (14).

Thromboembolic disease already has been discussed in this chapter, but pulmonary embolic disease may also be caused by intravascular tumor metastases, resulting in a clinical presentation indistinguishable from the more common venous thromboembolism. Hemoptysis is unusual, and symptoms of dyspnea and right heart failure predominate. Rarely, massive tumor embolism results in pulmonary infarction with hemoptysis. Pulmonary infarction due to malignant compression of pulmonary veins also has been reported (15).

DIAGNOSIS

The key element of diagnosis in cases of hemoptysis is the localization of bleeding to the lower respiratory tract. Although blood from the stomach usually has a low pH and blood from the respiratory tract a high pH, bleeding from the nasopharynx, larynx, or gastrointestinal tract may be difficult to distinguish clinically from true hemoptysis. Furthermore, bleeding from these sources may result in cough and the appearance of blood, which can be misinterpreted as hemoptysis. When there is doubt, a thorough examination of the nasopharynx, larynx, and upper gastrointestinal tract should be performed.

Once the lung has been identified as the source of bleeding, the next step is to localize the site of bleeding. Physical examination alone is not sensitive enough; a chest x-ray should be performed, and is often helpful in revealing a tumor or abscess. However, it can be misleading, as blood may be coughed into uninvolved portions of the lungs. Bronchoscopy is the surest way to visualize the source (or at least the segment) from which there is active bleeding. Flexible fiberoptic bronchoscopy is usually attempted first because it can be done relatively quickly at the bedside without general anesthesia, and can access more distal airways than the rigid bronchoscope. The latter has the advantages of greater suction capability, removal of clots or foreign bodies, and airway control that allows for patient ventilation, often necessary in cases of massive hemoptysis. Computed tomography (CT) scan has been compared with bronchoscopy in studies in which hemoptysis is the presenting problem. Patients with preexisting cancer constituted a small proportion of those studied. The CT scan is superior in identifying bronchiectasis, lung abscess, aspergilloma, and distal parenchymal abnormalities; however, the bronchoscope can obtain material that allows cytologic, histologic, and microbiologic diagnoses (16,17). In a recent study, it was suggested that CT may be the more efficient diagnostic tool (18). In patients with established malignancies, a CT scan may offer important information, as it can delineate peribronchial or mediastinal involvement of tumors that cannot be seen with a bronchoscope. Routine use of CT scan is not of proven benefit but should be considered in cases in which the chest radiographic findings are inconclusive, or to provide a more detailed anatomic localization of an abnormality for the bronchoscopist.

MANAGEMENT

The severity of hemoptysis determines the pace at which a workup should proceed. In a review of 10 years' experience at Duke University Medical Center, the mortality rate was 9% and 58% if blood loss was less than or more than 1000 mL per 24-hour period, respectively (1). A malignant cause for hemoptysis of greater than 1000 mL per 24 hours increased the mortality rate to 80%. Massive hemoptysis requires rapid intervention to guarantee that the patient has an adequate airway while attempting to control bleeding. If blood loss is minimal and sporadic, a more detailed evaluation can occur without immediate attention to resuscitative efforts. Early consultation with a pulmonary physician and thoracic surgeon is recommended.

Initial diagnostic studies should include chest radiograph, hematocrit, platelet count, blood urea nitrogen, serum creatinine, and coagulation panel. Oxygenation should be monitored by arterial blood gas determination or pulse oximetry, and adequate intravenous access established. Typed and cross-matched blood should be available in cases of significant bleeding. Mild sedation and judicious use of a cough suppressant can be employed, but excessive use compromises a patient's ability to clear the airway.

If oxygenation is compromised or the patient continues to bleed vigorously, elective intubation should be considered. The endotracheal tube should be large enough (7.5 or 8.0 mm) to allow passage of a bronchoscope. If it is known from which side the patient is bleeding, the patient should be placed in a lateral decubitus position with the bleeding side down to help minimize aspiration of blood into the good lung. Placement of a double-lumen endotracheal tube is sometimes necessary to allow separate ventilation of each lung while preventing aspiration of blood throughout the bronchial tree. The two small lumens preclude bronchoscopy with anything but a pediatric bronchoscope, and suctioning is limited because only small-caliber catheters can be passed distally. Newer-generation tubes with larger internal diameters may be less troublesome (19). The decision to intubate a patient with a terminal illness may be difficult. If bleeding can be localized and controlled quickly, a short period of intubation may not be unreasonable if it allows for improved quality of life. This would be unlikely for a patient in the later stages of a terminal illness, especially in the setting of massive hemoptysis. A number of treatment options are listed in Table 26.3 and discussed in the subsequent text. In the setting of fatal hemoptysis, exsanguination usually occurs within seconds with rapid loss of consciousness so that the patient is often unaware. If necessary, morphine or lorazepam can be used to overcome feelings of dyspnea and anxiety. The rapidity and amount of blood loss will however be disturbing for family members. Use of continuous oral suction and judicious placement of towels or blankets may help obscure the blood loss, but this is not a peaceful and clean way to die.

TABLE 26.3

MALIGNANCY-INDUCED HEMOPTYSIS TREATMENT OPTIONS

External beam radiotherapy
Brachytherapy
Bronchial artery embolization
Bronchoscopy
    Nd:YAG laser photocoagulation
    Electrocautery
    Argon plasma coagulation
    Cryotherapy
    Photodynamic therapy

Bronchoscopy

If bronchoscopy identifies the site of bleeding, several maneuvers can be done to stop or slow the bleeding. Bronchial lavage with iced saline (20), application of topical epinephrine (1:20,000), and topical thrombin and fibrinogen-thrombin solutions (21) all have been reported in small series to have varied success; however, they have not been evaluated in large numbers of patients in controlled studies. A pulmonary tamponade balloon can be inflated in the segmental bronchus leading to the site of bleeding, allowing time for stabilization of the patient and consideration of more definitive therapy (22). Bleeding from visible lesions in the trachea and proximal bronchi can be coagulated with a laser. This is particularly useful when the hemoptysis arises from an obstructing tumor, as both problems can be addressed simultaneously. In a series of 43 patients with advanced bronchogenic carcinoma (16 with concomitant hemoptysis), 38 were treated successfully (23). One patient died of continued tumor bleeding and aspiration of blood and two required tracheotomy to facilitate management of secretions. There was one pneumothorax, and one transient bronchial obstruction by a tumor fragment mobilized by laser therapy.

Radiotherapy

External beam radiation for 6–7 weeks is usually employed to attempt a cure for inoperable non–small cell carcinoma. In the palliative setting, therapy is delivered in the shortest time possible, with lower doses to achieve symptom relief while minimizing side effects: 8 Gy in 1 fraction, 20 Gy in 5 fractions, and 30 Gy in 10 fractions have all been used with success. Hemoptysis can be stopped in more than 80% of cases by using palliative radiotherapy (24), resulting in improvement in the quality of life (25). Although significant symptoms from radiation fibrosis are uncommon, there are reports of massive hemoptysis occurring long after, and attributed to, external beam radiotherapy (26). Such cases are rare, however,

probably because most patients succumb to their underlying cancer before significant vascular abnormalities develop. More recently, a Dutch group reported their experience with patients who had already received standard curative dose radiotherapy. Patients were re-treated using hypofractionated external beam radiotherapy (27). There were 28 patients in the series, 13 with hemoptysis. Hemoptysis ceased or was greatly diminished in all 13. In the whole group there were five cases of tumor-related fatal hemoptysis (17%) and one death attributed to a broncho-esophageal fistula (4%).

Endobronchial brachytherapy with Ir^{192} is another alternative. A detailed summary of the evolution of this modality is available for review (28). In recent years, high dose rates have been favored to decrease the time of treatment and permit outpatient rather than inpatient therapy (see Table 26.4). Gollins et al. (37) reported results in 406 patients. Of the 255 patients with hemoptysis, brachytherapy arrested the bleeding in 89% at 1.5 months, 84% at 4 months, and 77% at 12 months after the first treatment. The results were not as favorable for patients who received brachytherapy after failure of external beam radiation; 84%, 56%, and 25% of patients had resolution of hemoptysis 1.5, 4, and 12 months after brachytherapy, respectively. Although most patients died of their cancer during the study (mean survival was 173 days), control of hemoptysis was quite good. Massive hemoptysis as a terminal event occurred in 32 patients (8%). Potential complications of brachytherapy include mucositis, fistula formation, and fatal hemoptysis (43). The last event has a reported incidence of 1.4–30%. Recent studies have attempted to identify risk factors for brachytherapy-associated hemoptysis. Hennequin et al. (40) documented a 7.4% rate of hemoptysis in a series of 149 patients. Multivariate analysis indicated that tumor length and upper lobe location were risk factors for hemoptysis. In this series, 10 of 11 cases of hemoptysis were fatal; and all but one occurred in patients with progressive disease. Other studies have implicated high–dose rate brachytherapy (≥15 Gy) as a risk factor for fatal hemoptysis, particularly in patients who have already received external beam radiation (39,40). The risk of hemoptysis also appears to be related to direct contact of the applicator and the bronchial wall adjacent to

TABLE 26.4

HIGH–DOSE RATE ENDOBRONCHIAL BRACHYTHERAPY

Study	Year	Number of patients	Palliation[a] (%)	Severe complications[b] (%)
Seagren et al. (29)	1985	20	100	0
Macha et al. (30)	1987	56	74	0
Speiser (31)	1991	342	80	7
Bedwinek et al. (32)	1992	38	76	32
Sutedja et al. (33)	1992	31	71	42
Nori et al. (34)	1993	32	91	0
Pisch et al. (35)	1993	39	93	3
Zajac et al. (36)	1993	82	74	2
Gollins et al. (37)	1994	255	89	8
Chang et al. (38)	1994	76	87	4
Langendijk et al. (39)	1998	938	ND	48
Hennequin et. al. (40)	1998	149	ND	7.4
Hatlevoll et. al. (41)	1999	45	64	27
Escobar-Sacristan et. al. (42)	2004	81	85	1.2

ND, not described.
[a]Palliation, relief of cough, dyspnea, hemoptysis, or radiographic/bronchoscopic improvement.
[b]Severe complications, massive hemoptysis or fistula formation.
Modified from Villanueva AG, Lo TCM, Beamis JF. Endobronchial brachytherapy. *Clin Chest Med* 1995;16:445. with permission.

large vessels (44). With the introduction of spacing devices, direct contact with the mucosa can be avoided. Whether this significantly decreases the risk of bleeding remains to be seen. Brachytherapy has also been combined with bronchoscopic laser therapy in some centers (45,46). The Mayo Clinic reported results from 65 patients, 40 of whom had received prior laser therapy. In 24 patients with hemoptysis, bleeding resolved in 19. Response was poorer in patients who had received laser therapy, most likely because of more advanced disease (46). One comparison of brachytherapy and external beam radiotherapy for palliative treatment of non–small cell lung cancer has been published (47). Both methods were effective for the treatment of hemoptysis. Physician assessments at 4 weeks and 8 weeks found positive response rates of 90 versus 85% and 89 versus 78%, respectively, favoring external beam radiotherapy. Interestingly, patient assessment at 8 weeks favored external beam therapy to a greater degree (90 vs. 71%).

Bronchial Artery Embolization

Bronchial artery anatomy is quite variable but generally arises from the ventral surface of the descending aorta or as branches from the intercostal arteries at the level of T5 and T6. Intimate knowledge of this vascular anatomy is essential because the anterior spinal artery often arises from the bronchial arteries and inadvertent embolization could result in spinal cord infarction. Bronchiectasis, tuberculosis, and aspergilloma frequently result in hypertrophy of bronchial vessels, but there are often transpleural collaterals from other systemic vessels, such as the subclavian, internal mammary, or intercostal arteries, which must be identified. After angiographic identification of the vessels in question, a variety of agents (e.g., Gelfoam, polyvinyl alcohol particles, and metallic coils) can be injected selectively to stop blood flow. Initial success rates reported in the literature vary between 75% and 90%, with a re-bleeding rate of 15–30%. Hayakawa et al. (48) reported immediate (within 1 month) and long-term results for 63 patients. Of the 12 patients with hemoptysis due to neoplasm, bleeding was controlled in seven (58%). Long-term control was documented for four of these seven patients, with a median hemoptysis control period of 6 months (range, 0–9 months). All but one of the patients died within the 9-month follow-up period. Patients with bronchiectasis, inflammation, or idiopathic causes had immediate control in 94% of cases, with the median period of control lasting 15 months (range, 1–132 months) and a mortality rate of 11%. Recurrent bleeding can be treated with repeat embolization. Two recent series confirm the finding that the success rate for controlling hemoptysis of bronchial artery embolization is significantly less, and of shorter duration, in cases of lung cancer compared to nonmalignant conditions (49,50). Witt et al (51), in a small series, suggested that survival may be improved with bronchial artery embolization for malignancy-induced hemoptysis; however, this was based on a retrospective control group.

Other Modalities

There are reports of a number of other modalities that can be used to manage hemoptysis, such as Nd:YAG laser photocoagulation, electrocautery, cryotherapy, argon plasma coagulation (APC), and photodynamic therapy. Each has its advantages and disadvantages. Nd:YAG photocoagulation is effective but it requires expensive equipment, specialized training, and has the potential to cause thermal injury beyond the site of interest. It is generally used with a rigid bronchoscope. Electrocautery uses alternating current to coagulate and vaporize tissue.

Equipment is cheaper and can be used with a flexible fiberoptic bronchoscope. APC utilizes a catheter, which introduces high-frequency current to tissue without the need for direct contact. This too can be used with a fiberoptic bronchoscope. Cryotherapy probes use nitrous oxide or liquid nitrogen to freeze tissue. The repeated freeze–thaw cycle kills tissue. This is not a difficult technique but may require repeat bronchoscopy to complete the therapy as well as to remove dead tissue. Photodynamic therapy utilizes hematoporphyrins, which are taken up by tumor cells. This is given orally several days before bronchoscopic administration of light at particular wavelengths, which result in cell death. Treatment time therefore takes a number of days. In addition, the patient must avoid sun exposure, which may cause potential skin and ocular damage. Successful use of these modalities is largely anecdotal. They are discussed in more detail in a recently published review (52).

Surgery

The definitive therapy for massive hemoptysis is resection of the diseased portion of the lung; however, this is often precluded by the severity of the underlying lung disease. Similarly, massive hemoptysis from a bronchogenic carcinoma usually results from proximal endobronchial tumor, which is typically not amenable to surgical resection. Therefore, surgery is not an option for most palliative care patients.

CONCLUSION

Hemoptysis, in the setting of malignancy, can be a relatively minor problem or immediately life threatening. There are a number of diagnostic and therapeutic options that can be employed, but this depends on a given patient's clinical status and wishes for further intervention. Early consultation with pulmonary and/or thoracic surgery colleagues may be helpful in optimizing patient care.

References

1. Corey R, Hla KM. Major and massive hemoptysis: reassessment of conservative management. *Am J Med Sci* 1987;294:301–309.
2. Thompson AB, Teschler H, Rennard SI. Pathogenesis, evaluation, and therapy for massive hemoptysis. *Clin Chest Med* 1992;13:69 82.
3. Deffebach ME, Charan NB, Lakshminarayan S, et al. The bronchial circulation: small, but a vital attribute of the lung. *Am Rev Respir Dis* 1987;135:463–481.
4. Auerbach O. Pathology and pathogenesis of pulmonary arterial aneurysm in tuberculous cavities. *Am Rev Tuberc* 1939;39:99.
5. Awe RJ, Greenberg SD, Mattox KL. The source of bleeding in pulmonary aspergillomas. *Tex Med* 1984;80:58–61.
6. Carson JL, Kelley MA, Duff A, et al. The clinical course of pulmonary embolism. *N Engl J Med* 1992;326:1240–1245.
7. Horattas MC, Wright DJ, Fenton AH, et al. Changing concepts of deep venous thrombosis of the upper extremity: report of a series and review of the literature. *Surgery* 1988;104:561–567.
8. Kane GC, Sloane PJ, McComb B, et al. "Missed" inhaled foreign body in an adult. *Respir Med* 1994;88:551–554.
9. Miller RR, McGregor DH. Hemorrhage from carcinoma of the lung. *Cancer* 1980;46:200–205.
10. Panos RJ, Barr LF, Walsh TJ, et al. Factors associated with fatal hemoptysis in cancer patients. *Chest* 1988;94:1008–1013.
11. Davila DG, Dunn WF, Tazelaar HD, et al. Bronchial carcinoid tumors. *Mayo Clin Proc* 1993;68:795–803.
12. Allen MS. Malignant tracheal tumors. *Mayo Clin Proc* 1993;68:680–684.
13. Hansen CP, Holtveg H, Francis D, et al. Pulmonary hamartoma. *J Thorac Cardiovasc Surg* 1992;104:674–678.
14. Smith LJ, Katzenstein AA. Pathogenesis of massive pulmonary hemorrhage in acute leukemia. *Arch Intern Med* 1982;142:2149–2152.
15. Williamson WA, Tronic BS, Levitan N, et al. Pulmonary venous infarction secondary to squamous cell carcinoma. *Chest* 1992;102:950–952.
16. Set PA, Flower CDR, Smith IE, et al. Hemoptysis: comparative study of the role of CT and fiberoptic bronchoscopy. *Radiology* 1993;189:677–680.

17. McGuinness G, Beacher JR, Harkin TJ, et al. Hemoptysis: prospective high-resolution CT/bronchoscopic correlation. *Chest* 1994;105:1155–1162.

18. Revel MP, Fournier LS, Hennebicque AS, et al. Can CT replace bronchoscopy in the detection of the site and cause of bleeding in patients with large or massive hemoptysis. *AJR Am J Roentgenol* 2002;179:1217–1224.

19. Shivaram U, Finch P, Nowak P. Plastic endobronchial tubes in the management of life-threatening hemoptysis. *Chest* 1987;92:1108–1110.

20. Conlan AA, Hurwitz SS, Krige L, et al. Massive hemoptysis: review of 123 cases. *J Thorac Cardiovasc Surg* 1983;85:120–124.

21. Tsukamoto T, Sasaki H, Nakamura H, et al. Treatment of hemoptysis patients by thrombin and fibrinogen-thrombin infusion therapy using a fiberoptic bronchoscope. *Chest* 1989;96:473–476.

22. Saw EC, Gottlieb LS, Yokayama T, et al. Flexible fiberoptic bronchoscopy and endobronchial tamponade in the management of massive hemoptysis. *Chest* 1976;70:589–591.

23. Wolfe WG, Sabiston DC. Management of benign and malignant lesions of the trachea and bronchi with the neodymium-yttrium-aluminum-garnet laser. *J Thorac Cardiovasc Surg* 1986;91:40–45.

24. Awan AM, Weichselbaum RR. Palliative radiotherapy. *Hematol Oncol Clin North Am* 1990;4:1169–1181.

25. Langenduk JA, ten Velde GPM, Aaronson NK, et al. Quality of life after palliative radiotherapy in non-small cell lung cancer: a prospective study. *Int J Radiat Oncol Biol Phys* 2000;47:149–155.

26. Makker HK, Barnes PC. Fatal hemoptysis from the pulmonary artery as a late complication of pulmonary irradiation. *Thorax* 1991;46:609–610.

27. Kramer GW, Gans S, Ullmann E, et al. Hypofractionated external beam radiotherapy as retreatment for symptomatic non-small cell lung cancer: an effective treatment? *Int J Radiat Oncol Biol Phys* 2004;58:1388–1393.

28. Villanueva AG, Lo TCM, Beamis JF. Endobronchial brachytherapy. *Clin Chest Med* 1995;16:445–454.

29. Seagren SL, Harrell JH, Horn RA. High dose rate intraluminal irradiation in recurrent endobronchial carcinoma. *Chest* 1985;88:810–814.

30. Macha HN, Koch K, Stadler M, et al. New technique for treating occlusive and stenosing tumors of the trachea and main bronchi: endobronchial irradiation by high dose iridium-192 combined with laser canalization. *Thorax* 1987;42:511–515.

31. Speiser B. Advantages of high dose rate remote afterloading systems: physics or biology. *Int J Radiat Oncol Biol Phys* 1991;20:1133–1135.

32. Bedwinek J, Petty A, Bruton C, et al. The use of high dose rate endobronchial brachytherapy to palliate symptomatic endobronchial recurrence of previously irradiated bronchogenic carcinoma. *Int J Radiat Oncol Biol Phys* 1992;22:23–30.

33. Sutedja G, Baris G, Schaake-Koning C, et al. High dose rates brachytherapy in patients with local recurrences after radiotherapy of non-small cell lung cancer. *Int J Radiat Oncol Biol Phys* 1992;24:551–553.

34. Nori D, Allison R, Kaplan B, et al. High dose-rate intraluminal irradiation in bronchogenic carcinoma: techniques and results. *Chest* 1993;104:1006–1011.

35. Pisch J, Villamena PC, Harvey JC, et al. High dose-rate endobronchial irradiation in malignant airway obstruction. *Chest* 1993;104:721–725.

36. Zajac AJ, Kohn ML, Heiser D, et al. High-dose-rate intraluminal brachytherapy in the treatment of endobronchial malignancy. *Radiology* 1993;187:571–575.

37. Gollins SW, Burt PA, Barber PV, et al. High dose rate intraluminal radiotherapy for carcinoma of the bronchus: outcome of treatment of 406 patients. *Radiother Oncol* 1994;33:31–40.

38. Chang LF, Horvath J, Peyton W, et al. High dose rate afterloading intraluminal brachytherapy in malignant airway obstruction of lung cancer. *Int J Radiat Oncol Biol Phys* 1994;28:589–596.

39. Langendijk JA, Tjwa MKT, de Jong JMA, et al. Massive hemoptysis after radiotherapy in inoperable non-small cell lung carcinoma: is endobronchial brachytherapy really a risk factor? *Radiother Oncol* 1998;49:175–183.

40. Hennequin C, Tredaniel J, Chevret S, et al. Predictive factors for late toxicity after endobronchial brachytherapy: a multivariate analysis. *Int J Radiat Oncol Biol Phys* 1998;42:21–22.

41. Hatlevoll R, Karlsen KO, Skovlund E. Endobronchial radiotherapy for malignant bronchial obstruction or recurrence. *Acta Oncol* 1999;38:999–1004.

42. Escobar-Sacristan JA, Grande-Orive JI, Jimenez TG, et al. Endobronchial brachytherapy in the treatment of malignant lung tumors. *Eur Respir J* 2004;24:348–352.

43. Khanavkar B, Stern P, Alberti W, et al. Complications associated with brachytherapy alone or with laser in lung cancer. *Chest* 1991;99:1062–1065.

44. Hara R, Itami J, Aruga T, et al. Risk factors for massive hemoptysis after endobronchial brachytherapy in patients with tracheobronchial malignancies. *Cancer* 2001;92:2623–2627.

45. Lang N, Maners A, Broadwater J, et al. Management of airway problems in lung cancer patients using the neodymium-yttrium-aluminum-garnet (Nd-YAG) laser and endobronchial radiotherapy. *Am J Surg* 1988;156:463–465.

46. Schray MF, McDougall JC, Martinez A, et al. Management of malignant airway compromise with laser and low dose brachytherapy: the Mayo Clinic experience. *Chest* 1988;93:264–269.

47. Stout R, Barber P, Burt P, et al. Clinical and quality of life outcomes in the first United Kingdom randomized trial of endobronchial brachytherapy (intraluminal radiotherapy) vs. external beam radiotherapy in the palliative treatment of inoperable non-small cell lung cancer. *Radiother Oncol* 2000;56:323–327.

48. Hayakawa K, Tanaka F, Torizuka T, et al. Bronchial artery embolization for hemoptysis: immediate and long-term results. *Cardiovasc Intervent Radiol* 1992;15:154–158.

49. Swanson KL, Johnson CM, Prakash UBS, et al. Bronchial artery embolization- experience with 54 patients. *Chest* 2002;121:785–795.

50. Goh PY, Lin M, Teo N, et al. Embolization for hemoptysis: a six year review. *Cardiovasc Intervent Radiol* 2002;25:17–25.

51. Witt C, Schmidt B, Geisler A, et al. Value of bronchial artery embolization with platinum coils in tumorous pulmonary bleeding. *Eur J Cancer* 2000;36:1949–1954.

52. Kvale PA, Simoff M, Prakash UBS. Palliative care. *Chest* 2003;123:284s–311s.

CHAPTER 27 ■ AIRWAY OBSTRUCTION, BRONCHOSPASM, AND COUGH

JULIE A. BILLER

Disorders of the airways may produce debilitating or life-threatening symptoms in a diverse patient population. Therefore, health care providers, including generalists and those of many subspecialties, may be called on to diagnose and treat these disorders. Often, a multidisciplinary approach is needed. Airway obstruction, bronchospasm, stridor, and cough not only may produce symptoms that reduce the quality of life of the patients affected, but they can produce profound distress to the patients' families. In some situations, even our current best therapies do little to palliate symptoms. It is my hope that we shall see continued improvement in these areas. In this chapter, the diagnostic and current therapeutic approach to airway disorders are reviewed.

TRACHEOBRONCHIAL OBSTRUCTION

The tracheobronchial tree quite literally can be "between a rock and a hard place," resulting in airway obstruction. Obstruction may occur based on large exophytic endobronchial tumor causing intrinsic obstruction of the airway. On the other hand, mediastinal pathology can cause obstruction by extrinsic compression of the airways. Etiologies differ somewhat between the two modes of obstruction. *Intrinsic* obstruction is usually caused by primary malignancies arising from the airway epithelium. Two histologic types of tumors, squamous cell carcinoma and adenoid cystic carcinoma, constitute two thirds of the primary tracheal malignancies (1). The remaining third comprises a diverse group of tumors, both benign and malignant, detailed in Table 27.1. More commonly, the trachea can be a site of locally extensive disease, usually from organs in close proximity, such as the lung, larynx, thyroid, and esophagus. Intrinsic obstruction of the bronchial tree most frequently is seen in primary cancers of all histologic types. Approximately 5% of metastatic disease to the lungs is predominately endobronchial. Renal cell, colon, rectum, cervical, breast carcinomas, and malignant melanomas are the most common primary malignancies to give rise to endobronchial metastasis (2,3).

Extrinsic obstruction occurs when the airways are surrounded by firm tumor or encased by pathologically enlarged lymph nodes, usually caused by locally advanced disease arising from the lung, esophagus, and thyroid. Lymphoma, which can involve significant lymphadenopathy, is another cause of extrinsic compression. A variety of benign lesions that may imperil airway patency are listed in Table 27.1.

Evaluation

Patients with tracheobronchial obstruction usually present with complaints of dyspnea, hemoptysis, wheezing, or stridor, and sometimes with pneumonia or atelectasis. This constellation of symptoms has been described as the "tracheal syndrome" and is seen most commonly in proximal airway obstruction. Distal airway obstruction presents more commonly with obstructive pneumonitis; symptoms worsen when in the supine position (4). The onset of these obstructive symptoms can be insidious, and patients are often treated for other diseases, such as asthma or chronic obstructive pulmonary disease (COPD). Patients occasionally come to medical attention when pulmonary function tests obtained for other reasons suggest upper airway obstruction.

The evaluation of airway obstruction is primarily done through radiologic studies and bronchoscopy. Posteroanterior and lateral chest radiographs should be the first diagnostic study ordered. Grossly abnormal radiographs with a large central parenchymal mass or mediastinal mass/adenopathy causing tracheal narrowing or deviation rapidly raise concern for the patency of the airway. Unfortunately, there can be significant compromise to the airway but only subtle radiographic *changes*. Therefore, *close* attention must be paid to the tracheal air column. Often, abnormalities are more obvious on the lateral view.

Computed tomography (CT) scan of the neck and chest are extremely useful for a better definition of the airway anatomy, allowing accurate measurement of the diameter of the central airways to determine the extent of obstruction (2, 4). It is important in treatment planning to determine whether the obstruction is primarily intrinsic or extrinsic as treatment options are different. CT scan can often make this differentiation. In medically stable patients, pulmonary function testing, including spirometry and, most important, flow-volume loop, may identify upper airway obstruction quickly, inexpensively, and noninvasively. Frequently, such testing can localize whether the obstruction is extrathoracic or intrathoracic. Figure 27.1 A shows the typical flow-volume loop in a fixed airway obstruction. The most common causes of this type of lesion are tracheal stenosis, tumor (malignant or benign), goiter, fixation of vocal cords, and a large foreign body. Variable extrathoracic upper airway obstruction (Fig. 27.1B) affects primarily the inspiratory loop of the flow-volume curve. Common causes of this are bilateral vocal cord paralysis, epiglottis, vocal cord adhesions, and foreign body. Variable intrathoracic obstruction (Fig. 27.1C)

TABLE 27.1

ETIOLOGIES OF AIRWAY OBSTRUCTION

Intrinsic obstruction	Chondromas
Malignant	Hamartoma
Primary tumors	Lipoma
Tracheal	Leiomyoma
Squamous carcinoma	Granular cell myoblastoma
Adenoid cystic carcinoma	Granuloma 2 retained foreign body
Bronchogenic	Hemangiomas
Squamous	Postintubation strictures
Adenocarcinoma	Low-grade malignancy
Small cell	Carcinoid
Mixed morphology	Extrinsic obstruction
Metastatic	Malignant
Breast cancer	Lung
Melanoma	Lymphoma
Larynx	Esophageal
Esophagus	Thyroid
Renal cell	Benign
Colon	Fungal infection
Rectal	Reactive lymphadenopathy
Cervical	Bronchomalacia
Kaposi sarcoma (rarely obstructing)	Mediastinal fibrosis Vascular compression
Benign	Goiter
Papillomas	

affects primarily the expiratory loop of the flow-volume curve after the effort-dependent peak expiratory flow, which can be caused by intraluminal polypoid tumors or tracheomalacia.

To complete the evaluation of the patient with upper airway obstruction more invasive procedures may be necessary, which typically involve fiberoptic evaluation, including laryngoscopy or bronchoscopy. It may be necessary to have multiple subspecialists involved in complicated cases, including otolaryngologists, thoracic surgeons, pulmonologists, and anesthesiologists. Bronchoscopy may be performed for several reasons, principally to obtain pathologic material for diagnosis

or as a therapeutic maneuver (see the subsequent section on Therapy). This is especially important if small cell lung carcinoma is considered in the differential diagnosis as treatment differs significantly from other cell types. If there is any question about the adequacy of the airway, bronchoscopy is best performed by a thoracic surgeon in the operating room in the presence of an experienced anesthesiologist. During biopsy, the patient may have complications of airway obstruction or hemorrhage, which may endanger a marginal airway. Frequently, in this patient population, rigid bronchoscopy, with its better suction capabilities and ability to ventilate through the bronchoscope, is the procedure of choice.

Therapy

Patients who have airway obstruction because of primary malignancies of the trachea or larynx, benign strictures (such as postintubation tracheal stenosis or extrinsic compression secondary to goiter or lymphoma) should be referred to the appropriate specialist (surgeon, oncologist, or radiation oncologist) for evaluation of definitive therapy. Palliative therapeutic options (Table 27.2) for airway management in patients who are not candidates for definitive therapeutic procedures include airway stents, laser therapy, brachytherapy, photodynamic therapy (PDT), and tracheostomy. Some patients may be helped by using several of these modalities in combination.

For any palliative therapy to be attempted, the airway must be wide enough to allow passage of a rigid or flexible bronchoscope and still maintain oxygenation and ventilation. In the case of large exophytic tumors that compromise the patency of the central airways, the bronchoscopist can still usually pass a bronchoscope past the tumor. If this is not possible, a rigid bronchoscope may be used to "core out" the obstructing tumor, with its tip inserted in corkscrew fashion (1,2,5). If significant bleeding occurs, the rigid bronchoscope may be used to exert pressure and tamponade the bleeding. Ventilation can be maintained through the rigid bronchoscope, and it has a large suction channel to clear blood and tissue from the airways. Sometimes, it is necessary to pass a fiberoptic bronchoscope through the rigid bronchoscope to clear blood, secretions, or tissue fragments from the more distal airways. Some authors are strong

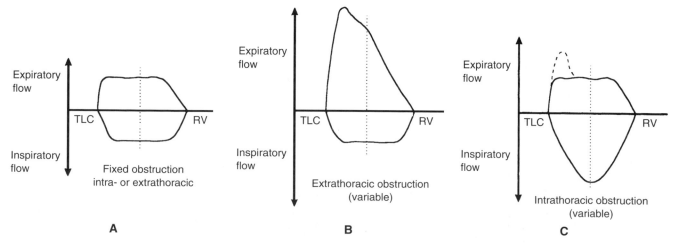

FIGURE 27.1. A: Maximal inspiratory and expiratory flow-volume curves in fixed obstruction. **B:** Extrathoracic variable obstruction. **C:** Intrathoracic variable obstruction. *Dashed line* represents a flow transient that is occasionally observed just before the plateau in intrathoracic obstruction. RV, residual volume; TLC, total lung capacity. (From Kryger M, Bode F, Antic R, et al. Diagnosis of obstruction of the upper and central airways. *Am J Med* 1976;61:85–93, with permission.)

TABLE 27.2

TREATMENT OPTIONS FOR CENTRAL OBSTRUCTING MALIGNANT AIRWAY LESIONS

Intrinsic	Extrinsic
External beam radiation	External beam radiation
Mechanical "core out"	Stent
Laser therapy	
Brachytherapy	
Cryotherapy	
Photodynamic therapy	
Stent	

Combination of treatment plans often necessary.

proponents of this technique (1,2,5). Although it requires expertise to reduce the risk of complications, such as tracheal perforation, hemorrhage, or rupture of the pulmonary artery, it does not need special equipment and usually requires only one endoscopic procedure. In a series from Mathisen and Grillo (5), 51 of 56 patients had significant improvement in airway obstruction after bronchoscopic "core out," and only two patients required a second procedure. The patients who did not improve had distal obstructing disease. Because a rigid bronchoscope is used to perform a "core out," it is best suited for large, central airway disease. Distal lesions or those obstructing the upper lobe orifices are less likely to be accessible with a rigid bronchoscope.

Another option for palliative resection of intrinsic obstructing lesions of the large airways is laser endobronchial resection (Figs. 27.2 and 27.3) (4). Lasers transform light energy to heat, which causes tissue coagulation and vaporization. With

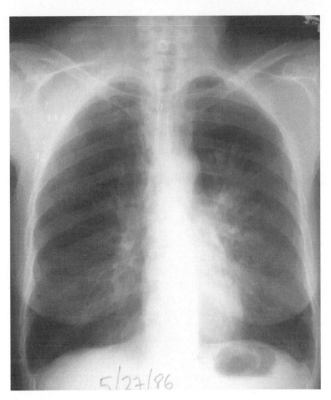

FIGURE 27.3. Chest radiograph of the same patient after laser resection of the tumor. Notice the resolution of volume loss and resolving pneumonitis.

advances in laser technology, this has become an increasingly popular modality over the past 20 years. Currently, the neodymium: yttrium, aluminum, garnet (Nd: YAG) laser is best suited for endobronchial resection (6). The light energy of the laser can be delivered through both rigid and flexible bronchoscopes. The wavelength of the laser is such that it is poorly absorbed by hemoglobin and water, resulting in deep tissue penetration. Because of high power output, it can thermally coagulate blood vessels, up to 2–3 mm in diameter, and vaporize tissue (7). There seems to be a preference toward rigid bronchoscopy because of its ability to ventilate the patient better and its improved suctioning abilities. However, there are many reports of the use of flexible fiberoptic bronchoscopic resections in patients unable to tolerate general anesthesia and rigid bronchoscopy (7–9). In some situations, both types of procedures may be performed in combination. The bronchoscope is passed into the airway and the base of the tumor is identified. The Nd:YAG laser is aimed at the base of the tumor parallel to the wall of the trachea. Using varying energy levels, pulsations of laser energy are used first to coagulate the tumor mass and then to vaporize the tissue. The tracheal wall is avoided to reduce the risk of perforation or hemorrhage. In addition to these complications, there is also risk of tracheoesophageal fistula formation, combustion and fire within the bronchoscope, and ocular damage to operating personnel if appropriate protective gear is not used (1). Other drawbacks to laser resection include the need for special equipment and its time-consuming nature. Most patients improve after the first endoscopic resection but may require multiple sessions to complete the excision.

Success rates are quite substantial with most patients having relief of symptoms or re-expansion of obstructed lung. In a series of 100 Nd:YAG-laser ablations performed on 40 patients, 22 patients were considered to have an excellent response to therapy and another 10 a fair response (10).

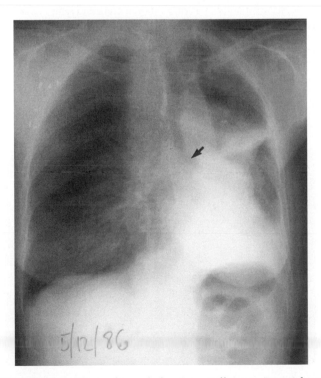

FIGURE 27.2. Chest radiograph showing cutoff airway (*arrow*) from obstructing tumor, significant volume loss of the left hemithorax, and postobstructive pneumonia.

Besides improving quality of life, some patients have prolonged survival from what would otherwise have been a fatal complication of their underlying disease.

Bronchoscopic brachytherapy is the placement of a radiation source in close proximity to an endobronchial tumor. *Brachytherapy*, or short-distance therapy, is in contrast with conventional, external beam radiation therapy delivered at a distance from the lesion. Brachytherapy is another modality to palliate locally extensive disease in the airways. Patients first undergo bronchoscopy to evaluate the extent of intraluminal tumor. A catheter is then advanced through a channel in the bronchoscope to the desired level, and the bronchoscope is removed. Correct placement of the catheter is verified by the reinsertion of the bronchoscope. The catheter is secured to the nasal orifice, and a radioactive source, usually iridium-192 or iodine-125, is placed in the catheter. Conventional-dose brachytherapy (50–120 cGy per hour) requires the catheter to remain inserted for 48–96 hours with the patient in a shielded room. High-dose brachytherapy (675 cGy per minute at 1 cm), delivered by a Gammaned II remote afterloading unit, has treatment duration of only a few minutes. No special radiation measures are needed for the patient after the afterloading unit is removed. Patients must have sufficient pulmonary reserve to undergo bronchoscopy and catheter placement. Brachytherapy *can* also be delivered by the insertion of radiation seeds or pellets into endobrachial lesions. Brachytherapy can improve symptoms of dyspnea and hemoptysis in approximately 90% of patients with stable airway disease (11). Because of the need for a stable airway, several studies combined laser-endobronchial resection with brachytherapy (5,12). High-dose brachytherapy was tolerated better with slightly improved survival compared with conventional-dose brachytherapy. Early complications to brachytherapy include airway obstruction secondary to mucous plugs requiring *therapeutic* bronchoscopy, radiation esophagitis, and laryngospasm. Long-term complications are more ominous, including fatal hemorrhage from fistula formation between airways and major blood vessels as well as airway esophageal fistula formation (12). Long-term survivors are at risk of airway stenosis at the site of laser or radiation therapy (9).

PDT is another option for the obstructed airway secondary to a malignant lesion. A sensitizing agent is administered intravenously 1–3 days before the treatment. The sensitizer is taken up by normal and tumor cells, although it is thought to be preferentially taken up by the tumor. An argon dye laser acts as the activating agent, treating endobronchial tumor with precision through the bronchoscope (2,13). After activation, tissue necrosis takes place from 3 to 10 mm deep. Usually follow-up bronchoscopy is needed for removal of necrotic material. Studies have found PDT to be effective in treating endobronchial tumor (13,14). A small prospective study comparing PDT to laser resection found both groups had similar symptomatic relief, but the PDT group had a longer time to treatment failure. There was one death felt to be from PDT (13). Complications from PDT can include airway edema and mucous plugging with atelectasis.

Freezing endoluminal tumor through cryotherapy is another option for palliative treatment of airway obstruction. Tumor cells are more sensitive to the extreme cold temperature (5). Cryotherapy probes can be passed through flexible or rigid bronchoscopes. The major drawback to cryotherapy is it does not cause immediate tumor sloughing (5,15).

Extrinsic compression of the airway is not amenable to the above mentioned therapies. Pressure from extraluminal tumor, vasculature, or luminal weakness (malacia) can cause the airways to narrow or collapse. Intraluminal pressure is needed to counteract these external forces. Over the past two decades, insertion of airway stents to maintain airway patency

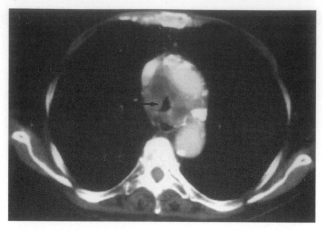

FIGURE 27.4. Tracheal compression (*arrow*) causing dyspnea in a 63-year-old woman. Biopsy of the tumor revealed squamous cell carcinoma.

has gained popularity as an effective palliative treatment for extrinsic compression. Stents can be inserted through rigid or flexible bronchoscopes. Their most impressive benefit is the immediate palliation of airway obstruction on placement of the stent (Figs. 27.4 and 27.5). Several different types of airway stents are available, including silicone stents (Dumon, Montgomery T-tube, Hood) or expandable metallic stents (Ultraflex, Gianturco, Wall, William Cook, etc.). Both types of stents are placed in a similar manner. The stents are compressed to an extremely small diameter within an introducer and are bronchoscopically inserted into the airway after the airway has been dilated with either a balloon or successively larger rigid bronchoscopes. When correct placement is verified, the stent is deployed, expanding to enlarge the airway. Ultraflex stents have a slightly different deployment apparatus that allows for better control during deployment (16).

Stents are available in varying diameters and lengths for use in the trachea and mainstem bronchi. However, none of the stents is without drawbacks. Silicone stents may migrate or may even be coughed completely out of the airway. Therefore, it is extremely important to place the appropriately sized stent, as migration usually is seen with stents that are too small (17). Silicone stents placed in the right mainstem bronchus may obstruct the orifice to the right upper lobe, putting the patient

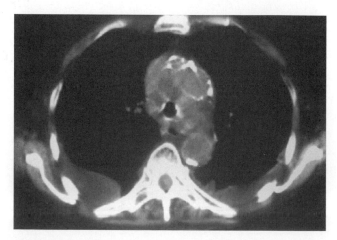

FIGURE 27.5. The same patient after placement of a stent into the trachea, which has increased the diameter of the airway and relieved her symptoms.

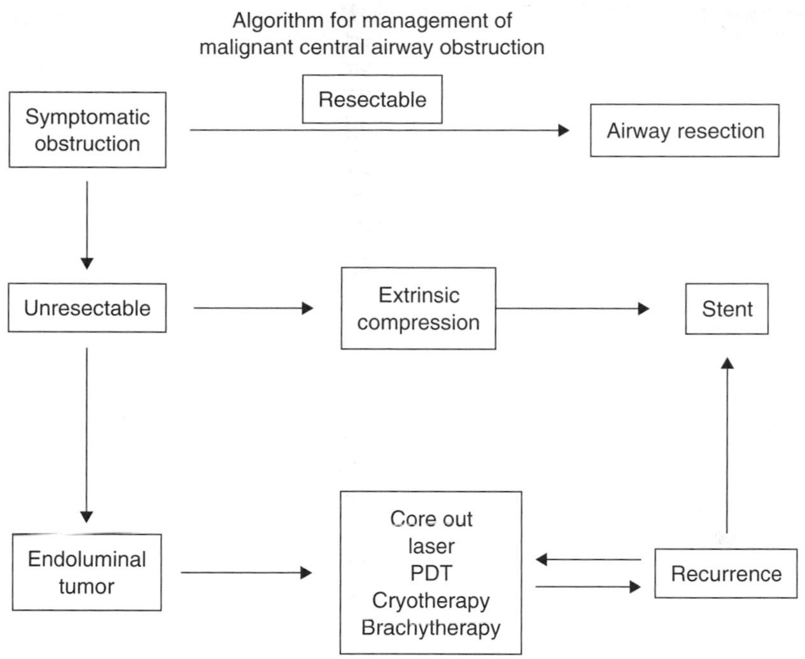

Algorithm for management of
malignant central airway obstruction

```
┌─────────────┐      ┌────────────┐
│ Symptomatic │──────│ Resectable │─────────────▶ ┌─────────────────┐
│ obstruction │      └────────────┘                │ Airway resection│
└─────────────┘                                     └─────────────────┘
       │
       ▼
┌─────────────┐      ┌──────────────┐
│ Unresectable│─────▶│  Extrinsic   │────────────▶ ┌───────┐
└─────────────┘      │ compression  │               │ Stent │
       │             └──────────────┘               └───────┘
       │                                                 ▲
       ▼             ┌──────────────┐                    │
┌─────────────┐      │  Core out    │      ┌────────────┐
│ Endoluminal │─────▶│   laser      │◀─────│ Recurrence │
│   tumor     │      │   PDT        │─────▶└────────────┘
└─────────────┘      │ Cryotherapy  │
                     │ Brachytherapy│
                     └──────────────┘
```

FIGURE 27.6. Algorithm for the management of central airway obstruction. Adapted from Wood D. Management of malignant tracheobronchial obstruction. *Surg Clin North Am* 2002;82(3):Figure 6, 640.

at risk for atelectasis and infectious complications. Patients may complain of halitosis after stent placement. Silicone stents are also believed to interfere with mucociliary clearance and pulmonary toilet (18). T-tube stents are placed in the trachea and usually require tracheostomy. A rare complication of stent placement is fatal erosion into a central vascular structure. Despite these potential drawbacks, silicone stents are well tolerated and quite successful in the treatment of extrinsic airway obstruction (19,20).

Expandable metallic stents are the latest type of stents to be used in the treatment of airway obstruction, but they have many drawbacks. Because these stents are made of loops of wire, they do not obstruct orifices of smaller airways, such as the opening of the right upper lobe, when placed in the right mainstem bronchus. Unfortunately, because of the loops, endobronchial tumor may grow through the stent and compromise the airway. The metallic stents have an irritant effect on the airways. Cough and granuloma formation are the most common complications (21,22). Some patients improve with inhaled corticosteroids and laser resection. Because of the tissue reaction, removal of the stents is difficult, often causing damage to the airways. There have been reports of fatal hemorrhage, broken suction catheters, stent migration, and stent breakage (23–25). The newer Ultraflex nitinol stent, which comes partially covered, may have less airway complications (16,22,26).

Lastly, some patients with upper airway obstruction may have relief of symptoms following tracheostomy, which is useful only in patents with laryngeal or very proximal tracheal obstruction. In patients with distal tracheal or small airway obstruction, the tracheostomy tube is not able to bypass the obstructing lesion. Recent improvements in tracheostomy tube technology can improve patient communication and decrease the risk of complications such as granulation tissue formation and bleeding. A recent study evaluated laser resection in malignant airway obstruction and found it a viable alternative to tracheostomy (27).

Tracheobronchial obstruction is a devastating complication from both malignant and nonmalignant disease. There are many possible therapies for palliation. These therapies are not mutually exclusive, and their use in combination should be encouraged. A multidisciplinary approach with appropriately

trained personnel is needed. Figure 27.6 gives an algorithm for the management of central airway obstruction.

STRIDOR

Stridor is loud, harsh breathing, particularly on inspiration. It occurs from obstructed airflow in the upper airway and large intrathoracic central airways. Stridor may indicate a pathologic narrowing of the airway, which is unable to maintain adequate oxygenation and ventilation of the patient. Therefore, evaluation and management of these patients should be done expediently. Treatment for stridor depends on the location of the obstruction and its etiology. When evaluating a patient presenting with stridor, it is useful to consider the airway as three areas or zones (15,28,29). The first is the *supraglottic zone*, which includes the nose, oral cavity, pharynx, and supraglottic larynx. This area is composed of soft tissues that are only loosely supported and hence more easily obstructed. Lesions in this area tend to cause stridor only on inspiration. The second is the *extrathoracic tracheal zone*, which is composed primarily of the glottis and subglottis. Because this area has more support, obstruction generally occurs more gradually. Lesions in this area may cause stridor both on inspiration and expiration known as *biphasic stridor*. Last is the *intrathoracic tracheal area*, which also includes the proximal portions of the mainstem bronchi. Stridor from this region may be primarily expiratory and may be confused with wheezing from distal intrathoracic airway obstruction. Of note, patients frequently deviate from these patterns of clinical presentations. The causes of stridor are numerous, some of which are listed in Table 27.3.

Evaluation

The tempo of evaluation of the patient presenting with stridor is determined by the acuity of the illness. Patients who present in severe respiratory distress with inadequate oxygenation or ventilation need the immediate establishment of an airway. Because they may have lesions that make intubation difficult or impossible, it is necessary to have available experienced

TABLE 27.3

CAUSES OF STRIDOR

Infection
  Tracheitis: bacterial or viral
  Epiglottitis
  Abscess: peritonsillar or retropharyngeal
  Viral laryngotracheobronchitis
Neoplasm
  See Table 27.1
Congenital
  Laryngomalacia
  Tracheomalacia/tracheal stenosis
  Vocal cord cysts/paralysis
  Webs
Trauma
  Facial
  Ingestion
  Inhalation injury
Postintubation
  Airway fracture
  Postsurgical
Neurological
  Central nervous system malformation
  Hypoxic encephalopathy
Other
  Foreign bodies (airway, esophageal)
  Psychogenic
  Exercise

personnel, including an anesthesiologist and otolaryngologist. Fiberoptic-assisted intubation may be necessary and also may be helpful in establishing the etiology of stridor.

In patients who appear stable, a brief history may help in differentiating the causes of stridor. Gradual onset of symptoms over weeks or months, especially if accompanied by constitutional symptoms, would suggest neoplasm. Stridor that occurs in hours or days, especially if the patient is febrile, is suspicious for an infectious etiology, such as epiglottis, croup, or abscess. A history of previous intubation is quite important because subglottic stenosis may not appear for months after a traumatic or prolonged intubation. Close questioning regarding episodes of choking or coughing while eating may raise the possibility of aspiration. Foreign body in either the airway or esophagus may cause stridor, especially in younger patients. Pressure exerted from an esophageal foreign body may partially obstruct the airway (30).

Physical examination of a patient with stridor typically begins with the examiner's unaided ear. Loud, noisy breathing is heard. The patient's respiratory rate, depth of respiration, use of accessory muscles of respiration, level of alertness, and evidence of cyanosis should be observed. Inability to handle oral secretions should be noted because it may suggest peritonsillar abscess, retropharyngeal hematoma or abscess, epiglottis, or foreign body.

Palpation of the airway should be performed to assess for crepitation, suggesting subcutaneous emphysema. A displaced trachea or firm mass could indicate tumor or goiter. Lymphadenopathy could suggest neoplasm. Auscultation of the entire airway may help localize the anatomical location of the lesion; so one should listen especially carefully over the larynx, extrathoracic trachea, and central chest.

Radiologic studies of the chest, as discussed earlier in this chapter, should be obtained to evaluate stridor in stable patients. In addition, anterior–posterior and lateral radiographs of the neck should be obtained. If more detailed imaging of the airway is needed, CT scans should be obtained. Spirometry with flow-volume loops, as discussed in evaluation of tracheobronchial obstruction, may be an important aid in evaluation of stridor.

Therapy

Stridor secondary to infectious etiologies requires treatment with appropriate antimicrobial therapy. *Haemophilus influenzae* is the most common bacterial cause of epiglottitis, although its incidence has been declining steadily. Respiratory syncytial virus infection may cause airway edema resulting in stridor. This infection is typically seen in children, although the virus has been recovered in immunocompromised adults. Treatment with the antiviral drug ribavirin may be considered in the acutely ill patient. Anaerobes, streptococcal species, and a wide assortment of less common agents may cause abscess formation, leading to airway obstruction. While waiting for the culture results, it is appropriate to treat the patient with broad-spectrum antibiotics.

Several therapies are available to stabilize the stridorous patient who is clinically decompensating. Heliox, a mixture of helium and oxygen, has been useful in improving oxygenation, ventilation, and decreasing work of breathing in patients with stridor from a wide variety of causes (31–35). These causes include postextubation edema, extrinsic compression from tumor, and status asthmaticus. Because heliox has a lower density than ambient nitrogen-oxygen gas mixture, there is decreased airway turbulence and airway resistance. The typical heliox mixture varies from helium 60% and oxygen 40% to maximum concentration of helium 80% and oxygen 20%. It can be delivered through a tight-fitting face mask, and relief of respiratory distress is often immediate. Treatment with high-dose i.v. corticosteroids should be started using methyl prednisolone 1 mg per kg every 6 to 8 hours. Racemic epinephrine 2.25%, 0.5 mL in 2.5 mL saline delivered through a handheld nebulizer as often as hourly, but usually every 3 to 4 hours, may be used especially for postextubation stridor (36).

Noninvasive mask ventilation (NIV) with continuous positive airway pressure or bilevel positive airway pressure may decrease the work of breathing and overcome large airway obstruction, although currently no studies have evaluated the efficacy of this therapy. NIV has been found to be effective in treating the respiratory failure associated with chronic obstructive lung disease (37). Close coordination with a respiratory therapist is needed if this therapy is initiated. Either a tight-fitting mask over the nose or nasal pillars applied to the nares may be used. Starting with a positive pressure of 5 cm H_2O it is titrated up to a maximum of 20 cm H_2O. Most patients are unable to tolerate higher pressures. If needed, supplemental oxygen and humidification can be "bled" into the positive pressure system. Finally, endotracheal intubation or tracheostomy should be considered in appropriate clinical situations for patients severely affected.

BRONCHOSPASM

Bronchospasm is the state of abnormal narrowing of the airways and is usually episodic. It can occur in many types of pulmonary disorders. Airflow is obstructed and becomes turbulent. Patients complain of dyspnea, wheezing, chest tightness, or pressure, although occasionally cough is the only symptom. Exacerbation of symptoms frequently occurs in the early hours of the morning, when the bronchial tone is normally increased. Wheezing is heard on auscultation of the chest, occasionally needing to be provoked by forced expiration or deep breathing. Expiration time is usually prolonged. Patients may use accessory muscles of respiration and pursed lip breathing.

Bronchospasm is the end result of airway narrowing, which is believed to be a consequence of a state of hyper-responsiveness of the airways to a wide variety of stimuli (38). More recently, airway inflammation has been considered of prime importance in the development of airway hyperactivity. The airway epithelium is thickened and friable, and microscopically there is infiltration with inflammatory cells, especially eosinophils and mast cells. Mucous glands are hyperplastic, and goblet cells are more numerous compared with normal persons (39). In severely affected persons, the airways may be plugged with excessive inflammatory secretions and desquamated epithelium (40).

Evaluation

The differential diagnosis for bronchospasm includes asthma, COPD, upper/large airway obstruction (see the section on Tracheobronchial Obstruction) congestive heart failure, gastroesophageal reflux, bronchiectasis, bronchiolitis (infectious or inflammatory, medication induced), lymphangitic tumor spread, or rarely, pulmonary embolism. Multiple etiologies for bronchospasm are common in an individual patient. The extent of evaluation depends on the complexity of an individual patient's medical condition. In a patient with a significant smoking history, chronic sputum production, and diffuse bronchospasm on examination, it is likely that an exacerbation of COPD explains the clinical situation. Obviously, in a patient who has a similar history but is immunocompromised, the diagnostic possibilities must be widened.

Chest radiographs should be obtained in patients presenting with bronchospasm. Bronchial wall thickening, flattened diaphragm, and increased retrosternal air space are consistent with hyperexpansion and air trapping and would support the diagnosis of asthma or COPD. In addition, the chest radiograph may reveal complications of obstructive lung disease, such as pneumonia, pneumothorax, or atelectasis.

A chest radiograph with no change from the patient's baseline film or with atelectasis or small pleural effusion should alert the clinician to possible pulmonary embolism. If the patient has a normal chest radiograph, a ventilation/perfusion (V/Q) scan should be obtained to assess for pulmonary embolism. The scan needs to be compared with the chest radiograph for accurate interpretation. A completely normal perfusion scan effectively excludes pulmonary embolism. Segmental perfusion defects in areas of normal ventilation define a high probability scan, which indicates an 85–90% probability of pulmonary embolism must be interpreted with care, as one of the few causes of false-positive scans is bronchospasm. Helical CT scanning of the chest may be more cost effective and more accurate than V/Q scanning in identifying clinically significant pulmonary emboli (41,42). With new CT scan protocols now including scanning the lower extremity helical CT scan can evaluate for deep vein thrombosis (DVT) at the same time (41).

New techniques are on the horizon for diagnosing pulmonary embolism. These include magnetic resonance imaging (MRI) (43). Numerous reviews in the literature discuss algorithms for pulmonary emboli (PE) (44). Again, if the clinical situation warrants further evaluation, noninvasive testing to detect lower extremity DVT or pulmonary angiography may need to be pursued.

Spirometry not only confirms airway obstruction but can suggest its anatomical location (upper *vs.* intrathoracic) and quantify the extent of airway obstruction. In addition, it may also be helpful in monitoring treatment *response*. Forced vital *capacity* (FVC) and forced expiratory volume at 1 second (FEV$_1$) are reduced in an obstructive lung defect with the reduction in FEV greater than that of FVC. In airway obstruction, the ratio of FEV$_1$ to FVC will be <70%. The severity of the obstructive defect is graded by the patient's percentage of predicted FEV$_1$ (70% or greater, mild; between 60 and 70%, moderate; between 50 and 60%, moderately severe; between 35 and 50%, severe; and <34%, very severe) (45).

The contour of the expiratory portion of a flow-volume loop shows concavity, which worsens with the extent of the obstructive lung defect. Patients with chronic obstructive lung disease have fixed airway obstruction but can have some degree of variability in FVC and FEV$_1$ during exacerbations. On the other hand, most patients with asthma should have normal or near-normal spirometry between episodes of illness. Spirometry often is obtained before or after use of inhaled bronchodilators. Patients who have at least a 15% improvement in FVC or FEV$_1$ and 200 mL absolute increase in FVC or FEV$_1$ are considered to have a significant immediate response. This group is considered to benefit most from inhaled bronchodilators and corticosteroids, although many studies have reported conflicting results regarding this issue (46). Patients who do not improve immediately after inhaled bronchodilators may have spirometric or clinical improvement with regular use; therefore, these medications should not be withheld.

Therapy

The goals of therapy in bronchospasm are to dilate the distal airways and reduce inflammation, hence relieving airway obstruction. There are many pharmacologic agents available to treat bronchospasm (Table 27.4). The severity of the patient's symptoms guides which of these medications are used and in what order. β-Adrenergic agonists (β-agonists) continue to be important pharmacologic agents to relieve bronchospasm. They can be administered in many forms: inhaled through metered-dose inhalers, inhaled through handheld nebulizers, taken orally, or injected subcutaneously or intravenously. Over the past decade, there has been a strong movement against using oral β-agonists as their efficacy is similar to the inhaled forms but with a higher incidence of side effects. Subcutaneous forms are used sparingly for emergency treatments. Intravenous administration of isoproterenol is no longer recommended (47).

β-agonists promote airway smooth-muscle relaxation. In addition, they increase mucociliary clearance and increase the secretion of electrolytes by the airways. Side effects include tremor, tachycardia, palpitations, hypokalemia, and hyperglycemia. Usually these side effects are most pronounced when the medications are first initiated and decreased over time. Patients with mild bronchospasm may be started on β-agonists alone to control symptoms. Given the inflammatory nature of asthma, patients with persistent symptoms should be treated with anti-inflammatory agents. Patients still use β-agonist medications on as-needed basis, as a rescue medication for mild or breakthrough symptoms. Some patients benefit by using a spacer device to improve delivery with metered-dose inhalers (48). The total dose of β-agonist should be 24 or fewer inhalations in a 24-hour period to prevent tachyphylaxis but in general practice patients are advised not to use β-agonists more than four to five times a day. Patients who do not find relief with use of β-agonists or who must increase their usual dose should be evaluated for additional therapies. The recent spate of literature on the safety of β-agonists found that mortality increased when patients were undertreated for asthma (49–52).

Anticholinergic agents act by decreasing parasympathetic bronchoconstriction of the airways. They are most useful

TABLE 27.4

THERAPY FOR BRONCHOSPASM

Medications		
β-agonists		
Albuterol (Proventil, Ventolin)	MDI	Two to three puffs up to q.i.d. not to exceed 24 puffs/d
	Neb	0.5–0.75 mL in 2.5 mL saline q.i.d. may increase frequency for severe symptoms
Levalbuterol (Xopenex)	MDI	One to two puffs q.i.d. not to exceed 12 puffs/d
Pirbuterol	MDI	Two to three puffs q.i.d. not to exceed 12 puffs/d
Anticholinergics		
Ipratropium bromide (Atrovent, Combivent—contains albuterol)	MDI	Two puffs up to q.i.d. not to exceed 12 puffs/d
	Neb	500 µg in 2.5 mL saline t.i.d. to q.i.d.
Tiotropium (Spiriva)	DPI	18 µg or one capsule daily
Nonsteroidal anti-inflammatory		
Cromolyn sodium (Intal)	MDI	Two to four puffs b.i.d. to q.i.d.
	Neb	1–2 mL (10–20 mg) b.i.d. to q.i.d.
Nedocromil sodium (Tilade)	MDI	Two puffs b.i.d. to q.i.d.
Long-acting β-agonist		
Formoterol (Foradil)	DPI	12 µg b.i.d.
Salmeterol (Serevent)	DPI	50 µg b.i.d.
Inhaled corticosteroids		
Beclomethasone (QVAR)	MDI	40, 80 µg One to two inhalations b.i.d.
Budesonide (Pulmicort)	Neb	0.25–0.50 mg b.i.d.
	DPI	Two to four inhalations b.i.d.
Flunisolide (Aerobid)	MDI	Two to four inhalations b.i.d.
Fluticasone (Flovent)	DPI	44, 110, 220 µg strengths One to two inhalations b.i.d.
Mometasone (Asmanex)	Spray DPI	One to two inhalations b.i.d.
Triamcinolone (Azmacort)	MDI	Two to four puffs t.i.d. to q.i.d.
Combination medications		
Advair (fluticasone/salmeterol)	DPI	100/50, 250/50, 500/50 One inhalation b.i.d.
Combivent (albuterol/ipratropium)	MDI	One to two inhalations q.i.d. 3 mL q.i.d.
Leukotriene receptor antagonists		
Montelukast (Singulair)	Oral	10 mg daily
Zafirlukast (Accolate)	Oral	20 mg b.i.d.
Zileuton (Zyflo)	Oral	600 mg up to q.i.d. monitor LFTs

MDI, metered-dose inhaler; Neb, through nebulizer; DPI, dry powder inhaler; LFTs, liver function tests.

in COPD, where parasympathetic activity is believed to be greater than normal. Ipratropium bromide and new dry powder tiotropium are the anticholinergic agents available for inhalational use in the United States. Because of studies showing ipratropium bromide may be more effective than β-agonists in promoting bronchodilation in patients with COPD, it is now the first agent used in maintenance therapy in COPD with persistent airway obstruction (53–55).

Corticosteroids are widely used in the treatment of bronchospasm and are the cornerstone of treatment of asthma (48). Patients with mild to moderate symptoms may benefit from inhaled corticosteroids. They are especially attractive because they act locally, with minimal absorption and limited toxicity. However, reports of hypothalamic-pituitary-adrenal axis suppression and cataract formation have been reported with the use of high-dose inhaled corticosteroids (56). In addition, patients should be cautioned that these medications must be used regularly and may take weeks for therapeutic effect. Therefore, corticosteroids should not be used as monotherapy for acutely symptomatic patients. Inhaled corticosteroids also may allow patients on systemic corticosteroid therapy to have their doses reduced or discontinued altogether (48). Patients with more serious symptoms or those in respiratory distress require systemic corticosteroids. These medications may take

up to 12 hours to have clinical effects. Prednisone, 0.5–1.0 mg per kg per 24 hours, may be used for 1–2 weeks and then gradually tapered. Seriously ill patients should receive methyl prednisolone, 1–2 mg per kg every 6–8 hours i.v., until improvement is noted. The i.v. dose may then be tapered over several days and the patient switched to oral corticosteroids. Peak flow meters along with physical examination and arterial blood gases help determine a patient's response to therapy.

Besides corticosteroids, cromolyn sulfate and nedocromil sodium are other inhaled anti-inflammatory agents. Their exact mode of action is unclear, but it is likely that they act as mast cell stabilizers. These medications are particularly useful in children for symptoms related to exercise or cold air and for patients with a strong allergic component to their bronchospasm. Again, patients must be educated to use these medications regularly because its maximal effects are not noted for 4–6 weeks. Since the mid-1990s, a new class of anti-inflammatory agents has been available for the treatment of asthma; leukotriene receptor antagonists (LTRAs). Leukotrienes are released within the airway following activation of inflammatory cells. They cause more airway inflammation with stimulation of their receptor sites in the airway. When the receptors are blocked, there is a reduction in airway inflammation and therefore mild bronchodilatation (48,56).

Theophylline, once a mainstay of therapy, has lost its place as a first-line therapy in the treatment of bronchospasm because of excessive toxicity and potential for serious drug interactions. It is still used in patients with COPD in an effort to augment respiratory muscle function and for its weak bronchodilator effects. In addition, it is used in corticosteroid-dependent asthmatics in hopes of decreasing their daily steroid dose (57). There has been a renewed interest in theophylline because of evidence it has an anti-inflammatory effect in the airways. Typically, patients are started on long-acting preparations at a dose of 400–900 mg per day to achieve serum levels of 8–12 U per mL. The dose must be individualized depending on concurrent medications, smoking history, and other medical problems such as congestive heart failure, as all of these change drug clearance.

There have been a few reports on the use of i.v. and inhaled magnesium sulfate for acute asthma exacerbations. So far, there has been no firm evidence of it efficacy (58,59).

LTRAs or modifiers are primarily used as add-on therapy in asthma and allergic rhinitis. Several studies have documented improvement in FEV$_1$ with use of these medications but with a lesser response as compared with long-acting β-agonists. Intravenous or nebulized magnesium sulfate has been reported to have positive effects in poorly controlled asthma.

Critically ill patients in respiratory failure secondary to bronchospasm who do not respond to maximal therapy, including intubation and mechanical ventilation, should be considered for bronchial muscle relaxation with inhalational anesthetics.

COUGH

Etiology

Cough is a protective, complex reflex that helps clear the airways of foreign material or excessive secretions. It can be an annoyance or severely debilitating when it occurs excessively or for a prolonged period of time. It is a common problem that translates into 30 million physician visits per year and millions of dollars spent on over-the-counter medications (60). It is so common a problem and sometimes frustrating to treat that the American College of Chest Physicians (ACCP) has just published a 292-page evidence-based practice guideline for care providers (61)!

The cough reflex is complicated and not fully understood. Suffice it to say that cough results from stimulation of cough receptors, which may be found in the larynx, respiratory epithelium, tympanic membranes, esophagus, pericardium, and sinus mucosa. Afferent impulses travel through the vagus, trigeminal, glossopharyngeal, and phrenic nerves to cough centers in the medulla. Efferent impulses travel through the vagus, phrenic, and spinal nerves to the glottis and respiratory muscles, which produce the high-velocity flow of air that defines a cough (62,63).

Evaluation

Cough is a common complaint in patients with advanced cancer. In the patient with cancer, cough may be secondary to endobronchial tumor, pericardial disease, vocal cord paralysis, or aspiration. Cough also may be due to complications of treatment, such as radiation pneumonitis or chemotherapy-induced interstitial lung disease (64). In addition, patients with underlying cancer may have all the same causes of cough found in the general population. The most common etiologies of chronic cough include upper airway cough syndrome (previously known as postnasal drip syndrome), asthma, and gastroesophageal reflux (65,66).

A detailed history and physical examination are most helpful in determining the cause of chronic cough (63). Chest radiographs should be obtained early in the evaluation of cough (67). In patients who chronically produce sputum or in whom there is a suspicion of interstitial lung disease, a high-resolution chest CT scan may be helpful. Of patients with interstitial lung disease, 10–15% have a normal chest radiograph. CT scan is very helpful in the evaluation of bronchiectasis.

Sinus imaging, including radiographs and CT scanning, are needed to evaluate for chronic sinus disease. Some authors recommend a trial of antihistamine decongestants (A/D) before pursuing sinus radiographic studies (60). Spirometry, before and after inhaled bronchodilators and methacholine challenge, help evaluate for asthma or chronic obstructive lung disease. Evaluation for gastroesophageal reflux disease can be undertaken with barium esophagography or 24-hour esophageal pH monitoring. Finally, if no cause has been found for chronic cough, bronchoscopy should be considered to evaluate for occult foreign body aspiration or small endobronchial lesions, such as carcinoid tumors or bronchogenic cancer, although studies have found this to be of low yield (65).

Therapy

Treatment of cough is most successful if it is tailored to a specific etiology. Upper airway cough syndrome may be well controlled with the use of A/D therapy. The literature suggests that first generation A/D preparations are more effective than the newer nonsedating formulations (68). Asthma therapy was discussed earlier in this chapter (see section on Therapy under Stridor). Gastroesophageal reflux disease is treated with H$_2$ receptor blockers or proton pump inhibitors along with lifestyle changes. In patients for whom no cause is found for their cough or it is due to airway involvement with tumor, empiric medical therapy is reasonable. Some patients obtain relief with the use of β$_2$-adrenergic agonists such as albuterol, two or three inhalations every 4–6 hours or 0.5 mL albuterol solution in 2 mL saline through a nebulizer every 4–6 hours.

For generations, opiates have been used and are variably effective antitussives (62,69). There is no evidence of superior antitussive effect with one preparation over another. Codeine, 15–30 mg every 4–6 hours, is a reasonable starting dose, with titration upward to control symptoms if the side effects are tolerable. Non-narcotic cough preparations, such as guaifenesin and dextromethorphan, benzonatate may be tried, although they have been only weakly effective. Research articles and the ACCP evidence-based clinical practice guidelines review the many conflicting studies evaluating over-the-counter and prescription cough medications (61,69,70).

Inhaled lidocaine is used to suppress cough during bronchoscopy. Animal studies and a few human studies suggest that lidocaine has an antitussive effect when inhaled through a nebulizer, probably acting on afferent C-fibers in the larynx and trachea. The dose is empiric; a starting dose is 5 mL of 2% lidocaine solution every 4 hours through a handheld nebulizer (62,64). Patients should be cautioned regarding anesthesia of the oropharynx and larynx, which puts them at risk for buccal injury or aspiration. The dose may be increased if needed, but there are no studies giving explicit guidelines for this therapy. Generally, during bronchoscopy, doses higher than 300 mg of lidocaine (15 mL of 2% solution) are avoided to decrease the risk of seizures, as there is significant systemic airway absorption of lidocaine.

In patients who have underlying chronic bronchitis, a trial of inhaled ipratropium bromide, two puffs four times a day, may diminish the cough (71). Finally, some patients respond to corticosteroids. Some of these patients have underlying asthma, whereas others may have other reasons for airway inflammation, such as chronic bronchitis, bronchiectasis, or radiation pneumonitis (72). Inhaled steroids such as flunisolide two puffs twice daily and triamcinolone two to four puffs four times a day may be tried as initial therapy or maintenance therapy after oral agents. Patients not responding to inhaled therapy should be tried on prednisone, 0.5–1.0 mg/kg/day for 2–4 weeks. If the cough subsides, the prednisone should be tapered to the lowest dose to control symptoms, or patients should be switched to inhaled steroids.

References

1. Mathisen DJ. Surgical management of tracheobronchial disease. *Clin Chest Med* 1992;13:151.
2. Wood D. Management of malignant tracheobronchial obstruction. *Surg Clin North Am* 2002;82:621–642.
3. Braman SS, Whitcomb ME. Endobronchial metastasis. *Arch Intern Med* 1995;135:543.
4. Chen K, Vawn J, Wenker O. Malignant airway obstruction: recognition and management. *J Emerg Med* 1998;16(1):83–92.
5. Mathisen DJ, Grillo HC. Endoscopic relief of malignant airway obstruction. *Ann Thorac Surg* 1989;48:469.
6. Lang N, Maners A, Broadwater J, et al. Management of airway problems in lung cancer patients using the neodymium-yttrium-aluminum-garnet (Nd-YAG) laser and endobronchial radiotherapy. *Am J Surg* 1988;156:463.
7. Turner J, Wang K, Endobronchial laser therapy. *Clin Chest Med* 1999;20(1):107–122.
8. Castro DJ, Saxton RE, Ward PH, et al. Flexible Nd:YAG laser palliation of obstructive tracheal metastatic malignancies. *Laryngoscope* 1990;100:1208.
9. Kao SJ, Shen CY, Hsu K. Nd-YAG laser application in pulmonary and endobronchial lesions. *Lasers Surg Med* 1986;6:296.
10. Parr GVS, Unger M, Trout RG, et al. One hundred neodymium-YAG laser ablations of obstructing tracheal neoplasms. *Ann Thorac Surg* 1984;38:374.
11. Marsh BR. Bronchoscopic brachytherapy. *Laryngoscope* 1989;99:1.
12. Schray MF, McDougall JC, Martinez A, et al. Management of malignant airway compromise with laser and low dose rate brachytherapy. *Chest* 1988;93:264.
13. Diaz-Jimenez J, Martinez-Ballaren J, Llunell A, et al. Efficacy and safety of photodynamic therapy versus Nd—YAG laser resection in NSCLC with airway obstruction. *Eur Respir J* 1999;14:800–855.
14. McCaughan J, Williams T. Photodynamic therapy for endobronchial malignant disease: a prospective fourteen year study. *J Thorac Cardiovasc Surg* 1997;114:940–946.
15. Lee P, Temm M, Chhajed P. Advances in bronchoscopy—therapeutic bronchoscopy. *JAPI* 2004;52:905–914.
16. Madden B, Datta S, Charokopes N. Experience with ultraflex expandable metallic stents in the management of endobronchial pathology. *Ann Thorac Surg* 2002;73:938–944.
17. Dumon JF. A dedicated tracheobronchial stent. *Chest* 1990;97:328.
18. Zarmini P, Melloin G, Chiesa G, et al. Self-expanding stents in the treatment of tracheobronchial obstruction. *Chest* 1994;106:86.
19. Bolliger CT, Probst R, Tschopp K, et al. Silicone stents in the management of inoperable tracheobronchial stenoses. *Chest* 1993;104:1653.
20. Gaer JA, Tsang V, Khaghani A, et al. Use of endobronchial silicone stents for relief of tracheobronchial obstruction. *Ann Thorac Surg* 1992;54:512.
21. Nashef SA, Dromer C, Velly JF, et al. Expanding wire stents in benign tracheobronchial disease: indications and complications. *Ann Thorac Surg* 1992;54:937.
22. Madden B, Park J, Sheth A. Medium-term follow-up after deployment of ultraflex expandable metallic stents to manage endobronchial pathology. *Ann Thorac Surg* 2004;78:1898–1902.
23. Hind CRK, Domaelly RJ. Expandable metal stents for tracheal obstruction: permanent or temporary? A cautionary tale. *Thorax* 1992;47:757.
24. Sawada S, Tanigawa N, Kobayaski M, et al. Malignant tracheobronchial obstruction lesions: treatment with Gianturco expandable metal stents. *Radiology* 1993;188:205.
25. Nomori H, Kobayashi R, Kodera K, et al. Indications for an expandable metallic stent for tracheobronchial stenosis. *Ann Thorac Surg* 1993;56:1324.
26. Wood DE, Liu Y, Vallieres E, et al. Airway stenting for malignant and benign tracheobronchial stenosis. *Ann Thorac Surg* 2003;76:167–174.
27. Palere V, Stafford F, Sammut M. Benefits of debulking with laser rather than going straight to trach. *Head & Neck* 2005;24:296–301.
28. Santamaria JP, Schafermeyer R. Stridor: a review. *Pediatr Emerg Care* 1992;8:229.
29. Stool SE. Stridor. *Int Anesthesiol Clin* 1988;26:19.
30. O'Hollaren MT, Everts EC. Evaluating the patient with stridor. *Ann Allergy* 1991;67:301.
31. Curtis JL, Mahlmeister M, Fink JB, et al. Helium-oxygen gas therapy use and availability for the emergency treatment of inoperable airway obstruction. *Chest* 1986;90:455.
32. Orr JB. Helium-oxygen gas mixtures in the management of patients with airway obstruction. *Ear Nose Throat J* 1988;67:866.
33. Skrinskas GJ, Hyland RH, Hutcheon MA. Using helium-oxygen mixtures in the management of acute airway obstruction. *Can Med Assoc J* 1983;R8:555.
34. Gluck E, Onorato DJ, Castriotta R. Helium-oxygen mixtures in intubated patients with status asthmaticus and respiratory acidosis. *Chest* 1990;98:693.
35. Gupta V, Cheifetz I. Heliox administration in the pediatric intensive care unit: an evidence-based review. *Pediatr Crit Care Med* 2005;6:204.
36. Schmitt G, Hall R, Wood LDH. Management of the ventilated patient. In: Murray JF Nadel JA, eds. *Textbook of respiratory medicine*. Philadelphia, PA: WB Saunders, 1992.
37. Kramer N, Meyer T, et al. Randomized, prospective trial of noninvasive positive pressure ventilation in acute respiratory failure. *Am J Respir Crit Care Med* 1995;151:1799.
38. Caramori G, Pandit A, Papi A. Is there a difference between chronic airway inflammation in chronic severe asthma and chronic obstructive pulmonary disease? *Curr Opin Allergy Clin Immunol* 2005;5:77.
39. Nadel JA. Regulation of bronchial secretion. In: Newball I-IH, ed. *Immunopharmacology of the lung*. New York: Marcel Dekker, 1983:109.
40. Saetta M, Stefano AD, Rosina C, et al. Quantitative structural analysis of peripheral airways and arteries in sudden fatal asthma. *Am Rev Respir Dis* 1991;143:138.
41. Gefter WB, Hatabu H, Holland GA, et al. Pulmonary thromboembolism: recent developments in diagnosis with CT and MR imaging. *Radiology* 1995;197:561–574.
42. Patel S, Kazerooni E. Helical CT For the evaluation of acute pulmonary embolism. *AJR Am J Roentgenol* 2005;185:135.
43. Spuentrup E, Katob M, et al. Molecular magnetic resonance imaging of pulmonary emboli with a fibrin-specific contrast agent. *Am J Respir Crit Care Med* 2005;172:494.
44. Roy P, Colombet I, et al. Systematic review and meta-analysis of strategies for the diagnosis of suspected pulmonary embolism. *BMJ* 2005;331:259.
45. Crapo RO, Morris AH, Gardner RM. Reference spirometric values using techniques and equipment that meet ATS recommendations. *Am Rev Respir Dis* 1981;123:859.
46. Mendella LA, Manfredi J, Warren CPW, et al. Steroid response in stable chronic obstructive pulmonary disease. *Ann Intern Med* 1982;96:17.
47. Stempel DA, Redding GJ. Management of acute asthma. *Pediatr Clin North Am* 1992;39:1311.
48. National Asthma Education and Prevention Program. *Expert panel report 2*. Bethesda, MD: National Institute of Health, Publication No. 97–405, April 1997.
49. Spitzer WO, Suissa S, Ernst P, et al. The use of beta-agonists and the risk of death and near death from asthma. *N Engl J Med* 1992;326:501.
50. Wong CS, Pavord ID, Williams J, et al. Bronchodilator, cardiovascular, and hypokalaemic effects of fenoterol, salbutamol, and terbutaline in asthma. *Lancet* 1990;336:1396.
51. Burrows B, Lebowitz MD. The beta-agonist dilemma. *N Engl J Med* 1992;326:560.
52. Poynter D. Fatal asthma–Is treatment incriminated? *J Allergy Clin Immunol* 1987;80:423.
53. Tashkin DP, Ashutosh K, Bleecker ER, et al. Comparison of the anticholinergic bronchodilator ipratropium bromide with metaproterenol in chronic obstructive pulmonary disease. *Am J Med* 1986;81:81.
54. Marlin GE, Bush DE, Berent N. Comparison of ipratropium bromide and fenoterol in asthma and chronic bronchitis. *Br J Clin Pharmacol* 1978;6:547.
55. Braun SR, Levy SF. Comparison of ipratropium bromide and albuterol in chronic obstructive lung disease: a three-center study. *Am J Med* 1991;21:28S.
56. Kamada AK, Szefler SJ, Martin RJ, et al. Issues in the use of inhaled glucocorticoids. *Am J Respir Crit Care Med* 1996;153:1739–1748.
57. Wrenn K, Slovis CM, Murphy F, et al. Aminophylline therapy for acute bronchospastic disease in the emergency room. *Ann Intern Med* 1991;115:241.
58. Gourgoulianisk KI, Chatziparasidis G, et al. Magnesium as a relaxing factor of airway smooth muscles. *J Aerosol Med* 2001;14:301.
59. Rowe B, Britzlaff J, Bourdan C, et al. Magnesium sulfate for treating exacerbations of acute asthma in the emergency department. *Cochrance Database Syst Rev* 2000;(2):CED0011490.
60. Pratter MR, Bartter T, Akers S, et al. An algorithmic approach to chronic cough. *Ann Intern Med* 1993;119:977.
61. Irwin RS, Baumann MN, Bolser DC, et al. Diagnosis and management of cough: ACCP evidence-based clinical practice guidelines. *Chest* 2006;129:1S–292S.
62. Fuller RW, Jackson DM. Physiology and treatment of cough. *Thorax* 1990;45:425.
63. Shuttair MF, Braun SR. Contemporary management of chronic persistent cough. *Mo Med* 1992;89:795.
64. Cowcher K, Hank GW. Long-term management of respiratory symptoms in advanced cancer. *J Pain Symptom Manage* 1990;5:320.

65. Poe RH, Israel RH, Utell MJ, et al. Chronic cough: bronchoscopy or pulmonary function testing? *Am Rev Respir Dis* 1982;126:160.
66. Irwin RS, Curley FJ, French CL. Chronic cough. *Am Rev Respir Dis* 1990;141:640.
67. Irwin RS, Curley FJ. The treatment of cough. A comprehensive review. *Chest* 1991;99:1477.
68. Pratter M. Chronic upper airway cough syndrome secondary to rhino sinus diseases. *Chest* 2006;129:635–715.
69. Irwin RS, Curley FJ, Bennett FM. Appropriate use of antitussives and protussives. A practical review. *Drugs* 1993;46:80.
70. Smith MB, Feldman W. Over-the-counter cold medications. A critical review of clinical trials between 1950 and 1991. *JAMA* 1993;269:2258.
71. Levy MH, Catalano RB. Control of common physical symptoms other than pain in patients with terminal disease. *Semin Oncol* 1985;12:411.
72. Puolijoki H, Lahdensuo A. Causes of prolonged cough in patients referred to a chest clinic. *Ann Med* 1989;21:425.

CHAPTER 28 ■ MANAGEMENT OF ADVANCED LUNG DISEASE INCLUDING PLEURAL AND PERICARDIAL EFFUSIONS

JOHN C. RUCKDESCHEL AND DARROCH W. O. MOORES

One of the most common, troubling problems for the patient with cancer is the development of a malignant effusion in any body cavity. When it occurs in the pleural cavity or the pericardium, this abnormal accumulation of fluid may cause severe symptoms or may even be life threatening. Although the development of a malignant pleural or pericardial effusion almost always indicates that the patient has incurable cancer, prompt recognition and diagnosis followed up by appropriate treatment can result in excellent palliation and a marked improvement in the patient's quality of life. In addition, it is critical that an accurate diagnosis is made to establish the malignant cause of the effusion, because patients with cancer can often develop an effusion from a benign cause such as radiation therapy, infection, chemotherapy, or heart failure.

PLEURAL EFFUSIONS

Incidence

In a general hospital patient population, 28–61% of all pleural effusions are malignant; the highest incidence is in the over-50 age-group (1–4). A malignant pleural effusion is the initial manifestation of cancer in 10–50% of patients (4,5). Eventually, about half of all patients with disseminated cancer develop a malignant pleural effusion (4). Overall, this is a highly significant clinical problem, resulting in approximately 100,000 malignant pleural effusions annually in the United States (6). Table 28.1 lists the frequency of the various tumor types that are associated with malignant pleural effusions. The tumor origin is not found in 15% of effusions. In such cases, the cell type is usually metastatic adenocarcinoma with the primary site unknown.

The appearance of a symptomatic, malignant, pleural effusion in a patient with known cancer significantly alters his or her quality of life. Although it is reported that up to 25% of patients with an effusion are asymptomatic, this may prove to be an overestimate if a careful history is elicited (7). In general, a prompt diagnosis accompanied by timely treatment of the effusion can markedly enhance the patient's functional status and should be considered early after the development of this common complication of advanced cancer.

Etiology and Pathophysiology

The pleura is a serous membrane that invests each lung to form a closed sac called the *pleural cavity*. There is a continuous passage of an almost protein-free fluid (protein content, 1.5 g per dL) through the pleural membrane that is attributable primarily to hydrostatic and colloid osmotic pressures. The net pressure in the parietal pleura is 9 cm H_2O, favoring movement of fluid into the pleural cavity, which is balanced with a net 10 cm H_2O pressure in the visceral pleura, favoring absorption of pleural fluid by the visceral capillaries. Therefore, the overall direction of movement of fluid is from the systemic circulation in the parietal pleura across the pleural cavity back into the pulmonary circulation in the visceral pleura. At any point of time, either pleural cavity has only 2–5 mL of fluid present, although as much as 5–10 L flow through this space in any 24-hour period (8,9). Any imbalance in these pressures that disturbs the normal equilibrium may lead to a net accumulation of fluid in the pleural cavity.

Traditionally, it has been held that the normal equilibrium may be interrupted, leading to the accumulation of an effusion. Some of the changes that may occur include the following:

- Increased capillary permeability due to inflammation from infection or tumor cell implantation
- Increased oncotic pressure of fluid in the pleural space due to inflammatory reaction from tumor cells or infection
- Decreased systemic oncotic pressure due to hypoalbuminemia from malnutrition
- Increased negative intrapleural pressure due to atelectasis, possibly because of tumor obstructing a bronchus
- Increased hydrostatic pressure in the pulmonary circulation, such as in congestive heart failure from cardiac or pericardial metastases

In addition, a malignant effusion may result from obstruction of the visceral or parietal lymphatic channels by tumor or radiation fibrosis (or a combination thereof), resulting in impaired absorption. Most malignant effusions are probably the result of a combination of factors, with an overall increase in fluid production and a decrease in absorption (3,10,11).

More recently, the role of vascular hyperpermeability as mediated by vascular endothelial growth factor (VEGF) has

TABLE 28.1

TUMOR CAUSES OF MALIGNANT PLEURAL EFFUSIONS FROM COLLECTED SERIES

Tumor type	Incidence (%)
Lung	35
Breast	23
Lymphoma/leukemia	10
Adenocarcinoma, unknown primary	12
Reproductive tract	6
Gastrointestinal tract	5
Genitourinary tract	3
Primary unknown	3
Other cancers	5

From Hausheer FH, Yarbro JW. Diagnosis and treatment of malignant pleural effusion. *Semin Oncol* 1985;12:54–75, with permission.

received increasing attention. Fidler's group at M. D. Anderson has demonstrated that pleural invasion by malignant cells expressing VEGF messenger ribonucleic acid (mRNA) is required for production of malignant effusions and that the effusions (but not tumor growth) could be abrogated by transfection of the cells with an antisense VEGF (12). PTK 787, a compound that blocks VEGF receptor tyrosine kinase phosphorylation (among other receptor tyrosine kinases), leads to reduced pleural fluid formation but not to reduced proliferation of the tumor cells (13). Several investigators have described increased levels of VEGF in the fluid of patients with malignant effusions (14–19) and the presence of increased FLT-1 VEGF receptors (fms-like tyrosine kinase receptor of VEGF) on mesothelial cells (15). A Dutch group has demonstrated that antibodies against VEGF or SU5416, a small molecule tyrosine kinase inhibitor, can also block production of both pleural and peritoneal fluid accumulation *in vitro* (20). Some studies have shown that VEGF levels can distinguish benign and malignant effusions (14–16) but there is some overlap seen (18). Although still in an early phase of understanding, the role of vascular hyperpermeability may explain why some agents that do not induce brisk fibrosis in the pleural space may still be useful in the treatment of malignant effusions (21).

Pleural effusions caused by malignancy usually result in an exudate with a high-protein content, although rare exceptions have been reported (1,5). However, transudative effusions (low protein) may occur as the indirect result of an advanced cancer, as in the patient with malnutrition and hypoalbuminemia, congestive heart failure due to cardiac failure, or liver disease secondary to metastases (3).

Clinical Presentation

The most critical initial step in evaluating the patient with a suspected malignant pleural effusion is to take a complete history and perform a careful physical examination. This simple step will usually exclude other causes of an effusion, such as heart failure or infection.

The clinical presentation of a malignant pleural effusion is almost always related to collapse of lung from the increased pleural fluid and the resulting initial symptom of exertional dyspnea. Later, resting dyspnea and orthopnea develop as the effusion increases in volume. A dry, nonproductive cough, a sense of heaviness in the chest, and occasionally pleuritic chest pain are also experienced. Nevertheless, an occasional patient

(<25%) will appear completely asymptomatic in the face of a significant effusion (11).

The physical findings of a malignant pleural effusion often include dullness to percussion of the affected hemithorax, decreased vocal fremitus, decreased breath sounds, egophony, and no demonstrable diaphragmatic excursion. Rarely, a very large effusion will result in a mediastinal shift with contralateral tracheal deviation and possibly even plethora or cyanosis from partial caval obstruction (3,7). Other signs and symptoms may be present initially but are usually related to the underlying primary tumor and not the effusion.

Diagnosis

The approach to the diagnosis and subsequent treatment of a patient with a suspected malignant pleural effusion is shown in Figure 28.1.

The initial screening consists of the posterior–anterior chest radiograph, including decubitus views, which will confirm the presence of free pleural fluid and will also suggest the presence of any loculated fluid. An upright posterior–anterior chest radiograph that demonstrates blunting of the costophrenic angle will detect 175–500 mL of fluid, whereas a decubitus view will show as little as 100 mL (22).

Computed tomography (CT) scan may play a role in the evaluation of patients with malignant pleural effusion. This is especially necessary if the hemithorax is opaque on chest radiograph, when a mesothelioma is suspected, or when the underlying primary tumor is unknown. However, a large effusion often obscures an underlying tumor in the lung, and CT scan may prove more useful after drainage of the effusion and lung re-expansion. Occasionally, chest ultrasonography may prove useful in differentiating between pleural fluid and pleural thickening (23), but its more common application is to localize small effusions to guide in thoracentesis (24).

After confirmation of a pleural effusion radiographically and after exclusion of any obviously nonmalignant causes, the next step is a diagnostic thoracentesis. In general, when a malignant effusion is suspected, only a small amount of fluid is withdrawn for diagnosis (at least 250 mL is needed for cytology). If the patient is symptomatic, enough fluid should be removed, slowly, to relieve symptoms but the chest should not be drained dry. Leaving a moderate amount behind makes insertion of a chest drainage tube easier.

The use of a disposable thoracentesis kit with a specially designed multihole catheter is preferred, because it tends to lessen the chance of complications such as a pneumothorax. Rapid removal of a large amount of fluid, especially over 1500 mL, is not advised, because this may result in life-threatening re-expansion pulmonary edema, a real and not infrequent complication of large-volume thoracenteses (25).

The fluid removed should be heparinized and sent to the lab for protein and lactic acid dehydrogenase (LDH) determinations and cytology. Other tests, including pH determination (for which the fluid must be collected in an anaerobic container), glucose level, cell count, and cultures with smears, are often obtained, although they are not necessary. With a malignant pleural effusion, the pH and glucose level are often low, but these are nonspecific findings (3). A malignant effusion is frequently hemorrhagic (erythrocyte count >100,000 per mm^3), but this is also nonspecific and occurs in only one third of cases (5). The Health and Public Policy Committee of the American College of Physicians has demonstrated that elevated levels of LDH or protein in the fluid and ratios of fluid to concurrent serum levels of LDH and protein are all that are required for the distinction of a transudate from an exudate (Table 28.2) (26). If the fluid is found to be a transudate, then malignancy is essentially excluded. An exudate

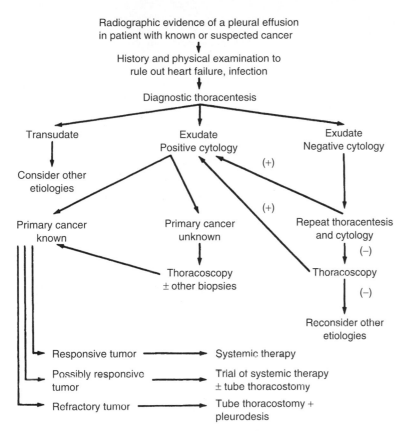

FIGURE 28.1. Approach to the diagnosis and treatment of malignant pleural effusions. +, study result is positive; —, study result is negative. (From Ruckdeschel JC. Management of malignant pleural effusion: an overview. *Semin Oncol* 1988;15:24–28, with permission.)

with a negative cytology result demands a second diagnostic thoracentesis with cytology, which will add approximately 6–11% more malignant diagnoses (3).

Cytology is the best method of diagnosing a malignant pleural effusion, although it is somewhat dependent upon tumor type, the experience of the cytopathologist, and the amount of fluid that is sent for cytologic analysis; at least 250 mL is preferred for the best yield (27). In patients with an effusion eventually proved to be malignant, the first cytology result will be positive in 53–59% of cases, rising to 65% when a second thoracentesis is performed (3). In some tumors, such as Hodgkin's disease, the rate of positive cytology results is relatively low at 23%, while with others, such as breast or lung cancer, the diagnosis rate is as high as 73% (3). A variety of immunocytochemical staining techniques and,

TABLE 28.2

DIAGNOSTIC TESTS CONFIRMING THE PRESENCE OF AN EXUDATE

Test	Positive predictive value (%)
1. Fluid LDH >200 international units	100
2. Fluid/blood LDH ratio >0.6	99
3. Fluid protein >3 g/dL	95
4. Fluid/blood protein ratio >0.5	99
(1), (2), or (4) above	99

LDH, lactic acid dehydrogenase.
Reprinted from Health and Public Policy Committee, American College of Physicians. Diagnostic thoracentesis and pleural biopsy in pleural effusions. *Ann Intern Med* 1985;103:799–802, with permission.

recently, cytogenetic markers have been added to complement the standard cytologic techniques. These methods have resulted in some increased diagnostic yield, although they often lack sensitivity and specificity, and also the laboratory expense is increased (3,10). We do not recommend using these tests outside of a clinical trial.

If the result of cytologic examination was negative, traditionally a blind pleural biopsy has been attempted, with some expectation of increased diagnostic yield. Although a blind biopsy may be a sensitive test in pleural tuberculosis because of its diffuse involvement, malignancies involving the pleura are commonly patchy in distribution, and a blind pleural biopsy usually adds little to the diagnosis. Although earlier series suggest that the pleural biopsy may be valuable in diagnosing malignancy in a patient with negative cytology results (3), a more recent direct comparison of pleural fluid cytology versus blind pleural biopsy casts doubt on its benefit. In this important series (28), cytology results were diagnostic of cancer in 71% of cases and suggestive in another 8%. Blind biopsy of the pleura gave positive results for malignancy in 45% of cases but provided a diagnosis in only 3% of cases where the cytology result was nondiagnostic.

Therefore, if two exudative pleural fluid cytology results are negative for malignancy, most clinicians now bypass the blind pleural biopsy and move promptly to video-assisted thoracoscopy (VATS), wherein visually directed pleural biopsies are readily obtained and the diagnostic yield is quite high. In large series, the diagnostic sensitivity of VATS with malignant pleural effusion is 97% (29). Although VATS is a surgical procedure usually requiring general anesthesia, the mortality and morbidity is quite low at 0.5% and 4.7%, respectively (30).

In addition to providing a high diagnostic yield of malignancy by directed biopsies during VATS, this procedure, when the ipsilateral lung is collapsed and the patient is under general anesthesia, permits direct definitive therapeutic intervention with lysis of adhesions, mechanical pleurodesis, pleurectomy, or talc poudrage, with a very low recurrence rate (31). Finally, when the fluid cytology result is positive but the primary site is unknown, VATS may be employed occasionally to obtain a larger amount of tissue for more definitive studies or to rule out the presence of a mesothelioma, especially when "adenocarcinoma, unknown primary" is the working diagnosis according to cytology. The advent of VATS has virtually eliminated the need for diagnostic open thoracotomy when a malignant effusion is suspected.

Prognosis

Once the diagnosis of a malignant pleural effusion has been made, the choice of therapy must be put in perspective with respect to the extent of the tumor, the condition of the host, and the prognosis. Virtually all of these patients have an incurable disease, so the treatment must be aimed at the most effective palliation for maximal, comfortable time outside of the hospital. For all patients, the overall mean survival time is 3–6 months. The mortality is as high as 54% at 1 month and rises to 84% at 6 months (11,32,33). Some malignant effusion patients with responsive tumors, such as breast cancer, may have a longer survival averaging 7–15 months (11); 20% have a 3-year survival (32). Ovarian cancer patients with a malignant effusion also have a longer expected mean survival of 9 months (23). Conversely, patients with lung cancer have a worse prognosis, with a mean survival of 2 months, and 66% will die by 3 months (11).

Treatment

Systemic Therapy

When the effusion is small and asymptomatic and the tumor is likely to be sensitive to systemic therapy, as with lymphoma, leukemia, breast cancer, ovarian cancer, small cell lung cancer, or germ cell tumors, the first line of therapy should be systemic chemotherapy or hormonal therapy, preceded by a "therapeutic" thoracentesis if the patient is symptomatic (7,10). When the tumor is relatively chemoresistant or has been shown to be so in the past, as with non–small cell lung cancer or pancreatic cancer, the choice then is for prompt tube thoracostomy followed up by intrapleural therapy if the patient has a reasonable life expectancy. In instances where the patient's outlook and performance status are poor, simple prolonged drainage by an indwelling catheter may be more appropriate.

Thoracentesis Alone

Thoracentesis alone may relieve symptoms briefly, but the fluid usually reaccumulates rapidly. In a study of 94 patients, the mean time for reaccumulation of the pleural effusion after thoracentesis was 4.2 days, and 97% had a recurrence of the fluid by 1 month (34). In addition, repeated thoracenteses carry the risk of empyema, pneumothorax, trapped lung from inadequate drainage and loculation of fluid, and the real possibility of progressive malnutrition from repeated removal of a large amount of the high-protein effusion fluid.

Radiation Therapy

Radiation therapy may occasionally be useful as primary therapy, but this is the case only when it is directed at paramalignant effusions caused by mediastinal lymphadenopathy and lymphatic obstruction. Improvement is uncommonly seen before 3 weeks, and therefore radiation has little application in the more acute symptomatic effusion.

Tube Thoracostomy Alone

Tube thoracostomy alone has been proposed as "effective" therapy for malignant effusions (3). But review of the results demonstrates that none of these older studies reliably supports the conclusion that chest tube drainage alone is efficacious in long-term control (3). Tube thoracostomy does appear quite useful in draining the pleural cavity and maintaining opposition of the pleural surfaces when a therapeutic agent is subsequently instilled into the chest for sclerotherapy.

Chronic Indwelling Chest Catheters

Soft silastic indwelling catheters can easily be placed under local anesthesia. Once placed, the patient or caregiver drains the pleural space periodically by connecting the catheter to a suction canister to provide relief from dyspnea or symptoms of pressure. When used long term (>6 weeks), these catheters can achieve spontaneous pleurodesis between 40 and 46% of the time (35–37). This rate of pleurodesis is substantially lower than that seen with a number of sclerosing agents (see subsequent text) but the catheters can be used in the setting of loculated effusions where sclerotherapy is not attainable. Results of treatment with the silastic catheter were compared with those obtained from chest tube drainage and sclerosis with doxycycline in 148 patients with malignant pleural effusion. Overall relief of symptoms and success rate were comparable in the two groups (37). The advantage for the silastic catheter group was the shortened hospitalization: 1 day versus 6.5 days, but the major disadvantage is the requirement that the catheter must stay in place for an extended period of time and may, therefore, not be well tolerated by the patient.

Recently, some enthusiasm has been expressed for the use of small-bore (8 French or 12 French) catheters for gravity drainage or even suction drainage of the pleural cavity followed by intracavitary sclerotherapy. The long-term results of this technique are still undetermined, although the selection of patients with free-flowing effusions can enhance the outcome significantly (38). These small-bore catheters can rapidly become occluded from debris and fibrin clots, and effective suction can usually be maintained in the pleural cavity for only a few hours. If, as per the general opinion, the visceral and parietal pleurae should be kept in direct opposition for a day or two after instillation of the sclerosing agent to obtain a pleurodesis, then it is unlikely that these small catheters will be as successful as larger chest tubes.

To achieve the best palliation, the pleural cavity should be drained completely and the lung fully expanded. This is best accomplished by closed tube thoracostomy. A no. 24 French or 28 French chest tube is usually inserted in the sixth or seventh interspace in the midaxillary line with the tube directed posterior to the lung to maximize drainage. Generally, the patient is given 3–6-mg morphine sulfate intravenously just before the procedure, to reduce pain and allay anxiety. The patient is positioned supine but turned up with the appropriate side of the chest elevated at 45–60 degrees, with the physician standing behind the patient. A brief thoracentesis is always performed first at the planned pleural entrance interspace to make sure that there is free aspiration of fluid. If no fluid is obtained, the chest tube entrance site must be altered to a place where fluid is readily obtained by thoracentesis. A small 2–3-cm skin incision is made 1.0–1.5 interspaces below the target interspace, and a subcutaneous tunnel is created bluntly with a clamp. Once the tube is inserted to a predetermined depth based on numerical markings on the tube itself, it is firmly sutured into place to the skin with heavy silk suture (0-silk or larger). The tube is then attached to an underwater seal drainage device at approximately 20 cm H_2O suction. If there is a very large effusion, all of it should not be drained immediately. Instead, 1000–1500 mL should be drained initially, and then the tube should be clamped for 30–60 minutes, draining approximately 1000 mL every 60 minutes until the chest is completely empty. More rapid drainage of a large pleural effusion encourages the development of the life-threatening problem of re-expansion pulmonary edema, a real and preventable phenomenon (25). Although some physicians use a trocar chest tube, the risks of laceration of the lung or even the heart or diaphragm are significant.

Chest radiographs are obtained immediately following the procedure and then daily as long as the tube is in place. The chest tube is left on suction for total drainage of the effusion and to encourage re-expansion of all possible lung. When a properly positioned chest tube is completely open and is on suction, essentially all of the fluid that is drainable will have drained within a few hours of insertion and certainly after overnight drainage. Likewise, all portions of the lung that are expandable and are not trapped will have expanded after overnight suction. Although some authors suggest waiting an indefinite period of time until the chest tube drainage has decreased to an arbitrary 100 mL per 24 hours (10), waiting this extra time is probably not necessary and may even lessen the chance of success. The prolonged presence of the tube irritating the pleural cavity may encourage loculations and lessen the eventual distribution and effectiveness of the sclerosing agent. Therefore, the decision when to instill the intracavitary agent should rest on the appearance of the chest radiograph and not the daily drainage. Usually, the best time to instill the sclerosing agent is the day after chest tube insertion.

Fibrinolytic Agents

If the chest radiograph taken the day after chest tube insertion shows apparent residual fluid, and especially if the fluid is thick or gelatinous, it may be worthwhile to try intrapleural instillation of urokinase 100,000 units in 100 mL 0.9% saline, clamping of the tube for 6 hours, and then resumption of suction for another 24 hours (39). This technique has been reported to improve drainage and lung expansion in loculated empyemas as well as with loculated malignant effusions with no side effects or systemic effects on coagulation or fibrinolysis (39,40).

Pleural Sclerotherapy

By far, the most common palliative treatment of malignant pleural effusions is drainage of the pleural space with re-expansion of the lung, followed by instillation of a chemical agent into the pleural cavity. It has been thought that the treatment works by causing a pleuritis designed to create a symphysis between the visceral and parietal pleurae (also called *pleurodesis by sclerotherapy*) to prevent reaccumulation of fluid in this space. As noted in the following text, this may not be the mechanism by which many sclerosing agents work, but rather it is their impact on production of various cytokines that impact on vascular permeability.

The most commonly used method to drain the effusion is with a chest tube, as described earlier (see the section Tube Thoracostomy). The complete drainage of the chest and full re-expansion of the lung are the major predictors of success. Another apparent determinant of the success in pleural sclerosis is the glucose level and the pH of the pleural effusion. Several authors have found that a low glucose level (<60 mg per dL) and pH (<7.20) in the malignant effusion result in a higher recurrence rate after attempted chemical pleurodesis as well as an overall shortened patient survival (41,42). Although interesting, the exact significance of these isolated reports is uncertain and probably should not influence the choice of agent or techniques employed.

Controversy abounds as to which is the most effective chemical sclerosing agent for malignant pleural effusions.

Comparison of the many published reports on various agents is often difficult because of the difference in reporting response rates, patient criteria, side effects, methods of evaluating results, and follow-up. The most widely followed set of guidelines to analyze results in the literature were those published by Hausheer and Yarbro (3). Many investigators have challenged whether the concept of complete and partial responses is relevant to the evaluation of pleurodesis (7). However, we believe that a simpler and more accurate means of assessing therapeutic efficacy is to follow the time to recurrence by comparing the chest radiograph taken before and after pleurodesis and removal of the chest tube. In many instances, the pleural effusion recurs or progresses, but re-treatment is not indicated because the patient has progressive disease elsewhere. For assessment of therapeutic efficacy, these cases still need to be counted as "failures." On the other hand, whether the progression is clinically meaningful—that is, needs re-treatment—is a significant issue in cost-effectiveness studies.

Mechanism of sclerosis. The mechanism of action of sclerosing agents appears to vary somewhat depending on the type of agent and the laboratory model tested. One of the earliest studies (43) employed the rabbit as the test animal and found that the pH of the solution instilled into the pleural cavity appeared to be an important determinant of success. The most acidic solutions tested, including unbuffered tetracycline (the most acidic being pH 2.5), were quite effective in creating a small polymorphonuclear-predominant effusion and resulted in complete pleural symphysis on postmortem examination of the animals. Other agents with higher, more neutral pHs, such as nitrogen mustard and quinacrine, had no significant effect on the rabbit pleurae in this study. However, a later study by the same group (44) using the same model but adding bleomycin and sodium hydroxide to the series test agents found that the pleural sclerosing effect was actually independent of pH and was more related to the increasing dosage of tetracycline, the only agent causing a pleural sclerosis in this model.

Clinical studies in humans have shown a significant discrepancy and lack of correlation with animal studies in the efficacy of sclerosing agents such as bleomycin. It has been demonstrated that bleomycin and even nitrogen mustard are highly effective in humans (3) despite the complete lack of effect in the rabbit model. Traditionally, it has been held that the rabbit model is of little relevance because of these discrepancies. It is possible that we are examining the measure of a wrong outcome. The presence or absence of pleural fibrosis (and all of its molecular findings such as a marked rise in basic fibroblast growth factor after talc pleurodesis (21)) may in fact be an epiphenomenon. If the full role of VEGF and related compounds is better elucidated, it may well be that the balance of permeability enhancing and suppressing factors caused by variations in tumor, inflammatory response, and "sclerosing" agent is, in fact, the key determinant in measuring the outcome of various clinical interventions. The various "sclerosing" agents and laboratory measures (e.g., pH and white blood cell count) will then need to be reassessed.

Technique of pleural sclerotherapy. The most common technique used to instill the sclerosing agent into the pleural cavity has developed primarily from convention and common usage (3,45–47) and not on the basis of rigorous studies. After complete drainage of the pleural cavity with a chest tube and re-expansion of the lung on suction, the tube is clamped and the patient is placed into the lateral decubitus position with the affected hemithorax upward to assure that all of the sclerosing agent initially drains into the chest. Most clinicians will administer a parenteral narcotic, such as morphine 3–6 mg, intravenously 10 minutes before the procedure to minimize the potential and unpredictable pain of the chosen sclerosing agent. Approximately 150-mg lidocaine (15 mL of a 1% solution without epinephrine) is instilled initially into the pleural cavity through the chest tube using a Luer-lock syringe and 22-gauge needle. It is allowed to remain for several minutes as local analgesia. The sclerosing agent dissolved in 50–100 mL 0.9% saline is then injected into the chest tube, and the tube is left clamped for 2 hours. The use of talc slurry requires a slightly different technique using a bulb syringe and a saline flush (48).

Usually the patient is then turned and repositioned every 15 minutes during the 2 hours to assure even distribution of the agent throughout the pleural cavity. However, when this patient repositioning maneuver was investigated carefully in a comparative clinical study, rotation of the patient during the time the chest tube was clamped offered no significant benefit to the success of the attempted pleurodesis (47). After 2 hours, the chest tube is unclamped and the tube is placed back on suction. The patient is followed up with daily chest radiographs to verify continued complete drainage of the pleural cavity. The chest tube is removed when the daily drainage drops to 100 mL or less (49) (or <50 mL per 8 hours), and the patient is discharged the same day, once a confirmatory radiograph has been taken after removal of the chest tube. Most physicians create a moderately long subcutaneous tunnel (1.0–1.5 interspaces) through which the chest tube is initially inserted, so that with tube removal the wound seals well without the need (and discomfort) for placing sutures to close the skin wound.

Sclerosing agents. Historically, a wide variety of agents have been instilled into the pleural space to create a pleurodesis (3,7). Table 28.3 lists most of the agents that have been described in the literature. These agents have differed greatly as to their effectiveness, side effects, availability, and even cost. Many are of only historical interest, whereas others, such as talc, bleomycin, and doxycycline, are in common use.

TABLE 28.3

INTRAPLEURAL SCLEROSING AGENTS

Tetracycline
Doxycycline
Minocycline
Bleomycin
Talc
Quinacrine
Nitrogen mustard
Doxorubicin
Radioisotopes (I-131, Y-90, P-32, AU-198)
Mitoxantrone
Corynebacterium parvum
Bacille Calmette-Guérin cell wall skeleton
OK432 (streptococcal preparation)
Silver nitrate
Eosinophil colony-stimulating factor
Interleukin-2
Thiotepa
5-Fluorouracil
Autologous blood
Cisplatin
Cytarabine
Mechlorethamine
Pirarubicin
Carboplatin
Mustine
Mepacrine
α, β, or γ interferon collagen

I-131, iodine 131; Y-90, yttrium-90; P-32, phosphorus-32; AU-198, gold-198.

TABLE 28.4

MALIGNANT PLEURAL EFFUSIONS: RESPONSE RATES OF CURRENTLY AVAILABLE THERAPY

Technique	Response rates (%)	
	Range	Mean
Tube thoracostomy alone	0–86	22
Tube thoracostomy drainage plus	—	—
Talc	72–100	96
Bleomycin	63–85	84
Tetracycline[a]	25–100	72
Doxycycline (30, 40)	73–95	84
Nitrogen mustard	27–95	44
Quinacrine	64–100	86
5-FU/Thiotepa	14–80	30
Doxorubicin (48)	18–24	24
Radioisotopes (AU-198, P-32, Y-90)	25–89	59
External radiation	—	—
Thoracoscopy with talc poudrage (32, 46–48)	87–95	92
Pleurectomy	88–100	98

5-FU, 5-fluorouracil; AU-198, gold-198; P-32, phosphorus-32; Y-90, yttrium-90.
[a]No longer clinically available after mid-1991; replaced with doxycycline.
From Hausheer FH, Yarbro JW. Diagnosis and treatment of malignant pleural effusion. *Semin Oncol* 1985;12:54–75, with permission.

Table 28.4 summarizes the efficacy of the most widely used sclerosing agents reported in the literature, comparing them with other methods of therapy designed to prevent the recurrence of malignant pleural effusions.

Tetracycline. As an agent for intrapleural sclerotherapy, tetracycline gained widespread acceptance and was preferred in the United States (49) and Europe (50). This agent demonstrated consistent efficacy, with a mean objective response (using the 1-g dose) of 69–85%, averaging 72% (3,45). It proved to be safe, effective, and quite inexpensive, and could be easily administered, with adverse reactions limited to fever (7–33%) and pain (17–62%) (3,30). Unfortunately, parenteral tetracycline is no longer commercially available.

Over the years, a variety of comparative clinical series, mostly nonrandomized, have been published with disparate methodology, patient selection, and response criteria, as well as retrospective analyses and variable results (3,45). Despite these limitations, most older studies comparing tetracycline with other agents such as nitrogen mustard, quinacrine, mustine, doxorubicin, bleomycin, and *Corynebacterium parvum* consistently demonstrated that tetracycline gave superior or at least equivalent results with much less toxicity (51). Of the few recent randomized larger trials, the series of Ruckdeschel et al. (52) and Johnson and Curzon (53) comparing intrapleural bleomycin and tetracycline showed a significantly better response to pleurodesis with bleomycin, with similar toxicity profiles. Nevertheless, tetracycline's ready availability and lower cost retained it as a preferred agent for pleurodesis of malignant effusions (49,50).

Doxycycline. Clinical studies with doxycycline have now accumulated, after the demise of parenteral tetracycline. Initially, most were nonrandomized trials (39,54–56). Doxycycline has consistently demonstrated effective results: response rates range from 73 to 95%, which is similar to those of bleomycin (Table 28.4). Its toxicity is similar to tetracycline and the pain on administration may be less. The 500-mg dosage of doxycycline empirically chosen for these preliminary studies was probably too low, because over one third of patients required repeat dosing for it to be effective (39). The major problem in using doxycycline, as noted in prior studies, is that it frequently requires several dosings for equal efficacy (57), and this seriously reduces its cost effectiveness because of the need for longer hospitalizations (58). Minocycline, another substitute for tetracycline, was reported in a small seven-patient study with results similar to tetracycline, and experience with this agent has been minimal.

Bleomycin. The most extensively studied cytotoxic chemotherapeutic agent used for intrapleural sclerotherapy is bleomycin. Not only does it play a significant role in the treatment of various solid tumors by parenteral administration, but also it has been shown to be highly effective in the palliative treatment of malignant pleural effusions, with response rates averaging 84% (3). Numerous nonrandomized studies have compared this agent with its primary competitor tetracycline, and most have suggested that there is no significant difference in efficacy or toxicity (51).

A few randomized trials of bleomycin versus tetracycline were performed, with varying results. Kessinger and Wigton (59), in their study of 41 patients, found no significant difference in the response rates using 89 units of bleomycin (67%) versus 500-mg tetracycline (61%), and both agents had similar toxicities. However, Ruckdeschel et al. (52), in their multi-institutional randomized study of 74 patients receiving either 60 units bleomycin or 1-g tetracycline intrapleurally, found the complete response rate at 1 month to be 64% (18/28) in the bleomycin arm and 33% (9/27) in the tetracycline arm. At 90 days, the complete response rate was 87% for bleomycin and 56% for tetracycline. Johnson and Curzon, in their randomized trial of 60 patients, found an 87% complete response rate at 90 days with bleomycin, compared with 56% with tetracycline (53). The acute toxicities of both drugs were similar, although there tended to be a higher incidence of pain in the tetracycline arm in both of the latter studies (52,53).

Although 45% of the intrapleural dose of bleomycin is absorbed (60), myelosuppression is not seen. However, since the plasma half-life of bleomycin increases with renal failure, systemic toxicity with alopecia and mucositis is possible and has rarely been reported in patients with renal failure (61). Therefore, caution is advised in using intrapleural bleomycin in patients with renal failure. Some have also recommended using the lower dose of 40 units per m^2 body surface area in the elderly because of their potential reduced plasma clearance of the drug (62).

The major disadvantage of bleomycin is its elevated cost in comparison with other agents such as doxycycline and talc. This has been the major impediment to its widespread use. However, if it proves to be a more effective agent resulting in reduced hospital stays, and if consistently only a single dose is required for sclerotherapy, the cost factor may be overcome and bleomycin may actually be less expensive overall. And it is important to remember that one additional hospital day would pay for any extra cost of this agent, if it is actually more efficient than less expensive agents.

D. K. Fuller (63) and Belani et al. (58) argue that bleomycin is more cost effective overall than talc, tetracycline, and doxycycline on the basis of their questionable *post hoc* comparative analyses of a variety of disparate clinical studies (often published many years apart) that commonly used inadequate doses of the test agent in the trials (i.e., 500-mg doxycycline instead of the current 1 g).

Talc

Talc insufflation. *Talc* is a generic term referring to a natural product containing the mineral talc (a trilayered

magnesium sheet silicate) found in talcose or soapstone, which is usually contaminated with chlorite and trace minerals (quartz, calcite, and dolomite) (64,65) The most important contaminant of talc is asbestos (fibers of actinolyte, amosite, anthophyllite, chrysolite, crocidolite, and tremolite), which has been linked to carcinogenesis. However, for clinical use, United States Pharmacopeia (USP) talc has been purified with particle sizes generally less than 50 μm. Most important, USP talc has been asbestos free for many years, although it still requires sterilization prior to use.

Talc is the oldest, cheapest, and perhaps the most effective agent in causing a pleurodesis. Talc was first used as a pleural sclerosant in 1935 by a Canadian surgeon, Norman Bethune, who insufflated talc into the pleural cavity of dogs and cats after creating a pneumothorax (66). After administration of talc, the resultant intense adhesive pleuritis, possibly accompanied by an adhesion-stimulating factor (64) obliterating the pleural space, is believed to be its primary clinical benefit in preventing the recurrence of malignant pleural effusions (65).

Insufflation of talc into the pleural cavity, or talc poudrage ("powdering"), is highly effective. Many studies demonstrate a response rate averaging 92% in malignant pleural effusions ranging from 87 to 95% (41,64,65,67). The primary disadvantage of talc poudrage is the requirement for thoracoscopy to be performed, usually with the patient under general anesthesia, to allow complete collapse of the lung to assure uniform distribution of the talc. An atomizer or bulb syringe is filled with dry talc, usually 2.5–5.0 g, and the talc is blown into the pleural cavity after ensuring that all loculations are removed. In select patients, the risks of this procedure are small, with low perioperative morbidity and mortality (64). However, many patients with malignant pleural effusions are debilitated and are poor candidates for an operative approach, or they are reluctant to have such a procedure because of their short life expectancy. In addition, thoracoscopic talc poudrage usually increases hospitalization time, adds surgical and anesthesia costs, and increases the potential for complications. Fortunately, several studies have suggested that similar results are possible with bedside talc slurry administration through a chest tube, obviating the need for the more invasive operative approach (3,48,68).

Talc slurry. Twenty-three years after the first described use of talc with an open thoracotomy, J. S. Chambers in 1958 reported the successful use of talc instilled through a tube thoracostomy to control a malignant pleural effusion (69). In subsequent studies (45,48,51,64,70), the administration of talc in a suspension or slurry has proved to be as efficacious as by poudrage (57,65,68), with response rates ranging from 72 to 100% and averaging 96% (3). The administration of talc slurry is generally performed at the bedside with 2–5-g of sterile USP talc suspended in 30–50-mL 0.9% saline solution in a bulb syringe instilled into a larger-bore chest tube after complete drainage of the pleural space.

Although the efficacy of talc is generally well recognized, concerns about its adverse effects and safety have slowed its use. The usual side effects reported are pain on administration in most patients (48), but this is readily manageable, as with other sclerosing agents. Fever also accompanies talc slurry administration 16–69% of the time, but it is usually short-lived (65). Talc empyema is reported in 0–11% of cases (65) and can be exceedingly difficult to treat effectively, because talc is a foreign body and cannot be removed from the site of infection: the pleural cavity.

However, more worrisome potential adverse effects are rare but can definitely occur, including talc microemboli to the brain (65); pulmonary complications of acute pneumonitis, pulmonary edema, and adult respiratory distress syndrome (71,72); and death (57,65). In the randomized trial, comparing talc poudrage to talc slurry (68), significant respiratory complications (14% vs. 6%) and death (8% vs. 4%), respectively, were seen, making this an uncommon but very significant toxicity. The definitive mechanism of respiratory complications is unknown, but it is probably related to the uptake of talc by the parietal pleural lymphatic system, with subsequent transport to the mediastinal lymph nodes and thoracic duct and hence to the systemic circulation. Talc administration has also been reported (65) to be associated with a variety of acute cardiovascular complications—arrhythmias, cardiac arrest, chest pain, myocardial infarction, and hypotension—but it is often difficult to attribute these effects specifically to the talc. Talc has also been compared with bleomycin (73,74), doxycycline (75), and silver nitrate (76) with talc usually performing somewhat better with respect to success of pleurodesis and somewhat worse with respect to side effects and severe toxicity.

A Cochrane Database Review (77) of 36 randomized trials of treatment for malignant pleural effusion demonstrated that pleurodesis was superior to tube drainage alone; that talc was the superior agent; and that talc administered by VATS was the most efficacious means of treatment. They did not detect an increased risk of death from talc (77).

Other Antineoplastic Agents

One of the first agents used intrapleurally to treat malignant effusions was the cytotoxic agent nitrogen mustard. This alkylating agent is highly reactive and loses its activity within minutes of contact with tissue. The response rates with nitrogen mustard varied greatly in various small series, from 27 to 95%, but averaged only 44% (3). When it was compared with other agents, the response rates were generally lower but the adverse reactions were much higher (3,45).

Many other chemotherapeutic agents have been described in various small series, including thiotepa, 5-fluorouracil, doxorubicin, combination cisplatin and cytarabine, etoposide, mitoxantrone, and mitomycin C (3,30,57). Generally, the results have been unimpressive and clearly are no better than those obtained with more common agents such as tetracycline or its derivatives or bleomycin (3). However, their systemic absorption by intrapleural administration is considerable and often leads to prolonged plasma levels and significant systemic toxicity, including myelosuppression. At present, the use of these agents in this context is investigational and is not generally recommended (10,30,57).

Biological Agents

Corynebacterium parvum. *Corynebacterium parvum* is an anaerobic gram-positive bacterium first described for intrapleural use to cause a pleurodesis in a trial in six patients in 1978 (78). *C. parvum* averaged response rates of 76% in single-agent studies but consistently demonstrated the same or worse response compared with bleomycin or tetracycline (46,57). *C. parvum* also has moderate toxicity, including fever (5%), pain (43%), cough (6%), and nausea (39%), and furthermore requires multiple instillations over a 2-day period. *C. parvum* offers no advantages as a pleural sclerosant and is also not available in the United States, resulting in its lack of current clinical use. Recently, staphylococcal super antigen has been tested as a sclerosant with promising activity, but results are preliminary (79).

Interferons and interleukins. The most recent attempt to use biological therapy for malignant pleural effusions involves the use of interferon-α, β, or γ with the intent to stimulate natural killer cells, in addition to their cytotoxic effects (57). The response rates have not been impressive, with only a 41% complete response in a series of 29 patients (80). Intrapleural administration of interferon is still in the investigational stage.

Several recent studies have investigated the use of recombinant interleukin-2 alone or in combination with lymphokine-activated killer cells in malignant pleural effusions from lung cancer (81,82). These preliminary studies have commonly shown the disappearance of the pleural effusion and occasionally the cancer cells themselves (82), but no serious side effects occurred. These studies are intriguing but require more study in larger patient groups.

Intrapleural radioisotopes. Finally, the use of intrapleural radioisotopes, especially radioactive gold and phosphorus, for control of malignant pleural effusions had a period of popularity beginning in 1951, when they were first described (83), until the late 1960s. The overall effectiveness of these agents was less than that of other available agents, with a mean response rate of 59% (3). The isotopes were also expensive and potentially hazardous to hospital personnel, patients needed to be isolated until the radioactive emissions were acceptably low, and special personnel and equipment were needed. Because of their relative ineffectiveness and their many disadvantages, radioisotopes are not currently recommended for pleural sclerotherapy and are of historical interest only (3).

Other agents. Recently, silver nitrate has been proposed as a sclerosing agent on the basis of animal models (79). In a randomized comparison to talc slurry, it appeared equally efficacious and of lesser toxicity (76).

Surgical Interventions

Pleurectomy. A thoracotomy with mechanical pleurodesis, or a pleurectomy to remove most of the parietal pleura, has occasionally been done in the past as a primary procedure for malignant effusions. Martini et al. (84) in 1975 reported the use of pleurectomy in 106 patients with malignant effusion and saw no recurrence in 100%, but there was a 9% mortality and a 23% rate of major complications: bleeding, air leaks, pneumonia, empyema, pulmonary embolus, respiratory insufficiency, and cardiac failure. Currently, this procedure should be considered for application only at the time of thoracotomy when a lung cancer is found to be unresectable with pleural metastases. Occasionally, a well-selected patient of good performance status and a long life expectancy, in whom all other attempts at control of the effusion have failed, might be considered a candidate for pleurectomy. The advent of videothoracoscopy now allows these procedures to be done, if necessary, in a minimally invasive manner, essentially making an open thoracotomy for this purpose a historical footnote.

Pleuroperitoneal shunt. Internal drainage of the malignant effusion into the abdomen using an implanted, valved, manually operated pump was initially described in 1984, with the most recent series reported in 1993 (85). Implantation of this device usually requires general anesthesia (occasionally, local anesthesia may be used in select patients) and the performance of a small thoracotomy and small celiotomy that are needed to implant the two limbs; the pump is implanted subcutaneously. Because the shunt must carry fluid from a negative-pressure area (the pleural cavity) to a positive-pressure area (the abdomen), major patient or family participation is necessary. For the shunt to function properly, manual pumping 100 times on five occasions per day is required. The shunt is occasionally an option in compliant, well-motivated patients with good performance status who have a trapped lung and an intractable effusion (5,10,46). Malfunction of the shunt over time, requiring its replacement, may further limit the usefulness of this device.

Videothoracoscopy. As experience with VATS grows, some investigators are now reporting series of successful VATS pleurectomy for malignant effusions. Waller et al. (86) performed a VATS parietal pleurectomy on 19 patients

(13 mesothelioma and 6 metastatic adenocarcinoma) with no operative deaths or major complications, and the median hospital discharge was on the fifth day. Another approach to VATS pleurectomy was described by Harvey et al. (87) that involved 11 selected patients with malignant pleural effusion, where they performed a parietal pleurectomy assisted by dissection of the pleura with a stream of water (hydrodissection). The effusion did not recur in any patient.

Another invasive technique. An innovative technique for approaching the lung cancer patient with pleural metastasis was described recently by Matsuzaki and associates (88). This approach took advantage of the antineoplastic effect of hyperthermia. The pleural cavity was irrigated using an extracorporeal circuit with a 43°C saline and *cis*-platinum solution for 2 hours in 12 patients with pleural metastases, who also underwent resection of their primary tumors. The pleural effusion was controlled in all 12 patients, and their median survival was 20 months, compared with 6 months in a cohort of seven matched control patients with pleural metastases. This report is preliminary but provocative, and the technique needs to be monitored as further work is reported.

Recurrent Effusions

The most perplexing and frustrating problem to deal with is the refractory pleural effusion in which the first attempt at pleural sclerotherapy has failed. In the past, a second attempt at tube thoracostomy followed up by intrapleural sclerotherapy was recommended, usually employing a different agent. If this second attempt failed, and if the patient had a good performance status and a reasonable estimated life span, then proceeding with VATS talc poudrage was considered an option. In most instances, the placement of a silastic catheter with prolonged external drainage has become the treatment of choice.

Recommendations

It is important to remember that the primary goal of therapy for a malignant pleural effusion is entirely palliative. The patient generally has a terminal disease with a very limited life span, usually counted in terms of a few months at best. The decision to treat and the actual treatment chosen must reflect the clinician's realistic understanding of the patient's overall prognosis and a desire to provide these terminally ill patients with the maximum possible comfortable time at home with the best quality of life. The timing of treatment is also critical. Waiting for "significant" symptoms to develop before draining a malignant effusion rarely improves the palliative benefits for the patient.

Our recommendations are as follows:

- In a patient with a chemosensitive tumor such as lymphoma, breast cancer, or small cell lung cancer, systemic therapy is the treatment of choice. If a thoracentesis is not needed for staging purposes, the patient can proceed directly to treatment if the effusion is asymptomatic, otherwise a therapeutic thoracentesis followed up by systemic treatment is preferred.
- In the patient with a less responsive or refractory solid tumor, all significant effusions should be drained and treated. We prefer standard chest tube drainage at present but await comparative data on small-bore catheters (89). Our choice of sclerosing agent is not clearly resolved, with bleomycin, doxycycline, and talc all having their proponents. Although the Cochrane analysis (77) demonstrates that talc poudrage at the time of thoracoscopy is the most effective at controlling effusions, it does not address cost-effectiveness issues and patient suitability for a surgical procedure. Our first choice is for a clinical trial.
- Talc is used whenever a second pleurodesis needs to be done for recurrent disease. Silastic catheter drainage has become the treatment of choice for loculated effusions or recurrent effusions in a patient with poor performance status. We almost never use pleuroperitoneal shunts.
- Our policy is increasingly moving to earlier use of thoracoscopy, in lieu of a second diagnostic thoracentesis. Being a cancer hospital the facilities for reducing adhesions, drawing the fluid, and initiating drainage all in one sitting are offered.

PERICARDIAL EFFUSIONS

Incidence

The appearance of a malignant pericardial effusion in patients with advanced cancer is not uncommon. In a collection of autopsy studies of patients with disseminated cancer, involvement of the heart and pericardium with metastatic malignancy is seen in up to 21% of cases (46,90–94), with the highest incidence occurring in patients with leukemia (69%), melanoma (64%), and lymphoma (24%) (94). Because a large number of patients with malignant pericardial effusions are asymptomatic, autopsy studies tend to have a higher incidence than in clinical series (95). In terms of the actual clinical impact of symptomatic pericardial effusions, there were 7000 patients who underwent pericardiectomy for all causes in US hospitals in 1993 (95). Generally, 25–50% of all patients requiring surgical pericardial drainage have proven malignant pericardial involvement (96–99). Because not all patients with a malignant pericardial effusion undergo a pericardiectomy, the total number of patients developing this complication of advanced cancer is much higher (100).

Etiology

Almost any tumor (except primary tumors of the brain) can metastasize to the pericardium and lead to an effusion (94). However, the most common tumors that involve the pericardium and heart are the same as with malignant pleural effusions: tumors of the lung and breast, lymphoma, and leukemia. These metastatic tumors account for almost 75% of all pericardial malignancies (101). When it metastasizes, melanoma frequently involves the heart, occurring in up to 50% of cases (100). Other malignancies that may spread to the pericardium to cause an effusion include gastrointestinal tumors and sarcomas. Primary tumors of the pericardium can cause effusions, but they are rare and include sarcomas, malignant teratomas, and mesotheliomas. Searching for the cause of a symptomatic pericardial effusion is critically important, because approximately 40% of patients with an underlying cancer have a nonmalignant cause of the effusion (100).

Pathophysiology

The pericardium, as it is commonly known, is actually the parietal pericardium. The visceral pericardium is a monocellular serosal layer constituting what is also known as the epicardium of the heart. Together, both pericardial layers constitute a serosal sac containing at any time 15–50 mL of low-protein fluid. The pericardium is flexible but relatively inelastic. It probably functions to mechanically protect the heart from outside friction, provide a barrier from inflammation, maintain cardiac position against gravitational forces and acceleration, and support the thinner heart chambers such as the atria and the right ventricle (101).

Like the pleurae, the fluid inside the pericardial sac is normally in a balanced steady state of secretion due to the serosal surface and reabsorption by the visceral (epicardium) and parietal pericardia. The increase in pericardial fluid that may lead to tamponade generally results from obstruction of the mediastinal lymphatic system, commonly by tumors, such as lung and breast cancers, that involve the mediastinal lymph nodes. Infiltration of the epicardium by tumor may block subepicardial venous flow, resulting in an outpouring of fluid into the pericardium. The parietal pericardium may also be infiltrated by tumor, resulting in increased fluid secretion. The result of blockage of pericardial fluid reabsorption, as well as often a net increase in secretion, may ultimately result in a symptomatic pericardial effusion (102,103). The role of VEGF or other growth factors modulating vascular permeability is unknown, with no reported series to date.

When fluid increases slowly, the pericardium will distend greatly, up to as much as 2 L, before the pericardium becomes tense. However, when the fluid accumulates more rapidly, the pericardium fails to stretch, pericardial pressure rises, and hemodynamic compromise may occur with as little an accumulation as 200 mL (104). The critical effect of this increase in pericardial pressure is impaired diastolic filling of the right side of the heart. The condition termed *cardiac tamponade* develops when there is "hemodynamically significant cardiac compression due to accumulating pericardial contents that evoke and defeat compensatory mechanisms" (105). On the basis of Starling's law, impaired diastolic filling will result in a depressed stroke volume and cardiac output. A greater volume of pericardial fluid and pressure causes an increase in ventricular diastolic pressure, which further impairs venous return, leading to a declining cardiac output. The autonomic nervous system responds to this decreased stroke volume and initially compensates by a release of catecholamines, resulting in an increased heart rate and arterial and venous vasoconstriction. The kidneys also respond to the decreased cardiac output by increasing sodium and fluid retention, leading to increased intravascular volume and venous pressure. Eventually, these compensatory mechanisms fail as intrapericardial pressure rises (often abruptly), resulting in a further decline in cardiac output with hypotension and circulatory collapse (104).

Clinical Presentation

Symptoms

Around two thirds of the patients with metastatic tumor involving the heart and pericardium will have no definite cardiovascular signs or symptoms (91), even when a careful history is taken. When the initial symptoms of a malignant pericardial effusion begin, they are often subtle and may be attributed to the underlying primary tumor. The actual development of symptoms depends on the rate at which the effusion accumulates, the actual effusion volume (and how close it is to causing maximal pericardial distention), and the underlying cardiac function, which itself may be impaired because of myocardial metastases or prior chemotherapy, as with doxorubicin (100,104). When the intrapericardial pressure increases sufficiently to impair diastolic ventricular filling, then symptoms begin to appear.

The most common and earliest symptom is dyspnea on exertion (93% of symptomatic patients), which may progress to dyspnea at rest as cardiac function is progressively compromised (91,100,105). Dyspnea is also the initial presenting symptom in patients with a malignant pleural effusion, a much more common complication of advanced cancer. A pleural effusion occasionally accompanies a malignant pericardial effusion, and this by itself may draw the attention away from the actual pericardial problem and confound the diagnosis. A comparison of the presenting signs and symptoms of pericardial and pleural effusions is found in Table 28.5 (90,105). Other common symptoms include chest pain or heaviness (63%), cough (30–43%), and weakness (26%) (94). Less common symptoms include peripheral edema, low-grade fever, dizziness, nausea, diaphoresis, and peripheral venous constriction. The presence of peripheral edema often leads unsuspecting clinicians to give diuretics, which significantly worsen the underlying physiologic problem. Cyanosis from decreased venous return and venous hypertension and agitation and tachypnea from low cardiac output and hypoxia are late manifestations of pericardial tamponade (100,104).

Signs

The classic signs associated with cardiac tamponade were described in 1937 by Claude Beck and are often referred to as *Beck's triad*: quiet heart sounds, hypotension, and venous distention (105). These signs remain the most commonly seen, although the muffled heart sounds may be more difficult to appreciate clinically. Unfortunately, all of these clinical signs appear late in the course of the physiologic deterioration. Therefore, waiting for them to develop before ordering diagnostic tests is inappropriate. Hypotension is found in 41–63% of patients, elevated venous pressure is seen in 50–63%, and resting tachycardia occurs in 68–89% (91). The venous pressure is almost always elevated in cardiac tamponade, although rarely it may be normal or low if the patient is hypovolemic. A central venous pressure greater than 15 mm Hg with hypotension is highly suggestive of tamponade.

The pathophysiologic effects of cardiac tamponade tend to exaggerate the normal fall in systolic blood pressure (usually less than 10 mm Hg) and stroke volume that occur with inspiration. The causes of this normal event are controversial but are thought to involve any or all of the following:

1. Inspiratory pooling of blood in the lungs with decreased filling of the left side of the heart
2. Increased right ventricular filling with leftward movement of the interventricular septum to cause reduced left ventricular filling and increased afterload
3. A fall in left ventricular stroke volume because of increased left ventricular transmural pressure
4. "Reverse thoracic pump" mechanism that is due to an inspiratory decrease of intracavitary left ventricular pressure relative to atmospheric pressure (104). Cardiac tamponade exaggerates this normal physiology and was termed by Kussmaul in 1873 as *pulsus paradoxus*. This term is a misnomer, because it refers to the accentuation of a normal phenomenon, not a reversal of it. Clinically, a patient is considered to have a pulsus paradoxus if the inspiratory drop in the systolic blood pressure is greater than 10 mm Hg. Although strongly associated with tamponade, a pulsus paradoxus may also be detected in other conditions such as pulmonary embolism, chronic obstructive lung disease, obesity, failure of the right side of the heart, and tense ascites.

Other signs, less frequent, that may be present include a narrowed pulse pressure, a visible increase in venous pressure on inspiration (Kussmaul's sign), hepatomegaly, hepatojugular reflux, peripheral edema, cyanosis, pericardial friction rub, arrhythmias, cold clammy extremities, low-grade fever, and ascites.

TABLE 28.5

COMPARISON OF THE PRESENTING SIGNS AND SYMPTOMS OF MALIGNANT
PLEURAL AND PERICARDIAL EFFUSIONS

Frequency	Pericardial	Pleural
Common	Dyspnea (exertion)	Dyspnea (exertion)
	Dyspnea (rest)	Dyspnea (rest)
	Chest pain or heaviness	Orthopnea
		Cough
	Cough	Percussion dullness
	Jugular venous distention	Egophony
		Percussion dullness
	Hypotension	
	Pulsus paradoxus	
	Resting tachycardia	
Uncommon	Cyanosis	Cyanosis
	Peripheral edema	Pleuritic chest pain
	Low-grade fever	Anorexia
	Distant heart sounds	
	Peripheral vasoconstriction	
	Narrowed pulse pressure	
	Kussmaul's sign	
	Low-voltage electrocardiogram (limb leads)	
	Electrical alternans	
	Hepatojugular reflux	
	Pleural effusion	

Adapted from Ruckdeschel JC. Malignant effusions in the chest. In: Kirkwood JM, Lotze MT, Yaska JM, eds. *Current cancer therapeutics*, 2nd ed. Philadelphia, PA: Churchill Livingstone, 1996:304–308, with permission.

Diagnosis

Radiographic

In a patient with cancer with or without symptoms, a change in the size and contour of the heart with clear lung fields on a standard chest radiograph should alert the clinician to consider the diagnosis of a pericardial effusion. The cardiac silhouette may resemble the so-called water-bottle heart with bulging of the normal contours. Nevertheless, a normal-size heart shadow does not exclude the presence of a pericardial effusion or even a life-threatening tamponade. A coexisting pleural effusion may be present in up to 70% of patients with pericardial effusion (91).

Chest CT scan obtained for staging or follow-up in a patient with cancer will reveal a pericardial effusion with more sensitivity than a standard chest radiograph (91). The chest CT scan may suggest a malignant pericardial process if the effusion has a high density, there is pericardial thickening, masses are contiguous with the pericardium, or there is an obliteration of the tissue planes between the mass and the heart. As a screening tool, however, chest CT scan has limited usefulness because of the blurring of the pericardial contents on the scan caused by continuous cardiac motion.

Another more invasive diagnostic procedure is catheterization of the right side of the heart, which can easily be done at the bedside in the intensive care unit. The passage of a flow-directed pulmonary artery catheter is a common critical care procedure that can establish the presence of a cardiac tamponade. The findings from this procedure in true tamponade are depressed cardiac output and the equalization of diastolic pressures in all heart chambers (105). Specifically, the right atrial mean, the right ventricular diastolic, and the pulmonary capillary wedge pressures all tend to equalize in tamponade and can be readily measured with the pulmonary artery catheter. However, if malignant pericardial effusion is suspected, catheterization of the right side of the heart is rarely necessary, because echocardiography is sensitive enough to establish a reliable diagnosis of tamponade noninvasively, thereby allowing for prompt pericardial decompression.

Electrocardiography

The electrocardiogram often has changes associated with a pericardial effusion, including tachycardia, atrial and ventricular arrhythmias, low-voltage QRS, and diffuse nonspecific ST and T-wave abnormalities. Electrical alternans is occasionally seen and consists of alternating large and small P wave and QRS complexes, caused by the increased rotary motion of the heart in the large fluid-filled pericardium. This interesting electrocardiographic abnormality generally resolves immediately with drainage of the effusion (92,105).

Echocardiography

The most sensitive and precise tool used to evaluate a pericardial effusion is echocardiography, usually in the two-dimensional mode (106). Any patient suspected of having an effusion deserves to have an echocardiogram. Not only is this examination rapid and noninvasive, but it can also be performed quickly at the patient's bedside even with the patient in a sitting position; the equipment is then available immediately to aid in the a diagnostic or therapeutic pericardiocentesis. Echocardiography is extremely sensitive and may detect as little as 15 mL of fluid, as well as identifying myocardial masses and even loculations of fluid.

Aside from its role in the diagnosis of a pericardial effusion, echocardiography is quite useful in assessing the hemodynamic consequences of the effusion. Cardiac tamponade is suggested by diastolic collapse of the right atrium or ventricle, inspiratory decrease in left ventricular dimensions, inspiratory increase in right ventricular dimensions, or failure of the inferior vena cava to collapse on inspiration (inferior vena cava plethora) (107,108). Prompt performance of an echocardiogram in a patient with a suspected effusion is quite important, because only 69% of patients with echocardiographic signs of tamponade are suspected of having a tamponade clinically prior to the study (109).

The most powerful predictor of the development of subsequent cardiac tamponade is the size of the effusion, because not all effusions will lead to hemodynamic compromise. Although the ready availability of echocardiography has allowed the earlier diagnosis of effusions in more patients, it may also have led to some overdiagnosis. Small effusions without symptoms are very rarely malignant and almost never require invasive evaluation or treatment.

Pericardial Fluid Examination

Percutaneous, ultrasound-guided pericardiocentesis can safely be performed in patients with larger effusions (>1 cm anterior clear space on echocardiogram). It will yield pericardial fluid for examination in approximately 90% of patients and will promptly and temporarily relieve tamponade (91,109). The fluid obtained should be sent to the lab for cytology and determination of LDH and total protein levels. If the patient has symptoms suggesting an infectious or rheumatologic cause of the effusion, other tests, such as glucose, cell count, and culture, should be added. This is rarely needed in the patient with an obvious intrathoracic malignancy. In a malignant pericardial effusion, the result of cytology will be positive for malignant cells in 65–90% of cases (110). False-negative cytologic results are frequently seen with lymphoma and mesothelioma. However, the lack of malignant cells in the effusion fluid obviously does not exclude the possibility of neoplastic pericarditis, and it is often necessary to obtain pericardial tissue for histology if a malignant diagnosis is still suspected.

Bloody ("crank-case oil" appearance) or serosanguineous fluid is associated with neoplastic pericarditis, but it may also be seen with idiopathic causes. Malignant effusions are bloody or serosanguineous in 76% of cases and serous in the rest (110). This bloody fluid never clots because it is defibrinated by the motion of the heart inside the pericardium in addition to the intrinsic, local fibrinolytic activity of the serosal lining of the pericardium (101).

Differential Diagnosis

Because up to 40% of patients with a symptomatic pericardial effusion and an underlying cancer will have a benign cause of the effusion and perhaps require a different treatment, it is important to find out the specific cause of the effusion (100). Of particular importance in the differential diagnosis is radiation-related pericardial effusion in patients who have received mediastinal radiation therapy (especially >4000 cGy) (111). From 7 to 30% of these patients may develop effusive or effusive-constrictive pericardial disease, usually within 24–36 months (occasionally within just a few weeks) of the radiotherapy (101,111). Purulent or tuberculous pericarditis is another possibility to consider, especially in the patient with cancer who is debilitated and febrile. Drug-induced pericarditis from agents, such as procainamide or hydralazine, or even from cancer chemotherapy drugs, such as doxorubicin (pericarditis-myocarditis syndrome) (112), may occasionally occur. Idiopathic (viral), uremic, hypothyroid, cholesterol, postmyocardial infarction, or autoimmune pericarditis are other considerations in the differential diagnosis (94). Generally, the pericardial fluid analysis together with the patient's

history will exclude most of the potential diagnoses and will pinpoint the actual cause of the effusion. In patients with cancer and evidence of a significant effusion of echocardiogram, we do not perform an intervening pericardiocentesis, but perform fluid analysis on the fluid removed at the time of treatment.

Prognosis

Although patients with cancer with cardiac tamponade from a malignant pericardial effusion usually are severely ill at presentation, prompt relief of the tamponade will often allow them to return to a surprisingly good functional status for significant time intervals. The quality and span of life depends largely on the histology of the malignancy and its extent. After surgical drainage of the pericardial effusion, patients with breast cancer have a mean survival of 8–18 months (113,114) and patients with lymphoma have a mean survival of 10 months (113). Patients with lung cancer fare somewhat worse, with a mean 3–5-month survival (98,113). However, the extended survival of these patients with advanced cancer with malignant pericardial effusions underscores the importance of tailoring the treatment for this complication to provide maximal benefit with the least chance of reaccumulation of the effusion.

Treatment

The choice of the optimal therapy for this problem is a controversial issue. The medical literature is filled with reports about various therapeutic options (Table 28.6) whose results vary as widely as the techniques. When these invasive techniques are compared, it is important to focus on the most recent reports, because the associated morbidity and mortality as well as the results generally improve with further experience. In the discussion that follows, each option in therapy will be discussed, but true comparative data among techniques are not currently available.

Pericardiocentesis

The earliest described method of nonsurgical drainage of the pericardium, performed by Schuh in 1840, was pericardiocentesis, which he used to relieve hemorrhagic effusion in 30 patients, of whom seven subsequently survived (115). As techniques have evolved and safety has improved, pericardiocentesis has remained the most common approach for diagnosis and therapy in patients with malignant pericardial effusions (111). It may be performed quickly under local anesthesia and is the initial procedure of choice in the emergency management of life-threatening tamponade.

TABLE 28.6

TREATMENT OPTIONS WITH MALIGNANT PERICARDIAL EFFUSIONS

Pericardiocentesis with or without catheter drainage
Intrapericardial sclerosis with chemicals or radioisotopes
Chemotherapy
Radiotherapy
Subxiphoid pericardiectomy ("window")
Left anterior thoracotomy with pericardiectomy
Median sternotomy with pericardiectomy
Videothoracoscopic pericardiectomy
Pericardioperitoneal shunt
Percutaneous balloon pericardiotomy

Pericardiocentesis is best performed from the subxiphoid approach, with the needle inserted between the xiphoid and the left costal arch at a 45-degree angle directed toward the left shoulder. This is the easiest and safest approach because there is a smaller chance of damaging a coronary artery. The patient is placed in the semi-Fowler's position so that most of the effusion is in the most dependent portion of the pericardium (116). In a true emergency, the needle can be advanced blindly or with electrocardiographic monitoring with the needle attached to a V lead. With continuous electrocardiographic monitoring, contact with the epicardium will be seen as an immediate ST segment elevation, often with premature ventricular contractions, warning the clinician to withdraw the needle. If bloody pericardial fluid is removed, it should not clot and generally has a hematocrit lower than that of intravascular blood. Whenever possible, a thoracic surgeon should be notified that pericardiocentesis will be performed in case a complication requiring immediate surgical drainage occurs.

Adding echocardiographic guidance to pericardiocentesis has increased the success rate in obtaining fluid for diagnosis and relieving symptoms to almost 97% and has decreased the complication rate (91,114). Major complications include coronary artery laceration, myocardial puncture, pneumothorax, trauma to abdominal organs (especially the liver), and even death. The complication rate in a series of pericardiocentesis using echocardiographic guidance is 2.4% with no deaths (114). The hazards of the procedure may be minimized if it is performed only on patients with a significant anterior clear space greater than 1 cm, using echocardiographic guidance, correcting thrombocytopenia before the procedure, and avoiding obviously loculated or posterior effusions (91,111,114).

Pericardiocentesis by itself is considered only an initial temporizing procedure to obtain diagnostic fluid and relieve symptoms. It is particularly useful in stabilizing a patient's condition before surgical drainage is performed. However, pericardiocentesis is not considered to be definitive treatment, because most (39–56%) malignant effusions will recur even after single or repeated taps (91,114). Insertion of a small no. 7 or no. 8 French multihole pigtail catheter over a guidewire into the pericardial space can be easily accomplished at the time of initial tap, to allow intermittent drainage over several days. Still, a large number of patients treated in this manner will require more definitive surgical drainage for long-term control of the effusion (91).

One word of caution is highlighted by two recent reports of large-volume pericardiocenteses on patients with tamponade. Wolfe and Edelman noted transient, severe, symptomatic systolic dysfunction in two women, lasting 1–2 weeks after they had undergone pericardiocentesis (650 mL bloody pericardial fluid removed from either patient) to relieve tamponade caused by a malignant pericardial effusion from metastatic breast cancer (117). Both patients were treated symptomatically and recovered gradually. Braverman and Sundaresan (116) reported a similar picture in a 27-year-old woman with pericardial tamponade from benign acute pericarditis who was noted to have global myocardial dysfunction after undergoing pericardiocentesis that removed 500 mL serous fluid. The cause of this phenomenon, which we have also seen, is not known, but it may relate to diminished coronary blood flow during the period of tamponade, leading to a degree of myocardial stunning that was eventually reversible.

Intrapericardial Sclerosis

The logical extension of pericardiocentesis with catheter drainage is injection of a sclerosing agent into the pericardium through the indwelling catheter to prevent a recurrence of the effusion, much like that practiced with malignant pleural effusions. Almost half of the pleural sclerosis agents listed in Table 28.3 have been used in various small series intrapericardially. Agents were chosen on the basis of their ability to cause irritation and/or their antitumor activity, but the mechanism of action of the successful agents is unknown.

Nitrogen mustard, thiotepa, and quinacrine were tried in the 1970s in small studies with fair results but with pain and substantial toxicity from bone marrow suppression, leading to abandonment of these agents. Intrapericardial tetracycline, the most widely used drug, has had a combined success rate of 85% in the two largest reports (118,119). Tetracycline was instilled in doses of 500 mg–1 g on several days in all patients (mean, 2.9 days), and the pericardial catheters remained in place for a mean of 8.8 days in one of the studies (118). Although a fairly effective agent with the expected toxicities of fever (18.7%), pain (9.9%), arrhythmias (12.1%), and catheter plugging (4.4%), tetracycline had the distinct disadvantage of requiring a long hospitalization. Tetracycline is no longer available, and the analog now used, doxycycline, has had a 100% success reported in one small series of seven patients, but they too required multiple instillations (120). The most recent series using pericardial sclerosis as primary management was larger, involving 85 patients, and had a 73% success rate in controlling the effusion for over 30 days (121). This group used tetracycline early in the series and doxycycline later, but as in prior reports, multiple instillations of drug were also necessary for success.

Bleomycin has also been used in very small series (a total of 15 patients in five series) with fairly good results and minimal toxicity, although such small patient series are difficult to interpret (114). Other anecdotal reports of cisplatin, teniposide, and fluorouracil have also appeared, although such small series preclude drawing any conclusions about efficacy and safety.

Immunostimulators interleukin-2 (122) and OK-432 (123) have also been employed by intrapericardial infusion to control malignant effusions. The results from these small series suggest that in two thirds of patients, the effusion can be controlled. However, this novel approach appears to offer no advantage over other agents.

One primary concern about the advisability of intrapericardial sclerosis is whether there is an increased risk of pericardial constriction in patients so treated. Lee et al. reported their favorable experience with intrapericardial sclerosis in 20 patients using mitomycin C, and had a 70% success rate (124). Soon afterward, however, the same group reported that, in one of their initially successful cases, the patient developed constrictive pericarditis 6 months later. They noted that this complication may occur if the patient survives long enough after pericardial sclerotherapy (125). Despite this concern, late pericardial constriction has not been commonly reported.

Intrapericardial radioisotopes, including gold and chromic phosphate, have been used (91,114). They are only partially effective even in radiosensitive tumors, and the logistical problems associated with them have precluded their use. In a novel approach, radioactive iodine (^{131}I) has been tagged to a monoclonal antibody (HMFG2) with intrapericardial administration, and the preliminary excellent results in a small series of four patients suggest that this technique bears further investigation (126).

Radiotherapy

External beam radiotherapy has been advocated for a variety of tumors with cardiac and pericardial involvement (127). In collected series (118), most patients underwent initial pericardiocentesis followed up by radiotherapy in the 1500–4000 cGy dose range, the threshold at which radiation pericarditis and myocarditis can appear (111,128). Approximately 67% of patients so treated will have a positive response, although the best results are found with lymphomas and leukemias (129). Pericardial inflammation is a complication of therapy and may lead to acute pericarditis or possibly late constriction. Generally, radiotherapy is recommended for patients with radiosensitive tumors without hemodynamic compromise who have not previously received radiotherapy (91).

Surgical Approaches

Because pericardial tamponade is predominantly a mechanical problem related to compression of the heart by an effusion, it is not surprising that the earliest attempts to treat this problem involved a surgical approach to drainage, and surgery has remained the preferred technique, although it has been considerably refined. In 1649, Jean Riolan first suggested trephination of the sternum to decompress a pericardial effusion compressing the heart, although the technique was not used until several centuries later (130). However, it was Napoleon's famous surgeon, Baron Dominique-Jean Larrey, who first used the subxiphoid approach to drain the pericardial cavity, considering this an easy operation with small risk. He believed, as we do today, that this most dependent portion of the pericardium was best, because the collection of fluid was more prominent and the heart was at the greatest distance away from the pericardium, with the least chance of a rhythm disturbance (131). Techniques have advanced during the intervening 150 years, although Larrey's approach is still favored.

The term *window* in reference to pericardial surgery was described first by Williams and Soutter in 1954 in their description of an anterior thoracotomy through which they created a small opening in the pericardium and held it open by suturing it to the lung (132). The term *subxiphoid pericardial window* was finally used by Fontanelle et al. in 1970, and that term has continued to the present (133).

Subxiphoid pericardiectomy ("window"). The most popular approach to surgical treatment of a malignant pericardial effusion is the subxiphoid pericardiectomy, which offers the distinct advantages of very low mortality (1% or less), 1% major morbidity, 100% immediate efficacy in relieving tamponade, and a long-term recurrence rate of 3–7% (41,91,111,134,135). Diagnostic accuracy is also excellent and approaches 100% because fluid and pericardial tissue are both removed and are sent for pathologic evaluation. A recent report involved 82 patients with malignant pericardial effusion who underwent subxiphoid pericardiectomy (135). No postoperative deaths were attributable to the surgical procedure, and there was only a 2.4% recurrence rate in the long term requiring further intervention.

Subxiphoid pericardiectomy may be performed in the operating room in 30–45 minutes on critically ill patients under local anesthesia. Often, general endotracheal anesthesia is used if there is no significant hemodynamic compromise or if the pericardium has been decompressed by pericardiocentesis. With general anesthesia, exposure is improved and a larger portion of pericardium may be removed because there is greater muscle relaxation. In addition, general anesthesia is necessary if there is extreme obesity or a narrow costal angle, or if there has been a previous upper midline incision. In fact, in these circumstances, it may be preferable to divert to a left anterior thoracotomy for the pericardiectomy.

For the subxiphoid approach, a short 4- to 6-cm midline incision is made, extending caudad from the xiphoid with entrance into the preperitoneal space after the linea alba has been opened. After fluid has been collected for cytology, the pericardium is explored with the finger to find tumor nodules and to break up loculations. Recurrence of the effusion is best prevented when a large 4 cm × 4 cm portion of pericardium

is removed for pathologic examination (91). Pericardial tubes can be then inserted anterior and posterior to the heart before the wound is closed. The tubes are left in place 2–3 days until the drainage is 50–100 mL per day. Commonly, patients are discharged home on the second or third postoperative day.

Occasionally, no obvious tumor nodules are seen on the pericardium when it is visualized directly through the wound. In this situation, the diagnostic yield may be improved with pericardioscopy using a rigid or flexible scope, which can be used to better inspect the rest of the pericardium to obtain directed biopsy specimens of suspected lesions (136). Three of 40 patients in the series of Millaire et al. had suspected malignancies confirmed by pericardioscopy alone at the time of surgery, which would have otherwise been missed (136).

Although the term *pericardial window* implies that the communication remains open to drain the pericardium, it is not clear that this is actually the mechanism of action. A subxiphoid pericardiectomy ("window") drains into the preperitoneal space, and probably it seals fairly soon. Sugimoto et al. (137) examined this question in following up their series of 26 patients who had undergone a subxiphoid pericardial window procedure. They found by echocardiography that there was thickening of the pericardium/epicardium and obliteration of the pericardial space. Autopsies of four patients who eventually died of their cancer a mean of 120 days after the procedure confirmed the fusion of the visceral and parietal pericardia. These workers concluded that the mechanism allowing success with this procedure is not the maintenance of a "window" draining the effusion continuously, but rather an inflammatory reaction causing fusion of the pericardium to the epicardium, obliterating the former space. They emphasized the necessity for keeping the pericardial space decompressed by suction postoperatively until the fluid drainage is minimal (<50 mL per 24 hours) to keep the two pericardial surfaces in opposition to allow fusion.

Left anterior thoracotomy and pericardiectomy. The left anterior thoracotomy for pericardiectomy can be performed quickly, has a low morbidity and mortality, and allows examination and biopsy of the contents of the left pleural cavity if desired. The procedure is performed through a 10-cm-long submammary incision entering the chest through the fifth intercostal space just lateral to the sternum. The pericardium is removed from just anterior to the left phrenic nerve over to the right mediastinal pleural reflection.

Some studies suggest that the amount of pericardium remaining after surgical drainage of the pericardium is directly related to the frequency of development of postoperative complications and recurrent effusion (98). Nevertheless, in collected series of pericardiectomy by left anterior thoracotomy (114), the overall success rate was 83% (freedom from recurrent effusion) and the mortality was 13%—not as favorable as the results with subxiphoid pericardiectomy. The other primary disadvantage of the left anterior thoracotomy is that it is a major thoracotomy requiring general anesthesia (114), and it may also be technically difficult to perform because of adhesions in the occasional patient with a lung cancer in the left pleural cavity who has been treated with radiotherapy (98,111,114).

Median sternotomy with pericardiectomy. The median sternotomy is an even more extensive procedure and gives very wide exposure to most of the pericardium. This approach is preferred only for constrictive pericardial disease, which may occur in the patient with cancer as the late result of radiation pericarditis, extensive tumor mass or cake, or possibly because of a late failure from a previous approach to pericardial drainage. Because of the risk of myocardial laceration and significant bleeding, most surgeons prefer to have cardiopulmonary bypass on standby when dealing with constrictive pericarditis.

One of the most important technical points in the performance of a pericardiectomy for constriction is to remove the pericardium over the left side of the heart first to prevent the acute pulmonary edema that may occur if the right side of the heart is decompressed first, which would allow increased blood flow to the constricted left ventricle (116). In addition, it is important to continue the pericardial resection down to include the cavae to release them; otherwise, the right-sided failure symptoms may persist postoperatively.

Thoracoscopic pericardiectomy (VATS pericardiectomy). The recent advent of videothoracoscopic surgery has allowed the surgeon to perform many procedures that were previously open procedures using this minimally invasive approach (138–140). Pericardiectomy for effusive disease has proved to be technically feasible with videothoracoscopy, with a recent series of 28 patients by Liu et al. demonstrating 100% long-term success, no significant morbidity, and 0% mortality (139).

Videothoracoscopy has the disadvantages of requiring the lateral decubitus position, increased operating time, and a double-lumen endotracheal tube. Also, the surgeon must have substantial videothoracoscopic experience to perform this procedure effectively and safely. These distinct disadvantages make VATS Pericardial window unsafe in the hemodynamically compromised patient. However, this approach is ideal in the patient with simultaneous pulmonary or pleural pathology that needs evaluation and treatment (such as with a pleural abrasion or talc poudrage), a recurrent or loculated pericardial effusion, previous heart surgery or subxiphoid pacemaker insertion, or a previous substernal esophagogastrostomy. The VATS pericardial window may also be performed from either the right side or the left side of the chest.

Pericardioperitoneal shunt. An additional alternative drainage method was reported by Wang et al. (141) in a small series of four patients. They used the Denver pleuroperitoneal shunt to drain the pericardium into the peritoneal cavity. They performed the procedure with the patients under local anesthesia; the mean hospital stay was 2.8 days in these shunt patients. Further results in larger groups of patients will be needed before any conclusions can be made about the efficacy and safety of this technique.

Percutaneous balloon pericardiotomy. In 1991 Palacios et al. reported a novel approach to drainage of pericardial effusions using a percutaneous balloon pericardiotomy (142). The pericardium is entered by a conventional subxiphoid pericardiocentesis. A guidewire is advanced into the pericardium, over which a Mansfield 20 mm × 3 cm dilating balloon is passed to a point where it straddles the pericardium and is then inflated to create a pericardial window. Usually the pericardial fluid drains into the pleural cavity, as indicated by a new pleural effusion. A catheter is then left in the pericardium until the drainage is minimal.

In their first 50 cases (143), successful, long-term decompression of the effusion was accomplished in 92%, with the rest requiring surgery on an urgent or emergent basis. A new left pleural effusion requiring treatment occurred in 16% of patients, and 4% required a chest tube for a pneumothorax. Another 11% developed a fever, but no pericardial infection was found. The current experience by this group includes 88 patients with a success rate of 88% (144). Experience with this new technique thus far is limited to just a few investigative groups. However, the results look promising, especially in patients with recurrent effusions, and this technique bears close observation over the next few years.

and breast and lymphoma/leukemia. The effusion can rapidly progress to tamponade and if unrecognized may lead to death. Prompt decompression of the effusion has been shown to markedly improve the quality and span of life. However, the optimal method of accomplishing this objective is not easily determined because of the difficulty in comparing the large number of nonrandomized series with heterogeneous patient populations employing various techniques and having varying criteria for successful clinical response. No treatment modality clearly emerges as the preferred technique. In addition, therapy to some extent must be individualized, depending on the tumor cell type and its sensitivity to chemotherapy or radiotherapy, the performance status of the host and expected length of survival, and whether the patient presents with pericardial tamponade. Our recommendations are as follows:

- In a patient without hemodynamic compromise and a chemosensitive tumor, such as lymphoma, leukemia, testicular cancer, or small cell lung carcinoma, systemic chemotherapy should be given. If symptoms or tamponade appears, then a pericardiocentesis should be performed, possibly followed up by subxiphoid pericardiectomy. If chemotherapy fails and the tumor is also radiosensitive, then radiotherapy should be considered as the next step.
- Patients with a symptomatic, suspected, or proven malignant pericardial effusion, a reasonable life expectancy (3 months or more), and no tamponade should be considered for an elective subxiphoid pericardiectomy. If tamponade and hemodynamic compromise are present, a decompressing pericardiocentesis should be performed, followed up by a subxiphoid pericardiectomy. If the institutional resources are such that surgical decompression is unavailable, a suitable approach would be intrapericardial sclerosis with bleomycin or doxycycline, although a higher failure rate should be expected.
- Very poor candidates for surgery, on the basis of comorbid disease, such as severe chronic obstructive pulmonary disease, should be considered primarily for intrapericardial sclerosis. Patients with a very short life expectancy (less than 1 month) should also be considered for intrapericardial sclerosis.
- In patients with a history of malignancy and who develop a pericardial effusion in which the diagnosis is uncertain, or when pericardial tissue is necessary for a histologic diagnosis, an operative intervention by the subxiphoid, videothoracoscopic, or left anterior thoracotomy approach is indicated.
- Videothoracoscopic pericardiectomy is indicated in the setting of coexisting pleural disease requiring evaluation and treatment or when a subxiphoid pericardiectomy is technically not advisable.
- Patients in whom chemotherapy, radiotherapy, or intrapericardial sclerosis has failed should be managed by surgical pericardiectomy.

In general, patients with pericardial involvement by their primary cancer have an incurable disease. Nevertheless, most patients with symptomatic effusions should be offered treatment, because they usually will respond rapidly and often quite remarkably to pericardial decompression and will have a meaningful period of palliation outside of the hospital at home.

Recommendations

A malignant pericardial effusion is a not uncommon complication of advanced cancers, particularly with cancer of the lung

References

1. Light RW, MacGregor MI, Luchsinger PC, et al. Pleural effusions: the diagnostic separation of transudates and exudates. *Ann Intern Med* 1972;77:507–513.

2. Tinney WS, Olsen AM. The significance of fluid in the pleural space: a study of 274 cases. *J Thorac Surg* 1945;14:248–252.

3. Hausheer FH, Yarbro JW. Diagnosis and treatment of malignant pleural effusion. *Semin Oncol* 1985;12:54–75.

4. Matthay RA, Coppage L, Shaw C, et al. Malignancies metastatic to the pleura. *Invest Radiol* 1990;25:601–619.

5. Fenton KN, Richardson JD. Diagnosis and management of malignant pleural effusions. *Am J Surg* 1995;170:69–74.

6. Lynch TE. The management of malignant pleural effusion. *Chest* 1993;103:385S–389S.

7. Ruckdeschel JC. Management of malignant pleural effusion: an overview. *Semin Oncol* 1988;15:24–28.

8. Agostini E. Mechanics of the pleural space. *Physiol Rev* 1972;52:57–128.

9. Black LF. The pleural space and pleural fluid. *Mayo Clin Proc* 1972;47:493–506.

10. Olopade OI, Ultmann JE. Malignant effusions. *CA Cancer J Clin* 1991;41:166–179.

11. Chernow B, Sahn SA. Carcinomatous involvement of the pleura. *Am J Med* 1977;63:695–702.

12. Yano S, Shinohara H, Herbst RS, et al. Production of experimental malignant pleural effusions is dependent on invasion of the pleura and expression of vascular endothelial growth Factor/Vascular permeability factor by human lung cells. *Am J Pathol* 2000;157(6):1892–1903.

13. Yano S, Herbst RS, Shinohara H, et al. Treatment for malignant pleural effusion of human lung adenocarcinoma by inhibition of vascular endothelial growth factor receptor tyrosine kinase phosphorylation. *Clin Cancer Res* 2000;6(3):957–965.

14. Lim SC, Jung SI, Kim YC, et al. Vascular endothelial growth factor in malignant and tuberculous pleural effusions. *J Korean Med Sci* 2000;15(3):279–283.

15. Thickett DR, Armstrong L, Millar AB. Vascular Endothelial Growth Factor (VEGF) in inflammatory and malignant pleural effusions. *Thorax* 1999;54(8):707–710.

16. Kraft A, Weindel K, Ochs A, et al. Vascular endothelial growth factor in the sera and effusions of patients with malignant and nonmalignant disease. *Cancer* 1999;85(1):178–187.

17. Momi H, Matsuyama W, Inoue K, et al. Vascular endothelial growth factor and proinflammatory cytokines in pleural effusions. *Respir Med* 2002;96(10):817–822.

18. Cheng DS, Lee YC, Rogers JT, et al. Vascular endothelial growth factor level correlates with transforming growth factor-ss isoform levels in pleural effusions. *Chest* 2000;118(6):1747–1753.

19. Zebrowski BK, Yano S, Liu W, et al. Vascular endothelial growth factor levels and induction of permeability in malignant pleural effusions. *Clin Cancer Res* 1999;5(11):3364–3368.

20. Verheul HM, Hoekman K, Jorna AS, et al. Targeting vascular endothelial growth factor blockade: ascites formation. *Oncologist* 2000;5(1):45–50.

21. Antony VB, Kamal MA, Godbey S, et al. Talc induced pleurodesis: role of basic fibroblast growth factor (bFGF). *Eur Respir J* 1997;10:4035.

22. Woodring JH. Recognition of a pleural effusion on supine radiographs: how much fluid is required? *Am J Roentgenol* 1984;142:59–64.

23. Doust BD, Baum JK, Maklad NF, et al. Ultrasonic evaluation of pleural opacities. *Radiology* 1975;114:135–140.

24. Ravin CE. Thoracentesis of loculated pleural effusions using grey scale ultrasonic guidance. *Chest* 1977;71:666–668.

25. Ratliff JL, Chavez CM, Jamchuk A, et al. Re-expansion pulmonary edema. *Chest* 1973;64:654–656.

26. Health and Public Policy Committee, American College of Physicians. Diagnostic thoracentesis and pleural biopsy in pleural effusions. *Ann Intern Med* 1985;103:799–802.

27. Leff A, Hopewell PC, Costello J. Pleural effusion from malignancy. *Ann Intern Med* 1978;88:532–537.

28. Nance KV, Shermer RW, Askin FB. Diagnostic efficacy of pleural biopsy as compared with that of pleural fluid examination. *Mod Pathol* 1991;4:320–324.

29. Boutin C, Astoul P, Seitz B. The role of thoracoscopy in the evaluation and management of pleural effusions. *Lung* 1990;168(Suppl):1113–1121.

30. Miles DW, Knight RK. Diagnosis and management of malignant pleural effusion. *Cancer Treat Rev* 1993;19:151–168.

31. LoCicero J III. Thoracoscopic management of malignant pleural effusion. *Ann Thorac Surg* 1993;56:641–643.

32. Roy RH, Can DT, Payne WS. The problem of chylothorax. *Mayo Clin Proc* 1967;42:457–467.

33. Van de Molengraft FJJM, Vooijs GP. Survival of patients with malignancy-associated effusions. *Acta Cytol* 1989;33:911–916.

34. Anderson CB, Philpott GW, Ferguson TB. The treatment of malignant pleural effusions. *Cancer* 1974;33:916–922.

35. Patz EF Jr, McAdams HP, Erasmus JJ, et al. Sclerotherapy for malignant pleural effusions: a prospective randomized trial of bleomycin vs doxycycline with small bore catheter drainage. *Chest* 1998; 113(5):1305–1311.

36. Pollak JS, Burdge CM, Rosenblatt M, et al. Treatment of malignant pleural effusions with tunneled long-term drainage catheters. *J Vasc Interv Radiol* 2001;12(2):201–208.

37. Putnam JB Jr, Light RW, Rodriguez RM, et al. A randomized comparison of indwelling pleural catheter and doxycycline pleurodesis in the management of malignant pleural effusions. *Cancer* 1999;86(10):1992–1999.

38. Walsh FW, Alberts WM, Solomon DA, et al. Malignant pleural effusions: pleurodesis using a small-bore percutaneous catheter. *South Med J* 1989;82:963–965.

39. Robinson LA, Fleming WH, Galbraith TA. Intrapleural doxycycline control of malignant pleural effusions. *Ann Thorac Surg* 1993;55:1115–1122.

40. Robinson LA, Moulton AL, Fleming WH, et al. Intrapleural fibrinolytic treatment of multiloculated thoracic empyemas. *Ann Thorac Surg* 1994;57:803–814.

41. Sanchez-Armegol A, Rodriguez-Panadero F. Survival and talc pleurodesis in metastatic pleural carcinoma, revisited. *Chest* 1993;104:1482–1485.

42. Sahn SA. Pleural effusions in cancer. *Clin Chest Med* 1993;14:189–200.

43. Sahn SA, Good JT Jr, Potts DE. The pH of sclerosing agents. *Chest* 1979;76:198–200.

44. Sahn SA, Good JT Jr. The effect of common sclerosing agents on the pleural space. *Am Rev Respir Dis* 1981;124:65–67.

45. Austin EH, Flye MW. The treatment of malignant pleural effusion. *Ann Thorac Surg* 1979;28:190–203.

46. Pass HI. Treatment of malignant pleural and pericardial effusions. In: DeVita VT Jr, Hellman S, Rosenberg SA, eds. *Cancer: principles and practice of oncology*, 4th ed. Philadelphia, pa: JB Lippincott Co, 1993:2246–2255.

47. Dryzer SR, Allen ML, Strange C, et al. A comparison of rotation and nonrotation in tetracycline pleurodesis. *Chest* 1993;104:1763–1766.

48. Webb WR, Ozmen V, Moulder PV, et al. Iodized talc pleurodesis for the treatment of pleural effusions. *J Thorac Cardiovasc Surg* 1992;103:881–886.

49. Sahn SA. Malignant pleural effusions. *Clin Chest Med* 1985;6:113–125.

50. McAlpine LG, Hulks G, Thompson NC. Management of recurrent pleural effusion in the United Kingdom: survey of clinical practice. *Thorax* 1990;45:699–701.

51. Fentiman IS. Diagnosis and treatment of malignant pleural effusions. *Cancer Treat Rev* 1987;14:107–118.

52. Ruckdeschel JC, Moores D, Lee JY, et al. Intrapleural therapy for malignant pleural effusions: a randomized comparison of bleomycin and tetracycline. *Chest* 1991;100:1528–1535.

53. Johnson CE, Curzon PGD. Comparison of intrapleural bleomycin and tetracycline in the treatment of malignant pleural effusion (abst). *Thorax* 1985;40:210.

54. Kitamura S, Sugiyana Y, Izumi T, et al. Intrapleural doxycycline for control of malignant pleural effusion. *Curr Ther Res* 1981;30:515–521.

55. Månsson T. Treatment of malignant pleural effusion with doxycycline. *Scand J Infect Dis* 1988;53(Suppl):29–34.

56. Seaton KG, Patz EF Jr, Goodman PC. Palliative treatment of malignant pleural effusions: value of small-bore catheter thoracostomy and doxycycline sclerotherapy. *AJR Am J Roentgenol* 1995;164:589–591.

57. Walker-Renard PB, Vaughan LM, Sahn SA. Chemical pleurodesis for malignant pleural effusions. *Ann Intern Med* 1994;120:56–64.

58. Belani CP, Einarson TR, Arikian SR, et al. Cost-effectiveness analysis of pleurodesis in the management of malignant pleural effusions. *J Oncol Manag* 1995;4:1–11.

59. Kessinger A, Wigton RS. Intracavitary bleomycin and tetracycline in the management of malignant pleural effusions: a randomized study. *J Surg Oncol* 1987;36:81–83.

60. Alberts DS, Chen HSG, Mayersohn M, et al. Bleomycin pharmacokinetics in man. II. Intracavitary administration. *Cancer Chemother Pharmacol* 1979;2:127–132.

61. Siegel RD, Schiffman FJ. Systemic toxicity following intracavitary administration of bleomycin. *Chest* 1990;98:507.

62. Trotter JM, Stuart JFB, McBeth F, et al. The management of malignant effusion with bleomycin (abst). *Br J Cancer* 1979;40:310.

63. Fuller DK. Bleomycin versus doxycycline: a patient-oriented approach to pleurodesis. *Ann Pharmacother* 1993;27:794.

64. Weissberg D, Ben-Zeev I. Talc pleurodesis: experience with 360 patients. *J Thorac Cardiovasc Surg* 1993;106:689–695.

65. Kennedy L, Sahn SA. Talc pleurodesis for the treatment of pneumothorax and pleural effusion. *Chest* 1994;106:1215–1222.

66. Bethune N. A new technic for the deliberate production of pleural adhesions as a preliminary to lobectomy. *J Thorac Surg* 1935;4:251–261.

67. Ohri SK, Oswal SK, Townsend ER, et al. Early and late outcome after diagnostic thoracoscopy and talc pleurodesis. *Ann Thorac Surg* 1992;53:1038–1041.

68. Dresler CM, Olak J, Herndon JE II, et al. Phased III intergroup study of talc poudrage vs talc slurry sclerosis for malignant pleural effusion. *Chest* 2005;127(3):909–915.

69. Chambers JS. Palliative treatment of neoplastic pleural effusion with intercostal intubation and talc instillation. *West J Surg* 1958;66:26–28.

70. Adler RH, Sayek I. Treatment of malignant pleural effusion: a method using tube thoracostomy and talc. *Ann Thorac Surg* 1976;22:8–15.

71. Rinaldo JF, Owens GR, Rogers RM. Adult respiratory distress syndrome following intrapleural administration of talc. *J Thorac Cardiovasc Surg* 1983;85:823–826.

72. Bondoc AY, Bach PB, Sklarin NT, et al. Arterial desaturation syndrome following pleurodesis with talc slurry: incidence, clinical features and outcome. *Cancer Invest* 2003;21(6):848–854.

73. Kennedy L, Harley RA, Sahn SA, et al. Talc slurry pleurodesis: pleural fluid and histological analysis. *Chest* 1995;107:1707–1712.

74. Haddad FJ, Younes RN, Gross JL, et al. Pleurodesis in patients with malignant pleural effusions: talc slurry or bleomycin? Results of a prospective randomized trial. *World J Surg* 2004;28(8):749–753.

75. Kuzdal J, Sladek K, Wasowski D, et al. Talc powder vs doxycycline in the control of malignant pleural effusion: a prospective, randomized trial. *Med Sci Monit* 2003;9(6):54–59.

76. Paschoalini Mda S, Vargas FS, Marchi E, et al. Prospective randomized trial of silver nitrate vs talc slurry in pleurodesis for symptomatic malignant pleural effusions. *Chest* 2005;128(2):684–689.

77. Shaw P, Agarwal R. Pleurodesis for malignant pleural effusions. *Cochrane Database Syst Rev* 2004;(1):CD002916.

78. Rossi GA, Felletti R, Balbi B, et al. Symptomatic treatment of recurrent malignant pleural effusions with intrapleurally administered *Corynebacterium parvum*: clinical response is not associated with evidence of enhancement of local cellular-mediated immunity. *Am Rev Respir Dis* 1987;135:885–890.

79. Ren S, Terman DS, Bohach G, et al. Intrapleural staphylococcal superantigen induces resolution of malignant pleural effusions and a survival benefit in non-small cell lung cancer. *Chest* 2004;126(5):1529–1539.

80. Rosso R, Rimoldi R, Salvati F, et al. Intrapleural natural beta interferon in the treatment of malignant pleural effusions. *Oncology* 1988;45:253–256.

81. Astoul P, Viallat JR, Laurent JC, et al. Intrapleural recombinant IL-2 in passive immunotherapy for malignant pleural effusion. *Chest* 1993;103:209–213.

82. Dianjun L, Yaorong W, Ziaodong Y, et al. Treatment of patients with malignant pleural effusions due to advanced lung cancer by transfer to autologous LAK cells combined with rIL-2 or rIL-2 alone. *Proc Chin Acad Med Sci Peking Union Med Coll* 1990;5:51–55.

83. Kent EM, Moses C. Radioactive isotopes in the palliative management of carcinomatosis of the pleura. *J Thorac Surg* 1951;22:503–516.

84. Martini N, Bains BS, Beattie EJ. Indications for pleurectomy in malignant pleural effusions. *Cancer* 1975;35:734–738.

85. Reich H, Beattie EJ, Harvey JC. Pleuroperitoneal shunt for malignant pleural effusion: a one-year experience. *Semin Surg Oncol* 1993;9:160–162.

86. Waller DA, Morritt GN, Forty J. Video-assisted thoracoscopic pleurectomy in the management of malignant pleural effusion. *Chest* 1995;107:1454–1456.

87. Harvey JC, Erdman CB, Beattie EJ. Early experience with videothoracoscopic hydrodissection pleurectomy in the treatment of malignant pleural effusion. *J Surg Oncol* 1995;59:243–245.

88. Matsuzaki Y, Shibata K, Yoshioka M, et al. Intrapleural perfusion hyperthermo-chemotherapy for malignant pleural dissemination and effusion. *Ann Thorac Surg* 1995;59:127–131.

89. Belani CP, Aisner J, Patz E. Ambulatory sclerotherapy for malignant pleural effusions (abst). *Proc Am Soc Clin Oncol* 1995;14:524.

90. Hawkins JW, Vacek JL. What constitutes definitive therapy of malignant pericardial effusion? "Medical" versus surgical treatment. *Am Heart J* 1989;118:428–432.

91. Theologides A. Neoplastic cardiac tamponade. *Semin Oncol* 1978;5:181–192.

92. Thurber DL, Edwards JE, Achor RWP. Secondary malignant tumors of the pericardium. *Circulation* 1962;26:228–241.

93. Lokich JJ. The management of malignant pericardial effusions. *JAMA* 1973;224:1401–1404.

94. Buzaid AC, Garewal HS, Greenberg BR. Managing malignant pericardial effusion. *West J Med* 1989;150:174–179.

95. National Center for Health Statistics. *National hospital discharge survey*. Hyattsville, MD, Vital and Health Statistics, No. 122 (PHS): NCHS, 1993;95–1783.

96. Miller JI, Mansour KA, Hatcher CR Jr. Pericardiectomy: current indications, concepts, and results in a university center. *Ann Thorac Surg* 1982;34:40–45.

97. Piehler JM, Pluth JR, Schaff HV, et al. Surgical management of effusive pericardial disease: influence of extent of pericardial resection on clinical course. *J Thorac Cardiovasc Surg* 1985;90:506–516.

98. Palatianos GM, Thurer RJ, Pompeo MQ, et al. Clinical experience with subxiphoid drainage of pericardial effusions. *Ann Thorac Surg* 1989;48:381–385.

99. Mills SA, Graeber GM, Nelson MG. Therapy of malignant tumors involving the pericardium. In: Roth J, Ruckdeschel JC, Weisenburger T, eds. *Thoracic oncology*, 2nd ed. Philadelphia, PA: WB Saunders, 1995:492–513.

100. Posner MR, Cohen GI, Skarin AT. Pericardial disease in patients with cancer—the differentiation of malignant from idiopathic and radiation-induced pericarditis. *Am J Med* 1981;71:407–413.

101. Spodick DH. Macrophysiology, microphysiology, and anatomy of the pericardium: a synopsis. *Am Heart J* 1992;124:1046–1051.

102. Miller AJ. Some observations concerning pericardial effusions and their relationship to the venous and lymphatic circulation of the heart. *Lymphology* 1970;3:76–78.

103. Pories WJ, Gaudiani VA. Cardiac tamponade. *Surg Clin North Am* 1975;55:573–589.

104. Spodick DH. The normal and diseased pericardium: current concepts of pericardial physiology, diagnosis and treatment. *J Am Coll Cardiol* 1983;1:240–251.

105. Beck CS. Acute and chronic compression of the heart. *Am Heart J* 1937;14:515–525.

106. Settle HP, Adolph RJ, Fowler NO, et al. Echocardiographic study of cardiac tamponade. *Circulation* 1977;56:951–959.

107. Himelman RB, Kircher R, Rockey DC, et al. Inferior vena cava plethora with blunted respiratory response: a sensitive echocardiographic sign of cardiac tamponade. *J Am Coll Cardiol* 1988;12:470–477.

108. Markiewicz W, Borovik R, Ecker S. Cardiac tamponade in medical patients: treatment and prognosis in the echocardiographic era. *Am Heart J* 1986;111:1138–1142.

109. Eisenberg MJ, Oken NK, Guerrero S, et al. Prognostic value of echocardiography in hospitalized patients with pericardial effusion. *Am J Cardiol* 1992;70:934–939.

110. Reyes VC, Strinden C, Banerji M. The role of cytology in neoplastic cardiac tamponade. *Acta Cytol* 1982;26:299–302.

111. Ruckdeschel JC, Chang P, Martin RG, et al. Radiation-related pericardial effusions in patients with Hodgkin's disease. *Medicine (Baltimore)* 1975;54:245–270.

112. Calabresi P, Chabner BA. Chemotherapy of neoplastic disease. In: Gilman AG, Rall TW, Nies AS, et al., eds. *The pharmacological basis of therapeutics*, 8th ed. New York: Pergamon Press, 1990:1241–1244.

113. Miller JI Jr. Surgical management of pericardial disease. In: Schlant RC, Alexander RW, O'Rourke RA, et al., eds. *The heart, arteries and veins*, 8th ed. New York: McGraw-Hill, 1994:1675–1680.

114. Press OW, Livingston R. Management of malignant pericardial effusion and tamponade. *JAMA* 1987;257:1088–1092.

115. Schuh F. Erfahrungen über die paracentere der brust und des herzbeutels. *Med Jahrb dkk. Öster -staates Wien* (Neuste Folge 24) 1841;33:388.

116. Braverman AC, Sundaresan S. Cardiac tamponade and severe ventricular dysfunction. *Ann Intern Med* 1994;120:442.

117. Wolfe MW, Edelman ER. Transient systolic dysfunction after relief of cardiac tamponade. *Ann Intern Med* 1993;119:42–44.

118. Davis S, Rambotti P, Grignani F. Intrapericardial tetracycline sclerosis in the treatment of malignant pericardial effusion. *J Clin Oncol* 1984;2:631–636.

119. Shepherd FA, Morgan C, Evans WK, et al. Medical management of malignant pericardial effusion by tetracycline sclerosis. *Am J Cardiol* 1987;60:1161–1166.

120. Kitamura S, Wagai F, Izumi T, et al. Treatment of carcinomatous pericarditis with doxycycline: intrapericardial doxycycline for control of malignant pericardial effusion. *Curr Therap Res* 1981;30:589–596.

121. Maher EA, Shepherd FA, Todd JRT. Pericardial sclerosis as the primary management of malignant pericardial effusion and cardiac tamponade. *J Thorac Cardiovasc Surg* 1996;112:637–643.

122. Lissoni P, Barni S, Ardizzoia A. Intracavitary administration of interleukin-2 as palliative therapy for neoplastic effusions. *Tumori* 1992;78:118–120.

123. Imamura T, Tamura K, Takenaga M, et al. Intrapericardial OK-432 instillation for the management of malignant pericardial effusion. *Cancer* 1991;68:259–263.

124. Lee LN, Yang PC, Chang DB. Ultrasound guided pericardial drainage and intrapericardial instillation of mitomycin C for malignant pericardial effusion. *Thorax* 1994;49:594–595.

125. Lin MT, Yang PC, Luh KT. Constrictive pericarditis after sclerosing therapy with mitomycin C for malignant pericardial effusion: report of a case. *J Formos Med Assoc* 1994;93:250–252.

126. Pectasides D, Stewart S, Courtney-Luck N, et al. Antibody-guided irradiation of malignant pleural and pericardial effusions. *Br J Cancer* 1986;53:727–732.

127. Cham WC, Freiman AH, Carstens HB, et al. Radiation therapy of cardiac and pericardial metastases. *Radiology* 1975;114:701–704.

128. Stewart JR, Cohen KE, Fajardo LF, et al. Radiation-induced heart disease: a study of 25 patients. *Radiology* 1967;89:302–310.

129. Terry LN, Kligerman MM. Pericardial and myocardial involvement by lymphomas and leukemias: the role of radiotherapy. *Cancer* 1970;25:1003–1008.

130. Riolan J. *Encheiridium anatomicum et pathologicum*. Lugdunum, Batavorum, Ex Officini Adriani, Wyngaarden. 1649:206–212.

131. Larrey D-J. *Clinique chirurgicale*, Vol. 2. Paris: Gabon, 1829:303–305, 315–321.

132. William C, Soutter L. Pericardial tamponade: diagnosis and treatment. *Arch Intern Med* 1954;94:571–584.

133. Fontanelle LJ, Cuello L, Dooley BN. Subxiphoid pericardial window. *Am J Surg* 1970;120:679–680.

134. Zwischenberger JB, Bradford DW. Management of malignant pericardial effusion. In: Pass HI, Mitchell JB, Johnson DH, et al., eds. *Lung cancer: principles and practice*. Philadelphia, PA: Lippincott–Raven, 1996:655–662.

135. Moores DWO, Allen KB, Faber LP, et al. Subxiphoid pericardial drainage for pericardial tamponade. *J Thorac Cardiovasc Surg* 1995;109:546–552.

136. Millaire A, Wurtz A, de Groote P, et al. Malignant pericardial effusions: usefulness of pericardioscopy. *Am Heart J* 1992;124:1030–1040.

137. Sugimoto JT, Little AG, Ferguson MK, et al. Pericardial window: mechanisms of efficacy. *Ann Thorac Surg* 1990;50:442–445.

138. Mack MJ, Aronoff RJ, Acuff TE, et al. Present role of thoracoscopy in the diagnosis and treatment of diseases of the chest. *Ann Thorac Surg* 1992;54:403–409.

139. Liu H-P, Chang C-H, Lin PJ, et al. Thoracoscopic management of effusive pericardial disease: indications and technique. *Ann Thorac Surg* 1994;58:1695–1697.

140. Georghiou GP, Stamler A, Sharoni E, et al. Video-assisted thoracoscopic pericardial window for diagnosis and management of pericardial effusions. *Ann Thorac Surg* 2005;80(2):607–610.

141. Wang N, Feikes JR, Mogensen T, et al. Pericardioperitoneal shunt: an alternative treatment for malignant pericardial effusion. *Ann Thorac Surg* 1994;57:289–292.

142. Palacios IF, Tuzcu EM, Ziskind AA, et al. Percutaneous balloon pericardial window for patients with malignant pericardial effusion and tamponade. *Cathet Cardiovasc Diagn* 1991;22:244–249.

143. Ziskind AA, Pearce AC, Lemmon CC, et al. Percutaneous balloon pericardiotomy for the treatment of cardiac tamponade and large pericardial effusions: description of techniques and report of first 50 cases. *J Am Coll Cardiol* 1993;21:1–5.

144. Ziskind AA, Rodriguez S, Lemmon CC, et al. Percutaneous balloon pericardiotomy for the treatment of malignant pericardial effusion: long term followup (abst). *Proc Annu Meet Am Soc Clin Oncol* 1994;13:a1494.

CHAPTER 29 ■ MANAGEMENT OF ADVANCED HEPATIC DISEASE

DANIEL Y. CHUNG AND DAVID A. SASS

Cirrhosis is a pathologically defined entity that is associated with a spectrum of characteristic clinical manifestations. Histologically, it represents a late stage of progressive hepatic fibrosis characterized by distortion of the hepatic architecture and the formation of regenerative nodules. This stage of advanced liver disease is generally deemed "irreversible" and the only therapeutic option may be liver transplantation. When patients with cirrhosis experience "decompensation," they are susceptible to a variety of complications and, as a result, they have a markedly reduced life expectancy. Cirrhosis was the tenth leading cause of death in the United States, according to a 2000 Vital Statistics Report, in which data was collected through 1998 and accounted for more than 25,000 deaths (1).

This chapter focuses on the medical management of patients with cirrhosis. Most of the chapter will deal with the specific management of cirrhotic-related complications. Mention will also be made of the indications for and evaluation of such patients for liver transplantation.

When treating patients with cirrhosis, it is important to first confirm the diagnosis. Thereafter, the physician should attempt to establish the etiology of the disease, assess severity, identify and treat any complications, and decide whether an evaluation for an orthotopic liver transplant (OLT) is indicated. Finally, family counseling regarding screening for genetic liver diseases, when appropriate, and administration of vaccines should also be offered.

CONFIRMING THE DIAGNOSIS OF CIRRHOSIS

Patients are diagnosed with cirrhosis in one of several ways:

1. They may have stigmata of chronic liver disease discovered on routine physical examination (Table 29.1)
2. They may undergo routine laboratory testing, radiologic testing [ultrasound, computerized tomography (CT) scan or magnetic resonance imaging], endoscopy (with the discovery of varices indicating portal hypertension), or an unrelated surgical procedure that incidentally leads to the diagnosis of cirrhosis
3. They may present with one of the life-threatening complications of decompensated cirrhosis *ab initio*
4. They may undergo a liver biopsy for further evaluation of abnormal liver enzymes and be found to have hepatic cirrhosis histologically
5. They may never come to clinical attention and be diagnosed at autopsy (up to 30–40% in older reviews) (2).

The gold standard for diagnosing cirrhosis is examining the explanted liver at autopsy or following liver transplantation where the architecture of the entire liver can be appreciated. In clinical practice, however, we usually rely on examination of a pathologic specimen obtained through transjugular or percutaneous liver biopsy. There have been numerous radiologic advances over the past several years, particularly with regard to CT scanning. These improvements include changes in scanner technology such as the ability to perform multiphasic contrast-enhanced studies as well as better intravenous contrast media. Nevertheless, none of the radiologic modalities has yet supplanted liver histology as the gold standard. However, liver biopsy is not always necessary to confirm a diagnosis of cirrhosis if the clinical, laboratory, and radiologic data strongly suggest the presence of cirrhosis, for example, a patient with ascites, severe coagulopathy, and a shrunken, nodular liver on ultrasound. In this instance, a liver biopsy may be hazardous as the coagulopathy may pose a significant bleeding risk.

DETERMINING THE CAUSE OF CIRRHOSIS

Determination of the cause of cirrhosis is important because it may influence treatment decisions and counseling of family members and may help predict complications [e.g., the development of hepatocellular carcinoma (HCC) is higher in patients with hemochromatosis and chronic hepatitis B than in other forms of cirrhosis]. A specific etiology can often be determined by way of history combined with serologic and histologic evaluation. The two most common causes in the United States are alcoholic liver disease and hepatitis C, together accounting for approximately half of those undergoing transplantation. When no apparent cause of cirrhosis is identified, the term "cryptogenic" is used (approximately 10–15% of cases). Many of the patients who were previously labeled as "cryptogenic" are now recognized as being cases of unrecognized nonalcoholic steatohepatitis (NASH). For a full classification of the many etiologies of cirrhosis and the best diagnostic tests, see Table 29.2.

ASSESSING THE SEVERITY OF THE DISEASE

Several prognostic tools have been developed to assess the severity of disease in patients with cirrhosis and the need

TABLE 29.1

STIGMATA OF CHRONIC LIVER DISEASE

Stigmata	Pathogenesis	Other facts
Cutaneous		
Spider angiomata (telangiectasias)	Unknown? related to sex-hormone metabolism	Usually on trunk, face, and upper limbs; not specific for cirrhosis
Palmar erythema	Altered sex-hormone metabolism	Not specific for cirrhosis; seen in hyperthyroidism, pregnancy, and rheumatoid arthritis
Jaundice (icterus)	Increased serum bilirubin (>2 mg/dL)	Yellow coloring of skin and mucous membranes. Differentiate jaundice from carotenemia by absence of yellow sclera in the latter
Nails and hands		
Muehrcke's nails	Unknown ? caused by hypoalbuminemia	Paired horizontal white bands separated by normal color. May be seen in other low albumin states
Terry's nails	Related to hypoalbuminemia	Proximal two third of nail plate is white and distal one third is red
Clubbing and hypertrophic osteoarthropathy	Unknown ? related to hypoxemia, right-to-left and portosystemic shunts	Neither feature is specific and can be seen in a variety of disorders
Dupuytren's contracture	Unknown ? related to free radical formation generated by oxidative metabolism of hypoxanthine	Thickening and shortening of the palmar fascia causing flexion deformities of the fingers, seen particularly in patients with alcoholic cirrhosis
Male sex organs		
Gynecomastia	Possibly caused by increased production of androstenedione from the adrenals	Rubbery or firm mass extending concentrically from the nipple in the male breast. Not specific for cirrhosis
Testicular atrophy	?more than one mechanism involved: either primary gonadal injury or suppression of hypothalamic-pituitary function	Impotence, infertility, loss of sexual drive and infertility. Not specific for cirrhosis
Features of portal hypertension		
Splenomegaly	Congestion of the red pulp	Splenic size does not correlate with portal pressures. Nonspecific
Ascites	Described in the text	Not specific
Caput medusae	Opening of the normally obliterated umbilical vein	Blood flow directed inferiorly away from the umbilicus
Cruveilhier–Baumgarten murmur	Collateral connections between portal system and remnant of umbilical vein	Venous hum auscultated with stethoscope over epigastrium
Fetor hepaticus	Increased concentrations of dimethylsulfide	Sweet, pungent smell of the breath, suggesting severe portosystemic shunting
Asterixis	Seen in hepatic encephalopathy ? mechanism	Bilateral but asynchronous flapping of outstretched, dorsiflexed hands. Not specific

for OLT. The Child-Turcotte-Pugh (CTP) classification, which was initially designed to stratify the risk of portocaval shunt surgery in patients with cirrhosis and variceal bleeding, has gained favor over the past decade as a simple method for determining the prognosis of patients with chronic liver disease (3) (see Table 29.3 for scoring system and survival rates). In 1997, the United Network for Organ Sharing (UNOS) established a CTP score of 7 or higher as the minimal listing criteria for eligibility of listing for OLT (4). On February 27, 2002, UNOS adopted the model for end-stage liver disease (MELD) score as an evidence-based means of organ allocation (5). MELD score is a severity score predictive of mortality in patients with chronic liver disease (6). It includes total serum bilirubin, international normalized ratio (INR) and serum creatinine:

$$MELD = 3.78 \times \log e \, [bilirubin \, (mg/dL)]$$
$$+ 11.2 \times \log e \, (INR)$$
$$+ 9.57 \times \log e \, [creatinine \, (mg/dL)]$$
$$+ 6.4$$

MELD was initially developed to predict the survival of patients undergoing transjugular intrahepatic portosystemic shunts (TIPS) (7) and was subsequently validated in patients with decompensated liver disease (6). Using the MELD model, patients are assigned a score on a continuous scale from 6 to 40,

TABLE 29.2

CAUSES OF CIRRHOSIS

Category	Cause	Diagnosis
Viral hepatitis	Chronic hepatitis B virus	HBSAg, HBCAb, HBV DNA
	Chronic hepatitis C virus	HCV Ab and HCV RNA
Alcoholic liver disease		History, liver biopsy
Autoimmune diseases	Autoimmune hepatitis	ANA, SMA, LKM, SPEP, quantit. Igs, liver biopsy
	Primary biliary cirrhosis	AMA, elevated IgM, liver biopsy
	Primary sclerosing cholangitis	ERCP, history of inflammatory bowel disease
Genetic liver diseases	Hereditary hemochromatosis	Iron saturation, ferritin, HFE genetic testing, liver biopsy
	Wilson's disease	Ceruloplasmin, 24-h urine copper, slit lamp exam for Kayser-Fleischer rings, liver biopsy
	α_1-antitrypsin deficiency	α_1-antitrypsin level, Pi type, liver biopsy
Venous outflow tract obstruction	Budd-Chiari syndrome	Venogram, liver biopsy
	Veno-occlusive disease	Liver biopsy
	Severe right-sided heart failure	Echocardiogram, right heart catheterization
Drugs, toxins, chemicals	For example, methotrexate, amiodarone	History
Pediatric biliary diseases (rare)	For example, Byler's disease, Alagille's syndrome, Indian childhood cirrhosis	History, cholestatic LFTs, liver biopsy
Pediatric metabolic liver diseases (rare)	For example, cystic fibrosis, galactosemia, glycogen storage disease, hereditary tyrosinemia and fructose intolerance	Abnormal enzyme levels, occasionally liver biopsy
Nonalcoholic steatohepatitis	—	Risk factors, liver biopsy
Cryptogenic	—	Diagnosis of exclusion

HBSAg, hepatitis B surface antigen; HBCAb, hepatitis B core antibody; HBV DNA, hepatitis B virus DNA; HCV Ab, hepatitis C antibody; HCV RNA, hepatitis C virus RNA; ANA, antinuclear antibody; SMA, antismooth muscle antibody; LKM, antiliver kidney microsomal antibody; SPEP, serum protein electrophoresis; quantit. Igs, quantitative immunoglobulins; ERCP, endoscopic retrograde cholangiopancreatogram; HFE, the gene for hereditary hemochromatosis; LFTs, liver function tests.

which equates to estimated 3-month survival rates from 90 to 7%, respectively (7). The MELD score has been shown to be useful in predicting short-term survival in groups of patients on the waiting list for OLT (8) as well as the risk of postoperative mortality (9). Once patients are listed for OLT, an updated MELD score is recalculated at varying intervals as a form of status recertification, according to the following schedule: every 12 months for those with a MELD ≤10; every 3 months for those with a MELD of 11–18; every month for those with a MELD of 19–24, and every week for those with a MELD of 25 or greater (http://www.optn.org/PoliciesandBylaws2/policies/docs/policy_8.doc).

TABLE 29.3

CHILD-TURCOTTE-PUGH SCORE TO ASSESS SEVERITY OF LIVER DISEASE

Points	1	2	3
Encephalopathy[a]	None	Grade 1–2	Grade 3–4
Ascites	Absent	Slight to moderate	Tense
Bilirubin (mg/dL)	1–2	2–3	>3
Albumin (g/dL)	>3.5	2.8–3.5	<2.8
Prothrombin time (seconds prolonged) or INR	1–4	4–6	>6
	<1.7	1.7–2.3	>2.3

Child's Class A: Score 5–6: well compensated disease (85–100% 1–2 year survival)
Child's Class B: Score 7–9: significant functional compromise (60–80% 1–2 year survival)
Child's Class C: Score 10–15: decompensated disease (35–45% 1–2 year survival)
[a]See Table 29.6 for grading of encephalopathy.
From: Conn HO. A peek at the Child-Turcotte classification. *Hepatology* 1981;1:673–676.

THE TRANSPLANT EVALUATION PROCESS

As soon as it has been determined that a patient is sick enough to require consideration for an OLT and that no other alternative treatments are available, a careful evaluation should be performed to assess the following:

1. Whether the patient would survive the operation and the immediate postoperative period
2. Whether the patient can be expected to comply with the complex medical and immunosuppressive regimen required post-transplantation
3. Whether the patient has any other comorbidities that would severely compromise graft or patient survival because of which transplantation would be futile and an inappropriate use of a scarce donor organ (10).

In assessing whether any given patient with cirrhosis is a suitable candidate for OLT, the evaluation process typically involves a multidisciplinary team including transplant hepatologists, transplant surgeons, transplant anesthesiologists, nurse coordinators, social workers, and transplant psychiatrists with expertise in substance abuse issues. Other consultants will also be called upon according to individual patient needs. The evaluation includes a thorough history and physical examination, a full psychosocial assessment, extensive laboratory testing, and abdominal imaging to exclude intra- as well as extrahepatic malignancies and to evaluate biliary and hepatic vascular anatomy. An extensive cardiopulmonary evaluation as well as age-appropriate screening is performed for various extrahepatic malignancies. On the basis of the pre-OLT evaluation testing, a multidisciplinary selection committee makes a decision regarding the candidacy for OLT listing. The natural history of disease should be compared with the expected survival after OLT. Current survival rates 1, 3, and 5 years after liver transplantation in the United States are 88, 80 and 75%, respectively (http://www.optn.org/latestdata/step2.asp).

MANAGEMENT OF SPECIFIC COMPLICATIONS

Ascites

Ascites, or the pathologic accumulation of fluid in the peritoneal cavity, is the most common major complication of cirrhosis. It is associated with a poor quality of life, increased risk of infection and renal failure, and a poor long-term outcome (11). Approximately 50% of patients with compensated cirrhosis will develop ascites over a 10-year period. Furthermore, only 50% of patients with cirrhosis survive 2–5 years after ascites onset, depending on the cause of liver disease (12). Cirrhosis accounts for 80% of all cases of ascites. Other etiologies are listed in Table 29.4. Defining the etiology of ascites and confirming that it is secondary to end-stage liver disease is critical, as successful treatment is dependent upon an accurate diagnosis.

The pathophysiology of ascites in liver disease involves splanchnic vasodilatation. In advanced stages of disease, arterial blood volume decreases and arterial pressure falls largely because of circulating vasodilators such as nitric oxide. There is a compensatory response of vasoconstrictors and anti-natriuretic factors leading to sodium and fluid retention. Intestinal capillary pressure and permeability are altered and the result is accumulation of abdominal fluid (11).

Patients with ascites frequently seek medical attention within a few weeks of onset. They often become intolerant of

TABLE 29.4

CAUSES OF ASCITES (AND THEIR FREQUENCIES)

Cirrhosis (81%)
Malignancy (10%)
Heart failure (3%)
Tuberculosis (1.7%)
Nephrogenic (dialysis ascites) (1%)
Miscellaneous (nephrotic syndrome, pancreatitis, biliary leak, fulminant hepatic failure) (each <1%)

Adapted from: Runyon BA. Approach to the patient with ascites. In: Yamada T, Alpers D, Owyang C, et al., eds. *Textbook of gastroenterology*. New York: J.B. Lippincott, 1995:927–52.

the abdominal distension leading to early satiety and shortness of breath. In the initial evaluation of patients with ascites, a careful history documenting risk factors for liver disease should be taken. Evidence of malignancy, cardiac disease, myxedema, renal disease, pancreatitis, and infections such as tuberculosis should all be ruled out as etiologies of ascites (12). In addition, more than one of these may be found in 5% of patients with ascites (13). Abdominal distension occurs if a moderate amount of ascites is present. Diagnosis can be made by percussing the flanks. Flank dullness can be detected if >1500 mL of fluid is present. If no flank dullness is present, the patient has a <10% chance of having ascites (14). A useful test for diagnosing ascites is examination for shifting dullness. The flank is percussed in the supine position and the air-fluid level marked. The patients are then turned on their side and percussion is again performed. If the air-fluid level shifts upward, it indicates that ascites is present. Other maneuvers such as the puddle sign and fluid wave have been described but their utility is often questioned (15). Many recommend some form of imaging in patients with ascites to not only confirm the presence of ascites but also to evaluate for cirrhosis and/or malignancy. Ultrasound of the abdomen is usually sufficient and can detect as little as 100 mL of fluid in the peritoneal cavity (12).

Abdominal paracentesis is recommended in the initial evaluation of patients with ascites. It is helpful not only in diagnosing the cause of ascites but also in ruling out suspected infection or peritonitis. A diagnostic paracentesis should be performed in patients with new onset of ascites and also in patients with known cirrhosis who are either admitted to the hospital or have unexplained clinical deterioration. Complications of paracentesis are surprisingly few. One percent of patients that are coagulopathic and undergoing paracentesis will develop abdominal wall hematomas, but coagulopathy should not preclude paracentesis unless there is apparent fibrinolysis or disseminated intravascular coagulation (DIC) (15). Perforation of the bowel occurs in fewer than 1 in 1000 cases (16). Many recommend performing paracentesis in the left lower quadrant, two fingerbreadths cephalad and medial to the anterior iliac spine, or generally at the site of maximal dullness. Cleansing and local anesthesia are used to prepare the site, and generally a 50-mL aspiration is sufficient to perform the necessary analysis. Bedside ultrasonography may be necessary to localize the optimal site for entry.

In general, cell count and differential, albumin, and total protein concentration should be analyzed on the initial specimen. Additional tests such as glucose, lactate dehydrogenase (LDH), amylase and cytology may be useful in certain clinical situations. It is useful to calculate the serum–ascites albumin gradient (SAAG) by subtracting the ascitic albumin level from the serum albumin concentration.

TABLE 29.5

DIFFERENTIAL DIAGNOSIS OF CAUSES OF ASCITES BASED ON SERUM–ASCITES ALBUMIN GRADIENT

SAAG >1.1 g/dL	SAAG <1.1 g/dL
Hepatic cirrhosis	Peritoneal carcinomatosis
Alcoholic hepatitis	Tuberculous peritonitis
Cardiac ascites	Pancreatic ascites
Massive liver metastases	Biliary ascites
Fulminant hepatic failure	Nephrotic syndrome
Portal vein thrombosis	Connective tissue disease (serositis)
Veno-occlusive disease	Chylous ascites
Budd-Chiari syndrome	—
Acute fatty liver of pregnancy	—
Myxedema	—
"Mixed" ascites	

SAAG, Serum-sscites albumin gradient
From: Runyon BA, Montana AA, Akriviadis EA, et al. The serum-ascites albumin gradient is superior to the exudate-transudate concept in the differential diagnosis of ascites. *Ann Int Med* 1992;117:215–220.

A value greater than or equal to 1.1 g per dL is indicative of portal hypertension. A SAAG of <1.1 g per dL suggests other etiologies of ascites (Table 29.5). If infection is suspected, a cell count and differential should be performed, as well as gram stain and culture. The inoculation of blood culture bottles has been shown to improve diagnostic yield (15). Spontaneous bacterial peritonitis (SBP) is diagnosed when greater than 250 neutrophils per mm^3 are present. An elevated LDH and a low ascitic glucose level may also be seen in SBP. Cytology is useful when peritoneal carcinomatosis is suspected. The sensitivity of cytology is 96.7% if three samples are taken and processed in a timely fashion (17).

The primary treatment of patients with ascites includes dietary sodium restriction and oral diuretics. The combination of these two therapies is effective in 90% of patients with cirrhosis and ascites (18). The recommended allowance for sodium is 2000 mg per day or 88 mmol per day. Fluid restriction should be reserved only for patients with dilutional hyponatremia (11). Measuring urinary sodium can also be of clinical utility; if patients do not lose weight despite elevated urine sodium, dietary noncompliance may be suspected. Conversely, if urinary sodium remains low, patients may require increased doses of diuretics. Typically, diuretic therapy consists of a single dose of oral furosemide and spironolactone at starting doses of 40 and 100 mg, respectively (15). Monotherapy with spironolactone has been shown to be superior to monotherapy with furosemide in a randomized clinical trial (19). Both are beneficial in combination as they work through different mechanisms and combination therapy with furosemide helps prevent hyperkalemia from spironolactone. If indicated, the dosages of both medications may be titrated upward every 3–5 days, maintaining the same dose ratio. Most agree that maximal doses should be 160 mg per day of furosemide and 400 mg per day of spironolactone. Amiloride may be substituted for spironolactone in patients who develop tender gynecomastia (20).

Patients with tense ascites or large-volume ascites can be a challenge to manage. A single paracentesis of 5 L or less may be performed safely without the infusion of volume expanders. Larger volumes can be removed with the infusion of intravenous albumin (8 g per L removed), which has been shown to decrease electrolyte and renal abnormalities, but has no effect on overall morbidity or mortality (21) After initial large-volume paracentesis, oral diuretics should be used as maintenance therapy to help prevent reaccumulation of fluid.

Refractory ascites is defined as a lack of response to maximal doses of diuretics (400 mg spironolactone and 160 mg furosemide) and a sodium-restricted diet. Approximately, 10% of patients will have refractory ascites (12). This definition also includes patients who cannot tolerate therapy secondary to side effects such as encephalopathy, electrolyte abnormalities, or azotemia. Refractory ascites carries with it an extremely poor prognosis. Therapeutic options for refractory ascites include serial large-volume paracentesis, TIPS, or liver transplantation. TIPS involves creation of an intrahepatic connection between the portal and hepatic vein, resulting in decompression of portal hypertension. TIPS and serial large-volume paracentesis have been compared in five large randomized controlled trials. Initial trials showed a survival benefit in patients receiving TIPS, but this has not been confirmed in subsequent trials (11). TIPS should be reserved for patients without severe liver failure or encephalopathy who either have loculated ascites or are unwilling to undergo serial paracentesis. Renal insufficiency, hyperbilirubinemia, advanced age, coagulopathy, and Child-Pugh class C have all been associated with increased mortality after TIPS and should be taken into consideration when deciding on therapeutic options.

Spontaneous Bacterial Peritonitis

SBP occurs in 10–30% of patients with ascites. It involves translocation of luminal bacteria to lymph nodes with resultant bacteremia and infection of ascitic fluid (11). Approximately one third of patients presenting with SBP have no signs or symptoms and physicians should have a low threshold for performing a diagnostic paracentesis to diagnose this potentially life-threatening condition. The diagnosis is confirmed by an ascitic fluid absolute neutrophil count of >250 per mm^3. Usually, ascites cultures will reveal a single organism (gram-negative rods or streptococcal species). Third-generation cephalosporins, such as cefotaxime, are first-line treatment for SBP. Five days of treatment is generally recommended, as a randomized controlled trial demonstrated no difference in 5 days of treatment as compared to 10 days (22). Oral ofloxacin has also been studied and has been shown to be as effective as parenteral cefotaxime in patients without vomiting or shock (23). Selected patients should have a follow-up paracentesis following treatment for SBP. It should be considered in patients who fail to improve clinically, have persistent leukocytosis or fever, or have findings suggestive of secondary peritonitis.

Because of high rates of recurrence, long-term antibiotic prophylaxis is recommended in patients with prior history of SBP. Prophylaxis is also recommended in patients with acute gastrointestinal bleeding and patients with ascitic fluid protein (AFP) levels <1 g per dL (15). Regimens with proven efficacy include norfloxacin 400 mg per day, ciprofloxacin 750 mg per week, and trimethoprim/sulfamethoxazole 5 times per week.

Hepatorenal Syndrome

The hepatorenal syndrome (HRS) involves the development of acute renal failure in patients with advanced liver disease. The underlying cause is unknown, but likely involves abnormalities in the arterial circulation due to endogenous vasoactive substances. The diagnosis is based on advanced chronic or acute renal failure in the absence of shock, bacterial infection, or nephrotoxic drugs. Patients with HRS also have

TABLE 29.6

GRADING SYSTEM OF HEPATIC ENCEPHALOPATHY

Grade	Level of consciousness	Personality and intellect	Neurologic signs	Electroencephalogram abnormalities
0	Normal	Normal	None	None
Subclinical	Normal	Normal	Psychomotor abnormalities	None
1	Inverted sleep pattern	Forgetfulness, mild confusion, agitation, irritability	Tremor, apraxia, incoordination, impaired handwriting	Triphasic waves (5 cycles/s)
2	Lethargy, slow responses	Disorientation as regards time, amnesia, decreased inhibitions, inappropriate behavior	Asterixis, dysarthria, ataxia, hypoactive reflexes	Triphasic waves (5 cycles/s)
3	Somnolence but rousability, confusion	Disorientation as regards place, aggressive behavior	Asterixis, hyperactive reflexes, Babinski signs, muscle rigidity	Triphasic waves (5 cycles/s)
4	Coma	None	Decerebration	Delta activity

From: Gitlin N. Hepatic Encephalopathy. In: Zakim D, Boyer TD, eds. *Hepatology: a textbook of liver disease*, 3rd ed, Vol 1. Philadelphia, PA: WB Saunders, 1996:605–17.

an absence of proteinuria and hematuria, do not improve with withdrawal of diuretics or plasma expansion, have low urinary sodium, and have normal renal morphology on ultrasound examination (15). There are two types described. In Type I there is rapid deterioration in renal function whereas type II has a more chronic gradual clinical course.

Several systemic vasoconstrictor therapies for HRS that may improve renal function by increasing the effective arterial blood volume have been studied. Octreotide in combination with midodrine (24) has been shown to be beneficial in a small series of patients. Terlipressin (not available in the United States) has also been shown to be beneficial in uncontrolled trials (25). Finally, liver transplantation is also considered an effective treatment for HRS and patients who are diagnosed should be referred for liver transplantation if they are appropriate candidates. Patients listed for transplantation may need to be on hemodialysis briefly as a "bridge" to surgery.

Hepatic Encephalopathy

Hepatic encephalopathy (HE) is a complex neuropsychiatric syndrome that may complicate chronic liver failure and is present to varying degrees in 50–70% of patients with cirrhosis. The clinical manifestations of this syndrome range from subtle abnormalities detectable only by psychometric testing to deep coma. Several grading systems have been proposed, but the one most often utilized is based on clinical and electroencephalographic abnormalities (Table 29.6). Most manifestations of HE are reversible with medical treatment. Some patients have progressive, debilitating syndromes, such as dementia, spastic paraparesis, cerebellar degeneration, and extrapyramidal movement disorders (26). Most theories explaining the pathogenesis of HE accept that nitrogenous products derived from the gut adversely affect brain function, and a large body of work points toward ammonia as a key factor (27). Abnormalities in glutaminergic, serotoninergic, γ-amino butyric acid (GABA), and catecholaminergic neurotransmission have also been invoked in experimental HE (28).

The management approach to HE first requires exclusion of other reasons for an altered mental status in individuals with cirrhosis. These conditions include, intracranial bleed or masses, post-ictal state, hypoglycemia and other metabolic encephalopathies, alcohol intoxication/withdrawal, and other toxic encephalopathies. Next, the suspicion for HE in patients with cirrhosis should prompt a search for precipitating factors. These are detailed in Table 29.7. Although hyperammonemia is frequently associated with HE, ammonia levels do not correlate with the grade of encephalopathy. Consequently, this measurement is of little clinical value in establishing the diagnosis or following up the progress of patients with HE (29).

TABLE 29.7

FACTORS PRECIPITATING HEPATIC ENCEPHALOPATHY IN PATIENTS WITH CIRRHOSIS

1. Drugs
   sedatives (benzodiazepines)
   narcotics (opiates)
   alcohol
2. Increased ammonia production or increased ammonia diffusion across blood-brain barrier:
   excess dietary protein intake
   gastrointestinal hemorrhage
   infection (including bacterial peritonitis)
   electrolyte derangements (hypokalemia)
   systemic metabolic alkalosis
   constipation (anorexia, fluid restriction)
3. Dehydration
   diarrhea
   vomiting
   hemorrhage
   azotemia
   diuretics or large-volume paracentesis
4. Portosystemic shunts: reduced hepatic metabolism of toxins because of diversion of portal blood
   surgical shunts
   transjugular intrahepatic portosystemic shunts
   spontaneous shunts
5. Vascular occlusion
   portal vein thrombosis
   hepatic vein thrombosis
6. Primary hepatocellular carcinoma

Specifics of treatment for those with HE include initial provision of supportive care, particularly intubation and mechanical ventilation for those hospitalized patients with advanced stages of HE. Next, it is critical to identify and remove precipitating factors (outlined in Table 29.7). Finally, medications are administered to reduce the production and absorption of nitrogenous load from the gut. Nonabsorbable disaccharides, such as lactulose are routinely ordered to decrease ammonia production in the gut. Lactulose can be administered as an oral liquid solution or as a retention enema. This agent works both by its cathartic effect and its increase in fecal nitrogen excretion by facilitating incorporation of ammonia into bacteria (28). The dose is usually adjusted to achieve two to three loose bowel movements per day. Other drugs used to combat HE, often in conjunction with nonabsorbable disaccharides, include antibiotics, such as neomycin, low-dose metronidazole, oral vancomycin, and rifaximin. Physicians should be aware of the potential for toxic side effects of these agents, namely, nephrotoxicity, ototoxicity, and peripheral neuropathy. The efficacy of experimental strategies involving ammonia fixation into the urea cycle using L-ornithine L-aspartate, benzoate, and zinc supplementation (30–32) are now being tested in clinical trials. There is no good clinical evidence supporting aggressive protein restriction in patients with HE and caution should be used when doing so, as individuals with cirrhosis already have a degree of protein calorie malnutrition.

Variceal Hemorrhage

Gastroesophageal variceal hemorrhage (VH) is perhaps the most devastating portal hypertension–related complication in patients with cirrhosis, occurring in up to 30% of such individuals during the course of their illness (33). VH is associated with substantial morbidity and mortality: 30–50% of each bleeding episode is fatal, and as many as 70% of survivors have recurrent bleeding within 1 year after the index hemorrhage (33,34). Management of patients with gastroesophageal varices includes the following:

1. Prevention of initial bleeding episode (*primary prophylaxis*)
2. Control of active VH
3. Prevention of recurrent bleeding after a first episode (*secondary prophylaxis*).

All patients with cirrhosis should undergo a staging endoscopy to evaluate for esophageal and gastric varices. For those with moderate to large varices who have never previously experienced a bleeding episode, primary prophylaxis using a nonselective beta (β) blocker, such as nadolol or propranolol, is prescribed to decrease the portal pressure and collateral flow. The dose can be titrated to decrease the resting heart rate by 25% and the systolic blood pressure to no lower than 90 mm Hg. The addition of long-acting nitrates to β-blockers has been shown to enhance their hemodynamic effect and reduce the risk of bleeding (35). For those patients who are intolerant of the side effects of β-blockers, endoscopic variceal band ligation is an accepted modality for primary prophylaxis. A recently published randomized controlled multicenter trial that evaluated variceal band ligation and propranolol for primary prophylaxis of VH found them to be similarly effective (36).

The treatment for acute variceal bleeding is usually given in an intensive care setting and is aimed at volume resuscitation, correction of coagulopathy, ensuring hemostasis with pharmacologic agents (such as somatostatin and its analog, octreotide), and endoscopic therapy. Antibiotics should be administered prophylactically to prevent SBP, especially in patients with ascites. Very often these patients require intubation

prior to an emergent endoscopy to protect their airway from aspirating gastric contents and blood. Variceal band ligation has become the procedure of choice in the management of active VH, as endoscopic sclerotherapy is a procedure associated with serious complications in 10—20% of patients (37). Balloon tamponade using a Sengstaken–Blakemore or Minnesota tube may be a life-saving, temporizing measure to control acute VH, (particularly from bleeding gastric varices) and to stabilize the patient by acting as a "bridge" to a TIPS. TIPS is a procedure performed by the interventional radiologist to acutely lower the portal pressure. It is employed as salvage therapy for patients with refractory VH who have failed endoscopic therapy or in cases of active gastric VH where endoscopic therapy cannot be applied. Shunt surgery is also reserved as salvage therapy for endoscopic failures. Survivors of a VH should be evaluated for OLT. Because there is a high risk of recurrence after the initial hemorrhage, preventive strategies (including a variety of pharmacologic, endoscopic, and interventional approaches) are required and should be tailored to the patient's clinical condition, surgical risk, and prognosis. Usually, this involves serial sessions of endoscopic band ligation in an effort to eradicate the varices.

Screening for Hepatocellular Carcinoma

Cirrhosis is a premalignant condition. It is our obligation to screen such individuals in the hope of an early diagnosis and detection of HCC at a treatable stage. The published figures for the development of HCC in a patient with cirrhosis is approximately 3% per annum (38) (with cirrhosis due to hepatitis B, hepatitis C and hemochromatosis being in the highest risk categories). Patients with most forms of chronic liver disease are not at an increased risk until cirrhosis develops with the exception of those with hepatitis B virus infection, who can develop HCC in the absence of cirrhosis (39). It is our practice at the University of Pittsburgh to perform semiannual α-fetoprotein (AFP) measurements along with an imaging study (ultrasound or triphasic CT scan). It is of note that AFP is elevated in only approximately 50% of HCCs and there is clearly no linearity between tumor size and AFP measurement. Treatment options for those diagnosed with HCC depend on the stage of the disease and are divided into surgical therapies (resection, cryoablation, and OLT) and nonsurgical therapies (ethanol injection, radiofrequency ablation, transarterial chemoembolization, chemotherapy, and radiation).

Hepatopulmonary Syndrome and Other Pulmonary Conditions

Hepatopulmonary Syndrome (HPS) is a progressive, debilitating complication of cirrhosis occurring in approximately 4–25% of OLT candidates (40). Patients present with a triad of cirrhosis, hypoxemia, and intrapulmonary vascular dilation. Workup for this diagnosis rests on establishing the PaO_2 on an arterial blood gas, a double contrast echocardiogram evaluating for microbubbles in the left cardiac chambers, and a 99mTC macroaggregated albumin lung perfusion scan to determine a shunt fraction. Complete resolution of HPS after OLT even in the setting of severe hypoxemia has been well documented (41).

Portopulmonary hypertension (PPH) refers to the development of pulmonary arterial hypertension in the setting of portal hypertension with or without liver disease. It is defined as a mean pulmonary artery pressure (PAP) >25 with a normal pulmonary capillary wedge pressure and an elevated pulmonary vascular resistance (42). Patients with a PAP

>40 mm Hg on echocardiography should undergo a right heart catheterization to confirm the diagnosis. Those with moderate to severe PPH have a high post-OLT mortality and surgery is contraindicated unless preoperative vasodilator agents, such as intravenous epoprostenol (43), are able to significantly lower the pulmonary pressures.

Hepatic hydrothorax is defined as the presence of a pleural effusion in a patient with cirrhosis and no evidence of underlying cardiopulmonary disease. It results from movement of ascitic fluid into the pleural space through diaphragmatic defects (usually right-sided) and the pleural fluid characteristics are those of a transudate. Management options include medical management of ascites and therapeutic thoracentesis (using a pigtail catheter). TIPS has been used successfully to manage the symptoms of hepatic hydrothorax in the setting of marked ascites (44); however, pleurodesis using talc or antibiotics usually fails.

Other Preventative Measures and General Health Maintenance Issues

1. *Hepatitis A and B vaccinations.* All patients with chronic or end-stage liver disease should be vaccinated against hepatitis A and B, as a superimposed acute viral infection of this nature could result in a fatal outcome in those with little functional hepatic reserve. We routinely check hepatitis A antibody (total or IgG) and a hepatitis B surface antibody to check on the immune status of a patient with cirrhosis prior to vaccinating.
2. *Abstinence from alcohol.* It is paramount for all patients with cirrhosis to completely abstain from alcohol, as any degree of alcohol ingestion can be hepatotoxic in such individuals. Also, many transplant programs will not list patients with alcohol-related cirrhosis until they have had a 6-month sobriety period, and some programs insist on active participation in an alcohol rehabilitation program.
3. *Osteopenia/osteoporosis management.* Osteoporosis and bone fractures are more common in patients with cirrhosis than in the general population. Cholestatic liver diseases, such as primary biliary cirrhosis and primary sclerosing cholangitis, in themselves are an added risk factor for bone disease because of malabsorption of fat-soluble vitamin D. Patients are screened with bone mineral densitometry dual-energy x-ray absorptiometry (DEXA), and a T-score of <−2.5 would be an indication for treatment. Hypoestrogenism and low testosterone in males may be contributing factors. Treatments include hormone replacement therapy, bisphosphonates or testosterone in those who are deficient. Vitamin D supplementation with an oral dose of 800 IU per day and 1–2 g per day of elemental calcium is also required.
4. *Pruritus.* Severe itching is a common symptom of chronic cholestatic liver diseases, particularly primary biliary cirrhosis. Cholestyramine (an ion exchange resin) and ursodiol are generally first-line therapies. For treatment of refractory cases, rifampin and the opioid receptor antagonists, naloxone or naltrexone, can be administered.
5. *Medications in patients with advanced liver disease.* Patients with cirrhosis should avoid any agent that has the potential to cause additional liver injury. This includes over-the-counter medications, such as high doses of acetaminophen, prescription drugs with hepatotoxic side effects, and certain herbal remedies. Although the exact amount of acetaminophen that is safe in cirrhosis is unknown, we recommend that patients use no more than 2 g per day (in divided doses). The nonsteroidal anti-inflammatory drugs are also relatively contraindicated in patients with cirrhosis for fear of precipitating renal failure.
6. *Surgery in patients with advanced liver disease.* Patients with liver disease who require surgery are at greater risk for surgical and anesthesia-related complications than those with a healthy liver. The magnitude of the risk depends on the type of liver disease and its severity, the surgical procedure, and the type of anesthesia (45). The most accurate predictor of outcome appears to be the patient's preoperative Child's classification. In one study evaluating patients with cirrhosis undergoing abdominal operations, the mortality was 10, 30 and 82% for Child's classes A, B, and C, respectively (46). All patients with known end-stage liver disease should be assessed for the presence of jaundice, encephalopathy, coagulopathy, ascites, electrolyte abnormalities, and renal dysfunction preoperatively, and following surgery they should be observed closely for hepatic decompensation. Patients with Child's B or C cirrhosis and who are candidates for OLT, may need to be evaluated for transplantation preoperatively in the event that their hepatic function decompensates postoperatively requiring OLT listing.

TRANSITIONING TO PALLIATIVE/END-OF-LIFE CARE

In those patients with liver failure who are deemed too sick to undergo transplantation and where there are clear medical contraindications to the transplant operation, physicians ought to view "palliation" as their major focus and aim for the delivery of end-of-life care rather than disease-directed therapies or curative efforts. Patients with Child's B or C cirrhosis require close monitoring and the burden of their care can be very heavy. Owing to the myriad of complications that occur, these patients are frequently admitted to the hospital and management of their medications and nutrition becomes challenging for the health care provider.

A combined team approach, between the patient's hepatologist, primary care physician, and a specialist in palliative care, will be paramount to improve the patient's quality of life and to ensure both patient and family satisfaction. Some have suggested that such a strategy to provide preoperative palliative care is also required in those awaiting OLT (47). The goals of treatment are directed chiefly at symptom control. In patients with decompensated cirrhosis, the main symptom is that of abdominal discomfort due to refractory ascites, which is also a leading indication for recurrent hospital admissions for large-volume paracenteses. In order to curtail hospital admissions, physicians may wish to consider the placement of a TIPS in such patients, realizing, of course, that this procedure may exacerbate encephalopathy.

It is essential for the primary care physician and palliative care team to explore patient and family attitudes toward advance directives, "do not resuscitate" orders, and other end-of-life issues and initiate such discussions early enough to allow full utilization of all available resources, including hospice services.

CONCLUSIONS

The care and monitoring of patients with end-stage liver disease can be very challenging indeed. These patients have a multitude of complications that may necessitate frequent admissions to the hospital. Careful management of liver-specific complications can maximize their survival, particularly those who are awaiting organ transplantation. Preventative health screening is equally important in the ongoing management of a patient with cirrhosis. Their care demands frequent outpatient clinic visits, routine laboratory monitoring, radiology and endoscopy scheduling, and a timely referral for OLT evaluation by both their primary care physicians in the community as well as their hepatologists. For those individuals where OLT is not a reasonable goal of care, the physician focus should shift to palliation and end-of-life care. Frequent communication by all the health care personnel involved is pivotal in the multidisciplinary treatment approach to such individuals.

References

1. Murphy SL. Deaths: final data for 1998. *Natl Vital Stat Rep* 2000; 48(11):1–105.
2. Haellen J, Norden J. Liver cirrhosis unsuspected during life. A series of 79 cases. *J Chronic Dis* 1964;17:951.
3. Pugh RNH, Murray-Lyon IM, Dawson JL, et al. Transection of the oesophagus for bleeding oesophageal varices. *Br J Surg* 1973;60(8):646–649.
4. Lucey MR, Brown KA, Everson GT, et al. Minimal criteria for placement of adults on the liver transplant waiting list: a report of a national conference organized by the American society of transplant physicians and the American association for the study of liver diseases. *Liver Transpl Surg* 1997;3:628–637.
5. Richmond VA. United Network for Organ Sharing. Allocation of liver policy. In: *United Network for organ donation*. 2002; http://www.UNOS.org/resources/policy.
6. Kamath PS, Wiesner RH, Malinchoc M, et al. A model to predict survival in patients with end-stage liver disease. [see comment]. *Hepatology* 2001;33(2):464–470.
7. Malinchoc M, Kamath PS, Gordon FD, et al. A model to predict poor survival in patients undergoing transjugular intrahepatic portosystemic shunts. [see comment]. *Hepatology* 2000;31(4):864–871.
8. Wiesner R, Edwards E, Friedman R, et al. Model for End-stage Liver Disease (MELD) and allocation of donor livers. [see comment]. *Gastroenterology* 2003;124(1):91–96.
9. Freeman RB, Wiesner RH, Edwards E, et al. Results of the first year of the new liver allocation plan. *Liver Transpl* 2004;10(1):7–15.
10. Murray KF, Carithers RL Jr. AASLD practice guidelines: evaluation of the patient for liver transplantation. *Hepatology* 2005;41(6):1407–1432.
11. Gines P, Cardenas A, Arroyo V, et al. Management of cirrhosis and ascites. [see comment]. *N Engl J Med* 2004;350(16):1646–1654.
12. Saadeh S, Davis GL. Management of ascites in patients with end-stage liver disease. *Rev Gastroenterol Disord* 2004;4(4):175–185.
13. Runyon BA, Montana AA, Akriviadis EA, et al. The serum-ascites albumin gradient is superior to the exudate-transudate concept in the differential diagnosis of ascites. *Ann Intern Med* 1992;117(3):215–220.
14. Cattau, EL Jr, Benjamin, SB, Knuff TE, et al. The accuracy of the physical examination in the diagnosis of suspected ascites. *JAMA* 1982;247(8):1164–1166.
15. Runyon BA. AASLD Practice Guidelines Committee. Management of adult patients with ascites due to cirrhosis. *Hepatology*, 2004;39(3):841–856.
16. Webster ST, Brown KL, Lucey MR, et al. Hemorrhagic complications of large volume abdominal paracentesis. *Am J Gastroenterol* 1996;91(2): 366–368.
17. Runyon BA, Hoefs JC, Morgan TR. Ascitic fluid analysis in malignancy-related ascites. *Hepatology* 1988;8(5):1104–1109.
18. Fogel MR, Sawhney VK, Neal EA, et al. Diuresis in the ascitic patient: a randomized controlled trial of three regimens. *J Clin Gastroenterol* 1981;1:73–80.
19. Perez-Ayuso RM, Arroyo V, Planas R, et al. Randomized comparative study of efficacy of furosemide versus spironolactone in nonazotemic cirrhosis with ascites. Relationship between the diuretic response and the activity of the renin-aldosterone system. *Gastroenterology* 1983;84(5 Pt 1):961–968.
20. Sharma P, Rakela J. Management of pre-liver transplantation patient–part 2. *Liver Transpl* 2005;11(3):249–260.
21. Gines P, Tito L, Arroyo V, et al. Randomized comparative study of therapeutic paracentesis with and without intravenous albumin in cirrhosis. *Gastroenterology* 1988;94(6):1493–1502.
22. Runyon BA, McHutchison JG, Antillon MR, et al. Short-course versus long-course antibiotic treatment of spontaneous bacterial peritonitis. A randomized controlled study of 100 patients. [see comment]. *Gastroenterology* 1991;100(6):1737–1742.
23. Navasa M, Follo A, Llovet JM, et al. Randomized, comparative study of oral ofloxacin versus intravenous cefotaxime in spontaneous bacterial peritonitis. [see comment]. *Gastroenterology* 1996;111(4):1011–1017.
24. Angeli P, Volpin R, Gerunda G, et al. Reversal of type 1 hepatorenal syndrome with the administration of midodrine and octreotide. *Hepatology*, 1999;29(6):1690–1697.
25. Moreau R, Durand F, Poynard T, et al. Terlipressin in patients with cirrhosis and type 1 hepatorenal syndrome: a retrospective multicenter study. [see comment]. *Gastroenterology* 2002;122(4):923–930.
26. Gitlin, N. Hepatic Encephalopathy. In: Zakim D, Boyer TD. *Hepatology: a textbook of liver disease*, Philadelphia, PA : WB Saunders, 1996:605–617.
27. Norenberg MD. Astrocytic-ammonia interactions in hepatic encephalopathy. *Semin Liver Dis* 1996;16(3):245–253.
28. Blei AT, Cordoba J. Practice Parameters Committee of the American College of Gastroenterology. Hepatic encephalopathy. *Am J Gastroenterol* 2001;96(7):1968–1976.
29. Clemmesen JO, Larsen FS, Kondrup J, et al. Cerebral herniation in patients with acute liver failure is correlated with arterial ammonia concentration. *Hepatology* 1999;29(3):648–653.
30. Riggio O, Merli M, Capocaccia L, et al. Zinc supplementation reduces blood ammonia and increases liver ornithine transcarbamylase activity in experimental cirrhosis. *Hepatology* 1992;16(3):785–789.
31. Marchesini G, Fabbri A, Bianchi G, et al. Zinc supplementation and amino acid-nitrogen metabolism in patients with advanced cirrhosis. *Hepatology* 1996;23(5):1084–1092.
32. Sushma S, Dasarthy S, Tandon RK, et al. Sodium benzoate in the treatment of acute hepatic encephalopathy: a double-blind randomized trial. *Hepatology* 1992,16(1):138–144.
33. North Italian Endoscopic Club for the Study and Treatment of Esophageal Varices. Prediction of first variceal hemorrhage with cirrhosis and esophageal varices. *N Engl J Med* 1988;319:983.
34. Graham D, Smith J. The course of patients after variceal hemorrhage. *Gastroenterology* 1981;80:800–809.
35. Garcia-Pagan JC, Feu F, Bosch J, et al. Propranolol compared with propranolol plus isosorbide-5-mononitrate for portal hypertension in cirrhosis. A randomized controlled study. *Ann Intern Med* 1991;114(10): 869–873.
36. Schepke M, Kleber G, Nurnberg D, et al. Ligation versus propranolol for the primary prophylaxis of variceal bleeding in cirrhosis. *Hepatology* 2004;40(1):65–72.
37. D'Amico G, Pagliaro L, Bosch J. Pharmacological treatment of portal hypertension: an evidence-based approach. [erratum in *Semin Liver Dis* 2000;20(3):399]. *Semin Liver Dis* 1999;19(4):475–505.
38. Colombo M, de Franchis R, Del Ninno E, et al. Hepatocellular carcinoma in Italian patients with cirrhosis. [see comment]. *N Engl J Med* 1991;325(10):675–680.
39. Beasley RP, Hwang LY, Lin CC, et al. Hepatocellular carcinoma and hepatitis B virus. A prospective study of 22, 707 men in Taiwan. *Lancet* 1981;2(8256):1129–1133.
40. Martinez GP, Barbera JA, Visa J, et al. Hepatopulmonary syndrome in candidates for liver transplantation. [see comment]. *J Hepatol* 2001;34(5):651–657.
41. Lange PA, Stoller JK. The hepatopulmonary syndrome. [see comment]. *Ann Intern Med* 1995;122(7):521–529.
42. Hoeper MM, Krowka MJ, Strassburg CP. Portopulmonary hypertension and hepatopulmonary syndrome. *Lancet* 2004;363:1461–1468.
43. Barst RJ, Rubin LJ, Long WA, et al., The Primary Pulmonary Hypertension Study Group. A comparison of continuous intravenous epoprostenol (prostacyclin) with conventional therapy for primary pulmonary hypertension. *N Engl J Med* 1996;334:296–302.
44. Gordon FD, Anastopoulos HT, Crenshaw W, et al. The successful treatment of symptomatic, refractory hepatic hydrothorax with transjugular intrahepatic portosystemic shunt. *Hepatology* 1997;25(6):1366–1369.
45. Friedman LS, Maddrey WC. Surgery in the patient with liver disease. *Med Clin North Am* 1987;71(3):453–476.
46. Mansour A, Watson W, Shayani V, et al. Abdominal operations in patients with cirrhosis: still a major surgical challenge. *Surg* 1997;122(4):730–735.
47. Rossaro L, Troppmann C, McVicar JP, et al. A strategy for the simultaneous provision of pre-operative palliative care for patients awaiting liver transplantation. *Transpl Int* 2004;17:473–475.

CHAPTER 30 ■ MANAGEMENT OF ADVANCED HEART FAILURE

RODNEY TUCKER AND BARRY K. RAYBURN

Heart failure is a chronic illness that is increasing in frequency and considered to be a major public health problem in the United States. It is primarily defined as a syndrome caused by the overall inadequate performance of the heart, leading to a constellation of clinical symptoms such as shortness of breath, fatigue, and swelling among others. The pathophysiology of heart failure involves a complex series of structural, functional, and biochemical events that are responsible for the overall progressive nature of the disease. The term *advanced heart failure* is most commonly used to describe symptomatic patients who have progressed to New York Heart Association (NYHA) Class IV or American Heart Association/American College of Cardiology (AHA/ACC) Stage D as described in this chapter and are receiving maximum medical therapies. The NYHA Class is based solely on symptoms with Class IV patients typically having heart failure symptoms at rest. The AHA/ACC Staging system, on the other hand, is based on stages of disease progression ranging from patients at potential risk for heart failure (Stage A) through patients with advanced heart failure, refractory to standard medical management (Stage D). Heart failure is responsible for most hospital admissions among the elderly and is one of the leading costs in the Medicare system. In addition, advanced heart failure has a worse prognosis than many cancers, with a one year mortality approximating 45% (1).

This chapter provides the basic epidemiology, pathophysiology, and natural history of heart failure with an emphasis on the advanced state. The rationale and complexity of the overall treatment is outlined, including pharmacotherapy as well as device therapy. The role of expanded services in supportive and palliative care as well as the role of the palliative medicine specialist as part of the care team is reviewed. Communication challenges that exist in caring for patients with an uncertain disease trajectory and the role of hospice as an option for care for patients with end-stage disease are highlighted.

EPIDEMIOLOGY

Despite substantial advances in the therapy for heart failure, it remains a common, morbid, and mortal condition. Current estimates suggest that approximately 5 million Americans suffer from heart failure with new cases being diagnosed at a rate of 550,000 per year (2). Both the incidence and prevalence figures are likely to continue to increase with estimates of an annual incidence of 800,000 by 2010 (3). Although improved survival from myocardial infarction has contributed in part to this rather dramatic increase in prevalent cases, this increase can be attributed chiefly to the "graying" of the American population. Heart failure disproportionately affects the elderly with the prevalence rising with each decade of life (Fig. 30.1). Between 1990 and 2000, the number of Americans aged 60 or over increased by 3.9 million with individuals over 85 years of age accounting for 1.1 million (4). Heart failure morbidity includes diminished functional capacity, complex drug regimens, and, for many patients with advanced heart failure, frequent hospitalizations. Cowie et al. studied hospitalizations in a community-based population and found that 59% of patients diagnosed with heart failure were admitted during the 19-month average follow-up period with many patients admitted multiple times (5). Heart failure mortality figures also remain high despite improvements in therapy. An important reality in the management of heart failure is that most of the patients with this diagnosis will ultimately die of it (6). Gross mortality estimates for patients with heart failure vary depending on a number of variables including demographic factors, comorbidities, underlying etiology, functional status, hemodynamic variables, and response to therapy. For example, severely symptomatic patients (NYHA Class IV) with an ischemic etiology and persistent elevation of right atrial pressure despite optimal medical management may have an annual mortality approaching 50%, whereas a relatively asymptomatic patient (NYHA Class I) with diastolic dysfunction due to underlying hypertension that is now controlled may have a mortality comparable to the general population with hypertension (7,8). In the context of this chapter, patients with "advanced" heart failure, by definition, are patients with a very high anticipated mortality. Although various models are available to predict mortality rates for individuals, such models often fail to accurately identify *which* patients with a specific set of characteristics are likely to die (9). Because of this difficulty, patients with heart failure are frequent "graduates" of hospice programs.

PATHOPHYSIOLOGY

The functional definition of heart failure is a clinical syndrome in which the heart is unable to meet the metabolic needs of the body (10). Several points are important in fully understanding this definition. First, heart failure is *not* a specific disease, but rather a clinical syndrome that results from any of a number of underlying diseases. An individual may recover from heart failure, although the underlying disease may still be present. Second, the definition of heart failure does not specify that the heart is weak. In fact, most cases of heart failure are the result of a combination of systolic and diastolic dysfunction, with

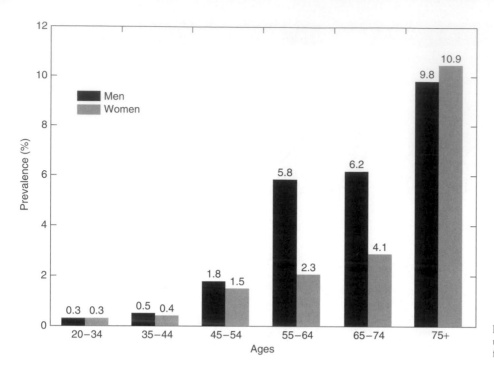

FIGURE 30.1. Prevalence of heart failure by age for men and women. Centers for Disease Control and NHBLI.

the latter predominating in up to 50% of the cases (8). Third, this definition avoids the term "congestive" because not all the manifestations of heart failure require congestion—or volume overload. Much of the symptom burden of heart failure results from a low cardiac output state.

There are two major pathophysiologic models that exist to explain the clinical manifestations of heart failure. The first and older of the two is a hydraulic model, which explains the relationships between flow and pressure in the cardiovascular system. Regardless of the predominance of systolic or diastolic dysfunction, an abnormal relationship between pressure and flow can result in elevated filling pressures on the right or left side of the heart coupled with low forward flow due to reduced contractility for any given filling pressure. The former phenomenon manifests as the congestive symptoms of edema, orthopnea, early satiety, and dyspnea, whereas the latter will manifest as fatigue, depression, anorexia, and also dyspnea due to muscle fatigue and inefficiency. Although this model

explains most of the symptoms of heart failure well, and can be used to model treatments such as diuresis and after-load reduction, it falls short of explaining the progressive nature of the syndrome and the high mortality despite the above-mentioned treatments. A more comprehensive model that has evolved and resulted in dramatic improvements in therapy is the neurohormonal model of heart failure. The central hypothesis of the neurohormonal model is that the hydraulic manifestations of heart failure lead to stimulation of various compensatory mechanisms that, in turn, are deleterious to cardiac function (Fig. 30.2). This model explains the relentlessly progressive nature of heart failure and has led to the development of several effective therapies as discussed in the following text. Besides neurohormones, other circulating factors such as inflammatory cytokines are involved in the clinical manifestations of heart failure and are included in this hypothesis.

Virtually any cardiac disease can ultimately result in heart failure. In the United States, the most common cause of heart

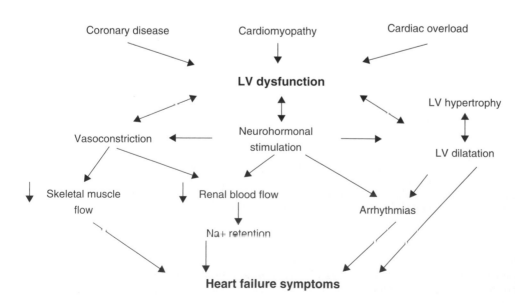

FIGURE 30.2. Schematic of the pathophysiology of heart failure illustrating the central role of neurohormonal activation. Adapted from Cohn JN, Pathophysiology of clinical heart failure. In: Hosenpud JD, Greenberg BH, eds. *Congestive Heart Failure*. New York: Springer-Verlang, 1994.

failure is coronary artery disease (11). Coronary disease may result in profound ventricular dysfunction through permanent loss of myocardium as in an infarct or through ischemia, a potentially reversible condition. Cardiomyopathies, hypertension, valvular heart disease, and congenital abnormalities account for the bulk of the remaining cases.

NATURAL HISTORY AND PROGNOSIS

As discussed in the preceding text, the mortality of heart failure remains high with advanced stage patients accounting for up to 50% annual mortality. Despite these rather ominous survival statistics, the clinical course of heart failure can be very protracted. A rather typical clinical course for an individual patient is illustrated in Figure 30.3. Patients are usually diagnosed with at least moderate symptoms. Following initiation of therapy, many patients improve significantly, and this improvement may be expected to last for a variable period of time. In some patients, this "plateau" of stability may be short-lived and in others it may continue for many years. In most of the patients, this stable phase will ultimately give way to a period of intermittent exacerbations characterized by frequent physician visits, changes in medical therapy, and hospitalizations. Although individual exacerbations may improve, the overall trend tends to be downhill with the time interval between exacerbations becoming shorter. Without further intervention, this course will ultimately lead to death from pump failure. Interventions at this advanced stage may temporarily reset the patient back onto a plateau, but will eventually lead to the same deterioration for most. For some patients, arrhythmias intercede in this clinical course, often at the earlier, less symptomatic stages, and result in sudden cardiac death. This latter phenomenon has led to the increased utilization of implantable defibrillators, which, in turn, may shift the mode of death toward progressive pump failure. The combination of a progressive natural history leading to death from pump failure and the unexpected possibility of sudden cardiac death at any point suggests that the role of supportive

care should ideally begin *early* in the patient's clinical course. Data from the Study to Understand Prognoses and Preferences for Outcomes and Risks of Treatment (SUPPORT) trial further support this idea (12). In this trial, over 1400 patients with heart failure were followed up. Thirty-eight percent died within the first year of follow-up. Clinicians caring for these patients estimated their 6-month survival at greater than 50% up to 3 days before their death. Therefore, the concept of using prognostic criteria to decide when to initiate supportive care may be flawed. End-of-life care is more typically provided to patients who have entered the downhill phase of their clinical course and have exhausted or opted out of therapies that could potentially return them to clinical stability. Such patients are usually characterized by NYHA Class III or IV symptoms and are in ACC/AHA Stage D.

HEART FAILURE THERAPY

Overview

Modern therapy for heart failure is a multifaceted approach to a complex clinical syndrome (Table 30.1). Therapy consists of education, pharmacotherapy, and for an increasing percentage of patients the use of electrical and mechanical devices. Education and basic pharmacotherapy provide the foundation upon which other therapeutic options are added in an individualized fashion. Our improved understanding of the pathophysiology of heart failure has led to comparable improvements in pharmacologic therapy. Most of the data regarding the treatment of heart failure have been obtained from patients in whom systolic dysfunction predominates. Fewer data exist for patients with primarily diastolic dysfunction. Where such data exist, they will be discussed but to a large extent the clinician is left with principles of management rather than specific data in managing patients with diastolic dysfunction.

Despite excellent data and rationale for various therapies in heart failure, an alarming number of patients are inadequately managed by either underutilization or, less commonly, overutilization of various therapies (13,14). This fact is significant for

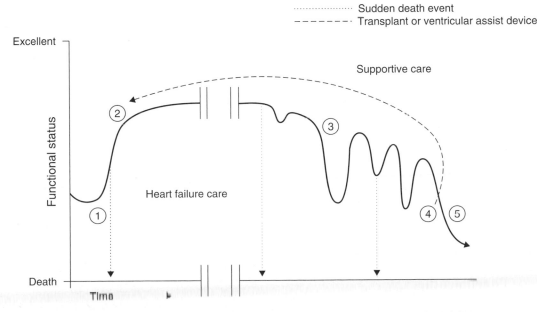

FIGURE 30.3. Progression of heart failure from initial presentation (1), through stabilization (2), progressive deterioration (3), and ultimately to death (5), unless alternate therapies are utilized (4). Redrawn with permission Renlund D, Goodlin S.

TABLE 30.1

HEART FAILURE THERAPY[a]

New York Heart Association class	Education	Pharmacotherapy	Device therapy	Other therapy
I	Natural history Dietary restrictions Exercise OTC medications Daily weights	ACE inhibitor or ARB β-blocker Diuretics (if needed)		Introduction to supportive care strategies
II	—	Consider digoxin	—	—
III	Reinforce the above Stricter dietary restrictions Encourage early contact for changes	Diuretics (possibly combination) Spironolactone Hydralazine/isosorbide in appropriate patients	Resynchronization Implantable defibrillator	Revisit role of supportive care Consider referral for advanced therapy
IV	—	Inotropic therapy or intravenous vasodilators in hospitalized patients	Ventricular assist device	Referral for advanced therapy in appropriate patients

ACE, angiotensin converting enzyme; ARB, angiotensin receptor blocker; OTC, over the counter.
[a]Pharmacotherapy applies primarily to patients with systolic dysfunction (see text).

the palliative care practitioner because of the possibility of patients being referred for end-of-life care whereas they may have significant therapeutic options. Data show that patients followed up by a physician specializing in the care of heart failure are more likely to be treated according to evidence-based guidelines than patients followed up by other specialists or by generalists (15,16). A patient referred for end-of-life care may warrant review by such a specialist, if available, to confirm the lack of therapeutic options.

Patient Education

All patients with heart failure should be educated as an integral part of their management. The specific role of disease management programs is discussed later in this chapter, but basic education is essential for all patients. Since volume management is a common problem in heart failure, all patients should be placed on a sodium-restricted diet. A typical limit is between 2 and 4 g of sodium per day. Fluid restrictions are also often employed, especially for patients with advanced heart failure or those suffering from hyponatremia. Weighing daily helps to monitor sudden changes in fluid volume, thus allowing for changes to be made in therapy before clinical symptoms worsen. Patients should also be encouraged to avoid certain types of medications—both prescription and over-the-counter. Decongestants can promote cardiac dysrhythmias in this susceptible population and should be avoided in most situations. The nonsteroidal anti-inflammatory drugs, by their nature, can lead to a reduction in renal blood flow, resulting in decreased response to diuretics and marked sodium retention. This phenomenon can happen with virtually all drugs in this class, including the newer cyclo-oxygenase-2 (COX-2) inhibitors (17).

Pharmacotherapy

Angiotensin Converting Enzyme Inhibitors

Activation of the renin-angiotensin system is a central feature in heart failure. This activation results in elevated levels of angiotensin II, which in turn causes vasoconstriction, sodium and water retention, and adverse cardiac remodeling (10). Angiotensin converting enzyme (ACE) inhibitors block the conversion of angiotensin I to angiotensin II, resulting in decreased levels of the latter in patients with heart failure. Multiple randomized clinical trials in patients ranging from NYHA Class IV to patients with asymptomatic left ventricular dysfunction have demonstrated improved patient outcomes with the use of ACE inhibitors (18). The use of ACE inhibitor may be limited by profound hypotension (although relative hypotension is common and often desirable in patients with heart failure), allergies to this class of medicines, and commonly a dry, persistent cough.

Angiotensin II Receptor Blockers

Alternate pathways for the production of angiotensin II exist, resulting in accumulation even in the presence of ACE inhibition. The development of angiotensin II receptor blockers allows for blockade at the level of the receptor. Studies on patients with heart failure have produced variable results, but overall suggest that the use of a receptor blocker as an alternate to an ACE inhibitor is likely comparable for most patients (10). Data do not yet support the routine use of this class of drug in addition to ACE inhibition and the weight of evidence still favors ACE inhibition as first-line therapy for tolerant patients. A major, significant trial of angiotensin II receptor blockade in patients with diastolic dysfunction (CHARM-Preserved) demonstrated a reduction in hospitalization but no change in mortality when compared with placebo (19).

β-Adrenergic Blockers

Beyond blockade of the renin-angiotensin system, the next major improvement in heart failure pharmacotherapy came with the use of β-adrenergic blocking drugs. With their predominant effect on the sympathetic stimulation seen in heart failure, β-adrenergic blockers have demonstrated an incremental improvement in mortality over ACE inhibition. β-blocker therapy is typically initiated at a very low dose and uptitrated gradually in patients who remain symptomatic despite ACE inhibition. Patients should also be well compensated from a volume perspective before the drug is started. Specific β-adrenergic blocking agents that have data supporting their use in heart failure include carvedilol, metoprolol succinate, and bisoprolol (20–23). These data support the use of β-adrenergic blocking agents in patients with NYHA Class II through Class IV symptoms (24). Other β-adrenergic blocking agents have been tested but have failed to demonstrate a benefit, suggesting that the effect may *not* be a class effect (25). Also, studies conducted before the routine use of ACE inhibitors failed to demonstrate a survival benefit (26). Therefore, whenever possible, clinicians should choose an appropriately studied agent for addition to background ACE-inhibitor therapy.

Spironolactone

The aldosterone blocking agent spironolactone has been studied and found to reduce mortality in a group of severely symptomatic (Class IV or recently Class IV) patients treated with ACE inhibitors (27). The side effect profile in this trial was acceptable; however, subsequent studies have demonstrated potentially more significant side effects and suggested possible overutilization (14).

Digoxin

Data from the Digoxin Investigation Group trial demonstrated that, although digoxin did not reduce overall mortality, it reduced rates of hospitalization generally as well as reduced rates of hospitalization specifically for symptoms of worsening heart failure (e.g., dyspnea and fatigue) among patients with a low ejection fraction (28). No effect was seen on mortality, and digoxin has no role in the management of patients with diastolic dysfunction.

Hydralazine and Nitrates

Initially studied as a means of after-load reduction, the combination of hydralazine and long-acting nitrates proved superior to placebo in decreasing mortality (29). Their use diminished dramatically in the ACE-inhibitor era, having been relegated as a backup strategy for intolerant patients. Recently, there has been a renewed interest in this form of therapy in the African-American population. The African-American Heart Failure Trial (AHeFT) demonstrated that the addition of BiDil, a combination drug containing hydralazine and isosorbide, reduced mortality in a group of African American patients already on conventional heart failure therapy (30).

Diuretics

These drugs are a necessary part of the treatment for heart failure in most of the patients. Ideally, diuretics need to be used as sparingly as possible because they tend to stimulate neurohormone production. Loop diuretics are typically used for management of volume status when patients are unable to maintain a euvolemic state with sodium restriction alone. For refractory patients, escalating doses of diuretics are appropriate rather than using an ineffective dose with increased frequency. If patients remain refractory, the addition of a second agent, typically a diazide such as metolazone, may result in markedly enhanced diuresis. Patients receiving combination diuretics are particularly susceptible to abnormalities in electrolytes.

Nesiritide

The newest drug in the pharmacotherapeutic armamentarium is nesiritide. This compound is identical to the naturally occurring B-type natriuretic peptide released from ventricular muscle tissue in response to stretch. The physiologic actions of this compound include balanced vasodilatation, natriuresis, improved diastolic relaxation, and an antifibrotic effect (31). This drug has a short half-life and is administered by continuous intravenous infusion in patients with decompensated heart failure due to volume overload refractory to diuretic therapy. Data demonstrate that nesiritide is superior to nitroglycerin in its ability to reduce wedge pressure and improve patient symptoms acutely (32). It is not an inotrope and does not have an associated risk of arrhythmias, making this agent potentially useful in patients with advanced heart failure without requiring extensive monitoring. Potential limitations include hypotension due to its vasodilatory properties and an elevation of serum creatinine in certain susceptible patients (33). The role of nesiritide in the outpatient setting or as a scheduled, intermittent infusion in patients with chronic heart failure continues to evolve.

Inotropic Therapy

The use of positively inotropic agents to treat patients with decompensated heart failure is a complex topic. Presently, two agents are commonly available for administration as intravenous infusions: the β-adrenergic agonist dobutamine and the phosphodiesterase inhibitor milrinone. Inotropic agents can improve hemodynamics in heart failure by forcing increased contractility of the failing myocardium. This can improve patient symptoms and assist in stabilizing decompensated patients. Unfortunately, a consequence of this type of therapy is an increased potential for serious arrhythmias and myocardial ischemia in susceptible patients. For this reason, inotropic therapy is typically reserved for short-term use in patients with severe decompensation in an effort to stabilize the clinical situation. Efforts at chronic use of oral versions of inotropic agents have resulted in excess mortality in the treatment group and no such agents are available in the United States. The practice of intermittent administration of inotropic agents or the routine use of low-dose inotropic agents in less severe heart failure has not been supported by clinical trials (34). Despite these data, the role and utility of inotropic agents in the setting of end-of-life care has not been extensively studied. While acknowledging that these agents cause a potential increase in overall mortality, it needs to be said that they may, nonetheless, have a palliative role in certain patients who are unable to leave the hospital owing to persistent decompensation despite other therapies.

Electrical Device-Based Therapies

An enormous surge in the use of electrical devices has occurred in the past decade. The use of biventricular pacemakers and implantable cardioverter-defibrillators is now so common that virtually any practitioner caring for patients with heart failure will be exposed to these devices. As patients transit from more aggressive care into end-of-life care, an understanding of the role and possible options for these devices is necessary for the clinician.

Biventricular Pacing

Some patients with left ventricular systolic dysfunction develop significant abnormalities of the conduction system or of mechanical-electrical coupling. This phenomenon, often characterized on the surface electrocardiogram by a widened QRS complex, results in ventricular dyssynchrony. In this situation, the ventricles do not maintain correct timing with respect to each other and lose some of the mechanical advantages of synchronous contraction. The placement of a biventricular pacing system with leads in the right ventricle and the lateral cardiac vein (to provide left ventricular pacing) can restore synchrony with resultant improvement in functional status and hospitalizations (35,36).

Implantable Cardioverter-Defibrillators

As noted in the preceding text, ventricular arrhythmias are a frequent cause of death among patients with heart failure. Despite various attempts, clinicians are poor at predicting which patients are likely to die in this manner. This fact has resulted in several large trials that indicate that many patients with heart failure due to systolic dysfunction who meet certain structural, electrical, and functional criteria benefit from the prophylactic placement of an implantable cardioverter-defibrillator (37,38). Since defibrillators are effective at preventing sudden cardiac death, an increasing number of patients will avoid this event and progress to advanced stages of pump failure. This will, in turn, increase the likelihood of patients coming to end-of-life care with an existing device in place. The proper management of these devices in the context of end-of-life care is an important point of discussion among patients, palliative care providers, and electrophysiologists responsible for their maintenance and programming. Patients may wish to discuss disabling the defibrillation feature of their device as a part of end-of-life care. The authors are also of the opinion that a discussion regarding this topic should be included for most patients before the initial implant of the device.

Mechanical Therapy

The other area of rapid development that is likely to impact practitioners caring for patients with heart failure at end of life are ventricular assist devices. These devices, best described as a "booster pump" for the left ventricle, were initially developed as a bridge to sustain critically ill patients until a heart became available for transplantation. Technological advances have led to smaller, more efficient, battery-operated implantable devices with relatively few mechanical problems. The success of these devices in the role as a bridge to transplantation led to the Randomized Evaluation of Mechanical Assistance for the Treatment of Congestive Heart Failure (REMATCH) trial, which studied the use of a left ventricular assist device in a population of patients who were ineligible for transplantation (39). When compared with standard medical therapy, it was seen that the use of a ventricular assist device resulted in improved mortality. This study led to the approval of the device for use in "destination" therapy in patients who are ineligible for transplant or chose not to undergo transplant. Although currently only affecting a small percentage of the overall heart failure population, these devices are likely to continue to advance technologically and will become more prevalent in the future.

SUPPORTIVE AND PALLIATIVE CARE IN ADVANCED HEART FAILURE

The terms *supportive care* and *palliative care* may be used interchangeably in the care of patients with advanced heart failure in describing the goals or components of care for these patients. *Supportive care* for those with advanced heart failure includes education about their disease and treatment options, benefits and side effects of various treatments, expected course of the illness, and resources for emotional and financial support. Formal supportive care programs may also include evaluations of symptom burden or patient distress and attempt to address these needs as well. These programs may be accessed at any time during the illness trajectory but they are particularly useful during acute treatment periods. *Disease management* and *collaborative care programs* are examples of

clinical models that provide comprehensive supportive care to patients with heart failure and their families.

The scope of *palliative care* encompasses supportive care and includes an emphasis on quality of life for patients with advanced illness such as heart failure. As the illness trajectory progresses, the goals of palliative care become a more integral part of the management of patients with heart failure. Improved quality of life is achieved by focusing on patient-directed goals of care, enhanced communication between patient, family, and health care team, conflict resolution, and comprehensive advanced care planning. An interdisciplinary approach to the sources of suffering in advanced heart failure requires a team composed of individuals with various training, such as physicians, psychologists, nurses, and chaplains. *Hospice* is one care option or model for patients in the last stage of their illness that incorporates an interdisciplinary team with expertise in end-of-life concerns. Comprehensive supportive care is a model that can assist patients as they transit to palliative goals of care through specialist-directed interdisciplinary management of illness and symptoms.

Disease Management and Collaborative Care

In managing patients with heart failure, there is a general consensus among various guidelines that counseling regarding diet (mainly fluid and sodium restriction), symptom management, risk factor modification, exercise, medication compliance, and discussions regarding illness course and prognosis should all be a part of the management strategy. Components of this strategy may be prioritized to different degrees according to the acuity at various points in the disease trajectory. Programs to assist in the *disease management* may include patient educational sessions, outpatient clinic follow-up programs staffed by nurses and educators, as well as home care models and protocols that have been developed in recent years. Examples of these programs have met with various degrees of success with particular improvements in hospital readmission rates, functional status, symptom management, and overall costs (40). However, many of the studies have not included sufficient numbers of patients with advanced or Stage IV heart failure to allow recommendations regarding this population, so these models warrant further study in the future.

Effective management of advanced or end-stage heart failure frequently requires discussion of care goals that may not have been emphasized as much in an earlier phase of the disease trajectory. An interdisciplinary team of professionals may need to be in place to coordinate good patient-directed outcomes. One such example of this type of coordinated care model is the MediCaring Collaborative Project, which emphasizes the importance of an interdisciplinary team coordinating care for patients with advanced illness. This model essentially incorporates the comprehensive aspects of palliative care within a managed care structure (41).

During the course of illness, patients with heart failure may be seen by a primary care physician in addition to a cardiologist as a consultant. Depending on the nature and acuity of the heart failure, the cardiologist may be the deciding authority for the patient's care to a large extent. Other medical specialists are often included in the patient's care team including a pulmonologist or endocrinologist depending on any comorbid conditions. Although referral for palliative care specialist services may be more commonplace in disease processes such as cancer or acquired immuno deficiency syndrome (AIDS), the role of the palliative medicine physician is appropriate in patients with heart failure (12,13).

Studies have shown that the physical and nonphysical needs of these patients are complex and dynamic as the disease progresses. The *collaborative care* team approach involving cardiologists, primary care physicians, and palliative medicine specialists is potentially the most beneficial in achieving appropriate patient-directed goals (44). Several models exist that emphasize appropriate referral for patients with palliative care needs in the inpatient as well as the outpatient setting (45). It may be beneficial to have a cardiac specialist lead the collaborative team but patient's preference may influence the choice of care team leader (46). Communication between care providers is a key component to the success of these models as the patient's condition deteriorates and goals of care change.

Symptom Burden and Comorbidities

The type and number of symptoms, severity, and impact on psychosocial well-being can approximate those of patients with advanced cancer. The most frequently noted symptoms include shortness of breath, difficulty with mobility, fatigue, cough, difficulty in sleeping, dry mouth, swollen extremities, as well as symptoms of pain, anxiety, depression and decreased sexual interest (47). Clearly, a high symptom burden impacts quality of life and management of these symptoms involves maximal management of the underlying heart failure with pharmacotherapy and other interventions (Table 30.2). Progression of the disease trajectory may be characterized by worsening anorexia and cachexia, confusion, and overall debility (48). Because of this progression, frequent discussions of goals of care and revision of the medical regimen to address the entire symptom burden are appropriate.

Although *shortness of breath* may be thought to be the most common symptom in patients with advanced heart failure, the incidence of pain and fatigue is quite high as well. Shortness of breath is treated with a combination of maximized diuretic therapy, nitrates, supplemental oxygen, inotropic therapy in some cases, as well as opioid therapy (49,50). Morphine sulfate is the most commonly studied opioid medication for relief from shortness of breath. Nonpharmacologic interventions such as cooling fans and relaxation techniques may also be beneficial in many patients.

Pain has been reported as a distressing symptom in up to 78% of patients in one series (51). SUPPORT reported significant percentages of patients with heart failure with severe pain while being hospitalized as well as after discharge (12). Although the etiology of the pain may be related to a cardiac source, the pain source may be related to comorbid conditions such as osteoarthritis, neuropathy, previous injuries and surgeries, or other interventions such as pacemakers or chest tubes. Treatment of these pain syndromes should be undertaken with these considerations in mind. Medications such as nonsteroidal anti-inflammatory medications and COX-2 inhibitors used routinely in the treatment of arthritis should be avoided in most cases owing to the potential for fluid retention

and exacerbation of the underlying failure secondary to their effects on renal function. Once again, this points to the potential need for appropriate dosing of opioid medications such as the codone compounds, morphine, and so on, depending on the severity of the pain syndrome in these patients.

Fatigue is a commonly listed complaint among patients with advanced stage heart failure and its treatment relates to the degree of success of the medical management of the underlying heart failure. Progressive fatigue and weakness as well as cachexia, anorexia, and weight loss all accompany advanced disease and signal a deteriorating condition (52). Treatment of any underlying comorbidities such as depression, disordered sleep patterns, hypothyroidism, and so on, is important, whereas low-dose psycho-stimulants may benefit a subset of patients. Resetting of goals of physical activity to match peak daily energy levels is an important issue that should be addressed in patients as their disease progresses.

Patients with advanced heart failure may have several comorbid conditions that require pharmacologic and non-pharmacologic interventions. Diabetes mellitus, hypertension, cholesterol disorders, chronic obstructive pulmonary disease, sleep apnea, renal insufficiency, osteoarthritis, and depression may accompany the heart failure diagnosis. With each comorbid condition, the potential benefits and side effects of certain groups of medications are to be considered as the underlying heart failure progresses. Many of the oral medications for diabetes mellitus for example, such as metformin, sulfonylureas, and the thiazolidinediones, will need dosage adjustment or discontinuance in late stage heart failure (53). Similar considerations should be given to certain antihypertensive medications, antiarrhythmics, and lipid lowering agents as well.

Depression ranks as one of the leading comorbid and unrecognized conditions in this group of patients. The symptoms of depression in advanced heart failure are essentially the same as with any other disease state and include labile emotions such as tearfulness, anhedonia, feelings of hopelessness, loss of appetite, decreased energy level, and even suicidal ideations. Several series have shown that depression is associated with poorer prognosis as well as higher readmission rates for hospitalization (54,55). Treatment of depression should be an integral part of the treatment plan, with the selective serotonin reuptake inhibitors being the preferred therapeutic agents.

Communication Challenges

As with most advanced and end-stage illnesses, communication between patients, families and caregivers, and health care professionals can be challenging. Communication in advanced heart failure is no exception and is influenced by several factors including the prognostic uncertainty of the course of the disease, lack of understanding on the part of the patients regarding their advanced disease prognosis, and lack of dialogue between patients and their providers about the end-of-life preferences. The complexity of treatments for patients with advanced heart failure in the setting of other comorbidities also provides communication challenges in negotiating goals of care.

As emphasized earlier in the chapter, communication about prognosis is challenging because of the unpredictable nature of the disease trajectory. Although the overall disease course is one of decline, it may be characterized by periods of stability and controlled symptom burden with fairly well-maintained functional status fluctuating with periods of significant symptom burden and decreased functional status. This prognostic uncertainty leads to confusion and reluctance on the part of many health care providers to provide the appropriate counseling regarding many end-of-life and advanced care planning issues.

TABLE 30.2

COMMON SYMPTOMS IN PATIENTS WITH ADVANCED CONGESTIVE HEART FAILURE

- Shortness of breath
- Fatigue
- Lower extremity swelling
- Decreased mobility
- Cough
- Dry mouth
- Pain, noncardiac and cardiac
- Difficulty sleeping
- Anxiety
- Depressed mood
- Decreased sexual interest
- Cachexia
- Confusion

Formal advanced care planning including dialogue regarding living wills, power of attorney for health care decision making, surrogate decision making, and life-support measures such as cardiac resuscitation and ventilator support should be incorporated into the overall care plan. For patients with heart failure, dialogue regarding patient preferences and goals of care with advanced technologies such as implantable cardiac defibrillators (ICD), pacemakers, infusional therapies, and left ventricular assist devices (LVAD) can be particularly complex. As emphasized in the Consensus Statement on Palliative and Supportive Care in Advanced Heart Failure published in 2004, more research in areas of prognostication and disease trajectory, outcomes of interventions to improve symptoms and quality of life, care coordination between systems of care, and communication skills is needed (56). The palliative care specialist can play an integral part in negotiating patient-directed goals of care and facilitating dialogue regarding the complex issues surrounding advanced heart failure.

ROLE OF HOSPICE

Although the concept of providing hospice care had been in existence for many years in the United Kingdom, the Medicare hospice benefit was not introduced in the United States until 1982. The hospice benefit was originally intended to provide a mechanism under Medicare by which patients could receive end-of-life services in their home or that of a loved one. Hospice provides a multidisciplinary team of professionals including physicians, nurses, home health aides, chaplains, social workers, and volunteers working in collaboration to provide for the needs of the patient and family during the last stage of an illness. The benefit includes the services of the team members noted above as well as prescription medications related to the terminal diagnosis and symptom management, medical equipment and supplies, and follow-up bereavement counseling services. A holistic approach in addressing potential sources of physical, emotional, psychosocial or spiritual suffering is the hallmark of hospice programs, which now may enroll patients in a variety of settings including long-term care facilities, assisted-living facilities, and dedicated palliative care units (57).

The Medicare eligibility guidelines require the patient's referring physician and hospice medical director to certify that the patient has a life expectancy of 6 months or less. The prognostic uncertainty of the disease trajectory in heart failure is often a barrier to hospice referral. The guidelines for prognosis are also included as part of the *Medical Guidelines for Determining Prognosis in Selected Non-cancer Diagnoses* published by the National Hospice and Palliative Care Organization (NHPCO) (58). These guidelines continue to be widely used by many hospice organizations but may be inadequate in the determination of prognosis of advanced heart failure considering the evolving natural history and treatment of advanced disease.

Historically, most of the patients enrolled in hospice programs have been those with advanced neoplastic disease. Although end-stage heart disease accounts for the largest number of noncancer patients admitted to hospice programs nationwide according to NHPCO, only approximately 11% of total patients enrolled in hospice programs carry this diagnosis (59). With the increasing incidence of the disease in an aging population, this percentage is likely to increase. In addition, medical directorship of hospice programs will likely be increasingly staffed by physicians with training in the principles of palliative medicine as well. Collaborative care and communication between the patient's primary physician, cardiologist, as well as the hospice medical director should be emphasized. Hospice organizations will be facing challenges to continually train nurses and others involved in the care

of these patients in the emerging treatments of heart failure including the palliative role of infusional inotropic agents and to develop protocols to address advanced technologies such as ICDs and LVADs that patients may have access to on admission to hospice.

CONCLUSIONS

Considering the increasing incidence of heart failure with particular emphasis on the advanced state in an aging population, the importance of comprehensive interdisciplinary management of these patients is paramount. Better understanding of the complex pathophysiology and progression of the disease has led to increasingly complex treatment regimens with both pharmacotherapy and device interventions. These treatment regimens have led to an increase in the number of patients who would be best managed at various points in their disease trajectories by teams of health care professionals. Through disease management or collaborative care programs, the role of each team member should be defined and correlated with corresponding patient education initiatives. With more complicated treatment regimens, significant communication challenges arise regarding disease trajectory, goals of care, and transitioning to an end-of-life setting. Therefore, the role of a collaborative team with a specialist in palliative medicine as a member will be beneficial during the advanced stage in particular. The advent of formal supportive care and palliative care programs in both inpatient and outpatient settings should allow greater access to these services in the future to complement the care of the patients' primary and specialty cardiology professionals. The role of hospice programs and services will continue to expand to serve this population, hopefully meeting the challenge of the increasingly complex goals and treatment regimens necessary for the palliative care of patients with advanced heart failure.

References

1. Jessup M, Brozena S. Heart failure. *N Engl J Med* 2003;348:2007–2018.
2. American Heart Association. *Heart disease and stroke statistics - 2005 update*. Dallas, TX: American Heart Association, 2005.
3. Berry C, Murdoch DR, McMurray JJ. Economics of chronic heart failure. *Eur J Heart Fail* 2001;3:283–291.
4. United States Bureau of the Census. *Profiles of general demographic characteristics 2000*. Washington, DC: United States Department of Commerce, 2001.
5. Cowie MR, Fox KF, Wood DA, et al. Hospitalization of patients with heart failure: a population-based study. *Eur J Heart Fail* 2002;23:877–885.
6. Malkin CJ, Channer KS. Life-saving or life-prolonging? Interpreting trial data and survival curves for patients with congestive heart failure. *Eur J Heart Fail* 2005;7:143–148.
7. Cowburn PJ, Cleland JG, Coats AJ, et al. Risk stratification in chronic heart failure. *Eur J Heart Fail* 1998;19:696–710.
8. Frigerio M, Aguggini G. Diastolic heart failure. *Ital Heart J* 2004;5(Suppl 6):48S–54S.
9. Levenson JW, McCarthy EP, Lynn J, et al. The last six months of life for patients with congestive heart failure. *J Am Geriatr Soc* 2000;48:S101–S109.
10. Colucci WS, Braunwald E. Pathophysiology of heart failure. In: Zipes DP, Libby P, Bonow RO, eds. *Braunwald's heart disease: a textbook of cardiovascular medicine*, 7th ed. Philadelphia, PA: Elsevier, 2005; 509–638.
11. Hunt SA, Baker DW, Chin MH, et al. ACC/AHA guidelines for the evaluation and management of chronic heart failure in the adult: executive summary a report of the American College of Cardiology/American Heart Association Task Force on Practice Guidelines (Committee to Revise the 1995 Guidelines for the Evaluation and Management of Heart Failure): Developed in collaboration with the international society for heart and lung transplantation; endorsed by the heart failure society of America. *Circulation* 2001;104:2996–3007.
12. The SUPPORT Principal Investigators. A controlled trial to improve care for seriously ill hospitalized patients. The study to understand prognoses and preferences for outcomes and risks of treatments (SUPPORT). *JAMA* 1995;274:1591–1598.
13. Butler J, Arbogast PG, Daugherty J, et al. Outpatient utilization of angiotensin-converting enzyme inhibitors among heart failure patients after hospital discharge. *J Am Coll Cardiol* 2004;43:2036–2043.

14. Juurlink DN, Mamdani MM, Lee DS, et al. Rates of hyperkalemia after publication of the Randomized Aldactone Evaluation Study. *N Engl J Med* 2004;351:543–551.
15. Edep ME, Shah NB, Tateo IM, et al. Differences between primary care physicians and cardiologists in management of congestive heart failure: relation to practice guidelines. *J Am Coll Cardiol* 1997;30:518–526.
16. Philbin EF, Weil HF, Erb TA, et al. Cardiology or primary care for heart failure in the community setting: process of care and clinical outcomes. *Chest* 1999;116:346–354.
17. Bleumink GS, Feenstra J, Sturkenboom MC, et al. Nonsteroidal anti-inflammatory drugs and heart failure. *Drugs* 2003;63:525–534.
18. Brown NJ, Vaughan DE. Angiotensin-converting enzyme inhibitors. *Circulation* 1998;97:1411–1420.
19. Yusuf S, Pfeffer MA, Swedberg K, et al. Effects of candesartan in patients with chronic heart failure and preserved left-ventricular ejection fraction: the CHARM-Preserved Trial. *Lancet* 2003;362:777–781.
20. MERIT-HF Investigators. Effect of metoprolol CR/XL in chronic heart failure: metoprolol CR/XL randomised Intervention trial in congestive heart failure (MERIT-HF). *Lancet* 1999;353:2001–2007.
21. CIBIS-II Investigators. The Cardiac Insufficiency Bisoprolol Study II (CIBIS-II): a randomised trial. *Lancet* 1999;353:9–13.
22. Hjalmarson A, Goldstein S, Fagerberg B, et al. Effects of controlled-release metoprolol on total mortality, hospitalizations, and well-being in patients with heart failure: the Metoprolol CR/XL randomized intervention trial in congestive heart failure (MERIT-HF). MERIT-HF Study Group. *JAMA* 2000;283:1295–1302.
23. Packer M, Bristow MR, Cohn JN, et al. The effect of carvedilol on morbidity and mortality in patients with chronic heart failure. U.S. Carvedilol Heart Failure Study Group. *N Engl J Med* 1996;334:1349–1355.
24. Packer M, Fowler MB, Roecker EB, et al. Effect of carvedilol on the morbidity of patients with severe chronic heart failure: results of the carvedilol prospective randomized cumulative survival (COPERNICUS) study. *Circulation* 2002;106:2194–2199.
25. Beta-Blocker Evaluation of Survival Trial Investigators. A trial of the beta-blocker bucindolol in patients with advanced chronic heart failure. *N Engl J Med* 2001;344:1659–1667.
26. Waagstein F, Bristow MR, Swedberg K, et al. Beneficial effects of metoprolol in idiopathic dilated cardiomyopathy. Metoprolol in Dilated Cardiomyopathy (MDC) Trial Study Group. *Lancet* 1993;342:1441–1446.
27. Pitt B, Zannad F, Remme WJ, et al. The effect of spironolactone on morbidity and mortality in patients with severe heart failure. Randomized Aldactone Evaluation Study Investigators. *N Engl J Med* 1999;341:709–717.
28. DIG Investigation Group. The effect of digoxin on mortality and morbidity in patients with heart failure. The Digitalis Investigation Group. *N Engl J Med* 1997;336:525–533.
29. Cohn JN, Archibald DG, Ziesche S, et al. Effect of vasodilator therapy on mortality in chronic congestive heart failure. Results of a Veterans Administration Cooperative Study. *N Engl J Med* 1986;314:1547–1552.
30. Taylor AL, Zeische S, Yancy C, et al. Combination of isosorbide dinitrate and hydralazine in blacks with heart failure. *N Engl J Med* 2004;351:2049–2057.
31. Rayburn BK, Bourge RC. Nesiritide: a unique therapeutic cardiac peptide. *Rev Cardiovasc Med* 2001;2(Suppl 2):S25–S31.
32. Publication Committee for the VMAC Investigators (Vasodilatation in the Management of Acute CHF). Intravenous nesiritide vs nitroglycerin for treatment of decompensated congestive heart failure: a randomized controlled trial. *JAMA* 2002;287:1531–1540.
33. Sackner-Bernstein JD, Skopicki HA, Aaronson KD. Risk of worsening renal function with nesiritide in patients with acutely decompensated heart failure. *Circulation* 2005;111:1487–1491.
34. Cuffe MS, Califf RM, Adams KF Jr, et al. Short-term intravenous milrinone for acute exacerbation of chronic heart failure: a randomized controlled trial. *JAMA* 2002;287:1541–1547.
35. Abraham WT, Fisher WG, Smith AL, et al. Cardiac resynchronization in chronic heart failure. *N Engl J Med* 2002;346:1845–1853.
36. Bristow MR, Saxon LA, Boehmer J, et al. Cardiac-resynchronization therapy with or without an implantable defibrillator in advanced chronic heart failure. *N Engl J Med* 2004;350:2140–2150.
37. Bardy GH, Lee KL, Mark DB, et al. Amiodarone or an implantable cardioverter-defibrillator for congestive heart failure. *N Engl J Med* 2005;352:225–237.
38. Moss AJ, Zareba W, Hall WJ, et al. Prophylactic implantation of a defibrillator in patients with myocardial infarction and reduced ejection fraction. *N Engl J Med* 2002;346:877–883.
39. Rose EA, Gelijns AC, Moskowitz AJ, et al. Long-term mechanical left ventricular assistance for end-stage heart failure. *N Engl J Med* 2001;345:1435–1443.
40. Quaglietti SE, Atwood JE, Ackerman L, et al. Management of the patient with congestive heart failure using outpatient, home, and palliative care. *Prog Cardiovasc Dis* 2000;43:259–274.
41. Lynn J, Wilkinson A, Cohn F, et al. Capitated risk-bearing managed care systems could improve end-of-life care. *J Am Geriatr Soc* 1998;46:322–330.
42. Thorns AR, Gibbs LM, Gibbs JS. Management of severe heart failure by specialist palliative care. *Heart* 2001;85:93–93.
43. Hauptman PJ, Havranek EP. Integrating palliative care into heart failure care. *Arch Intern Med* 2005;165:374–378.
44. Davidson PM, Paull G, Introna K, et al. Integrated, collaborative palliative care in heart failure service experience 1999–2002. *J Cardiovasc Nurs* 2004;19:68–75.
45. Rabow MW, Dibble SL, Pantilat SZ, et al. The comprehensive care team: a controlled trial of outpatient palliative medicine consultation. *Arch Intern Med* 2004;164:83–91.
46. Wotton K, Borbasi S, Redden M. When all else has failed: nurses' perception of factors influencing palliative care for patients with end-stage heart failure. *J Cardiovasc Nurs* 2005;20:18–25.
47. Anderson H, Ward C, Eardley A, et al. The concerns of patients under palliative care and a heart failure clinic are not being met. *Palliat Med* 2001;15:279–286.
48. Pritzker MR. Chronic heart failure and the quality of life. *N Engl J Med* 1999;340:1511–1511.
49. Johnson MJ, McDonagh TA, Harkness A, et al. Morphine for the relief of breathlessness in patients with chronic heart failure–a pilot study. *Eur J Heart Fail* 2002;4:753–756.
50. Jennings AL, Davies AN, Higgins JP, et al. Opioids for the palliation of breathlessness in terminal illness. *Cochrane Database Syst Rev* 2001;4:CD002066.
51. McCarthy M, Lay M, ddington-Hall J. Dying from heart disease. *J R Coll Physicians Lond* 1996;30:325–328.
52. Anker SD, Sharma R. The syndrome of cardiac cachexia. *Int J Cardiol* 2002;85:51–66.
53. Masoudi FA, Wang Y, Inzucchi SE, et al. Metformin and thiazolidinedione use in medicare patients with heart failure. *JAMA* 2003;290:81–85.
54. Faris R, Purcell H, Henein MY, et al. Clinical depression is common and significantly associated with reduced survival in patients with non-ischaemic heart failure. *Eur J Heart Fail* 2002;4:541–551.
55. Jiang W, Alexander J, Christopher E, et al. Relationship of depression to increased risk of mortality and rehospitalization in patients with congestive heart failure. *Arch Intern Med* 2001;161:1849–1856.
56. Goodlin SJ, Hauptman PJ, Arnold R, et al. Consensus statement: palliative and supportive care in advanced heart failure. *J Card Fail* 2004;10:200–209.
57. Zambroski CH. Hospice as an alternative model of care for older patients with end-stage heart failure. *J Cardiovasc Nurs* 2004;19:76–83.
58. National Hospice Organization Standards. *Medical guidelines for determining prognosis in selected non-cancer diseases.* Arlington, VA: National Hospice Organization, 1996.
59. National Hospice and Palliative Care Organization. Hospice facts and figures. www.nhpco.org; 2003.

CHAPTER 31 ■ MANAGEMENT OF HYPERCOAGULABLE STATES AND COAGULOPATHY

KENNETH D. FRIEDMAN AND THOMAS J. RAIFE

Hemostasis is carefully balanced: hemostatic plugs form at inappropriate openings in the vascular network, but thrombus extension is limited, so the remainder of the vascular highway remains fluid. Many disease processes can undermine this wondrous balance, either by stimulating inappropriate occlusion of intact blood vessels or by failure of hemostatic plug formation at sites of vascular wall breakdown. This chapter reviews clinical approaches to both pathologic thrombosis and failure of hemostasis, with an eye toward practical measures in a palliative care setting.

THROMBOTIC DISORDERS

Thrombosis can be considered a pathologic clot formation, occurring either in an inappropriate location or to an inappropriate extent. This review mainly focuses on venous thromboembolic (VTE) disease. Risk factors for the development of thrombosis are many, and the prevalence of thrombosis increases with age and the severity of predisposing conditions. A high proportion of hospice patients are on warfarin sodium, reflecting the high rate of thrombotic complications in this patient population (1). The presenting symptoms of some arterial and most venous thrombotic events are vague. A high index of suspicion and specific testing for confirmation are required. Therapeutic intervention is undertaken with an understanding of the opposing risks of thrombotic progression on the one hand and the hemorrhagic potential of anticoagulation on the other. Studies of the value of various diagnostic protocols, the efficacy and safety of specific interventions, and the risk of bleeding or recurrent thrombosis have led to the development of clinical pathways for diagnosis, and have defined "acceptable" rates for complications such as bleeding and recurrent thrombosis. However, these studies have largely been conducted in patients with expected survival of 3 months or longer, and the principles defined in them may not fully translate to the palliative care setting (2,3). The palliative care physician must integrate acute care principles with specific end-of-life goals and expectations to arrive at an appropriate palliative care plan for thrombosis.

Mechanism Underlying Thrombotic Risk

Cancer is a well-established risk factor for VTE. Thrombosis is a major cause of morbidity in patients with neoplastic disease, and is reported to be clinically evident in 11–15% of patients being treated for malignancy. Risk for thrombosis increases with disease progression. One study of hospice patients with cancer revealed a 50% prevalence of thrombosis, often associated with poor mobility and low albumin level (4). Thrombosis has been observed in up to 50% of patients with cancer at autopsy (2,3). The most thrombogenic tumors include ovarian, brain, pancreatic, gastric, and colorectal neoplasms. Breast carcinoma has a relatively low risk, but the risk rises with certain hormonal manipulations (5).

Mechanisms of cancer-induced activation of the coagulation mechanism have been attributed to aberrant expression of tissue factor by tumors or reactive endothelium, tumor-derived procoagulant factors that can activate factor X on malignant cells, dysfunctional prothrombotic hematopoietic clones, hyperviscosity, and inflammatory mechanisms (6,7). Proinflammatory cytokines such as tumor necrosis factor-α and interleukin-1β induce expression of tissue factor on endothelial cells (8). These mechanisms may explain why patients with cancer are at increased risk for development of disseminated intravascular coagulation (DIC), which sometimes presents as localized thrombosis. Finally, a host of chemotherapeutic drugs, hormonal manipulations, and stasis resulting from vascular compression add to thrombotic risk (5).

Many other advanced disease states are complicated by thrombosis. The incidence of stroke and venous thrombosis is as high as 4% in severe heart failure (9). Hepatic dysfunction increases risk of thrombosis in part through decreased hepatic clearance of activated coagulation factors. Inflammatory reactions and acute phase responses are common to many disease states; the actions of inflammatory cytokines and elevated levels of factor VIII, fibrinogen (10,11), and platelets all tip the hemostatic balance toward thrombosis. Additional risk factors include the presence of central venous catheters (6,12) and venous stasis associated with immobilization due to pain and debilitation.

Although most thrombotic events that complicate the care of debilitated patients are venous, arterial thrombosis is also a potential problem. Arterial events are generally attributed to atherosclerotic disease, with formation of platelet-fibrin thrombi. Hypotension may worsen the progression of vascular ischemia in the face of preexisting arterial disease. Polycythemia vera and essential thrombocythemia are the predisposing factors in arterial and venous thrombosis. Finally, embolic venous thrombi may cross into the arterial circulation through cardiac shunts and present as "paradoxical" arterial emboli in patients with patent foramen ovale.

Evaluation of the Patient with Venous Thrombosis

The presenting signs and symptoms of VTE are often nonspecific, and the problem may be particularly pronounced in the palliative care setting. Alternative causes of extremity swelling include nonthrombotic vascular obstruction, heart failure, renal insufficiency, hypoalbuminemia, lymphatic obstruction, neurologic factors, and hypothyroidism. Similarly, the sensation of breathlessness may stem from anxiety, cardiac failure, tumor invasion, infection, and obstructive pulmonary disease. Conversely, edema in unusual sites may indicate venous thrombosis in palliative care patients. Upper extremity edema may be due to axillary or mediastinal metastasis, catheter-related thrombosis, or venous thrombosis. Hepatic vein thrombosis may present as worsening hepatic failure or sudden onset of ascites (2). Detection of VTE disease is important because it can be successfully treated. Treatment not only reduces the risk of fatal pulmonary embolism (PE) but it can also reduce leg pain, immobility, and symptoms of breathlessness (13). Bilateral asymmetric leg edema was the most common presenting finding in one study of hospice patients with advanced cancer who later developed VTE (13). Investigation of symptoms consistent with thrombosis is strongly recommended in patients in whom antithrombotic therapy may be considered.

Noninvasive studies are the diagnostic tools of choice, because contrast venography and conventional pulmonary angiography (the reference standards) are inconvenient, costly, and associated with substantial morbidity. Quantitation of fibrin D-dimer (the plasmin-derived degradation product of cross-linked fibrin clot) may be insufficient for exclusion of VTE in patients with cancer (14). Although one study observed a satisfactory negative predictive value in patients with cancer (15), another study reported that the negative predictive value of the SimpliRED bedside D-dimer test was only 79% in patients with cancer versus 97% in a more general population of ambulatory patients (16,17).

Clinical approaches that include noninvasive imaging studies are recommended for the evaluation of suspected VTE (18,19). Compression ultrasonography may be the best study for the diagnosis of proximal deep vein thrombosis (DVT) in the terminal patient. It is simple, highly accurate, and fast when done by experienced personnel. The sensitivity for proximal leg DVT is reported at over 97%, with specificity reported at 92–100%. Compression ultrasonography is significantly less useful in the evaluation of thrombosis below the knee (2,19).

Spiral computed tomography (CT) (computed tomographic pulmonary angiography) is rapidly replacing lung scintigraphy (also known as *ventilation/perfusion scan*) as the diagnostic procedure of choice for noninvasive evaluation of patients with suspected PE. Although, a "normal" scintigraphy report effectively excludes the diagnosis of PE and a "high-probability" report is sufficient for diagnosing a patient with a moderate to high clinical suspicion of PE, the technique is nondiagnostic in approximately two thirds of patients (20). Pulmonary disease and tumor in the lung degrade the diagnostic yield of lung scintigraphy studies.

Spiral CT scan has a high sensitivity for detection of PE in central pulmonary vessels (sensitivity and positive predictive value approach 95%), and advances using multidetector CT scan have improved visualization of subsegmental pulmonary vessels (21). Recent evidence supports the safety of withholding anticoagulation therapy based on a negative spiral CT

scan study (22). CT scan is also useful for uncovering alternative sources of pulmonary symptoms in patients with advanced disease, because the images provide details of lung parenchyma, mediastinum, and pleura. Concerns about CT scan include the lingering questions regarding sensitivity for detection of embolism in subsegmental pulmonary arteries, the occasional misinterpretation of studies, the requirement for intravenous injection of a significant iodine-contrast dye load, and the high cost of the study (23).

Utilization of these diagnostic techniques in the palliative care setting has not been extensively evaluated. A survey of palliative care physicians in the United Kingdom revealed that only 60–80% of responding physicians would use tests to confirm a clinically suspected VTE (24). One palliative care group's protocol is to establish the degree of clinical suspicion, and if high, to obtain leg ultrasonography. When PE is suspected and the leg ultrasound is inconclusive, spiral CT scan is obtained. Pulmonary scintigraphy is reserved for patients in whom dye load is contraindicated (25).

Treatment of the Patient with Venous Thrombosis

The American College of Chest Physicians periodically updates its recommendations for the management of VTE in the nonpalliative care setting (26). The goals of treatment of VTE are to prevent death from progressive PE and to minimize the postphlebitic symptoms of pain, swelling, and dyspnea. Thrombolytic therapy is usually considered overly aggressive for palliative care. Anticoagulation is the mainstay of therapy and is instituted immediately to inhibit new clot formation while intrinsic fibrinolytic mechanisms reopen obstructed blood vessels. Anticoagulation is then continued on a long-term basis to prevent recurrent thrombosis. In a general population of patients, the duration of anticoagulation therapy is stratified according to the patient's risk for recurrence (26).

The main complication of anticoagulation therapy is hemorrhage, and assessment of the risks of hemorrhage should be undertaken before instituting anticoagulation (Table 31.1). Absolute contraindications include significant active bleeding or severe bleeding tendency. Relative contraindications include recent bleeding, recent surgery, moderate to severe bleeding tendency, thrombocytopenia, active peptic ulcer disease, uncontrolled hypertension, and severe renal or liver disease. Central nervous system hemorrhage is a particular concern in patients with metastatic cancer in the brain, especially from melanoma, choriocarcinoma, or renal cell carcinoma. However, several authors advocate the safety of anticoagulation in the setting of nonhemorrhagic metastatic disease to the central nervous system when close control of anticoagulation is maintained (27,28). When hemorrhagic risk contraindicates anticoagulation therapy or anticoagulation has been proved to be insufficient to prevent thrombotic progression, inferior vena cava (IVC) filter devices can be inserted to preserve lung function and prevent death due to acute PE.

Heparin drugs have been the mainstay of initial anticoagulation therapy owing to their immediate onset of action (29). Their anticoagulant effect is achieved by promoting the inhibitory activity of antithrombin. Heparin drugs have been subdivided into unfractionated heparin (UFH), low-molecular-weight heparins (LMWH) derived by depolymerization of UFH, and synthetic pentasaccharides (fondaparinux).

LMWH preparations offer several important pharmacologic advantages over UFH (29) and have become the primary medication used for initial management of VTE disease. Many large clinical trials have demonstrated that LMWH is equivalent in safety and efficacy to UFH in the management of acute

TABLE 31.1

CONTRAINDICATIONS AND RELATIVE RISK FACTORS FOR HEMORRHAGIC COMPLICATIONS OF ANTICOAGULANT THERAPY

Contraindications
    Significant active bleeding (gastrointestinal or
        elsewhere)
    Recent major surgery or central nervous system
        procedure
    Severe bleeding tendency
Factors conferring increased bleeding risk
    Preexisting abnormality of hemostasis
        Thrombocytopenia
        Concomitant use of platelet-inhibiting drugs
        Coagulopathy
    Recent hemorrhagic episode
    Recent major surgery
    Comorbid disease states
        Advanced disease
        Active peptic ulcer disease
        Uncontrolled hypertension
        Severe renal or hepatic disease
    Central nervous system metastasis
    Heavy ethanol use
    Advanced age

VTE and that it is safe for use in outpatient community-based care (30). A recent meta-analysis of randomized trials revealed that LWMH is more effective and safer then UFH, but whether LMWH is superior in the subset of patients with cancer has not been formally evaluated (31). Similar to UFH, LMWH is a parenteral medication, but depolymerization results in a longer half-life, greater bioavailability, and more predictable pharmacodynamics. For the average patient with VTE, these pharmacologic advantages translate into weight-adjusted dosing once or twice daily without a requirement for laboratory monitoring. These advantages also render LMWH an appropriate agent for outpatient use. Other potential advantages include reduced risks for development of osteoporosis (32) and heparin-induced thrombocytopenia (HIT) (33). The main disadvantages of LMWH are increased cost and a more prolonged anticoagulant effect that is less reversible with protamine sulfate. Among patients with cancer, one study found a trend toward increased thrombus recurrence with once-daily dosing of enoxaparin compared to twice-daily dosing (34); however, the potential benefit of twice-daily dosing must be balanced against inconvenience and cost when considering the care of patients in a palliative care setting. Multiple LMWH preparations are available and the dosing schedules for each were largely empirically determined. The dosing schedule should appropriately match the LMWH preparation being used. Because LMWH is cleared by the kidney, in patients with renal insufficiency (creatinine greater than 2 mg per dL or estimated creatinine clearance of under 30 mL per minute) use of UFH or dose modification of LMWH with monitoring of levels is advisable. Although target levels of LWMH have not been established through therapeutic trials, a target peak level of 0.6–1.0 antifactor Xa units per mL measured 3–4 hours after subcutaneous administration of LMWH has been recommended (26).

UFH may still be used for the initial management of VTE in some patients. Its main advantages are low cost, short half-life, and reversibility by administration of protamine sulfate. The main disadvantages of UFH are its wide dose–response variability, narrow therapeutic window, and the need for

parenteral administration. Other complications include the rare but serious immunologic condition HIT (35) and the risk of osteoporosis with very long term heparin therapy (32). UFH is usually given by continuous infusion (36), but subcutaneous administration every 12 hours has also been used. The therapeutic dose is determined empirically. Algorithms for prescriptive dose adjustment are based on frequent monitoring of anticoagulant effect (29). The sensitivity of the activated partial thromboplastin time (aPTT) to heparin effect varies widely between laboratories; it is advisable to consult the local laboratory to learn the recommended therapeutic range. The aPTT is a less useful yardstick of heparin effect in patients who have "heparin resistance," which is defined as requirement of over 40,000 units of UFH per day to achieve a therapeutic range aPTT. Either direct heparin assessment by "antifactor Xa" assays (therapeutic range 0.35–0.70 U per mL) or use of LMWH is recommended in this setting.

The first synthetic pentasaccaride anticoagulant, fondaparinux, was recently approved for initial treatment of VTE, with randomized trials demonstrating noninferiority to LMWH and UFH (37,38). Like LMWH, fondaparinux requires subcutaneous administration and is cleared by the kidney. Potential advantages include a longer half-life (17–21 hours) allowing once-daily administration, and emerging experience suggests a potential use in patients with a history of HIT.

After achieving initial anticoagulation, long-term anticoagulation (secondary prophylaxis) is undertaken to prevent recurrence of VTE. Warfarin sodium derivatives (e.g., Coumadin) are frequently chosen for this phase of care (26), but LMWH should be considered in some settings (see subsequent text). Coumadin and other oral vitamin K antagonists inhibit hepatic synthesis of multiple coagulation factors. The onset of oral anticoagulant effect is delayed until previously synthesized coagulation factors are cleared. Therefore, "loading" doses do not overcome the long half-life of circulating clotting factors. Because of this delay, heparin drugs are usually used concurrently with initial oral anticoagulation to provide protection before the onset of oral anticoagulation effect. Current recommendations suggest that heparin drugs be maintained for at least 5 days and continued for 2 days after laboratory studies confirm that adequate oral anticoagulation has been established.

Management of oral anticoagulation is complex owing to the narrow therapeutic window, multiple drug interactions, interindividual differences in hepatic metabolism, and the shifting intensity of anticoagulation due to changes in diet (39). The therapeutic intensity of oral anticoagulation requires laboratory monitoring. A prothrombin time (PT)-based international normalized ratio (INR) target of 2.5 is suggested in most settings, but a higher target of 3.0 is suggested for patients with many types of mechanical heart valves (40). The typical initial dose of warfarin sodium is 5 mg per day in acute care patients, but initial doses may need to be lower in chronically ill patients, patients with poor nutrition, patients on medications that are known to increase oral anticoagulant effect, and in the elderly. Owing to individual variation in anticoagulant effect, ongoing monitoring of individual patient response and dose adjustment are required. Initially, INR monitoring and dose adjustment are performed daily, with monitoring intervals lengthened as the dose requirement is empirically established. Weekly evaluation may be prudent for at least the first 6–12 weeks of therapy, the time when the highest rate of hemorrhage occurs (41). In general patient populations, the risk of bleeding with INRs in the therapeutic range is between 2 and 3%, but patients with cancer are at increased risk for bleeding complications (2). Adverse events may be avoided through more frequent monitoring (28,42). Outcome data are scant in the palliative care literature. In this setting, oral

TABLE 31.2

GUIDELINES FOR REVERSAL OF WARFARIN SODIUM ANTICOAGULATION

INR	Urgency of reversal	Recommendation
<5.0	1–2 d	Decrease or discontinue warfarin sodium until INR improves
	12–24 h	Discontinue warfarin sodium
		Consider vitamin K_1: 2.5 mg orally
	As soon as possible	Discontinue warfarin sodium
		Vitamin K_1: 5–10 mg i.v.[a]
		Fresh frozen plasma (at least 15 mL/kg)
5.0–9.0	1–3 d	Discontinue warfarin sodium until INR improves
	12–24 h	Discontinue warfarin sodium
		Vitamin K_1: 2.5–5.0 mg orally or 2.0–4.0 mg subcutaneously
	As soon as possible	Discontinue warfarin sodium
		Vitamin K_1: 10 mg i.v.[a]
		Fresh frozen plasma (at least 15 mL/kg)
		Consider prothrombin-complex concentrate or recombinant factor VIIa for life-threatening bleeds
>9.0	1–3 d	Discontinue warfarin sodium
		Vitamin K_1: 2.5–5.0 mg orally or subcutaneously
	12–24 h	Discontinue warfarin sodium
		Vitamin K_1: 2.5–5.0 mg orally or 10 mg subcutaneously
		Consider fresh frozen plasma (at least 15 mL/kg)
	As soon as possible	Discontinue warfarin sodium
		Vitamin K_1: 10 mg i.v.,[a] consider repeat doses
		Fresh frozen plasma (at least 15 mL/kg)
		Consider prothrombin-complex concentrate or recombinant factor VIIa for life-threatening bleeds

INR, international normalized ratio.

[a] i.v. Vitamin K_1 should be administered slowly; rare anaphylactic reactions have occurred.

Modified from Pineo GF, Hull RD. The use of heparin, low-molecular-weight heparin, and oral anticoagulants in the management of thromboembolic disease. In: Portenoy R, Bruera E, eds. *Topics in palliative care*, Vol. 4. New York: Oxford University Press, 2000:185,201–205, with permission.

anticoagulation may be more problematic owing to changes in diet, gastrointestinal (GI) or hepatic disturbances, changes in medications, or the need to discontinue anticoagulation to accomplish other invasive interventions without untoward risk of bleeding. One small hospice audit revealed a high incidence of oral anticoagulation–related hemorrhagic events, and found that external bleeding was quite distressing to the patients and their caregivers (1,43). Tight INR control was somewhat helpful, but required frequent INR monitoring (averaging once every 2.4 days), adding a considerable burden to dying patients.

Management of a patient with an INR above the target value requires consideration of the degree of INR elevation and patient's intrinsic risk of hemorrhage (Table 31.2). In patients who are not bleeding, dose adjustments may be sufficient. Low-dose oral vitamin K_1 can be used to shorten the time required for reestablishing the target INR level (44). In a bleeding patient, coagulation factor replacement in the form of fresh frozen plasma (FFP) transfusion speeds up correction of the INR (39,45). Bleeding patients who are unable to tolerate the volume load of plasma transfusion may be treated with prothrombin-complex concentrates (26) or recombinant factor VIIa; however, the complexity and expense of these measures should be carefully considered in the palliative care setting.

LMWH has also been evaluated for the long-term anticoagulation of patients. LMWH offers two advantages. The first is improved efficacy of LMWH over oral anticoagulation in patients with cancer. In such patients, the annual rate of recurrent thrombosis while on oral anticoagulation is much higher than in other populations, and may be as high as 27% (31). In a randomized trial, assignment to long-term LMWH rather than

oral anticoagulation was shown to reduce the rate of recurrent VTE by half without an increase in major bleeding events (46). The second advantage is the simplicity of use of LMWH, including absence of laboratory monitoring requirements and dietary or drug interactions, which offers significant advantages for the terminally ill patient. The recommended dose is generally similar to that used during initial anticoagulation therapy, and once-daily dosing may be sufficient for long-term secondary prophylaxis (46).

Duration of anticoagulation is determined by the risk of recurrence (26). Three to 6 months of anticoagulation is recommended for the general patient with a reversible short-term risk factor, a minimum of 6 months for the patient with idiopathic VTE, and 12 months to an indefinite period for the patient with a significant long-term risk factor. In terminally ill patients with persistent risk factors (such as cancer), the decision to continue anticoagulation should be regularly revisited because it is unclear at what point the reduction in risk of thrombotic recurrence justifies the logistical burden of anticoagulant therapy and the ongoing risk of hemorrhage. When the care plan is for comfort measures only or if the patient is rapidly failing, continued anticoagulation may be inappropriate (2).

Recurrence of venous thrombosis in the face of anticoagulation appears to be a particular problem in patients with cancer or the antiphospholipid antibody syndrome (18,47). A patient who develops thrombosis with a subtherapeutic INR may be retreated with UFH or LMWH for 5–7 days and then continued on oral anticoagulation with the usual target INR of 2.5. For the patient who is already in the therapeutic INR range at the time of thrombosis, possible measures include aiming for a higher INR of 3–4.5 (and accepting the higher risk for bleeding events), switching to long-term LMWH, or considering IVC filter placement (48).

An IVC filter is not an alternative to anticoagulation, but placement of a filter may prolong life by prevention of acute PE. IVC filters reduce the short-term risk of PE, but they do so at the expense of increased risk for progressive leg thrombosis and postphlebitic syndrome (49). Placement of an IVC filter should be reserved for patients with active bleeding or a high risk of bleeding, or for patients who develop recurrent thrombosis despite anticoagulant therapy. In the latter setting, concurrent anticoagulation should also be considered; thrombotic complications occurred in one sixth of patients with cancer who had a filter placed (27). Because of the expense and morbidity associated with IVC filters, their use in the palliative care setting should be carefully considered.

Catheter-Related Thromboses

Eliminating venipuncture clearly increases a patient's comfort level. As a result, central venous catheters are commonly used in patients with cancer and other chronic illness for administration of medications, transfusions, and laboratory monitoring. These devices are associated with a number of complications, including increased risk for infection and thrombosis (12). Thrombus may obstruct a line tip, form a sleeve around the intravascular portion of the catheter, or obstruct the veins of the arm, neck, or mediastinum.

Intralumenal catheter obstruction is common, but low-dose thrombolytic therapy, instilled as a single dose (or occasionally as repeated doses), is usually effective in opening a tip thrombosis. Streptokinase, urokinase, and tissue plasminogen activator have been used for this purpose (12). Inability to draw from a line (so called "ball-valve" effect) may be due to obstruction, but venography reveals that approximately 40% of these problems are attributable to nonthrombotic, local mechanical effects.

Vein thrombosis is a common complication of central lines. The incidence of venous thrombosis is unclear, ranging from 12–74% of lines; however, most thrombotic episodes are asymptomatic. Symptoms of central vein thrombosis may be nonspecific, including arm, neck, or head swelling, headache, arm pain or numbness, prominent surface venous pattern of the arm, or erythema. Owing to the smaller size of the upper extremity veins, symptomatic PE is a rare complication (12). Objective imaging is necessary to confirm the diagnosis. Although anatomic limitations reduce the sensitivity of sonography to only 54–100%, the high specificity of sonography (estimated at 94–100%) makes a positive study useful (50). Repeated ultrasound, spiral CT scan or contrast venography may be useful in some patients.

Optimal therapy of central vein thrombosis is uncertain because comparative prospective trials have not been performed. Catheter removal should be considered if the line is nonfunctional, but anticoagulation without line removal is acceptable in patients in whom continued use of the line is desired. Currently, anticoagulation therapy is modeled from studies of DVT of the leg. Initial management using an immediate acting anticoagulant such as LMWH is followed by longer-term oral anticoagulation or continued LMWH (12). Superior vena cava filters have rarely been placed in patients in whom anticoagulation is not an option. Older open-label prospective randomized studies have shown the utility of prophylaxis with very-low-dose (1 mg per day) warfarin sodium or daily subcutaneous dalteparin 2500 IU, but these data have been called into question by the more recent studies (12,51). Given the risk of excessive oral anticoagulation in patients with anorexia and the inconvenience of prophylactic LMWH, prophylaxis against thrombosis is not recommended for patients with central venous catheters (12,52).

HEMORRHAGIC DISORDERS

Bleeding occurs in up to 10% of patients with advanced cancer (10). When visible, and especially when massive, it can cause considerable anxiety for the patient, family, and health care providers (6). It may present as simple bruising or petechia on the skin, or as blood loss from mucosal or tumor surfaces. Bleeding may lead to debilitation from anemia and serve as a reminder of the uncontrolled and progressive course of illness. Patients may be unsettled by specific complications associated with bleeding in certain locations, such as chronic cough or dyspnea related to pulmonary bleeding. In addition, episodic low volume bleeding may herald a more catastrophic hemorrhagic event. The clinical approach to these situations requires a balanced consideration of the underlying causes of bleeding (Table 31.3), the available therapeutic modalities, and the patient's palliative care goals.

Mechanisms of Hemorrhagic Risk

Vascular Integrity

The loss of vascular wall integrity underlies all bleeding events. Multiple factors conspire to destroy vascular integrity in the terminally ill patient. Local tumor invasion in the GI tract is associated with 12–17% of cases of GI hemorrhage in patients with cancer (53). Chest wall breast carcinoma, endobronchial lung cancer, and locally invasive head and neck or cervical cancer can all cause local hemorrhage. Mucositis may be induced by nonsteroidal anti-inflammatory drugs, stress, peptic ulcer disease, local infection, or as a result of chemotherapy or radiation treatment. Finally, primary vascular defects may be involved, as in amyloidosis or vitamin C deficiency.

TABLE 31.3

MECHANISMS OF HEMORRHAGIC RISK

Loss of vascular integrity
    Tumor surface bleeding
    Tumor erosion into a major vessel
    Mucositis (stress, drug related, acid peptic disease,
        chemotherapy induced, radiation therapy induced)
Platelet defects
    Thrombocytopenia
        Marrow proliferative failure (myelophthisis,
            drug-induced, radiation therapy-induced,
            viral, vitamin deficiency)
        Accelerated platelet clearance (disseminated
            intravascular coagulation, sepsis,
            immunologic, hypersplenism)
    Platelet function defects (drug-induced, uremic,
        paraprotein effect)
Coagulation defects
    Vitamin K deficiency (decreased intake or bowel flora
        production, malabsorption, oral
        anticoagulant-induced)
    Liver disease
    Disseminated intravascular coagulation
    Accelerated fibrinolysis
    Coagulation inhibitors (heparin drugs, autoimmune)

Platelet Function

Failure of hemostatic mechanisms may allow minor defects of vascular integrity to become manifest. Many factors can result in thrombocytopenia or diminished platelet function. Platelet counts above 50,000 per mm^3 are generally well tolerated in the absence of trauma (54), and significant risk of spontaneous hemorrhage is rare in clinically stable patients until counts fall below 10,000 per mm^3 (54).

Failure of marrow production is a very common mechanism of thrombocytopenia. Extensive marrow replacement by tumor (myelophthisis) occurs early in leukemia, but is a sign of advanced metastatic disease in solid tumors. Peripheral blood abnormalities that are supportive of a diagnosis of myelophthisis include pancytopenia and the presence of circulating neutrophil precursors, nucleated red blood cells, and "teardrop" red cells. Marrow failure is an anticipated complication of many antineoplastic drugs and may complicate radiation therapy. Other causes of marrow failure include vitamin deficiency (B$_{12}$ or folate), hypothyroidism, viral infections, and adverse medication effects. If required, marrow failure can be confirmed by bone marrow biopsy. Platelet-selective cytopenias and disorders characterized by shortened platelet survival are characteristic of some drug-induced complications. Infection, DIC, hypersplenism, and autoimmune phenomena are among the potential underlying mechanisms of thrombocytopenia. The approach to diagnosis and treatment of thrombocytopenia in the palliative care setting requires judgment as to potential benefits in relation to the discomfort, cost, and risk to the patient.

Medication-related inhibition of platelet function should be considered in the bleeding patient because adjusting medications may be a relatively simple means of restoring platelet function in some patients in the palliative care setting (55). Aspirin and most nonsteroidal anti-inflammatory drugs exert antiplatelet-effect due to cyclo-oxygenase inhibition. In addition, these agents increase the risk of gastric erosion and bleeding. Continued use of antiplatelet agents (such as clopidorgel) in a patient with vascular disease should be questioned if the patient develops significant bleeding complications.

Coagulation Defects

Abnormalities of the coagulation mechanism such as vitamin K deficiency, hepatic disease, and DIC should be considered in a palliative care patient with bleeding (56).

Vitamin K is a fat-soluble factor required for hepatic synthesis of multiple coagulation proteins. Oral anticoagulants produce their effect through inhibition of vitamin K metabolism. Nutritional deficiency of vitamin K occurs when there is impairment of either dietary intake or bowel flora synthesis of vitamin K. Disruption of both mechanisms is common (55). In addition, malabsorption disorders such as bowel resection/bypass and biliary obstruction and the use of cholestyramine may undermine fat-soluble vitamin absorption. Supportive laboratory evidence includes a prolonged PT with a normal or less prolonged aPTT and normal fibrinogen and platelet levels. The PT should correct after 1:1 mixing with normal plasma, and the abnormalities should improve with vitamin K$_1$ administration.

Liver dysfunction contributes to bleeding in a variety of ways. The liver produces most coagulation proteins and is a reservoir for vitamin K. In addition to impaired synthetic capacity from parenchymal liver disease, liver dysfunction may cause portal hypertension with resulting thrombocytopenia from hypersplenism and GI bleeding due to esophageal or rectal varices.

Owing to its short half-life, factor VII levels fall early in the course of liver disease, resulting in prolongation of the PT, which should correct in a 1:1 mix with normal plasma. Mildly elevated fibrin degradation products may reflect defective hepatic clearance. The aPTT is typically less prolonged than the PT, and levels of fibrinogen and platelets are variable. Other clinical or biochemical evidence should support the diagnosis of hepatic disease. In the patient with severe liver disease, responsiveness to vitamin K$_1$ administration is generally limited.

DIC is a secondary coagulation disturbance associated with many disorders. Frequently, DIC is associated with cancer. Other causes include trauma, burns, sepsis, and prolonged circulatory insufficiency. DIC is characterized by activation of both procoagulant and fibrinolytic pathways. Activation of these pathways results in consumption of platelets and coagulation factors, intravascular deposition of fibrin, and simultaneous release of fibrin degradation products, and destabilization of hemostatic plugs (57). The thrombotic spectrum of DIC includes large vessel thrombosis and microvascular thrombosis with multiorgan failure. The hemorrhagic spectrum ranges from asymptomatic laboratory abnormalities, to increased bruising, reoccurrence of bleeding at sites of prior trauma, or even spontaneous mucosal bleeding. The diagnosis of DIC rests on clinical suspicion supported by laboratory abnormalities including prolonged PT and aPTT, decreased fibrinogen and platelets, and a positive test for fibrin split products or D-dimer.

Clinical Approaches to the Bleeding Patient

The cause and severity of bleeding define the spectrum of available interventions. The patient's anticipated life expectancy, quality of life, care setting, and palliative care goals may narrow the spectrum. The potential benefits of intervention (Table 31.4) must be weighed against the consequences. In addition to general supportive measures, the care plan may entail avoidance of interventions that increase bleeding risk, local measures to treat bleeding, and systemic interventions to improve hemostasis.

General Supportive Measures

It is helpful to identify patients who are at particular risk for massive bleeding. Tumors likely to present bleeding problems include fungating tumors of the head and neck, gynecologic tumors, and tumors close to major vessels. Patients on antithrombotic therapy and those with severe liver disease or marrow failure are also at increased risk for hemorrhage. Massive bleeding can be extremely distressing to patients and caregivers alike. Panic responses and calls to emergency medical personnel may result in the initiation of inappropriate interventions. If a risk for catastrophic bleeding exists, sensitive anticipatory conversations involving the care provision team serve to empower caregivers to act compassionately and appropriately if massive bleeding develops (45,58). Patients with hematemesis should be placed in the left lateral position to reduce respiratory compromise. The use of dark-colored towels and basins helps make blood loss less evident and reduces anxiety associated with bleeding. It may be helpful to have prefilled syringes containing sedative medication (e.g., 2.5–5 mg of midazolam hydrochloride) available for subcutaneous or intravenous administration in the event of catastrophic hemorrhage (58).

Local Measures

Local interventions to control hemorrhage include compression dressings, application of materials to improve hemostasis, and special procedures to occlude bleeding vessels (45). Packing is useful in areas such as the nose, rectum, or vagina. Pressure through use of balloon catheters or posturing is of additional benefit in areas of small capillary or venous

TABLE 31.4

PALLIATIVE MANAGEMENT OF THE BLEEDING PATIENT

General supportive measures
    Identify the patient at risk
    Establish open communication of issues of care
    Generate care plan
        Consider measures for catastrophic bleeding
        Use of sedatives (midazolam hydrochloride)
        Revisit as required by patient course
Local measures
    Packing
    Compressive dressings and postures
    Topical hemostatics (collagen, thrombin, fibrin gel, antifibrinolytics)
    Topical astringents or vasoconstrictors (silver nitrate, alum, formaldehyde, cocaine, epinephrine)
Special techniques
    Endoscopic interventions (cauterization, sclerosis, ligation)
    Interventional radiology (vascular embolization)
    Palliative radiotherapy
    Palliative surgery (vascular ligation)
Systemic interventions
    Discontinue antiplatelet and antithrombotic medications
    Vitamin K administration
    Antifibrinolytic medication (tranexamic acid, ε-aminocaproic acid)
    Transfusion support
        Platelets or plasma for hemostatic support
        Red cells for symptomatic anemia
    Desmopressin
    Somatostatin analogs (octreotide acetate)

Modified from Gagnon B, Mancini I, Pereira J, et al. Palliative management of bleeding events in advanced cancer patients. *J Palliat Care* 1998;14:50–54.

bleeding. Choice of topical agents to further improve hemostasis is generally based on local factors, cost, and individual considerations. Topical cocaine has been used with nasal packing. Acetone may similarly improve the efficacy of vaginal packing. Purified gelatin in the forms of compressed packed foam (Gelfoam), sterile sponge dressings, or sterile powdered bovine-derived collagen provides surfaces for formation of a hemostatic clot. Bovine thrombin can be applied topically in powder form to dressings or directly onto oozing surfaces. It can also be used in solution to moisten dressings (59). Topical fibrin sealant derived from human plasma can be applied directly to bleeding surfaces (60). Aluminum astringents, such as 1% alum solution, have been applied in the form of continuous bladder irrigation. Aluminum hydroxide complexed with sulfated sucrose (sucralfate) is an active ulcer healing drug, which has been used successfully for control of esophagitis, rectal or vaginal bleeding; 1 g of sucralfate tablet dispersed in water-soluble gel (e.g., K-Y jelly), can be applied to bleeding sites once or twice daily. Cauterizing and vasoconstrictive agents are alternative approaches for controlling hemorrhage. Formaldehyde solutions have been used to control hematuria (61) and may control bleeding associated with radiation proctitis (62). Silver nitrate cauterization is commonly used for nasal bleeding. Epinephrine (as a 0.002% solution) may be used to induce vasoconstriction. Epinephrine

use in combination with lidocaine is discouraged (45), but if combination medication is used, the lidocaine doses should not exceed 7 mg per kg (59).

Special Techniques

Specific local interventions include endoscopic or intravascular application of hemostatic measures and use of radiotherapy to induce vascular sclerosis. The spectrum of endoscopic procedures includes cauterization and electrically induced coagulation, application of sclerosing agents and ligation of esophageal varices, and topical or injection application of hemostatic agents (45). In addition to inconvenience, the risks of endoscopic procedures include worsened bleeding through physical trauma and perforation of viscera.

In a subset of patients, vascular embolization performed by interventional radiology has been used for a variety of bleeding indications (56). Embolic particles include metal coils and gelatin sponges. The technique is restricted to vascular beds in which catheters can be easily guided. Vascular access is usually obtained through an axillary or femoral approach, the blood vessels supplying the bleeding area are identified angiographically, and then the hemostatic agent is inserted into the vessel. Embolization therapy is well established in the treatment of head and neck, pelvic, GI, and pulmonary neoplasm-associated bleeding. Complications include the need for mild sedation during the procedure, embolization of vascular beds not affected by tumor, bleeding at the site of vascular access, and a "postembolization" syndrome characterized by discomfort, malaise, and fever after vascular occlusion of a large tumor mass. Palliative radiation therapy may be used to control hemorrhage from head and neck, gynecologic, GI, bladder, and other tumors (56). The optimal method of treatment remains controversial. Prior therapy in the same radiation field increases the risk of adverse events and limits the utility of this approach in some patients. (For further discussion of this area see Chapter 49.)

Systemic Interventions

Systemic interventions include augmentation of platelet or coagulation mechanisms and inhibition of fibrinolytic mechanisms. Alternatively, some medications may improve vascular or other responses to bleeding. Red blood cell transfusion may palliate the symptoms of anemia.

In the bleeding patient with a platelet count under 50,000 per mm³, platelet transfusion may temporarily help control bleeding. Prophylactic platelet transfusions are used in the care of patients with marrow failure and severe thrombocytopenia with platelet counts between and 20,000 per mm³. The use of a 10,000 per mm³ threshold for prophylaxis appears to have a similar safety for a 20,000 per mm³ threshold (54); however, bleeding may occur with platelet counts over 20,000 per mm³ when associated with vascular and anatomic abnormalities (63). Platelet transfusion therapy is complicated by the short survival of transfused platelets. Although the mean platelet life span is 9.5 days in normal individuals, platelet survival may be less than 3 days in patients with stable platelet counts near 20,000 per mm³ owing to marrow hypoplasia (64). In the palliative care setting, marrow failure is often a chronic problem and a single platelet transfusion is unlikely to raise the platelet count for more than a few days. The limited role and complications associated with platelet transfusions should be discussed with the patient by the care providing team to arrive at an appropriate care plan. Prophylactic platelet transfusion (or trial of growth factors such as interleukin 11) is generally not warranted in a palliative care setting (2). However, palliation with limited platelet transfusions may be considered when symptoms of bleeding are distressing, such as painful hematomas, headache, disturbed vision due to recent hemorrhage, and continuous oral, GI, or genitourinary tract bleeding (65). (For more extensive comments see Chapter 6.)

The treatment of coagulopathy should be based on the underlying mechanism, the extent of coagulation disturbance, and the urgency for correction of the defect. Vitamin K deficiency and oral anticoagulation effect usually respond to vitamin K_1 within 24 hours. Vitamin K_1 is available as 5-mg oral tablets; subcutaneous administration is preferable in patients in whom malabsorption is a factor. Chronic administration (such as 5 mg twice per week) may be required to maintain the effect. Intravenous infusion of vitamin K_1 is discouraged except in emergencies because of rare reports of anaphylactoid reactions (59); infusion rates of under 1 mg per minute may decrease the risk of such reactions (45). For rapid correction of the coagulopathy of vitamin K deficiency, transfusion of FFP is the mainstay of therapy (55). FFP may also provide temporary improvement for bleeding patients with liver disease or malignancy-associated DIC. Although FFP contains all necessary coagulation proteins, transfusion of FFP may be considered excessive in the palliative care setting. In DIC, some recommendations have been made for the use of heparin to control thrombin-generated consumption of platelets and coagulation factors, but its use in this setting remains controversial (55,57).

Desmopressin is an analog of the posterior pituitary hormone vasopressin. 1-Deamino-[8-D-arginine] vasopressin (DDAVP) has been used extensively in the management of patients with mild deficiency of coagulation factor VIII (mild hemophilia A) or von Willebrand factor (type I von Willebrand disease) because levels of these proteins rise approximately two- to threefold after administration of this agent (66). DDAVP has also been used successfully in patients with acquired defects of platelet function resulting from uremia, cirrhosis, and aspirin. It has also proved useful for management of variceal bleeding, possibly due to splanchnic vasoconstriction and decreasing portal pressures. DDAVP is administered as either an intravenous infusion (0.3–0.4 µg per kg over 20 minutes) or through nasal inhalation (a single 150 µg application for weight under 50 kg, and two applications for larger patients). Common side effects include mild facial flushing and headache. Water retention with hyponatremia can occur owing to the potent antidiuretic effect of desmopressin. Excessive administration of fluids should be avoided.

Antifibrinolytic agents prevent clot lysis by blocking the binding sites of plasmin and its activators in plasma or saliva. Among these agents, tranexamic acid is ten times more potent than ε-aminocaproic acid and has a longer half-life (66). These drugs are rapidly absorbed from the GI tract and excreted in the urine, and both have dose-related nausea, vomiting, and diarrhea as the main toxicities. A dose of tranexamic acid of 1.5 g, followed up by 1 g three times per day, or ε-aminocaproic acid started at 5 g, followed up by 1 g four times per day, was used in one palliative care study (67). Fourteen of 16 patients had cessation of tumor-associated bleeding, with most having a complete control of hemorrhage within 4 days. Treatment was continued for up to 54 days and bleeding was not reported after cessation of the therapy. Topical administration of these agents was described in this study and in several case series of oral surgery (56). Although antifibrinolytic agents have been used in patients with thrombocytopenic bleeding, results of studies have not been consistent. One placebo-controlled trial did not demonstrate benefit in a population of patients with aplastic anemia or myelodysplasia, but two small studies with aminocaproic acid showed some effect on control of hemorrhage (67). Antifibrinolytic therapy is generally avoided in the treatment of upper urinary tract hemorrhage as ureteral clots may obstruct urinary flow. Systemic antifibrinolytic therapy increases the risk of thrombosis and should be used very cautiously in DIC.

Systemic interventions are occasionally used to alter the physiologic responses to bleeding. An example is the use of the somatostatin analog octreotide acetate in patients with GI bleeding (56). Although mostly used in the treatment of acute upper GI bleeding, at least one successful use in a palliative care setting is reported (58). It was suggested that octreotide acetate results in decreased splanchnic blood flow, reduced venous pressures, cytoprotection, and suppression of gastric acid secretion. The recommended dose was 50–100 µg administered subcutaneously every 12 hours, increased according to clinical response to a maximum of 600 µg per day. Continuous infusion by either intravenous or subcutaneous route is a possible alternative (56). Adverse effects are dose dependent, and include nausea, abdominal discomfort, and diarrhea.

Massive or ongoing bleeding will exacerbate anemia in chronically ill patients. Anemia may present as poor tolerance to exercise or chronic fatigue. Arbitrary thresholds for transfusion support often fail to take into account the particular situation of a patient, and anemia is often better tolerated by younger individuals and patients without comorbidities of cardiopulmonary or vascular diseases. Decisions regarding either indirect support of red cell production with growth factors (such as erythropoietin) or direct transfusion of red blood cells should be consistent with the goals of care for the patient. Response to growth factors is generally slow, and a trial of transfusion may be more appropriate. If within a day or two of transfusion there is no improvement in fatigue, dyspnea, or associated symptoms, further transfusion will probably be unhelpful (2). (For more extensive comments see Chapter 6.)

References

1. Johnson MJ. Problems of anticoagulation within a palliative care setting: an audit of hospice patients taking warfarin. *Palliat Med* 1997;11:306–312.
2. Davis MP. Hematology in palliative medicine. *Am J Hosp Palliat Med* 2004;21:445–454.
3. Kirkova J, Fainsinger RL. Thrombosis and anticoagulation in palliative care: an evolving clinical challenge. *J Palliat Care* 2004; 2:101–104.
4. Johnson MG, Sproule MW, Paul J. The prevalence and associated variables of deep venous thrombosis in patients with advanced cancer. *Clin Oncol* 1999;11:105–110.
5. Linenberger ML, Wittkowsky AK. Thromboembolic complications of malignancy: Risks. *Oncology* 2005;19:853–861.
6. Dicato M, Ries F, Duhem C. Bleeding and coagulation problems. In: Klastersky J, Schimpf J, Senn H-J, eds. *Handbook of supportive care in cancer*, New York: Marcel Dekker Inc, 1995.
7. Gordon S. Cancer cell procoagulants and their implications. *Hematol Oncol Clin North Am* 1992;6:1359–1374.
8. Bevilacqua MP, Pober JS, Majeau GR, et al. Recombinant tumor necrosis factor induces procoagulant activity in cultured human vascular endothelium: characterization and comparison with the actions of interleukin-1. *Proc Natl Acad Sci U S A* 1996;83:4533–4537.
9. Lip GY, Gibb CR. Does heart failure confer a hypercoagulable state? Virchow's triad revisited. *J Am Coll Cardiol* 1999;33:1424–1426.
10. Koster T, Blann AD, Breit E, et al. Role of clotting factor VIII in effect of von Willebrand factor on occurrence of deep-vein thrombosis. *Lancet* 1995;345:152–155.
11. Koster T, Rosendall FR, Reitsma PH, et al. Factor VII and fibrinogen levels as risk factors for venous thrombosis: a case-control study of plasma levels and DNA polymorphisms–the Leiden Thrombophilia Study (LETS). *Thromb Haemost* 1994;71:719–722.
12. Rosovsky RP, Kuter DJ. Catheter-related thrombosis in Cancer patients: pathophysiology, diagnosis, and management. *Hematol Oncol Clin North Am* 2005;19:183–202.
13. Kirkova J, Oneschuk D, Hanson J. Deep vein thrombosis (DVT) in advanced cancer patients with lower extremity edema referred for assessment. *Am J Hosp Palliat Med* 2005;22:145–149.
14. Gomes MP, Deitcher SR. Diagnosis of venous thromboembolic disease in cancer patients. *Oncology* 2003;17:126–135.
15. ten Wolde M, Kraaijenhagen RA, Prins MH, et al. The clinical usefulness of D-dimer testing in cancer patients with suspected deep venous thrombosis. *Arch Intern Med* 2002;162:1880–1884.
16. Lee AYY, Julian JA, Levine MN, et al. Clinical utility of a rapid whole-blood D-dimer assay in patients with cancer who present with suspected acute deep venous thrombosis. *Ann Intern Med* 1999;131:417–423.

17. Wells PJ, Brill-Edwards P, Stevens P, et al. A novel and rapid whole-blood assay for D-dimer in patients with clinically suspected deep vein thrombosis. *Circulation* 1995;91:2184–2187.
18. Lee AYY. Treatment of venous thromboembolism in cancer patients. *Thromb Res* 2001;102:V195–V208.
19. Perrier A, Desmarais S, Miron M-J, et al. Non-invasive diagnosis of venous thromboembolism in outpatients. *Lancet* 1999;353:190–195.
20. The PIOPED Investigators. Value of ventilation/perfusion scan in acute pulmonary embolism. Results of the prospective investigation of pulmonary embolism diagnosis (PIOPED). *JAMA* 1990;263:2753–2759.
21. Russo V, Piva T, Lovato L, et al. Multidetector CT: a new gold standard in the diagnosis of pulmonary embolism? State of the art and diagnostic algorithms. *Radiol Med* 2005;109:49–61.
22. Moore LK, Jackson WL, Shorr AF, et al. Meta-analysis: outcomes in patients with suspected pulmonary embolism managed with computed tomographic pulmonary angiography. *Ann Intern Med* 2005;141:866–874.
23. Rathbun SW, Raskob GE, Whitsett TL. Sensitivity and specificity of helical computed tomography in the diagnosis of pulmonary embolism: a systematic review. *Ann Intern Med* 2000;132:227–232.
24. Johnson MJ, Sherry K. How do palliative care physicians manage venous thromboembolism? *Palliat Med* 1997;11:462–468.
25. Merminod T, Zulian GB. Diagnosis of venous thromboembolism in cancer patients receiving palliative care. *J Pain Symptom Manage* 2000;19:238–239.
26. Buller HR, Agnelli G, Hull RD, et al. Antithrombotic therapy for venous thromboembolic disease. The seventh ACCP Conference on antithrombotic and thrombolytic therapy. *Chest* 2004;126:401S–428S.
27. Ihnat DM, Mills JL, Hughes JD, et al. Treatment of patients with venous thromboembolism and malignant disease: should vena cava filter placement be routine? *J Vasc Surg* 1998;28:800–807.
28. Bona RD, Hickey AD, Wallace DM. Efficacy and safety of oral anticoagulation in patients with cancer. *Thromb Haemost* 1997;78:137–140.
29. Hirsh J, Warkentin TE, Shaughnessy SG, et al. Heparin and low-molecular-weight heparin mechanisms of action, pharmacokinetics, dosing, monitoring, efficacy and safety. *Chest* 2001;119:64S–94S.
30. Wells PJ, Kovacs MJ, Bormanis J, et al. Expanded eligibility for outpatient treatment of deep venous thrombosis and pulmonary embolism with low-molecular-weight heparin. *Arch Intern Med* 1998;158:2001–2003.
31. Lee AYY, Levine MN. Venous thromboembolism and cancer: risks and outcomes. *Circulation* 2003;107:117–121.
32. Monreal M, Lafoz E, Olive A, et al. Comparison of subcutaneous unfractionated heparin with a low molecular weight heparin (Fragmin) in patients with venous thromboembolism and contraindications to coumarin. *Thromb Haemost* 1994;71:7–11.
33. Warkentin TE, Levine MN, Hirsh J, et al. Heparin-induced thrombocytopenia in patients treated with low-molecular-weight heparin or unfractionated heparin. *N Engl J Med* 1995;332:1330–1335.
34. Merli G, Spiro TE, Olsson C-G, et al. Subcutaneous enoxaparin once or twice daily compared with intravenous unfractionated heparin for treatment of venous thromboembolic disease. *Ann Intern Med* 2001;134:191–202.
35. Warkentin TE, Chong BH, Greinacker A. Heparin-induced thrombocytopenia-towards consensus. *Thromb Haemost* 1998;79:1–7.
36. Pineo GF, Hull RD. The use of heparin, low molecular weight heparin, and oral anticoagulants in the management of thromboembolic disease. In: Portenoy R, Bruera E, eds. *Topics in palliative care*, Vol. 4. New York: Oxford University Press, 2000.
37. Buller HR, Davidson BL, Decousus H. Subcutaneous fondaparinux versus intravenous unfractionated heparin in the initial treatment of pulmonary embolism. *N Engl J Med* 2004;349:1695–1702.
38. Buller HR, Davidson BL, Decousus H, et al. Fondaparinux or enoxaparin for the initial treatment of symptomatic deep venous thrombosis: a randomized trail. *Ann Intern Med* 2004;14:867–873.
39. Gage BF, Fihn SD, White RH. Management and dosing of warfarin therapy. *Am J Med* 2000;109:481–488.
40. Salem DN, Stein PD, Al-Ahmed A, et al. Antithrombotic therapy in valvular heart disease—native and prosthetic: the seventh ACCP conference on antithrombotic and thrombolytic therapy. *Chest* 2004;126:457S–482S.
41. Fihn SD, McDonell M, Martin D, et al. Risk factors for complications of chronic anticoagulation. *Ann Intern Med* 1993;118:511–520.
42. Prandoni P. Antithrombotic strategies in patients with cancer. *Thromb Haemost* 1997;78:141–144.
43. Johnson MJ. Problems of anticoagulation within a palliative care setting—correction. *Palliat Med* 1998;12:463–463.
44. Patel RJ, Witt DM, Saseen JJ, et al. Randomized, placebo-controlled trail of oral phytonadione for excessive anticoagulation. *Pharmacotherapy* 2000;2:1159–1166.
45. Pereira J, Phan T. Management of bleeding in patients with advanced cancer. *Oncologist* 2004;9:561–570.
46. Lee AYY, Levine MN, Baker RI. Low-molecular weight heparin versus a coumarin for the prevention of recurrent venous thromboembolism in patients with cancer. *N Engl J Med* 2003;349:146–153.
47. Khamashta MA, Cuadrado MJ, Mujic F, et al. The management of thrombosis in antiphospholipid-antibody syndrome. *N Engl J Med* 1995;332:993–997.
48. Lee AYY. Management of thrombosis in cancer: primary prevention and secondary prophylaxis. *Br J Haematol* 2004;128:291–302.
49. Decousus H, Leizorovicz A, Parent F, et al. A clinical trial of vena caval filters in the prevention of pulmonary embolism in patients with proximal deep-vein thrombosis. *N Engl J Med* 1998;338:409–415.
50. Mustafa BO, Rathbun SW, Whitsett TL, et al. Sensitivity and specificity of ultrasonography in the diagnosis of upper extremity deep vein thrombosis: a systematic review. *Arch Intern Med* 2002;162:401–404.
51. Heaton DC, Han DY, Indere A. Minidose (1 mg) warfarin as prophylaxis for central vein catheter thrombosis. *Intern Med J* 2002;32:84–86.
52. Geerts W, Pineo GF, Heit JA, et al. Prevention of venous thromboembolism: the seventh ACCP conference on antithrombotic and thrombolytic therapy. *Chest* 2004;126:338S–400S.
53. Schnoll-Sussman F, Kurtz RC. Gastrointestinal emergencies in the critically ill cancer patient. *Semin Oncol* 2000;27:270–283.
54. Slichter SJ. Relationship between platelet count and bleeding risk in thrombocytopenic patients. *Transfus Med Rev* 2005;18:153–167.
55. Raife TJ, Rosenfeld SB, Lentz SR. Bleeding from acquired coagulation defects and antithrombotic therapy. In: Simon TL, Dzik WH, Snyder FL, et al, eds. *Rossi's principles of transfusion medicine*, 3rd ed. Philadelphia, PA: Lippincott Williams & Wilkins, 2002.
56. Pereira J, Mancini I, Bruera E. The management of bleeding in advanced cancer patients. In: Portenoy R, Bruera E, eds. *Topics in palliative care*, Vol. 4. New York: Oxford University Press, 2000.
57. Levi M. Current understanding of disseminated intravascular coagulation. *Br J Haematol* 2004;124:567–576.
58. Gagnon B, Mancini I, Pereira J, et al. Palliative management of bleeding events in advanced cancer patients. *J Palliat Care* 1998;14:50–54.
59. McEvoy GK. *AHFS Drug Information 2004*. Bethesda, MD: American Society of Health-System Pharmacists Inc, 2004.
60. Mankad PS. The role of fibrin sealants in surgery. *Am J Surg* 2001;182:21S–28S.
61. White RH, Sawczuk I. Hematuria. In: Walsh TD, ed. *Symptom control*. Cambridge, MA: Blackwell Scientific Publications, 1989.
62. Roche B, Chautems R, Marti MC. Application of formaldehyde for treatment of hemorrhagic radiation-induced proctitis. *World J Surg* 1996;20:1092–1094.
63. Bernstein SH, Vose JM, Tricot G, et al. A multicenter study of platelet recovery and utilization in patients after myeloablative therapy and hematopoietic stem cell transplantation. *Blood* 1998;91:3509–3527.
64. Hanson SR, Slichter SJ. Platelet kinetics in patients with bone marrow hypoplasia: evidence for a fixed platelet requirement. *Blood* 1985;66:1105–1109.
65. Lassauniere JM, Bertolino M, Hunault M, et al. Platelet transfusion in advanced hematologic malignancy: a position paper. *J Palliat Care* 1996;12:38–42.
66. Mannucci PM. Hemostatic drugs. *N Engl J Med* 1998;339:245–253.
67. Dean A, Tuffin P. Fibrinolytic inhibitors for cancer-associated bleeding problems. *J Pain Symptom Manage* 1997;13:20–24.

CHAPTER 32 ■ UROLOGIC ISSUES IN PALLIATIVE CARE

DAVID A. KUNKLE, STEVEN J. HIRSHBERG, AND RICHARD E. GREENBERG

The management of patients with a progressive medical disease should permit them to live the remainder of their lives to their fullest potential, maximizing both the quality and quantity of life. The development of complications related to the genitourinary system is not uncommon in these patients. Although some of these problems may merely be considered minor annoyances, others are quite serious and can potentially undermine a patient's quality of life. The most serious complications may, in fact, reduce life expectancy.

Commonly, classification of genitourinary problems differentiates the urinary tract into upper and lower systems. The upper urinary tract refers to those organs proximal to the ureterovesical junction. The lower urinary tract pertains to the bladder, prostate, and urethra. This chapter discusses the diagnosis and management of both the upper and the lower urinary tract pathology. Specifically, the matters of irritative voiding symptoms, bladder outlet obstruction, upper urinary tract obstruction, hematuria, and priapism are addressed with regard to the palliative care patient.

IRRITATIVE VOIDING SYMPTOMS

The complex of irritative voiding symptoms refers to the symptoms of urinary frequency, urgency, and dysuria. These symptoms are common in patients seeking urologic evaluation. Rarely, they are the first indication of a severe underlying problem. In addition to symptomatic relief, the management must focus on identifying and treating the underlying disorder (Table 32.1). Investigations may be warranted and modified on the basis of clinical presentation and patient prognosis.

Infection

Urinary tract infection is one of the most common conditions treated by physicians. Typical signs of lower urinary tract infection (simple cystitis) include urinary frequency, urgency, dysuria, foul-smelling urine, hematuria, and suprapubic tenderness. Many cases of urinary tract infection in hospitalized or hospice patients are iatrogenic, secondary to urinary tract manipulation (most often by urethral catheters). When evaluating a patient who presents with acute onset of new irritative voiding symptoms, urinary tract infection should be among the first diagnoses considered. A urinalysis, including both dipstick and microscopic analysis, should be performed before starting empiric antibiotic therapy. Those patients who are either hospitalized, institutionalized, or who have recently

been discharged from such a facility should also have a urine culture and sensitivity performed. The potential virulence of the bacterial flora associated with these facilities justifies early culture. Likewise, a patient with recent urinary tract instrumentation, including urethral catheterization, who develops signs of urinary tract infection should also have a urine culture done at initial evaluation.

When obtaining urine specimens from patients who appear to have failed the appropriate antibiotic therapy, it is particularly important to ensure proper collection of the specimen. This especially holds true for debilitated patients and those with significant functional impairments who may not be able to properly collect a clean-catch specimen. If the patient is unable to appropriately collect urine for urinalysis or urine culture, a catheterized specimen may be necessary before continuing or modifying treatment. Additionally, when specimens are collected from patients with either an indwelling catheter or condom catheter, one must take care in interpreting the results. Urine from these patients is almost always colonized with bacteria, and, consequently, the finding of bacteriuria alone does not necessarily indicate active urinary tract infection, although a negative culture under these circumstances is often considered adequate to rule out infection. In the setting of chronic indwelling catheter with urinary bacterial colonization, the decision to treat with antimicrobials may, in part, be determined by the presence or absence of symptoms.

Patients who develop recurrent or relapsing symptomatic infections should undergo further evaluation to rule out structural abnormalities and urinary obstruction. Stasis of urine flow at any level of the urinary tract predisposes an individual to urinary infection by creating a favorable environment for bacterial proliferation. Urinary obstruction may occur in the setting of anatomic abnormalities, obstructing stone or neoplasm, or bladder outlet obstruction. Additional factors contributing to urinary tract infection include diabetes mellitus and immunosuppression as a result of cancer or its therapies. Other patients at particular risk for urinary tract infection include those on chronic steroid therapy and those infected with the human immunodeficiency virus.

Initial evaluation of patients with recurrent urinary tract infections should include measurement of a postvoid bladder residual to rule out the presence of a large volume of residual urine. Although there is no absolute volume of urine to be considered abnormal following urination, an excess of approximately 150–200 mL should prompt therapy to improve bladder emptying. This can be determined by catheterizing a patient once he has voided to completion. As an alternative, the postvoid residual may be measured by ultrasound imaging,

TABLE 32.1

IRRITATIVE VOIDING SYMPTOMS

Differential diagnosis/Etiologies	Commonly used pharmacologic agents (*dosing*)
Atrophic vaginitis	Oral anticholinergics
Bladder neoplasm	Oxybutynin (*Ditropan/Ditropan XL*) (5 mg orally, may titrate)
Chemical irritants	Tolterodine (*Detrol/Detrol LA*) (2–4 mg orally, may titrate)
Cyclophosphamide cystitis	Trospium (*Sanctura*) (20 mg orally—once or twice daily)
Detrusor instability	Solifenacin (*Vesicare*) (5 mg orally daily)
Eosinophilic cystitis	Hyoscyamine (*Levsin*) (0.125 mg orally/sublingual, may titrate)
Extrinsic bladder compression/pelvic mass	Darifenacin (*Enablex*) (7.5 or 15 mg orally)
Interstitial cystitis	Belladonna and opium (suppository)
Intravesical foreign body/calculus	Phenazopyridine (*Pyridium*) (200 mg orally three times daily)
Neurogenic bladder	
Radiation cystitis	
Vulvar cancer	
Ureteral calculus	
Urethral caruncle	
Urethral diverticulum	

which should include measurements of bladder volume both before and after voiding. A newer option for assessment of residual urine is the Bladder Scan device (Diagnostic Ultrasound, Bothell, WA), a portable ultrasound unit, which can be used at the bedside shortly following urination. Additional studies may include renal ultrasound to exclude hydronephrosis, and intravenous pyelogram (IVP) or noncontrast computed tomography (CT) scan evaluation for calculi, hydronephrosis, or diverticuli. Urine culture and sensitivity are considered mandatory when infections do not resolve with empiric antibiotic therapy.

Tumor-Related Symptoms

Although significantly less common than urinary tract infection, tumor invasion in the bladder is capable of causing irritative voiding symptoms. Tumor invasion may originate from within the bladder, such as in the setting of urothelial carcinoma, or extravesically from within the pelvis. A genitourinary tumor that commonly presents with irritative voiding symptoms is carcinoma *in situ* of the bladder. Although carcinoma *in situ* may be completely asymptomatic, it more commonly presents with irritative voiding symptoms. On the other hand, low-grade papillary lesions of the bladder or upper tracts usually have insidious onset and may be completely asymptomatic. Common malignancies originating outside of the bladder include tumors of the ovary, cervix, uterus, rectum, prostate, and colon.

The distinction between tumor invasion and urinary tract infection can usually be made on the basis of the history and several tests. Although the symptomology may be quite similar, direct tumor invasion is more likely to have an insidious onset and also likely to be associated with gross hematuria. All patients with irritative voiding symptoms should undergo a detailed urinalysis (dipstick and microscopic analysis of urine sediment). If a urinary tract infection is excluded by urinalysis and urine culture (when indicated), other etiologies should be considered. The differential diagnosis for noninfectious causes of bladder irritability includes bladder or ureteral calculi (secondary to irritation caused by a calculus in the intramural portion of the distal ureter), foreign bodies, and tumors. Like urinary tract infection, these diseases may produce pyuria on routine urinalysis. However, unless there is concurrent urinary tract infection, urine should be sterile when examined in the setting of these noninfectious etiologies. One notable exception is in the case of sterile pyuria associated with genitourinary tuberculosis.

Any patient with new-onset irritative voiding symptoms and sterile urine should have a voided urinary cytology. Although not necessarily diagnostic of a urothelial tumor, a positive urine cytology is particularly helpful in diagnosing carcinoma *in situ* of the bladder. However, a negative cytology does not exclude malignancy because of its relatively low sensitivity for detecting low-grade superficial papillary transitional cell carcinomas of the bladder or upper tracts. Overall, urinary cytology has been reported to have a sensitivity of 38.0% and a specificity of 98.3% with improved sensitivity for higher-grade malignancy (1). Other recent advances in the early diagnosis of carcinoma *in situ* include various urinary markers (e.g., nuclear matrix protein-22, hyaluronic acid-hyaluronidase, BTA-Stat, urinary bladder cancer antigen), which are still under investigation as to their clinical usefulness.

Patients who develop irritative voiding symptoms associated with microscopic or gross hematuria with negative urine cultures also deserve additional evaluation. The accepted evaluation for these patients includes evaluation for upper and lower urinary tract pathology. Traditionally this has included cystoscopy, urine cytologic evaluation, and intravenous urography. In patients with an advanced medical illness, in whom diagnosis of urothelial cancer may not change the overall management, this algorithm may be modified. With the development of fiber optics and flexible cystoscopes, office or bedside cystoscopy may be performed with minimal discomfort. Renal and bladder ultrasound, which can now be performed with relative ease, can detect solid tumors of the kidney or large tumors in the bladder; it would be unlikely, however, to diagnose a small tumor of the urothelium. Additionally, newer techniques in CT scan, with spiral scans and three-dimensional reconstruction, enable detailed evaluation of the entire urinary system with minimal morbidity.

The initial treatment of a tumor that directly invades the bladder wall and causes irritative voiding symptoms should include transurethral resection of the bladder tumor (TURBT). Depending on the extent of tumor, this may be carried out on an outpatient basis, although some form of anesthesia, usually spinal or general, is required. Transurethral resection entails using a special cystoscope (resectoscope) with a cutting "loop."

By the application of an electrical current, the loop essentially cuts through bladder tissue. This loop is used to resect the abnormal urothelium and the underlying layers (submucosa and muscularis) of the bladder. The diagnostic value of TURBT further supports its acceptance as the procedure of choice for the initial evaluation of all bladder tumors. If a full thickness resection is performed, the depth of tumor invasion and the degree of differentiation can be determined with a single procedure.

Patients who persist with disabling irritative voiding symptoms after TURBT may be treated symptomatically. Anticholinergic drugs such as oxybutynin, tolterodine, and solifenacin are commonly used to treat symptoms of urinary frequency, urgency, and nocturia. These drugs may be started at low doses and then titrated based upon their affect. Caution must be used in those patients who also have a component of bladder outlet obstruction or bowel obstruction because their anticholinergic action may aggravate urinary retention and gastrointestinal dysmotility. A careful observation of voiding and bowel elimination patterns during treatment is required in these patients. At times, a fine balance between irritative voiding symptoms and urinary retention must be obtained. In severe cases, anticholinergic therapy can be used to purposely induce retention, allowing the patient to be effectively managed with intermittent catheterization. In addition, there is a relative contraindication to the use of anticholinergic therapy in patients with closed angle glaucoma. However, if patients maintain routine pharmacologic therapy for this condition, there should be little chance of clinical deterioration (2).

Urinary analgesic drugs, the most well known of which is phenazopyridine (Pyridium), may offer some symptomatic benefit to patients with irritative voiding symptoms. It is converted from its inactive to its active form within the urinary tract. At times, a combination of this treatment and an anticholinergic medication may be particularly helpful in relieving symptoms.

Radiation Cystitis

It is not uncommon for patients to develop irritative voiding symptoms after external beam or interstitial radiation therapy to the pelvis. Radiation therapy is often used to treat genitourinary, gynecologic, and gastrointestinal tumors. Acute radiation cystitis after external beam radiation is characterized by dysuria, frequency of urination, nocturia, and rarely, hematuria. Dean and Lytton (3) evaluated patients after pelvic irradiation and found that 21% reported urologic symptoms. However, in only 2.5% were these truly related to the radiation itself; in most cases, the symptoms were attributable to recurrent or persistent tumor. Newer methods of delivering external beam radiation therapy such as intensity modulated radiation therapy (IMRT) offer the hope of increasing treatment doses while minimizing side effects.

Symptoms usually begin to develop after exposure to 3000 cGy, and there is an increased incidence of cystitis in those patients receiving >6000–6500 cGy. Patients who experience persistent symptoms after completion of radiation fall into the category of chronic radiation cystitis. A history of open bladder surgery, in the subset of patients who receive higher doses of radiation, appears to be an independent risk factor for the development of chronic radiation cystitis.

The associated symptom complex frequently determines measures used to treat acute radiation cystitis. To address symptoms, pharmacotherapy with phenazopyridine or anticholinergic medications, either alone or in combination, are frequently administered. However, those patients who are refractory to these symptomatic treatments can become debilitated and experience a marked decline in quality of life due to severe urinary frequency, urgency, dysuria, nocturia, and at times, urge incontinence. Approaches to treating patients with intractable symptoms are limited to procedures that divert the urine stream. Occasionally, diversion of the urine with a urethral catheter improves symptoms, although frequently the bladder discomfort is actually exacerbated by catheter irritation. Alternatives to catheter drainage, which have been used with limited success, include small suprapubic catheters and bilateral percutaneous nephrostomy diversion.

Invasive approaches aimed at diverting the urine or enlarging the bladder require a major abdominal surgery. A potential deterrent to any surgery involving the bladder in patients with radiation cystitis is the damaging effects of the radiation itself. Risks of peri- or postoperative complications for augmentation cystoplasty or urinary diversion are dramatically increased in patients with irradiated bowel or bladder due to underlying radiation-induced vasculitis.

Augmentation cystoplasty involves enlarging the bladder by surgically incorporating a patch of small bowel, colon, or stomach at the dome of the bladder. Urinary diversion requires constructing either a urostomy with external appliance or a continent diversion by means of a catheterizable pouch or orthotopic neobladder. Similarly, these procedures require the use of segments of small bowel or large bowel, both of which may have been irradiated. If palliative urinary diversion is entertained, the bladder itself does not necessarily need to be removed. In fact, cystectomy should probably be avoided because of the increased surgical risks after radiation therapy. Although surgical diversion and bladder augmentation are considered in this discussion for the sake of completeness, few patients within the palliative care population are actually considered as candidates for this intervention because of the associated surgical risks and the time required for convalescence.

Chemical Cystitis

Several agents that are administered intravesically for the treatment of either superficial or multifocal transitional cell carcinoma of the bladder or carcinoma in situ can be potentially toxic and irritating. All of these agents have the potential to cause a chemical cystitis to varying degrees.

The most common and the most effective medication used for intravesical treatment of noninvasive bladder carcinoma is bacillus Calmette-Guérin (BCG). A standard course of BCG therapy involves weekly bladder instillations for 6 weeks. Depending on the clinical response and the physician's preference, maintenance therapy may continue after the initial 6-week regimen. Symptoms of urinary frequency, dysuria, and hematuria may develop after two or three instillations and last for approximately 2 days after each treatment. These symptoms are an expected consequence of the immune stimulation and inflammatory reaction that are thought to be essential components of the tumor-suppressive action of BCG (4). Lamm et al. (5) reviewed the complications of BCG therapy in 1278 patients and found that 91% developed dysuria, 90% had urinary frequency, and 43% reported hematuria. These symptoms seemed to increase with both the duration and frequency of treatments. Although BCG is available in several strains, the local irritative symptoms were not limited to any particular strain.

In patients undergoing a 6-week course of therapy, symptoms can usually be well controlled with the combination of phenazopyridine and anticholinergic medications. Although there have not been any randomized or controlled studies of these medications, several investigators with over 2600 patients support their routine use for symptomatic relief (6). For those patients refractory to this regimen, or in those patients who continue with maintenance therapy, treatment with isoniazid, diphenhydramine, acetaminophen, and nonsteroidal anti-inflammatory medications may be helpful. Treatment is usually continued for the duration of symptoms and may be given prophylactically for 3 days starting on the morning of BCG administration. Because all these agents have a different mechanism of action, they are frequently used in combinations, and doses are titrated until a maximal effect is obtained. A rare complication of treatment with BCG is the development of a nonfunctional contracted bladder, which occurs in approximately 0.2% of cases. Because contracted bladders do not tend to develop in patients with severe irritative symptoms who were treated with prophylactic isoniazid, early treatment with antituberculous medication may be helpful in preventing this disabling complication.

Local irritative side effects are seen somewhat less frequently with other intravesical chemotherapeutic regimens. Agents used for intravesical treatment of bladder cancer include triethylenethiophosphoramide (thiotepa), etoglucid (epodyl), mitomycin C, doxorubicin, and interferon-α. Mitomycin C has been associated with chemical cystitis in 10–15% of patients and, in rare cases, can lead to a contracted bladder. Doxorubicin has also been associated with chemical cystitis and defunctionalized bladders. Treatment of cystitis due to these agents is similar to that due to BCG except that antituberculous medications have no effect on the irritative symptoms caused by these agents.

Systemic administration of certain cytotoxic drugs can also lead to irritative symptoms. These symptoms are commonly associated with cyclophosphamide and ifosfamide (oxazaphosphorine alkylating agents), busulfan (1, 4-dimethanesulfonayoxybutane), and methenamine mandelate (7). Such symptoms may be avoided through the concomitant administration of mesna during chemotherapy. Mesna is a chelating agent that binds acrolein, a toxic byproduct of phosphamides, thereby decreasing its toxic effects.

In rare cases, irritative voiding symptoms can be refractory to conservative therapies. If the suffering from unrelieved symptoms is severe, urinary diversion may be contemplated. The standard form of urinary diversion with the lowest risk of short-term morbidity is the ileal conduit (see section on Radiation Cystitis). This procedure requires general anesthesia, major intra-abdominal surgery, and a minimum 5- to 7-day postoperative recovery. Although it is an alternative for those patients who have experienced a marked loss of independence and quality of life, the risks associated with the procedure must be weighed against the possible benefits.

OUTLET OBSTRUCTION

One of the most common problems of the urinary tract in men is bladder outlet obstruction, which can result from either benign or malignant processes. In men, the most common organ to impede bladder emptying is the prostate gland. Bladder outlet obstruction may also occur as a direct consequence of tumor extension or other pathology arising from the rectum or urethra. In addition, a lesion of the ovary, cervix, or uterus may be the cause in women. The ultimate consequence to the patient with obstructive uropathy, without intervention, is renal failure secondary to chronic urinary retention. This condition progresses more rapidly if there is concomitant urinary infection, a situation not uncommon in patients who fail to adequately empty their bladder.

A careful history may disclose the lesion responsible for urinary retention. Physiologically, failure to empty the bladder indicates failure to generate adequate detrusor pressure to overcome urethral resistance. This may result from primary detrusor failure (e.g., associated with diabetes mellitus or sacral plexus injury) or from bladder outlet obstruction at or distal to the bladder neck. A detailed urologic history relating symptoms before the episode of urinary retention may clarify the underlying problem. Patients who complain of urinary frequency, urgency, nocturia, and a slow urinary stream frequently have obstruction as the underlying etiology of their urinary retention. In contrast, patients who report a slow stream, impaired bladder sensation, increasing intervals between voids, and decreased urgency are more likely to have primary detrusor failure. Because the management of these two disorders differs significantly, it is obviously critical to make this distinction before initiating therapy (Table 32.2).

Nonsurgical Treatment

Whereas the initial management of urinary retention secondary to benign prostatic hyperplasia (BPH) may warrant a period of catheter drainage and an empiric trial of α-antagonist medications (terazosin, doxazosin, alfuzosin, or tamsulosin), bladder outlet obstruction secondary to malignant disease is less likely to respond to this approach. Deconditioning and immobility are additional complicating factors in the terminally ill; debilitation may decrease the likelihood of

TABLE 32.2

MANAGEMENT OPTIONS FOR OBSTRUCTIVE UROPATHY

Bladder outlet obstruction	Upper tract urinary obstruction
Nonsurgical	Internal ureteral stenting
α-Antagonist pharmacotherapy	Percutaneous nephrostomy drainage
5-α Reductase inhibitors	Open surgical urinary diversion
Androgen deprivation therapy	Self-expanding ureteral stents
Indwelling Foley catheter	
Clean intermittent catheterization	
Suprapubic catheter drainage	
Surgical	
Transurethral resection of the prostate	
Laser prostatectomy	
Transurethral microwave thermotherapy	
Transurethral needle ablation of the prostate	
High-frequency radio wave ablation of the prostate	
Transurethral vaporization of the prostate	
Urethral stenting	

recovery of adequate bladder detrusor function. Those patients with BPH who fail initial conservative measures (α-blockers and bladder rest) after an adequate time period (e.g., 1 to 2 weeks) may be candidates for alternative measures. These options, which are all invasive to an extent, include chronic urethral or suprapubic bladder drainage, intermittent catheterization, and surgical procedures such as urethral stenting, urinary diversion, or surgical resection of the obstructing tissue. In patients with malignant disease, these approaches should be considered earlier in the course of treatment of the patient.

Hormonal Manipulation

A nonsurgical approach to patients with obstruction due to prostate carcinoma involves hormonal manipulation. This modality should be especially considered for those patients not previously treated in this fashion. Up to 72% of patients with advanced prostate cancer may have symptoms of bladder outlet obstruction (8). Surya and Provet (9) suggest that androgen deprivation may be preferable to surgery as the initial mode of therapy in this group of patients. Androgen deprivation may be accomplished by means of surgical bilateral orchiectomy or "medical orchiectomy" with luteinizing hormone releasing hormone (LHRH) analogs (leuprolide or goserelin) or diethylstilbestrol. In those patients with advanced disease who are to be initiated on LHRH analogs, a recent bone scan should be available to rule out significant occult bony disease in the vertebral column. After initiation of treatment with LHRH agonists, a luteinizing hormone and consequent testosterone surge may occur within the first 2 weeks of therapy; therefore patients with significant vertebral metastases, whether occult or overt, are at significant risk for spinal cord compression. For similar reasons, patients with bone pain may have increased analgesic needs shortly after beginning treatment with LHRH analogs. To reduce the potential for these adverse events, the authors recommend that all patients be started on antiandrogen therapy (flutamide, bicalutamide, nilutamide) before initiation of LHRH agonist therapy to avoid this testosterone flare phenomenon. At a minimum, patients with documented bony disease in the cervical, thoracic, or lumbar axial skeleton should be started on an antiandrogen 7 days before commencing therapy with LHRH analogs. Patients who fail to void 2 to 3 weeks after reduction of serum testosterone to castrate levels usually require surgical intervention or prolonged catheter drainage. It is notable that, in patients with advanced prostate cancer receiving androgen deprivation therapy, the development of obstructive uropathy has been shown to result in significantly reduced survival (10).

Clean Intermittent Catheterization

For the medically ill patient who does not wish to undergo a surgical procedure or who is deemed medically unfit to tolerate surgery, clean intermittent catheterization (CIC) and chronic indwelling catheterization represent common options for adequate bladder decompression. These options are best suited for those with urinary retention secondary to detrusor failure as opposed to outlet obstruction. CIC has been the nonsurgical treatment of choice to empty the bladder ever since Lapides introduced the concept in the late 1960s (11). CIC enables a motivated patient to avoid a chronic indwelling urethral catheter, thereby decreasing the attendant risks of infection, stricture, epididymitis, and symptoms associated with a dysfunctionalized bladder. Once a patient is placed on an adequate CIC schedule, bladder residuals must be monitored so that upper tract deterioration due to storing urine at high pressures is avoided. Common findings on routine urinalysis in those patients on CIC include pyuria and bacteriuria.

Those patients with systemic evidence of infection (i.e., fever, flank pain, and leukocytosis) should receive appropriate antimicrobial treatment. However, in the absence of these symptoms, the use of broad-spectrum antibiotic therapy in an attempt to sterilize the urine should be avoided because of the potential to develop resistant bacterial species. In patients with recurrent urosepsis, however, chronic antibiotic prophylaxis using low-dose antibiotics or urinary antiseptic drug regimens may be considered. Sterile intermittent catheterization may also alleviate problems of recurrent infections in those patients with clinical symptoms. Other issues that must be addressed before initiating CIC, especially in chronically ill patients, are sufficient manual dexterity and an adequate urethral channel to perform catheterization.

Indwelling Catheters

Although the use of indwelling catheters is usually limited to acute urinary retention, the benefits and risks of chronic catheterization in the medically ill patient must be carefully weighed. Frequently, a permanent urethral catheter is the most appropriate method of management in the patient with a very short life expectancy. Because these catheters can be changed at relatively long intervals, they may also be the modality of choice for patients who are technically difficult to catheterize or who are unable to catheterize themselves because of functional impairments. Urethral catheters are relatively simple devices, but may cause significant discomfort in patients who experience bladder spasms. These patients may leak urine around the catheter and experience intense suprapubic discomfort. Treatment for this predicament may include oral anticholinergic medications or suppositories containing belladonna and opium. Other problems with long-term catheterization include obstruction of urine drainage secondary to calcification of the catheter itself, calcification of the catheter balloon, urethral stricture, urethritis, epididymitis, urosepsis, and urethral erosion. Although placement of a suprapubic catheter avoids urethral trauma and irritation and decreases the risk of urosepsis, significant complications may still occur.

Surgical Treatment

Transurethral Resection of the Prostate

During a transurethral resection of the prostate (TURP), benign or malignant prostatic tissue is resected using an electrocautery loop. Although the procedure itself is usually limited to 1 hour, potential exists for the development of significant complications, especially in patients with underlying cardiac disease. TURP has the potential to create large fluid shifts by the absorption of irrigation fluid through prostatic venous channels during resection. In a patient with underlying cardiac disease, this may cause congestive heart failure in an otherwise compensated patient. Other inherent risks associated with this procedure include bleeding, which has the potential to be significant during resection of a large gland; urinary tract infection; urethral stricture; dilutional hyponatremia; bladder perforation; erectile dysfunction; postoperative hydronephrosis; and urinary incontinence. Newer potassium-titanyl-phosphate (KPT) and holmium lasers are now available for vaporization of the prostate due to BPH. These devices offer decreased surgical morbidity and decreased postoperative catheter times when compared to standard TURP.

In patients who fail other treatments, TURP remains the gold standard for removal of obstructing prostatic tissue. Several newer techniques, however, have been developed for resecting, evaporating, or coagulating the obstructing prostate. These newer techniques include electrosurgical vaporization of the prostate, transurethral needle ablation, microwave therapy, and high-frequency radio wave ablation. Several of these "minimally invasive" devices are now approved by U.S. Food and Drug Administration (FDA) for treatment of benign disease but no major studies have examined their use in patients with malignant disease of the prostate. Overall, these alternative methods seem to promise a rapid relief of symptoms with relatively low morbidity. However, long-term data to support sustained results for these techniques is still being collected. The role of these treatments for palliation has yet to be defined.

Palliative Transurethral Resection of the Prostate

Bladder outlet obstruction may occur because of prostate cancer, and it has been estimated that 25–35% of patients on a watchful waiting treatment plan for prostate cancer may ultimately require TURP (12). An alternative to a standard TURP, in which all of the prostatic tissue is removed out to the surgical capsule, is the "channel" TURP performed for palliation. Channel TURP is defined as a TURP performed to alleviate obstructive voiding symptoms in the patient with advanced or previously treated cancer. It may also refer to a TURP performed to remove obstructing prostatic tissue without necessarily resecting all of the tissue to the surgical capsule. Advantages of channel TURP as against traditional TURP arise from performing a more limited operation with less associated operative morbidity. The risk of urinary incontinence is of particular concern during resection of malignant prostatic tissue, which may cause alteration of normal anatomic landmarks and may directly invade the external urethral sphincter.

Mazur and Thompson (13) reviewed 41 patients with known prostate cancer who underwent channel TURP. All these patients were able to void after the procedure, although 22% of their patients eventually required additional procedures at a minimum of 15 months after the initial resection. The patients who were totally incontinent were those with malignant invasion of the external sphincter, which required intentional resection of this tissue to relieve obstruction. Crain et al. similarly reviewed their experience with 24 palliative TURPs performed in 19 patients with locally advanced prostate cancer (12). They found that, compared with patients undergoing TURP for benign disease, those treated with palliative TURP were more likely to have failure of initial voiding trial and require reoperation, chronic drainage, and recatheterization. They concluded that TURP may be performed for palliation in patients with advanced prostate cancer with a significant improvement in urinary symptoms. They also found that these patients sustain the increased rates of postoperative urinary retention and reoperation. It should be noted that potential exists for dissemination of tumor cells through prostatic venous channels when TURP is performed in the setting of prostate cancer; however, there are no definitive studies that demonstrate worse outcomes for patients undergoing palliative TURP.

Postbrachytherapy Transurethral Resection of the Prostate

Urinary retention has been noted in 1.5–22% of patients receiving brachytherapy for locally confined prostate cancer, with postimplant TURP rates ranging from 0 to 8.7% (14). Usually, TURP is delayed until 6 months after implantation to allow most of the required radiation to be delivered to the prostate. Because TURP will remove some of the implanted seeds, delaying intervention allows delivery of 90% of the intended radiation. Studies examining TURP performed after prostatic brachytherapy have found rates of postoperative urinary incontinence varying from 0 to 18% (14,15).

Urethral Stents

Recent advances with novel materials have led to the creation of self-expanding metal stents for placement into multiple organ systems, including the urinary tract. Several reports have suggested that these devices may be promising, especially for a patient with a limited life expectancy who wishes to remain free of catheters and external urine collection devices. Insertion of the stent itself is a relatively simple procedure and can usually be performed with local anesthesia and a minimal amount of sedation. Morgentaler and DeWolf (16) reviewed their experience with self-expanding prostatic stents in 25 patients with symptomatic bladder outlet obstruction. Twenty-one of the 25 patients had urinary retention and the remaining 4 had either bladder neck contractures or severe symptoms of BPH. All patients underwent insertion of the Gianturco-Z stent (Cook Inc., Bloomington, IN). Initially, 95% of the patients were able to void. However, at a longer follow-up, the success rate had declined to 75% because of stent migration in several patients. The authors theorized that the high rate of stent migration was due to improper selection of stent length.

Additional studies (17–19) have evaluated different stents [UroLume Wallstent (American Medical Systems, Minnetonka, MN) and Titan intraprostatic stent]. The patients enrolled in these studies mainly suffered from BPH and not prostatic carcinoma. Overall, there was an almost 100% return of voiding function. However, a long-term follow-up has shown that although these stents often need to be removed or replaced, symptomatic improvements are acceptable (20). The patients who failed to void were found to have detrusor failure secondary to chronic urinary retention. Symptoms after stent insertion were similar to those seen initially after TURP, namely, urinary frequency, urgency, and hematuria. Failures in these studies were usually due to either improper stent length or migration of the stent. Complications were minor, and patients who required stent removal were able to have it performed without excessive difficulty. Other studies, with small numbers of patients, have used stents in patients with prostate cancer with similar short-term results (21). Therefore, with improvement of stent sizing and insertion technique, intraprostatic stents hold significant promise for treating urinary outflow obstruction in the medically ill patient with bladder outlet obstruction.

UPPER TRACT OBSTRUCTION

Extrinsic ureteral obstruction may occur in the setting of bulky pathology in the pelvis and retroperitoneum or as a manifestation of metastatic disease. It is the responsibility of the physician to provide the patient with appropriate information to make an informed decision concerning aggressive or conservative therapy for this situation. In a patient with limited life expectancy and poor quality of life, conservative therapy may allow death to occur in a manner that is foreseen and suitable to the patient. Patients who have exhausted all primary treatments and continue to have progressive obstruction despite optimal therapy will likely receive limited benefit from urinary diversion. Furthermore, patients with severe, unrelenting, and unmanageable pain seldom show improvement of these symptoms after urinary diversion. Because untreated bilateral ureteral obstruction inevitably leads to renal failure, uremia, and death, both the patient and physician must understand that the decision to withhold treatment is an acceptance of this clinical progression. The clinical manifestations of renal failure and uremia include fatigue, decreased appetite, nausea, uremic coma, and eventually, death. In a patient suffering from end-stage malignancy, this may be an acceptable sequence of events. The potential for success and durable response after treatment for ureteral obstruction depends mainly on the extent of the underlying pathology and whether there remain any valid treatment options for the primary disease.

Internal Ureteral Stents

Endoscopic retrograde stenting is a means of providing internal urinary diversion; when performed for malignant ureteral obstruction, it may be a technically challenging procedure and occasionally may be impossible. Other common disadvantages of internal stents are the need for frequent stent changes, insufficient relief of obstruction, and return of obstruction upon stent removal. It has been noted that internal ureteral stents have a high failure rate in the presence of extrinsic compression, with success rates of 37–47% described for their use in the treatment of malignant obstruction (22). When used successfully, indwelling stents must be changed every 3 to 6 months to prevent encrustation and subsequent obstruction; changing of stents may need anesthesia, and it subjects the patient to recurrent procedures.

External Urinary Diversion

With the widespread use of modern percutaneous drainage techniques, those patients who are acceptable candidates for diversion of the urine stand an improved chance of experiencing significant clinical improvement with minimized morbidity. Before the 1970s, urinary diversion required an open surgical procedure to divert the flow of urine from the kidneys. These procedures were problematic because most patients with malignant ureteral obstruction were often poor surgical candidates because of their underlying nutritional, hematologic, and immunologic status. In the early 1970s, Grabstald and McPhee (23) studied 218 patients who underwent open nephrostomy for malignant ureteral obstruction. They discovered a major life-threatening complication rate of 45%. There was a 3% operative mortality rate, and 43% of these patients did not leave the hospital. A later study by Meyer et al. (24) showed that 30% of patients undergoing open urinary diversion died within 52 days of surgery, and the overall median survival was only 3.3 months. Therefore, open nephrostomy subjects the patient to significant operative and perioperative risks, without durable responses.

As a result of these outcomes, open surgical procedures have been supplanted by less-invasive techniques. Percutaneous nephrostomy tube placement may now be considered as another alternative to endoscopic stenting or in cases of stent failure. It is important to note the more invasive nature of percutaneous urinary diversion compared to internal stenting and the potential for tube dislodgement; both of these factors, along with the need for external collection of diverted urine, may negatively impact the patient's quality of life. Studies have shown a limited response after percutaneous nephrostomy. Keidan et al. (25) showed that although renal function improved in 85% of patients, the median survival was only 13 weeks, and 55% of the patients required additional hospitalizations for urosepsis and additional procedures. Kinn and Ohlsen (26) noted that the survival period after urinary diversion was 7.9 months for patients with prostate cancer patients and 5.3 months for those with advanced bladder cancer. On the other hand, a study by Gasparini et al. (27) revealed much better results, albeit in a patient population that included many patients with newly diagnosed disease. They showed that 77% of patients undergoing either percutaneous nephrostomy (68%) or cystoscopic stent insertion (32%) could be discharged from the hospital. The mean survival time after urinary diversion was 75 weeks, and one patient lived as long as 4.7 years. There appeared to be a survival advantage in those patients who had not previously undergone hormonal therapy or chemotherapy. Also, in contrast to earlier studies of open urinary diversion, there were no perioperative deaths or cardiac, pulmonary, or hemorrhagic complications. Wilson et al. (28) demonstrated survival times that were improved almost four times in those patients who received percutaneous nephrostomy for gynecologic malignancy as opposed to those with primary bladder cancer. Overall palliative percutaneous urinary diversion may be performed in the setting of malignant ureteral obstruction with minimal procedural morbidity and is effective in improving renal function. However, long-term survival remains limited and is a function of the patient's primary pathology.

The decision to manage a patient with malignant ureteral obstruction by means of internal ureteral stents or percutaneous nephrostomy must be determined individually on the basis of the patient's clinical status and their requests. Ku et al. (22) performed a retrospective comparison of patients with malignant ureteral obstruction receiving either internal ureteral stenting or percutaneous nephrostomy tube drainage. They did not note any significant difference in the overall stent-related or catheter-related complications or any difference in the incidence of fever or acute pyelonephritis. The incidence of failed urinary diversion due to obstruction was significantly higher in those patients treated with stents (11%) compared with those treated with nephrostomy (1.3%). Other studies (29) have demonstrated an inferior quality of life associated with long-term management of nephrostomy tubes.

An additional option for the patient who successfully undergoes percutaneous nephrostomy and returns to a normal lifestyle is the potential for internalization of the nephrostomy tube. This requires placing a ureteral stent into the ureter through an antegrade approach through the nephrostomy tract. The ureteral stent thus internalized would then be managed similar to the stent that was placed endoscopically as primary treatment. Alternatively, a nephroureteral stent can be placed through the flank and into the bladder. This tube can then be capped, thereby allowing antegrade flow of urine from the kidney into the bladder without the need for an external drainage bag. This tube can then be changed in the interventional radiology department rather than the operating room.

Self-Expanding Ureteral Stents

Finally, as with urethral obstruction secondary to malignancy, there have been reports of the use of self-expanding metal stents for the treatment of ureteral obstruction. Lugmayr and Pauer (30) studied 23 patients who had undergone insertion of the Wallstent device for malignant ureteral obstruction. They were successful in implanting the device in 97% of patients, and 83% of the stented ureters remained patent after 30 weeks. Because 81% of patients survived at least 6 months, the patency rate appeared comparable to survival rates. Therefore, expanding ureteral stents may offer a viable option for treating the obstructed ureter, although this option has not been studied as extensively as internal ureteral stents and percutaneous urinary diversion.

HEMATURIA

General Considerations

Two commonly used methods of detecting blood in urine are the microscopic urinalysis and the urine dipstick test (UDT). The UDT works through a peroxidase reaction (i.e., the peroxidase-like activity of hemoglobin causes the oxidation of a chemical indicator within the dipstick and thereby changes its color). Intact red blood cells are not required for oxidation and false-positive readings may be caused by hemoglobinuria or myoglobinuria. Although the presence of intact red cells usually causes punctate discoloration of the dipstick rather than the uniform discoloration commonly seen with hemoglobinuria, confirmation of red cells is required. Therefore, all patients with a positive UDT require microscopic analysis to confirm the presence of red blood cells. UDTs have been shown to have a sensitivity of >90% for hematuria when properly used (31). Although some controversy exists as to whether hematuria should be defined as >0–2 or 0–4/5 red blood cells per high-power microscopic field, clearly a value of >5 red blood cells per high-power field should be considered significant. Evaluation is warranted by the finding of microscopic hematuria from two of three properly collected urine specimens. If a patient is considered high risk for urologic disease, then one sample is sufficient.

Gross hematuria refers to the presence of blood in the urine that can be seen with the unaided eye. It is important to confirm the presence of red blood cells once dark urine is seen. There are multiple other potential causes of discoloration within a urine specimen. Some of the more common causes of discolored urine include concentrated urine and systemic administration of flutamide, phenazopyridine, sulfasalazine, phenolphthalein (seen with the use of some over-the-counter laxatives), nitrofurantoin, metronidazole, methylene blue, bilirubinuria, and vitamin B complex.

Often, the location of urinary tract bleeding can be determined by careful history alone. The history should identify the presence or absence of pain, the color of the blood (bright red versus tea color versus light pink), the presence or absence of clots, and the timing of the presence of the hematuria in the urine stream. Also, hematuria must be differentiated from urethral bleeding, which usually presents as either blood at the urethral meatus or spotting on the sheets or undergarments with a clear voided urinary stream. Bright red blood usually implies that bleeding is from either the prostate or the bladder, whereas darker blood more commonly originates from the upper urinary tract. Bleeding only upon initiation of the urinary stream (initial hematuria) that is followed by clear urine implies that the bleeding originates distal to the level of the bladder neck or prostate. The presence of blood throughout the urine stream (total hematuria) usually implies that bleeding is from the kidney, ureter, or bladder, whereas terminal hematuria (blood mainly at the end of urination) may also signal a disease process near either the bladder neck or prostatic urethra.

The evaluation of confirmed hematuria (Fig. 32.1) may include urine culture (in those patients with concurrent pyuria); voided or catheterized urine cytology; an imaging study to evaluate the kidneys, ureters, bladder, and urothelium; and cystoscopy to evaluate the urethra, prostate, and bladder urothelium. In patients with known urinary tract pathology, the assessment of patients with new-onset hematuria may be modified, especially if previously performed studies have been negative. Because of the tendency of urothelial malignancies to recur, onset of hematuria within 6 months of initial evaluation should prompt consideration of repeating the studies mentioned in the preceding text.

With regard to diagnostic imaging, the study that has classically been considered the gold standard for imaging the urinary system, in spite of its technical limitations, is the IVP. If the ureters are not visualized completely, additional studies may be warranted. Retrograde pyelography, which is used to identify lesions of the collecting system, may be performed at the time of cystoscopic evaluation to better evaluate or possibly localize upper urinary tract pathology.

Ultrasound imaging can be considered as an alternative to IVP in patients at increased risk from exposure to contrast material, including those with azotemia, diabetes mellitus, or history of contrast allergy. Ultrasound is unable to visualize the collecting system unless it is significantly dilated and is not sensitive for detecting abnormalities of the urothelium. Real-time ultrasound is relatively sensitive for detecting calcifications within the renal parenchyma and collecting system, but it does not clarify the clinical significance of such calcifications unless there is significant hydronephrosis, which, in turn, may depend in part on the hydration status of the patient. If ultrasound is utilized, it should be coupled with a plain abdominal radiograph (a "kidney–ureter–bladder" film) to examine the remainder of the collecting system for calcifications that could result in urinary obstruction (e.g., ureteral calculus) or hematuria.

Computed tomographic imaging of the abdomen and pelvis has assumed a more important role in the screening evaluation for urologic pathology. CT scans are much more sensitive than IVP for detecting certain types of pathology (e.g., renal masses), although they may be less likely to detect subtle obstruction. With spiral CT scanners being common now, this technology is becoming more useful for obtaining large amounts of information in a short period of time. Spiral scanning allows not only narrow "cuts" through the kidney for the detection of stones <5 mm, but with newer software programs and multidetector CT scanners, three-dimensional reconstruction of the entire urinary tract with excellent detail is also possible. A potential benefit of IVP over CT scan is that it is a functional and dynamic study, which can be tailored to an individual patient when desired. During a CT scan, there is less control over the technique. Despite this drawback, spiral CT scans undoubtedly hold a significant place in the imaging of the urinary system, offering consistently high-quality images without overlying bowel or stool with the added benefit of avoiding a bowel prep. Alternatively, magnetic resonance imaging (MRI) with gadolinium may be used for evaluation of renal pathology with excellent detail in those patients who are unable to receive intravenous contrast for CT scan or IVP evaluation. However, MRI is not considered as sensitive as CT scan for detection of urinary calculi.

Asymptomatic Lower Tract Hematuria

Causes of asymptomatic microscopic hematuria (Table 32.3) range from minor, insignificant findings that require no intervention to lesions that are immediately life threatening. Statistically, most microscopic hematuria of a urologic etiology are clinically asymptomatic and arise from the lower urinary tract. The most prevalent cause in men is benign prostatic enlargement. Asymptomatic microscopic hematuria rarely, if ever, leads to a significant decrease in the patient's hemoglobin level or contributes to iron deficiency anemia. The clinical significance of microscopic hematuria lies in its potential significance as a sign of occult urinary tract pathology.

If the detection of urinary tract pathology is unlikely to alter the overall management of the patient, the standard algorithm for evaluating hematuria may be individualized. Cystoscopy is an invasive procedure and can be avoided if an obvious cause for the hematuria is detected. For example, if IVP or ultrasound demonstrates a large renal tumor, additional invasive procedures may not be necessary. Although it is possible that a patient could have a second malignancy or other bladder pathology (i.e., transitional cell carcinoma of the bladder), further evaluation may not necessarily be in the best interests of the patient.

If the source of microscopic hematuria is not detected by imaging studies and cystoscopy is contemplated, the benefits

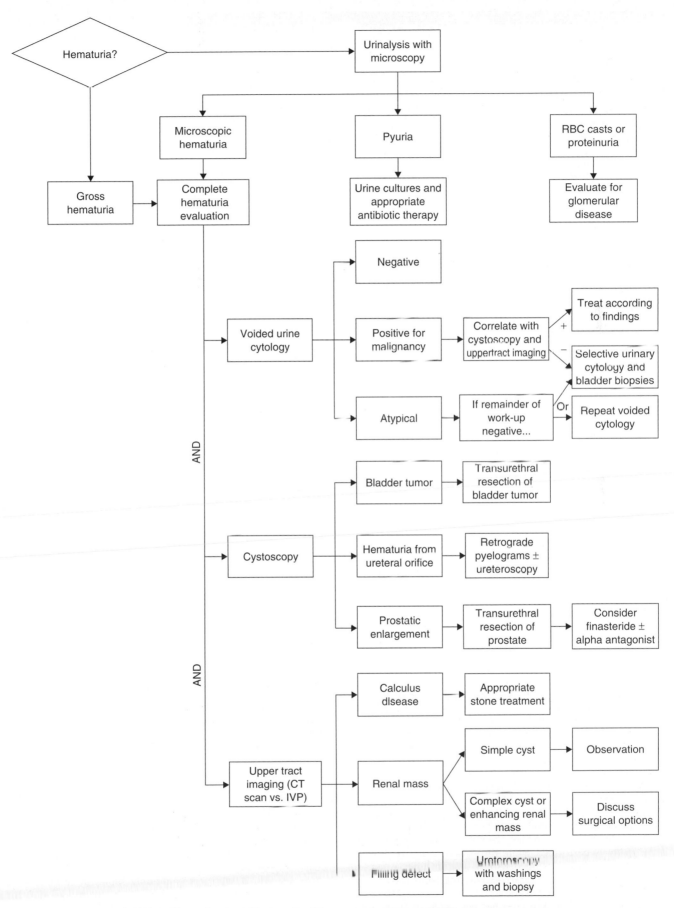

FIGURE 32.1. The evaluation of hematuria. CT, computed tomography; IVP, intravenous pyelogram.

TABLE 32.3

CAUSES OF HEMATURIA

Glomerular causes	Renal causes
Primary glomerulonephritis	Arteriovenous malformations/fistulas
Focal glomerular sclerosis	Infarct
IgA nephropathy	Medullary sponge kidney
Membranoproliferative glomerulonephritis	Papillary necrosis
Postinfectious glomerulonephritis	Polycystic kidney disease
Rapidly progressive glomerulonephritis	Renal trauma
Secondary glomerulonephritis	Renal tumors
Cryoglobulinemia	Renal vein thrombosis
Hemolytic-uremic syndrome	Upper urinary tract infection
Medication-induced nephritis	**Extrarenal causes**
Systemic lupus erythematosus	Benign prostatic enlargement
Thrombotic thrombocytopenic purpura	Calculus disease
Vasculitis	Cyclophosphamide cystitis
Hereditary	Foreign body
Alport's syndrome	Indwelling ureteral stent
Fabry's disease	Indwelling urethral catheter
Thin glomerular basement membrane	Lower urinary tract infection
disease	Radiation cystitis
	Trauma to ureter, bladder, urethra
	Tumor of ureter, bladder, prostate, urethra

and risks of cystoscopy must be assessed. Flexible cystoscopy may approach risk and discomfort levels associated with simple urethral catheterization, and the process takes <60 seconds for completion. However, both flexible and rigid cystoscopy can potentially cause urinary retention in a patient with well-compensated bladder outlet obstruction. Additionally, patients with BPH who are likely to have delicate dilated veins on the surface of the prostate as the etiology of their hematuria may be at risk for the development of significant bleeding after this invasive procedure. Patients undergoing cystoscopy are also at risk for development of urinary infection because of urinary tract instrumentation and appropriate empiric antibiotic prophylaxis should be administered.

Asymptomatic gross hematuria may be managed similar to microscopic hematuria on an elective basis. Patients who experience gross hematuria should be advised to increase their fluid intake and avoid strenuous activity. In the patient who does not experience significant voiding difficulties, the evaluation of this disorder may proceed electively, in a similar fashion to that already described.

Asymptomatic Upper Tract Hematuria

As with bleeding from the lower urinary tract, the same evaluation algorithm should be applied when there is asymptomatic bleeding from the upper tract (i.e., urinalysis, imaging study, cystoscopy, and, possibly, culture). Unlike asymptomatic bleeding from the lower urinary tract, imaging studies may be more useful than cystoscopy to determine the site of bleeding. For most patients with microscopic hematuria originating in the upper tracts, cystoscopy is usually normal. In patients with gross hematuria and no symptoms (gross painless hematuria), cystoscopy may be able to lateralize the lesion if the study is performed while the patient is actively bleeding. Once the bladder is filled with irrigation fluid, a "jet" of blood-tinged urine may be seen emanating from the ureteral orifice on the side of the pathology.

Although bleeding itself does not necessarily warrant therapy, the pathology causing the bleeding may require treatment.

Common etiologies for upper tract bleeding include renal masses, tumors of the renal pelvis and ureter, stones, and papillary necrosis. Once the site of the bleeding is determined either by imaging studies or cystoscopy, further diagnostic techniques, such as retrograde pyelography, selective ureteral catheterization for cytology, or ureteroscopy, can be entertained. The discussion of further therapy for each pathologic condition in an asymptomatic patient is beyond the scope of this chapter.

Symptomatic Lower Tract Hematuria

Symptomatic hematuria, though less common than asymptomatic hematuria, is yet obviously more clinically significant. The spectrum of symptomatology in patients with gross hematuria ranges from no change in the voiding pattern to acute urinary retention caused by bladder outlet obstruction from clots. Most cases of gross hematuria are alarming, but relatively few patients actually require immediate intervention. As previously noted, patients with new-onset gross hematuria should be told to avoid strenuous activities and increase fluid intake. Increased urine production may dilute the blood in the bladder and reduce the formation of clots. Patients taking antiplatelet medications should temporarily discontinue use of these agents in order to support the hemostatic process and minimize additional bleeding. A patient is unlikely to develop significant voiding difficulties in the absence of blood clots. If clots are indeed passed, significant bleeding should be assumed and the physician should anticipate the need for intervention. As the concentration of blood increases and larger clots form, a patient eventually develops clot urinary retention.

The first step in treating a patient with clot urinary retention is to place a large catheter into the bladder and evacuate all blood clots. Preferably, a 22F or larger catheter is used. It is nearly impossible to evacuate clots through 16F or 18F urethral catheters, which are most commonly found in catheter kits, as it is not uncommon to irrigate 200–300 mL or more of clot from the bladder. It is also advisable to insert a three-way catheter, if available, so that continuous bladder irrigation

(CBI) can be started if needed. Analogous to increasing the urine flow rate, CBI dilutes the concentration of blood in the urine, thereby helping to prevent new clot formation. After inserting the catheter and irrigating the bladder free of clots, the cause of the hematuria should be assessed, as described in the section General Considerations. In rare cases, when the bladder cannot be cleared of clot through an irrigating catheter, the patient may need operative intervention, with insertion of a resectoscope and manual clot evacuation with syringes or special equipment. In these patients, one should obtain a complete blood count and coagulation studies to exclude an underlying hematologic problem. Unlike microscopic hematuria, gross hematuria can frequently lead to anemia and may potentially require transfusion. This is especially true of patients debilitated by chronic disease and those who are just completing chemotherapy or radiation therapy, who may have decreased bone marrow reserves.

The management of patients who present with gross hematuria can usually be temporized with catheter drainage. Once imaging studies are performed, a differential diagnosis is formulated. When studies of the upper tracts are normal, the pathology is likely to reside within either the prostate or the bladder. Cystoscopy should be able to localize bleeding from the lower urinary tract and aid in the development of a treatment plan for disorders of either the prostate or the bladder. If bleeding is discovered in the prostate during cystoscopy, it may be difficult to control with fulguration (electrocoagulation) alone. More commonly, when bleeding is discovered emanating from the prostate or bladder neck, prostatic tissue must be resected, with subsequent electrocoagulation of the friable area. Bleeding in this area can be diffuse, and hemostasis may be aided after completion of the procedure by placing a urethral catheter on traction, which causes compression and tamponade of vessels in the prostate and bladder neck. Once the acute situation is resolved, some patients may develop recurrent or chronic hematuria secondary to prostatic bleeding. There have been several reports indicating the efficacy of finasteride in these patients to decrease the extent and number of recurrent episodes of hematuria (32,33). Studies have indicated that treatment with finasteride induces a reduction in the density of prostatic microvessels, thereby helping to reduce bleeding (34). It should be noted that these studies were performed on patients with benign prostatic disease, and not prostate cancer. Despite this, finasteride is a generally well-tolerated medication and is often used empirically in this situation.

Bleeding that originates from within the bladder is termed *hemorrhagic cystitis* and, as already discussed, commonly occurs from either radiation therapy or chemotherapeutic agents. Unlike radiation therapy, hematuria that results from chemotherapeutic medications is not necessarily associated with irritative voiding symptoms. The chemotherapeutic agents most commonly associated with hemorrhagic cystitis are cyclophosphamide and its analogs. The reported incidence of hemorrhagic cystitis after cyclophosphamide therapy ranges from 2 to 40% (35). The compound acrolein is the active metabolite of cyclophosphamide that actually causes the bladder damage produced by cyclophosphamide (36,37). Mesna (2-mercaptoethane sulfonate) was developed specifically to bind to acrolein and thereby reduce the harmful effects of this by-product (38). Mesna is now given routinely when a patient is treated for malignancy with cyclophosphamide.

As described previously, the hematuria caused by radiation is commonly associated with dysuria, frequency, and urgency. Hemorrhagic cystitis can follow external beam or interstitial radiation treatment of primary genitourinary (prostate and bladder) malignancies, cancers of the cervix or rectum, or other pelvic lesions. The spectrum of hematuria secondary to radiation therapy also ranges from microscopic bleeding to bleeding severe enough to require transfusion of blood products. The time course of the development of hematuria ranges from months to years after the initiation of radiation therapy. Reported frequency of bladder hemorrhage after pelvic irradiation ranges from 2.5 to 12%, and there is often no correlation between the extent of treatment and development of severe hematuria (35).

The damaging effects of radiation therapy on the bladder are similar to those found in other organs. The clinically significant symptoms in all organs are mediated through vascular damage. Radiation therapy induces a progressive endarteritis, which leads to hypovascular, hypocellular, and hypoxic tissue. Tissue breakdown occurs because of the inability of radiated tissue to replace normal collagen and cellular losses. If chronic, these changes may eventually result in fibrosis (39). These derangements may also cause an irradiated bladder to be extremely susceptible to injury and slow to heal when injured. Unlike bleeding resulting from cyclophosphamide treatment, there are no prophylactic measures yet available that can be employed to prevent bladder damage. Once radiation hemorrhagic cystitis occurs, aggressive symptomatic intervention should be initiated, and further radiation exposure should be minimized.

As with other types of gross hematuria, initial management of radiation- or chemotherapy-induced cystitis involves insertion of a large urethral catheter. Removal of all clots is paramount for success in eventually clearing the urine. All subsequent therapies are enhanced in a bladder free of clots because clot evacuation reduces naturally occurring fibrinolysins, which may act through the clotting cascade to perpetuate bleeding. If initial conservative management with catheter drainage and CBI fails, one must consider alternative therapies to control hemorrhage. Several topical agents may be applied intravesically to aid in cessation of bleeding. Before proceeding with these therapies, cystoscopy should be performed to rule out an upper tract source of bleeding and to fulgurate any obvious bleeding sites.

Empiric therapy may be initiated with ε-aminocaproic acid (amicar) given either orally, parenterally (40), or intravesically (41). ε-Aminocaproic acid reduces fibrinolysis by inhibiting plasminogen activator substances. This drug has been used extensively for idiopathic hematuria (42) and hematuria of unknown etiology associated with sickle cell disease (43). Although there have not been any controlled or randomized studies on the use of ε-aminocaproic acid for treatment of hematuria, studies and clinical experience substantiate its use for severe hemorrhagic cystitis. Initially given either parenterally or orally, a loading dose of 5 g is followed up by hourly doses of 1.00–1.25 g. Maximal response is usually achieved in 8–12 hours. Patients who initially respond to the parenteral route can then be shifted to the oral route for maintenance therapy. Maintenance therapy includes taking the total daily dosage (6–8 g) divided into four doses. When given intravesically, 200 mg of ε-aminocaproic acid is added to each liter of 0.9% saline, and this mixture is administered as CBI. A side effect of ε-aminocaproic acid is the formation of thick, tenacious clots, which can become difficult for the patient to pass spontaneously and are extremely difficult to irrigate in patients with catheters. Administering ε-aminocaproic acid to patients with bilateral upper tract bleeding is relatively contraindicated because thick clots in the renal pelvis or ureters can lead to upper tract obstruction, clot colic, and potentially even renal failure.

Silver nitrate 0.5–1.0% mixed in sterile water may be administered into the bladder for treatment of acute bleeding. Rather than being run as CBI, this drug is instilled for 10–20 minutes, following which the bladder is emptied. In certain refractory cases, multiple instillations may be required (44).

One percent alum has also shown some efficacy in treating hemorrhagic cystitis. Unlike silver nitrate, the 1% solution is usually given through CBI (45,46). Although somewhat effective, the rates of success are variable. The advantage of alum, apart from allergy, lies in the fact that its administration is safe and requires no anesthesia.

The most efficacious and probably the most toxic treatment for hemorrhagic cystitis is intravesical formalin. Formalin is the aqueous solution of formaldehyde. Formalin acts by fixing the bladder mucosa by cross-linking proteins, thereby preventing necrosis, sloughing, and blood loss. Studies have shown that formalin is up to 80% effective in arresting bladder hemorrhage (47–49). Formalin is available as 37 or 40% aqueous formaldehyde, which is diluted with sterile water to yield final concentrations of 10% formalin (3.7% formaldehyde) or 1% formalin (0.37% formaldehyde). Formalin administration is painful and requires regional or general anesthesia. It is administered in concentrations ranging from 1.0–10%, starting at the lowest and progressing to higher concentrations only as clinically indicated. The bladder is usually filled to capacity using gravity drainage under no more than 15 cm per H_2O pressure. Bladder instillation usually occurs for 10–14 minutes (50).

Risks of formalin administration include damage to the bladder and upper tracts. Reflux of formalin to the ureters and kidneys can lead to fibrosis, obstruction, hydronephrosis, and renal papillary necrosis. A cystogram should be performed before formalin administration to rule out vesicoureteral reflux. In those patients who are shown to have reflux, ureteral balloon catheters may be utilized to prevent retrograde flow of formalin. Also, the procedure can be performed in the reverse Trendelenburg position to minimize reflux. Through its ability to cross-link proteins within the wall of the bladder, administration of formalin can lead to a decrease in bladder capacity and, in extreme cases, a nonfunctional, contracted bladder. Patients must be advised of these potential risks and formalin therapy must be reserved only for those cases of hemorrhagic cystitis that are truly refractory to all other medical treatments.

Two other nonsurgical therapies for hemorrhagic cystitis deserve mention. There have been several reports (51–54) on the use of hyperbaric oxygen therapy for radiation-induced hemorrhagic cystitis. More recent studies have similarly reported long-term success with this modality of treatment (55,56). Hyperbaric oxygen induces hyperoxia, by which increased tissue concentrations of oxygen are attained owing to the increased dissolved oxygen in the serum. This condition results in neovascularization and secondary growth of healthy granulation tissue. Therefore, hyperbaric oxygen tends to reverse the ischemic process caused by radiation therapy. Additionally, hyperoxia itself induces vasoconstriction, which may have a direct effect on bleeding from the bladder mucosa. A response rate of 82% across multiple series is reported for treatment of radiation-induced hemorrhagic cystitis with hyperbaric oxygen (54). A greater therapeutic response rate has been noted in those patients who receive treatment within 6 months of onset of hematuria (57).

Finally, there have been reports on the use of conjugated estrogens for treatment of hemorrhagic cystitis. Although the mechanism is unknown, there is a suggestion that estrogens may decrease capillary fragility. Liu et al. (58) reported on five consecutive cases in which bleeding from both radiation therapy and cyclophosphamide administration was successfully treated with conjugated estrogens. A follow-up study by Miller et al. (35) showed that six of seven patients treated with oral estrogens for hemorrhagic cystitis improved sufficiently to avoid further invasive therapy. Although no standard doses or length of therapy have been established, the usual starting dose of conjugated estrogens used is 2.5 mg twice daily. After an adequate response has been achieved, the dose can be tapered. Final doses in the range of 1.25 mg daily are reported, which can sometimes be weaned to 0.625 mg

daily. It should be noted that conjugated estrogens are well known to induce cardiovascular complications at high doses. Although no thromboembolic or cardiovascular complications occurred in the two studies mentioned, the long-term safety of estrogens at moderate to high doses is unknown. However, in a terminally ill patient, the benefits of estrogen therapy might outweigh the risks if the significant bleeding associated with hemorrhagic cystitis could be managed in this manner.

For those patients who do not respond to oral or intravesical medical therapy, there are more invasive means of reducing bleeding from the bladder. Selective embolization of branches of the hypogastric arteries may be performed in those terminally ill patients who are poor candidates for a major surgical procedure. Performed through a vascular access, this procedure may require only local anesthesia. The technique works optimally when arteriography demonstrates a discreet vessel responsible for the bleeding; unfortunately, this clinical scenario is unusual. If the entire bladder urothelium appears to be involved, the anterior branches of both hypogastric arteries may be occluded. Complications of embolization include claudication of the gluteal muscles, temporary lower extremity paralysis, and even necrosis of the bladder (59).

Some patients fail conservative measures and may require surgery to control the bleeding. Unfortunately, many of these patients are poor surgical candidates because of ongoing hemorrhage and coagulopathy. These patients, who usually undergo urinary diversion, and at times cystectomy, universally do poorly.

Symptomatic Upper Tract Hematuria

Symptomatic bleeding from the upper urinary tract is usually manifest as clot colic, or the acute onset of flank pain secondary to acute ureteral obstruction. Clinically, clot colic mimics renal colic secondary to stones. Differentiating the two can sometimes be difficult, especially because clot colic in the presence of complete ureteral obstruction can present without overt hematuria.

The history and selective imaging studies may assist in the diagnosis of acute ureteral obstruction. Acute onset flank pain in an elderly person who has no history of kidney stones is more likely caused by clot or tumor. Likewise, upper urinary tract obstruction without evidence of calcifications on IVP or ultrasound is more likely secondary to clot or tumor.

Occasionally, upper tract bleeding may be severe enough to require transfusion of blood products. Patients who have undergone renal procedures such as percutaneous nephrostomy or renal biopsy may experience gross hematuria because of an arteriovenous fistula. Those with chronic indwelling ureteral stents are at risk for stent erosion into iliac vessels. These conditions may produce rapid blood loss and, occasionally, may result in exsanguination.

Unlike bleeding from the lower urinary tract, there are only a few noninvasive measures that may benefit the patient with symptomatic upper tract bleeding. As in lower tract bleeding, forced diuresis by increasing oral and intravenous fluids may help dilute the blood in the urine sufficiently to prevent clot formation. The administration of ε-aminocaproic acid can be considered, although as noted previously, upper tract bleeding is a relative contraindication for the use of this treatment because it may result in large tenacious clots that can produce ureteral obstruction. Therefore, ε-aminocaproic acid must be used with caution for upper tract bleeding.

For patients who continue to develop clot colic from persistent upper urinary tract bleeding, most methods to stop the bleeding generally require invasive intervention. If no pathology is seen on imaging studies, including IVP or CT scan, an arteriogram may be warranted to exclude an arteriovenous fistula. It is important to visualize the iliac vessels at arteriography in order to diagnose potential fistula with the ureter in those patients with indwelling stents and severe hematuria. This procedure may be able to identify the area of bleeding so that selective embolization or vascular stenting can be performed.

If all studies, including the arteriogram, are normal, one may be faced with the difficult question of whether to surgically remove a kidney or the ureter. In this situation, cystoscopy may be extremely helpful in lateralizing the pathology. Once lateralized, ureteroscopy can often be employed as a diagnostic and even therapeutic tool. Advances in endoscopic equipment have enabled not only visualization of previously unreachable areas but also biopsy and fulguration of suspicious lesions. Despite these advances, there remain rare instances of highly symptomatic upper tract bleeding that are elusive to diagnosis. It is a particularly difficult decision to remove a kidney and the ureter without a confirmed etiology. In this situation, a patient must be very symptomatic and must have failed all other more conservative means.

Patients with advanced renal cell carcinoma and metastatic disease may also develop bleeding and clot formation. Palliative measures may include radiation therapy or chemotherapy. Because the prognosis in these patients is very poor and surgery to remove the primary tumor does not impact positively on survival, it is again crucially important to document the degree of bleeding and the relative morbidity arising from the bleeding. Only when bleeding and clot colic impact negatively on quality of life should patients be considered for palliative nephrectomy. Statistically, metastatic tumors are much more common than primary renal cell carcinomas in terminally ill patients.

PRIAPISM

Although an extremely uncommon oncologic complication, priapism can present severe morbidity for an affected patient. *Priapism* refers to a sustained, painful, penile erection not induced by sexual stimulation. If left untreated, priapism eventually leads to fibrosis and impotence. Although impotence is not generally of paramount concern in the palliative care patient, the severe pain caused by priapism is certainly relevant. Priapism in the oncology patient may have multiple causes including vascular congestion from hematologic malignancies, direct invasion of tumor into the corporal bodies, or disruption of penile venous outflow from a pelvic mass. Regardless of the cause, the treatment of malignant priapism is aimed at treating the primary tumor and may include chemotherapy, radiation, or a combination of therapies (60).

CONCLUSIONS

The ultimate goal with all urologic complications in patients with progressive medical diseases is to maximize the quantity of life without jeopardizing or negatively impacting the quality of life. Urologic complications in these patients may arise from benign or malignant disease processes or as a consequence of treatments for an underlying malignancy. With the armamentarium of imaging studies, medications, and surgical interventions, the physician treating these patients should strive to allow them to live the remainder of their lives to their fullest capacity.

References

1. Planz B, Jochims E, Deix T, et al. The role of urinary cytology for detection of bladder cancer. *Eur J Surg Oncol* 2005;31:304.
2. Frank MG, Park R. The drug-induced glaucomas. *N J Med* 1974;71:470.
3. Dean RJ, Lytton B. Urologic complications of pelvic irradiation. *J Urol* 1978;119:64.
4. Lamm DL. Complications of bacillus calmette-guerin immunotherapy. *Urol Clin North Am* 1992;19:565.
5. Lamm DL, Stogdill VD, Stogdill BJ, et al. Complications of bacillus calmette-guerin immunotherapy in 1,278 patients with bladder cancer. *J Urol* 1986;135:272.
6. Lamm DL, Van Der Meijden PM, Morales A, et al. Incidence and treatment of complications of bacillus calmette-guerin intravesical therapy in superficial bladder cancer. *J Urol* 1992;147:596.
7. deVries CR, Freiha FS. Hemorrhagic cystitis: a review. *J Urol* 1990;143:1.
8. Forman JD, Order SE, Zinreich ES, et al. The correlation of pretreatment transurethral resection of prostatic cancer with tumor dissemination and disease-free survival. *Cancer* 1986;58:1770.
9. Surya BV, Provet JA. Manifestations of advanced prostate cancer: prognosis and treatment. *J Urol* 1989;142:921.
10. Oefelein MG. Prognostic significance of obstructive uropathy in advanced prostate cancer. *Urology* 2004;63:1117.
11. Lapides J, Diokno AC, Silber SJ, et al. Clean, intermittent self-catheterization in the treatment of urinary tract disease. *J Urol* 1972;107:458.
12. Crain DS, Amling CL, Kane CJ. Palliative transurethral prostate resection for bladder outlet obstruction in patients with locally advanced prostate cancer. *J Urol* 2004;171:668.
13. Mazur AW, Thompson IM. Efficacy and morbidity of "channel" TURP. *Urology* 1991;38:526.
14. Flam TA, Peyromaure M, Chauveinc L, et al. Post-brachytherapy transurethral resection of the prostate in patients with localized prostate cancer. *J Urol* 2004;172:108.
15. Kollmeier MA, Stock RG, Cesaretti J, et al. Urinary morbidity and incontinence following transurethral resection for the prostate after brachytherapy. *J Urol* 2005;173:808.
16. Morgentaler A, DeWolf WC. A self-expanding prostatic stent for bladder outlet obstruction in high risk patients. *J Urol* 1993;150:1636.
17. Kaplan SA, Merrill DC, Mosely WG, et al. The titanium intraprostatic stent: the United States experience. *J Urol* 1993;150:1624.
18. Guazzoni GG, Bergamashi F, Montorsi F, et al. Prostatic Urolume Wallstent for benign prostatic hyperplasia patients at poor operative risk: clinical, uroflowmetric and ultrasonographic patterns. *J Urol* 1993;150:1641.
19. Milroy E, Chapple CR. The Urolume stent in the management of benign prostatic hyperplasia. *J Urol* 1993;150:1630.
20. Anjum MI, Chari R, Shetty A, et al. Long term clinical results and quality of life after insertion of a self-expanding flexible endourethral prosthesis. *Br J Urol* 1997;80:885.
21. Konety BR, Phenlan MW, O'Donnell WF, et al. Urolume stent placement for the treatment of postbrachytherapy bladder outlet obstruction. *Urology* 2000;55:721.
22. Ku JH, Lee SW, Jeon HG, et al. Percutaneous nephrostomy versus indwelling ureteral stents in the management of extrinsic ureteral obstruction in advanced malignancies: Are there differences? *Urology* 2004;64:895.
23. Grabstald H, McPhee M. Nephrostomy and the cancer patient. *South Med J* 1973;66:217.
24. Meyer JE, Yatsuhashi M, Green TH. Palliative urinary diversion in patients with advanced pelvic malignancy. *Cancer* 1980;45:2698.
25. Keidan RD, Greenberg RE, Hoffman JP. Is percutaneous nephrostomy for hydronephrosis appropriate in patients with advanced cancer? *Am J Surg* 1988;156:206.
26. Kinn AC, Ohlsen H. Percutaneous nephrostomy—a retrospective study focused on palliative indications. *APMIS* 2003;(Suppl)109:66.
27. Gasparini M, Carroll P, Stoller M. Palliative percutaneous and endoscopic urinary diversion for malignant ureteral obstruction. *Urology* 1991;38:408.
28. Wilson JR, Urwin GH, Stower MJ. The role of percutaneous nephrostomy in malignant ureteral obstruction. *Ann R Coll Surg Engl* 2005;87:21.
29. Fallon B, Onley L, Culp DA. Nephrostomy in cancer patients to do or not to do? *Br J Urol* 1980;52:237.
30. Lugmayr H, Pauer W. Self-expanding metal stents for palliative treatment of malignant ureteral obstruction. *AJR Am J Roentgenol* 1992;159:1091.
31. Messing EM, Young TB, Hunt VB, et al. The significance of asymptomatic microhematuria in men 50 or more years old: findings of a home screening study using urine dipsticks. *J Urol* 1987;137:919.
32. Foley SJ, Soloman LZ, Wedderburn AW, et al. A prospective study of the natural history of hematuria associated with benign prostatic hyperplasia and the effect of finasteride. *J Urol* 2000;163:496.
33. Sieber PR, Rommel FM, Huffnagle HW, et al. The treatment of gross hematuria secondary to prostatic bleeding with finasteride. *J Urol* 1998;159(4):1232–1233.
34. Hochberg DA, Basillote JB, Armenakas NA, et al. Decreased suburethral prostatic microvessel density in finasteride treated prostates: a possible mechanism for reduced bleeding in benign prostatic hyperplasia. *J Urol* 2002;167:1731.
35. Miller J, Burheld GD, Moretti KL. Oral conjugated estrogen therapy for treatment of hemorrhagic cystitis. *J Urol* 1994;151:1348.
36. Cox PJ. Cyclophosphamide cystitis and bladder cancer: a hypothesis. *Eur J Cancer* 1979;15:1071.
37. Cox PJ. Cyclophosphamide cystitis—identification of acrolein as the causative agent. *Biochem Pharmacol* 1979;28:2045.

38. Brock N, Pohl J, Stekar J. Detoxification of urotoxic oxazaphosphorines by sulfhydryl compounds. *J Cancer Res Clin Oncol* 1981;100:311.

39. Scheonrock GJ, Ciani P. Treatment of radiation cystitis with hyperbaric oxygen. *Urology* 1986;27:271.

40. Stefanini M, English HA, Taylor AE. Safe and effective, prolonged administration of epsilon aminocaproic acid in bleeding from the urinary tract. *J Urol* 1990;143:559.

41. Singh I, Laungani GB. Intravesical epsilon aminocaproic acid in management of intractable bladder hemorrhage. *Urology* 1992;40:227.

42. Nash DA Jr, Henry AR. Unilateral essential hematuria. Therapy with epsilon aminocaproic acid. *Urology* 1984;23:297.

43. Black WD, Hatch FE, Acchiardo S. Aminocaproic acid in prolonged hematuria of patients with sicklemia. *Arch Int Med* 1976;136:678.

44. Kumar APM, Wrenn EL Jr, Jayalakshmamma B, et al. Silver nitrate irrigation to control bladder hemorrhage in children receiving cancer therapy. *J Urol* 1976;116:85.

45. Mukamel E, Lupu A, deKernion JB. Alum irrigation for severe bladder hemorrhage. *J Urol* 1986;135:784.

46. Goel AK, Rao MS, Bhagwat AG, et al. Intravesical irrigation with alum for the control of massive bladder hemorrhage. *J Urol* 1985;133:956.

47. Kumar S, Rosen P, Grabstald H. Intravesical formalin for the control of intractable bladder hemorrhage secondary to cystitis or cancer. *J Urol* 1975;114:540.

48. Fair WR. Formalin in the treatment of massive bladder hemorrhage: techniques, results, and complications. *Urology* 1974;3:573.

49. Firlit CF. Intractable hemorrhagic cystitis secondary to extensive carcinomatosis: management with formalin solution. *J Urol* 1973;110:57.

50. Donahue LA, Frank IN. Intravesical formalin therapy for hemorrhagic cystitis: analysis of therapy. *J Urol* 1989;141:809.

51. Weiss JP, Mattei DM, Neville EC, et al. Primary treatment of radiation-induced hemorrhagic cystitis with hyperbaric oxygen: 10-year experience. *J Urol* 1994;151:1514.

52. Norkool DM, Hampson NB, Gibbons RP, et al. Hyperbaric oxygen therapy for radiation-induced hemorrhagic cystitis. *J Urol* 1993;150:332.

53. Rijkmans BG, Bakker DJ, Dabhoiwala NF, et al. Successful treatment of radiation cystitis with hyperbaric oxygen. *Eur Urol* 1989;16:354.

54. Corman JM, McClure D, Pritchett R, et al. Treatment of radiation induced hemorrhagic cystitis with hyperbaric oxygen. *J Urol* 2003;169:2200.

55. Matthews R, Rajan N, Josefson L, et al. Hyperbaric oxygen therapy for radiation induced hemorrhagic cystitis. *J Urol* 1999;161:435.

56. Del Pizzo JJ, Chew BH, Jacobs SC, et al. Treatment of radiation induced hemorrhagic cystitis with hyperbaric oxygen: long term followup. *J Urol* 1998;160:731.

57. Chong KT, Hampson NB, Corman JM. Early hyperbaric oxygen therapy improves outcome for radiation-induced hemorrhagic cystitis. *Urology* 2005;65:649.

58. Liu YK, Harty JI, Steinbock GS, et al. Treatment of radiation or cyclophosphamide induced hemorrhagic cystitis using conjugated estrogen. *J Urol* 1990;144:41.

59. Sieber PR. Bladder necrosis secondary to pelvic artery embolization: case report and literature review. *J Urol* 1994;15:422.

60. Russo P. Urologic emergencies in the cancer patient. *Semin Oncol* 2000;27:284.

CHAPTER 33 ■ MANAGEMENT OF RENAL FAILURE

W. SCOTT LONG

Renal failure (RF) is a multisystem disease that complicates the course of treatment of patients with cancer, both in the early and late stages. Because even modest degrees of RF may increase mortality, independent of comorbidity (1–3), its early detection and treatment are crucial for supporting the patient. This chapter first presents the incidence of RF in patients with cancer, followed by a discussion of its causes, workup, and treatments. The second part of the chapter deals with the care of patients with cancer who are dying of RF when curative therapy is no longer desired and/or possible.

Definitions and criteria for acute renal failure (ARF) abound, though without a consensus (4,5). It is a general opinion, however, that ARF denotes the onset of serious dysfunction over a few days and may be at least partially reversible if treated early. Chronic renal failure (CRF) results from irreversible parenchymal damage of longer duration. No clearly defined time limit signals the transition from ARF to CRF. The term "end-stage renal disease" (ESRD) most often implies CRF requiring dialysis for patient survival.

The perspective in this chapter is primarily medical. However, care of patients and families entails not only clinical and ethical expertise but also education, emotional support, guidance, patience, and responsibility at each step. From the perspective of supportive oncology "medical care" includes an integrated plan of multidisciplinary care, appropriate here as elsewhere in the practice of oncology, for the benefit of patients, their families, and clinicians. Willing collaboration among clinicians with recognition of individual strengths and limitations improves both provision and acceptance of care.

INCIDENCE AND CAUSES OF RENAL FAILURE IN PATIENTS WITH CANCER

Epidemiology of RF has changed over the recent decades (5–9). Due in large part to scientific and technological advances, a greater awareness of basic health care measures and, in this country, a presumption of universal health care regardless of age and cost, the population of patients with cancer has aged and their comorbidities increased. Mortality rates of 40–70% in critically ill patients with ARF of all etiologies have shown too little change, although surveys point to improved survival of patients with ARF in trauma, obstetric, and postoperative cases (6–8). In one large study, one third of patients with ARF were treated in intensive care units (ICUs) and the mortality

was found to be 70% compared to a mortality of 18–43% when treated in other parts of the hospital (10).

Malignancy in conjunction with ARF is associated with worse prognosis (11,12) and dialysis is withheld in such cases (13). Among patients with cancer, incidence of RF generally ranges from 15–50% depending upon the study design and definition of RF (12,14–16). ARF occurs in a third to a half of patients with hematologic tumors and in those undergoing bone marrow transplant (BMT) (14,17,18); incidence in multiple myeloma is somewhat less (19).

Renal cell carcinoma (RCC) is cancer of the kidney, urothelial sites, or metastatic renal deposits. In one study, ARF occurred in 33 of 259 patients undergoing surgery for RCC (20). Renal metastases are not uncommon in autopsied patients with cancer, although neither metastases nor parenchymal infiltration by leukemias and lymphomas is often associated with RF (21).

Acting over greater distances, circulating tumor antigens may promote pathological changes, most commonly membranous glomerulopathies (especially in stomach, colon, and lung cancer) and minimal change glomerulopathy and focal glomerulosclerosis in hematologic tumors (21,22). Lymphomas and multiple myeloma have been associated with acute interstitial nephritis (23).

Vascular effects of tumors can produce RF through disseminated intravascular coagulation (DIC), hemolytic uremic syndrome (HUS), and thrombotic thrombocytopenic purpura (TTP). These may arise from distant tumors, associated conditions like sepsis, and therapies directed against cancer. DIC occurs from pancreatic, gastric, prostate, and trophoblastic tumors, as well as from acute promyelocytic leukemia. HUS and TTP appear in patients with mucinous gastric adenocarcinoma and carcinomas of pancreas and prostate (21,22,24). Large-caliber vessels are also involved, for example, in renal vein thrombosis in RCC.

A single type of tumor may compromise renal function through several pathways. For example, multiple myeloma produces renal damage through the toxic effects of light-chain absorption in proximal tubular cells, obstruction due to intratubular coagulation of myeloma proteins and cellular debris, parenchymal precipitation of calcium phosphate crystals (nephrocalcinosis), and deposition of amyloid (19). Sepsis, often found in myeloma, favors ARF and carries a poor prognosis, whatever its setting (8,10,11).

Iatrogenic RF was identified in 40–55% of patients with hospital-acquired renal insufficiency or failure (8,10,11). Anticipating and minimizing unwanted effects of the disease and therapies on renal function are key steps in protecting patients from RF and its complications. Evaluation of baseline renal function identifies patients already at risk, signals the need for specific preventive measures, and guides the treatment of evolving renal compromise, if it arises.

Medications commonly used in patients with cancer can cause ARF. Aminoglycosides, amphotericin B, and radiocontrast agents are notoriously nephrotoxic (8,11,21). ß-lactam and sulfonamide antibiotics, nonsteroidal anti-inflammatory drugs (NSAIDs), thiazide diuretics and furosemide, allopurinol, phenytoin, and cimetidine have produced ARF through allergic interstitial nephritis (23). NSAIDs, angiotensin converting enzyme inhibitors, angiotensin receptor blockers, calcineurin inhibitors, amphotericin B, interleukin-2, and radiocontrast dyes can reduce renal perfusion (21,25,26). Injury from radiocontrast agents is promoted by increased age (>60), diabetes mellitus, preexistent renal disease, decreased extracellular fluid (ECF) volume, and high doses of contrast (21). The recent use of acetylcysteine in patients with chronic renal insufficiency (27) as well as the use of nonionic contrast dyes and careful hydration before any dye exposure have reduced renal injury by contrast dyes. Imaging techniques not requiring the use of contrast dyes, for example, magnetic resonance imaging (MRI), are helpful in patients susceptible to renal damage (28).

Chronic and acute comorbidities often exacerbate renal insult in patients with cancer, especially in the elderly with decreasing renal reserve and other common illnesses like diabetes mellitus and hypertension. Age alone has been identified as an independent risk factor for RF in many studies (6,8,29), though not in all (10,11). In the elderly, decreased glomerular filtration rate (GFR), diminished muscle mass, prolonged bed rest, and reduced ECF volume may produce a falsely "normal" creatinine and thus overestimate real GFR. In this population, an approximation of GFR rate by the Modification of Diet in Renal Disease (MDRD) formula (30) can be done for obtaining a more reliable guide to dosing of potential nephrotoxins, so long as one can reasonably assume a steady state serum creatinine level. This assumption does not hold in patients with an evolving ARF (28,30).

Some chemotherapeutic and immunosuppressive agents create dose-related renal damage with such regularity that routine precautions are mandatory. In common with risk factors associated with the "usual suspects" mentioned in the preceding text, renal damage is often exacerbated by these agents in patients already at risk with volume depletion due to vomiting, diarrhea, third-spacing of fluid (e.g., capillary leak syndrome associated with interleukin-2, hepatorenal syndrome) and in patients with preexistent renal compromise.

Cisplatin, methotrexate, ifosfamide, streptozotocin, and mitomycin C are among the most nephrotoxic chemotherapeutic compounds in frequent use, as is interleukin-2 among the antineoplastic biologic agents. In addition, the immunosuppressive agents, cyclosporin A and FK306 (tacrolimus), produce both acute and chronic insults to renal function. Antineoplastic agents produce RF by various means including vasoconstriction, direct tubular toxicity, tubular obstruction, microangiopathy, and capillary leak. They should be used with renoprotective measures before, during, and after administration (21,25,31).

BMT, used to treat hematologic malignancies and solid tumors, is associated with ARF in one third to one half of patients. In a recent meta-analysis of six studies, 42–84% of 1211 patients developed ARF with greater rates found in those receiving allogeneic cells. Patients in ARF had increased risk of death; and 83–100% of those requiring dialysis died (18). Interventions during BMT could lead to the development of ARF. During marrow ablation and reduction of malignant cells, chemotherapy and whole body radiation may precipitate tumor lysis syndrome (TLS). Immunosuppression promotes infection with sepsis. ARF may be further favored by nephrotoxic compounds such as aminoglycosides and amphotericin B. Loss of volume through vomiting and diarrhea triggered by chemotherapy promote ARF through decreased renal perfusion. Shielding the kidneys during whole body irradiation can mitigate short- and long-term renal injury. The incidence of many of these insults in BMT can be reduced by routine precautions, for example, i.v. hydration, alkaline diuresis, allopurinol, and leucopheresis. Later, serious RF can develop months after BMT owing to graft versus host disease and its therapies. Still later, HUS/TTP may produce ARF (16,21).

DIAGNOSIS OF RENAL FAILURE

Rising azotemia during routine testing of asymptomatic patients may be the first indication of renal insufficiency or failure. Note that in evolving ARF, the equation elaborated by the MDRD Study for estimation of GFR does not produce accurate values because serum creatinine levels lag behind deteriorating renal function. (During the recovery phase, a similar offset between serum creatinine and renal function occurs in the opposite direction.)

Recalling that modest degrees of RF may increase mortality, independent of comorbidity (1–3), the physician begins to search for causes, measure the rate, and correct the consequences of evolving RF. Delayed consultations with nephrologists—or none—lead to worse outcomes for patients with RF (32).

Physiologically, ARF falls into three well-known categories: prerenal, renal [also called *parenchymal failure, intrinsic failure*, or *acute tubular necrosis (ATN)*], and postrenal. Most studies of ARF report hospital experience. Of 748 hospitalized patients with ARF of all etiologies, approximately 50% had ATN, 25% had prerenal, 13% had acute-on-chronic, and 10% had postrenal causes (33). ATN is predominant in patients in the ICU. Community-based studies show a relative increase in prerenal and postrenal failure and lower incidence of ATN in patients hospitalized for community-acquired ARF (10,34). Patients in nonoliguric RF (>400 cc per day) generally fare better because volume overload is less problematic (10,11,29). Overall, ATN is associated with higher mortality that ARF with prerenal or postrenal causes (10).

Prerenal failure indicates that one or more precipitating causes of failure are "upstream" from the kidney. A history of ECF depletion, decreases in daily weight and in fluid intake/output, and an examination revealing poor skin turgor, dry oral mucosa, dry axillae, resting tachycardia, and orthostatic pulse and pressure suggest prerenal failure. Patients with prerenal failure tend to produce small amounts of concentrated urine with low sodium content. The ratio of plasma blood urea nitrogen (BUN) to creatinine in prerenal failure is usually ≥20. Urinary indices (e.g., fractional excretion of sodium) can be helpful but not diagnostic, especially in elderly patients with decreased concentrating ability, patients with preexistent renal insufficiency, or in patients who were on diuretics recently.

Urinary sediments in prerenal failure are generally free of cellular debris other than clear hyaline tubular casts. In ATN, "active" or "busy" sediments show epithelial cells, cellular debris, and tubular casts, but may contain no casts. Red cell casts suggest glomerulonephritis; tubular casts of leukocytes occur in allergic interstitial nephritis (e.g., due to penicillins, cephalosporins, NSAIDs, and allopurinol).

In postrenal failure, increased backpressure caused by ureteral obstruction due to tumor, lymphadenopathy, retroperitoneal fibrosis, or prostatic disease compromises renal circulation and GFR, produces hypoxia and, if uncorrected, results in RF. Renal vein thrombosis in RCC causes similar problems.

Identified prerenal or postrenal failure does not preclude parenchymal damage. In addition to the laboratory tests mentioned in preceding text, imaging with ultrasound, computed tomography, and MRI, often used early to rule out postobstructive lesions, also describe the size and number of kidneys with estimation of cortical thickness to identify preexistent disease. New techniques for diagnosis, especially for early diagnosis of ATN, are being developed (28). Renal biopsy to guide therapy needs consideration if there are no obvious causes for parenchymal damage or if aspects of history, examination, and laboratory data suggest other causes of RF (e.g., glomerular, interstitial, or vascular disease) for which specific treatments exist. Some consider the presence of a terminal illness or renal neoplasm as a contraindication for renal biopsy (35).

TREATMENT OF RENAL FAILURE AND ITS COMPLICATIONS

Therapies for RF in patients with cancer can be divided into two overlapping groups. The first group of therapies is based on the judgment that quantity and quality of life at risk are worth the great effort that is made to save or prolong it significantly. In this first group, therapy aims to correct the underlying pathophysiology and its consequences and to optimize the patients' health and comfort. The second group of therapies of "care only" is brought into play when active curative therapy is no longer sought or possible, and comfort and quality of life become the predominant goals. During the evolution of RF and/or cancer, the categorization of patients into these groups may change.

Active treatment of some problems caused by RF may be required soon after detection to protect the patient's status during further workup and therapy and to prevent evolution of renal damage into long-lasting compromise or death. Treatments chosen depend on the severity of signs and symptoms, comorbidity, the desired and side effects of each agent or intervention, and the overall goals of the patient and family.

Nondialytic Therapy

Azotemia, metabolic offsets (e.g., hyperkalemia, acidosis), and, in many cases, volume overload characterize untreated RF. Most patients with ARF are not dialyzed except in the ICU (9,10,29,34). Table 33.1 gives an overview of nondialytic measures taken to protect patients from the dangers of ARF.

Volume overload most often occurs in patients with oliguric failure unresponsive to cautious fluid challenge. Diuretics (e.g., mannitol, furosemide) and vasodilators (e.g., low-dose dopamine) may convert oliguric to nonoliguric failure in some patients during the early phase of ARF but have not been found to reduce the duration of ATN and the likelihood of dialysis or to improve survival (36). Medications to correct other aspects of ARF (e.g., sodium bicarbonate for acidosis or for urinary alkalinization) may promote volume overload and pulmonary edema. Oxygen should be used to counteract hypoxia in pulmonary edema. Increasing venous capacitance with morphine sulfate (MS) and some other vasodilators may help gain time in the most urgent cases of volume overload. Pulmonary edema requires correction with hemodialysis or hemofiltration unless rapidly resolved by conservative measures. In less urgent cases, restriction of salt (<2 g per day) and water (<1 L per day) intake, as well as loop diuretics in nonoliguric failure, protects patients from fluid overload. The gut also may be used to excrete fluid through the promotion of diarrhea with poorly reabsorbed carbohydrates like sorbitol or lactulose; as much as 4–5 L per day can be lost by such methods.

Metabolic acidosis due to decreased acid excretion in RF and rising acid production in hypercatabolism exerts multiple

NONDIALYTIC MANAGEMENT OF ACUTE RENAL FAILURE

Volume overload	Place patient in upright position.
	Restrict salt (1–2 g/d) and water (<1 L/d) intake.
	Use loop diuretics, especially in a nonoliguric patient.
	Oliguric patients may benefit from increase in venous capacitance through administration of nitrates, furosemide, or morphine (monitor for retention).
Metabolic acidosis	$NaHCO_3$ infusion (if volume status allows) to maintain pH >7.2 and HCO_3^- >15 mM/L.
	Limit protein intake, generally 0.6–1 g/kg body weight/d (adjusted for BUN) unless patient is severely catabolic.
Hyperkalemia	Control K^+ intake in diet, generally to <40 mEq/d; no K^+ supplements or K^+-rich medications.
	Avoid K^+-sparing diuretics.
	Redistribute K^+ from extracellular to intracellular fluid: glucose + insulin, $NaHCO_3$ infusion, Ca^{2+} gluconate, β_2 agonist inhalation.
	Promote K^+ excretion: cation exchange resins.
Hyponatremia	Restrict free water intake to <1 L/d.
	Avoid hypotonic infusions.
Hyperphosphatemia	Minimize dietary phosphate and phosphate-rich enemas (e.g., Fleet's); use phosphate binders, e.g., calcium salts, $Al(OH)_3$.
Hypocalcemia	Provide calcium salts (gluconate or carbonate, the latter if bicarbonate needed).
Hypermagnesemia	Avoid magnesium-based antacids.
Nutrition	Limit protein intake, generally to 0.6–1g/kg body weight/d (adjusted for BUN), unless patient is severely catabolic.
	Provide parenteral or enteral nutrition in severely catabolic patients or those with a lengthy course.
	Provide calories as carbohydrate, ~100 g/d.

BUN, blood urea nitrogen.

deleterious effects including neurological and cardiovascular deterioration. Acidosis can be controlled by oral or intravenous bicarbonate replacement to bring bicarbonate above 15 mEq per L. Monitoring protects patients from adverse consequences of bicarbonate loads, such as hypocalcemia, hypokalemia, alkalosis, and volume overload. In urgent cases, usually in conjunction with other metabolic offsets, acidosis requires dialysis (e.g., for bicarbonate <10 mEq per L or pH below 7.20). In less severe acidosis, diets low in protein (approximately 0.5 g/kg body weight/day) and high in carbohydrates (approximately 100 g per day) diminish acid production.

Hyperkalemia may accompany RF of all causes, but rapid accumulation of K^+ in ECF is especially threatening with tissue destruction (e.g., TLS). Hyperkalemia and its treatment are best monitored with plasma levels and electrocardiographic changes. When $[K^+]$ is approximately 7 mEq per L, high T-waves and depressed S-T segments occur, followed by intraventricular conduction blocks and loss of P-waves when $[K^+]$ is approximately 8 mEq per L, leading to ventricular standstill. Emergent correction of hyperkalemia and follow-up measures to maintain plasma $[K^+]$ at safe levels are described in standard medical texts and manuals.

Hypercalcemia (>14 mg per dL or 3.5 mmol per L, corrected for albumin) is a common metabolic emergency in patients with cancer with both hematologic and solid tumors (37), especially in multiple myeloma. Myeloma patients with serum $[Ca^{2+}]$ >11.5 mg per dL, corrected for protein binding, had a significantly higher incidence of RF (49%) than those with lower $[Ca^{2+}]$ (10%) (38). Of 50 patients seen for hypercalcemia in hospital setting, cancer was the cause in 41, half of these due to lung cancer (39). Although bisphosphonates figure prominently in the therapy of hypercalcemia, their known nephrotoxicity must be kept in mind (26). Further discussion of hypercalcemia and its treatment in patients with cancer is found in Chapter 34.

Hyperuricemia (>15 mg per dL) in patients with cancer is primarily the result of TLS found in both hematologic and solid tumors (14,40,41). It can occur spontaneously and should be sought before therapy in patients at risk. Diagnosis of acute uric acid nephropathy in TLS is suggested by appropriate history and laboratory values. At uric acid levels >20 mg per dL, crystals form in the renal medulla to cause obstruction and inflammation, promoting RF. Sludge of uric acid crystals and amorphous material in the renal pelvis and ureters may add a postrenal component. Urinary amorphous or crystalline urates are not diagnostic.

Prevention of hyperuricemia and other metabolic problems in TLS is preferable to treatment. Such measures given before, during, and after chemotherapy consist of vigorous intravenous hydration with loop diuretics, allopurinol, and, in patients not already hyperphosphatemic, urinary alkalinization. Alkalinization must be avoided in hyperphosphatemic patients because alkaline urine favors nephrocalcinosis to create or worsen RF. Thiazide diuretics promote urate reabsorption and are not used. Even without sodium bicarbonate or acetazolamide, hydration may produce fluid overload, especially in oliguric RF. In such cases, hemodialysis is necessary, sometimes on a daily basis, to reduce urate quickly.

Hyperphosphatemia (>5 mg per dL or >1.67 mmol per L), like hyperuricemia, is particularly threatening in TLS. Not only is it associated with nephrocalcinosis, but concomitantly lowered $[Ca^{2+}]$ may present problems in neuromuscular, cardiac, and central nervous system function. In severe cases, usually associated with other metabolic problems, hyperphosphatemia requires dialysis. Mild to moderate elevations of serum phosphate concentrations are commonly found in RF because of decreased renal phosphate clearance and increased release of cellular phosphates in acidosis. In these conditions, hyperphosphatemia is usually controlled by phosphate-binding antacids (e.g., aluminum hydroxide), by reduced intake including parenteral phosphate, and by avoidance of phosphate-rich enemas (e.g., Fleet enemas). Magnesium-containing antacid should not be used because magnesium accumulates in RF.

In many patients, infection precipitates RF, exacerbates established RF, and threatens renal recovery. Sepsis in patients with ARF is associated with increased mortality (6,8,14,29, 33). Insults to body integrity are superimposed on the compromised immune system in RF by the use of urinary catheters, intravascular devices, and intubation. During workup of a serious suspicion of infection, one should begin on antibiotics that are chosen to minimize further renal damage and adjusted for ARF and its concurrent therapies, such as dialysis (42).

Some antibiotics can complicate RF. For example, penicillin G promotes seizure activity, whereas K^+ penicillin with 3 mEq per million units contributes to hyperkalemia. Trimethoprim, cefoxitin, cefotetan, and cimetidine may cause spuriously high creatinine levels. Tetracyclines promote uremia through their effects on protein metabolism. Antibiotics both filtered and secreted (e.g., penicillins, cephalosporins, trimethoprim, and sulfonamides) achieve higher concentrations in tubular fluid and urine than those dependent on GFR alone (e.g., aminoglycosides) and are often associated with allergic interstitial nephritis (23). Aminoglycosides and amphotericin B are well-known nephrotoxins.

Nutritional support in patients with cancer with RF partially offsets the consequences of protein catabolism and other metabolic dysfunctions, decreased intake, and increased loss (e.g., through dialysis) of nutrients. In a prospective study, severe malnutrition was found in 130 of 309 patients with cancer and ARF; malnutrition showed a significant correlation with complications (e.g., sepsis), mortality, and length of stay in the hospital. Of particular relevance to this chapter, 75 of these patients had cancer (43).

The overall goal of nutrition in such patients is maintenance of protein stores and lean body mass with their consequent benefits. In many patients with cancer, comorbidities (e.g., sepsis, multiorgan system failure) determine the energy needs rather than RF itself. Estimation of basal energy expenditure (BEE), for example, by Benedict-Harris equations and, where possible, measurement of actual energy expenditures, guides the prescription of nutritional supplementation. Generally, slight underprescription is better for patients than overfeeding, which promotes CO_2 production and hyperlipidemia. Such estimations have shown that only rarely do patients with RF need more than 30% BEE. Patients with limited or moderate catabolism should receive supplements to provide energy at approximately 25–30 kcal/kg body weight/day. In those in severe hypercatabolic states (e.g., sepsis or multiple organ dysfunction), the target rates are nearer to 25–35 kcal/kg/day (44,45).

Enteral routes, preferred for physiologic reasons (the gut's barrier and immune functions), the quality of life, and economy, are associated with better survival (3). For patients with complications who are in ICUs, nutritional supplements often start 2–4 days after uremic control, that is, after the ebb period of ARF when nutrition may in fact promote increased oxygen need and exacerbate RF. For optimal nutritional support, the managing physician needs to collaborate with a nephrologist, a nutritionist, a pharmacist, and nurses.

Finally, despite the many reasons aggressive nutritional supplementation should promote greater well-being and quicker healing in patients with ARF, clinical studies have not consistently shown improved renal function or longer patient survival with provision of nutritional supplements (45).

Hematological problems in RF include anemia and coagulopathies. Anemia, common even in early RF (34), often has several causes: bleeding, blood loss through dialysis or surgery, and diminished erythropoietin synthesis in damaged kidneys. Hemostasis and transfusions provide acute repletion; erythropoietin supports chronic repletion where appropriate.

Coagulopathies in uremic patients though resulting primarily from platelet dysfunction could also occur because of anemia, coagulation factor abnormalities (e.g., von Willebrand factor), and thrombocytopenia, as well as other coagulopathies due to comorbid conditions including cancer. Coagulation is usually measured as bleeding time (normally 6–9 minutes); risk of hemorrhage becomes significant with bleeding time >10 minutes. Temporary or partial correction of coagulopathy in preparation for invasive procedures like renal biopsy can be effected by several means, including infusion of cryoprecipitate, synthetic vasopressin, and infused or oral estrogens (46).

Gastrointestinal bleeding occurs in up to one third of patients with RF, usually owing to stress ulcers. It is most often mild but can be life threatening (10). Its role in mortality has decreased with improved prophylaxis and therapy, primarily by the use of proton pump inhibitors and H_2 blockers.

Uremic encephalopathy, as with many clinical consequences of uremia, shows great variations among patients but is generally worse when azotemia develops rapidly. Anorexia, insomnia, and restlessness along with decreased attention and mentation characterize the first phase. In untreated encephalopathy, emotional lability, decreased ability to think, vomiting, and lethargy follow. The most severe consequences are agitated confusion, dysarthria, and bizarre behavior, proceeding to stupor, coma, and death (47). Convulsions appear in this phase; in two early studies, the incidence of seizures varied from 5–38% (48,49). The differential diagnosis of such neurologic changes includes paraneoplastic encephalopathies, other metabolic disorders (e.g., liver dysfunction), and medication-induced changes in neurologic function (e.g., confusion associated with opioids, benzodiazepines, or NSAIDs). Normeperidine, penicillins, and theophylline have all been associated with seizures. Quiet surroundings, reassurance, and reorientation by a small number of familiar caregivers help patients in the early stages of uremic encephalopathy. Medication is often needed. The drug of choice for treating confusion is haloperidol, to which sometimes a benzodiazepine is added to calm the patient. Many psychotropic medications (see the section Adjustment of Medication) can be given safely to patients with RF; however, dosing regimens must be monitored and individualized for the desired effect (50). Advancing neurologic symptoms despite treatment are among the main indicators for initiation of dialysis in appropriate patients.

Dialysis

The discussion here focuses primarily on dialysis [also called *renal replacement therapy (RRT)*] for ARF. The percentage of patients who receive RRT varies with the site of treatment: 13% in one small study of community ARF (34), 15–36% in general hospital studies (8,10), and 48–64% in ICU studies (9,29), although in one large study of ICU patients with ARF, only 5% needed RRT (3). Patients requiring RRT have significantly lower survival rates than those who do not require RRT (3,9,10,18). The statistics among patients with cancer are grim. Survival in dialyzed patients with myeloma was approximately 70% (19), in hematologic malignancies it was less than a third (24), and in patients post-BMT survival it was <15% (18).

In patients with ARF not controlled by conservative measures, dialysis is used to correct the signs and symptoms of uremia, including electrolyte and acid–base imbalances; to remove fluid overload; to "make room" for other therapies that include nutrition, blood products, and intravenous medications; to mitigate immune and metabolic abnormalities; and

TABLE 33.2

INDICATIONS FOR DIALYSIS

Volume overload resistant to diuretics and fluid restriction with impending or symptomatic pulmonary congestion, especially if therapeutic infusion needed (e.g., nutrition, medication)

Metabolic acidosis pH <7.2 despite bicarbonate infusion or intolerance of its volume load

Hyperkalemia with K^+ >6.5 mEq/L despite other interventions or >5.5 mEq/L with ECG changes

Uremic signs including severe changes in cognition, awareness; seizures or myoclonus, asterixis; pericarditis or pericardial effusion; bleeding; ileus, nausea/vomiting

ECG, electrocardiogram.

to protect the patient prophylactically from emergent complications. Since rapid onset of ARF minimizes homeostatic adjustments found in CRF, timely initiation of dialysis for patients with ARF is often critical.

Table 33.2 summarizes the commonly used criteria for initiation of dialysis. Criteria for urgent dialysis vary among nephrologists and institutions. Rapid development of uremic signs and symptoms like pericarditis, encephalopathy, hemorrhage, or vomiting are critical reasons for beginning RRT. In oncology patients, TLS, which causes sudden elevation of K^+, uric acid, phosphate, and decreased urine output, may require immediate dialysis (51,52).

Most patients with ARF either respond to dialysis or die within a month or two of its initiation. Most survivors of ARF live without dialysis, although some have persistent renal insufficiency, and a few (1–3%) require dialysis for ESRD (8,19,33,34,38). The last figure for ESRD rises to 10–14% in survivors of dialysis in the ICU (33). In one recent study of hospital-acquired renal insufficiency designed to catch minimal offsets in renal function, 19% of dialyzed patients died, 39% recovered normal renal function, 39% were discharged with increased creatinine levels and 3% were in ESRD requiring ongoing dialysis (8). In contrast, the rates of reversible RF in patients with myeloma is <10% in most studies although two small studies showed 43% and 75% of patients were able to discontinue dialysis (19).

Techniques for RRT include intermittent hemodialysis (IHD), slow continuous renal replacement therapy (CRRT), and peritoneal dialysis (PD) (51–53). Different techniques may be used sequentially in a patient; for example, maintenance therapy with IHD or PD after emergent correction by CRRT or IHD. (PD is rarely used in adult ARF; it is used more commonly in neonates and small infants and much more widely in the treatment of CRF.) All dialysis for ARF requires daily assessment of patients by nephrologists and intensivists as part of interdisciplinary care.

IHD is an efficient means of altering the composition and volume of ECF. In patients with life-threatening volume overload or changes in ECF composition, it is often the method of choice. This technique, which is associated with rapid shifts in electrolytes, can promote cardiac arrhythmias or hypotension, which in turn may cause further renal injury. IHD is poorly tolerated in patients with cardiovascular instability or multiorgan system failure (51–53).

CRRT offers the advantages of hemodynamic stability coupled with control of ECF volume and composition in cancer patients with multiple problems, including cardiovascular instability, hypercatabolism, and the need for large volumes of fluids (e.g., medication and nutrition). However, these therapies require indwelling intravascular catheters, patient immobility, intensive nursing care, and careful control of coagulation for days at a time. Some authors favor a hybrid measure called *slow low efficient daily dialysis (SLEDD)* in treating ARF (53). It is a longer therapy with the smoother physiological control of CRRT, the shorter durations, a better control of weight, easier nursing requirements, and the economic advantages of IHD.

In the last 10–15 years, use of CRRT has increased greatly although not all are convinced of its superiority over IHD (53). Also there is ongoing debate over the dose and timing for optimal dialysis and the advantages of synthetic or modified cellulosic ("biocompatible") over cellulosic dialysis ("bioincompatible") membranes in IHD (3,9,29,36).

Sometimes difficult decisions must be made concerning initiation, withholding, or withdrawal of dialysis. Much of the work on decision about dialysis in recent years has focused on patients with ESRD, their families, surrogates, and caregivers (54); but some of the same issues concern patients on dialysis afflicted by ARF (13,55).

Clinical guidelines for initiation, withholding, and withdrawal of dialysis in ARF or CRF were published in 2000 with support from eight major organizations for the benefit of physicians, nurses, administrators, and patients involved in providing or receiving care for RF (56).

The nine recommendations proposed are:

1. Sharing decision making between physicians and patients (or surrogates)
2. Providing education about clinical options
3. Associating prognoses and quality of life
4. Obtaining informed consent or refusal for initiation, withholding, or withdrawal of dialysis
5. Signing of advance directives, if not previously accomplished
6. Acknowledging the potential for conflict and the importance of its resolution
7. Withholding or withdrawing dialysis in appropriate situations (e.g., nonrenal terminal illness)
8. Using time-limited trials of dialysis
9. Knowing the importance of palliative care throughout a patient's care.

Initiation of dialysis in patients with cancer with ARF has elicited a variety of responses (57). Some authors propose that palliative intervention including dialysis for symptoms associated with uremia is appropriate under any of the following circumstances:

1. The clinician feels symptoms will be controlled or performance status will improve with therapy.
2. The patient strongly wishes the therapy to be started, even if not recommended.
3. The patient has a prognosis of >2 months and a Karnofsky score of ≥50% (58).

In many cases of ARF, it is reasonable to try dialysis for 1–2 months, sometimes longer, before reconsideration. Some clinicians hesitate to use dialysis for patients with metastatic or nonresectable solid tumor or hematologic tumors refractory to treatment, especially with an expected survival of less than 2 years (59,60). Further, clinicians must consider the cost, available resources, institutional guidelines, and individual patients' clinical circumstances in these decisions (61,62).

In cancer patients with ARF, the physicians concerned must balance factors for and against dialysis, including the following:

1. Desires of patient and family concerning treatment
2. The patient's "baseline" state before ARF and the likelihood of benefiting from proposed dialysis

3. The probable course of the patient's underlying malignancy and its response to antineoplastic therapy

This task is difficult. First, a patient's choice may change with education and experience. Second, for caregivers prognosis is a complicated endeavor, as discussed in Chapter 42. Estimation of a patient's baseline state involves not only the evaluation of tumor, its stage, and its predicted response to planned therapy, but also a patient's comorbidities, performance status, and psychosocial issues. Finally, physicians and other clinicians should be clear about their own experiences and personal philosophies in order to articulate their reasons and feelings about using or not using dialysis. Collaborating caregivers should arrive at a consensus so that patient and family are not confused by multiple opinions. Optimally these decisions synthesize individual patients' data, clinical experience with the disease and the opinions and feelings of all involved: patients, families, surrogates, and clinical caregivers.

If a decision to begin dialysis for RF in a patient with cancer is made, clearly stated clinical goals, including a timetable for reconsidering dialysis, should be accepted by all the people involved. If the situation permits—and it often does not—patient and family may want time to consider options and to ask for further guidance from the physician and other caregivers. In any event, timely decisions must be made. Absence of consensus among patient, family, and caregivers presents great problems. Identification of advance directives and of the decision maker among patient, family, and/or surrogate is important. Empathy, along with identification of and appropriate responses to crucial differences in styles and content (and, in some unfortunate cases, legal constraints), may help resolve these difficult problems (63,64).

The same factors for initiation of dialysis pertain to its withdrawal, and for all those involved. In general, advanced age, multiple organ system failure, and chronic diseases like dementia or cancer often favor withdrawal from dialysis (63–65).

CARE OF PATIENTS WITH CANCER DYING OF RENAL FAILURE

Referral to hospice is appropriate for patients wishing to die at home or outside the hospital, for example, in an inpatient hospice unit. In recent years, the number and percentage of hospice patients dying of nonmalignant diseases have increased; in this group, one can include patients with cancer dying "early" of RF. The National Hospice and Palliative Care Organization has drawn up guidelines for hospice admission for patients dying of nonmalignant disease. All patients referred to hospice must meet the following requirements:

1. The patient and/or family know that the patient's condition is life-limiting.
2. They have chosen to pursue goals of comfort rather than treatment for cure.
3. In addition, the patient should have documented clinical progression of disease and/or recent impairment of nutritional status related to the terminal illness.
4. The renal-specific criteria are as follows:
   (a) Creatinine clearance <10 mL per minute or serum creatinine >8 mg per dL
   (b) ESRD in patients discontinuing or refusing dialysis, and "therefore with uremia, oliguria, intractable hyperkalemia, uremic pericarditis, hepatorenal syndrome, or intractable fluid overload"
   (c) Poor prognosis indicated by "mechanical ventilation, malignancy of other organ systems, chronic

lung disease, advanced cardiac disease, advanced liver disease, sepsis, immunosuppression/acquired immunodeficiency syndrome, albumin <35 mg per/l, cachexia, platelet count $<25 \times 10^9$; age >75 years, disseminated intravascular coagulation, gastrointestinal bleeding" (66)

Most of the discussion on palliative care in patients with RF who are off dialysis has concerned those with ESRD (54, 67,68); few relate to care of those in ARF with dialysis refused, withheld, or withdrawn (13). In many cases, the latter will need the symptom control related to ongoing disease processes, for example, pain, dyspnea, nausea and vomiting, delirium and, in some of those sufficiently awake, anxiety and existential anguish. In ICUs, decisions to refuse or discontinue dialysis are often accompanied by cessation of other life-sustaining measures, for example, mechanical ventilation, total parenteral nutrition, and i.v. medications like antibiotics and pressors (55). For these patients, the course is often short, and the major renal issues concern adjustment of dosing regimens for medication important for symptom control (see subsequent text).

Under some conditions dialysis may continue or be initiated in patients who have given up therapies of curative intent. Reasons may include maintenance of a clinical condition required to reach specific goals, for example, settlement of legal, financial, professional, and/or family issues. Sometimes components of RRT are used to alleviate specific symptoms, for example, ultrafiltration to remove volume overload. Definition of goals and time limits for extension of RRT are helpful to all concerned. Some patients with cancer dying of RF not requiring dialysis have a longer course as explained in the preceding text, and their symptoms will approach those found in ESRD. For such patients, the most severe symptoms are constipation, insomnia, dry mouth, pain, and itching; the most common symptoms are lack of energy, drowsiness, paresthesias, pain, and dry mouth (69). At the very end of life the most frequent symptoms recorded were pain, agitation, myoclonus, dyspnea, and agonal breathing and fever occurring in 20–40% of patients; diarrhea, dysphagia, and nausea were less frequent (69,70).

Treatment of many of these symptoms commonly found in patients with cancer is detailed in other chapters in this text. The potential dyspnea in patients dying of RF deserves a separate comment. Many patients off dialysis fear the desperate shortness of breath associated with volume overload. Before withdrawal, patients should be dialyzed to dry weight to protect them from pulmonary congestion. Thirst is uncommon, and overload is not usually a threat if caregivers do not confuse a dry mouth with thirst and give excess fluids rather than good mouth care. If pulmonary congestion does occur, oxygen, opioids, and vasodilators can often control the problem. In a few cases, it may be expedient to use retained access for ultrafiltration.

The remainder of this chapter concerns two issues: adjustment of analgesic, anticonvulsant, and psychotropic medications, which play major roles in symptom control at the end of life, and discussion of a "good" renal death.

Adjustment of Palliative Medication

Many texts have been written to guide dose and schedule modification in patients with RF, treated with or without various forms of RRT (e.g., references (71,72)). For newer medications, medical literature and manufacturers' educational material must be used.

First, some general guidelines are provided:

1. Therapeutic preferences and related issues are best discussed with competent patients or their decision-makers before discontinuation of dialysis. As stressed in the guidelines, patients with renal problems should be encouraged to consider advance directives long before reaching this stage.

2. Significant interindividual variations in pharmacological parameters and subjective response exist in persons with normal renal function. Complications of RF, such as changes in fluid compartment size, reduced renal metabolism, effects of uremic toxins on other physiologic systems, changes in plasma binding, and other comorbidities, are superimposed on age-related changes in many patients with cancer. Medications need readjustment for each patient's responses, especially as uremia deepens. (This observation also applies to dying patients entering prerenal failure with limited fluid intake but without preexisting renal disease.)

3. Medication regimens should be kept as simple as possible. Dosage adjustments for patients usually become less important at the very end of life. Medications with wide therapeutic ranges are helpful because most terminally ill patients do not want to have blood drawn to check drug levels, and most physicians do not want to prescribe medications that may complicate dying.

4. Other interventions should be as noninvasive as possible. Nonoral delivery is possible with many classes of medications relevant to end of-life care, including opioids, NSAIDs, phenothiazines, benzodiazepines, anticonvulsants, antihistamines, antiemetics, scopolamine, dexamethasone, and proton pump inhibitors (73). Increased use of subcutaneous, intravenous, transdermal, rectal, buccal (now "orally dissolvable tablets"), and other routes minimizes injections. Subcutaneous delivery of medication is less painful than intramuscular injections and can be used intermittently through a percutaneous button or continuously through a pump to avoid repeated injections. This route is less effective in patients with anasarca. Retention of central access, where possible, provides an intravenous route for medication.

5. Sedation is considered desirable by and for some patients at the end of their lives, especially if symptom control is elusive. One must ask to know.

Table 33.3 presents medications commonly used in symptom palliation. The reader must remember that these are only guidelines and that all medications must be adapted to the clinical situation of each patient with close follow-up.

Pain can be frequent and severe in patients dying of CRF or ARF (68,74). "Renal" deaths are often considered painless; but comorbidities and their treatments, prolonged hospitalization, decreased mobility can all make dying more miserable for patients and their families if pain is inadequately treated. In addition, specifically related to long-standing renal disease, pains associated with bone changes and calciphylaxis may be present. The latter results from rapidly progressive, painful deposition of calcium deposits in skin (75).

Opioids with their large interindividual variations in metabolic processing and clinical effects are the mainstay of treatment for severe pain. MS is the most frequently used strong opioid, although in many situations other strong opioids may be as effective and offer other advantages (76). Hepatic metabolism produces morphine-6-glucuronide (M6G) and morphine-3-glucuronide (M3G). Both are excreted primarily through the kidney and have been shown to accumulate in patients in RF. M6G is considered analgesic and in some studies more potent than the parent morphine; it has also been implicated in respiratory depression and sedation in some patients. M3G is associated with hyperactivity and central excitation, once again not in all studies (76,77). Accumulation of these two glucuronides may place patients

TABLE 33.3

PALLIATIVE MEDICATION IN RENAL FAILURE

Initial doses

Morphine sulfate 5–10 mg p.o. OR 2–3 mg sq q4h p.r.n. moderate–severe pain
Hydromorphone 2–3 mg p.o. OR 0.4–0.6 mg sq q4h p.r.n. moderate–severe pain
Oxycodone 5–10 mg p.o. q4h p.r.n. moderate–severe pain
Codeine 15–30 mg p.o. q4h p.r.n. mild–moderate pain
Acetaminophen 325–650 mg p.o./p.r. q4h p.r.n. mild pain
Lorazepam 0.5–1 mg p.o./i.m./i.v./topical q6h p.r.n. anxiety
Diazepam 2–5 mg p.o./i.m./i.v. q8h p.r.n. anxiety
Haloperidol 1–3 mg p.o. OR 0.5–1.5 mg sq q8h p.r.n. nausea/vomiting or p.r.n. agitated confusion
The lower dose (or in some cases half the lower dose) should be tried in frail and/or elderly patients

Routine doses

MORPHINE SULFATE, HYDROMORPHONE, OXYCODONE, CODEINE

Reduced renal excretion of morphine sulfate and codeine and/or their metabolites in RF requires dose reduction during routine
   administration (71):
   for GFR >50 mL/min, give 100% dose in normal patients
   10–50 mL/min, give 75% dose in normal patients
   <10 mL/min, give 50% dose in normal patients
Compared to morphine and codeine, fewer data exist on dosing of oxycodone and hydromorphone and/or their metabolites in
   RF, but their retention in RF suggests use of the same guidelines based on GFR for initial doses
These three levels of dose reduction should also be used if changing renal function is superimposed upon already prescribed
   opioid analgesia
In all patients with RF receiving opioids, continued monitoring for effect and safety is imperative

ACETAMINOPHEN

Acetaminophen is adjusted in RF by extending the dosing interval; for the three levels of GFR given above, the intervals are
   q4h, q6h and q8h (71)
The other medications listed above can be given without dose adjustment in patients with RF although monitoring for effect
   and safety is always important

RF, renal failure; GFR, glomerular filtration rate.

with RF at increased risk for adverse effects of opioids such as respiratory depression, cognitive deficits, obtundation, hyperexcitability, confusion, myoclonus, and nausea (15,78). In patients with RF no longer on dialysis, for example, those with GFR of 10–50 mL per hour, dose reduction generally starts at approximately 50% of a dose used for patients with normal renal function, and with a 75% reduction for patients with GFR <10 mL per minute (71,72). In both cases, morphine is titrated to the needs and responses of individual patients.

Effects of metabolite accumulation in RF have not been as well studied in hydromorphone, oxycodone, methadone, and codeine. Hydromorphone-3-glucuronide accumulation in patients with RF is associated with hyperalgesia, respiratory stimulation, and neuroexcitation (79). Oxycodone, methadone, and codeine and/or their metabolites accumulate in RF. Review of opioids in RF reveals how incomplete and often conflicting the literature is in general, and recommendations for use in RF vary (74,80). Avoidance of long-acting preparations, opioids with longer half-lives, and transdermal formulations promotes better immediate control of opioid effects and side effects in imminently dying patients.

Analgesia for neuropathic pain may include tricyclic antidepressants, anticonvulsants, and other agents, most—but not all—of which undergo hepatic metabolism and are excreted in feces so that very little adjustment is necessary for use in RF (74). Nortriptyline and desipramine, tricyclic antidepressants with fewer anticholinergic side effects than amitriptyline, are used for dull, burning dysesthesias. They can be continued without dose adjustment as long as the patient can take oral medication; parenteral amitriptyline is now available for continued neuropathic coverage. Carbamazepine and phenytoin, anticonvulsants used for lancinating neuropathic pain, can be given without dose adjustment. Gabapentin, an anticonvulsant widely used for burning dysesthesias and lancinating pains, needs dose reduction commensurate with GFR: reduction of usual dose by 50% when GFR is 10–50 mL per minute and by 75% with GFR ≤10 mL per minute (67,72).

NSAIDs for bony pain may become more relevant in the terminal phase when nephrotoxicity is not important. However, even with protection of the gastric mucosa, these uremic patients are at greater risk for gastritis and hemorrhage made worse by their antiplatelet effects. The same risk occurs with the oral or subcutaneous use of corticosteroids for bony pain, although in some orchidectomized patients with prostate carcinoma, small doses (1–2 mg twice a day) of dexamethasone may offer good analgesia with few risks. Neither the common NSAIDs (excepting ketorolac and diclofenac) nor steroids (e.g., dexamethasone) need dose adjustment in patients dying of RF (71,72). Combinations of NSAIDs, corticosteroids, and any other drugs with potential to increase bleeding risks should be avoided. For gastroprotection, H_2 blockade is given orally or intravenously in reduced doses for patients with RF, whereas proton pump inhibitors and misoprostol need no dose adjustment (67,71,72).

In addition to opioids and NSAIDs, steroids and bisphosphonates diminish incident pain due to bony metastases and can be administered by either parenteral or oral routes. Although their nephrotoxicity is no longer a concern in patients dying of RF, doses of bisphosphonates need reduction depending on GFR to avoid complications due to hypocalcemia, such as seizures and tetany.

Phenytoin and phenobarbital are the primary anticonvulsants in terminal patients with ESRD. Compared to phenytoin, phenobarbital has the wider therapeutic range, is more sedating and can be given by oral, subcutaneous, intravenous, or intramuscular routes. Carbamazepine is an alternative choice for tonic-clonic seizures, as well as for less frequently noted partial and complex partial seizures. These three agents can be given without dose reduction (67), although some authors recommend reduction of phenobarbital by 25% of its usual dose in patients with ESRD (71) Unfortunately, carbamazepine exists only in oral formulations; in some situations one could try rectal administration although other parenteral agents may be preferable and more successful.

Pentobarbital is used for agitated delirium at the end of life and can be given at its usual doses while the dose of thiopental for the same purpose is reduced by 25%. In any event, no substitute exists for close observation of patients with cautious titration for an effective dose. Parenteral benzodiazepines like diazepam or midazolam may become the preferred alternative at the end of life, especially if questions of allergy arise for any of the anticonvulsants mentioned in preceding text.

Benzodiazepines are also used to relieve anxiety and treat myoclonus intrinsic to uremia and/or from accumulation of opioids and their metabolites. In general, benzodiazepines with shorter half-lives and/or no clinically active metabolites (e.g., lorazepam, oxazepam, and temazepam) are preferred to diazepam, with its longer half-life, unless sedation or seizure control are specifically sought. Benzodiazepines can be given initially without dose adjustment (50) and then titrated to effect. Like barbiturates they may cause respiratory depression.

Midazolam, a benzodiazepine with a short half-life, administered intravenously, subcutaneously, or intramuscularly, is helpful in patients with myoclonus, anxiety, terminal agitation, and, in some cases, seizures. In patients dying of RF, 50% of the normal dose is started and then titrated to effect (71,72). For patients with multifocal myoclonus, an initial dose of 2–5 mg subcutaneously every hour is recommended until myoclonus is controlled, followed by continuous pump-delivered subcutaneous or intravenous doses. The same approach and initial dose may be used for moribund patients with grand mal seizures. Increased delivery is often necessary because of midazolam's marked tachyphylaxis.

Agitated confusion is common and particularly troubling for patients with cancer dying of RF. Among drugs to treat confusion, haloperidol is the drug of choice and generally, a second helpful high-potency antipsychotic, it undergoes extensive hepatic metabolism and can generally be given without dose adjustment. Benzodiazepines may be used in conjunction with antipsychotics to promote calm; and at the end of life diazepam may be preferred over the shorter-acting lorazepam. However, midazolam is also useful. In patients with i.v. access, midazolam 2.5 mg infused over 2 minutes can produce emergency sedation during a catastrophic terminal event. Sedation is often preferable if agitated confusion cannot be corrected. In patients with uncontrolled suffering at the very end of life and after careful discussion with family, midazolam, propofol, or the barbiturates pentobarbital and thiopental can produce a welcome deep sedation (81).

A Good Death in Renal Failure

Many patients, families, and clinicians have collaborated to explore their ideas and feelings about a good death from RF. An important recent study surveyed patients with chronic disease [cancer, ESRD, chronic obstructive pulmonary disease (COPD), congestive heart failure (CHF)], recently bereaved family members from a veterans administration (VA) population, and caregivers drawn from professional organizations (total $N = 1462$) (82). Attributes of a good death were identified as follows:

1. Symptom management and personal care
2. Preparation for the end of life
3. Achieving a sense of completion in patients' lives
4. Treatment preferences
5. Treating the patient as a whole person
6. Relationship between patients and professionals

Good pain control was the attribute of a good death that ranked first in all four groups (patients, family, physicians, and other caregivers). Being at peace with God was essentially of equal importance to pain control for patients. These findings stress the importance of care delivered by an interdisciplinary treatment team (IDT) in order to address both the tangible and intangible needs of patients and families.

Most studies of death due to RF focus on patients in ESRD (54,83), but many similar issues are relevant in deaths from ARF. Four papers from the same group, two studies (69,84) and two case reports (85,86), detail the experience of patients in ESRD after they were withdrawn from dialysis. The earlier, smaller study ($N = 18$) quantitated the quality of death in 11 prospectively studied patients with five-point scores of the following parameters:

1. Duration of dying after stopping dialysis
2. Presence of physical suffering
3. Consideration of psychosocial issues (e.g., decision-making process, level of awareness, involvement of family and friends)

The category of "good death" (score >10/15) included 7 of the 11 patients. The remaining four patients' courses after discontinuation of dialysis were compromised by "varying degrees of pain, confusion, agitation, social unrest, and a longer than average survival."

In their second study (69), an interdisciplinary team from the same group reported a mixed retrospective–prospective study of the course after discontinuation of dialysis in 131 patients with ESRD enrolled in eight dialysis clinics. Three quarters of the fully studied 79 patients had three to seven comorbidities, and 12% had malignancies. Median time to death after dialysis discontinuation was 6 days in 126 patients; the average was 8 days. Some patients lived for 30–46 days, and ten debilitated patients lived less than 2 days. Caregivers or families felt that treatment was effective in the final 24 hours of life for 93% of patients. Nonetheless, among the same patients, pain occurred in 42% (severe in 5%), agitation in 30% (severe in 1%), myoclonus in 28% (severe in 4%), and dyspnea/agonal breathing in 25% (severe in 3%). Pain medication was used at least once after stopping dialysis in 87% of patients. Although none needed ultrafiltration for pulmonary edema, 22% used oxygen. In this study the authors have raised the question whether the treatment can be considered acceptable or effective on the basis of these numbers. Nonetheless, in a follow-up study, the conclusion was that the majority of patients had a very good (38%) or a good (47%) death according to their scoring system (87). Cohen et al. have more recently discussed measures of the quality of dying in ESRD based on five characteristics (88):

1. Pain control
2. Nonpain symptoms
3. Advance care planning
4. Peacefulness
5. Duration of dying

This same group has described the function of the Renal Palliative Care Initiative (RCPI) relating goals and experiences with advance care planning, assessment of symptoms and guidelines for their treatment, the use of morbidity and mortality conferences, use of local hospice services and bereavement care for survivors (83). The principles and practice of the RPCI are well illustrated in two cases of dialysis withdrawal, detailing all the major issues from the perspectives of family and clinicians (85,86).

Certainly not all problems have been resolved. Issues remaining include more effective education of caregivers and of patients, families, and surrogates; development of IDT work for dying patients with RF and their families; continued clinical studies of symptom control in RF; and a smooth transition with continuity of care as patients move from active treatment seeking cure to palliative care involving the dialysis team in collaboration with hospice. Nonetheless, the progress over the last 10 years for patients and families, as well as for their caregivers, has been significant and its impetus encouraging.

SUMMARY

RF is a multisystem disease, which occurs commonly in patients with cancer and increases their morbidity and mortality. In the specialized world of contemporary medicine, the most important functions of the oncologist with regard to RF in addition to treatment are prevention, referral, and collaboration—prevention in designing and providing therapy to minimize occurrence and exacerbation of RF, referral to a nephrologist when renal function is deteriorating, and collaboration with patient, family, and other clinicians throughout the patient's course of treatment. Collaboration is often difficult because of the different expertise, experience, and expectations of those involved. Knowledge, patience, practice, and a steady focus on the needs and desires of the patients and their families are all important to effective care.

References

1. Chertow GM, Levy EM, Hammermeister KE, et al. Independent association between acute renal failure and mortality following cardiac surgery. *Am J Med* 1998;104:343.
2. Levy EM, Viscoli CM, Horwitz RI. The effect of acute renal failure on mortality. A cohort analysis. *JAMA* 1996;275:1489.
3. Metnitz PGH, Krenn CG, Steltzer H, et al. Effect of acute renal failure requiring renal replacement therapy on outcome in critically ill patients. *Crit Care Med* 2002;30:2051.
4. Mehta RL, Chertow GM. Acute renal failure definitions and classification: time for change? *J Am Soc Nephrol* 2003;14:2178.
5. Schrier RW, Wang W, Poole B, et al. Acute renal failure: definitions, diagnosis, pathogenesis, and therapy. *J Clin Invest* 2004;114:5.
6. Turney JH, Marshall SH, Brownjohn AM, et al. The evolution of acute renal failure, 1956–1988. *QJM* 1990;74:83.
7. McCarthy JT. Prognosis of patients with acute renal failure in the intensive-care unit: a tale of two eras. *Mayo Clin Proc* 1996;71:117.
8. Nash K, Hafeez A, Hou S. Hospital-acquired renal insufficiency. *Am J Kidney Dis* 2002;39:930.
9. Mehta RL, Pascual MT, Soroko S, et al. Spectrum of acute renal failure in the intensive care unit: the PICARD experience. *Kidney Int* 2004;66:1613.
10. Liaño F, Pascual J. The Madrid Acute Renal Failure Study Group. Epidemiology of acute renal failure: a prospective, multicenter, community-based study. *Kidney Int* 1996;50:811.
11. Hou SH, Bushinsky DA, Wish JB, et al. Hospital-acquired renal insufficiency: a prospective study. *Am J Med* 1983;74:243.
12. Rasmussen HH, Pitt EA, Ibels LS, et al. Prediction of outcome in acute renal failure by discriminant analysis of clinical variables. *Arch Intern Med* 1985;145:2015.
13. Wenger NS, Lynn J, Oye RK, et al. Withholding versus withdrawing life-sustaining treatment: patient factors and documentation associated with dialysis decisions. *J Am Geriatr Soc* 2000;84:S75.
14. Lanore JJ, Brunet F, Pochard F, et al. Hemodialysis for acute renal failure in patients with hematologic malignancies. *Crit Care Med* 1991;19:346.
15. Tiseo PJ, Thaler HT, Lapin J, et al. Morphine-6-glucuronide concentrations and opioid-related side effects: a survey in cancer patients. *Pain* 1995;61:47.
16. Zager RA. Acute renal failure in the setting of bone marrow transplantation. *Kidney Int* 1994;46:1443.
17. Zager RA, O'Quigley J, Zager BK, et al. Acute renal failure following bone marrow transplantation: a retrospective study of 272 patients. *Am J Kidney Dis* 1989;13:210.
18. Parikh CR, McSweeney P, Schrier RW. Acute renal failure independently suggests mortality after myeloablative allogeneic hematopoietic cell transplant. *Kidney Int* 2005;67:1999.
19. Bladé J, Rosiñol L. Management of myeloma patients with renal failure. In: Gahrton G, Durie BGM, Samson DM, eds. *Multiple myeloma and related disorders*. London: Arnold, 2004:339.
20. Campbell SC, Novick AC, Streen SB, et al. Complications of nephron sparing surgery for renal tumors. *J Urol* 1994;151:1177.
21. Kapoor M, Chan GZ. Malignancy and renal disease. *Crit Care Clin* 2001;17:571.
22. Mead P, Morley AR. Diseases of the kidney secondary to malignant disease. In: Jamison RL, Wilkinson R, eds. *Nephrology*. London: Chapman & Hall, 1997:674.
23. Kodner CM, Kudrimoti A. Diagnosis and management of acute interstitial nephritis. *Am Fam Physician* 2003;67:2527.
24. Fer MF, McKinney TD, Richardson RL, et al. Cancer and the kidney: renal complications of neoplasms. *Am J Med* 1981;71:704.
25. Olyaei AJ, de Mattos AM, Bennett WM. Nephrotoxicity of immunosuppressive drugs: new insights and preventive strategies. *Curr Opin Crit Care* 2001;7:384.
26. Perazella MA. Drug-induced renal failure: update on new medications and unique mechanisms of nephrotoxicity. *Am J Med Sci* 2003;325:349.
27. Tepel M, van der Giet M, Schwarzfeld C, et al. Prevention of radiographic contrast agent-induced reductions in renal function by acetylcysteine. *N Engl J Med* 2000;343:180.
28. Dagher PC, Herget-Roenthal S, Ruehm SG, et al. Newly developed techniques to study and diagnose acute renal failure. *J Am Soc Nephrol* 2003;14:2188.
29. Brivet FG, Kleinknecht DJ, Loirat P, et al. Acute renal failure in intensive care units—causes, outcome, and prognostic factors of hospital mortality: a prospective, multicenter study. *Crit Care Med* 1996;24:192.
30. Levey AS, Bosch JP, Lewis JB, et al. A more accurate method to estimate glomerular filtration rate from serum creatinine: a new prediction equation. *Ann Intern Med* 1999;130:46.
31. Kintzel PE. Anticancer drug-induced kidney disorders. Incidence, prevention and management. *Drug Saf* 2001;24:19.
32. Mehta RL, MacDonald B, Gabbai F, et al. Nephrology consultation in acute renal failure: does timing matter? *Am J Med* 2002;113:456.
33. Liaño F, Pascual J. Outcomes in acute renal failure. *Semin Nephrol* 1998;18:541.
34. Feest TG, Round A, Hamad S. Incidence of severe acute renal failure in adults: results of a community based study. *Br Med J* 1993;306:481.
35. Andreucci VE, Fuiano G, Stanziale P, et al. Role of renal biopsy in the diagnosis and prognosis of acute renal failure. *Kidney Int* 1998;53 (Suppl 66):S91.
36. Esson ML, Schrier RW. Diagnosis and treatment of acute tubular necrosis. *Ann Intern Med* 2002;137:744.
37. Stewart AF. Hypercalcemia associated with cancer. *N Engl J Med* 2005;352:373.
38. Alexanian R, Barlogie B, Dixon D. Renal failure in multiple myeloma: pathogenesis and prognostic implications. *Arch Intern Med* 1990;150:1693.
39. Kim GH, Lim CS, Han JS, et al. Clinical characteristics of hypercalcemia (Abstract). *Kidney Int* 1992;39:1066.
40. Flombaum CD. Metabolic emergencies in the cancer patient. *Semin Oncol* 2000;27:322.
41. Kalemkerian GP, Darwish B, Varterasian ML. Tumor lysis syndrome in small cell carcinoma and other solid tumors. *Am J Med* 1997;103:363.
42. deLalla F. Antibiotic therapy and microbiologic considerations in the intensive care unit. *Kidney Int* 1998;53(Suppl 66):S87.
43. Fiaccadori E, Lombardi M, Leonardi S, et al. Prevalence and clinical outcome associated with preexisting malnutrition in acute renal failure: a prospective cohort study. *J Am Soc Nephrol* 1999;10:581.
44. Toigo G, Aparicio M, Attman P-O, et al. Expert working group report on nutrition in adult patients with renal insufficiency (Part 2 of 2). *Clin Nutr* 2000;19:281.
45. Druml W, Mitch WE. Nutritional management of acute renal failure. In: Brady HR, Wilcox CS, eds. *Therapy in nephrology and hypertension. Companion of Brenner and Rector's The kidney*, 2nd ed. London: WB Saunders, 2003:753.
46. Schetz MRC. Coagulation disorders in acute renal failure. *Kidney Int* 1998;53(Suppl 66):S96.
47. Fraser CL, Arieff AI. Nervous system complications in uremia. *Ann Intern Med* 1988;109:143.
48. Swann RC, Merrill JP. The clinical course of acute renal failure. *Medicine* 1953;32:215.
49. Locke S, Merrill JP, Tyler HR. Neurologic complications of acute uremia. *Arch Intern Med* 1961;108:519.
50. Cohen LM, Tessier EG, Germain MJ, et al. Update on psychotropic medication use in renal disease. *Psychosomatics* 2004;45:34.
51. Ventkatesan J, Shapiro JI, Hamilton RW. Dialysis considerations in the patient with acute renal failure. In: Henrich WL, ed. *Principles and practice of dialysis*, 2nd ed. Baltimore, MD: Lippincott Williams & Wilkins, 1999:366.

52. D'Intini V, Bellomo R, Ronco C. Renal replacement methods in acute renal failure. In: Davison AM, Cameron JS, Grünfeld J-P, et al., eds. *Oxford textbook of clinical nephrology*, 3rd ed. Oxford: Oxford University Press, 2005:1495.

53. Van Biesen W, Vanholder R, Lameire N. Dialysis strategies in critically ill acute renal failure patients. *Curr Opin Crit Care* 2003;9:491.

54. Moss AH. Patient selection for dialysis, the decision to withdraw dialysis, and palliative care. In: Brady HR, Wilcox CS, eds. *Therapy in nephrology and hypertension. Companion of Brenner and Rector's The kidney*, 2nd ed. London: WB Saunders, 2003:875.

55. Brody H, Campbell ML, Faber-Langendoen K, et al. Withdrawing intensive life-sustaining treatment—recommendations for compassionate clinical management. *N Engl J Med* 1997;336:652.

56. Galla JH. Clinical practice guideline on shared decision-making in the appropriate initiation of and withdrawal from dialysis. *J Am Soc Nephrol* 2000;11:1340–1342.

57. Epstein AC. Should cancer patients be dialyzed? *Semin Nephrol* 1993;13:315.

58. Sobel BJ, Casciato DA, Lowitz BB. Renal complications. In: Casciato DA, Lowitz BB, eds. *Manual of clinical oncology*, 2nd ed. Boston, MA: Little, Brown and Company, 1988:462.

59. Hirsch DJ, West ML, Cohen AD, et al. Experience with not offering dialysis to patients with a poor prognosis. *Am J Kidney Dis* 1994;23:463.

60. Lowance DC. Factors and guidelines to be considered in offering treatment to patients with end-stage renal disease: a personal opinion. *Am J Kidney Dis* 1993;21:679.

61. Hamel MB, Phillips RS, Davis RB, et al. Outcomes and cost-effectiveness of initiating dialysis and continuing aggressive cared in seriously ill hospitalized adults. *Ann Intern Med* 1997;127:195.

62. Chertow GM. Dialysis: cost effective "SUPPORT" for patients with acute renal failure. *Am J Kidney Dis* 1998;31:545.

63. Moss AH. Managing conflict with families over dialysis discontinuation. *Am J Kidney Dis* 1998;31:868.

64. Bowman KW, Singer PA. End of life care in dialysis. In: Levinsky N, ed. *Ethics and the kidney*, Oxford: Oxford University Press, 2001:110.

65. Mailloux LU, Bellucci AG, Napolitano B, et al. Death by withdrawal from dialysis: a 20-year clinical experience. *J Am Soc Nephrol* 1993;3:1631.

66. Lynn J. Serving patients who may die soon and their families: the role of hospice and other services. *JAMA* 2001;285:925.

67. Cohen LM, Reiter GS, Poppel DM, et al. Renal palliative care. In: Addington-Hall JM, Higginson IJ, eds. *Palliative care for non-cancer patients*. Oxford: Oxford University Press, 2001:103.

68. Weisbrod SD, Carmody SS, Bruns FJ, et al. Symptom burden, quality of life, advance care planning and the potential value of palliative care in severely ill haemodialysis patients. *Nephrol Dial Transplant* 2003;18:1345.

69. Cohen LM, Germain M, Poppel DM, et al. Dialysis discontinuation and palliative care. *Am J Kidney Dis* 2000;36:140.

70. DeVelasco R, Dinwiddie LC. Management of the patient with ESRD after withdrawal from dialysis. *ANNA J* 1998;25:611.

71. Aronoff GR, Berns JS, Brier ME, et al., *Drug prescribing in renal failure. Dosing guidelines for adults*, 4th ed. Philadelphia, PA: American College of Physicians, 1999.

72. Olyaei AJ, de Mattos AM, Bennett WM. Drug usage in dialysis patients. In: Nissenson AR, Fine RN, eds. *Clinical dialysis*, 4th ed. New York: McGraw-Hill, 2005:891.

73. Hanks G, Roberts CJC, Davies AN. Principles of drug use in palliative medicine. In: Doyle D, Hanks G, Cherny N, et al., eds. *Oxford textbook of palliative medicine*, 3rd ed. Oxford: Oxford University Press, 2004:213.

74. Kurella M, Bennett WM, Chertow GM. Analgesia in patients with ESRD: a review of available evidence. *Am J Kidney Dis* 2003;42:217.

75. Llach F. The evolving patterns of calciphylaxis: therapeutic considerations. *Nephrol Dial Transplant* 2001;16:448.

76. Lötsch J. Opioid metabolites. *J Pain Symptom Manage* 2005;29:S10.

77. Penson RT, Joel SP, Gloyne A, et al. Morphine analgesia in cancer pain: role of the glucuronides. *J Opioid Manage* 2005;1:83.

78. Ashby M, Fleming B, Wood M, et al. Plasma morphine and glucuronide (M3G and M6G) concentrations in hospice inpatients. *J Pain Symptom Manage* 1997;14:157.

79. Murray A, Hagen N. Hydromorphone. *J Pain Symptom Manage* 2005; 29:S57.

80. Dean M. Opioids in renal failure and dialysis patients. *J Symptom Manage* 2004;28:497.

81. Rousseau P. Palliative sedation in the management of refractory symptoms. *J Supp Onc* 2004;2:181–186.

82. Steinhauser KE, Christakis NA, Clipp EC, et al. Factors considered important at the end of life by patients, family, physicians, and other caregivers. *JAMA* 2000;284:2476.

83. Poppel DM, Cohen LM, German MJ. The renal palliative care initiative. *J Palliat Med* 2003;6:321.

84. Cohen LM, McCue JD, Germain M, et al. Dialysis discontinuation. A good death? *Arch Intern Med* 1995;155:42.

85. Cohen LM, Poppel DM, Cohn GM, et al. A very good death: measuring quality of dying in end-stage renal disease. *J Palliat Med* 2001;4:167.

86. Cohen LM, German MJ, Poppel DM. Practical considerations in dialysis withdrawal. *JAMA* 2003;289:2113.

87. Cohen LM, Germain MJ, Poppel DM, et al. Dying well after discontinuing the life-support treatment of dialysis. *Arch Intern Med* 2000;160: 2513.

88. Cohen LM, Germain MJ. Measuring quality of dying in end-stage renal disease. *Semin Dial* 2004;17:376.

Two pertinent books came to my attention after this chapter was written:

(1) Chambers EJ, Germain M, Brown E, eds. *Supportive care for the renal patient*. New York: Oxford University Press, 2005.

(2) Cohen EP, ed. *Cancer and the kidney*. New York: Oxford University Press, 2005.

CHAPTER 34 ■ HYPERCALCEMIA

HOWARD SU-HAU YEH AND JAMES R. BERENSON

INTRODUCTION

Background and Epidemiology

Hypercalcemia of malignancy (HCM), characterized by high serum levels of calcium, is the leading malignancy-related metabolic complication in hospital practice and it is recognized as an oncologic emergency. This life-threatening incidence is reported in up to 10.9% of hospitalized patients (1–4). HCM is a condition that results from disruption of calcium homeostasis because of bone resorption secondary to skeletal invasion or indirectly through the production of endocrine factors. HCM can be divided into osteolytic hypercalcemia, where increased calcium results from the marked activity of osteoclastic bone resorption and humoral hypercalcemia, in which increased calcium is secondary to systemic secretion of parathyroid hormone protein (PTH). Among patients with HCM, approximately 20% of cases are due to osteolytic HCM and 80% are caused by humoral HCM. Nearly 10 to 20% of patients with various solid tumors and hematologic malignancies are affected by HCM at some point during the course of their disease (5). In solid tumors, lung and breast cancers are associated with 67% of cases of HCM (2,6,7). Among hematologic malignancies, HCM occurs most commonly in patients with multiple myeloma (MM) with a prevalence of approximately 30% before the widespread use of bisphosphonates. In general, HCM usually develops either at the initial stages of cancer or late in the natural history of the disease. Patients diagnosed with HCM typically have more advanced disease, are more likely to have distant metastases and renal failure, and generally have a poor prognosis (3,8).

Differential Diagnosis of Hypercalcemia

Hypercalcemia is an elevation in unbound, ionized serum calcium concentration. In the presence of hypercalcemia, it is crucial to distinguish between primary hyperparathyroidism and HCM. HCM should be suspected in patients with unexplained hypercalcemia and a low serum PTH concentration. Patients with parathyroid hormone-related protein (PTHrP)-induced hypercalcemia typically have advanced malignancy.

The diagnosis of humoral HCM can be confirmed by demonstrating a high serum concentration of PTHrP, using immunoradiometric assay (IRMA) (9). Serum PTHrP concentrations are low and undetectable in patients with primary hyperparathyroidism and in normal subjects. There is no difference in measuring serum PTHrP from assays that detect primarily amino-terminal or carboxyl-terminal epitopes of PTHrP. The main concern with the two types of assays is that patients with renal insufficiency may have high serum PTHrP values when a carboxy-terminal assay is used.

Nonetheless, some argue that the IRMA test can be time-consuming and costly for screening purposes. Therefore, one may consider using the formula described by Lind et al. (10) as a screening tool:

$$[serum \ chloride \ (mmol/l) - 84] \\ \times [albumin \ (g/l) - 15]/serum \ phosphate \ (mmol/l)$$

Values under 400 predict a malignancy, whereas values over 500 predict a parathyroid origin. This formula enables one to classify 97% of patients with cancer and 96% of patients with primary hyperparathyroidism, after excluding 5% of patients of borderline hypercalcemia that fall between the values of 400 and 500. The use of the formula is an inexpensive and easy tool to screen for a preliminary cause of HCM.

Clinical Presentation

The primary causal factor of HCM is the release of calcium into the blood from increased bone resorption that is uncoupled from bone formation, as typically occurs in patients with advanced malignancies. The excess serum calcium results in polyuria and gastrointestinal disturbances. Polyuria impairs reabsorption of sodium, potassium, and magnesium by the proximal tubules, causing hypovolemia and dehydration, which further compromise the glomerular filtration rate. The decreased glomerular filtration rate then leads to increased sodium resorption (and associated increased calcium resorption) in the proximal tubule, creating a positive feedback cycle of compromised kidney function and increasing serum calcium (5).

Normal levels of serum calcium (corrected for the concentration of serum albumin) range from 2.0 to 2.7 mmol per L (8.0 to 10.8 mg per dL) (11). Above this range, subtle symptoms of anorexia, nausea, constipation, and altered mental status begin to present. Moderate elevations of corrected serum calcium (CSC) levels at approximately 3.0 mmol per L (12 mg per dL) can lead to renal insufficiency and deposit of excess calcium in tissues. Severe HCM [CSC levels of ≥ 3.8 mmol per L (≥ 15 mg per dL)] may present with severe nausea and vomiting, dehydration, renal insufficiency, and clouding or loss of consciousness. This condition requires immediate intervention as coma and cardiac arrest may occur at these CSC levels.

Although HCM can present with either subtle or dramatic symptoms, symptom development, and severity in an individual patient do not always strictly correlate with serum calcium levels and may depend more on the rapidity with which HCM develops in the patient (5,12).

Prognosis of HCM

Median survival in the setting of HCM generally ranges from 1 to 3 months (6,7,13–15). Patients with high levels of calcium seem to have a shorter life span (4,15). Patients with high serum PTHrP concentrations also have shorter median survival times (16,17). When serum PTHrP concentration is above 12 pmol per L, it is often associated with both a lesser response rate to bisphosphonate therapy and more rapid recurrence rate of hypercalcemia (16,18,19). Those who respond to intravenous (i.v.) bisphosphonate therapy may have a significantly better outcome, although survival duration remains short (53 vs. 19 days) (19).

Mechanisms of Disease

HCM is primarily driven by increased osteoclast-mediated bone resorption. Osteoclasts are activated by cell-to-cell contact with osteoblasts and bone marrow stromal cells. Tumor cells produce circulating soluble factors such as PTHrP, tumor necrosis factor-α, and prostaglandin E, among others (20) These factors, along with the macrophage colony-stimulating factor, induce osteoblasts and stromal cells to express the receptor activator of nuclear factor kappa B (RANK) ligand (RANKL) (21). Membrane-bound RANKL binds to and stimulates RANK expressed by osteoclast progenitors and promotes osteoclast differentiation and activation (20). The subsequent bone-degrading osteoclast activity results in the release of calcium and several soluble growth factors, including Interleukin-6 (IL-6) and transforming growth factor-β, which in turn can stimulate tumor cell growth, thereby perpetuating a cycle of bone destruction. In addition, PTHrP stimulates increased renal tubular calcium reabsorption, resulting in further increased serum calcium levels.

The potent stimulatory effects of RANKL on osteoclastogenesis are usually counteracted by secreted osteoprotegerin (OPG), which acts as a safeguard mechanism for bone destruction (20,22–24). OPG is produced by many cell types. *In vitro* and *in vivo* osteoclast differentiation from precursor cells is blocked in a dose-dependent manner by recombinant OPG. OPG also binds to tumor necrosis factor–related apoptosis-inducing ligand (TRAIL). Therefore, RANKL and OPG are important regulators produced by the marrow microenvironment, and the ratio of RANKL to OPG regulates osteoclast formation and osteoclast activity. In malignant tumors, the upregulation of the cellular machinery (osteoclasts) and molecular pathways (RANKL/RANK/OPG) result in tumor-associated hypercalcemia, osteolysis, pathologic fractures, and severe pain.

IL-6 is also known to stimulate osteoclast formation and causes mild hypercalcemia (25). Greenfield et al. have shown that IL-6 is a downstream effector of the action of PTH on the bone. They have also suggested that IL-6, in turn, promotes PTHrP-mediated hypercalcemia and bone resorption and this cytokine can act at later stages in the osteoclast lineage (26).

Additionally, calcitriol (1,25-dihydroxyvitamin D3) may also be a cause of HCM, particularly in a variety of B-cell malignancies (27). As reported in an M.D. Anderson Cancer Center study, calcitriol is believed to be the cause of almost all cases of hypercalcemia in Hodgkin's disease and approximately one third of cases in non-Hodgkin's lymphoma.

Calcitriol-induced hypercalcemia has also been described in patients with lymphomatoid granulomatosis lymphoma (28). Calcitriol may also be associated with hypercalcemia in the setting of chronic granulomatous diseases. This aspect is of therapeutic interest because glucocorticoids and noncalcemic vitamin D analogs may be possible treatment options for counteracting this pathophysiologic mechanism.

CURRENT TREATMENT OPTIONS

Intravenous Hydration

Adequate hydration with normal saline is the key to the initial management of HCM. High serum calcium levels lead to inadequate urine concentrating ability by the nephron tubules; this results in polyuria, hypovolemia, and dehydration. Restoring normal blood volume through aggressive IV rehydration is critical and improves the glomerular filtration rate and, along with sodium, increases renal excretion of excess serum calcium (29). Patients often receive inadequate fluids initially, which does not allow either adequate rehydration or successful excretion of the excessive calcium. Use of loop diuretics following rehydration at this stage may be required (but must be carefully monitored) to counteract fluid overload, especially in those patients who are also at the risk of developing congestive heart failure (30). Careful monitoring of serum and urine electrolytes is also necessary in these patients as they often require replacement during intravenous hydration and diuretic therapies. However, given that HCM tends to worsen with the progression of the underlying cancer, increased calcium diuresis provides only transient relief. Effective treatment of HCM also requires pharmacologic agents to treat the underlying cause of increased calcium release from bone.

Early Inhibitors of Osteoclast-Mediated Bone Resorption

The primary pharmacologic approach for the treatment of HCM has been to decrease the rate of bone resorption. Early treatments tended to use non–bone-specific agents that researchers found lower the serum calcium. However, these treatments lacked the potency of bone-specific agents such as the bisphosphonates that were developed later. One of the first treatments for HCM was oral phosphate, which lowers serum calcium levels both by preventing dietary calcium absorption and by inhibiting osteoclast-mediated bone resorption. The major side effect of phosphate therapy is persistent diarrhea; and, therefore, phosphate therapy should not be used in patients with impaired renal function because calcification of soft tissues can lead to death from organ failure (11). Calcitonin was another early agent used for treatment of HCM. Calcitonin counteracts hypercalcemia by interfering with osteoclast maturation at several points in the differentiation pathway and by simultaneously increasing renal calcium excretion (11). The onset of action of calcitonin is rapid (within 30 minutes) although the response tends to abate within 48 hours because of downregulation of the calcitonin receptors by osteoclasts. In addition, corticosteroids are known to be a highly effective treatment for calcitriol-mediated hypercalcemia, particularly among patients with Hodgkin's disease and non-Hodgkin's lymphomas with HCM. Time to response is generally within 1 to 4 days. However, corticosteroids are not as effective in nonhematologic cancers (31). Finally, gallium nitrate and plicamycin (also known as mithramycin) were both originally used as anticancer agents and were later found to decrease serum calcium levels through cytotoxic effects on osteoclasts (11). Although these agents are effective in lowering serum calcium levels in patients with HCM, they also carry significantly higher risks of toxicity than the newer, highly effective bisphosphonate drug class (32).

Bisphosphonates

Bisphosphonates are the current standard of care in the treatment of HCM (see Table 34.1). They are nonhydrolyzable analog of inorganic pyrophosphate that bind avidly to hydroxyapatite crystals and are subsequently released during the process of bone resorption. The released bisphosphonate is taken up by osteoclasts and inhibit the cell's activity and survival. Once internalized, bisphosphonates are cytotoxic to osteoclasts and the more potent bisphosphonates interfere with intracellular signaling pathways required for osteoclast activity and survival. The first-generation bisphosphonates— clodronate and etidronate—were introduced clinically more than three decades ago (11). Although these agents are relatively weak inhibitors of bone resorption, they have some clinical utility for treating HCM. Several of the recently developed more potent nitrogen-containing bisphosphonates including pamidronate, zoledronic acid, and ibandronate are more effective for treating HCM. Pamidronate was approved in 1991 for treatment of HCM. Although pamidronate is the standard of care in the United States, zoledronic acid has recently been approved by the U.S. Federal Drug Administration (FDA) (in 2001) for treatment of HCM and shown to be more effective than pamidronate (see following text). Ibandronate has been recently approved in Europe for the treatment of HCM but is not yet approved for use in the United States.

Zoledronic acid represents the latest generation of bisphosphonates. In preclinical studies in the *in vivo* thyroid-parathyroidectomized (TPTX) rat model of vitamin D_3–induced hypercalcemia and *in vitro* mouse-calvaria cultures, zoledronic acid was shown to be more potent than both pamidronate and ibandronate (33). In fact, zoledronic acid is the most potent bisphosphonate tested to date, proving to be between 87- and 940-fold more potent than pamidronate

disodium in decreasing bone resorption in *in vivo* models of hypercalcemia (33). Figure 34.1 represents the relative potencies of these bisphosphonates in inhibiting hypercalcemia induction in rats and reducing calcium release in bone resorption in *in vitro* assays (35).

In a dose-finding study, 33 patients with hypercalcemia were administered one of four escalating doses of i.v. zoledronic acid with a median infusion time of 30 minutes. Doses as low as 0.02 and 0.04 mg/kg of body weight (i.e., 1.2 mg and 2.4 mg for a 60-kg individual) effectively normalized serum calcium. After a single administration of 0.04 mg per kg zoledronic acid, 93% of patients experienced a return to normocalcemia within 2 to 3 days, and 78% of evaluable patients maintained normocalcemia throughout the 32 to 39 days of the trial. The only clinically detectable side effect was a transient fever that occurred in 30% of patients (36).

A second dose-escalation phase I trial was conducted to evaluate the effect of zoledronic acid on biochemical markers of bone resorption in patients with bone metastases. A single 1- to 16-mg infusion of zoledronic acid was administered. This trial showed a dose-response relationship of zoledronic acid with bone resorption markers. Zoledronic acid was well tolerated at all dose levels (37).

Zoledronic acid (4 or 8 mg) is superior to pamidronate disodium (90 mg) in treating patients with moderate to severe HCM. On the basis of the results of the early single-arm dose-escalation studies, two randomized, parallel, phase III trials were designed to test the efficacy of 4 or 8 mg of IV zoledronic acid compared with 90-mg pamidronate in normalizing serum calcium levels in patients with moderate to severe HCM (38). These international studies were the largest prospective, randomized, comparative clinical trials conducted comparing two different bisphosphonates in the treatment of HCM. Total enrollment was 287 patients, 275 of whom were evaluable for efficacy. Patients were randomly assigned to receive either zoledronic acid (4 or 8 mg) through a 5-minute infusion or pamidronate disodium (90 mg) through a 2-hour infusion. The primary endpoints were to define the proportion of patients with normalized serum calcium at day 10 and the duration of response. Treatment groups were well balanced for all baseline disease characteristics. Overall, 59% of patients

TABLE 34.1

TYPES OF BISPHOSPHONATES

	Relative potency	Dose (mg)	Mode of administration	Adverse effects
Non-nitrogen Clodronate	1	1600	Oral	Hypersensitivity, renal insufficiency, hypocalcemia, hyperkalemia, hyperparathyroidism, hypocalcemia, abdominal pain, arthralgia.
Single nitrogen Pamidronate	20	90	2 h i.v.	Fever in 20% hypophosphatemia, hypocalcemia, hypomagnesemia, loss of appetite, nausea, vomiting
Ibandronate	857	6 50	1 h i.v. Oral	Rash, abdominal pain, constipation, diarrhea, dyspepsia, nausea, arthralgia, back pain, dizziness, headache
Two nitrogens Zoledronic acid	16,700	4	15 min i.v.	Minor; fever, rarely hypocalcemia, hypophosphatemia, loss of appetite, nausea, vomiting

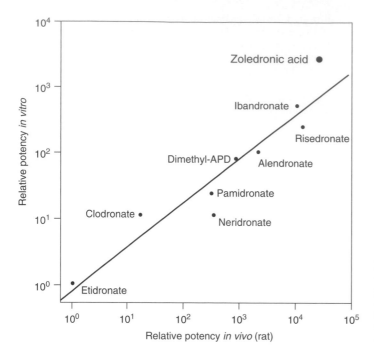

FIGURE 34.1. Relative potencies of bisphosphonates in inhibition of calcium release *in vitro* versus inhibition of hypercalcemia induction in a rat HCM model. Reprinted with permission from McCloskey EV, MacLennan IC, Drayson MT, et al. A randomized trial of the effect of clodronate on skeletal morbidity in multiple myeloma. MRC Working Party on Leukaemia in Adults. *Br J Haematol* 1998;100(2):317–325.

were male, with a mean age of 59 years (range, 21 to 87) and a mean baseline CSC of 3.47 mmol per L (38).

Both zoledronic acid doses (4 and 8 mg) proved superior to the pamidronate disodium dose (90 mg) as shown in Table 34.2 (38). The mean patient CSC in each treatment group is represented graphically in Fig. 34.2 (38). Zoledronic acid yielded a more rapid and sustained decrease in CSC than did pamidronate. By day 10, normocalcemia was achieved by 88% of patients treated with 4-mg zoledronic acid versus only 70% of patients treated with pamidronate ($P = .002$). Moreover, Kaplan-Meier estimation of time to relapse showed that zoledronic acid maintains normocalcemia significantly longer than pamidronate disodium (Fig. 34.3) (38). The median response duration was almost twice as long (30 days) for 4-mg zoledronic acid than for pamidronate (17 days; $P = .001$) (35). There was no significant difference in response rate between the 4- and 8-mg zoledronic acid group, implying that 4 mg of IV zoledronic acid is a sufficient dose.

The most commonly reported adverse events of zoledronic acid included fever, anemia, nausea, constipation, and diarrhea. These occurred with similar frequency between the zoledronic acid and pamidronate disodium groups. Although renal adverse events were reported more frequently in the zoledronic group than the pamidronate disodium group, there were no differences in the National Cancer Institute's clinical toxicity criteria grade 3 or 4 for serum creatinine between treatment groups (38). Moreover, subsequent randomized clinical studies comparing these two drugs among patients with bone metastases who received long-term treatment every 3 to 4 weeks suggest that zoledronic acid (at a recommended dose of 4 mg through 15-minute infusion) and pamidronate disodium (90 mg through 2-hour infusion) have similar renal safety profiles (38). The higher 8-mg dose showed unfavorable effects on renal function when administered on a monthly basis and is not used clinically.

Osteonecrosis of the Jaw

Osteonecrosis of the jaw (ONJ) is a newly reported complication that may result from long-term use of zoledronic acid or pamidronate treatment for patients with MM and other malignancies (40–43). The frequency with which this complication occurs in patients with cancer receiving bisphosphonate therapy is unknown. However, it appears that there is a higher risk of this complication among patients receiving these drugs.

TABLE 34.2

NORMALIZATION OF SERUM CALCIUM LEVELS BY TREATMENT WITH ZOLEDRONIC ACID OR PAMIDRONATE DISODIUM IN PATIENTS WITH HCM

Agent	Patients with normalized CSC, % day 4 (onset)	Patients with normalized CSC, % day 10	Median days to relapse
90-mg pamidronate	33.3	69.7	17
4-mg zoledronic acid	45.3*	88.4*	30*
8-mg zoledronic acid	55.6*	86.7*	40*

*$P < 0.05$, as compared with pamidronate.
Data from Major P, Lortholary A, Hon J, et al. Zoledronic acid is superior to pamidronate in the treatment of hypercalcemia of malignancy: a pooled analysis of two randomized, controlled clinical trials. *J Clin Oncol* 2001;19:558–567.

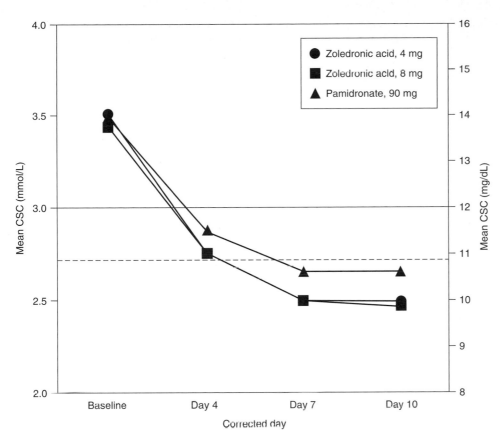

FIGURE 34.2. Mean corrected serum calcium (CSC) at baseline and Days 4, 7, and 10 after treatment of hypercalcemia with zoledronic acid 4 mg, zoledronic acid 8 mg, or pamidronate 90 mg. Reprinted with Permission from Major P, Lortholary A, Hon J, et al. Zoledronic acid is superior to pamidronate in the treatment of hypercalcemia of malignancy: a pooled analysis of two randomized, controlled clinical trials. *J Clin Oncol* 2001;19(2):558–567.

Most cases are associated with exposed mandibular bone with minimal symptoms but infrequently patients may require more extensive intervention including surgical procedures to treat this problem. It is now recommended that patients receiving bisphosphonates, including most patients with myeloma, should be evaluated early on in their treatment for dental problems and encouraged to maintain excellent dental hygiene. It should be noted that there is no evidence that discontinuation of the bisphosphonate or replacement with other bisphosphonates changes the course of this complication.

Prophylactic Bisphosphonates

In the studies evaluating the effects of bisphosphonates on skeletal complications among patients with breast cancer with lytic bone metastases, prevention of hypercalcemia has been demonstrated. In one study, Theriault et al. (44) assessed the efficacy of pamidronate in reducing skeletal morbidity in 372 breast cancer patients with osteolytic bone metastases, receiving hormonal therapy. Patients were randomized to receive double-blinded treatment with either 90 mg of

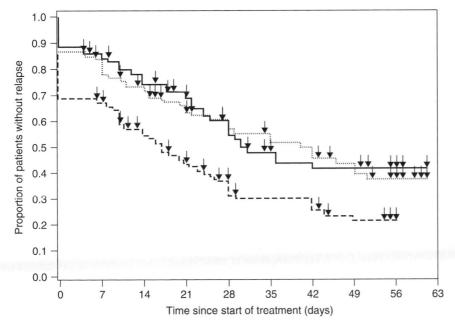

FIGURE 34.3. Kaplan-Meier estimation of time to relapse of hypercalcemia after treatment with (—) zoledronic acid 4 mg (median, 30 days), (----) zoledronic acid 8 mg (median, 40 days), or (—) pamidronate 90 mg (median, 17 days). Arrows denote censored time. Zoledronic acid 4 mg versus pamidronate, $P = .001$; zoledronic acid 8 mg versus pamidronate, $P = .007$. Reprinted with Permission from Major P, Lortholary A, Hon J, et al. Zoledronic acid is superior to pamidronate in the treatment of hypercalcemia of malignancy: a pooled analysis of two randomized, controlled clinical trials. *J Clin Oncol* 2001;19(2):558–567.

pamidronate (through a 2-hour infusion) or placebo every 4 weeks for 24 treatment cycles. Among 371 evaluable patients, hypercalcemia was significantly lower in patients treated with pamidronate than in patients treated with placebo at 24 months. In another similar study by Hortobágyi et al., 380 women with breast cancer and at least one lytic bone lesion who were receiving chemotherapy were randomly assigned to a monthly injection of pamidronate or placebo (45). Over the course of 1 year, the incidence of episodes of severe hypercalcemia was reduced by approximately half in the pamidronate-treated group. There were also lower incidence of pathologic fractures, bone pain, and spinal cord compression in both studies.

Bisphosphonate in the Hospice Setting

There is a paucity of studies on hospice patients using bisphosphonates. One small study was conducted using etidronate in the hospice setting. The report showed reduction in opiate use, improvement in pain control and preservation of cognitive function (46). Control of the rate of hypercalcemia development is unknown. As bisphosphonates remain a relatively expensive therapy in patients with cancer, more studies are needed to evaluate the cost-effectiveness of this treatment in the hospice setting.

Emerging Therapeutic Approaches

In animal models, passive immunization using antisera raised against rat PTH-like peptide [PLP-(1–34)] and rat PTH-(1–84)] have been studied (47). After immunization, plasma calcium in the tumor-bearing animals rapidly normalized and remained within the normal range for several days. These changes were associated with increased survival of the tumor-bearing rats. Similarly, monoclonal antibodies to PTHrP are being evaluated. The neutralizing effect of the antisera has shown specific reduction of serum calcium in the tumor-bearing animals (48). At present, however, both passive immunization and monoclonal antibodies to PTHrP are not available to patients.

A noncalcemic analog of calcitriol in the T lymphocyte cell line was studied at the University of Tokyo (49). This study demonstrated that the analog is capable of reducing PTHrP concentrations in vitro by approximately 50%. This compound suppresses both cell proliferation and PTHrP gene expression through binding to the vitamin D receptor that is overexpressed in T cells lines. Whether the noncalcemic analog of calcitriol will prove to be effective in patients remains to be determined.

Recently, OPG has been shown to inhibit osteoclast formation and activity by inhibiting RANK-RANKL signaling in a murine model of humoral HCM (47). The study showed that OPG treatment significantly returned osteoclast activity to sub-physiological range but had no effects on tumor size, tumor-induced cachexia or PTHrP levels. These studies suggest a therapeutic potential for OPG as well as inhibitors of RANK signaling in the prevention and treatment of HCM. Ongoing early clinical trials suggest that inhibitors of RANK-RANKL may significantly reduce bone loss in patients with cancer.

It is possible that the development of antibodies to OPG may occur in patients treated with OPG resulting in the prevention of its normal anti-bone resorptive function. To avoid potential problems with the use of OPG analogs, a recombinant form of RANKL, RANK-Fc, which is an antagonist of RANKL-RANK signaling, has been recently developed and consequently inhibits both bone disease and myeloma growth in a murine SCID-hu model of human myeloma (50). This recombinant protein is now being evaluated in clinical trials among patients with metastatic bone disease.

Aklilu et al. recently identified that the Ras signaling pathway is involved in PTHrP production by tumors. Treatment with Ras inhibitors in vitro produced a significant reduction in PTHrP mRNA expression of PTHrP and a significant decrease in cell proliferation. Treatment in mice bearing tumors with these inhibitors resulted in a significant decrease in plasma PTHrP and near normalization of serum calcium (51). This study indicates that Ras processing inhibitors may also be candidates for therapeutic agents to treat HCM.

CONCLUSION

HCM is a serious, often life-threatening skeletal complication. The goals of treatment for HCM are to control the underlying disorder, restore adequate hydration, increase urinary excretion of calcium, and inhibit osteoclast activity in bone. Zoledronic acid is a new, highly potent, nitrogen-containing bisphosphonate that has been recently approved for the treatment of HCM and represents a significant clinical advance in HCM treatment. The success rate is over 90%. The increased potency of zoledronic acid observed in preclinical models of HCM translated into improved clinical efficacy in the management of HCM, compared with pamidronate, the previous standard of care. Two randomized comparative trials demonstrated that zoledronic acid was superior to pamidronate disodium, safe and well tolerated. Furthermore, the recommended faster infusion time of 15 minutes of this newer agent represents a great advance over early bisphosphonate treatments for management of HCM, which required infusion times as long as 24 hours (52,53).

As our understanding of the pathophysiology of HCM continues to increase, therapies will continue to evolve, offering new and more effective options for the management of HCM. In preclinical trials, subcutaneous injection of either OPG or antibodies against PTHrP or RANKL normalized serum calcium levels in animal models of HCM, without evidence of the nephrotoxicity that occasionally complicates the use of IV bisphosphonates (47,49,54). The antagonist of RANKL, RANK-Fc, is currently being evaluated in clinical trials among patients with metastatic bone disease (50). Moreover, inhibition of the signaling pathway, Ras-Raf MAPK-ERK, has been demonstrated to decrease PTHrP production and normalization of calcium of tumor-bearing animals (51). Ras-processing inhibitors are currently in clinical development. However, it remains to be seen whether these advances will eventually translate into more effective therapies for the management and treatment of HCM and how they will compare with the IV bisphosphonates.

References

1. Rosol TJ, Capen CC. Mechanisms of cancer-induced hypercalcemia. *Lab Invest* 1992;67(6):680–702.
2. O'Rourke NP, McCloskey EV, Kanis JA. Tumour induced hypercalcemia: a case for active treatment. *Clin Oncol* 1994;6(3):172–176.
3. Vassilopoulou-Sellin R, Newman BM, Taylor SH, et al. Incidence of hypercalcemia in patients with malignancy referred to a comprehensive cancer center. *Cancer* 1993;71:1309–1312.
4. Heath DA. Hypercalcemia in malignancy. *BMJ* 1989;298(6686):1468–1469.
5. Bajorunas DR. Clinical manifestations of cancer-related hypercalcemia. *Semin Oncol* 1990;17:16–25.
6. Fisken RA, Heath DA, Bold AM. Hypercalcemia: a hospital survey. *Q J Med* 1980;49:405–418.
7. Firkin F, Seymour JF, Watson AM, et al. Parathyroid hormone-related protein in hypercalcemia associated with hematological malignancy. *Br J Haematol* 1996;94(3):486–492.

8. Grill V, Martin TJ. Hypercalcemia. In: Rubens RD, Mundy GR, eds. *Cancer and the skeleton*. London: Martin Dunitz Ltd, 2000:75–89.

9. Ratcliffe WA, Hutchesson AC, Bundred NJ, et al. Role of assays for parathyroid-hormone-related protein in investigation of hypercalcaemia. *Lancet* 1992;339(8786):164–167.

10. Lind L, Ljunghall S. Serum chloride in the differential diagnosis of hypercalcemia. *Exp Clin Endocrinol* 1991;98(3):179–184.

11. Mundy GR. Hypercalcemia. In: *Bone remodeling and its disorders*, 2nd ed. London: Martin Dunitz Ltd, 1999;107–122.

12. Poe CM, Radford AI. The challenge of hypercalcemia in cancer. *Oncol Nurs Forum* 1985;12:29–34.

13. Stewart AF, Horst R, Deftos LJ, et al. Biochemical evaluation of patients with cancer-associated hypercalcemia: evidence for humoral and nonhumoral groups. *N Engl J Med* 1980;303:1377–1383.

14. Mundy GR, Ibbotson KJ, D'Souza SM, et al. The hypercalcemia of cancer: clinical implications and pathogenic mechanisms. *N Engl J Med* 1984;310:1718–1727.

15. Won C, Decker DA, Drelichman A, et al. Hypercalcemia in head and neck carcinoma: incidence and prognosis. *Cancer* 1983;52(12):2261–2263.

16. Wimalawansa SJ. Significance of plasma PTH-rp in patients with hypercalcemia of malignancy treated with bisphosphonate. *Cancer* 1994;73(8):2223–2230.

17. Pecherstorfer M, Schilling T, Blind E, et al. Parathyroid hormone-related protein and life expectancy in hypercalcemic cancer patients. *J Clin Endocrinol Metab* 1994;78(5):1268–1270.

18. Gurney H, Grill V, Martin TJ. Parathyroid hormone-related protein and response to pamidronate in tumour-induced hypercalcaemia. *Lancet* 1993;341(8861):1611–1613, 37–39.

19. Ling PJ, A'Hern RP, Hardy JR. Analysis of survival following treatment of tumour-induced hypercalcaemia with intravenous pamidronate (APD). *Br J Cancer* 1995;72(1):206–209.

20. Roodman GD. Biology of osteoclast activation in cancer. *J Clin Oncol* 2001;19:3562–3571.

21. Suda T, Kobayashi K, Jimi E, et al. The molecular basis of osteoclast differentiation and activation. *Novartis Found Symp* 2001;232:235–247; discussion 247–250.

22. Simonet WS, Lacey DL, Dunstan CR, et al. Osteoprotegerin: a novel secreted protein involved in the regulation of bone density. *Cell* 1997;89:309–319.

23. Yasuda H, Shima N, Nakagawa N, et al. Identity of osteoclastogenesis inhibitory factor (OCIF) and osteoprotegerin (OPG): a mechanism by which OPG/OCIF inhibits osteoclastogenesis *in vitro*. *Endocrinology* 1998;139:1329–1337.

24. Guise TA. Molecular mechanisms of osteolytic bone metastases. *Cancer* 2000;88:2892–2898.

25. Greenfield EM, Shaw SM, Gornik SA, et al. Adenyl cyclase and interleukin 6 are downstream effectors of parathyroid hormone resulting in stimulation of bone resorption. *J Clin Invest* 1995;96(3):1238–1244.

26. de la Mata J, Uy HL, Guise TA, et al. Interleukin-6 enhances hypercalcemia and bone resorption mediated by parathyroid hormone-related protein *in vivo*. *J Clin Invest* 1995;95(6):2846–2852.

27. Seymour JF, Gagel RF. Calcitriol: the major humoral mediator of hypercalcemia in Hodgkin's disease and non-Hodgkin's lymphomas. *Blood* 1993;82(5):1383–1394.

28. Scheinman SJ, Kelberman MW, Tatum AH, et al. Hypercalcemia with excess serum 1,25 dihydroxyvitamin D in lymphomatoid granulomatosis/angiocentric lymphoma. *Am J Med Sci* 1991;301(3):178–181.

29. Davis KD, Attie MF. Management of severe hypercalcemia. *Crit Care Clin* 1991;7:175–190.

30. Davidson TG. Conventional treatment of hypercalcemia of malignancy. *Am J Health Syst Pharm* 2001;58(Suppl 3):S8–S15.

31. Ralston SH, Gallacher SJ, Patel U, et al. Cancer-associated hypercalcemia: morbidity and mortality. *Ann Intern Med* 1990;112(7):499–504.

32. Zojer N, Keck AV, Pecherstorfer M. Comparative tolerability of drug therapies for hypercalcaemia of malignancy. *Drug Saf* 1999;21:389–406.

33. Green JR, Müller K, Jaeggi KA. Preclinical pharmacology of CGP 42'446, a new, potent, hetcrocyclic bisphosphonate compound. *J Bone Miner Res* 1994;9:745–751.

34. McCloskey EV, MacLennan IC, Drayson MT, et al. A randomized trial of the effect of clodronate on skeletal morbidity in multiple myeloma. MRC Working Party on Leukaemia in Adults. *Br J Haematol* 1998;100(2):317–325.

35. Data on file. Basel, Switzerland, Novartis Pharma AG, 2000.

36. Body JJ, Borkowski A, Cleeren A, et al. Treatment of malignancy-associated hypercalcemia with intravenous aminohydroxypropylidene diphosphonate. *J Clin Oncol* 1986;4:1177–1183.

37. Berenson JR, Vescio R, Henick K, et al. Phase I open label, dose ranging, safety trial of rapid intravenous zoledronic acid, a novel bisphosphonate, in cancer patients with osteolytic bone metastases. *Cancer* 2001;91:144–154.

38. Major P, Lortholary A, Hon J, et al. Zoledronic acid is superior to pamidronate in the treatment of hypercalcemia of malignancy: a pooled analysis of two randomized, controlled clinical trials. *J Clin Oncol* 2001;19:558–567.

39. Major P, Lortholary A, Hon J, et al. Zoledronic acid is superior to pamidronate in the treatment of hypercalcemia of malignancy: a pooled analysis of two randomized, controlled clinical trials. *J Clin Oncol* 2001;19(2):558–567.

40. Ruggiero SL, Mehrotra B, Rosenberg TJ, et al. Osteonecrosis of the jaws associated with the use of bisphosphonates: a review of 63 cases. *J Oral Maxillofac Surg* 2004;62:527.

41. Migliorati CA. Bisphosphonates and oral cavity avascular bone necrosis. *J Clin Oncol* 2003;21:4253.

42. Lugassy G, Shaham R, Nemets A, et al. Severe osteomyelitis of the jaw in long-term survivors of multiple myeloma: a new clinical entity. *Am J Med* 2004;117:440.

43. Durie BG, Katz M, McCoy J, et al. Osteonecrosis of the jaws in myeloma: time dependent correlation with Aredia®and Zometa®use (abstract). *Blood* 2004;104:216a.

44. Theriault RL, Lipton A, Hortobagyi GN, et al. Pamidronate reduces skeletal morbidity in women with advanced breast cancer and lytic bone lesions: a randomized, placebo controlled trial. Protocol 18 Aredia Breast Cancer Study Group. *J Clin Oncol* 1999;17:846–854.

45. Hortobágyi GN, Theriault RL, Lipton A, et al. Long-term prevention of skeletal complications of metastatic breast cancer with pamidronate. Protocol 19 Aredia Breast Cancer Study Group. *J Clin Oncol* 1998;16:2038–2044.

46. Gloth FM III. Use of a bisphosphonate (etidronate) to improve metastatic bone pain in three hospice patients. *Clin J Pain* 1995;11(4):333–335.

47. Henderson J, Bernier S, D'Amour P, et al. Effects of passive immunization against parathyroid hormone (PTH)-like peptide and PTH in hypercalcemic tumor-bearing rats and normocalcemic controls. *Endocrinology* 1990;127(3):1310–1380.

48. Kukreja SC, Shevrin DH, Wimbiscus SA, et al. Antibodies to parathyroid hormone-related protein lower serum calcium in athymic mouse models of malignancy-associated hypercalcemia due to human tumors. *J Clin Invest* 1988;82(5):1798–1802.

49. Inoue D, Matsumoto T, Ogata E, et al. 22-Oxacalcitriol, a noncalcemic analogue of calcitriol, suppresses both cell proliferation and parathyroid hormone-related peptide gene expression in human T cell lymphotrophic virus, type I-infected T cells. *J Biol Chem* 1993;268(22):16730–16736.

50. Sordillo EM, Pearse RN. RANK-Fc: a therapeutic antagonist for RANK-L in myeloma. *Cancer* 2003;97(3 Suppl):802–812.

51. Aklilu F, Park M, Goltzman D, et al. Induction of parathyroid hormone-related peptide by the ras oncogene: role of ras farnesylation inhibitors as potential therapeutic agents for hypercalcemia malignancy. *Cancer Res* 1997;57:4517–422.

52. Flores JF, Rude RK, Chapman RA, et al. Evaluation of a 24-hour infusion of etidronate disodium for the treatment of hypercalcemia of malignancy. *Cancer* 1994;73:2527–2534.

53. Meunier PJ, Chapuy MC, Delmas P, et al. Intravenous disodium etidronate therapy in Paget's disease of bone and hypercalcemia of malignancy. Effects on biochemical parameters and bone histomorphometry. *Am J Med* 1987;82:71–78.

54. Capparelli C, Kostenuik PJ, Morony S, et al. Osteoprotegerin prevents and reverses hypercalcemia in a murine model of humoral hypercalcemia of malignancy. *Cancer Res* 2000;60(4):783–787.

CHAPTER 35 ■ METABOLIC DISORDERS IN THE CANCER PATIENT

IRENE M. O'SHAUGHNESSY AND ALBERT L. JOCHEN

Endocrine disorders occur in individuals with advanced malignancy under various circumstances. Cancer may produce effects through the excess production of hormones, cytokines, and growth factors—the so-called paraneoplastic syndromes (Table 35.1). Conversely, cancer or its metastases may interfere with the normal function of endocrine organs, resulting in hormone-deficiency states. Most commonly, patients may have a metabolic disorder such as diabetes, thyroid dysfunction, or hyperparathyroidism that predates the diagnosis of their malignancy or is diagnosed incidentally during the course of their malignancy. This chapter discusses the most common paraneoplastic syndromes and hormone-deficiency states associated with malignancy, as well as the management of diabetes and thyroid disease in the patient with cancer.

ENDOCRINE PARANEOPLASTIC SYNDROMES

Inappropriate Antidiuresis

The differential diagnosis of hyponatremia in the patient with cancer is similar to that in the general population and includes hepatic and cardiac failure, renal disease, overdiuresis, factitious hyponatremia associated with hyperglycemia, and other conditions. In the syndrome of inappropriate antidiuretic hormone (SIADH), hyponatremia results from the overproduction of arginine vasopressin (AVP) by the posterior pituitary gland in response to a stimulus by tumor cells, by the actual production of AVP or AVP-like peptides by tumor cells, or as a side effect of medications that are able to stimulate AVP production.

Epidemiology

The most common malignancies causing SIADH are small cell lung cancer and carcinoid tumors; SIADH is also seen with cancers of the esophagus, pancreas, duodenum, colon, adrenal cortex, prostate, thymomas, and lymphomas. In one series, the incidence of clinically significant SIADH was 9% among 523 patients with small cell lung cancer. A larger fraction of patients had milder abnormalities in AVP metabolism without hyponatremia. Therefore, approximately one half of patients had abnormal renal handling of water loads that were subclinical (1,2). Another study found that 41% of patients with all types of lung cancers and 43% of patients with colon cancer

had significantly elevated levels of AVP without evidence of clinically significant SIADH (3). Hyponatremia is also a common electrolyte disorder in patients hospitalized with acquired immunodeficiency syndrome (AIDS) and AIDS-related complex (ARC). Often it is associated with gastrointestinal losses or SIADH and an increase in morbidity and mortality (4).

Clinical Features

The clinical features of hyponatremia depend on the degree of hyponatremia and the rate of its development. Most patients with chronic hyponatremia are asymptomatic. Generally, symptoms do not occur until the serum sodium falls below 115–120 mEq per L (5). When they occur, the signs and symptoms of SIADH are caused by water intoxication (i.e., hypo-osmolality and hyponatremia) and are manifested as confusion, lethargy, seizures, or coma. Occasionally, patients may present with focal neurologic deficits.

Diagnosis

Because most cases of SIADH are asymptomatic, the diagnosis is usually first suspected by noting a low serum sodium on routine chemistries. Other causes of hyponatremia, such as hypovolemia, hypervolemia (occurring in renal or hepatic disease or cardiac failure), hypothyroidism, and adrenal insufficiency, must be excluded before the diagnosis of SIADH can be considered. Urine chemistries show urinary osmolality that is greater than serum osmolality and a high urinary sodium concentration (Table 35.2). Medications commonly used by patients with cancer associated with SIADH include morphine sulfate, vincristine sulfate, cyclophosphamide, phenothiazines, and tricyclic antidepressants. Most drugs cause SIADH by stimulating posterior pituitary secretion of AVP.

Treatment

The treatment of SIADH is determined by the rate of development of hyponatremia and the presence of neurologic sequelae (Table 35.3). If the patient is symptomatic and has a serum sodium level below 130 mEq per L, fluid restriction to 800–1000 mL per 24 hours is effective in slowly raising serum osmolality over a period of 3–10 days. Acute hyponatremia with neurologic symptoms has a mortality rate of 5–8% and warrants more aggressive treatment. For patients with

TABLE 35.1

COMMON PARANEOPLASTIC SYNDROMES

Syndrome	Tumor type
Inappropriate antidiuresis (hormone vasopressin)	Lung cancer, all types
Cushing's syndrome (adrenocorticotropic hormone, corticotropic hormone)	Lung cancer, all types
Hypocalcemia	Bone metastases
Hypophosphatemia ("phosphatonin")	Mesenchymal tumors
Hyperthyroidism (human chorionic gonadotropin)	Lung cancer, all types
Gynecomastia (estrogens, follicle-stimulating hormone, luteinizing hormone)	Lung cancer, all types
Calcitoninemia (calcitonin)	Medullary carcinoma of the thyroid, lung cancer, breast cancer
Acromegaly (growth hormone, growth hormone–releasing hormone)	Carcinoids, pheochromocytoma, pancreatic cancer

more severe hyponatremia, the intravenous administration of hypertonic saline (3% saline at a rate of 0.1 mg/kg/minute) and furosemide may be necessary (6). Careful monitoring of vital signs and urinary losses of sodium and potassium is indicated. Rapid correction of severe hyponatremia has been associated with central pontine myelinosis, which presents with quadriparesis and bulbar palsy 1–2 days after hyponatremia is corrected. A safe rate of correction in severe hyponatremia is 0.5–1.0 mEq/L/hour until the sodium concentration reaches 125 mEq per L (7,8).

Fluid restriction is not feasible in some patients who require long-term treatment of SIADH. In these patients, medications, including demeclocycline hydrochloride, lithium carbonate, and urea, have been tried. Demeclocycline is the drug of choice and causes partial nephrogenic diabetes insipidus by inhibiting the formation of AVP-induced cyclic adenosine monophosphate in distal tubules. It is initially administered orally in divided doses of 900–1200 mg per day and then reduced to maintenance doses of 600–900 mg per day. Side effects are mainly gastrointestinal, although hypersensitivity and nephrotoxicity can occur. Similar to demeclocycline hydrochloride, lithium carbonate also causes a reversible, partial form of nephrogenic diabetes insipidus but is less effective. Urea acts as an osmotic diuretic and allows the patient to maintain a normal fluid intake. Urea can be administered intravenously or orally. When given by mouth, the usual dosing is 30 g of urea dissolved in 100 mL of orange juice or water once daily (9).

CUSHING'S SYNDROME

Endogenous Cushing's syndrome is due to one of three causes: overproduction of glucocorticoid by a primary adrenal

TABLE 35.2

DIAGNOSIS OF SYNDROME OF INAPPROPRIATE ANTIDIURESIS

Plasma sodium level below 135 mEq/L
Urine osmolality greater than serum osmolality
Elevated urine sodium (>20 mEq/L)
Normal extracellular fluid volume
Rule out other causes of euvolemic hyponatremia

neoplasm, excessive production of adrenocorticotropic hormone (ACTH) by a pituitary adenoma, or a paraneoplastic syndrome in which either ACTH or corticotropin-releasing hormone (CRH) are produced ectopically by the tumor. A number of tumors are capable of producing ACTH, its prohormone "big ACTH," or proopiomelanocortin (POMC) (Table 35.4). The POMC gene is located at p23 on the short arm of chromosome 2 near N-myc oncogene at p24. Normally the expression of the POMC gene is influenced by glucocorticoids, which suppress transcription, and CRH, which stimulates transcription through cyclic adenosine monophosphate. The activation of alternative steroid-insensitive promoters may result in ectopic ACTH production that is insensitive to glucocorticoid suppression. Pituitary cells and some tumors produce the normal 1200-base mRNA transcript; however, some nonpituitary tissues produce either a larger or smaller POMC mRNA transcript. Alternative post-transcription processing of POMC gives rise to a large number of biologically active peptides in addition to ACTH. These include pro-ACTH and a number of different peptides containing melanocyte-stimulating hormone (MSH) (α-MSH, ACTH, pro-ACTH, β-MSH, τ-lipotropin, β-lipotropin, τ-MSH, N-POMC, pro-τ-MSH), all of which can lead to generalized hyperpigmentation (10,11). Radioimmunoassays differ in their abilities to detect aberrant ACTH. The immunoradiometric assay for ACTH is able to distinguish between ACTH and its larger precursors, pro-ACTH, and POMC (12).

Epidemiology

Ectopic ACTH is most frequently secreted by lung carcinomas. A number of other tumor types are also capable of producing this syndrome (Table 35.4). In the general population, approximately 65% of patients with Cushing's syndrome have pituitary adenomas producing ACTH (Cushing's disease), 20% have primary adrenal tumors, and 14% have ectopic ACTH. Therefore, ectopic ACTH production is the least common of the three major causes in the general population.

Clinical Features of Ectopic Adrenocorticotropic Hormone Syndrome

Manifestations of the ectopic ACTH syndrome include hypokalemia, hyperglycemia, edema, muscle weakness (especially proximal) and atrophy, hypertension, and weight loss. Features

TABLE 35.3

USUAL TREATMENT OF HYPONATREMIA

Treatment	Dosage	Uses
Fluid restriction	800–1000 mL limit/24 h	Serum sodium <130 mEq/L and symptomatic Acute and chronic hyponatremia
Hypertonic saline (3% saline)	0.1 mg/kg/min	Rarely used Acute severe hyponatremia (mental status changes, coma)
Demeclocycline	Initial dose: 900–1200 mg/d in divided doses Maintenance: 600–900 mg/d	Chronic hyponatremia
Lithium carbonate (rarely used)	600–900 mg p.o. daily	Chronic hyponatremia Significant toxicity
Urea (rarely used)	30 g in 100 mL orange juice or water daily	Chronic hyponatremia

typically seen in long-standing pituitary or adrenal Cushing's syndrome (e.g., central obesity, plethoric facies, cutaneous striae, "buffalo hump," and hyperpigmentation) are less common in highly malignant tumors such as small cell lung carcinoma but occur more frequently in more indolent tumors such as carcinoids, thymomas, and pheochromocytomas.

Diagnosis

The biochemical diagnosis of Cushing's syndrome is suggested by an elevated 24-hour urinary-free cortisol (>100 μg per 24 hours). The other principal screening test is the overnight low-dose dexamethasone suppression test. The test is positive when 1 mg of dexamethasone given at midnight is unable to suppress the following 8:00 AM cortisol to <5 μg per dL. Failure of cortisol to suppress after high-dose dexamethasone (8 mg at midnight) suggests either ectopic ACTH or a primary adrenal tumor (13). These two are differentiated by measuring plasma ACTH. In primary adrenal tumors, ACTH levels are below 20 pg per mL, whereas in ectopic ACTH levels are generally >100–200 pg per mL and frequently are elevated above 1000 pg per mL. Inferior petrosal sinus sampling of ACTH is useful in confirming the diagnosis of pituitary Cushing's syndrome (14), but it is rarely indicated in the patient with advanced malignancy secreting ectopic ACTH.

Difficulties arise in differentiating those rare tumors producing ectopic CRH from the more common ectopic ACTH production; CRH stimulates release of pituitary ACTH. The clinical presentation and biochemical results are identical for ectopic CRH and ACTH. The prognosis and therapy are identical for the two disorders.

TABLE 35.4

TUMORS ASSOCIATED WITH ECTOPIC ADRENOCORTICOTROPIC HORMONE/CORTICOTROPIC HORMONE SYNDROME

Small cell lung carcinoma
Thymoma
Pancreatic islet cell tumor
Carcinoid tumors (lung, gut, pancreas, ovary)
Medullary carcinomas of the thyroid
Pheochromocytomas

Treatment of Ectopic Adrenocorticotropic Hormone Syndromes

Where possible, the treatment of ectopic ACTH syndrome should be directed primarily at the tumor. Palliative treatment of Cushing's syndrome involves inhibition of steroid synthesis. Drugs successfully used include aminoglutethamide, metyrapone, mitotane, ketoconazole, and octreotide acetate (15). Rarely, bilateral adrenalectomy is considered.

Aminoglutethamide blocks the first step in cortisol biosynthesis. At higher doses, it inhibits production of glucocorticoids, mineralocorticoids, and androgens, whereas at lower doses it primarily inhibits the conversion of androgens to estrogens, contributing to its efficacy in the treatment of postmenopausal breast cancer. At the higher doses required to treat ectopic ACTH syndrome, many patients experience sedation, ataxia, and skin rashes. Metyrapone inhibits 11-β-hydroxylase and 18-hydroxylase, resulting in adrenal atrophy and necrosis. It is a toxic drug with significant gastrointestinal side effects, including anorexia, nausea, vomiting, and diarrhea, and central nervous system (CNS) toxicity, including lethargy and somnolence. For these reasons, it is used as second-line therapy.

Ketoconazole acts mainly on the first step of cortisol biosynthesis but also inhibits the conversion of 11-deoxycortisol to cortisol. It can cause rare but significant reversible hepatotoxicity and is associated with nausea and vomiting.

Octreotide acetate, a long-acting analog of somatostatin, can reduce ectopic ACTH secretion. It must be injected, is expensive, and is only partially effective in most patients. The efficacy of these treatments can be monitored by 24-hour urine cortisol measurements. As levels return to normal and then fall below normal, replacement with glucocorticoids and mineralocorticoids in physiologic doses similar to patients with Addison's disease is frequently necessary. In cases of stress, these patients require stress doses of glucocorticoids (e.g., hydrocortisone 100 mg intravenously every 8 hours).

HYPERCALCEMIA

Malignancies are frequently associated with disorders of calcium metabolism, including hypercalciuria and hypercalcemia, and are the most common cause of hypercalcemia in hospitalized patients. After primary hyperparathyroidism, they are the second most common cause overall. Malignancies produce hypercalcemia by one of three mechanisms. Neoplasms may secrete parathyroid hormone-related protein (PTHrP), which, although distinct from PTH, has sufficient amino-terminal homology with PTH to mimic its effects on PTH receptors. This is the most common mechanism subserving malignancy-associated hypercalcemia, accounting for 80% of all cases (16). PTHrP is produced most commonly by squamous cell cancers (head, neck, lung, and esophagus), renal cell carcinoma, and breast cancer. Metastases with extensive localized bone destruction constitute the second most common mechanism of tumor-related hypercalcemia. Finally, hematologic neoplasms (e.g., multiple myeloma and lymphoma) cause hypercalcemia by releasing osteoclast-activating cytokines, and occasionally (in lymphomas), 1,25-dihydroxy-vitamin D. Patients with malignancy may also have hypercalcemia from a cause unrelated to their cancer. In particular, hypercalcemia from primary hyperparathyroidism is a common disorder in the general population.

Most cancer-related hypercalcemia complicates an advanced malignancy that is already diagnosed and associated with a poor prognosis. Rarely, the tumor is occult and requires an extensive workup to unmask it. The features of advanced cancer typically dominate the presentation, with weight loss, anorexia, fatigue, and pain from bone metastases. The hypercalcemia is more acute and severe (often >14 mg/dL) than is typical for primary hyperparathyroidism and is more likely to cause nausea, vomiting, dehydration, and changes in mentation (hypercalcemic crisis). When possible, treatment is directed toward the primary tumor. Hypercalcemic crisis is treated medically (Table 35.5). Patients with severe hypercalcemia are typically dehydrated, with resultant diminished urine output. This further exacerbates the hypercalcemia by reducing the ability of the kidneys to eliminate calcium in the urine. Therefore, the first step in treating hypercalcemia is vigorous hydration to reestablish urine output and calciuresis. After adequate rehydration, loop diuretics such as furosemide can be used to further promote a calciuric diuresis. This therapy has the advantage of working rapidly (over hours) but is limited by incomplete calcium-lowering effects and the need for intravenous fluids. Calcitonin injections are often used concomitantly with hydration because of their rapid action, although their efficacy is somewhat limited by modest calcium-lowering effects and by tachyphylaxis. Intravenous infusion of a bisphosphonate, either pamidronate or zoledronate, is the most consistently effective treatment of cancer-related hypercalcemia, although the infusion has a delay in of 1–2 days in the onset of action. A single infusion will normalize calcium

levels in most patients with a persistent duration of action lasting a few weeks to several months. Increased bone resorption by PTHrP-activated osteoclasts is the mechanism subserving most cancer-related hypercalcemia and intravenous bisphosphonates effectively block this pathway. Therefore, the usual therapy in hypercalcemic crisis is to begin rapid onset, partially effective therapy with hydration and calcitonin, while giving an infusion of a bisphosphonate that will have potent calcium-lowering effects in a day or two. Other therapies are used in selected cases of hypercalcemia. For example, glucocorticoids are useful calcium-lowering agents in hematologic malignancies and in hypercalcemia mediated by vitamin D intoxication. Many other therapies, commonly used in the past, have been supplanted by the safety and potency of bisphosphonates. These include intravenous and oral phosphates, gallium nitrate, plicamycin, and indomethacin.

HYPOCALCEMIA

Hypocalcemia is an uncommon paraneoplastic syndrome occurring primarily in patients with bony metastases. It occurs most commonly in association with osteoblastic metastases of the breast, prostate, and lung; its incidence is approximately 16% (17). Tetany is a rare complication of tumor-associated hypocalcemia. The etiology of the hypocalcemia is not understood. Ectopic calcitonin secretion from the underlying tumor has been rarely implicated. Acute hypocalcemia is treated by i.v. calcium gluconate or calcium chloride (Table 35.6). Vitamin D and calcium supplements are the therapeutic mainstays of all forms of chronic hypocalcemia.

ONCOGENIC HYPOPHOSPHATEMIC OSTEOMALACIA

Oncogenic hypophosphatemic osteomalacia, an acquired form of adult-onset, vitamin D–resistant rickets, is associated with mesenchymal tumors, often benign, that occur in soft tissues or bones (18). These tumors are also referred to as *ossifying mesenchymal tumors, giant cell tumors of bone, sclerosing hemangioma,* or *cavernous hemangioma*. This syndrome has been rarely reported with other cancers, such as lung and prostate. The clinical syndrome can precede the

TABLE 35.5

USUAL TREATMENT OF HYPERCALCEMIC CRISIS

Treatment	Dosage	Advantages	Disadvantages
Rehydration	As needed	Rapid action	None
Saline diuresis (optional)	150–200 mL/h of normal saline with or without 40 mg/d furosemide	Rapid action	Partial response, risk of fluid overload
Calcitonin (optional)	200 units SQ q 6 h	Rapid action	Partial response, tachyphylaxis
Pamidronate	60 or 90 mg i.v. over 4 h	Potent, normalizes calcium in over 90% of cases. Prolonged response.	1–2 day delay in action
Zoledronate	4 mg i.v. over 30 min	Potent, normalizes calcium in over 90% of cases. Prolonged response.	1–2 day delay in action
Prednisone (in select cases)	60 mg daily	Suitable for oral outpatient therapy	Effective only in select patients, for example, some hematologic malignancies

TABLE 35.6

MANAGEMENT OF HYPOCALCEMIA

Acute symptomatic hypocalcemia (tetany)

1. 10% calcium gluconate (90 mg of elemental calcium/10 mL ampule)
   - Dilute 2 × 10-mL ampules of calcium gluconate in 50–100 mL of D5 solution. Infuse 2 mg/kg body weight over 5–10 min; or 10% calcium chloride (272 mg of elemental calcium/10 mL ampule)
   - Dilute 1 × 10-mL ampule in 50–100 mL of D5 solution. Infuse 2 mg/kg over 5–10 min.
2. Following rapid loading infusion, reduce to a slower infusion of 15 mg/kg of calcium gluconate mixed with D5 infused over 6–12 h.

Chronic hypocalcemia

1. Oral elemental calcium 1–2 g in 2–3 divided doses
2. Vitamin D replacement (approximate doses only)
   - 1,25-Dihydroxyvitamin D: 0.25–2.0 μg/d
   - Vitamin D: 25,000–100,000 IU/d

discovery of the tumor by several years. Clinical and laboratory features include osteomalacia, severe phosphaturia, renal glycosuria, hypophosphatemia, normocalcemia (normal parathyroid hormone levels), and increased alkaline phosphatase. The proposed mechanisms for this syndrome include inhibition of the conversion of 25-hydroxyvitamin D to 1,25-dihydroxyvitamin D and through a substance produced by the tumor with a phosphaturic effect, "phosphatonin." A candidate gene for "phosphatonin" has recently been described—fibroblastic growth factor 23 (19). Treatment is directed at surgical resection of the underlying tumor. When this is not possible, treatment with high doses of vitamin D and phosphate is often required.

HYPERURICEMIA

Uric acid is a metabolite of purine catabolism. Hyperuricemia can be present in a mild form resulting from high turnover of cancer cells in large tumors, or in an acute form as a component of the tumor lysis syndrome. The tumor lysis syndrome is a complication of anticancer therapy in which abrupt necrosis of a bulky tumor releases large amounts of intracellular ions and other metabolites. The resulting metabolic abnormalities include hyperuricemia, hyperphosphatemia, hypocalcemia, and acute renal failure. The tumor lysis syndrome is observed most commonly in pediatric patients and young adults with lymphomas or leukemias, but is also occasionally recognized in older patients with solid tumors. The hyperuricemia results from rapid release and catabolism of purine-containing intracellular nucleic acids. Plasma levels of uric acid exceed secretory pathways and uric acid crystals precipitate in the renal tubules producing acute renal failure.

Tumor lysis syndrome can usually be prevented by identifying patients at risk before initiating chemotherapy. Risk factors include large, actively growing tumors (especially lymphomas) that are expected to be sensitive to cytotoxic therapy, patients with preexisting renal insufficiency, and patients with preexisting elevations in uric acid levels. In patients with these risk factors, allopurinol and intravenous hydration can be initiated prior to cytotoxic therapy. In hyperuricemia resistant to allopurinol, the urate oxidase enzyme rasburicase can be used to rapidly normalize uric acid levels. Rasburicase infused intravenously (0.2 mg/kg/day) converts uric acid to the more soluble compound allantoin, decreasing uric acid levels by 86% within 4 hours (20). Clinical features of tumor lysis syndrome include lethargy, nausea and vomiting from hyperuricemia; spasms, seizures, and tetany from hypocalcemia; and oliguric

renal failure. Laboratory findings include hyperphosphatemia, hyperkalemia, azotemia, hyperuricemia, and hypocalcemia. Supportive care and monitoring in an intensive care unit is required. In patients with oliguric renal failure, hemodialysis is indicated for uncontrolled hyperkalemia, persistent hyperphosphatemia complicated by symptomatic hypocalcemia, or hypervolemia.

HYPERTHYROIDISM

Most commonly, human chorionic gonadotropin (hCG) is secreted by trophoblastic or germ cell tumors (21). Because of its evolutionary homology with the thyroid-stimulating hormone (TSH), hCG has intrinsic thyrotropic action. Overt hyperthyroidism usually occurs with large tumors secreting large quantities of hCG, such as gestational trophoblastic disease (e.g., choriocarcinoma, hydatidiform mole) and testicular tumors. The hyperthyroidism resolves with surgical resection of the underlying tumor. When necessary, treatment of the hyperthyroidism is achieved by using antithyroid drugs such as propylthiouracil or methimazole.

GYNECOMASTIA

Gynecomastia is defined as *palpable breast tissue in men* (22) and may be caused by drugs that lower testosterone levels (23), including alkylating agents, vinca alkaloids, and nitrosureas. Antiemetics, such as metoclopramide and phenothiazines, may produce gynecomastia by stimulating prolactin production. Alternatively, tumor production of gonadotropins or estrogens may result in gynecomastia; these include adrenal and testicular tumors and hepatomas. Tumors that produce hCG can stimulate estrogen production by interstitial and Sertoli cells of the testes, resulting in gynecomastia. The approach to the treatment of gynecomastia includes treatment of the underlying tumor and, if implicated, cessation of drugs known to cause gynecomastia.

Treatment of gynecomastia with antiestrogens and androgens such as tamoxifen citrate, clomiphene citrate, topical dihydrotestosterone, and danazol is generally unsuccessful. For more severe cases, long-term management with liposuction and subcutaneous mastectomy may be necessary. Low-dose radiation therapy has been used with some success for the treatment of painful gynecomastia.

CALCITONINEMIA

Calcitonin is a polypeptide hormone produced by the C cells of the thyroid. It diminishes the release of calcium from bone and increases the excretion of urine calcium, sodium, and phosphate. Interestingly, no clinical syndromes are associated with tumor production of calcitonin except for one reported case of a patient with small cell carcinoma with hypercalcitoninemia and hypocalcemia (24). Calcitonin plays an important role as a tumor marker in monitoring patients with medullary carcinoma of the thyroid and in the diagnosis of multiple endocrine neoplasia type 2, a familial disorder characterized by medullary carcinoma of the thyroid, parathyroid adenomas, and pheochromocytoma. In addition to medullary thyroid carcinoma, a number of other cancers have been associated with elevations in calcitonin, including small cell (48–64%) and other lung cancers, carcinoid, breast cancer, colon cancer (24%), and gastric cancer (38%). With the exception of medullary thyroid carcinoma, the clinical usefulness of serum calcitonin levels as a tumor marker remains undetermined (25).

ACROMEGALY

Most cases of acromegaly result from overproduction of growth hormone by pituitary tumors. Growth hormone elevations may also result from production of growth hormone–releasing hormone by tumors, particularly pancreatic islet-cell tumors and bronchial carcinoids. Treatment of this paraneoplastic syndrome is directed at the treatment of the underlying tumor. Occasionally, growth hormone–releasing hormone secretion responds to administration of long-acting somatostatin analogs (26).

CARCINOID SYNDROME

Carcinoid tumors are of neuroendocrine origin and are usually (74% of the time) found in the gastrointestinal tract with the most common locations being the small bowel, the appendix, and the rectum. Other gastrointestinal sites include the esophagus, bile ducts, pancreas, and liver. They are also found outside the gastrointestinal tract in the larynx, thymus, lung, breast, ovary, urethra, and testis.

The classic carcinoid syndrome is characterized by flushing, diarrhea, and bronchospasm. Less frequent signs and symptoms associated with carcinoid tumors include coronary artery spasms leading to angina pectoris, pellagra, endocardial fibrosis, arthropathy, and hypotension (Table 35.7). Cardiac symptoms can be particularly disabling in some patients, manifesting primarily as right-sided heart failure. Cardiac disease is caused by fibrous deposits on the endocardial surface of the right side of the heart, particularly on the tricuspid and pulmonary valves. This leads to valvular insufficiency or stenosis (27,28). Because of the drainage of bronchial carcinoids into the pulmonary veins, these tumors cause fibrous deposits on the mitral valve.

Acute symptoms in the carcinoid syndrome are due primarily to the production of 5-hydroxytryptophan (serotonin), although secretion of other hormones, such as bradykinin, hydroxytryptamine, and prostaglandins, may also play a role. Useful biochemical markers include measurement of serum 5-hydroxytryptophan and 24 hour urine collections for the serotonin metabolite 5-hydroxyindoleacetic acid.

The peak incidence of carcinoid tumors is in the sixth and seventh decades. Carcinoid tumors are slow growing and tend to metastasize to regional lymph nodes and the liver. Because

TABLE 35.7

SYMPTOMS AND COMPLICATIONS OF CARCINOID TUMORS

Symptoms of carcinoid syndrome	Flushing, diarrhea, wheezing, hypotension, cyanosis, arthralgias
Complications of carcinoid tumors	Right-sided heart failure Left-sided heart failure (rare) Intestinal obstruction Biliary obstruction Gastrointestinal bleeding Pellagra

of their indolent nature, prognosis tends to be very good for most patients. A recent large survey of over 8000 patients with carcinoid syndrome demonstrated a median 5-year survival of 50% (29). Patients with the most common type of carcinoid tumor, localized to the small bowel, had a 5-year survival of 80%.

Surgery is the mainstay of treatment for localized tumors. Debulkment of primary tumors remains an option for patients with metastatic involvement of regional lymph nodes or the liver. The medical treatment of the carcinoid syndrome is directed at inhibiting serotonin synthesis and at blocking its effects peripherally. Different drugs can be used to accomplish these goals (30), albeit with variable and inconsistent results. Antiserotonin agents such as cyproheptadine hydrochloride and methysergide can ameliorate the diarrhea. For long-term treatment, cyproheptadine hydrochloride is the preferred medication because of the risk of retroperitoneal, cardiac, and pulmonary fibrosis associated with methysergide. Antidiarrheal agents such as loperamide hydrochloride and diphenoxylate hydrochloride also can be quite helpful in controlling the diarrhea. Flushing appears to be due to the secretion of histamine. The administration of a combination of H_1 and H_2 histamine receptor antagonists can often control this symptom. Somatostatin analogs such as octreotide acetate are the most commonly used medications used to control symptoms of carcinoid syndrome and are effective in controlling the symptoms of flushing and diarrhea in up to 75% of patients (26). Local control of metastatic disease in the liver can also be attempted with radiofrequency ablation and arterial chemoembolization (31).

Carcinoid syndrome associated with bronchial carcinoid tumors has distinctive features. Many patients experience improvement in symptoms with glucocorticoids or phenothiazines.

ENTEROENDOCRINE TUMORS OTHER THAN CARCINOID

Recently, there has been an increased recognition and characterization of the heterogeneous group of rare gastroenteropancreatic neuroendocrine neoplasms. They vary in terms of their degree of malignancy and their biological behavior and clinical course. They may be quite small or large and bulky. Depending on their cell type, they can produce a number of different endocrine syndromes. These include hypoglycemia (insulinoma), Zollinger Ellison syndrome (gastrinoma), watery diarrhea, hypokalemia-achlorhydria (VIPoma), glucagonoma syndrome (glucagonoma), and so on. The primary treatment for both cure and palliation is surgery. However, they are also treated with drugs or agents that target the tumor's specific product or its effects. Most of these tumors show some response to somatostatin analogs. Because of their slow growth, patients often survive for many years with these tumors (32).

EXTRAPANCREATIC TUMOR HYPOGLYCEMIA

Tumors most likely to cause hypoglycemia are of mesodermal origin, such as fibrosarcomas and mesotheliomas, or of epithelial origin, such as hepatomas, adrenal cortical carcinomas, and gastrointestinal adenocarcinomas. Hypoglycemia usually occurs in the late stages of malignancy. The mechanism by which hypoglycemia occurs involves a combination of impaired hepatic glucose production and increased peripheral glucose utilization. Many patients have poor nutritional status, with depleted stores of the glycogen and protein needed to sustain hepatic glycogenolysis and gluconeogenesis. Hepatic damage from metastases further limits the ability to sustain gluconeogenesis. In most patients, however, hypoglycemia results predominantly from increased peripheral glucose utilization, raising the possibility of production of hormones with insulin-like properties. Insulin levels, as well as levels of insulin-like growth factor I and growth hormone, are low, whereas insulin-like growth factor II (IGF-II) levels are usually normal. Recent work has focused on the tumor production of an abnormally processed variant of IGF-II, "big IGF-II." This variant is not measured in usual radioimmunoassays for IGF-II but possesses normal biological activity. It is likely that "big IGF-II" accounts for many or most cases of tumor hypoglycemia (33,34).

Symptoms of hypoglycemia result from neuroglycopenia (confusion, seizures, and coma) or from activation of the adrenergic nervous system (sweating, palpitations, hunger, and tremors). The presence of tumor-associated hypoglycemia is established by demonstrating a low serum glucose level (<40–50 mg%) in a patient with symptoms of hypoglycemia who responds to oral or intravenous glucose. No further diagnostic workup is necessary. The primary treatment is nutritional support, either oral or intravenous. For immediate relief of symptomatic hypoglycemia, glucose is given as an intravenous bolus of 50% dextrose and then continued as a drip of 10% glucose. Refractory hypoglycemia can be treated with the counterregulatory hormones glucagon or cortisone.

SOMATOSTATIN ANALOGS

Somatostatin was first discovered as a hypothalamic hormone-inhibiting growth hormone secretion (35,36). It is now known that it is secreted at multiple sites throughout the human body. Somatostatin has physiologic effects on multiple endocrine and exocrine secretions (37). In the pituitary, the secretion of growth hormone, prolactin, and thyrotropin is inhibited. In the gastrointestinal tract, somatostatin inhibits the secretion of cholecystokinin, gastric inhibitory peptide, gastrin, motilin, neurotensin, and secretin. The secretion of glucagon, insulin, and pancreatic polypeptide is inhibited in the pancreas. In the CNS, somatostatin acts as a neurotransmitter in distinct pathways and as a neuromodulator, modulating the release of other neurotransmitters such as serotonin and acetylcholine. Somatostatin also inhibits a number of exocrine secretions such as amylase from the salivary glands, hydrochloric acid and pepsinogen by gastrointestinal mucosa, pancreatic enzymes and bicarbonate from the pancreatic acini, and bile by the liver. It also regulates gastrointestinal motility.

Two distinct effects of somatostatin have made it very useful in the treatment of certain cancers that express somatostatin receptors. Somatostatin has been shown to inhibit the growth of both normal and tumorous cells by inhibiting cell division and triggering cell death by apoptosis (38,39). In patients with growth hormone–secreting pituitary tumors, somatostatin has been shown to reduce tumor size by 10–25% in approximately 50% of cases (40). Because a variety of endocrine tumors express somatostatin receptors, it is also used in the treatment of a number of paraneoplastic syndromes, as already mentioned. Because of its short plasma half-life, natural somatostatin has limited therapeutic potential. The first two longer acting and more potent somatostatin analogs developed were octreotide and lanreotide, but only octreotide is available in the United States. An intermediate acting form of octreotide is administered subcutaneously every 8 hours and a long-acting form is administered by intramuscular injection every 28 days (41). Radiolabeled somatostatin analogs have also been used as either tumor tracers or therapeutic agents (42).

Because of its potent antisecretory effects, somatostatin analogs are among the few oncologic agents that are continued in patients with paraneoplastic syndromes in spite of tumor progression (43). The most common side effects are a direct consequence of somatostatin's numerous actions on the endocrine and exocrine systems. Side effects are primarily gastrointestinal and include diarrhea, abdominal pain, flatulence, biliary tract abnormalities, and nausea and vomiting. More serious adverse effects include cholecystitis and ascending cholangitis (44).

ENDOCRINE DISEASES IN PATIENTS WITH CANCER

Malignancies often occur in patients with preexisting medical conditions such as diabetes mellitus and thyroid disease. Treatment of these conditions must continue during and after treatment of the malignancy and during palliative care. In each condition, goals of treatment must be reevaluated with prognosis of the underlying malignancy in mind.

DIABETES MELLITUS

Standard guidelines for the treatment of both type 1 and type 2 diabetes mellitus can generally be followed in the patient with cancer; however, the appropriateness of "tight control" needs to be addressed in these patients. On the basis of results of the Diabetes Control and Complications Trial (45), it is accepted that intensive insulin treatment of type 1 diabetes results in a decrease in microvascular complications. These results have been extrapolated to type 2 diabetes mellitus (46); however, in the patient with cancer with a limited life expectancy, intensive insulin therapy to prevent long-term complications is not a reasonable goal. The major complication of intensive insulin therapy is an increased risk of hypoglycemia. In patients with malignancies and poor nutrition, the risk of hypoglycemia is further increased. Additionally, intensive insulin treatment requires frequent blood glucose monitoring, which may place a further burden on the patient and his or her caregivers. Sulfonylurea agents are frequently included in treatment regimens for type 2 diabetes. In the cancer population with suboptimal nutrition, recent weight loss, or impaired kidney or liver function, these agents should be used with extreme caution. Severe prolonged hypoglycemia can result from the use of sulfonylurea drugs. Many patients with type 2 diabetes previously treated with these agents can have their diabetic medication discontinued because of normalization of blood glucose levels secondary to weight loss and poor calorie intake.

Diets should be tailored to meet the needs of the individual patient. Patients with poor appetite and decreased oral intake should be allowed to liberalize their diets from the traditional "diabetic diet." Patients may experience early satiety and mechanical problems with chewing and swallowing; nutritional supplementation with commercial products may be necessary. Consultation with a registered dietitian is helpful when devising an appropriate diet for the patient with cancer who has diabetes.

In summary, when choosing an appropriate treatment for diabetes mellitus in the cancer population, reasonable goals should be chosen. An attempt should be made to avoid symptomatic hyperglycemia, to decrease the risk of hypoglycemia, and to provide the patient with as many dietary choices as possible.

DIABETES AND GLUCOCORTICOID THERAPY

Glucocorticoids are used as adjunctive therapy in a number of chemotherapeutic regimens. Frequently they are given in high doses and/or intermittently. The use of steroids can increase blood glucose in patients with preexisting diabetes or can cause new hyperglycemia in patients with previously normal blood glucose. The latter is referred to as steroid-induced diabetes. In those individuals without diabetes, the risk of steroid-induced diabetes is increased with a family history of diabetes, increasing age, obesity, and increasing glucocorticoid dose (47). Glucocorticoids cause hyperglycemia by a number of different mechanisms. They increase hepatic glucose production and inhibit insulin-stimulated glucose uptake in peripheral tissues (48). They also have a direct effect on beta cell function although this is less well understood (49).

Glucocorticoids differ in their effects on carbohydrate metabolism. With hydrocortisone, produced by the adrenal glands, as a reference point, the synthetic steroids prednisone and dexamethasone are 3.5–4 times and 30 times more potent than hydrocortisone in decreasing carbohydrate metabolism, respectively (50).

The effect of glucocorticoids on carbohydrate metabolism is transient and reversible. This has been demonstrated in patients on alternate day steroids whose blood glucose levels were higher on the day they received steroids (51). There is a characteristic pattern of hyperglycemia caused by steroids. The fasting glucose is minimally elevated with exaggerated postprandial hyperglycemia. When steroids are dosed once a day, the blood glucose peak usually occurs 8–12 hours later (52). Following discontinuation of steroids, blood glucose usually returns to baseline within 2–3 days.

The treatment of diabetes in the face of glucocorticoid therapy can be challenging. Whereas diet therapy is important, when used alone, it is rarely effective in controlling hyperglycemia caused by high-dose steroids (53). Oral sulfonylurea agents are occasionally effective, particularly in patients with lower fasting blood glucose levels (<200 mg per dL.) However, most patients will need insulin and, in many cases, large doses of insulin. For patients receiving high doses of glucocorticoids in the hospital, a variable-rate intravenous insulin infusion should be considered (54). This is particularly useful for the patient receiving intravenous pulse steroids because insulin requirements can change rapidly throughout the day. Regular insulin is used exclusively in intravenous infusions.

For the patient receiving subcutaneous insulin, the two most common regimens consist of NPH insulin twice daily at breakfast and supper, and insulin glargine once daily at bedtime or in the morning. For patients whose blood glucose levels are >200 mg per dL, a reasonable starting dose of "basal" insulin is 0.3 units per kg, with the expectation that rapid increases in dosage may be necessary in the subsequent 2–3 days on the basis of the blood glucose response. When using NPH insulin, two thirds of the dose is administered in the morning and one third before supper. Regular insulin or a rapid acting insulin analog is given premeal if the patient is eating or every 6 hours if the patient is NPO (52). Correction dose insulin therapy, also known as *supplemental insulin*, should be administered before meals and at bedtime in the patient who is eating or every 4–6 hours in the patient who is NPO. Blood glucose levels should be reviewed on a daily basis and the scheduled insulin doses revised if correction doses are frequently required. Alternate day steroids require alternate day insulin regimens.

EUTHYROID SICK SYNDROME

Severe illness, whether acute or chronic, can cause changes in thyroid physiology, leading to what has been referred to as the *euthyroid sick syndrome* (55). Changes can occur in levels of total thyroxine (T_4) and, to a lesser extent, free thyroxine and TSH levels. T_4 is decreased because of its decreased binding to its serum transport proteins. The decrease in triiodothyronine (T_3) results from inhibition of 5'-deiodinase, the enzyme that converts T_4 to T_3. Low T_4 levels are associated with a higher mortality rate; TSH levels are generally helpful in distinguishing euthyroid sick syndrome from pituitary hypothyroidism. In addition, free thyroxine levels are usually normal.

ADRENAL INSUFFICIENCY

Because of the vascular nature of the adrenal cortex, the adrenal glands are common sites of metastatic disease. Typically, adrenal metastases are found incidentally during abdominal computed tomography and magnetic resonance imaging scans and are usually of no functional significance. In a minority of cases, bilateral adrenal cortical destruction is sufficiently advanced to impair normal functioning and result in deficient production of cortisol (56). Symptoms of adrenocortical deficiency overlap with typical symptoms of advanced malignancy and include weight loss, fatigue, nausea, anorexia, and hypotension. Either hyponatremia or hyperkalemia heightens suspicion for the presence of adrenal insufficiency.

The ACTH stimulation test is the most direct diagnostic study used to exclude adrenocortical insufficiency. A normal test contains the following three elements: a morning basal cortisol of at least 7–9 µg per dL, an increase >7 µg per dL 30 minutes after administration of 0.25 mg intravenous ACTH, and a maximum response to intravenous ACTH of 18–20 µg per dL or higher.

Severely symptomatic adrenal insufficiency (*adrenal crisis*) is treated with intravenous saline and stress doses of hydrocortisone, 100 mg intravenously every 8 hours, tapered to a chronic oral maintenance dose of 20 mg every morning and 10 mg every evening. Patients with concomitant aldosterone deficiency resulting in hyperkalemia may also require the addition of the oral aldosterone analog fludrocortisone acetate (0.05–0.20 mg daily).

OSTEOPOROSIS IN THE PATIENT WITH CANCER

Osteoporosis has become a serious public health concern, leaving patients at risk for low trauma fractures of the hip, vertebrae, ribs, wrist, pelvis, and humerus. Patients with cancer may be at risk for osteoporosis because of preexisting factors such as age, low body weight, tobacco use, and family history of osteoporosis. Their risk may be further increased by the administration of glucocorticoids, immobilization or inactivity, and hypogonadism.

Postmenopausal women with osteoporosis should be treated according to current National Institutes of Health (NIH) consensus guidelines (57,58). The approach to the premenopausal woman with osteoporosis is less well defined. Women with a history of malignancy are at risk for osteoporosis for a number of reasons, including premature menopause. Significant bone loss can occur within the first year after the onset of amenorrhea in patients treated with chemotherapy, including aromatase inhibitors, for breast cancer (59). Maintenance of adequate calcium and vitamin D intake is essential but may not be adequate to maintain bone density. Oral bisphosphonates, such as alendronate and risedronate, have been used with some success in the prevention of bone loss in patients with breast cancer (60). Many patients with cancer experience chemotherapy-induced nausea, vomiting, or gastrointestinal difficulties, which may preclude the use of oral bisphosphonates. Intravenous bisphosphonates such as pamidronate and zoledronate have been shown to be safe and efficacious in the prevention of bone loss in patients with premenopausal breast cancer receiving chemotherapy (61).

Though osteoporosis is considered a "woman's disease," men are also clearly at risk. Certain malignancies are associated with an increased risk of osteoporosis in both men and women, such as multiple myeloma. Recently, there has also been growing concern regarding the increased risk of osteoporosis in the patient with prostate cancer who is treated with androgen deprivation therapy (ADT). Because sex hormones are a major contributing factor for the maintenance of bone density in men, androgen deprivation has a major impact on bone loss and increased risk for fracture (62). ADT can take several forms. It may either be achieved surgically through bilateral orchiectomy or medically, usually with luteinizing hormone-releasing hormone (LHRH) agonist therapy. Studies indicate that men treated with ADT for prostate cancer lose bone mass to the extent of 4–10%, and are at increased risk for fracture (63).

Given the known risk for bone loss in men treated with ADT for prostate cancer, men need a careful clinical evaluation including a comprehensive medical history and diagnostic workup, which will detect most risk factors for osteoporosis. Patients with prostate cancer who have musculoskeletal complaints should receive a prompt evaluation. If bony metastases are present, they should be treated with acute radiation therapy or surgical intervention, as needed. Currently, the indications for obtaining a bone mineral density (BMD) test in men are the following: vertebral abnormalities identified on x-ray that are indicative of osteoporosis, low bone mass, or vertebral fracture; long-term glucocorticoid use; diagnosis of hyperparathyroidism; monitoring of osteoporosis treatment. However, many experts now recommend that, for patients with prostate cancer being treated with ADT, a baseline dual-energy x-ray absorptiometry (DEXA) scan be obtained before initiation of ADT. If the baseline test is normal, a DEXA should be repeated every 1–2 years after the patient has received at least 1 year of ADT.

Men with abnormal bone density test results should be counseled on lifestyle changes including smoking cessation, regular weight bearing exercise, and reduction in alcohol intake if excessive. Those individuals diagnosed with low bone density (sometimes referred to as osteopenia) or osteoporosis should begin dietary intake of calcium at 1200 mg per day and supplemental vitamin D 400 IU per day. In addition, pharmacologic interventions may be indicated (64). Bisphosphonates are the most widely used medications for the prevention and treatment of osteoporosis in men. Alendronate is the only bisphosphonate that is FDA approved for the general treatment of osteoporosis in men, although both risedronate and alendronate are approved for the treatment of glucocorticoid-induced osteoporosis in both men and women. Bisphosphonates have two potential uses for men with advanced prostate cancer. They may help maintain bone mass and they may delay skeletal progression of the cancer. Intravenous forms of bisphosphonates such as pamidronate and zoledronic acid are indicated for the treatment of bone metastases. Other agents currently under investigation include estrogen, bicalutamide (a competitive inhibitor of androgen action with little effect on circulating testosterone levels), and raloxifene, a selective estrogen receptor modulator (SERM), currently indicated for the prevention of osteoporosis in postmenopausal women.

References

1. Hansen M, Hammer M, Humer L. Diagnostic and therapeutic implications or ectopic hormone production in small cell lung cancer. *Thorax* 1980;35:101.
2. Comis RL, Miller M, Ginsberg SJ. Abnormalities in water homeostasis in small cell anaplastic lung cancer. *Cancer* 1980;45:2414.
3. Odell WD, Wolfsen AR. Humoral syndromes associated with cancer. *Annu Rev Med* 1978;29:379–406.
4. Tang WW, Kaptein EM, Feinstein EI, et al. Hyponatremia in hospitalized patients with the Acquired Immunodeficiency Syndrome (AIDS) and the AIDS-Related complex. *Am J Med* 1993;94:169.
5. Sorensen JB, Andersen MK, Hansen HH. Syndrome of inappropriate secretion of antidiuretic hormone (SIADH) in malignant disease. *J Intern Med* 1995;238:97.
6. Hantman D, Rossier B, Zohlman R. Rapid correction of hyponatremia in the syndrome of inappropriate secretion of antidiuretic hormone: an alternative treatment to hypertonic saline. *Ann Intern Med* 1973;78:870.
7. Sterns RH. Severe symptomatic hyponatraemia: treatment and outcome. *Ann Intern Med* 1987;107:656.
8. Ayus JC, Olivero JJ, Frommer JP. Rapid correction of severe hyponatraemia with intravenous hypertonic saline solution. *Am J Med* 1982;72:43.
9. Decaux G, Brimioulle S, Genette F. Treatment of the syndrome of inappropriate secretion of antidiuretic hormone by urea. *Am J Med* 1980;69:99.
10. Hale AC, Besser GM, Rees LH. Characterisation of pro-opiomelanocortin derived peptides in pituitary and ectopic adrenocorticotrophin secreting tumors. *J Endocrinol* 1986;108:49.
11. Tanaka K, Nicolson WE, Orth DN. The nature of immunoreactive lipotropins in human plasma and tissue extracts. *J Clin Invest* 1978;62:94.
12. Raff H, Findling JW, Aron DC. A new immunoradiometric assay for corticotropin evaluated in normal subjects and patients with Cushing's syndrome. *Clin Chem* 1989;35:596.
13. Tyrell JB, Findling JW, Aron DC, et al. An overnight high-dose dexamethasone suppression test for rapid differential diagnosis of Cushing's syndrome. *Ann Intern Med* 1986;104:180.
14. Oldfield EH, Chrousos GP, Schulte HM, et al. Preoperative lateralization of ACTH-secreting pituitary microadenomas by bilateral and simultaneous inferior petrosal venous sinus sampling. *N Engl J Med* 1985;312:100.
15. Pierce ST. Paraendocrine syndromes. *Curr Opin Oncol* 1993;5:639.
16. Wysolmersk JJ, Broadus AE. Hypercalcemia of malignancy: the central role of parathyroid hormone-related protein. *Annu Rev Med* 1994;45:189.
17. Raskin P, McClain CJ, Medsger TA. Hypocalcemia associated with metastatic bone disease. *Arch Intern Med* 1973;132:539.
18. Salassa RM, Jowsey J, Arnaud C. Hypophosphatemic osteomalacia associated with "nonendocrine" tumors. *N Engl J Med* 1970;283:65.
19. Quarles DL, Drezner MK. Pathophysiology of X-linked hypophosphatemia, tumor-induced osteomalacia, and autosomal dominant hypophosphatemia: a perPHEXing problem. *J Clin Endocrinol Metab* 2001;86:494–496.
20. Goldman SL, Holcenberg JS, Finklestein JZ, et al. A randomized comparison between rasburicase and allopurinol in children with lymphoma or leukemia at high risk for tumor lysis. *Blood* 2001;97:2998.
21. Caron P, Salandini AM, Plantavid M. Choriocarcinoma and endocrine paraneoplastic syndromes. *Eur J Med* 1993;2:499.
22. Glass AR. Gynecomastia. *Endocrinol Metab Clin North Am* 1994;23:825.
23. Thompson DF, Carter JR. Drug-induced gynecomastia. *Pharmacotherapy* 1993;13:37.
24. Gropp C, Havemann K, Scheuer A. Ectopic hormones in lung cancer patients at diagnosis and during therapy. *Cancer* 1980;46:347.
25. Silva OL, Broder LE, Doppman JL, et al. Calcitonin as a marker for bronchogenic cancer: a prospective study. *Cancer* 1979;44:680.
26. Lamberts SW, van der Lely AJ, de Herder WW. Octreotide. *N Engl J Med* 1996;334:246.
27. Pellikka PA, Tajik AJ, Khandena BK, et al. Carcinoid heart disease. Clinical and echocardiographic spectrum in 74 patients. *Circulation* 1993;87:1188–1196.

28. Anderson AS, Karuss D, Lang R. Cardiovascular complications of malignant carcinoid disease. *Am Heart J* 1997;134:693–702.
29. Modlin IM, Sander A. An analysis of 8305 cases of carcinoid tumors. *Cancer* 1998;79:813–829.
30. Gregor M. Therapeutic principles in the management of metastasizing carcinoid tumors: drugs for symptomatic treatment. *Digestion* 1994; 55(Suppl 3):60.
31. Diaco DS, Hajarizadeh H, Mueller CR. Treatment of metastatic carcinoid tumors using multimodality therapy of octreotide acetate, intra-arterial chemotherapy and hepatic arterial chemoembolization. *Am J Surg* 1995;169:523.
32. Warner RRP. Enteroendocrine tumors other than carcinoid: a review of clinically significant advances. *Gastroenterology* 2005;128:1668.
33. Phillips LS, Robertson DG. Insulin-like growth factors and non-islet cell tumor hypoglycemia. *Metabolism* 1993;42:1093.
34. Zapf J. Role of insulin-like growth factor II and IGF binding proteins in extrapancreatic tumor hypoglycemia. *Horm Res* 1994;42:20.
35. Reichlin S. Somatostatin. *N Engl J Med* 1983;309:1495.
36. Reichlin S. Somatostatin. *N Engl J Med* 1983;309:1556.
37. Krantic S, Goddard I, Saveanu A, et al. New modalities of somatostatin actions. *Eur J Endocrinol* 2004;151:643.
38. Bevan JS. Clinical review: the antitumoral effects of somatostatin analog therapy in acromegaly. *J Clin Endocrinol Metab* 2005;90:1856.
39. Lamberts SWJ, Reubi J-C, Krenning EP. The role of somatostatin analogues in the control of tumor growth. *Semin Oncol* 1994;21:61.
40. Newman CB, Melmed S, George A, et al. Octreotide as primary therapy for acromegaly. *J Clin Endocrinol Metab* 1998;83:3034.
41. Delaunoit T, Rubin J, Neczyporenko F, et al. Somatostatin analogues in the treatment of gastroenteropancreatic neuroendocrine tumors. *Mayo Clin Proc* 2005;80:502.
42. DeJong M, Valkema R, Jamar F, et al. Somatostatin receptor-targeted radionuclide therapy of tumors: preclinical and clinical findings. *Semin Nucl Med* 2002;32:133.
43. Oberg K, Kvols L, Caplin M, et al. Consensus report on the use of somatostatin analogs for the management of neuroendocrine tumors of the gastroenteropancreatic system. *Ann Oncol* 2004;15:966.
44. Freda PU. Somatostatin analogs in acromegaly. *J Clin Endocrinol Metab* 2002;87:3013.
45. DCCT Research Group. Epidemiology of severe hypoglycemia in the diabetes control and complications trial. *Am J Med* 1991;90:450.
46. UK Prospective Study (UKPDS) Group. Intensive blood-glucose control with sulphonylureas or insulin compared with conventional treatment and risk of complication in patients with type 2 diabetes (UKPDA 33). *Lancet* 1998;352:837–853.
47. Ruiz JO, Simmons RL, Callender CO, et al. Steroid diabetes in renal transplant recipients: pathogenic factors and prognosis. *Surgery* 1973;73:759.
48. Boyle PJ. Cushings disease, glucocorticoid excess, glucocorticoid deficiency, and diabetes. *Diabetes Rev* 1993;1:301.
49. Kalhan SC, Adam PAJ. Inhibitory effect of prednisone on insulin secretion in man: model for duplication of blood glucose concentration. *J Clin Endocrinol Metab* 1975;41:600.
50. Conn JW, Fajans SS. Influence of adrenal cortical steroids on carbohydrate metabolism in man. *Metabolism* 1956;5:114.
51. Greenstone MA, Shaw AB. Alternate day corticosteroid causes alternate day hyperglycemia. *Postgrad Med J* 1987;63:761.
52. Clement S, Braithwaite SS, Magee MF, et al. Management of diabetes and hyperglycemia in hospitals. *Diabetes Care* 2004;27:553.
53. Miller MB, Neilson J. Clinical features of the diabetic syndrome appearing after steroid therapy. *Postgrad Med J* 1964;40:660.
54. Hirsch IB, Paauw DS. Diabetes management in special situations. *Endocrinol Metab Clin North Am* 1997;26:631.
55. Docter R, Krenning EP, de Jong M. The sick euthyroid syndrome: changes in thyroid hormone serum parameters and hormone metabolism. *Clin Endocrinol* 1993;39:499.
56. Redman BG, Pazdur R, Zingas AP. Prospective evaluation of adrenal insufficiency in patients with adrenal metastasis. *Cancer* 1987;60:103.
57. NIH Consensus development panel on osteoporosis prevention, diagnosis, and therapy. *JAMA* 2001;285:785.
58. Rosen CJ. Postmenopausal osteoporosis. *N Engl J Med* 2005;353:595.
59. Ganz PA, Greendale GA. Menopause and breast cancer: addressing the secondary health effects of adjuvant chemotherapy. *J Clin Oncol* 2001;19:3303.
60. Delmas PD, Balena R, Confravreux E, et al. Bisphosphonate risedronate prevents bone loss in women with artificial menopause due to chemotherapy of breast cancer: a double-blind, placebo controlled study. *J Clin Oncol* 1997;15:955.
61. Fuleihan GE, Salamoun M, Mourad YA, et al. Pamidronate in the prevention of chemotherapy-induced bone loss in premenopausal women with breast cancer: a randomized controlled trial. *J Clin Endocrinol Metab* 2005;90(6):3209.
62. Shahinian VB, Kuo YF, Freeman JL, et al. Risk of fracture after androgen deprivation for prostate cancer. *N Engl J Med* 2005;352:154.
63. Preston DM, Torrens JI, Harding P, et al. Androgen deprivation in men with prostate cancer is associated with an increased rate of bone loss. *Prostate Cancer Prostatic Dis* 2002;5:304.
64. Amin S, Felson DT. Osteoporosis in men. *Rheum Dis Clin North Am* 2001;27:19.

CHAPTER 36 ■ HEADACHE AND OTHER NEUROLOGIC COMPLICATIONS

WENDY C. ZIAI

Intracranial pathology can result in a variety of distressing symptoms. Fortunately, the underlying cause can often be identified and treated, and the accompanying symptoms commonly respond to supportive measures. This chapter is divided into two sections. The first deals with headache and other symptoms of intracranial pathology and reviews their pathogenesis and management strategies. Although nausea and vomiting are common in patients with intracranial pathology, this topic is covered elsewhere. The second section reviews cancer-related neurologic syndromes, such as brain metastasis, base of skull metastasis, and cerebrovascular disease; oncologic interventions and supportive care strategies are outlined for each.

SYMPTOMS OF INTRACRANIAL PATHOLOGY

Headache

Assessment

Principles of headache assessment used for the general medical population can be useful for patients with a cancer history, with one important exception: headache in a patient with cancer may be the presenting symptom of a serious complication of the disease or its treatment which compels an early and thorough assessment for a structural disease. This assessment begins by confirming the onset, duration, progression, and focality of the headache. Pain characteristics include qualitative descriptors, severity, exacerbating and relieving features, associated symptoms, and the outcome of analgesic drugs or other therapies. Although prior headache history is important, the burden of proof is to rule out a new and serious cause of headache; brain metastasis can present with a headache similar to a previously experienced benign headache (1).

Cancer or its treatment can cause headache in a variety of ways. Some processes are considerably more likely to occur at particular points along the course of the disease. For example, approximately 90% of patients who die of melanoma have central nervous system metastases at autopsy; disseminated metastases are less likely to occur until regional metastases have developed. Therefore, the cancer history, extent of known disease, and prior treatments should be determined for all patients with cancer and a headache.

The physical examination of the patient with cancer and a headache begins with a general physical examination and screening neurologic examination, including examination of the ocular fundi, range of motion of the cervical spine, and assessment for meningismus. Provocation of the pain by the examiner can be informative: an underlying pathologic process is usually not far from the area of tenderness. Sites of pain indicated by the patient should be inspected and palpated. The examiner should palpate over facial sinuses, bony skull prominences, the occipitonuchal junction, and neck arteries. The orbits should be gently palpated and examined for proptosis. If the patient's pain is provoked by any of these maneuvers, the pain referral pattern should be noted.

Although comprehensive investigations can help identify cancer-related causes of headaches, the extent of investigation should be guided according to the clinical situation. Bone scintigram, computed tomography (CT) of the head with fine bone windows, magnetic resonance imaging (MRI), and spinal fluid examinations are all commonly used in headache assessment. Blood tests can include serum hemoglobin, blood gas levels, and sedimentation rate.

Head pain usually originates from intracranial or extracranial pain-sensitive structures. Nociceptive input from these sites arises by displacement, distention, or inflammation of vascular structures, sustained contraction of muscles, or direct pressure on nerves. Alternatively, head pain may start from nonnociceptive mechanisms arising from damage to peripheral or central pain pathways that subserve the head.

Anatomy of Head Pain

Pain-sensitive structures in the head include the fifth, ninth, and tenth cranial nerves (CNs); the upper three cervical nerves; and the great venous sinuses and their tributaries from the surface of the brain. In addition, all the tissues covering the cranium including skin, muscles, blood vessels, especially the arteries, and periosteum of the skull are pain sensitive. The cranial bones, diploic and emissary veins, brain parenchyma, parts of the dura, most of the pia mater and arachnoid, and the ependymal lining of the ventricles and choroid plexus, are insensitive to pain.

Nociceptive input from supratentorial structures, including the superior surface of the tentorium cerebelli, causes pain to be felt anterior to a line drawn from the ears across the top of the head. Damage to these structures activates branches of the trigeminal nerve. Nociceptive input from infratentorial structures, including the inferior surface of the tentorium cerebelli, causes pain posterior to this line and is conveyed by sensory fibers in the fifth, seventh, ninth, and tenth CNs and the upper three cervical nerves (2).

Primary and Secondary Headaches

Primary headaches, migraines, tension-type headaches, cluster headaches, and others are the most frequent types of headache in western society. They are functional disorders that, by definition, are characterized by the absence of a structural lesion. In contrast, secondary headaches are symptomatic of an underlying disease, either an intracranial lesion or a systemic process. The International Headache Society has provided a comprehensive classification of headache that identifies eight groups of secondary headaches (3) (Table 36.1). Although a temporal relationship between the headache and the underlying disorder is usually apparent, the diagnosis can be challenging because of the high prevalence and similar features of primary headaches.

The incidence of headache in patients with primary or metastatic brain tumors is approximately 50% (4). Headache is a presenting symptom in 30–60% of adult patients with brain tumor, and 60–70% of patients develop headache during the course of this illness (4). Headache is not commonly an isolated symptom of intracranial tumors, only 8% in one prospective Italian study (5). Primary and metastatic brain tumors had a similar incidence of headache in a New York–based study (1), although other studies report a higher occurrence of headache in primary than in metastatic tumors (4,5). The median duration of headache at diagnosis, ranging from 3.5 weeks in the New York study (1) to 15.7 months in a study from Bangkok (4), may depend on socioeconomic factors, such as access to neurosurgical expertise and early neuroradiological detection.

Factors reported to influence the incidence of headache in patients with brain tumors include tumor location, rate of growth, increased intracranial pressure (ICP), size of the enhancing lesion, amount of midline shift, and a history of previous headache (1). Headache occurs more commonly in infratentorial (64–84%) than supratentorial (34–60%) tumors (2,4) and is especially common with midline and basal tumors (95 and 70%, respectively). Slow-growing tumors such as low-grade supratentorial astrocytomas and neuroepithelial tumors (including gangliogliomas, dysembryoplastic neuroepithelial tumors, and pleomorphic xanthoastrocytomas) have a low headache incidence but are frequently associated with seizures (2). Faster-growing tumors, particularly high-grade

gliomas, have been reported to cause headaches in approximately one-half of patients but a lower incidence of seizures.

The classic brain-tumor headache is characterized by its progressively increasing severity, frequency, and duration; early morning awakening; disappearance after rising; association with nausea and vomiting; and aggravation by exertion, sneezing, coughing, or Valsalva's maneuver. This syndrome is actually uncommon, occurring in only 17–28% of patients (2). In reality, no single headache pattern is typical of a brain tumor. The most common headache profile is bifrontal, often worse ipsilaterally, dull, nonthrobbing, and aching in nature. These characteristics are similar to a tension-type headache. The pain is usually mild to moderate, intermittent, and relieved by simple analgesics in approximately one-half of patients. Severe headaches are reported by approximately 40% of patients, and 45% indicate that headache is the worst symptom. Also, 30–70% of patients experience nocturnal headache, and only 18–36% report early morning headache. Positional changes, either supine to standing or standing to supine, induce or aggravate the headache in 20–32%; in 18–23% of patients, the headache worsens with Valsalva's maneuvers. Nausea and vomiting are associated with headache in 36–48% of patients (2,4).

Brain-tumor headaches may mimic primary headaches. Forsyth and Posner (1) found that tumor headaches were similar to tension-type headaches in 77% of patients; 9% of patients had migraine-like headaches and 14% had other types. In one study of patients with cancer and a significant history of prior headache, 78% experienced new headaches associated with their brain tumor (2). The brain-tumor headache may be similar to the patient's prior headache but is generally more severe, frequent, or associated with new symptoms or abnormal signs.

The location of the headache in relation to tumor site, the presence of raised ICP, and the localizing value of focal headache depend on the mechanism by which the headache is produced. Two mechanisms commonly account for headache in patients with brain tumor:

1. Direct traction or distortion of pain-sensitive structures by the tumor mass
2. Distant traction through extensive displacement of brain tissue, either directly by the mass (e.g., herniation syndromes) or by hydrocephalus caused by obstruction of cerebrospinal fluid (CSF) pathways (2).

Direct traction accounts for the localizing value of headaches in patients without raised ICP. Supratentorial tumors not associated with raised ICP often produce bilateral headache in the frontal region (85%). Unilateral headache is present in 28–53% (2,4), and the headache usually lateralizes to the side of the tumor. With the exception of cerebellopontine-angle tumors, which are more likely to produce symptoms by the compression of adjacent CNs, posterior fossa tumors often present with occipital or neck pain as the first symptom.

The headache of increased ICP tends to be severe, aching, and constant; is unrelieved by simple analgesics; is worse in the morning and with Valsalva's maneuvers; and is associated with nausea or vomiting. It is most commonly located in the frontal region, either bifrontal or vertex, or in the neck alone. Occasionally, increased ICP accounts for the surprising occurrence of occipital headaches in association with a supratentorial tumor or frontal headache together with a posterior fossa tumor. Sudden-onset headache or rapid exacerbation of headache may represent hemorrhage into a tumor, pituitary apoplexy, or intraventricular tumor such as colloid cyst of the third ventricle causing obstruction of CSF and increased ICP. Severely increased ICP can ultimately result in life-threatening cerebral herniation syndromes and sudden death.

TABLE 36.1

SECONDARY CAUSES OF HEADACHE

Head trauma
Vascular disorders
Nonvascular intracranial disorder
Substances or their withdrawal
Noncephalic infection
Metabolic disorder
Disorder of cranium, neck, eyes, ears, nose, sinuses, teeth, mouth or other facial structures, cranial neuralgias, nerve trunk pain, and deafferentation pain
Headache not classifiable

Adapted from Olesen J. Headache classification committee of the International Headache Society: classification and diagnostic criteria for headache disorders, cranial neuralgias, and facial pain. *Cephalalgia* 1988;7(Suppl 8):1, with permission.

INTRACRANIAL PATHOLOGY: ANALGESIC STRATEGIES

Management strategies for patients with pain from intracranial pathology derive from general principles of supportive care and focus on both oncologic and analgesic interventions (Table 36.2). The use of surgery to manage symptoms from intracranial pathology is limited to highly selected patients to relieve specific syndromes that are refractory to more conservative treatment. For example, rare patients undergo resection of a large cerebellar metastasis to reduce severe headache, despite the presence of other, less symptomatic, metastatic lesions. Others are offered shunt insertion for hydrocephalus or percutaneous aspiration of a tumor cyst through an Ommaya reservoir, if relief of mass effect on initial aspiration results in a significant relief of symptoms. Radiotherapy is frequently effective relieving pain or other symptoms from metastatic disease, even if the primary tumor is relatively radiation resistant (6). If the goal of treatment is limited to symptom control alone, patients are generally candidates for radiotherapy if life expectancy is greater than 2 months and symptoms are not easily managed with more conservative means.

Chemotherapy can be palliative for metastatic intracranial disease from specific tumor primaries, including breast (7), small cell carcinoma of the lung (8), testes (9), and others. Hormonal therapy can be well tolerated and can be effective in shrinking metastatic disease in patients with breast or prostate cancer who have not been previously exposed to such treatment.

The role of corticosteroids to manage symptoms from intracranial pathology requires particular emphasis. An empiric course over a few days can be used to establish efficacy. Dexamethasone, the preferred agent, is available in oral and parenteral formulations and generally lacks mineralocorticoid (salt-retaining) effect, but has an increased risk of hyponatremia which may lead to increased edema generation. Nonfluorinated corticosteroids such as prednisone may have less risk of causing myopathy (10). The dose–effect relationship of dexamethasone is a controversial subject, and the optimum dose for tumor-related cerebral edema has not been established. Comparison of 4-, 8- and 16-mg per day dexamethasone (Decadron) therapy in 89 patients with CT-proved brain metastasis, no signs of impending herniation, and Karnofsky scores of 80 or less showed the same degree of improvement in Karnofsky score over 1 week and more frequent

toxicity in the 16-mg per day group over 4 weeks (11). Another study of 12 patients with brain metastasis treated with high-dose dexamethasone for 48 hours reported complete responses in only 3 patients, partial response in 1, and no response in 8 (12). Other reports support the use of steroid doses much higher than the conventional 4 mg every 6 hours, up to 96 mg over 24 hours, suggesting that the ideal dexamethasone dose should be established for each individual patient (13). Other therapies which may contribute to reducing brain edema include prevention of overhydration, severe hypertension, and seizures; use of furosemide; and, in severe situations, use of osmotherapy with mannitol or hypertonic saline and surgery when consciousness is impaired or brain herniation is imminent (14).

In patients with brain tumor, cushingoid facies predict the presence of steroid myopathy (10). Other side effects of steroids include hyperglycemia, present in nearly 50% treated over a long period (14), cataracts, osteoporosis, and dose-dependent neuropsychiatric effects, seen in 18.5% of patients at doses greater than 12 mg per day Decadron (80 mg per day prednisone) (15). The side effects can become disabling over time. To reduce the risk of side effects, the lowest effective dose of steroid should be identified by methodical titration upward or downward.

NEUROPATHIC PAIN DUE TO CENTRAL NERVOUS SYSTEM DISEASE

Central pain is defined as pain associated with a lesion of the central nervous system, particularly of the spinothalamic tract or thalamus (16). Central pain must be differentiated from other types of neuropathic pain associated with lesions of the peripheral nervous system and from nociceptive pain associated with ongoing stimulation of nociceptors by a tissue-damaging lesion. Current theories of central pain postulate selective deafferentation of the spinothalamic tract over prior concepts of thalamic pain as the more likely underlying mechanism (17).

Many types of structural lesions in the brain and spinal cord can cause central pain. Although the type, duration, and size of the lesion can influence the tendency to produce central pain, similar lesions may or may not be painful or may produce different types of pain (16). Only a few patients with susceptible lesions actually develop central pain. The locations of the most painful lesions are in the spinal cord, lower brain stem, and ventral posterior part of the thalamus (16). The most common causes of these lesions are spinal cord trauma and cerebrovascular accidents. Interestingly, intracranial and spinal tumors have a low prevalence of central pain and the few described cases refer to expansive lesions in the contralateral parietal cortex, not thalamic tumors (17). Several patients have reported central pain due to meningioma. In a series of 49 patients with thalamic tumors, only one had central pain (18).

The diagnosis of central pain depends on a detailed neurologic history and examination along with laboratory investigations, including CT scans or MRI, CSF analysis, neurophysiologic testing, and other tests as appropriate. Symptoms characteristic of central pain are rarely psychogenic in origin (16).

The onset of central pain may be immediate or delayed, first appearing years after the original problem. Although the pain typically has a burning, tingling, or "pins and needles" quality, it may be superficial, deep, or both. It is not always dysesthetic and can have a variety of descriptors in the same or different regions. The sensation is often unlike any prior experience and

---

TABLE 36.2

MANAGEMENT STRATEGIES FOR PAIN FROM INTRACRANIAL PATHOLOGY

Oncologic interventions
Radiation therapy: conventional, radiosurgery
Surgery: resection, shunt insertion, percutaneous aspiration of cyst
Chemotherapy

Analgesic interventions
Pharmacotherapy: opioids, anticonvulsants, antidepressants, corticosteroids
Physical measures
Psychologic measures
Neurolytic or anesthetic procedures
Neurostimulatory procedures
Acupuncture

is typically difficult to describe (16). The pain may be triggered by physical activity, stress, loud noise, vibrations, weather changes, altered muscle or visceral function, or seizures. It is usually constant, varies in severity from mild tingling to unbearable, and may have more than one element; commonly, a severe intermittent component is superimposed on constant pain. Central pain is usually permanent, although transient pain in patients with spinal cord injury and complete cessation of pain either spontaneously or after the occurrence of new lesions have been reported (16). Although not necessary for its development, central pain is usually associated with a sensory deficit in the same area as the pain. Hypesthesia to temperature is the most common finding. Sensory deficits are consistent with the site of the known lesion; for example, ventral posterior thalamic lesions may be associated with a hemibody sensory loss, and low brainstem infarcts may produce a crossed, dissociated sensory loss.

The management of central pain is based largely on clinical experience. Treatment modalities include pharmacotherapy, sensory stimulation, neurosurgical procedures, and sympathetic blockade (19). The first-line drugs are antidepressants with noradrenergic properties, specifically amitriptyline hydrochloride, which appears to be the most effective but also has the most side effects. Other medications have been found to be effective in randomized controlled trials for central pain, including intravenous lidocaine (20), intravenous morphine (21), oral lamotrigine (19), and gabapentin (22). Carbamazepine and other membrane-stabilizing drugs may be useful as second agents for the treatment of central pain, although carbamazepine at doses up to 800 mg per day in one study did not produce significant pain relief compared with placebo (23). The best central pain response to antidepressants is seen in post-stroke patients, whereas antiepileptic drugs (AEDs) seem to be most effective for paroxysmal central pain (19). Nonsteroidal anti-inflammatory drugs and oral opioids generally have a weak or no effect. A range of other therapies are used, including γ-aminobutyric acid (A) agonists (e.g., diazepam [Valium]), intrathecal (IT) baclofen, clonidine, neuroleptics, systemically administered local anesthetics, and naloxone hydrochloride (19). Patients with brain injury should be treated for motor spasticity which can contribute to chronic pain with resultant loss of function. Stimulation techniques include low- and high-frequency transcutaneous electrical nerve stimulation, spinal cord stimulation, and deep brain stimulation. Motor-cortex stimulation, a relatively new technique, is reported to benefit certain forms of intractable pain (24). Transection of spinal nerves (e.g., dorsal root entry zone lesions) or cordotomies are offered to patients primarily with intractable cancer-related pain and have limited temporal effectiveness of about 1 year before recurrence which is more difficult to manage (25).

CRANIAL NEURALGIAS

Cranial neuralgias are of particular significance to the patient with cancer, as they frequently lead to a diagnosis of base of skull or neck metastases. Also, the frequent response of these pain syndromes to a regimen containing selected adjuvant analgesics (e.g., anticonvulsants) highlights the value of prompt diagnosis. Trigeminal and glossopharyngeal neuralgias are characterized by paroxysmal lancinating pain in the face or throat and neck, respectively. Pain lasts from a few seconds to a minute or two, with frequent recurrence. The pain is often spontaneous at onset, but it may be initiated by sensory stimuli such as touch or tickle applied to certain trigger areas; movements such as chewing or talking can also precipitate pain. Other features, such as continuous dull aching, burning, or pressure pain, are often reported (26). The differential diagnosis includes disorders of the jaw, teeth, sinuses, base of skull, and neck. Although these neuralgias are most commonly idiopathic, the onset of cranial neuralgia in a patient with a cancer history mandates a search for metastatic disease. Numb chin syndrome, involving facial and oral numbness in the distribution of the mental nerve, has been associated with a metastatic etiology in 89% of patients (27). Radiologic studies include CT scan or MRI with views of the base of skull and sinuses. Plain radiographs or tomograms of the skull base may show abnormalities. CSF analysis may be abnormal in patients with associated leptomeningeal metastases (LM).

SEIZURES

A seizure may be defined as an episode of uncontrolled motor, sensory, or psychological activity caused by the sudden excessive discharge of cerebral cortical neurons (28), followed by a postictal phase of metabolic cerebral depression lasting a variable period. The first appearance of any seizure during adulthood, with or without a localizing aura, is sufficiently suspicious to warrant an investigation for neoplasm.

Generalized or focal seizures occur in 20–50% of patients with brain tumors (28). The occurrence of a seizure depends on the tumor site, type, and infiltration or expansive properties. In patients with supratentorial tumors, seizures are a presenting symptom in up to half of patients (29). The highest seizure incidences occur with oligodenrogliomas (92%), astrocytomas (70%), meningiomas (67%), and glioblastomas (37%) (29). In patients with slow-growing chronic tumors, the seizure incidence is as high as 75% and may predate other symptoms for years (29). Focal seizures are associated with tumors involving the motor cortex, the sensory cortex, or the temporal lobe. Temporal lobe gliomas typically produce psychomotor seizures, with or without olfactory hallucinations (uncinate fits); abnormal visual or auditory perception; déjà vu phenomenon; or automatic behavior (28). Parietal lobe tumors may cause generalized or focal sensory seizures, and occipital lobe neoplasms have been associated with an aura of flashing lights, but not formed images. Infratentorial tumors and neoplasms involving only the white matter are not commonly associated with seizures.

In patients with intracerebral metastases, the occurrence of seizures at presentation or during the course of illness was 27% in one series of 470 patients (30). The most common primary sites were melanoma (67% incidence of seizures), lung (48%), breast (32%), and unknown primary tumor (55%). With the exception of malignant melanoma and choriocarcinoma, metastatic brain neoplasms are less likely to cause seizures than primary brain tumors. The presence of multiple metastases or combined brain and LM are the conditions most frequently associated with seizures. Seizures associated with cerebral metastases are usually of the simple or complex partial type.

Seizures can be an indication of tumor progression or recurrence. Other etiologies, such as electrolyte disturbances (e.g., hyponatremia), drug interactions, and noncompliance with anticonvulsants may predispose to late development of seizures. *Status epilepticus*, defined as a persistent seizure (usually considered to last longer than 5 minutes) or repeated seizures without interictal return of consciousness, is a neurologic emergency. Acute management begins with assurance of the airway, ventilation, and perfusion. Blood should be sampled for urgent electrolyte screen and other appropriate tests, and intravenous glucose should typically be given (usually 50 mL of a 50% solution) before any results are known. The typical treatment protocol involves the intravenous administration of a benzodiazepine, such as lorazepam or diazepam, followed by intravenous loading with phenytoin (PHT) or valproate sodium. Persistent seizure activity beyond 7–10 minutes is an indication for continuous electroencephalographic monitoring and to start general anesthetic procedures, with intubation followed by a short-acting barbiturate (pentobarbital sodium), or continuous infusion of midazolam or propofol (28). The minimal dose of anesthetic agents required to stop electrographic seizures is generally recommended. Although focal continuous epilepsy (epilepsy partialis continua) is also treated promptly, this syndrome is less injurious to the patient and is usually treated without the high-dose intravenous drugs administered for generalized status (28).

The routine use of prophylactic anticonvulsants in patients with brain tumor is generally recommended only in patients who present with seizures and in those undergoing craniotomy. Even the evidence that prophylactic antiepileptics prevent postoperative seizures is not consistent (31), although the American Academy of Neurology has a practice guideline that it is appropriate to taper and discontinue prophylactic anticonvulsants after the first postoperative week in patients who have not had a seizure (32). No published data show efficacy of anticonvulsants in preventing seizures beyond the postoperative phase in patients with malignant primary or metastatic brain tumors who have never had a seizure (33). In one study, a 10% incidence of late seizures in patients with brain metastases was noted, regardless of whether prophylactic PHT was given (34); however, serum anticonvulsant levels were subtherapeutic in two thirds of the patients who developed seizures. Two randomized prospective studies with over 130 patients found no significant benefit of prophylactic anticonvulsants in preventing late seizures over placebo or no treatment in patients with brain tumor who had no prior history of seizures (35,36). A meta-analysis of over 400 patients found no AED benefit at 1 week and at 6 months, regardless of neoplastic type (33). One study suggested that patients with cerebral metastases from melanoma should probably receive prophylactic anticonvulsants due to the higher risk of seizures (up to 50%) in this group and a high risk of seizures in those not treated with prophylaxis (37%) (37). The most commonly prescribed drug is PHT, in doses of 300–400 mg per day which, along with carbamazepine, phenobarbital, and the newer anticonvulsant oxcarbazepine, induces P450 enzymes in the liver and may lead to increased metabolism of chemotherapeutic agents with similar metabolism and conversely lower anticonvulsant levels due to their increased metabolism (31). For patients undergoing chemotherapy with a history of seizures, better choices may include valproate sodium, gabapentin, lamotrigine, topiramate, levetiracetam, and zonisamide which are not enzyme inducers (31) (see Table 36.3 for main indications and doses of AED).

Concomitant use of dexamethasone also increases the required dose of AEDs such as PHT and reduces the bioavailability of dexamethasone (38). Toxic PHT levels may occur with frequent dosage adjustments and can produce side effects of nystagmus and ataxia. More serious complications from PHT include erythema multiforme and Stevens-Johnson syndrome, which have been associated with concomitant whole brain radiation therapy (WBRT) (39); myopathy (40); immunosuppressive effects specifically targeted against cell-mediated immunity (41); hepatoxicity; hyperkinetic movement disorder; and osteomalacia (28).

Discontinuation of seizure prophylaxis in patients with a benign tumor and preoperative seizures has been recommended only for patients with complete excision of a benign tumor who remain seizure free after 12 months. The risk of relapse remains at least 35% if the patient has had previous seizures (42).

SINGULTUS (HICCUPS)

Singultus (hiccups) is a forceful involuntary inspiration caused by a spasmodic contraction of the diaphragm that terminates with the sudden closure of the glottis. The closure of the glottis results in the characteristic hiccup sound. Hiccups serve no known physiologic function (43) and are usually a transient benign disorder that resolves without medical therapy. Chronic hiccups may reflect underlying pathology, including a lesion that irritates the peripheral vagus or phrenic nerves, drug toxicity, metabolic abnormalities, infection, and intracranial disease. Rarely, chronic hiccups are psychogenic.

The mechanism of hiccup may involve dysfunction of peripheral components or central connections of the reflex arc. The afferent neural pathway is composed of sensory branches of the phrenic and vagus nerves as well as dorsal sympathetic afferents from T6 through T12. The principal efferent limb, which produces the diaphragmatic contraction, includes motor fibers of the phrenic nerve and efferent branches to the glottis and external intercostal muscles (inspiratory). There is reciprocal inhibition of the expiratory intercostal muscles. The separate innervation of right and left hemidiaphragms and the long course of the two phrenic nerves, each of which contacts various organs, account for the large variety of reported mechanisms for hiccup. Hiccups may be bilateral or unilateral; most of these occur in the left diaphragm. The central control of hiccups, although not yet fully defined, is believed to include a supraspinal center that is integrated with the respiratory center output to respiratory motor neurons in the spinal cord (44). Experimental electrical stimulation of the medulla in cats has demonstrated the generation of hiccup-like responses in the medullary reticular formation lateral to the nucleus ambiguus, just rostral to the obex (45). Cells in the nucleus raphe magnus containing the inhibitory neurotransmitter γ-aminobutyric acid may be the source of inhibitory inputs to the hiccups reflex arc. The reported rate of repetitive hiccups is between 4 and 60 per minute; the most common rate is 17–20 per minute—not surprisingly, similar to the respiratory rate (43).

Central nervous system causes of hiccups include parenchymal lesions within the medulla and local pathology causing medullary compression. Both these lesions can produce dysfunction at the level of the vagal nucleus and the nucleus tractus solitarius (43). It has also been suggested that central nervous system conditions causing hiccups may release the normal inhibitory tone on the hiccup reflex arc (43). Specific lesions of the medulla include neoplasms, syringomyelia, infarction (often the territory of the posterior inferior cerebellar artery), and infections, including meningitis, encephalitis, neurosyphilis, and human immunodeficiency virus encephalopathy. Compressive lesions causing hiccups include neoplasms, hematomas, cavernomas, and bleeding into the fourth ventricle (46). Most lesions develop slowly, are located near the dorsolateral aspect of the medulla, and extend toward the obex (46).

Identification of serious underlying causes of hiccups depends on their duration, severity, and associated conditions. Benign hiccups may last up to 48 hours and are usually related to gastric distension, alcohol ingestion, or emotional factors. Persistent hiccups are defined as a hiccup episode lasting longer than 48 hours but less than 1 month, and intractable hiccups persist longer than a month. Both are assumed to have an organic etiology until proven otherwise by extensive medical and laboratory investigations.

Neurogenic hiccups may require urgent management. Some patients experience severe fatigue as a result of sleep deprivation. Others develop respiratory irregularity or even respiratory arrest, probably related to a lesion at the medullary respiratory control centers (46). When respiratory difficulties occur, associated brain stem symptoms or signs are usually present. With the exception of intubated patients or those with a tracheotomy, hiccups alone do not produce any significant

TABLE 36.3

ADULT DOSES OF OLD- AND NEW-GENERATION ANTIEPILEPTIC DRUGS AND MAIN INDICATIONS IN SEIZURE DISORDERS

Antiepileptic drug	Main indication in seizure disorders	Adult loading and maintenance dose
FIRST-GENERATION AEDs		
Benzodiazepines		
Lorazepam	SE	Lorazepam: 0.1 mg/kg at 2 mg/min i.v. (SE)
Midazolam	Partial and generalized seizures	Midazolam: 0.3 mg/kg at 4 mg/min i.v. (SE); maintenance: 0.08–0.4 mg/kg/hr (SE)
Diazepam		Diazepam: 0.2 mg/kg at 5 mg/min i.v. (SE)
PHT/phosphenytoin	Partial seizures (with and without secondary generalization); primary generalized TC seizures; SE	Loading dose PHT (i.v./p.o.): 15–20 mg/kg at 50 mg/min i.v. or 15–20 mg/kg PHT equivalents (PE) at 150 mg PE/min Maintenance (i.v./p.o.): 300–400 mg/d. Goal serum level of 10–20 ug/mL or free level 1–2 µg/mL
Carbamazepine	Partial seizures (with and without secondary generalization); primary generalized TC seizures	Loading dose (p.o.): 400 mg (in 2 divided doses) on day 1; increase by 200 mg daily at 1 to 2 week intervals. Maintenance (p.o.): 600–1200 mg/d. Goal serum level of 6–12 µg/mL
Valproic acid	Partial and generalized seizures; SE	Loading dose (i.v./p.o.): 15–20 mg/kg Maintenance (i.v./p.o.): 600–1000 mg/d (monotherapy); 1500–3000 mg/d (combination therapy). Goal serum level of 50–100 µg/mL
Phenobarbital	Partial and generalized seizures (not effective against absence seizures); SE	Loading dose (i.v./p.o.): 15–20 mg/kg at 100 mg/min Maintenance (i.v./p.o.): 120–250 mg/d. Goal serum level of 20–40 µg/mL
Ethosuxamide	Absence seizures, CSWS	Maintenance (p.o.): 500–2000 mg/d. Goal serum level of 40–100 µg/mL
SECOND-GENERATION AEDs		
Gabapentin	Partial seizures (with and without secondary generalization)	Maintenance (p.o.): 900–1800 mg/d (doses up to 6000 mg/d have been used)
Lamotrigine	Partial and generalized seizures (may aggravate severe myoclonic epilepsy of infancy)	Maintenance (p.o.): 100–200 mg/d (if on valproate); 200–600 mg/d (not on valproate)
Oxcarbazepine	Partial seizures (with and without secondary generalization) and primary generalized TC seizures	Maintenance (p.o.): 600–2400 mg/d
Levetiracetam	Partial and probably generalized seizures	Maintenance (p.o.): 1000–3000 mg/d
Topiramate	Partial and generalized seizures (efficacy against absence seizures not proven)	Maintenance (p.o.): 400 mg/d (in two divided doses)
Tiagabine	Partial seizures (with and without secondary generalization)	Maintenance (p.o.): up to 56 mg/d (lower if not on inducers)
Pregabalin	Partial seizures (with and without secondary generalization)	Maintenance (p.o.): 150–600 mg/d
Zonisamide	Partial and probably generalized seizures	Maintenance (p.o.): 300–400 mg/d
Vigabatrin	Infantile spasms (West syndrome). Partial seizures (with and without secondary generalization) refractory to all other AEDs	Maintenance (p.o.): 2000–3000 mg/d
Felbamate	Severe epilepsies, particularly Lennox-Gastaut syndrome, refractory to all other AEDs	Maintenance (p.o.): 1800–3600 mg/d

AED, antiepileptic drug; SE, status epilepticus; PHT, phenytoin; TC, tonic-clonic; CSWS, continuous spike-waves during slow sleep.
Adapted from Perucca E. An introduction to antiepileptic drugs. *Epilepsia*, 2005;46(Suppl 4):31–37; with permission.

ventilatory effect because the glottis closes almost immediately after the onset of diaphragmatic contraction (44).

The management of hiccups includes physical, pharmacologic, and surgical interventions. Initial therapy should focus on elimination or treatment of the underlying cause. Physical stimulation of afferent nerve endings or certain end organs may interrupt the hiccup reflex arc. Traditional remedies include swallowing sugar, breathing into a bag, and breath holding. Physiologically, the hiccup reflex is inhibited by high arterial carbon dioxide tension.

Pharmacologic measures for hiccups are supported by anecdotal experience. Numerous classes of drugs have been used, including antipsychotics, tricyclic antidepressants, anticonvulsants, antiarrhythmics, central nervous system stimulants, muscle relaxants, inhalation agents, local anesthetics, and gastric motility agents. The most commonly used and the most consistently effective agent is chlorpromazine, a centrally acting major tranquilizer and dopamine antagonist. It is especially effective when given as an intravenous bolus (47). The second drug of choice is metoclopramide, a gastric motility agent and dopamine antagonist (47). Other valuable agents include the anticonvulsants carbamazepine, PHT, and valproic acid and the antispasmodic baclofen. Baclofen with gabapentin as an add-on therapy has been recommended for hiccups in the palliative care population (47). Surgical interventions are reserved for intractable hiccups that fail to respond to physical or pharmacologic therapy. Phrenic nerve transection, crushing, or anesthetic blockade may be complicated by severe respiratory impairment, especially if both the phrenic nerves are disrupted. In addition, such a procedure may fail to relieve hiccups (47). Phrenic nerve surgery is therefore a last resort and should be preceded by a local anesthetic block to assess the efficacy and the potential respiratory compromise from diaphragmatic paralysis (47). Vagus nerve stimulation has been recently reported with complete resolution of spasms following posterior fossa stroke (48).

NEUROLOGIC IMPAIRMENTS CAUSED BY INTRACRANIAL PATHOLOGY

Focal neurologic symptoms such as weakness, numbness, incoordination, and visual impairment can interfere significantly with function. If correctly diagnosed, treatment of the underlying cause or measures to accommodate the deficit may be possible. Several complex neurologic syndromes and specific neuropsychiatric conditions deserve emphasis because of the high degree of impairment and the clinical difficulty in making a correct diagnosis.

Patients with bifrontal disease may appear to the family as lacking initiative and sparkle. Speech is sparse or nonexistent (*mutism*), and yet the patient is fully aware of the conversation around him or her. There may be urinary urgency or incontinence ("unwitting wetting"); a shuffling, wide-based gait; and an apparent slowness of thought processes. Damage to both the frontal lobes can result from radiation therapy or from multiple bilateral metastases, hydrocephalus, leptomeningeal tumor, cerebrovascular disease, or other causes. Findings on examination that support the diagnosis include bilateral grasp reflexes, snout reflex, positive glabellar tap, presence of bilateral palmomental reflexes, and apraxic gait. The patient may be cognitively intact and able to later recall details of events that occurred while he or she was sick. Understanding that the lack of motivation is neurologic, rather than psychological, may help the family cope with the patient's condition.

In the nondominant parietal syndrome, there is denial of illness and the patient may believe that he or she

should be able to manage alone at home despite severe impairment. Brain metastases and cerebrovascular disease are the most common causes. The diagnosis of a nondominant parietal syndrome is confirmed by identifying focal sensory or motor deficits (usually affecting the left side of the body), hemianopsia, dressing, and constructional apraxia, agnosia, and denial of body parts (neglect). The overall management and rehabilitation strategies are similar to those used for other neuropsychologic impairments. The prognosis for improvement is poor as a result of the patient's lack of insight.

Intracranial pathology can also cause delirium and specific disorders of mood or perception. Delirium is an acute organic disorder of attention and cognition. Thinking, perception, memory, and psychomotor status may be disturbed in the delirious patient (35). In contrast to dementia, delirium is acute and potentially reversible. Delirium involves a wide differential diagnosis in which toxic and metabolic disorders are prominent. In addition to neoplasm, many other structural disorders may be responsible, including hydrocephalus, stroke, subdural hematoma, cranial arteritis, and trauma. Delirium may also be caused by seizures. New onset of delirium requires prompt assessment for treatable causes.

Personality changes, including depression, euphoria, loss of inhibition, and impulsive behavior, may also reflect intracranial disease, including raised ICP secondary to a space-occupying lesion. Temporal lobe lesions have been noted to produce bizarre thinking and immature emotional behavior. The diagnosis of these conditions, particularly the organic mood disorders, may be challenging given the high prevalence of primary psychiatric disorders in the cancer population.

CANCER-RELATED NEUROLOGIC SYNDROMES

Brain Metastases

Clinically evident brain metastases occur in 20–30% of patients with systemic cancer and are found at autopsy in up to 50% (49). Two thirds of these patients will have neurologic symptoms during life (50). Metastases are the most common malignant tumor of the brain and have an annual incidence three times that of primary brain tumors (49). The three most common cancers that metastasize to the brain are lung, breast, and melanoma.

Brain metastases tend to be a late finding; evidence of other metastatic disease is usually present. Only 19% of 201 patients with brain metastases studied at the Memorial Sloan-Kettering Cancer Center lacked evidence of systemic metastases on initial evaluation (50). The interval between diagnosis of the primary malignancy and the discovery of brain metastases depends on the tumor type. Small cell lung cancer, for example, metastasizes early; there is an 11% incidence of silent metastases at diagnosis (51). Other tumors, such as breast carcinoma, typically develop brain metastases late, once disseminated disease is present (51). In addition to the primary cancer, factors that influence brain metastases include age and gender (52). Some tumors, such as breast or renal cancers, tend to cause single lesions, whereas others, such as melanoma, lung cancer, and tumors of unknown origin, are more likely to cause multiple metastases (53). In patients with lung cancer and melanoma, men have a greater predilection to develop brain metastases than women, perhaps reflecting the more common site of melanoma in men on the head, neck, and trunk; for lung cancer, explanations for this observation are lacking (52). Certain metastatic brain tumors are prone to hemorrhage: melanoma, choriocarcinoma, renal cell carcinoma, and bronchogenic carcinoma (52). Skull metastases occur with cancers of the breast and prostate (53).

The distribution of brain metastases is proportional to cerebral blood flow as well as brain weight (52). The cerebral hemispheres receive 85% of cerebral blood flow and are the site of approximately 80% of brain metastases. The posterior fossa, the recipient of 15% of cerebral flow, is the site in 20% of metastases (16% in the cerebellum and 3% in the brainstem) (52). The predilection of gastrointestinal and pelvic malignancies to metastasize to the posterior fossa suggests a route of dissemination through Batson's plexus, which may receive venous drainage from the pelvic organs, but the evidence for this is not conclusive.

The location of brain metastases is frequently at the gray–white matter interface or at vascular borders called "watershed zones;" the latter account for one third of the total brain volume, but two thirds of brain metastases (54). In these regions, the blood vessels rapidly branch into end capillaries and may act as a trap for metastatic cell emboli.

The most common presenting symptoms are headache, weakness, and behavioral changes (53). Patients usually have focal findings, which onset over days to weeks and have a progressive course. Although focal signs often suggest the site of metastases, false localizing signs may occur as a result of compression of distant structures by shifts caused by increased ICP. These signs may cause a perplexing constellation of symptoms and signs. Generalized neurologic dysfunction caused by raised ICP may present in an acute or gradual manner.

Headache is the most common initial complaint. It occurs in half of patients with a single brain metastasis, and almost all these patients manifest other signs or symptoms. Patients with multiple or cerebellar metastases have a higher incidence of headache (52,53). Papilledema occurs in less than one fourth of patients with brain metastases. Focal weakness, the second most common presenting symptom, is reported in approximately 40% of patients, although examination reveals weakness in up to two thirds (53). Mental or behavioral changes, an initial finding in 30% of patients, may reflect multiple brain metastases or focal lesions causing raised ICP or hydrocephalus. One study reported that three fourths of patients with brain metastasis failed to score normally on standard mental status tests (55). Seizures, either focal or generalized, are the first signs in 15–20% of patients. Occasionally, transient neurologic events occur with complete resolution; excluding seizures, acute onset of symptoms was reported in less than 10% of patients. The complaint of gait ataxia can result from a posterior fossa tumor, a large frontal lobe lesion, or hydrocephalus. These patients may lack significant unsteadiness on examination. Other presenting symptoms include sensory disturbance and vision loss, typically hemianopsia. The onset of neurologic dysfunction may be insidious, over weeks or months. Intratumoral hemorrhage may cause an acute worsening of preexisting, slowly evolving symptoms.

A study of the diagnostic value of neurologic evaluation for the prediction of intracranial metastases in 68 patients with cancer and a new or changed headache found intracranial metastases in 32% (56). Independent predictors of intracranial metastases were headache duration ≤10 weeks, emesis, and pain that is not of tension type. Other features of the neurologic examination did not contribute to the prediction model.

The most sensitive diagnostic test for brain metastases is gadolinium-enhanced MRI which should be considered for any patient with cancer and an unexplained neurologic disturbance. It is also indicated for neurologically asymptomatic patients undergoing attempted curative treatment of a primary tumor with high metastatic potential to brain, such as lung cancer or metastatic melanoma (53). Gadolinium-enhanced MRI reveals multiple metastases in approximately 70% of patients, compared to 50% with CT scan (57). Features that suggest a metastatic lesion include spherical shape with "ring" enhancement, location at gray–white matter junction, and vasogenic edema.

Evaluation of the status of the systemic cancer is important in determining the appropriate therapy for an intracranial metastasis. Factors that affect the choice of treatment modality for brain metastases include patient age, size, number and location of the metastasis, neurologic status, patient performance status, extent of the primary tumor, other sites of metastatic disease, and response to prior therapy (52). Therapeutic options include surgery, radiation therapy (either focal or whole brain), chemotherapy, and targeted small molecule therapy (58). Supportive treatment alone may be appropriate for patients near death with disseminated disease.

The prognosis for patients with brain metastases depends on many of the same factors mentioned in the preceding text that determine treatment: age, performance status [often determined by the use of the Karnofsky performance status (KPS) score], type of primary tumor, number of brain metastases (single or multiple), and the extent of extracranial disease activity (59).

For patients treated with WBRT, the death rate from neurologic progression of metastases is similar to that of systemic disease (60). Two thirds of patients with serious neurologic dysfunction and one third of patients with moderate dysfunction obtain relief or improvement of symptoms (52). The standard dose is 3000 cGy in 10 fractions (300 cGy per treatment), although regimens vary depending on the center. Protracted radiation therapy regimens (2000 cGy in 20 fractions) have previously been advised when anticipated survival is >1 year owing to a lesser rate of later neurologic complications associated with this regimen (61). Accelerated radiation therapy may be used to achieve rapid palliation in patients whose condition is deteriorating quickly. Prophylactic cranial irradiation is advocated for newly diagnosed patients with cancer and a high risk of developing brain metastases especially for small cell lung cancer for which increased survival advantage and reduction in the rate of brain metastases has been demonstrated (59).

Radiosurgery, which delivers a very high dose of radiation to a small target, has undergone an exponential growth in use and is an alternative to surgery, especially for tumors which are inaccessible or in eloquent brain regions (59). Several reviews of this modality demonstrate comparable survival and local control to combined surgical resection and WBRT and superior local control to surgery alone (59). From a systematic review of randomized trials on patients with cancer and brain metastases, for patients with a single brain metastasis and minimal or absent extracranial disease, surgical excision followed by WBRT improves survival compared with WBRT alone and reduces brain-tumor recurrence, but not survival compared with surgery alone (62). In patients with one to three newly diagnosed brain metastases not operated on, there is a possible small survival benefit of using a radiosurgery boost and WBRT compared to WBRT alone, but only for single metastases (63). The role of WBRT after radiosurgery remains controversial. Altered WBRT dose-fractionation schedules compared with standard fractionation schedules (3000 cGy in ten fractions or 2000 cGy in five fractions) did not change the overall survival or functional neurologic improvement (62). Addition of radiosensitizers or chemotherapy to WBRT has not been shown statistically significant benefits in survival or time to neurologic progression (62). One multicenter analysis by Auchter et al. (64) demonstrated a survival and functional independence advantage of radiosurgery alone over surgical resection plus WBRT with a decrease in deaths from central nervous system progression. Factors influencing the efficacy of radiosurgery include size and shape of the lesion, number of tumors, and nature of the primary tumor. In general, well-demarcated, spherical tumors of small volume (<4 cm), without invasion deep into the brain tissue, respond best to radiosurgery. The risk for distant recurrences increases significantly when more than three metastases are treated in one patient. Radiosurgery treatment for metastases secondary to melanoma and renal cell carcinoma has been associated with high quality of life even in the presence of multiple metastases, compared with patients with lung cancer, who have a significantly shorter life expectancy. Relative contraindications to stereotactic radiosurgery (SRS) include large tumors, hemorrhagic tumors, and tumors producing significant mass effect. Conventional treatment with surgery followed by WBRT is then recommended (Table 36.4).

Of patients who exhibit an initial clinical response to radiotherapy, approximately 80% maintain clinical improvement at 3 months and 60% are stable at 6 months (51). Two thirds of patients who show a major response to radiotherapy die of systemic disease and only 15% die solely as a result of neurologic deterioration (53). The extent of systemic cancer is, therefore, a strong prognostic indicator in patients with brain metastases. The presence of liver or lung metastases predicts poor survival in patients who develop brain metastases.

Surgical interventions in patients with brain metastases encompass procedures to relieve ICP, biopsy to establish diagnosis (principally in patients with an unknown primary), and resection of metastatic lesions. Surgical resection is considered in patients with a single brain metastasis in an accessible location and limited systemic disease (life expectancy >2 months) although removal of significant mass lesions causing mass effect or shunting for hydrocephalus may provide significant quality of life benefit even in patients with worse prognostic factors (59). Unfortunately, only approximately 25% of patients with brain metastases fulfill these indications, as only half of brain metastases are single, and half of single metastases are excluded on account of the inaccessibility of the tumor, extensive systemic disease, or other factors. An additional benefit of surgical intervention is tissue diagnosis; in one study, 11% of patients in one study did not have metastatic tumors despite suggestive radiographic findings (65).

For most patients, WBRT with corticosteroids remains the treatment of multiple brain metastases. Chemosensitive tumors such as small cell lung cancer (SCLC), breast, and germ-cell tumors may benefit from additional chemotherapy, although the role of chemotherapy as initial treatment or salvage therapy is unclear (59). Regression of brain metastases from chemosensitive tumors has occurred after systemically administered cytotoxic chemotherapy (7–9).

Leptomeningeal Metastases

The syndrome of LM (also known as *meningeal carcinomatosis* or *lymphomatous/leukemic meningitis*) refers to diffuse or multifocal seeding of the leptomeninges by systemic cancer, most commonly by hematogenous spread, either arterial or venous (66). LM are identified at autopsy in up to 8% of patients with systemic cancer. The most frequent cancers to metastasize to the leptomeninges are solid tumors, notably breast, lung, melanoma, and gastrointestinal cancers, as well as lymphomas (malignant high-grade non-Hodgkin's) and acute leukemias (lymphocytic) (66). Primary brain tumors account for 10–32% of cases in some series. The duration from the discovery of the primary malignancy to the diagnosis of leptomeningeal involvement is very broad, from 3 months to 6 years in some series (67). A rising incidence of LM may reflect an increased overall survival of many cancers (68).

Two characteristic features suggest a diagnosis of leptomeningeal cancer. First, neurologic dysfunction appears at multiple levels of the neuraxis in the absence of brain or spinal epidural metastases on radiographic examination. The patient may present with a variety of complaints and tends to accumulate new symptoms over weeks as the disease progresses. Second, neurologic signs tend to be much more prominent than symptoms. Although most patients initially complain of symptoms in one anatomic area, examination reveals signs of neurologic abnormality in two or more areas in more than 80% of patients (69).

Symptoms referable to the brain are the initial complaint in approximately half of patients, with headache being the single most frequent initial symptom; headache is reported by one third of patients at presentation (66). The headache can occur in a variety of locations, including bifrontal, diffuse, or radiating from the occipital region into the neck. Nausea or vomiting, light-headedness, and cognitive disturbances are associated features. Changes in mental status alone are a common finding and eventually occur in 80% of patients; these changes are characterized by lethargy, confusion, and memory deficit. Other common cranial symptoms and signs include lateralized weakness, seizures, CN palsies (most commonly diplopia, hearing loss, and facial weakness) and papilledema. Spinal symptoms due to the involvement of the spinal cord or exiting nerve roots and meninges include weakness (lower or upper motor neuron), sensory loss (dermatomal or segmental), pain, ataxia, fecal incontinence, and urinary retention. Occasionally, asymptomatic urinary retention occurs.

The diagnosis of LM is based on clinical findings and CSF analysis (Table 36.5). The finding of malignant cells in the CSF is the diagnostic gold standard; positive cytology is eventually found in 90% of patients, although three or more examinations of large volumes of CSF may be required (67). Associated CSF findings include increased opening pressure, elevated protein, decreased glucose, and lymphocytosis. The CSF levels of these components can vary if sampled at different levels of the neuraxis, with some patients showing positive cytology only if sampled from the ventricular system (67). After two negative lumbar punctures for CSF cytology, it has been recommended to proceed to ventricular or lateral cervical CSF analysis (66). Recommended workup for LM includes contrast-enhanced MRI of the brain and spine, followed by the evaluation of CSF for cell count, chemistry, and cytopathology if a lumbar puncture can be safely performed. MRI can detect up to 50% of cases with false-negative lumbar punctures (70). Contrast-enhanced T1-weighted sequences in more than one plane should be included. A normal study does not exclude the diagnosis owing to a 30% incidence of false-negative results (71). A CSF flow scan is recommended to further define the extent of the disease and to determine whether other therapies should be considered. Cytology may be supplemented by flow cytometry, immunohistochemical studies, protein studies, and polymerase chain reaction (PCR) (72). A pathologic diagnosis of cancer with the clinical syndrome of LM can also make this diagnosis (66). When cytology is nondiagnostic and disease is identified on imaging without an identified primary cancer, then a leptomeningeal and/or brain biopsy is indicated (72).

Treatment of LM is aimed at prolonging survival and improving or stabilizing neurologic disability. Untreated, LM from a variety of tumor types have a median survival of 4–6 weeks (70). With standard treatment, which is always palliative, survival ranges from 4 to 10 months (69). Treatment of LM due to solid tumors is less successful than that due to leukemia and lymphoma (72). The main modality of treatment for LM has been IT chemotherapy for patients in good risk groups, with focal external beam radiotherapy to sites of symptomatic and bulky disease or to the entire neuraxis. This is usually combined with optimal

TABLE 36.4

OUTCOME FROM RANDOMIZED STUDIES OF WHOLE BRAIN RADIATION THERAPY, SURGERY, SURGERY + RADIOTHERAPY AND RADIOSURGERY FOR BRAIN METASTASES

Treatment modality	Single or multiple brain metastases
WBRT	Single brain metastases *Median survival (mo)*
Mintz et al. (3000 cGy/10 fr)[a]	6.3
Vecht et al. (4000 cGy/20 fr b.i.d.)[b]	6
Patchell et al. (3600 cGy/12 fr)[c]	3.5
WBRT	Multiple brain metastases *Median survival (mo)*
Horton et al.[d]	3.5
Surgery	Single brain metastases
Patchell et al.[e]	*Median survival (mo)* 9.9 (vs. 11.0: Surgery + WBRT)
Surgery	Multiple brain metastases
No randomized studies found	
WBRT + Surgery	Single brain metastases *Median survival (mo)*
Mintz et al. (3000 cGy/10 fr)[a]	5.6
Vecht et al. (4000 cGy/20 fr b.i.d.)[b]	10
Patchell et al. (3600 cGy/12 fr)[c]	9.2
WBRT + Surgery	Multiple rain metastases *Median survival (mo)*
KPS ≥70; age <65; controlled primary tumor No extracranial disease[f]	6.0 (vs. 13.5 with single metastasis)
All other situations[f]	4.1 (vs. 8.1 with single metastasis)
KPS <70[f]	2.3
Radiosurgery	Single brain metastases *Median survival (mo)*
SRS + WBRT[g]	6.5 (vs. 4.9 with WBRT alone)
Radiosurgery	Multiple brain metastases *Median survival (mo)*
SRS + WBRT (2–4 metastases)[h]	11 (vs. 7.5 with WBRT alone)
SRS + WBRT (2–3 metastases)[i]	5.3 (vs. 6.7 with WBRT alone—abstract)

WBRT, whole brain radiation therapy; SRS, stereotactic radiosurgery, KPS, Karnofsky performance score.
[a]Mintz AH, Kestle J, Rathbone MP, et al. A randomized trial to assess the efficacy of surgery in addition to radiotherapy in patients with single brain metastasis. *Cancer* 1996;78:1470–1476.
[b]Vecht CJ, Haaxma-Reiche H, Noordijk EM, et al. Treatment of single brain metastasis: radiotherapy alone or combined with neurosurgery? *Ann Neurol* 1993;33:583–90.
[c]Patchell RA, Tibbs PA, Walsh JW, et al. A randomized trial of surgery in the treatment of single metastases to the brain. *N Engl J Med* 1990;322:494–500.
[d]Horton J, Baxter DH, Olson KB, et al. The management of metastases to the brain by irradiation and corticosteroids. *Am J Roentgenol Radium Ther Nucl Med* 1971;3:334.
[e]Patchell RA, Tibbs PA, Regine WF, et al. Postoperative radiotherapy in the treatment of single metastases to the brain. *JAMA* 1998;280(17):1485–1489.
[f]Lutterbach J, Bartlet S, Ostertag C. Long-term survival in patients with brain metastases. *J Cancer Res Clin Oncol* 2002;128:417–425.
[g]Andrews DW, Scott CB, Sperduto PW. et al. Whole brain radiation therapy with or without stereotactic radiosurgery boost for patients with one to three brain metastases: phase III results of the RTOG 9508 randomized trial. *Lancet* 2004;363:1665–72.
[h]Kondziolka D, Patel A, Lunsford LD. et al. Stereotactic radiosurgery plus whole brain radiotherapy versus radiotherapy alone for patients with multiple brain metastases. *Int J Radiat Oncol Biol Phys* 1999;45:427–434.
[i]Sperduto PW, Scott C, Andrews D. et al. Preliminary report of RTOG 9508: a phase III trial comparing whole brain irradiation alone versus whole brain irradiation plus stereotactic radiosurgery for patients with two or three unresected brain metastases (abstract). *Int J Radiat Oncol Biol Phys* 2000;48:113.

treatment of the systemic cancer and symptomatic treatment including corticosteroids, CSF shunting, and anticonvulsants as needed (72). Craniospinal radiation, used for the treatment of leukemic meningitis, is associated with significant systemic toxicity. In general, systemic chemotherapy fails because of poor CSF penetration (66). IT chemotherapy, delivered by an Ommaya reservoir, or by lumbar puncture, results in high CSF drug levels without systemic dose-limiting toxicity.

Base of Skull Metastases

The base of the skull includes the temporal, sphenoid, and occipital bones (including the clivus) as well as the bony orbit. Base of skull metastases are most commonly secondary to tumors of the breast, lung, and prostate. Other tumors that may metastasize to the skull base include head and neck tumors, lymphoma, and other tumors that metastasize to the

TABLE 36.5

EVALUATION OF LEPTOMENINGEAL DISEASE: SIGNS/SYMPTOMS AND INVESTIGATIONS

Signs and symptoms	Incidence
LOCALIZING SYMPTOMS/SIGNS	
Cranial neuropathies (common—CN III, IV, VI, VII, VIII)	9–22%
Radiculopathy (back pain)	1–14%
Myelopathy	2–6%
Cauda equina syndrome	2–3%
Mononeuritis	Rare
Bilateral internuclear ophthalmoplegia	Rare
Urinary and fecal retention	Rare
Ischemic symptoms/stroke	Rare
NONLOCALIZING SYMPTOMS/SIGNS	
Headache	10–31%
Sensory	30%
Nausea/vomiting	15%
Weakness	3–36%
Visual—diplopia, blurred vision, papilledema	2–32%
Ataxia	3–15%
Meningismus	2–13%
Encephalopathy	2–10%
Seizure	1–5%
Fever	Rare
Other (DI, stroke, myoclonus, apnea, diencephalic syndrome)	Rare

Evaluation	Findings
Physical and neurologic exam	Characteristic neurologic findings as in the preceding text
MRI of brain and spine + gadolinium	Enhancement of leptomeninges, ventricular surface, CNs, or spinal roots in linear or nodular pattern
	Communicating hydrocephalus
	Parenchymal mass
CSF examination (high volume, serial lumbar punctures)	Increased protein (most cases)
Routine studies	Decreased glucose (25–30%)
Cytology	Lymphocytic pleocytosis (50%)
Flow cytometry—cell surface markers, DNA, RNA	Eosinophilia
Immunocytochemistry	Elevated opening pressure (50%)
Tumor markers	Malignant cells (cytopathology)
Polymerase chain reaction	Monoclonal cell population (flow cytometry)
	Tumor markers (CEA, LDH, βhCG, B2MG, MBP, VEGF, others)
BIOPSY	
Adjunctive studies	
Electromyography/nerve conduction studies	Distinguish radiculopathy vs. peripheral neuropathy; define extent of disease
Nerve biopsy	Direct nerve infiltration
Myelography (if MRI contraindicated)	Thickening and nodularity of nerve roots; extradural mass effect; CSF flow block
Workup for primary tumor (if no prior history of cancer) or for extraneural recurrence (with history of cancer)	

CN, cranial nerve; DI, diabetes insipidus; MRI, magnetic resonance imaging; CSF, cerebrospinal fluid; CEA, carcinoembryonic antigen; LDH, lactic dehydrogenase; βhCG, β-human chorionic gonadotrophin; B2MG, B_2-microglobulin; MBP, myelin basic protein; VEGF, vascular endothelial growth factor.
Adapted from Kesari S, Batchelor TT, Leptomeningeal metastases. *Neurol Clin North Am* 2003;21:25–66; with permission.

bone. The median interval from the primary tumor diagnosis to the onset of neurologic signs was 23 months in one study; two thirds of patients had metastatic disease elsewhere when the base of skull metastases were diagnosed (73). Several discrete neurologic syndromes have been described, characterized by the dysfunction of CNs as they pass through bony foramen.

Common areas include the bony orbit, parasellar region, middle cranial fossa, jugular foramen, occipital condyle, clivus, and sphenoid sinus. Base of skull metastases may present with head pain, CN palsies, or both. Treatment is usually effective and includes pharmacologic analgesic interventions (usually nonsteroidal anti-inflammatories with opioids) and focal radiation therapy. Resectability of tumors invading the base of skull depends on histologic type and patient performance status; usual contraindications include brain invasion and the involvement of the internal carotid artery or cavernous sinus (68). Recovery of the CN function tends to be slow.

CEREBROVASCULAR DISEASE IN PATIENTS WITH CANCER

After metastases, cerebrovascular lesions are the next most common neurologic finding at autopsy in patients with cancer. In one autopsy series, 14.6% of patients had cerebrovascular lesions (74); of these, approximately half had clinical symptoms of cerebrovascular disease during life. The usual risk factors in the general population for stroke, including age, hypertension, coronary artery disease, and diabetes, may be less important in this population than the pathophysiologic effects of neoplastic disease and its treatment, although this issue remains controversial (74,75).

Hemorrhagic cerebrovascular events are more common than ischemic events in the cancer population (74). Cerebral metastases and coagulation disturbances, including thrombocytopenia and leukostasis, are the usual causes of intracerebral hemorrhage (ICH) in patients with cancer. The reported overall incidence of hemorrhage from an intracranial tumor is 1–15% (76). One neurosurgical series demonstrated an overall tumor hemorrhage rate of 14.6%, of which 5.4% were classified as macroscopic and 9.2% as microscopic (77). As a cause of spontaneous ICH, however, tumor-induced ICH is not a common etiology (only 2% of 461 autopsy cases in one study) (78).

Among all tumor types, those with the highest incidence of bleeding are metastatic melanoma, renal cell carcinoma, germ-cell tumors (particularly choriocarcinoma), and bronchogenic carcinoma. The latter is the most common cause because lung cancer is responsible for the majority of brain metastasis (79). Simultaneous hemorrhage into multiple brain metastases occurs frequently (79). The usual presentation mimics an acute vascular event, such as a hypertensive hemorrhage or ruptured berry aneurysm. Headache, progressive obtundation, seizures, and focal neurologic signs are reported in two thirds of patients with cancer and intracranial hemorrhage. Hypertensive hemorrhages may be distinguished from intratumoral bleeding by the presence of a history of high blood pressure and the location of the hemorrhage in the basal ganglia in 90% of cases. Hypertensive hemorrhage is a relatively rare cause of ICH in the patient with cancer (74). Neoplastic aneurysms, although uncommon, are another cause of intracranial hemorrhage in patients with cancer.

Coagulopathy may be an indirect effect of the tumor or may result from iatrogenic causes, including chemotherapy-related thrombocytopenia and treatment with warfarin sodium. Disease-related coagulopathy may be consumptive, such as disseminated intravascular coagulation (DIC). Neurologic complications from the latter disorder may be either ischemic or hemorrhagic, including intracerebral bleed and subdural hematoma. Coagulopathy-induced intraparenchymal hemorrhage is most commonly associated with hematologic malignancies, especially acute leukemia. Eighteen percent of patients with acute myelocytic leukemia (AML) and 8% of patients with acute lymphocytic leukemia (ALL) have ICH found at autopsy (80). The hemorrhage is often large and fatal in AML, yet small and may be asymptomatic in ALL (79) Patients with solid tumors and thrombocytopenia have a low incidence of ICH except when the platelet count falls below 10,000 per µL; coagulopathy-related ICH in this population, which may be due to DIC, liver dysfunction, or cancer

therapy, usually occurs as a terminal event (76). DIC with ICH is a common cause of death in acute promyelocytic leukemia (81). Anticoagulant-induced intracranial hemorrhage is not common. DIC can present with encephalopathy, even in the absence of abnormalities in blood-clotting parameters or low platelets. The onset of symptoms may be gradual from coagulopathy-induced ICH, compared to an acute presentation from hemorrhage into a metastatic tumor.

Suspected intratumoral hemorrhage should be investigated with CT scan or MRI. Management is primarily medical and includes ensuring airway control, treatment of severe hypertension, management of elevated ICP, corticosteroids (for tumor edema only), reversal of hemostatic abnormalities (if possible), and antitumor therapy (if appropriate). Surgical evacuation of the hematoma should be considered in select patients depending on hematoma location and size, patient status, and correctable hematologic abnormalities. An intraventricular catheter may be placed for the management of hydrocephalus or increased ICP. Spontaneous ICH in acute promyelocytic leukemia has been reduced significantly with prophylactic heparin, chemotherapy, and transretinoic acid (82,83).

In patients with leukemia, another cause of ICH is hyperleukocytosis (elevation of the peripheral blast count to greater than 100,000 per mm^3 in AML or 140,000 per mm^3 in ALL), which causes early death secondary to ICH in a reported 15% of patients (84). Clinically, such patients develop multiple intraparenchymal hemorrhages, occasionally associated with intraventricular or subarachnoid hemorrhage. Chemotherapy and leukophoresis to lower the peripheral blast count can reduce, but not eliminate, the risk of ICH (74). Leukostasis can also be treated with radiation therapy (1200–2400 cGy) (70). Blood hyperviscosity can be treated with plasmapheresis or phlebotomy for polycythemia vera (79).

Causes of cerebral infarction in patients with cancer include atherosclerosis, nonbacterial thrombotic endocarditis (NBTE), cerebral DIC, venous sinus thrombosis, infection, tumor embolism, and treatment complications. From autopsy studies, atherosclerosis is the most common cause of cerebral infarction in patients with cancer, but most strokes were asymptomatic (77%) (74). NBTE was the most common cause of symptomatic stroke (27% of strokes), followed by intravascular coagulation (24%) and atherosclerosis (15%). A retrospective review of all ischemic strokes diagnosed in patients with cancer at Memorial Sloan-Kettering Cancer Center from 1997 to 2001 confirmed 96 strokes with median age 67 years and 61.5% male gender (75). The vascular risk profile was similar to most large stroke series except for a low incidence of atrial fibrillation. The most common primary tumor was lung cancer in 30% of cases, followed by brain and prostate cancer (9% each). The majority of strokes were embolic (54%) and only 22% were atherosclerotic (large vessel 10%; small vessel 12%); only 3% were attributed to NBTE which was likely underestimated owing to the lack of transesophageal echocardiogram (TEE) evaluation (75). There was no significant relationship between stroke-specific treatment and survival which had a median of 4.5 months.

NBTE causes cerebral infarction by either intravascular microthrombosis or embolism from fibrin and platelet deposition on heart valves (74). NBTE is most commonly associated with adenocarcinoma, especially mucin-producing carcinomas of the lung or gastrointestinal tract. The clinical presentation is usually an acute onset of focal neurologic signs, most frequently aphasia, which either stabilize or progressively worsen. A diffuse encephalopathy also commonly accompanies focal signs. Systemic bleeding, venous thrombosis, and pulmonary embolism are part of the spectrum of coagulopathy that may accompany NBTE. NBTE is best diagnosed with TEE demonstrating valvular vegetations in the setting of negative blood cultures (85). The treatment focuses on the underlying cause of the syndrome; heparin has been shown to improve symptoms from cerebral ischemia but carries the risk of intracerebral and systemic bleeding.

Radiation of the head and neck for treatment of Hodgkin's disease, head and neck carcinomas, breast cancer, and primary brain tumors can produce accelerated carotid atherosclerosis, causing symptomatic carotid occlusive disease from 6 months to decades after radiation therapy. The total dose is usually greater than 50 Gy, and accelerated atherosclerotic disease is limited to vessels within the irradiated area. There is no association with generalized atherosclerosis beyond concurrent patient-related factors, such as cigarette smoking. The process is accelerated with concurrent hypercholesterolemia (86). The presentation mimics non–radiation-related atherosclerosis and may include transient ischemic attacks, infarction, amaurosis fugax, or seizures. Cerebral angiography shows occlusion or extensive stenosis disproportionately affecting the common carotid artery. Although carotid endarterectomy (with or without a patch) remains the standard treatment for this complication, carotid stenting appears to be a safe and efficient treatment even for severe radiation-induced stenosis (87). Another complication of neck radiation is acute rupture of the carotid artery (which usually occurs after resection of head and neck malignancies), in which necrosis of the skin flap and surgical wound infection have occurred. Although low-dose heparin may reduce the risk of infarction, the prognosis is poor because of potential exsanguination or infarction if the carotid artery is ligated (88).

Thrombosis of cerebral venous sinuses or large cortical veins in patients with cancer may be either a metastatic or a nonmetastatic complication. In both cases, the superior sagittal sinus is most frequently involved. Metastatic tumor directly causes sagittal sinus thrombosis by either external compression or infiltration of the sinus, which results in stasis or a nidus around which a thrombus may form (89). Nonmetastatic sagittal sinus occlusion may be caused by local injury to the sinus, but is more likely related to a hypercoagulable state of malignancy. Metastatic involvement of the sagittal sinus is seen in lymphoma and some solid tumors, such as neuroblastoma and lung cancer. Nonmetastatic venous thrombosis is less common and occurs in patients with hematologic malignancies; it is usually associated with advanced disease. Clinically, nonmetastatic sagittal sinus thrombosis usually presents as an acute onset of seizures, which may be accompanied by encephalopathy and focal signs if infarction has occurred (85). Metastatic sagittal sinus thrombosis presents with subacute signs of increased ICP, such as headache and vomiting; cerebral infarction can also occur. Diagnosis is best made by MRI, magnetic resonance venography, or coronal views during enhanced CT scan. When patients present early in their disease, prognosis is usually good, often with spontaneous recovery. Patients with advanced disease have a poor prognosis. The benefit of heparin in the cancer population is not certain, given the risk of major hemorrhage. Cranial irradiation is indicated for metastatic sagittal sinus thrombosis.

Cerebral hemorrhage or infarction can also occur as complications of treatment of neoplastic disease. Chemotherapy such as asparaginase (superior sagittal sinus thrombosis), mitomycin, and others have been associated with a variety of cerebral complications, either hemorrhagic or ischemic (85,90).

CONCLUSION

Symptoms from neurologic complications of malignancy are common and serious and can be difficult to diagnose. Because of their prevalence and potential for effective palliation, intracranial manifestations of malignancy and their management deserve the attention of all cancer health care providers.

References

1. Forsyth PA, Posner JB. Headaches in patients with brain tumors: a study of 111 patients. *Neurology* 1993;43:1678–1683.
2. Forsyth PA, Posner JB. Intracranial neoplasms. In: Oleson J, Hansen P, Welch KMA, eds. *The headaches.* New York: Raven Press, 1993:705.
3. Olesen J. The International Classification of Headache Disorders, 2nd edition: application to practice. *Funct Neurol* 2005;20(2):61–68.
4. Suwanwela N, Phanthumchinda K, Kaoropthum S. Headache in brain tumour: a cross-sectional study. *Headache* 1994;34:435.
5. Vazquez-Barquero A, Ibanez FJ, Herrera S, et al. Isolated headache as the presenting clinical manifestation of intracranial tumors: a prospective study. *Cephalalgia* 1994;14:270–272.
6. Coia LR. The role of radiation therapy in the treatment of brain metastases. *Int J Radiat Oncol Biol Phys* 1992;23:229.
7. Rosner D, Nemoto T, Lane WW. Chemotherapy induces regression of brain metastases in breast carcinoma. *Cancer* 1986;58:832.
8. Kristensen CA, Kristjansen PE, Hansen HH. Systemic chemotherapy of brain metastases from small cell lung cancer: a review. *J Clin Oncol* 1992;10:1498.
9. Spears WT, Morphies VG II, Lester SG, et al. Brain metastases and testicular tumors: long term survival. *Int J Radiat Oncol Biol Phys* 1992;22:17.
10. Dropcho EJ, Soong SJ. Steroid-induced weakness in patients with primary brain tumors. *Neurology* 1991;41:1235.
11. Vecht CJ, Hovestadt A, Verbiest HB, et al. Dose-effect relationship of dexamethasone on Karnofsky performance in metastatic brain tumors: a randomized study of doses 4, 8, and 16 mg per day. *Neurology* 1994;44(4):675.
12. Wolfson AH, Snodgrass SM, Schwade JG, et al. The role of steroids in the management of metastatic carcinoma to the brain. A pilot prospective trial. *Am J Clin Oncol* 1994;17(3):234.
13. Lieberman A, Lebrun Y, Glass P, et al. Use of high dose corticosteroids in patients with inoperable brain tumors. *J Neurol Neurosurg Psychiatry* 1977;40:678.
14. Kaal ECA, Vecht CJ. The management of brain edema in brain tumors. *Curr Opin Oncol* 2004;16:593–600.
15. Brown ES, Chandler PA. Mood and cognitive changes during systemic corticosteroid therapy. Primary care companion. *J Clin Psychiatry* 2001;3:17–21.
16. Beric A. Central pain and dysesthesia syndrome. In: Backonja MM. ed. *Neurol Clin* 1998;16(4):899.
17. Amancio EJ, Peluso CM, Santos AC, et al. Central pain due to parietal cortex compression by cerebral tumor: report of 2 cases Arq. *Neuropsiquiatr* 2002;60(2-B):487–489.
18. Tovi D, Schisano G, Lilequist B. Primary tumours of the region of the thalamus. *J Neurosurg* 1961;18:730.
19. Nicholson BD. Evaluation and treatment of central pain syndromes. *Neurology* 2004;62(5 Suppl 2):S30–S36.
20. Attal N, Gaudé V, Brasseur L, et al. Intravenous lidocaine in central pain: a double-blind, placebo-controlled, psychophysiological study. *Neurology* 2000;54:564–574.
21. Attal N, Guirimand F, Brasseur L, et al. Effects of IV morphine in central pain: a randomized placebo-controlled study. *Neurology* 2002;58:554–563.
22. Tai Q, Kirshblum S, Chen B, et al. Gabapentin in the treatment of neuropathic pain after spinal cord injury: a prospective, randomized, double-blind, crossover trial. *J Spinal Cord Med* 2002;25:100–105.
23. Leijon G, Boivie J. Central post-stroke pain–a controlled trial of amitriptyline and carbamazepine. *Pain* 1989;36:27–36.
24. Nguyen JP, Lefaucher JP, Le Guerinel C, et al. Motor cortex stimulation in the treatment of central and neuropathic pain. *Arch Med Res* 2000;31(3):263.
25. Finnerup NB, Yezierski RP, Sang CN, Burchial KJ, Jensen TS. Treatment of spinal cord injury pain. Pain Clinical Updates. *IASP* 2001;9(2):1–17, Available at: http://www.iasp-pain.org/PCU01-2.html.
26. Rushton JG, Stevens JC, Miller RH. Glossopharyngeal (vagoglossopharyngeal) neuralgia. *Arch Neurol* 1981;38:201.
27. Lossos A, Siegal T. Numb chin syndrome in cancer patients: etiology, response to treatment and prognostic significance. *Neurology* 1992;42:1181.
28. Victor M, Ropper AH. *Adams and victor's principles of neurology*, 7th ed. New York: McGraw-Hill, 2001.
29. Morris HH, Estes ML. Brain tumors and chronic epilepsy. In: Wyllie E. ed. *The treatment of epilepsy: principles and practice,* Philadelphia, PA. Lea and Febiger, 1993:659.
30. Oberndorfer S, Schmal T, Lahrmann H, et al. The frequency of seizures in patients with primary brain tumors or cerebral metastases. An evaluation from the Ludwig Boltzmann Institute of Neuro-Oncology and the Department of Neurology, Kaiser Franz Josef Hospital Vienna. *Wien Klin Wochenschr* 2002;114(21–22):911–916.

31. El Kamar FG, Posner JB. Brain metastases. *Semin Neurol* 2004;24(4): 347–362.

32. Glantz MJ, Cole BF, Forsyth PA, et al. Practice parameter: anticonvulsant prophylaxis in patients with newly diagnosed brain tumors. Report of the Quality Standards Subcommittee of the American Academy of Neurology. *Neurology* 2000;54(10):1886–1893.

33. Sirven JI, Wingerchuk DM, Drazkowski JF, et al. Seizure prophylaxis in patients with brain tumors: a meta-analysis. *Mayo Clin Proc* 2004;79(12):1489–1494.

34. Cohen N, Strauss G, Lew R, et al. Should prophylactic anticonvulsants be administered to patients with newly diagnosed cerebral metastases? A retrospective analysis. *J Clin Oncol* 1988;6:1621.

35. Glantz M, Friedberg M, Cole B, et al. Double-blind, randomized, placebo-controlled trial of anticonvulsant prophylaxis in adults with newly diagnosed brain metastases. *Proc Am Soc Clin Oncol* 1994;176(abst 492).

36. Weaver S, Forsyth P, Fulton D, et al. A prospective randomized trial of prophylactic anticonvulsants in patients with primary or metastatic brain tumors and without prior seizures: a preliminary analysis of 67 patients. *Neurology* 1995;45(Suppl 4):A263(abst 371P).

37. Byrne TN, Cascino TL, Posner JB. Brain metastases from melanoma. *J Neurooncol* 1983;1:313.

38. Chalk JB, Ridgeway K, Brophy TR, et al. Phenytoin impairs the bioavailability of dexamethasone in neurological and neurosurgical patients. *J Neurol Neurosurg Psychiatr* 1984;47:1087.

39. Delattre J, Safai B, Posner JB. Erythema multiforme and Stevens-Johnson syndrome in patients receiving cranial irradiation and phenytoin. *Neurology* 1988;38:194.

40. Barclay CL, McLean M, Hagen N, et al. Severe phenytoin hypersensitivity with myopathy: a case report. *Neurology* 1992;42:4303.

41. Bardana EJ, Gabourel JD, Davis G, et al. Effects of phenytoin on man's immunity. Evaluation of changes in serum immunoglobulins, complements, and antinuclear antibody. *Am J Med* 1983;74:289.

42. Agbi CB, Bernstein M. Seizure prophylaxis for brain tumour patients: brief review and guide for family physicians. *Can Fam Physician* 1993;39: 1153.

43. Loft LM, Ward RF. Hiccups. A case presentation and etiologic review. *Arch Otolaryngol Head Neck Surg* 1992;118:1115.

44. Davis JN. An experimental study of hiccup. *Brain* 1970;93:851.

45. Oshima T, Sakamoto M, Tatsuta H, et al. GABAergic inhibition of hiccup-like reflex induced by electrical stimulation in medulla of cats. *Neurosci Res* 1998;30(4):287.

46. Musumeci A, Cristofori L, Bricolo A. Persistent hiccup as presenting symptom in medulla oblongata cavernoma: a case report and review of the literature. *Clin Neurol Neurosurg* 2000;102:13.

47. Smith HS, Busracamwongs A. Management of hiccups in the palliative care population. *Am J Hosp Palliat Care* 2003;20(2):149–154.

48. Payne BR, Tiel RL, Payne MS, et al. Vagus nerve stimulation for chronic intractable hiccups. Case report. *J Neurosurg* 2005;102(5):935–937.

49. Boring CC, Squires TS, Tong T. Cancer statistics. *CA Cancer J Clin* 1993;43:7.

50. Cairncross JG, Kim J-H, Posner JB. Radiation therapy of brain metastases. *Ann Neurol* 1980;7:529–541.

51. O'Neill BP, Ruchner JC, Cotley RJ, et al. Brain metastatic lesions. *Mayo Clin Proc* 1994;69:1062.

52. Sawaya R, Ligon BL, Bindal RK. Management of metastatic brain tumours. *Ann Surg Oncol* 1994;1:169.

53. Posner JB. *Neurologic complications of cancer, Contemporary neurology series*, vol. 45. Philadelphia, PA: FA Davis Co, 1995;3:77.

54. Hwang TL, Close TP, Grego JM, et al. Predilection of brain metastases in the gray and white matter junction and vascular border zones. *Cancer* 1996;77:1551.

55. Young DF, Posner JB, Chu F, et al. Rapid-course radiation therapy of cerebral metastases: results and complications. *Cancer* 1974;34:1069.

56. Christiaans MH, Kelder JC, Arnoldus EPJ, et al. Prediction of intracranial metastases in cancer patients with headache. *Cancer* 2002;94:2063–2068.

57. Akeson P, Larsson EM, Kristofferson DT, et al. Brain metastases: comparison of gadodiamide injection-enhanced MR imaging at standard and high dose, contrast-enhanced CT, and non-contrast-enhanced MR imaging. *Acta Radiol* 1995;36:300.

58. Katz A, Zalewski P. Quality-of-life benefits and evidence of antitumour activity for patients with brain metastases treated with gefitinib. *Br J Cancer* 2003;89(S2):S15–S18.

59. Kaal EC, Niel CG, Vecht CJ. Therapeutic management of brain metastasis. *Lancet Neurol* 2005;4(5):289–298.

60. Gaspar L, Scott C, Rotman M, et al. Recursive partitioning analysis (RPA) of prognostic factors in three radiation therapy oncology group (RTOG) brain metastases trials. *Int J Radiat Oncol Biol Phys* 1997;37:745.

61. DeAngelis LM, Delattre JW, Posner JB. Radiation-induced dementia in patients cured of brain metastases. *Neurology* 1989;39:789.

62. Tsao MN, Lloyd NS, Wong RK, Rakovitch E, Chow E, Laperriere N, et al. The Supportive Care Guidelines Group of Cancer Care Ontario's Program in Evidence-based Care. Radiotherapeutic management of brain metastases: a systematic review and meta-analysis. *Cancer Treat Rev* 2005;31(4):256–273.

63. Andrews DW, Scott CB, Sperduto PW, et al. Whole brain radiation therapy with or without stereotactic radiosurgery boost for patients with one to three brain metastases; phase III results of the RTOG 9508 randomised trial. *Lancet* 2004;363:1665–1672.

64. Auchter RM, Lamond JP, Alexander E, et al. A multi-institutional outcome and prognostic factor analysis of radiosurgery for resectable single brain metastasis. *Int J Radiat Oncol Biol Phys* 1996;35:27.

65. Patchell RA, Tibbs PA, Walsh JW, et al. A randomized trial of surgery in the treatment of single metastases to the brain. *N Engl J Med* 1990;322:484.

66. Chamberlain MC. Leptomeningeal metastases: a review of evaluation and treatment. *J Neurooncol* 1998;37:271.

67. Wasserstrom WR, Glass JP, Posner JB. Diagnosis and treatment of leptomeningeal metastases from solid tumours: experience with 90 patients. *Cancer* 1982;49:759.

68. Maroldi R, Ambrosi C, Farina D. Metastatic disease of the brain: extra-axial metastases (skull, dura, leptomeningeal) and tumour spread. *Eur Radiol* 2005;15(3):617–626.

69. Grant R, Naylor B, Greenberg HS, et al. Clinical outcome in aggressively treated meningeal carcinomatosis. *Arch Neurol* 1996;51:457.

70. Posner JB. Leptomeningeal metastases. In: Posner JB. ed. *Neurological complications of cancer*. Philadelphia, PA: FA Davis Co, 1995:143.

71. Freilich RJ, Krol G, DeAngelis LM. Neuroimaging and cerebrospinal fluid cytology in the diagnosis of leptomeningeal metastasis. *Ann Neurol* 1995;38:51–57.

72. Kesari S, Batchelor TT. Leptomeningeal metastases. *Neurol Clin North Am* 2003;21:25–66.

73. Greenberg HS, Deck MDF, Vikram B, et al. Metastases to the base of the skull: clinical findings in 43 patients. *Neurology* 1981;31:530.

74. Graus F, Rogers LR, Posner JB. Cerebrovascular complications in patients with cancer. *Medicine* 1985;64:16.

75. Cestari DM, Weine DM, Panageas KS, et al. Stroke in patients with cancer: incidence and etiology. *Neurology* 2004;62(11):2025–2030.

76. Destian S, Sze G, Krol G, et al. MR imaging of hemorrhagic intracranial neoplasms. *AJNR Am J Neuroradiol* 1988;9:115.

77. Kondziolka D, Bernstein M, Resch L, et al. Significance of hemorrhage into brain tumours: clinicopathological study. *J Neurosurg* 1987;67:852.

78. Hirano A, Matsui T. Vascular structures in brain tumours. *Hum Pathol* 1975;6(5):611–621.

79. Quinn JA, DeAngelis LM. Neurologic emergencies in the cancer patient. *Semin Oncol* 2000;27(3):311.

80. Hersh EM, Bodey GP, Nies BA, et al. Causes of death in acute leukemia: a ten year study of 414 patients from 1954–1963. *JAMA* 1965;193:105.

81. Cordonnier C, Vernant JP, Brun B, et al. Acute promyelocytic leukemia in 57 previously untreated patients. *Cancer* 1985;55:18.

82. Drapkin RL, Gee TS, Dowling MD, et al. Prophylactic heparin therapy in acute premyelocytic leukemia. *Cancer* 1978;41:2484.

83. Castaigne S, Chromienne C, Daniel MT, et al. All-*trans* retinoic acid as a differentiation therapy for acute promyelocytic leukemia: I, clinical results. *Blood* 1990;76:1704.

84. Schiff D, Batchelor T, Wen PY. Neurologic emergencies in cancer patients. *Neurol Clin* 1998;16:449.

85. Rogers LR. Cerebrovascular complications in cancer patients. *Neurol Clin* 2003;21:167–192.

86. Loftus CM, Biller J, Hart MN, et al. Management of radiation-induced accelerated carotid atherosclerosis. *Arch Neurol* 1987;44:711.

87. Houdart E, Mounayer C, Chapot R, et al. Carotid stenting for radiation-induced stenosis: a report of 7 cases. *Stroke* 2001;32(1):118.

88. Razack MS, Saho K. Carotid artery hemorrhage and ligation in head and neck cancer. *J Surg Oncol* 1982;19:189.

89. Sigsbee B, Deck MDF, Posner JB. Non-metastatic superior sagittal sinus thrombosis complicating systemic cancer. *Neurology* 1979;29:139.

90. Wall JG, Weiss RB, Norton L, et al. Arterial thrombosis associated with adjuvant chemotherapy for breast carcinoma: a cancer and leukemia Group B Study. *Am J Med* 1984;87:501.

CHAPTER 37 ■ MANAGEMENT OF SPINAL CORD AND CAUDA EQUINA COMPRESSION

SHARON M. WEINSTEIN

EPIDEMIOLOGY

The spine is the most frequent site of bony involvement in patients with malignant metastases (1). The major complications of spinal neoplasm are pain and neurologic injury. Compression of neural structures may be caused directly by the tumor mass or by the displacement of bony fragments into the spinal canal. Tumor of the vertebral bodies has been demonstrated in 25–70% of patients with metastatic cancer (2), and spinal metastases are present in 40% of patients who die from cancer (3). Metastatic lesions from other primary malignancies are three to four times as common as primary bony tumors of the spine (4).

Each year in the United States, approximately 20,000 patients with cancer are treated for malignant epidural compression (EC) of the spinal cord and/or cauda equina. It has been estimated that EC affects 5–10% of adult solid tumor patients and 5% of pediatric solid tumor patients (5,6). These percentages are corroborated by autopsy series (4,7).

Half of all patients initially presenting with EC are not known to have cancer at the time that pain or neurologic deficits begin (8). Therefore, it is common for EC to be the presenting symptom of malignancy.

The distribution of spinal tumors reflects the prevalence of primary malignancies as well as the physiology of metastasis. Multiple myeloma is the most common primary bone tumor, representing 10–15% of malignant epidural spinal disease. Osteogenic sarcoma is the second most common primary spinal tumor, usually affecting children and adolescents. Fifty percent of chordomas affect the sacrococcygeal bones and 35% affect the base of the skull. Chondrosarcoma and Ewing's sarcoma are other bone tumors that may be primary in the vertebrae, although this is rare.

Primary tumors of the breast, lung, and prostate commonly spread to the spinal column. The spine is also a frequent site of metastasis of a nonspinal primary osteogenic sarcoma. Spinal metastases are less common in renal carcinoma, melanoma, soft tissue sarcoma, Ewing's sarcoma, germ cell tumors, neuroblastoma; and carcinomas of the head and neck, thyroid, and bladder. Rarely, malignant neoplasms of the brain, pancreas, liver, or ovary affect the bony spinal column.

Ten percent of symptomatic spinal metastases originate from unknown primary tumors (3). Some malignancies spread to the intraspinal space without directly affecting the bone. Lymphoma and neuroblastoma often invade the spinal canal through the intervertebral foramina. Ewing's sarcoma, as well as osteosarcoma, may be primary in the epidural space. Primary epidural tumors are rare.

By location in the spinal column, thoracic metastases are estimated to occur twice as frequently as lumbar metastases and four times as frequently as cervical metastases (2). Almost two thirds of metastatic spinal lesions present clinically in the thoracic region (9), although in some autopsy series, lesions of the lumbar spine have been most prevalent (3). The level of spinal involvement varies with the tumor type. Breast and lung tumor metastases are equally distributed throughout the spine. Prostate, renal, and gastrointestinal metastases are more often found in the lower thoracic, lumbar, and sacral levels. Tumors of the uterus and uterine cervix most commonly spread to the lower lumbar and sacral spine. Pancoast tumors of the apex of the lung extend directly into the cervicothoracic spine in 25% of cases (9), often by intraforaminal extension. Multiple noncontiguous levels of spinal tumor are present in 10–38% of cases (10); this pattern is relatively less common in patients with lung cancer (8).

EC is caused by the direct extension of the tumor from the vertebral body in 85–90% of cases (9). In pediatric patients, EC due to tumor of the posterior elements is more likely, and intraforaminal spread of tumor from paraspinal sites also occurs more frequently than in adults (10). It is noted, however, that tumor metastases in the epidural space seldom breach the dura (3,11).

The prevalence of EC varies according to the tumor type. In one series of 103 patients with lung cancer, 26% with squamous histology, 9% with adenocarcinoma, and 14% with small cell tumors had spinal cord compression (12). The prevalence of all neurologic complications in this series was approximately 40%.

Breast cancer accounts for almost one fourth of EC diagnosed in cancer hospitals. Vertebral metastases are identified in 60% of patients with breast cancer, and multiple levels of compression are common. EC is rarely the initial presentation or an early finding in breast cancer (13).

Approximately 7% of patients with prostate cancer develop EC. EC was noted in 12.2% of patients with poorly differentiated tumors and 2.9% of those with well-differentiated tumors (14). The average time from initial prostate cancer diagnosis to EC is 2 years, although it is shorter in stage D2. In approximately 30% of prostate cancer patients with EC, it is the initial manifestation of the cancer (15).

Renal cell carcinomas may also cause EC secondary to bony metastasis. Testicular cancer rarely metastasizes to bone but may grow into the spinal canal from the retroperitoneal space. Malignant melanoma may produce EC from vertebral disease, but intradural and leptomeningeal involvement are probably more common. Head and neck cancers rarely metastasize beyond the cervical lymph nodes; approximately 80% of distant metastases are detected within 2 years of initial diagnosis. Therefore, a patient with head and neck cancer presenting with EC after 2 years should be evaluated for a second primary malignancy. EC occurred at all levels of the spine in one small series of patients with head and neck cancers (16).

Esophageal cancers may rarely cause EC by direct invasion to the thoracic spinal column (17). Carcinoid tumors are associated with neurologic complications in <20% of cases; the most frequent is EC due to spinal metastases, generally a late complication.

In plasmacytoma and multiple myeloma, EC is usually due to bony collapse, occurring in >10% of patients. Hodgkin's disease and non-Hodgkin's lymphomas are associated with a 5% incidence of EC, usually in the presence of extranodal or extensive nodal disease. The thoracic spine is most often involved, in many cases by intraforaminal spread of tumor (18). Patients with EC due to lymphoma are at high risk for meningeal disease. Cerebrospinal fluid (CSF) examination should be considered along with spinal imaging, as concurrent meningeal lymphoma is common and affects the antineoplastic treatment regimen. Vertebral compression fracture with radicular pain is a rare presenting sign of acute leukemia (19).

EC is the presenting sign of cancer in up to 30% of pediatric cases. The time interval to presentation with EC may be twice as long in children without a known cancer, compared to those already diagnosed with malignancy (20). Children without a cancer history presenting with EC are often initially misdiagnosed (6). EC is the most frequent neurologic complication of Ewing's sarcoma (21).

DIFFERENTIAL DIAGNOSIS

The differential diagnosis of back pain and neurologic dysfunction secondary to EC includes benign tumors; it is interesting to note that meningiomas occur frequently in patients with breast cancer (2). Given its high prevalence, coexisting nonmalignant disease of the spine may affect as many as 30% of patients with EC (22). Degenerative, inflammatory, and infectious processes affect the spinal structures (23). Soft tissue injuries causing back pain are very common. Trauma is the most common cause of back pain in children; other nonmalignant conditions such as Scheuermann's disease and scoliosis (24) also present in this age-group. Back pain in patients with cancer may be a secondary symptom caused by vertebral osteoporosis owing to radiation therapy or corticosteroids.

Spinal cord or cauda equina dysfunction may be related to direct tumor or treatment effects, without EC. Leptomeningeal disease, intradural extramedullary or intramedullary spinal cord disease, paraneoplastic necrotizing myelopathy, and myelopathy induced by radiation or intrathecal chemotherapy should be considered if no epidural compressive lesion is found. Myelopathy is a late complication of radiation; epidural lipomatosis may be caused by corticosteroid therapy. Vascular events of the spinal cord may occur in association with tumor masses.

PATHOGENESIS OF NEUROLOGIC DYSFUNCTION AND PAIN

The high incidence of metastasis to the vertebrae, despite their poor blood supply, is explained by their specific physiologic features. The vertebrae have a large capillary capacity, promoting local stasis of blood. The walls of the vascular sinusoids are discontinuous and intersinusoidal cords form *cul-de-sacs* for tumor. Tumor products and the products of bone resorption act to stimulate tumor growth (25). Monocytes producing interleukin-1 may promote resorption of normal bone (2). Metastases may occur more commonly in previously damaged bone (26).

Batson's plexus is a valveless system of epidural veins in which blood may flow rostrally or caudally. On Valsalva's maneuver, this system drains the viscera and may be a route of metastatic spread. Tumor also reaches the bone through the arteries, lymphatics, and by direct extension.

Epidural tumor produces dysfunction of neural structures by direct compression and by secondary demyelination, ischemia, and tissue edema. Inflammation may change vascular permeability and disrupt the blood–spinal barrier at the tumor site. The release of excitatory amino acids by injured neurons further promotes ischemia and injury.

In the initial stage of epidural cord compression, there may be white matter edema and axonal swelling with normal blood flow. These changes are due to direct compression or venous congestion. Over time, progressive compression decreases blood flow and disturbs vascular autoregulation, leading to the development of vasogenic edema. Spinal cord infarction may result from the interruption of venous outflow or occlusion of small arteries or from the interruption of the major arterial supply to the spinal cord (including the artery of Adamkiewicz) or radicular arteries in the intervertebral foramina.

A necrotic cavity, usually located in the ventral portion of the posterior columns or dorsal horn, has been visualized on magnetic resonance imaging (MRI) (10). The effects of cord compression may also be due to coup or contrecoup injury, which is not easily predicted on the basis of the tumor location in relation to the spinal cord. Demyelination as a mechanism of neural dysfunction (5) is supported by pathologic examinations, which demonstrate greater demyelination of white matter than gray matter, a pattern that does not conform to arterial supply. Animal experiments indicate that a more rapid ischemic change produces a greater degree of irreversible neurologic injury (27,28). Similar observations have been made in the human spinal cord.

Pain due to malignancy of the spine may result from activation of afferent nociceptive neurons by mechanical distortion and inflammatory mediators (nociceptive pain) or from neural dysfunction (neuropathic pain). Nociceptors innervate the periosteum of bone, soft tissues (ligaments and muscles), facet articular cartilage, dura mater, nerve root sheaths, and blood vessels. Vertebral collapse and structural instability can give rise to mechanical pain through injury to these structures, which worsens during spine loading and weight shifting. There may be secondary myofascial pain as well. Neuropathic pain results from altered peripheral and central neural activity that may be induced by injury of the nerve roots, axonal injury, or other processes such as deafferentation (loss of primary sensory input).

PATIENT EVALUATION

Although it is widely recognized that pain is often the first symptom of spinal neoplasm, accurate assessment of back and neck pain in the patient with cancer may be challenging to even the experienced clinician. A complete history and physical examination, including thorough neurologic examination, are essential to localize the underlying pathology. Proper clinical localization is necessary to choose diagnostic and therapeutic interventions correctly (Table 37.1). The importance of obtaining a detailed understanding of the spinal lesion(s) and relationship to symptoms cannot be overemphasized.

TABLE 37.1

PATTERNS OF SPINAL TUMOR INVOLVEMENT

Bone
    Bone alone
        Single site
        Multiple contiguous sites
        Multiple noncontiguous sites
    Bone and paraspinal soft tissues
    Bone, paraspinal tissues, and viscera
    Bone and nerve roots
    Bone and epidural space (without thecal compression)
    Bone and epidural spinal cord compression
    Bone and epidural cauda equina compression
Epidural
    Intraforaminal
        Isolated
        Local extension
    Epidural and spinal cord compression
        Single site
        Multiple contiguous sites
        Multiple noncontiguous sites
    Epidural and cauda equina compression
        Single site
        Multiple contiguous sites
        Multiple noncontiguous sites
Diffuse

Inadequate evaluation increases the likelihood of otherwise preventable neurologic compromise. In a retrospective survey of patients with cancer presenting with back pain, misdiagnosis was attributed to poor history, inadequate examination, and insufficient diagnostic evaluation (29). In a review of cancer pain consultations performed by a neurology-based pain service, the comprehensive evaluation of pain led to an identification of new malignant involvement in 65% of cases (30). This underscores the importance of thorough clinical evaluation.

History

Up to 95% of adult and 80% of pediatric patients with EC present with pain (10,31). The difference in pain prevalence between adults and children may reflect greater difficulty in the pain assessment of and the underreporting of pain in children. Pain may precede other symptoms and signs of EC by 1 year (10). This interval may vary by tumor type; it is generally shorter for lung cancer than breast cancer (32). Overall, patients experience pain for an average of 4–5 months before presentation (3).

Pain may be local at the site of pathology or referred in a nonradicular or radicular (dermatomal) distribution or have combined features. Radicular or root pain is reported in 90% of lumbosacral EC, 79% of cervical, and 55% of thoracic cord compression (32). Radicular pain may be bilateral in thoracic lesions and is often described as a tight band around the chest or abdomen. It is important to note that radicular pain may be experienced in only one part of a dermatome. When a nerve root lesion produces chest or abdominal pain, the complaint may be mistakenly identified as referred pain of visceral origin. Radicular lesions are usually associated with segmental findings on examination. Nonradicular referred pain may be associated with vague paresthesias and tenderness at the painful site. Pain may be continuous at rest and markedly

aggravated by body movements (incident pain). Although local pain from a vertebral lesion is worsened with loading due to upright posture, pain due to EC is often greatly increased by lying supine. A lesion confined to the vertebral body may also produce nonradicular referred pain. Disease at C7 may refer pain to the interscapular region, and pain due to disease at L1 may be referred to the iliac crests, hips, or sacroiliac region. Sacral disease often causes midline pain radiating to the buttocks, which is made worse with sitting. Radicular pain, in particular, may be paroxysmal, spontaneous, or provoked by movement or sensory stimulation. Valsalva's maneuver may produce or aggravate both local and radicular pain. Pain on neck flexion or straight leg raising implies dural traction. Lhermitte's sign (electric shock–like pain) is a symptom of spinal cord dysfunction. Compression of the cervical spinal cord rarely produces funicular pain, which is pain referred to the lower extremities, thorax, or abdomen as a band of paresthesias. "Pseudoclaudication" of legs may be an isolated lumbar root symptom (2).

The neurologic findings associated with EC also vary. There can be extensive epidural tumor with no neurologic findings on examination. Upper motor neuron weakness may occur with lesions of the spinal cord (above the L1 vertebral body). This finding is present in 75% of patients with EC at diagnosis (9). Sensory changes occur in approximately half of patients at presentation, including paresthesias and sensory loss, which can be segmental or below the level of injury. Sensory complaint without pain is exceedingly rare. Bladder and bowel dysfunction are evident in more than half of patients on presentation with EC; constipation usually precedes urinary retention or incontinence (2).

Examination

The physical examination begins with the observation of posture, spinal curvature, symmetry of paraspinal muscles, extremities, and skin. The practitioner may appreciate tenderness of the spinous processes on palpation or percussion, although this may not correlate with the level of spinal disease. Gibbus deformity and vertebral misalignments are frequently palpable; actual crepitus of the spine is unusual. Tenderness or spasm of the paraspinal muscles may also be noted. Urinary retention may be demonstrated by bladder percussion. Laxity of the anal sphincter may be apparent on digital rectal examination. Specific areas of sacral or coccygeal tenderness may be identified by external palpation, rectal, or pelvic examination.

Spinal maneuvers to elicit pain should be performed carefully. Thoracic and abdominal radicular pain may be provoked on lateral flexion and rotation of the trunk. Increased pain on neck flexion and straight leg raise sign may be "pseudomeningeal" signs of dural traction due to epidural tumor. If neck rigidity is present, the examiner should use extreme caution with range-of-motion maneuvers. Muscle spasm may be triggered by bony instability of the cervical spine, and forced movements may dislodge bony fragments, causing acute spinal cord or brainstem injury.

The neurologic examination reveals positive findings in most patients with EC. The examination should include assessment of mental status, cranial nerves, motor function, reflexes, sensation, coordination, and gait. Proximal lower extremity weakness may be initially evident only as difficulty in rising from a chair. Although weakness due to upper motor neuron dysfunction is usually associated with increased tone and hyperreflexia, acute "spinal shock" can cause a flaccid areflexic paralysis. In the subacute phase of recovery from spinal shock, "mass reflexes" appear consisting of flexor spasms, hyperhydrosis, and piloerection due to autonomic dysfunction. Lower motor neuron weakness may be accompanied by flaccidity, atrophy, muscle fasciculations, and hyporeflexia. A cervical lesion can produce segmental hyporeflexia in the arm or arms and increased reflexes below. Lesions above the pyramidal decussation of the corticospinal tracts in the lower brainstem may be associated with loss of contralateral abdominal reflexes; lesions below the decussation produce loss of ipsilateral abdominal reflexes. Segmental motor dysfunction due to thoracic nerve root disease may produce asymmetric abdominal muscle contraction and loss of abdominal reflexes. Beevor's sign (upward movement of the umbilicus on attempted flexion of the trunk) indicates a lesion at or near the T10 level. Lesions of the roots of the upper lumbar plexus produce hip flexion weakness and a dropped knee-jerk reflex; lesions of the roots to the lower lumbar plexus may produce foot drop and diminished ankle-jerk reflex. Loss of bulbocavernosus and anal reflexes may accompany conus and cauda equina lesions (2).

Although the sensory examination may help in determining the level of epidural disease, EC results in a broad variation of sensory dysfunction, with incomplete lesions being the rule. The level of reduced sensation may be determined to be up to five segmental levels below, or one to two segments above, the level of cord compression. A sensory level on the trunk sparing the sacral dermatomes may occur in up to 20% of patients with thoracic or high lumbar compression (2). Suspended partial sensory levels or unilateral bands of sensory loss may be seen with spinal cord lesions up to the brainstem. Facial numbness may be due to upper cervical lesions. Lesions of the upper thoracic nerve roots may result in Horner syndrome, with autonomic dysfunction of the face and upper extremity. Compression of the conus of the spinal cord may produce sensory loss in the saddle area (buttocks and perineum) without lower extremity symptoms or signs.

Gait ataxia is an uncommon isolated sign of spinal cord compression. Other unusual features are signs of raised intracranial pressure; facial paresis, lower extremity fasciculations, or sciatica with cervical tumor; nystagmus with thoracic tumor; spinal myoclonus; an inverted knee-jerk reflex; and "painful legs and moving toes" (10).

Diagnostic Evaluation

The selection of specific imaging tests is guided by the clinical presentation. Several imaging methods are available to confirm EC. Because the correct interpretation of symptomatic and asymptomatic lesions on diagnostic imaging studies requires a thorough knowledge of the patient's clinical presentation, it is strongly recommended that clinicoradiographic correlation be made by the examining physician. In each individual case, the "neurologic urgency" for further diagnostic tests must be modified according to the potential for treatment, the patient's condition, and overall prognosis (Fig. 37.1).

Plain radiographs confirm tumor and assess structural stability of the spinal elements. In the patient with cancer at risk for spinal metastases with neck, shoulder, or upper extremity pain, flexion and extension views of the cervical spine should not be forced. Although plain radiographs are >90% sensitive and 86% specific for demonstrating abnormalities in the patient with symptomatic spinal metastases, autopsy series suggest that up to 25% of spinal lesions are invisible on radiography (2). False negatives occur because of mild degree of pathology, poor visualization (e.g., the first thoracic vertebra), or because the abnormality is missed on interpretation. The false-positive rate for interpreting collapsed vertebrae as malignant may be as high as 20% (33).

It is estimated that a 30–50% change in bone mass is needed before plain films become abnormal (31). On anterior/posterior view, spinal radiographs may show pedicle erosion (the "winking owl" sign), increased interpeduncular

distance, paraspinal widening, or paraspinal soft tissue shadow. On lateral view, vertebral collapse (wedging of the body), scalloped bodies, disc space destruction, a narrow spinal canal, hypertrophied facets, and disc calcification may be seen. Oblique views are needed to discriminate spondylolytic osteophytic encroachment from tumor causing foraminal abnormality (5). Vertebral collapse and pedicle erosion >50% are especially predictive of EC. On plain radiography, multiple vertebral involvement is noted in up to 86% of patients with spinal tumor (5) and in >30% of patients with EC.

Computed tomography (CT) scan may be useful to better delineate pathology using restricted fields of view (2). CT is superior to other imaging techniques for demonstrating cortical bone architecture (4). Before the availability of MRI, CT scan in combination with myelography was considered the gold standard for demonstrating the level and extent of epidural disease. CT myelography may be considered if the index of suspicion for epidural disease is high and other imaging studies are normal or if MRI cannot be interpreted or performed. Lumbar puncture should precede cervical puncture in most cases. Injection of air to supplement contrast medium may better image a CSF block. If the upper and lower extent of the block cover a long spinal segment, myelography may be repeated after treatment to determine if multiple discrete lesions are present and to better define radiotherapy portals. If repeated imaging is anticipated, oil-based contrast medium may be used to allow for follow-up radiographic imaging without repeated punctures. Another advantage of myelography over other diagnostic imaging tests is the collection of CSF for analysis. However, there is a risk of worsening neurologic function after dural puncture in the patient with partial CSF block, due to the "coning" of the spinal cord as pressure below the block is relieved. This risk may be as high as 15% (2,10). It is therefore recommended that under these conditions, corticosteroids be administered before dural puncture.

Radionuclide bone scintigrams reveal a 5–10% change in bone tissue (31). Bone scintigrams are more sensitive than radiographs except in multiple myeloma (10). They are not as specific as radiographs in identifying the level of EC. False positives may be due to nonmalignant skeletal conditions and false negatives, due to lytic lesions, for example, myeloma or solid tumors such as lung and melanoma, and prior radiation therapy. If the entire skeleton is involved by tumor, no contrast in the radionuclide uptake can be appreciated. New technology of immunoscintigraphy may prove to be more sensitive (2).

MRI is now considered by many experts to be the imaging procedure of choice for EC. MRI without contrast enhancement may eliminate the need for other imaging studies. MRI sensitivity and specificity rival that of CT myelography and are better with contrast. In the patient with back pain and radicular symptoms but no bony tumor on plain radiograph, gadolinium-enhanced MRI is indicated to identify intraforaminal disease such as that which occurs in lymphoma and some solid tumors (31). Double-dose gadolinium-enhanced MRI may increase the accuracy. MRI with and without contrast excludes vertebral metastases, paravertebral lesions, EC, intramedullary tumor, and many leptomeningeal processes. Fat suppression and T_2 weighting, not supplemented by addition of contrast, may improve the detection of myeloma lesions (34). In previously irradiated bone, MRI signal intensity is increased and gadolinium contrast enhancement is decreased.

In the cancer patient with back pain and suspected EC, complete spine MRI is indicated when there is a high risk of noncontiguous or skip lesions. A full spine sagittal "screening" image to identify targets for more detailed imaging is suggested (5). Often, the cervical spine is not imaged because it adds significantly to sequencing time. Failure to identify multiple levels of EC may compromise radiotherapy

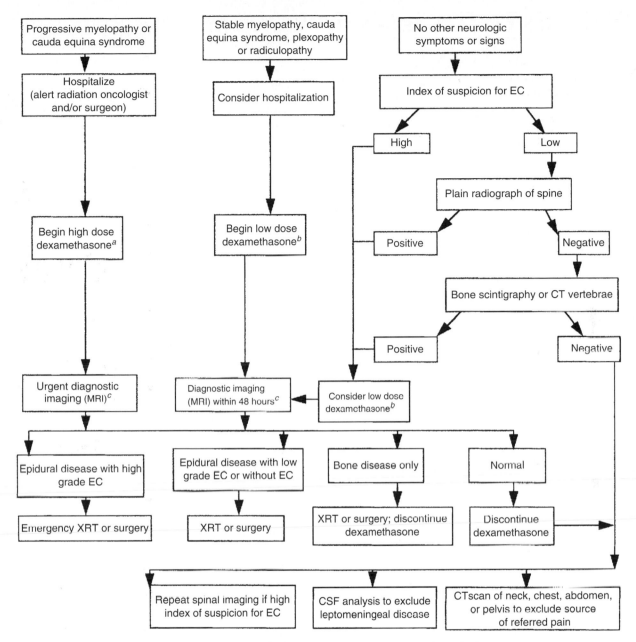

FIGURE 37.1. Patient with cancer and with back or neck pain—candidate for radiotherapy or surgery. CSF, cerebrospinal fluid; CT, computed tomography; MRI, magnetic resonance imaging; EC, epidural compression of the spinal cord and/or cauda equina; XRT, external beam radiotherapy. [a]High-dose dexamethasone, 100 mg followed by 24 mg q6h with taper over weeks. [b]Low-dose dexamethasone, 20 mg followed by 4 mg q6h with taper over weeks. [c]MRI, suggest sagittal screening of vertebral column with expanded imaging of affected areas or CT myelography (see text). (Data from Foley KM. Pain syndromes in patients with cancer. In: Portenoy RK, Kanner RM, eds. *Pain management: theory and practice.* Philadelphia, PA: FA Davis Co, 1995:195; and Posner, JB. *Neurological complications of cancer, contemporary neurology series,* Vol. 45. Philadelphia, PA: FA Davis Co, 1995:112, with permission.)

if untreated lesions become symptomatic and are detected at a later time. The cost-effectiveness of sagittal screening studies for identifying treatable lesions has not yet been determined. In patients with claustrophobia or severe pain in the supine position, conscious sedation or general anesthesia may be required to complete the MRI. The risk of sedation or anesthesia for MRI must be weighed against the risks of alternative imaging procedures, such as CT myelography, for each individual patient. Newer tumor-imaging techniques may add to the diagnostic evaluation of patients with spinal malignancies in future.

CSF examination is not required for the diagnosis of epidural tumor, and as noted in the preceding text, dural puncture may pose some risk to the patient with EC and should therefore be avoided. If performed, CSF analysis may show elevated protein with normal glucose and, rarely, pleocytosis in the patient with EC.

The patient presenting with EC and an unknown primary tumor generally undergoes a battery of tests to identify the primary neoplasm. At times, biopsy of a vertebral, epidural, or paraspinal lesion is needed to determine the primary tumor histology.

MANAGEMENT OF ACUTE SPINAL CORD OR CAUDA EQUINA COMPRESSION

Pharmacologic Interventions

Corticosteroids are the mainstay of pharmacologic therapy for acute EC. The administration of these agents prevents lipid peroxidation of neuronal cell membranes, ischemia, and increased intracellular calcium (35). Vasogenic edema in EC has been demonstrated to be responsive to corticosteroids. Cytotoxic edema may also play a role. Alternative steroids and other agents to treat edema, such as mannitol, may be used.

The timing of administration and dosage of corticosteroids may affect neurologic outcome, and there is some evidence for a therapeutic window (2,35). Better analgesic effect of higher-dose regimens has been demonstrated in one study (36). Many authors favor a prolonged course of high-dose corticosteroids, for example, the equivalent of a bolus of 100 mg dexamethasone followed by 96 mg per day in divided doses, tapered over a few weeks for high-grade EC, and a lower dosage, for example, 20 mg dexamethasone followed by 16 mg per day in divided doses with a taper for low-grade EC (2,5,36).

High-dose therapy may be more analgesic, but increases the risk of side effects. Side effects depend on the duration of drug administration, cumulative dose, and regimen. In one prospective study of patients with EC treated with high-dose corticosteroids, it was noted that depressive symptoms and neuropsychiatric disorders were more common than in similar patients not receiving such treatment (37). Suppression of the hypothalamic-pituitary-adrenal axis occurs with sustained dosing; it is suggested that dosing be readministered after withdrawal in situations of severe physiologic stress. Steroid-induced osteoporosis may be reversible in the young (38). Other withdrawal symptoms, including *Pneumocystis* infection, have been reported. Corticosteroids are metabolized by the cytochrome P-450 system, which has implications for drug interactions with anticonvulsants and other medications; this potential interaction with anticonvulsants may be the least with valproate sodium (35). Clinicians should be aware that rapid administration of steroids causes severe burning pain in the perineum; therefore, it is preferable that doses not be given as intravenous push. Except in emergency situations, corticosteroids should be held before making the cancer diagnosis if lymphoma is suspected because of the immediate oncolytic effect, which would impede diagnosis.

Virtually all patients presenting with EC have severe pain requiring opioid analgesics. Practitioners should be prepared to titrate an opioid analgesic to effect; this may require high doses, especially in patients with neurologic involvement (39).

Nonpharmacologic Interventions

Radiation Therapy

Radiation therapy for EC is chosen to inhibit tumor growth, restore and preserve neurologic function, treat pain, and improve quality of life. The course of external beam radiotherapy (XRT) for spinal metastases and EC depends on the radiosensitivity of the tumor and its extent. Currently, XRT is considered by many clinicians to be the primary treatment for EC. The course may be accelerated for patients in severe pain. The spinal section routinely treated includes two vertebral segments above and below a single site of neurologic compression. Anterior/posterior portals are set to include the vertebral body, especially in low thoracic and lumbar lesions.

Fields are also designed to accommodate paravertebral tumor. A single port field can be used in very ill patients affected by cachexia. As there are no known predictive factors for epidural progression with multiple sites of spinal disease, the decision to treat asymptomatic noncontiguous sites depends on clinical judgment. In addition to the clinical condition of the patient, factors to be considered include the type of tumor, presence of vertebral collapse, and anticipated future difficulty in matching radiation portals. Special techniques are required to re-irradiate. XRT alone is more than 85% effective for EC in radiosensitive tumors (3). Motor improvement is seen in 49% and stabilization of function in another 31% of patients. However, <50% of patients regain their lost function (3). The possibility of progression to EC may be reduced by irradiating bony lesions. It is uncertain whether radiation treats micrometastases or prevents them. The response to XRT may be delayed in some cases; the factors accounting for this observation are not well understood (2). Brachytherapy can be used for adjacent paraspinal masses and may prevent EC (40).

Surgery

Surgical intervention for EC may be performed for the following:

1. To establish the cancer diagnosis when it is in doubt and when tissue is required for histologic examination
2. To achieve surgical cure for a primary neoplasm
3. To treat prior irradiated radioresistant tumor with symptomatic progression of EC
4. To decompress neural structures and stabilize the spine
5. To halt a rapid clinical deterioration (2–4,22).

The specific goals of surgery are to resect pathology, restore load-bearing capacity, decompress neural structures, achieve stability, treat pain, and improve quality of life. Length of survival may be extended with improvement in functional status.

A long-awaited multicenter study recently concluded by Patchell et al. showed superior clinical outcomes for first-line decompressive surgery combined with postoperative radiotherapy compared to radiotherapy alone in patients with spinal cord displacement due to tumor compression. Criteria for the study entry included single-level compression, <48 hours paraplegia at the worst, prognosis of at least 3 months, and good overall condition. Patients with highly radiosensitive malignancies were excluded from participation. Study patients were treated with corticosteroids and randomized to receive 30 Gy of radiotherapy within 24 hours or surgical decompression within 24 hours followed by the same radiotherapy within 14 days of surgery. Better clinical outcomes were demonstrated for both primary (ability to walk) and secondary endpoints. The secondary endpoints included survival time; continence; requirement for opioid and corticosteroid medications; and function as assessed with formal functional rating scales (Frankel Functional Scale, American Spinal Injury Association Motor Score). More surgical patients retained the ability to walk ($p = .012$) and those able to walk at the time of enrollment retained this ability longer, having received surgery (median 153 vs. 54 days, $p = .024$). Continence, muscle strength, and functionality were significantly better in the surgical group ($p = .016$, $p = .001$, and $p = .0006$, respectively). A nonsignificant trend toward longer survival was also observed in the surgical group. Duration of hospitalization showed no difference. The results observed during the clinical trial were sufficient to meet early termination criteria, and enrollment was halted. The study supports primary surgical intervention for patients with characteristics similar to those studied (41). For patients with more complex malignant neurologic involvement and those with a higher degree of comorbidity, individualized risk/benefit analyses may favor nonsurgical treatment (42).

Many factors affect the choice of the surgical technique, including tumor location, tumor extent, integrity of adjacent segments, and general debility. In vascular tumors such as renal and thyroid, operative intervention may be preceded by vascular embolization. Tumor decompression and stabilization may be achieved through either an anterior vertebrectomy or a laminectomy. Posterior decompression through wide laminectomy is generally followed by stabilization to prevent kyphosis (2,43–45). New posterolateral techniques are being developed for specific EC syndromes in advanced patients with cancer.

In one thorough retrospective study (46) of 110 patients after aggressive surgical intervention for spinal metastases, 82% of patients showed improvement in pain relief and ambulatory status. The goals of the treatment were identified as gross total resection of tumor and spine reconstruction. Half of the patients had prior treatment and were deteriorating clinically. The "traditional" criteria for surgery, such as relapse after radiation therapy and the determination of histology, were expanded to include gross tumor resection for radioresistant or solitary lesions and for spinal stabilization. In this series, more complex surgical instrumentation was used than previously reported. Most patients received ongoing systemic therapy, partly confounding the analysis of long-term outcomes. The complication rate of 48% correlated with age older than 65, prior spinal treatment, and the presence of paraparesis. These factors also correlated with greater morbidity and poorer survival. However, in this series, nearly half of the patients were alive at 2 years, an improvement over prior studies that had compared the posterior surgical laminectomy and radiation therapy to radiation therapy alone. This improvement in survival was noted in patients with more advanced cancer and prior treatment. These authors concluded on the basis of prior reports (47,48) and the data from this series that the anterior surgical approach with stabilization may improve outcomes and suggested further definition of the subset of patients that might benefit from early anterior resection and spinal stabilization.

Early reviews of surgical outcomes have confirmed higher morbidity and mortality in patients with prior spine irradiation, age older than 70 years, and those with poor performance status at the time of surgery (49). In one reported series, the factors predictive of shorter survival were poorer preoperative neurologic status (leg strength grade 3/5 or weaker), anatomical site of the primary carcinoma (lung or colon cancer), and multiple vertebral body involvement. These authors consider surgical intervention contraindicated if two or more of those factors are present (48). Several authors have suggested that a limited posterolateral approach to tumor resection be reserved for patients with expected survival <6 months (46,50). Few data are available with regard to surgical intervention for lateral epidural or intraforaminal disease. In a recent experience, a small group of patients, not considered candidates for major surgical procedures, benefited from limited resection of lateral epidural tumor. Surgery was preceded by careful correlation of symptoms with tumor mass, and good outcomes were recorded in all eight patients (50). This experience again supports careful consideration in each case until the criteria for primary surgical intervention are more fully delineated. Clearly, further refinement of surgical approaches depends on precise neuroanatomic localization of neoplastic involvement (Table 37.1).

The complication rate for spinal surgery may be as high as 30% in patients who have undergone prior XRT (3). Coagulopathy and exogenous anticoagulants increase the risk of hematoma at the operative site. Difficult wound healing, infection, bony instability, nonfusion, displacement of implants, and other complications may occur.

There has been a steady evolution in the concepts and execution of surgical management for EC. In choosing primary surgical versus radiotherapeutic intervention, the prognosis for neurologic improvement and expected impact on functional status must be considered. In some series, radiation therapy has been shown to be equally effective to laminectomy and radiation, but with <50% neurologic improvement overall (9). *De novo* anterior–posterior resection with spine stabilization may result in better outcomes than laminectomy and radiation or radiation alone, as surgical complications are generally manageable, survival is improved (although the 2-year survival for lung cancer may be 10% and for colorectal cancer, only 17%), and patients may remain ambulatory longer (46). The data are as yet insufficient to draw final conclusions regarding pain and quality-of-life outcomes in all patients, but as discussed in the preceding text, there is a subset of patients presenting with single-level spinal cord displacement that will benefit from primary surgical intervention. The decision to recommend initial radiation therapy versus surgical intervention must be individualized, especially in those patients with more complex presentations. To date, the cauda equina syndrome has not been well studied. It has been suggested that without bony instability, the speed of progression of neurologic deficit and radiosensitivity of the tumor are the main factors to consider in determining primary antineoplastic treatment with either surgery or radiation. Severe deficits generally hold a poor prognosis independent of treatment.

Nonsurgical stabilization of the bony spine can be accomplished with a cervical collar or body bracing. The patient with cancer, neck pain, and suspected cervical spine disease should be placed in a collar while diagnostic evaluation is being conducted.

ONGOING CARE

Pain Management

Extended corticosteroid administration (i.e., for the duration of life in patients with EC and short prognosis) has not been well studied but is common in clinical practice. This practice should be discouraged unless there is evidence of ongoing steroid-reversible neurologic deficits due to the high risk of steroid toxicities discussed in the section "Pharmacologic Interventions" (51).

Guidelines for the use of nonsteroidal anti-inflammatory medications, opioid analgesics, and adjuvant analgesics for neuropathic pain have been published in recent years (52–56). Chronic opioid therapy is often required for persistent pain after treatment of EC. Cases have been reported in which patients with EC required prolonged high-dose intrathecal infusion of opioid and local anesthetic to obtain adequate analgesia (57,58). Radionuclides are discussed in other chapters.

Neuroablative procedures are considered when the benefit-to-risk ratio favors analgesia over the potential for further neurologic compromise. Destruction of the nervous tissue may be accomplished by anesthetic or surgical means. Chemical epidural neurolysis may be chosen to effect single or multiple nerve root interruption. Intrathecal neurolysis would be anticipated to achieve analgesia over a wider territory and may be selected when the epidural space is compromised. Both approaches entail the risk of acute neurologic deterioration, which may be irreversible (59). Neurosurgical ablation of nerve roots (rhizotomy) involves major surgery and is less often indicated in very sick patients. Midline myelotomy may be indicated in patients with severe midline sacral pain and bladder or bowel compromise due to tumor of the sacrum. Spinothalamic tractotomy or cordotomy, although more easily performed as a percutaneous procedure, is not generally useful for pain in association with spine disease or EC. Hypophysectomy for diffuse painful metastatic bone disease may yield success rates as high as 90% in some endocrine-responsive tumors (60).

Integration of pharmacologic and nonpharmacologic analgesic therapies is needed for most patients with EC. A multidisciplinary approach to pain management and rehabilitation of patients with resected sacral chordoma has been reported (61).

Rehabilitation

Each patient's rehabilitation program must be individually tailored and continually reassessed and modified. For some patients, comprehensive care may be best accomplished in a formal inpatient rehabilitation setting (62). Specific rehabilitation goals are to improve ambulation, achieve weight bearing and transfers, restore bladder and bowel function, and protect the skin. The family is included in learning how to assist the patient with severely impaired mobility.

Spinal orthotics stabilize the spine and may decrease spinal pain by limiting motion. Physical therapy techniques for pain relief include massage, ultrasound, and transcutaneous electrical nerve stimulation.

Approximately 50% of patients require urinary catheterization before and after XRT for EC (3). Sexual dysfunction may be treatable with physical and medical interventions.

A number of medical problems common to the cancer population may limit aggressive rehabilitation efforts. Organ failure due to the disease or its treatment, hemodynamic instability, poor nutrition, cancer cachexia, and multiple physical and psychological symptoms may complicate rehabilitation. An active exercise program may have to be modified. Weakness due to spinal cord or nerve root compression may be complicated by peripheral neuropathy or myopathy, which are common complications of antineoplastic treatment. The skin of many patients with cancer is relatively more prone to breakdown and infection. Skin care and protection are essential, especially in the bedridden patient.

Chronic musculoskeletal problems may occur in children after spine irradiation during growth, due to the development of secondary spinal deformities. The risk of fracture in osteoporotic or tumor-laden bones should be carefully evaluated before initiating a mobility program. In patients who are paraparetic or paraplegic, prophylactic fixation of upper extremity lesions may be considered to aid mobility and weight bearing. In bedridden patients with multiple impending fractures, positioning and transfers must be undertaken with great caution.

The goals of physical medicine and rehabilitation in the patient with EC range from active programs to supportive and palliative care (63). Preventive rehabilitation therapy is directed toward achieving maximal functional restoration in patients who are cured or are in stable remission from their cancer. Continued encouragement for the effort required in aggressive rehabilitation is needed for a progressive decline in function due to advancing disease. For patients with limited prognosis, usually considered as <6 months' life expectancy, family participation receives more emphasis. The needs of the patient tend toward more dependent care as the cancer progresses. Palliative rehabilitation interventions are intended to provide comfort to the patient in the terminal stages of illness, and as noted in the preceding text, include the family.

Psychological Interventions

Ongoing psychological support of the patient with metastatic spine disease is essential. Issues of loss of independence and function require careful attention. Families often benefit from emotional support for anticipatory grieving. Professional assistance may be indicated as the burden of care increases with a patient's progressing disease. The palliative care team will often assist with complex therapeutic decision analysis and provide psychosocial support in this setting.

CLINICAL OUTCOMES

The potential for the recovery of function in patients with tumor involvement of the spine and associated neurologic structures varies by tumor type (primary or metastatic), the number of vertebrae involved, the nature and degree of neurologic involvement, the oncologic status, and the general medical condition. In most series, approximately 50% of patients with metastatic spine tumors are ambulatory at presentation, 35% are paretic, and 15% are plegic (2). Up to 30% of patients with weakness become plegic within the first week of presentation (5). The prognosis for regaining ambulatory status in patients with EC who begin therapy while being ambulatory is 75%; prognosis declines to 30–50% for patients who begin therapy while being paretic, and to 10% for those who begin therapy while being plegic (31). The duration of neurologic symptoms before treatment also affects the prognosis for neurologic recovery. If paraplegia has been present for days or if urinary retention is present for >30 hours, the likelihood of recovery is decreased (64). Rapidly progressing symptoms confer a worse prognosis.

Patients who remain unable to ambulate after irradiation treatment for EC have a particularly poor prognosis for survival, owing to the complications of paresis and more advanced disease. Survival rates for patients with EC are 40% at 1 year if ambulatory before and after radiation treatment, whereas patients who are nonambulatory before and ambulatory after treatment have a survival rate of 30% at 1 year and 20% at 3 years. Prognosis falls to 7% at 1 year for patients who are nonambulatory after treatment (3).

Response to treatment for EC and survival vary with the nature of the malignancy. In patients with prostate cancer, the response to the treatment of neurologic complications depends on whether the patient has received prior hormonal therapy. Better response to hormonal manipulation correlates with longer survival. The median survival of patients with prostate cancer after diagnosis with EC is 6 months; only 34% survive at least 1 year (65). Renal cancer is poorly radioresponsive and median survival time after diagnosis with EC is <4 months (66). Hemorrhagic complications of spinal surgery for metastatic renal tumor may be avoided by preoperative embolization (67). In testicular cancer, chemotherapy is effective for untreated lesions or for responsive tumors (68), but radiation and surgery may be considered if the disease is not chemoresponsive (66). Up to 75% of patients with melanoma and EC respond to radiation therapy (69–71). Patients with carcinoid tumor and EC have a median survival of 6 months. Ambulatory status may be preserved with radiation in up to 90% of patients with carcinoid tumors (17). In myeloma, long-term survival is common. In a series of patients with multiple myeloma, the 1-year survival was 100% and the median survival 37 months after EC was diagnosed (72). Solitary plasmacytomas are generally irradiated and surgically removed. Patients with multiple myeloma often receive radiation therapy to maximum spinal cord tolerance before surgical intervention is considered. Most lymphomas respond to chemotherapy and radiation. In pediatric patients, surgery may be preferred for radioresistant sarcomas and small cell tumors (Ewing's sarcoma, neuroblastoma, lymphoma, and germ cell tumors) presenting with rapid neurologic deterioration. A trend toward extended survival has been shown after surgical decompression in Ewing's sarcoma. Many small cell tumors respond to chemotherapy or radiation. Younger age may confer greater risk of radiation complications (73). Complete resection of primary spinal extraosseous epidural Ewing's sarcoma may be difficult. The 18-month survival was <40% in a small series of patients with this unusual malignancy (74).

In a recent series, median survival after first presentation with spinal cord compression was noted to be 2.9 months (75). Less than half of patients treated for EC are alive after 2 months (9). EC is an indicator of poor prognosis. Definitive intervention for EC must therefore be considered in the context of the patient's overall disease status. Systemic antineoplastic therapy may at times precede or entirely supplant intervention targeted at EC. For patients with very advanced cancer, the burden of diagnostic evaluation and intervention to reverse EC often outweighs minimal potential gains in function. Although few studies of quality of life have been conducted in this population, pain control should remain a high priority regardless of prognosis. Given limited available data, clinicians caring for patients with spinal neoplasm must work in a coordinated interdisciplinary fashion to carefully select those interventions that will achieve therapeutic goals for each individual patient and family.

References

1. Loeser JD. Neurosurgical approaches in palliative care. In: Doyle D, Hanks GWC, MacDonald N, eds. *Oxford textbook of palliative medicine.* Oxford: Oxford University Press, 1993:221.
2. Posner JB. *Neurologic complications of cancer, Contemporary neurology series,* vol 45. Philadelphia, PA: FA Davis Co, 1995:112.
3. Perrin RG, Janjan NA, Langford LA. Spinal axis metastases. In: Levin VA, ed. *Cancer in the nervous system.* New York: Churchill Livingstone, 1996:259.
4. Byrne TN, Waxman SG. *Spinal cord compression: diagnosis and principles of management, Contemporary neurology series,* vol 33. Philadelphia, PA: FA Davis Co, 1990.
5. Grant R, Papadopoulos SM, Greenberg HS. Metastatic epidural spinal cord compression. *Neurol Clin* 1991;9(4):825.
6. Klein SL, Sanford RA, Muhlbauer MS. Pediatric spinal epidural metastases. *J Neurosurg* 1991;74:70.
7. Barron KD, Hirano A, Araski S, et al. Experiences with metastatic neoplasms involving the spinal cord. *Neurology* 1959;9:91.
8. Stark RJ, Henson RA, Evans SJW. Spinal metastases: a retrospective survey from a general hospital. *Brain* 1982;105:189.
9. Obbens EAMT. Neurological problems in palliative medicine. In: Doyle D, Hanks GWC, MacDonald N, eds. *Oxford textbook of palliative medicine.* Oxford: Oxford University Press, 1993:460.
10. Byrne TN. Spinal metastases. In: Wiley RG, ed. *Neurologic complications of cancer.* New York: Marcel Dekker Inc, 1995:23.
11. Harrington KD. Metastatic disease of the spine. In: Harrington KD, ed. *Orthopedic management of metastatic bone disease.* St. Louis: Mosby, 1988:309.
12. Misulis KE, Wiley RG. Neurological complications of lung cancer. In: Wiley RG, ed. *Neurologic complications of cancer.* New York: Marcel Dekker Inc, 1995:295.
13. Anderson NE. Neurological complications of breast cancer. In: Wiley RG, ed. *Neurologic complications of cancer.* New York: Marcel Dekker Inc, 1995:319.
14. Kuban DA, El-Mahdi AM, Sigfred SV, et al. Characteristics of spinal cord compression in adenocarcinoma of the prostate. *Urology* 1986;28:364.
15. Flynn DF, Shipley WU. Management of spinal cord compression secondary to metastatic prostatic carcinoma. *Urol Clin North Am* 1991;18:145.
16. Moots PL, Wiley RG. Neurological disorders in head and neck cancers. In: Wiley RG, ed. *Neurologic complications of cancer.* New York: Marcel Dekker Inc, 1995:353.
17. Hagen NA. Neurological complications of gastrointestinal cancers. In: Wiley RG, ed. *Neurologic complications of cancer.* New York: Marcel Dekker Inc, 1995:395.
18. Friedman M, Kim TH, Panahon AM. Spinal cord compression in malignant lymphoma: treatment and results. *Cancer* 1976;37:1485.
19. Ribeiro RC, Pui CH, Schell MJ. Vertebral compression fracture as a presenting feature of acute lymphoblastic leukemia in children. *Cancer* 1988;61:589.
20. Jennings MT. Neurological complications of childhood cancer. In: Wiley RG, ed. *Neurologic complications of cancer.* New York: Marcel Dekker Inc, 1995:503.
21. Molloy PT, Phillips PC. Neurological complications of sarcomas. In: Wiley RG, ed. *Neurologic complications of cancer.* New York: Marcel Dekker Inc, 1995:417.
22. Galasko CSB, Sylvester BS. Back pain in patients treated for malignant tumours. *Clin Oncol* 1978;4:273.
23. Kanner RM. Low back pain. In: Portenoy RK, Kanner RM, eds. *Pain management: theory and practice, Contemporary neurology series,* vol 48. Philadelphia, PA: FA Davis Co, 1996:126.
24. Sty JR, Wells RG, Conway JJ. Spine pain in children. *Semin Nucl Med* 1993;23(4):296.
25. Manishen WJ, Sivananthan K, Orr FW. Resorbing bone stimulates tumor cell growth. A role for the host microenvironment in bone metastasis. *Am J Pathol* 1986;123:39.
26. Powell N. Metastatic carcinoma in association with Paget's disease of bone. *Br J Radiol* 1983;56:582.
27. Tarlov IM, Klinger H. Spinal cord compression studies. II: time limits for recovery after acute compression in dogs. *Arch Neurol Psychiatry* 1954;71:271.
28. Gledhill RF, Harrison BM, McDonald WI. Demyelination and remyelination after acute spinal cord compression. *Exp Neurol* 1973;38:472.
29. Burger EL, Lindeque BG. Sacral and non-spinal tumors presenting as backache: a retrospective study of 17 patients. *Acta Orthop Scand* 1994;65(3):344.
30. Gonzales GR, Elliott KJ, Portenoy RK, et al. The impact of a comprehensive evaluation in the management of cancer pain. *Pain* 1991;47(2):141.
31. Hewitt DJ, Foley KM. Neuroimaging of pain. In: Greenberg JO, ed. *Neuroimaging.* New York: McGraw-Hill, 1995:41.
32. Gilbert RW, Kim JH, Posner JB. Epidural spinal cord compression from metastatic tumor: diagnosis and treatment. *Ann Neurol* 1978;3:40.
33. Wong DA, Fornasier VL, MacNab I. Spinal metastases: the obvious, the occult, and the imposters. *Spine* 1990;15:1.
34. Rhamouni A, Divine M, Mathieu D, et al. Detection of multiple myeloma involving the spine: efficacy of fat-suppression and contrast-enhanced MR imaging. *AJR Am J Roentgenol* 1993;160(5):1049.
35. Vecht CJ, Verbiest HBC. Use of glucocorticoids in neuro-oncology. In: Wiley RG, ed. *Neurologic complications of cancer.* New York: Marcel Dekker Inc, 1995:199.
36. Greenberg HS, Kim JH, Posner JB. Epidural spinal cord compression from metastatic tumor: results with a new treatment protocol. *Ann Neurol* 1980;8:361.
37. Breitbart W, Stiefel F, Kornblith AB, et al. Neuropsychiatric disturbances in cancer patients with epidural spinal cord compression receiving high dose corticosteroids: a prospective comparison study. *Psychooncology* 1993;2:233–245.
38. Pocock NA, Eisman JA, Dunstan CR, et al. Recovery from steroid induced osteoporosis. *Ann Intern Med* 1987;107:319.
39. Yoshioka H, Tsuneto S, Kashiwagi T. Pain control with morphine for vertebral metastases and sciatica in advanced cancer patients. *J Palliat Care* 1994;10(1):10.
40. Armstrong JG, Fass DE, Bains M, et al. Paraspinal tumors: techniques and results of brachytherapy. *Int J Radiat Oncol Biol Phys* 1991;20:787.
41. Patchell RA, Tibbs PA, Regine WF, et al. Direct decompressive surgical resection in the treatment of spinal cord compression caused by metastatic cancer: a randomised trial. *Lancet* 2005;366:643–648.
42. Gerber DE, Grossman SA. Does decompressive surgery improve outcome in patients with metastatic epidural spinal-cord compression? *Nat Clin Pract Neurol* 2006;2:10–11.
43. Galasko CSB. Orthopaedic principles and management. In: Doyle D, Hanks GWC, MacDonald N, eds. *Oxford textbook of palliative medicine.* Oxford: Oxford University Press, 1993:274.
44. Findlay GFG. Adverse effects of the management of malignant spinal cord compression. *J Neurol Neurosurg Psychiatry* 1984;47:761.
45. McBroom R. Radiation or surgery for metastatic disease of the spine? *Soc Med Curr Med Lit—Orthop* 1988;1:97.
46. Sundaresan N, Sachdev VP, Holland JF, et al. Surgical treatment of spinal cord compression from epidural metastasis. *J Clin Oncol* 1995;13(9):2330.
47. Sioutos PJ, Arbit E, Meshulam BS, et al. Spinal metastases from solid tumors: analysis of factors affecting survival. *Cancer* 1995;76(8):1453.
48. Siegal T, Siegal TZ. Surgical decompression of anterior and posterior malignant epidural tumors compressing the spinal cord: a prospective study. *Neurosurgery* 1985;17:424–432.
49. Sundaresan N, Digiacinto GV, Hughes JEO, et al. Treatment of neoplastic spinal cord compression: results of a prospective study. *Neurosurgery* 1991;29:645.
50. Weller SJ, Rossitch E Jr. Unilateral posterolateral decompression without stabilization for neurological palliation of symptomatic spinal metastases in debilitated patients. *J Neurosurg* 1995;82(5):739.
51. Reid IR, King AR, Alexander CJ, et al. Prevention of steroid-induced osteoporosis with (3-amino-1-hydroxypropylidene)-1,1-bisphosphonate (APD). *Lancet* 1988;1:143.

52. Portenoy RK. Pharmacologic management of chronic pain. In: Fields HL, ed. *Pain syndromes in neurologic practice*. New York: Butterworth–Heinemann, 1990:257.

53. Payne R, Weinstein SM, Hill CS. Management of cancer pain. In: Levin VL, ed. *Cancer in the nervous system*. New York: Churchill Livingstone, 1996:411.

54. World Health Organization. *Cancer pain relief and palliative care*. Geneva: World Health Organization, 1990.

55. Jacox A, Carr DB, Payne R, et al. *Management of cancer pain, Clinical practice guideline no 9*, AHCPR Publication No 94–0592. Rockville, MD: Agency for Health Care Policy and Research, U.S. Department of Health and Human Services, Public Health Services, March 1994.

56. American Pain Society. *Principles of analgesic use in the treatment of acute pain and cancer pain*, 5th edn. Glenview, IL: American Pain Society, 2003.

57. Payne R, Cunningham M, Weinstein SM, et al. Intractable pain and suffering in a cancer patient. *Clin J Pain* 1995;11:70.

58. Aguilar JL, Espachs P, Roca G, et al. Difficult management of pain following sacrococcygeal chordoma: thirteen months of subarachnoid infusion. *Pain* 1994;59(2):317.

59. Morgan RJ, Steller PH. Acute paraplegias following intrathecal phenol block in the presence of occult epidural malignancy. *Anesth* 1994;49(2):142.

60. Waldman SD, Feldstein LS, Allen ML. Neuroadenolysis of the pituitary: description of a modified technique. *J Pain Symptom Manage* 1987;2:45.

61. Watling C, Allen RR. Treatment of neuropathic pain associated with sacrectomy. *Proceedings of the 48th Annual Scientific Meeting of the American Academy of Neurology*, San Francisco, CA, 1996 (abst).

62. Schlicht LA, Smelz JK. Metastatic spinal cord compression. In: Garden FH Grabois M, eds. *Cancer rehabilitation. Physical medicine and rehabilitation. State of the art reviews*, vol 8(2). Philadelphia, PA: Hanley and Belfus, 1994:345.

63. Garden FH, Gillis TA. Principles of cancer rehabilitation. In: Braddom RL, ed. *Physical medicine and rehabilitation*. Philadelphia, PA: WB Saunders, 1996:1199.

64. Bach F, Larsen BH, Rohde K, et al. Metastatic spinal cord compression: occurrence, symptoms, clinical presentation and progression in 398 patients with spinal cord compression. *Acta Neurochir (Wien)* 1990;107(1–2):37–43.

65. Delattre JY, Krol G, Thaler HT, et al. Distribution of brain metastases. *Arch Neurol* 1988;45:741.

66. Fadul CE. Neurological complications of genitourinary cancer. In: Wiley RG, ed. *Neurologic complications of cancer*. New York: Marcel Dekker Inc, 1995:388.

67. Sundaresan N, Choi IS, Hughes JEO, et al. Treatment of spinal metastases from kidney cancer by presurgical embolization and resection. *J Neurosurg* 1990;73:548.

68. Cooper K, Bajorin D, Shapiro W, et al. Decompression of epidural metastases from germ cell tumors with chemotherapy. *J Neurooncol* 1990;8:275.

69. Rate WR, Solin LJ, Turrisi AT. Palliative radiotherapy for metastatic malignant melanoma: brain metastases, bone metastases, and spinal cord compression. *Int J Radiat Oncol Biol Phys* 1998;15:859.

70. Herbert SH, Solin LJ, Rate WR, et al. The effect of palliative radiation therapy on epidural compression due to metastatic malignant melanoma. *Cancer* 1991;67:2472.

71. Henson JW. Neurological complications of malignant melanoma and other cutaneous malignancies. In: Wiley RG, ed. *Neurologic complications of cancer*. New York: Marcel Dekker Inc, 1995:333.

72. Spiess JL, Adelstein DJ, Hines DJ. Multiple myeloma presenting with spinal cord compression. *Oncology* 1988;45:88.

73. Mayfield JK, Riseborough EJ, Jaffe N, et al. Spinal deformities in children treated for neuroblastoma. *J Bone Joint Surg* 1981;63:183.

74. Kaspars GJ, Kamphorst W, et al. Primary spinal epidural extraosseous Ewing's sarcoma. *Cancer* 1991;68:648.

75. Loblaw DA, et al. A population-based study of malignant spinal cord compression in Ontario. *Clin Oncol (R Coll Radiol)* 2003;15:211–217.

CHAPTER 38 ■ NEUROMUSCULAR DYSFUNCTION AND PALLIATIVE CARE

DIANNA QUAN, JAMES W. TEENER, AND JOHN T. FARRAR

The neuromuscular disorders experienced by patients with cancer may cause weakness, fatigue, muscle cramps, sensory loss, pain, or dysesthesias. To determine the etiology of these symptoms accurately and formulate a treatment strategy, physicians need a logical approach to assessment. First, a careful history is taken and a neurologic examination is performed to identify potential neuromuscular dysfunction presenting as part of the complex set of symptoms that occur with cancer. Second, a specific diagnosis is established through laboratory testing or appropriate consultation. Finally, appropriate evidence-based therapy is prescribed. This approach is explored in the subsequent text with reference to common cancer-associated neuromuscular diseases.

The term *neuromuscular* refers to both the muscle and the peripheral nervous system, including anterior horn cells, dorsal root ganglia, sensory and motor spinal nerve roots, plexi, peripheral nerves, and neuromuscular junctions. Patients with cancer can develop neuromuscular deficits due to compression or invasion of these structures by neoplasm, paraneoplastic effects of cancer, or toxic effects of antineoplastic therapies, including chemotherapy or radiation.

A careful history and examination of the patient help the practitioner differentiate a neuromuscular problem from a central nervous system (CNS) or non-neurologic problem. The tempo of symptom onset is important. Weakness or sensory dysfunction that develops abruptly may indicate a vascular injury in the central or peripheral nervous system, tumor impingement on neural structures, or fulminant autoimmune or inflammatory process. Patients with new and rapidly progressive neuromuscular symptoms require immediate attention. Regardless of tempo of onset, symptoms should be assessed in the context of the location and type of underlying malignancy, previous or current treatments and medications, and underlying comorbid conditions.

The nature and distribution of symptoms offer further diagnostic clues. For example, weakness of one side of the body may suggest a CNS lesion, whereas symmetrical weakness of distal leg and hand muscles is more likely caused by neuropathy. Proximal weakness is more typical of myopathies or defects of neuromuscular transmission. Both positive (e.g., tingling or pain) and negative (e.g., numbness) sensory complaints may occur with nervous system injury. A sensory level or sensory loss below a particular dermatome is typical of spinal cord compression, whereas foot and hand numbness in a "stocking and glove" pattern is more typical of a neuropathy. Reflexes are usually brisk when weakness is caused by a CNS lesion and reduced in cases of neuropathy. Deep tendon reflexes are often normal in myopathy but the magnitude of the reflex motor response may be reduced if the myopathy is severe.

If the history and physical examination are not definitive, other diagnostic procedures should be used. Electrodiagnostic studies, especially nerve conduction studies (NCS) and needle electromyography (EMG) can frequently help to localize the problem to nerve, muscle, or neuromuscular junction. Depending on the symptoms, additional laboratory studies, such as creatine phosphokinase level, hemoglobin A1C, 2-hour 75 g glucose tolerance test, thyroid function tests, vitamin B_{12} level, Lyme antibody titers, HIV, cryoglobulins, or serum protein electrophoresis with immunofixation electrophoresis may identify a specific contributing cause. Even when the primary diagnosis is clear, identifying other treatable related factors may allow intervention to slow further deterioration.

Table 38.1 presents common symptoms of neuromuscular disorders. Some of the symptoms, such as fatigue or diffuse weakness, are not specific for neuromuscular disease. Others, such as muscle tenderness, focal pain or sensory loss, may lead to an anatomic localization.

Treatment strategies for neuromuscular disorders fall into two categories: etiologic and symptomatic. With our current state of knowledge, complete reversal of the underlying disease with effective etiologic therapy is rare. When available, etiologic treatments for the specific disease entity are described in the subsequent text. Symptomatic therapy, which is becoming more effective, is presented as a separate section. One important general point is that damaged tissues may require higher levels of nutrients and cofactors to support the maximum degree of recovery. Although there are no specific data, appropriate nutrition and supplementation of vitamins and trace minerals are likely to be important components in the treatment of all oncology-related neuromuscular disorders.

We do not specifically discuss any alternative or complementary therapeutic approaches because there is inadequate evidence to support the use of any of these particular treatments in this set of disorders. However, use of these treatments continues to increase and should be documented and reviewed in the course of caring for all patients with oncology-related neuromuscular disease (1).

TABLE 38.1

COMMON SYMPTOMS OF NEUROMUSCULAR DYSFUNCTION

	Focal weakness	Diffuse weakness	Numbness/ Dysesthesia	Focal pain	Muscle cramps	Myalgias	Fatigue
Polyneuropathy	+	+	+	+	+	−	+
Mononeuropathy	+	−	+	+	+	−	−
Sensory neuropathy	−	−	+	−	−	−	−
Motor neuropathy	+	−	−	−	+	−	+
Plexopathy	+	−	+	+	+	−	−
Radiculopathy	+	−	+	+	+	−	−
NMJ defect	−	+	−	−	−	−	+
Myopathy	−	+	−	+	+	+	+

+, common; −, uncommon; NMJ, neuromuscular junction.
Most symptoms also have a large number of non-neuromuscular causes.

SPECIFIC NEUROMUSCULAR DISORDERS

Neuropathy

Neuropathy is the most frequently encountered neuromuscular complication of cancer. Although neurotoxic chemotherapy is most commonly implicated, neuropathy may also be caused by direct extension or metastatic tumor infiltration of the nerve, or by remote (paraneoplastic) effects of cancer. Nerve involvement may be focal or widespread, and resulting symptoms and signs may be focal or diffuse. Dysesthetic pain, numbness, and weakness are frequent complaints. Fatigue and muscle cramps also may be troublesome. Reflexes are generally reduced or absent in affected areas.

It is useful to categorize neuropathies according to the distribution of the problem and the primary neurologic modalities affected: sensory, motor, or sensorimotor. Neuropathy may be further classified according to the predominant pathology: axonal loss, demyelination, or neuron cell body death. Although one deficit may predominate, both sensation and strength are usually involved to some degree in most neuropathies. Disorders that exclusively affect either sensation or strength are most often caused by lesions of the dorsal root ganglion cells or anterior horn cells, respectively, and therefore are described most accurately as neuronopathies.

The evaluation of neuropathy usually involves an EMG and NCS. These tests confirm the extent and distribution of nerve involvement and help differentiate primary neuronal or axonal injury from injury to the myelin sheathe. A careful history, neurologic examination, and high-quality electrodiagnostic testing will provide guidance for choosing other necessary tests. Nerve biopsy is occasionally indicated to help differentiate direct tumor invasion (which may be amenable to chemotherapy or radiation) from inflammation, radiation damage, amyloid deposition, or demyelination. Spinal magnetic resonance imaging (MRI) may reveal structural lesions, such as metastases, that can cause patterns of sensory and motor dysfunction that mimic peripheral neuropathy. In addition, spinal nerve root enhancement is often noted following the administration of gadolinium in patients with inflammatory demyelinating neuropathies. Examination of cerebrospinal fluid (CSF) reveals an elevated protein level in most patients with inflammatory demyelinating neuropathies. CSF may also be subjected to cytologic examination to search for evidence of malignancy involving the spinal subarachnoid space. It is also important to identify potential non-neoplastic causes of neuropathy. A useful general algorithm for evaluation of neuropathy has been presented by Brown (2).

The primary treatment of neuropathy should be directed at the specific underlying cause, if one can be identified. The palliative treatment of neuropathy depends primarily on the predominant symptom (e.g., weakness, sensory loss, pain) and is discussed in the Symptomatic Treatments section.

Cancer-Related Neuropathies

A group of clinically significant sensorimotor neuropathies not related to chemotherapy may accompany or even precede the diagnosis of cancer. Causes to consider in this setting include direct infiltration by tumor, amyloid deposition, and remote effects of cancer. The pathogenesis of neuropathy may remain unknown in some cases, despite extensive investigations. Electrodiagnostic testing is essential to help quantify the degree and pattern of involvement and to distinguish between demyelination and axonal injury. Some processes such as vasculitis or demyelination may have focal, multifocal, or symmetrical presentations. The pattern and tempo of involvement can provide important information to guide further evaluation. Common clinical patterns of neuropathy are presented in the subsequent text.

Polyneuropathy

Axonal Polyneuropathy

Idiopathic neuropathy. Patients with malignancy often develop a mild, symmetrical idiopathic sensorimotor polyneuropathy. This neuropathy typically presents with numbness and tingling in the feet. Symptoms may progress to more widespread sensory disturbances, as well as distal leg and hand weakness. NCS confirm an axonal neuropathy; CSF protein may be normal or, rarely, slightly elevated. The etiology of this typically mild neuropathy is uncertain and is likely to be multifactorial. Predisposing factors may include chemotherapeutic agents, weight loss, malnutrition, and organ failure.

Amyloid neuropathy. Patients with systemic amyloidosis due to plasma cell dyscrasia may develop a polyneuropathy that is predominantly sensory and typically involves small, unmyelinated or thinly myelinated fibers. Autonomic dysfunction is an early and prominent feature. The diagnosis is made by detection of amyloid material on nerve biopsy or may be inferred if amyloid is detected in other locations such as bone marrow or fat pad aspirate. Even among these patients, however, genetic causes should be considered. Nearly, 10% of patients with suspected AL amyloidosis were noted to have familial amyloid polyneuropathy in one series (3). Failure to identify a genetically mediated neuropathy may result in unnecessary treatment of monoclonal gammopathy.

Paraneoplastic neuropathy. Paraneoplastic polyneuropathy is rare. One of the more common and well-studied syndromes is related to an antineuronal autoantibody referred to as anti-Hu. These antibodies are associated with small cell lung cancer, breast cancer, gynecological, and other malignancies. The syndrome is more properly characterized as a sensory neuronopathy, but may be clinically indistinguishable from a symmetrical sensory polyneuropathy in its initial stages. More recently described anti-CV2 antibodies may be present in small cell lung cancer, thymoma and other tumors and have been associated with mixed axonal and demyelinating polyneuropathies. Symptoms may be predominantly sensory, motor, or mixed (4).

Tumor infiltration. Widespread metastatic infiltration of nerves or spinal nerve roots by tumors, such as lymphoma or melanoma, may result in a confluent multifocal neuropathy that is indistinguishable from a length-dependent, symmetrical sensorimotor polyneuropathy. In some patients with non-Hodgkin's lymphoma (and much less commonly Hodgkin's disease), tumor infiltration of nerve roots and nerves has been detected on nerve biopsy (5). This has been termed *neurolymphomatosis*. These patients may respond to antineoplastic treatment.

Demyelinating Polyneuropathy

Acute inflammatory demyelinating polyneuropathy (Guillain-Barré Syndrome). Guillain-Barré syndrome has been associated with Hodgkin's lymphoma and solid tumors, particularly those involving the lung (5,6). Patients suspected of having this disorder require immediate hospitalization for monitoring their respiratory vital capacity and cardiac function. The rate of progression and severity of this disease is highly variable; at worst, patients can become quadriplegic and ventilator dependent within days. Less severely affected patients may have onset of sensory loss, dysesthesia, or weakness over a few weeks. Autonomic involvement can lead to fatal cardiac arrhythmias if not detected, making cardiac monitoring imperative during the initial period. Although untreated symptoms typically reach a nadir within 6 weeks, early treatment with intravenous immunoglobulin or plasmapheresis hastens recovery and may result in better long-term outcome. Patients with cancer appear to respond to the same therapies used for non–cancer-related Guillain-Barré syndrome.

Chronic inflammatory demyelinating polyradiculoneuropathy. Chronic inflammatory demyelinating polyradiculoneuropathy (CIDP) is rarely associated with cancer. Demyelinating neuropathies occur in patients with monoclonal gammopathies (7). A predominantly motor demyelinating neuropathy can be identified in up to 50% of patients with osteosclerotic myeloma. Most patients have elevated levels of monoclonal IgG or IgA lambda. The neuropathy may occur as part of a syndrome consisting of polyneuropathy, organomegaly, endocrinopathy, monoclonal gammopathy, and skin changes (POEMS). These neuropathies may improve markedly with treatment of the tumor (7).

Paraproteinemic neuropathy. In some patients with Waldenstrom's macroglobulinemia or monoclonal gammopathy of undetermined significance, an IgM antibody directed against myelin-associated glycoprotein (MAG) can be detected in serum and in the myelin sheath. These patients have a predominantly sensory demyelinating neuropathy (7). The pattern of weakness and sensory loss may be symmetrical or asymmetrical, and NCS reveal classic demyelinating electrophysiology. CSF protein is frequently elevated. Remissions are reported after treatment of the tumor; the neuropathy may sometimes respond to corticosteroids or intravenous immunoglobulin, although the improvement is typically modest. Recent promising anecdotal data is also available for rituximab in this situation (8).

Focal Neuropathy

Isolated mononeuropathies also may develop in patients with cancer. Causes to consider in this setting include compression neuropathies, invasion of neural structures by tumor, vasculitis, or focal presentations of demyelinating neuropathies. The tempo of onset and clinical setting provide guidance for further evaluation and management.

Compression Neuropathy

Peroneal neuropathies at the fibular head typically develop in bedbound patients with weight loss. Loss of the usual fatty cushion predisposes the peroneal nerve to compression at this site. Nutritional, metabolic, and microcirculatory factors also may contribute to this neuropathy. Other nerves such as the ulnar nerve at the elbow may be similarly affected. Chronic arm and hand edema due to prior lymph node dissection may also predispose patients to median nerve compression at the wrist (carpal tunnel syndrome). Focal compression neuropathies generally improve with simple measures, such as careful positioning to avoid further trauma and padding of vulnerable areas such as the elbow and fibular head (9).

Tumor Infiltration

Other focal neuropathies arise when malignant cells invade nerves and cause axonal degeneration. Cranial neuropathies, resulting from invasion of these nerves as they traverse the subarachnoid space are common. Lumbar puncture and contrast-enhanced MRI of the affected area may demonstrate tumor. In cases where repeated lumbar punctures are nondiagnostic, nerve biopsy should be considered to provide histologic confirmation of tumor, especially if further antineoplastic therapy is an option.

Vasculitic Neuropathy

Peripheral nerves may be damaged by a cancer-associated vasculitis, which often causes either an acute or chronic sensorimotor polyneuropathy. The disorder may also begin as a painful mononeuropathy or mononeuritis multiplex and become confluent. Small cell cancer and adenocarcinoma of the lung, renal cell carcinoma, lymphoma, endometrial, and prostate cancer have all been associated with vasculitic neuropathy. Other lymphoproliferative disorders may be associated with cryoglobulinemic neuropathy, which may have a focal, or distal and symmetrical presentation. NCS demonstrate evidence of axonal damage. The diagnosis is confirmed by demonstration of lymphocytic infiltration and necrosis of blood vessels on nerve or muscle biopsy. Treatment with corticosteroids or other immunosuppressants may result in symptomatic improvement (10,11).

Chemotherapy-Related Neuropathy

Chemotherapeutic agents are among the most common causes of neuropathy in patients with cancer. A wide variety of chemotherapeutic agents has been associated with the development of neuropathy. Patients receiving vinca alkaloids, platinum-based agents, and taxanes may develop symptoms although the severity is highly variable. Other drugs toxic to peripheral nerves include suramin, thalidomide, cytosine arabinoside, etoposide, ifosfamide, and 5-fluorouracil (12). Less commonly used agents such as misonidazole and dolostatin-10 have also been reported to result in neuropathy (13,14).

Vinca alkaloids, especially vincristine are a frequent cause of chemotherapy-induced neurotoxicity. Vincristine routinely causes a peripheral neuropathy when used at the usual weekly doses of 1.4 mg per m^2 or greater (15). Paresthesias may first become noticeable in the fingers. The first clinical sign is usually loss of ankle reflexes. Although mild sensory loss does not warrant a reduction in dosage, weakness may develop rapidly and is a dose-limiting side effect when severe. Signs of impending motor involvement include cramps and mild clumsiness. Weakness typically reverses when the dose is reduced or the drug is stopped; paresthesias take longer to disappear, and mild sensory deficits may persist. Occasionally, patients develop prolonged or permanent dysfunction. Less commonly peripheral neuropathy may occur with vinorelbine tartrate and vinblastine (12). In most cases of vinca alkaloid neuropathy, electrodiagnostic studies demonstrate a symmetrical sensorimotor polyneuropathy with predominant axonal involvement.

Cisplatin may begin to cause neurotoxicity or ototoxicity at a cumulative dose of approximately 300 mg per m^2, and more than 50% of patients who receive 600 mg per m^2 develop symptoms (16). The neuropathy is usually symmetrical and predominantly sensory; decreases in vibratory, light touch, and pinprick sensation are accompanied by progressive loss of deep tendon reflexes. The loss of proprioception may result in sensory ataxia. Despite discontinuation of the drug, neuropathic symptoms may continue to increase for weeks before stabilizing, a phenomenon known as "coasting." Recovery occurs over months, but is often incomplete. Weakness is rare in all but the most severely affected patients. Similar symptoms are reported with carboplatinum, but are less frequent than with cisplatin (12). Oxaliplatin, a newer platinum derivative, mainly causes a completely or partially reversible sensory neuropathy at high cumulative doses. Acral, perioral, and pharyngeal dysesthesias, cramps, and stiffness may occur. Neuromyotonia related to peripheral nerve hyperexcitability has been observed on electrodiagnostic examination of oxaliplatin treated patients (17).

Paclitaxel and docetaxel commonly cause a symmetrical, predominantly large fiber sensory or sensorimotor polyneuropathy at usual doses. Pain, tingling, and numbness may begin within 1–3 days after a single high-dose treatment. The feet and distal legs are affected first, but sensory changes in the hands and face may present earlier than in other toxic neuropathies. Weakness and autonomic abnormalities occasionally develop (18,19). Coasting occurs but most symptoms eventually improve when the drug is discontinued. Neurotoxicity may limit treatment, particularly with high-dose regimens. Risk factors for the development of neuropathy include an earlier neuropathy, high doses (>250 mg per m^2), prolonged length of treatment, and possibly older age (20).

Combinations of multiple neurotoxic agents may result in cumulative peripheral nerve injury beyond that expected with the individual agents. For example, paclitaxel may cause a more severe neuropathy than usual in patients previously treated with cisplatin (21). Those with underlying nerve problems, such as diabetic neuropathy or Charcot Marie-Tooth disease may also be especially predisposed to developing neuropathy from chemotherapy. Any patient with suspected chemotherapy-related neuropathy should also undergo a complete evaluation to identify other contributing causes of neuropathy, either related to the cancer itself or to underlying treatable conditions. It is occasionally useful to follow electrodiagnostic markers of nerve dysfunction prospectively to identify impending nerve disease early in the course of chemotherapy. Somatosensory-evoked responses are generally affected early, followed by a reduction in sensory amplitudes on NCS (22). NCS are a more reliable measure and can be performed serially to monitor the degree of nerve injury.

Treatment consists mainly of limiting a patient's exposure to the offending medication. Numerous agents including amifostine, glutamine, and glutathione have been studied for their potential neuroprotective effects (23–28). Amifostine is a broad-spectrum cytoprotector against both ionizing radiation and chemotherapy and is approved in the United States for cytoprotection in cisplatin-related nephrotoxicity. It is not specifically indicated for neurotoxicity with cisplatin, but has been reported to reduced cisplatin-related peripheral neuropathy in some settings (24). In small clinical trials glutathione and glutamine have shown neuroprotective effects in platinum-based and paclitaxel regimens, respectively; however, neither agent is used in routine clinical practice presently (23,26–28). Numerous other cytokines and growth factors have been studied but have yet to demonstrate consistent effects in clinical and preclinical testing (29). Symptomatic therapy is discussed in the Symptomatic Treatments section.

Neuronopathy

Paraneoplastic processes preferentially attack nerve cell bodies. The cell bodies of motor and sensory neurons are found in the anterior horn of the spinal cord and the dorsal root ganglia, respectively. Damage to the cell bodies of these neurons produces a lesion that is most accurately called a *neuronopathy*. Patients presenting with exclusively sensory or motor dysfunction should be evaluated for the presence of neuronopathy. Symptomatic therapy depends on the predominant symptoms and is discussed in the Symptomatic Treatments section.

Motor Neuronopathy

Subacute motor neuronopathy. Motor neuron disease has been associated with several types of lymphoproliferative disorders, including Waldenstrom's macroglobulinemia, multiple myeloma, chronic lymphocytic leukemia, follicular cell lymphoma, and Hodgkin's disease (30). Patients may have symptoms of upper and lower motor neuron weakness that are clinically indistinguishable from amyotrophic lateral sclerosis (ALS). Electrodiagnostic studies usually demonstrate widespread denervation. Anecdotal reports of ALS in this setting suggest that some patients may improve after treatment of the malignancy (30). At this time, however, there is insufficient epidemiologic or scientific data to support a definite link between motor neuron disease and cancer, and extensive cancer screening in patients with motor neuron disease is not routinely warranted.

Paraneoplastic Encephalomyelitis

Motor neuron involvement is seen as a feature of paraneoplastic encephalomyelitis, which is typically associated with a sensory neuronopathy; however, neurons at any level of the nervous system, including the motor neurons of the anterior horn, may also be affected. Patients may develop concomitant confusion and memory disturbances, weakness, and sensory loss or dysesthesia. When paraneoplastic encephalomyelitis is caused by small cell lung cancer, the anti-Hu antibody is sometimes present. Treatment of the underlying tumor is the therapy of choice but is helpful only in a minority of patients (31).

Sensory Neuronopathy

The so-called *subacute sensory neuronopathy*, often referred to as a *sensory neuropathy*, is the most widely recognized neuromuscular paraneoplastic syndrome (32). Patients typically present with numbness, dysesthesias, paresthesias, gait disturbance, and occasionally, aching pain. The findings can be asymmetric. A sensory ataxia due to loss of proprioception is typical and can be severe. Electrodiagnostic studies show markedly decreased or absent sensory nerve action potentials, findings consistent with damage to dorsal root ganglia. Motor NCS are frequently normal.

Patients who develop sensory neuronopathy without a known cancer require a detailed and sometimes repeated search for underlying malignancy. Small cell lung cancer is by far the most commonly associated cancer; breast, ovarian, uterine, and gastrointestinal carcinomas also must be considered. The presence of anti-Hu antibodies is highly suggestive of the presence of a small cell lung cancer. In approximately 70% of patients with an anti-Hu antibody, there is evidence of CNS or lower motor neuron involvement as well (33). In these patients, an immune mechanism has been supported by the identification of a complement-binding IgG antibody that binds to an antigen found in the tumor and a 35–38-kD brain nuclear protein (34). Treatment of the underlying tumor may result in stabilization of the sensory neuronopathy or, in rare cases, improvement (31). Some patients can learn to adapt to the sensory ataxia by using visual cues, but in severe cases, function is permanently lost and patients may become wheelchair bound. Intravenous immunoglobulin and plasmapheresis have not been demonstrated to be efficacious in the few reported clinical trials.

Radiculopathies

In patients with cancer, new onset of symptoms referable to spinal nerve roots should prompt an urgent evaluation of the spinal column. Paraspinal tumor masses can cause acute and rapid spinal cord compression leading to paraplegia. Tumors originating from the spinal column commonly compress nerve roots as well as the spinal cord. Pain is usually the first symptom of compressive radiculopathy. Other symptoms and signs vary, with neurologic deficits presenting in the dermatomal or myotomal distribution supplied by the involved spinal nerve roots.

Patients with cancer may be especially susceptible to reactivation of herpes zoster infection (shingles). A skin eruption in a dermatomal distribution, often over the trunk, is an early feature. Severe pain is present in the acute phase and may persist for months or years following the skin rash (postherpetic neuralgia). Involvement of motor nerve roots is uncommon but can occasionally produce severe weakness in the distribution of the affected myotomes.

Radiculopathy may also be caused by leptomeningeal tumor. Meningeal carcinomatosis or lymphomatosis can cause radicular pain, sensory loss, weakness, and areflexia. Signs of meningeal irritation, such as meningismus and headache, may be present. Leptomeningeal spread is possible with many tumors but is most common with cancers of breast, lung, and gastrointestinal tract, melanoma, and lymphoma. A tumor invading multiple spinal roots can produce a polyradiculopathy that clinically resembles a severe sensorimotor polyneuropathy.

Contrast-enhanced MRI is the initial step in the evaluation of a patient with suspected meningeal carcinomatosis or lymphomatosis. Thickened enhancing nerve roots may be seen, particularly when the cauda equina is affected. If an MRI is contraindicated, myelography sometimes demonstrates multiple nodular defects on nerve roots. Unless the MRI is unequivocally positive, the next step should be a spinal fluid examination. In nearly all cases of meningeal carcinomatosis or lymphomatosis, the spinal fluid proves to be abnormal. Spinal fluid cytology may provide a specific diagnosis, but repeated sampling may be required. In one study, 50% of patients had false-negative CSF cytology at the initial lumbar puncture, but the CSF almost always had some abnormality (35). Most experts suggest performing at least three lumbar punctures separated by several days, if initial cytologies are negative. Electrodiagnostic studies can confirm a radiculopathy and may also help to identify a confounding or coexisting peripheral neuropathy. Rarely, a meningeal or nerve root biopsy is needed if a high degree of suspicion remains despite an unrevealing noninvasive evaluation. Meningeal tumors can sometimes be controlled for a time with radiation and intrathecal or intracerebroventricular chemotherapy; however, long-term prognosis is grim.

Plexopathies

The diagnosis of plexopathy in the patient with cancer may be challenging. Because of proximity to frequently used radiation ports, the brachial and lumbar plexi are susceptible to radiation injury. Differentiating between recurrent cancer and radiation-induced plexopathy can be difficult and has obvious implications for therapy. As with all peripheral nerve injury, plexopathies usually present with both positive (e.g., tingling) and negative (e.g., numbness) sensory complaints and weakness of the involved limb. In general, malignant plexopathy is more often painful than radiation-induced plexopathy, but this is not always the case. A radiographic or tissue diagnosis is strongly recommended before proceeding with additional antitumor therapy.

Other causes of plexopathy are rare. Idiopathic brachial plexopathy has been reported in patients with Hodgkin's disease (36). Brachial plexopathy can complicate a lymphedematous shoulder, and lumbosacral plexopathy can occur after psoas muscle hemorrhage or abscess. Regional intra-arterial infusion of chemotherapeutic agents may produce local neurotoxicity manifesting as brachial or lumbosacral plexopathies.

Diagnostic studies are required to confirm the diagnosis. Electromyographic data can help localize the lesion and, in some cases, suggest an etiology. Radiation-induced plexopathy tends to be associated with more diffuse injury on EMG and with myokymia (rhythmic, repetitive spontaneous discharges). Myokymia occurs frequently in patients with radiation-induced plexopathy but has not been reported in those with malignant plexopathy. MRI may reveal a mass in the region of the plexus or enhancement along the nerve trunks. Positron emission tomography (PET) has been used as a means to increase diagnostic accuracy in cases of suspected malignant plexopathy. Lesions with high glycolytic rates suggest tumor rather than radiation injury. However, this technology is not available at all centers and its specificity in distinguishing tumor from radiation-induced injury remains to be demonstrated (37). Occasionally, the etiology of a plexopathy cannot be established noninvasively, and exploration of the plexus with biopsy is required.

The treatment of plexopathy is difficult. In patients with malignant plexopathy, radiotherapy may provide pain relief.

Neurologic signs may not improve, however, and pain can persist and become a difficult management problem. Radiation-induced plexopathy is generally less painful but is slowly progressive and eventually causes significant disability. There is no specific primary treatment.

Brachial Plexopathies

Brachial plexopathies are typically unilateral. The most common causes are local extension or metastatic spread of breast or lung cancer. Lymphoma, sarcoma, melanoma, and other types of cancer less commonly invade the brachial plexus. Patients with malignant brachial plexopathy typically experience severe pain that radiates from the shoulder girdle into the medial arm and hand (38). The lower nerve trunk of the brachial plexus is usually most involved, producing hand weakness, atrophy, and sensory disturbances that may mimic an ulnar neuropathy. Horner syndrome is seen in up to 50% of patients.

Radiation may induce a brachial plexopathy when given at a dose greater than 6000 cGy. Brachial plexopathy is a late manifestation of radiation therapy, and onset has been reported from 3 months to 26 years after treatment. The upper nerve trunk of the plexus is the most common area of involvement. Unlike neoplastic plexopathies, paresthesias, hypesthesia, heaviness, and weakness of the arm predominate over pain. In some series, exacerbation of arm lymphedema is more common with radiation plexopathy, but others have noted no difference in lymphedema among malignant and radiation plexopathy cases (38,39). Clinical features that help distinguish malignant from radiation-induced plexopathy are pain severity (worse with neoplasm), presence of Horner syndrome (with neoplasm), lymphedema (more common after radiation), and distribution of the arm weakness (proximal with radiation injury and more distal from neoplastic invasion).

Lumbosacral Plexopathies

Lumbosacral plexopathies are most commonly caused by direct extension of intra-abdominal neoplasms, such as colorectal or cervical cancer, or by radiation. Pain is a frequent early feature, and the upper, lower, or entire nerve plexus can be affected. The plexopathy is frequently slowly progressive, and bilateral symptoms may be seen. Computed tomography or MRI scanning of the region of the lumbosacral plexus typically demonstrates the responsible mass. A biopsy is required only if there has been no previous tissue diagnosis.

Radiation-induced lumbosacral plexopathy generally presents as slowly progressive weakness; pain occurs in 50% of patients. Like radiation-induced brachial plexopathy, lumbosacral plexopathy may follow radiation by months to years. Myokymia is seen on electrodiagnostic studies in 50% of patients.

Neuromuscular Junction Disorders

Myasthenia Gravis

Myasthenia gravis results in fatigue and weakness due to a post-synaptic defect of neuromuscular transmission. Although most patients do not have an associated malignancy, approximately 10% of patients with myasthenia gravis have a thymoma. Conversely, 30% of patients with thymoma develop myasthenia gravis. The diagnosis is confirmed by the presence of anti-acetylcholine receptor antibodies or electrodiagnostic testing. Patients with thymoma require resection or treatment of the tumor, although not all have relief of associated fatigue and weakness. Immunomodulating treatments such as steroids, plasma exchange, azathioprine, or mycofenylate mofetil, among others also may be required.

In some patients with myasthenia gravis and thymoma, a coexistent syndrome of neuromuscular hyperexcitability or dysautonomia may be present (32,40). Neuromuscular hyperexcitability can manifest electrodiagnostically as continuous involuntary motor unit activity (stiff-person syndrome) or myokymia and neuromyotonia (Isaac's syndrome). Clinically, patients with stiff-person syndrome develop muscle stiffness and painful muscle spasms that are triggered by a sudden startling stimulus. Anti-glutamic acid decarboxylase (GAD) antibodies are found in most of the patients with stiff-person syndrome and may be seen in up to 22% of patients with thymoma, some of whom may be asymptomatic (41). Loss of GABAergic inhibition to motor neurons due to the presence of anti-GAD antibodies is suspected in most cases, although antibodies to presynaptic amphiphysin protein have also been described. Stiff-person syndrome may be observed in thymoma without concomitant myasthenia gravis. The syndrome also occasionally occurs with Hodgkin's lymphoma and plasmacytoma.

Patients with Isaac's syndrome also complain of stiffness and cramps, but myokymia or muscle twitching, and hyperhydrosis can be additional prominent features. Antibodies against voltage-gated potassium channels or ganglionic acetylcholine receptors may be seen. Neuromyotonia as a paraneoplastic syndrome may occur without associated myasthenia gravis Thymomas are the most common associated tumors, but Hodgkin's lymphoma, small cell lung cancer, and breast cancer are also seen.

A few individuals with thymoma, with or without myasthenia gravis, may develop concomitant autonomic neuropathy. These individuals are sometimes found to have antibodies to ganglionic acetylcholine receptor antibodies. The treatment for these muscle hyperexcitability and autonomic syndromes associated with thymoma is similar to the treatment for myasthenia gravis. Plasma exchange, intravenous gammaglobulin, and steroids have all had anecdotal positive effect.

Lambert-Eaton Myasthenic Syndrome

Although Lambert-Eaton Myasthenic Syndrome (LEMS) is rare, 50–70% of patients with the disorder have cancer. Among these, 80% have a small cell lung cancer. There have been case reports of LEMS in many other types of cancer, but these associations may be incidental. The cause of LEMS is IgG antibodies directed against the presynaptic voltage-sensitive calcium channels of the motor and autonomic nerve terminals. These antibodies interfere with the voltage-dependent release of acetylcholine at the neuromuscular junction and in autonomic nerves. Calcium channel antibody titers can be measured in the serum of patients with LEMS. The immunologic stimulus is probably the voltage-sensitive calcium channel of the carcinoma cells. Patients younger than 40 years of age are more likely to suffer from an autoimmune rather than a paraneoplastic process. The syndrome occurs more frequently in men than in women (approximately a 2:1 ratio), and cancer is the cause more often in men (70%) than in women (25%).

Proximal muscle weakness in patients with LEMS is typical, and there may be mild myalgias and tenderness of the muscles. Bulbar and ocular muscles are rarely affected and typically not to the degree seen in myasthenia gravis. Patients may complain of severe fatigue and weakness, but on examination often have only mild demonstrable weakness. Occasionally, strength may improve after exercise but then declines further with sustained activity. Deep tendon reflexes tend to be reduced or absent at rest but may increase if tested immediately after a brief, strong contraction of the appropriate muscle. Most patients complain of dry mouth, and some patients have other autonomic manifestations, including impotence, hypotension, and constipation. Fewer than 10% of patients with LEMS demonstrate ganglionic acetylcholine receptor antibodies. The mechanism of dysautonomia is probably different from that seen in patients with concomitant myasthenia gravis and autonomic neuropathy (42)

The diagnosis of LEMS can be confirmed through electro-diagnostic studies. Regular motor NCS often show reduced amplitudes because of impaired release of acetylcholine. A small decrement is seen with repetitive stimulation at low rates; however, with high rates of stimulation or immediately after a brief contraction of the muscle, the motor amplitudes markedly increase to at least double their resting size (most likely because of an increase in the concentration of calcium in the nerve terminals leading to increased acetylcholine release). In questionable situations, the diagnosis can be confirmed with single-fiber EMG.

Therapy for LEMS should be tailored to the individual patient on the basis of clinical severity, the presence of underlying malignancy or other disease, and life expectancy. Once a diagnosis of LEMS has been confirmed, an extensive search for malignancy must be carried out. Computed tomography scanning of the chest and sometimes bronchoscopy are recommended. If small cell lung cancer is identified, initial therapy should aim at treating the cancer. Weakness associated with LEMS frequently improves with effective cancer therapy, and often no further treatment is needed (43). Pyridostig-mine 30–120 mg every 4–6 hours usually does not produce significant symptomatic improvement, but rare patients may benefit. Immunotherapy with plasma exchange, intravenous immunoglobulin, corticosteroids, or azathioprine may be used if the weakness is severe and unresponsive to less aggressive therapy. The orphan drug 3,4-diaminopyridine improves strength and lessens autonomic symptoms in most patients with LEMS (44).

As with myasthenia gravis, drugs that adversely affect neuromuscular transmission should be avoided. These include the aminoglycosides, β-blockers, calcium channel blockers, and antiarrhythmics such as quinine sulfate, quinidine sulfate, or procainamide hydrochloride. Neuromuscular blocking agents typically used during intubation have an exaggerated and prolonged effect in patients with LEMS.

Myopathy

Except for the local invasion of myofascial structures, primary muscle dysfunction associated with cancer most often arises as a remote effect, thought to be due to autoimmune or toxic metabolites. The best known example is dermato-myositis. Some cancer therapies, particularly corticosteroids, can also cause a myopathy. The loss of muscle tissue from reduced activity and poor nutrition is common. Myopathy should be suspected in the patient with progressive weakness, especially if proximal, and no sensory symptoms. Most pathologic myopathies are associated with an elevated crea-tinine phosphokinase. Myopathy can often be confirmed by EMG, and a muscle biopsy may help further to define the syndrome. Treatment usually involves therapy directed toward the specific underlying disorder. There are few symptomatic therapies.

Inflammatory Myopathies

Historically, there has been considerable confusion regarding the relationship between cancer and the inflammatory myopathies. Whereas some studies have demonstrated an increased incidence of neoplasm in patients with both polymyositis and dermatomyositis, others found no such relationship. Currently, little evidence suggests that either inclusion-body

myositis or polymyositis is associated with cancer; however, there does appear to be an increased incidence of malignancy in patients with dermatomyositis, particularly among older patients. Approximately 25% of patients with dermatomyositis had a known malignancy at presentation, or a malignancy was detected soon after the diagnosis of dermatomyositis (45).

The distinction between polymyositis and dermatomyositis is based on the presence or absence of the characteristic skin manifestations of dermatomyositis. These include a purplish (heliotrope) periorbital rash and a more widespread erythematous pruritic scaly rash over extensor surfaces and sun-exposed areas. The pathologic findings on muscle biopsy also differ substantially, usually allowing a distinction to be made between types of inflammatory myopathies.

Dermatomyositis associated with malignancy usually responds to immunosuppressive therapy with oral corticos-teroids, such as prednisone at 40–60 mg per day for at least 1–2 months, followed by a slow taper. The daily dose can be reduced by 5 mg every week until 30 mg per day, with further tapering at only 2.5 mg per week. Relapse frequently occurs after early or rapid reduction in steroid doses. Other immunosuppressive agents, including methotrexate, cyclophosphamide, chlorambucil, and azathioprine, have been used, most typically in patients who do not respond to corticosteroids or cannot tolerate their side effects. Intravenous immunoglobulin at a total dose of 2 g per kg divided over several days also was demonstrated to be effective (46). Treatment of the underlying tumor also may result in improvement of the myositis.

Cancer-Related Muscle Necrosis

Cancer-related muscle necrosis, a rare, rapidly progressive, fatal muscle degeneration, has been linked to small cell lung cancer and to gastrointestinal, breast, and bladder cancers (47). This disorder presents with a rapidly progressive weakness that spreads from the limbs to involve bulbar and respiratory muscles. Electrodiagnostic studies demonstrate changes typical of myopathy. On muscle biopsy, there is profound muscle-fiber necrosis with little or no inflammation. In general, no treatment has proved helpful.

Carcinoid Tumor–Associated Myopathy

Carcinoid tumors may cause muscle damage and progressive proximal weakness, perhaps related to secretion of serotonin or other substances by the tumor (48). Most histopathologic changes are nonspecific, with preponderance of type I fibers and type II fiber atrophy. The symptoms sometimes improve with a serotonin antagonist such as cyproheptadine hydrochloride or methysergide.

Steroid-Induced Myopathy

Corticosteroids often produce a myopathy, which can be progressive and often affects the proximal muscles preferentially. The weakness typically has an insidious onset, but may occasionally be sudden. Despite profound weakness, the serum creatinine phosphokinase is typically normal or only mildly elevated, and EMG may or may not reveal myopathic changes. Muscle biopsy may demonstrate the nonspecific finding of type II muscle-fiber atrophy. Necrosis and regenerating fibers are rarely seen. Susceptibility to steroid myopathy varies widely. Patients who develop significant cushingoid body habitus seem to be more at risk (49). The fluorinated corticosteroids, such as dexamethasone, betamethasone, or triamcinolone, are more often implicated in the development of steroid myopathy.

Patients often improve with a reduction in the steroid dose. Strength in some patients who are receiving a fluorinated drug improves if therapy is changed to a nonfluorinated steroid, such as prednisone or hydrocortisone. Physical exercise can also help maintain muscle strength and maximize function.

SYMPTOMATIC TREATMENTS

Primary treatment of the oncologic or neuromuscular lesion should be provided if feasible and appropriate for the patient's medical condition and goals. In some cases, this strategy may halt or reverse neurologic deficits and possibly provide some degree of symptom control. Purely symptomatic therapies are often needed as well, and become the major interventions for those who cannot benefit from primary therapy.

Pharmacologic

Aside from muscular cramps, symptoms involving the peripheral nervous system are predominantly neuropathic in origin, specifically sensory loss, paresthesias, dysesthesias, and pain. Pain is usually the most compelling symptom, and management can be challenging. Opioid drugs, combined with nonopioid and adjuvant analgesic drugs, are commonly administered. The adjuvant analgesics are particularly important in the treatment of neuropathic pain, which overall is less responsive to the opioids than other types of pain.

Occasional patients with medically refractory pain may be candidates for an anesthetic, neurostimulatory, or neurosurgical intervention. The decision to undertake an invasive therapy must carefully consider potential risks and benefits and relies on a comprehensive assessment of the patient.

Muscle cramps can be particularly troublesome in patients with cancer. Although cramps are often thought of as nonspecific, in reality they typically point to underlying neuromuscular or metabolic dysfunction. In a published study of 50 patients with cancer who complained of muscle cramps, examination and evaluation of the patient led to a specific etiology in 82% (50). Peripheral neuropathy was identified in 22 of the patients, nerve root or plexus lesions in 17 patients, and polymyositis in two patients. Hypomagnesemia was thought to account for muscle cramps in one patient. Therefore, muscle cramps typically mark the presence of an identifiable and often previously unsuspected neurologic disorder.

Cramps are most effectively eliminated by treating the underlying cause. Unfortunately, this is rarely possible in patients with cancer, except when cramps are due to calcium abnormalities. Cramps occasionally may be successfully treated using agents thought to stabilize muscle membrane, such as quinine sulfate, or a number of antiepileptic medications. Quinine sulfate appears to be most effective in treating nocturnal cramps, whereas antiepileptic medication should be tried for daytime cramping. Strict attention to adequate hydration and electrolyte balance are also critical. Other agents, such as benzodiazepines, antispasticity drugs (e.g., baclofen, tizanidine hydrochloride), anti-inflammatory agents, or narcotics, have not been shown to be effective, but some have sedating properties that may help patients sleep more readily (51).

The mainstays of pharmacologic treatment for positive neuropathic symptoms (e.g., dysesthesias, paresthesias, radiating pain) are anticonvulsants and tricyclic antidepressants (51). Less well studied are baclofen, the benzodiazepines, oral anesthetic agents, and α-adrenergic blockers (52,53). Numbness or sensory loss does not respond to medication and can only be reduced by addressing the primary neurotoxic process and allowing injured nerves to recover.

The following important principles are generally applicable. Choose each medication carefully, considering both the intended effects and potential side effects. If potential side effects are significant, start with a very low dose, increasing slowly every few days to allow patients to become tolerant to the side effects. Newer medications may have fewer side effects and can be titrated more rapidly. Increase the dose of each medication until the desired effect is achieved, until side effects become unmanageable, or until high therapeutic drug levels are obtained. Give each medication an adequate trial before considering it a failure or success, as some drugs may require several weeks to reach their maximum efficacy. Even when treating the same symptoms in different patients, it is important to remember that each patient's response to individual analgesic agents may be different. Given the wide difference in mechanism of action of the adjuvant medications, a number of different agents may need to be tried sequentially before an effective one is found.

A number of new anticonvulsants have been introduced in the last decade, several of which have better safety profiles than those of existing medications. The introduction of these new drugs has resulted in increased treatment options for neuropathic pain. Currently, gabapentin has become the drug of first choice because of its low side-effect profile and relative lack of interaction with other medications. Although there are no published clinical trials in patients with cancer, two excellent, double-blind, randomized, placebo-controlled clinical trials have been published showing efficacy and safety in post-herpetic neuralgia and diabetic neuropathy (54,55). Clinical trials are ongoing in a number of agents and both duloxetine (an antidepressant) and pregabalin (an anticonvulsant) have received U.S. Food and Drug Administration (FDA) approval for use in either post-herpetic neuralgia or diabetic neuropathy (56,57). On the basis of animal data (58) and the number of registered clinical trials currently available (59), a number of the other newer agents also show similar promise.

Other techniques that have been used for pain or other neuromuscular symptoms include heat, cold, massage, transcutaneous electrical nerve stimulation, and acupuncture. The available literature is generally inconclusive about the efficacy of these alternative and complementary therapies, but the importance of research in this area is generally recognized. In 1998, the National Center for Complementary and Alternative Medicine was established as one of the centers comprising the National Institutes of Health, and numerous clinical trials are currently being funded to study complementary and alternative treatments for symptoms related to cancer (59).

Rehabilitation

Rehabilitation should play an important role in the treatment of any neuromuscular complication of cancer. There is increasing evidence that monitored exercise can improve muscle strength and endurance while reducing the complications of joint contractures, disuse atrophy, joint stiffness, osteoporosis, and pain. In a study of 301 patients terminally ill with cancer, an increase in the Barthel mobility index from 12 to 19 out of a possible total of 47 was achieved with a supervised program of rehabilitation in the hospice setting. The Barthel mobility index consists of a subset of mobility elements from the standard Barthel Index, an instrument that rates functional capacity in activities of daily living. The rehabilitation program was thought to be effective by most patients and their families (60). In another study, a supervised program of active resistance and endurance exercise was shown to maintain and even increase muscular strength in patients with neuromuscular disease (61). Although the special features of neuromuscular disease in patients with cancer were not addressed specifically in these studies, it is reasonable to conclude that supervised rehabilitation efforts, particularly physical therapy, can be effective in maximizing the function of patients suffering from neuromuscular complications of cancer.

Over time, weakness can lead to contractures of the affected joint. Regular stretching exercises may prevent this complication. For patients with severe weakness from any cause, splinting in a neutral position also may be needed to prevent contractures. In addition to exercise, appropriate devices can increase patient function. Orthotic braces may allow a weak joint to function more normally. For example, molded ankle-foot orthotics, which stabilize the ankle in a neutral position and eliminate foot drop, can help a patient maintain ambulation.

Significant loss of proprioception often results in gait instability. A cane or walker can provide additional stability, which often helps patients feel more secure. Walking should be encouraged, because gait tends to improve as the brain adapts to a reduced level of proprioceptive input. Use of a cane, walker, or even wheelchair should be encouraged to allow continued independence. Reduced sensation in the hands produces difficulty with fine manipulation, such as buttoning a shirt. Special devices can be created to improve hand and finger function. A trained occupational therapist is best qualified to evaluate and fit patients for such assistive devices.

Psychological

Cognitive interventions, such as relaxation, imagery distraction, reframing, hypnosis, and biofeedback, can be helpful in managing pain and improving function. Because the success of these techniques is highly dependent on the patient's ongoing commitment to use them, the clinician must try to identify techniques that are best suited for a patient's specific needs and personality. Many cancer treatment centers now offer ongoing support groups and cancer-specific psychological therapy that may be helpful to patients.

SUMMARY

Through a logical approach guided by the physical examination and selected additional studies, the etiology of most neuromuscular complications of cancer can be determined. In many cases, therapy aimed at the specific etiology is effective. Symptomatic therapies should always be considered to enhance function and reduce discomfort. Although many of the neuromuscular manifestations of cancer lack effective primary therapy, significant palliation should be possible in most patients.

References

1. Cassileth BR. Complementary and alternative cancer medicine. *J Clin Oncol* 1999;17:44–52.
2. Brown MJ. Evaluating the perplexing neuropathic patient. *Semin Neurol* 1987;7:1.
3. Lachmann HJ, Booth DR, Booth SE. Misdiagnosis of hereditary amyloidosis as AL (primary) amyloidosis. *N Engl J Med* 2002;346:1786–1791.
4. Antoine J-C, Honnorat J, Camdessanché J-P. Paraneoplastic anti-CV2 antibodies react with peripheral nerve and are associated with a mixed axonal and demyelinating peripheral neuropathy. *Ann Neurol* 2001;49:214–221.
5. Kelly JJ, Karcher DS. Lymphoma and peripheral neuropathy: a clinical review. *Muscle Nerve* 2005;31:301–313.
6. Klingon DG. The Guillain-Barré syndrome associated with cancer. *Cancer* 1965;18:157.
7. Cocito D, Durelli L, Isoardo G. Different clinical, electrophysiological and immunological features of CIDP associated with paraproteinaemia. *Acta Neurol Scand* 2003;108:274–280.
8. Renaud S, Gregor M, Fuhr P, et al. Rituximab in the treatment of polyneuropathy associated with anti-MAG antibodies. *Muscle Nerve* 2003;27:611–615.
9. Dawson DM, Hallett M, Millender LH. *Entrapment neuropathies*, 2nd ed. Boston: Little, Brown and Company, 1990:156.
10. Oh SJ, Slaughter R, Harrell L. Paraneoplastic vasculitis neuropathy. A treatable neuropathy. *Muscle Nerve* 1991;14:152.
11. Vincent D, Dubas F, Hauw JJ, et al. Nerve and muscle microvasculitis in peripheral neuropathy: a remote effect of cancer? *J Neurol Neurosurg Psychiatry* 1986;49:1007.
12. Dropcho EJ. Neurotoxicity of cancer chemotherapy. *Semin Neurol* 2004;24:419–426.
13. Grigsby PW, Winter K, Wasserman TH, et al. Irradiation with or without misonidazole for patients with stages IIIB and IVA carcinoma of the cervix: final results of RTOG 80-05. Radiation therapy oncology group. *Int J Radiat Oncol Biol Phys* 1999;44:513–517.
14. Pitot HC. Phase I trial of Dolastatin-10 (NSC 376128) in patients with advanced solid tumors. *Clin Cancer Res* 1999;5:525–531.
15. Casey EB, Jelliffe AM, LeQuesne PM, et al. Vincristine neuropathy—clinical and electrophysiological observations. *Brain* 1973;96:69.
16. Krarup-Hansen A, Helweg-Larsen S, Hauge EN, et al. Examination of distal involvement in cisplatin-induced neuropathy in man. *Brain* 1993;116:1017–1041.
17. Wilson RH, Lehky T, Thomas RR, et al. Acute oxaliplatin-induced peripheral nerve hyperexcitability. *J Clin Oncol* 2002;20:1767–1774.
18. Freilich RJ, Balmaceda C, Seidman AD, et al. Motor neuropathy due to docetaxel and paclitaxel. *Neurology* 1996;47:115–118.
19. Jerian SM, Sarosy GA, Link CJ. Incapacitating autonomic neuropathy precipitated by taxol. *Gynecol Oncol* 1993;51:277–280.
20. Donehower RC, Rowinsky EK. An overview of experience with Taxol in the U.S.A. *Cancer Treat Rev* 1993;19(Suppl C):63.
21. Cavaletti G, Bogliun G, Marzorati L, et al. Peripheral neurotoxicity of taxol in patients previously treated with cisplatin. *Cancer* 1995;75:1141–1150.
22. Bird SJ, Kaji R, Mollman J. Sensory evoked potentials are a sensitive indicator of cisplatin neuropathy. *Neurology* 1989;39:263.
23. Hoekman K, van der Vijgh WJF, Vermorken JB. Clinical and preclinical modulation of chemotherapy-induced toxicity in patients with cancer. *Drugs* 1999;57:133–155.
24. Planting AS, Catimel G, de Mulder PH, et al. EORTC Head and Neck Cooperative Group. Randomized study of a short course of weekly cisplatin with or without amifostine in advanced head and neck cancer. *Ann Oncol* 1999;10:693–700.
25. Koukourakis MI. Amifostine in clinical oncology: current use and future applications. *AntiCancer Drugs* 2002;13:181–209.
26. Vahdat L, Papadopoulous K, Lange D, et al. Reduction of paclitaxel-induced peripheral neuropathy with glutamine. *Clin Cancer Res* 2001;7:1192–1197.
27. Cascinu S, Catalano V, Cordella L, et al. Neuroprotective effect of reduced glutathione on oxaliplatin-based chemotherapy in advanced colorectal cancer. *J Clin Oncol* 2002;20:3478–3483.
28. Smyth JF, Bowman A, Perren T, et al. Glutathione reduces the toxicity and improves quality of life of women diagnosed with ovarian cancer treated with cisplatin: results of a double-blind randomized trial. *Ann Oncol* 1997;8:569–573.
29. Cavaletti G, Zanna C. Current status and future prospects for the treatment of chemotherapy-induced peripheral neurotoxicity. *Eur J Cancer* 2002;38:1832–1837.
30. Gordon PH, Rowland LP, Younger DS, et al. Lymphoproliferative disorders and motor neuron disease: an update. *Neurology* 1997;48:1671–1678.
31. Graus F, Keime-Guibert F, Rene R, et al. Anti-Hu-associated paraneoplastic encephalomyelitis: analysis of 200 patients. *Brain* 2001;124:1138–1148.
32. Vernino S, Auger RG, Emslie-Smith AM, et al. Myasthenia, thymoma, presynaptic antibodies, and a continuum of neuromuscular hyperexcitability. *Neurology* 1999;53:1233–1239.
33. Dalmau J, Graus F, Rosenblum MK. Anti-Hu-associated paraneoplastic encephalomyelitis/sensory neuronopathy: a clinical study of 71 patients. *Medicine (Baltimore)* 1992;71:59.
34. Graus F, Ramon R. Paraneoplastic neuropathies. *Eur Neurol* 1993;33:279.
35. Wasserstrom W, Glass JP, Posner JB. Diagnosis and treatment of leptomeningeal metastases from solid tumors: experience with 90 patients. *Cancer* 1982;49:759.
36. Lachance DH, O'Neill BP, Harper CM, et al. Paraneoplastic brachial plexopathy in a patient with Hodgkin's disease. *Mayo Clin Proc* 1991;66:97.
37. Ahmad A, Barrington S, Maisey M, et al. Use of positron emission tomography in evaluation of brachial plexopathy in breast cancer patients. *Br J Cancer* 1999;79:478–482.
38. Kori S, Foley KM, Posner JB. Brachial plexus lesions in patients with cancer: 100 cases. *Neurology* 1981;31:45.
39. Thomas JE, Colby MY. Radiation-induced or metastatic brachial plexopathy? A diagnostic dilemma. *JAMA* 1972;222:1392.
40. Vernino S, Cheshire WP, Lennon VA. Myasthenia gravis with autoimmune autonomic neuropathy. *Auton Neurosci* 2001;88:187–192.
41. Vernino S, Lennon VA. Autoantibody profiles and neurological correlations of thymoma. *Clin Cancer Res* 2004;10:7270–7275.
42. Vernino S, Adamski J, Kryzer TJ, et al. Neuronal nicotinic ACh receptor antibody in subacute autonomic neuropathy and cancer-related syndromes. *Neurology* 1998;50:1806–1813.
43. Chalk CH, Murray NM, Newsom-Davis J, et al. Response of the Lambert-Eaton myasthenic syndrome to treatment of associated small-cell lung carcinoma. *Neurology* 1990;40:1552.

44. Sanders DB, Howard JF, Massey JM. 3,4-Diaminopyridine in Lambert-Eaton myasthenic syndrome and myasthenia gravis. *Ann N Y Acad Sci* 1993;681:588.
45. Callen JP. Myositis and malignancy. *Curr Opin Rheumatol* 1994;6:590.
46. Dalakas MC, Illa I, Dambrosia JM, et al. A controlled trial of high dose intravenous immune globulin infusions as treatment for dermatomyositis. *N Engl J Med* 1994;329:1993.
47. Brownell B, Hughes JT. Degeneration of muscle in association with carcinoma of the bronchus. *J Neurol Neurosurg Psychiatry* 1975;38:363.
48. Swash M, Fox KP, Davidson AR. Carcinoid myopathy: serotonin-induced muscle weakness in man. *Arch Neurol* 1975;32:572.
49. Khaleeli AA, Edwards RHT, Gohil K, et al. Corticosteroid myopathy: a clinical and pathologic study. *Clin Endocrinol* 1983;18:155.
50. Steiner I, Siegal T. Muscle cramps in cancer patients. *Cancer* 1989;63:574.
51. Siegal T. Muscle cramps in the cancer patient: causes and treatment. *J Pain Symptom Manage* 1991;6:84–91.
52. Lussier D, Huskey AG, Portenoy RK. Adjuvant analgesics in cancer pain management. *Oncologist* 2004;9:571–591.
53. Cersosimo RJ. Oxaliplatin-associated neuropathy: a review. *Ann Pharmacother* 2005;39:128–135.
54. Backonja M, Beydoun A, Edwards KR, et al. Gabapentin for the symptomatic treatment of painful neuropathy in patients with diabetes mellitus. *JAMA* 1998;280:1831–1836.
55. Rowbotham M, Harden N, Stacey B, et al. Gabapentin for the treatment of postherpetic neuralgia. *JAMA* 1998;280:1837–1842.
56. Lesser H, Sharma U, LaMoreaux L, et al. Pregabalin relieves symptoms of painful diabetic neuropathy: a randomized controlled trial. *Neurology* 2004;63:2104–2110.
57. Freynhagen R, Strojek K, Griesing T, et al. Efficacy of pregabalin in neuropathic pain evaluated in a 12-week, randomised, double-blind, multicentre, placebo-controlled trial of flexible- and fixed-dose regimens. *Pain* 2005;115:254–263.
58. Lynch JJ III, Wade CL, Zhong CM, et al. Attenuation of mechanical allodynia by clinically utilized drugs in a rat chemotherapy-induced neuropathic pain model. *Pain* 2004;110:56–63.
59. Anonymous, http://www.clinicaltrials.gov/, National Library of Medicine, The U.S. National Institutes of Health, September 8, 2005.
60. Yoshioka H. Rehabilitation for the terminal cancer patient. *Am J Phys Med Rehabil* 1994;73:199–206.
61. Vignos PJ. Physical models of rehabilitation in neuromuscular disease. *Muscle Nerve* 1983;6:323.

CHAPTER 39 ■ COGNITIVE DISORDERS: DELIRIUM AND DEMENTIA

JOHN L. SHUSTER JR.

Dementia and delirium are classified in the most recent edition of the *Diagnostic and Statistical Manual of Mental Disorders* (DSM-IV) (1) as cognitive disorders, because both are characterized by deficits in cognition or memory that lead to clinically significant distress or disability. To merit a cognitive disorder diagnosis, changes in memory and cognition must represent a significant change from the patient's previous level of functioning, differentiating these disorders from mental retardation and pervasive developmental disorders which typically have their onset in infancy or childhood (1).

DEFINITIONS

Both dementia and delirium produce a range of cognitive deficits, including, but not limited to, deficits in memory. A cognitive disorder characterized exclusively by memory impairment or dysfunction would be properly diagnosed as an *amnestic disorder* (1). Amnestic disorders, which may be transient or chronic, are further classified according to their etiology, if known (i.e., whether the memory impairment results from a known general medical condition or is the consequence of substance use, abuse, or dependence). Focal impairment of memory typically results from injury to one or more of the structures that mediate memory storage and retrieval, such as the mammillary bodies, hippocampus, and fornix. Examples of problems that can lead to amnestic disorder include vascular or hypoxic brain injury, herpes and other causes of encephalitis; closed or penetrating head injuries, and Korsakoff's syndrome due to chronic alcohol exposure and thiamine deficiency. Medications (anticonvulsants, intrathecal methotrexate, chronic use of sedative-hypnotics) and toxic exposures (lead, mercury, carbon monoxide, organophosphate insecticides, and solvents) have also been associated with amnestic disorders (1).

Dementia is a syndrome of multiple cognitive deficits, including memory dysfunction, tending to develop gradually over a period of time as the result of an underlying medical condition. Memory impairment, although not the only deficit seen in dementia, is usually the prominent feature, especially in the early stages of the disease.

Delirium also produces a broad range of cognitive deficits and results from the effect of an underlying medical condition on the functioning of the brain. Relatively rapid onset (over a period of hours to days) and prominence of a disturbance in consciousness (the so-called "clouding of consciousness") are key features of delirium. Lipowski defines delirium as "a transient organic mental syndrome of acute onset, characterized by global impairment of cognitive functions, a reduced level of consciousness, attentional abnormalities; increased or decreased psychomotor activity, and a disordered sleep–wake cycle" (2).

DISTINGUISHING DEMENTIA FROM DELIRIUM

Differentiating the cause of pervasive cognitive disturbance in the palliative care setting is sometimes a challenging task, especially when the patient is at high risk for either disorder (e.g., the elderly patient with advanced or terminal disease). Obtaining a clear and reliable history of the patient's recent baseline mental status is the key to this differential diagnosis. In a patient with no history of memory or other cognitive disturbance before the onset or exacerbation of a medical illness, complication, or drug exposure, the diagnosis of delirium is most likely, because the course of onset and progression is usually much longer with dementia. In many instances, however, the course of an emerging delirium in a palliative care patient is prolonged compared with the typical course of delirium emerging in the acute hospital or critical care setting, because the rate of onset of delirium is primarily determined by the severity and speed of progression of the underlying and causative medical disorder or disorders. Similarly, a presentation with prominent disturbance in consciousness is atypical of dementia, at least in the early or middle stages of the disease course. The relatively quick onset of delirium (often with rapid crescendo to severe cognitive impairment and behavioral changes), the prominence of disturbed consciousness, and correlation with some abrupt change in the patient's medical condition are the main features distinguishing delirium from dementia. When feasible, obtaining an electroencephalogram can be helpful in this differential diagnosis. Prominence of slow waves (δ and θ) on the tracing and disruption of the α rhythm are characteristic of delirium. These findings can help in differentiating delirium from dementia and other psychiatric disturbances (3,4).

Comorbidity of Dementia and Delirium

Delirium is a common complication of dementia, especially as dementia advances. Any brain injury, especially one as profound as most causes of dementia, lowers the threshold for developing delirium in response to a given toxic, metabolic, or infectious insult. History is again the guide here, as a sudden deterioration in a demented patient, particularly if associated with agitation or other manifestations of distress, should be considered an episode of comorbid delirium until proved otherwise. Resolution of the delirious episode may restore the patient's mental state and functioning back to the best recent baseline level, but is unlikely to improve cognition further owing to the underlying dementia.

DEMENTIA

The burden of suffering in advanced dementia is not trivial. One of the recommendations of the 2004 NIH State-of-the-Science Conference on Improving End-of-Life Care was that patients dying of dementia need to become a high priority for future research on palliative and end-of-life care (5). Patients with dementia frequently die in states of suffering and distress. Aminoff and Adunsky used the Mini Suffering State Examination (MSSE) to serially assess the suffering of patients with dementia admitted to a geriatric medicine ward (6,7). Suffering levels were high at baseline—41% and 35% were rated with high and intermediate levels of suffering, respectively, at admission. MSSE scores increased as death approached. In the last week before death, 63% of patients had high levels and 93% had at least intermediate levels of suffering on the MSSE. Most of the patients (71.8%) were rated as "not calm" in the last week of life (7). Symptom burden in end-stage delirium is high, including confusion and agitation (present in 83% of a series of 170 patients), incontinence (72%), pain (64%), depressed mood (61%), and constipation (59%) (8). Pain, shortness of breath, skin breakdown, depression, fearfulness, anxiety, and agitation are commonly present in advanced dementia (9).

Advanced dementia is a major problem and a major cause of death in the nursing home setting. Shuster et al. found that 61.4% of patients in a Veterans Affairs nursing home had a dementia diagnosis, and that 67.2% of those with dementia had advanced to the point of qualification for hospice admission (10). Approximately two thirds of patients with dementia die in the nursing home setting, but their end-of-life care is often perceived by bereaved family caregivers as lacking in basic quality (i.e., inadequate pain control; poor communication) (11).

Prevalence and Epidemiology

Alzheimer's disease (AD) accounts for more than half of all cases of dementia in the United States (12). Either alone or as a comorbid condition with AD, vascular (multi-infarct) dementia accounts for the great majority of dementias not diagnosed as AD (12,13). The incidence of dementia increases with age. Between 2% and 4% of the population over 65 have dementia due to AD, with the prevalence increasing to 20% or more among those aged 85 and older (1).

Presentation of Advanced Dementia

The common causes of dementia are incurable and invariably lead to the death of the patient. Treatment is palliative from the time of diagnosis. Care largely involves helping patients and families cope with relentlessly progressive debility, manifest in terms of declining cognition, diminished intake and consequences of poor nutrition, frequent infections, and loss of capacity for self-care and mobility. The course of advancing dementia varies greatly among individuals and the loss of functional capacities does not progress in a uniform

---

TABLE 39.1

MANIFESTATIONS OF ADVANCED DEMENTIA

Neurocognitive
Progressive worsening of memory and other cognitive deficits
Confusion and disorientation become profound
Behavioral changes: agitation, combativeness, resistance to care, apathy
Progressive deterioration of speech, ability to communicate; patient eventually becomes incoherent, mute, unresponsive

Functional
Independent mobility progressively lost; patient becomes bed-bound
Capacity for self-care and performance of independent activities of daily living progressively lost; patient becomes totally dependent

Nutritional
Progressive loss of appetite
Progressive loss of capacity to swallow; ability to eat independently almost invariably declines
Aspiration increasingly becomes a risk

Complications
Bowel and bladder incontinence
Fevers and infections (e.g., pneumonia, urinary tract infections, sepsis)
Decubitus ulcers
Weight loss and malnutrition

Adapted from Shuster JL. Palliative care for advanced dementia. *Clin Geriatr Med* 2000;16:373–386, with permission.

---

or predictable way. However, there are consistent patterns of signs, symptoms, and functional loss that herald the final stages of dementia (Table 39.1) (14).

Evaluation for Hospice Eligibility

Given that most dementias are incurable, the only available treatments are palliative, and advancing dementia invariably leads to death, it would seem that end-stage dementia is a natural fit for hospice care. Access to hospice care has been improving in recent years for patients with dementia, but this patient population is clearly still underserved by hospice and palliative care programs (14–16). This is largely due to the difficulty in predicting mortality in end-stage dementia with accuracy, because the eligibility for admission to hospice care in the United States is based on a medical prediction of mortality within 6 months.

The National Hospice and Palliative Care Organization (NHPCO) has prepared a set of model hospice admission guidelines for noncancer diagnoses, including dementia (17). The intent of these guidelines is to help clinicians identify a population of patients very likely to die within 6 months if a given disease runs its normal course. For dementia, the guidelines are based on the Functional Assessment Staging (FAST) scale (18). Eligibility for hospice care under these guidelines requires that the patient be at or beyond the most advanced stage (Stage 7) measured by this instrument. This phase of a dementing illness would be characterized by inability to walk, dress, or bathe independently, bowel and bladder incontinence, and loss of all capacity for meaningful communication. Presence of any of a number of common complications of advanced dementia can strengthen the case for hospice eligibility (e.g., aspiration pneumonia, pyelonephritis, septicemia, multiple decubitus ulcers, recurrent fevers, weight loss, hypoalbuminemia) (17).

By the time dementia progresses to the point that the patient is considered eligible for hospice care in the United States, the patient and family have typically dealt with the consequences of dementia for years. Many important decisions about the goals and direction of care (e.g., decisions about tube feedings, aggressiveness of treatment with antibiotics) may have already been made without the participation of the palliative care team. Care provided directly to the patient may be limited to physical symptom control, comfort, and prevention of complications that can produce suffering. Patients with dementia rated 7 or higher on the FAST scale are beyond the capacity to benefit from much of the psychological, social, interpersonal, and spiritual care that characterizes palliative care and hospice. Although family members can still benefit greatly from the care of the hospice or palliative care team, the current system of determining hospice eligibility does not facilitate making all the benefits of palliative care available to patients with dementia.

Not only does the 6-month prognosis requirement of the NHPCO criteria serve as a hindrance to providing palliative care through hospice before the patient's ability to benefit more directly, the criteria leave much to be desired in terms of their capacity to predict 6-month mortality in patients with dementia. Studies using the NHPCO eligibility guidelines for dementia show that the guidelines have a positive predictive value (as measured by the proportion of hospice-eligible patients who died within 6 months) of only approximately 35% (10,19).

Multiple barriers impede access to hospice and palliative care for patients with advanced dementia. Retrospective review of deaths from dementia reveal that only approximately 10% of deaths were anticipated 3 months in advance, contributing to extremely low rates of hospice referral (16). Additionally, some of the components of excellent palliative care and hospice, such as careful attention to nutrition, meticulous nursing care, and management of infections and other secondary complications of dementia, can prolong survival. Although these interventions may be consistent with goals and preferences of patients and families, they complicate end-of-life care for demented patients if hospice programs avoid admission or recertification of these patients for fear of regulatory scrutiny if patients survive longer than 6 months (14).

Treatment

The goal of palliative care is to achieve the best quality of life for patients and their families. Palliative care interventions typically focus on providing assurance of nonabandonment to patients and families, aggressive symptom control, assistance with specific life goals, integration of the end-of-life experience and assistance with losses, grief, and bereavement (14). Given the advanced state of dementia when most patients come to the attention of palliative care, symptom-control measures are often the most helpful interventions available.

Agitation and restlessness are among the most common and most troublesome complications of advancing dementias. Determination of specific causes of restlessness, including untreated delirium, pain/discomfort, or depression should be the first step in management. Behavioral interventions (e.g., reassuring contact with familiar others; familiar environmental

cues; soothing music) and determination and correction of any precipitants of agitated behavior, if patterns of behavior exist, can be very helpful (20). Pharmacologic interventions for agitation in dementia include cholinesterase inhibitors and memantine (see subsequent text), antipsychotics (see subsequent text), anticonvulsants (e.g., valproate, carbamazepine, gabapentin), benzodiazepines, serotonergic antidepressants (particularly citalopram and trazodone), buspirone, and β-blockers (20). Preliminary evidence suggests that valproate may slow the progression of AD (21). Benzodiazepines should be used with caution, because paradoxical disinhibition (and worsening agitation) is common when patients with dementia are treated with these drugs. "Sundowning"—a pattern of increased agitation occurring in the evening—should lead to the consideration of the presence of delirium (due to the characteristic sleep/wake cycle disruption), sleep disturbances, or the timing of medication administration (22).

Advancing dementia is often complicated by hallucinations, ranging from pleasant or reassuring perceptions of the presence of absent or deceased friends and relatives to disturbing, frightening, or bizarre experiences. Although antipsychotic medication should be used for the treatment of disturbing hallucinations, these phenomena are often poorly responsive to pharmacotherapy and, if problematic, should also be managed with support, reassurance, and distraction/redirection. Generally, progressive memory loss leads to delusional thoughts, commonly manifest as accusations by the patient, that family members or other caregivers are stealing from the patient (when items have simply been misplaced), delusional beliefs that family members are impostors, or delusional accusations of marital infidelity. Family members may need particular support to cope with delusional accusations by the demented patient. Delusions and hallucinations are predictors of more rapid progression of dementia (23).

Although depression is a common complication of the early to middle stages of dementia, patients are typically unable to generate complaints of depressed mood or accurately guide therapy by reporting target symptoms by the time they are treated in a palliative care setting. Antidepressants may be effective in reducing agitation and restlessness, which may be the only manifestations of depression a patient with advanced dementia is able to demonstrate. Additionally, it is advisable to maintain antidepressant therapy as long as it is safe and well tolerated if it has been determined to be beneficial earlier in the course of dementia.

Pain is a common complication of advanced dementia and there is no evidence that demented patients suffer less with pain simply because they are unable to complain about it (24). Pain behaviors and reporting may be reduced as a consequence of impairments in memory, verbal capacity, motivation, and complex thinking. Further, any degeneration of the central nervous system that involves the sensory cortex or structures that relay, process, or mediate pain signals could produce, distort, or otherwise complicate pain in ways that might well amplify the pain experience and the suffering that pain causes (14,24). For example, patients with vascular dementia would be at higher risk for other cerebrovascular lesions (e.g., thalamic infarctions), which could produce distressing and treatment-refractory central pain syndromes. Those who care for patients with advanced dementia should therefore be especially vigilant to screen for pain and potentially painful comorbid conditions.

Course and Prognosis

The course of dementias, even the course of cases of AD, varies greatly. In the typical case of AD, cognitive deterioration as measured by the Mini-Mental State Examination (MMSE) (25) is in the range of 3–4 points lost per year. The average duration from onset of symptoms to death is 8–10 years, with the end stage of the illness lasting as long as 2 to 3 years (1). Neurodegenerative changes of dementia do not cause death directly, but death occurs as a consequence of secondary complications (e.g., infections; poor nutrition, and immobility leading to organ system failure). Most older patients with dementia have comorbid medical problems, which can often accelerate the course of the patient's terminal illness, depending on their severity and reversibility.

PALLIATIVE CARE CONTROVERSIES

Decisions and Goals of Care

One of the core elements of good palliative care is the emphasis on collaboration with the patient and family in determining the goals of care and the priority of various possible intervention in light of those goals. Because many of the palliative goals of care are more subjective in nature than goals that might be pursued earlier in the course of an illness, the preferences, values, and priorities of the patient are actively sought and integrated into plans of care and resulting actions. Unfortunately, by the time most patients receive palliative care for dementia, their cognitive impairment precludes any meaningful participation in this process. Further, it is relatively uncommon for patients with dementia to have discussed their preferences, values, and priorities with the individual who will serve as their designated or default proxy for healthcare-related decision making. Although the ideal situation would involve incremental decision making over the long course of a dementing illness, allowing maximal participation of the patient in the process as long as possible and permitting professional caregivers and proxy decision makers to understand trends in the patient's preferences, values, and priorities, this is seldom the case. The more proxy decision makers understand the patient's perspective on decisions (e.g., antibiotic therapy; nutritional support or tube feeding, cardiopulmonary resuscitation, transfers to other settings for treatment of acute or emergent problems), the more likely they will be to understand their role as speaking on behalf of the patient and as the individual who best knows the patient's preferences, values, and priorities as opposed to perceiving themselves as holding their loved one's life in their hands. This process works best as a dialogue continuing over time and across several sessions. Exploration of the meaning of decisions to forego life-prolonging therapies and

the burden on the proxy decision maker should be pursued in combination with gentle but clear information about of the burden of continuing such therapies, always in the context of the patient's preferences, values, and priorities, to the extent that they are known.

THE ROLE OF CHOLINESTERASE INHIBITORS AND MEMANTINE

Cholinesterase inhibitors are a relatively new class of drugs. The theoretical basis for their use results from the understanding of AD as a gradual loss of central cholinergic function caused by the progressive death of cholinergic neurons. These drugs are approved for use in mild to moderate AD for the purpose of slowing the rate of cognitive loss and have been demonstrated to be beneficial for this purpose (26). Commonly used agents in this class include donepezil, galantamine, and rivastigmine. Tacrine, the first drug in this class to be approved, is seldom used because of the risk of hepatotoxicity. These agents appear to offer little or no benefit in terms of cognitive preservation once AD has reached the advanced stages, and are expensive compared to most medications used in hospice care. From this perspective, cholinesterase inhibitors would seem to be of no use in patients once they have progressed to the point of hospice eligibility.

There is, however, an emerging body of evidence which suggests that cholinesterase inhibitors are effective in preventing the emergence of agitation and other problematic behaviors in dementia (when long-term therapy is maintained) as well as in reducing these behaviors when cholinesterase inhibitor therapy is initiated for this purpose (26–34). The frequency, magnitude, and durability of such beneficial effects of these agents remain to be determined.

The role of memantine, an N-methyl-D-aspartate (NMDA) antagonist, in palliative care is also unclear. Memantine is approved and has been shown to be effective in the treatment of moderate to severe dementia (35). Antagonism at the NMDA receptor is believed to slow the progression of dementia by blocking the activity of the excitatory neurotransmitter glutamate. Like cholinesterase inhibitors, memantine appears to reduce agitation and other problematic behaviors in dementia (29,35,36), but the evidence for these beneficial effects should be considered preliminary.

Table 39.2 summarizes the evidence for the use of cholinesterase inhibitors and memantine in advanced and terminal dementias. For now, use of these agents for control of agitation and behavioral symptoms of dementia in the hospice and palliative care setting remains a clinical cost/benefit

TABLE 39.2

COMPARISON OF CHOLINESTERASE INHIBITORS AND MEMANTINE IN THE PALLIATIVE CARE OF DEMENTIA

| Drug | Progression Effectively Slowed in | | | Effective in AD | Effective in other dementias | Reduces PBD emergence[a] | Improves PBD after emergence[a] | Improves ADL functioning[a] |
	Early/Mild dementia	Moderate dementia	Advanced dementia					
Donepezil	X	X		X	?	X	X	
Galantamine	X	X		X	?	X	?	?
Rivastigmine	X	X		X	?	X	?	
Memantine		X	X	X	?	X	X	X

AD, Alzheimer's disease; PBD, problematic behaviors in dementia (e.g., agitation, restlessness, combativeness); ADL, activities of daily living; X, evidence or reports of effectiveness; ?, effectiveness unclear.
[a]In advanced-stage dementia.
Most data come from small studies or sub analyses of larger data sets from studies with cognition as the primary outcome (26–36).

decision. However, when a patient with dementia develops an acute increase in agitation or other problematic behaviors after discontinuation of either cholinesterase inhibitors or memantine, reinitiation of therapy is reasonable.

Antipsychotic Medications for Agitation

Antipsychotic medications are some of the best studied, most reliably effective, and most controversial treatments for agitation in dementia (20,37,38). Because of their risk of short- and long-term side effects and because of a history of nursing homes using these drugs without a clear clinical indication, language in the Omnibus Budget Reconciliation Act 1987 specifically regulates the use of neuroleptics. In the nursing home setting, these agents are generally reserved for therapy targeted at agitation, delirium, or psychosis complicating dementia and are used at the lowest effective doses and reassessed frequently for side effects and need for maintenance therapy. Because most of these agents are FDA approved only for the treatment of psychotic disorders, agitated dementia is an "off-label" indication for neuroleptics. The newer atypical antipsychotic drugs have come into wide use for this purpose because of their relatively low risk of extrapyramidal side effects in older patients.

In 2005, the U.S. Food and Drug Administration (FDA) issued a Public Health Advisory (39) suggesting that treatment with atypical antipsychotics may increase the risk of mortality in agitated patients with dementia. The advisory reported that 15 of 17 placebo-controlled trials of atypical antipsychotics (5106 patients total) showed increased mortality—mostly due to cardiac and infectious causes—among treated patients compared to those in placebo groups. The advisory estimated a 1.6–1.7-fold increase in mortality risk associated with atypical antipsychotic treatment for behavioral disturbances in dementia, and suggested that mortality risk might also be increased if older neuroleptic drugs are used for this indication. Since this time, the FDA has required that manufacturers of atypical antipsychotics include this finding in the form of a "black box" warning in the prescribing information for each of these drugs.

It is important to note that this warning only pertains to the use of atypical antipsychotics for behavioral disturbances in dementia and is not generalizable to nondemented patient populations. Additionally, this Public Health Advisory does not necessarily imply that use of atypical antipsychotics for other approved and off-label indications is associated with increased mortality risk. Antipsychotic medications are the mainstay of treatment for delirium (see subsequent text). Delirium is very commonly comorbid with advanced dementia, although differentiating delirium in the setting of advanced dementia can be challenging (40). Delirium is also clearly associated with increased risk of mortality (see subsequent text), so decisions about antipsychotic treatment of possible delirium in patients with dementia should consider the mortality risk of leaving delirium untreated as well as the risk of treatment. Preliminary evidence from a case–control study of demented nursing home residents comparing residents who did or did not die during the study period suggests that agitation itself is associated with increased mortality risk, and that patients who died were significantly less likely to have been exposed to antipsychotic medications (12 vs. 37% in the group that did not die) (41).

Given all the available evidence, it is advisable to reserve antipsychotics, especially atypical agents, for the treatment of agitated patients with dementia who do not respond to the alternative treatments listed in the preceding text or for whom other treatments are contraindicated. In agitation caused by delirium or agitation in the patient with dementia who is actively dying, the risk/benefit decisions will likely lean in the direction of treatment with antipsychotic medication, consistent with palliative goals of care.

DELIRIUM

Delirium develops as a consequence of a physical illness, metabolic disturbance, or medication side effect that causes widespread cerebral dysfunction (1,42). Demonstrable changes in cerebral metabolism occur as a consequence of delirium. Any condition that compromises the brain's supply of glucose or oxygen, disturbs the balance of the brain's environment (e.g., fever, infections, electrolyte imbalances), or grossly disturbs brain functioning (e.g., tumors, strokes, seizures, withdrawal states, brain injuries, effects of drugs) can produce delirium. In patients with advanced or terminal illnesses, multiple potential causes of delirium are the rule and not the exception.

The characteristic features of delirium involve a disturbance in consciousness and cognition that develops over a relatively short period of time. Consciousness is typically clouded, with prominent disturbances in attention. Cognitive disruption can be subtle in mild delirious states, but can also be widespread to global in more severe cases, including disturbances in memory, orientation, language, thinking, and speech. Affective and perceptual disturbances, including hallucinations, illusions, and delusions, are also common. A diagnosis of delirium requires the identification or strong suspicion of one or more general medical conditions as causative factors. The features of delirium usually emerge over a period of hours to days, although this course may be more prolonged depending on the time course of the underlying problems. Other common, but not universal, features of delirium include the following:

1. A rapidly fluctuating course of the severity of symptoms, which may cause the patient's presentation to vary as often as hour to hour
2. Alterations in arousal and psychomotor functioning (e.g., agitation)
3. Disturbances in the sleep–wake cycle (typically daytime sleepiness and increased arousal at night)

Delirium is easy to recognize when patients are agitated and restless, but all the impairments in consciousness and cognition can be seen in the absence of agitation (42–44). These cases of so-called quiet delirium can be difficult to detect without close examination for cognitive disturbance.

Delirium is not only common in the palliative care setting, it is a cause of substantial suffering to patients and families (42,43). Because delirium produces an acute disturbance of cognition, patients are typically unable to reliably report the distress they may experience while delirious. Further, formation of memories of the delirious experience may be fragmentary, at best (a blessing in most cases). Although recall of the experience may be incomplete after delirium resolves, interviews of patients after delirium clearly reveal that retained memories of the experience cause substantial distress (43). Whether the patient demonstrates agitation while delirious appears to make no difference in terms of the resulting distress. Clearly, there is also a significant burden of distress on families and caregivers who witness the apparent suffering caused by delirium (42,43). Education of family (and professional caregivers unaccustomed to caring for delirious patients) is very important. Because it produces a dramatic and relatively abrupt change in the patient's behavior, witnesses often misinterpret delirium as an episode of psychosis or willful bad behavior. Information should be provided about the probable cause of the delirious episode, the plans for intervention and care, and the likelihood of resolution of the delirium.

Prevalence and Epidemiology

The prevalence of delirium is very low in community samples (1). Rates of delirium are directly correlated with rates of medical illnesses, and delirium is very common in the presence of any serious medical illness (2). Hospitalized patients have a higher likelihood of being delirious than medically healthy patients in the community, and patients in critical care settings are substantially more likely to become delirious than patients on medical wards. Delirium is quite common at the end of life, especially in the days and hours immediately preceding death. Rates of delirium in excess of 80% have been reported for patients in the days just before death (45–47). Morita et al. reported that the percentage of patients who were cognitively able to communicate meaningfully diminished from 43% 5 days before death to 28% 3 days before death and only 13% in the last day of life (48).

Age increases the risk of developing delirium. In patients older than 65, 10% are delirious on hospital admission and another 10–15% develop delirium before discharge (1). Other risk factors for developing delirium include polypharmacy, fever, hypoxia, uremia, hepatic insufficiency, anemia, infections, hypoalbuminemia, dehydration, brain tumors, immobility, underlying neurologic disorders, and reduced acuity of hearing or vision (42,49).

Differential Diagnosis

A number of conditions may mimic, produce, or exacerbate delirium, and these are summarized in Table 39.3. Any concurrent medical diagnosis, medication, or poorly controlled symptom can also complicate the picture and make the delirious patient worse. Table 39.4 lists medications commonly associated with delirium.

Caraceni and Grassi's textbook on delirium in palliative medicine contains an excellent overview of the neurobiology, neurochemistry, and pathophysiology of delirium (50).

TABLE 39.3

DIFFERENTIAL DIAGNOSIS OF DELIRIUM (ALTERNATIVE CAUSES OF AGITATION AND CONFUSION)

Amnestic disorder
Anger
Anxiety
Bladder distention
Brain injury (especially frontal lobe injury)
Constipation
Dementia and other degenerative brain disorders
Depression
Dyspnea
Fear
Interpersonal conflict
Nausea
Pain
Personality disorder
Psychosis
Seizure (or pre-epileptic neuroelectrical disturbance)
Substance intoxication
Substance withdrawal

Adapted from Shuster JL Jr. Delirium, agitation, and confusion at the end of life. *J Palliat Med* 1998;1:177–186., with permission.

TABLE 39.4

MEDICATIONS COMMONLY ASSOCIATED WITH DELIRIUM

Antibiotics (especially intravenous)
Anticholinergic drugs
Anticonvulsants
Antiemetics
Antihistamines
Antispasmodics
Corticosteroids
Digoxin
Dopamine agonists
Muscle relaxers
Opiates
Psychotropic drugs
    Tricyclic antidepressants
    Psychostimulants
    Low-potency antipsychotic drugs
    Sedative-hypnotics
Anticancer drugs
    L-Asparaginase
    Bleomycin
    Capecitabine
    Carmustine
    Cisplatin
    Carboplatin
    Cytarabine
    Fludarabine
    5-Fluorouracil
    Ifosfamide
    Interferon
    Interleukin α
    Interleukin-2
    Methotrexate
    Paclitaxel
    Procarbazine
    Thiotepa
    Trimetrexate
    Vinblastine
    Vincristine

Evaluation

Careful serial assessment of cognition is crucial to the detection of delirium at the end of life. Clinical screening instruments such as the Mini-Mental State Exam (25), the Confusion Assessment Method (51), or the Nursing Delirium Screening Scale (52) can be valuable in the detection of cognitive decline and delirium. These instruments are easy to learn to use and can be administered serially to screen for delirium.

The evaluation and workup of the delirious patient in palliative care should be guided by the goals of care and the overall condition of the patient. If the patient develops a quiet delirium (essentially a gradual loss of cognition and awareness) as part of the active dying process and agitation or other complications do not emerge, active evaluation and intervention may not be indicated. On the other hand, if the onset of delirium is sudden and unexpected or significantly precedes the anticipated time of the patient's death, a more vigorous evaluation may be appropriate.

Evaluation should be focused on a search for potentially reversible causes of delirium. This search should be generally limited to relatively noninvasive measures with high diagnostic yield leading to specific interventions judged to have high likelihood of benefit.

A substantial proportion of cases of delirium seen in the terminally ill are at least potentially reversible (45,53). Commonly reversible causes include toxicity of medications (e.g., anticholinergic drugs, accumulation of neurotoxic opiate metabolites) and dehydration. Withdrawal states are another important consideration in delirium at the end of life. Other factors which can precipitate or cause delirium and are likely remediable include pain, sepsis, fecal impaction, and bladder distention.

TREATMENT

A four-stage management approach to delirium in palliative care is outlined in Table 39.5. First, given the high prevalence of delirium in advanced and terminal illness, efforts should be made to avoid precipitating cognitive decline (by exercising caution with medications to avoid medications commonly associated with confusion) while maintaining environmental reminders and soothing contact with others for the patient whose functional status is declining. Serial screening for cognitive decline can help detect delirium in early stages and facilitate treatments aimed at reversing cognitive disturbance.

Once delirium emerges, treatment should be aimed at restoring cognitive functioning to the highest possible level and not simply at controlling agitation. This goal is achieved by seeking out and treating reversible causes of delirium, intervening early with antipsychotic medications, and providing a soothing balance of reassuring frequent contact with others while avoiding overstimulation. Finally, in the patient whose agitated delirium does not respond to therapeutic intervention and whose survival is measured in hours to days, agitation is controlled by palliative sedation by infusion of benzodiazepines or other sedatives.

Medications to treat delirium are summarized in Table 39.6. Antipsychotic drugs are the mainstay of treatment for delirium in terminal illness (42,46). Standard antipsychotic drugs (e.g., chlorpromazine, haloperidol), have long been accepted as effective treatments for delirium. Haloperidol is widely used to treat delirium and is considered the antipsychotic medication of choice in palliative care (42,44,46). Newer (atypical) antipsychotics are also useful in the treatment of delirium, although these are less thoroughly studied. These drugs have

TABLE 39.5

TREATMENT GOALS FOR DELIRIUM IN PALLIATIVE CARE

1. *Prevention of cognitive decline*:
   (a) Use caution with medications known to cause confusion
   (b) Maintain familiar surroundings for the patient
   (c) Use hearing aids or glasses, if indicated
   (d) Strive to prevent common complications of terminal illness which can precipitate delirium
2. *Early detection of cognitive decline*:
   (a) Screening of cognitive function serially (due to frequency of delirium in palliative care setting)
   (b) Aim to simplify intervention by early detection
3. *Early intervention for confusion, delirium*:
   (a) Find and treat reversible causes
   (b) Pharmacologic intervention—antipsychotic drugs
   (c) Titrate personal contact, reorientation efforts to patient response (avoiding abandonment and overstimulation)
   (d) Restore the patient to meaningful cognitive connection with family and friends
4. *Comfort sedation when patient is actively dying and agitated delirium cannot be reversed*:
   (a) Pharmacologic intervention—sedative drugs
   (b) Ease the dying of the patient who would otherwise die in a state of suffering

fewer extrapyramidal side effects and may eventually prove to be advances in the treatment of delirium at the end of life (54,55). As with older neuroleptics, average doses in the range of 50% of those required for psychosis are usually effective for delirium, but full antipsychotic doses may be required in some cases.

Benzodiazepines, especially lorazepam, are sometimes used in the treatment of delirium, either alone or in combination with neuroleptics (42,46). Benzodiazepines are ineffective for delirium (44) and interfere with the goal of restoring a patient's cognition. Primary management of delirium with

TABLE 39.6

MEDICATIONS FOR DELIRIUM IN PALLIATIVE CARE

Agent (class)	Dose range (mg)	FREQ	Routes	Notes
Antipsychotics				
Haloperidol	0.5–2.0	b.i.d.-q.i.d.[a]	p.o., i.v., i.m., s.c.	(Goal is reversal of cognitive impairment)
Chlorpromazine	25–100	b.i.d.-q.i.d.[a]	p.o., i.m., s.q.	
Olanzapine	5–10	q.h.s.-b.i.d.	p.o., s.l.	
Risperidone	1–2	b.i.d.-q.i.d.[a]	p.o.	
Quetiapine	25–200	b.i.d.[a]	p.o.	
Ziprasidone	20–80	b.i.d.	p.o., i.m.	
Benzodiazepines				(Goal is sedation for
Lorazepam	[b]	[b]	i.v., s.l.	refractory, agitated
Midazolam	[b]	[b]	i.v., s.l.	delirium in the actively dying patient)

FREQ, frequency.
[a]May require a higher dose or more frequent dosing.
[b]Dose varies, titrated to effect.

benzodiazepines should be reserved for cases when sedation, whether temporary or of longer duration, is the desired outcome.

Prognosis

Since its initial description by the ancient Greeks, delirium has been recognized as an indicator of mortality (2). A recent flurry of literature indicates that delirium is an independent predictor of mortality, increased inpatient length of stay, and other poor patient outcomes (56–62). This appears to be the case whether the setting of care is the general hospital (56–58), an intensive care unit (59,60), or a nursing home (61,62). Recovery from delirium is associated with improved survival compared with persistent delirium (57,63,64). Even patients whose acute cognitive disturbance does not reach the full diagnostic threshold for delirium as defined in DSM-IV (subsyndromal delirium) are at risk for poorer outcomes, including increased risk of mortality (65).

PALLIATIVE CARE CONTROVERSIES

Decisions and Goals of Care

Delirium presents the same issues and challenges about decision making, agency, and shaping goals of care as discussed in the section on dementia, with the added complication of the typically faster course of development of delirium. Without much lead time to prepare for the need to make important strategic and situational decisions about the goals of care, proxy decision makers often feel even more distressed in their role.

Palliative Sedation

Palliative sedation (also called "intentional sedation," "terminal sedation," "comfort sedation," or "controlled sedation for refractory suffering") has been defined as "the use of sedative medications to relieve intolerable and refractory distress by the reduction of patient consciousness" (66). Agitated delirium unresponsive to more conservative therapies in the dying patient is a common indication for palliative sedation. Palliative sedation is controversial because it treads closely to euthanasia in the opinion of some. A conservative perspective would view palliative sedation as a therapy of last resort to provide relief from severe and refractory distress and suffering (e.g., treatment-refractory agitated delirium) when more conservative interventions have failed or would most likely fail to provide comfort and relief and failure to act would most likely allow uncontrolled suffering to complicate the patient's death. When severe and intolerable suffering cannot be otherwise controlled in the dying patient, relief is provided through palliative sedation by reducing or eliminating awareness of the suffering. Most practitioners of palliative medicine would be comfortable with such a definition, provided the following criteria are met:

1. The patient has a terminal illness (i.e., the patient would be eligible for admission to hospice).
2. The patient's dying is imminent (i.e., the patient is actively dying and death is likely to occur in a matter of hours to days; with or without sedation).
3. Therapy aimed at emphasizing comfort over awareness is consistent with the goals of care articulated by the patient or the patient's surrogate.

4. Informed consent to proceed with palliative sedation is obtained from the patient or (in most cases) from the patient's surrogate.

Decisions to initiate palliative sedation typically require a family conference to ensure that intervention is consistent with the goals of care articulated by the patient or the patient's surrogate, that proper education and opportunity to ask questions is provided, and that informed consent is obtained.

Close supervision and monitoring of the patient is necessary to ensure that sedating medications administered for palliative sedation are effective in producing restful comfort, do not fall short of this goal and leave symptoms, suffering, and distress untreated, and are not administered in doses exceeding those needed to reliably achieve the goal of restful comfort. Frequent monitoring of patient response and subsequent dose adjustment are necessary to ensure that palliative sedation is and remains effective. For this reason, palliative sedation is usually administered in the inpatient setting, although it can be provided in the home hospice setting if adequate professional clinical staff supervision is available in the home to monitor patient response and manage medication dose adjustments.

A thorough discussion of palliative sedation, including the ethical Principle of Double Effect and medications used in palliative sedation, is contained in Chapter 57. The ethical issue of euthanasia and assisted suicide and distinctions between these and palliative sedation is contained in Chapter 64.

It is not clear whether earlier detection and intervention in the palliative care setting would reduce the incidence of refractory delirium necessitating palliative sedation in the active dying phase to any substantial degree. However, given the prevalence of delirium in the days and hours near death, the apparent suffering of agitated delirious patients, and the toll that deciding to initiate palliative sedation takes on caregivers and families, aggressive screening for early cognitive decline and prompt intervention to reverse delirium is good care. If interventions are successful, restoring the patient's capacity to communicate meaningfully with family and friends at a time when every moment is precious is a most valuable gift to be able to give.

References

1. American Psychiatric Association. *Diagnostic and statistical manual of mental disorders*, 4th edn. Washington, DC: American Psychiatric Press, 1994.
2. Lipowski ZJ. *Delirium: acute confusional states*. New York: Oxford University Press, 1990.
3. Koponen H, Partanen J, Paakkonen A, et al. EEG spectral analysis in delirium. *J Neurol Neurosurg Psychiatry* 1989;52:980–985.
4. Jenssen S. Electroencephalogram in the dementia workup. *Am J Alzheimers Dis Other Demen* 2005;20:159–166.
5. Sachs GA. Key factors affecting those dying with dementia. *NIH state-of-the-science conference on improving end-of-life Care*, Program and Abstracts, 2004:23–27. Bethesda, MD.
6. Aminoff BZ, Purits E, Noy S, et al. Measuring the suffering of end-stage dementia: reliability and validity of the mini-suffering state examination. *Arch Gerontol Geriatr* 2004;38:123–130.
7. Aminoff BZ, Adunsky A. Dying dementia patients: too much suffering, too little palliation. *Am J Alzheimers Dis Other Demen* 2004;19:243–247.
8. McCarthy M, Addington-Hall J, Altmann D. The experience of dying with dementia: a retrospective study. *Int J Geriatr Psychiatry* 1997;12:404–409.
9. Volicer L, Hurley AC, Blasi ZV. Scales for evaluation of end-of-life care in dementia. *Alzheimer Dis Assoc Disord* 2001;15:194–200.
10. Shuster JL, Rice K, Tucker M, Allen RS. Hospice eligibility guidelines in a VA long term care facility: Rates of hospice eligibility and prediction of six-month mortality. Presented at National Hospice and Palliative Care Organization *1st National conference on access to hospice and Palliative Care*, August 2, 2005, St. Louis, MO.
11. Teno JM, Clarridge BR, Casey V, et al. Family perspectives on end-of-life care at the last place of care. *JAMA* 2004;291:88–93.
12. Evans DA, Funkenstein HH, Albert MS, et al. Prevalence of Alzheimer's disease in a community population of older persons. Higher than previously reported. *JAMA* 1989;262:2551–2556.

13. Tomlinson BE, Blessed G, Roth M. Observations on the brains of demented old people. *J Neurol Sci* 1970;11:205–242.

14. Shuster JL. Palliative care for advanced dementia. *Clin Geriatr Med* 2000;16:373–386.

15. Hanrahan P, Luchins DJ. Access to hospice programs in end-stage dementia: a national survey of hospice programs. *J Am Geriatr Soc* 1995;43:56–59.

16. Mitchell SL, Morris JN, Park PS, et al. Terminal care for persons with advanced dementia in the nursing home and home care settings. *J Palliat Med* 2004;7:808–816.

17. National Hospice Organization Medical Guidelines Task Force. *Medical guidelines for determining prognosis in selected non-cancer diseases.* Arlington, VA: National Hospice Organization, 1995.

18. Reisberg B. Functional assessment staging (FAST). *Psychopharmacol Bull* 1988;24:653–659.

19. Mitchell SL, Kiely DK, Hamel MB, et al. Estimating prognosis for nursing home residents with advanced dementia. *JAMA* 2004;291:2734–2740.

20. Gray KF. Managing agitation and difficult behavior in dementia. *Clin Geriatr Med* 2004;20:69–82.

21. Tariot PN. Valproate use in neuropsychiatric disorders in the elderly. *Psychopharmacol Bull* 2003;37(Suppl 2):116–128.

22. Martin J, Marler M, Shochat T, et al. Circadian rhythms of agitation in institutionalized patients with Alzheimer's disease. *Chronobiol Int* 2000;17:405–418.

23. Scarmeas N, Brandt J, Albert M, et al. Delusions and hallucinations are associated with worse outcome in Alzheimer disease. *Arch Neurol* 2005;62:1601–1608.

24. Farrell MJ, Katz B, Helme RD. The impact of dementia on the pain experience. *Pain* 1996;67:7–15.

25. Folstein MF, Folstein SE, McHugh PR. "Mini-mental state". A practical method for grading the cognitive state of patients for the clinician. *J Psychiatr Res* 1975;12:189–198.

26. Masterman D. Cholinesterase inhibitors in the treatment of Alzheimer's disease and related dementias. *Clin Geriatr Med* 2004;20:59 68.

27. Gray KF. Managing agitation and difficult behavior in dementia. *Clin Geriatr Med* 2004;20:69–82.

28. Wynn ZJ, Cummings JL. Cholinesterase inhibitor therapies and neuropsychiatric manifestations of Alzheimer's disease. *Dement Geriatr Cogn Disord* 2004;17:100 108.

29. Forchetti CM. Treating patients with moderate to severe Alzheimer's disease: implications of recent pharmacologic studies. *Prim Care Companion J Clin Psychiatry* 2005;7:155–161.

30. Gauthier S, Feldman H, Hecker J, et al. Donepezil MSAD Study Investigators Group. Efficacy of donepezil on behavioral symptoms in patients with moderate to severe Alzheimer's disease. *Int Psychogeriatr* 2002;14:389–404.

31. Paleacu D, Mazeh D, Mirecki I, et al. Donepezil for the treatment of behavioral symptoms in patients with Alzheimer's disease. *Clin Neuropharmacol* 2002;25:313–317.

32. Wilkinson DG, Hock C, Farlow M, et al. Galantamine provides broad benefits in patients with 'advanced moderate' Alzheimer's disease (MMSE < or = 12) for up to six months. *Int J Clin Pract* 2002;56:509–514.

33. Cummings JL, Schneider L, Tariot PN, et al. Reduction of behavioral disturbances and caregiver distress by galantamine in patients with Alzheimer's disease. *Am J Psychiatry* 2004;161:532–538.

34. Johannsen P. Long-term cholinesterase inhibitor treatment of Alzheimer's disease. *CNS Drugs* 2004;18:757–768.

35. Gauthier S, Wirth Y, Mobius HJ. Effects of memantine on behavioural symptoms in Alzheimer's disease patients: an analysis of the Neuropsychiatric Inventory (NPI) data of two randomised, controlled studies. *Int J Geriatr Psychiatry* 2005;20:459–464.

36. Areosa SA, Sherriff F, McShane R. Memantine for dementia. *Cochrane Database Syst Rev* 2005;CD003154.

37. Snowden M, Sato K, Roy-Byrne P. Assessment and treatment of nursing home residents with depression or behavioral symptoms associated with dementia: a review of the literature. *J Am Geriatr Soc* 2003;51:1305–1317.

38. Tariot PN, Profenno LA, Ismail MS. Efficacy of atypical antipsychotics in elderly patients with dementia. *J Clin Psychiatry* 2004;65(Suppl 11):11–15.

39. http://www.fda.gov/cder/drug/advisory/antipsychotics.htm, 2005.

40. Lewis LM, Miller DK, Morley JE, et al. Unrecognized delirium in ED geriatric patients. *Am J Emerg Med* 1995;13:142–145.

41. Allen RS, Burgio LD, Fisher SE, et al. Behavioral ███████ nursing home residents with dementia at the ████ 2005;45:661–666.

42. Shuster JL Jr Delirium, agitation, and confusion ████ *Med* 1998;1:177–186.

43. Breitbart W, Gibson C, Tremblay A. The deli███ recall and delirium-related distress in hospitalized ████ spouses/caregivers, and their nurses. *Psychosoma.* ████

44. Breitbart W, Marotta R, Platt MM, et al. A double-blind trial of haloperidol, chlorpromazine, and lorazepam in the treatment of delirium in hospitalized AIDS patients. *Am J Psychiatry* 1996;153:231–237.

45. Bruera E, Miller L, McCallion J, et al. Cognitive failure in patients with terminal cancer: a prospective study. *J Pain Symptom Manage* 1992;7:192–195.

46. Breitbart W, Bruera E, Chochinov H, et al. Neuropsychiatric syndromes and psychological symptoms in patients with advanced cancer. *J Pain Symptom Manage* 1995;10:131–141.

47. Conill C, Verger E, Henriquez I, et al. Symptom prevalence in the last week of life. *J Pain Symptom Manage* 1997;14:328–331.

48. Morita T, Tei Y, Inouye S. Impaired communication capacity and agitated delirium in the final week of terminally ill cancer patients: prevalence and identification of research focus. *J Pain Symptom Manage* 2003;26:827–834.

49. Inouye SK, Charpentier PA. Precipitating factors for delirium in hospitalized elderly persons. *JAMA* 1996;275:852–857.

50. Caracini A, Grassi L. *Delirium: acute confusional states in palliative medicine.* New York: Oxford University Press, 2003.

51. Inouye SK, van Dyke CH, Alessi CA, et al. Clarifying confusion: the confusion assessment method. *Ann Intern Med* 1990;113:941–948.

52. Gaudreau JD, Gagnon P, Harel F, et al. Fast, systematic, and continuous delirium assessment in hospitalized patients: the nursing delirium screening scale. *J Pain Symptom Manage* 2005;29:368–375.

53. Lawlor PG, Gagnon B, Mancini IL, et al. Occurrence, causes, and outcome of delirium in patients with advanced cancer: a prospective study. *Arch Intern Med* 2000;160:786–794.

54. Schwartz TL, Masand PS. The role of atypical antipsychotics in the treatment of delirium. *Psychosomatics* 2002;43:171–174

55. Friedlander MM, Brayman Y, Breitbart WS. Delirium in palliative care. *Oncology* 2004;18:1541–1550.

56. McCusker J, Cole M, Abrahamowicz M, et al. Delirium predicts 12-month mortality. *Arch Intern Med* 2002;162:457–463.

57. McCusker J, Cole M, Dendukuri N, et al. The course of delirium in older medical inpatients: a prospective study. *J Gen Intern Med* 2003;18:696–704.

58. Leslie DL, Zhang Y, Holford TR, et al. Premature death associated with delirium at 1-year follow-up. *Arch Intern Med* 2005;165:1657–1662.

59. Ely EW, Shintani A, Truman B, et al. Delirium as a predictor of mortality in mechanically ventilated patients in the intensive care unit. *JAMA* 2004;291:1753–1762.

60. Lin SM, Liu CY, Wang CH, et al. The impact of delirium on the survival of mechanically ventilated patients. *Crit Care Med* 2004;32:2254–2259.

61. Pitkala KH, Laurila JV, Strandberg TE, et al. Prognostic significance of delirium in frail older people. *Dement Geriatr Cogn Disord* 2005;19:158–163.

62. Marcantonio ER, Kiely DK, Simon SE, et al. Outcomes of older people admitted to postacute facilities with delirium. *J Am Geriatr Soc* 2005;53:963–969.

63. Lundstrom M, Edlund A, Karlsson S, et al. A multifactorial intervention program reduces the duration of delirium, length of hospitalization, and mortality in delirious patients. *J Am Geriatr Soc* 2005;53:622–628.

64. Milbrandt EB, Kersten A, Kong L, et al. Haloperidol use is associated with lower hospital mortality in mechanically ventilated patients. *Crit Care Med* 2005;33:226–229.

65. Cole M, McCusker J, Dendukuri N, et al. The prognostic significance of subsyndromal delirium in elderly medical inpatients. *J Am Geriatr Soc* 2003;51:754–760.

66. Cherny NI, Portenoy RK. Sedation in the management of refractory symptoms: guidelines for evaluation and treatment. *J Pall Care* 1994;10:31–38.

T3

CHAPTER 40 ■ DEPRESSION AND ANXIETY

KIMBERLY MILLER AND MARY JANE MASSIE

Emotional distress is a normal response to a catastrophic event such as the diagnosis of cancer or any other life-threatening medical disease. The diagnosis of cancer induces stresses that are caused by the patient's perceptions of the disease, its manifestations, and the stigma commonly attached to this disease. For most individuals, the primary fear is a painful death. Patients also fear becoming disabled and dependent, having altered appearance and changed body function, and losing the company of those close to them. Each of these fears is accompanied by a level of psychological distress that varies from patient to patient. This variability is related to medical factors (e.g., site and stage of illness, treatments offered, course of the cancer, and the presence of pain); psychological factors (e.g., prior adjustment, history of losses, coping ability, emotional maturity, the disruption of life goals, and the ability to modify plans); cultural, spiritual and social factors (e.g., availability of emotional support from family, friends, and coworkers); and financial stability (1). Understanding these factors allows the clinician to predict and manage distress that exceeds a threshold arbitrarily defined as normal. The presence of intolerable or prolonged distress that compromises the usual function of the patient requires evaluation, diagnosis, and management.

NORMAL RESPONSES TO THE STRESS OF CANCER

Individuals who receive a diagnosis of cancer, or who learn that relapse has occurred or that treatment has failed, often show a characteristic emotional response: a period of initial shock and disbelief, followed by a period of turmoil with mixed symptoms of anxiety and depression, irritability, and disruption of appetite and sleep. The ability to concentrate and carry out usual daily activities is impaired, and thoughts about the diagnosis and fears about the future may intrude (2). These normal responses to crisis or transitional points in cancer resemble the response to stress associated with other threatened or actual losses.

These symptoms usually resolve over days to weeks with support from family, friends, and a physician who outlines a treatment plan that offers hope. Interventions beyond those provided by physicians, nurses, and social workers are generally not required, unless symptoms of emotional distress interfere with function or are prolonged or intolerable. Prescribing a hypnotic (e.g., zolpidem) for insomnia and anxiolytics (e.g., a benzodiazepine, such as alprazolam or lorazepam) to reduce anxiety can help the patient through this crisis period.

Some patients continue to have high levels of depression and anxiety (both are usually present, although one may predominate) that persist for weeks or months. This persistent reactive distress is not adaptive, often impairs social or occupational functioning and frequently requires psychiatric treatment. These disorders are classified in the current *Diagnostic and Statistical Manual of Mental Disorders Fourth Edition (DSM-IV)* (3) as adjustment disorders with depressed mood, anxiety, or mixed anxiety and depressed mood, depending on the predominant manifestation. For these patients, mental health professionals working in oncology use short-term supportive psychotherapy, which offers emotional support, provides information to help the patient adapt to the crisis, emphasizes past strengths, and supports previously successful ways of coping. Anxiolytic or antidepressant drugs are prescribed as indicated and as symptoms improve, medication can be reduced and discontinued. Having the patient talk with another patient who has been through the same treatment is often a helpful adjunct.

PREVALENCE OF PSYCHIATRIC DISORDERS IN PATIENTS WITH CANCER

There are many myths about the psychological problems of patients with life-threatening illness. The assumptions may range from "all patients are in distress and require psychiatric treatment" to "distress is part of the cancer experience and people cope in their own way over time." One of the first efforts in the field of psycho-oncology was to obtain objective data on the type and frequency of psychological problems in patients with cancer.

Using criteria from the *Diagnostic and Statistical Manual of Mental Disorders Third Edition (DSM-III)* (4) classification of psychiatric disorders, the Psychosocial Collaborative Oncology Group (PSYCOG) determined the psychiatric disorders in 215 randomly selected hospitalized and ambulatory adult patients with cancer in three cancer centers (5). Although slightly over half (53%) the patients evaluated were adjusting normally to stress, the remainder (47%) had clinically apparent psychiatric disorders. Of the 47% with psychiatric disorders, over two thirds (68%) had reactive or situational anxiety and depression (adjustment disorders with depressed or anxious mood), 13% had a major depression, 8% had an organic mental disorder, 7% had a personality disorder, and 4% had a preexisting anxiety disorder. The authors concluded that nearly 90% of the psychiatric disorders observed were reactions to, or manifestations of, disease or treatment.

Interestingly 39% of those who received a psychiatric diagnosis were experiencing significant pain. Although in contrast, only 19% of patients who did not receive a psychiatric diagnosis had significant pain. The psychiatric diagnosis of the patients with pain was predominately adjustment disorder with depressed or mixed mood (69%); however, it is of note that 15% of patients with significant pain had symptoms of major depression. In a study of cancer pain syndromes, unmanaged pain emerged as a causal factor in patient's reports of increased anxiety (6).

Both data and clinical observation suggest that the psychiatric symptoms of patients who are in pain (i.e., acute anxiety, depression with despair, agitation, irritability, unco-operative behavior, anger, and inability to sleep may occur) must initially be considered a consequence of uncontrolled pain symptoms. Feelings of hopelessness, helplessness, and occasionally suicidal ideation occur when the patient believes that pain represents disease progression. These symptoms are not labeled as a psychiatric disorder unless they persist after pain is adequately controlled. Clinicians should manage pain (7) and then reassess the patient's mental state after pain is controlled, to determine whether the patient has a psychiatric disorder.

IMPACT OF DEPRESSION AND ANXIETY ON THE MANAGEMENT OF PATIENTS WITH CANCER

The timely diagnosis and effective management of depression and anxiety in patients with cancer contribute not only to an improvement in quality of life but also enhanced patient involvement in treatment. A meta-analysis of the effects of depression and anxiety on compliance with medical treatment suggests that patients who are depressed are three times more likely to be noncompliant than patients who are not depressed (8). Additionally, depression may impair patients' capacity to understand and process information about their prognosis.

SCREENING FOR PSYCHOLOGICAL DISTRESS IN PATIENTS WITH CANCER

The presence of psychological distress can have a significant impact on patients' lives. However despite this understanding, in the context of a busy oncology clinic, the focus on psychological symptoms is not paramount. Coupled with clinic time pressure is many patients' concern that alerting their health care providers to their psychological distress may divert their physicians from pursuing the most aggressive cancer regimen. To address this issue, brief pencil and paper screening measures or a visual analog scale measuring psychological distress can rapidly identify patients whose levels of distress warrant further evaluation (9). Teaching oncology staff members to use brief, semi-structured interviews can improve their recognition of anxiety and depressive symptoms.

PREVALENCE OF DEPRESSION IN PATIENTS WITH CANCER

In Massie's review of over 150 studies, the prevalence of major depression in patients with cancer ranged from 0% to 38% and the prevalence of depression spectrum syndromes ranged from 0% to 58% (10). Most of this variance can be attributed to the lack of standardization of methodology and diagnostic criteria. For example, in a study of 152 patients with cancer, Kathol et al. found a 13% difference (25% vs. 38%) in the prevalence of depression depending on the diagnostic system used (11).

The clinical rule of thumb is that 25% of patients with cancer are likely depressed enough at some point in the course of disease to warrant evaluation and treatment. Advanced disease has been correlated with a higher prevalence of depression in several studies. The reported prevalence of depression in patients with advanced cancer has been found to be as high as 26% (10,12). Greater physical disability is associated with a higher prevalence of depression.

DIAGNOSIS OF DEPRESSION IN PATIENTS WITH CANCER

The diagnosis of depression in physically healthy people depends heavily on the presence of somatic symptoms, including anorexia, fatigue, insomnia, and weight loss; however, these indicators are of less value as diagnostic criteria for depression in patients with cancer, as they are common to both cancer and depression. In patients with cancer, the diagnosis of depression must depend on psychological (i.e., dysphoric mood, feelings of helplessness and hopelessness, loss of self-esteem, feelings of worthlessness or guilt, anhedonia, and thoughts of death or suicide) not somatic symptoms. Table 40.1 outlines the differential diagnosis of depression.

TABLE 40.1

DIFFERENTIAL DIAGNOSIS OF DEPRESSION

Diagnosis	Features
Major depression	2 wk depressed mood, anhedonia, hopelessness, helplessness, guilt, worthlessness, suicidal ideation, personal history of depression, family history of depression
Mood disorder due to general medical condition	Evidence of direct physiologic effect of general medical condition (e.g., hypothyroidism)
Substance-induced mood disorder	Evidence of mood disturbance developed during intoxication/withdrawal from substance or medication use (e.g., interferon)
Delirium	Disturbance of consciousness, change in cognition, perceptual disturbances
Adjustment disorder with depression	Depressed mood, tearfulness or hopelessness in response to identifiable stressor (e.g., diagnosis of cancer)

Mood Disorder Due to Cancer, Other Medical Conditions, or Substances

When evaluating patients who are depressed, it is imperative to determine whether organic factors underlie the depressive syndrome. A depressive syndrome caused by the direct physiologic effects of cancer is called *mood disorder due to cancer* in the current *DSM-IV* nosology. The key feature of this disorder is a prominent and persistent depressed mood that resembles a major depression. The presence of encephalopathy precludes the diagnosis of mood disorder due to cancer unless depression had been diagnosed before confusional symptoms developed. The patient with a delirium due to cancer may have cognitive

TABLE 40.2

DRUGS ASSOCIATED WITH DEPRESSIVE SYMPTOMS

Generic name	Brand name
Acyclovir	—
Amphetamine-like drugs	—
Anabolic steroids	—
Anticonvulsants	—
Baclofen	Lioresal
Barbiturates	—
Benzodiazepines	—
β-Adrenergic blockers	—
Bromocriptine	Parlodex
Clonidine	Catapres
Cycloserine	Seromycin
Dapsone	—
Digitalis glycosides	—
Diltiazem	Cardizem
Disopyramide	Norprace
Disulfiram	Antabuse
Ethionamide	Trecator-SC
Etretinate	Tegison
HMG-CoA reductase inhibitors	—
Isoniazid INH	—
Isosorbide	Isordil
Isotretinoin	Accutane
Levodopa	Dopar
Mefloquine	Lariam
Methyldopa	Aldomet
Metoclopramide	Reglan
Metrizamide	Amipaque
Metronidazole	Flagyl
Nalidixic acid	Neggram
Narcotics	—
Nifedipine	Procardia
Nonsteroidal anti-inflammatory drugs	—
Norfloxacin	Noroxin
Ofloxacin	Floxin
Phenylephrine	NeoSynephrine
Procaine derivatives	—
Reserpine	Serpasil
Sulfonamides	—
Thiaziades	—
Thyroid hormones	—
Trimethoprim-sulfamethoxazole	Bactrim

HMG-CoA, hydroxy-3-methylglutaryl/coenzyme A reductase inhibitors.
Adapted from Craig TJ, Abeloff MD. Psychiatric symptomatology among hospitalized cancer patients. *Am J Psychiatry* 1974;131:1323.

deficits, such as disorientation, poor memory or decreased concentration, fluctuating level of consciousness, and altered perceptions, including hallucinations and delusions. Tumor involvement of the central nervous system, metabolic disturbances (i.e., hypothyroidism, hyperparathyroidism, adrenal insufficiency, folate and B$_{12}$ deficiencies), and the presumed organic processes associated with carcinoma of the pancreas may be contributing factors to the mood disorder.

DSM-IV defines disturbances in mood due to the direct physiologic effects of a substance (i.e., a drug of abuse or a medication) as a *substance-induced mood disorder*. This diagnosis would be appropriate when depression is related to drug therapies (Table 40.2), including anticancer drugs (Table 40.3). There are several reports of exogenously administered cytokines, such as interferon-α and interleukin-2 causing depression. These cytokine therapies have been shown to be associated with significant depressive symptoms in 30–50% of patients (13).

The evaluation of every patient who is depressed and has cancer should include a consideration of medical, endocrinologic, and neurologic problems in addition to screening for depressive symptoms. Many clinicians prefer to use an easily reproducible instrument [e.g., the Mini-Mental State Examination (MMSE)] (14) to document elements of the patient's mental status at the time of the initial evaluation and subsequent evaluations. All such brief instruments have limitations because they assess only selected aspects of cognition. The MMSE can easily and quickly be administered at the bedside and detects impairments in cognition (e.g., orientation, memory, concentration, language, and comprehension). It provides a numerical score out of 30, while accounting for educational level. A change in cognition, especially if acute, should raise suspicion of a nonpsychiatric etiology of concurrent depressive symptoms.

If the depressive disorder is believed to be caused by a medical condition or by a drug, the clinician should first attempt to treat the condition or change the drug. Often, antidepressants are started concurrently in an effort to alleviate symptoms or because the clinician anticipates that the depression that complicates the underlying disorder will not be relieved by addressing the medical condition alone. Only when the primary cause of the depression cannot be corrected (e.g., the chemotherapeutic agent must be continued), should the antidepressant therapy be initiated.

Depression with Psychotic Features

Although rare, depression accompanied by delusions, hallucinations, or grossly disorganized behavior is sometimes

TABLE 40.3

ANTICANCER DRUGS ASSOCIATED WITH DEPRESSION

Drug
Corticosteroids
Vinblastine
Vincristine
Vinorelbine
Interferon
Procarbazine
Asparaginase
Tamoxifen
Cyproterone

encountered in patients who are medically ill. In this population, the presence of depressive symptoms (e.g., flat affect, lack of interest in daily activities) coupled with psychotic symptoms more often reflect a delirium, and before the diagnosis of depression with psychotic features is made, the presence of the underlying organic causes of these mental status changes should be explored. When psychotic features are present, an antipsychotic and an antidepressant are usually started concurrently. High-potency typical antipsychotics (e.g., haloperidol) and novel antipsychotics (e.g., olanzapine and risperidone) are usually preferred to treat all forms of psychosis, including those associated with delirium and dementia. High-potency typical neuroleptics and risperidone have the lowest rate of seizures (15).

Depression in the Elderly

Older individuals are at increased risk for depression and suicidal acts, whether physically healthy or not. In addition to the loss of good health, the elderly patient with cancer often has sustained other losses, including physical ability (e.g., vision and hearing loss) and financial stability. Grief after the death of a spouse or friends may be unresolved, and self-esteem may be damaged through retirement or changed social standing. Although the clinical presentation of depression can be similar to that described for younger adult patients, other presentations are more typical of this phase of life. For example, the chief complaint may be cognitive, such as poor memory or concentration. By taking a thorough history and by interviewing relatives or friends to document the patient's history, the clinician learns that depressive features may antedate the cognitive complaints. When asked specific questions, the patient often says "I don't know" instead of attempting to answer. Objective testing (e.g., with the MMSE) often reveals better results than those expected on the basis of subjective complaints. This constellation is typical of the clinical syndrome *depressive pseudodementia* and often responds well to treatment with antidepressants.

Suicide

Suicidal ideation requires careful assessment to determine whether the patient has a depressive illness or is expressing a wish to have ultimate control over intolerable symptoms. Thoughtful clinical judgment is required to make this differentiation, especially in the patient with advanced disease. Factors that place a patient with cancer at risk for suicide (Table 40.4) include poor prognosis and advanced illness, depression and hopelessness, uncontrolled pain, delirium, history of poor impulse control or psychiatric illness, previous suicide attempts or family history of suicide, history of recent death of friends or spouse, current or previous alcohol or substance abuse, physical and emotional exhaustion, and social isolation. Other risk factors include male gender; advanced age (sixth and seventh decades), and the presence of fatigue.

Although few patients with cancer commit suicide, they may be at somewhat greater risk than the general population (16). Factors such as poor prognosis, delirium, uncontrolled pain, depression, and hopelessness often occur in a patient with advanced disease, increasing the risk of suicide. Hopelessness is an even stronger predictive factor than depression itself (17). Studies exploring the desire for early deaths have found that 1.4–17% of terminally ill patients with cancer who wish to have their lives end naturally or by suicide or euthanasia. Figures range depending on the assessment tools used and populations studied (18).

TABLE 40.4

SUICIDE RISK FACTORS IN PATIENTS WITH CANCER

Related to mental status
  Suicidal ideation
  Lethal plans
  Depression and hopelessness
  Delirium and disinhibition
  Psychotic features
  Loss of control and impulsivity
  Irrational thinking
Related to cancer
  Uncontrolled pain
  Advanced disease and poor prognosis
  Exhaustion and fatigue
  Site of cancer (oropharyngeal, lung, gastrointestinal, genitourinary, breast)
  Medication effects (steroids)
Related to history
  Previous suicide attempts
  Psychopathology
  Substance abuse (alcohol)
  Recent loss (spouse or friends)
  Poor social support
  Older male
  Family history of suicide

The management of the patient with cancer and suicidal tendencies includes maintaining a supportive therapeutic relationship; conveying the attitude that much can be done to improve the quality, if not the quantity, of life even if the prognosis is poor; and actively eliciting and treating specific symptoms (e.g., pain, nausea, insomnia, anxiety, fatigue, and depression). The most useful psychotherapeutic modalities are based on a crisis intervention model using cognitive techniques (e.g., giving back a sense of control by helping the patient to focus on that which can still be controlled) and supportive methods, sometimes involving family and friends. One should keep in mind that the partner and other family members are also at increased risk for suicide and that they also often require evaluation and support.

When considering the need to hospitalize a patient with suicidal tendencies, evaluation of the risk factors (Table 40.4), including the presence of a plan and its lethality, and associated intent, ensues. If the patient with suicidal tendencies does not have any physiologic factors contributing to their psychiatric presentation, admitting the patient to a psychiatric unit may be indicated. However, during the palliative phase, when patients are too ill to be psychiatrically hospitalized, they may be admitted to oncology wards, where a 24-hour companion can be provided. Companions can provide constant observation, monitor the suicidal risk, and reassure the patient. Need for observation is evaluated daily; companions are discontinued when the patient is no longer suicidal and is judged to be in control and able to act rationally. Similarly, companions or nurses can be provided in hospice settings as well as in the home to ensure patient safety.

TREATMENT OF DEPRESSION

Before planning an intervention, the patient should be evaluated for a history of depressive episodes and substance abuse; family psychiatric history, including depression and suicide; concurrent life stresses; losses secondary to cancer (e.g., financial, social, and occupational) and the availability of social support. An assessment of the patient's personal experience with cancer deaths, of the meaning of illness, and of the patient's understanding of the medical situation (including prognosis) is essential. Patients with cancer who are depressed are usually treated with a combination of supportive psychotherapy and antidepressants; electroconvulsive therapy (ECT) is used less often.

Psychological Treatment

Evidence from meta-analyses has shown that psychologic treatments effectively treat anxiety and depression in patients with cancer (19–21). The goals of psychotherapy are to reduce emotional distress and to improve morale, coping ability, self-esteem, sense of control, and resolve problems. Patients with cancer are often referred for, or request for, psychiatric consultation at times of crisis in illness—at the time of initial diagnosis or recurrence, at the beginning of any new treatment, when standard or experimental treatments fail, or when patients perceive themselves as dying. The referral is often an emergency and, because of the acute crisis, the patient often readily accepts an intervention.

Psychotherapy may be delivered to the patient individually, in a group setting or in sessions with their partner and/or family. Various models of psychotherapy may be used in the psycho-oncology population (e.g., psychoeducational, supportive, grief, existential, cognitive behavioral, interpersonal, psychodynamic, life narrative, dignity conserving, and meaning-centered). These models have been reviewed elsewhere (22). A flexible approach, using principles from several different models, allows a personalized treatment plan for the patient. Often, 4–15 sessions are required to treat the acute problem, although studies have shown that a greater effect size occurs in delivering 8 versus 4–7 hours of counseling (20). Patients consider their recent losses (good health, body integrity, self-esteem, family support, presumed longevity, financial security, and opportunity for job satisfaction) in the context of a past history of loss or success, and are helped to chart a future direction that incorporates life and body alterations brought on by the diagnosis of a chronic life-threatening illness.

Psychoeducational interventions that provide patients and family members information about the illness and its treatment can lead to reductions in anxiety and depression. Educational interventions, such as clarifying information and explaining emotional reactions to the patient, family, and staff, are useful.

Cognitive techniques are also useful to help the patient correct misconceptions and exaggerated fears. Patients are encouraged to consider an array of different possible explanations or outcomes for their situation and then to determine which aspects they can still improve. These techniques have been developed specifically for patients with cancer (23). These approaches provide patients with a sense of control over their situation and help the individual to avoid focusing only on the worst eventualities. Behavioral interventions include relaxation training through progressive muscular relaxation, guided imagery, massage, hypnosis or meditation together with activity scheduling, exposure, and systematic desensitization.

Emotional support is also provided. Listening to the patient carefully and allowing the patient to express feelings, fears, and anger in a nonjudgmental setting is often therapeutic. Legitimization of the difficulty of the situation and of the right to be upset reduces the fear of being perceived as weak or inappropriate. Reassurances should be realistic and consistent with the available knowledge of the situation. The desire of patients to maintain hope is, of course, respected, as are the defense mechanisms of denial, repression, and regression, as long as these do not interfere with diagnostic or therapeutic

processes or with important personal matters that must be addressed. As the patient's history of loss is explored, the clinician identifies and reinforces the patient's successful ways of coping. At the termination of psychotherapy, patients are reassured to hear that the clinician is available for future visits if symptoms recur or if the disease worsens (1). Supportive–expressive group therapy (SEGT) has proved to improve anxiety and depression in randomized controlled trials in patients with advanced cancer (24).

Another important aspect of the treatment of the patient with cancer who is depressed is social support provided by family, friends, and community or religious groups. Although family is enlisted to provide emotional support, family members must be encouraged to minimize family conflicts, which are an additional emotional burden and can be addressed more appropriately after the patient's depression has resolved. This process may also identify vulnerable family members who cannot provide emotional support and indeed may also need psychosocial help. These family members are encouraged to seek individual or group support for themselves. Often, this may only occur after their loved one is deceased and supporting family members with a grief therapy model, either individually or in a group, may be helpful.

As a patient enters the terminal phase of their illness, the focus will shift to existential, spiritual, and relationship themes. At this time, implementing themes from dignity conserving and meaning-centered psychotherapies, both developed from an existential model, are useful (25).

Drug Therapies

Antidepressants

Although there are many reports of the efficacy of antidepressants in depressed patients with cancer, there are few randomized placebo-controlled trials. This observation reflects the difficulty in conducting controlled studies of drugs in medically ill patients with cancer. Nonetheless, there is much clinical experience with antidepressant drugs in this population. A specific antidepressant is often chosen on the basis of its side effect profile. The antidepressant agents that are better tolerated in patients with comorbid depression and medical conditions are the newer agents, including selective serotonin reuptake inhibitors (SSRIs) and the novel or mixed action antidepressants. Tricyclic antidepressants (TCAs), psychostimulants, mood stabilizers such as lithium carbonate and the monoamine oxidase inhibitors (MAOIs) are used for selected patients (Table 40.5).

Selective serotonin reuptake inhibitors. The SSRIs (fluoxetine, sertraline, paroxetine, fluvoxamine, citalopram and escitalopram) and novel antidepressants are considered first-line treatment because they are better tolerated, have fewer sedative and autonomic effects, and have a safe cardiac profile. The most common side effects are nausea, headache, somnolence or insomnia, sexual dysfunction and a brief period of increased anxiety. These drugs can cause appetite suppression that usually lasts a period of several weeks, but the anorectic properties of these drugs are not a limiting factor in this population. All SSRIs are equally efficacious, with depressive symptoms improving after 2 to 4 weeks of a therapeutic dose (Table 40.5 for recommended dosing). Although the SSRIs share a similar side effect profile, there are some clinically relevant differences. Fluoxetine, for example, has the longest half-life (5 weeks), resulting in little if any risk of SSRI discontinuation syndrome with abrupt withdrawal. Due to the relative short half-life (24 hours) of the other SSRIs, patients are at risk of developing significant psychiatric, neurologic, gastrointestinal or flu-like symptoms after abrupt withdrawal. Paroxetine leads to the most anticholinergic side effects of

TABLE 40.5

ANTIDEPRESSANT MEDICATIONS USED IN PATIENTS WITH CANCER

Drug	Starting daily dosage, mg (p.o.)	Therapeutic daily dosage, mg (p.o.)	Comments
Newer agents			
Serotonin reuptake inhibitors			
Fluoxetine	5–10	20–60	Stimulating; long half-life
Sertraline	25	50–200	Relatively few drug interactions
Paroxetine	5–10	10–60	More anticholinergic side effects, more weight gain
Escitalopram	5–10	10–20	Relatively few drug interactions
Citalopram	10	10–60	Relatively few drug interactions
Fluvoxamine	25	50–300	More sedating, more drug interactions
Others			
Trazodone	25–50	150–300	Sedating, orthostatic hypotension, rare priapism
Bupropion	75–100	150–450	Stimulating, risk for seizures, minimal effect on weight and sexual functioning; useful for smoking cessation
Venlafaxine	18.75–37.5	75–300	Treats neuropathic pain; causes elevated blood pressure at higher doses
Mirtazapine	15	15–45	Sedating, anxiolytic, antiemetic, appetite stimulating; available in orally disintegrating tablet
Duloxetine	20	40–60	Treats diabetic neuropathy, pain syndromes
Tricyclic antidepressants			
Amitriptyline	10–25	50–150	
Imipramine	10–25	50–200	
Desipramine	10–25	50–150	Least sedating tricyclic antidepressant
Nortriptyline	10–25	50–150	Least anticholinergic tricyclic antidepressant; blood levels must be checked
Psychostimulants			
Dextroamphetamine	2.5 at 8 a.m. and noon	5–60	Insomnia, anxiety, tremor, tachycardia, hypertension, seizures, confusion, delirium
Methylphenidate	2.5 at 8 a.m. and noon	5–60	Insomnia, anxiety, tremors, tachycardia, hypertension, seizures, confusion, delirium
Modafinil	50–100 a.m.	100–400	Similar side effects as other stimulants, but less frequent; better tolerated than other stimulants; more costly

the SSRIs and causes the most weight gain. Fluvoxamine and paroxetine are more sedating, whereas fluoxetine is the most stimulating; the former are often chosen for patients who are highly anxious, although the latter is used for patients suffering from anergic depression. Sertraline, citalopram and escitalopram have fewer drug interactions, whereas fluvoxamine has the most and this feature often limits its use. Musselman et al. have demonstrated that paroxetine, started at the time interferon-α is started, reduces the incidence of depression (26). Additionally, citalopram, sertraline, fluoxetine, and mirtazapine have been shown to treat interferon-α induced depression in clinical trails (27,28). However, many of the patients in these trials had hepatitis C, rather than cancer, as their primary medical diagnosis.

Novel and mixed action antidepressants. The novel and mixed action antidepressants (venlafaxine, duloxetine, bupropion, trazodone, and mirtazapine) differ from the SSRIs in their mechanism of action, resulting in their different side effect profiles. Venlafaxine and duloxetine are serotonin/norepinephrine uptake inhibitors, with venlafaxine inhibiting serotonin reuptake at lower doses, thereby sharing some of the side effects of the SSRIs, while inhibiting norepinephrine reuptake at higher doses. At higher doses, usually greater than 225 mg daily,

venlafaxine may contribute to hypertension. Both duloxetine and venlafaxine have been shown to improve neuropathic pain.

Bupropion is primarily a noradrenergic agent that increases dopamine reuptake at higher doses. Its stimulating effects may be beneficial to the patient with cancer who is depressed and fatigued. Bupropion has fewer gastrointestinal side effects than the SSRIs, and tends to cause constipation more frequently than nausea, vomiting, or diarrhea. It increases the risk of seizures at higher doses and should be used in caution with patients with seizure disorders or organic brain pathology. Furthermore, it may assist in smoking cessation and has minimal effect on weight or sexual functioning. Although rare, it may contribute to confusion or psychotic symptoms in a patient who is delirious due to its effect on dopamine.

Trazodone may be used for its sedating properties and in low doses (50–100 mg at bedtime) is helpful in the treatment of the depressed cancer patient with insomnia. Trazodone has been associated with priapism and therefore should be used with caution in men. Mirtazapine is a noradrenergic and specific serotonergic antidepressant. It has low affinity for muscarinic, cholinergic, and dopaminergic receptors, but a high affinity for H_1 histaminic receptors. It antagonizes

$5HT_2$ and $5HT_3$ receptors, resulting in increased serotonin release through $5HT_1$. It is through these mechanisms that the common features of sedation, anxiolysis, appetite stimulation, and antiemesis occur. Because it can cause weight gain, it may be advantageous for patients with anorectic-cachectic cancer but is not a good choice for those who are gaining weight from steroids or chemotherapy. It is, therefore, an appropriate and useful antidepressant in the psychooncology or palliative care setting. Venlafaxine, trazodone, mirtazapine, trazodone, and SSRIs are useful in managing hot flashes (29,30).

Tricyclic antidepressants. TCAs antagonize muscarinic, cholinergic, H_1-histaminic, and α-1-adrenergic receptors, contributing to the side effects of confusion, dry mouth, constipation, urinary retention, sedation, weight gain, and orthostatic hypotension. TCAs are still used in the oncology setting for both adults and children with cancer, especially when comorbid neuropathic pain is present. Dosing is typically initiated at 10–25 mg at bedtime, especially in debilitated patients, and the dose is increased by 25 mg every 1–2 days until beneficial effect is achieved.

The choice of TCA depends on the nature of the depressive symptoms, medical status, and side effects of the specific drug. The patient who is depressed is agitated and has insomnia benefits from the use of a TCA that has a sedating effect, such as amitriptyline or doxepin. Patients with psychomotor slowing benefit from use of the compounds with the least sedating effect, such as nortriptyline or desipramine. The patient who has stomatitis secondary to chemotherapy or radiotherapy, or who has slow intestinal motility or urinary retention, should not receive a TCA.

Patients who are unable to swallow pills may be able to take an antidepressant in an elixir, intramuscular form or rectal suppository form. Robinson and Owen have comprehensively reviewed alternative routes of administration in medically ill and surgical patients (15).

Imipramine, doxepin, amitriptyline, desipramine, and nortriptyline are used frequently in the management of neuropathic pain in patients with cancer. Dosing is similar to that in the treatment of depression. Analgesic efficacy, if it occurs, is usually observed at a dose of 50–150 mg daily; higher doses occasionally are needed. Although the initial assumption was that analgesic effect resulted indirectly from the effect on depression, it is now clear that these tricyclics have a separate specific analgesic action, which is probably mediated through several neurotransmitters.

Elderly and children. When treating depression in the elderly, medications are started at a low dose, and the dosage is increased more slowly than with a younger adult patient. Also, drugs with few anticholinergic effects are preferred due to greater sensitivity of the elderly to anticholinergic complications (e.g., delirium, urinary retention, and cardiac arrhythmias).

There are no controlled studies to support the efficacy of antidepressants in medically ill children with depression. Nevertheless, clinicians often find it helpful to prescribe antidepressants to treat depression. However, due to recent "black box" warnings associating SSRIs with suicidal thinking in children and adolescents, close monitoring is essential. As in the elderly, these drugs are started at a low dose (31).

Lithium carbonate. Patients who have been receiving lithium for bipolar affective disorder before cancer should be maintained on it throughout cancer treatment, although close monitoring is necessary when the intake of fluids and electrolytes is restricted, such as during the preoperative and postoperative periods. The maintenance dose of lithium may need reduction in seriously ill patients. Lithium should be prescribed with caution in patients receiving cisplatin due to potential nephrotoxicity of both drugs. Lithium may also be used as prophylaxis for corticosteroid-induced mood disorder (32), although antipsychotics such as haloperidol, olanzapine, and risperidone are also frequently used.

Monoamine oxidase inhibitors. If a patient has responded well to an MAOI for depression before treatment for cancer, its continued use is warranted. Most psychiatrists, however, are reluctant to start patients with cancer who are depressed on MAOIs because the need for dietary restriction is poorly received by patients who already have dietary limitations and nutritional deficiencies secondary to cancer illness and treatment. Medication interactions (e.g., meperidine) and associated risk of hypertensive crisis and death significantly limit their use.

Psychostimulants. In patients with cancer, the psychostimulants (i.e., dextroamphetamine, methylphenidate, and modafinil) promote a sense of well-being, decrease fatigue, improve concentration and attention, and stimulate appetite. An advantage of these drugs is their rapid effectiveness. Psychostimulants can potentiate the analgesic effects of opioid analgesics and are commonly used to counteract opioid-induced sedation. Occasionally they can produce nightmares, agitation, insomnia, and even psychosis. At higher doses, they can cause tachycardia or hypertension. They also may lower the seizure threshold. These side effects occur less commonly with modafinil.

Treatment with dextroamphetamine and methylphenidate is usually initiated at a dose of 2.5 mg at 8 a.m. and noon and modafinil is started at 50 to 100 mg each morning. The dose can be titrated upward, depending on response and tolerability. Patients can be maintained on psychostimulants for long periods (e.g., >1 year) and if tolerance develops, dose adjustments can be made.

Antipsychotics. Antipsychotics are started with antidepressants when patients are experiencing depression with psychotic features, and may be used in patients with preexisting bipolar disorder or anxiety as a symptom of depression. Unlike the benzodiazepines, antipsychotics do not cause respiratory depression or confusion, and are therefore useful in anxious patients with cancer who often have altered mental states. High potency typical antipsychotics (e.g., haloperidol) or atypical antipsychotic medications (e.g., olanzapine and risperidone) are usually preferred because of their low anticholinergic potential, which reduces the risk of delirium and other anticholinergic side effects. These antipsychotics are less sedating and lower the seizure threshold less than low potency antipsychotics (e.g., chlorpromazine) and are preferable when the risk of seizures is a concern. Some patients are unable to take oral medication. The typical antipsychotics, haloperidol, and chlorpromazine are available in intravenous form. Olanzapine is available in a disintegrating wafer and risperidone has a similar formulation. Atypical antipsychotic medications that are used less frequently in the oncology or palliative care settings are quetiapine, ziprasidone and aripiprazole. Quetiapine is a sedating atypical antipsychotic that may also cause orthostatic hypotension. Ziprasidone is available intramuscularly and may prolong QT interval. Aripiprazole causes minimal sedation. These three atypical antipsychotics and risperidone can cause weight gain. Ziprasidone has the lowest risk. Olanzapine can cause considerable weight gain.

Electroconvulsive Therapy

ECT is indicated for patients with cancer who are depressed and have significant contraindications to or are refractory to antidepressants, or have depression with psychotic or suicidal features. Although the use of ECT in patients with brain tumors was once believed to be contraindicated because of the risk of brain herniation, there are numerous case reports describing safe and effective use of ECT in such patients (33).

Complementary and Alternative Medicine

Some 80% of patients with cancer use complementary and alternative medicine (CAM) treatments. Some alternative treatments (acupuncture; relaxation; guided imagery; yoga; meditation; massage; tai chi; biofeedback; music, art, movement, and aroma therapies) are offered as adjuncts to traditional cancer care aimed at improving quality of life and decreasing symptoms of anxiety and depression, with no promise of cure. Other therapies such as shark cartilage, colonics, herbal remedies, and high-dose vitamin therapies do not improve quality of life and may be harmful. Some remedies are highly toxic (34).

The Memorial Sloan-Kettering Cancer Center has a Web site (http://www.mskcc.org/aboutherbs) on which it provides unbiased scientific reviews about potential drug interactions and adverse effects of some 135 herbal and botanical agents relevant to patients with cancer (35).

PREVALENCE OF ANXIETY IN PATIENTS WITH CANCER

Cancer disrupts the social roles of patients, their interpersonal relationships, and the ways in which they view their future; most people who have cancer are both fearful and sad. In a recent cross-sectional observational study of 178 patients with cancer, almost half had significant anxiety, but the rate of anxiety disorder and its subtypes was 18%, comparable to that in the general population (36).

Most studies of psychiatric symptoms in patients with cancer have reported a higher prevalence of mixed anxiety and depressive symptoms than anxiety alone. Correlations between measures of depression and anxiety on both clinician-rated (36) and self-report measures (37) are high. In all likelihood, this observation indicates that these measures tap a common psychological trait: negative affect (37).

Anxiety increases with the diagnosis of cancer, peaks before surgical interventions, and frequently remains high thereafter, declining gradually during the first postoperative years. Anxiety increases as cancer progresses, and psychological health declines along with the decline in physical status. Chemotherapy administration is a source of anxiety that may develop into a conditioned anticipatory response, which may persist for years after the cessation of the chemotherapy. Radiotherapy treatment is also associated with increased anxiety, accompanied by concerns about increased body vulnerability and worries about whether the radiation will cause further damage. The anxiety experienced during chemotherapy and radiation therapy may paradoxically increase at the termination of treatment, as patients feel unprotected, see their physician(s) less often, and worry about the effectiveness of treatment. Patients who are participating in clinical trials and feel that they have been randomized to a less aggressive treatment modality may also experience increased anxiety.

DIAGNOSIS OF ANXIETY IN PATIENTS WITH CANCER

A small percentage of patients with cancer have anxiety disorders that antedate the diagnosis of cancer and are exacerbated by the stress associated with cancer diagnosis or treatment. For most patients, anxiety symptoms are reactions to cancer and its treatment and are associated with feelings of foreboding, apprehension, or dread. Although anxiety symptoms can be either cognitive or somatic, the most salient symptoms are usually somatic and include tachycardia, shortness of breath, sweating, abdominal distress, and nausea. Loss of appetite, diminished libido, and insomnia, symptoms also associated with depression, are common in patients with anxiety, as are feelings of hyperarousal and irritability. In patients with panic attacks, symptoms related to increased autonomic discharge increase dramatically.

In addition to somatic symptoms, the anxious patient with cancer is often plagued by recurrent unpleasant thoughts about cancer, including fears of death, disfigurement, disability, and dependency. The thinking style of the anxious patient is characterized by overgeneralization and catastrophizing; negative outcomes seem inevitable, and patients view themselves as helpless in a hopeless situation. Anxious patients may see their environment as threatening and are often motivated to flee, a reaction that commonly precipitates treatment refusals or demands for premature hospital discharge.

Table 40.6 outlines the differential diagnosis of anxiety.

TABLE 40.6

DIFFERENTIAL DIAGNOSIS OF ANXIETY

Diagnosis	Features
Anxiety disorder due to general medical condition	Evidence of direct physiologic effect of general medical condition causing anxious symptoms (e.g., hyperthyroidism)
Substance-induced anxiety disorder	Evidence anxiety develop during substance intoxication/withdrawal from substance or medication use (e.g., dexamethasone)
Delirium	Disturbance of consciousness, change in cognition, perceptual disturbances
Adjustment disorder with anxiety	Nervousness, worry, jitteriness in response to identifiable stressor (e.g., learning of cancer recurrence)
Major depression	2 wk depressed mood, anhedonia, hopelessness, helplessness, guilt, worthlessness, suicidal ideation, family history of depression, personal history of depression
Anxiety disorders	
■ Post-traumatic stress disorder	Reexperiencing trauma, avoidance/numbing, increased arousal
■ Generalized anxiety disorder	Excessive worry about many things
■ Panic disorder	Panic attacks ± agoraphobia
■ Specific phobia	Fear of specific object or situation (e.g., claustrophobia in magnetic resonance imaging)
■ Obsessive compulsive disorder	Obsessions and compulsions

Phobias, Panic Disorder, Generalized Anxiety Disorder, and Post-traumatic Stress Disorder

Phobias, panic disorder, post-traumatic stress disorder (PTSD), and generalized anxiety disorder may antedate the diagnosis of cancer or first appear as patients are diagnosed and undergo cancer treatment. Because they cause extreme distress and have the potential to interfere with adequate medical management, it is important to accurately diagnose and treat these anxiety disorders.

There is a range of phobias that can be exacerbated by exposure to the medical environment—phobias about needles, blood, hospitals, and doctors are common. The common characteristic of all phobias is extreme anxiety on exposure to a feared object(s) or situation(s), and a persistent anxiety in the anticipation of these situations. Agoraphobia (the most common phobia in the general population) and claustrophobia may appear de novo in patients who are confined in the frightening hospital environment without their usual environmental supports. Patients who require magnetic resonance imaging or radiation therapy, or who must be confined in intensive care or reverse-isolation settings, frequently experience increased anxiety (38).

Panic disorder can present in the context of a cancer diagnosis. In contrast to phobias, in which there is a clearly defined situation or object of dread, panic disorder often presents as sudden, unpredictable episodes of intense discomfort and fear, accompanied by shortness of breath, diaphoresis, tachycardia, feelings of choking or being smothered, and thoughts of impending doom. Symptoms of a preexisting panic disorder may intensify during cancer treatment; severe untreated symptoms may result in abrupt termination of cancer treatment. In contrast to panic disorder, generalized anxiety disorder is characterized by continuous and pervasive worry, difficulty in controlling the worry or apprehension, and the presence of symptoms of autonomic hyperactivity and hypervigilance.

In addition to heightened psychological distress associated with cancer treatment, some patients with cancer may experience the symptoms characteristic of PTSD after the completion of treatment. Younger age, less education, and lower income are associated with more PTSD symptoms as well as more advanced disease and lengthier hospitalizations (39).

Anxiety Disorder Due to Cancer, Other Medical Conditions, or Substances

Anxiety in patients with cancer may be caused or exacerbated by medications used to treat cancer or other conditions, abnormal metabolic states, or uncontrolled pain. Physical symptoms associated with specific cancers (such as dyspnea in patients with primary or secondary cancer in the lung) can also cause significant anxiety. Anxiety may also be conditioned by events related to chemotherapy or radiation therapy. The DSM-IV (3) has included the diagnostic categories of anxiety disorder due to a medical condition (e.g., cancer) and substance-induced anxiety disorder.

Some drugs, such as the corticosteroids, can produce anxiety, and others (e.g., antipsychotics) can cause restlessness and agitation that is described as anxiety by the patient. Akathisia produced by antipsychotics, including dopamine blocking antiemetics (e.g., metoclopramide and prochlorperazine), is frequently misdiagnosed as anxiety or agitation. Drug intoxication (e.g., cocaine) and withdrawal symptoms (e.g., from alcohol, benzodiazepines, or opioids) also have anxiety as a common symptom. Bronchodilators, β-adrenergic drugs, and psychostimulants (including caffeine) can cause anxiety, irritability, and tremulousness. Thyroid replacement medication can produce symptoms of anxiety, especially when the dosage is being adjusted (40).

Metabolic disturbances such as hypoglycemia, hypoxia, and undetected anemia may be manifested by symptoms of anxiety, restlessness, and agitation, followed by confusion and disorientation. Encephalopathy associated with systemic infection and the remote effects of specific tumors (pancreatic, thyroid, pheochromocytoma, and parathyroid) may also result in high levels of anxiety. Some patients with central nervous system neoplasms report anxiety as a prominent symptom.

Chemotherapy and radiation therapy can be associated with increased anxiety. Repeated exposures to highly emetogenic chemotherapeutic agents may lead to the development of anticipatory nausea and vomiting (ANV), a conditioned response to environmental cues (e.g., the sight of the hospital or the smell of the alcohol swabs) that surround the chemotherapy experience. ANV may be linked to a preexisting anxiety diathesis and may persist for years after the cessation of chemotherapy. Patients undergoing radiation therapy may experience a level of apprehension and anxiety that may persist as treatment progresses. Worsening side effects and the fear associated with the cessation of treatment may perpetuate the anxiety. The psychological distress associated with radiation therapy may exceed the physical distress resulting from the treatment itself.

Anxiety as a Manifestation of Other Psychiatric Disorders

In the medically ill, anxiety may be a manifestation of either depression or delirium. Increasingly, depression and anxiety are viewed as syndromes existing on a continuum; there is an overlap in the symptomatology between these two mood states. Depression may be distinguished from anxiety by the presence of the psychological symptoms such as hopelessness, anhedonia, worthlessness, and suicidal ideation. Delirium frequently has anxiety or restlessness as a prominent feature but is distinguished from anxiety by the presence of disorientation, impaired memory and concentration, fluctuating level of consciousness, and altered perceptions, including hallucinations and delusions.

TREATMENT OF ANXIETY

The most effective management of anxiety in patients with cancer is multimodal, including psychotherapy, behavioral therapy, and pharmacologic management. During the initial evaluation of the patient's symptoms, both emotional support and information are given to the patient. Exploration of the patient's fears and apprehensions about disease progression, upcoming procedures, or psychosocial concerns often alleviates a substantial degree of the anxiety. Patient concerns usually include death, physical suffering, increased dependence, loss of dignity, changes in social role functioning, spiritual matters, and worry about finances or employment.

Psychological Treatment

Relatively short-term psychological interventions have proved to be effective in reducing the distress associated with cancer (41). The efficacy of psychological treatments without the use of drugs depends on the duration and severity of the patient's anxiety. In the case of mild to moderate anxiety, the use of psychological techniques alone may be sufficient. In addition to effectively treating distress in patients presenting with anxiety, a meta-analysis of psychological interventions suggests that these interventions, such as cognitive-behavioral techniques, can effectively prophylax against the development of anxiety in patients diagnosed with cancer (19).

Careful patient selection is important for the success of psychological approaches. Patients with cancer most likely to benefit from psychological interventions are those who have anxiety that has not been controlled by other means, have a need for self-control and are reluctant to take medication, and have experienced or acknowledge the efficacy of such approaches. Individuals who are poor candidates for psychological approaches are those who have delirium or dementia, are disinterested or demonstrate noncompliance in learning to use psychological techniques, and have a history of serious psychiatric illness.

In general, the most effective treatment programs for anxiety include a variety of supportive, behavioral, cognitive-behavioral, and psychoeducational techniques, delivered individually or in a group setting.

Psychoeducational interventions are particularly useful for anxious patients with cancer who have difficulty understanding information about their prognosis, planned procedures or treatments. Providing information about predictable side effects as patients begin surgical, chemotherapeutic, or radiotherapeutic interventions, helps to normalize the experience and reduce anxiety. Similarly, explaining the predictable emotional phases associated with cancer may alleviate anxiety. Providing information to a patient's family can improve the coping of family members, which in turn enhances the patient's sense of support.

The rationale for the use of behavioral techniques, including relaxation training, guided imagery, or hypnotherapy, is the substitution of more adaptive behavior (e.g., increased coping ability) for less adaptive behavior (e.g., anxiety). Progressive relaxation involves instructing the patient to sequentially relax parts of the body through either tensing and relaxing the muscle groups (active muscle relaxation) or through concentrating on relaxing parts of the body without tensing the muscles (passive muscle relaxation). Both approaches are effective in reducing anxiety, although in medically debilitated patients passive relaxation may be more manageable. Hypnosis can be effective in the management of psychological distress associated with procedures and in the management of treatment-related side effects such as ANV and pain. Desensitization, response prevention, thought stopping, modeling, and distraction are other behavioral techniques that may be useful in the management of anxiety and phobias.

Behavioral techniques are effective in the treatment of ANV. As noted previously, ANV appears to be correlated with preexisting trait anxiety and with state anxiety at the time of chemotherapy infusions (42). Progressive muscle relaxation helps to decrease nausea and vomiting, as well as anxiety, in patients who are receiving emetogenic chemotherapy. An approach to ANV that combines behavioral approaches and a cognitive approach in which the patient's thoughts and feelings about chemotherapy are explored and modified may be most effective (23).

Individual psychotherapy, including cognitive-behavioral approaches, can be effective in the treatment of cancer-related anxiety (43). According to the cognitive-behavioral model, emotional distress arises or continues because of maladaptive beliefs and thinking patterns. Patients are encouraged to identify these maladaptive thoughts, reconsider them more logically, and experiment with alternative viewpoints and behaviors that give them greater control over their situation. Adjuvant psychological therapy is a structured cognitive-behavioral intervention that teaches patients to identify negative thoughts; to rehearse impending stressful events and implement ways of handling them more effectively; to plan and carry out practical activities that create a sense of mastery; and to express feelings openly to one's partner. Self-esteem is increased as patients identify personal strengths.

Group interventions have also been shown to reduce psychologic distress in patients with cancer (43). These interventions have benefited patients in all stages of cancer and with a variety of cancer diagnoses. In one study, patients who participated in support groups for at least a year reported less tension than did controls (44). The techniques employed in these groups included fostering a sense of supportive commonality among the members, education, emotional support, stress management, coping strategies, and behavioral training.

Pharmacologic Treatment

Although a significant percentage of patients with advanced cancer receive antianxiety drugs, the severity of symptoms is the most useful guide in deciding whether a pharmacological approach to the management of anxiety should be tried. Patients with mild reactive anxiety may benefit from either supportive measures or behavioral measures alone.

For patients who experience persistent apprehension and anxiety, the first-line drugs are the benzodiazepines (Table 40.7). Lorazepam (0.5–2 mg three times daily) and alprazolam (0.25–1 mg three times daily) are useful for anxiety, nausea, and panic. Both lorazepam and alprazolam have been shown in controlled trials to reduce postchemotherapy nausea and vomiting, as well as ANV (45). Benzodiazepines have amnestic properties; when given before chemotherapy or a procedure, this effect may reduce the likelihood of a conditioned aversion developing. A longer-acting benzodiazepine, such as clonazepam (0.5–1.0 mg twice daily), may provide more consistent relief of anxiety symptoms and have mood-stabilizing effects as well. The short- to medium-acting benzodiazepines as well as the nonbenzodiazepine hypnotics (zolpidem 10–20 mg qhs, zaleplon 10 mg qhs, or zopiclone) may be effective for insomnia. Low dose antipsychotics such as haloperidol (0.5–1 mg qhs), olanzapine (2.5–5.0 mg qhs) or risperidone (0.5–2 mg qhs) may be more effective for the patient who is both anxious and confused. For patients with compromised hepatic function, the use of shorter-acting benzodiazepines, such as lorazepam, oxazepam, and temazepam, is preferred. These drugs are metabolized by conjugation with glucuronic acid and have no active metabolites.

Drowsiness and somnolence are the most common adverse effects of benzodiazepines. Reductions in dose and the passage of time eliminate these effects. Mental status changes, such as impaired concentration, memory, or delirium, may result from benzodiazepine usage and are more common in elderly patients, those with advanced disease, and those with impaired hepatic function.

Structurally different from other anxiolytics, buspirone (5–20 mg t.i.d.) is useful for patients with generalized anxiety disorder as well as those in whom there is the potential for benzodiazepine abuse. Buspirone is not effective on an as-needed basis: its effects are not apparent for 1–2 weeks. Additionally, patients who have been prescribed benzodiazepines in the past may find that buspirone does not alleviate their anxiety as effectively as benzodiazepines.

For the treatment of panic disorder and agoraphobia, benzodiazepines, and antidepressant medications (TCAs, SSRIs, and MAOIs) have demonstrated effectiveness. Although alprazolam rapidly blocks panic attacks, withdrawal can be difficult after prolonged use. Although MAOIs are effective in the management of panic disorder and depression, the risk of hypertensive crisis from concomitant ingestion of drugs (e.g., opioids) or tyramine-containing foods make these medications less desirable for patients with cancer.

TABLE 40.7

ANTIANXIETY DRUGS USED IN PATIENTS WITH CANCER

Drug	Approximate dose equivalent	Starting daily dose, mg (p.o.)	Comments
Benzodiazepines			
Temazepam	15	15–30 q.h.s.	Short acting
Oxazepam	10	10–15 t.i.d.	Short acting
Alprazolam	0.25	0.25–1.00 t.i.d.	Useful for nausea, short acting
Lorazepam	1	0.5–2.0 t.i.d	Useful for nausea short acting, preferred in hepatic disease
Diazepam	5	2.5–10 b.i.d.	Longer half-life
Clonazepam	0.5	0.25–1.00 b.i.d.	Longer half-life, mood stabilizing
Antihistamines	—	—	—
Hydroxyzine	10	10–50 t.i.d.	Sedating, may cause confusion
Diphenhydramine	25	25–50 t.i.d.	Sedating, may cause confusion
Hydrochloride	—	—	—
Neuroleptics	—	—	—
Chlorpromazine	12.5	25 b.i.d.	Sedating anticholinergic; lowers seizure threshold
Haloperidol	0.5	0.5–2.0 b.i.d.	More EPS, not sedating
Olanzapine	2.5	2.5–10 qhs	Sedating, appetite stimulation, weight gain, ? hyperglycemia
Risperidone	0.5	0.5–2.0 b.i.d.	Not sedating, some EPS >6 mg daily dose
Quetiapine	25	25–100 qhs	Sedating, orthostatic hypotension
Ziprasidone	—	20–80 b.i.d.	QT prolongation, not sedating, no weight gain
Aripiprazole	—	10–20 daily	No sedation, minimal weight gain; some EPS
Other	—	—	—
Buspirone	—	5–10 t.i.d.	May take 2–4 wk to be effective
Zolpidem tartrate	—	10–20 qhs	—
Zaleplon	—	10–20 qhs	Short duration of action
Zopidone	—	2–3 qhs	Unpleasant taste

b.i.d., twice daily; qhs, at bedtime; t.i.d., three times daily.

In anxious patients with severely compromised pulmonary function, the use of benzodiazepines that suppress central respiratory mechanisms may be unsafe. A low dose of an antihistamine (e.g., hydroxyzine, 10–50 mg t.i.d.) can be useful for these individuals. Alternatively, opiates, such as morphine, are used in this setting.

CONCLUSION

Depression and anxiety are common symptoms in palliative care settings. These symptoms warrant evaluation and the use of pharmacological and psychosocial interventions to relieve suffering. Psychological distress should not be regarded as an unavoidable consequence of cancer and other severe, life-threatening illnesses.

References

1. Payne DK, Massie MJ. Anxiety and depression. In: Berger AM, Portenoy RK, Weissman DE, eds. *Principles and practice of palliative care and supportive oncology*, 2nd edn. Philadelphia, PA: Lippincott Williams & Willkins, 2002:577.
2. Massie MJ, Holland JC. Overview of normal reactions and prevalence of psychiatric disorders. In: Holland JC, Rowland JH, eds. *Handbook of psychooncology: psychological care of the patient with cancer*. New York: Oxford University Press, 1989:273.
3. American Psychiatric Association. *Diagnostic and statistical manual of mental disorders*, 4th edn. Washington, DC, 1994.
4. American Psychiatric Association. *Diagnostic and statistical manual of mental disorders*, 3rd edn. Washington, DC, 1980.
5. Derogatis LR, Morrow GR, Fetting J, et al. The prevalence of psychiatric disorders among cancer patients. *JAMA* 1983;249:751.
6. Portenoy RK, Payne DK, Jacobsen PB. Breakthrough pain: characteristics and impact in patients with cancer pain. *Pain* 1999;81:129.
7. Breuera E, Portenoy R, eds. *Cancer pain assessment and management*. New York: Cambridge University Press, 2003.
8. DiMatteo MR, Lepper HS, Croghan TW. Depression is a risk factor for noncompliance with medical treatment: a meta-analysis of the effects of anxiety and depression on patient adherence. *Pain* 2000;24:2101.
9. Trask PC. Assessment of depression in cancer patients. *J Natl Cancer Inst Monogr* 2004;32:80.
10. Massie MJ. Prevalence of depression in patients with cancer. *J Natl Cancer Inst Monogr* 2004;32:57.
11. Kathol R, Mutgi A, Williams J, et al. Diagnosis of major depression according to four sets of criteria. *Am J Psychiatry* 1990;147:1021.
12. Hotopf M, Chidgey J, Addington-Hall J, et al. Depression in advanced disease: a systematic review. *Palliat Med* 2002;16:81.
13. Capuron L, Ravaud A, Miller A, et al. Baseline mood and psychosocial characteristics of patients developing depressive symptoms during interleukin-2 and/or interferon-alpha cancer therapy. *Sci Dir Brain Behav Immun* 2004;18:205–213.
14. Folstein MF, Folstein S, McHugh PR. Mini-mental state: a practical method for grading the cognitive state of patients for the clinician. *J Psychiatr Res* 1975;12:189.
15. Robinson MJ, Owen JA. Psychopharmacology. In: Levenson J, ed. *The American psychiatric publishing textbook of psychosomatic medicine*. Washington, DC: American Psychiatric Press, 2004:871.
16. Breitbart W. Suicide in cancer patients. In: Holland JC, Rowland JH, eds. *Handbook of psychooncology: psychological care of the patient with cancer*. New York: Oxford University Press, 1989:291.
17. Chochinov HM, Wilson KG, Enns M, et al. Depression, hopelessness, and suicidal ideation in the terminally ill. *Psychosomatics* 1998;39:366.
18. Tiernan E, Casey P, O'Boyle C, et al. Relations between desire for early death, depressive symptoms and antidepressant prescribing in terminally ill patients with cancer. *J R Soc Med* 2002;95:386.
19. Sheard T, Maguire P. The effect of psychological interventions on anxiety and depression in cancer patients: results of two meta-analyses. *Br J Cancer* 1999;11:1770.
20. Devine EC, Westlake SK. The effects of psychoeducational care provided to adults with cancer: meta—analysis of 166 studies. *Oncol Nurs Forum* 1995;22:1369.
21. Meyer TS, Mark MM. Effects of psychological interventions with adult cancer patients: a meta—analysis of randomized experiences. *Health Psychol* 1995;14:101.
22. Miller K, Kissane D. In Bruera Ed. Palliative medicine (in press).

23. Moorey S, Greer S. In: Paul G, ed. *Cognitive behavior therapy for people with cancer*, Oxford: Oxford University Press, 2002.

24. Cunningham AJ, et al. A randomized controlled trial of the effects of group psychological therapy on survival in women with metastic breast cancer. *Psychooncology* 1998;7:508.

25. Breitbart W, Gibson C, Poppito S, et al. Psychotherapeutic interventions at the end of life: a focus on meaning and spirituality. *Can J Psychol* 2004;49:366–372.

26. Musselman DL, Lawson DH, Gumnick JF, et al. Paroxetine for the prevention of depression induced by high-dose interferon alfa. *N Engl J Med* 2001; 344.

27. Creed F, Olden KW. Gastrointestinal disorders. In: Levenson, J, ed. *Textbook of psychosomatic medicine*. Washington, DC. The American Psychiatric Publishing, 2004:473.

28. Beratis S, Katrivanou A, Georgiou S, et al. Major depression and risk of depressive symptomatology associated with short-term and low-dose interferon—alpha treatment. *J Psychosom Res* 2005;38:15.

29. Pansini F, Albertazzi P, Bonaccorsi G, et al. Tazodone: a non-hormonal alternative for neurovegetative climacteric symptoms.. *Clin Exp Obstet Gynecol* 1995;22:341.

30. Hoda D, Perez DG, Loprinzi CL. Dilemas in breast disease—hot flashes in breast cancer survivors. *Breast J* 2003;9:431.

31. Rosenstein DL, Pao M, Cai J. Psychopharmacologic management in oncology. In: Abraham J, ed. *Bethesda handbook of clinical oncology*. Philadelphia, PA: Lippincott Williams & Wilkins, 2005:527.

32. Sirois, Francois. Steroid psychosis: a review. *Gen Hosp Psychiatry* 2003; 25:27–33.

33. Patkar AA, Hill KP, Weinstein SP, et al. ECT in the presence of brain tumor and increased intracranial pressure: evaluation and reduction of risk. *JECT* 2000;16:189–197.

34. Markman M. Safety issues in using complementary and alterative medicine. *J Clin Oncol* 2002;20:S39–S41.

35. Mitka M. Website showcases science-based information on herbs, other supplements. *JAMA* 2003;289:829.

36. Stark D, Kiely M, Smith A, et al. Anxiety disorders in cancer patients: their nature, associations, and relation to quality of life. *J Clin Oncol* 2002;20(14):3137–3148.

37. Weisman A, Worden J. The emotional impact of recurrent cancer. *J Psychosoc Oncol* 1986;3:5.

38. Munro A, Biruls R, Griffin A, et al. Distress associated with radiotherapy for malignant disease: A quantitative analysis based on patients perceptions. *Br J Cancer* 1989;60:370.

39. Jacobson PB, Widows MR, Hann DM, et al. Posttraumatic stress disorder symptoms after bone marrow transplantation for breast cancer. *Psychosom Med* 1998;62:366–371.

40. Massie MJ, Greenberg D. Oncology. In Levenson J, ed. *APPI textbook of psychosomatic medicine*. Washington, DC: American Psychiatric Press, 2004:597.

41. Trijsburg R, Van Knippenbert F, Rijpma W. Effects of psychological treatment on cancer patients: a critical review. *Psychosom Med* 1992;54:489.

42. Andrykowski M. The role of anxiety in the development of anticipatory nausea in cancer chemotherapy: a review and synthesis. *Psychosom Med* 1990;52:458.

43. Fawzy F, Fawzy N, Arndt L, et al. Critical review of psychosocial interventions in cancer care. *Arch Gen Psychiatry* 1995;52:100.

44. Spiegel D, Bloom J, Yalom I. Group support for patients with metastatic cancer. *Arch Gen Psychiatry* 1981;38:527.

45. Greenberg D, Surman O, Clarke J, et al. Alprazolam for phobic nausea and vomiting related to cancer chemotherapy. *Cancer Treat Rep* 1987;71: 549.

CHAPTER 41 ■ SUBSTANCE ABUSE ISSUES IN PALLIATIVE CARE

STEVEN D. PASSIK, MEGAN OLDEN, KENNETH L. KIRSH, AND RUSSELL K. PORTENOY

INTRODUCTION

Chemical dependency in patients at the end of life raises complex clinical challenges. Particularly alarming is the sharp increase in controlled prescription drug abuse in the United States in the past decade (1). Physicians and other medical staff need to be continually mindful of the potential for substance abuse and diversion in the palliative care setting. The severity of substance-related problems varies significantly: some patients exhibit minor difficult behaviors, such as escalating drug dosages without informing their physicians or using analgesics to treat symptoms other than those intended. At the other end of the continuum, some patients present to the palliative care team with a known history of, or current substance dependence on, illicit drugs or prescription medications that requires aggressive drug control on the part of the treatment team. Proper identification, assessment, and clinical management of the entire spectrum of substance-related problems are critically important for optimal treatment of patients in palliative care settings.

Clinicians must balance the obligation to be thorough in assessing potential opioid abuse or diversion with the duty to ensure that patients' pain is not undertreated. Regulatory pressures only add to this burden, leading some physicians to believe that they must avoid being duped by those abusing prescription pain medications at all costs. Although it is tempting to reduce the clinical implications of patient behavior to dichotomous labels of "addiction" or "not addiction," this oversimplification is not in the patient's best interests. In fact, pain management can be adapted to address the multiple possibilities that might be behind the problematic behaviors noted in an assessment. Physicians can assert control over prescriptions without necessarily ceasing to prescribe controlled substances entirely. Although these situations invariably defy simple solutions, knowledgeable clinicians can implement strategies to simultaneously address the need for compassionate care and management of problematic drug use.

PREVALENCE

Approximately half the individuals aged 15 to 54 in the United States have used illegal drugs at some point in their lives and an estimated 6–15% have a current or past substance use disorder of some type (2–7). In less than a decade, sharp increases in the rate of controlled prescription drug abuse have been noted, with rates climbing by nearly 94%, from 7.8

million in 1992 to 15.1 million in 2003 (1). As a result of the high prevalence of substance abuse in the US population and the association between drug abuse and life-threatening diseases such as acquired immunodeficiency syndrome (AIDS), cirrhosis, and some types of cancer (8–12), patients with substance abuse–related issues are encountered commonly in palliative care settings. In diverse patient populations with progressive life-threatening diseases, the presence of a current or past drug problem complicates the management of the underlying disease and can undermine palliative treatment. The balance between the therapeutic use of potentially abusable drugs and the abuse of these drugs must be understood to optimize care.

The rapid rise in controlled prescription drug abuse is of particular concern for the palliative care team. When misused, prescription opioids and central nervous system depressants and stimulants can be deadly. In 2002, controlled prescription drugs were implicated in 30% of drug-related emergency-room deaths and in at least 23% of emergency department admissions (1). Contrary to past data suggesting that most controlled prescription drug abusers were regular or experienced users, approximately one third of abusers in 2000 were new users of controlled prescriptions, according to data from the National Center of Addiction and Substance Abuse (1). Between the years 1992 and 2003, there has been a 225% increase in new opioid abusers, a 150% increase in new tranquilizer abusers, a 127% increase in new sedative abusers, and a 171% increase in new stimulant abusers (1). Particular regions of the country, most notably the south and west, have been hardest hit.

The growing rates of abuse of controlled prescription drugs raise questions about the prevalence of substance abuse in patient populations with cancer and how palliative care physicians can best address the needs of their patients. Despite its prevalence in the general population, substance abuse appears to be very uncommon within the tertiary care population with cancer. In a 6-month period in 2005, fewer than 1% of inpatient and outpatient consultations performed by the psychiatry service at Memorial Sloan-Kettering Cancer Center (MSKCC) were requested for substance abuse–related issues and only 3% of patients who were referred to the psychiatry department were subsequently diagnosed with a substance-abuse disorder of any type (13). This prevalence is much lower than the frequency of substance-abuse disorders in society at large, in general medical populations, and in emergency medical departments (2,6,14–16). A 1983 study of the Psychiatric Collaborative Oncology Group, which assessed psychiatric diagnoses in ambulatory patients with cancer from

TABLE 41.1

DSM-IV DIAGNOSTIC CRITERIA FOR SUBSTANCE ABUSE AND SUBSTANCE DEPENDENCE

Criteria for substance abuse[a]

A maladaptive pattern of substance use leading to clinically significant impairment or distress, as manifested by one (or more) of the following, occurring within a 12-month period:

Recurrent substance use resulting in a failure to fulfill major role obligations at work, school, or home (e.g., repeated absences or poor work performance related to substance use; substance-related absences, suspensions, or expulsions from school; neglect of children or household)

Recurrent substance use in situations in which it is physically hazardous (e.g., driving an automobile or operating a machine when impaired by substance use)

Recurrent substance-related legal problems (e.g., arrests for substance-related disorderly conduct)

Continued substance use despite having persistent or recurrent social or interpersonal problems caused or exacerbated by the effects of the substance (e.g., arguments with spouse about consequences of intoxication, physical fights)

The symptoms have never met the criteria for substance dependence for this class of disorder.

Criteria for substance dependence[a]

A maladaptive pattern of substance use, leading to clinically significant impairment or distress, as manifested by three (or more) of the following, occurring at any time in the same 12-month period:

Tolerance, as defined by either a need for markedly increased amounts of the substance to achieve intoxication or desired effect or markedly diminished effect with continued use of the same amount of the substance

Withdrawal, as manifested by either the characteristic withdrawal syndrome for the substance or the same (or a closely related) substance taken to relieve or avoid withdrawal symptoms

The substance is often taken in larger amounts over a longer period than was intended

There is persistent desire or unsuccessful effort to cut down or control substance use

A great deal of time is spent in activities necessary to obtain the substance (e.g., visiting multiple physicians or driving long distances), use the substance (e.g., chain smoking), or recover from its effects

Important social, occupational, or recreational activities are given up or reduced because of substance use

The substance use is continued despite knowledge of having a persistent or recurrent physical or psychological problem that is likely to have been caused or exacerbated by the substance (e.g., current cocaine use despite recognition of cocaine-induced depression, or continued drinking despite recognition that an ulcer was made worse by alcohol consumption)

[a]From American Psychiatric Association. *Diagnostic and statistical manual for mental disorders—III*. Washington, DC: American Psychiatric Association, 1983.

several tertiary care hospitals (15), also found a low prevalence of substance-related disorders. Following structured clinical interviews, fewer than 5% of 215 patients with cancer met the Diagnostic and Statistical Manual for Mental Disorders (DSM) 3rd Edition criteria for a substance-use disorder (17) (Table 41.1).

The relatively low prevalence of substance abuse among patients with cancer treated in tertiary care hospitals may reflect institutional biases or a tendency for patients to underreport in these settings. Many drug abusers are poor, feel alienated from the health care system, may not seek care in tertiary centers, and may be reluctant to acknowledge the stigmatizing history of drug abuse. For these reasons, the low prevalence of drug abuse in cancer centers may not be representative of the true prevalence in the cancer population overall. In support of this conclusion, the findings of a 1995 survey of patients admitted to a palliative care unit indicate alcohol abuse in more than 25% of patients (18). Additional studies are needed to clarify the current epidemiology of substance abuse and dependence in patients with cancer and others with progressive medical diseases. These patients can be adequately and successfully treated only when their substance problems are noted by staff and their needs addressed.

DEFINITIONS OF ABUSE AND DEPENDENCE

Both epidemiologic studies and clinical management depend on an accepted, valid nomenclature for substance abuse

and dependence. Unfortunately, this terminology is highly problematic. The pharmacologic phenomena of tolerance and physical dependence are commonly confused with abuse and true substance dependence as defined by the *DSM-IV* (Table 41.1), and the definitions applied to medical patients have been developed from experience with substance-abusing populations. The clarification of this terminology is an essential step in improving the diagnosis and management of substance abuse in the palliative care setting (Table 41.2).

Tolerance

Tolerance is a pharmacologic property defined by the need for increasing doses to maintain effects (19,20). An extensive clinical experience with opioid drugs in the medical context has not confirmed that tolerance causes substantial problems (21,22).

TABLE 41.2

SUBSTANCE ABUSE DEFINITIONS IN THE MEDICALLY ILL

Tolerance	The need for increasing doses to maintain analgesic effects
Addiction	Continuing and compulsive use despite physical, psychological, or social harm.
Physical dependence	Presence of withdrawal following abrupt dose reduction

Although tolerance to a variety of opioid effects, including analgesia, can be reliably observed in animal models (23), and tolerance to nonanalgesic effects, such as respiratory depression and cognitive impairment (24), occurs routinely in the clinical setting, analgesic tolerance seldom interferes with the clinical efficacy of opioid drugs. Indeed, most patients attain stable doses associated with a favorable balance between analgesia and side effects for prolonged periods; dose escalation, when it is required, usually heralds the appearance of a progressive painful lesion (25–31). Unlike tolerance to the side effects of opioids, clinically meaningful analgesic tolerance, which would yield the need for dose escalation to maintain analgesia in the absence of progressive disease, appears to be a rare phenomenon. Clinical observation also fails to support the conclusion that analgesic tolerance is a substantial contributor to the development of substance dependence.

Physical Dependence

Physical dependence is defined solely by the occurrence of an abstinence syndrome (withdrawal) following abrupt dose reduction or administration of an antagonist (19,20,32). There is great confusion among clinicians about the differences between physical dependence and true substance dependence. Physical dependence, like tolerance, has been suggested to be a component of substance dependence (33,34), and the avoidance of withdrawal has been postulated to create behavioral contingencies that reinforce drug-seeking behavior (35). These speculations, however, are not supported by experience acquired during opioid therapy for chronic pain. Physical dependence does not preclude the uncomplicated discontinuation of opioids during multidisciplinary pain management of nonmalignant pain (36), and opioid therapy is routinely stopped without difficulty in the patients with cancer whose pain disappears following effective antineoplastic therapy. Indirect evidence for a fundamental distinction between physical dependence and substance dependence is even provided by animal models of opioid self-administration, which have demonstrated that persistent drug-taking behavior can be maintained in the absence of physical dependence (37).

Addiction

The terms *addiction* and *addict* are particularly troublesome. These labels are often inappropriately applied to describe both aberrant drug use (reminiscent of the behaviors that characterize active abusers of illicit drugs) and phenomena related to tolerance or physical dependence. The labels "addict" and "addiction" should never be used to describe patients who are only perceived to have the capacity for an abstinence syndrome. These patients must be labeled "physically dependent." Use of the word "dependent" alone also should be discouraged, because it fosters confusion between physical dependence and psychological dependence, a component of substance dependence. For the same reason, the term *habituation* should not be used. It is recommended that the *DSM-IV* (17) terms *substance abuse* and *substance dependence* be applied as appropriate.

Definitions of "substance abuse" and "substance dependence" must be based on the identification of drug-related behaviors that are outside of cultural or societal norms. The ability to categorize questionable behaviors (e.g., consuming a few extra doses of a prescribed opioid, particularly if this behavior was not specifically prescribed by the clinician, or using an opioid drug prescribed for pain as a nighttime hypnotic) as nonnormative presupposes that there is certainty about the parameters of normative behavior. In fact, even experienced pain clinicians disagree on the interpretation of varied drug-taking patterns. In a recent survey, pain clinicians expressed significant individual differences in the perception of which behaviors were the most problematic when asked to rank order a list of aberrant drug-taking behaviors (38). In general, physicians rated illegal behaviors as the most aberrant, followed by alteration of the route of delivery and self-escalation of dose.

Unfortunately, there are few empirical data in medically ill populations that define the meaning of specific drug-related behaviors in relation to substance-use disorders or future drug abuse; as a result, the boundaries of normative behavior remain ill-defined. The confusing nature of normative drug taking was highlighted in a pilot survey performed in 2000 at MSKCC, which revealed that inpatients with cancer harbor attitudes supporting misuse of drugs in the face of symptom management problems and that women with human immunodeficiency virus (HIV) (at MSKCC for palliative care) engage in such behaviors commonly (39). The prevalence of such behaviors and attitudes among the medically ill raises concern about their predictive validity as a marker of any diagnosis related to substance abuse. Clearly, there is a need for empirical data that illuminate the prevalence of drug-taking attitudes and behaviors in different populations of medically ill patients.

The core concepts used to define substance dependence also may be problematic as a result of changes induced by a progressive disease. Deterioration in physical or psychosocial functioning caused by the disease and its treatment may be difficult to separate from the morbidity associated with drug abuse. This may particularly complicate efforts to evaluate the concept of "use despite harm," which is critical to the diagnosis of substance abuse or dependence. For example, the nature of questionable drug-related behaviors can be difficult to discern in the patient who develops social withdrawal or cognitive changes following brain irradiation for metastases. Even if impaired cognition is clearly related to the drugs used to treat symptoms, this outcome might only reflect a narrow therapeutic window, rather than a desire on the patient's part for these psychic effects.

Definition of Substance Dependence in the Medically Ill

Previous definitions that include phenomena related to physical dependence or tolerance cannot be the model terminology for medically ill populations who receive potentially abusable drugs for legitimate medical purposes. A more appropriate definition of substance dependence notes that it is a chronic disorder characterized by "the compulsive use of a substance resulting in physical, psychological or social harm to the user and continued use despite that harm" (40). Although this definition was developed from experience in substance-abusing populations without medical illness, it appropriately emphasizes that substance dependence is, fundamentally, a psychological and behavioral syndrome. Any appropriate definition of substance abuse or dependence must include the concepts of loss of control over drug use, compulsive drug use, and continued use despite harm.

Even appropriate definitions of substance dependence will have limited utility, however, unless operationalized for a clinical setting. The concept of "aberrant drug-related behavior" is a useful first step in operationalizing the definitions of substance abuse and dependence, and recognizes the broad range of behaviors that may be considered problematic by prescribers. Although the assessment and interpretation of these behaviors can be challenging, as discussed previously, the occurrence of aberrant behaviors signals the need to reevaluate and manage drug taking, even in the context of an appropriate medical indication for a drug.

If drug-taking behavior in a medical patient can be characterized as aberrant, a "differential diagnosis" for this behavior can be explored. That a patient has a true substance-dependent disorder is only one of several possible explanations. The challenging diagnosis of pseudoaddiction must be considered if the patient is reporting distress associated with unrelieved symptoms. In the case of pseudoaddiction, behaviors such as aggressively complaining about the need for higher doses, or occasional unilateral drug escalations indicate desperation caused by pain and disappear if pain management improves.

Alternatively, impulsive drug use may indicate the existence of another psychiatric disorder, diagnosis of which may have therapeutic implications. Patients with borderline personality disorder can express fear and rage through aberrant drug taking and behave impulsively and self-destructively during pain therapy. Passik and Hay (41) reported a case in which one of the more worrisome aberrant drug-related behaviors, forging of a prescription for a controlled substance, was an impulsive expression of fears of abandonment, having little to do with true substance abuse in a borderline patient. Such patients are challenging and often require firm limit-setting and careful monitoring to avoid impulsive drug taking.

Similarly, patients who self-medicate for anxiety, panic, depression or even periodic dysphoria and loneliness can present as aberrant drug takers. In such instances, careful diagnosis and treatment of these problems can at times obviate the need for such self-medication. Occasionally, aberrant drug-related behavior appears to be causally related to a mild encephalopathy, with confusion about the appropriate therapeutic regimen. This may be a concern in the treatment of the elderly patient. Low doses of neuroleptic medications, simplified drug regimens, and help organizing medications can address such problems. Rarely, problematic behaviors indicate criminal intent, such as when patients report pain but intend to sell or divert medications.

These diagnoses are not mutually exclusive. A thorough psychiatric assessment is critically important, both in the population without a prior history of substance abuse and the population of known abusers, who have a high prevalence of psychiatric comorbidity (42,43).

In assessing the differential diagnosis for drug-related behavior, it is useful to consider the degree of aberrancy (Table 41.3). The less aberrant behaviors (such as aggressively complaining about the need for medications) are more likely to reflect untreated distress of some type, rather than

TABLE 41.3

DEGREES OF ABERRANCE IN DRUG-TAKING BEHAVIOR[a]

Mildly aberrant	Requests for specific pain medication
	Aggressive complaints about the need for medication
	Using drugs prescribed for a friend or family member
	Frequent prescription losses
	Hoarding drugs
More highly aberrant	Forging prescriptions
	Obtaining drugs from nonmedical source
	Sale of prescription drugs
	Crushing sustained-release tablets for snorting or injecting

[a]From Passik SD, Kirsh KL, Whitcomb L, et al. Pain clinicians' rankings of aberrant drug-taking behaviors. *J Pain Palliat Care Pharmacother* 2002;16:39–49.

substance dependence–related concerns. Conversely, the more aberrant behaviors (such as injection of an oral formulation) are more likely to reflect true substance dependence. Although empirical studies are needed to validate this conceptualization, it may be a useful model when evaluating aberrant behaviors.

EMPIRICAL STUDIES USING THE ABERRANT DRUG-TAKING CONCEPT

Several studies have investigated the usefulness of considering aberrant drug taking as occurring on a continuum. Although the studies performed to date all involve small samples, they have shown that conceptualizing aberrant drug taking in this way has important implications for clinicians. The first study examined the relationship between aberrant drug-taking behaviors and compliance-related outcomes in patients with a history of substance abuse receiving chronic opioid therapy for nonmalignant pain. Dunbar and Katz (44) examined outcomes and drug taking in 20 patients with diverse histories of drug abuse who underwent a year of chronic opioid therapy. During the year of therapy, 11 patients were adherent with the drug regimen and 9 were not. The authors examined patient characteristics and aberrant drug-taking behaviors that differentiated the two groups. The patients who did not abuse the therapy were abusers of solely alcohol (or had remote histories of polysubstance abuse), were participating in 12-step programs, and had good social support. The patients who abused the therapy were polysubstance abusers, were not participating in 12-step programs, and had poor social support. The specific behaviors that were recorded more frequently by those who abused the therapy were unscheduled visits and multiple phone calls to the clinic, unsanctioned dose escalations, and acquisition of opioids from more than one source.

A second study examined the relationship between aberrant drug taking and the presence or absence of a psychiatric diagnosis of substance-use disorder in pain patients. Compton et al. (45) studied 56 patients seeking pain treatment in a multidisciplinary pain program who were referred for "problematic drug taking." The patients all underwent structured psychiatric interviews, and the sample was divided between those qualifying and those not qualifying for psychiatric diagnoses of substance-use disorders. The authors then examined the subjects' reports of aberrant drug-taking behaviors on a structured interview assessment. The patients who qualified for a substance-use disorder diagnosis were more likely to have engaged in unsanctioned dose escalations, received opioids from multiple sources, and reported a subjective impression of loss of control of their prescribed medications.

Passik and researchers at a major cancer center (39) examined the self reports of aberrant drug-taking attitudes and behaviors in samples of patients with cancer ($n = 52$) and patients with AIDS ($n = 111$) on a questionnaire designed for the purposes of the study. Reports of past drug use and abuse were more frequent than present reports in both groups. Current aberrant drug-related behaviors were seldom reported, but attitude items revealed that patients would consider engaging in aberrant behaviors, or would possibly excuse them in others, if pain or symptom management were inadequate. It was found that aberrant behaviors and attitudes were endorsed more frequently by the women with AIDS than by male and female patients with cancer. Overall, patients greatly overestimated the risk of substance dependence during pain treatment. Experience with this questionnaire suggests that patients both with cancer and AIDS respond in a forthcoming fashion to drug-taking behavior questions and describe attitudes and behaviors which may be highly relevant to the diagnosis and management of substance-use disorders.

These studies help clarify the meanings ascribed by clinicians to the various behaviors that occur during long-term administration of a potentially abusable drug. Ultimately, such studies may define the true "red flags" in a given population.

Far too often, anecdotal accounts shape the way clinicians view drug-related behaviors. Some behaviors are regarded almost universally as aberrant despite limited systematic data to suggest that this is the case. Consider, for example, the patient who requests a specific pain medication, or a specific route or dose. Although this behavior may reflect a patient who is knowledgeable and assertive—favorable characteristics in other contexts—it is often greeted with suspicion on the part of practitioners. Other behaviors may be common in medically ill non–substance-abusing populations, and although aberrant, they may have little predictive value for true substance dependence. For example, the finding that many non–substance-abusing patients with cancer use anxiolytic medications prescribed for a friend or other (39) more than likely reflects the undertreatment and underreporting of anxiety in patients with cancer than true-substance abuse.

RISK OF SUBSTANCE ABUSE AND DEPENDENCE IN THE MEDICALLY ILL

Opioid administration in patients with cancer having no prior history of substance abuse is only rarely associated with the development of significant substance abuse or dependence (46–58). Indeed, concerns about abuse in this population are now characterized by an interesting paradox: although the lay public and inexperienced clinicians still fear the development of substance abuse or dependence when opioids are used to treat cancer pain, specialists in cancer pain and palliative care widely believe that the major problem related to potential abuse is not the phenomenon itself, but rather the persistent undertreatment of pain driven by inappropriate fear that it will occur.

The very sanguine experience in the cancer population has contributed to a desire for a reappraisal of the risks and benefits associated with the long-term opioid treatment of chronic nonmalignant pain (31,59). The traditional view of this therapy is negative, and early surveys of substance abusers, which noted that a relatively large proportion began their abuse as patients on medication administered opioid drugs for pain (60–62), provided some indirect support for this perspective. The most influential of these surveys recorded a history of medical opioid use for pain in 27% of white male addicts and 1.2% of black male abusers (62).

Surveys of substance-abusing populations, however, do not provide a valid measure of the liability associated with chronic opioid therapy in medically ill populations without known drug abuse. Prospective patient surveys are needed to define this risk accurately. Studies of relatively short-term opioid exposure have been reassuring. The Boston Collaborative Drug Surveillance Project evaluated 11,882 inpatients who had no prior history of substance abuse and were administered an opioid while hospitalized; only 4 cases of substance abuse or dependence could be identified subsequently (63). A national survey of burn centers could find no cases of abuse in a sample of more than 10,000 patients without prior drug abuse history who were administered opioids for pain (64), and a survey of a large headache clinic identified opioid abuse in only 3 of 2369 patients admitted for treatment, most of whom had access to opioids (65). These surveys do not, however, define

the risk of substance abuse or dependence during long-term, open-ended opioid therapy. Other supporting data derive from surveys of patients with cancer and postoperative patients, which indicate that euphoria, a phenomenon believed to be common during the abuse of opioids, is extremely uncommon following administration of an opioid for pain; dysphoria is observed more typically, especially in those who receive meperidine (66).

The inaccurate perception that opioid therapy inherently yields a relatively high likelihood of substance abuse or dependence has encouraged assumptions that are not supportable given the current understanding of substance abuse. Perhaps most important, the relevance of a genetically determined predisposition to substance abuse (67) tends to be minimized or dismissed by such a view. A more critical evaluation of the extant literature (28–31,67–69) actually yields little substantive support for the view that large numbers of individuals with no personal or family history of substance abuse or dependence, no affiliation with a substance-abusing subculture, and no significant premorbid psychopathology will develop abuse or dependence *de novo* when administered potentially abusable drugs for appropriate medical indications.

RISK IN PATIENTS WITH CURRENT OR REMOTE DRUG ABUSE

There is very little information about the risk of substance abuse or dependence during, or after, the therapeutic administration of a potentially abusable drug to patients with a current or remote history of substance abuse or dependence. Anecdotal reports have suggested that successful long-term opioid therapy in patients with cancer pain or chronic nonmalignant pain is possible, particularly if the history of substance abuse or dependence is remote (44,70,71). Indeed, a 1992 study showed that patients with AIDS-related pain could be successfully treated with morphine whether or not they were substance users or nonusers. The major group difference found in this survey was that substance users required considerably more morphine to reach stable pain control (72).

These data are reassuring but do not obviate the need for caution. For example, although there is no empirical evidence that the use of short-acting drugs or the parenteral route is more likely to lead to problematic drug-related behaviors than other therapeutic approaches, it may be prudent to avoid such therapies in patients with histories of substance abuse.

CLINICAL MANAGEMENT

Aberrant drug-taking among patients with advanced illnesses (with or without a prior history of substance abuse) represents a serious and complex clinical occurrence. Perhaps the more difficult situations involve the patient who is actively abusing illicit or prescription drugs or alcohol concomitantly with medical therapies. Whether the patient is an active drug abuser, has a history of substance abuse, or is not complying with the therapeutic regimen, the clinician should establish structure, control, and monitoring so that they can prescribe freely and without prejudice.

Multidisciplinary Approach

A multidisciplinary team approach is usually optimal for the management of substance abusers in the palliative care setting. If available, mental health professionals with specialization in the substance abuse can be instrumental helping palliative care team members develop strategies for management and patient treatment compliance. Providing care to these patients can lead to feelings of anger and frustration among staff. Such feelings can unintentionally compromise pain management and contribute to feelings of isolation and alienation by the patient. A structured multidisciplinary approach can be effective in helping the staff better understand the patient's needs and develop effective strategies for controlling pain and aberrant drug use simultaneously. Staff meetings can be helpful in establishing treatment goals, facilitating compliance, and coordinating the multidisciplinary team.

Assessment

The first member of the medical team (frequently a nurse) to suspect problematic drug taking or a history of drug abuse should alert the patient's palliative care team, thereby beginning the multidisciplinary assessment and management process (73). A physician should assess the potential of withdrawal or other pressing concerns and begin involving other staff (i.e., social work and/or psychiatry) to initiate the planning of management strategies (Table 41.4). Obtaining as detailed as possible a history of the duration, frequency, and desired effect of drug use is crucial. Frequently, clinicians avoid asking patients about substance abuse because of fear that they will anger the patient or that they are incorrect in their suspicion of abuse. This stance can contribute to continued problems. Empathic and truthful communication is always the best approach.

The use of a careful, graduated interview can be instrumental to assess drug use. This approach entails starting the assessment interview with broad questions about the role of drugs (e.g., nicotine, caffeine) in the patient's life and gradually becoming more specific in focus to include illicit drugs. Such an approach is helpful in reducing denial and resistance.

This interviewing style may also assist in the detection of coexisting psychiatric disorders. Comorbid psychiatric disorders can significantly contribute to aberrant drug-taking behavior. Studies suggest that 37–62% of alcoholics have one or more coexisting psychiatric disorders and the patient's drug history may be a clue to comorbid psychiatric disorders (e.g., drinking to quell panic symptoms). Anxiety, personality disorders, and mood disorders are the

most commonly encountered (7,43,75). The assessment and treatment of comorbid psychiatric disorders can greatly enhance management strategies and reduce the risk of relapse.

Prescreening Patients

Assessment tools have been developed for chronic pain populations for the purpose of evaluating the likelihood of problematic drug use during therapy. In the most recent effort, Butler et al. tested a screening measure for patients suffering from chronic pain (74). An initial 24-item self-administered Screener and Opioid Assessment for Patients with Pain (SOAPP) was validated in a sample of 175 chronic nonmalignant pain patients, 95 of whom were available for a 6-month follow-up. From these results, a 14-item short form was derived that has adequate psychometrics and shows promise as a way to screen chronic pain patients who might be at risk for substance abuse and dependence. The applicability of this instrument, or others developed for this purpose, in populations with medical illness remains to be determined in future studies.

The Four A's for Ongoing Monitoring

On the basis of extensive clinical experience, four domains have been proposed as most relevant for ongoing monitoring of patients with chronic pain on opioids. These domains have been summarized as the "Four A's" (analgesia, activities of daily living, adverse side effects, and aberrant drug-taking behaviors) (76). The monitoring of these outcomes over time should inform therapeutic decision-making and provide a framework for documentation. A checklist tool has been developed to aid in monitoring of the Four A's (77) (Table 41.5).

Development of a Treatment Plan—General Considerations

Clear treatment goals are essential in managing aberrant drug-related behaviors. Depending on the history, a complete remission of the patient's substance use problems may not be a reasonable goal. The distress of coping with a life-threatening

---

TABLE 41.4

SCREENING FOR SUBSTANCE ABUSE AND TREATMENT RECOMMENDATIONS

Assessment guidelines

Use graduated interview approach beginning with broad questions about substances such as nicotine or caffeine and becoming more specific

Assess for comorbid psychiatric disorders, such as anxiety, personality disorders, and mood disorders

Consider diagnostic instruments, such as Screener and Opioid Assessment for Patients with Pain (74)

Treatment recommendations

General	Listen and accept patient's report of distress
	Use behavioral and nonopioid interventions for pain when possible
	Consider drugs with slower onset and longer duration (e.g., transdermal fentanyl and modified-release opioids). Note that higher doses may be needed for adequate pain control in patients with a history of abuse or dependence
	Frequently assess adequacy of symptom and pain control
Outpatients	Limit amount of drug dispensed per prescription
	Make refills contingent on clinic attendance
	Consider urine toxicology screenings to assess usage
	Involve family members and friends in the treatment plan
Inpatients	Consider placing the patient in a private room near the nurses' station
	Consider daily urine collection

TABLE 41.5

FOUR A'S FOR ONGOING MONITORING

Analgesia	Document and monitor patient's pain, using scales such as a 0–10 pain rating scale. Although listed as the first "A," analgesia is not necessarily to be considered the most important outcome of pain management. An alternate view is how much relief it takes for a patient to feel that their life is meaningfully changed so they can work toward the attainment of their own goals.
Activities of daily living	Monitor patient's typical level of daily activities and psychosocial functioning to observe increases over time. The second 'A' concerning activities of daily living refers to quality of life issues and functionality. It is necessary that patients understand that they must comply with all of their recommended treatment options so that they are better able to return to work, avocation and social activities.
Adverse effects	Strive for highest analgesia with most benign side-effect profile. Patients must also be made aware of the adverse side effects inherent in the treatment of their pain condition with opioids and other medications. Side effects must be aggressively managed so that sedation and other side effects do not overshadow the potential benefits of drug therapy. The most common side effects of opioid analgesics include constipation, sedation, nausea and vomiting, dry mouth, respiratory depression, confusion, urinary retention, and itching.
Aberrant behaviors	Be aware of aberrant behaviors suggestive of drug use, such as multiple "lost" prescriptions or unauthorized dose escalations. Patients must be educated through agreements, or other means, about the parameters of acceptable drug taking. Even an overall good outcome in every other domain might not constitute satisfactory treatment if the patient is not compliant with the contract in worrisome ways. Dispensing pain medicine in a highly structured fashion may become necessary for some patients who are in violation or constantly on the fringes of appropriate drug taking.

illness and the availability of prescription drugs for symptom control can undermine efforts to maintain control over comorbid substance abuse or dependence (78). For some patients, "harm reduction" may be a better model. It aims to enhance social support, maximize treatment compliance, and contain harm done through episodic relapse.

Several elements are key in this approach. First, clinicians must establish a relationship based on empathic listening and accept the patient's report of distress. Second, it is important to use nonopioid and behavioral interventions for pain when possible, but not as substitutes for appropriate pharmacologic management. Third, specific aspects of drug selection and dosing should be informed by a history of problematic drug use. For example, a history of active opioid abuse usually means that higher doses may be needed more rapidly than commonly observed in patients who are opioid-naive. Underdosing may lead to a degree of persistent pain that drives the patient's attempts to self-medicate. The use of medications with slow onset and longer duration (e.g., transdermal fentanyl and modified-release opioids) should be considered in those with substance-use disorders. Patients who are perceived to be at high risk should not be given short-acting opioids for breakthrough pain. Finally, the team should make plans to frequently reassess the adequacy of pain and symptom control.

Urine Toxicology Screening

Clinicians must control and monitor drug use in all patients, a daunting task in some active abusers. In some cases, a major issue is compliance with treatments for the underlying disease, which may be so poor that the substance abuse actually shortens life expectancy by preventing the effective administration of primary therapy. Prognosis may also be worsened by the use of drugs in a manner that negatively interacts with therapy or predisposes to other serious morbidity. The goals of care can be very difficult to define when poor compliance and risky behavior appears to contradict a reported desire for disease-modifying therapies.

Urine toxicology screening has the potential to be a useful tool to the practicing clinician both for diagnosing

potential abuse problems as well as monitoring patients with an established history of abuse. However, a 2000 chart review of the ordering and documentation of urine toxicology screens suggests that urine toxicology screens are employed infrequently in tertiary care centers (79). In addition, when urine tests are ordered, documentation tends to be inconsistent regarding the reasons for ordering as well as any follow-up recommendations based on the results. Indeed, the chart review found that nearly 40% of the charts surveyed listed no reason for obtaining the urine toxicology screen and the ordering physician could not be identified nearly 30% of the time. Staff education efforts can help to address this problem.

The Patient with Advanced Disease

Managing substance abuse in patients with advanced medical illness may be particularly challenging. Although clinicians may be tempted to overlook a patient's use of illicit substances or alcohol, viewing these behaviors as a last source of pleasure for the patient, drug use that is out of control may have a highly deleterious impact on palliative care efforts. Aberrant drug-related behaviors may be associated with poor symptom control, distress, increased stress for family members, family concern over the misuse of medication, poor compliance with the treatment regimen, and diminished quality of life. Complete abstinence from drugs of abuse may not be a realistic outcome, but reduction in use can certainly have positive effects for the patient (80).

Outpatient Management

There are a number of additional strategies for promoting treatment adherence in an outpatient setting. A written contract between the team and patient helps to provide structure to the treatment plan, establishes clear expectations of the roles played by both parties, and outlines the consequences of aberrant drug taking. The inclusion of spot urine toxicology screens in the contract can be useful in maximizing treatment compliance. Expectations regarding follow-up visits and management of drug supply also should be stated. For example, clinicians may wish to limit the amount of drug dispensed per prescription and make refills contingent upon clinic attendance. The clinician may consider the requirement for joint management by a specialist in substance abuse or required attendance at a 12-step program. With the patient's consent, the clinician may wish to contact the patient's sponsor and make him or her aware that the patient is being treated for a chronic illness that requires medications (e.g., opioids). This action will reduce the potential for stigmatization of the patient as being noncompliant with the ideals of the 12-step program. Finally, clinicians should involve family members and friends in the treatment to help bolster social support and functioning. Becoming familiar with the family may help the team to identify family members who are themselves drug abusers and who may potentially divert the patient's medications. Mental health professionals can help family members with referrals to drug treatment and codependency groups as a way to help the patient receive optimal medical care.

Inpatient Management

The management of patients with active substance-abuse problems who have been admitted to the hospital for treatment of a life-threatening illness is based on the guidelines discussed in the preceding text for outpatient settings. These guidelines aim to promote the safety of patients and staff, contain manipulative behaviors by patients, enhance the appropriate use of medication for pain and symptom management, and communicate an understanding of pain and substance abuse management. First, the patient's drug use needs to be discussed in an open manner. It may be necessary to reassure the patient that steps will be taken to avoid adverse events such as drug or alcohol withdrawal. In some challenging cases, it would be best to admit a patient several days in advance of a planned procedure for stabilization of the drug regimen.

If the patient is actively abusing drugs, it is often best to place the patient on the unit in a private room, if possible, near the nurses' station. This aids in monitoring the patient and may discourage attempts to leave the hospital for the purchase of illicit drugs. Further, the team should require visitors to check in with nursing staff prior to visitation. In some cases, it may be necessary to search the packages of visitors in order to stem a patient's access to drugs. Depending on the severity of the problem, the clinician should consider ordering daily urine collection, which may or may not be sent for random toxicology analysis. In all cases, pain and symptoms should be frequently assessed.

Management approaches should be tailored to reflect the clinician's assessment of the severity of drug abuse. Open and honest communication between the clinician and the patient throughout the admission reassures the patient that these guidelines were established in their best interest.

In some cases, these guidelines fail to curtail aberrant drug use despite repeated interventions by staff. At that point, the patient should be considered for discharge. This appears to be necessary only in the most recalcitrant of cases. The clinician should involve members of the staff and administration for discussion about the ethical and legal implications of such a decision.

Methadone

Oral methadone can be used safely and effectively as an analgesic (80–84). Once-daily methadone is rarely useful as an analgesic and patients receiving maintenance methadone for opioid dependence cannot obtain pain relief merely by increasing their dose. Indeed, practitioners sometimes assume that patients receiving methadone from a maintenance program do not need further pain medication, but this is simply not true (85,86). Methadone can be used for pain management by increasing the dose and dividing it during the day. Alternately, an entirely separate pharmacologic therapy can be chosen and incorporated into the patient's treatment plan.

Alcohol

Patients with life-threatening illness who are dependent on alcohol require careful assessment and management. When these patients are not identified and are admitted to the hospital, alcohol withdrawal can be an unexpected complication. Patients at the end of life can also inadvertently experience withdrawal symptoms if they decrease their alcohol intake as their physical condition declines. Withdrawal symptoms may be mistaken for simple anxiety when the full extent of the patient's use of alcohol is not known (87). The first symptoms of withdrawal usually manifest a few hours following the cessation of alcohol intake and often consist of tremors, agitation, and insomnia. In mild to moderate cases, these symptoms lessen within 2 days. Patients with terminal illness are more likely than the physically healthy to progress from these milder symptoms to a state of delirium characterized by autonomic hyperactivity, hallucinations, incoherence, and disorientation (73). Delirium tremens (DTs) occur in approximately 5–15% of patients in alcohol withdrawal (88), typically within the first 72–96 hours of withdrawal. Severe DTs is a medical emergency and requires prompt treatment.

In surgical settings, alcohol withdrawal can cause up to a threefold increase in postoperative mortality when unrecognized and not addressed (89,90). Because patients with cancer who abuse alcohol are already at high risk for delirium postoperatively due to poor nutrition, prior head trauma, and other causes of brain injury, the impact of severe alcohol withdrawal may be life-threatening (73).

The extreme vulnerability of patients who are terminally ill necessitates that potential withdrawal symptoms be managed aggressively and prevented whenever possible (89). To date no research exists to determine the best approach to treat acute alcohol withdrawal in the palliative care setting; in its absence, basic management steps, such as the use of hydration, benzodiazepines, and in some cases, neuroleptics, should be taken to manage alcohol withdrawal syndrome (73,87). The administration of a vitamin-mineral solution is indicated, including parenteral thiamine 100 g for 3 days before switching to oral administration to prevent the development of Korsakoff's syndrome. A daily dose of folate 1 mg should also be given throughout treatment (73).

Patients in Recovery

Pain management with patients in recovery presents a unique challenge. Depending on the structure of the recovery program (e.g., Alcoholics Anonymous, methadone maintenance programs), a patient may fear ostracism from the program's members or have intense fear regarding susceptibility to relapsing into substance-abuse behaviors. Nonopioid therapies should be optimized, which may require referral to a pain center or other specialists (85). If opioids are required, therapy should be structured based on a thorough assessment, the goals of care, and the life expectancy of the patient. In some cases, it is necessary to use opioid management contracts, random urine toxicology screens, and occasional pill counts. If possible, attempts should be made to include the patient's recovery program sponsor in order to garner their cooperation in monitoring of the patient.

CONCLUSION

The effective management of patients who engage in aberrant drug-related behavior necessitates a comprehensive approach that recognizes the biological, chemical, social, and psychiatric aspects of substance abuse and provides practical means to manage risk, treat pain effectively and assure patient safety. An accepted nomenclature for substance abuse and dependence, and an operational approach to the assessment of patients with medical illness, are prerequisites to an accurate definition of risk in populations with and without histories of substance abuse. Unfortunately, there are very limited data relevant to risk assessment in the medically ill. Also, there is almost no information about the risk of less serious aberrant drug-related behaviors, the risk of these outcomes in populations that do have a history of abuse, or the risk associated with the use of potentially abusable drugs other than opioids.

References

1. National Center on Addiction and Substance Abuse at Columbia University. Under the counter: the diversion and abuse of controlled prescription drugs in the U.S., July 2005.
2. Colliver JD, Kopstein AN. Trends in cocaine abuse reflected in emergency room episodes reported to DAWN. *Public Health Rep* 1991;106:59–68.
3. Warner LA, Kessler RC, Hughes M, et al. Prevalence and correlates of drug use and dependence in the United States. Results from the National Comorbidity Survey. *Arch Gen Psychiatry* 1995;52:219–229.
4. Kessler RC, Chui WT, Demler O, et al. Prevalence, severity, and comorbidity of 12-month DSM-IV disorders in the National comorbidity survey replication. *Arch Gen Psychiatry* 2005;62:617–627.
5. Kessler RC, Berglund P, Demler O, et al. Lifetime prevalence and age-of-onset distributions of DSM-IV Disorders in the National comorbidity survey replication. *Arch Gen Psychiatry* 2005;62:593–602.
6. Groerer J, Brodsky M. The incidence of illicit drug use in the United States, 1962–1989. *Br J Addict* 1992;87:1345.
7. Regier DA, Farmer ME, Rae DS, et al. Comorbidity of mental disorders with alcohol and other drug abuse. *J Am Med Assoc* 1990;264:2511–2518.
8. Wells KB, Golding JM, Burnam MA. Chronic medical conditions in a sample of the general population with anxiety, affective, and substance use disorders. *Am J Psychiatry* 1989;146:1440.
9. Smith-Warner SA, Spiegelman D, Yaun S, et al. Alcohol and breast cancer in women: a pooled analysis of cohort studies. *J Am Med Assoc* 1998;279:535–540.
10. Blot WJ. Alcohol and cancer. *Cancer Res* 1992;52:S2119–S2123.
11. Thun MJ, Peto R, Lopez AD, et al. Alcohol consumption and mortality among middle-aged and elderly U.S. adults. *N Engl J Med* 1997;337:1705–1714.
12. Room R, Babor T, Rehm J. Alcohol and public health. *Lancet* 2005;365:519–530.
13. Yu, DK. Review of Memorial Sloan-Kettering Counselling Center Database (Unpublished) 2005.
14. Burton RW, Lyons JS, Devens M, et al. Psychiatric consults for psychoactive substance disorders in the general hospital. *Gen Hosp Psychiatry* 1991;13:83.
15. Derogatis LR, Morrow GR, Fetting J, et al. The prevalence of psychiatric disorders among cancer patients. *J Am Med Assoc* 1983;249:751.
16. Regier DA, Meyers JK, Dramer M, et al. The NIMH epidemiologic catchment area program. *Arch Gen Psychiatry* 1984;41:934.
17. American Psychiatric Association. *Diagnostic and statistical manual for mental disorders—III*. Washington, DC: American Psychiatric Association, 1983.
18. Bruera E, Moyano J, Seifert L, et al. The frequency of alcoholism among patients with pain due to terminal cancer. *J Pain Symptom Manage* 1995;10(8):599.
19. Dole VP. Narcotic addiction, physical dependence and relapse. *N Engl J Med* 1972;286:988.
20. Martin WR, Jasinski DR. Physiological parameters of morphine dependence in man–tolerance, early abstinence, protracted abstinence. *J Psychiatr Res* 1969;7:9.
21. Portenoy RK. Opioid tolerance and efficacy: basic research and clinical observations. In: Gebhardt G, Hammond D, Jensen T, eds. *Proceedings of the VII World congress on pain, progress in pain research and management*, Vol. 2. Seattle, WA: IASP Press, 1994:595.
22. Foley KM. Clinical tolerance to opioids. In: Basbaum AI, Besson J-M, eds. *Towards a new pharmacotherapy of pain*. Chichester: John Wiley and Sons, 1991:181.
23. Ling GSF, Paul D, Simantov R, et al. Differential development of acute tolerance to analgesia, respiratory depression, gastrointestinal transit and hormone release in a morphine infusion model. *Life Sci* 1989;45:1627.
24. Bruera E, Macmillan K, Hanson JA, et al. The cognitive effects of the administration of narcotic analgesics in patients with cancer pain. *Pain* 1989;39:13.
25. Twycross RG. Clinical experience with diamorphine in advanced malignant disease. *Int J Clin Pharmacol Ther Toxicol* 1974;9:184.
26. Kanner RM, Foley KM. Patterns of narcotic drug use in a cancer pain clinic. *Ann N Y Acad Sci* 1981;362:161.
27. Chapman CR, Hill HF. Prolonged morphine self-administration and addiction liability: evaluation of two theories in a bone marrow transplant unit. *Cancer* 1989;63:1636.
28. Meuser T, Pietruck C, Radruch L, et al. Symptoms during cancer pain treatment following WHO guidelines: a longitudinal follow-up study of symptom prevalence, severity, and etiology. *Pain* 2001;93:247–257.
29. McCarberg BH, Barkin RC. Long-acting opioids for chronic pain: pharmacotherapeutic opportunities to enhance compliance, quality of life, and analgesia. *Am J Ther* 2001;8:181–186.
30. Aronoff GM. Opioids in chronic pain management: is there a significant risk of addiction? *Curr Rev Pain* 2000;4:112–121.
31. Zenz M, Strumpf M, Tryba M. Long-term opioid therapy in patients with chronic nonmalignant pain. *J Pain Symptom Manage* 1992;7:69.
32. Redmond DE, Krystal JH. Multiple mechanisms of withdrawal from opioid drugs. *Annu Rev Neurosci* 1984;7:443–478.
33. World Health Organization. Technical Report no. 516, Youth and Drugs. Geneva: World Health Organization, 1973.
34. American Psychiatric Association. *Diagnostic and statistical manual for mental disorders—IV*. Washington, DC: American Psychiatric Association, 1994.
35. Wikler A. *Opioid dependence: mechanisms and treatment*. New York: Plenum Press, 1980.
36. Halpern LM, Robinson J. Prescribing practices for pain in drug dependence: a lesson in ignorance. *Adv Alcohol Subst Abuse* 1985;5:184.
37. Dai S, Corrigal WA, Coen KM, et al. Heroin self—administration by rats: influence of dose and physical dependence. *Pharmacol Biochem Behav* 1989;32:1009.
38. Passik SD, Kirsh KL, Whitcomb L, et al. Pain clinicians' rankings of aberrant drug-taking behaviors. *J Pain Palliat Care Pharmacother* 2002;16:39–49.
39. Passik S, Kirsh KL, McDonald M, et al. A pilot survey of aberrant drug-taking attitudes and behaviors in samples of cancer and AIDS patients. *J Pain Symptom Manage* 2000;19:274–286.
40. Rinaldi RC, Steindler EM, Wilford BB, et al. Clarification and standardization of substance abuse terminology. *J Am Med Assoc* 1988;259:555.
41. Hay J, Passik SD. The cancer patient with borderline personality disorder: suggestions for symptom-focused management in the medical setting. *Psychooncology* 2000;9:91–100.
42. Khantzian EJ, Treece C. DSM—III psychiatric diagnosis of narcotic addicts. *Arch Gen Psychiatry* 1985;42:1067.
43. Grant BF, Stinson FS, Dawson DA, et al. Prevalence and co-occurrence of substance use disorders and independent mood and anxiety disorders. *Arch Gen Psychiatry* 2004;61:807–816.
44. Dunbar SA, Katz NP. Chronic opioid therapy for nonmalignant pain in patients with a history of substance abuse: report of 20 cases. *J Pain Symptom Manage* 1996;11:163.
45. Compton P, Darakjian J, Miotto K. Screening for addiction in patients with chronic pain with "problematic" substance use: evaluation of a pilot assessment tool. *J Pain Symptom Manage* 1998;16:355–363.
46. Jorgensen L, Mortensen M-J, Jensen N-H, et al. Treatment of cancer pain patients in a multidisciplinary pain clinic. *Pain Clinic* 1990;3:83.
47. Moulin DE, Foley KM. Review of a hospital-based pain service. In: Foley KM, Bonica JJ, Ventafridda V, eds. *Advances in pain research and therapy, Second International Congress on Cancer Pain*. Vol 16, New York: Raven Press, 1990:413.
48. Schug SA, Zech D, Dorr U. Cancer pain management according to who analgesic guidelines. *J Pain Symptom Manage* 1990;5:27.
49. Schug SA, Zech D, Grond S, et al. A long-term survey of morphine in cancer pain patients. *J Pain Symptom Manage* 1992;7:259.
50. Ventafridda V, Tamburini M, DeConno F. Comprehensive treatment in cancer pain. In: Fields HL, Dubner R, Cervero F, eds. *Advances in pain research and therapy, proceedings of the fourth world congress on pain*, Vol 9, New York: Raven Press, 1985:617.
51. Ventafridda V, Tamburini M, Caraceni A, et al. A validation study of the WHO method for cancer pain relief. *Cancer* 1990;59:850.
52. Walker VA, Hoskin PJ, Hanks GW, et al. Evaluation of WHO analgesic guidelines for cancer pain in a hospital-based palliative care unit. *J Pain Symptom Manage* 1988;3:145.
53. World Health Organization. *Cancer pain relief and palliative care*. Geneva: World Health Organization, 1990.
54. Health and Public Policy Committee. American College of Physicians. Drug therapy for severe chronic pain in terminal illness. *Ann Intern Med* 1983;99:870.
55. Agency for Health Care Policy and Research, U.S. Department of Health and Human Services. *Clinical practice guideline number 9: management*

of cancer pain. Washington, DC: U.S. Department of Health and Human Services, 1994.

56. Ad Hoc Committee on Cancer Pain, American Society of Clinical Oncology. Cancer pain assessment and treatment curriculum guidelines. *J Clin Oncol* 1992;10:1976.

57. American Pain Society. *Principles of analgesic use in the treatment of acute pain and cancer pain.* Skokie, IL: American Pain Society, 1992.

58. Zech DFJ, Grond S, Lynch J, et al. Validation of the World Health Organization Guidelines for cancer pain relief: a 10 year prospective study. *Pain* 1995;63:65.

59. Portenoy RK. Opioid therapy for chronic nonmalignant pain: current status. In: Fields HL, Liebeskind JC, eds. *Progress in pain research and management, Pharmacological approaches to the treatment of chronic pain: new concepts and critical issues,* Vol. 1. Seattle, WA: IASP Publications, 1994:247.

60. Kolb L. Types and characteristics of drug addicts. *Ment Hyg* 1925;9:300.

61. Pescor MJ. The Kolb classification of drug addicts. *Public Health Rep* Suppl 155: 1939.

62. Rayport M. Experience in the management of patients medically addicted to narcotics. *J Am Med Assoc* 1954;156:684.

63. Porter J, Jick H. Addiction rare in patients treated with narcotics. *N Engl J Med* 1980;302:123.

64. Perry S, Heidrich G. Management of pain during debridement: a survey of U.S. burn units. *Pain* 1982;13:267.

65. Medina JL, Diamond S. Drug dependency in patients with chronic headache. *Headache* 1977;17:12.

66. Kaiko RF, Foley KM, Grabinski PY, et al. Central nervous system excitatory effects of meperidine in cancer patients. *Ann Neurol* 1983;13:180.

67. Grove WM, Eckert ED, Heston L, et al. Heritability of substance abuse and antisocial behavior: a study of monozygotic twins reared apart. *Biol Psychiatry* 1990;27:1293.

68. Gardner-Nix JS. Oral methadone for managing chronic nonmalignant pain. *J Pain Symptom Manage* 1996;11:321.

69. Potter JS, Hennessy G, Borrow JA, et al. Substance use histories in patients seeking treatment for controlled-release oxycodone dependence. *Drug Alcohol Depend* 2004;76:213–215.

70. Macaluso C, Weinberg D, Foley KM. Opioid abuse and misuse in a cancer pain population [Abstract]. *J Pain Symptom* 1988;3:S24.

71. Gonzales GR, Coyle N. Treatment of cancer pain in a former opioid abuser: fears of the patient and staff and their influence on care. *J Pain Symptom Manage* 1992;7:246.

72. Kaplan R, Slywka J, Slagle S, et al. A titrated analgesic regimen comparing substance users and non-users with AIDS-related pain. *J Pain Symptom Manage* 2000;19:265–271.

73. Lundberg JC, Passik SD. Alcohol and cancer: a review for psycho-oncologists. *Psychooncology* 1997;6:253–266.

74. Butler SF, Budman SH, Fernandez K, et al. Validation of a screener and opioid assessment measure for patients with chronic pain. *Pain* 2004; 112:65–75.

75. Penick E, Powell B, Nickel E, et al. Comorbidity of lifetime psychiatric disorders among male alcoholics. *Alcohol Clin Exp Res* 1994;18:1289–1293.

76. Passik SD, Weinreb HJ. Managing chronic nonmalignant pain: overcoming obstacles to the use of opioids. *Adv Ther* 2000;17:70–80.

77. Passik SD, Kirsh KL, Whitcomb LA, et al. A new tool to assess and document pain outcomes in chronic pain patients receiving opioid therapy. *Clin Ther* 2004;26:552–561.

78. Passik SD, Portenoy RK, Ricketts PL. Substance abuse issues in cancer patients: part 2: evaluation and treatment. *Oncology (Huntingt)* 1998; 12:729–734.

79. Passik S, Schreiber J, Kirsh KL, et al. A chart review of the ordering and documentation of urine toxicology screens in a cancer center: do they influence patient management? *J Pain Symptom Manage* 2000;19:40–44.

80. Passik S, Theobald D. Managing addiction in advanced cancer patients: why bother? *J Pain Symptom Manage* 2000;19:229–234.

81. Ripamonti C, Groff L, Brunelli D, et al. Switching from morphine to oral methadone in treating cancer pain: what is the equianalgesic dose ratio? *J Clin Oncol* 1998;16:3216–3221.

82. Mercadante S, Sapio R, Serretta M, et al. Patient-controlled analgesia with oral methadone in cancer pain: preliminary report. *Ann Oncol* 1996; 7:613–617.

83. Carrol E, Fine E, Ruff R, et al. A four-drug pain regimen for head and neck cancers. *Laryngoscope* 1994;104:694–700.

84. Lawlor P, Turner K, Hanson J, et al. Dose ratio between morphine and methadone in patients with cancer pain: a retrospective study. *Cancer* 1998;82:1167–1173.

85. Parrino M. *State methadone treatment guidelines,* Treatment Improvement Protocol (TIP) 1 DHHS Publication No. (SMA) 93–1991. Rockville, MD: Center for Substance Abuse Treatment, 1993.

86. Zweben JE, Payte JT. Methadone maintenance in the treatment of opioid dependence: a current perspective. *West J Med* 1990;152:588–599.

87. Myrick H, Anton RF. Treatment of alcohol withdrawal. *Alcohol Health Res World* 1998;22:38–43.

88. Sonne NM, Tonnesen H. The influence of alcoholism on outcome after evacuation of subdural haematoma. *Br J Neurosurg* 1992;6:125–130.

89. Maxmen JS, Ward NG. Substance-related disorders. In: *Essential psychopathology and its treatment.* New York, NY: WW. Norton and Company, 1995:132–172.

90. Spies CD, Nordmann A, Brummer G, et al. Intensive care unit stay is prolonged in chronic alcoholic men following tumor resection of the upper digestive tract. *Acta Anaesthesiol Scand* 1996;40:649–656.

ISSUES IN PALLIATIVE CARE

CHAPTER 42 ■ EPIDEMIOLOGY AND PROGNOSTICATION IN ADVANCED CANCER

ELIZABETH B. LAMONT AND NICHOLAS A. CHRISTAKIS

One meaning of *prognosis* is a physician's estimate of the future course of a patient's disease and especially of their survival. Prognoses are important to physicians and patients in all phases of cancer care, and they inform both medical and nonmedical decisions. In early-stage disease, prognoses help physicians and patients to weigh the likely benefit of given therapies (e.g., adjuvant chemotherapy). In advanced stage disease, prognoses may be of additional importance, as they may herald a switch from primarily curative or life-prolonging care to primarily palliative care and in so doing set off a cascade of both clinical and personal decisions. Despite its importance and ubiquity, reliable prognostication in advanced disease is not straightforward. Numerous studies have revealed substantial optimistic bias in physicians' prognoses for their patients terminally ill with cancer. It seems likely that this optimistic bias may contribute to the short survival observed in patients referred for hospice care and to other types of decisions doctors and patients make near the end of life. Research that is focused on improving physicians' prognostic abilities is therefore of critical importance to palliative care.

PROGNOSTIC INACCURACY

Although prognosis is a central element of a significant amount of oncologic research, formal and explicit prognostication is not often required in the clinical care of patients with cancer. Nevertheless, there are two instances in the care of patients with advanced cancer where physicians are asked explicitly to prognosticate when they are enrolling patients on experimental chemotherapy protocols, and when they are referring patients for hospice care. Each therapy has discrete and opposite eligibility requirements pertaining to survival—that is, to be considered for enrollment on phase I experimental chemotherapy protocols, patients typically must have an estimated survival of longer than 3 months. To be considered for enrollment for hospice care under the Medicare Hospice Benefit, patients must have an estimated survival of less than 6 months. Because of these formal requirements, physicians' ability to determine fine gradations in survival among patients in their last 6 months of life may mean the difference between aggressive and palliative care.

Optimism in Formulating Prognoses

How good are physicians at determining which patients are in their last 6 months of life? The answer may be found in disparate sources of literature, that is, literature pertaining to both aggressive and palliative therapies for patients with advanced cancer. From the experimental chemotherapy literature; Janisch et al. analyzed survival data from 349 patients with advanced cancer after enrollment in phase I therapies (1). Overall, they found that the median survival was 6.5 months, well above the requisite 3 months described in most eligibility requirements. However, 25% died within 3 months (i.e., inconsistent with the prognostic standard), although very few of those with a performance status of more than 70 died before 3 months. Given the low clinical response rates associated with phase I therapies, it is unlikely that survival was enhanced by the therapies themselves. Therefore, results from this study suggest that physicians enrolling patients on phase I protocols are generally able to predict which patients have longer than 3 months to live. An alternate explanation is that other eligibility requirements, such as performance status and laboratory tests, select patients with longer than 3 months to live, obviating the utility of the physicians' prognostic assessment. Because the study was not designed to test physicians' prognostic accuracy, it is difficult to draw strong conclusions about the actual role of physicians' prognostication.

Within the palliative care literature, there are several studies specifically designed to determine physicians' prognostic accuracy in predicting survival of patients admitted to hospice programs (2–8). Investigators in these studies have measured physicians' prognostic accuracy by comparing patients' observed survival to their predicted survival (these predictions are not necessarily ones communicated to patients; rather, they are ones physicians formulate for themselves). Results of the studies, summarized in Table 42.1, show that, in aggregate, physicians' overall survival estimates tended to be incorrect by a factor of approximately three, always in the optimistic direction.

Studies of physicians' abilities to predict survival of patients terminally ill with cancer are not limited to patients in palliative care settings but have also been evaluated in ambulatory patients undergoing anticancer therapy. Mackillop and Quirt measured oncologists' prognostic accuracy in the care of their

TABLE 42.1

SUMMARY OF STUDIES COMPARING PHYSICIANS' ESTIMATED SURVIVAL TO PATIENTS' ACTUAL SURVIVAL

Primary investigator	Reference	Year	Number of doctors	Number of patients	Median estimated survival (wk)	Median actual survival (wk)	Estimated survival/Actual survival
Parkes	(2)	1972	NR	168	4.5[a]	2.5[a]	1.8
Evans	(3)	1985	3	42	NR	NR	3.2[c]
Heyse-Moore	(4)	1987	NR	50	8	2	4
Forster	(5)	1988	3	108	7[b]	3.5	2
Maltoni	(6)	1994	4	100	6	5	1.2
Christakis	(7)	2000	343	468	NR	3.4	5.3[c]

NR, not reported.
[a]Values estimated from graph in paper.
[b]Seven weeks calculated through statement in paper that survival was overestimated by 3.4 weeks on average.
[c]Ratio of mean estimated survival/mean survival.

ambulatory patients with cancer by asking them to first predict patients' likelihood of cure and then to estimate the duration of survival for those whose likelihood of cure was zero (9). At the 5-year point, patients who were alive and disease-free were termed "cured;" the dates of death of the incurable patients also were determined. The researchers reported that oncologists were highly accurate in predicting cure. That is, for subgroups of patients (not individual patients) the ratio of the observed cure rate at 5 years to the predicted cure rate was quite high, at 0.92. However, the same oncologists had difficulty predicting the length of survival of individual incurable patients. They predicted survival "correctly" for only one third of patients, with the errors divided almost equally between optimistic and pessimistic.

Optimism in Communicating Prognoses

Once a prognosis has been formulated, a physician must decide how to communicate it. This is the distinction between foreseeing and foretelling the patient's future (10). Although, as noted in the preceding text, there is unconscious optimism in the prognoses physicians formulate regarding the survival

of their patients' with advanced cancer, there is also additional—and conscious—optimism in the prognoses physicians subsequently communicate to their patients. For example, one study asked physicians referring patients terminally ill with cancer for hospice care, how long they thought the patient had to live and also what prognosis, if any, they would provide to their patient if the patient inquired (11). It found that the median survival the physicians would communicate to patients was 90 days, their median formulated survival was 75 days, and the median observed survival was 24 days. This study revealed that the prognoses patients hear from their physicians may be more optimistic than what their physicians actually believe, which again is more optimistic than what actually occurs. Figure 42.1 shows the relationship between these three types of prognoses (communicated, formulated, and observed).

In sum, although physicians are asked to foresee gradations of survival in patients with advanced cancer enrolling in certain therapies (either aggressive or palliative), they are able to do so accurately less than a third of the time and, when in error, they generally tend to overestimate survival. This overestimation in formulated survival is compounded by an overestimation of communicated survival. Therefore, through their physicians' stepwise prognostic errors, patients with advanced-stage cancer may become twice removed from the reality of their survival, both times toward a falsely optimistic prognosis.

PROGNOSTIC ACCURACY

Within palliative care, there is a growing literature focused on identifying predictors of survival of patients with advanced cancer that might aid physicians in their prognostic estimates for similar patients. This literature is motivated not only by the centrality of prognosis to the care of such patients but also by physicians' inability to prognosticate accurately and their discomfort in doing so. Multiple prospective and retrospective cohort studies have consistently identified three broad classes of survival predictors: patients' performance status, patients' clinical signs and symptoms, and physicians' clinical predictions. New research seeks to increase the predictive yield of these clinical factors through models of increasing complexity that integrate these elements with each other and with new elements into easy-to-use composite measures. Additional new research in the broader oncologic arena of translational research seeks to exploit survival aspects of new biological markers [i.e., molecular (e.g., BCR-ABL

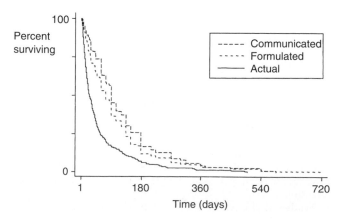

FIGURE 42.1. Relationship between physicians' communicated and formulated prognoses and the actual survival of their patients with advanced cancer after referral to hospice palliative care. (From Lamont EB, Christakis NA. Prognostic disclosure to patients with cancer near the end of life. *Ann Intern Med* 2001;134(12):1096–1105, with permission.)

TABLE 42.2

KARNOFSKY PERFORMANCE STATUS SCALE

Value	Level of functional capacity
100	Normal, no complaints, no evidence of disease
90	Able to carry on normal activity; minor signs or symptoms of disease
80	Normal activity with effort; some signs or symptoms of disease
70	Cares for self, unable to carry on normal activity or to do active work
60	Requires occasional assistance, but is able to care for most needs
50	Requires considerable assistance and frequent medical care
40	Disabled, requires special care and assistance
30	Severely disabled, hospitalization is indicated although death is not imminent
20	Hospitalization is necessary, very sick, active supportive treatment necessary
10	Moribund, fatal processes progressing rapidly
0	Dead

rearrangement in chronic myelogenous leukemia (12), EGFR mutations in non–small cell lung cancer (13))].

Performance Status

A performance status is a global measure of a patient's functional capacity. Because it has been consistently found to predict survival in patients with cancer, it is frequently used as a selection criteria for patients entering clinical trials and also as an adjustment factor in the subsequent analyses of treatment effect (14). Several different metrics have been developed to quantify performance status, and among them, the Karnofsky performance status (KPS) is the most often used. The KPS ranges from values of 100, signifying normal functional status with no complaints or evidence of disease, to zero, signifying death. The complete spectrum of values for the KPS scale is reproduced in Table 42.2.

Multiple studies have reported associations between survival of patients' with cancer and their performance status (1,3,6,15–28). The direction of the association is positive—that is, as a patient's performance status declines, so, too, does their survival. The magnitude of the association is described differently in different studies depending on the statistical methods used, but several studies report that among patients enrolled in palliative care programs, a KPS of less than 50% suggests a life expectancy of fewer than 8 weeks (3,6,15,17,28,29). The association between KPS value and survival in patients with advanced cancer enrolled in palliative care programs is described in Table 42.3.

Patients' Signs and Symptoms

Patients' clinical signs and symptoms have also been studied with respect to survival in advanced cancer. The usefulness of such indicators, even in preference to biological details of a patient's condition, was first outlined in a classic paper by Alvan Feinstein in 1966 (32,33). Recently, at least two groups have engaged this topic in their systematic reviews of prognostic factors in advanced cancer (34,35). In examining 136 different variables from 22 studies; Vigano et al. found that, after performance status; specific signs and symptoms were the next best predictors of patient survival (34). The presence of dyspnea, dysphagia, weight loss, xerostomia, anorexia, and cognitive impairment had the most compelling evidence for independent association with patient survival in these studies. Table 42.3 contains the range of median survivals for the various symptoms reported in univariate analyses from these and other studies.

For example, numerous investigators have documented that dyspnea is inversely associated with survival in this patient population (15,17,27,36,37). The presence of dyspnea is associated with a survival of fewer than 30 days according to work by Maltoni et al. (15). Other investigators have described dyspnea as doubling the hazard of death (36). Similarly, others have shown inverse associations between dysphagia and survival (15,17,37,38), with Maltoni et al. describing an associated median survival of fewer than 30 days (15). Anorexia, confusion, and xerostomia are also inversely associated with survival, with median survival times of fewer than 60 days (15,29,30). These findings suggest that for patients with advanced cancer such as those referred to palliative care programs; the presence or absence of these symptoms may help physicians to estimate patient survival (Table 42.4).

Several groups of investigators have evaluated associations between biological markers (i.e., laboratory values) and survival in advanced patients with advanced cancer. For example, in their retrospective analysis of 339 phase I chemotherapy

TABLE 42.3

PREDICTORS OF SURVIVAL WITH ADVANCED CANCER UNDER PALLIATIVE CARE

Index	Value	Median survival (d)	References
Karnofsky performance status	10–20	7–16	(3,6,15,17,28–30)
	30–40	8–50	
	≥50	50–90	
Anorexia	Present	≤58	(15,29,30)
Confusion	Present	≤38	(29,30)
Dysphagia	Present	<30	(15)
Dyspnea	Present	<30	(15)
Xerostomia	Present	<50	(30)
Leukocytosis	>8500 cells/μL	≤30	(31)
Doctor estimate	3 mo	30	(2,4,7)

TABLE 42.4

PREVALENCE OF SYMPTOMS AT THE END OF LIFE ACCORDING TO MEMORIAL SYMPTOM ASSESSMENT SCALE (MSAS)

	Inpatients ($n = 66$)[a] %	Hospice enrollees ($n = 192$)[b] %	Community dwelling decedents ≥ age 65 ($n = 969$)[c] %
Diseases represented	Metastatic cancer or stage IV lymphoma	Cancer	All (cancer and noncancer)
Respondent	Patient (self-report)	Hospice staff	Family care giver
Ascertainment, time period	Prospective, during hospital admission	Prospective, during hospice enrollment	Retrospective, during last week of life
Symptom			
Physical			
Lack of energy	83	—	92
Pain	78	86	60
Dry mouth	82	—	76
Drowsiness	74	—	82
Nausea	61	30	—
Poor appetite	61	—	84
Feeling bloated	36	—	—
Unpleasant taste	50	25	—
Constipated	48	46	44
Weight loss	29	—	—
Dizziness	29	—	—
Vomiting	41	—	—
Cough	52	—	—
Shortness of breath	38	—	60
Itchiness	24	10	—
Diarrhea	24	—	—
Difficulty swallowing	24	—	—
Psychologic			
Feeling worried	61	—	33
Difficulty sleeping	55	—	—
Feeling sad	55	—	43
Difficulty concentrating	50	42	—
Feeling nervous	41	—	23
Feeling irritable	29	38	36
Mean # symptoms/pt (mean ± SD)	10.60 ± 3.74	—	—

[a]Tranmer JE, Heyland D, Dudgeon D, et al. Measuring the symptom experience of seriously ill cancer and noncancer hospitalized patients near the end of life with the Memorial symptom assessment scale. *J Pain Symptom Manage* 2003;25(5):420–429.
[b]Kutner JS, Kassner CT, Nowels DE. Symptom burden at the end of life: hospice providers' perceptions. *J Pain Symptom Manage* 2001;21(6):473–480.
[c]Tilden VP, Tolle SW, Drach LL, et al. Out-of-hospital death: advanced care planning, decedent symptoms, and caregiver burden. *J Am Geriatr Soc* 2004;52:532–539.

patients with advanced cancer at the University of Chicago; Janisch et al. found that among routine pretreatment laboratories, only platelet count elevation and serum albumin depression were associated with shorter survivals in a multivariate model that included KPS (1). Among a sample of 207 consecutive advanced non–small cell lung patients; Muers et al. found that in addition to performance status and symptoms, lymphocyte count, albumin, sodium, and alkaline phosphatase were all predictive of survival (39). Similarly, Maltoni et al. examined 13 hematologic and urinary parameters at baseline and every 28 days in a group of 530 patients in Italian palliative care centers (31). In a multivariate model that included performance status, the investigators describe high total white blood cell count, low lymphocyte percentage, and low pseudocholinesterase as associated with diminished survival. Their Kaplan-Meier curves suggest that patients with elevated white blood cell counts (>8500 cell/μL) had median survivals of 1 month or less. The Janisch, Meurs, and Maltoni results are consistent; Janisch et al. (1) found a strong correlation between platelet count and absolute neutrophil count and therefore dropped absolute neutrophil count from the final model. There may be a similar degree of correlation between albumin and pseudocholinesterase, both serum proteins. From these studies one can conclude that there appear to be negative associations between survival and bone marrow parameters (e.g., platelets, white blood cells) as well as positive associations between survival and synthetic parameters (e.g., serum proteins) in this patient population.

Physicians' Clinical Predictions

As noted previously, numerous studies suggest that physicians' predictions regarding patients' survival in palliative care programs are frequently incorrect and that the direction of the error is almost always optimistic. However, the overly optimistic estimates *are* correlated with actual survival (6,7,40). That is, although physicians are not well-calibrated with respect to survival (i.e., they are systematically optimistic), they nevertheless, have discriminatory abilities (8,41). They are able to order patients in terms of how sick they are or how long they have to live. This fact suggests that physicians' clinical predictions may be a useful, but not exclusive, source of information regarding patient survival. Therefore, integration of clinical predictions with other known prognostic factors may be beneficial in predicting patient survival. For example, Muers et al. found that the addition of physician clinical prediction to their previously mentioned prognostic model (that contained performance status, symptoms, and laboratory values) improved the model's predictive power (39). This suggests that physicians are able to measure and quantify factors relevant to survival that are unmeasured by the previously mentioned factors. Similarly, Knaus et al. in their Study to Understand Prognoses and Preferences for Outcomes and Risks for Treatments patients, found that multivariate regression models that included physicians' prognostic estimates were more accurate than the models without the physician input (42). Hence, although it is true that statistical models can be more accurate than human intuition alone, it is also true that physicians provide valuable prognostic information that, thus far, has not been captured in the objective models (39,42,43). Such integrated models hold the greatest promise for improving physicians' predictive accuracy in patients with advanced cancer. Maltoni et al. explicitly combined this information with other known predictors of patient survival in their predictive tool (44).

Integrated Models

Investigators have also sought to model patient survival by combining and interacting these previously identified clinical predictors. Bruera et al. described a parsimonious model that combined three independently predictive elements (dysphagia, weight loss, cognitive failure) (38). They reported that the presence of all three poor prognostic factors among patients with advanced cancer admitted to palliative care predicted death within 4 weeks, with a sensitivity of 0.74 and a specificity of 0.71. In this study, this measure performed better than physicians' clinical estimates of survival.

Using data from the National Hospice Study; Reuben et al. evaluated the initial performance status and symptomatology of 1592 terminal patients with cancer admitted to hospice care and found that interacting the two survival predictors led to better prognostic modeling (17). That is, the survival associated with a given performance status depended on the number and type of additional symptoms. For example, patients with an initial KPS of 50% or more and no symptoms had a median survival of 172 days. This survival decreased to 125 days when dyspnea was also present at the initial evaluation. The survival decreased to 67 days when dyspnea, dysphagia, weight loss, and xerostomia were all present at the initial evaluation.

The most recent generation of studies describe integrated models that combine these and other prognostic variables into a single prognostic score. For example, Morita et al. developed a regression model predicting survival from performance status and certain clinical signs and symptoms (37). Coefficients from the regression were then transformed into partial scores, and summing the values of each partial score led to a final score termed the *Palliative Prognostic Index* (PPI). After developing the PPI in a sample of 150 patients, the investigators then tested the approach on a second sample of 95 patients, finding that the PPI predicted 3-week survival with sensitivity of 83% and a specificity of 85% and 6-week survival with sensitivity of 79% and a specificity of 77%. Table 42.5 contains a description of the PPI scoring system and Table 42.6 a summary of predictive relevance of PPI scores. Several other groups have developed similar scoring systems that rely on integration of all or some of the previously described classes of prognostic indicators of patients with advanced cancer and under palliative care (26,30,44). Such scoring systems need to be sensitive to a variety of methodologic concerns (33,41,45–47). Further research is ongoing to determine if these scoring systems are useful in the clinical care of patients with cancer and if they are applicable to patients who are not yet enrolled in palliative care programs or who are dissimilar from such patients (48). With respect to the clinical usefulness of the scoring systems, treating physicians will need to determine if the tools' test characteristics (e.g., sensitivity

TABLE 42.5

DESCRIPTION OF THE COMPONENTS OF THE PALLIATIVE PROGNOSTIC INDEX: A SCORING SYSTEM FOR SURVIVAL PREDICTION OF TERMINALLY ILL CANCER PATIENTS

Prognostic domains	Partial score value
Performance status	
10–20	4.0
30–50	2.5
≥60	0
Clinical symptoms	
Oral intake	1.0
Moderately reduced	2.5
Severely reduced	0
Normal	1.0
Edema	3.5
Dyspnea at rest	4.0
Delirium	

The scores from each prognostic domain are added, and the sum total is associated with a likelihood of survival either <3 weeks or >6 weeks.
From Morita T, Tsundoa J, Inoue S, et al. The palliative prognostic index: a scoring system for survival prediction of terminally ill cancer patients. *Support Care Cancer* 1999;7:128–133, with permission.

and specificity) fall above certain minimum thresholds for use in clinical decisions. Because of the issue of "zero time" (33,49) (i.e., the analytical impact of the selection of the time at which measurement of survival begins), many of the algorithms that rely on KPS, symptoms, or laboratory values obtained *after* referral to hospice may not be applicable to patients with advanced cancer *before* referral to hospice.

Prognostic Consultations

Another way for physicians to improve the accuracy of their prognostic estimates is to elicit prognostic estimates from disinterested colleagues. Through informal, "curbside" consultations or through more formal avenues such as tumor boards, physicians may find colleagues helpful in determining patient prognoses. This recommendation stems in part from results of several studies revealing that survival predictions averaged across physicians are more accurate than a prediction from a single physician (50,51) and from

TABLE 42.6

MEDIAN SURVIVAL OF PATIENTS ACCORDING TO PALLIATIVE PROGNOSTIC INDEX SCORE[a]

Palliative prognostic index score	Median survival (d)
0.0–2.0	90
2.1–4.0	61
<4.0	12

[a]Median survival value was estimated from survival curve in paper.
From Morita T, Tsundoa J, Inoue S, et al. The palliative prognostic index: a scoring system for survival prediction of terminally ill patients with cancer. *Support Care Cancer* 1999;7:128–133.

TABLE 42.7

MEDIAN SURVIVALS FROM STUDIES THAT INCLUDE UNTREATED PATIENTS

Tumor site	Histology	Dx stage	Median survival[a]	N[a]	References
Breast	NR	NR	2.3 y	1022	(50)
Colon	Adenocarcinoma	IV	5 mo	12	(56,57)
Gastric	Adenocarcinoma	IV	5 mo	30	(59)
Head and neck	Squamous cell	IV/recurrent	4 mo	808	(51)
Lung	Non–small cell	IIIb/IV	5.3 mo	57	(53)
			5.9 mo	150	(54)
Liver	Hepatocellular	NR	1 mo	127	(52,55)
Pancreas	Adenocarcinoma	NR	3 mo	39	(58)

Dx, diagnosis; NR, not reported.
[a]Values pertain to the subset of untreated patients.

results of studies that show that disinterested physicians may provide more accurate predictions (7) than physicians with an emotional or other stake in the outcome of a patient's care. This technique may improve predictive accuracy and minimize optimistic bias by enhancing the "signal-to-noise ratio" in predictions or by decreasing "ego bias."

Other Sources of Prognostic Information

Other sources of information regarding survival in advanced cancer are studies that include patients with cancer who do not undergo anticancer therapy. Both natural history studies and randomized therapy trials that include a "best supportive care" arm describe patients who do not undergo anticancer therapy. Typically, natural history studies are single institution case series of untreated patients with mortality follow up. For example, Kowalski and Carvalho described the survival pattern of patients with recurrent or metastatic squamous cell carcinoma of the head and neck (52). The median survival they report is 4 months. Others have looked at this issue in breast cancer (53) and hepatocellular cancer (54). Survival information can also be found by examining the survival of patients on the "best supportive care" arms of randomized clinical trials [e.g., trials in advanced non–small cell lung cancer (55,56), hepatocellular cancer (57), stage IV colon cancer (58,59), stage IV pancreatic cancer (60), stage IV gastric cancer (61)]. Table 42.7 contains a description of results of some of these trials (52–61).

CONCLUSION

Prognostication in advanced cancer is a difficult task that may become easier as physicians become more comfortable with the process and as researchers begin to develop better clinical prediction tools. Such efforts will help abate the pervasive and systematic optimism in both the formulated and communicated prognoses physicians develop near the end of life. Ultimately, such improvement might be evident through increasing survival times after referral to palliative care programs. As physicians' predictive accuracy improves, survival after referral to hospice may approach physicians' ideal of 3 months (62) rather than the current survival of 3 or 4 weeks (7,63). More broadly, however, such improvement may provide patients with a better understanding of their expected survival and thereby allow them to make informed medical and social choices regarding their treatment path at the end of life; whether curative or palliative (64).

ACKNOWLEDGMENT

This chapter was supported in part by a grant from the National Institutes of Health (EBL, grant #K07 CA93892 to Elizabeth Lamont, MD, MS).

References

1. Janisch L, Mick R, Schilsky RL, et al. Prognostic factors for survival in patients treated in phase I clinical trials. *Cancer* 1994;74:1965–1973.
2. Parkes EM. Accuracy of predictions of survival in later stages of cancer. *BMJ* 1972;2:29–31.
3. Evans C, McCarthy M. Prognostic uncertainty in terminal care: can the Karnofsky index help? *Lancet* 1985;1:1204–1206.
4. Heyse-Moore LH, Johnson-Bell VE. Can doctors accurately predict the life expectancy of patients with terminal cancer? *Palliat Med* 1987;1:165–166.
5. Forster LE, Lynn J. Predicting life span for applicants to inpatient hospice. *Arch Intern Med* 1988;148:2540–2543.
6. Maltoni M, Nanni O, Derni S, et al. Clinical prediction of survival is more accurate than the Karnofsky performance status in estimating life span of terminally ill cancer patients. *Eur J Cancer* 1994;6:764–766.
7. Christakis NA, Lamont EB. Extent and determinants of error in doctors' prognoses in terminally ill patients: prospective cohort study. *BMJ* 2000;320:469–473.
8. Glare P, Virik K, Jones M, et al. A systematic review of physicians' survival predictions in terminally ill cancer patients. *BMJ* 2003;327:195–200.
9. Mackillop WJ, Quirt CF. Measuring the accuracy of prognostic judgements in oncology. *J Clin Epidemiol* 1997;50:21–29.
10. Lamont EB, Christakis NA. Some elements of prognosis in terminal cancer. *Oncology* 1999;13:1165–1170.
11. Lamont EB, Christakis NA. Prognostic disclosure to cancer patients near the end of life. *Ann Intern Med* 2001;134:1096.
12. Kantarjian H, Sawyers C, Hochhaus A, et al. Hematologic and cytogenetic responses to imatinib mesylate in chronic myelogenous leukemia. *N Engl J Med* 2002;346:645–652.
13. Lynch TJ, Bell DW, Sordella R, et al. Activating mutations in the epidermal growth factor receptor underlying responsiveness of non-small-cell lung cancer to gefitinib. *N Engl J Med* 2004;350(21):2129–2139.
14. Zubrod GC, Schneiderman M, Frei E, et al. Appraisal of methods for the study of chemotherapy in man: comparative therapeutic trial of nitrogen and mustard and triethylene thiophosphoramide. *J Chronic Dis* 1960;11:7–33.
15. Maltoni M, Pirovano M, Scarpi E, et al. Prediction of survival or patients terminally ill with cancer. *Cancer* 1995;75:2613–2622.
16. Christakis NA. Timing of referral of terminally ill patients to an outpatient hospice. *J Gen Intern Med* 1994;9:314–320.
17. Reuben DB, Mor V, Hiris J. Clinical symptoms and length of survival in patients with terminal cancer. *Arch Intern Med* 1988;148:1586–1591.
18. Coates A, Porzsolt F, Osoba D. Quality of life in oncology practice: prognostic value of EORTC QLQ-C30 scores in patients with advanced malignancy. *Eur J Cancer* 1997;33:1025–1030.
19. Allard P, Dionne A, Potvin D. Factors associated with length of survival among 1081 terminally ill cancer patients. *J Palliat Care* 1995;11:20–24.
20. Rosenthal MA, Gebski VJ, Kefford RF, et al. Prediction of life-expectancy in hospice patients: identification of novel prognostic factors. *Palliat Med* 1993;7:199–204.

21. Loprinzi CL, Laurie JA, Wieand S, et al. Prospective evaluation of prognostic variables from patient-completed questionnaires. *J Clin Oncol* 1994;12:601–607.

22. Yates JW, Chalmer B, McKegney P. Evaluation of patients with advanced cancer using the Karnofsky performance status. *Cancer* 1980;45:2220–2224.

23. Mor V, Laliberte L, Morris JN, et al. The Karnofsky performance status scale. *Cancer* 1984;53:2002–2007.

24. Hyde L, Wolf J, McCracken S, et al. Natural course of inoperable lung cancer. *Chest* 1973;64:309–312.

25. McCusker J. The terminal period of cancer: definition and descriptive epidemiology. *J Chronic Dis* 1984;37:377–385.

26. Shimozuma K, Sonoo H, Ichihara K, et al. The prognostic value of quality-of-life scores: preliminary results of an analysis of patients with breast cancer. *Surg Today* 2000;30:255–261.

27. Pirovano M, Maltoni M, Nanni O, et al. A new palliative prognostic score: a first step for the staging of terminally ill cancer patients. *J Pain Symptom Manage* 1999;17:231–239.

28. Morita T, Tsundoa J, Inoue S, et al. Validity of the palliative performance scale from a survival perspective. *J Pain Symptom Manage* 1999;18:2–3.

29. Llobera J, Esteva M, Rifa J, et al. Terminal cancer: duration and prediction of survival time. *Eur J Cancer* 2000;36:2036–2043.

30. Tamburini M, Brunelli C, Rosso S, et al. Prognostic value of quality of life scores in terminal cancer patients. *J Pain Symptom Manage* 1996;11:32–41.

31. Maltoni M, Pirovano M, Nanni O, et al. Biological indices predictive of survival in 519 Italian terminally ill cancer patients. *J Pain Symptom Manage* 1997;13:1–9.

32. Feinstein AR. Symptoms as an index of biological behavior and prognosis in human cancer. *Nature* 1966;209:241–245.

33. Feinstein AR. *Clinical judgement*. Baltimore, MD: Williams & Wilkins, 1967.

34. Vigano A, Dorgan M, Buckingham J, et al. Survival prediction in terminal cancer patients: a systematic review of the medical literature. *Palliat Med* 2000;14:363–374.

35. Chow E, Harth T, Hruby G, et al. How accurate are physicians' clinical predictions of survival and the available prognostic tools in estimating survival times in terminally ill cancer patients? A systematic review. *Clin Oncol* 2001;13:209–218.

36. Hardy JR, Turner R, Saunders M, et al. Prediction of survival in a hospital-based continuing care unit. *Eur J Cancer* 1994;30A:284–288.

37. Morita T, Tsundoa J, Inoue S, et al. The palliative prognostic index: a scoring system for survival prediction of terminally ill cancer patients. *Support Care Cancer* 1999;7:128–133.

38. Bruera E, Miller MJ, Kuehn N, et al. Estimate of survival of patients admitted to a palliative care unit: a prospective study. *J Pain Symptom Manage* 1992;7:82–86.

39. Muers MF, Shevlin P, Brown J, et al. Prognosis in lung cancer: physicians' opinions compared with outcome and a predictive model. *Thorax* 1996;51:894–902.

40. Vigano A, Dorgan M, Bruera E, et al. The relative accuracy of the clinical estimation of the duration of life for patients with end of life cancer. *Cancer* 1999;86:170–176.

41. Justice AC, Covinsky KE, Berlin JA. Assessing the generalizability of prognostic information. *Ann Intern Med* 1999;16:515–524.

42. Knaus WA, Harrell FE, Lynn J, et al. The SUPPORT prognostic model. Objective estimates of survival for seriously ill hospitalized adults. *Ann Intern Med* 1995;122:191–203.

43. Lee KL, Pryor DB, Harrell FE, et al. Predicting outcome in coronary disease. Statistical models versus expert clinicians. *Am J Med* 1986;80:553–560.

44. Maltoni M, Nanni O, Pirovano M, et al. Successful validation of the palliative prognostic score in terminally ill cancer patients. *J Pain Symptom Manage* 1999;17:240–247.

45. Feinstein AR, Wells CK, Walter SD. A comparison of multivariable mathematical methods for predicting survival. I. Introduction, rationale, and general strategy. *J Clin Epidemiol* 1990;43:339–347.

46. Walter SD, Feinstein AR, Wells CK. A comparison of multivariable mathematical methods for predicting survival. II. Statistical selection of prognostic variables. *J Clin Epidemiol* 1990;43:349–359.

47. Wells CK, Feinstein AR, Walter SD. A comparison of multivariable mathematical methods for predicting survival. III. Accuracy of predictions in generating and challenge sets. *J Clin Epidemiol* 1990;43:361–372.

48. Glare PA, Eychmueller S, McMahon P. Diagnostic accuracy of the palliative prognostic score in hospitalized patients with advanced cancer. *J Clin Oncol* 2004;22(23):4823–4828.

49. Feinstein AR, Pritchett JA, Schimpff CR. The epidemiology of cancer therapy. *Arch Intern Med* 1969;123:232–344.

50. Christakis NA. *Death foretold: prophecy and prognosis and medical care*. Chicago: University of Chicago Press, 1999.

51. Poses RM, Bekes C, Winkler RL, et al. Are two (inexperienced) heads better than one (experienced) head? *Arch Intern Med* 1990;150:1874–1878.

52. Kowalski LP, Carvalho AL. Natural history of untreated head and neck cancer. *Eur J Cancer* 2000;36:1032–1037.

53. Johnstone PA, Norton MS, Riffenburgh RH. Survival of patients with untreated breast cancer. *J Surg Oncol* 2000;73:273–277.

54. Attali P, Prod'homme S, Pelletier G, et al. Prognostic factors in patients with hepatocellular carcinoma. *Cancer* 1987;59:2108–2111.

55. Cellerino R, Tummarello D, Guidi F, et al. A randomized trial of alternating chemotherapy versus best supportive care in advanced non–small cell lung cancer. *J Clin Oncol* 1991;9:1453.

56. Anderson H, Hopwood P, Stephens RJ, et al. Gemcitabine plus best supportive care (BSC) verses. BSC in inoperable non–small cell lung cancer—a randomized trial with quality of life as the primary outcome. *Br J Cancer* 2000;83:447–453.

57. CLIP Group. Tamoxifen in treatment of hepatocellular carcinoma: a randomised controlled trial. *Lancet* 1998;352:17–20.

58. Cunningham D, Glimelius B. A phase III study of irinotecan versus best supportive care in patients with metastatic colorectal cancer who have failed 5-fluorouracil therapy. *Semin Oncol* 1999;26:6–12.

59. Scheithauer W, Rosen H, Krnek GV, et al. Randomised comparison of combination chemotherapy plus supportive care with supportive care alone in patients with metastatic colorectal cancer. *BMJ* 1993;306:752–755.

60. Keating JJ, Johnson PJ, Cochrane AM, et al. A prospective randomized trial of tamoxifen and cyproterone acetate in pancreatic carcinoma. *Br J Cancer* 1989;60:789–792.

61. Glimelius B, Ekstrom K, Hoffman K, et al. Randomized comparison between chemotherapy plus best supportive care with best supportive care in advanced gastric cancer. *Ann Oncol* 1997;8:163–168.

62. Christakis NA, Iwashyna TJ. Attitude and self-reported practice regarding prognostication in a national sample of internists. *Arch Intern Med* 1998;158:2389–2395.

63. Christakis NA, Iwashyna TJ. The impact of individual and market factors on the timing of initiation of hospice terminal care. *Med Care* 2000;38:528–541.

64. Weeks JC, Cook EF, O'Day SJ, et al. Relationship between cancer patients' predictions of prognosis and their treatment preferences. *JAMA* 1998;279:1709–1714.

CHAPTER 43 ■ EPIDEMIOLOGY AND PROGNOSTICATION IN NONCANCER DIAGNOSES

DANIEL L. HANDEL AND JOYSON KARAKUNNEL

Prognostication of illness is an important part of helping health care providers in guiding treatment. Yet, the ability of health care professionals to provide this information is extremely difficult and often erroneous (1). The progression of illness has been well studied and broadly characterized by four "trajectories of an illness." These trajectories have been characterized in functional graphs, with each of the four trajectories having the following unique properties: baseline commencement, shape, and duration (2,3). Therefore, death can occur in the following ways:

1. Unexpectedly (sudden death)
2. Predictably following a steady functional decline (cancer)
3. Following a deteriorating baseline that is punctuated with health crises, each of which is followed by a partial recovery to a lower level of function (chronic illness) (2–5)
4. As the result of a long-term low level of function followed by a gradual decline through even poorer health (neurodegenerative disorders such as dementia) (6) (Fig. 43.1)

Cancer's relatively predictable functional decline can often be anticipated by the patient and the family and is well known in the hospice environment. Sudden death is by its nature unanticipated, with little opportunity for planning or anticipatory grieving. However, the family does not undergo prolonged periods of functional decline and issues brought by intermittent health crises that are common in chronic illness. In chronic illness, the gradual functional decline can be interrupted by sudden, precipitous downturns, from which the patient commonly recovers to a new and lower functional baseline. These peaks and valleys are often unpredictable and can be extremely frightening for the patient and family. This course will often end unexpectedly with a fatal event occurring during one of these valleys. The fourth and final characterization of the illness trajectory begins with a low functional level that inexorably declines to death. The function in this type of degenerative illness is chronically at a low baseline level, never recovering significantly to an improved baseline. Patients or families often endure significant suffering as functional declines dictate difficult health care decisions. The emphasis of this chapter will be on diseases that fall into the latter two categories, namely, those characterizing chronic and neurodegenerative illnesses. Chronic disease has become a growing problem in our society as treatment options expand and people survive longer with serious illness. Many of these illnesses are chronic and debilitating. Stroke is the number three killer in the United States, with an incidence of more than 700,000 strokes per year, making stroke the leading cause of debilitating disease in the United States (7). Cardiovascular disease accounts for 1 in 2.6 deaths in the United States (7). Together, these diseases account for most hospitalizations in the United States (7). The economic burden is also overwhelming to society (7). The incurability of many of these illnesses makes recovery from the diseases very unlikely. In fact, the "trajectory of illness" for these illnesses demonstrates that patients have a slow decline with little or no overall improvement before the fatal event.

Health care providers try to accurately predict the course of these illnesses. Prognostication is an important tool used by health care providers. It helps provide information for families and patients on the likely course of illness and guidance in establishing reasonable goals of care. The establishment of a likely course of the illness and goals of care facilitates informed decision making about potential treatments and interventions. In addition, good prognostication can help guide the critically important process of determining hospice appropriateness and eligibility. The decision to pursue hospice can benefit not only the patient but also society. Patients with chronic illnesses, as mentioned previously, are faced with repeated decisions regarding hospitalizations and treatments that fail to improve function or meaningfully impact medical outcomes. Prognostication and appropriate medical decision making can help alleviate the societal and personal burdens resulting from futile medical treatments.

Yet, health care providers should use caution when evaluating data that is available from several different studies (8) (Table 43.1). The limitations of these predictions are factors that hinder a provider's ability to determine the appropriate counsel and therapy at any given point in the illness. Regardless of the setting or illness, these clinical predictions are not uniformly effective (1,9,10). In addition, health care workers often give more optimistic predictions than warranted by the data (11). But there are several prognostic tools that can help in patient evaluations: the Karnofsky Performance Status Scale (KPS) (12,13) (Table 43.2), the New York Heart Association (NYHA) Functional Classification (14), the Functional Assessment Staging (FAST) scale (which can be used for a variety of symptoms) (15), and the index of activities of daily living (ADL) (16). For noncancerous illnesses, the best prognostic factors tend to be either disease-specific factors

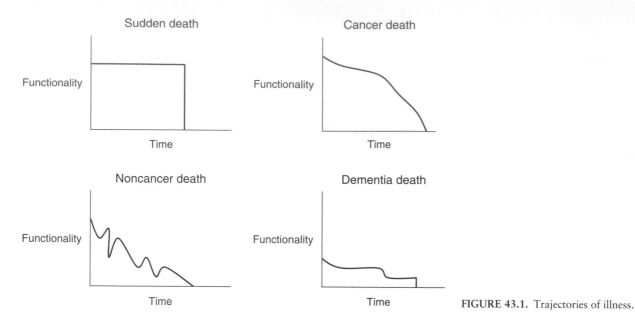

FIGURE 43.1. Trajectories of illness.

TABLE 43.1

LIMITATIONS OF PROGNOSIS STUDIES

1. Limited number of large studies with hospice patients. Most outcome measures do not include the 6-month definition of terminal illness adopted by medicare.
2. Clinical judgment should be applied to individual patients during the course of hospice as most studies look at large number of subjects *who may have significant interindividual differences*
3. Prognostication studies do not look at home-based patients
4. Studies analyze data from all stages of disease but there is limited data on prognosis in end-stage patients
5. Prognosis studies evaluate standard medical therapy vs. natural course of disease so the actual prognosis with noncurative therapy may be much longer than that predicted by prior prognosis studies that compared survival times encountered in standard medical therapy and natural course of disease
6. Hospice may prolong noncancer-related illness due to improved patient compliance, symptom control, and prevention of complications

Adapted from National Hospice Organization. *Medical guidelines for determining prognosis in selected non-cancer diseases.* Arlington, VA: National Hospice Organization, 1996.

TABLE 43.2

KARNOFSKY PERFORMANCE STATUS SCALE

Able to carry on normal activity and to work; no special care needed	100	Normal, no complaints; no evidence of disease
	90	Able to carry on normal activity; minor signs or symptoms of disease
	80	Normal activity with effort; some signs or symptoms of disease
Unable to work; able to live at home and care for most personal needs; varying amount of assistance needed	70	Cares for self; unable to carry on normal activity or to do active work
	60	Requires occasional assistance, but is able to care for most of his personal needs
	50	Requires considerable assistance and frequent medical care
Unable to care for self; requires equivalent of institutional or hospital care; disease may be progressing rapidly	40	Disabled; requires special care and assistance
	30	Severely disabled; hospital admission is indicated although death not imminent
	20	Very sick; hospital admission necessary; active supportive treatment necessary
	10	Moribund, fatal processes progressing rapidly
	0	Dead

TABLE 43.3

MEDICARE HOSPICE GUIDELINES—GENERAL CRITERIA

The patient should meet all the following criteria (20)
  I. The patient's condition is life limiting, and the patient and/or family have been informed of this determination
    A. A "life-limiting condition" may be due to a specific diagnosis, a combination of diseases, or there may be no specific diagnosis defined
  II. The patient and/or family have elected treatment goals directed toward relief of symptoms, rather than cure of the underlying disease
  III. The patient has *either* of the following
    A. Documented clinical progression of disease
      1. Progression of the primary disease, multiple emergency department visits, or inpatient hospitalizations over the prior 6 months
      2. For patients who do not qualify under 1, 2, or 3, a recent decline in functional status may be documented
        a. Functional decline should be recent, to distinguish patients who are terminal from those with reduced baseline functional status due to chronic illness. Diminished functional status may be documented by *either* of the following (21,22)
          1. Karnofsky performance status of $\leq 50\%$
          2. Dependence in at least three of six activities of daily living
    B. Impaired nutritional status related to the terminal process (23)
      1. Unintentional, progressive weight loss >10% over the prior 6 months
      2. Serum albumin <2.5 gm/dL may be a helpful prognostic indicator, but should not be used in isolation from other factors in I–III above

Adapted from National Hospice Organization. *Medical guidelines for determining prognosis in selected non-cancer diseases.* Arlington, VA: National Hospice Organization, 1996.

such as arterial blood gas levels and left-ventricular function in congestive heart failure (CHF) or global functional indicators (6-minute walk test or quality of life indicators) (17,18). The Medicare/Medicaid Hospice Benefit provides both general and disease-specific guidelines for patients who are referred to hospice. The *Medical Guidelines for Determining Prognosis in Selected Non-Cancer Disease* (19) is organized to provide general, functional indicators to assist in the assessment for hospice eligibility, coupled with specific, disease-specific guidelines that apply to particular diseases. Excerpts from these guidelines will be shared throughout this chapter to detail some important considerations in evaluating the needs and hospice appropriateness of specific conditions. It should be noted that these are not rules but rather guidelines to assist the health care provider in determining hospice eligibility. General guidelines are listed in Table 43.3.

In palliative medicine, prognosis is mainly used to guide decision making and to facilitate preparation for anticipated changes. It is also common in palliative care to give estimates in term of life events that the patient may be anticipating, that is, birthday, graduation, wedding, and so on. When answering such questions, health care providers should answer questions directly and honestly, be open about areas of uncertainty, and offer answers of hope. In cases where these goals seem to conflict with each other, the artistic practitioner openly communicates accurate information while continuing to support hope within the patient or the family. It is also important to emphasize that patients can sometimes postpone death until after an important anticipated event (such as a wedding or holiday) (24).

CONGESTIVE HEART FAILURE

CHF is a chronic illness that is associated with severe morbidity as well as mortality. Hospital admissions for patients with heart failure have risen from 1985 to 1995 (25). As therapies allow individuals to live longer, heart failure has become an illness of the elderly. Large trials such as the Framingham Heart Study have unfortunately not shown a decrease in overall death rates (26) despite therapeutic advances. Currently, because there is no curative treatment for end-stage heart failure, treatment remains palliative in nature.

Heart failure patients often endure multiple symptoms during the course of the illness and face recurrent hospitalizations. This dramatic increase in health care utilization places physical, emotional, and financial burdens on the patients, families, and society. The number of heart failure patients that comprise the hospice population is approximately 10% according to the Standards and Accreditation Committee and Medical Guidelines Task Force (8). This relatively low rate may partly be due to the lack of recognition of end stage CHF as a life-limiting disease.

Heart failure is a chronic disease that occurs after several different causes such as myocardial infarction, valvular disease, and arrhythmias. Several risk factors such as advanced age and uncontrolled blood pressure also add to the increased likelihood of developing CHF. Symptoms of heart failure stem from the decreasing functionality of the heart to maintain adequate perfusion to the body. Many symptoms such as breathlessness and edema are treated symptomatically with diuretics. The management of heart failure employs more preventive then curative strategies. For example, early control of blood pressure and angiotensin-converting enzyme (ACE) inhibitor treatment are important therapies that have been shown to increase survival in high-risk individuals. But once CHF progresses into the advanced stages, these preventative strategies are far less helpful; symptom management in advanced heart failure management mostly improves quality of life and functional outcomes. The clinical course of heart failure follows the classical trajectory of chronic illness. There is a gradually declining functional baseline, interrupted by points of crises, followed by aggressive revival to a new functional baseline that is typically lower than that previously experienced.

Functional indicators provide the most accurate measure of prognostication (25). Cardiopulmonary testing is the most

TABLE 43.4

MEDICARE HOSPICE GUIDELINES—CONGESTIVE HEART FAILURE

I. Symptoms of recurrent congestive heart failure *at rest*
   A. These patients are classified as New York Heart Association Class IV
   B. *Ejection fraction of 20% or less* is helpful supplemental objective evidence, but should not be required
II. Patients should have been *optimally treated* previously with diuretics and vasodilators, preferably angiotensin-converting enzyme inhibitors (27)
   A. The patient experiences persistent symptoms of congestive heart failure despite attempts at maximal medical management with diuretics and vasodilators
   B. "Optimally treated" means that patients who are not on vasodilators have a medical reason for refusing these drugs, for example, hypotension or renal disease
   C. Although newer β-blockers with vasodilator activity, for example, carvedilol, have recently been shown to decrease morbidity and mortality in chronic congestive heart failure, they are not included in the definition of "optimal treatment" at this time
III. In patients with refractory, optimally treated congestive heart failure as defined above, each of the following factors have been shown to decrease survival further, and therefore may help in educating medical personnel as to the appropriateness of hospice for cardiac patients (28)
   A. Symptomatic supraventricular or ventricular arrhythmias that are resistant to antiarrhythmic therapy
   B. History of cardiac arrest and resuscitation in any setting
   C. History of unexplained syncope
   D. Cardiogenic brain embolism, that is, embolic CVA of cardiac origin
   E. Concomitant human immunodeficiency virus disease

Adapted from National Hospice Organization. *Medical guidelines for determining prognosis in selected non-cancer diseases.* Arlington, VA: National Hospice Organization, 1996.

accurate measure of determining functional status but this may not necessarily be the most practical method in the advanced heart failure patient population. Guidelines which can be useful in guiding the health care provider in determining prognosis include the following: The *Medical Guidelines for Determining Prognosis in Selected Non-Cancer Disease for Congestive Heart Failure* (Table 43.4), the NYHA classification (Table 43.5) which is the most commonly used, the Minnesota living with Heart Failure questionnaire (29), and the Kansas City Cardiomyopathy questionnaire (30). These guidelines complement a practitioner's clinical judgment in determining the severity of disease.

Prognostic criteria are derived from several large heart failure trials (9,31). Yet, the evidence for prognostication is limited from these trials because of underrepresentation of women, elderly, and nonwhite individuals, as well as the propensity for such trials to focus on less advanced CHF (32). Hospice is currently employed very late in the course of this illness. This is partly because of the inability to make an accurate prognosis (33). Medicare provides guidelines for prognosis on the basis of data from clinical heart failure trials which may help resolve some of this uncertainty. Involving

palliative care early in CHF is likely to alleviate symptoms and may result in improved drug compliance, fewer hospital stays, and decreased psychosocial suffering. In fact, this may provide a transition for the patient into the hospice setting (19).

HUMAN IMMUNODEFICIENCY VIRUS

Human immunodeficiency virus (HIV) is the causative virus of acquired immunodeficiency syndrome (AIDS). According to the World Health Organization (WHO), there were 40 million people living with HIV/AIDS, 3 million HIV-/AIDS-related deaths, and 5 million new infections in 2003 worldwide. AIDS therapy and research has progressed significantly since the time that HIV was first discovered. Currently, there are multiple medications and a multitude of treatment regimens. But these advances in treatment can also produce greater side effects and pain (34).

AIDS is a disorder that is characterized by a pathologically lowered T-cell immunity. It is currently treated with the highly active antiretroviral therapy (HAART) regimen with success

TABLE 43.5

NEW YORK HEART ASSOCIATION FUNCTIONAL CLASSIFICATION

Class I	Patients with cardiac disease, but without resulting limitation of physical activity. Ordinary physical activity does not cause undue fatigue, palpitation, dyspnea, or anginal pain
Class II	Patients with cardiac disease resulting in slight limitation of physical activity. They are comfortable at rest. Ordinary physical activity results in fatigue, palpitation, dyspnea, or anginal pain
Class III	Patients with marked limitation of physical activity. They are comfortable at rest. Less than ordinary activity causes fatigue, palpitation, dyspnea, or anginal pain
Class IV	Patients with cardiac disease resulting in inability to carry on any physical activity without discomfort. Symptoms of heart failure or of the anginal syndrome may be present even at rest. If any physical activity is undertaken, discomfort is increased

TABLE 43.6

MEDICARE HOSPICE GUIDELINES—HIV

The following factors are correlated with early mortality
  I. CD4$^+$ count
    A. Patients whose CD4$^+$ count is below 25 cells/μL, measured during a period when the patient is relatively free of acute illness, may have a prognosis of <6 months, but should be followed clinically and observed for disease progression and decline in recent functional status
    B. Patients with CD4$^+$ count above 50 cells/μL who are followed by an experienced AIDS practitioner probably have a prognosis longer than 6 months unless there is a non–HIV-related coexisting life-threatening disease
  II. Viral load
    A. Patients with a persistent HIV ribonucleic acid (viral load) of >100,000 copies/mL may have a prognosis of <6 months
    B. Patients with lower viral loads may have a prognosis of <6 months if
      1. They have elected to forego antiretroviral and prophylactic medication
      2. Their functional status is declining
      3. They are experiencing complications listed in IV below

  III. Life-threatening complications with median survival
    A. Central nervous system lymphoma   2.5 months
    B. Progressive multifocal leukoencephalopathy   4 months
    C. Cryptosporidiosis   5 months
    D. Wasting (loss of 33% lean body mass)   <6 months
    E. Mycobacterium avium complex bacteremia, untreated   <6 months
    F. Visceral Kaposi's sarcoma unresponsive to therapy   6-month mortality 50%
    G. Renal failure, refuses, or fails dialysis   <6 months
    H. Advanced AIDS dementia complex   6 months
    I. Toxoplasmosis   6 months
  IV. The following factors have been shown to decrease survival significantly and should be documented if present
    A. Chronic persistent diarrhea for 1 year, regardless of etiology
    B. Persistent serum albumin <2.5 gm/dL
    C. Concomitant substance abuse
    D. Age >50
    E. Decisions to forego antiretroviral, chemotherapeutic, and prophylactic drug therapy related specifically to HIV disease
    F. Congestive heart failure, symptomatic at rest

AIDS, acquired immunodeficiency syndrome; HIV, human immunodeficiency virus.

but resistance is becoming more widespread in the current therapeutic regimens. In addition, HIV is characterized by many concurrent infections because of the lowered immune status of patients. These infections not only lead to more symptoms but also to recurrent hospitalizations and further declining status. There can also be concurrent depression and psychosocial issues as the patient faces low points during the course of the illness.

Disease progress is monitored by viral load as well as functional measures. Patients with concurrent illnesses (such as lymphoma, tuberculosis, cervical cancer, and other opportunistic malignancies) have worse overall prognoses. In addition, several HIV-related malignancies have not seen a decrease with the introduction of the HAART therapy (34). Currently, Medicare guidelines provide an acceptable measure of determining life expectancy among individuals with HIV and eligibility for hospice (Table 43.6). These guidelines are based on the natural history of HIV as well as medical criteria (lab values or comorbidities) that have been well characterized in the determination of prognosis (35–37). HIV treatment has undergone vast improvements in therapy resulting in a change in the course of this disease; with these improvements the illness has changed from a rapidly terminal illness (over months) to a chronic disease (over years to decades).

CHRONIC OBSTRUCTIVE PULMONARY DISEASE

Chronic obstructive pulmonary disease (COPD) is the development of narrowing of airways that is not fully reversible (20). There are nearly a quarter million deaths due to COPD in the United States every year (21). This illness follows a similar path of functional decline to other chronic, progressive illnesses. Superimposed on this course of gradual decline, there are often periods of unexpected and sudden downturns. These are often followed by a return to a gradually declining functional baseline.

COPD is an inflammatory disease that individuals are at increased risk of in industrialized countries. This is mainly due to the increased irritants in the air. Individuals complain of increasing shortness of breath and require frequent bronchodilator therapy. COPD patients often experience acute exacerbations that require extremely aggressive therapy and possible ventilator support. This course of slowly worsening respiratory function is commonly mirrored by declines in forced expiratory volume in one second (FEV$_1$), forced vital capacity (FVC), and other measures of pulmonary obstruction. Patients die most often during periods of acute exacerbations, but may also succumb to the underlying, slowly progressive pulmonary insufficiency or to comorbid conditions.

Prognosis of COPD can be difficult to determine as illness severity has significant interindividual clinical differences during the disease course. Medicare has tried to alleviate some of the concerns by proposing guidelines for individuals who have COPD and who may be candidates for terminal care (Table 43.7). These guidelines are based on several clinical trials that have examined the prognosis of COPD (22,23,27). In addition, several other methods are being employed to try to increase precision for the predication of life expectancy. Greater focus on exercise performance testing and other functional indicators have improved prognostic accuracy. Other predictors for increased risk and poor prognosis have been determined by multivariate analysis of epidemiologic studies (21). Even with many of these guidelines, life expectancy predictions often prove incorrect (1).

RENAL DISEASE

End-stage renal disease (ESRD) is due to many causes and can be identified by several factors (Table 43.7). With the aging of the US population and advancements in medical care, there is an increased use of hemodialysis for individuals at ages that would not have heretofore even been considered (28). The increased mortality rate (24%) in this population of ESRD patients is higher than that of some types of cancer (28). It is clear that ESRD is both a chronic, incurable illness (except through transplantation) and a condition that carries a relatively high death rate.

Renal failure can be secondary to an underlying primary illness (cancer, CHF, cirrhosis) but it can also be the primary illness. It is associated with abnormally elevated blood urea nitrogen (BUN) and creatinine. Patients with chronic renal failure commonly experience fatigue and pain while also complaining about the large number of medications and time required for hemodialysis and related procedures. These prolonged dialysis visits and the multitude of medication further challenges the patient's quality of life. Pain and depression are common comorbidities as the course of dialysis is continued.

Prognosis of dialysis patients is extremely difficult to predict owing to risk factors that may have a substantial effect on the overall course (Table 43.7). Large studies have examined the relative impact of these risk factors and criteria that stratify these individuals as having a worse prognosis (38,39). Studies have indicated that it is the functional status and not comorbidities that best predicts response to chronic dialysis (40). So, importance should be placed on functional tests such as the KPS (Table 43.2).

Medicare provides guidelines for hospice eligibility (Table 43.7) in patients with renal failure. It should be kept in mind that dialysis is considered a life-prolonging intervention and so does not support the goals of hospice (when used for the hospice-qualifying diagnosis of ESRD). When the burdens associated with dialysis outweigh its benefits, the ESRD patient who elects to stop dialysis and pursue aggressive palliative care can usually be kept comfortable, through carefully managed symptoms. So, prognosis is not the solitary or most accurate predictor of a patient's need for palliative care; instead, symptoms and their impact on quality of life should prompt the palliative care consultation.

LIVER DISEASE

Chronic liver disease and cirrhosis are major causes of death in the United States. In 2003, chronic liver disease and cirrhosis were jointly ranked as the 12th cause of death, accounting for 24,000 deaths. The disease process leads to neither a sudden nor an anticipated death, but instead to a chronic illness interspersed with health crises. The patient must not only face the burdens of the disease but also simultaneously entertain the possibility of a liver transplantation. Cirrhosis and many chronic liver diseases have no known cure except for liver transplantation. As medical progress in many other disease states results in increased longevity, there follows an increase in the illnesses that can lead to liver disease. As the demand for liver transplantation increases, there is also an increasing shortage of livers that are available for patients on the transplant list (41).

Chronic liver disease can be caused by a variety of disorders, such as hepatitis, alcoholism, and genetic causes. The patient initially presents with pain or abnormal lab values. The patient develops edema, ascites, and pruritus as the disease progresses. In an effort to alleviate these symptoms, patients are diuresed and this can sometimes aggravate renal failure. Survival of patients with cirrhosis is decreased as patients begin to develop infections, renal failure, and further complications (42). Psychosocial distress may develop owing to ongoing uncertainty about the likelihood and availability of a liver transplantation.

Severity of illness for patients is mainly determined by criteria that are used to evaluate the patients for liver transplantation. Some of these evaluation methods are Child-Turcotte-Pugh (CTP) and Model for End-Stage Liver Disease (MELD) (43). These criteria are mainly of significance for transplantation. Prognosis is extremely difficult to establish in liver disease individuals (1). Medicare provides guidelines that can help a practitioner determine eligibility for hospice (Table 43.8). One of the most important criteria is that the patient may not be appropriate or eligible for transplantation. The guidelines for prognosis are results from studying the liver transplant and end-stage cirrhotic liver populations (44–46) and, therefore, may have limited applicability to other populations with chronic liver disease. Palliative consultation should be considered early in the course of this disease. Further research should be conducted to determine better prognostic measures for liver disease.

PALLIATIVE MEDICINE IN NEUROLOGIC DISORDERS
Epidemiology

Neurologic disorders are among the leading causes of death in the United States. Stroke results in 60 deaths per 100,000 in the western world. Multiple sclerosis (MS) and Parkinson's disease have high rates of prevalence, significantly chronic courses with a high symptom burdens, and both result in premature death. In both these illnesses, death often results from acute intercurrent illness, such as pneumonia, as a complication of the progressive neurologic deterioration. There is also a significant group of rare and highly lethal neurologic diseases, including amyotrophic lateral sclerosis (ALS), Huntington's disease, multiple systems atrophy (MSA), muscle disorders, and central nervous system (CNS) infections that cause, as a group, significant morbidity and mortality. These neurologic disorders broadly comprise three groups, on the basis of their time course and duration. Diseases of the most aggressive group, including progressive stroke and Creutzfeldt-Jakob disease often lead to death within days to weeks. The chronic progressive group of diseases, such as ALS, Huntington's disease, Alzheimer's disease, and muscular dystrophies, often lead to death in months to years. Whereas disease trajectories

TABLE 43.7

MEDICARE HOSPICE GUIDELINES—CHRONIC OBSTRUCTIVE PULMONARY DISEASE AND RENAL DISEASE

Chronic obstructive pulmonary disease

I. Severity of chronic lung disease documented by the following
  A. Disabling dyspnea at rest, poorly or unresponsive to bronchodilators, resulting in decreased functional activity
  B. FEV_1, after bronchodilator, <30% of predicted, is helpful supplemental objective evidence, but should not be required if not already available
  C. Progressive pulmonary disease
    1. Increasing visits to emergency departments or hospitalizations for pulmonary infections and/or respiratory failure
    2. Decrease in FEV_1 on serial testing of >40 mL/y is helpful supplemental objective evidence, but should not be required if not already available
II. Presence of cor pulmonale or right heart failure
  A. These should be due to advanced pulmonary disease, not primary or secondary to left heart disease or valvulopathy
III. Hypoxemia at rest on supplemental oxygen
  A. pO_2 ≤55 mm Hg on supplemental oxygen
  B. Oxygen saturation ≤88% on supplemental oxygen
IV. Hypercapnia
  A. pCO_2 ≥50 mm Hg
V. Unintentional progressive weight loss >10% of body weight over the preceding 6 months
VI. Resting tachycardia >100/min in a patient with known severe chronic obstructive pulmonary disease

Renal disease

I. Laboratory criteria for renal failure
  A. Creatinine clearance of <10 mL/min (<15 mL/min for patients with diabetes)
  B. Serum creatinine >8.0 mg/dL (>6.0 mg/dL for patients with diabetes)
  Notes
    1. Creatinine clearance may be estimated by using the following formula, thereby avoiding a 24-h urine collection
      Ccreat = (140 − age in y) (body weight in kilogram)/(72) (serum creat in mg/dL); multiply by 0.85 for women
    2. Blood urea nitrogen values are not used in the determination of critical renal failure, because they can be extremely elevated from prerenal azotemia due to dehydration, hypovolemia, or other causes
II. Clinical signs and syndromes associated with renal failure
III. The following clinical signs are used as criteria for beginning dialysis. For patients with end-stage renal disease who are not to be dialyzed, the following may help define hospice appropriateness
  A. Uremia: clinical manifestations of renal failure
    1. Confusion, obtundation
    2. Intractable nausea and vomiting
    3. Generalized pruritus
    4. Restlessness, "restless legs"
  B. Oliguria: urine output <400 mL/24 h
  C. Intractable hyperkalemia: persistent serum potassium >7.0 not responsive to medical management
  D. Uremic pericarditis
  E. Hepatorenal syndrome
  F. Intractable fluid overload
IV. In hospitalized patients with acute renal failure, these comorbid conditions predict early mortality
  A. Mechanical ventilation
  B. Malignancy—other organ systems
  C. Chronic lung disease
  D. Advanced cardiac disease
  E. Advanced liver disease
  F. Sepsis
  G. Immunosuppression/acquired immunodeficiency syndrome
  H. Albumin <3.5 gm/dL
  I. Cachexia
  J. Platelet count <25,000
  K. Age >75
  L. Disseminated intravascular coagulation
  M. Gastrointestinal bleeding

FEV_1, forced expiratory volume in one second.

TABLE 43.8

MEDICARE HOSPICE GUIDELINES—LIVER DISEASE

The patient should not be a candidate for liver transplantation
  I. Laboratory indicators of severely impaired liver function
     Patients with this degree of impairment have a poor prognosis. The patient should show *both* of the following
     A. Prothrombin time prolonged to >5 s over control
     B. Serum albumin <2.5 gm/dL
 II. Clinical indicators of end-stage liver disease
     The patient should show at least one of the following
     A. Ascites, refractory to sodium restriction and diuretics, or patient noncompliant
        1. Maximal diuretics generally used: spironolactone 75–150 mg/d plus furosemide ≥40 mg/d
     B. Spontaneous bacterial peritonitis
        1. Median survival 30% at 1 year; high mortality even when infection is cured initially if liver disease is severe or accompanied by renal disease
     C. Hepatorenal syndrome
        1. In patient with cirrhosis and ascites, elevated creatinine and blood urea nitrogen with oliguria (400 mL/d), and urine sodium concentration <10 mEq/L
        2. Usually occurs during hospitalization; survival generally days to weeks
     D. Hepatic encephalopathy, refractory to protein restriction and lactulose or neomycin, or patient noncompliant
        1. Manifested by decreased awareness of environment, sleep disturbance, depression, emotional lability, somnolence, slurred speech, obtundation
        2. Physical examination may show flapping tremor of asterixis, although this finding may be absent in later stages
        3. Stupor and coma are extremely late-stage findings
     E. Recurrent variceal bleeding
        1. Following initial variceal hemorrhage, one third died in hospital, one third experienced repeat hemorrhage within 6 wk; two thirds survived <12 mo
        2. Patient should have hemorrhaged *despite therapy* or refused further therapy, which currently includes the following
           a. Injection sclerotherapy or band ligation, if available
           b. Oral β-blockers
           c. Transjugular intrahepatic portosystemic shunt
III. The following factors have been shown to worsen prognosis and should be documented if present
     A. Progressive malnutrition
     B. Muscle wasting with reduced strength and endurance
     C. Continued active alcoholism, that is, >80 g ethanol/d
     D. Hepatocellular carcinoma
     E. Hepatitis B surface antigen positivity

National Hospice Organization. *Medical guidelines for determining prognosis in selected non-cancer diseases.* Arlington, VA: National Hospice Organization, 1996.

do vary, this group of diseases often leads to progressive decline in function and ultimately to death. A third group of diseases, including stroke, some cases of MS and Parkinson's disease, and persistent vegetative state lead to chronic disability.

Amyotrophic Lateral Sclerosis (ALS-Lou Gehrig's Disease)

ALS is the most common degenerative motor neuron disorder in adults, with an incidence of approximately 2/100,000 per year and a prevalence of 6–7 per 100,000. The mean age of onset is slightly <60 years, with most cases beginning in or after the fourth decade of life. Only 10% of cases survive >10 years, and the average duration of disease is 3–4 years. Unfortunately, no treatments prolong survival significantly in this disease.

This disease often presents with muscular fasciculation, weakness, and slowly progressive paresis of the voluntary muscles. A significant minority of patients have bulbar symptoms such as dysarthria (poorly articulated speech) or dysphagia (impaired swallowing) at initial presentation. Hyperreflexia and spasticity are also noted as the disease progresses, owing

to involvement in upper motor neurons (as well as peripheral nerve wasting). The main symptoms of ALS are produced, either directly or indirectly, from the motor neuron degeneration. Symptoms such as weakness and atrophy, fasciculations, spasticity, dysarthria, dyspnea (from hypoventilation), and dysphagia are caused directly from neuronal death. Symptoms such as sleep disturbance, drooling, abnormal secretions, psychologic disturbances (commonly reactive depression and anxiety), and pain are indirect consequences of neuronal degeneration. Cognitive function is usually spared, along with sphincter control and sensation. The symptom burden of this illness is high, and symptoms can often be improved but not resolved.

Palliative care is best initiated early in the course of this illness and continues throughout the disease trajectory up to bereavement counseling. Because of the multitude and burden of symptoms and the relatively rapid course of the disease, many disciplines within the palliative care team are needed. Critical abnormalities of swallow, speech, and respiratory function often herald the final stage of this disease, as death often results from respiratory or infectious complications. A retrospective review of ALS deaths provides reassuring evidence that 90% of patients died peacefully, with no choking deaths noted (47). The terminal events of this disease are heavily influenced by the types of interventions chosen by patients, such as ventilator support. When patients are not artificially ventilated, a gradual hypercapnia ensues, with declining alertness into coma and eventual death. Many patients with ALS choose to die at home and with aggressive symptom management; this is often possible. As with other progressive chronic illnesses, early palliative intervention is highly advantageous.

Stroke

Stroke encompasses a heterogeneous group of diseases that result in the interruption of blood flow to the brain. This includes such diverse conditions as brain infarct, intracranial hemorrhage, subarachnoid hemorrhage, and vasculitides, and vascular dissections. Stroke incidence varies from 0.75 per 1000 in the fourth decade to 9 per 1000 in the seventh decade of life. Stroke deaths remain near 30 per 100,000 per year in the United States.

Typical symptoms of stroke include paresis, disturbances of sensation (hypoesthesia) and special senses (diplopia, blindness, hemianopia), cognitive deficits (loss of consciousness, agitation), vomiting, and headache. The brain infarct can result from emboli from the heart, major head and brain arteries, and aorta or it can more often result from primary thrombosis of brain vessels in diabetes or peripheral vascular disease.

One of every two to three cases will present as a "stroke-in-evolution," with progression of symptoms after presentation. Approximately one in ten cases will develop severe clinical symptoms requiring urgent transfer to an intensive, tertiary care setting. Several factors are known to affect outcome, including functional score at presentation, prior stroke history, level of consciousness, and level of social support (48). Older age is a predictor of more severe strokes, as are other comorbid factors. Even in the face of healthier lifestyles, an increase in stroke rates and stroke severity is anticipated because of increasing longevity.

Several subtypes of stroke pose significant palliative problems and have greater likelihood of fatal outcomes. Basilar artery thrombosis results in infarction of the midbrain centers controlling breathing and circulation. This is a highly lethal type of stroke, and survivors often suffer significant disability, including locked-in syndrome. Selective arterial thrombolysis can be utilized in some cases, decreasing mortality by one half. Profound brain stem dysfunction often results in deep coma or loss of brain stem reflexes and often precedes death within days to weeks.

Brain stem infarction may result in "locked-in" syndrome (as discussed subsequently), where the patient is quadriplegic and yet fully alert. Eye movements are intact, but no other voluntary movement is possible. Because there is no cognitive dysfunction, patients can experience the discomfort of being "locked in" an unmoving body while being "locked out" of the outside world. The key to management of these patients is early recognition of the condition and the provision of effective methods of communication and stimulation. Recent technologic advances have made successful modes of communication possible.

Malignant middle cerebral artery infarction results from large infarctions from this major intracerebral artery. They often cause large space-occupying lesions that threaten brain stem herniation, resulting in mortality rates of 70 to 80%. Decompressive surgery can lessen mortality by >50%, and the resulting disability may not be more severe than that of other major stroke populations. However, left-sided strokes may cause major problems with global aphasia and hemiplegia.

Severe intracerebral hemorrhage results from bleeds of >50 mL of blood and portends a grave prognosis. The gravest prognoses accompany bleeds of 100 mL or more or with the comorbidities of liver dysfunction and coagulopathies.

Taken as a whole, this family of stroke diseases represents a major category that requires management of many symptoms. At least half of stroke patients report significant pain, which can result from the stroke injury or from secondary problems such as pressure ulcers or joint contractures. Equally common are cognitive impairment (most often confusion) and urinary incontinence. A decrease or loss of consciousness is often present initially and may proceed to coma. Behaviors of distress (grimacing, flexed posture, writhing, and grunting) and autonomic signs may then be the only clues to pain. Secretions are often problematic in the final stages before death and can be managed with appropriate medications and suctioning.

Multiple Sclerosis

MS is the most frequent inflammatory disorder to cause demyelination of the CNS. Its cause is still unknown, although the past decade has brought significant advances in therapy, including immunomodulatory approaches. Whereas survival is prolonged for most patients, some subgroups of MS patients have more aggressive disease, characterized by an unremitting course that causes significant functional limitations and greater mortality rates. Mortality rates increase remarkably as neurologic deficits increase. Common causes of death include complications of chronic illness such as infection, pulmonary embolism, and renal insufficiency. Suicide rates are high (up to 15% in some series) because of the burden of neurologic disabilities and resulting loss of autonomy. Pain occurs in most cases, more commonly in late disease. Painful dysesthesias, paroxysms of neuritic pain, and painful spasms are common sources of pain. Chronic central pain from lesions of the spinothalamic tract is also common, often resulting in burning sensations. Headache is also common in MS. Depression and cognitive changes are encountered and become more prevalent as disease progresses. Depression relates both to the extent of CNS involvement and the amount of steroid treatment. Pseudobulbar symptoms of pathologic crying or laughter may respond to selective serotonin reuptake inhibitors (SSRIs) or to tricyclic antidepressant medication.

Parkinson's Disease

Parkinson's disease is also an example of a degenerative neurologic disease with a long chronic course. Because there is no cure for this disease, and because there is a mounting burden of neurologic disabilities as the disease progresses, there is a need for palliative approaches to ease suffering. As disability worsens and response to therapy lessens, goals of care become relevant to most patients. Motor symptoms are very common early problems, whereas neuropsychiatric symptoms of depression, confusion, and hallucinations become more prevalent as disease progresses (49). Pain is a common problem in end-stage Parkinson's disease, due to severe stiffness and immobility (50). Constipation can also be a major source of suffering in later stages of disease. Dementia becomes increasingly frequent in advanced disease.

Dementia

Dementia is characterized by failing memory and the decline in generalized cognitive abilities in the face of clear consciousness and is among the most common diagnoses in chronic care settings. Dementias are more common in late life, and, in a

TABLE 43.9

MAJOR CAUSES OF PROGRESSIVE DEMENTIAS

Senile dementia, Alzheimer type[a]	50%
Diffuse Lewy body disease[a]	Rare
Parkinson's disease[a]	2%
Multi-infarct dementia	20%
Communicating hydrocephalus	5%
Alcoholic-posttraumatic	5%
Huntington's	5%
Intracranial mass lesions	5%
Uncommon: chronic drug abuse; degenerative dementias (spinocerebellar, amyotrophic lateral sclerosis, multiple sclerosis, Pick's, Wilson's); metabolic (hypothyroid, liver, nutritional); static dementia	8%

[a]symptomatic treatment available.
Adapted from Marshall F. In: Andreoli E, Carpenter CCJ, Griggs R et al., eds. *Cecil essentials of medicine*, 6th ed. Philadelphia, PA: WB Saunders, 2004.

series of reports involving more than 15,000 persons over the age of 60 years, the incidence of moderate or severe dementia was found to be 4.8% (51). There are >4 million patients with dementia in the United States, one third of whom have moderate to severe intellectual impairment. With the aging of western populations, it is anticipated that this family of diseases will increase in prevalence and severity over time. Whereas dementia can have multiple etiologies, it is rarely curable. Table 43.9 shows the major causes of progressive dementias.

TABLE 43.10

BEHAVIOR AND FUNCTIONAL (ADL) PROBLEMS CITED BY FAMILIES OF DEMENTED PATIENTS

Behavior	Families reporting occurrence (%)
Memory disturbance	100
Catastrophic reactions	87
Demanding or critical behavior	71
Night waking	69
Hiding things	69
Communication difficulties	68
Suspiciousness/paranoia	63
Making accusations	60
Meals	60
Daytime wandering	59
Bathing	53
Hallucinations	49
Delusions	47
Physical violence	47
Incontinence	40
Cooking	33
Hitting/aggressive behaviors	32
Driving	20
Smoking	11
Inappropriate sexual behavior	2

Adapted from Rabins PV, Mace NL, Lucas MJ. The impact of dementia on the family. *JAMA* 1982;248:333.

Behavioral issues of dementia are noted in Table 43.10. Patients initially present with one or more of these symptoms, which often worsen insidiously. Memory changes are most commonly first noticed for recent happenings. Less often, emotional disturbances such as depression or anxiety may be prominent early symptoms. Progression is usually slow and gradual; however, the symptom burden often increases dramatically during the course of the illness. Functional status appears to be the main predictor of survival in this disease. The onset of inability to ambulate independently heralds the final stage of this disease. Inability to feed oneself, severe dysphagia, food rejection, or recurrent aspiration pneumonia also indicates advanced disease (52). National Hospice Organization (NHO) criteria include the following:

1. Advanced disease (unable to walk independently and/or hold a meaningful conversation)
2. Onset of medical complications (aspiration, pneumonia, decubitus ulcers, etc.)

In the terminal phase, the patient may lose all ability to speak, move, or think. This "late vegetative phase" is associated with diffuse slowing of electroencephalographic brain waves and brain atrophy on imaging exams. Most Alzheimer's disease patients die in a helpless state of intercurrent illnesses.

PEDIATRIC DISEASES

Children who are appropriate for palliative care have different diseases compared to adult palliative care patients. Pediatric palliative care serves a wide range of diseases which fall broadly into categories of cancer, inherited congenital disorders, pulmonary diseases, and metabolic or neurologic diseases. Pediatric palliative programs work hard to admit patients as terminal diagnoses are made, so as to follow the children and their families throughout the trajectory of the illness. Consequently, the length of stay may be longer than in adult programs. In pediatric programs, the emphasis is commonly on minimizing symptoms while continuing life-prolonging interventions. It is more common for pediatric palliative programs to simultaneously prepare patients and families for the likelihood of death while continuing aggressive life-prolonging treatments.

The common final pathway in the terminal phase of incurable pediatric solid tumors, much as in adult cancers, involves disease-related symptoms and wasting syndromes. Pediatric patients with cancer are aggressively treated and often suffer greater treatment-related symptoms than adults. Pain is a commonly reported symptom, with an overall prevalence approximating 50% in many pediatric cancer case series reports. Pain that cannot be relieved using conventional treatment is intractable pain. Intractable pain that continues despite unconventional or novel treatments is known as *refractory pain*. This is rarely encountered in pediatric palliative care and may require treatments that cause sedation in order to manage pain and suffering in such circumstances. Collins (53) reports an incidence of 6% refractory pain in a series of pediatric cancers. He notes that neuropathic pain is often the reason for the refractory nature of the disease-related pain. Such conditions include spinal cord compression, nerve root invasion, leptomeningeal involvement, and plexus or peripheral nerve invasion. Instruments for symptom measurement must be developmentally appropriate in addition to being tailored to the clinical presentation. Preverbal children require behavioral measurement tools for pain and other symptoms.

Other common symptoms encountered by children with terminal illness include nausea, vomiting, lack of appetite, cough, drowsiness, nervousness, worrying, insomnia, irritability, sadness, itching, and dry mouth (54). Seizures may be of recent onset or a long-standing problem. They may be a direct complication of the terminal process (brain tumor extension or metastases) or may result from a metabolic derangement associated with the underlying terminal condition. Recent reviews emphasize the success of aggressive management in such situations (55). Spinal cord compression, as in adults, has the best results when managed expectantly and before loss of ambulation occurs. Terminal dyspnea (an uncomfortable difficulty in breathing) can result from a number of etiologies and is best managed with noninvasive supplemental ventilation, low-dose benzodiazepines and opioids (56), and cognitive-behavioral strategies (57).

Children with congenital deformities incompatible with life comprise another group served by palliative care. These children often have significant neurologic impairments, inability to feed, and impaired consciousness. Common symptoms are those mentioned earlier and also include abnormal secretions, or vomiting. These infants are commonly morphologically abnormal. Parental guilt is often an issue that requires significant education and counseling. The clinical course may be variable but is often days to weeks.

Pediatric AIDS has, similar to adult AIDS, been largely transformed from a virulent and lethal disease into a chronic illness with the advent of potent HAART. However, HAART remains somewhat less effective in children compared to similar regimens for adults. Pediatric acquisition of HIV infection remains most often through mother to infant transmission during pregnancy, delivery, or nursing. The best prevention strategy for vertical transmission of the virus (from mother to infant) remains antiretroviral prophylaxis during times of risk. The use of zidovudine (ZDV) prophylaxis during the latter two trimesters of pregnancy and delivery effectively reduced transmission by one half (58).

Symptoms of this disease in children are at least as myriad as those of adult AIDS patients. The Center for Disease Control and Prevention's (CDC's) classification system for HIV infected children reflects the stage of HIV disease and its prognosis (59). With the advent of improved therapy, more children are living into their teens and carry the burden of this chronic disease. They live with a chronic, life-limiting illness and should have palliative care available from the time of diagnosis through death. In this way, a team-oriented approach devoted to improve quality of life can support the child and family through challenging treatments and progressive illness. During the final stage of illness, many (although not all) children wish to know that they are dying and make explicit plans for their death and burial.

CONCLUSIONS

Since the development of palliative care, the study of the epidemiology of disease has contributed to the education and preparation of patients and families facing incurable illnesses while also guiding health care providers in the management of common problems. Likewise, knowledge of common symptoms and signs that herald the final stages of disease can empower health care systems to plan effective processes that lessen suffering while limiting wasted resources. Symptoms of terminal disease often stem from both disease-specific problems (e.g., dyspnea of lung cancer) as well as complications of therapy (e.g., chemotherapy-induced nausea and vomiting). Future advances in palliative medicine will likely involve a more thorough understanding of the nature, timing, and causation of symptoms and problems associated with advanced, incurable illness. Further incorporation of integrative philosophy into palliative medicine will bring a stronger focus on the patient with the illness to augment the personal strengths of that individual in coping with illness and dying.

References

1. Fox E, Landrum-McNiff K, Zhong Z, et al. Evaluation of prognostic criteria for determining hospice eligibility in patients with advanced lung, heart, or liver disease. SUPPORT Investigators. Study to understand prognoses and preferences for outcomes and risks of treatments. *JAMA* 1999;282:1638–1645.
2. Glaser BG, Strauss AL. *Awareness of dying*. Chicago: Aldine Publishing, 1965.
3. Glaser BG, Strauss AL. *Time for dying*. Chicago: Aldine Publishing, 1968.
4. Field MF, Cassel CK. *Approaching Death: Improving care at the end of life*. Washington, DC: National Academy Press, 1997.
5. Lynn J. Perspectives on care at the close of life. Serving patients who may die soon and their families: the role of hospice and other services. *JAMA* 2001;285:925–932.
6. Doyle D. *Oxford textbook of palliative medicine*, 3rd ed. Oxford: Oxford University Press, 2004;xxv, 1244.
7. American Heart Association. *Noteworthy numbers from Heart Disease and Stroke Statistics*. 2002.
8. National Hospice Organization. *Medical guidelines for determining prognosis in selected non-cancer diseases*. Arlington, VA: National Hospice Organization, 1996.
9. Support principal investigators. A controlled trial to improve care for seriously ill hospitalized patients. The study to understand prognoses and preferences for outcomes and risks of treatments (SUPPORT). *JAMA* 1995;274:1591–1598.
10. Alvarez-Fernandez B. Estimating prognosis for nursing home residents with advanced dementia. *JAMA* 2004;292:1553; author reply 1553–1554.
11. Parkes C. Accuracy of predictions of survival in later stages of cancer. *Br J Cancer* 1972;2:29–31.
12. Mor V, Laliberte L, Morris JN, et al. The Karnofsky performance status Scale. An examination of its reliability and validity in a research setting. *Cancer* 1984;53:2002–2007.
13. Evans C, McCarthy M. Prognostic uncertainty in terminal care: can the Karnofsky index help? *Lancet* 1985;1:1204–1206.
14. American Heart Association science advisory, assessment of functional capacity in clinical and research applications. *Circulation* 2000;102:1591–1597.
15. Reisberg B. Functional Assessment Staging (FAST). *Psychopharmacol Bull* 1988;24:653–659.
16. Katz S, Ford AB, Moskowitz RW, et al. Studies of illness in the AGED. The index of ADL: a standardized measure of biological and psychosocial function. *JAMA* 1963;185:914–919.
17. Witte KK, Nikitin NP, Parker AC, et al. The effect of micronutrient supplementation on quality-of-life and left ventricular function in elderly patients with chronic heart failure. *Eur Heart J* 2005;26(21):2238–2244.
18. Puhan MA, Scharplatz M, Troosters T, et al. Respiratory rehabilitation after acute exacerbation of COPD may reduce risk for readmission and mortality—a systematic review. *Respir Res* 2005;6:54.
19. Campbell DE, Lynn J, Louis TA. Medicare program expenditures associated with hospice use. *Ann Intern Med* 2004:269–277.
20. Barnes PJ. Chronic obstructive pulmonary disease. *N Engl J Med* 2000;343:269–280.
21. Hansen-Flaschen J. Chronic obstructive pulmonary disease: the last year of life. *Respir Care* 2004;49:90–97; discussion 97–98.
22. Anthonisen NR. Prognosis in chronic obstructive pulmonary disease: results from multicenter clinical trials. *Am Rev Respir Dis* 1989;140:S95–S99.
23. Hodgkin JE. Prognosis in chronic obstructive pulmonary disease. *Clin Chest Med* 1990;11:555–569.
24. Phillips DP, Smith DG. Postponement of death until symbolically meaningful occasions. *JAMA* 1990;263:1947–1951.
25. Hauptman PJ, Havranek EP. Integrating palliative care into heart failure care. *Arch Intern Med* 2005;165:374–378.
26. Jessup M, Brozena S. Heart failure. *N Engl J Med* 2003;348:2007–2018.
27. Traver GA, Cline MG, Burrows B. Predictors of mortality in chronic obstructive pulmonary disease. *Am Rev Respir Dis* 1979;119:895–902.
28. Weisbord SD, Carmody SS, Bruns FJ, et al. Symptom burden, quality of life, advance care planning and the potential value of palliative care in severely ill haemodialysis patients. *Nephrol Dial Transplant* 2003;18:1345–1352.
29. Rector TS, Cohn JN. Pimobendan Multicenter Research Group. Assessment of patient outcome with the Minnesota living with heart failure questionnaire: reliability and validity during a randomized, double-blind, placebo-controlled trial of pimobendan. *Am Heart J* 1992;124:1017–1025.
30. Soto GE, Jones P, Weintraub WS, et al. Prognostic value of health status in patients with heart failure after acute myocardial infarction. *Circulation* 2004;110:546–551.
31. Reyes AJ. Angiotensin-converting enzyme inhibitors in the clinical setting of chronic congestive heart failure. *Am J Cardiol* 1995;75:50F–55F.
32. Goodlin SJ, Hauptman PJ, Arnold R, et al. Consensus statement: palliative and supportive care in advanced heart failure. *J Card Fail* 2004;10:200–209.

33. Levenson JW, McCarthy EP, Lynn J, et al. The last six months of life for patients with congestive heart failure. *J Am Geriatr Soc* 2000;48:S101–S109.

34. Harding R, Karus D, Easterbrook P, et al. Does palliative care improve outcomes for patients with HIV/AIDS? A systematic review of the evidence. *Sex Transm Infect* 2005;81:5–14.

35. Mellors JW, Rinaldo CR Jr, Gupta P, et al. Prognosis in HIV-1 infection predicted by the quantity of virus in plasma. *Science* 1996;272:1167–1170.

36. Moore RD, Chaisson RE. Natural history of opportunistic disease in an HIV-infected urban clinical cohort. *Ann Intern Med* 1996;124:633–642.

37. Kitahata MM, Koepsell TD, Deyo RA, et al. Physicians' experience with the acquired immunodeficiency syndrome as a factor in patient's survival. *N Engl J Med* 1996;334(11):701–706.

38. Chertow GM, Christiansen CL, Cleary PD, et al. Prognostic stratification in critically ill patients with acute renal failure requiring dialysis. *Arch Intern Med* 1995;155:1505–1511.

39. United States Renal data system. Comorbid conditions and correlations with mortality risk among 3399 hemodialysis patients. *Am J Kidney Dis* 1992;20:32–38.

40. Smith C, Da Silva-Gane M, Chandna S, et al. Choosing not to dialyse: evaluation of planned non-dialytic management in a cohort of patients with end-stage renal failure. *Nephron Clin Pract* 2003;95:c40–c46.

41. Huo TI, Wu JC, Lin HC, et al. Evaluation of the increase in model for end-stage liver disease (DeltaMELD) score over time as a prognostic predictor in patients with advanced cirrhosis: risk factor analysis and comparison with initial MELD and Child-Turcotte-Pugh score. *J Hepatol* 2005;42:826–832.

42. Gines P, Cardenas A, Arroyo V, et al. Management of cirrhosis and ascites. *N Engl J Med* 2004;350:1646–1654.

43. Narain P, Rubenstein LZ, Wieland GD, et al. Predictors of immediate and 6-month outcomes in hospitalized elderly patients. The importance of functional status. *J Am Geriatr Soc* 1988;36:775–783.

44. Christensen E, Andersen PK, Fauerholdt L, et al. Updating prognosis and therapeutic effect evaluation in cirrhosis with Cox's multiple regression model for time-dependent variables. *Scand J Gastroenterol* 1986;21:163–174.

45. Albers I, Hartmann H, Bircher J, et al. Superiority of the Child-Pugh classification to quantitative liver function tests for assessing prognosis of liver cirrhosis. *Scand J Gastroenterol* 1989;24:269–276.

46. D'Amico G, Morabito A, Pagliaro L, et al. Survival and prognostic indicators in compensated and decompensated cirrhosis. *Dig Dis Sci* 1986;31:468–475.

47. Neudert C, Olicer D, Wasner M, et al. The course of the terminal phase in patients with amyotrophic lateral sclerosis. *J Neurol* 2001;248:612–616.

48. Kwakkel G, Wagenaar RC, Kollen BJ, et al. Predicting disability in stroke-a critical review of the literature. *Age Ageing* 1996;25:479–489.

49. Hoehn MM, Yahr MD. Parkinsonism: onset, progression, and mortality. *Neurology* 1967;17:427–442.

50. Quinn NP, Lang AE, Koller WC, et al. Painful Parkinson's disease. *Lancet* 1986;1:1366–1369.

51. Terry RD, Katzman R. Senile dementia of the Alzheimer type. *Ann Neurol* 1983;14:497.

52. Stern Y, Tang MX, Albert MS, et al. Predicting time to nursing home care and death in individuals with Alzheimer's disease. *JAMA* 1997;277:806–812.

53. Collins JJ, Grier HED, Kinney HC, et al. Control of severe pain in terminal pediatric malignancy. *J Pediatr* 1995;126(4):653–657.

54. Collins JJ, Devine TD, Dick GS, et al. The MSAS: validation study in children aged 10–18. *J Pain Symptom Manage* 2000;19(5):363–377.

55. Scott RC, Besag FM, Neville BG. Buccal midazolam and rectal diazepam for treatment of prolonged seizures in childhood and adolescence: a randomized trial. *Lancet* 2002;353:623–626.

56. Boyd KJ, Kelly M. Oral morphine as symptomatic treatment of dyspnea in patients with advanced cancer. *Palliat Med* 1997;11:277–281.

57. Corner J, Planth H, Hern R, et al. Non-pharmacological interventions for breathlessness in lung cancer. *Palliat Med* 1996;10(4):299–305.

58. Schaffer N, Chuachoowong R, Mock PA, et al. Bangkok Collaborative Perinatal HIV Transmission Study Group. Short-course zidovudine for perinatal HIV-1 transmission in Bangkok, Thailand: a randomized controlled trial. *Lancet* 1999;354:795–802.

59. Centers for Disease Control and Prevention. Revised classification system for human immunodeficiency virus infection in children less than 13 years of age. *MMWR Morb Mortal Wkly Rep* 1994;43(53):1–10.

CHAPTER 44 ■ DEFINITIONS AND MODELS OF PALLIATIVE CARE

J. ANDREW BILLINGS

In the past decade, palliative care has emerged as a recognized entity in American medicine, although its definition, scope, structure, clinical methods, and value remain poorly understood.

Palliative care clinicians face two troublesome issues in introducing themselves to a patient, family, or health care professional. First, the term *palliative care service* is still unfamiliar to many people. A simple, straightforward, concise explanation is called for, yet just a few words rarely suffice. Other specialists—for example, a cardiologist ("a heart doctor") or an orthopedist ("a bone surgeon")—are unlikely to be asked to define their field of expertise in more than a couple of terms, nor feel challenged by such an undertaking, yet this task regularly confront the palliative care clinician.

Second, a full explanation of palliative care, at least as defined by many in the field, necessarily refers to death, a potentially frightening topic that the patient and family, as well as the palliative care clinician, may wish to avoid, particularly in the first moments of an intake interview. The clinician, before broaching such difficult matters as end-of-life care, wants to first listen to the patient and family (1) and understand their perspectives and information preferences, while avoiding "saying something wrong." A nuanced description of palliative care services, especially for strangers facing dying, is a challenge. Phrases such as "terminal care," "life-threatening illness," "life-limiting illness," or even "seriously ill" may stick in the clinician's mouth. One searches for euphemisms in these opening moments, yet struggles to establish a relationship that is based on authenticity and measured frankness. Moreover, regardless of the simplicity and immediate acceptability of our explanations, patients and families will become familiar with the notion of palliative care as it becomes more widely available, just as they now are with hospice. Regardless of any name we chose, laypersons will associate palliative care services with death, and hence giving up, hopelessness, suffering, and other regularly shunned notions.

To complicate this awkward situation, interpretations of the meaning of palliative care and of its scope vary within the palliative and larger health care communities, reflecting the evolving nature of this not-yet-fully formed young field (2,3). The scope of palliative medicine remains an issue for debate, ranging from absurdly broad definitions as "alleviation of symptoms," "improving quality of life," or treating patients "not responsive to curative treatment" or with "complex and serious illness" to extremely narrow notions of "care in the final months of life" or a subspecialty of oncology. Approaches to identifying a final phase of life during which palliative care is appropriate—a time of "transition"—have not been clinically useful (4–7). Such differences in definition reflect frank disagreement about the appropriate scope of the field and have important implications for its future. Differences also exist across countries, and hence the focus in this chapter is on the United States, where the distinction between palliative care and hospice is a particularly important issue. The bewildering lack of consensus may be viewed generously as an early stage in the development of a field that still is formulating some of its most basic features.

Until 2004, the United States lacked elementary guidelines for palliative care programs—structure and scope of services, criteria for judging adequacy of services, standards for professional staffing and training, and so forth (8). A major step forward in the development of the field is contained in the *Clinical Practice Guidelines for Quality Palliative Care* (9), developed by the National Consensus Project for Quality Palliative Care (www.nationalconsensusproject.org), a group of over 100 representatives from the palliative care community. Along with a useful definition, discussed in the subsequent text, the document includes an overview of the field and seven domains of practice—structure and process of care; physical psychological, social, religious, spiritual, existential, cultural, ethical and legal aspects of care; and care of the imminently dying patient—each associated with specific criteria. These guidelines incorporate important previous documents, including recommendations from a variety of professional organizations in medicine and nursing, national standards developed from other countries, reports from the Institute of Medicine, *Standards of Practice for Hospice Programs* (10) from the National Hospice and Palliative Care Organization, and Initial Voluntary Program Standards for Fellowships Training in Palliative Medicine (11).

Any description of palliative care and the hospice movement should hark back to Cicely Saunders, who developed the first modern palliative care program at St. Christopher's Hospice in London (12). She described the fundamental hospice philosophy or hospice approach to care—skilled care that addressed physical, psychosocial, and spiritual needs of the patient and family—that forms the basis for palliative care programs throughout the world. Many current programs characterize themselves as a "hospice" or may use that word to indicate a freestanding unit where dying persons reside and receive care, similar to St. Christopher's Hospice. The word "hospice," however, had unacceptable connotations in French-speaking Canada, leading Balfour Mount around 1973 to coin the term *palliative care* for describing his new program at the Royal Victoria Hospital in Montreal (13), the first hospice-like unit based in an academic teaching hospital (14). "Palliative care" and the related term *palliative medicine* have become the labels of choice throughout the world for programs based on the hospice philosophy, and as discussed more fully in the subsequent text, are now being used increasingly in the United States (15–22) where hospice programs constituted a first wave of the hospice movement in this program, followed by the second wave of palliative care. "Palliative care" overlaps with "terminal care," "death-and-dying," "hospice," "end-of-life care," "thanatology," "comfort care" (23), care of "patients who may die soon and their families" (24), "supportive care" (25,26) (this term sometimes refers to comfort care, as well as to support of the compromised host or critically ill patient, particularly those suffering adverse effects of cancer treatment), and, more recently, "hospice palliative care" (21). The diversity of meanings of these terms and their unfamiliarity to many persons can bewilder patients, family members, and colleagues in the health professions.

It is worth noting here that the scope of a field need not have sharp borders, defining exclusive territory. A variety of specialists have distinctive expertise, for instance, in pain medicine, but the existence of the specialty of pain medicine does not undermine or exclude these other fields or require that they delegate particular clinical activities to specialists.

Seeking a definition for palliative care is not an idle exercise in wordsmithing, but an essential search to clarify the nature of the field. This chapter attempts to provide clarification and to stimulate further discussion about the definition and standards for palliative care.

COMMON DEFINITIONS OF PALLIATIVE CARE

... the meaning of a word is its use in the language (27).

"To palliate" literally means "to cloak." This phrase can be used to describe measures that ease suffering—that alleviate without curing—but also can connote glossing over or even giving a deceptively attractive appearance to a significant underlying problem. Therefore, for clinicians, palliation can be viewed disapprovingly as merely covering up problems. Terms such as *comfort measures only* or *palliation only* suggest withholding, passivity, or giving up, whereas "best supportive care" at least suggests high quality and action. However, as currently used in American medicine, "palliative care" has become a widely accepted term for an approach to the management of a terminal illness that focuses on symptom control and support rather than on cure or life prolongation.

Anticancer treatments, such as chemotherapy or radiation, that are used to improve quality of life without an expectation of prolonging life may be described as having "palliative intent." Interventions that were previously dismissed as ineffective in terms of such outcomes as survival, disease-free survival, tumor response, or performance status can still be valued in terms of relief of specific symptoms, psychosocial well-being, and quality of life. Such usages of the term importantly underscore the lack of clear boundaries between treatment of an underlying disease and the alleviation of symptoms. If palliative care is to assist patients at all phases of care, including a patient waiting for a transplant who is seeking a cure or life prolongation, we should avoid the vague distinctions about "curative," "life-prolonging," "improving quality of life" and about the intent or effect of conventional treatments or what we do not do, while focusing on our "value added."

Two widely cited definitions of "palliative care" deserve note. First, the World Health Organization (WHO), in its 1990 publication *Cancer Pain Relief and Palliative Care*, defined the term as "the active total care of patients whose disease is not responsive to curative treatment" (28).

This definition is not very helpful to patients and should be offensive to medical colleagues, who, it implies, deal only with inactive or partial care or with curative treatment! The term *active* is presumably included here to dispel notions that palliative care is passive or focused simply on avoiding interventions but seems to add little to the definition. What is inactive care? Palliative care clinicians certainly cannot claim special expertise in the vast number of diseases that do not respond to curative treatment. Also, ideally, our definition should focus on the positive aspects of the work, such as helping patients and families live well or promoting their quality of life. Here, the emphasis on failure—"not responsive to curative treatment"—seems unnecessarily gloomy but perhaps is fairly gentle and acceptably euphemistic. The commonly stated but problematic distinctions between palliation and curative or life-prolonging (or "life-extending") treatment (or treatment with "aggressive intent") are not invoked.

One strength of the WHO definition is the assertion that palliative care should address all forms of suffering (28): "total care." Related terms are "total pain or suffering," "holistic care," "total palliative care," and "multidimensional care." Unfortunately, such claims can sound a bit overinflated or unrealistically ambitious. *Holism* is a bankrupt term, a notion that should serve as a red light that often signals nonsense. It has lost its cachet in thoughtful social science circles (29), and the term is now regularly used synonymously with *alternative* or *complementary* medicine. Therefore, holism, rather than implying a multifaceted, inclusive vision of health and illness, often stands for an unproven or idiosyncratic approach to care and a rejection of mainline medicine. A derogatory term, *symptomatologists*, has been introduced by Kearney (30) and might be used to describe caregivers who limit their attention to physical complaints but do not address the overall suffering of the person (31). *Comprehensive care* is a preferable term, especially because it already has established meaning in health services literature and avoids pretentious or confusing implications of the other terms (32). Other characteristics of palliative care that might be related to or subsumed by the term *comprehensive* are "interdisciplinary," "coordinated," "integrated," "accessible," "case management," "disease management," and perhaps "humanistic" care.

This WHO definition and related definitions are followed by a longer attempt at clarification:

> "Control of pain, of other symptoms, and of psychological, social, and spiritual problems is paramount. The goal of palliative care is achievement of the best possible quality of life for patients and their families. Many aspects of palliative care are also applicable earlier in the course of the illness, in conjunction with anticancer treatment" (28).

These additional assertions are helpful, although they do not clearly distinguish palliative care from other clinical fields. Many clinicians recognize the importance of comfort and support in terminal disease as well as in nonterminal disease. Arguably, all of medicine can be viewed as seeking the goal of quality of life. Moreover, the association of palliative care solely with cancer is misleading.

A second definition of palliative care, used by the authors of *The Oxford Textbook of Palliative Medicine*, first published in 1993, has also been widely cited:

> "The study and management of patients with active, progressive, far-advanced disease for whom the prognosis is limited and the focus of care is the quality of life" (33).

This definition is more concise and more precise than the WHO phrases. By choosing a word such as "focus," it avoids making palliative care a conflicting or totally separate approach from "conventional," "curative," "aggressive," or "life-prolonging" measures. As discussed later, the distinction between hospice and other forms of care, as established in the United States by the Medicare Hospice Benefit, is clinically bizarre and creates a false dichotomy, suggesting that palliation can occur only in exclusion of other forms of treatment. A Canadian Palliative Care Association definition also stresses that palliative care "may be combined with therapies aimed at reducing or curing the illness, or it may be the total focus of care" (34). Indeed, palliative care has been termed elsewhere as *simultaneous care* (35) and must embrace all the "high-tech," expensive, "aggressive" measures that can enhance patient and family well-being at the end of life (36). Certainly, palliative care should not be consigned to the final days of life when other approaches are abandoned. Moreover, as John Rowe stresses:

> *"Real quality of care for these [dying] patients is not more care or even less care, but the right care... This concept... doesn't rely on emerging data from molecular biology. It is not considered to be on the cutting edge by many of our faculty. But it is, in my mind, the essence of what all of us who are physicians swore when we took the Hippocratic oath" (37).*

The Oxford text definition also suffers from jargon and confusing terminology. Who does not have a "limited" (or "unlimited") prognosis? Is this designation preferable to "incurable" or "terminal?" Who is going to attend to the subtle distinction about the disease being both active and progressive? Where is the family in this explication?

None of these definitions is brief or clear enough to answer a patient's or family member's questions: what does palliative care mean? Or, what does a palliative care service do? Indeed, the definitions may be too abstruse and too vague even for clinicians or health care policy experts who are familiar with the jargon.

PROBLEMATIC PRECEPTS OF PALLIATIVE CARE

A variety of guidelines and position statements on the care of the dying are available, as referenced in the National Consensus Project Guidelines (9). Definitions of palliative care are sometimes accompanied by precepts or clarifications (38,39). When viewed critically, many of these are meaningless, silly, grandiose, inappropriate for a health care discipline, or simply inaccurate. Although palliative care may be the standard bearer for some important aspects of modern medicine—particularly a focus on alleviating and preventing suffering, an emphasis on comprehensive care, and the use of interdisciplinary teams—many slogans should be quickly recognized as inappropriate for a discussion of a clinical specialty, regardless of its scope or the sense of mission of its advocates. Here, we should be mindful of Doyle's admonition "never to believe that we have a monopoly on care, concern, or compassion," and of hospice's tendency to "self-righteousness" (40).

Some terms and phrases that are used in definitions, precepts, and public statements about palliative care—for instance, "patient-centered care," "care *versus* cure," "whole person care," "treating the person, not the disease," "compassion," "skill," "dignity," "the art and science of caring," "recognition of patient values," or "culturally sensitive services"—may suggest important standards distinguishing good from bad palliative care but do not constitute essential parts of a definition. They may also imply that palliative care has a special claim on particular virtues. These terms simply muddy the waters and engender misgivings from even those sympathetic to the new field. For instance, although palliative care should certainly be tailored to the needs and wishes of the patient and family, this feature does not distinguish it from other fields of medicine any more than do skill or compassion. Quality of life is a concern in all areas of medicine, and any

intelligent approach to assessing quality of life requires an understanding of patients' knowledge about their condition and potential management strategies, their values, and their personal cost-benefit calculations.

The term *dignity* (as in "death with dignity") is often used, although it seems vague and potentially laden with the care providers' values (41,42). As one physician reported, "I have never been particularly dignified in the sense that so many people use that word, nor have I even cared much about it. I am not sure I will want to pursue this quality when I am dying, let alone have my care significantly influenced by other caregivers' notions of what constitutes a dignified death." Similar concerns can be raised about such terms as "develop a sense of awe," "allow natural death," "find meanings for life," or "develop a sense of worthiness," all of which may be appropriate goals for some patients, not for others. Nonetheless, spiritual issues, such as meaning, hope, transcendence, connectedness, and purpose, deserve a great deal of attention in palliative care services.

We also often read that hospice or palliative care "affirms life and regards dying as a natural process." But what does it mean not to affirm life? Do other clinicians disapprove of life or truly regard dying as an abnormal process? Ideology seems to be subtly creeping into a clinical definition. Certainly, palliative care clinicians may be less likely than other clinicians to view death as a failure or as an inevitable enemy, and may be more likely to see positive opportunities for growth and reconciliation in the face of dying. They also probably acknowledge dying more openly than many colleagues, but these attitudes cannot be definitions, any more than a proclivity to favor cardiac catheterization or surgical approaches for managing ovarian cancer defines, respectively, a cardiologist or a gynecologic oncologist.

Likewise, we regularly read that hospice or palliative care "neither hastens nor postpones death," which appears to be a statement of ideology or intentions, perhaps reflecting an aversion to euthanasia or, tellingly, to life-prolonging treatment. This maxim may reflect some of the religious orientation of the hospice movement and even its distant historical background of seeking to save souls, but does not seem appropriate for defining a field of health care. Regardless, the statement has no empirical basis and does not reflect the obvious fact that hospice or palliative care practices often postpone or hasten death. For instance, patients who are eating poorly, losing weight, and becoming progressively weakened and who then receive careful mouth care, vigorous nutritional support, expert pain control, and other comfort measures are likely to live longer (and wish to keep living longer) with these palliative interventions. Likewise, vigorous application of opioid analgesics or sedatives to treat a patient's severe pain, dyspnea, emotional suffering, or terminal distress may cause drowsiness and reduced intake of food and fluids, as well as predispose to aspiration and therefore potentially hasten death.

Finally, notions of "artificial" (as in "artificial nutrition"), "natural" (as in "allow natural death"), or "extraordinary" (as in "extraordinary measures") do not hold up under fundamental philosophical or clinical scrutiny.

HOSPICE AND PALLIATIVE CARE IN THE UNITED STATES: A PARTING OF WAYS OR A NEW COALITION?

> *"Competition is greatest between those who occupy the same position in the economy of nature" (43).*

Hospice in the United States may be viewed as the first wave of the hospice movement. In the 1960s, volunteer hospice programs brought the hospice approach to scattered communities, focusing on home care and cancer. In the early 1980s, with the institution of the Hospice Medicare Benefit that provided funding for hospice programs, the hospice movement grew dramatically, reaching a major portion of patients dying with cancer and a significant number of persons terminally ill with noncancer diagnoses. Hospice became a widely recognized feature of the health care industry. Opportunities exist for substantial growth of hospice programs, even within the current model of care (44), but around the turn of the century, when lengths of stay in hospice declined, the movement reached a point where its impact seemed confined to care in the community in the last few weeks of life, leading to new ideas about promoting the hospice approach. Palliative care is a second wave of the hospice movement, embracing the hospice philosophy of care—the "gold standard" for end-of-life care—and seeking to bring this approach to a wider group of patients than currently served by hospice programs in this country. Palliative care also seeks more actively to integrate the hospice approach into clinical practice rather than promoting a totally separate care system for selected dying persons and their families. Most palliative care practitioners in this country have not forsaken hospice, but rather are trying to apply the model more broadly and also more sensibly than currently fostered by federal and state hospice regulations and by health care insurance. All hospice care can be viewed as a segment of palliative care.

In the United States, hospice has come to mean specifically a governmentally regulated organization or program for dying persons and their families (37), typically focusing on home care and limited to patients with the following:

- An expected prognosis of 6 months or less if the disease runs its usual course
- A focus on comfort measures—this is sometimes (but not always) defined by hospice programs as a desire to forego a variety of "aggressive" and often expensive management approaches (usually including cardiopulmonary resuscitation; blood product replacement; acute care hospitalization; and some forms of radiotherapy, surgery, and chemotherapy), at least insofar as these treatment modalities are being used in an attempt to cure or prolong life rather than to palliate symptoms
- A general preference for care at home (except where inpatient hospice is available and specifically sought)
- A capacity to acknowledge a desire a focus on comfort care, as indicated by signing an enrollment form or having the form signed by a proxy
- Health insurance that covers hospice, unless the patient or family is willing to pay for services or the hospice program will provide free services

Many hospice programs also require that the patient have a primary caregiver—someone to oversee care and to be readily available to the patient in the home. Typically, although not necessarily, the primary caregiver lives in the home. Other eligibility requirements, which one hears about occasionally from patients or family members but are not embodied in federal hospice regulations or the Patient Self-Determination Act, are that the patient and family agree to forego cardiopulmonary resuscitation, calls for emergency services, and/or further hospitalization.

Moreover, as documented for home care patients with amyotrophic lateral sclerosis, although hospice staff may be perceived as more knowledgeable and empathetic than conventional home care clinicians, hospice may provide fewer hours of formal care, particularly home health aide time (45). Therefore, patients and families are often forced to choose between hospice care with insufficient home health aide support and a conventional home care approach that includes significantly more home health aide hours but less capability of providing state-of-the-art end-of-life care.

Hospice programs in the United States have more and more been boxed in by the eligibility requirements created by Medicare and other insurers and by the limitations on reimbursement that make it difficult for them to cover increasingly expensive and widely utilized treatments or provide as much home health aide time as conventional programs (46–49). Many programs have become extremely cautious with admission or recertification in the face of the threat posed by an unsympathetic and perhaps ill-conceived government audit that scrutinizes long-stay patients and those with noncancer diagnoses. Hospice programs have therefore been increasingly relegated to care in the last few weeks of life (50,51). At the same time, health maintenance organizations and insurers have attempted to "unbundle" hospice services, providing and paying for only part of the hospice package (e.g., home nursing without social service, chaplaincy, volunteers, or bereavement care).

Eligibility requirements that may make sense from a fiscal vantage for the government or insurance programs in designing the hospice benefit or in running a program under the current reimbursement scheme make little sense to a clinician concerned with overall care of the dying and their families. For instance, many patients who are receiving purely "comfort care" and seem appropriate for hospice-like services can be expected to live for years. Many "aggressive" or "high-tech" or simply expensive interventions are appropriate for patients in the very late phases of a terminal illness and should not be foregone just to qualify for comprehensive hospice home care services. The use of antiretroviral regimens or of treatments to prevent blindness from cytomegalovirus in far-advanced acquired immunodeficiency syndrome would be common examples. Similarly, patients who may be ineligible for some hospice programs because they do not have a primary caregiver may still want to receive care at home and can benefit greatly from the support offered by hospice. Patients who need the greater home health aide hours offered by conventional home care programs and therefore choose to forego hospice enrollment may wish a palliative care approach. Patients who are aversive to the word "hospice" or who are reluctant to sign forms that redefine their insurance benefits or who have difficulty acknowledging that they are imminently facing death may benefit from and should be able to receive palliative services.

Much to the dismay of palliative care providers, hospice in the United States has become a program for imminently dying persons, caring for many patients only in the last few days or week of life (5). Only a small proportion (roughly 20%) of dying persons are cared for by hospice programs in this country. Palliative care seeks involvement with patients and families as soon as the diagnosis of a life-threatening illness is confirmed, occasionally even earlier, as commonly conveyed in Figure 44.1. While undergoing curative or life-prolonging treatments, they regularly experience physical and psychosocial distress related to their underlying condition or its management. Indeed, patients with complex chronic, but not necessarily life-threatening conditions, benefit from approaches focused on comfort and support. Palliative care specialists may be needed to address such distress. Palliative care is not just for the imminently dying, nor should hospice be (52).

In the United States, the greatest threat to hospice from palliative care would seem to be the possibility that the hospice philosophy will be distorted and supplanted by the newer programs. Palliative care teams, as a generality, differ significantly from hospice teams in this country. Hospice grew up as a grassroots, counterculture, community based, nurse-led, and somewhat antiphysician, antiacademic movement with a strong emphasis on psychosocial care, spirituality, avoiding inappropriate interventions, using simple

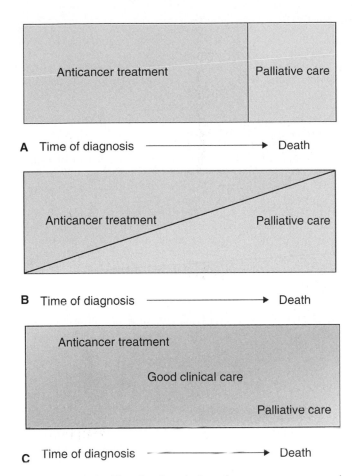

FIGURE 44.1. A: The drawing depicts the common pattern of acknowledging approaching death only in the last days of life. **B:** The drawing depicts integration of palliative care at the time of diagnosis and increased use as the disease progresses (after World Health Organization). **C:** The drawing conveys the lack of a clear boundary between anticancer treatment and palliative care.

measures for comfort, and "letting go." It retains much of this flavor today. Palliative care, on the other hand, is developing in academic centers and therefore is more "evidence-based," centered in hospitals, and often focused on inpatient care and consultation, led by physicians who see themselves as specialists, and sympathetic to a full range of treatment options in advanced illness. Notably, none of the definitions of palliative care cited earlier in this paper includes interdisciplinary care as a basic feature. ["Interdisciplinary" in some settings is used unself-consciously to describe the collaboration of two specialists (e.g., a neurologist and oncologist) but is used here to describe the breadth of the hospice team.] Therefore, social workers, chaplains, bereavement counselors, and volunteers—all required in hospice—play an uncertain role in the future of palliative care (53), although their importance has been reinforced in the Clinical Practice Guidelines for Quality Palliative Care (9). A pain- or symptom-control team that does not provide comprehensive, interdisciplinary care to patients and families may provide a needed service, but should not be confused with the ideal of palliative care. Similarly, although the impact of conventional cancer treatments on quality of life and symptom control deserves much more study, palliative cancer therapy alone is not palliative care (54). Until clear standards (as contrasted with guidelines) are established for palliative care programs, including minimum criteria for the structure of the service, valid, professionally recognized credentialing of

clinicians, and accountability for standards of quality care, any program can say, "We do that," and apprehension is inevitable that palliative care will dilute or distort the hospice philosophy and reverse the gains from the establishment of certified hospice programs in this country over the past three decades.

Hospices rightly object to terms such as "hospice-like" care because so many conventional home care programs have claimed to provide services that are equal to that of hospice but in fact do not offer many of the standard benefits of hospice, including interdisciplinary care, specially trained and supported clinicians, volunteer and bereavement services, and free medications and durable medical equipment. At the same time, some home care or hospice programs are establishing "bridge" or "prehospice" programs or specialized home care services for particular advanced diseases (e.g., heart failure, stroke) that are paid for under conventional home care and avoid some of the difficulties posed by hospice admission or recertification requirements. Bridge programs represent an effort within hospice and home care organizations to extend some hospice services to patients and family that currently are not enrolled in hospice, including patients for whom conventional home care reimbursement is more favorable (e.g., for covering repeated hospitalizations or expensive interventions). These programs may also facilitate earlier and more appropriate transfers to hospice, although this sometime stated goal has not been documented. Such bridge programs may be presented as hospice-like, but they have not been systematically studied in such a way as to assess their impact or allow a meaningful comparison with hospice care. Similar questions arise with palliative care services, which lack meaningful standards of care or accreditation of providers. Bridge programs and palliative care programs both exemplify, in part, an attempt to extend the hospice philosophy of care to more patients and families, while sidestepping the regulatory constraints of certified hospice programs, as well as the current limitations of hospice services.

Proposals from within the hospice community have attempted to deal with the constrictive hospice eligibility requirements. The National Hospice and Palliative Care Organization's Committee on the Medicare Hospice Benefit and End of Life Care has proposed that the 6-month prognosis requirement be eliminated and that alternate eligibility models be piloted. MediCaring (55) is an alternative program, using a hospice-like approach for patients with serious or complex chronic illnesses.

Many opportunities remain for cooperation among palliative care programs and hospice. Briefly, hospice is generally the home care program of choice for eligible dying patients and families. Palliative care programs provide a conduit for wider education about and earlier referrals to hospice. Insofar as many palliative care services are based in hospitals, they are generally better able than hospice programs to participate in the key treatment decisions, including the transition to comfort care, which often occur in the inpatient setting. Palliative care programs tend to be based in academic institutions and can provide broader training of physicians and other health care professionals about good end-of-life care, which includes hospice care. Few academic palliative care programs will want to start their own home hospice programs, and most will want to work closely with hospices in a variety of communities to ensure continuity of excellent care when patients are being cared for at home. Hospices are needed as training sites for students in the health professions (56). Additionally, although a great strength of hospice in the United States has been its emphasis on quality home care and the management of chronic, progressive, fatal disease, palliative medicine can contribute to care in a variety of other settings—the acute care hospital, including the intensive care unit and the emergency ward, as well as offices and extended care facilities—and has a role in deaths from acute conditions.

PALLIATIVE CARE AS A SPECIALTY

Finlay (57) suggests distinguishing the following:

- The "palliative approach" or philosophy of care, which may be viewed as a core basis of clinical work
- "Palliative interventions" that include common approaches to alleviating suffering in clinical care and are used by many clinicians
- "Specialist palliative care," which is the domain of clinicians with accredited training and implies minimum program and professional standards

(A similar distinction exists between the hospice approach or philosophy of care and hospice programs.)

Therefore, palliative care is a discipline or body of expertise and an approach to care that should infuse all medical services. Most palliative care will be provided by generalists and by specialists in established medical disciplines, such as oncology or cardiology. Some of the expertise required to provide palliative care, such as radiation therapy, interventional cardiology, or intensive care, will remain the domain of specialists in other fields. However, just as a primary care physician does not need to be a cardiologist to help a patient with congestive heart failure, a clinician does not need to be a palliative care specialist to care for terminally ill persons. Conversely, cardiologists are available to both clinicians and patients for consultation and referral, typically for helping ensure that the best possible care is being provided and to offer specialized services, where desirable. Likewise, palliative care programs and palliative medicine specialists provide the consultation and referral opportunities that will allow for broader clinical education and research in the field, and for state-of-the-art care for more terminally ill patients and their families.

Much of the discussion in this chapter, then, is meant to define specialist palliative care services. A palliative care specialist, such as a palliative medicine specialist or a palliative care nurse practitioner, is a clinician with distinctive training in this field who works in conjunction with a specially trained, interdisciplinary palliative care team. A large literature documents unmet needs of terminally ill patients and their families, as well as a lack of expertise of both generalists and other specialists in meeting these needs (21,22,58–61), so a case can easily be made for a separate discipline of palliative care that entails such features as the following:

- Diagnostic and management skills and the ability to act as a consultant to other clinicians for a multitude of illnesses and complex conditions, including syndromes that are usually seen only in the late phases of an illness
- Expertise in the pharmacologic basis for alleviating suffering, as well as in nonpharmacologic approaches
- Communication skills—widely recognized as challenging and beyond the everyday competency of most clinicians—that reflect expertise in the psychological, social, and spiritual aspects of care for patients and families, including bereavement care
- Caring for seriously ill patients in the home or other alternatives to the acute care hospital
- Team care
- Educating generalists and other specialists about palliative care
- Conducting research in palliative care

Palliative medicine has been recognized as a specialty in the United Kingdom since 1987, in Australia and New Zealand since 1988, and more recently in Canada. A variety of criteria have been cited as the requisites for identifying a distinct discipline: "a defined need, a separate and specific body of knowledge, skills, and attitudes, a shared set of principles, public acceptance, defined standards of practice, a literature devoted to the field and a research base" (58). As a fledgling field in the United States, palliative care now can boast of multiple clinical centers and training programs; a variety of fine textbooks (62), journals, and educational conferences; a small research enterprise, and a well-established board (the American Board of Hospice and Palliative Medicine) and professional organization (the American Academy of Hospice and Palliative Medicine) with a well-attended annual meeting and journal (the Journal of Palliative Medicine). The Supreme Court ruling on legalization of physician-assisted suicide has been interpreted as acknowledging a right to "good palliative care." Certainly, the justification for a new field would include an ability to address unmet patient and family needs, offer expertise with difficult cases and unfamiliar treatment methods, train health professional students and graduate clinicians, and carry out research. Recent deliberations by the American Board of Internal Medicine suggest that palliative medicine will soon be a recognized specialty under the Accreditation Council on Graduate Medical Education.

Many of the values and skills embodied in the notion of palliative care are more readily identified with generalist or primary care practice than with specialist or consultive practice. If palliative care practitioners are specialists, they **cannot** delineate their work as the following:

- Organ- or organ-system based (e.g., nephrologists principally take care of the kidney, neurologists the nervous system),
- Disease-based (e.g., oncologists principally take care of cancer), or
- Age-based (e.g., pediatricians provide general medical care to children)

However, palliative care includes (if is not exclusively about) end-of-life care, directed to dying persons and their families at all phases of terminal illness. It cannot be a subset of oncology or any other subspecialty because palliative care deals with every failing vital organ and a variety of diseases occurring at all ages. Similarly, although palliative medicine may be developing primarily as hospital consultation service (17) and might be viewed as an inpatient specialty, analogous to "intensivists" or "hospitalists," the bulk of patients requiring palliative care are outpatients most of the time. A focus only on institutional care would undermine a comprehensive approach and contribute to further fragmentation of end-of-life care.

Palliative care practitioners, then, are like generalists, providing comprehensive, accessible, first-line care, but only to a subset of patients and their families—those facing a life-threatening illness. This approach is similar to how geriatricians may define themselves as generalists for the elderly.

Regardless of the orientation of palliative care practitioners as specialists or generalists, they need to interface effectively with patients, families, and health care providers who have a variety of needs, wishes, and resources. They need to work closely and comfortably with clinical colleagues who provide the bulk of preterminal care. For instance, when a skilled, dedicated primary care provider is managing a case, the palliative care practitioner might act solely as a consultant, providing advice directly to the referring physician. Only part of the palliative care team—for instance, the social worker, chaplain, or volunteer—might become directly involved with the patient or family, complementing the work of the primary care doctor. On the other hand, if the patient is being followed, for instance, by a neurosurgeon who views his or her job as largely completed after recovery from surgery, the patient, family, and health care providers may prefer that the palliative care team assume a primary care role or major leadership role, taking responsibility for not only the management of the terminal illness but also for coordinating the input of the specialists, ensuring good communication, and overseeing general medical management. For a patient undergoing chemotherapy or radiation for a cancer, care might be comanaged with the oncologist or radiation therapist; the palliative care clinician might share some responsibility for symptom management but perhaps take a dominant role in supervising home care services or providing psychosocial and spiritual support.

From this perspective, palliative care in the United States must be flexible and collaborative (63), yet retain some responsibility for ensuring coordination of comprehensive care and, at times, providing a full range of appropriate services. Palliative care programs must have the capability of offering a spectrum of consultative and primary care services. A simple consultative approach that focuses on symptoms, particularly physical symptoms, without addressing broader psychosocial and spiritual aspects of patient and family suffering—exemplified by some pain services or pain and symptom-control teams—is neither state-of-the-art symptom control nor palliative care.

A few arguments against establishing a separate specialty of care deserve note. One concern is that terminally ill persons will become recognized as a distinct class of patients who are referred to specialists, thereby reducing the skills of generalists and other clinicians in the care of these patients, while isolating the patients from their usual health care team. Second, most of the needs of the dying are shared with other patients with "life-threatening and complex" diseases, and a smarter approach to reforming the health care system might embrace these constituents.

TYPES OF PALLIATIVE CARE PROGRAMS

In the United States currently, palliative care programs can be divided into those that are covered under a hospice benefit and those, generally labeled as palliative care services, that rely on conventional channels of reimbursement and possibly also hospice reimbursement. Programs can also be divided up according to the sites in which care is offered and whether staffing at the site is provided directly by a dedicated hospice/palliative care team or by usual clinical staff in consultation with such a team.

For state and federal certification, hospice programs are obliged to provide both home care and limited acute inpatient care. Home care may include nursing home care, and indeed, some hospices provide primarily nursing home care. Residential facilities or boarding houses run by hospice programs may provide home care in a special setting where the hospice benefit is used to pay for medical-nursing services, whereas room and board is covered by the patient or sources other than health insurance. Home care under hospice may include brief periods of "continuous care," which involves around-the-clock presence of nurses or home health aides who address a need for more intensive service. Respite care, typically offered in a nursing home setting, may also be available. Acute inpatient care may be provided: in scattered hospital beds; in a dedicated inpatient unit located in a hospital, extended care facility, or nursing home; or less frequently, in a freestanding inpatient hospice unit. Acute hospital days under hospice generally constitutes a small fraction (<5%) of the total days in hospice. Rare hospice programs in this country offer day care.

Palliative care programs in this country may assume similar configurations as provided under the hospice benefit but now generally consist of inpatient consultation teams, dedicated inpatient units of various sizes in acute care hospitals or extended care facilities, ambulatory care clinics, and specialized home care programs (including "bridge" services affiliated with a hospice). Eligibility for palliative care services tends to be much broader than under the Medicare Hospice Benefit but may include less attention to psychosocial and spiritual issues or home care, and lack appropriate reimbursement.

Most care in hospice is provided in consultation with and under the orders of a primary care physician, although a hospice medical director or other hospice physician may direct care in some programs. In palliative care, the option for primary care management of patients also exists.

ELEMENTS OF A DEFINITION

Palliative care is characterized by the following four features (Table 44.1):

1. Focusing on a particular clinical condition, variously defined as *"serious, chronic illness," "life-threatening illness,"* or *"end-of-life care."* Unlike hospice in this country, the field does not need to specify a prognosis. In describing itself as caring for the dying, euphemisms should be avoided, but a definition need not be so blunt as to frighten patients and their families (e.g., speaking about "incurable" or "terminal" disease) nor be so kindly as to become hopelessly vague (e.g., describing patients as "advanced"). For health care colleagues, *"terminal illness"* or *"end-of-life care"* are relatively clear notions and allow flexibility to participate in the earlier phases of "active, progressive" fatal conditions that eventually become "far-advanced." For patients and families, *"life-threatening illness"* may be the most appropriate and acceptable descriptor, although this term includes conditions, such as acute trauma, that are not typically within the palliative care domain.
2. Employing a distinct method of evaluation and management, a special expertise:
   - *Comprehensive* (meaning addressing all forms of suffering)
   - *Interdisciplinary* (or collaborative) care
   The terms are included here because of their importance in distinguishing the mission of this field. Admittedly, most clinical disciplines do not specify a method of care except for the generally understood distinction between medical and surgical specialties. Within a field,

TABLE 44.1

ELEMENTS DEFINING PALLIATIVE CARE AS A NEW SPECIALTY

Element	Sample term
Directed toward a particular clinical condition	*Life-threatening illness; serious, chronic illness; end-of-life care*
Employing a distinct method of evaluation and management	*Comprehensive, interdisciplinary care*
Applied to a particular set of patients	*Patient and family; the bereaved*
Focused on a specific management goal	*Promoting quality of life; alleviating and preventing suffering; living as well as possible in the face of a serious illness; comfort care*

we may hear about a "minimally invasive surgeon" or an "interventional radiologist," but all palliative care is comprehensive in scope and interdisciplinary in practice.

3. Directing care to the *patient and the family* and, by implication, extending care into the period of bereavement.

4. Focusing on a specific management goal: *promoting quality of life* (or *alleviating and preventing suffering* or, particular for patients and families, *living as well as possible*). This goal need not exclude other goals, including cure or remission. Just because you have a cardiologist does not mean that you cannot have a gastroenterologist. MacDonald summarized this concept nicely as a fourth phase of cancer prevention (64). Alternative terms that may be more acceptable to patients and families are *"comfort care"* or *"supportive care,"* although the former tends to imply passivity and withholding, as suggested by "comfort measures only," whereas the latter is regularly used to designate treatments clearly aimed at prolonging or sustaining life.

Hence, palliative care is comprehensive, interdisciplinary care for patients living with a life-threatening illness and for their families, and focusing on promoting quality of life. Key elements for helping the patient and family live as well as possible in the face of a serious condition include ensuring physical comfort, psychosocial and spiritual support, information sharing and establishing a treatment plan reflective of patient values and goals, and provision of coordinated services across sites of care.

This explication does not mention anything about supporting the service providers, an essential feature of any palliative care program, yet one that does not seem to deserve inclusion in a brief definition statement. The definition also does not specifically address the components of an interdisciplinary team and, like other definitions in the preceding text, does not specifically mention volunteers or bereavement services.

The National Consensus Project defined palliative care first in terms of its goals, although these goals—relieving suffering, enhancing quality of life, optimized function, personal growth—are not unique to the field:

> The goal of palliative care is to prevent and relieve suffering and to support the best possible quality of life for patients and their families, regardless of the stage of the disease or the need for other therapies. Palliative care is both a philosophy of care and an organized, highly structured system for delivering care. Palliative care expands traditional disease-model medical treatments to include the goals of enhancing quality of life for patient and family, optimizing function, helping with decision-making and providing opportunities for personal growth. As such, it can be delivered concurrently with life-prolonging care or as the main focus of care (9).

WHAT DO YOU SAY?

For statements that are intended primarily for clinicians and other health professionals, I speak of "comprehensive care, provided by an interdisciplinary team, for patients and families living with a life-threatening or terminal illness, particularly those aspects of care focused on living as well as possible with a serious condition." I might then go on to clarify:

> In alleviating suffering and promoting quality of life, major concerns are pain and symptom management, psychosocial and spiritual support, shared decision-making and advance care planning to address patient's values and goals, and coordination of care across multiple sites, including arranging for excellent services in the community. We also provide bereavement support for the family.

In talking with patients as a consultant, I might say:

> Palliative care is a special service to help patients and their families live as well as possible in the face of a serious or life-threatening illness. We offer a coordinated team approach—the team includes a nurse practitioner, social worker, chaplain, and physicians—who work with your current health care providers to ensure, insofar as you need it, that you and your family have access to excellent pain control and other comfort measures, get the information you want to participate in decisions about your care, receive emotional and spiritual support and practical assistance, obtain expert help in planning for care outside the hospital, continue getting good services in the community, and overall enjoy life as best you can. We try to coordinate and tailor a package of services that best suits your values, beliefs, wishes, and needs in whatever setting you are receiving care.

STANDARDS

Discussions about definitions, philosophies, or precepts can be useless if not translated into meaningful, robust standards of practice. Two kinds of standards are commonly applied: program standards, which describe the organization and delivery of palliative care services, and professional standards, which apply to the training and skills of members of the palliative care team.

Program Standards

In hospice, Medicare regulations not only provide guidance about hospice eligibility, as described in the preceding text, but also identify the members of the interdisciplinary team, prescribe regular team meetings, and indicate how services are reimbursed (65). As scant as these regulations may seem, they have been generally successful in establishing significant minimum standards for hospice programs. No standards of this sort exist for palliative care programs in this country, although the National Consensus Project *Guidelines* could readily be adopted for such a purpose. For now, anyone can use the term *palliative care service* to describe a program. Patients, families, clinicians, administrators, regulators, and policy makers have no guarantee of a minimal standard of service when referring to such a program.

Professional Standards

Disappointingly few meaningful standards exist for physician participation in a hospice or palliative care program. Anyone with a medical license can serve as a hospice medical director. Certification programs in medical and nursing aspects of palliative care (the American Board of Hospice and Palliative Medicine, the Palliative Care Nursing Society) have been developed and continue to improve. Unfortunately, the initial board examination for physicians set an extremely low standard, but the American Board of Hospice and Palliative Medicine, after certifying roughly 800 physicians, has revised its examination procedure to conform better to current standards of educational testing. Recertification is required after 10 years. The board has also worked to establish palliative medicine as a recognized medical speciality, a process that is anticipated to be completed in 2007. Fellowship training will eventually be a requirement for certification. Fellowship standards have already been established.

Do definitions and standards matter? A few examples drawn from "real life" suggest relevant issues:

- A pathologist with a deep commitment to end-of-life care but no clinical training after medical school becomes a hospice medical director.

- A long-standing palliative care program in a predominantly rural region has never had a medical director, regular physician oversight, or even routine opportunities for the clinical staff to obtain medical consultation on their patients.
- An academic palliative care program includes no regular participation from the chaplaincy and provides no organized bereavement services.
- A clinical fellowship program in palliative care enrolls only patients with cancer, whereas another serves only patients and families who meet the admission requirements for hospice in the United States.

CONCLUSION

Throughout the world now, palliative care is developing as an area of special clinical competence. The field is growing rapidly in the United States (66) and is progressing quickly to become a recognized medical specialty here. Palliative care has attracted clinicians from disparate backgrounds and interests, and hence the field currently embraces a diversity of views about its scope, goals, and methods. This diversity is a virtue. Where different viewpoints and expertise are shared, cross-fertilization occurs, and untested assumptions are challenged. However, diversity implies disagreement or conflict within the field and hence confusion for those trying to understand it on a simpler level. Diversity currently also means lack of meaningful standards. A major challenge today for palliative care is to avoid orthodoxy, yet move ahead with greater unanimity about the nature of the field and with improved standards for palliative care professionals and programs.

ACKNOWLEDGMENT

Dr. Billings is a Soros Faculty Scholar of the Open Society Institute Project on Death in America, and was supported in part by the Robert Wood Johnson Foundation. Portions of this paper were originally published as Billings JA. What is palliative care? *J Palliat Med* 1998;1:73–81.

References

1. Von Gunten CF, Ferris F, Weissman DE. *Fast facts and concepts #38. Discussing hospice.* April 2001. End-of-Life Physician Education Project. Available at http://www.eperc.mcw.edu.
2. Van Kleffens T, Van Baarsen B, Hoekman K, et al. Clarifying the term "palliative" in clinical oncology. *Eur J Cancer Care* 2004;13:263–271.
3. Levy MH. Supportive oncology-palliative care: what's in a name. *Semin Oncol* 2005;32:131–133.
4. Downing GM, Braithwaite DL, Wilde JM. Victoria BGY palliative care model–a new model for the 1990s. *J Palliat Care* 1993;9:26–32.
5. Christakis NA, Escarce JJ. Survival of medicare patients after enrollment in hospice programs. *N Engl J Med* 1996;335:172–178.
6. Lynn J, Harrell F Jr, Cohn F, et al. Prognoses of seriously ill hospitalized patients on the days before death: implications for patient care and public policy. *New Horiz* 1997;5:56–61.
7. Christakis NA, Lamont EB. Extent and determinants of error in doctors' prognoses in terminally ill patients: prospective cohort study. *BMJ* 2000; 320:469–473.
8. Ferris FD. Standards and guidelines. Do they matter? *J Pal Med* 2004; 7:750–752.
9. National Consensus Project for Quality Palliative Care. *Clinical practice guidelines for quality palliative care.* 2004. www.nationalconsensusproject. org.
10. National Hospice and Palliative Care Organization. *Standards of practice for hospice programs.* Alexandria, VA: National Hospice and Palliative Care Organization, 2000. Available at www.nhpco.org.
11. Billings JA, Block SD, Finn JW, et al. Initial voluntary program standards for fellowship training in palliative medicine. *J Palliat Med* 2002;5: 23–33.
12. Clark D. Originating a movement: Cicely Saunders and the development of St. Christopher's Hospice, 1957–1967. *Mortality* 1998;3:43–63.
13. Mount BM. The Royal Victoria Hospital Palliative Care Service: a Canadian experience. In: Saunders C Kastenbaum R. eds. *Hospice care on the international scene*, New York: Springer-Verlag, 1997:73–85.
14. Glare P. Palliative care in teaching hospitals: achievement or aberration? *Prog Palliat Care* 1998;6:4–9.
15. Walsh TD. Continuing care in a medical center: The Cleveland Clinic Foundation Palliative Care Service. *J Pain Symptom Manage* 1990;5:273–378.
16. Weissman DE, Griffie J. The palliative care consultation service of the medical college of Wisconsin. *J Pain Symptom Manage* 1994;9:474–479.
17. Weissman DE. Consultation in palliative medicine. *Arch Intern Med* 1997;157:733–737.
18. Pawling-Kaplan M, O'Connor P. Hospice care for minorities: an analysis of a hospital-based inner city palliative care service. *Am J Hosp Care* 1989;13–13.
19. Gomez CF. Hospice and home care: opportunities for training. In: *ABIM committee on evaluation of clinical competence. Caring for the dying: identification and promotion of physician competency.* Philadelphia, PA: American Board of Internal Medicine, 1996:27–30.
20. *Pioneer programs in palliative care: nine case studies.* New York: Milbank Memorial Fund, 2000:73–91.
21. Foley KM, Gelband H, eds. *Improving palliative care for cancer: summary and recommendations.* Washington, DC: National Academy Press, 2001.
22. Cassell CK, Foley KM. *Principles for care of patients at the end of life: an emerging consensus among the specialties of medicine.* New York: Milbank Memorial Fund, 1999.
23. Bascom PB. A hospital-based comfort care team: consultation for seriously ill and dying patients. *Am J Hosp Palliat Care* 1997;14:57–60.
24. Lynn J. Serving patients who may die soon and their families. The role of hospice and other services. *JAMA* 2001;285:925–932.
25. Carlson RW, Devich L, Frank RR. Development of a comprehensive supportive care team for the hopelessly ill on a university hospice medical center. *JAMA* 1988;259:378–383.
26. Berger AM, Portenoy RK, Weissman DE. Preface. In: Berger A, Portenoy RK, Weissman DE, eds. *Principles and practice of supportive oncology*, Philadelphia, PA: Lippincott Williams & Wilkins, 1998:19–20.
27. Wittgenstein L. *Philosophical investigation: the English text of the third edition*, Anscombe GEM, translator. New York: Macmillian Publishing, 1958:20.
28. World Health Organization. *Cancer pain relief and palliative care*, Technical Report Series 804. Geneva, Switzerland: World Health Organization, 1990:11.
29. Phillips DC. *Holistic thought in social science.* Stanford, CA: Stanford University Press, 1976.
30. Kearney M. Palliative medicine—just another specialty? *Palliat Med* 1992;6:39–39.
31. Cassell ES. The nature of suffering and the goals of medicine. *N Engl J Med* 1982;306:639–645.
32. Carlson RW, Devich L, Frank RR. Development of a comprehensive supportive care team for the hopelessly ill on a university hospice medical center. *JAMA* 1988;259:378–383.
33. Doyle D, Hanks GWC, MacDonald N. Introduction. In: Doyle D, Hanks GWC, MacDonald N, eds. *Oxford textbook of palliative medicine*, Oxford: Oxford University Press, 1993:3.
34. Ferris FD, Cummings I, eds, The Canadian Palliative Care Association. *Palliative care: toward a consensus in standardized principles of practice. First phase working document.* Ottawa: Canadian Palliative Care Association, 1995:12.
35. Meyers FJ, Linder J. Simultaneous care: disease treatment and palliative care throughout the illness. *J Clin Oncol* 2003;21:1412–1415.
36. Dush DM. High-tech, aggressive palliative care: in the service of quality of life. *J Palliat Care* 1993;9:37–41.
37. Rowe JW. Health care myths at the end of life. *Bull Am Coll Surg* 1996;81:11–18.
38. *Making promises: a vision of a better system.* Washington, DC: Americans for Better Care of the Dying, 1998 http://www.abcd-caring.org/tools/actionguides.htm.
39. Task Force on Palliative Care, Last Acts Campaign, Robert Wood Johnson Foundation. Precepts of palliative care. *J Palliat Med* 1998;1:109–112.
40. Doyle D. Facing the 1990's: special issues. *Hosp Update* 1990;2:1–9.
41. Street AF. Construction of dignity in end-of-life care. *J Palliat Care* 2001;17:93–101.
42. Chochinov HM, Hack T, Hassard T, et al. Dignity therapy: a novel psychotherapeutic intervention for patients near the end of life. *J Clin Oncol* 2005;23:5520–5525.
43. Darwin C. The origin of species.
44. Balsano AE, Cella PM. *The changing role of hospice and its fit in an integrated delivery system, Hospital technology special report 15(8). AHA hospital technology series.* Chicago, IL: American Hospital Association, 1996.
45. Krivickas LS, Shockley L, Mitsumoto H. Home care of patients with amyotrophic lateral sclerosis (ALS). *J Neurol Sci* 1997;152(Suppl 1):S82.
46. Billings JA. The hospice medicare benefit: an appraisal at 15 years—introduction to a series. *J Palliat Med* 1998;2:123–125.
47. Kinzbrunner BM. Hospice: 15 years and beyond in the care of the dying. *J Palliat Med* 1998;2:127–137.

48. Walsh D. The medicare hospice benefit: a critique from palliative medicine. *J Palliat Med* 1998;2:147–149.

49. Byock I. Hospice and palliative care: a parting of ways or a path to the future. *J Palliat Med* 1998;2:165.

50. *Facts and figures on hospice care in America.* Arlington, VA: National Hospice and Palliative Care Organization, 2000 http://www.nhpco.org/files/public/facts figures feb04.pdf.

51. United States General Accounting Office. *More beneficiaries use hospice but for fewer days of care,* (GAO/HEHS-00-182). Washington, DC: General Accounting Office, 2000.

52. Cleary JF, Carbone PP. Palliative medicine in the elderly. *Cancer* 1997;80:1335–1347.

53. Billings JA, Pantilat S. Survey of palliative care programs. *J Palliat Med* 2002;4:309–314.

54. Porzsolt F, Tannock I. Goals of palliative cancer therapy. *J Clin Oncol* 1993;11:378–381.

55. Skolnick AA. MediCaring project to demonstrate, evaluate innovative end-of-life program for chronically ill. *JAMA* 1998;279:1511–1512.

56. Billings JA, Block SD. Palliative care in undergraduate medical education: status report and future directions. *JAMA* 1997;278:733–738.

57. Finlay IG, Jones RVH. Definitions in palliative care. *BMJ* 1995;311:754.

58. Field MJ, Cassel CK, eds. Committee on Care at the End of Life, Division of Health Care Services, Institute of Medicine. *Approaching death: improving care at the end of life.* Washington, DC: National Academy Press, 1997:9–10.

59. The SUPPORT Principal Investigators. A controlled trial to improve care for seriously ill hospitalized patients. *JAMA* 1989;274:1591–1598.

60. Schroeder SA. The legacy of SUPPORT. *Ann Intern Med* 1999;131:780–782.

61. American Society of Clinical Oncology. Cancer care during the last phase of life. *J Clin Oncol* 1998;16:1986–1996.

62. Quill TE, Billings JA. Palliative care textbooks come of age. *Ann Intern Med* 1998;129:590–594.

63. MacDonald N. Oncology and palliative care: the case for co-ordination. *Cancer Treat Rev* 1993;19(Suppl A):29–41.

64. MacDonald N. Palliative care: the fourth phase of cancer prevention. *Cancer Detect Prev* 1991;15:253–255.

65. Final rule, Medicare program hospice care. Department of Health and Human Services. Health Care Financing Administration regulation Part 418. Federal register. December 18, 1983, Volume 48 No. 243.

66. Billings JA, Pantilat S. Palliative medicine fellowship programs in the United States: year 2000 survey. *J Palliat Med* 2000;3:391–396.

CHAPTER 45 ■ HOSPICE

MARTHA L. TWADDLE

END-OF-LIFE CARE

For each of us, the sounds of our time passing are amplified in our feelings and emotions, in our fears and anxieties, in our loves and our guilts, in our thoughts, beliefs, and hopes. It is to these that we must listen if we are to hear the sounds of time passing and if we are to capture the meaning of those sounds. However, we can neither listen for and to, nor can we really hear, the sounds of our time and others' time passing if we are fragmented, scattered, and drawn here and there under the force of untold stresses, through one distraction after another. David Roy (1)

National data reports tell us that over 80% of those who die in the United States do so after a lengthy, progressively debilitating illness (2). In essence, over 80% of the time, the outcome of the disease is predictable, but it is likely that the timing of the outcome is not. In the oncology model, the trajectory of the illness has changed over the recent decades to increasingly be one of a chronic progressively debilitating illnesses, punctuated by acute exacerbations with temporary recoveries. Like nonmalignant illness, oncology patients may likely experience more frequent exacerbations in their final months and years, these crises coming closer and closer together with less and less time or capacity for an interval sustained recovery. These frequent exacerbations may be related directly to the malignant illness or are oft times caused by associated morbidities or infections. This pattern of closely occurring crises focuses the health care teams on "rescue" behaviors and may obscure their perspective as to the overall pattern of decline. Unlike nonmalignant illnesses, more has been clarified as to the pattern of far-advanced malignant diseases, characteristically punctuated by a precipitous decline in functional status, with the trajectory toward death more typically predictable, or at the least, recognizable (3).

PATIENT AND FAMILY GOALS MAY LACK SYNERGY WITH MODERN HEALTH CARE

The data also tell us that when faced with approaching death, modern Americans prefer to maximize the time with those activities that are meaningful to them and speak to the integrity of their individual well-being (4–8). Unfortunately, with encroaching illness, the time spent in organizing resources, navigating the complexity of health care systems, and receiving institutional-based "care" through procedures, tests, and products tends to overwhelm the energies of individuals and families. When given the choice, most patients likely would not elect to focus their last days and energies on interactions with health care systems. But the operative phrase within the that statement is "when given the choice." Informed consent regarding procedures is the standard of care in health care; however, discussions that might provide opportunity to decline further disease-focused interventions without risk of abandonment, real or perceived, are not yet common practice (9–12).

In the disease-management model, resources are focused on the eradication of the disease and prolongation of life. The goals and resources of care are focused on disease intervention. The physician, nurse, and others work in the warrior roles of fighting disease and within this context, see death as failure, and the lack of disease-interventional treatments as "doing nothing." It is normative for a physician who has exhausted all protocols in fighting a malignancy to say "I have nothing left to offer you" when in fact, an armamentarium of supportive care modalities may be available and of benefit. The warriors of health care do not typically have the perspective to ask the questions that would thereby generate the choices. This may not be for any lack of empathy on their part, but rather attests to the emphasis of their training and practice, the finely honed intervention skills that are prioritized within the highly technologic, science-based environment of health care centers.

PALLIATIVE CARE COMPLEMENTS TREATMENTS

Palliative care by definition and practice is not an alternative, *per se*, to this approach, but rather represents the foundation of good medical care (13). This approach views the patient as a whole person in the context of his or her family and his or her community and seeks to understand the cultural, social, spiritual, and psychological aspects that will influence the provision or acceptance of professional medical care. The emphasis of palliative care is to clarify the goals of care in the light of how the individual defines the quality and meaning of his or her life. With the goals defined and documented, care ideally moves from crisis intervention to crisis avoidance, resources for support and advocacy are defined earlier in the illness, and discussions of the burden and benefit of interventions are recurrently pursued. Palliative care is thereby a continuum of supportive care that ideally begins at the time of a potentially life-limiting diagnosis and actively supports the patient and family throughout the course of illness, however long that journey may be (14–16) (Fig. 45.1).

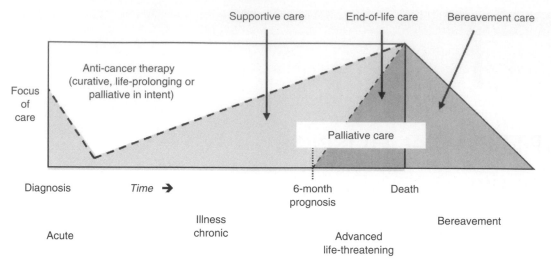

FIGURE 45.1. Diagram of the continuum of palliative care through hospice (with permission).

HOSPICE CULMINATES THE CONTINUUM

Within this continuum of palliative care, and most often at its end, is hospice, which is best defined as the most intensive, refined form of palliative care. Hospice is a philosophy of care that recognizes that the disease is not curable, that time is limited to months at best and that symptom control and quality of life are preeminent goals. In this paradigm, *all* interventions and therapies must have immediate, tangible benefit to the patient and family, consistent with their personally defined goals. Hospice views death as an expected outcome within a discrete time frame. It offers a support system to patients, families, and professionals that affirms the outcome of death not as failure, but its heralded approach as opportunity to maximize quality so that the patient might live well until death. Recognizing the time limitations of life allows patients and families to prioritize the activities and interactions that have meaning, to seek closure personally and practically, and

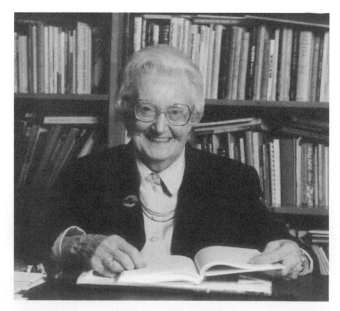

FIGURE 45.2. Dame Cicely Saunders of Great Britain is credited as launching the modern concept of hospice care.

to have an opportunity to "leave a legacy," if so desired, or to have some focused intent as to how or even in what manner one will be remembered after death.

ROOTS OF HOSPICE CARE

Hospice is a term with deep history. Originally places of safety for travelers on pilgrimage throughout the ancient Middle East (c 400 AD), these centers of "hospitality" evolved into the earlier hospitals of Europe, oft times operated and staffed by religious orders. Dame Cicely Saunders of Great Britain is credited as launching the modern concept of hospice care (17) (Fig. 45.2). Dame Saunders initially practiced as a nurse during World War II, but a back injury forced her to redirect her career to medical social work. In this context, she cared for and befriended a young man, David Tasma, a 40-year-old dying of inoperable cancer. Visiting him frequently in hospital, she witnessed how his symptoms were controlled by the administration of morphine and noted particularly how, when free of pain, he "had time to sort out who he was, dying at the age of 40, and coming from the Warsaw ghetto. Of course, leaving nobody behind and feeling he had made no impression on the world for ever having lived in it. But as we were talking, he said he would leave me something in his will, he had insurance, and he said, 'I'll be a window in your home.' And the idea of openness to everybody who might come, openness to every future challenge, really stems from that gift, which was, I think, the founding gift of the whole hospice movement, made by David Tasma, who thought his name would never mean anything to anybody" (18).

THE EXPANSION OF THE BRITISH MODEL OF HOSPICE

The original concept of hospice in England, sparked into being by Dame Saunders and David Tasma's gift, was care for those with advanced cancer provided in an institutional setting, in essence, a specialty hospital. St. Christopher's hospice opened in 1967 and in this setting, Dame Saunders pioneered the application of the scientific approach to the care of the dying, establishing many of the current best practices of palliative medicine, in particular, the around-the-clock administration of analgesic therapy to control pain symptoms. Dame Saunder's trainees further developed hospice in the world.

awareness of death and the recognition of the patient's coping mechanisms through her observational studies published in *Death and Dying* in 1969 (21). In keeping with the grassroots psychology of the American, hospice programs were established at the community level, often by professional volunteers, to provide an alternative to institutional-based dying. The early pioneers of hospice in the United States were vocal in their condemnation of "modern" health care's inattention to the needs of dying patients and their families and sought to establish health care systems that existed outside of the mainstream in reaction to this deficit. Within the United States, terminally ill patients with diagnoses other than cancer were increasingly served by hospice programs: by 2003, 51% of patients were admitted with noncancer diagnoses, with the most common being end-stage heart disease (22). The New Haven program brought together hospice leaders and advocates in the late 1970s to establish guidelines for the operations of hospice programs in the United States. This led to the development of the National Hospice Organization, now the National Hospice and Palliative Care Organization (NHPCO). The mission of this membership organization that represents the nation's hospice programs is "to lead and mobilize social change for improved care at the end of life" (23).

Through the involvement and advocacy of such leaders, the United States Congress authorized the Medicare Hospice Benefit (MHB) in 1982. This entitlement benefit addresses the types of services provided within hospice care, the persons eligible to elect the benefit and the payment system that supports the care. Hospice programs throughout the United States moved to become medicare certified by adhering to these federal guidelines. Medicaid and commercial insurance developed similar guidelines and hospice programs thereby could bill and receive insurance dollars to support care. The medicare benefit is divided into periods, the initial being two 90-day periods with an unlimited number of 60-day increments to follow. Each benefit period requires physician recertification around prognosis and goals of care (24,25).

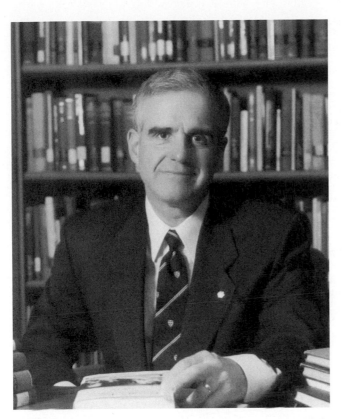

FIGURE 45.3. Dr. Balfour Mount is credited for having coined the term "palliative medicine" to describe the medical discipline of hospice care.

- Dr. Robert Twycross established the World Health Organization's Collaborating Center for Hospice/Palliative Care at the Sir Michael Sobell House in Oxford. A prolific writer and erudite teacher, he has written and published extensively on pharmacologic interventions in pain and symptom management.
- Dr. Balfour Mount (Fig. 45.3), a urologic surgeon at McGill University, is credited with having coined the term "palliative medicine" to describe the medical discipline of hospice care. His work at the Royal Victoria Hospital in Montreal helped moved forward the integration of this care model throughout North American and, along with Dr. Josephina Magno, contributed substantially to the formation in 1988 of the Academy of Hospice Physicians which later evolved to the American Academy of Hospice and Palliative Medicine (AAHPM) (19).
- Florence Wald, PhD, Dean of the Graduate School of Nursing at Yale University, opened the New Haven Connecticut Hospice in 1974. This was a sentinel event for hospice, the introduction of the hospice care model into the United States; and the form of hospice care being delivered in the home setting, a model that is most common within the United States to this day. Early models of inpatient hospice care were established at Calvary Hospital and St. Luke's-Roosevelt Hospital in New York City; however, the model that has grown prolifically in the United States has been home care (20).

GROWTH WITHIN THE UNITED STATES

The growth of hospice in the United States found fertile soil in the work of Dr. Elizabeth Kubler-Ross, who raised the

THE BUSINESS OF HOSPICE CARE

As is typical with any philosophical approach that moves to a business model, hospice care in America has been challenged by the tension between its philosophy and what is economically feasible to support. In truth, the MHB was one of the first capitated insurance programs and also, one of the most successful. With a flat per diem rate of roughly a hundred dollars, the hospice program is responsible to provide the professional care of nurses, social workers, chaplains, and therapists in an interdisciplinary team structure. The per diem also covers all the medications, therapies, and procedures related to the hospice diagnosis and any durable medical equipment necessary to care for the patient. The MHB also specifically calls for the involvement of volunteers to provide support to the patient and family. The benefit requires the participation of a hospice medical director to oversee the medical management and, along with the primary attending physician, to certify the patient has a life expectancy of 6 months or less if the disease follows its normal course. Clinical care provided by a physician in the domain of either primary care or palliative medicine is not part of the per diem and is reimbursed through established billing protocols that cover physician services. The benefit also requires a minimum of 12 months of bereavement support for the survivors of the deceased; the per diem payment does not continue through that time period (Table 45.1) (26).

The MHB also requires and covers three other levels of care. The General Inpatient Benefit (GIP) was established

TABLE 45.1

COMPARISON OF HOME HEALTH AND HOSPICE REQUIREMENTS AND SERVICES.

	Home health	Hospice
Eligibility	Any diagnosis	Any diagnosis
	Need to have a skilled need (this can be nursing or therapy)	No such requirement
	Need to be homebound	No such requirement
Site of care delivery	Can only be provided in the home or assisted living (not skilled, LTCF or hospital)	Many sites of care-home, LTCF, ALF, hospital, adult day care, etc.)
Certification	Only one medical director certifies	Need two physicians to certify
	60-day certification periods	Certification periods are three 90 days and then 60 days
Care management	Physician directed, prescriptive	Interdisciplinary team directed
Services covered	Payment does not include meds or DME.	Does include meds and DME
	Includes supplies related to admitting diagnosis	Includes supplies related to admitting diagnosis plus general care (diapers, skin care, etc.)
	Can only be provided in the home or assisted living (not skilled, LTCF or hospital)	Many sites of care-home, LTCF, ALF, hospital, adult day care, etc.)
Levels of care	N/A	Four different levels of care-routine home care, respite, continuous care, and inpatient
Hours of coverage	Varies from agency to agency. Most will direct patient to ER after hours.	24 hour on call support
Physician reimbursement	*Referring physician* may bill for accumulation of 30-min increments of "oversite" care. *Medical director* is salaried if has no medical practice.	*Referring physician* bills insurance with a GW or GV modifier. *Consulting physicians* bill hospice program. *Hospice medical director* receives administrative salary or stipend.

LTCF, long-term care facility; ALF, assisted living facility; DME, durable medical equipment; N/A, not applicable; ER, emergency room.

to address the short-term needs of hospice patients when an acute condition precluded the safe delivery of care in any other setting. Under this portion of the benefit, the hospice patient could be hospitalized for acute symptom exacerbations, sudden breakdown of caregiving support, and physical, psychologic, or existential issues around dying that would be best managed in an inpatient setting. The goal of the GIP benefit is to stabilize or resolve the issue(s) that led to inpatient care and return the patient to a less acute setting. No more than 20% of the hospice's overall patient days can be at the GIP level of care. Continuous care is available to address high acuity situations in the home setting that require additional care in a low-tech environment for a finite period of time. By definition, the hospice team is providing continuous care to the patient; a minimum of 8 hours must be nursing care. The MHB also provides respite care, a 5-day provision that is allowed as often as necessary to ease caregiving strain. Under this provision, the patient is typically transferred from a home to a nursing home or other inpatient facility for a finite period of time, and a small per diem rate goes for room and board as well as to cover all medications and equipment related to the hospice diagnosis supplied within the facility. Most commercial insurance programs mimic the MHB, but with variations that require hospice programs to negotiate and clarify the scope of coverage.

The MHB is a capitated reimbursement program. The Center for Medicare and Medicaid Services (CMMS) determines the adjusted cap amount and works through contracted fiscal intermediaries to distribute the funds for hospice services. The Medicare fiscal intermediary is responsible to calculate each hospice's cap amount by multiplying the adjusted cap by the number of medicare beneficiaries who elected to receive hospice care from each hospice during a 12-month period

ending with September 30 of each year. If in excess of the cap, each hospice must refund medicare payments in excess of this aggregated cap amount (24).

CHALLENGES AND LIMITATIONS TO ACCESS

The challenges of fully utilizing hospice care exist more in its business model than philosophy. Given the regulatory issues and cost constraints, most hospice programs accept patients who have made the decision to forego further disease-related treatments and disease-modifying therapies, consistent with the medicare regulations. Many programs accept only those patients who overtly acknowledge that death is imminent; have caregivers in place and systems available to support them safely in the home setting until death. Despite the steady growth in the utilization of hospice services in the United States, increasing from 340,000 in 1994 to 885,000 in 2002, to an estimated 950,000 in 2003, the median length of stay in hospice programs in 2003 was only 22 days, with 37% of hospice patients dying within 7 days or less of accessing hospice support. In a study of referral patterns, those patients referred by oncologist typically have the shortest length of stay in hospice care, as opposed to patients referred from primary care practitioners (27).

INCREASING ACCESS—THE NATIONAL AGENDA

Despite the financial and regulatory limitations of hospice care, larger hospice programs in the United States have sought ways to increase access and provide the fullness of support to patients who are grappling with the decisions of foregoing further disease-modifying treatment. The NHPCO and the National Association of Home Care and Hospice (NAHC) have focused many resources on improving access to care, particularly for underserved patients. Increasingly, hospice programs accept patients who are still receiving disease-modifying treatments with palliative intent, who have not yet established a "Do Not Attempt Resuscitation Order" or who do not have a caregiver living with them. Hospice programs will increasingly underwrite such therapies as palliative radiation or palliative chemotherapy if the goals of care are clearly for enhanced quality of life and symptom management, and if the treatments have little, if any, associated morbidity. The developments within the field of oncology of improved supportive therapies that may slow the progression of the disease with little, if any, dose-limiting side effects have fueled the discussions further regarding continuing such therapies in the setting of hospice. Although great variations exist in the field of hospice as to eligibility around admissions, the overarching theme is to enhance access and stretch the model of care beyond confines that limit its utilization (28).

PEDIATRIC HOSPICE CARE

The pediatric population, currently underserved by hospice, benefits significantly from this enhanced access model. Approximately 100,000 children die each year in the United States, eclipsed by the approximately 1 million who suffer from progressive chronic illnesses (29). Programs specific to the needs of these children and their families are few, particularly for the child who is dying. The adult model of hospice care is insufficient and challenged greatly by the inclusion of children. Late referrals for hospice, lack of pediatric trained hospice staff, and much higher costs associated in caring for children and for the bereavement care of the parents and siblings reflect the inadequacies of the present paradigm. Research and research dollar allocation specific to this area are meager and yet the need for specialized education and research is urgent. Insurance benefits for hospice care for children are often inadequate or nonexistent.

In October of 2001, the Children's International Project on Palliative/Hospice Services issued a white paper of specific recommendations for change and improvement in the care of children living with life-threatening conditions (30). The Institute of Medicine's *When Children Die; Improving Palliative and End-of-Life Care for Children and their Families* reinforced the best model to approach the care for these children is palliative care (31). The cessation of supportive modalities such as fluids and many medications is typically not feasible for a child; palliative care allows continued active physical support with intensive psychosocial spiritual care for the child and their parents. Bereavement care for parents following the death of a child is critically important. Morbidity and mortality increases in this circumstance, particularly for the mother who has experience the death of her child (32).

DOES HOSPICE MEAN GIVING UP?

The philosophical barriers regarding access to hospice care are matters of ongoing debate. Physicians and patients will argue that accepting hospice support is "giving up." There is, however, a substantive difference in acceptance of a terminal diagnosis and resignation to the illness. Acceptance confers that the reality is acknowledged, and plans, attitudes, and priorities are adjusted given this reality. Patients live within this new reality—with new limitations. Resignation confers passivity,

an inactive waiting. Although some individuals may live their lives and their last days in this manner, it is not the imposed paradigm for those receiving a terminal diagnosis or choosing the support of hospice care. Many in hospice care speak of hope, and would likely define that as trust and reliance in the people and process of support as opposed to hope as an expectation of fulfillment (cure) (33). In hospice, these individuals and families are *hopeful* in living well despite advanced disease, seeking active supportive care to enhance their living in the time they have left. There are, in addition, a percentage of patients who survive hospice care, discharged after a period in hospice with stabilization of their disease process, if not improvement in their condition. These patients are most often those with noncancer diagnoses and a higher functional status (34).

HOSPICE OUTCOMES ARE POSITIVE

The reported satisfaction ratings of hospice care are extremely high, and the testimonials of individuals who access hospice support further fuel the passion of its advocates (6,35,36). The data also suggests that the well-being and survival of the survivors themselves is directly impacted by hospice support. A 2003 retrospective cohort study by Dr. Nicholas Christakis matched over 30,000 couples who used hospice care with an equal number who did not. The results suggested strongly that hospice care might attenuate the ordinarily increased mortality following the death of a spouse, particularly so for women (37).

Along with high satisfaction ratings of hospice care are significant cost savings. The cost of provisioning care to patients choosing palliative care or hospice support services is significantly less compared to those expenditures for patients who pursue a disease-intervention model until death (38,39). This is particularly significant because medicare recipients tend to consume the highest percentage of their health care dollars in the weeks and months just prior to death, in large part due to the utilization of intensive care services (40). Of concern is the recently cited trend toward the increasingly aggressive treatment of cancer patients in the weeks just before death, which is reflected in higher utilization of emergency rooms and intensive care units (41). In a study of over 8700 medicare patients, mean and median costs were lower for patients enrolled in hospice care. The lower costs, however, were not associated with a shorter time frame until death; in fact, the patients in hospice care tended to live longer than matched controls that did not elect hospice care (42).

THE GROWTH OF MEDICAL PROFESSIONALISM IN HOSPICE CARE

A significant shift in hospice care has occurred gradually throughout the 1990s and is ongoing. This is best defined as the reintegration of hospice into the mainstream of health care. The integration has occurred through many routes. President Clinton's health care reform proposals of 1993 recognized hospice care as an accepted part of the health care continuum. Hospital systems have increasingly recognized the benefits in terms of clinical outcomes, patient satisfaction, and cost savings achieved through the integration of hospice services (43). The Medicare Hospice General Inpatient Benefit allows patients to activate their hospice benefit, whereas still hospitalized; in essence, discharging them from the acute care admission and readmitting them to hospice care with a paper shuffle, as opposed to any physical changes in setting. Hospices and hospitals often have partnered in these arrangements to facilitate hospice patients receiving inpatient care and also accessing a revenue stream that can help support the care (44,45). These integrative models have been further developed on the national level through the encouragement and mentoring of NHPCO, NAHC, and the Center for Advancement of Palliative Care (CAPC) (46). CAPC has taught and mentored several different models for the integration of palliative care and hospice into the hospital/institution settings through its national meetings and training sites. Leaders from NHPCO, CAPC, AAHPM, and the Hospice and Palliative Nursing Association (HPNA), along with the now defunct Last Acts Project collaborated to create the *National Consensus Project in Quality Palliative Care* which was published in April 2004, providing institutions and agencies with best practice guidelines in palliative care (13). Intrinsic to these guidelines is the idea of the continuum of palliative and hospice care and the defining presence of the interdisciplinary team. In addition, the compilation of over 1400 references was a sizable advancement toward establishing the evidence base of palliative care in the United States.

CONCLUSION

Hospice, as a vital support system for end-of-life care for patients and families, is steadily integrating into traditional health care. As the medical community and the public become increasingly aware of the benefits of hospice, the phrase "There's nothing more I can offer you" will become a relic of the past. The utilization of the palliative care continuum, the emphasis on access to care, and the expansion of insurance and regulatory guidelines will allow more patients and families who face life-limiting illnesses to experience the fullness of hospice support. Hospice care clearly promotes the concept of "live until you die" by actively supporting patients and families with attention to the physical, psychologic, social, cultural, and spiritual aspects of care. Patients who elect hospice care may live longer than those who forego this support, and yet their health care costs are significantly less. Ongoing support for families in bereavement promotes wellness and opportunities for healing; and positively protects against the raised mortality risk of the bereaved.

WEB-BASED RESOURCES

American Academy of Hospice and Palliative Medicine (AAHPM)
    http://www.aahpm.org
American Board of Hospice and Palliative Medicine (ABHPM)
    http://www.abhpm.org
Center for Advancement of Palliative Care (CAPC)
    http://www.capc.org
End-of-Life Palliative Educational Resource Center (EPERC)
    http://www.eperc.mcw.edu
National Association of Homecare (NAHC)
    http://www.nahc.org
National Consensus Project (NCP)
    http://www.nationalconsensusproject.org
National Hospice and Palliative Care Organization
    http://www.nhpco.org/templates/1/homepage.cfm
Pediatric Palliative Care
    http://www.nhpco.org/files/public/ChIPPSCallforChange. pdf
    http://aappolicy.aappublications.org/cgi/content/full/ pediatrics;106/2/351
    http://www.whocancerpain.wisc.edu/eng/16_3-4/resources. html

References

1. Roy D. Palliative care in a technological age. *J Palliat Care* 2004;20:267–268.
2. Pickle L, Mungiole M, Jones GK, et al. *Atlas of United States mortality.* US Department of Health and Human Services. Publication (PHS) 97–1015, 1996.
3. Teno JM, Weitzen S, Fennell ML, et al. Dying trajectory in the last year of life: does cancer trajectory fit other diseases? *J Palliat Med* 2001;4:457–464.
4. McSkimming S, London M, Lieberman C, et al. Improving response to life-threatening illness. *Health Prog* 2004;1:26–56.
5. Steinhauser KD, Clipp EC, McNeilly M, et al. In search of a good death: observations of patients, families, and providers. *Ann Intern Med* 2000;132:825–832.
6. Teno JM, Clarridge BR, Casey V, et al. Family perspectives on end-of-life care at the last place of care. *JAMA* 2004;291:88–93.
7. Steinhauser KE, Christakis NA, Clipp EC, et al. Preparing for the end of life: preferences of patients, families, physicians, and other care providers. *J Pain Symptom Manage* 2001;22:727–737.
8. Steinhauser KE, Christakis NA, Clipp EC, et al. Factors considered important at the end of life by patients, family, physicians and other care providers. *JAMA* 2000;284:2476–2482.
9. Lamont EB, Christakis NA. Prognostic disclosure to patients with cancer near the end of life. *Ann Intern Med* 2001;134:1096–1105.
10. Casarett D, Crowley R, Stevenson C, et al. Making difficult decisions about hospice enrollment: what do patients and families want to know? *J Am Geriatr Soc* 2005;53:249–254.
11. The SUPPORT principle investigators. A controlled trial to improve care for seriously ill hospitalized patients. The study to understand prognoses and preferences for outcomes and risks of treatments (SUPPORT). *JAMA* 1995;274:1591–1598.
12. Baker R, Wu AW, Teno JM, et al. Family satisfaction with end-of-life care in seriously ill hospitalized adults. *J Am Geriatr Soc* 2000;48 (5 Suppl):S61–S69.
13. National Consensus Project for Quality Palliative Care. *Clinical practice guidelines for quality palliative care.* Brooklyn, NY: National Consensus Project, 2004.
14. Von Gunten CF. Secondary and tertiary palliative care in US hospitals. *JAMA* 2002;287:875–881.
15. Selwyn PA, Forstein M. Overcoming the false dichotomy of curative vs palliative care for late-stage HIV/AIDS: "let me live the way I want to live, until I can't". *JAMA* 2003;290:806–814.
16. Meyers FJ, Linder J. Simultaneous care: disease treatment and palliative care throughout illness. *J Clin Oncol* 2003;21:1412–1415.
17. Clark D. *Cicely Saunders—founder of the hospice movement.* Oxford: Oxford University Press, 2002.
18. Curriculum Emanuel LL, von Gunten CF, Ferris FD, eds. *The Education in Palliative and End-of-life Care (EPEC) curriculum:* © The EPEC Project Chicago, IL: Northwestern University, Feinberg School of Medicine. 1999, 2003.
19. Holman GH, Forman WB. On the 10TH anniversary of the organization of the American Academy of Hospice and Palliative Medicine (AAHPM): the first 10 years. *Am J Hosp Palliat Care* 2001;18:275–278.
20. Buck J. Home hospice versus home health. *Nurs Hist Rev* 2004;12:25–46.
21. Kubler-Ross E. *On death and dying.* New York: Macmillan, 1969.
22. Hospice facts and figures. NHPCO. Available at: http://www.nhpco.org/files/public/Hospice_Facts_110104.pdf. Accessed September 1, 2005.
23. Mission and vision. NHPCO. Available at: http://www.nhpco.org/i4a/pages/index.cfm?pageid=3288. Accessed June 10, 2005.
24. Lurvey A, Cope J. The medicare hospice benefit. United Government Services, LLC. March 18, 2004. Available at: http://www.medicarenhic.com/cal_prov/billing%5Chospicebenefit_0304.htm. Accessed June 10, 2005.
25. Part 418—Hospice Care. Code of federal regulations. Title 42 public health. Available at: http://www.washingtonwatchdog.org/documents/cfr/title42/part418.html. Accessed June 11, 2005.
26. Hospice Facts and Statistics. National Association for Home Care & Hospice. 2004. Available at: http://www.nahc.org/NAHC/Research/04HPC_Stats.pdf. Accessed June 15, 2005.
27. Lamont EB, Christakis NA. Physician factors in the timing of cancer patient referral to hospice palliative care. *Cancer* 2002;94:2733–2737.
28. Jennings B, Ryndes T, D'Onofrio C, et al. Access to hospice care: expanding boundaries, overcoming barriers. *Hastings Cent Rep Spec Suppl* 2003;2:S3–S9, S9–S13, S15–S21.
29. Schmidt LM. Pediatric hospice care: coming of age? *Caring* 2003;22(5):20–22.
30. A Call for Change: recommendations to improve the care of children living with life-threatening conditions. 2001. Children's International Project on Palliative/Hospice Services. http://www.nhpco.org/files/public/ChIPPSCallforChange.pdf. Accessed September 14, 2005.
31. Board on Health Science Policy. When children die: improving palliative and end-of-life care for children and their families. 2002. http://www.nap.edu/catalog/10390.html Accessed September 14, 2005.
32. Li J, Pright DH, Mortensen PB, et al. Mortality in parents after death of a child in Denmark: a nationwide follow up study, *Lancet* 2003, 361(9355):363–367.
33. Tulsky J. Hope and hubris. *J Palliat Med* 2002;5:339–341.

34. Kutner JS, Blake M, Meyer SA. Predictors of live hospice discharge: data from the National Home and Hospice Care Survey (NHHCS). *Am J Hosp Palliat Care* 2002;19:331–337.

35. Casarett DJ, Hirschman KB, Crowley R, et al. Caregivers' satisfaction with hospice care in the last 24 hours of life. *Am J Hosp Palliat Care* 2003;20:205–210.

36. Miceli PJ, Mylod DE. Satisfaction of families using end-of-life care: current successes and challenges in the hospice industry. *Am J Hosp Palliat Care* 2003;20:360–370.

37. Christakis NA, Iwashyna TJ. The health impact of health care on families: a matched cohort study of hospice use by decedents and mortality outcomes in surviving, widowed spouses. *Soc Sci Med* 2003;57:465–475.

38. Elsayem A, Swint K, Fisch M, et al. Palliative care inpatient service in a comprehensive cancer center: clinical and financial outcomes. *Clin Oncol* 2004;22:2008–2014.

39. Campbell ML, Frank RR. Experience with an end-of-life practice at a university hospital. *Crit Care Med* 1997;25:197–202.

40. Harrison JP, Ford D, Wilson K. The impact of hospice programs on US hospitals. *Nurs Econ* 2005;23:78–84.

41. Earle CC, Neville BA, Landrum MB, et al. Trends in the aggressiveness of cancer care near the end of life. *J Clin Oncol* 2004;22:315–321.

42. Pyenson B, Connor S, Fitch K, et al. Medicare cost in matched hospice and non-hospice cohorts. *J Pain Symptom Manage* 2004;28:200–210.

43. Higginson IJ, Finlay IG, Goodwin DM, et al. Do hospital-based palliative teams improve care for patients or families at the end of life? *J Pain Symptom Manage* 2002;23:96–106.

44. Dunlop RJ, Hockey JM. *Hospital-based palliative care teams: the hospital-hospice interface*. NY: Oxford University Press, 1998.

45. Meier DE. When pain and suffering do not require a prognosis: working toward meaningful hospital-hospice partnership. *J Palliat Med* 2003;6:109–115.

46. Center for Advancement of Palliative Care. http://www.capc.org, 2005.

CHAPTER 46 ■ MULTIDIMENSIONAL PATIENT ASSESSMENT

J. CAMERON MUIR, MARY WHEELER, JENNIFER CARLSON, AND NANCY W. LITTLEFIELD

INTRODUCTION/BACKGROUND

From the earliest times in medicine, there has been a significant emphasis on the relief of suffering. As Hippocrates said: "I will use treatment to help the sick". . . and "to help, or at least to do no harm" (1). From the time of Hippocrates (approximately 500 BC) through the 19th century, the focus of health care has been on the relief of suffering associated with injury and disease. However, during the last half of the 19th century, the 20th century, and into the 21st century, health care has been largely focused on disease and has inadequately addressed care for the person. As a result, the disease has been treated, although the suffering that the patient is experiencing is often left unaddressed. It has only been during the past 25 years, that there has been a resurgence of the ethic of palliative care. This resurgence is most likely due to recognition of the limits of the current curative model of care: although we have become more proficient at staving off death, it will still occur 100% of the time (2). It is through a skilled multidimensional patient assessment (MDPA) that the various elements of suffering can be identified and addressed from diagnosis of a cancer, through treatment and into remission, or at disease progression, and on until death.

In this chapter, we will review the components of a multidimensional patient screening and assessment, which is often also referred to by the patient/family as "holistic or whole person" care. Particular emphasis will be placed on the role of an interdisciplinary team (IDT), and a distinction will be made between the traditional "medical model" and the interdisciplinary "biopsychosocial-spiritual model" of care, which is so well modeled in the field of hospice and palliative care. The different components of the MDPA will then be described with particular emphasis on knowing how and when to integrate other disciplines' skills and assistance.

INTERDISCIPLINARY ASSESSMENT

There is a growing appreciation that a patients' experience of their advanced illness is complex: from physical symptoms, to coping, finance, caregiver burden, social/family changes, and spiritual concerns. And furthermore, that no one person—regardless of their professional discipline—will be able to manage all of these issues (3–5). In fact, attempts to do so may result in either harm to the health care provider through exhaustive efforts to deal with everything "myself" leading to stress and burnout (6,7); or harm to the patient and family, because the health care provider either completely misses an

issue due to lack of skill in that area, or by trying to do something that they are not adequately trained to do.

Each health care discipline has expertise and skills in providing care to the patient and family and in identifying their specific needs, and clarifying goals of treatment within a holistic framework. One might ask: "What discipline is most appropriate for performing an initial assessment?" Although there is little data to support an answer to this question, there is some anecdotal evidence from evaluation of the systems currently in place and what seems to work. There are two predominant models of care provided in health care: the traditional "medical" model, and the interdisciplinary/palliative care model. There are significant differences between the two models of care (8,9).

The traditional medical model is the predominant model of health care and can be characterized as disease focused with the physician as the leader. Physicians run most ambulatory clinics that see patients with "problem lists" and "chief complaints"; a history is taken, and then a physical examination is performed. Based upon clinical findings, patients undergo diagnostic testing in an attempt to reveal a diagnosis for which some form of therapy is instituted to cure or at least improve the disease. This model often fails to take two critical elements into account: the nonphysical needs of the patient and family, and the fact that the vast majority of medical diseases in the 21st century are chronic, often progressive diseases that ultimately cannot be cured, only palliated. In the medical model, the primary mode of communication between health care providers is often the written chart note, with the involvement of other medical specialists, as well as other professional disciplines; this system is often haphazard and uncoordinated.

The interdisciplinary/palliative care model is team driven with the focus of care being the patient and family, rather than the disease (10,11). Table 46.1 provides an overview of the discipline-specific components of a typical interdisciplinary assessment. Interdisciplinary care recognizes that the discipline that often spends the greatest amount of time with a patient and family is usually the nurse, and the nurse is also equipped with the broadest assessment skills. The nursing assessment in palliative care, whether performed in a unit, or in an ambulatory or community setting, is of paramount importance.

The nurse coordinates the plan of care for the patient and family as well as the IDT, which can include physicians, social workers, and pastoral caregivers among others (13). The nurse should have good physical assessment skills, a strong knowledge of current innovations in pain and symptom management, as well as astute psychological and spiritual

TABLE 46.1

COMPONENTS OF THE INTERDISCIPLINARY TEAM ASSESSMENT

Nursing	System review
	Pain and other symptoms
	Function
	Patient/family learning needs
Social work	Current mental status
	Patient/family perception of disease/illness
	Values of patient/family
	Goals
	Patient/family feelings and stressors
	Suicide risk
	Children's issues/concerns
	Financial issues/consideration
	Pain
Chaplain	Patient coping strengths
	Hopes, goals, and expectations
	Indicators of spiritual distress
	Patient/family needs
	Pain
Physician (12)	Pain and other symptoms
	Goals of care/advance care planning
	Illness trajectory and prognostic assessment and communication
	Psychosocial spiritual needs
	Patient support system
	Assess discharge planning issues

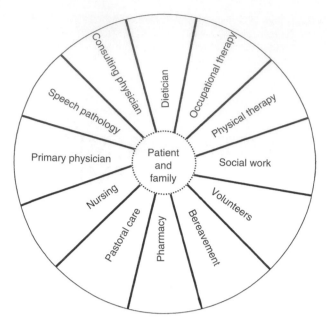

FIGURE 46.1. Multidisciplinary team. (From Krammer LM, Muir JC. Gooding-Keller N, et al. Palliative care and oncology opportunities for oncology nursing. *Oncol Nurs Updates* 1999;3(6):1–12, with permission.)

evaluation strategies to ensure the plan of care is congruent with the goals of the patient and family. The nurse is often in a position to develop the strongest therapeutic relationship with the patient and family.

The nurse works with the patient and family using skilled compassion and concern; empowering the patient to exercise control in decision making where possible, which can only enhance the patient's sense of control. The nurse continually reassesses the patient and family's goals, treatment preferences, coping abilities, and support needs. The nurse is the conduit for information, critical assessments, and evaluation of the patient and family goals within the IDT. The physician can provide expertise about the disease, treatment options, risks and benefits, likely outcomes, and symptom management interventions. In addition, they can help to anticipate critical decisions, and guide and support the patient and family through the process. In order to assess patient and family coping, and identify individual strengths and community resources a social worker is essential to the team. In addition, they are also most adept to evaluating and negotiating financial and insurance resources. Pastoral care can be invaluable in helping to understand the patient's spiritual strengths and concerns, and assist the patient and family in maintaining/reframing hope and establish meaning in the setting of advanced disease.

A key element of interdisciplinary palliative care is a strong emphasis on coordination of care. This is most commonly achieved through team meetings, where different disciplines verbally communicate each of their assessments in order to synthesize a comprehensive care plan that will meet the patient and family needs. For an IDT to be most effective, candid communication between team members is vital.

The distinction between interdisciplinary and multidisciplinary practice is critical. In the traditional multidisciplinary team, care of the patient is directed by the physician (Fig. 46.1). Many other members of the health care team may be involved

in the delivery of care; however, efforts are often uncoordinated and fragmented.

The primary mode of communication between disciplines is the medical chart (14). The result is often ineffective communication between professions, lack of accountability, and a tendency for each discipline to independently develop their own patient care goals. To contrast, in an interdisciplinary model, leadership is shared and communication between team members is collaborative (15).

Although individual health care providers may have discipline-specific goals as part of the plan of care, it is

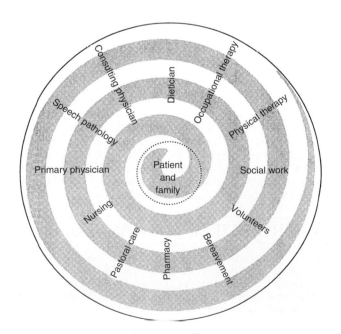

FIGURE 46.2. Interdisciplinary team. (From Krammer LM, Muir JC. Gooding-Keller N, et al. Palliative care and oncology opportunities for oncology nursing. *Oncol Nurs Updates* 1999;3(6):1–12, with permission.)

essential that the team remains focused on the patient-driven goals; communication between team members will be more effective if the focus of team interaction remains on the patient and family. Maintaining this focus is more successful when the team allows time to discuss the challenges individual professionals are facing in association with the patient and family, and if the team regularly reviews the plan of care. This model allows for team members to directly interact with the patient and family, and to provide consultation to one another, in order to achieve the goals identified by the patient and family (Fig. 46.2). Therefore, the sum (from the patient's point of view) is greater than the individual parts (16,17).

INTERDISCIPLINARY COMMUNICATION AND COLLABORATION

The most elegant of assessment will not benefit the patient, the family, or the IDT unless the information is communicated to all that need to know. Collaborative communication has been defined as working together cooperatively, sharing responsibility for problem solving, conflict management, decision making, communication and coordination (18). Open communication is linked with positive attitudes toward work, increased job satisfaction, increased job performance, increased job retention (19), decreasing cost of care (20). However, clinicians receive little education about how to effectively communicate with each other (21).

We communicate to team members what we feel is important. Physicians and nurses often use knowledge from the biomedical model of health and illness in assessment (22), and social workers often use the biopsychosocial-spiritual perspective (23). Nurses' communication is narrative and descriptive, whereas the physicians' communication is problem or need focused (21). Interruptions and distractions can negatively affect the process and contribute to clinicians forgetting to share pertinent information (21). There may be so much information that it is difficult to determine what is critical (21). Deficient communication creates conditions for acrimony, frustration, distrust, and can lead to inferior care and increased risk of error (24). Issues that impede effective communication include multiple service providers and a lack of standardized documentation (25).

Nursing and physician communication has been studied more than other interactions between the members of the IDT. Physicians state that they recognize the importance of nursing knowledge, but do not necessarily make use of it (22). Nurses complain that there is not enough information and physicians complain that there is too much information (25). Different disciplines require and use different information to provide optimal care (25).

The patient record serves as the most consistent source of patient specific health care data. It is where numerous clinicians go to find valid and reliable information. It also serves as the legal record for patient care (21). Verbal communication is less structured than written, but may be the primary way that information is transmitted (21). When choosing what to communicate, the situation, background, assessment, recommendations (SBAR) model may be used. Communicating information using this model provides the following:

- Information about the patient's current situation
- A context for the patient's current situation
- An assessment of the current problem
- A recommendation that addresses the patient's needs

In addition to what is said, how it is said impacts collaboration. Verbal communication styles are important, and studies show that health care can be improved by using an attentive style of

---

TABLE 46.2

COMMUNICATION STYLES

Attentive style (20):
- Make it obvious that you are listening to each other
- Refrain from participating in other activities that interrupt communication
- Provide verbal feedback to summarize precisely what other say
- Use appropriate eye contact
- Provide an opportunity to discuss the issues
- Offer an opportunity to reflect and correct misunderstandings

Contentious style (20):
- Argumentative
- Challenging
- Being overly precise to the extent that conversation focuses on unimportant points

Dominant (20):
- Speaking frequently/monopolizing the conversation
- Speaking strongly
- "Take charge" manner

Assertive style (21):
- Being organized in thought
- Possessing technical competence
- Possessing social competence
- Seeking common understanding, ownership, and value from all team members

---

communication. These desired behaviors are not new and can be taught. It is recommended to avoid a contentious style, which is argumentative and challenging or a dominant style, which doesn't allow others to participate (20). Descriptions of some of the communication styles are presented in Table 46.2.

The IDT may be comprised of members of different generations. The Silent Generation was born between 1922 and 1942, the Baby Boomers were born between 1943 and 1960, Generation X was born between 1961 and 1980, and Generation Y was born in 1981 and later. Communication styles between generations may be different. If your team communicates using an electronic medical record, members of the Silent Generation and Baby Boomers may need more training and a different type of training than Generations X and Y (26). Health care professionals can anticipate that computers and related technology will become essential as a vital communication tool (27).

Tips to improve communication are not unique to end-of-life care. Table 46.3 can be seen for specific recommendations. Members of the IDT share the same goal of providing excellent care. Our challenge is to make the most of all interactions, utilizing the best knowledge and abilities of all team members that lead to positive patient outcomes (28)

COMPONENTS OF A MULTIDIMENSIONAL PATIENT ASSESSMENT

There are a number of sources describing elements of a multidimensional patient assessment (2).

History of Illness and Treatment Responses

The initial elements of the MDPA parallel that of the traditional medical model. The assessment begins with an illness history that begins with determination of the primary

TABLE 46.3

SUGGESTIONS TO IMPROVE COMMUNICATION AND COLLABORATION

- Work at developing relationships based on mutual respect
- Assume you are on the same team
- Recognize equality among professionals
- Be prepared for conflict
- Discuss preferred methods for communication
- Know what you need to find out or report
- Agree upon an approach to family members
- Report clinically essential information and explain your finding in the appropriate context
- Describe pertinent environmental and economic factors that may help to explain the patient's condition
- Turn a conversation into an opportunity to collaborate

From Burke M, Boal J, Mitchell R. Communicating for better care. *Am J Nurs* 2004;104(12):40–47 (24).

diagnosis and course of treatment. In addition, attention should be paid to assessing the therapies that have been utilized and not only their impact on the disease, but also their impact on the patient's symptoms from the disease, and what therapies have exacerbated or ameliorated these symptoms (29). One must also elicit information about other illnesses and therapies that the patient has that may be important contributors to suffering and complicate subsequent therapies. One should have information on the extent/stage of disease, and familiarity with the diagnostic testing that confirmed the extent of disease.

Physical Assessment

The physical assessment is designed to screen for the presence of physical symptoms contributing to suffering. To ascertain the "subjective" symptom burden, one must inquire as to their presence and severity. Specific assessment tools can assist in the screening for multiple symptoms (30–33). The Edmonton Symptom Assessment Scale (Table 46.4) with the accompanying System Graph for clinical tracking (Fig. 46.3) (30) is a concise, user-friendly palliative care assessment tool. Use of these tools may be helpful in building a therapeutic relationship by reminding that patient that relief of their suffering is important. The physical assessment also includes understanding how symptoms impair function, sleep, movement, eating, mood, and so forth. In addition to the core physical assessment of both the nurse and physician, there are a number of other disciplines whose input can be critical. Physical and occupational therapy assessments may reveal deficits and provide interventions that can be essential to maintaining functional capacity, ensuring patient safety, conserving energy, and decreasing fatigue. A speech therapy assessment can provide valuable information regarding swallowing function, while a nutritional assessment by a dietitian can aid in determining caloric intake needs thereby reducing cancer-related cachexia.

It is important to emphasize that most symptoms have physical, emotional, spiritual, and functional components. For example, dyspnea can be due to airway impingement by tumor, coupled with an emotional fear of suffocating; this in turn, leads to limits on activity and the patient asks, "what have I done to deserve this?" Each symptom should be thoroughly assessed to determine both the physiologic/pathologic etiologies and the nonphysical components so as to guide appropriate therapies.

TABLE 46.4

EDMONTON SYMPTOM ASSESSMENT SCALE

version date: December 11, 2002
Edmonton Symptom Assessment Scale (ESAS)
Date of completion: _____   Time: _____

Please circle the number that best describes:

No pain										Worst possible pain
0	1	2	3	4	5	6	7	8	9	10

Not tired										Worst possible tiredness
0	1	2	3	4	5	6	7	8	9	10

Not nauseated										Worst possible nausea
0	1	2	3	4	5	6	7	8	9	10

Not depressed										Worst possible depression
0	1	2	3	4	5	6	7	8	9	10

Not anxious										Worst possible anxiety
0	1	2	3	4	5	6	7	8	9	10

Not drowsy										Worst possible drowsiness
0	1	2	3	4	5	6	7	8	9	10

Best appetite										Worst possible appetite
0	1	2	3	4	5	6	7	8	9	10

Best feeling of well being										Worst possible feeling of well being
0	1	2	3	4	5	6	7	8	9	10

No shortness of breath										Worst possible shortness of breath
0	1	2	3	4	5	6	7	8	9	10

Other problem

ESAS completed by:
☐☐ Patient ☐☐ Health professional
☐☐ Family ☐☐ Assisted by family or health professional

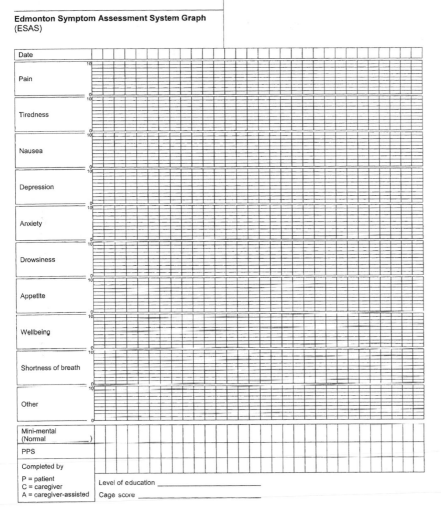

Capital Health

Edmonton Symptom Assessment System Graph
(ESAS)

Date

Pain

Tiredness

Nausea

Depression

Anxiety

Drowsiness

Appetite

Wellbeing

Shortness of breath

Other

Mini-mental
(Normal   )

PPS

Completed by

P = patient
C = caregiver
A = caregiver-assisted

Level of education _____

Cage score _____

CH-0208 May 2001

FIGURE 46.3. Edmonton Symptom Assessment System Graph (ESAS). (From http://www.palliative.org/PC/ClinicalInfo/AssessmentTools/ESAS.pdf with permission.)

The assessment of cognitive function is particularly important and can be readily determined through the Folstein Mini Mental state examination (MMSE) (Table 46.5). It is important to determine whether a patient has either acute (e.g., delirium) or chronic cognitive deficits (e.g., dementia) that would impair decision-making capacity (DMC) and/or safety. Some geriatric and palliative care programs utilize the MMSE as part of routine clinical practice for all patients.

Decision-Making Capacity

Important in the many facets of care surrounding terminal disease is patient autonomy or self-determination. Ensuring patient autonomy through life limiting illness, dictates that a person who possesses the ability to make one's own decision or DMC, should be allowed to do so (1). When patients find themselves on the journey from diagnosis to advanced disease, there are numerous decisions that the individuals should be allowed to choose if they have the ability to do so. For most, decisions will span a wide continuum that will include types and length of treatment, where treatments should take place, whether or not to enter a clinical trial and to decisions regarding advance care planning such as living wills, durable power of attorney for health care and resuscitation wishes.

Whether an individual has the ability to dictate his treatment preferences including the right to forgo life-sustaining treatment, and the method by which that right can be exercised, will fundamentally be dependent on whether or not the patient has the DMC to make the decision. Historically, when a patient disagreed with treatment plan options, especially if that disagreement would lead to the death of the patient, DMC was questioned and often left in the hands of the court for final determination. Today, if there is question of an individual's DMC, the care team should make every effort to determine if there are reversible causes contributing to perceived lack of capacity. Chemical imbalances, reactions to aggressive treatment and even the stress of treatment can alter sound decision making. Of importance in the assessment of DMC is the understanding that it is not an all (has capacity) or nothing (lacks capacity) process. Indeed, some individuals may have the capacity to make certain kinds of decision and not others and therefore have a capacity that varies by the nature of the decision. They may have the capacity to make particular decisions at some times, but not others, and therefore a capacity that varies by time. An example would be attributes of capacity necessary to make decisions about routine blood tests or payment of the phone bill but lack the attributes as to whether chemotherapy

TABLE 46.5

MINI MENTAL STATE EXAMINATION

Category	Question	Score
Orientation	Name the day/date/month/season/year	5
	Name the floor/hospital/town/state/country	5
Registration	Name three objects and have patient repeat them immediately	3
Attention	Serial 7's or spell "world" backwards or days of week backwards	5
Recall	Ask the patient to name three objects stated above after 3 min	3
Language and praxis	Point to a pencil and watch and ask the patient to name them	2
	Ask patient to repeat the following: "No ifs, ands, or buts"	1
	Follow a three-stage command:	3
	"Take a paper in your right hand, fold it in half, and put it on the floor"	
	Read and obey the following sign: "Close your eyes"	1
	Write a sentence	1
	Copy this design: intersecting pentagons	1
Total		30

CLOSE YOUR EYES

Folstein MF, Folstein SE, McHugh PR. "Mini-mental state". A practical method for grading the cognitive state of patients for the clinician. *J Psychiatr Res* 1975;12(3):189–198.

should be discontinued. A complete and thorough MMSE at the time of admission will help to determine the patient's baseline DMC and will set the foundation for any subsequent changes that occur through the course of disease. When the results of clinical exams fail to achieve clarity about individual decision-making capacity, a court judge can make the final determination of competence (34). Such determination should always serve the purpose of protecting the authority of the patient to control his own life in a way that supports his own values.

Information sharing—a key part of the MDPA is assessing the patient's wishes and desires for the sharing of information. Although, western medical ethics emphasizes autonomy, truth telling, and informed consent, it is important to recognize that not all cultures and practices agree with this approach. Robert Buckman, MD has written a helpful six-step protocol for communicating difficult information (35).

In this method, one must remember to ask the patient how much they know about their disease with an open-ended question such as: "What is your understanding of your disease," followed by active listening. But then to follow up this question with a second, perhaps more important question that is again open-ended: "How much do you want to know about your disease," followed by active listening. When one is still not certain about how to proceed in the sharing of information, a follow-up question that is useful is, "If I have some important information to share about your medical condition, with whom would you want me to share it?"

Psychological Assessment

A psychological assessment should be done to evaluate mood and coping. It is important for team members to develop a sense of familiarity with each of these areas—and most importantly to recognize when there are issues that need further assessment and/or intervention by another health care discipline. Most palliative care and hospice teams rely heavily on social workers to provide education to the health care team, and expertise in detailed assessments of mood and coping. When the initial assessment of the social worker or nurse suggest significant needs, then referral to a mental health provider can be helpful. Social workers generally have a well-developed network of mental health providers in the community that can be called upon for counselling (individual, group, couples), support groups, and potentially pharmacologic therapy.

The assessment of mood is vital in the palliative and supportive oncology arena (36). Anxiety and depression are common among patients with cancer. Depression is common in advanced cancer and often undiagnosed and untreated (36,37). Many clinicians believe that it is "normal" to be depressed when one has advanced cancer. Although, it is true that depression is common in advanced cancer, it is not normal and significant depression warrants both pharmacologic and nonpharmacologic therapy. Involvement of a mental health provider to provide further assessment and intervention may be beneficial. The health care provider must always be alert to the possibility of significant depression leading to suicidal ideation (38). If this is suspected, one must make an immediate assessment of whether or not the patient has a plan to act upon this idea, and whether they will "contract for safety" (let someone know if they feel that they might act on their plan). In any case, the presence of suicidal ideation requires prompt intervention. If the skills for this intervention are not present in the palliative care or oncology team, then psychiatric consultation is critical.

The diagnosis of advanced cancer is often devastating to a patient and their family (39). There are a number of responses that a person can have to this threat to their personhood including fear, anger, avoidance, denial, intellectualization, intense grieving, and existential questioning. All of these coping mechanisms are normal and may be adaptive and beneficial to the patient and family at that particular time. It is imperative that the health care provider continually assesses the emotional coping of patients and families to determine when there may be problematic coping. It is helpful to assess not only current coping strategies used by the patient and family, but also strategies used in the past. This will assist the team to anticipate ineffective coping styles and to develop individualized strategies for the patient and the family members. General open-ended questions (e.g., "people often feel a number of different emotions as they are living with cancer, what are you feeling?") followed by active listening can be very helpful. With good psychosocial support from the cancer care team, most patients can effectively live with their cancer as they reach acceptance and, ideally, peace with their illness and their life.

Social Assessment

In the MDPA, it is important to keep in mind that the patient and family, rather than the disease, are the primary focus of care. One needs to glean a basic understanding of the patient's family and family dynamics, their culture, and community, and relevant information about their finances. The social worker, often in conjunction with the nurse, can help to obtain critical social information.

Each patient and family will experience illness within the context of his or her particular world view. Being sick, even slightly, can be a disabling experience, both physically and psychologically, with attendant feelings of loss of control and helplessness becoming paramount. This is particularly so in terminal illness. For example, the change of role within the family can become a critical issue; perhaps the patient who is the primary income generator is unable to work and therefore unable to provide materially; or the main family caregiver is too ill to continue lifelong habits of looking after other family members. For the entire family there are often major adjustments to be made; financial, social, and emotional adaptations will occur with varying effectiveness. In order to open communication and provide whole person care, the patient and family must be integral members of the team and therefore involved in treatment decisions and in development of an appropriate care plan (40).

A patient's entire family system is affected by the diagnosis of a life-threatening illness (41,42). The patient's relationship to the world changes with the news that life span has been defined, therefore altering family interactions (43). The patient's roles within the family—as a provider, a caregiver, a parent, a spouse, or a sexual partner—may be

challenged (41–43). Therefore the particular issues and needs of family members, in addition to the patient, must also be assessed. Furthermore, because care may be provided by family members in the home setting, the family should also be consulted with and educated about the diagnosis, treatment options, the illness trajectory, symptom burden/treatment and caregiving—with the patient's permission (43).

What constitutes "family" will vary for patients. It is vital to determine who the patient considers to be "family" or "community of care," who they wish to be included in decision making, and whom they identify as their means of support. Family units can be comprised of the traditional nuclear and extended family, but also may be a same sex couple, members of a religious order, members of an ethnic/cultural community, or, simply, a group of friends. Focused discussion with the patient should occur upfront to determine who they identify as "family," with whom they wish to share information, and how much and what type of detail they wish to share.

Social workers use the genogram or family tree to facilitate understanding of a particular family's structure and dynamics. The genogram helps to identify the family structure in a clear and comprehensive way. It highlights relationships, strengths and weaknesses, and can often clarify some of the family norms around disease/illness and coping. Gathering the information to develop a genogram also facilitates the partnership between the health care team and the patient and family. The information gleaned should be documented in the medical record and reassessed periodically.

As discussed earlier, the importance of addressing advanced care planning for the patient and family is critical (44), and is best addressed early in the course of illness, and frequently reassessed, rather than left for discussion at 3 AM in the ER when a crisis occurs. Early discussions regarding prognosis, likely course of the disease, events to anticipate, and clarifying advance directives (e.g., living wills and/or designation of a durable power of attorney for health care), all can serve to mitigate subsequent dilemmas, increase control, and lessen angst. This helps patients and their families to prepare for changes in the patient's condition and facilitates open communication between the patient, family, and the health care team (41). This type of communication minimizes the sense of abandonment that many patients fear and helps facilitate a sense of control (42,45).

It is important to determine specific cultural or other particular practices of the patient and family in order to be sensitive and respectful. If the health care provider encounters an unfamiliar culture, custom, or tradition, they should use this as an opportunity to learn about it from the patient and family or from a local expert. This will not only enhance the health care provider's knowledge base and skill set, but also show significant respect for the patient and family that will help to build a therapeutic relationship (46). The social worker or chaplain is often an initial resource for these issues.

A critical component of the social assessment is to determine patients' financial issues or concerns. Often, medications are expensive and not covered by insurance resulting in either significant out-of-pocket-expenses for the patient or lack of adherence to a medication regimen. Finally, one should always be aware of the burden that many patients and families feel as they are going through their illness. The SUPPORT study found that 31% of all families spent most or all of their savings on the treatment of their terminal illness, with 29% reporting loss of the major source of income (47). Both nurses, and, in particular, social workers, can be extraordinarily helpful in determining the family resources and potential concerns.

Spiritual Assessment

Patients often ask that their health care professional be familiar with, assess, and care for all elements of their disease, which includes care for their spiritual needs. Not to be confused with religion, spiritual care focuses on supporting the patient's understanding of who they are and what place their life holds in the reality of their disease and the context of their world.

In NHS-Scotland's Guidelines for Spiritual and Religious Care offers a clear description of the difference of the two terms:

- *Religious Care.* Care that is given in the shared context of shared values beliefs, values, and lifestyles that are shared within a faith community.
- *Spiritual Care.* Care that is given in one-to-one relationships, is completely centered around the person and makes no assumptions about personal conviction or life orientations (48).

A spiritual assessment can provide another link to a better understanding of a patient's suffering (49). The fundamental component of the spiritual assessment is to listen to the patient to determine the *meaning* of this illness to them. This may, or may not, have anything to do with formal religion, but may reflect more of a struggle over the patient's own issues of "ultimate concern": fears about the future for both themselves and their loved ones; desire to not be a burden to their family members; issues of loss of control, independence, hope, and their changing role within their family, community, or workplace; fears about their own death and the questions around dying.

A spiritual assessment can provide important information on how the patient is coping with the serious illness and inward suffering. A specially trained pastoral care provider is an invaluable member of the team in this regard. Questions regarding one's life purpose and meaning that are discussed in a safe and respected place can contribute to a greater sense of autonomy during disease progression (48). For many, these concerns, if not assessed and addressed, grow and can lead to spiritual crisis where feelings of guilt, unworthiness, hopelessness, and abandonment fulminate. One must ask open-ended questions like: "How have you tried to make sense of what is happening to you?" or "What are some of the things that give you a sense of hope?" (2), and then be prepared to listen to the response to understand the patient's sense of meaning. Additional questions that help to elicit ones state of purpose: "What are the things that help to bring you rest during difficult days?" and "Where do you look to find sources of positive energy or hope?" are often helpful. Incomplete or unattended spiritual care may lead to a crisis of the spirit which can be demonstrated in uncontrolled or exaggerated symptoms, expressions of guilt and despair, lack of focus and control and further feelings of loss (48).

In addressing *religious* care, the IDT should be well informed of the landscape of religious diversity within their communities and have resources available to them to bring specific traditions to the patient. Outside of the hospice spiritual care provider, the patient's own religious leader or members of their own faith community may be a useful source of strength to the patient and family (50) and information about a particular faith tradition for the health care team. The skillful spiritual care provider on the IDT can be extremely effective in assessing and facilitating the resources necessary to meet the unique spiritual and religious care needs.

Practical Assessment

The final area of assessment is the practical assessment (51). Essential to the practical assessment is communication and collaboration. Communication begins with discussing patient and family needs. Issues to consider here are whether or not the patient will need help at home in the form of a formal caregiver, the home environment, medication administration, safety and cultural issues that impact the patient's and family's actions. Collaboration with appropriate agencies that provide care in the home setting will be an invaluable assistance to patients and their families.

Many factors impact the patient's need for a caregiver and to what extent the caregiver will be able to provide care or support. In a private home the primary caregiver may be with the patient 24 hours/day, but be frail or ill and unable to physically provide hands-on care. Although this type of caregiver can contact others in the case of an emergency, they may require assistance from other family members, private hired nursing assistants, or aides from a home health agency. These auxiliary caregivers can assist in terms of activities of daily living. For example, shopping for food, food preparation, bathing, dressing, and hygiene.

Planning for likely changes in patient function can help to reduce the chance of a crisis developing. Nurses are particularly skilled at anticipating the practical problems that may befall the person with advanced disease. In addition, a nursing assistant is trained to assist the patient in activities of daily living while developing a relationship that allows for detection of subtle changes in the patient that can prevent hospitalization when treated early. A nursing assistant can be assigned through a home health agency for a few hours a day or the patient and family may choose to privately hire an aide for shift work or as a live-in.

A patient who lives, or is moving to an Assisted Living Facility (ALF), may need to make arrangements for personal care as well. This should be determined by assessing the patient's physical needs and communicating with the facility's staff to coordinate what services are available to deliver the appropriate care.

A discussion with the patient and family regarding the home environment and the patient's mobility will be paramount to arranging for appropriate transportation, and durable medical equipment such as hospital beds, wheelchairs or walkers. Include in the assessment the patient's endurance, physical ability to climb stairs, as well as the home environment that might have narrow hallways or cluttered areas causing a fire hazard. An evaluation by a home health agency may need to be coordinated to thoroughly assess the home setting and safety issues. Consider that a social worker may be needed to assist in placement issues if the patient can no longer climb stairs due to weakness or shortness of breath or if confusion/forgetfulness prevent the patient from safely living alone.

A major concern involving the practical assessment is the patient's ability to administer medications safely. Evaluate the patient's learning ability, including whether they can read, comprehend simple instructions and their stress level that can affect comprehension. Determine what teaching needs exist regarding their medications. Consider the following: can the patient get the prescriptions filled? Do they have transportation to the pharmacy or someone to go for them? Do they have money to pay for the prescriptions? Is their eyesight poor? Can they read the labels? Can they open the bottles? Do they need someone to fill pillboxes to prevent duplication or missed doses? If they can't read, do they need color or symbols on the labels to provide simple instruction? Do they need the medication administration instructions written in layman's terms?

Assisting the patient and family to anticipate their growing needs includes the evaluation of safety related to the use of oxygen if applicable in the home setting. Patients and families need to understand the risks and proper care to provide the prescribed amount of oxygen and to prevent accidents. Collaboration with a home health agency that can evaluate the home setting and reinforce teaching is essential to providing safe care.

Cultural influences must be included as part of the practical assessment. Every practitioner must be sensitive to different cultures that can influence how a patient and family respond to conversations regarding prognosis, instructions, and support. It is impossible to be knowledgeable about all cultures. Therefore, open dialogue and carefully worded questions can allow a practitioner to ascertain the aspects of a culture that may provide barriers between the health care establishment and a patient and their family. In many cultures, it is inappropriate for certain family members to provide hands-on care even though they are more than capable. A Medical Power of Attorney (MPOA) may have been established, however, to confirm who is to be approached with issues concerning prognosis, test results, the plan of care and possible end-of-life issues. Do not assume the spouse is the point of contact. Not taking the time to consider a patient's ethnicity could lead to offending the patient and/or the family and limiting or ruining the professional relationship.

The practical assessment allows the practitioner to anticipate needs as the patient's condition declines. Discussing possible scenarios and communicating the plan for when conditions develop, allow the patient and family to feel in control when so much is out of their control. Anticipating patient and family needs provides time to make arrangements before a crisis develops. Communication and collaboration will be core to developing a trusting relationship that will assist in reducing stress to some degree as a patient nears the end of life.

SUMMARY AND CONCLUSIONS

As medical technologies and therapies have converted many illnesses into chronic conditions that people have to live with for months or perhaps years, it is important to remember that medical illness affects every aspect of individual and family life. In the setting of palliative and supportive oncology, there are a number of domains of whole patient assessment that should be obtained on the initial visit that are, perhaps, different from those currently obtained in the traditional medical model. Although these additional domains of assessment may seem overwhelming both in time and emotion for one clinician, it is what our patients and their families are expecting. Therefore, it is imperative that our training in oncology nursing, social work, and medicine (surgical, radiation, and medical oncology) have the principles of "Primary Palliative Care" that are embodied in the MDPA as core competencies in clinical practice (2).

Furthermore, each professional, regardless of discipline-specific training, must learn to more fully respect and collaborate with our colleagues in other disciplines, to integrate their assessments, share the burden of the issues that will be revealed, and ultimately achieve better outcomes for our patients and families in terms of whole person care. Ultimately, through this effort, the health care provider will also find, that, through interdisciplinary teamwork, "the sum is greater than the individual parts", leading to greater personal and professional satisfaction for all clinicians involved in palliative and supportive oncology.

References

1. Johnson AR, Siegler M, Winslade WJ. *Clinical ethics: indications for medical interventions*, 3rd ed. New York: McGraw-Hill, 1992:15.
2. American Medical Association's Institute for Ethics. *Trainers guide, education for physicians on end-of-life care (EPEC project)*, Gaps in end-of-life care, 1999:1–20.
3. Mount BM. The problem of caring for the dying in a general hospital; the palliative care unit as a possible solution. *Can Med Assoc J* 1976;115(2):119–121.
4. McHugh M, West P, Assatly C, et al. Establishing an interdisciplinary patient care team: collaboration at the bedside and beyond. *J Nurs Adm* 1996;26(4):21–27.
5. Skobel SW, Cullom BA, Showalter SE. When a nurse is not enough: why the hospice interdisciplinary team may be a nurse's best gift. *Am J Hosp Palliat Care* 1997;14(4):201–204.
6. Abeloff MD. Burnout in oncology–physician heal thyself [editorial; comment]. *J Clin Oncol* 1991;9(10):1721–1722.
7. Axelson JA, Clark RH. Burnout syndrome among oncologists [letter; comment]. *J Clin Oncol* 1992;10(2):346.
8. Saunders JM, McCorkle R. Models of care for persons with progressive cancer. *Nurs Clin North Am* 1985;20(2):365–377.
9. Byock IR. Conceptual models and the outcomes of caring. *J Pain Symptom Manage* 1999;17(2):83–92.
10. Cummings I. The interdisciplinary team. In: Doyle D, Hanks GWC, MacDonald N, eds. *Oxford textbook of palliative medicine*, 2nd ed. Oxford: Oxford University Press, 1998:20–30.
11. Ahles TA, Martin JB. Cancer pain: a multidimensional perspective. *Hosp J* 1992;8(1–2):25–48.
12. Weissman DE. Consultation in palliative medicine. *Archives Intern Med* 1977;157:733–737.
13. Abrahm JL. Promoting symptom control in palliative care. *Semin Oncol Nurs* 1998;14(2):95–109.
14. Fernandez RD, Spragley F. Strengthen your care continuum by targeting charting excellence. *Nurs Manage* 2004;35(10):25–29.
15. Krammer LM, Muir JC, Gooding-Keller N, et al. Palliative care and oncology: opportunities for oncology nursing. *Oncol Nurs Updates* 1999;3(6):1–12.
16. Grumbach K, Bodenheimer T. Can health care teams improve primary care practice? *JAMA* 2004;291(10):1246–1251.
17. Bower P, Campbell S, Bojke C, et al. Team structure, team climate and the quality of care in primary care: an observational study. *Qual Saf Health Care* 2003;12(4):273–279.
18. Boyle DK, Kochinda C. Enhancing collaborative communication of nurse and physician leadership in two intensive care units. *J Nurs Adm* 2004;34(2):60–70.
19. Amos MA, Hu J, Herrick CA. The impact of team building on communication and job satisfaction of nursing staff. *J Nurses Staff Dev* 2005;21(1):10–16.
20. Coeling HVE, Cukr PL. Communication styles that promote perceptions of collaboration, quality, and nurse satisfaction. *J Nurs Care Qual* 2000;14(2):63–74.
21. Beyea SC. Improving verbal communication in clinical care. *AORN J* 2004;79(5):1053–1057.
22. Coombs M. Medical hegemony in decision-making—a barrier to interdisciplinary working in intensive care? *J Adv Nurs* 2004;46(3):245–252.
23. Reese DJ, Sontag MA. Successful interprofessional collaboration on the hospice team. *Health Soc Work* 2001;26(3):167–173.
24. Burke M, Boal J, Mitchell R. Communicating for better care. *Am J Nurs* 2004;104(12):40–47.
25. Street AB, Blackford J. Communication issues for the interdisciplinary community palliative care team. *J Clin Nurs* 2001;10(5):643–650.
26. Hu J, Herrick C, Hodgin KA. Managing the multigenerational nursing team. *Health Care Manag* 2004;23(4):334–340.
27. Miller PA, Carlton KH. Technology as a tool for health care collaboration. *Comput Nurs* 1998;16(1):27–29.
28. Lindeke LL, Sieckert AM. Nurse-physician workplace collaboration. *Online J Issues Nurs* 2005;10(1):1–7, (web address for article www.medscape.com/viewarticle/499368.
29. World Health Organization. *Cancer pain relief and palliative care: report of the WHO expert committee*, Technical bulletin 804. Geneva: WHO,1990.
30. Bruera E, Kuehn N, Miller MJ, et al. The Edmonton Symptom Assessment System (ESAS): a simple method for the assessment of palliative care patients. *J Palliat Care* 1991;7(2):6–9.
31. Portenoy RK, Thaler HT, Kornblith AB, et al. The memorial symptom assessment scale: an instrument for the evaluation of symptom prevalence, characteristics and distress. *Eur J Cancer* 1994;30A(9):1326–1336.
32. Holland JC. Preliminary guidelines for the treatment of distress. *Oncology (Huntingt)* 1997;11(11A):109–114; discussion 115 117.
33. Gammon J. Which way out of the crisis? Coping strategies for dealing with cancer. *Prof Nurse* 1993;8(8):488–493.
34. Furrow BR, Greaney TL, Johnson SH, et al. *Health law: cases, materials and problems*, 4th ed. St. Paul, MN: West Publishing Co., 2001:171–172.

35. Knapp ER, DelCampo RL. Developing family care plans: a systems perspective for helping hospice families. *Am J Hosp Palliat Care* 1995;12(6):39–47.

36. Cleeland CS, Ryan KM. Pain assessment: global use of the brief pain inventory. *Ann Acad Med Singapore* 1994;23(2):129–138.

37. Breitbart W. Psycho-oncology: depression, anxiety, delirium. *Semin Oncol* 1994;21(6):754–769.

38. Valente SM, Saunders JM, Cohen MZ. Evaluating depression among patients with cancer. *Cancer Pract* 1994;2(1):65–71.

39. Buckman R. Communication in palliative care: a practical guide. In: Doyle D, Hanks GW, MacDonald N, eds. *Oxford textbook of palliative medicine*. Oxford: Oxford University Press, 1998.

40. Martinez J, Wagner S. Hospice care. In: Groenwald SH, Frogge MH, Goodman M, et al. eds. *Cancer nursing: principles and practice*, 4th ed. Boston, MA: Jones and Bartlett, 1997:1531–1549.

41. Weggel JM. Palliative care: new challenges for advanced practice nursing. *Hosp J* 1997;12:43–56.

42. Goetschius SK. Nursing and end-of-life care: exploring family roles. *Innov breast cancer care* 1998;4:9–12.

43. Teno JM, Nelson HL, Lynn J. Advance care planning. Priorities for ethical and empirical research. *Hastings Cent Rep* 1994;24(6):S32–S36.

44. Task Force on Cancer Care at the End-of-life. Cancer care during the last phase of life. *J Clin Onc* 1998;16:1986–1996.

45. Neuberger J. Introduction: cultural issues in palliative care. In: Doyle D, Hanks GWC, MacDonald N, eds. *Oxford textbook of palliative medicine*, 2nd ed. Oxford: Oxford University Press, 1998:777–785.

46. Covinsky KE, Goldman L, Cook EF, et al. The impact of serious illness on patients' families. SUPPORT Investigators. Study to understand prognoses and preferences for outcomes and risks of treatment. *JAMA* 1994;272(23):1839–1844.

47. Highfield MF. Spiritual assessment across the cancer trajectory: methods and reflections. *Semin Oncol Nurs* 1997;13(4):237–241.

48. Gordon T, Mitchell D. A competency model for the assessment and delivery of spiritual care. *Palliat Med* 2004;18:646–651.

49. Handzo RG. Chaplaincy: a continuum of caring. *Oncology (Huntingt)* 1996;10(9 Suppl):45–47.

50. Emanuel EJ, Fairclough DL, Slutsman J, et al. Assistance from family members, friends, paid care givers, and volunteers in the care of terminally ill patients. *N Engl J Med* 1999;341(13):956–963.

51. Cherny NI, Catane R. Palliative medicine and the medical oncologist. Defining the purview of care. *Hematol Oncol Clin North Am* 1996;10(1):1–20.

CHAPTER 47 ■ CROSS-CULTURAL ISSUES

JAMES L. HALLENBECK

People experience both health and illness in cultural contexts. A better understanding of culture helps the clinician avoid certain common pitfalls, thereby improving the chances of good outcomes. Very sick and dying patients in our society are often dependent upon care from people of very different cultural backgrounds, making cross-cultural misunderstandings and conflict common. Following an introductory discussion of culture and ethnicity and their relation to palliative care, this chapter will explore cultural issues in palliative care from a framework of three interrelated concepts—cultural sensitivity, competence, and effectiveness (1). Cultural sensitivity refers to an awareness of cultural influences on beliefs, practices, communication styles, and system issues as they affect the patient, the family, and the clinician. Cultural competence refers to skills and behaviors that serve to decrease cross-cultural conflict and improve care outcomes. Finally, the chapter will conclude with a discussion of the effectiveness of various interventions that might be used to improve care across cultures.

WHAT IS CULTURE?

Various definitions of culture exist in the literature. Helman defines culture as "a set of guidelines (both explicit and implicit) which individuals inherit as members of a particular society, and which tells them how to view the world, how to experience it emotionally, and how to *behave* in it in relation to other people, to supernatural forces or gods, and to the natural environment" (2). This definition suggests culture, as a *noun*, exists as a pervasive set of guidelines shaping the individual. Culture, as a *verb*, is in fact more than an inheritance; it is a dynamic *process* wherein people interact with each other and thereby actively create an ever-changing world experience. Culture can also be viewed as a complex and overlapping set of descriptors, adjectives and adverbs, giving meaning, shading, and even texture to various patterns of human organization and behavior.

IMPORTANCE OF CULTURE TO PALLIATIVE CARE

Recent American national consensus guidelines identified cultural aspects of care as one of the eight domains of palliative care, highlighting their importance (3). Criteria under this domain are outlined in Table 47.1. Although the criteria list is short, it suggests a broad array of concerns to be addressed: knowledge of and sensitivity to cultural backgrounds, awareness regarding cultural influences on bioethics and communication skills, and system issues. At both the clinician and the program level the challenge is taking such a list and translating it into discrete skills and actions that will result in more culturally effective care. Before considering specific interventions, let us consider why culture is so important in palliative care.

We live in an increasingly pluralistic society, although the extent of diversity varies dramatically by geographic region. Pluralism exists not only in terms of ethnicity but other cultural attributes. National and geographic origin, current home (geographic location, urban/rural), gender, sexual orientation, marital status, family, professional and community roles, religion, economic and educational status—these cultural attributes and others contribute to our cultural personae (4). Social factors associated with these attributes can create barriers to care, limiting the availability and effectiveness of palliative care for certain populations. Pluralism also exists among health care workers (5). When people become chronically ill, they are more likely to come under the care of clinicians and others from very different backgrounds than their own (6,7). Relationships in such situations are often imposed. That is, health care workers, whether physicians working in an intensive care unit or nurse's aides in a nursing home, and patients have limited choices as to who will care for whom. Because hands-on care, such as that provided by nurse's aides, is devalued in our society, immigrant and underclass workers make up a substantial portion of this workforce. These workers have little choice but to accept positions at the bottom of the social ladder, which in our society includes the provision of the most intimate care for chronically ill and dying patients. Conversely, patients and families are increasingly dependent upon care provided by such workers. Imposed relationships at such a fragile stage in the life cycle can create a problematic environment. Efforts to understand each other are not only desirable, but also essential.

Although culture lurks in the background of all human experience, it comes alive and overt during transition periods in the human life cycle. Death and dying are obviously major transitions and as such are heavily invested with culture. Cultural transitions are often marked by ritual and rites wherein meaning is expressed and created through particular behaviors. Beyond this, ritual is used to change reality or at least to create a particular human expression of reality. Rites and rituals related to palliative care are most obvious in considering death and dying practices (8). More subtle may be myriad behaviors, some of a very personal nature, that are used to cope with transitions in chronic illness. For example, ritual is involved in the process of making a person a patient in a hospital. Wristbands and hospital gowns serve ritual purposes

TABLE 47.1

CULTURAL ASPECTS OF CARE

National Consensus Project Criteria

The cultural background, concerns, and needs of the patient and their family are elicited and documented

Cultural needs identified by team and family are addressed in the interdisciplinary team care plan

Communication with patient and family is respectful of their cultural preferences regarding disclosure, truth-telling and decision making

The program aims to respect and accommodate the range of language, dietary, and ritual practices of patients and their families

When possible, the team has access to and utilizes appropriate interpreter services

Recruitment and hiring practices strive to reflect the cultural diversity of the community

From Clinical Practice Guidelines for Quality Palliative Care, National Consensus Project, 2004.

beyond mere technical efficiency. The ritual use of wigs or caps after hair loss through chemotherapy is another example that may serve the purpose of maintaining a certain image of self (in addition to keeping one's head warm). Conversely, "going bald" after hair loss may serve a ritual purpose of declaring acceptance as a new member of a class of cancer patients. Clinicians also engage in ritual behavior. For example, death pronouncement is more a ritual than a diagnosis of death (9). The importance of ritual as a cultural activity related to dying (and birth) is highlighted by Grimes in his book, *Deeply into the Bone—Reinventing Rites of Passage.*

> "If we do not birth and die ritually, we will do so technologically, inscribing technocratic values in our very bones. Technology without ritual (or worse, technology *as* ritual) easily degenerates into knowledge without respect." (8, p13).

Culture shapes how we relate to and communicate about major aspects of life, including serious and chronic illness. As discussed further in the subsequent text, if clinicians, patients, and families approach illness from differing cultural perspectives, miscommunication is almost inevitable, barring serious efforts to compensate for such differences. Finally, culture is inexorably intertwined with society and the health care system. It would be a mistake to view "culture" as a disembodied set of beliefs and practices, somehow separate from the social and organizational forces that shape our lives. As will be discussed at the end of the chapter, understanding this relationship and effecting systemic change may be one of the most effective ways to improve cross-cultural outcomes.

ETHNICITY

Most clinician training regarding culture has focused on ethnicity, as have many palliative care texts and articles (10). The tendency in many such texts is to describe beliefs and practices of particular ethnic groups relative to health care. Lipson, for example, provides overviews of how 24 ethnic groups construct illness, relate to symptoms such as pain, decision-making, relations with clinicians, preparations for dying, grief practices, and death rites, among others (11). Although this and similar texts may be helpful to clinicians struggling to care for patients from very foreign ethnic groups,

some caution is in order. Excessive reliance on such texts risks stereotyping by underestimating the extent of cultural diversity within ethnic groups (12). Culture tends to be portrayed more as a determinant *thing*, such as a genetic code, rather than an active *process* of social engagement. An exclusive focus on ethnicity and associated beliefs and practices also tends to narrowly define culture and limits the ability to appreciate other important aspects of culture (5,13). Problematic, cross-cultural encounters between individuals and health care systems may too easily be ascribed to differences in belief systems, with inadequate attention to social forces associated with ethnicity such as those arising from poverty or racism. As a case in point, a follow-up analysis of support study population demonstrated that African Americans (among other nonwhite groups) were more likely than Caucasians to die in acute care hospitals (odds ratio 1.88) (14). Other studies have suggested that as a group, African Americans are more likely to desire aggressive, life-prolonging care, and less likely to complete written advance directives (15). Whereas all this may be true, it would be a mistake to *assume* a connection between the probability of dying in the hospital and ascribed cultural beliefs of African Americans. Other demographic variables correlated with African American ethnicity, such as higher population densities in urban areas, proximity to hospitals, or socioeconomic factors such as poverty, might play as great or a greater role than beliefs. As a practical matter it is far easier to classify people by ethnicity than to sort out the influences of related and overlapping factors such as these.

Still, ethnicity is a useful starting point for considering the forces that affect care, as long as one understands that considerably more than "beliefs and practices" are at work. Correlated with ethnicity are important factors such as immigrant status, educational background, socioeconomic status, geographic and demographic distribution relative to health care resources, communication styles, and other social roles (4,16). Space does not allow for a detailed discussion of all these factors, although they undeniably affect clinician interactions with patients and families in profound ways. If seeking to learn more about a particular ethnic group, the clinician will likely be disappointed by a traditional Medline search. Although some good books are available, few journal articles are specific to cultural aspects of particular ethnic groups. In contrast, the Internet is a particularly rich source for material with a number of Web sites specializing in this area. A selected list of Internet references is listed in Table 47.2.

Cultural sensitivity requires an awareness of and respect for differences. This is far easier said than done. As one anthropologist put it, "culture hides much more than it reveals, and strangely enough what it hides, it hides most effectively from its own participants (17)". This statement suggests that examination of one's own culture, a form of cultural self-reflection, is a natural starting point for increasing cultural sensitivity. Such reflection is furthered by contrasting one's understanding and assumptions with those of other cultural groups. Of particular importance is contrasting differing understandings of illness, medical systems, and styles of communication. To a degree such reflection can be stimulated by formal medical education. Unfortunately, medical curricula have rarely included cultural aspects of care, despite studies calling for such inclusion. A study in 1992 queried 126 medical schools regarding possible courses in "cultural sensitivity." Of 98 respondents only 13 schools reported offering such courses and all but one were elective. Fifty-nine schools indicated that they had incorporated cultural sensitivity in other courses such as courses on medical ethics (18). A systematic review of the literature from 1963 to 1998 published in 1999 found 17 reports of curricula meeting search criteria (19). Thirteen

TABLE 47.2

INTERNET REFERENCES

Internet links for Cross-Cultural Issues in Health

The Center for Cross-Cultural Health. Links to multiple other cross-cultural web sites.
http://www.crosshealth.com/links.htm

The Cross-Cultural Health Care Program. Specializes in issues related to medical interpreters and other cultural competency issues. http://www.xculture.org

Stanford Geriatric Education Center. Specializing in ethnogeriatrics. Includes on-line training modules on cross-cultural communication. http:/sgec.stanford.edu/

Ethnomed: Ethnic Medicine Information from Harborview Medical Center. Contains health care information pertinent to health care of recent immigrants.
http:/www.ethnomed.org

CultureMed. From SUNY, this web site promotes culturally competent health care for immigrants and refugees. Superb bibliographies.
http://www.sunyit.edu/library/html/culturedmed/

International Association for Hospice and Palliative Care. Leading international hospice and palliative care organization for a more global perspective.
http://www.hospicecare.com/

of these programs were in North America and 11 were exclusively for students in year 1 and 2 of medical school. The focus of most of the content was on ethnicity, attitudes, health beliefs, and language barriers. Only one program is reported to have considered anthropological and sociological theories (20). The lack of breadth and the apparent lack of depth of training suggested in this review are discouraging. However, there are some encouraging signs of change. Carrillo et al. published a description of a course for medical students and residents consisting of four 2-hour modules covering *basic concepts, core cultural issues, understanding the meaning of the illness, determining the patient's social context, and negotiating across cultures*, which seems to be more in keeping with recent anthropologic and sociologic trends (21). In an intervention designed to assist internal medicine programs in the United States in improving palliative care education, Weissman found that teaching regarding cross-cultural issues was high on the list of unmet needs of residency training programs (22). In response to this, a module on addressing cross-cultural concerns was developed (23). This suggests that physicians are generally interested in improving their training in cultural issues, which bodes well for future educational efforts.

CULTURE OF BIOMEDICINE AND PALLIATIVE CARE

In keeping with the notion of cultural self-reflection, let us consider biomedicine as a culture, particularly as it has evolved in the United States and the relation between biomedicine and palliative care. Originating in western Europe, the evolution of biomedicine has been guided by complex historical, religious, philosophical, and economic forces (24). Biomedicine has now become, arguably, the dominant medical system throughout the world, being integrated, or at least coexisting, with numerous other medical systems. Insight into cultural aspects of biomedicine is critical for the practitioner trying to work with individuals across cultures.

Although sharing with other medical systems a fundamental charge to heal the sick, biomedicine's emphasis in recent decades has been increasingly to fix broken bodies (24, 25). Pursuing a western rationalist belief that the *good* is best approached through scientific inquiry, biomedicine has developed a mechanistic approach to care. Through a progressively refined and reductionist understanding of the origins of illness, labeled *disease*, the hope (and the myth) of biomedicine is to eliminate physical disease entirely. Although suffering is not entirely ignored in biomedicine, it does take second place to biology as an issue of concern in that it is often presumed that suffering will disappear once disease has been eliminated. This belief that suffering is derivative to biological malfunctioning is naïve on two fronts. First, it simply takes no account of aspects of suffering not arising from the body (26,27). Second, almost too obviously, biomedicine to date has failed to eliminate disease. Given our continuing mortality, inevitably the elimination of one illness must, by default, increase the probability of becoming ill and eventually dying from something else. Therefore, suffering continues. Indeed, biomedicine "creates" new forms of illness and associated suffering, as the field of supportive oncology, dealing in large part with the sequelae of oncologic treatment, is ample testimony. The evolution of palliative and supportive care, pain clinics, and hospices as social phenomena on the margin of biomedicine can be understood in part as reactions to the failure of this dominant myth of biomedicine (Table 47.3).

Biomedicine is unusual as a medical system in its inattention to any concept of a "life force" (28,29). Most other medical systems include some notion of a life force and commonly frame the understanding of health and illness in terms of balance and imbalance between aspects of energy (often positive and negative) that give rise to a life force (13). Examples include Chinese (yin-yang) and Hispanic (hot-cold), among others. A medicine that identifies healing as a process of *balancing* seems philosophically closer to the spirit of palliative care than a medicine based on *cure* and is arguably more relevant when cure is no longer possible. Balance need not be approached solely in terms of energy. For example, palliative approaches to congestive heart failure and skin disorders often emphasize a balance between wetness and dryness.

Biomedical culture influences our behavior as clinicians at more intimate levels as well. Our cultural personae as clinicians are shaped to a large degree by innumerable small interactions with teachers and peers. For example, in learning to *take* a history, clinicians come to understand that the Social History should primarily focus on behavioral risk factors for disease, such as alcohol intake and sexual activity, not the social network of the patient. Nor is there even a section

TABLE 47.3

TENSIONS IN THE CULTURE OF BIOMEDICINE

Individualism	⟷ Reductionism
Autonomy	Paternalism
Disease in the individual body	Mechanistic/technologic approach to illness
Consumerism	Bureaucratization
Egalitarianism	⟷ Capitalism
Health care as a right	Health care as commodity

Lacking in modern biomedicine:

Focus on suffering as primary object of medicine

Inclusion of a concept of a life force in model

Illness as something transcending the individual

for a Personal History of the patient as a *person*. Such a bias is a reflection of the biomedical emphasis on disease and relative neglect of more social aspects of illness. With chronic or terminal illness, preventive health care, emphasized in the traditional H&P, becomes less relevant and the social network upon which the patient increasingly relies becomes more relevant. Insensitive application of a biomedically oriented approach to care risks neglect of social and cultural aspects of the patient's illness, which tend to grow in importance with progressive severity and chronicity of illness.

Palliative care, working at the margin of biomedicine, constitutes a radical challenge to many of biomedicine's tenets. The emphasis in palliative care is on the person and family as the unit of care. Attention to suffering and quality of life assumes primacy in care provision. It should come as little surprise that resistance to such an approach has been engendered by many in biomedicine. Resistance is less a conscious opposition to palliative goals of care (nobody is *against* relief of suffering) and more a reflection of a cross-cultural conflict between the traditional biomedical culture and the evolving subculture of palliative care.

BIOETHICS, BIOMEDICINE, AND CROSS-CULTURAL ENCOUNTERS IN PALLIATIVE CARE

The relevance of bioethical concerns to palliative care should be obvious. It is more difficult to appreciate that bioethics are the product of western biomedicine and as such are prone to cultural biases. The national consensus guidelines list three topics more commonly discussed as bioethical issues as "cultural preferences": disclosure, truth telling, and decision making. Other topics such as hydration and nutrition could be added to this list. Such topics do indeed raise ethical concerns. However, to address the ethics of such concerns as being separate from the diverse belief and value systems shaping "cultural preferences" is to risk cultural insensitivity. Therefore, the practice of bioethics must be informed by a consideration of intrinsic cultural biases as the first step in the development of a culturally sensitive bioethics.

Anthropologic critiques of bioethics are limited, but raise important issues of concern (30). Often noted as "ethnocentric" positions of bioethics are the following:

- The dominance of abstract ethical "principles" as prime movers for decision making, based on tenets of western philosophy.

Classically four such principles are identified—autonomy, beneficence, nonmaleficence, and justice. The process of using abstract principles as prime movers betrays a cultural bias. So too does the choice of specific principles. For example, *interdependence*, valued by so many non-western cultures as a principle for decision making, might be posited as the counterweight to autonomy, rather than justice (31,32).

- A tendency to make such abstractions "practical" through the practice of consultations on ethics, especially in the United Sates.
- Codification of such abstractions in a plethora of laws, regulations, and policies, reflecting the bureaucratic and litigious tendencies of American society.
- The dominance of autonomy as a guiding principle (33,34)
- Suffering as a derivative, not a primary concern of ethics.

An almost unassailable insistence on surrogate decision making as the only proper vehicle for deciding a course of action for patients lacking capacity derives from the dominance of autonomy as a principle of bioethics. The anthropologic basis for the primacy of surrogate decision making and substituted judgment, in which the proxy is supposed to decide as if he or she were the patient is highly questionable (35). Even a cursory examination of decision making for incapacitated patients across world cultures would find very few examples of groups espousing surrogate decision making as a guiding value. One could argue that the primacy given to surrogate decision making reflects the limited view of a very small subculture of western bioethicists (and the courts and many policy makers who seem to share this view) (6).

CULTURAL COMPETENCE

The prior section on cultural sensitivity stressed the importance of an appreciation and respect for differences among cultural groups. Such awareness is an important step in moving toward cultural competence and effectiveness, but is inadequate in and of itself. Cultural competence requires the acquisition of new skills and behaviors to address differences identified through greater sensitivity and awareness. The term cultural competence, which has become broadly accepted in the literature, is somewhat unfortunate in that it implies that clinicians are either *competent* or *incompetent* in their practices, when in fact cultural competence should be understood as existing along a broad spectrum of abilities; one does not *become* culturally competent, the best one can do is to *improve* one's competency. In this section the issue of nondisclosure will be discussed as an example of a skill used to address a bioethical issue in a culturally sensitive manner and then the broader issue of cross-cultural communication will be addressed.

EXAMPLE OF NONDISCLOSURE

The scene is well known to most clinicians. A relative requests that the clinician not inform a patient of some bad news such as a diagnosis of cancer or a terminal prognosis (36,37). Such a request appears to conflict with autonomy as a guiding principle and multiple health care policies that stress the importance of informed consent. The dilemma is doubly difficult because the request is that clinicians either not talk to or blatantly lie to the patient, inhibiting open communication that might resolve the issue.

A narrowly applied bioethics could do serious harm in such a case. Rigidly insisting that the patient has "the right to know" could both alienate family members and damage the patient by forcing undesired information. Anecdotal case reports suggest that some patients, if bluntly told of their prognosis, will in fact lose the will to live, as families sometimes warn. Orona suggests a possible resolution to the problem based on a twist of logic, which recognizes that autonomy can be reframed as a choice *not* to act independently but to defer to others (33). The trick is how to identify such a choice on the part of the patient without giving undesired information. Skill must be used in exploring the understandings of the patient and the family and then negotiating a resolution.

At the simplest level the clinician should state and demonstrate *respect* in the face of such a request (23,38). Recalling that family-based decision making and nondisclosure are common worldwide, and recognizing that courage is often needed to make such a request in the face of a powerful health care system that generally disapproves of nondisclosure, may help the clinician engender respect.

Exploration of the context may begin with the person(s) making the request for nondisclosure. Why are they making this request? How do they understand the roles of participants, both in the family and among clinicians, relative to care? What do they fear might happen if the person knew? What are their hopes?

Just as cultures are not monoliths, neither are families. It is quite possible for a family to believe the patient does not want to know, when in fact he or she does. The clinician might then inquire how the family and specifically the patient have dealt with similar situations in the past. The clinician might ask questions such as, *"Do you think or know that she would agree with this? Have you discussed this approach with her? How has she dealt with similar situations in the past?"*

Exploration is not a one-way street; it is not the same as *taking* a history. Clinicians are advised to share their (often equally foreign) biomedical viewpoints as well as the dilemmas being confronted, including policies that require informed consent. For example, beyond the mundane (getting consent forms signed), clinicians may admit that they too wish only the best for the patient. One might say that in one's experience some people even in cultures that practice nondisclosure really want to know and that if this were so, nondisclosure might cause the patient distress and this would bother the clinician. The clinician might explain that he or she values truth telling and could not lie if asked a question directly. Hopefully, finding the presumed common ground of wishing the best for the patient will foster some mutual understanding.

The clinician will probably want to explore the patient's understanding and concerns. The intent and desire to explore the patient's wishes regarding disclosure without coercion may be explained to family members. At a simple level one may simply need to confirm that the patient wishes to "defer" decision making to the family, although a richer exploration is encouraged. What to do if the patient states that she wants to know the truth or to be in charge should be worked out before such an encounter. Most clinicians will want to be clear on certain ground rules such as not lying. If the patient requests to be informed, rather than simply be told, the clinician may change roles and facilitate improved communication between the patient and family.

Dealing with difficult dilemmas in real life cannot be done as prescriptively as the preceding text might imply. The preceding text is presented to offer the clinician some guidance as to how to explore and negotiate such a situation and to illustrate an approach to conflict resolution.

INTERCULTURAL COMMUNICATION

As the prior discussion highlights, good communication is critical to the practice of medicine in general and palliative care in particular (39). Generic communication skills in palliative care, such as the ability to listen or give bad news, will not be discussed here. A number of recent texts explore intercultural communication in health care (40,41). Cultural aspects of communication specific to palliative care are beginning to be addressed in the literature and will be discussed further here (38,42).

The most obvious cultural communication barrier is language. Communication will be largely ineffective and prone to serious misunderstanding without competent translation. Relying on family members as translators, although sometimes unavoidable, is problematic, as messages between clinician and patient may be filtered (43). Using family members as translators also puts both patients and family members in awkward positions. They may be forced to discuss sensitive topics inappropriate for their family roles. *Role conflict*, in which new social roles conflict with established roles, may result. For example, in using a bilingual child as a translator, as is common, there may be a role reversal between the patient/parent and the child in which the parent becomes dependent upon the child. Professional medical translators, where available, are generally recommended although their use does not eliminate communication challenges (44). Skilled interpreters can do more than translate words. They may act as "cultural guides," facilitating broader understanding (45).

In considering language as a cultural barrier, the tendency is to view the other's language as the problem, something that needs only to be *translated*. More difficult is recognition of the barriers intrinsic to the language of biomedicine. The language of biomedicine emphasizes scientific, technologic, and cognitive concerns and tends to neglect more human concerns such as emotion. Patients and families often attempt to express their concerns through this biomedical language, trying to speak to us in our peculiar, foreign tongue. For example, distress in witnessing a family member near death may be expressed as a demand for some medical intervention such as intravenous hydration. In part, this may be because people have become familiar with the bias of biomedicine to focus on *doing* rather than *feeling*. In hearing such a demand, clinicians are prone to hear and respond to the technical aspects of the communication and ignore the affective subtext of distress (46). Therefore, the specialized language of biomedicine can pose particular communication challenges for those attempting to address more human concerns, as palliative care leaders have rightfully advocated is necessary. A specific communication skill of particular value in palliative care is to learn to recognize and address the subtext of a message both in terms of affect and underlying cultural values.

Cross-cultural communication in palliative care is particularly difficult because key content issues, such as serious illness, difficult decisions, and dying, are very sensitive for many people. Discussion of certain topics may frankly be taboo. In many cultures and for many people, words have power. To speak of illness or dying is to increase the chance of illness or death occurring. Carrese, discussing Navajo difficulties with western bioethics, quotes a Navajo medicine man:

In my practice, when I'm working with the patient, I am very careful of what I say, because any negative words could hurt the patient. So, with Western medicine, a doctor could be treating a patient, and he can mention death, and that is sharper than any needle (47).

Communication is far more than simple transmission of data from one source to another. Without some understanding of the context within which communication occurs, mutual understanding is impossible. A branch of anthropology has focused on intercultural communication, based largely upon the pioneering work of anthropologist Edward Hall (17). Hall recognized that cultural contexts are not inert boxes within which communication exists, but important aspects of communication itself. Hall and others have identified some cultures as being relatively high and others as relatively low in context (48). High-context cultures tend to depend more on the context of the situation than on verbal expression for communication. Context refers to things such as *who* is speaking to *whom*, the setting for the discussion, relationships between participants (including issues such as dominance, trust, or mistrust), the physical use of space and shared meanings. Nonverbal communication is closely linked to context. Context may be imbedded in verbal communication as well. The very different meanings in two expressions for dying, "kick the bucket" and "passing on," derive from shared contextual meanings (49). High context people tend to become offended by overly direct verbal communication and a lack of attention to relationship building by low-context individuals. In contrast, low-context cultures and individuals tend to stress direct verbal communication. Low-context people may become frustrated by vagueness and lack of direction in discussions with high-context individuals. Much of what is important to high-context people is frankly invisible to low-context people.

Biomedicine, arising from a western, predominantly northern European scientific tradition, is very low in context. Although such a low-context approach may serve well where efficiency is needed and accurate transmission of data is required across cultures and languages, it becomes problematic when dealing with the more human issues, which commonly arise in palliative care.

Just as cultures may be higher or lower in context, so too can different human activities. Very personal, taboo, or dangerous activities tend to be highly imbedded with context. Serious illness and dying are very personal and dangerous activities and therefore are intrinsically high in context. Major communication problems arise when clinicians practicing within the world of biomedicine use low-context communication strategies in dealing with patients and families experiencing illness as high-context events. Very direct, scientifically oriented communication, emphasizing reason over emotion, as typical of western biomedicine, can easily clash with more indirect, contextual styles typical of many cultural groups. Low-context clinicians in dealing with high-context encounters, may benefit from first identifying encounters as such. Hints to a high-context encounter include much indirectness in the conversation and the involvement of multiple participants. Requests for nondisclosure, previously discussed, typically occur in high-context encounters. Although the low-context tendency is to "get down to business" and resolve an issue quickly, perhaps by too directly emphasizing the patient's right to know, this approach often backfires when inadequate attention has been paid to relationship building, which is usually critical to the resolution of high-context problems. The low-context clinician may need to slow down and build new relationships before negotiating a specific course of action. Adjusting one's speed of communication, using spatial positioning and surroundings to convey intended meanings, and building relationships, are examples of explicit high-context communication skills.

EXPLANATORY MODELS AND ILLNESS NARRATIVES

Serious and life-limiting illnesses pose threats to personhood (25,50,51). People tend to live optimistically, creating life stories that end with everyone living "happily ever after." Serious illnesses are radical interruptions in these stories. Sick individuals and the others involved, struggle to make some sense of this negation, to fill in the blank by interpreting illnesses and eventually incorporating them into revised life stories. In revising their stories people tend to fall back on traditional patterns and understandings. These understandings of illness often differ significantly from biomedical understandings.

Kleinman introduced the term *explanatory model* as a means of exploring different understandings of illness (52,53). "Explanatory models are the notions that patients, families, *and practitioners* have about a specific illness episode" (52, p121) (italics mine). As this quotation points out, clinicians also have their own explanatory models for illness, most typically revolving around the concept of *disease*. Kleinman has suggested that eliciting a patient's explanatory model (and reciprocally reflecting and sharing one's one model) can further mutual understanding and help form a basis for collaborative decision-making (52, p227–251). He writes that in the face of illness two questions seem to dominate—*why* did this happen and *what* should be done about it. Specific

TABLE 47.4

EXPLANATORY MODEL QUESTIONS

What—do you call the problem, do you think the illness does, do you think the natural course of the illness is, do you fear?
Why—do you think this illness or problem has occurred?
How—do you think the sickness should be treated, do you want us to help you?
Who—should you turn to for help and who should be involved in decision-making? What are their roles in your illness?

questions useful in eliciting an explanatory model are included in Table 47.4.

Such an exploration should consist of "*empathic listening, translation,* and *interpretation*" (52, p228). In more recent writings Kleinman explicitly warned against using the explanatory model as a form of interrogation:

"I meant the explanatory models technique to be a device that would privilege meanings, especially the voices of patients and families, and that would design respect for difference. I intended it to be a *modus operandi* to get at what is at stake in suffering. I saw explanatory models as a methodology for clinical self-reflexivity, for pressing against biomedical crystallizations, for laying hold of the sources of clinical miscommunication. I wanted to encourage the use of open-ended questions, negotiation, and listening, not the usual mode of clinical interrogation" (28, pp8–9).

The preceding passage suggests that Kleinman understood the explanatory model technique as a means to enhance both cultural sensitivity and competence in clinical encounters.

Exploring explanatory models is critical for effective communication. This is a process not only of listening to the patient, but of sharing and interpreting the clinician's explanatory model of the patient's illness. Such exploration serves as a basis for collaboration and negotiation as to goals and choices. More concretely, exploration itself is often therapeutic.

EXAMPLE OF THE USE OF THE EXPLANATORY MODEL IN PALLIATIVE CARE

Consider the following common dilemma: a patient with cancer does not want to take an opioid you believe would be helpful in managing the patient's pain. Although it might be tempting to simply explain common misperceptions regarding opioid management, exploration of explanatory models might be more productive in the long run, as outlined in Table 47.5.

As this hypothetical example shows, there are areas of overlap and difference in the two models. In the process of exploring the model the clinician comes to understand that far more is involved than clearing up misunderstandings of addiction. The patient is struggling with whether or not the pain can or should be relieved. Statements made reflect spiritual and psychologic distress, which might best be addressed by others.

Kleinman points out that explanatory models are not complete accounts of illness in and of themselves. They are part of broader *illness narratives*, which in turn are actively created out of rich life experiences in response to a disruption in life stories—a process of *integration* in the face of the disintegrating forces of illness (50,51). This process of healing

TABLE 47.5

PATIENT AND PHYSICIAN EXPLANATORY MODELS OF PAIN

Question	Patient's model	Clinician's model
Why do you think you are in pain?	The cancer (superficial level)	The cancer (superficial level)
	I deserve to suffer for mistakes I have made in the past (deeper level)	A combination of nociceptive and neuropathic pain, due to nerve compression (deeper, biomedical level)
What do you think the natural course of your illness and pain will be?	There isn't much that can be done about it. The pain and my illness will worsen until I die. The situation is hopeless	While this is a terminal illness, this particular pain syndrome seems eminently treatable. The patient could feel much better
What do you think would happen if you took morphine?	I would just get addicted, which would make matters worse	The pain would improve. The patient would not become addicted, although certain side effects such as constipation would need to be managed
Who should be involved in dealing with your pain?	It is really up to God. Perhaps this is also a test for me to see how I handle all this. I wonder if I'm up to it	Whereas there is a physical cause for the pain, it is also clear that the patient is struggling with other issues. Perhaps others on our team could be of help

work in the face of certain unalterable realities of illness seems to get to the heart of what palliative care is all about.

CULTURAL EFFECTIVENESS

An American Academy of Pediatrics position paper stated, "[W]hereas cultural competence and cultural sensitivity refer to the provider's attributes, the term culturally effective health care refers to the interaction between the provider and patient" (54). This statement, although reasonably pointing beyond individual provider characteristics, is unsatisfying as a definition for cultural effectiveness. Here, cultural effectiveness will refer to outcomes resulting from provider or health care system interventions in response to efforts reflecting cultural sensitivity and competence. The question, quite simply, is what interventions result in *effective* change for the better?

One systematic review of 34 educational initiatives found that most studies of courses on cultural sensitivity and competence demonstrated measurable changes in attitudes and skills over short to intermediate time ranges (55). However, this review found only three studies demonstrating improved patient satisfaction and no articles addressing patient health outcomes such as access to or provision of care. None of the reviewed studies was specific to palliative care. Obviously, more research is needed.

Interventions that might be effective could work at either interpersonal or system levels. As the referenced review demonstrates, courses addressing knowledge, attitudes, and skills, can

clearly affect the clinician. Despite a lack of studies, it seems highly probable that such courses also improve patient and family satisfaction, to the extent they result in more sensitive and effective communication. Where particular tensions exist between clinicians and particular patient populations, as where most providers are from a different ethnic or religious group than are most patients, targeted educational interventions addressing such tensions would seem particularly important.

The bigger challenge seems to be to identify interventions that would likely improve access to care and clinical outcomes for underserved groups. This is a major challenge for palliative, supportive, and hospice care programs, as a number of studies have demonstrated underutilization and barriers to care for minority groups and special populations (4,56–60). A partial list of at-risk populations that would likely benefit from special attention is presented in Table 47.6. It is not hard to imagine that these groups, among others, might have very special palliative needs that currently are poorly addressed within existing systems of care. Hospice and palliative care organizations are rightly concerned that the care they provide too often is for those in privileged classes.

Whereas a variety of macroscopic social forces, related to patient demographics and health care system factors, undoubtedly serve as barriers to good palliative and supportive care these should not prohibit system changes at a local level. Table 47.7 provides a partial list of interventions that local programs might consider. Of note, formal training becomes a system change, when it is required and monitored. A community needs assessment might start with a review of patients historically served by the program and then a study of cultural groups in the program's catchment area to identify underserved populations. Outreach to and collaborative problem solving with leaders of underserved populations might then improve access and hopefully outcomes for patients.

TABLE 47.6

SPECIAL AT-RISK OR UNDERSERVED POPULATIONS

Immigrants and refugees
The homeless and the impoverished
People with histories of substance abuse
People with chronic mental illness
People with developmental and other disabilities
People with sexual identity issues
The incarcerated

SUMMARY

Culture is all around us and yet for the most part, we are blind to it. We may recognize culture in others, very different from ourselves; it is far more difficult to be aware of how our own culture invisibly influences our own thoughts, actions, and organizations. It is the very ubiquitous nature of culture that makes it so difficult to move from good intentions to action.

TABLE 47.7

SUGGESTIONS FOR PROGRAMMATIC CHANGES TO IMPROVE CULTURAL EFFECTIVENESS

Inclusion of cultural sensitivity and competency training as a
staff requirement
Staff recruitment, reflecting community diversity
Community needs assessment
Identify and make accessible resources useful in meeting the
needs of target populations including:
Internet resources
Local community agencies and support groups
Library of relevant books, journals, educational material
Establishment of policies and procedures addressing
translation needs
Inclusion of a cultural assessment as part of routine patient
and family assessment
Outreach efforts to disadvantaged groups with palliative care
needs:
Partnerships and educational efforts with community
organizations
Brochures and educational material linguistically and
culturally appropriate for target populations

The temptation is to rest on our intentions or to narrowly circumscribe "cultural competence" with isolated educational courses. As has been demonstrated admirably elsewhere in the palliative care movement, the most effective changes are likely to result from systemic changes that institute new patterns of care.

ACKNOWLEDGMENT

Work is supported by the Department of Veterans Affairs, VA Palo Alto Health Care System.

References

1. Crawley LM, Marshall PA, Lo B, et al. Strategies for culturally effective end-of-life care. *Ann Intern Med* 2002;136(9):673–679.
2. Helman C. *Culture health and illness*, 3rd ed. London: Butterworth-Heineman, 1994.
3. *Clinical practice guidelines for quality palliative care*. Brooklyn: National Consensus Project for Quality Palliative Care, 2004.
4. Oliviere D, Monroe B, eds. *Death, dying and social differences*. New York: Oxford University Press, 2004.
5. Koenig B. Cultural diversity in decisionmaking about care at the end of life. In: Field M, Cassel C, eds. *Approaching death: improving care at the end of life (Institute of Medicine)*. Washington, DC: National Academy Press, 1997.
6. Hallenbeck J, Goldstein MK. Decisions at the end-of-life: cultural considerations beyond medical ethics. *GENERATIONS*. 1999;23(1):24–29.
7. Barker JC. Cultural diversity–changing the context of medical practice. *West J Med* 1992;157(3):248–254.
8. Grimes R. *Deeply into the bone—reinventing rites of passage*. Berkley, CA: University of California Press, 2000.
9. Hallenbeck J. Palliative care in the final days of life—"they were expecting it at any time". *JAMA* 2005;293(18):2265–2271.
10. Braun K, Pietsch J, Blanchette P. *Cultural issues in end-of-life decision making*. Thousand Oaks, CA: Sage Publications Inc, 2000.
11. Lipson JG, Minarik PA, Dibble SL, University of California San Francisco. School of Nursing. *Culture and nursing care: a pocket guide*. San Francisco, CA: UCSF Nursing Press, 1996.
12. Gunaratnam Y. Culture is not enough—a critique of multi-culturalism in palliative care. In: Small N, ed. *Death, gender and ethnicity*. London: Routledge, 1997:166–186.
13. Good B. *Medicine, rationality, and experience: an anthropological perspective*. New York: Cambridge University Press, 1994.
14. Pritchard RS, Fisher ES, Teno JM, et al. Influence of patient preferences and local health system characteristics on the place of death. SUPPORT

Investigators. Study to Understand Prognoses and Preferences for Risks and Outcomes of Treatment. *J Am Geriatr Soc* 1998;46(10):1242–1250.
15. Eleazer GP, Hornung CA, Egbert CB, et al. The relationship between ethnicity and advance directives in a frail older population. *J Am Geriatr Soc* 1996;44(8):938–943.
16. Field D, Hockey J, Small N, eds. *Death, gender and ethnicity*. New York: Routledge, 1997.
17. Hall E. *The silent language*. New York: Anchor, 1990.
18. Lum C, Korenman S. Cultural-sensitivity training in U.S. medical schools. *Acad Med* 1994;69:239–241.
19. Loudon R, Anderson P, Sing Gill P, Greenfield S. Educating medical students for work in culturally diverse societies. 1999.
20. Wells K, Benson M, Hoff P. Teaching cultural aspects of medicine. *J Med Educ* 1985;60(6):493–495.
21. Carrillo JE, Green AR, Betancourt JR. Cross-cultural primary care: a patient-based approach. *Ann Intern Med* 1999;130(10):829–834.
22. Weissman D. Personal Communication.
23. Hallenbeck J. Cross-cultural issues in end-of-life care. In: Weissman DE, Ambuel B, Hallenbeck J, eds. *Improving end-of-life care: a resource guide for physician education*. 3rd ed. Madison, WI: Medical College of Wisconsin, 2000.
24. Fabrega H. *Evolution of sickness and healing*. Berkeley, CA: University of California Press, 1997.
25. Hahn R. *Sickness and healing—An anthropological perspective*. New London: Yale University Press, 1995.
26. Cassell E. *The nature of suffering: and the goals of medicine*. New York: Oxford University Press, 1991.
27. Byock IR. The nature of suffering and the nature of opportunity at the end of life. *Clin Geriatr Med* 1996;12(2):237–252.
28. Kleinman A. *Writing in the margin: discourse between anthropology and medicine*. Berkeley, CA: University of California Press, 1995.
29. Brady E, ed. *Healing Logics—culture and medicine in modern health belief systems*. Logan: Utah State University Press, 2001.
30. Marshall PA, Koenig B. Bioethics in anthropology: perspectives on culture, medicine and morality. In: Sargent C, Johnson T, eds. *Handbook of medical anthropology—contemporary theory and method*. Westport, CT: Greenwood, 1996:349–373.
31. Bowman K. Communication, negotiation, and mediation: dealing with conflict in end-of-life decisions. *J Palliat Care* 2000;(Suppl 16):S17–S23.
32. Chan HM. Sharing death and dying: advance directives, autonomy and the family. *Bioethics* 2004;18(2):87–103.
33. Orona C, Koenig B, Davis A. Cultural aspects of nondisclosure. *Camb Q Healthc Ethics* 1994;3:338–346.
34. Frank G, Blackhall L, Michel V, et al. A discourse of relationships in bioethics: patient autonomy and end-of-life decision making among elderly Korean Americans. *Med Anthro Q* 1998;12(4):403–423.
35. High D. Families' roles in advance directives. *Hastings Cent Rep* 1994; 24(Suppl 6):S16–S18.
36. Charlton R. The dilemma of truth disclosure: stoke-on trent, England. *Am J Hosp Palliat Care* 1997;14(4):166–168.
37. Muller J. Ethical dilemmas in cross-cultural context. *West J Med* 1992;1992 (157):323–327.
38. Hallenbeck J. Intercultural differences and communication at the end of life. *Prim Care* 2001;28(2):401–413.
39. von Gunten CF, Ferris F, Emanuel L. Ensuring competency in end-of-life care. *JAMA* 2000;284(23):3051–3057.
40. Krept G, Kunimoto E. *Effective communication in multicultural health care settings*. Thousand Oaks, CA: Sage Publications Inc, 1994.
41. Luckman J. *Transcultural communication in health care*. Albany: Delmar, 2000.
42. Kogan S, Blanchette P, Masaki K. Talking to patients about death and dying: improving communication across cultures. In: Braun K, Pietsch J, Blanchette P, eds. *Cultural issues in end-of-life decision making*. Thousand Oaks, CA: Sage Publications Inc, 2000:305–325.
43. Chan A, Woodruff R. Comparison of palliative care needs of English and non-English speaking patients. *J Palliat Care* 1999;15(1):26–30.
44. Rivadeneyra R, Elderkin-Thompson V, Cohen Silver R, et al. Patient centeredness in medical encounters requiring an interpreter. *Am J Med* 2000;108:470–474.
45. Yeo G. Ethical considerations in Asian and Pacific island elders. *Clin Geriatr Med* 1995;11:139–152.
46. Suchman AL, Markakis K, Beckman HB, et al. A model of empathic communication in the medical interview. *JAMA* 1997;277(8):678–682.
47. Carrese J, Rhodes L. Western bioethics on the Navajo reservation. *JAMA* 1995;274:826–829.
48. Porter R, Samovar L. An introduction to intercultural communication. In: Porter R, Samovar L, eds. *Intercultural communication*. 8th ed. Belmont, MA: Wadsworth, 1997:5–26.
49. Lee W. That's Greek to me: between a rock and a hard place in intercultural encounters. In: Samovar L, Porter R, eds. *Intercultural communication*. 8th ed. Belmont, MA: Wadsworth; 1997:213–216.
50. Frank A. *The wounded storyteller—body, illness, and ethics*. Chicago, IL: University of Chicago Press, 1995.
51. Becker G. *Disrupted lives—how people create meaning in a chaotic world*. Berkeley, CA: University of California Press, 1999.
52. Kleinman A. *The illness narratives - suffering healing and the human condition*. New York: Basic Books, 1988.

53. Hallenbeck J. The explanatory model. *J Palliat Med* 2003;6(6):931.
54. Culturally effective pediatric care: education and training issues. American Academy of Pediatrics Committee on Pediatric Workforce. *Pediatrics* 1999;103(1):167–170.
55. Beach MC, Price EG, Gary TL, et al. Cultural competence: a systematic review of health care provider educational interventions. *Med Care Apr* 2005;43(4):356–373.
56. Jennings B, Ryndes T, Donofrio C, et al. Access to hospice care: expanding boundaries, overcoming barriers. *Hastings Cent Rep Spec Suppl* 2003; 33(2):S3–S59.
57. Reese DJ, Melton E, Ciaravino K. Programmatic barriers to providing culturally competent end-of-life care. *Am J Hosp Palliat Care* 2004;21(5): 357–364.
58. Kessler D, Peters TJ, Lee L, et al. Social class and access to specialist palliative care services. *Palliat Med* 2005;19(2):105–110.
59. Greiner KA, Perera S, Ahluwalia JS. Hospice usage by minorities in the last year of life: results from the National Mortality Followback Survey. *J Am Geriatr Soc* 2003;51(7):970–978.
60. Moller D. *Dancing with broken bones—portraits of death and dying among inner-city poor.* New York: Oxford University Press, 2004.

CHAPTER 48 ■ COMMUNICATION DURING TRANSITIONS OF CARE

JAMES A. TULSKY AND ROBERT M. ARNOLD

Palliative care aims to meet the disparate needs of patients and families during a time of life-limiting illness. Good communication is indispensable to uncovering patient and family needs and individually negotiating the goals of care. Everyone defines a good death differently (1), and whether a patient's suffering is caused by pain, nausea, unwanted medical intervention, or spiritual crisis, the common pathway to treatment is through a provider who is able to elicit these concerns and is equipped to help the patient and family address them.

Good communication brings real and tangible benefits. In patients with cancer, the number and severity of unresolved concerns has been shown to predict high levels of emotional distress and future anxiety and depression (2,3). Conversely, considerable evidence suggests that improved physician–patient communication correlates with improved health outcomes, patient satisfaction, and emotional well-being (4–6). For example, primary care patients exhibit decreased anxiety, and are more satisfied with their physicians if they discuss advance care planning (7). Communication itself appears to be therapeutic, as simply telling one's story may improve objective health outcomes (8). Finally, families who are better prepared for their loved one's deaths may experience less difficult bereavement.

This chapter is designed to

1. Review recent literature concerning health care provider communication
2. Survey basic communication issues relevant to palliative care, particularly the role of affect in communication
3. Give the reader practical advice regarding some of the common topics that arise when caring for patients with life-limiting illness—giving bad news, discussing advance care planning, introducing palliative care, and talking about prognostic issues.

HEALTH CARE PROVIDERS DO NOT COMMUNICATE WELL

Unfortunately, the general quality of communication between health care providers and patients with life-limiting disease is suboptimal. Studies show that the discussion of bad news frequently does not meet patient needs or falls short of expert recommendations (9–11). Both physicians and nurses tend to underestimate and not elicit cancer patients' concerns (12), and commonly do not attend to patients' affect or even recognize their emotional cues (13,14). Rather than using facilitative communication techniques, such as open-ended questions or empathic responses when inquiring about psychosocial issues, they often block discussion of these issues by changing the subject or not attending to patients' emotional states (15). Even in a hospice setting, one study revealed that only 40% of patient concerns were elicited (16). As a result, patients with cancer tend to disclose fewer than 50% of their concerns (15,16), which leads further to physicians' inaccurate assessments of patient distress (17). Two large studies of audio-recorded oncology visits with terminally ill patients found that physicians only dedicated a small percentage of their time to health-related, quality of life issues, including psychosocial concerns, frequently missed opportunities to address issues that seemed to be most important to patients, and did not often check for patient's understanding (18,19). Finally, physicians rarely talk with seriously ill patients about their goals, values, or even treatment decisions (20–22). A significant gap exists between the idealized model of provider–patient communication at the end of life and the reality of practice.

WHAT CAUSES POOR COMMUNICATION?

Why is the "state-of-the-art" so poor? First, health care providers are not selected for their communication skills. Expertise in cognitive areas is not always positively correlated with empathy or an interest in understanding another person's experience. Medical education emphasizes cognitive teaching techniques and cognitive material rather than the psychoemotional–spiritual aspects of care. Second, until recently there has been little training regarding communication skills in general, not to mention communication about these difficult topics. For example, in a survey of over 3200 oncologists, few had any formal training in end-of-life care or communication skills. Oncology programs are not alone in devoting little attention to this subject. At both the medical school and residency level, inadequate attention is given to care of the dying (23). Among graduating students at two medical schools, only 48% said they had adequate role models for how to discuss end-of-life issues. At another school, 41% of medical students on a medicine rotation and 73% on a surgery rotation had never observed a staff physician talk with a dying patient. Happily, educational interventions have improved this situation; over 60% of medical students now report "adequate" training on end-of-life care. Unfortunately, these interventions continue to focus on cognitive aspects of care. Students report that death is still viewed as a loss not to be discussed and that they are discouraged from showing their emotions (24). Finally, physicians have difficulty inquiring directly about the emotional status of dying patients because of their feelings about the patient or their own mortality. We will particularly focus on this issue.

Considerable evidence suggests that physicians' personal feelings toward their patients are important to the doctor–patient relationship (25), and many have suggested that physicians' emotional responses to their dying patients may interfere with their care (26). Physicians dealing with dying patients are not objective observers. They are active participants whose beliefs and feelings influence the interaction. For example, a study of surrogate decision making found that physicians' predictions of their patients' wishes regarding life-sustaining treatment were closer to their own choices than to the choices expressed by their patients (27).

Caring for the dying may elicit significant stress in physicians and a variety of reactions, including guilt ("If only I'd convinced him to get that screening colonoscopy."), impotence ("There's nothing I can do for her."), failure ("I messed up. I'm a bad doctor."), loss ("I'm really going to miss this person."), resentment ("This patient is going to keep me in the hospital all night."), and fear ("I know they're going to sue me.") (28). According to Spikes and Holland, many physicians have unconscious feelings of omnipotence and troublesome responses stem from a physician's need to preserve his or her image as a "powerful healer" who can master any situation (26). Feeling that he or she has failed the dying patient, a physician may respond by acting defensively, wishing that the patient would die (to avoid dealing with the patient), or by treating too aggressively (to ensure that "everything has been done to save the patient").

Empathizing with a dying patient often evokes anxiety about physician's own mortality. Physicians respond by withdrawing from terminally ill patients, avoiding threatening topics (15,29), employing blocking behaviors that distance them from addressing affective concerns of patients (30), or falsely reassuring them that "everything is OK (26)."

Empirical data support these claims about physicians' anxieties regarding death. Physicians score higher on death anxiety scales than other professional groups (31). They also find caring for terminally ill patients stressful. For example, in a survey of 598 oncologists, 56% reported being burned out and 53% attributed these feelings to continuous exposure to fatal illness (32). When caring for dying patients, physicians often report sadness, helplessness, failure, disappointment, and loneliness (33). These feelings, particularly if unrecognized, may affect patient care. Residents who are more burned out endorse more negative attitudes and behaviors related to patient care (34). Conversely, residents who report better personal well-being score higher on empathy scales (35). A study of 25 pediatric residents explored the relationship between their orientation toward death and their response to a clinical vignette. Residents with a high death threat and anxiety scores were more likely to adopt avoidance and denial strategies for dealing with the vignette (36).

Although these issues are profound, awareness of their own emotional responses to caring for dying patients can help physicians begin to focus more objectively on the effect of their behavior on the patient.

BASIC COMMUNICATION SKILLS

Talking to dying patients is just like, and completely unlike, all other communication with patients. Whether one is explaining the implications of hypertension, or talking about impending death, basic principles of good communication are useful. The primary difference between these communication tasks is the meaning of the conversation to the patient and the provider, and the attendant level of emotional significance. When the situation is more likely to make the patient (or physician) feel vulnerable, sad, or inadequate, one should focus extra attention on the task. In this section, we will address basic communication skills that are universal to all encounters.

A little effort spent on advance preparation can have a tremendous impact on the quality of the encounter. Whenever possible, important medical information, particularly bad or sad news, should be delivered during a scheduled meeting. This allows patients to prepare themselves for the type of information they will hear and to make sure that appropriate family members or friends are present. It also allows the physician to allocate the necessary time to the encounter and to come prepared with basic medical information and anticipating the most likely questions regarding treatment options, prognosis, and resources for support and guidance.

Communication best occurs face-to-face. Telephones accentuate physical communication difficulties and there is no opportunity to employ the benefits of nonverbal communication. Given that over 50% of communication is nonverbal, both parties operate at a disadvantage if they cannot see each other. The physician should sit at eye level and within reach of the patient. If possible, one's pager or cellular phone should be turned off, or at least put on a quiet mode, and one should avoid interruptions.

Increasingly, we encounter non-English-speaking patients. One must absolutely employ the assistance of an interpreter in such settings. However, it is equally important to avoid using family members as interpreters. Not only does this run the risk of faulty translation or reinterpretation of the physician's statements, it also places family members into the uncomfortable position of being the physician's and patient's spokesperson. The common practice of using bilingual young children as translators is particularly problematic. Most hospitals and health care facilities in regions with high numbers of immigrants employ professional translators or maintain lists of language skills among facility staff members.

Regarding the dialogue itself, considerable data exist from the medical and psychological literature to support certain general techniques that allow more accurate assessment of anxiety and depression and increased disclosure of concerns (13,37). One should maintain good eye contact, ask open-ended rather than closed-ended questions, focus on the patient's concerns as well as the agenda for the visit, respond to the patient's affect, ask about the patient's life outside of medicine, attend to psychosocial issues, and ensure that nonverbal behavior signifies attentiveness (Table 48.1) In contrast, disclosure of concerns is inhibited by closed-ended or leading questions,

TABLE 48.1

GENERAL COMMUNICATION SKILLS TO ENHANCE DISCLOSURE OF CONCERNS

Maintain good eye contact
Ask open-ended rather than closed-ended questions
Focus on the patient's concerns as well as the agenda for the visit
Observe and respond to the patient's affect
Ask about the patient's life outside of medicine and attend to psychosocial issues
Ensure that nonverbal behavior signifies attentiveness

focusing on physical aspects of illness, and offering of advice and premature reassurance (13).

One core precept is not to assume that one knows what is on the patient's agenda. For example, while many patients will want to discuss end-of-life issues, approximately 25% will not. This may have to do with cultural particularities or with how individuals cope with illness. Physicians are not very good at predicting which patients want more and which patients want less information. Instead of assuming one should ask. For example, on a first visit one could say, "I want to touch base with you about how you want me to handle information we get about your illness. Some patients want to know everything that is going on with their illness, the good and the bad. Other people do not want as much information and want me to speak more generally. And some would really prefer I do not discuss bad news with them but want me to discuss these issues with their family. Which kind of person do you think you are?"

Another important precept of communication is to "ask before telling." Patients often carry misperceptions or incomplete information obtained from the popular media, folklore, or friends and family. It is easier to deal with this information if it is discussed directly. Thus, it is usually helpful to ask patients about their understanding of their illness before educating them. Furthermore, one study of intensive care unit (ICU) family conferences observed that allowing families more opportunity to speak may improve family satisfaction (38).

WHAT IS EFFECTIVE COMMUNICATION AT THE END OF LIFE?

According to dying patients, family members and health care providers, goals for communication at the end of life include talking with patients in an honest and straightforward way, being willing to talk about dying, giving bad news in a sensitive way, listening to patients, encouraging questions from patients, and being responsive to patients' readiness to talk about death (39). Patients want physicians to achieve a balance between being honest and straightforward and not being discouraging. For some this requires leaving open the possibility that unexpected "miracles" might happen, discussing outcomes other than a cure that can offer patients hope and meaning, and helping patients prepare for the losses they may experience. Patients cope better when physicians emphasize what can be done, explore realistic goals and discuss day-to-day living (40). Although patients must receive adequate information to make informed choices, they wish to receive that information in an emotionally supportive way (41). Patients want to discuss emotional concerns but are frequently unwilling to bring them up spontaneously and may need to be prompted (42).

This may sound impossible. How can one be honest and be hopeful? How can one ensure informed consent and let patients decide they do not want to hear all the information? While many models have been proposed (43–47) they have in common several principles:

1. Given that patients vary greatly in their desire for information and participation in decision making, one should assess patients' preferences for communication as part of the medical encounter (48,49). One cannot presume to "intuit" patient's wants and needs, therefore one should ask.
2. One should give information nontechnically and in brief, understandable pieces. This allows the physician to constantly reassess the patient's verbal or nonverbal reaction to the information, as well as their desire for more information.

3. Patients and their family members may have different goals and needs for information, thus one needs to assess each person in a group conversation.
4. While doctors focus on medical treatments and dying, patients focus on function and relationships. Therefore, treatments should be discussed within the framework of the patient's goals rather than in abstraction.
5. Attention to the affective component of the conversation is as important as the cognitive aspects. Thus all models stress the critical role of empathy in communication. In the rest of this chapter we will focus on the role of emotions in such discussions.

THE ROLE OF AFFECT

Most difficulties in communication at the end of life are the result of inattention to affect. *Affect* refers to the feelings and emotions associated with the content of the conversation. Feelings such as anger, guilt, frustration, sadness, and fear modify our ability to hear, to communicate, and to make decisions. For example, after hearing bad news, most patients are so overwhelmed emotionally that they are unable to comprehend very much about the details of the illness or a treatment plan. Some studies have shown that emotion affects processing; people who are in negative moods may pay more attention to how messages are given than to the content of the messages (50). Thus when patients are experiencing high levels of negative affect and caregivers do not ameliorate this affect, patients may be less likely to receive the health care providers' messages. Unfortunately, conversations between doctors and patients often transpire only in the cognitive realm; emotion is frequently not acknowledged or handled directly and physicians miss opportunities to do so (51).

Dealing with Physicians' Emotions

Physicians, as well as patients, experience many emotions as they care for people approaching the end of life. In addition to its effect on their own communication, physician affect plays an important role in patients' reactions to medical information. In one study women were randomly assigned to view a video of an oncologist, who was portrayed as either worried or not worried, presenting mammogram results. Those watching the "worried" physician received less information, experienced higher anxiety levels and perceived the situation as more severe compared with those watching the "nonworried" physician (52).

For physicians, the first step toward managing feelings of loss, helplessness, or anxiety is to acknowledge that they exist, and to recognize that they are normal. When experiencing a strong emotion while interacting with a patient, one should ask oneself, "Where is this coming from?" Although it may be a result of what the physician brings to the encounter (e.g., one's own sense of mortality or how it makes one think of his grandmother who died), it may also be a clue into what the patient is feeling. Thus many doctors report, feeling anxious when talking with a patient who has an anxiety disorder, or feeling overly sad when talking with a depressed patient. If the physician gets a sense that he or she is reflecting the patient's emotion it may help to ask the patient about this (e.g., "I wonder if you're feeling sad?").

If the emotion is a result of the physician's reaction to the encounter, the next step is to discuss this with colleagues or confidants. In most cases, however, patients do not benefit from hearing such thoughts. When considering sharing such feelings with a patient, a good rule of thumb is to ask oneself, "Am I doing this for me or for the patient?" If the answer is truly the latter, then it may be appropriate to share.

Dealing with Patients' Emotions

One barrier to engaging patient affect is the fear of being unable to manage the emotional response. This section will describe an approach to handling emotions that is also likely to further elicit the sorts of patient concerns described earlier.

The primary goal when responding to emotions is to convey a sense of empathy. Empathy is the sense that "I could be you," and is what patients are usually feeling when they comment about a physician who really cared for them (53). Empathy can be expressed either verbally or nonverbally. The eponym SOLER is used to identify the following nonverbal behaviors that have been shown to reflect empathy:

1. Facing the patient Squarely indicates involvement and interest in the patient's story.
2. Adopting an Open body position is a sign that you are open to the patient.
3. Leaning toward the patient reflects intimacy and flexibility to the patient's position.
4. Eye contact reflects attention in North American cultures, although it is impolite in other cultures; and
5. One should maintain a relaxed and natural body posture (54).

Robert Smith has created a useful mnemonic to recall four basic techniques to use when confronted by patient emotions, NURS (Name, Understand, Respect, and Support) (55). This discussion adds a final "E" for Explore (Table 48.2). Naming the emotion serves to acknowledge the feeling and to demonstrate that it is a legitimate area for discussion. Statements such as, "That seems sad for you," can serve this purpose well, although one needs to be careful not to inappropriately label the patient. Therefore, naming is often best done in a quizzical fashion that does not presuppose the emotion (e.g., "Many people would feel angry if that happened to them. I wonder if you ever feel that way?").

Expressing a sense of understanding normalizes the patient's emotion and conveys empathy. However, expressing understanding must be done cautiously to prevent a response such as, "How can you possibly understand what I'm going through? Have you ever had a stroke?" A typical statement might be, "Although I've never shared your experience, I do understand that this has been a really hard time for you."

Respect reminds us to praise patients and families for what they are doing and how they are managing with a difficult situation. Offering respect defuses defensiveness and makes people feel good about themselves and more capable of handling the future. A useful statement might be, "I am so impressed with how you've continued to provide excellent care for your mother as her dementia has progressed."

Support is essential to helping people in distress not to feel alone. Simple statements such as, "I will be there with you throughout this illness," can be tremendously comforting. Health care providers ought not to feel the entire support burden on their shoulders—support offered can include other members of a team. For example, "We will send a nurse to your home to check in on you in a couple of days and if you'd like, I could ask the chaplain to visit you."

Finally, patients will frequently make statements that deserve further exploration. For example, a patient may say, "After you gave me the results of the test, I thought that this is going to be it." A simple response such as, "Tell me more," may help reveal the patient's fears and concerns about cancer that will be helpful in planning future treatment.

Hope in the Context of Palliative Care

Physicians struggle to promote hope in the patient with advanced disease and to support a positive outlook, fearing that discussing death may decrease the patient's hopefulness (39,56,57). As a result, they frequently convey prognosis with an optimistic bias or do not give this information at all. This is relevant to treatment choices; patients with more optimistic assessments of their own prognosis are more likely to choose aggressive therapies at the end of life (58). In turn, fearing the loss of hope, patients frequently cope by expressing denial, and may be unwilling to hear what is said.

It is not clear if health care providers can either steal or instill hope. However, they can provide an empathic, reflective presence that will help patients draw strength from their existing resources. Physicians should recognize that it is not their job to "correct" the patient's hope for a miracle. The key question is whether the hope is interfering with appropriate planning and behavior. A patient who has completed his will and said his good-byes, but is still hoping for a miracle is different from a patient who is making long-term investments and does not plan for custody of a minor child despite a 3-month prognosis.

Physicians can respond in several ways (in addition to demonstrations of empathy discussed earlier). Acknowledging the hope may allow the physician and the patient to "hope for the best but prepare for the worst." They can also recognize that people hope for many different things and leave space for patients to hope for outcomes and futures that are more likely to occur. One might say, "I know you are hoping that your disease will be cured. Are there other things that you want to focus on?" Or, "If we cannot make that happen, what other shorter term goals might we focus on?" Finally, one can ask about what tasks are left undone as a way to get patients to begin to think in a shorter time course.

Managing Conflict

Conflict occurs frequently in discussions about end-of-life care. In one study of 102 consecutive cases of decisions to limit life-sustaining care in ICUs at an academic medical center, conflict of some type was described in 78% of cases and clinician-family conflict occurred nearly half the time (59). Although often avoided by clinicians and patients, conflict managed well can be productive (60). However, when clinicians engage in behaviors such as denying the conflict, assuming they know the whole story or the other party's intentions, repeatedly trying to convince the other party and ignoring their own strong emotions, they are likely to exacerbate the problem. Useful tools to address conflict include many of the communication techniques already described: active listening, empathizing, reframing, explaining, and self-disclosure. Back and Arnold have described a stepwise approach to addressing conflicts that recognizes the emotional content of these situations and

---

TABLE 48.2

NURSE-ING AN EMOTION

Name the emotion
Understand the emotion
Respect or praise the patient
Support the patient
Explore what underlies the emotion

Fischer GS, Tulsky JA, Arnold RM. Communicating a poor prognosis. In: Portenoy RK, Bruera E, eds. *Topics in palliative care*, Vol. 4. New York: Oxford University Press, 2000.

focuses on interests, rather than positions (60). They encourage clinicians to:

1. Notice the conflict
2. Prepare themselves by getting into a ready state of mind, examine what has happened and their feelings and decide on the purpose of working through the conflict
3. Find a nonjudgmental starting point
4. Reframe emotionally charged issues
5. Respond empathically
6. Look for options that meet the needs of both parties
7. Get help if no satisfactory agreement can be reached

Such an approach will likely achieve a resolution in most cases and improve relationships with patients, family members, and other clinicians.

PRACTICAL SUGGESTIONS FOR SPECIFIC SITUATIONS

Communicating Bad News

Communicating bad news draws upon the skills discussed previously (see the section What is Effective Communication at the End of Life?). Many protocols exist for the delivery of bad news, however, the behaviors tend to be grouped into several key domains: preparation, content of message, dealing with patient responses, and ending the encounter (Table 48.3) (11). The primary elements of preparation have been addressed above (see the section Basic Communication Skills).

Content of Message

Knowledge of what the patient already knows or believes is extremely valuable to have, before revealing bad news to

---

TABLE 48.3

KEY ELEMENTS OF DELIVERING BAD NEWS

Preparation
Find out what patient knows and believes
Find out what patient wants to know
Suggest a supportive person accompany the patient
Learn about the patient's condition
Arrange the encounter in a private place with enough time

Content
Get to the point quickly
Fire "warning shot" (e.g., "I have bad news.")
State the news clearly, simply, and sensitively
Avoid false reassurance
Make truthful, hopeful statements
Provide information in small chunks

Handle patient's reactions
Inquire about meaning of the condition for the patient
NURSE expressed emotions
Assure continued support

Wrap-up
Set up a meeting within next few days
Offer to talk to relatives/friends
Suggest that patients write down questions
Provide a way to be reached in emergencies
Assess tendency to commit suicide

Fischer GS, Tulsky JA, Arnold RM. Communicating a poor prognosis. In: Portenoy RK, Bruera E, eds. *Topics in palliative care*, Vol. 4. New York: Oxford University Press, 2000.

---

a patient. This allows the physician to begin the explanation from the patient's perspective, aligning oneself with the patient and making communication more efficient and effective. The time that a test is ordered is a good time to assess this. One might ask, "Is there anything that you are particularly concerned about?" If the patient mentions a serious illness that might be present, the physician can follow-up by asking what the patient's specific fears and concerns are.

When prepared to deliver the content of the message, the physician should begin by firing a brief "warning shot," and then stating the news in clear and direct terms. One should avoid spending any time "beating around the bush," before sharing the news. After this brief exchange, the physician should remain silent and allow the patient an opportunity for the news to sink in. One can strike an empathic pose, maintain comfortable eye contact, and perhaps use a nonverbal gesture such as reaching out and touching the patient's hand. However, silence is imperative to allow the patient an opportunity to process the information, formulate a response, and to experience his or her emotions. Physicians who feel uncomfortable during this silent phase need to appreciate that the discomfort is rarely shared by the patient, who is engrossed in thought about the meaning of the news and thoughts about the future. Furthermore, very little that is said by the physician at this time will be remembered by the patient, so it is best not to say it at all. If the patient makes no verbal response after, perhaps, two minutes, it can be useful to check in: "I just told you some pretty serious news, do you feel comfortable sharing your thoughts about this?"

Dealing with the Response

The remainder of the conversation should be spent primarily dealing with the patient's response. This includes using the SOLER and NURSE skills to legitimize and empathize with the patient's experience. It is also important to explore the meaning the news has for the patient and to achieve a shared understanding of the disease and it's implications. For example:

MD: What is most troubling to you about having cancer?
PT: It's a death sentence—my mother died from cancer, my brother died from cancer. I guess it's my turn now.
MD: Given your experience, I can see how this is really scary for you. And cancer can be very serious. However, in your case, there are a lot of treatment options, and you have a good chance of surviving with this disease.
PT: So this won't kill me?
MD: I certainly hope not. And, I'll be there with you every step of the way fighting this illness.

Hopeful messages need to be tailored to patients' specific concerns, particularly addressing patient misconceptions and fears. Once patients' concerns have been explored, patients can be reassured more effectively. When effective treatment is available, this fact should be explained. When the treatment options are poor, hope may be found by alleviating the patients' worst fears. Doctors may reassure patients that they will not be abandoned during their illness, that the doctor will remain available if things get worse, that everything will be done to maintain patients' comfort, and that they will continue to watch for new treatment developments. Often people find hope and strength from their religious or spiritual beliefs, from having their individuality respected, from meaningful relationships with others, and from finding meaning in their lives. Exploring these with the patient over time may help to foster realistic hope. Although physicians may have a desire to make an overly reassuring statement to the patient right after revealing the diagnosis, hopeful statements that are truthful and that are made after taking the time to first explore the patient's concerns are more likely to be accepted by the patient. One can offer a realistic sense of hope, whether biomedical ("We'll keep our eyes open for new treatments and discuss them as they become available") or psychosocial ("I look forward to talking with you more about how we can help you live everyday as fully as possible, despite this illness").

Patients may have specific questions about further tests, treatment options, and prognosis. It is important to respond to these seriously. However, many patients will suffer difficulties in comprehension in such emotionally challenging situations. Information, particularly a plan, is helpful, as it allows the patient to reconceptualize the future as a safer, more predictable place. The exact details matter less than the clarity of the plan and the reassurance that the physician will be available. Giving simple, focused bits of information, using nonvague language that patients can understand, carefully observing the patient's verbal and nonverbal reactions to what is said, and most importantly, avoiding information-packed speeches helps.

Ending the Encounter

The clinician must end the encounter in a way that leaves the patient feeling supported and with some sense of hope. Support can be provided through meeting patients' immediate health needs and risks. One must treat pain and palliate other symptoms. Patients should be asked how they plan to cope with the news, and if their response raises any concerns about suicide this should be asked about directly and addressed. One should try to minimize aloneness through statements of nonabandonment and referral to other resources, such as support groups, counselors, or pastoral care.

Lastly, one should provide a specific follow-up plan: "I'd like you to keep a list of questions so I can answer them for you on our next visit this Tuesday. We'll talk about all your options again at that time... Okay? And please feel free to call me." The physician needs to remember that the goal of this conversation is not to leave a happy patient. That is rarely possible (or even desirable) after delivering bad news. Instead, one hopes to leave a patient who feels supported and cared for, and can look forward to a specific plan of action.

Advance Care Planning

Discussions about advance care planning encompass many goals. These include preparing for death and dying, exercising control, relieving burdens placed on loved ones, helping patients make decisions consistent with their values, and leaving patients feeling supported and understood (61). The first step in preparing to discuss advance care plans is deciding upon the appropriate goals for the discussion. What one hopes to accomplish will vary depending on the clinical situation (62). Advance care planning includes many different tasks: informing the patient, eliciting preferences, identifying a surrogate decision maker, and providing emotional support. Frequently, one cannot accomplish all of this in one conversation and focusing on the goals of the discussion allows the physician to tailor the encounter. Advance care planning is completed as a process over time that allows patients an opportunity for thoughtful reflection and interaction with others.

For a healthy, older patient, physicians might establish whom the patient would like to appoint as a health care surrogate. They might ask whether the patient already has a written advance directive and explore the patient's thoughts about dying and the general views about life-sustaining treatments. For a patient with a life-limiting chronic illness, the doctor might also discuss the patient's attitudes about

specific interventions that are likely to occur (e.g., mechanical ventilation in severe chronic obstructive pulmonary disease). Finally, for a patient who will soon die, the doctor will shift the focus from future treatment in hypothetical scenarios to establishing what the goals should be for care provided in the present. In all cases, advance care planning can help patients prepare for death, discuss their values with their loved ones, and achieve a sense of control (61). It can help build trust between doctors and their patients, so that when difficult treatment decisions arise, doctors, patients, and their loved ones can communicate openly and achieve resolution.

Initiating the Conversation

There are a number of ways to begin the discussion. Often physicians can relate the topic to a recent serious event such as a hospitalization. Another way to begin is to ask about experiences with relatives or friends who have died. Many patients are likely to have observed serious illness closely, and perhaps have had loved ones in some of the situations which the physician is describing. They are likely to have much information and misinformation about end-of-life care and are likely to have thought about their own deaths. Opening a discussion in this manner can naturally lead to a discussion about how decisions were made and what the patient thought of that particular death. This will provide valuable insights into the patient's own values.

Providing Information

Patients must have adequate information to make informed decisions. It helps to start by asking patients what they understand about their medical illness. If the patient's condition is more serious than what he or she realizes, then the physician will need to shift focus. The physician will want to put off discussing advance care planning, focusing the discussion instead on explaining to the patient the seriousness of his or her condition.

Studies indicate that patients are more interested in what the expected health outcome will be than in details about the interventions themselves (63,64). The primary reason for patients to consider withholding treatments is to avoid an outcome judged by them to be worse than death (65). The other reason is that the burden of the treatment, on themselves or their loved ones, outweighs the potential benefit. Therefore, patients should achieve an understanding of the impact of common, life-sustaining interventions on one's quality of life. In contrast, vivid descriptions of the nature of the treatments themselves (e.g., intubation, cardioversion, ICU care) may alarm patients and be less helpful.

Eliciting Preferences

Patients state preferences after learning about potential options and evaluating these in light of their personal values. Values refer to deeply held beliefs such as a desire for personal independence or the importance of a religious practice. By exploring patients' values and goals, clinicians can help them clarify their specific preferences. Sometimes one can ask explicitly about such values (e.g., "What makes life worth living for you?"). Alternatively, values may be elicited in the process of asking about specific treatment preferences. For example, after a patient makes a statement about end-of-life care (e.g., "I'd never want to be on one of those machines"), the clinician may respond by simply asking, "Why?" The answer to this question (e.g., "Because I never want to be a burden on my family or society") may uncover a patient's core values that will impact greatly on treatment decisions.

Identifying what conditions the patient would find unacceptable can also help clarify a patient's preferences. A useful question is, "Can you imagine any situations in which life would not be worth living (66)?" This question can be followed by asking what the patient would be willing to forgo in order to avoid such states.

For many patients, dealing with uncertainty is the most difficult aspect of decision making. When doctors ask patients if they would want a particular treatment, like a ventilator, patients will often state that the treatment should be provided "if it will help me, but if it won't help me, don't do it." Statements like this ignore the reality that physicians are often uncertain about the outcome. Everyone responds to uncertainty differently, and the patient's approach to this issue should be discussed explicitly as well. For example, one may ask, "What if we are not sure whether we will be able to get you off the breathing machine?" Depending on the patient's answer to this question, the doctor can explore what the chance of success needs to be in order to pursue aggressive treatment. Some patients will state that any possibility of recovery is worth pursuing while others will refuse curative treatment when the likelihood of recovery drops below a particular threshold (58). Some patients are comfortable using numbers talking about probabilities, others are less quantitatively facile (67,68). The patient's preferences should dictate the extent to which numbers are used in this discussion. Many patients will be satisfied, leaving it to the judgment of the physician and family members, with only general instructions. The option of a treatment trial is also a useful way to provide clarity in the face of uncertainty.

It is impossible to elicit meaningful preferences for every intervention in every possible situation. By focusing on a patient's values and goals, the physician can then help the patient make decisions about current or future treatments that are consistent with those goals. Discussions should move back and forth from preferences to reasons and values to information and back again, ensuring that the patient understands the implications of his or her stated preferences, and that the doctor understands the patient's values. In this way, when the physician is faced with an unanticipated clinical situation, he or she can use the patient's stated values and goals to help determine the appropriate course of action. In such discussions, it is frequently worthwhile to inquire specifically about some controversial treatments such as artificial nutrition and hydration. This is particularly true in states that require the patients' specific directive to withhold these treatments.

Patients and physicians often use vague terms that ought to be avoided. For example, a statement that a treatment should be continued as long as "quality of life is good" begs further clarification. How does the patient (or his or her surrogate, or the physician) define a good quality of life? In fact, it is always important to ensure that the patient and physician have a shared understanding of the conversation and its implications. Similarly, medical jargon should be avoided, one should always define technical terms, and patients must be encouraged to ask questions.

Choosing Surrogate Decision Makers

Identifying who is to act as the patient's health care proxy may be the most important outcome of a conversation about advance care planning. Does the patient wish this to be a single individual or an entire family? Given the literature demonstrating poor concordance between patient preferences and surrogate perceptions of those preferences, the clinician would be wise to stress the need for the patient to communicate with the selected proxy decision maker (69). Patients should also be asked how much leeway their proxies should have in decision making (70). Should proxies adhere strictly to patients' stated preferences, or ought they to have more flexibility when making actual decisions?

These discussions can be emotionally difficult, even when they are welcome. It is important to draw upon the emotion-handling skills described earlier (see the section Role of Affect) and to acknowledge patient's feelings of sadness, fear, or anger, when they come up, and to validate those feelings by stating your understanding of their reaction. The physician can admit that the discussion can be difficult and support the patient by stating how helpful he or she has been in helping to understand his or her preferences. Another way doctors can provide support to patients is to assure them that they will do whatever they can to meet their goals (such as comfort) and to articulate what some of those things might be. In this way, doctors can assure patients that they will continue to care for them, even if they are in a condition in which they would not want life-sustaining treatment.

Communicating over the Transition

It is possible that the greatest communication challenges face physicians and patients as they discuss progression of disease, the transition from curative therapy to palliation and the referral to hospice care. Such times of transition involve the recognition of loss, redefinition of self-concept and social role, and great emotional stress. Patients are likely to feel sadness, anger, and denial. Physicians frequently have difficulty with such discussions because they feel a sense of failure, are worried that patients will feel abandoned, or that they will be overcome in the conversation by anxiety or despair. Furthermore, they may have their own unresolved issues about mortality or fear the patient's anticipated emotional response.

Again, it is useful to identify the goals of these conversations. They include eliciting emotional, psychologic and spiritual concerns, and providing empathic and practical support. Of course, it is also important to help patients acknowledge their illness and to make appropriate health care decisions, such as enrolling in hospice. However, conversations should not be dominated by the physician's agenda, and patients must be given ample space to make decisions according to their own timetables. Physicians should employ behaviors that promote the sharing of concerns by patients, and avoid behaviors such as reassurance that inhibit such sharing. See Table 48.4 for useful, open-ended questions with which one can initiate such conversations.

As patients respond to these questions, the physician should continue to focus on the psychosocial and spiritual aspects of their illness and not allow the biomedical issues to dominate. It is important to avoid false reassurance. A particular form

---

TABLE 48.4

OPEN-ENDED QUESTIONS TO INITIATE CONVERSATIONS ABOUT DYING

"What concerns you most about your illness?"
"How is treatment going for you (your family)?"
"As you think about your illness, what is the best and the worst that might happen?"
"What has been most difficult about this illness for you?"
"What are your hopes (your expectations, your fears) for the future?"
"As you think about the future, what is most important to you (what matters the most to you)?"

Lo B, Quill T, Tulsky J. Discussing palliative care with patients. *Ann Intern Med* 1999;130:744–749.

of response that can be extremely effective at these times is the "wish statement (71)." These are particularly effective in response to statements that appear to demonstrate significant denial of the severity of illness. For example:

> PT: I'm going to get better. I know that this new chemotherapy they're offering at the university will make the difference.
> MD: I wish that there was a treatment that would make this cancer go away.
> PT: You mean that you don't think it will work.
> MD: It's hard to come to terms with this, but, unfortunately, I don't believe it would help you overcome your cancer.
> PT: I was afraid you might say that. What do we do now?
> MD: There's a lot that we can do. Let's talk about what goals are most important for you right now.

The wish statement allows the doctor to demonstrate empathy toward the patient and to align herself with the patient's hopes. Yet, at the same time it implicitly conveys the message that certain goals are unrealistic. In this way, the physician can address the patient's denial without losing the therapeutic alliance.

Dreaded Questions

Finally, it is useful to consider several of the questions that many physicians find most difficult to answer (e.g., "Why me?" "How long do I have to live?"). Responding to such questions draws upon the many skills described in this chapter and it is useful to keep several additional points in mind. The most important thing a physician can do is remain curious. One should not assume that one knows what the question is "really" about. A patient who is asking, "How long do I have?" may be wondering if she is going to live until Christmas, whether reports she has heard that the disease is fatal are accurate, or whether she is going to get out of the hospital. Acknowledge the question, but make sure you understand it before trying to answer (e.g., "That is a really tough question. What are you concerned about?"). It is also important to recognize that it is not necessarily the physician's job to solve the problem. Physicians do not have the answers to questions such as "Why me?" and may not be able to diminish the feelings of sadness and loss. What one can do is to acknowledge and normalize the feelings. In allowing the patient to be heard, the physician may decrease the patient's sense of being alone in their disease, and thus decrease their suffering. (An illustrative example is to imagine you have had a very bad day at work. When you come home and start to tell your family, how would you feel if they started to brainstorm different solutions to the problem? Most individuals would prefer their loved ones to acknowledge their day—"sounds like it was a really tough day"—rather than try to solve their problem.)

Having anticipated replies can be useful and several examples follow (45):

> PT: How long do I have to live?
> MD: I wonder if it is frightening not knowing what will happen next, or when.

This response acknowledges that underlying such a question is tremendous emotion, most likely fear. It will be important for the physician to give a factual response to this question. However, the patient will not be prepared to hear this response until the doctor has addressed his or her emotional concerns. The suggested answer above allows patients to speak about their fears and worries. When the physician needs to use a more factual response, the following is a way of being honest while maintaining hope: "On average, a person in your situation lives up to 3 to 4 months, but some people have much less time, and others may live over a year. I would now take care of any practical or family matters that you wish to have completed before you die, but continue to hope that you are one of the lucky people who gets a bit more time."

> FM: Does this mean you're giving up on him?
> MD: Absolutely not. But tell me, what do you mean by giving up?

Suggesting that a patient receives palliative care risks conveying a sense of abandonment. Physicians must be emphatic that palliative care and hospice are active forms of care that meet patients' varying goals at the end of life. However, further exploration of patients' or family's concerns about abandonment are important to understanding their perceptions and attitudes toward care at the end of life.

> Patient: "Are you telling me that I am going to die?"
> Physician: "I wish that were not the case, but it is likely in the near future. I am also asking, how would want to spend the remaining time if it were limited?"

This wish statement helps the physician identify with the patient's loss. The following sentence is an attempt by the physician to reframe the patient's understanding of the situation. He has acknowledged that the patient is dying, but now he seeks to understand what the patient's goals might be in light of this new information. Creating new goals in this way provides an outlet for the patient's hope.

Bereavement

Palliative care does not end when a patient dies. An awareness of bereavement can help one communicate with family and loved ones after the loss. Bereaved people ought to be encouraged to tell their stories of loss, including describing details of the days and weeks around the death of their loved one. Similarly, family members and friends benefit by recalling earlier positive memories of the person. Physicians can explore how the bereaved person has responded to the grief ("How have things been different for you because your husband died?"), and identify their social support and coping resources. One should not overlook the frequently enormous practical ramifications of loss such as financial difficulties, the need to leave a home, and transportation. Finally, physicians need to be aware that a significant minority of patients, 10–20%, have difficulty regaining their normal functioning after the loss. This syndrome—complicated grief—seems distinct from depression and is characterized by excessive rumination and preoccupation with the dead individual (72).

Good communication skills are central to the provision of palliative care. The fundamentals of such communication are listening, recognizing one's own affective responses, attending to patients' emotional needs, and achieving a shared understanding of the concerns at hand. Specific tasks, such as delivering bad news, discussing advance care planning, helping patients through the transition to hospice care, and responding to difficult questions, require using these skills to ensure that patients' concerns are elicited and addressed, and they are informed and feel supported.

References

1. Steinhauser KE, Christakis NA, Clipp EC, et al. Factors considered important at the end of life by patients, family, physicians, and other care providers. *JAMA* 2000;284:2476–2482.

2. Heaven CM, Maguire P. The relationship between patients' concerns and psychological distress in a hospice setting. *Psychooncology* 1998;7(6):502–507.

3. Parle M, Jones B, Maguire P. Maladaptive coping and affective disorders among cancer patients. *Psychol Med* 1996;26(4):735–744.

4. Bertakis KD, Roter D, Putnam SM. The relationship of physician medical interview style to patient satisfaction. *J Fam Pract* 1991;32(2):175–181.

5. Kaplan SH, Greenfield S, Ware JE, Jr. Assessing the effects of physician-patient interaction on the outcomes of chronic disease. *Med Care* 1989;27:S110–S127.

6. Roter DL, Hall JA, Kern DE, et al. Improving physicians' interviewing skills and reducing patients' emotional distress. A randomized clinical trial. *Arch Intern Med* 1995;155(17):1877–1884.

7. Tierney WM, Dexter PR, Gramelspacher GP, et al. The effect of discussions about advance directives on patients satisfaction with primary care. *J Gen Intern Med* 2001;16:32–40.

8. Smyth JM, Stone AA, Hurewitz A, et al. Effects of writing about stressful experiences on symptom reduction in patients with asthma or rheumatoid arthritis: a randomized trial. *JAMA* 1999;281(14):1304–1309.

9. Butow PN, Kazemi JN, Beeney LJ, et al. When the diagnosis is cancer: patient communication experiences and preferences. *Cancer* 1996;77(12):2630–2637.

10. Friedrichsen MJ, Strang PM, Carlsson ME. Breaking bad news in the transition from curative to palliative cancer care-patient's view of the doctor giving the information. *Support Care Cancer* 2000;8(6):472–478.

11. Ptacek JT, Eberhardt TL. Breaking bad news. A review of the literature. *JAMA* 1996;276(6):496–502.

12. Goldberg R, Guadagnoli E, Silliman RA, et al. Cancer patients' concerns: congruence between patients and primary care physicians. *J Cancer Educ* 1990;5(3):193–199.

13. Maguire P, Faulkner A, Booth K, et al. Helping cancer patients disclose their concerns. *Eur J Cancer* 1996;32A(1):78–81.

14. Butow PN, Brown RF, Cogar S, et al. Oncologists' reactions to cancer patients' verbal cues. *Psychooncology* 2002;11(1):47–58.

15. Maguire P. Improving communication with cancer patients. *Eur J Cancer* 1999;35(10):1415–1422.

16. Heaven CM, Maguire P. Disclosure of concerns by hospice patients and their identification by nurses. *Palliat Med* 1997;11(4):283–290.

17. Ford S, Fallowfield L, Lewis S. Doctor-patient interactions in oncology. *Soc Sci Med* 1996;42(11):1511.

18. Detmar SB, Muller MJ, Wever LD, et al. The patient-physician relationship. Patient-physician communication during outpatient palliative treatment visits: an observational study. *JAMA* 2001;285(10):1351–1357.

19. Gattellari M, Voigt KJ, Butow PN, et al. When the treatment goal is not cure: are cancer patients equipped to make informed decisions? *J Clin Oncol* 2002;20(2):503–513.

20. Emanuel LL, Barry MJ, Stoeckle JD, et al. Advance directives for medical care—a case for greater use. *N Engl J Med* 1991;324(13):889–895.

21. Tulsky JA, Chesney MA, Lo B. How do medical residents discuss resuscitation with patients? *J Gen Intern Med* 1995;10(8):436–442.

22. Tulsky JA, Fischer GS, Rose MR, et al. Opening the black box: how do physicians communicate about advance directives? *Ann Intern Med* 1998;129(6):441–449.

23. Billings JA, Block S. Palliative care in undergraduate medical education. Status report and future directions. *JAMA* 1997;278(9):733–738.

24. Rhodes-Kropf J, Carmody SS, Seltzer D, et al. "This is just too awful; I just can't believe I experienced that." Medical students' reactions to their "most memorable" patient death. *Acad Med* 2005;80(7):634–640.

25. Smith RC, Zimny EM. Physicians' emotional reactions to patients. *Psychosomatics* 1988;29(4):392–397.

26. Spikes J, Holland J. The physician's response to the dying patient. In: Strain JJ, Grossman S, eds. *Psychological care of the medically ill: a primer in liaison psychiatry*. New York: Appleton-Century-Crofts, 1975:138–148.

27. Schneiderman LJ, Kaplan RM, Pearlman RA. Do physicians own preferences for life-sustaining treatment influence their perceptions of patients' preferences? *J Clin Ethics* 1993;4:28–33.

28. Quill TE, Townsend P. Bad news: delivery, dialogue, and dilemmas. *Arch Intern Med* 1991;151(3):463–468.

29. The AM, Hak T, Koeter G, et al. Collusion in doctor-patient communication about imminent death: an ethnographic study. *BMJ* 2000;321(7273):1376–1381.

30. Maguire P. Barriers to psychological care of the dying. *BMJ* 1985;291:1711–1713.

31. Benoliel JQ. Health care delivery: not conducive to teaching palliative care. *J Palliat Care* 1988;4(1&2):41–42.

32. Whippen DA, Canellos GP. Burnout syndrome in the practice of oncology: results of a random survey of 1,000 oncologists. *J Clin Onc* 1991;9:1916–1920.

33. Schaerer R. Suffering of the doctor linked with death of patients. *Palliat Med* 1993;7:27–37.

34. Shanafelt TD, Bradley KA, Wipf JE, et al. Burnout and self-reported patient care in an internal medicine residency program. *Ann Intern Med* 2002;136(5):358–367.

35. Shanafelt TD, West C, Zhao X, et al. Relationship between increased personal well-being and enhanced empathy among internal medicine residents. *J Gen Intern Med* 2005;20(7):612–617.

36. Neimeyer GJ, Behnke M, Reiss J. Constructs and coping: physicians' response to patient death. *Death Educ* 1983;7:245–264.

37. Fogarty LA, Curbow BA, Wingard JR, et al. Can 40 seconds of compassion reduce patient anxiety? *J Clin Onc* 1999;17(1):371–379.

38. McDonagh JR, Elliott TB, Engelberg RA, et al. Family satisfaction with family conferences about end-of-life care in the intensive care unit: increased proportion of family speech is associated with increased satisfaction. *Crit Care Med* 2004;32(7):1484–1488.

39. Wenrich MD, Curtis JR, Shannon SE, et al. Communicating with dying patients within the spectrum of medical care from terminal diagnosis to death. *Arch Intern Med* 2001;161(6):868–874.

40. Clayton JM, Butow PN, Arnold RM, et al. Fostering coping and nurturing hope when discussing the future with terminally ill cancer patients and their caregivers. *Cancer* 2005;103(9):1965–1975.

41. Parker PA, Baile WF, de Moor C, et al. Breaking bad news about cancer: patients' preferences for communication. *J Clin Oncol* 2001;19(7):2049–2056.

42. Detmar SB, Aaronson NK, Wever LD, et al. How are you feeling? Who wants to know? Patients' and oncologists' preferences for discussing health-related quality-of-life issues. *J Clin Oncol* 2000;18(18):3295–3301.

43. Baile WF, Glober GA, Lenzi R, et al. Discussing disease progression and end-of-life decisions. *Oncology* 1999;13(7):1021–1031.

44. Larson DG, Tobin DR. End-of-life conversations: evolving practice and theory. *JAMA* 2000;284(12):1573–1578.

45. Lo B, Quill T, Tulsky J. Discussing palliative care with patients. *Ann Intern Med* 1999;130(9):744–749.

46. Parle M, Maguire P, Heaven C. The development of a training model to improve health professionals' skills, self-efficacy and outcome expectancies when communicating with cancer patients. *Soc Sci Med* 1997;44(2):231–240.

47. von Gunten CF, Ferris FD, Emanuel LL. The patient-physician relationship. Ensuring competency in end-of-life care: communication and relational skills. *JAMA* 2000;284(23):3051–3057.

48. Hagerty RG, Butow PN, Ellis PA, et al. Cancer patient preferences for communication of prognosis in the metastatic setting. *J Clin Oncol* 2004;22(9):1721–1730.

49. Pfeifer MP, Mitchell CK, Chamberlain L. The value of disease severity in predicting patient readiness to address end-of-life issues. *Arch Intern Med* 2003;163(5):609–612.

50. Bohner G, Chaiken S, Hunyadi P. The role of mood and message ambiguity in the interplay of heuristic and systematic processing. *Eur J Soc Psychol* 1994;24(1):207–221.

51. Levinson W, Gorawara-Bhat R, Lamb J. A study of patient clues and physician responses in primary care and surgical settings. *JAMA* 2000;284(8):1021–1027.

52. Shapiro DE, Boggs SR, Melamed BG, et al. The effect of varied physician affect on recall, anxiety, and perceptions in women at risk for breast cancer: an analogue study. *Health Psychol* 1992;11(1):61–66.

53. Spiro HM. What is empathy and can it be taught? In: Spiro HM, ed. *Empathy and practice of medicine: beyond pills and the scalpel*. New Haven: Yale University Press, 1993:7–14.

54. Egan G. *The skilled helper: a problem-management and opportunity-development approach to helping*, 7th ed. California, CA: Brooks/Cole, 2002.

55. Smith RC, Hoppe RB. The patient's story: integrating the patient- and physician-centered approaches to interviewing. *Ann Intern Med* 1991;115(6):470–477.

56. Christakis NA. *Death foretold: prophecy and prognosis in medical care*. Chicago, IL: University of Chicago Press, 2000.

57. Delvecchio MJ, Good BJ, Schaffer C, et al. American oncology and the discourse on hope. *Cult Med Psychiatry* 1990;14(1):59–79.

58. Weeks JC, Cook EF, O'Day SJ, et al. Relationship between cancer patients' predictions of prognosis and their treatment preferences. *JAMA* 1998;279(21):1709–1714.

59. Breen CM, Abernethy AP, Abbott KH, et al. Conflict associated with decisions to limit life-sustaining treatment in intensive care units. *J Gen Intern Med* 2001;16(5):283–289.

60. Back AL, Arnold RM. Dealing with conflict in caring for the seriously ill: "it was just out of the question." *JAMA* 2005;293(11):1374–1381.

61. Singer PA, Martin DK, Lavery JV, et al. Reconceptualizing advance care planning from the patient's perspective. *Arch Intern Med* 1998;158:879–884.

62. Teno JM, Lynn J. Putting advance-care planning into action. *J Clin Ethics* 1996;7:205–213.

63. Frankl D, Oye RK, Bellamy PE. Attitudes of hospitalized patient toward life support: a survey of 200 medical inpatients. *Am J Med* 1989;86:645–648.

64. Pfeifer MP, Sidorov JE, Smith AC, et al. The discussion of end-of-life medical care by primary care patients and physicians: a multicenter study using structured qualitative interviews. *J Gen Intern Med* 1994;9:82–88.

65. Patrick DL, Starks HE, Cain KC, et al. Measuring preferences for health states worse than death. *Med Decis Making* 1994;14(1):9–18.

66. Pearlman RA, Cain KC, Patrick DL, et al. Insights pertaining to patient assessments of states worse than death. *J Clin Ethics* 1993;4(1):33–41.

67. Mazur DJ, Hickam DH. Patients' interpretations of probability terms. *J Gen Intern Med* 1991;6(3):237–240.

68. Woloshin KK, Ruffin MT, Gorenflo DW. Patients' interpretation of qualitative probability statements. *Arch Fam Med* 1994;3:961–966.

69. Seckler AB, Meier DE, Mulvihill M, et al. Substituted judgment: how accurate are proxy predictions? *Ann Intern Med* 1991;115(2):92–98.

70. Sehgal A, Galbraith A, Chesney M, et al. How strictly do dialysis patients want their advance directives followed? *JAMA* 1992;267(1):59–63.

71. Quill TE, Arnold RM, Platt F. "I wish things were different": expressing wishes in response to loss, futility, and unrealistic hopes. *Ann Intern Med* 2001;135(7):551–555.

72. Lichtenthal WG, Cruess DG, Prigerson HG. A case for establishing complicated grief as a distinct mental disorder in DSM-V. *Clin Psychol Rev* 2004;24(6):637–662.

CHAPTER 49 ■ PALLIATIVE RADIATION THERAPY

ANDREA BEZJAK, PETER KIRKBRIDE, AND REBECCA WONG

INTRODUCTION

Palliative radiotherapy (RT) is radiation treatment administered to improve symptoms and relieve suffering. Half the patients who are diagnosed with cancer will receive RT at some point in the course of their disease, with a variety of intents—curative, radical, adjuvant, palliative, or prophylactic; these terms are defined in Table 49.1. An estimated 40–50% of all RT courses are palliative in nature (1), although that figure may underestimate palliative RT usage as it does not include high-dose "curative" treatments that are also used for tumor control or the prevention and relief of distressing symptoms rather than expectations of cure. In this chapter, we will define what is meant by "palliative RT," review the rationale for its use, and discuss the evidence on which current palliative practice is based by answering the basic questions of "What, Why, Who, When, How, and Where." As background, the reader may refer to the "Rules For The Practice of Radiation Therapy" (2) (Table 49.2) which are based on the ethical principles used to guide the practice of medicine.

What is Palliative Radiotherapy?

Therapeutic radiation is part of the electromagnetic spectrum; it consists of high-energy photons generated from a series of complex interactions in a linear accelerator (x-rays), or directly from the nucleus of a radioactive isotope such as cobalt 60 (γ rays). Unlike "brachytherapy," in which radioactive sources are placed directly into or close to the tumor in the patient's body, external beam RT is delivered from an outside source to the patient's body. Definitions of these and other commonly used terms are contained in Table 49.3. Radiation can cure many radiosensitive cancers, although high doses are required to eradicate all tumor cells. Typically 66–70 Gray (Gy) or more are delivered in daily treatments or "fractions" (often of 1.8 or 2 Gy per fraction) over 6–8 weeks. Side effects of RT are related to normal tissue injury and include both "acute" (during or shortly after completion of RT, e.g., mucositis, diarrhea) and "chronic" (months to years after RT, e.g., fibrosis). It is the normal tissue tolerances that limit the doses of RT that can be safely delivered. Therefore, when the cancer cannot be cured and the goal of treatment is symptom relief, it is logical to administer a lower dose of RT over a shorter period of time.

The time between RT fractions allows normal tissue cells to repair and regenerate. It also allows for previously fraction-resistant tumor cells to become more radiosensitive by becoming oxygenated or by moving to a different phase in the cell cycle. The use of smaller daily fractions (2 Gy or less) also significantly reduces the risk of late complications of RT such as fibrosis or necrosis. Higher RT doses lead to more acute effects, which are virtually unavoidable in curative treatment. In the palliative population, the same extent of acute effects would not be acceptable, as they would negatively affect quality of life over a time that may represent a substantial proportion of the patients remaining life span. As a result, in palliative RT complete tumor ablation is not the goal; symptom relief can be produced with fewer number of larger RT fractions; and the late effects which take several months or years to develop, are less relevant to a population with a short life expectancy. Consequently, palliative RT is typically administered using lower total doses (frequently 8–30 Gy), larger daily fraction sizes (3–10 Gy per fraction), and shorter total treatment times (1 day–2 weeks) than curative RT. The resultant side effects are less intense (due to lower total doses) and less prolonged (due to shorter overall treatment time). The actual effect on the tumor is greater than the same total dose administered in conventional 2-Gy fractions (as the biological dose is greater for larger fraction sizes).

Why Should We Consider Palliative Radiotherapy?

Palliative RT is widely used for a variety of oncological problems. It is effective not only for the relief of cancer-related pain and symptoms but is also well tolerated with relatively mild local side effects. The traditional indications for palliative RT are illustrated in Table 49.4. In general, palliative RT can be used to treat both primary tumors and metastases provided the lesion being irradiated is directly responsible for a symptom. The potential benefits need to be balanced against the expected side effects of RT, as well as expected responses to alternative palliative measures. If the patient's symptoms are pharmacologically well controlled, it is not always necessary to irradiate. Then one needs to consider other clinical benefits from RT, such as a decrease in opioid requirements, and the resultant reduction in drug side effects such as constipation.

Typically, palliative RT causes only mild and transient side effects due to the lower total RT doses commonly employed. In addition, it is usually tolerated well by all but the most infirm of patients. However, as many side effects develop post-RT, those caring for patients after RT need to be counseled accordingly.

TABLE 49.1

DEFINITIONS OF TERMS USED TO DESCRIBE THE INTENT OF RADIATION THERAPY

Curative	Goal of treatment is elimination of tumor and cure of the patient
Radical	Refers to intensity of treatment and dose of radiation: high-dose radiation treatment given with the intent of eradicating cancer from area being irradiated
Adjuvant	A form of treatment used in conjunction with primary therapy implemented to aid the principal treatment regimen (e.g., radiation after complete surgical resection of all known cancer to prevent or minimize the risk of local recurrence)
Palliative	Treatment that aims to relieve or alleviate symptoms, not cure
Prophylactic	Any treatment regimen given with preventative intent. Examples include prophylactic cranial radiation (to prevent brain metastases by eliminating possible microscopic tumors in the brain) and prophylactic radiation of bone metastases (to minimize the risk of fracture)

Who Should Receive Palliative Radiotherapy?

The essential axiom of palliative RT is its use in patients who have local symptoms attributable to the presence of a malignant tumor, although patients at risk of symptom development may also benefit. There are few contraindications to palliative RT. Many patients deemed not suitable for radical treatment due to poor performance status, coexisting medical conditions, or extensive disease, may benefit from palliative RT. For example, patients with poor lung function and limited respiratory reserve unable to undergo surgery or radical RT may still benefit from low-dose thoracic RT with its lower risk

TABLE 49.2

RULES FOR THE PRACTICE OF RADIATION THERAPY

Palliative radiotherapy should be part of a comprehensive program of care

The decision to recommend palliative radiotherapy should be based on a thorough assessment of the patient

The decision to recommend palliative radiotherapy should be based on objective information

The risk-benefit analysis should include consideration of all aspects of the patient's well-being

The short-term risks and benefits of palliative radiotherapy are more important than those that may or may not occur in the future

The decision to use palliative radiotherapy should be consistent with the values and preferences of the patient

The patient should be involved in the treatment decision to the extent that she or he wishes

Time is precious when life is short

Delays in starting palliative radiotherapy should be as short as reasonably achievable

Courses of palliative radiotherapy should be no longer than necessary to achieve their therapeutic goal

Palliative and curative goals should not be considered mutually exclusive

Palliative radiotherapy should consume no more resources than necessary

Mackillop WJ. The principles of palliative radiotherapy: a radiation oncologist's perspective. *Can J Oncol* 1996;6(1 Suppl):5–11 with permission.

of toxicity. Similarly, patients with collagen vascular diseases, who often experience exaggerated and severe reactions to radical RT, may be considered for palliative RT, although the risk-benefit ratio of the treatment needs to be thoroughly discussed.

Radiation may not be appropriate for bed-bound patients in the final stages of their illness, as they may not live long enough to experience its benefit. If a patient's poor condition is a consequence of severe pain and/or large doses of opioid analgesia, it may be possible to achieve meaningful benefit, although symptom relief may take between 1 and 4 weeks. In such situations, the use of the "one-stop-shop" approach, where a patient can be assessed, his/her treatment planned, and treatment rendered with a single fraction all on the same visit, may be useful (3).

There is a common misapprehension that patients who have received RT cannot be re-treated in the same area. There is no doubt that if a patient has previously received radical treatment, it may be challenging or even impossible to administer a second high-dose course to the same area. However, in the palliative situation, the risk of late RT complications is less of an issue. As a result, it may be feasible to administer low-dose RT to a previously treated area. Depending upon tumor location, it is possible to repeat lose-dose treatments. Although some patients may benefit, it is not always clear whether additional RT is beneficial after failure to derive a positive response from an initial course of palliative RT. Reirradiation issues are further discussed in the section that follows.

When Should Palliative Radiotherapy Be Given?

Radiotherapeutic Emergencies

A true radiotherapeutic emergency occurs when failure to deliver treatment within a few hours or days could result in death or catastrophic irreversible damage. Severe pain, although distressing to the patient, is not an emergency, but should be treated with great urgency. As RT cannot produce immediate pain relief, pharmacologic measures are essential while RT is being organized and delivered. Table 49.5 lists indications for emergency RT in a large academic cancer center in Canada, the Princess Margaret Hospital, Toronto. In these circumstances, the patient should be seen by a radiation oncologist on the same day the lesion is diagnosed, and appropriate treatment should be started promptly.

TABLE 49.3

DEFINITIONS OF COMMON RADIOTHERAPY TERMS

External beam radiation	Radiation delivered from an outside source, external to the patient's body (noninvasive)
Linear accelerator	A radiotherapy machine used to produce and deliver radiation in the form of x-rays. Radiation is in the form of photon or electron beams and can be of various energies. Term is often abbreviated to LINAC
Brachytherapy	An internal treatment with sealed radioactive sources placed in direct contact with the tumor. Optimizes the dose of radiation delivered to the target tissue while minimizing the dose to surrounding healthy tissue. "Brachy" is Greek for short distance
Radioactive isotope	Naturally occurring elements that emit radiant energy (i.e., cobalt-60, radium-226, cesium-137). Isotopes have the same number of protons in their nuclei (same atomic number) but have different numbers of neutrons (different mass number). Because isotopes have unstable nuclei, they attempt to stabilize by giving off ionizing radiation
Fraction	The term *fraction* indicates the number of individual radiation treatments required to complete the treatment regimen (i.e., 2000 cGy/5 fractions indicates five individual radiation treatments over a period of 5 days with a total dose of 2000 cGy, or 400 cGy/fraction)
Hypofractionated radiation	A radiotherapy regimen utilizing fewer fractions than the standard course of treatment. Higher doses per fraction are characteristic of this type of radiotherapy. Often used in the palliative setting or if a high localized dose is needed (i.e., stereotactic radiosurgery, afterloading brachytherapy)
Hyperfractionated radiation	A radiotherapy regimen utilizing an increased number of fractions than the standard course of treatment. Smaller doses per fraction are characteristic of this type of radiotherapy
Stereotactic radiation	Stereotactic implies precise positioning in three-dimensional space. Stereotactic radiosurgery is a radiation therapy technique utilizing a large number of narrow, highly focused beams, which are aimed from various directions and meet precisely at a specific predetermined point (e.g., when treating the brain, multiple beams circle the head and meet at a specified point). This can be done using gamma-knife or high-energy linear accelerator
Radiosurgery	Stereotactic technique that delivers RT in a single fraction
Gamma-knife	High-intensity, multisource irradiation (using 201 cobalt-60 collimated beams) typically used on small target areas to deliver high dose of radiation to a small area. Today, this highly focused radiation is primarily used for stereotactic radiosurgery
Cyberknife	X-ray and computer program–guided lightweight linear accelerator used for stereotactic radiotherapy. Provides targeted radiation to any anatomic location with minimal exposure to surrounding skin. Computer program—generated analysis of tumor shape and location before treatment in addition to compensatory abilities for patient movement during treatment

Although RT should be administered without delay, relief may not be immediate. The time taken for the benefits of RT to be observed depends on the situation but is rarely less than a few days. With the exception of a few very radiosensitive tissues and cells (e.g., lymphocytes), RT does not cause immediate cell death. Rather, it leads to the failure of cell division, and subsequently cell death at the next scheduled division. As a result, both the beneficial effects and the acute toxicities of RT take several days to manifest. Although not the norm, when treating bone metastases, large-fraction wide-field treatment such as half-body irradiation (HBI) occasionally produces same-day benefits.

TABLE 49.4

INDICATIONS FOR THE USE OF PALLIATIVE RADIOTHERAPY

Pain relief (bone metastases, lung cancer causing chest pain, tumors causing nerve root and soft tissue infiltration)
Control of bleeding (hemoptysis, vaginal and rectal bleeding)
Control of fungation and ulceration
Relief of impending or actual obstruction (esophagus, large airways, rectum)
Shrinkage of tumor masses causing symptoms (e.g., brain metastases, skin lesions)
Oncologic emergencies (spinal cord compression, superior vena cava obstruction)

TABLE 49.5

SITUATIONS REQUIRING THE EMERGENCY USE OF RADIATION THERAPY, PROVIDED NO OTHER TREATMENT IS APPROPRIATE[a]

Established spinal cord compression
Established superior vena cava obstruction
Life-threatening lower airway obstruction
Life-threatening hemorrhage
The following are critical complications of radio-responsive tumors:
Ocular compression with blindness
Peripheral nerve compression, including cauda equina syndrome, with established motor dysfunction
Life-threatening renal insufficiency caused by kidney infiltration or ureteric obstruction
Life-threatening mass brain lesion
Malignant hypercalcemia refractory to other measures where radiotherapy constitutes appropriate definitive treatment
Progression of cancer documented following decision to treat with radiation therapy

[a]As identified by The Department of Radiation Oncology. Toronto, Canada: Princess Margaret Hospital, 1998.

Treatment of Symptoms

There is no threshold of symptom severity that a patient needs to cross to require palliative RT. When treating small or large volume tumors, RT is equally useful whether the disease is producing mild or severe symptoms with little difference in palliative effect, although side effects are usually greater with large volume irradiation. In some instances, as in patients with pain from multiple bone metastases, it may be more appropriate to treat with analgesics as this may give better overall relief with less side effects than RT. Additionally, some patients may become completely pain free if their analgesics are adjusted appropriately. In those circumstances, it may be possible to defer RT.

Prevention of Symptoms

In a situation where a patient has an incurable cancer that is asymptomatic, treatment may be deferred until symptoms arise, although this should be discussed with the patient. A randomized clinical trial by Falk et al. (4), supports this approach in the management of lung cancer. Two hundred thirty patients with incurable lung cancer and no symptoms requiring immediate RT were randomized for immediate palliative RT (17 Gy in 2 fractions) or observation with RT at the time of symptomatic progression. After a 6-month follow-up, patients who received immediate RT were no more likely to be free of chest symptoms (i.e., cough, dyspnea) or to survive than patients in the observation arm. Additionally, one third of patients in the observation arm never required RT (or chemotherapy). Therefore, the use of RT to prevent potential symptoms (of lung cancer) is not supported by evidence. Many radiation oncologists have admitted the use of palliative RT to "give hope" (5) as many patients are unhappy about a "wait-and-watch" approach and would prefer to receive active treatment. In such cases, the benefits may be minimal and patients may still be exposed to side effects. Despite the lack of evidence, prophylactic palliative RT may be used if the physician feels the patient is at high risk of developing a clinically significant morbidity such as fracture, cord compression, airway obstruction, or superior vena cava compression.

Retreatment with Radiation

Patients, who have previously received RT, whether palliative or radical, may develop new symptoms related to tumor in the same anatomical area. As palliative RT may provide symptom relief, further reirradiation should be considered although questions frequently arise as to the feasibility of further RT to a previously irradiated area. Due consideration to three key factors helps address this question: what is the residual tolerance of the normal structures? How likely is the disease to respond? How do the risks and benefits of retreatment with RT compare to other symptom management options?

Normal tissue tolerance refers to the relationship between dose levels and the risk of developing significant long-term side effects. Normal tissue tolerances are unique to each anatomic structure. For example, small bowel tolerance is in the order of 45 Gy in 1.8- to 2-Gy fractions, with an expected 5% patient population risk of serious small bowel serious complications (e.g., bowel obstruction). The risk of toxicity escalates with increasing doses. Normal tissue tolerance is further affected by treatment volume and underlying medical conditions. Some normal tissue repairs occur with the passage of time although many of the changes due to high-dose RT, such as fibrosis, vascular changes, and depletion of parenchymal cells, are permanent. Therefore, previous RT doses, even if remote, need to be considered, when assessing the risk of reirradiation.

How the symptom and the disease are likely to respond to reirradiation are important factors in considering reirradiation.

Palliative RT provides symptom relief by a complex and poorly understood mechanism that includes, but is not limited to, killing tumor cells, leading to a reduction in tumor volume. Patients who previously responded well to RT are expected to respond again, although possibly with a lower probability and durability of response. At the cellular level, previously irradiated areas may represent an environment with a greater proportion of resistant cancer cells, and regions of hypoxia that may lead to an attenuated response.

Finally, alternative treatment options should always be considered, so as to select the approach with the least side effects and the best likelihood of benefit. Literature describing the effectiveness of reirradiation is typically scant and confined to retrospective reviews. Patients administered reirradiation represent a minority of those initially treated. The selection criteria for reirradiation are generally not well described, making generalization difficult. Altered fractionation (lower dose per fraction) has been used in an attempt to lower the risk of late effects (6), although evidence to support its superiority is limited.

The evidence regarding reirradiation for specific clinical indications (bone metastases, brain metastases, lung cancer) is described in corresponding sections of this chapter. In all of the common indications for palliative RT, only highly specific patients are offered reirradiation. Patient selection is typically based on the feasibility of delivering a reasonable dose and volume, the predictability of acceptable risks of late toxicities and favorable performance status and life expectancy. The low risk of generally observable late effects is likely the combination of a meticulous planning technique, choice of dose fractionation, exclusion of patients at high risk of developing toxicities, and, in cases such as brain metastases, the shorter life expectancy that limits the manifestation of late effects. Despite these limitations, reirradiation has a definitive role in providing symptom relief in selected patients and should be considered where appropriate.

"Opportunity Costs"

Although individual RT treatments often take only 10–20 minutes to deliver, time spent traveling and waiting for treatment can add up to several hours. A protracted course of RT, especially for patients living some distance from the treatment center, may occupy most of their waking hours. One needs to remember that "time is precious when life is short" (2). For each patient, the benefits of treatment need to be compared with the cost of "lost opportunities" for them to spend their remaining days as they choose (7). In many situations, it appears likely that large single fractions are as efficacious as longer courses (see next section). Even if they were not, it may still be appropriate in patients when the "opportunity cost" of a 2-week treatment would be extremely high. Reduction in palliative benefit would be minimal at most, and concerns about the duration of the effect of single treatments are probably not relevant in patients with extremely limited prognosis.

How Much Radiation Should Be Given?

Fractionation schedules for palliative RT have evolved based on clinical experiences rather than exact science. Experimental treatment models have been developed and continue to be refined, increasing the understanding of total dose effect, fraction size, and treatment time on radical course RT outcomes. Until recently, minimal literature has been published on how these variables influence noncurative RT. Many palliative fractionation regimes exist due to physician personal preference and are often based on a variety of influences such as departmental policies, machine availability, training, and concern about acute and late side effects (8).

Initially, schedules were developed pragmatically by physicians who realized the following:

1. A full radical dose of radiation was inappropriate in a patient who could not be cured
2. Symptoms could be significantly relieved by smaller total doses
3. Shorter treatment times were more convenient for patients and their families

Most of the basis of palliative RT can be traced to recommendations from 1948 that "a useful palliative dosage was one half or better still two thirds of a tumor lethal dose" (9). Within the last 10–15 years, there have been more controlled clinical trials and increased research comparing different palliative prescriptions for various clinical scenarios.

Where in the Body Can Palliative Radiotherapy Be Effective?

The following sections deal with the sites most commonly irradiated palliatively. Non–small cell lung cancer (NSCLC) is the primary tumor most commonly treated with palliative intent. Bone and brain are the most common sites of metastatic disease for most cancers and occupy a large workload percentage of a typical RT department. RT can also be useful to palliate pelvic disease, lymph node metastases, and spinal cord compression. Although liver metastases are common, they are less often palliated with RT because of the toxicity of irradiating large volumes of hepatic tissue and lack of palliative benefit in all but the most radio-responsive tumors. Recently, there have been more studies documenting the role of radical RT doses in good prognosis patients for solitary or few liver metastases, in which RT can produce local control.

Lung Cancer

Lung cancer is the most common cancer in North America and the most common cause of cancer deaths in both men and women. Most patients either present with stage IV (metastatic and incurable) disease or develops metastases some time after the initial diagnosis. Although advances have been made with palliative chemotherapy, palliative RT continues to play an important role in the management of intrathoracic (and extrathoracic) disease, including endobronchial or extrinsic lesions causing atelectasis, postobstructive pneumonia, shortness of breath, cough, hemoptysis, pain, and large airway obstruction. Not surprisingly, RT is not effective in relieving shortness of breath resulting from widespread or parenchymal disease, pleural effusion, or lymphangitic carcinomatosis. Symptoms due to nerve compression (e.g., superior sulcus/Pancoast tumors and intercostal neuropathic pain) are more difficult to palliate and may require high doses of RT aimed at tumor eradication.

The relevant issues in assessing palliation in patients with lung cancer are the following:

1. Symptom relief, including the rapid onset of symptom relief; the degree of relief (partial or complete improvement), and the duration of symptom relief
2. Whether the patient has only one symptom or a conglomerate of symptoms (e.g., hemoptysis is easier to palliate than dyspnea)
3. The toxicity of treatment
4. Any change in the patient's performance status

Obviously the interplay between these issues is complex, and most research studies only attempt to measure some of these variables.

Numerous palliative RT trials have been performed; the more recent ones are highlighted in Table 49.6 (10–14). Most of the dose-fractionation schedules demonstrated considerable symptom palliation. Many studies have suggested that less protracted radiation protocols (including 17 Gy in 2 fractions 1 week apart and 10 Gy in a single fraction) (11) provide better palliation (i.e., equivalent symptom control with less toxicity and less burden to the patient and family). In a recent Norwegian study comparing short, intermediate and long schedules of 17 Gy per 2 fractions, 42 Gy per 15 fractions and 50 Gy per 25 fractions, there was no difference in quality of life, symptom response or survival among the three study arms (15). In the shorter treatment protocols, approximately 80–85% of patients reported improvement in hemoptysis while 60% reported improvement in cough and two thirds reported pain improvement. On an average, symptom relief lasted for at least 50% or more of the patient's survival time. A few studies, on the other hand, have documented a longer duration of symptom control with the more protracted fractionation: in the Dutch trial by Kramer et al. (16), palliation in the 10×3 Gy arm was more prolonged than in 2×8 Gy. Similarly, a recently published study by Erridge et al. (17) demonstrated superior symptom control with a more protracted course, consisting of 30 Gy per 10 fractions as compared to 10 Gy single fraction. It should be noted, however, that defining and analyzing symptom palliation in lung cancer is complex, as the effectiveness of palliative radiation may be related to initial symptom severity (18). Timing of the assessment is also important (19) as a standard definition of palliation is lacking. These methodological concerns may be contributing factors to some of the disparities seen in various studies.

Although the primary goal of palliative RT is symptom control, survival is another relevant outcome. Until the mid-1990s, there was no suggestion of a survival difference with any of these palliative regimens (10–12). Subsequent studies have reported that higher RT doses may result in longer survival times in patients with good performance status. This was initially documented in the 1996 report of the Medical Research Council study (13), in which patients with good performance status treated with 39 Gy per 13 fractions had a 2-month survival advantage compared to patients treated with 17 Gy per 2 fractions. Similar findings were seen in a Canadian randomized study of 20 Gy in 5 fractions versus 10 Gy single fraction, in which symptom control was equivalent but a 2-month survival difference favored the fractionated arm (14). In addition, the Dutch study (16) also reported significantly better 1-year survival times of 19.6% as compared to 10.9% for 30 Gy per 10 fractions versus 16 Gy per 2 fractions.

Differences observed in these clinical trials are of interest, but can be incorporated in recommending palliative RT in clinical practice. Chest symptoms such as cough, hemoptysis, and superior vena cava (SVC) obstruction caused by tumor mass are likely to improve with short or intermediate RT fractionation schedules, with mild to modest toxicity. External beam RT remains the gold standard form of palliative RT for lung cancer. For patients with previous external beam RT and cases where the tumor is causing obstruction of a major airway, direct insertion of radioactive sources into the bronchial lumen (endobronchial brachytherapy) may be considered. The response rates vary between 70 and 90% in appropriately selected patients (20).

Retreatment with irradiation in patients with locally progressive disease following previous radical RT is a relatively common and challenging problem. A study by Gressen et al. (21) involving 34 patients undergoing retreatment produced results representative of other studies. The median initial RT dose was 59 Gy (range 32–66), the duration between initial and subsequent treatment was 15 months (range 3–156),

TABLE 49.6

SELECTED RANDOMIZED CLINICAL TRIALS OF PALLIATIVE RADIATION FOR LUNG CANCER

Author, year, reference	Number of patients randomized	Treatment comparison	Primary/Secondary end points	Results
MRC 1991 (10)	369	17 Gy/2 fr vs. 30 Gy/10 fr (option of 27 Gy/6 fr)	Clinician assessment of symptoms, daily diary card by patient	Improvement in: hemoptysis (81–86%), cough (56–65%); median duration of palliation >50% of survival; median survival 6 mo
MRC 1992 (11)	235	17 Gy/2 fr vs. 10 Gy/1 fr	As MRC 1991	Palliation of symptoms same in two arms for ≥50% survival
Macbeth (MRC) 1996 (13)	509	17 Gy/2 fr vs. 39 Gy/13 fr	Rotterdam symptom checklist, MRC patient diary	2 fr had more rapid symptom palliation; 13 fr had longer survival (7- vs. 9-mo median)
Ball 1997 (12) (Australia)	200	20 Gy/5 fr ±5 FU 1 g/d ×5 d	Symptom relief	RR 29% vs. 16%; survival same; toxicity greater in chemo arm
NCIC CTG SC.15 Bezjak 2000 (14)	231	20 Gy/5 fr vs. 10 Gy single fr	Patient diary at 1 mo, QLQ-C30, LCSS	Similar palliation; 2-mo survival advantage to fractionated arm
Sundstrom et al. 2004 (15)	407	17 Gy/2 fr vs. 42 Gy/15 fr vs. 50 Gy/25 fr	Clinician assessments-baseline to 54 wk post-RT; QLQ-C30 and QLQ-LC13	Symptom relief (dyspnea, cough, and hemoptysis) were equivalent; no significant differences in survival
Kramer et al. 2005 (16)	297	30 Gy/10 fr vs. 16 Gy/2 fr	Rotterdam symptom checklist	Both were equally effective; palliation in 3 Gy/10 fr more prolonged with less worsening symptoms and a significantly better 1-y survival
Erridge et al. 2005 (17)	149	10 Gy/1 fr vs. 30 Gy/10 fr	Physician assessed total symptom score, HADS, Spitzer's QOL index	Significantly more patients achieved complete resolution of symptoms and palliation of chest pain and dyspnea with 30 Gy/10 fr

CR, complete regression; CXR, chest x-ray; fr, fraction; LCSS, lung cancer symptom score; MRC, medical research council; NCIC CTG, National Cancer Institute of Canada Clinical Trials Group; PR, partial regression; EORTC QLQ-C30, European Organization for Research and Treatment of Cancer Quality of Life Questionnaire-Core 30; EORTC QLQ-LC13, European Organization for Research and Treatment of Cancer Quality of Life Questionnaire-Lung Cancer 13; RTOG, Radiation Therapy Oncology Group; RT, radiotherapy; HADS, Hospital Anxiety and Depression Score; RR, response rate.

and the median retreatment dose was 30 Gy (6–38 Gy). On the whole, the overall estimated symptom response rate between studies was favorable with 83% for hemoptysis, 65% for cough, 60% for dyspnea, and 69% for pain. Late complications were low, with an overall estimated symptom response rate of 3%.

Bone Metastases

RT remains the gold standard for palliation of painful bone metastases. Randomized trials have provided concrete scientific evidence supporting the validity of RT. Fractionation schedules examined include single 8 Gy, 20 Gy per 5 fractions, 30 Gy per 10 fractions, and 50 Gy in 25 fractions. Direct comparison is problematic as various study endpoints have been utilized including a variety of measurement tools, measurement time frames and a lack of consideration of analgesic usage (22). More recently, consensus has been reached among international investigators on a common set of endpoints to be employed in clinical trials of radiation for bone metastases which are indeed being reported in the current generation of randomized trials (23).

Despite difficulties with direct comparisons of trial results, there is strong evidence of the palliative benefit of radiation for bone metastases. Pain response was reported in 30–70%

of trial patients. Complete pain relief at 1 month was seen in 25% of patients (24). Two large randomized studies, published in 1999, reported equivalent response rates in both single 8 Gy and fractionated schedules (25,26), but higher retreatment rates in the single fraction arm: the Bone Pain Trial Working Party reported 23% retreatment in single fraction and 10% in fractionated arm (25), and Steenland et al. (26) reported those rates to be 25 and 7% respectively. A meta-analysis comparing single fraction RT to more protracted schedules (27) confirmed that the equivalent response rates between single and fractionated RT were seen when all the relevant trials were pooled. Its conclusion was that single fraction RT should be recommended for its convenience and ease of administration, given no advantage of fractionated RT in pain relief of uncomplicated bone metastases; there was insufficient data to comment on its effectiveness in treatment of complicated bone metastases, that is metastases at risk of fracture, or causing nerve or cord compression. The conclusion of the meta-analysis is supported by the most recently published Radiation Therapy Oncology Group (RTOG) trial of nearly 900 patients with painful bone metastases from breast or prostate cancer (23), in which there were no differences in response rates at 3 months between single 8 Gy (15% complete response, 50% partial response) and 30 Gy per 10 fractions (18 and 48% respectively). That trial, like others before, documented a higher rate of retreatment in single fraction arm—18% of patients were re-treated, as compared to 9% of patients in the 30 Gy arm; this may be in part because of a somewhat shorter duration of pain relief from single 8 Gy, and in part because of more willingness to repeat RT after 8 Gy than after 30 Gy. Subsequent pathologic fracture rates did not differ while acute toxicity was greater in the fractionated arm.

RT is typically used in the treatment of bone metastases causing pain, threatening nerve or cord compression or at risk of pathologic fracture. "Wide-field" RT, consisting of HBI or radioactive isotopes, is used in the treatment of symptomatic areas for patients with widespread bony disease. Response rates and duration are comparable to those achieved with local radiation, although a study by Zelefsky et al. (28) suggests superior duration and retreatment results may occur from fractionated HBI. At present, the efficacy of strontium-89, either alone or in conjunction with local radiation, is confined to the treatment of prostate bone metastases because of its affinity for osteoblastic lesions. Evidence exists regarding strontium-89s benefit to both the treatment of painful metastases and the prevention of future lesions. Currently research is going on with a focus on newer isotopes such as rhenium-186 and samarium-153.

Reirradiation of previously treated bone metastases can be effective, with response rates of 50% and response durability of 5 months. In a study by Hayashi et al. (29), initial pain relief, relief duration ($\geq$4 m), performance status [Eastern Cooperative Oncology Group (ECOG) $\leq$2] and solitary bone metastases were prognostic of a favorable response. An international trial led by NCIC Clinical Trials Group is currently addressing the efficacy of and optimal dose fractionation (8 Gy single or 20-Gy fractionated RT) for painful bone metastases reirradiation.

Palliative RT side effects for bone metastases vary depending on the anatomic location of treatment. Nausea and vomiting may be common, particularly in patients receiving treatment to the thoracolumbar spine. The incidence of acute side effects, especially emesis, is similar for both single fraction and multifraction treatment regimes in studies utilizing five HT3 antagonists. The risk of developing complications within the treated bone appears minimal. Peat et al. (30) reported no differences in the numbers of fractures or incidences of paraplegia developing in a treated area. HBI-related toxicity tends to increase with dose, ranging from 30 to 60% gastrointestinally, 20–40% hematologically, and occasional pulmonary toxicity. Strontium-89 trials have reported no significant gastrointestinal toxicity while hematologic effects, although not uncommon, are usually mild.

It is not standard practice to prophylactically irradiate all bone metastases, whether painful or not, although benefits may arise from RT if there exists a risk of fracture. Criteria defined in orthopaedic literature (31) targets lesions for which surgery should be considered, but RT may also be of benefit. These include lytic lesions >2.5 cm in diameter involving the cortex. Although pain relief occurs in 70–80% of patients with breast cancer receiving RT to lytic bone metastases, radiologic reossification rates are 17–31% (32). Of 59 patients with nonfractured lesions treated primarily with RT, 4 developed subsequent pathologic fractures, two of which occurred during the time of radiation. Of these 59 patients, 39 were classified as high risk. The fractures that did occur, developed during treatment. Therefore, RT may be effective for initial management of high-risk bone metastases from breast cancer. Nevertheless, it would seem prudent that both the radiation oncologist and orthopaedic surgeon assess patients at risk for pathologic fractures. If fracture does occur, most patients will receive "adjuvant" radiation, although the merit of this practice has never been validated. Regimes utilized in this situation are based on those used to treat pain, but it is not clear whether the shorter hypofractionated regimes are as effective as longer courses in producing reossification. There may exist a subset of patients who do not require additional radiation following surgery. This may include patients who are completely ambulatory and pain free following surgery and possess a poor prognosis due to their underlying malignancy.

Brain Metastases

Solitary brain metastases can be treated by surgical resection. Three small randomized trials compared resection followed by radiation to RT alone (33–35), with two reporting improved survival in the surgical arms. Whole brain RT (WBRT) has been shown to reduce the risk of local recurrence at the surgical site in addition to elsewhere in the brain (34). An alternative to surgical resection is stereotactic radiation (SRT), also known as radiosurgery, or "gamma-knife" (after the specific treatment unit). SRT consists of multiple external beams from multiple directions. This allows for the ability to concentrate the radiation dose to a limited area of the brain. Small trials have produced impressive results for SRT and WBRT versus WBRT alone although the results have not been reproduced in multicenter settings (36). An RTOG trial (37) randomized 333 patients with one to three brain metastases to WBRT alone or WBRT followed by a SRT boost. Patients with single brain metastasis treated with stereotactic boost versus WBRT alone showed a survival advantage of 4.9 versus 6.5 months respectively. Patients in the SRT arm were more likely to have stable or improved performance status at 6 months' follow-up (43%) than patients treated with WBRT alone (27%). As a result, WBRT followed by SRT is considered to be standard practice for patients with single unresectable brain metastasis, and a consideration for patients with two to three brain metastases (38). Due to the potential for long-term side effects of WBRT, many oncologists and patients appear to be opting for stereotactic body radiation therapy (SBRT) only. In practice, many oncologists and patients, at least in some countries (notably United States) appear to be forgoing WBRT and treating patients with SBRT alone, arguing for potential long-term adverse effects of WBRT. However, these patients frequently develop subsequent brain metastases. It is not clear what the normal tissue effects of repeated courses of SRT are, and whether the practice of withholding WBRT is justified. The American Society for Therapeutic Radiology and Oncology (ASTRO) has recently summarized the current evidence on the role of radiosurgery for brain metastases (38).

Most patients with brain metastases present with multiple metastases and are not candidates for limited radiation. Whole brain external beam RT is usually recommended, although steroids alone may be an option for patients with very limited life expectancy (39). The prevention of neurologic deterioration is a frequently cited justification for RT in asymptomatic patients although its benefit in asymptomatic patients has not been established. RT fractionation schedules utilized include 40 Gy in 20 fractions, 30 Gy in 10 fractions, 20 Gy in 5 fractions, and 17 Gy in 2 fractions. Studies comparing RT schedules (40,41) report no difference in response rate and survival, although a quicker response was seen with shorter fractionation schedules. Neurologic symptom relief was reported in 50–90% of patients whereas 50% of patients experienced functional improvement and median survival was 15–20 weeks. The distinction between steroid effect versus RT was not made (42). Additionally, most of the assessments were completed by medical personnel rather than by direct patient report. Furthermore, purposive patient selection for RT is of utmost importance. This issue is clearly evident in a study by Priestman et al. comparing 12 Gy in 2 fractions to 30 Gy in 10 fractions (41). At the 1-month follow-up assessment, one third of the 533 patients randomized were gravely ill or deceased.

Improvements in palliative brain RT outcomes continue, particularly with patients possessing longer life expectancies. A recursive partitioning model has been derived from an RTOG study and the analysis of patient outcomes. This model has identified three prognostic strata based on patient age, performance status, and the presence or absence of extracranial cancer (43). Patients under 60 years of age, with a Karnofsky performance status of 80–100, and no cancer elsewhere, possess the best prognosis (strata I, 7 months median survival). Patients lacking one of the above criteria fall into an intermediate prognosis group (strata II), and those not satisfying two or more criteria have a poor outcome and are less likely to benefit from treatment (strata III). If treatment is indicated for patients in strata III, a short course of palliative RT is usually employed. For strata I and strata II, more aggressive treatments being explored include accelerated or hyperfractionated RT, combining WBRT with systemic agents such as temozolomide, and the utilization of radiosensitizers such as motexafin gadolinium (44). Some of these strategies show promising results although the full benefit will not been known until after the completion and maturation of current randomized clinical trials.

Patients previously treated with WBRT can be considered for reirradiation, although the literature describes highly selected patients. In a study by Guiney et al. (45) of 89 patients representing 3% of patients treated with WBRT initially, 27% reported complete symptom resolution after second course of RT (typically 20 Gy, following initial 30 Gy.) Neurologic function class and performance status improvement occurred in 40 and 30% respectively while median duration of response was modest at 2.75 months. Treatment was well tolerated, with only one case of late radiologic change. These results support the efficacy of well-selected patients although life expectancy still tends to be short. As a result, the relative benefit of reirradiation in the context of a short life expectancy has to be considered.

Advanced Pelvic Malignancies

RT is commonly employed in patients with locally advanced, inoperable, or recurrent rectal and gynecologic cancers who develop distressing symptoms such as pain, bleeding, and mucous discharge. Although effective in a significant number of cases, minimal published data exists detailing the probability of benefit, or appropriate fractionation. A review of RT for recurrent rectal cancer estimates that 70–90% of patients received initial benefit for pain relief, with 23–50% experiencing symptom control for 6 months. As a range of doses were utilized, it was not possible to assess the optimal regime, or discern any difference in symptom relief between lower and higher doses (46). A subsequent report from the Peter MacCallum Cancer Institute (47) found no significant dose response effect between the radical group (50–60 Gy) and high-dose palliative group (45 Gy) for patients with residual disease postresection.

Treatment approaches vary and range from large fractions of up to 10 Gy, often repeated at intervals (48) to more conventionally fractionated high-dose treatment, such as the 50 Gy in 25 fractions (49). An RTOG study of 10 Gy fractions administered with the radiosensitizer misonidazole suggested a 41% increased risk of grade 3/4 complications in those who survived 12 months (50). Nevertheless, the use of large single fractions remains commonplace, especially for patients with poor performance status or with limited life expectancy. Other regimes commonly used include 20 Gy in 5 fractions, 30 Gy per 10 fractions, and 40 Gy per 16 fractions. For patients with

good performance status and no disease outside the pelvis, doses up to 50 Gy can be employed.

With recent advances in surgical techniques, combination chemoradiotherapy may render patients previously considered inoperable, resectable with a more favorable outcome (51). Similarly, aggressive combination of external beam RT surgery and intraoperative RT has provided favorable results and should be considered in patients with localized disease (52).

Retreatment of symptomatic pelvic tumors is particularly challenging. Because life expectancy is frequently protracted in the absence of life-threatening distant disease, they present as a major source of morbidity and suffering. These patients have a greater need for treatment that would provide symptom control, but are also at risk of late toxicities that may further compromise quality of life. Mohiuddin et al. (53) described the experience of Kentucky University in retreating 103 patients with rectal cancer. Initial RT doses were high with a median dose of 50.4 Gy (range 30–74.2 Gy). The interval between courses of treatment was relatively long, being 19 m (range 2–86 m). Retreatment doses were median 34.8 Gy (range 15–49.2 Gy). Combination RT and chemotherapy (fluorouracil, 5FU) was used at the time of retreatment in all patients. Palliative response rates were high for bleeding (80%), pain relief (33%), and mass effect (20%). Late complications in the form of ≥Gd 3 chronic diarrhea in 17% of cases.

Lymph Node Metastases

Involvement of lymph glands by metastatic cancer is common. They may cause airway or nerve pain, patient distress due to appearance or interference with normal daily activities. One of the most significant complications of malignant lymphadenopathy is superior vena caval obstruction (SVCO). SVCO causes facial and neck swelling, headache, dyspnea, chest wall vein distention, and occasionally syncope. It is usually because of compression of the SVC by mediastinal lymphadenopathy. Most cases (80%) are due to malignancy, with the most common underlying diagnosis being lung cancer (60–70%). Other causes include lymphoma, germ cell tumors, and breast cancer.

Although not considered to be an oncologic emergency, SVCO can cause distressing symptoms and should be treated urgently. Lymphoma and small cell lung cancers causing SVCO are normally treated with chemotherapy. In the case of NSCLC, RT is the treatment of choice, although intraluminal stents are increasingly being used, especially for patients who progress during or after their RT.

The radiation dose regimes employed for SVCO will depend on the underlying histology and the intent of treatment. Patients with lymphoma and germ cell tumors may be treated as part of a curative protocol, using radical doses of RT given in conventional daily fractions. Most patients with NSCLC will be treated with palliative intent although occasionally it may be appropriate to use a curative regime. Doses tend to be similar to those used for locally advanced NSCLC (see the section Lung Cancer), although some oncologists use larger than normal fractions for the initial few treatments, if the patient is very symptomatic, to expedite response. Response rates between 40 and 90% (22,54,55) have been reported depending on underlying histology, treatment regime, and patient population.

Other lymph node masses causing pain or distress can be treated by short courses of palliative RT, usually 20–30 Gy in 5–10 fractions. Unsightly or painful lesions in the skin or subcutaneous tissue can be managed similarly. Response rates vary, depending on the underlying histology, but are probably in the order of 50–70%. Sometimes only a small reduction in the actual volume of the malignant mass occurs, but this can still lead to significant symptom relief.

Spinal Cord Compression

Spinal cord compression is one of relatively few oncologic emergencies. Prompt recognition, diagnosis, and treatment may avert neurologic deterioration and prevent paralysis. Spinal cord compression is usually due to the extension of vertebral metastases into the epidural space or paravertebral tumors. It may also be the result of vertebral collapse, with bony fragments causing cord compression. Up to 90% of patients with vertebral metastases experience pain before any neurologic changes. Any worsening of back pain in a patient known to have or be at risk for developing bone metastases should be assessed promptly. Unfortunately, patients frequently do not bring symptoms to the attention of their physician early enough. Many present hours after they have lost the use of their limbs, bladder, and/or bowel. If paraplegia has been present for more than 24–48 hours, it may be impossible to reverse the neurologic damage. The most important predictor of neurologic recovery is the ambulatory status at time of treatment of cord compression. Of patients who are ambulatory 89% remain so after treatment, 53% of patients with paresis (weakness) become ambulant, and only 10% of patients with paraplegia (bilateral loss of leg power, i.e., bedridden) regain their mobility after treatment (56).

A randomized trial has been reported (57) in which 101 patients with spinal metastatic disease causing cord compression were randomized to surgery (decompression and stabilization) followed by RT, or RT alone (30 Gy per 10 fractions). Significant advantages to the surgical arm were reported with greatly improved rates of mobility (median ambulation time 126 vs. 35 days) and neurologic recovery (56 vs. 19% of nonambulatory patients regained ability to walk). It will be interesting to see if the recent publication of this trial will affect practice and lead to increasing consideration of surgical resection as initial treatment of a larger proportion of patients with cord compression.

Evidence for the role of RT in spinal cord compression has been summarized in practice guidelines (58). Palliative RT is preferred over surgical decompression in patients who possess radiosensitive tumors (e.g., lymphoma, myeloma); have a limited life expectancy (days to a few weeks), and would find surgery to be too burdensome; possess extensive vertebral or epidural metastasis where surgery stabilization would not be possible; present long after the loss of neurologic function and have continuing pain in the region of the cord compression and are not candidates for surgery due to their debility; or other contraindications. As with bone metastases, typical palliative treatment plans for spinal cord compression are 20 Gy in 5 fractions over 1 week or 30 Gy in 10 fractions over 2 weeks. Maranzano et al. (59) reported a randomized trial of two hypofractionated schedules—8 Gy ×2 versus 30 Gy split course RT, with similar outcomes in the two study arms (pain relief in 56–59%, ability to walk in 68–71%). If complete paraplegia is present for a considerable time before presentation, there is little hope of neurologic recovery. Palliative RT may be reserved to manage pain in the future, should it become a problem.

Treatment of the spinal cord in patients who have had previous spinal radiation presents a frequent clinical dilemma. If neurologic status is threatened and surgery is not advisable, reirradiation may indeed be appropriate. Many radiation oncologists use a smaller fraction size to minimize the risk of late complications, specifically radiation myelitis. The risk of radiation-induced paralysis cannot be completely dismissed and needs to be put into perspective of almost definite tumor-induced paralysis if treatment is withheld. In an already paraplegic patient, attention to maximum cord tolerance is not a concern. If pain is present, the patient can be treated with the required dosage of palliative radiation for pain control without regard for the already damaged spinal cord.

What After Radiotherapy?

Acute side effects are common and although self-limiting they nevertheless require symptomatic management as they may impair the patient's well-being. They usually occur after the treatment has finished and can cause considerable anxiety if a patient is not informed of them. Common acute effects, their time course, and recommendations for management are shown in Table 49.7. In addition, many patients receiving RT will complain of fatigue during and after their course of treatment. The exact etiology of this is unknown but is probably multifactorial.

RT late complications, which occur months or years after treatment, are usually not relevant to many patients receiving palliative treatment. However, the radiation oncologist still needs to be mindful of the risks of inducing irreversible problems, such as myelitis, lung fibrosis, and renal failure, especially in patients who might have a long life expectancy, such as those with metastatic breast cancer.

Unlike high-dose radical treatments, low-dose palliative RT is not necessarily a "once-only" treatment. Therefore, if a patient treated for painful bony metastases develops recurrent pain in the irradiated area several months later, retreatment may be possible and should be discussed with the responsible radiation oncologist.

Where Do We Go From Here?

Traditionally, palliative RT has not attracted the same focus as curative efforts in regard to research and development. Significant progress has been made in recent years secondary to coordinated efforts at the institutional level (3,61), professional organizations and funding agencies. Barriers remain in getting patients to undergo treatment that could potentially benefit them. Health services research provides invaluable tools to help identify gaps in care delivery and address potential barriers. Huang et al. demonstrated variations in access to RT in relation to how far patients lived from RT facilities (62). Recognition of the role of RT, timely referrals by health care professionals, adequacy in the planning of resources to minimize waiting times and public education regarding palliative RT are some areas of focus on to maximize symptom relief through optimal RT modality usage.

Technologic advances have advanced how radical RT is being delivered with improved target delineation, dose escalation, and normal tissue sparing. While the application of these tools have been more selective in palliative RT, advances in how modern technology can help expand the ability to palliate is actively being investigated. Planning computed tomography scan provides enhanced anatomic detail over conventional fluoroscopic planning and optimal modality usage in preparation of palliative treatments is being addressed (46). Stereotactic RT, previously exclusive to selected brain metastases, is now being applied to other areas such as spine and paraspinal tumors (63), allowing one to spare the spinal cord. Similarly, the use of more sophisticated techniques including conformal RT and intensity modulated RT now offers the opportunity to deliver retreatment to previously irradiated areas. Retreatment, previously considered unsafe, now allows for further improvement of symptoms. The boundary between what is potentially curable and incurable is now being challenged through the ability to safely escalate dose with more sophisticated planning techniques combined with chemotherapy and surgery.

Advances in clinical trial methodology have provided us with a new generation of high quality trials to guide evidence-based care. The incorporation of quality of life outcomes, the use of validated symptom measurement tools and the

TABLE 49.7

ACUTE SIDE EFFECTS OF RADIATION THERAPY

Site	Symptoms	Time course	Management
General	Fatigue	Most pronounced after completion of RT; gets better with time	Same as for cancer-related fatigue (60)
Skin	Erythema	Settles within 3 wk of completion of therapy	None, or 1% hydrocortisone for skin irritation if skin surface unbroken
	Skin breakdown	Occurs only after higher dose XRT but if severe may last for several weeks	If only dry desquamation ("peeling"), no specific therapy except as above. If skin breaks down and begins to become ulcerated and weepy (moist desquamation), skin care like for a burn is required to prevent secondary infection
Abdomen	Nausea and vomiting	May occur after first treatment and persist for several days after completion of therapy	Antiemetics are used either as prophylaxis or as therapy for established emesis
	Diarrhea	Occurs usually late in protracted course of XRT or after completion of short course of treatment	Prevention with low-fiber diet may be all that is required. Established diarrhea best treated with simple antidiarrheas (e.g., Lomotil, Imodium)
	Dysuria, frequency	Timing as above for diarrhea	Exclude UTI by culturing MSU. If no bacterial infection, increase fluid intake, consider cranberry juice or Pyridium
Head and neck	Painful inflammation of mouth, pharynx (mucositis)	Occurs during later stages of protracted course of XRT, may persist for 2–3 wk after completion of therapy	Soft diet. Treat any secondary infection such as oral candidiasis. In severe cases, local anesthetic solution may be required
Thorax	Dysphagia (esophagitis)	As above	Soft diet, analgesics. Patients may benefit from antacids to prevent reflux
Head	Alopecia	Occurs over a few days after starting treatment	No specific therapy. Patients should be reassured that hair will regrow

MSU, midstream urine; UTI, urinary tract infection; RT, radiotherapy; XRT, x-ray radiotherapy.

need for common definitions and outcome measures have become widely recognized and frequently incorporated in most contemporary palliative trials. Ongoing developments will provide us with increasingly more versatile tools to test new hypothesis and challenge empirical practices. The clinical significance and validation of quality of life measures, contemporary concepts such as quality adjusted life years, utilities, economic analysis (64) and patient preferences (65) are the focus of active investigation on how to best incorporate these concepts into palliative trials. These tools may become useful in the palliative arena allowing us to tackle constructs and create outcome measures previously difficult to measure using traditional methods.

Novel interventions and strategies are most likely to succeed when based on a solid understanding of the underlying mechanisms and pathophysiology. Translational research bridges the gap between the bench and the bedside and is likely a crucial link to future advances. Explicit attempts to incorporate secondary translational hypothesis into clinical trials are currently under way in trial groups such as the Symptom Control Group of the National Cancer Institute of Canada Clinical Trials Group (NCIC CTG). Efforts to improve integration between translational and clinical research is ongoing.

Palliative RT is being recognized as a unique area of expertise deserving of our dedication and commitment. Coordination of these efforts through organization at the clinical and research levels has resulted in significant improvements in recent years. Future advances are likely to occur from an improved understanding of technologic applications, research methods, translational research and patterns of care.

ACKNOWLEDGMENTS

The authors are grateful to Ms. Katy Burrows, PROP Research Analyst, for her assistance in the preparation of this chapter and to the Allan Kerbel Symptom Control Fund for support of the Palliative Radiation Oncology Program.

References

1. Janjan NA. An emerging respect for palliative care in radiation oncology. *J Palliat Med* 1998;1(1):83–88.
2. Mackillop WJ. The principles of palliative radiotherapy: a radiation oncologist's perspective. *Can J Oncol* 1996;6(1 Suppl):5–11.
3. Danjoux C, Szumacher E, Andresson L, et al. Palliative radiotherapy at Toronto Sunnybrook Regional Cancer Center: the rapid response radiotherapy program. *Curr Oncol* 2000;7(1):52–56.
4. Falk SJ, Girling DJ, White RJ, et al. Immediate versus delayed palliative thoracic radiotherapy in patients with unresectable locally advanced non-small cell lung cancer and minimal thoracic symptoms: randomised controlled trial. *BMJ* 2002;325(7362):465.
5. Maher EJ, Timothy AR, Squire CJ. Audit: the use of radiotherapy for NSCLC in the UK. *Clin Oncol (R Coll Radiol)* 1993;5:72–79.
6. Thames HDJ, Whithers HR, Peters LJ, et al. Changes in early and late radiation responses with altered dose fractionation: implications for dose-survival relationships. *Int J Radiat Oncol Biol Phys* 1982;8(2):219–226.
7. Munro AJ, Sebag-Montefiore D. Opportunity cost—a neglected aspect of cancer treatment. *Br J Cancer* 1992;65(3):309–310.
8. Crellin AM, Marks A, Maher EJ. Why don't British radiotherapists give single fractions of radiotherapy for bone metastases? *Clin Oncol (R Coll Radiol)* 1989;1:63–66.
9. Patterson R. *The treatment of malignant disease by radium and x-rays.* London: Edward Arnold & Co, 1948.
10. Medical Research Council. Inoperable non-small-cell lung cancer (NSCLC): A Medical Research Council randomised trial of palliative radiotherapy

with two fractions or ten fractions. Report to the Medical Research Council by its Lung Cancer Working Party. *Br J Cancer* 1991;63(2):265–270.

11. Medical Research Council. A Medical Research Council (MRC) randomised trial of palliative radiotherapy with two fractions or a single fraction in patients with inoperable non-small-cell lung cancer (NSCLC) and poor performance status. Medical Research Council Lung Cancer Working Party. *Br J Cancer* 1992;65(6):934–941.

12. Ball D, Smith J, Bishop J, et al. A phase III study of radiotherapy with and without continuous-infusion fluorouracil as palliation for non-small-cell lung cancer. *Br J Cancer* 1997;75(5):690–697.

13. Macbeth FR, Bolger JJ, Hopwood P, et al. Randomized trial of palliative two-fraction versus more intensive 13-fraction radiotherapy for patients with inoperable non-small cell lung cancer and good performance status. Medical Research Council Lung Cancer Working Party. *Clin Oncol (R Coll Radiol)* 1996;8(3):167–175.

14. Bezjak A, Dixon P, Brundage M. Characteristics of lung cancer patients entered on a Canadian palliative radiotherapy study (National Cancer Institute of Canada Clinical Trials Group (NCIC CTG) SC.15 study). *Lung Cancer* 2000;29(Suppl 1):171.

15. Sundstrom S, Bremnes R, Aasebo U, et al. Hypofractionated palliative radiotherapy (17 Gy per two fractions) in advanced non-small-cell lung carcinoma is comparable to standard fractionation for symptom control and survival: a national phase III trial. *J Clin Oncol* 2004;22(5):801–810.

16. Kramer GW, Wanders SL, Noordijk EM, et al. Results of the Dutch National Study of the palliative effect of irradiation using two different treatment schemes for non-small-cell lung cancer. *J Clin Oncol* 2005;23(13):2962–2970.

17. Erridge SC, Gaze MN, Price A, et al. Symptom control and quality of life in people with lung cancer: a randomised trial of two palliative radiotherapy fractionation schedules. *Clin Oncol (R Coll Radiol)* 2005;17(1):61–67.

18. Hopwood P, Stephens RJ. Symptoms at presentation for treatment in patients with lung cancer: implications for the evaluation of palliative treatment. The Medical Research Council (MRC) Lung Cancer Working Party. *Br J Cancer* 1995;71(3):633–636.

19. Stephens RJ, Hopwood P, Girling DJ. Defining and analysing symptom palliation in cancer clinical trials: a deceptively difficult exercise. *Br J Cancer* 1999;79(3–4):538–544.

20. Barton R, Kirkbride P. Special techniques in palliative radiation oncology. *J Palliat Med* 2000;3(1):75–83.

21. Gressen EL, Werner-Wasik M, Cohn L, et al. Thoracic reirradiation for symptomatic relief after prior radiotherapeutic management for lung cancer. *Am J Clin Oncol* 2000;23(2):160–163.

22. Wu JS, Bezjak A, Chow E, et al. Primary treatment endpoint following palliative radiotherapy for painful bone metastases: need for a consensus definition? *Clin Oncol (R Coll Radiol)* 2002;14(1):70–77.

23. Hartsell WF, Scott CB, Bruner DW, et al. Randomized trial of short-versus long-course radiotherapy for palliation of painful bone metastases. *J Natl Cancer Inst* 2005;97(11):798–804.

24. McQuay HJ, Collins SL, Carrol D, et al. Radiotherapy for the palliation of painful bone metastases. *Cochrane Database Syst Rev* 2000(2):CD001793.

25. Bone Pain Trial Working Party. 8 Gy single fraction radiotherapy for the treatment of metastatic skeletal pain: randomized comparison with a multifraction schedule over 12 months of patient follow-up. *Radiother Oncol* 1999;52:111–121.

26. Steenland E, Leer JW, van Houwelingen H, et al. The effect of a single fraction compared to multiple fractions on painful bone metastases: a global analysis of the Dutch Bone Metastasis Study. *Radiother Oncol* 1999;52:101–109.

27. Wu JS, Wong R, Johnston M, et al. Meta-analysis of dose-fractionation radiotherapy trials for the palliation of painful bone metastases. *Int J Radiat Oncol Biol Phys* 2003;55(3):594–605.

28. Zelefsky MJ, Scher HI, Forman JD, et al. Palliative hemiskeletal irradiation for widespread metastatic prostate cancer: a comparison of single dose and fractionated regimens. *Int J Radiat Oncol Biol Phys* 1989;17(6):1281–1285.

29. Hayashi S, Hoshi H, Iida T. Reirradiation with local-field radiotherapy for painful bone metastases. *Radiat Med* 2002;20(5):231–236.

30. Peat I, Spooner D, Hardwick M, et al. The Birmingham-Leicester pain study. *Clin Oncol (R Coll Radiol)* 2000;12:328–332.

31. Beals RK, Lawton GD, Snell WE. Prophylactic internal fixation of the femur in metastatic breast cancer. *Cancer* 1971;28:1350–1354.

32. Keene JS, Sellinger DS, McBeath AA, et al. Metastatic breast cancer in the femur: a search for the lesion at risk of fracture. *Clin Orthop* 1986;203:282–288.

33. Mintz AH, Kestle J, Rathbone MP, et al. A randomized trial to assess the efficacy of surgery in addition to radiotherapy in patients with a single cerebral metastasis. *Cancer* 1996;78(7):1470–1476.

34. Patchell RA, Tibbs PA, Walsh JW, et al. A randomized trial of surgery in the treatment of single metastases to the brain. *N Engl J Med* 1990;322(8):494–500.

35. Vecht CJ, Haaxma Reiche H, Noordijk EM, et al. Treatment of single brain metastasis: radiotherapy alone or combined with neurosurgery? *Ann Neurol* 1993;33(6):583–590.

36. Kondziolka D, Patel A, Lunsford LD, et al. Stereotactic radiosurgery plus whole brain radiotherapy versus radiotherapy alone for patients with multiple brain metastases. *Int J Radiat Oncol Biol Phys* 1999;45(2):427–434.

37. Andrews DW, Scott CB, Sperduto PW, et al. Whole brain radiation therapy with or without stereotactic radiosurgery boost for patients with one to three brain metastases: phase III results of the TROG 9508 randomized trial. *Lancet* 2004;363(9422):1665–1672.

38. Mehta MP, Tsao MN, Whelan TJ, et al. The American Society for Therapeutic Radiology and Oncology (ASTRO) evidence-based review of the role of radiosurgery for brain metastases. *Int J Radiat Oncol Biol Phys* 2005;63(1):37–46.

39. Bezjak A, Adam J, Panzarella T, et al. Radiotherapy for brain metastases: defining palliative response. *Radiother Oncol* 2001;61(1):71–76.

40. Haie-Meder C, Pellae-Cosset B, Laplanche A, et al. Results of a randomized clinical trial comparing two radiation schedules in the palliative treatment of brain metastases. *Radiother Oncol* 1993;26(2):111–116.

41. Priestman TJ, Dunn J, Brada M, et al. Final results of the Royal College of Radiologists' trial comparing two different radiotherapy schedules in the treatment of cerebral metastases. *Clin Oncol (R Coll Radiol)* 1996;8(5):308–315.

42. Millar BA, Bezjak A, Tsao M, et al. Defining the impact and contribution of steroids in people receiving whole-brain irradiation for cerebral metastases. *Clin Oncol (R Coll Radiol)* 2004;16:339–344.

43. Gaspar L, Scott C, Murray K, et al. Validation of the RTOG recursive partitioning analysis (RPA) classification for brain metastases. *Int J Radiat Oncol Biol Phys* 2000;47(4):1001–1006.

44. Carde P, Timmerman R, Mehta MP, et al. Multicenter phase Ib/II trial of the radiation enhancer motexafin gadolinium in patients with brain metastases. *J Clin Oncol* 2001;19(7):2074–2083.

45. Wong WW, Schild SE, Sawyer TE, et al. Analysis of outcome in patients reirradiated for brain metastases. *Int J Radiat Oncol Biol Phys* 1996;34(3):585–590.

46. Haddad P, Wong RK, Levin W, et al. Computed tomographic simulation in palliative radiotherapy: the Princess Margaret Hospital experience. *Clin Oncol (R Coll Radiol)* 2004;16(6):425–428.

47. Guiney MJ, Smith JG, Worotniuk V, et al. Results of external beam radiotherapy alone for incompletely resected carcinoma of rectosigmoid or rectum: Peter McCallum Cancer Institute experience 1981–1990. *Int J Radiat Oncol Biol Phys* 1999;43(3):531–536.

48. Hodson DI, Malaker K, McLellan W, et al. Hypofractionated radiotherapy for the palliation of advanced pelvic malignancy. *Int J Radiat Oncol Biol Phys* 1983;9(11):1727–1729.

49. Gallagher MJ, Richter MP. Radiotherapeutic management of pelvic recurrence in patients with rectal and rectosigmoid carcinoma. *Am J Clin Oncol* 1984;7:115.

50. Spanos WJ Jr, Wasserman T, Meoz R, et al. Palliation of advanced pelvic malignant disease with large fraction pelvic radiation and misonidazole: final report of RTOG phase I/II study. *Int J Radiat Oncol Biol Phys* 1987;13(10):1479–1482.

51. Wong R. Unresectable rectal cancer. Can neoadjuvant chemoradiotherapy achieve a cure? 2004;3(2):24–27.

52. Willett CG, Gunderson LL. Palliative treatment of rectal cancer: is radiotherapy alone a good option? *J Gastrointest Surg* 2004;8(3):277–279.

53. Mohiuddin M, Marks G, Marks J. Long-term results of reirradiation for patients with recurrent rectal carcinoma. *Cancer* 2002;95(5):1144–1150.

54. Hoskin PJ, Yarnold JR, Roos DR, et al. Radiotherapy for bone metastases. *Clin Oncol (R Coll Radiol)* 2001;13:88–90.

55. Rodrigues CI, Njo KH, Karim AB. Hypofractionated radiation therapy in the treatment of superior vena cava syndrome. *Lung Cancer* 1993;10(3–4):221–228.

56. Maranzano E, Latini P. Effectiveness of radiation therapy without surgery in metastatic spinal cord compression: final results from a prospective trial. *Int J Radiat Oncol Biol Phys* 1995;32(4):959–967.

57. Patchell RA, Tibbs PA, Regine WF, et al. Direct decompressive surgical resection in the treatment of spinal cord compression caused by metastatic cancer: a randomized trial. *Lancet* 2005;366:643–648.

58. Loblaw DA, Laperriere NJ. Emergency treatment of malignant extradural spinal cord compression: an evidence-based guideline. *J Clin Oncol* 1998;16(4):1613–1624.

59. Maranzano E, Bellavita R, Rossi R, et al. Short-course versus split-course radiotherapy in metastatic spinal cord compression: results of a phase III, randomized, multicenter trial. *J Clin Oncol* 2005;23(15):3358–3365.

60. National Comprehensive Cancer Network. *Cancer-related fatigue: clinical practice guidelines in oncology—version 2*. 2005; available at www.nccn.org.

61. Kirkbride P. A dedicated palliative radiation oncology program: The Princess Margaret Hospital experience [Abstract]. *Clin Oncol (R Coll Radiol)* 2000;12:329.

62. Huang J, Zhou S, Groome P, et al. Factors affecting the use of palliative radiotherapy in Ontario. *J Clin Oncol* 2001;19(1):137–144.

63. Bilsky MH, Yamada Y, Yenice KM, et al. Intensity-modulated stereotactic radiotherapy of paraspinal tumors: a preliminary report. *Neurosurgery* 2004;54(4):823–830; discussion 830–831.

64. van den Hout WB, van der Linden YM, Steenland E, et al. Single- versus multiple-fraction radiotherapy in patients with painful bone metastases: cost-utility analysis based on a randomized trial. *J Natl Cancer Inst* 2003;95(3):222–229.

65. Shakespeare TP, Lu JJ, Back MF, et al. Patient preference for radiotherapy fractionation schedule in the palliation of painful bone metastases. *J Clin Oncol* 2003;21(11):2156–2162.

CHAPTER 50 ■ PALLIATIVE CHEMOTHERAPY

ERIC M. CHEVLEN

INTRODUCTION—WHAT IS PALLIATIVE CHEMOTHERAPY?

In the early days of medical oncology, the term *palliative chemotherapy* would have been considered by many to be an oxymoron at best, a cruel jest at worst. Chemotherapy was widely seen, and not completely without justice, as a toxic assault upon a dying patient in the attempt, usually vain, to prolong his miserable life by a few extra weeks. This perception was coeval with the science itself. The first effective chemotherapy for any malignancy was reported in 1948 by Sidney Farber et al. They treated 16 children with acute leukemia. Only five entered remission, and the longest of these remissions was a paltry 6 weeks. Most of the children he treated experienced toxicity without benefit. Yet, that experience in treating acute leukemia in children proved to be the springboard from which modern chemotherapy has jumped. Now, three fourths of children with leukemia can be cured of their disease and go on to enjoy a normal life.

Although that progress in the management of childhood leukemia is certainly admirable, it does not address the semantic challenge of the term "palliative chemotherapy." Clearly, modern chemotherapy of childhood leukemia is not simply palliative; its goal is cure. It does not conform to the World Health Organization definition of palliative care: "the active total care of patients whose disease is not responsive to curative treatment." Of course, under this definition, any chemotherapy in which cure is not the goal or expected outcome would be considered palliative chemotherapy. Such a definition is clearly too broad for our purposes. It would include almost all chemotherapy now used to treat cancer, since only a minority of cancer cases is expected to be cured by chemotherapy.

Confounding the problem of defining "palliative chemotherapy" is the fact that the Medicare Hospice Benefit pays for drugs "used primarily for the relief of pain and symptom control related to the individual's terminal illness." With this in mind, some medical oncologists have argued that any chemotherapy that is not curative in intent is, by default, palliative chemotherapy, and should be a covered service for hospice patients. Hospices have understandably resisted this interpretation, both because it is contrary to the *prima facie* understanding of hospice care, and because the high cost of most chemotherapy would quickly bankrupt any hospice attempting to pay for it with the fixed per diem reimbursement it currently receives from Medicare, about $107 per day.

In the first edition of this book, the term "chemotherapy" seemed less problematic than the term "palliative," but this is no longer the case. In 1909, when Paul Ehrlich concocted the first effective drug therapy for syphilis, an inorganic compound based on arsenic, the term "chemotherapy" was used to distinguish synthesized medications from those derived from plant or animal products. Now that most pharmacotherapy is synthesized, the term "chemotherapy" has come to mean the drug therapy of cancer in particular, in contradistinction to treatment of cancer by surgery or radiation therapy. But even here, the term is unclear. For example, tamoxifen is a synthesized chemical used to treat cancer, but most oncologists would refer to it as "hormone therapy" rather than chemotherapy. Strontium-89 chloride is a simple two-atom chemical used to treat cancer, but most oncologists would refer to it as a variant of radiation therapy, rather than chemotherapy. Some treatments straddle categories. The monoclonal antibody rituximab, for example, is an immunotherapy, but it is a chimeric molecule, part murine, and part human, produced in a laboratory in a cell suspension culture derived from a third mammal, the hamster. Is it not also a chemotherapy? When a radioactive element is affixed to a monoclonal antibody, as in the case of yttrium-90 radiolabeled ibritumomab tiuxetan (Zevalin), does it thereby become radiation therapy?

Clearly, as the science of treating cancer advances, the lexicography will scurry along after it, but never quite keep up with it. For the purpose of this discussion, palliative chemotherapy refers to the administration of medications that kill or suppress growth of cancer cells, when used to ameliorate the symptoms caused by an incurable malignancy. Although they may reasonably be called *forms of chemotherapy*, this chapter will not discuss the palliative use of hormonal agonists or antagonists, nor will it discuss the palliative use of injectable radionuclides except in the context of radioimmunoconjugates.

USUAL RATIONALE FOR CHEMOTHERAPY USE

Chemotherapy can be used as adjuvant, curative, or palliative treatment, depending on the type and stage of malignancy. When used in the latter two circumstances, its effect is usually described by response rate. Response rate primarily refers to objective measurements of changes in cancer size, sites of metastatic disease, and measurable serologic or other markers of tumor activity.

Adjuvant chemotherapy refers to systemic treatment administered after all gross evidence of disease has been controlled by surgery or radiation therapy, but when the possibility of cancer recurrence is high. Adjuvant chemotherapy is given with the intent of completely eradicating any undetectable cancer cells that may be present. The benefit-to-toxicity ratio of adjuvant chemotherapy is extremely important. Most medical oncologists do not suggest very toxic or potentially lethal adjuvant chemotherapy if the likelihood of cancer recurrence is low and the percentage of patients likely to benefit is also low (i.e., residual cancer cells may not be killed with the treatment). In this instance, the treatment may harm more patients than it helps. Yet the individual with the cancer can have a very different perspective regarding this issue. Patients are often willing to undergo adjuvant therapies of prolonged duration and endure significant impairment in their quality of life (QOL) for a relatively small increase in the likelihood of cure (1). An additional benefit of adjuvant chemotherapy is the positive psychological effect of "doing something" to decrease the risk of cancer recurrence. Medical oncologists are wise, however, to keep in mind the distinction between "doing something" and "doing something beneficial" (2).

The goal of curative chemotherapy is to eradicate all cancer completely and to prevent its recurrence. Diffuse large cell lymphoma, testicular cancer, and Hodgkin's disease are just three of several different kinds of malignancies for which chemotherapy has been shown to provide the possibility of cure in the nonadjuvant setting. Chemotherapy should be recommended in most circumstances for highly chemotherapy-responsive cancers. Maintenance chemotherapy (that is, treatment continued for prolonged or indefinite periods of time after complete response is obtained) has been shown to be of no benefit for a number of chemotherapy-curable or highly chemosensitive cancers (testicular cancer, small cell lung cancer, ovarian cancer, lymphomas, and Hodgkin's disease).

Chemotherapy used in conjunction with another anticancer therapy can be palliative if it decreases treatment-related morbidity, even if it does not improve the chance of cure. For example, anal or laryngeal carcinoma can often be locally controlled or cured with aggressive surgery. This success, however, comes with significant morbidity—the need for colostomy or loss of voice. Organ function can be maintained for patients with these and other malignancies by combined chemotherapy and radiation therapy. It is anticipated that more malignancies will be treated with these organ-sparing treatments in the future.

Chemotherapy as a single modality may also be given with no expectation of curing the cancer. In such a situation, the goal of treatment is symptom reduction, life prolongation, or the combination of the two. Whereas, most patients will accept potentially curative therapy almost regardless of the toxicity it carries, the emotional response to noncurative therapy is quite different. The patient quite rightly asks what price in side effects he must pay for life prolongation, and how much life prolongation is he likely to get for this price? All the more so, when the therapeutic goal is the more modest one of symptom reduction without life prolongation, the patient asks if the same symptom control might be achieved with less toxic therapy. The good medical oncologist asks himself the same questions.

Not surprisingly, those noncurative chemotherapies which have a high response rate and which yield a clinically significant prolongation of life also reduce cancer-related symptoms, and improve the overall QOL. The reason is self evident: the symptoms were due to the cancer, and reducing the cancer reduces the symptoms. Examples of this are initial treatment of metastatic breast cancer or extensive stage small cell lung cancer.

It is not the intent of this chapter in a textbook of palliative care and supportive oncology to discuss curative therapies, adjuvant therapies, or even dramatically life-prolonging palliative therapies. These mainstays of medical oncology are better discussed in standard textbooks of medical oncology and in oncology journals. Rather, this chapter focuses on the more problematic situation. The question concerning poorly responsive cancers addressed here are twofold:

1. May chemotherapy improve QOL even if it does not prolong survival?
2. May chemotherapy prolong survival and still not diminish QOL?

The tacit assumption of this approach is that chemotherapy may have an anticancer effect too small to greatly prolong survival, but still have enough anticancer activity and low-enough toxicity to improve QOL.

PATIENT ACCEPTANCE OF THE NEED FOR CHEMOTHERAPY

After recovering from the initial shock of a cancer diagnosis, patients appear to be quite willing to accept chemotherapy's side effects in an attempt to control the malignancy. In a study of 100 patients with cancer, Slevin reported the differences between patients' attitudes toward either mild or intensive chemotherapy (3). This information was compared to a similar survey of doctors, nurses, and a control group matched to the patients for age, sex, and occupation. Study participants were asked to consider various probabilities of cure, prolongation of life, and relief of symptoms necessary for them to accept toxicities associated with mild and aggressive treatments. Patients with cancer were more likely than the other groups to accept intensive and toxic treatments for an extremely small probability of cure, prolongation of life, or symptom relief. For example, 53% of patients with cancer would undergo a very toxic chemotherapeutic regimens for a 1% chance of cure, and 42% would accept the same regimen for a 3-month prolongation of life. In contrast, only 20% of the matched control subjects would accept the treatment for a 1% chance of cure, and the same percentage would accept it for a 3-month prolongation of life. The respective endorsement by medical oncologists was only 10% for each question. The control group was also less likely to accept the treatment-related side effects, and wanted more potential benefits for any particular risk. Medical oncologists were more likely to accept aggressive treatments than general practitioners. Oncology nurses' scores fell between those of the generalists and the control group. Radiation oncologists were the least likely of any group to accept treatment. After 3 months of actual treatment, the same questionnaire was readministered to patients. Their responses were essentially unchanged. This important study indicates that individuals' attitudes change dramatically when they actually receive the diagnosis of cancer; when the situation is real, rather than hypothetical, more risks are taken. Patients younger than 40 years of age are even more likely to undergo chemotherapy for extremely little predicted chance of symptomatic or longevity benefit (4). These studies bring to mind the Siberian gulag-inspired observation of Alexander Solzhenitsyn in *A Day in the Life of Ivan Denisovich*: "A warm man can never understand a cold one."

CHEMOTHERAPY RESPONSIVENESS OF MALIGNANCIES

The likelihood of palliative chemotherapy benefit varies among cancer types. Malignancies with moderate to high sensitivity to

TABLE 50.1

METASTATIC AND INCURABLE CANCERS WITH MODERATE TO HIGH RESPONSE RATE

Bladder cancer
Breast cancer
Cervical/endometrial cancer
Chronic lymphocytic leukemia
Chronic myelogenous leukemia
Colon cancer
Esophageal cancer
Head and neck cancer
Multiple myeloma
Low-grade non-Hodgkin's lymphoma (most subtypes)
Ovarian cancer
Prostate cancer (hormone therapy)
Small cell lung cancer

chemotherapy are listed in Table 50.1. Anticipated chemotherapy response rates are in the 30 to 80% range. The primary goal of chemotherapy for these incurable, locally advanced or metastatic cancers is to achieve a partial or complete tumor response and to prolong progression-free and overall survival.

Metastatic or locally advanced cancers that have low expected response rates to chemotherapy are listed in Table 50.2. Partial responses to chemotherapy of less than 25%, usually of short duration, have been reported for these malignancies. Complete responses are extremely rare. The oncologist can recommend chemotherapy of limited proven benefit, investigational treatments, or nonchemotherapeutic palliative supportive care as reasonable alternatives for patients with these malignancies. Most cancer specialists have anecdotal experience of an occasional patient's unexpected excellent response in these chemotherapy-resistant cancers. One is cautioned not to base treatment of the average patient on the anecdotal (and at times inexplicable or coincidental) outcome of an individual patient.

Some chemotherapeutic agents have received U.S. Food and Drug Administration (FDA) approval primarily because they have improved QOL. A number of treatment studies report decreased pain, or other symptomatic improvement, induced

TABLE 50.2

INCURABLE CANCERS WITH LOW RESPONSE RATES TO CHEMOTHERAPY

Adrenal carcinoma
Adult sarcomas
Almost all malignancies in patients with poor performance status (Eastern Cooperative Oncology Group 3 or 4)—see text
Carcinoid tumor
Gastric cancer
Hepatoma/biliary cancers
Kidney cancer
Melanoma
Mesothelioma
Most previously treated cancers
Non–small cell lung cancer
Prostate cancer (chemotherapy)
Thyroid cancer

by chemotherapy, despite little or no objective tumor response. Hypotheses to explain this phenomenon include alteration in the local milieu of the neoplasm and inhibition of production of circulating cytokines responsible for many adverse symptoms associated with malignancies (5,6). Changes in growth factor production could result in tumor growth inhibition, as opposed to tumor shrinkage. Decreased inflammatory responses induced by many chemotherapeutic drugs or antikinins have led to their widespread use in rheumatologic diseases. Similar local environment alterations may occur at tumor sites with a decrease in tumor-associated symptoms, but without necessarily influencing tumor size.

THE PHYSICIAN'S IMPACT ON TREATMENT CHOICES

The physician has considerable influence in the patient's decision about starting or continuing chemotherapy. Although most of adult patients with cancer in one report ($N = 439$) wanted "all" information to be given, only 69% wanted to participate in the therapeutic decision-making. Twenty-five percent wanted the physician to make all of the decisions. This latter group consisted of predominantly older and sicker men (7). Although patients tend to accept their physicians' advice, this is not universal. A better-informed and educated patient, or a patient who believes that his physician is ambivalent about a recommendation, is more likely to decide independently (8).

Oncologists should not feel obligated to offer chemotherapy to every patient with malignancy. A group of patients for whom the predicted toxicity of treatment should preclude consideration of chemotherapy can be defined (see the section Prognostic Factors). Other patients may fall into a gray zone in which the benefit to toxicity ratio of treatment is less clear.

The practice of giving subtherapeutic doses of chemotherapy primarily to prevent patients from believing their cases are hopeless is strongly discouraged. This is more likely to reflect the physician's discomfort in dealing with a terminally ill patient than it is to address the patient's psychological needs. A more compassionate and an ethical approach is to review the medical situation with the patient and family, and to provide them with an informed assessment of possible treatment choices. Usually, this will include nonchemotherapy palliative care. This is especially true near the end of life. Patient and family desires for open communication and participation in decision making, which may be tempered by cultural differences, must be considered in these discussions.

Investigational studies of newer chemotherapy or palliative treatments are considerations when no proven beneficial anticancer treatment exists. The patient and family should understand that the benefit of investigational treatment is unproved; it may cause more harm than good. Patients and families may mistakenly believe that "no chemotherapy" means "no need for the physician to follow up and treat the patient" or "nothing more can be done." Unfortunately, some medical oncologists share that mistaken belief. Palliative care should be offered as a positive intervention, rather than just the absence of chemotherapy. Future visits should be scheduled with the physician who is supervising the patient's care. Visits should be at intervals that meet the physical and psychological needs of the patient and family. Even when it seems likely that the patient will be too sick to keep any more appointments, they should be scheduled nonetheless. Such scheduling provides a message of ongoing concern for the welfare of the patient and caregivers.

DISCUSSING PALLIATIVE CHEMOTHERAPY WITH PATIENTS

Patients and families often request statistics regarding the likelihood of tumor response, expected duration of response, possible treatment-related toxicities, and average survival prolongation that may occur with chemotherapy. This information may have significant impact on the decision to accept a recommended trial of chemotherapy. In addition to giving an honest reply, the physician should respond to these inquiries by trying to learn if there are specific factors leading to the question. What questions and decisions need to be addressed in the patient's or family's lives? Is there a contemplated retirement, a reunion, a special upcoming event, or significant unfinished business that must be completed? Are there fears about dying, or spiritual issues that need interventions from the physician or other supportive caregivers?

Patients and families often misconstrue a survival estimate on the basis of published or personal experiences as a precise number to live or die by. For example, a physician's statement that the median survival is 6 months is frequently misunderstood by the patient and family to mean that the patient has 6 months to live. Similarly, an expected "20% response rate to treatment" for a published cohort of patients may be misconstrued by the patient to mean that he specifically has a 20% chance of responding to the same treatment. The patient must be informed that statistics refer to groups of patients and not individuals. Oftentimes, patients or their families insist on a numeric answer concerning therapeutic efficacy or expected longevity. They may honestly be informed with such phrases as, "I expect the time would more likely be measured in weeks than in months," or "There is a reported response rate of 60%, which lasts on average for 4 months." This is an opportunity to discuss possible scenarios and alternatives to the question, "What if a response does not occur?" Although these replies are not very precise—indeed, it is very difficult for a reply to these questions to be both honest and precise—they at least give the patients information to correct gross misconceptions about their prognoses. It is possible to have these difficult discussions and still impart hope for comfort, maintenance of functionality for as long as possible, and finally, a death without uncontrolled pain or loss of dignity.

Patients often fear becoming a burden to their loved ones. It is unwise to deny the possibility that the patient will become a burden, for it is true. But the patient may be reminded that many we have loved most in our lives, such as children and parents, have been burdens to us from time to time. Every person, at one time or another in his life is *useless*. But no person is ever *worthless*. The family needs the opportunity to show its love by bearing this burden, and the patient wrongs them not to allow this opportunity. There is truth in the proverb "Even more than the calf wants to suck, the cow wants to suckle." Also important is the reassurance that the physician will continue to care for the patient and family, even if chemotherapy is no longer used.

When patients and their families are provided with the best possible prognostic information, decisions frequently differ from those made when less information is imparted. Patients with metastatic colon and lung cancer who believed that they had a significant chance of dying within 6 months were less likely to choose a possible life-extending therapy over comfort care (9). When informed that the likelihood of 6-month survival was 90, 75, 50, 25, or 10%, the likelihood that the patient would choose a life-extending therapy was decreased to 51, 29, 29, 31, and 21%, respectively. In this study, patients, as compared to their physicians, more commonly overestimated their chance of surviving 6 months. For example, whereas 50% of physicians believed that a patient group would have a 6-month survival, only 12.5% of patient members of that group thought that they would survive less than 6 months. Physician estimates of prognosis were more accurate than the patient's own estimates, as evidenced by the fact that only 45% of the patient group was alive at 6 months. If chemotherapy is chosen by mutual agreement between the patient and physician, their attitude should be that all that is necessary will be done to assure that the particular patient will benefit from the treatment, even if the response rate is reported to be relatively low. This optimistic approach after a realistic discussion is appropriate and of great psychological benefit to the patient and the family, as well as the physician and other members of the health care team.

PROGNOSTIC FACTORS

A composite of patient and disease-related factors will help determine if chemotherapy is a reasonable treatment option. Probably the single most important factor (other than tumor type) that determines possible benefit-to-toxicity ratio of chemotherapy is the performance status (PS) or activity level of the patient. Two measures used to quantify this are the Eastern Cooperative Oncology Group (ECOG) and Karnofsky scales (Table 50.3). Because the ECOG scale offers the rater only five choices, although the Karnofsky scale offers ten (ignoring the bizarre inclusion of 0% = dead on a performance scale), it is not surprising that there is less interobserver variability with use of the ECOG scale (10). Moreover, at least in the case of lung cancer, the ECOG scale has a somewhat better prognostic capability (11). Regardless of the cause of debility (malignancy or other comorbid medical illness), a severely weakened patient with a restricted PS (ECOG 3 or 4; Karnofsky<50%) is more likely to experience excessive toxicities from chemotherapy than a beneficial response. It is worth emphasizing, however, that the data correlating benefit of chemotherapy and PS derive mostly from studies of *cytotoxic* chemotherapy. As more targeted (and therefore less toxic) therapies are developed, the range of PS values for which chemotherapy will prove reasonable will doubtless expand.

The sites of metastatic spread may allow better predictions of the potential initial response to chemotherapy as well as overall prognosis. For example, breast cancer metastatic to the skin, bone, and lymph nodes is usually more responsive to chemotherapy than are liver or pulmonary lymphangitic metastases. Chemotherapy "sanctuary sites," such as the brain and other central nervous system structures, are usually least responsive to systemic cytotoxic treatments.

Numerous other prognostic features exist for specific malignancies. Data are increasingly available to support genetic aberrations, biochemical markers, and even psychometric assessments as predictive of short- and long-term prognosis for malignancies, as well as the likelihood of response to chemotherapy (12). Patients whose cancers are refractory to ongoing chemotherapy are less likely to respond to second or subsequent chemotherapy treatments. Similarly, cancers that have recurred within 6 months of cessation of chemotherapy are less likely to respond to retreatment with the same chemotherapy than are those that recur after a longer disease-free period. Absent routinely curative therapies, however, prognostication must remain, at best, predictive rather than prophetic (13).

IS AGE AN INDEPENDENT PROGNOSTIC FACTOR?

Low PS is clearly a risk factor for poor outcome of cancer chemotherapy, and PS is at least somewhat related to age.

TABLE 50.3

EASTERN COOPERATIVE ONCOLOGY GROUP AND KARNOFSKY PERFORMANCE STATUS SCALES

Eastern Cooperative Oncology Group	Karnofsky scale
0: Fully active, able to carry on all predisease performance without restriction	100%: normal, no complaints, no evidence of disease
1: Restricted in physically strenuous activity but ambulatory and able to carry out work of a light or sedentary nature, that is, light housework, office work	90%: able to carry on normal activity; minor signs or symptoms of disease 80%: normal activity with effort; some signs or symptoms of disease
2: Ambulatory and capable of all self-care but unable to carry out any work activities; up and about more than 50% of waking hours	70%: cares for self; unable to carry on normal activity or to do active work 60%: requires occasional assistance, but is mostly able to care for himself
3: Capable of only limited self-care, confined to bed or chair more than 50% of waking hours	50%: requires considerable assistance and frequent medical care 40%: disabled, requires special care and assistance
4: Completely disabled, cannot carry on any self-care; totally confined to bed or chair	30%: severely disabled, hospitalization indicated; death not imminent 20%: very sick, hospitalization necessary, active supportive treatment necessary 10%: moribund, fatal processes, progressing rapidly 0%: dead

However, the impact of age *per se* on the outcome of chemotherapy is far less clear.

We do know that elderly patients are less likely to be offered chemotherapy than younger patients. For example, a report based on the Surveillance, Epidemiology, and End Results (SEER)-Medicare database showed that women over 80 years old were less likely to receive adjuvant chemotherapy for stage II ovarian cancer than women aged 65 to 69. Survival was better in women receiving chemotherapy. Controlling for other factors, mortality was not associated with increasing age (14). Similarly, a study of women over 50 years old who were eligible for adjuvant chemotherapy of breast cancer by consensus guidelines showed that increasing age was associated strongly with a decreasing likelihood of receiving a recommendation in favor of chemotherapy. This study was conducted at a tertiary referral center, the kind of facility seldom criticized as being overly timid in its treatment. Patient age correlated with treatment recommendation even when the data were adjusted for comorbidity scores. Moreover, this reduced recommendation of chemotherapy was not a reflection of patient preference; the authors found that patient acceptance of chemotherapy did not vary with age (15).

Reduced use of chemotherapy for elderly patients is not limited to the adjuvant setting, and not limited to the treatment of poorly responsive tumors. A retrospective study of patients with limited stage small cell lung cancer revealed that patient age, quite independent of PS and comorbidity score, correlated with intensity of treatment. But multivariate analysis showed no significant association of age or comorbidity score with treatment response and survival (16).

The astute reader will note that these data concerning chemotherapy and the elderly derive from retrospective studies. If, as noted in the preceding text, the elderly are less likely than the young to be offered chemotherapy, then the outcome information really pertains to that particular subset of the elderly population selected for treatment, rather than to elderly patients in general. It is quite possible that oncologists are selecting elderly patients for chemotherapy on clinical grounds not being recognized in the retrospective studies.

QUALITY OF LIFE

QOL measurements were infrequently recorded or reported during the first four decades of modern chemotherapy trials. QOL measurements refer to a quantitative evaluation of numerous qualitative parameters that are believed to be core values in day-to-day enjoyment of life. A frequently cited definition of QOL is that of the World Health Organization: "QOL is defined as an individual's perception of their position in life in the context of the culture and value systems in which they live and in relation to their goals, expectations, standards, and concerns. It is a broad ranging concept affected in a complex way by the person's physical health, psychological state, level of independence, social relationships, and their relationship to salient features of their environment." Health-related QOL is a subset of specific QOL end points relating to the health of an individual.

As stated previously, QOL assessments are increasingly reported as independently assessed variables in clinical trials. Multiple QOL scales of varying complexity have been developed (17). Examples of parameters measured include pain and pain relief, fatigue, malaise, psychologic distress, nausea and vomiting, physical functioning, treatment-related symptoms and toxic effects, body image, sexual functioning, memory, concentration, economic impact of the disease, and global QOL (18). These QOL inventories may be used in conjunction with the more commonly used measurements of chemotherapy-induced toxicities to better assess overall patient tolerance to the drug regimen administered.

A patient's QOL is a subjective parameter that can be misjudged by the health care provider and a patient-appointed surrogate (19). Even worse, a patient's low QOL as assessed by others, or even by himself, may be mistaken for a life not worth living. Malignancy- or treatment-induced debilities may be better tolerated by individuals with previous disabilities. Younger, more active patients may have significant difficulties with a functional compromise. The loss of hair for one patient may be more psychologically debilitating than a decrease in mobility for another. Each patient and situation is unique, and QOL is an experience that can change dramatically over time.

At times, logistic QOL issues, as opposed to health-related QOL issues, become quite important in the patient's decision to accept or reject a chemotherapeutic regimens. Length of treatment, impact on family life, or travel distance to the treatment center may weigh more heavily on decisions for chemotherapy than do actual drug-related toxicities. With the development of more effective antinausea therapies, distress due to nausea and vomiting have been replaced by distress over fatigue and psychosocial impact of cancer as a chief worry of cancer patients (20). More research is required to define these complex QOL issues accurately. By now, oncologists and palliative care specialists know that they cannot measure pain by looking at a patient; pain is a subjective phenomenon. Similarly, the health care team must remember that QOL too is a subjective phenomenon, and cannot be measured except by patient report.

An assumption by the health care team that a marked improvement in QOL with a slight decrease in overall survival would be in the best interest of the patient with cancer may not be shared by the patient. In a study of health values of the seriously ill, patients and their self-designated medical decision-making surrogates were independently interviewed (19). The patients had a variety of chronic debilitating diseases with an anticipated median 6-month mortality rate of 50%. All patients had significant disease-related debility. Patients were evaluated for time trade-off. They were asked the hypothetical question, "If you could live one year at your current level of function and health, how much time would you trade for a shorter survival in excellent health?" Approximately, one third of the patients would not give up any time at their present level of debility in exchange for even 1 week less of life but in excellent health. At the other extreme, 9% preferred living 2 weeks or less in excellent health to 1 year in their current state of health. Only 2% of patients described their current health as no better than death. On average, only 3.2 months would be returned for the prospect of an absolutely healthy life instead of 1 year at the patient's current state of disability. In general, patients rated their current state of health as better than did their designated surrogates. If surrogates were to make decisions for patients, those surrogates were more likely to give up survival time for improved health. This study emphasizes that others cannot predict patients' health values accurately, even those closest to them emotionally. In general, patients accept making great sacrifices to live the maximum amount of time. When sequential interviews with the same patient were possible, the value of being alive, even in poor health, increased with time. That is, the longer the patient survived, the less likely he was to trade time alive for better health.

PALLIATIVE CHEMOTHERAPY—SPECIFIC EXAMPLES

It would be a fool's errand to include in this chapter an extensive discussion of the chemotherapy of cancers for which the benefit of chemotherapy is indisputable. There is no lack of textbooks and journals to guide the clinician treating good PS patients with such diagnoses as lymphoma, breast cancer, small cell lung cancer, and myeloma. Rather, the discussion in the following text will focus on those malignancies for which the benefit of chemotherapy is often not obvious. By definition, the benefit of the therapies discussed will be modest, but not entirely nugatory.

Pancreatic Cancer

Pancreatic cancer holds a place of pride in this discussion, if one may so anthropomorphize a rapidly progressive relentless cancer, because it was the first malignancy for which the FDA approved a treatment on the basis of improved QOL rather than response rate or prolonged survival. In 1985, a three-way randomized trial had proved that neither bolus 5-fluorouracil (5-FU) plus doxorubicin nor that combination plus mitomycin (MMC) was better than bolus 5-FU alone in the treatment of metastatic pancreas cancer (21). For 12 years after that report, bolus 5-FU remained the standard therapy, although there was no evidence that it prolonged survival or even improved QOL. Then, a prospectively randomized study comparing gemcitabine to 5-FU showed an improved QOL with gemcitabine, although there was no difference in survival between the two treatments (22). The FDA approved gemcitabine hydrochloride for the palliative treatment of pancreatic cancer in May 1996, thereby ushering in a new era in medical oncology. Gemcitabine hydrochloride was the first chemotherapy drug cleared for marketing by the FDA based on a unique clinical end point assessing the effect of the drug on measured disease-related symptoms; that end point is called *clinical benefit response*. No longer would response rate or survival be the only criteria of approval for chemotherapy; the importance of QOL as a legitimate end point in cancer chemotherapy could no longer be ignored.

Of course, it is nearly miraculous that bolus 5-FU ever helps treat *any* cancer. It is an S-phase specific antimetabolite with a remarkably short half-life. Since only a small percentage of cancer cells are in S-phase at any particular moment, the potential target of this chemotherapy is quite limited. Recent studies reflect the recognition of this fact, and use 5-FU by continuous infusion, or replace it altogether with a congener of much longer half-life (23). It is conceivable, therefore, that 5-FU might have some usefulness in treating pancreatic cancer if it were given by prolonged infusion. This concept was tested in a prospectively randomized trial comparing protracted venous infusion of (PVI) of 5-FU with PVI plus MMC (24). Neither treatment yielded a high response rate, although the combination therapy was statistically superior in response rate to the single agent. The monotherapy evoked a meager 8.4% response rate, and the combination was a little better at 17.6%. The overall survival did not differ significantly between the two groups. Global QOL improved significantly after 24 weeks of treatment compared with baseline for patients receiving 5-FU plus MMC, although there was no statistically significant difference in QOL between arms. How one is to interpret the researchers' report of an improved average QOL appearing only after nearly half of the cohort of treated patients have died remains problematic.

Prostate Cancer

Hormone-refractory metastatic prostate cancer serves as an example of some of the difficulties in clinical decision making when chemotherapy is given for palliation of symptoms. Prostate cancer is usually a disease of older men, many of whom have significant comorbidities. Assessing treatment response is often difficult, because most patients have metastases primarily in bone, a site in which a decrease in tumor size is difficult to prove. Drop in serum prostate specific antigen (PSA) level is often used as a substitute for measurable reduction in tumor size. Reductions of more than 50% in PSA levels correlate with improved survival and symptom control; smaller declines have not been shown to be clinically meaningful (25).

Despite these difficulties, well-designed phase III studies have shown a benefit of palliative chemotherapy in patients with hormone-refractory prostate cancer. Glucocorticoids used as a single agent after failure of androgen-ablative therapy are somewhat useful (26,27). Mitoxantrone hydrochloride plus hydrocortisone or prednisone yielded modest improvements in QOL measurements compared to glucocorticoid alone (28,29). On the other hand, a chemically similar drug, the anthracycline epirubicin, did not improve QOL in patients with hormone-refractory prostate cancer, even when combined with medroxyprogesterone (30). Suramin, with or without hydrocortisone, demonstrated pain improvement and delay in disease progression, but with no benefit in overall QOL (31). Those patients receiving the lowest dose of suramin enjoyed a better QOL than did those on higher doses, but this may well be a sign of the toxicity of the higher doses, rather than the palliative benefit of the lower dose (32).

The combination of mitoxantrone plus prednisone did not remain the standard of care very long. A prospectively randomized study compared it to the combination of docetaxel and prednisone (33). The latter not only improved QOL more than did the mitoxantrone plus prednisone combination. Docetaxel plus prednisone also prolonged survival more than the older combination. Many consider it the current standard of care. An attempt to improve on that combination by combining docetaxel with estramustine improved survival by an average of about 2 months compared with mitoxantrone plus prednisone, but did so at the cost of an increased rate of adverse events (34).

Colon Cancer

Treatment standards are rapidly evolving for patients with metastatic and recurrent colon cancer. Until recently, the combination of bolus or brief infusion 5-FU plus leucovorin (5-FU/LVR) was the standard treatment for this disease. But as the motto of the nursing journal declares, "Times change, and we must change with them."

The improvement in treatment of colon cancer came in logical steps. First, it was demonstrated that adding irinotecan to the old standard bolus 5-FU/LVR improved the outcome. A randomized trial in previously untreated patients compared irinotecan alone to 5-FU/LVR and to the combination of all

three agents. The triple-agent therapy significantly improved both progression-free and overall survival, without adversely affecting overall QOL (35). This is known as the IFL, or Saltz, regimen (Table 50.4).

Subsequent studies retained the clearly useful irinotecan, but delivered the 5-fluorouracil as a continuous infusion rather than a bolus (36). The irinotecan-containing treatment yielded higher response rates, longer survival, and better QOL than the infusional 5-FU/LVR alone. This regimen, which has two minor dose variations, is known as the Douillard regimen (after its first author, a Frenchman) or the AIO regimen (after the German group that developed the infusional schedule, the Arbeitsgemeinschaft Internische Onkologie). A variation of this regimen using a longer infusion of 5-FU is known as FOLFIRI (37) (Table 50.4). Although these are important, if not dispositive, advantages of infusional therapy, this treatment has the disadvantage of the inconvenience and complications associated with ambulatory pump therapies.

Combining oxaliplatin with infusional 5-FU/LVR gives us the regimen known as FOLFOX. There are several variations of the regimen, such as FOLFOX 4 and FOLFOX6, which differ by the dose and schedule of the components (Table 50.4). FOLFOX4 significantly improved the response rate and relapse-free survival rate as compared with infusional 5-FU/LVR alone (38). However, the overall survival, which can be greatly affected by subsequent therapies, did not differ between these two treatments. The QOL was not impaired by the more effective therapy, despite its greater rate of diarrhea and neuropathy.

After both FOLFOX and FOLFIRI were shown to be active treatments in colon cancer, the logical next step was to compare the two regimens head-to-head. In the trial comparing FOLFOX6 to FOLFIRI, patients randomized to one treatment would receive the other upon disease progression (39). There was no significant difference between the two arms in response rate, time to first progression, or overall survival. The side effect profile of the two regimens differed, but no specific QOL assessment was done.

One of the major detractions, of course, of both FOLFOX and FOLFIRI is the need for the patient to have secure venous access and to wear a portable infusion pump. Capecitabine, an orally administered fluoropyrimidine with a half-life

TABLE 50.4

DRUG COMBINATIONS FOR TREATMENT OF COLON CANCER

AIO regimen (folic acid, 5-FU, irinotecan)	Irinotecan (80 mg/m^2) as a 30-min infusion d 1; leucovorin (500 mg/m^2) as a 2-h infusion d 1; followed by 5-FU (2–2.3 g/m^2) intravenous bolus through ambulatory pump over 24 h weekly × 6 repeated every 8 wk.
Douillard regimen (folic acid, 5-FU, irinotecan)	Irinotecan (180 mg/m^2) as a 2-h infusion d 1; leucovorin (200 mg/m^2) as a 2-h infusion d 1 and 2; followed by a loading dose of 5-FU (400 mg/m^2) IV bolus, then 5-FU (600 mg/m^2) through ambulatory pump over 22 h d 1 and 2 every 2 wk.
FOLFOX4 regimen (oxaliplatin, leucovorin, 5-FU)	Oxaliplatin (85 mg/m^2) as a 2-h infusion d 1; leucovorin (200 mg/m^2) as a 2-h infusion d 1 and 2; followed by a loading dose of 5-FU (400 mg/m^2) IV bolus, then 5-FU (600 mg/m^2) through ambulatory pump over 22 h d 1 and 2 every 2 wk.
FOLFOX6 regimen (oxaliplatin, leucovorin, 5-FU)	Oxaliplatin (85–100 mg/m^2) as a 2-h infusion d 1; leucovorin (400 mg/m^2) as a 2-h infusion d 1; followed by a loading dose of 5-FU (400 mg/m^2) IV bolus on d 1, then 5-FU (2400–3000 mg/m^2) through ambulatory pump over 46 h every 2 wk.
FOLFIRI regimen (folic acid, 5-FU, irinotecan):	Irinotecan (180 mg/m^2) as a 2-h infusion d 1; leucovorin (400 mg/m^2) as a 2-h infusion d 1; followed by a loading dose of 5-FU (400 mg/m^2) IV bolus on d 1, then 5-FU (2400–3000 mg/m^2) through ambulatory pump over 46 h every 2 wk.
IFL (or Saltz) regimen (irinotecan, 5-FU, leucovorin)	Irinotecan (125 mg/m^2), 5-FU (500 mg/m^2) IV bolus, and leucovorin (20 mg/m^2) IV bolus weekly for 4 out of 6 wk.

IV, intravenous.

considerably longer than that of 5-FU, provides a higher response rate with a more favorable toxicity profile than does bolus 5-FU plus leucovorin (40). Naturally, capecitabine is being tested as a substitute for 5-FU/LVR in both the FOLFOX and FOLFIRI regimens.

A different paradigm in the palliative treatment of colorectal cancer is the use of bevacizumab, a monoclonal antibody directed against vascular endothelial growth factor (VEGF). Because its side effect profile is quite distinct from that of cytotoxic chemotherapy, it makes a natural addition to the chemotherapies mentioned in the preceding text. When combined with bolus 5-FU/LVR, it improves response rate, progression-free survival, and overall survival (41). Its use in combination with infusional 5-FU and with oxaliplatin and irinotecan is the subject of ongoing study.

Another monoclonal antibody, cetuximab, targets the receptor for which VEGF is the ligand. It has been studied and FDA approved for use in irinotecan-refractory patients. Curiously, the antibody was more effective when combined with irinotecan, although all the subjects in the study had previously failed on irinotecan (42). The combination significantly prolonged progression-free survival, but QOL was not specifically measured. An acne-like rash is a frequent side effect of this therapy.

Non–Small Cell Lung Cancer

The old era of grim pessimism in the palliative chemotherapy of non–small cell lung cancer (NSCLC) has yielded to a new era of grim optimism. In other words, there has been clear progress in the chemotherapy of America's number one cancer killer, but it has been achingly slow.

There is now enough evidence that chemotherapy doublets can reasonably be offered to most good PS patients with advanced NSCLC. First-line treatment with gemcitabine plus cisplatin is better than cisplatin alone in regards to response rate, progression-free survival, and overall survival (43). The pivotal trial comparing the two approaches found no difference in QOL between the two arms. Another phase III study compared gemcitabine-cisplatin to etoposide-cisplatin. Gemcitabine-cisplatin provided a significantly higher response rate and a delay in disease progression without impairing QOL in patients with advanced NSCLC (44).

Gemcitabine-cisplatin is certainly not the only doublet to have shown usefulness in the palliative chemotherapy of NSCLC. In general, the doublets based on carboplatin or cisplatin are reasonable alternatives. These include cisplatin plus vinorelbine, cisplatin plus paclitaxel, cisplatin plus docetaxel, carboplatin plus paclitaxel, and the triplet combination of cisplatin plus vinblastine plus MMC (45). For patients who are not candidates for platinum-based therapies, the combination of paclitaxel and gemcitabine is a reasonable alternative. A trial comparing this combination to paclitaxel plus carboplatin found little difference between the two (46).

The median age of advanced NSCLC patients is 68 years and rising. How best to treat them is not clear. On the one hand, a retrospective review showed that response rate, toxicity, and survival in fit, elderly NSCLC patients receiving platinum-based treatment was similar to that of younger patients. On the other hand, patients 70 years old or older have more comorbidities and can expect more leukopenia and neuropsychiatric toxicity from the chemotherapy. For elderly patients, or patients with PS2, treatment with single-agent chemotherapy is probably preferable (45).

Two cytotoxic drugs have shown benefit for second-line chemotherapy of NSCLC. Despite its low response rate, docetaxel significantly prolongs survival in this cohort of patients more than best supportive care (BSC) (47). Moreover, use of the chemotherapy is associated with improvement in several measurements of QOL (48). More recently, pemetrexed has joined docetaxel in being FDA approved for use as a second-line agent in NSCLC. When compared to docetaxel, it was found to have clinically equivalent efficacy. However, the toxicity of pemetrexed was substantially less than that of the taxane, making it a more attractive choice.

A new class of drugs has joined the classical chemotherapy agents for NSCLC. This class is the tyrosine kinase inhibitors (TKIs). Only two, gefitinib (Iressa) and erlotinib (Tarceva), are available for NSCLC so far, but there will surely be more in the future. All anticancer drugs try to exploit some difference between normal and malignant cells. Most cytotoxic agents exploit the fact that normal cells can recover from damage done by chemotherapy more quickly and completely than can malignant cells. Also, a higher proportion of cancer cells are somewhere in the cycle of cell proliferation than is true of most benign cells. In other words, cytotoxic agents try to take advantage of a *kinetic* difference between benign and malignant cells. The TKIs, in distinction, take advantage of the fact that they inhibit a vital process prevalent in many cancer cells, but far less often expressed in normal cells. The TKIs, then, target a *physiologic* distinction between normal and malignant cells.

Many malignant cells, including those of NSCLC, express an increased number or mutated form of the epidermal growth factor receptor (EGFR) (49). Because these receptors are members of the HER (human epidermal receptor) family, they are known as HER1/EGFR. The intracellular domain of this receptor is a tyrosine kinase. Phosphorylation of the tyrosine kinase triggers a signal cascade that eventuates in changed genome expression. Gefitinib and erlotinib bind to the tyrosine kinase domain at the ATP-binding site, thereby robbing the tyrosine kinase of its energy source.

The objective response rate to these drugs is low, but some of the well-documented responses have been nigh miraculous. Erlotinib's reported response rate is only 8% above that of placebo, not much different than that of gefitinib. Both agents have a favorable impact on symptoms, but erlotinib was also found to prolong survival of previously treated lung cancer patients, although gefitinib was not. There seems to be little reason to start a new patient on gefitinib. The main toxicity of erlotinib is rash and diarrhea. However, these are seldom severe enough to cause discontinuation of therapy. Curiously, erlotinib does not enhance the activity of cisplatin-gemcitabine chemotherapy, but it does have beneficial activity as a single agent in previously treated lung cancer (50).

Breast Cancer

In the initial treatment of locally advanced or metastatic breast cancer, the relatively high response rate and beneficial impact on overall survival leave little doubt as to the treatment's palliative benefit. Less obvious, however, are the benefits of such therapies when used after first-line therapies fail.

Because their toxicity is generally low and thereby their therapeutic index is high, it is not surprising that second-line hormonal therapy can improve QOL in breast cancer patients. A study of 177 women whose breast cancer progressed on tamoxifen citrate found that responses to subsequent hormonal therapy correlated well with sustained or improved QOL (51).

The data concerning the palliative benefit of chemotherapy for breast cancer progressing after initial chemotherapy are less compelling. In 1999, Campora et al. noted that the median survival for metastatic breast cancer had not varied for 50 years, remaining in the range of 2.0 to 3.5 years (52). In their retrospective analysis of treatments in the pretaxane era, the likelihood of benefit of chemotherapy after failure of first-line anthracycline-containing therapy was never more than 15%.

The availability of the taxanes has changed the approach to patients with recurrent breast cancer refractory to anthracycline chemotherapy. Docetaxel has been compared to MMC plus vinblastine sulfate; it produces a longer time to progression, greater overall survival, and a similar impact on QOL (53). Studies comparing its palliative benefits to those of vinorelbine tartrate give mixed results. One study found that both taxanes, paclitaxel and docetaxel, were similar in benefit to vinorelbine tartrate, with the latter being less expensive (54). Another study found that docetaxel was better than paclitaxel and vinorelbine tartrate, both in alleviation of malignancy-related symptoms and cost-effectiveness (55).

Several approaches to overcome the limitations of palliative chemotherapy for recurrent breast cancer have been tried. The first approach is to use single agents sequentially rather than in combination. In a randomized trial, patients treated with single-agent epirubicin hydrochloride followed by single-agent MMC had similar survival but less treatment-related toxicity and better QOL, as compared with those treated with cyclophosphamide plus epirubicin hydrochloride plus fluorouracil followed by the combination of MMC plus vinblastine sulfate (56).

Another way to reduce treatment toxicity is to discontinue treatment after remission is achieved. This method seems less promising than the use of sequential single agents. A prospective randomized trial compared treating women with recurrent breast cancer with cyclophosphamide plus methotrexate plus 5-FU plus prednisone continuously versus the same drugs given for three cycles and then repeated for another three cycles on evidence of disease progression (57). QOL improved for both groups during the initial three cycles of chemotherapy; after that, intermittent therapy was associated with worse scores for physical well-being, mood, appetite, and QOL.

Finally, a herald of future therapies is the use of trastuzumab, a monoclonal antibody approved to treat metastatic breast cancer. It is targeted against HER2, a marker that is up regulated in a minority of cases of breast cancer. Addition of trastuzumab to the chemotherapy for women whose tumors overexpress HER2 yields a significant survival advantage. Moreover, its use improves QOL scores (58).

Radioimmunotherapy of Lymphoma

Lymphomas are usually sensitive to both chemotherapy and radiation therapy. Unfortunately, despite the high initial response rate, many patients relapse and eventually become refractory to further chemotherapy. Radioimmunotherapy is a novel way of treating these patients (59). It has been so successful in heavily pretreated patients, that it is being investigated as an initial therapy.

The target of radioimmunotherapy is the CD20 antigen, present on the surface of more than 90% of B-cell non-Hodgkin's lymphoma. The antigen is not expressed on hematopoietic stem cells, plasma cells, or nonhematopoietic tissues. Monoclonal antibodies directed against CD20 have been developed, and their use without radioactive conjugates is now a standard part of the chemotherapy of lymphoma.

In radioimmunotherapy, a radioactive atom is conjugated to the monoclonal antibody. Two types of radioimmunotherapy of lymphoma are now available, using yttrium-90 (Zevalin) or iodine-131 (Bexxar). The monoclonal antibody moiety binds the drug to the surface of the lymphoma cell. In addition to the anticancer toxicity caused by the antibody itself, the radioactive element causes damage to the DNA of the malignant cell. Yttrium-90 is a pure beta emitter with a mean path length in tissue of 2.5 mm. Iodine-131 emits most of its energy as beta irradiation, and has a mean path length in tissue of 0.3 mm. Thus, these agents are able to deliver their radiation energy in a targeted fashion, substantially sparing normal tissue from their toxic effect. The drugs may suppress marrow and the immune system, but have little other subjective toxicity.

WHEN TO INITIATE PALLIATIVE CHEMOTHERAPY

When curative therapy is not a realistic goal, as is the case in most adult metastatic malignancies, then multiple factors must be weighed regarding the time to initiate systemic anticancer therapy. The goal of palliative chemotherapy must be to relieve or prevent tumor-induced symptoms and/or to prolong survival.

Because any symptom caused directly or indirectly by the neoplasm can potentially be ameliorated by an effective chemotherapeutic regimen, patients who are symptomatic from malignancy or are expected to become symptomatic soon should be considered for treatment. Chemotherapy as the sole treatment has been used effectively to palliate emergencies such as superior vena cava syndrome, epidural spinal cord compression, or airway obstruction due to chemosensitive tumors. When these emergencies occur in patients whose tumors are more resistant to chemotherapy, they are more appropriately managed with a local treatment such as radiotherapy or surgery.

A difficult choice is whether to delay noncurative chemotherapy for the asymptomatic patient with low volume of disease in nonvital areas, because some tumor types may display indolent growth. These patients may experience no signs or symptoms from their malignancy for prolonged periods of time. In these circumstances, especially for cancers with low expected response rates to chemotherapy, the benefit to toxicity ratio of therapy may be more heavily weighted toward the toxicity side. Forestalling initial cytotoxic treatment then becomes an attractive alternative. Treatment can be withheld with close monitoring of the patient and initiated once symptomatic progression is evident or anticipated to occur soon.

A primary concern for this "watch and wait" approach is that a patient can move from "too well to treat" to "too sick to treat" quickly and unexpectedly. This is especially problematic if the patient desires a trial of chemotherapy. Treatment could be withheld, and then unexpected severe problems may prevent the patient from receiving chemotherapy, thereby missing the elusive "window of opportunity." The possibility also exists that a malignancy may demonstrate a decreased response to treatment with increased tumor size. Delay of chemotherapy theoretically allows for the potential development of more chemotherapy-resistant cells.

Prospective trials for most types of incurable malignancies do not permit a definite recommendation regarding whether to initiate treatment at the time of diagnosis or "watch and wait" for the asymptomatic patient. A candid discussion of options is essential in making this decision. Some patients would be psychologically distressed with a delay of therapy. If there are objective parameters to follow for tumor response to treatment, two to three courses of treatment with reevaluation for response is a reasonable approach. Treatment could continue for regressive disease or be discontinued or changed for tumor progression. If toxicities from treatment are severe, attenuation, change, or cessation of treatment are alternatives to consider. The case of stable disease is more problematic. Slowly growing tumors refractory to chemotherapy may not demonstrate apparent growth until after many months of treatments. It may be impossible to judge if the cancer is just displaying a slow growth phase or if the treatment is keeping the disease "in check." This is especially true with the recently available TKIs. One must be cautious when attributing stable disease to chemotherapy "response," but clearly a cancer that is not growing or causing difficulties is better than one that is. If the treatment is not causing significant side effects, it would be reasonable to discuss with the patient the possibility of continuing the treatment until the time of disease progression versus discontinuing treatment and resuming it at the time of progression.

The decision to treat the asymptomatic patient becomes even more difficult if there is no disease that can be followed for response to treatment, and the response rate to chemotherapy is relatively low. Prospective follow-up studies from baseline can then only report on disease progression. A "watch and wait" policy for the patient without symptoms or followable disease, with reservation of treatment until the disease becomes measurable or symptomatic, is one option. The other choice is a finite number of chemotherapy cycles (4–8 months), unless previous clinical trials have determined optimal duration of treatment.

SUMMARY

The goal of therapy for patients with incurable cancer must be either prolongation of life or reduction of symptoms. Ideally, the goal should be both. Chemotherapy may be part of the overall palliative plan.

Chemotherapy has improved dramatically since the days of Sidney Farber (see the section Introduction—What is Palliative Chemotherapy?). It is likely to improve much more in coming years. The improved therapeutic index may come as a result of an increase in drug efficacy, or a decrease in drug toxicity. Targeted therapies hold out the promise of achieving both types of improvement. It is likely, therefore, that many patients who today are quite reasonably not offered chemotherapy as part of their palliative treatment will in the future be appropriate candidates for palliative chemotherapy.

Until that long-awaited halcyon day arrives, the oncologist—to say nothing of the patient and his family—must deal with the harsh reality of our pre-magic bullet era. Clearly, our being knowledgeable clinicians is necessary. Just as clearly, being knowledgeable is not sufficient for the task before us. As much as knowledge, we need wisdom. Oncologists must act with wisdom to identify which patient is likely to benefit from the marginally beneficial treatments in today's armamentarium. When appropriate, we must have the courage to truthfully inform the patient that, despite his anguished hopes, there is in fact no chemotherapy that will prolong his life or reduce his symptoms.

The etymology of the word "compassion" teaches us that its core meaning is "to suffer with." Perhaps that is why compassion is often the most difficult trait of all to bring to the encounter with the patient dying of cancer. In truth, it is the ultimate challenge of our calling, brought to bear even as the patient is facing the ultimate challenge of his life. We must have the compassion always to see our patient as a person, not a case. We must never abandon him, never shun him because he reminds us of our inadequacies. Even if—especially if—all our knowledge and experience are feckless against his intractable symptoms, we can and must provide the ministry of presence. Even as he is ceasing to be, we must perdure in being, and suffering, with him.

References

1. Kirkwood JM, Manola J, Ibrahim J, et al. A Pooled Analysis of Eastern Cooperative Oncology Group and intergroup trials of adjuvant high-dose interferon for melanoma. *Clin Cancer Res* 2004;10(5):1670–1677.

2. Cella D. What do global Quality-of-Life questions really measure? Insights from Hobday et al and the "Do Something" Rule. *J Clin Oncol* 2003; 21(16):3178–3179.

3. Slevin ML, Stubbs L, Plant HJ, et al. Attitudes to chemotherapy: comparing views of patients with cancer with those of doctors, nurses, and general public. *BMJ* 1990;300(6737):1458–1460.

4. Bremnes RM, Andersen K, Wist EA. Cancer patients, doctors and nurses vary in their willingness to undertake cancer chemotherapy. *Eur J Cancer* 1995;31A(12):1955–1959.

5. Korn EL, Arbuck SG, Pluda JM, et al. Clinical trial designs for cytostatic agents: are new approaches needed? *J Clin Oncol* 2001;19(1):265–272.

6. Miller KD, Sweeney CJ, Sledge GW Jr. Redefining the target: chemotherapeutics as antiangiogenics. *J Clin Oncol* 2001;19(4):1195–1206.

7. Blanchard CG, Labrecque MS, Ruckdeschel JC, et al. Information and decision-making preferences of hospitalized adult cancer patients. *Soc Sci Med* 1988;27(11):1139–1145.

8. Siminoff LA, Fetting JH. Factors affecting treatment decisions for a life-threatening illness: the case of medical treatment of breast cancer. *Soc Sci Med* 1991;32(7):813–818.

9. Weeks JC, Cook EF, O'Day SJ, et al. Relationship between cancer patients' predictions of prognosis and their treatment preferences. *JAMA* 1998;279(21):1709–1714.

10. Roila F, Lupattelli M, Sassi M, et al. Intra and interobserver variability in cancer patients' performance status assessed according to Karnofsky and ECOG scales. *Ann Oncol* 1991;2(6):437–439.

11. Buccheri G, Ferrigno D, Tamburini M. Karnofsky and ECOG performance status scoring in lung cancer: a prospective, longitudinal study of 536 patients from a single institution. *Eur J Cancer* 1996;32A(7):1135–1141.

12. Buccheri G, Ferrigno D. Prognostic factors. *Hematol Oncol Clin North Am* 2004;18(1):187–201.

13. Chevlen E. The limits of prognostication. *Duquesne Law Rev* 1996;35(1): 337–354.

14. Hershman D, Fleischauer AT, Jacobson JS, et al. Patterns and outcomes of chemotherapy for elderly patients with stage II ovarian cancer: a population-based study. *Gynecol Oncol* 2004;92(1):293–299.

15. DeMichele A, Putt M, Zhang Y, et al. Older age predicts a decline in adjuvant chemotherapy recommendations for patients with breast carcinoma: evidence from a tertiary care cohort of chemotherapy-eligible patients. *Cancer* 2003;97(9):2150–2159.

16. Ludbrook JJ, Truong PT, MacNeil MV, et al. Do age and comorbidity impact treatment allocation and outcomes in limited stage small-cell lung cancer? A community-based population analysis. *Int J Radiat Oncol Biol Phys* 2003;55(5):1321–1330.

17. Moinpour CM. Measuring quality of life: an emerging science. *Semin Oncol* 1994;21(5 Suppl 10):48–60.

18. Michael M, Tannock IF. Measuring health-related quality of life in clinical trials that evaluate the role of chemotherapy in cancer treatment. *CMAJ* 1998;158(13):1727–1734.

19. Tsevat J, Cook EF, Green ML, et al. Health values of the seriously ill. SUPPORT investigators. *Ann Intern Med* 1995;122(7):514–520.

20. Carelle N, Piotto E, Bellanger A, et al. Changing patient perceptions of the side effects of cancer chemotherapy. *Cancer* 2002;95(1):155–163.

21. Cullinan SA, Moertel CG, Fleming TR, et al. A comparison of three chemotherapeutic regimens in the treatment of advanced pancreatic and gastric carcinoma. Fluorouracil vs fluorouracil and doxorubicin vs fluorouracil, doxorubicin, and mitomycin. *JAMA* 1985;253(14):2061–2067.

22. Burris HA III, Moore MJ, Andersen J, et al. Improvements in survival and clinical benefit with gemcitabine as first-line therapy for patients with advanced pancreas cancer: a randomized trial. *J Clin Oncol* 1997;15(6): 2403–2413.

23. Schilsky RL. Pharmacology and clinical status of capecitabine. *Oncology (Huntingt)* 2000;14(9):1297–1306.

24. Maisey N, Chau I, Cunningham D, et al. Multicenter randomized phase III trial comparing protracted venous infusion (PVI) fluorouracil (5-FU) with PVI 5-FU plus mitomycin in inoperable pancreatic cancer. *J Clin Oncol* 2002;20(14):3130–3136.

25. Small EJ, McMillan A, Meyer M, et al. Serum prostate-specific antigen decline as a marker of clinical outcome in hormone-refractory prostate cancer patients: association with progression-free survival, pain end points, and survival. *J Clin Oncol* 2001;19(5):1304–1311.

26. Fossa SD, Slee PH, Brausi M, et al. Flutamide versus prednisone in patients with prostate cancer symptomatically progressing after androgen-ablative therapy: a phase III study of the European organization for research and treatment of cancer genitourinary group. *J Clin Oncol* 2001;19(1): 62–71.

27. Nishimura K, Nonomura N, Yasunaga Y, et al. Low doses of oral dexamethasone for hormone-refractory prostate carcinoma. *Cancer* 2000; 89(12):2570–2576.

28. Kantoff PW, Halabi S, Conaway M, et al. Hydrocortisone with or without mitoxantrone in men with hormone-refractory prostate cancer: results of the cancer and leukemia group B 9182 study. *J Clin Oncol* 1999; 17(8):2506–2513.

29. Tannock IF, Osoba D, Stockler MR, et al. Chemotherapy with mitoxantrone plus prednisone or prednisone alone for symptomatic hormone-resistant prostate cancer: a Canadian randomized trial with palliative end points. *J Clin Oncol* 1996;14(6):1756–1764.

30. van Andel G, Kurth KH, Rietbroek RL, et al. Quality of life assessment in patients with hormone-resistant prostate cancer treated with epirubicin or with epirubicin plus medroxy progesterone acetate - is it feasible? *Eur Urol* 2000;38(3):259–264.

31. Small EJ, Meyer M, Marshall ME, et al. Suramin therapy for patients with symptomatic hormone-refractory prostate cancer: results of a randomized phase III trial comparing suramin plus hydrocortisone to placebo plus hydrocortisone. *J Clin Oncol* 2000;18(7):1440–1450.

32. Ahles TA, Herndon JE, Small EJ, et al. Quality of life impact of three different doses of suramin in patients with metastatic hormone-refractory prostate carcinoma: results of Intergroup O159/Cancer and Leukemia Group B 9480. *Cancer* 2004;101(10):2202–2208.

33. Tannock IF, de WR, Berry WR, et al. Docetaxel plus prednisone or mitoxantrone plus prednisone for advanced prostate cancer. *N Engl J Med* 2004;351(15):1502–1512.

34. Petrylak DP, Tangen CM, Hussain MH, et al. Docetaxel and estramustine compared with mitoxantrone and prednisone for advanced refractory prostate cancer. *N Engl J Med* 2004;351(15):1513–1520.

35. Saltz LB, Cox JV, Blanke C, et al. Irinotecan Study Group. Irinotecan plus fluorouracil and leucovorin for metastatic colorectal cancer. *N Engl J Med* 2000;343(13):905–914.

36. Douillard JY, Cunningham D, Roth AD, et al. Irinotecan combined with fluorouracil compared with fluorouracil alone as first-line treatment for metastatic colorectal cancer: a multicentre randomised trial. *Lancet* 2000;355(9209):1041–1047.

37. Andre T, Louvet C, Maindrault-Goebel F, et al. CPT-11 (irinotecan) addition to bimonthly, high-dose leucovorin and bolus and continuous-infusion 5-fluorouracil (FOLFIRI) for pretreated metastatic colorectal cancer. GERCOR. *Eur J Cancer* 1999;35(9):1343–1347.

38. de GA, Figer A, Seymour M, et al. Leucovorin and fluorouracil with or without oxaliplatin as first-line treatment in advanced colorectal cancer. *J Clin Oncol* 2000;18(16):2938–2947.

39. Tournigand C, Andre T, Achille E, et al. FOLFIRI followed by FOLFOX6 or the reverse sequence in advanced colorectal cancer: a randomized GERCOR study. *J Clin Oncol* 2004;22(2):229–237.

40. Cassidy J, Twelves C, Van CE, et al. First line oral capecitabine therapy in metastatic colorectal cancer: a favorable safety profile compared with intravenous 5-fluorouracil/leucovorin. *Ann Oncol* 2002;13(4):566–575.

41. Kabbinavar FF, Hambleton J, Mass RD, et al. Combined analysis of efficacy: the addition of bevacizumab to fluorouracil/leucovorin improves survival for patients with metastatic colorectal cancer. *J Clin Oncol* 2005;23(16):3706–3712.

42. Cunningham D, Humblet Y, Siena S, et al. Cetuximab monotherapy and cetuximab plus irinotecan in irinotecan-refractory metastatic colorectal cancer. *N Engl J Med* 2004;351(4):337–345.

43. Sandler AB, Nemunaitis J, Denham C, et al. Phase III trial of gemcitabine plus cisplatin versus cisplatin alone in patients with locally advanced or metastatic non-small-cell lung cancer. *J Clin Oncol* 2000;18(1):122–130.

44. Cardenal F, Lopez-Cabrerizo MP, Anton A, et al. Randomized phase III study of gemcitabine-cisplatin versus etoposide-cisplatin in the treatment of locally advanced or metastatic non-small-cell lung cancer. *J Clin Oncol* 1999;17(1):12–18.

45. Pfister DG, Johnson DH, Azzoli CG, et al. American Society of Clinical Oncology treatment of unresectable non-small-cell lung cancer guideline: update 2003. *J Clin Oncol* 2004;22(2):330–353.

46. Kosmidis P, Mylonakis N, Nicolaides C, et al. Paclitaxel plus carboplatin versus gemcitabine plus paclitaxel in advanced non-small-cell lung cancer: a phase III randomized trial. *J Clin Oncol* 2002;20(17):3578–3585.

47. Shepherd FA, Dancey J, Ramlau R, et al. Prospective randomized trial of docetaxel versus best supportive care in patients with non-small-cell lung cancer previously treated with platinum-based chemotherapy. *J Clin Oncol* 2000;18(10):2095–2103.

48. Dancey J, Shepherd FA, Gralla RJ, et al. Quality of life assessment of second-line docetaxel versus best supportive care in patients with non-small-cell lung cancer previously treated with platinum-based chemotherapy: results of a prospective, randomized phase III trial. *Lung Cancer* 2004;43(2):183–194.

49. Arteaga C. Targeting HER1/EGFR: a molecular approach to cancer therapy. *Semin Oncol* 2003;30(3 Suppl 7):3–14.

50. Fuster LM, Sandler AB. Select clinical trials of erlotinib (OSI-774) in non-small-cell lung cancer with emphasis on phase III outcomes. *Clin Lung Cancer* 2004;6(Suppl 1):S24–S29.

51. Bernhard J, Thurlimann B, Schmitz SF, et al. Defining clinical benefit in postmenopausal patients with breast cancer under second-line endocrine treatment: does quality of life matter? *J Clin Oncol* 1999;17(6):1672–1679.

52. Campora E, Gardin G, Gasco M, et al. Metastatic breast cancer patients failing first-line, anthracycline-containing chemotherapy: is further therapy of benefit? *Anticancer Res* 1999;19(4C):3429–3432.

53. Nabholtz JM, Senn HJ, Bezwoda WR, et al. Prospective random-ized trial of docetaxel versus mitomycin plus vinblastine in patients with metastatic breast cancer progressing despite previous anthracycline-containing chemotherapy. 304 Study Group. *J Clin Oncol* 1999;17(5):1413–1424.

54. Leung PP, Tannock IF, Oza AM, et al. Cost-utility analysis of chemotherapy using paclitaxel, docetaxel, or vinorelbine for patients with anthracycline resistant breast cancer. *J Clin Oncol* 1999;17(10):3082–3090.

55. Launois R, Reboul-Marty J, Henry B, et al. A cost-utility analysis of second-line chemotherapy in metastatic breast cancer. Docetaxel versus paclitaxel versus vinorelbine. *Pharmacoeconomics* 1996;10(5):504–521.

56. Joensuu H, Holli K, Heikkinen M, et al. Combination chemotherapy versus single-agent therapy as first- and second-line treatment in metastatic breast cancer: a prospective randomized trial. *J Clin Oncol* 1998;16(12):3720–3730.

57. Coates A, Gebski V, Bishop JF, et al. Improving the quality of life during chemotherapy for advanced breast cancer. A comparison of intermittent and continuous treatment strategies. *N Engl J Med* 1987;317(24):1490–1495.

58. Osoba D, Slamon DJ, Burchmore M, et al. Effects on quality of life of combined trastuzumab and chemotherapy in women with metastatic breast cancer. *J Clin Oncol* 2002;20(14):3106–3113.

59. Hernandez MC, Knox SJ. Radiobiology of radioimmunotherapy: targeting CD20 B-cell antigen in non-Hodgkin's lymphoma. *Int J Radiat Oncol Biol Phys* 2004;59(5):1274–1287.

CHAPTER 51 ■ PALLIATIVE SURGERY

ALEXANDRA M. EASSON

Palliative surgery may be an important part of the management of patients with advanced cancer. Appropriate and timely surgical referral can alleviate or prevent significant pain and other distressful symptoms in the context of multidisciplinary palliative care. Palliation means "affording relief, not cure... to reduce the severity of" (1). Palliative surgery may therefore be defined as "interventions where the major goal is the relief of symptoms and suffering, not the prolongation of life, for patients for whom there is no chance of cure" (2,3). Palliative procedures may be beneficial for patients in whom death is imminent, but such procedures may also be helpful for patients with indolent or recurrent disease in whom death is months or years away.

Like conventional surgery, palliative surgery encompasses a wide spectrum of procedures, with differing levels of invasiveness, requirements for anesthesia, inherent technical difficulty, and attendant risks. Palliative surgery does not connote any degree of diminishment of care. If anything, palliative surgery may provide more aggressive care recognizing the value of procedural interventions leading to symptom relief and enhanced quality of life. Care and preparation is required to select the patients who will experience improved quality of life and relief of symptoms with acceptable morbidity. In addition, because surgical interventions offer local tumor control only, the potential benefits of local treatment must be put in context with the disease process as a whole. The conditions for which palliative surgical procedures are useful may be only one of many that cause distress and suffering for the patient. Pharmacologic symptom management and other supportive measures must therefore remain an important adjunct before, during, and after surgical intervention.

This chapter will outline some of conditions for which palliative surgery can and should be considered. It will then discuss the decision-making approach that a surgeon should undertake before embarking on a palliative surgical procedure.

Two types of procedures may be indicated in palliative patients:

1. Palliative, in which the goal of the intervention is the relief of symptoms
2. Supportive in which the procedure is a technical intervention done as part of a multidisciplinary treatment plan (Table 51.1)

PALLIATIVE SURGICAL PROCEDURES

A surgical intervention can be described as any invasive procedure that treats patients. The spectrum of palliative surgical procedures is therefore broad and includes procedures performed by percutaneous, endoscopic, laparoscopic and open techniques.

Tumor Resection

Complete Resection

Tumor resection of a local recurrence or a metastasis may be appropriate. Soft tissue tumors may result in difficult wound problems because of pain, ulceration, or fistula formation causing odor, discharge, or bleeding. Examples include ulcerating breast tumors; eroding head and neck

---

TABLE 51.1

EXAMPLES OF PALLIATIVE SURGICAL PROCEDURES

PALLIATIVE (INTERVENTION AS TREATMENT)
Tumor resection: pain, bleeding, fistulas
  Complete resection
  Debulking
  Amputation
Relief of obstruction
  Resection
  Bypass
  Percutaneous drainage
  Ablative therapy, dilatation, stent placement
Drainage of effusions
  Ascites
  Pleural effusions
  Pericardial effusions
Bony metastases
  Impending fractures
  Pathologic fractures
  Spinal instability
  Spinal cord or cauda equina compression
Neurosurgical techniques
  Peripheral neurectomy
  Hypophysectomy
  Cordotomy
Surgical castration
  Tumor embolization

SUPPORTIVE (PART OF MULTIDISCIPLINARY CARE)
Biopsy
Vascular access (for systemic agents)
Nutritional support

tumors; enterocutaneous or perineal fistulas draining bile, stool, or urine; and bulky axillary or inguinal nodal metastases causing progressive lymphedema and limited function. Surgical resection, if negative margins can be obtained, may result in significantly improved quality of life. The patient may already have had several attempts at local tumor control which may increase the complexity and potential morbidity of any planned local resection. For example, resection of a tumor through irradiated tissue may require the transfer of a soft tissue and/or muscle flap from an unirradiated area. Resection of recurrent anal cancer after failed chemo-radiation may require a two-team approach, where the surgical oncologist removes the tumor and a plastic surgeon fills the perineal defect with a gracilis or rectus abdominis muscle soft tissue flap.

For the patient who presents with metastatic disease, surgery may be an important part of gaining control of the local disease even if cure is not possible. Once a tumor has infiltrated a nerve root, surgery is unlikely to be helpful, so palliative surgical intervention may be warranted to prevent difficult symptoms despite distant metastases. Radical palliative resections such as esophagectomy, pancreaticoduodenectomy (4), and pelvic exenteration have been described for the purposes of local symptom control (5,6). In select patients, improvements in quality of life can be dramatic even if survival is not lengthened.

Debulking

Surgical resection should generally not be performed unless a complete resection can be achieved, as the tumor will simply recur. For some tumors, however, incomplete or debulking resections are appropriate, such as for slow-growing tumors (e.g., metastatic carcinoid or thyroid cancer), or when effective antitumor therapy can be given postoperatively to treat the residual tumor (ovarian cancer).

Amputation

Amputation may be necessary for extremity lesions such as soft tissue sarcomas and melanomas. It is usually a secondary procedure after failed limb-conserving therapy; unless it is absolutely necessary for palliation of pain, fungation or prevention of major hemorrhage. Amputation should be avoided in the presence of metastatic disease (7).

Relief of Obstruction

Mechanical obstruction of an organ or viscus is common in patients with advanced cancer and can cause significant pain and distress that is difficult to palliate without relief of the obstruction. Extrinsic compression or intrinsic tumor growth may obstruct the respiratory, gastrointestinal, biliary, vascular, or urologic systems partially or completely, acutely or chronically. Recognition of the symptoms of impending obstruction followed by early intervention may prevent a sudden life-threatening crisis. Relief from obstruction may allow many months of symptom-free survival and is generally most successful when there is a single site rather than multiple sites of obstruction.

The symptoms resulting from obstruction will depend on the site of obstruction and the organ involved. Treatment involves identifying the site and type of obstruction, by direct visualization or radiologic imaging, and should generally be initiated when the patient is symptomatic. Before acting to relieve the obstruction, it is important to confirm that symptoms are in fact due to obstruction. For example, bronchial obstruction is only one of many causes of shortness of breath. Furthermore, treatment to relieve the obstruction should only be done if the obstructive symptoms significantly

contribute to the patient's overall distress and symptom burden.

A variety of procedures may be used to relieve obstructive symptoms (2). Percutaneously placed gastric, biliary, or bladder drains may effectively decompress obstructed viscera, but require the additional care of an external drainage catheter. Endoscopic and/or fluoroscopic placement of stents through an obstructed lumen may also provide effective relief. Internal stents, long used in the biliary tree, esophagus, bronchus, and ureters, are now available for the small bowel, colon and rectum, and major blood vessels. More invasive techniques to manage obstruction include surgical bypass and/or tumor resection, by either minimally invasive or open techniques. These often provide the best long-term relief of obstruction but require a general anesthetic and are accompanied by a higher risk of morbidity and death.

Surgical Resection

Surgical resection is effective if the tumor causing the obstruction can be resected with negative margins even in the presence of metastatic disease. This is generally most applicable to obstructions of the gastrointestinal tract (8). Retrospective studies support palliative gastric resection for the relief of symptoms (9). Small or large bowel obstructions occur in 5–43% of patients with advanced primary or metastatic intra-abdominal malignancy. Symptoms include abdominal cramping and pain, nausea and vomiting, and constipation. The passage of liquid stool does not rule out obstruction, as it may be due to overflow. Peritonitis suggests a strangulated bowel loop or perforation and is an indication for emergency surgery. If there is a history of malignancy or previous surgery, a nasogastric tube is initially inserted for decompression. A computed tomography (CT) scan of the abdomen is recommended if the obstruction does not resolve to determine the site(s) and type of obstruction. Surgical resection is most effective if there is one site of obstruction. Benign causes of obstruction are found in 3–48% of patients with a history of malignant disease, and the postoperative mortality is similar (10%) to those patients without a history of malignancy. The most common causes of nonmalignant obstruction include adhesions, internal herniation (perhaps around a stoma), and radiation enteritis. Patients with multiple sites of obstruction in the small bowel usually have carcinomatosis. Symptoms of obstruction in these patients are often multifactorial and are rarely an acute event, alternating between complete and partial obstruction (10). The results of surgery for patients with carcinomatosis are poor and considerable clinical skill must be exercised by the surgeon in deciding whether or not the patient would benefit from an attempt at a surgical resection (8). Good prognostic factors include the following:

1. A well-nourished patient
2. Early stage of disease
3. Low-grade initial lesion and
4. Long interval from the first operation (11)

Poor prognostic criteria include the following:

1. Intestinal dysmotility due to carcinomatosis
2. Cachectic, older patients
3. Ascites requiring frequent drainage
4. Low serum albumin
5. Previous radiotherapy to the abdomen or pelvis
6. Palpable intra-abdominal masses, liver, and distant metastases
7. Multiple levels of bowel obstruction with prolonged transit time and
8. Poor performance status (10)

Malignant bowel obstruction in the large colon is usually due to one site of obstruction, and patients will often benefit from a surgical procedure. The tumor should be resected if possible, but a bypass or stoma will also provide effective symptom relief.

Surgical Bypass

Several enteroenterostomies to bypass areas of obstruction may be performed in the small and large bowel if resection is not possible to restore intestinal continuity. If this is not possible, a diverting ostomy may be performed proximal to the obstructed segment. Patients require at least 100 cm of small bowel to maintain nutrition without parenteral supplementation, and proximal stomas may case postoperative complications due to high fluid outputs. In the large bowel, a colostomy will relieve unresectable distal colonic obstruction, but will not prevent bleeding, pain, and discharge from the retained tumor.

Obstructions of the biliary tree are managed by percutaneous biliary drainage with or without stent placement, endoscopic stent placement or with a surgical bypass procedure. While internal–external percutaneous drains offer easy access in case of tube blockage, many patients do not like having an external tube to care for. Endoscopic stenting is effective, but may block, often resulting in readmission due to sepsis and requiring stent changes every few months. Four randomized trials comparing endoscopic stent insertion versus surgical bypass allow some broad conclusions to be made (12). Both techniques are effective in initial drainage of the biliary tree and improvement of symptoms. Endoscopic stenting has a lower early morbidity and mortality rate compared to surgical bypass, and therefore is more suitable for sick and debilitated patients. However, late complications of cholangitis and recurrent jaundice are high with endoscopic stenting, so repeat procedures may be required every 3–6 months. Patients expected to live longer than 6 months may therefore be more suitable for surgical bypass.

Percutaneous Drainage

Percutaneously placed gastrostomy tubes may be placed to relieve obstructive symptoms for patients with bowel obstruction due to carcinomatosis who are not candidates for surgical bypass. This will avoid the uncomfortable long-term placement of a nasogastric tube in patients unfit for surgery.

Ureteric obstruction due to pelvic malignancy may be relieved by percutaneous placement of nephrostomy catheters and is highly successful in relieving the pain of obstruction and returning renal function to normal. However, the role of treatment of ureteric obstruction in palliative patients is not defined and will vary according to the performance status and wishes of the patient. The results for most patients are quite poor, yet there are those for whom intervention will result in several months of productive life in which to accomplish expressed goals. In one retrospective study of patients with advanced malignancy, 86% of patients had significant cancer-related symptoms after endoscopic or percutaneous diversion and 51% required repeat interventions. Furthermore, the average survival was 5 months, with 50% of that time spent in hospital (13). In another study, 58% required a second procedure after internal drainage, but useful life was achieved in 84% of patients (14). Indications for intervention include bilateral hydronephrosis, unilateral ureteric obstruction with renal insufficiency, or pyelonephritis. Contraindications include asymptomatic patients unless the function of the contralateral kidney is of concern, or patients with rapidly progressive disease for which no other therapy is planned.

Ablative Therapy, Dilatation, Stent Placement

Local ablation using laser, electrocautery, cryotherapy, or photodynamic therapy can provide immediate relief of symptoms in easily accessed areas such as the trachea, esophagus, and rectum (2,15,16). These modalities are generally applied through a rigid or flexible endoscope with or without general anesthesia, and results of obstruction are generally equivalent, achieving relief of symptoms in most patients with minimal morbidity. Because obstruction recurs within weeks due to tumor regrowth, the time between treatments can be extended if the ablation is followed by the insertion of a stent or by intraluminal radiation. Endoscopic dilatation is effective in the esophagus, with a low complication rate (perforation in 5%), but must also be repeated every 3–4 weeks.

Stenting is becoming an effective option for palliation. Stents range from a rigid tube, placed with a rigid endoscope, to self-expanding wire stents inserted by flexible endoscopy or radiologic guidance. Covered wire stents reduce the incidence of tumor in-growth, but are associated with an increased incidence of migration and occlusion. Stents can be placed in the bronchus, duodenum, esophagus, bronchus, biliary tree, and colon; the site of obstruction must be relatively short and fixed.

Drainage of Effusions

An accumulation of fluid in the abdomen, pleural space, or pericardium is common in patients with cancer. A new effusion may be malignant or nonmalignant, even in patients with known metastatic disease. An initial diagnostic tap of fluid for the presence of malignant cells is usually indicated. Nonmalignant effusion usually requires treatment of the underlying medical condition, but surgical intervention may be required.

A malignant effusion occurs in three settings:

1. The presence of a small amount of fluid may render a patient noncurable, altering the treatment course but not causing enough symptoms to warrant intervention.
2. There may be an anticancer treatment to which the effusion will respond; the goal of treatment is symptom palliation and increased survival using investigational therapies such as the instillation of a biologic agent or chemotherapy with or without cytoreductive surgery (17–20).
3. In most cases, a malignant effusion occurs in the context of known metastatic disease for which treatment is given without expectation that survival will be altered.

In this palliative context, surgical drainage is not necessary unless the effusion causes significant symptoms that would be relieved by drainage of the fluid.

Ascites

Malignant ascites is defined as clinically evident and abnormal fluid accumulation within the abdominal cavity associated with a disseminated malignancy in the absence of hepatic cirrhosis (21). Most of patients with intra-abdominal malignancy will accumulate fluid in their abdomen due to a variety of processes, including vascular and lymphatic compression from liver metastases, portal hypertension from tumor infiltration of the liver parenchyma, decreased protein levels from cancer cachexia and malnutrition, and secretion by peritoneal tumor deposits (22). Cancers of the ovary, pancreas, breast, colon, and rectum, and of unknown origin are the most common causes of malignant ascites in palliative patients (21,22). Malignant cells within the ascitic fluid can be identified by cytology in only 60% of patients, despite this criterion being considered the gold standard for diagnosis (23); the diagnosis is confirmed when intra-abdominal cancer is identified by radiologic imaging, laparotomy, or laparoscopy. Although patients with ovarian cancer live significantly longer than patients with other tumors because of the availability of more effective anticancer therapies, the development of malignant ascites generally heralds a poor prognosis. As fluid builds up, patients will experience increased abdominal girth causing discomfort, anorexia, nausea, early satiety, dyspnea, and fatigue. For 15–71% of these patients, the increasing intra-abdominal pressure due to massive fluid accumulation causes significant symptoms which significantly affects their quality of life (21). Massive swelling of the entire lower half of the body is common when hepatic metastases compress the inferior vena cava (IVC syndrome), and may cause patients to be bedridden.

Medical therapy, such as a diuretic and restriction of sodium and fluid intake, may be helpful for central ascites. Repeated therapeutic paracentesis (percutaneous drainage) is most commonly used. Up to 5 liters of fluid may be drained at one time through a needle in the abdominal wall. Patients may require drainage two to three times per week, and often become very symptomatic prior to drainage. Peritoneovenous shunts, constructed of a plastic drainage tube with one end in the abdominal cavity and the other end inserted into the jugular vein, are now rarely used in malignant ascites because of a 25–49% complication rate (e.g., blockage, infection) and a high 30-day mortality rate (24). More recently, permanent indwelling peritoneal catheters, similar to peritoneal dialysis catheters, have been used (25–27). Percutaneous catheters can be managed by nurses or caregivers at home, which is important as patients become less mobile near the end of their lives (28). In patients with IVC syndrome causing severe ascites and anasarca, radiologic placement of expandable metallic IVC stents provide significant relief (29).

Pleural Effusion

Fifty percent of patients with cancer form pleural effusions; of these, only 40% are malignant. The most common primary tumors causing malignant effusions are lung, breast, lymphoma, and unknown primary (30). Initial cytology from a diagnostic tap will be positive in 66% of malignant effusions; repeat cytology or pleural biopsy will increase the diagnostic yield to 73–90% (31). Patients experience dyspnea (50–75%), chest pain (25%), and cough (25%). Simple thoracentesis, done blindly or with ultrasound guidance, offers rapid but temporary relief of symptoms as the effusion will recur in 98% of patients, and symptoms will recur in 82% of patients by 30 days. An external drainage catheter followed by pleurodesis is 70–80% effective as a single procedure (32,33). In this technique, a sclerosing agent (talc, silver nitrate) is instilled at the bedside to cause adhesion of the pleural surfaces once chest tube drainage is <100 mL per day. Outpatient catheter placement to straight drainage will offer effective palliation often without the need for hospital admission or a sclerosing agent (34,35). Early thorascopic or open drainage of the pleural cavity with or without decortication is advocated by some to reduce the rate of recurrence (36). Malignant pleural effusions may recur after pleurodesis due to the following:

1. Inadequate initial drainage
2. Ineffective sclerosing agent
3. Insufficient contact between pleural surfaces due to scarring, adhesions, or fibrin deposition or
4. lack of complete lung expansion due to intraparenchymal disease (tumor, radiation).

Options for treatment include thoracoscopy or open surgical drainage if not previously attempted, pleuroperitoneal shunts, or indwelling pleural catheters.

Pericardial Effusion

Malignancy accounts for 50% of pericardial effusions requiring treatment and most often occur as a late manifestation of breast, lung, gastrointestinal tract cancer, as well as sarcoma and lymphoma (37). Asymptomatic effusions, seen in 1–20% of patients with cancer at autopsy, do not require treatment. Symptoms include dyspnea, cough, chest pain, palpitations, weakness, and dizziness. Patients may present with pericardial tamponade, which is acutely life-threatening; these patients have anxiety, chest pain, and dyspnea, and are often leaning forward in an attempt to get comfortable.

Percutaneous drainage, pericardiocentesis, is the initial procedure used when tamponade is suspected. Tamponade, requiring a general anesthetic in this setting, may be fatal. Malignant effusions will recur in 90% at 3 months; therefore further treatment is required unless death is imminent (37). Percutaneous insertion of a drainage catheter using ultrasound guidance is an effective minimally invasive option (38). Sclerosis is effective in 75% of patients at 3 months (39). Other options involve creating a window either by thoracoscopy or thoracotomy to allow the fluid to drain to another body cavity.

Bone Metastases

Pain is the most common presentation of skeletal metastases, occurring in two third of patients with radiologically evident metastases. Radiation, systemic anticancer therapy and pain medication are the usual first lines of management. Surgery may be indicated when one of the following conditions arises:

1. Impending fracture
2. Pathologic fracture
3. Spinal instability or
4. Spinal cord or cauda equina compression

Impending Fracture

By the time a lytic bony metastasis is visible on an x-ray, considerable destruction of the bony cortex has occurred, incurring a risk of fracture. For large lesions, radiation therapy alone may temporarily weaken the bone and increase fracture risk. Primary surgical stabilization of the bone, followed by radiation, may be advantageous as internal fixation is easier when the bone is intact. Surgeons are attempting to define which patients with bone metastases would benefit from surgery to prevent fractures (40). In 1989, Mirels proposed a scoring system to estimate the risk of pathologic fracture based on four features: the size and site of a bony metastasis, the severity of pain, and its lytic versus blastic nature as determined on x-ray (Table 51.2) (41). Each item was given a score between 1 and 3, and a total score derived by summing the individual scores; total scores therefore ranged from 4–12 points. Treatment recommendations based on the risk of fracture could therefore be made. This system has been validated by Damron et al. and appears to predict the fracture risk better than clinical judgment alone, independent of the level of clinical experience (42). A recent randomized trial of radiation versus surgery for bony metastases of the femur recommended surgery to prevent fracture if the axial cortical involvement was >30 mm; otherwise, radiation therapy was recommended (43).

Pathologic Fracture

The most common site of pathologic fracture is the long bone of the femur, but a fracture can occur in any bone. In one series of patients with breast cancer, surgical treatment of bone fractures decreased pain in 77% and increased function in 65% of patients (44). Unlike after trauma, most of these fractures will not heal normally; this results in a high rate of fixation failure after surgical stabilization. In one series, the overall failure rate of fixation was 11%, and it was 20–24% in diaphyseal and distal femur fractures, resulting in additional operations, complications, and loss of function (45). Advances

TABLE 51.2

RISK OF PATHOLOGIC BONY FRACTURES: MIRELS' RATING SYSTEM AND TREATMENT RECOMMENDATIONS

Mirels' rating system

Feature		Score
Site	Upper extremity	1
	Lower extremity	2
	Peritrochanteric	3
Nature of lesion	Blastic	1
	Mixed lytic and blastic	2
	Lytic	3
Size (relative proportion of bone width involved with tumor)	<1/3	1
	1/3–2/3	2
	>2/3	3
Pain	Mild	1
	Moderate	2
	Functional limitation	3

Treatment recommendations

Risk of fracture	Score total	
Impending	≥9	Prophylactic stabilization
Borderline	8	Consider stabilization
Not impending	≤7	Nonoperative care

The scores for each item are added for each patient to produce a score point total (42).

are being made in the surgical treatment of cancer-related pathologic fractures. These include intermedullary fixation or bone prostheses rather than splinting to allow rapid return to function, and hardware that provides permanent support rather than depending on the bone to heal for strength; such improvements have reduced failure rates to 2% (40). Local radiation 12–14 days postoperatively does not interfere with fracture healing provided the fracture is adequately stabilized.

Spinal Instability

Spinal instability may result from widespread vertebral metastases and cause pain so severe that the patient is unable to sit, stand, or walk. No discrete vertebral fracture is seen; rather there is destruction of bone with vertebral collapse. Surgical stabilization of the spine may provide pain relief, through either an anterior or posterior approach.

Spinal Cord or Cauda Equina Compression

Spinal cord or cauda equina compression occurs in 5–20% of patients with vertebral metastases. Pain is usually first felt, frequently localized to the site of disease, followed by motor dysfunction, weakness, paresthesia, and sensory loss. When spinal cord compression is suspected, urgent investigation with magnetic resonance imaging or CT myelography is critical; once the diagnosis is made, immediate treatment must be offered to preserve lower extremity and sphincter function. Most spinal metastases are located in the vertebral body, anterior to the spinal cord. Surgical decompression historically consisted of a laminectomy alone (removal of the posterior element spinal column only); this procedure did not always relieve the compression and resulted in spinal instability with increasing kyphosis, increasing pain, and neurologic deficit. Therefore standard treatment of cord compression usually consists of corticosteroids and radiation, with surgical decompression offered to select patients. However, current surgical management involves circumferential decompression by removing the tumor through an anterior approach, and if needed, immediate operative spinal stabilization. This procedure was recently compared with radiation therapy in a randomized trial (46). This trial had to be stopped early (after 101 patients) because significantly more patients in the surgery group regained the ability to walk than in the radiation group (62 vs. 19%). It remains to be seen how quickly this trial will impact the clinical management of these patients.

Neurosurgical Procedures

Neurosurgical procedures for pain relief are currently less commonly used because of the effectiveness of pharmacologic and percutaneous techniques. However, open procedures may be considered when all else has failed to control pain, the severity of the pain warrants surgery, and there are no medical contraindications to the procedure.

Peripheral Neurectomy

For patients with cancer, neurosurgical pain relief procedures are usually ablative, involving division or destruction of the nerves responsible for the pain. The lowest or most peripheral point relative to the location of the pain is usually the most appropriate site for the procedure. A procedure should be undertaken only if disruption of the nerve is likely to help in pain control. Nociceptive pain is the most responsive to ablative techniques; however, the presence of pain in addition to nociceptive pain should not rule out the procedure, as the ablative techniques may provide enough pain control to enable effective pharmacologic management of the remaining pain (47). Because both motor and sensory fibers overlap in a single nerve, even select division of a nerve may result in significant motor and sensory disturbances.

Destruction of the nerves may be done by a variety of modalities, including destruction by radiofrequency ablation, chemical neurolysis, or open techniques. Chest wall pain due to a paraspinal tumor involving a nerve at or distal to the neural foramen may be effectively relieved by peripheral neurectomy, as the resulting motor loss is relatively insignificant (47). Benefit from ablation of the trigeminal or glossopharyngeal nerves in patients with head and neck cancers is also reported (48).

Neurolytic celiac plexus blockade (NCPB) has been shown to prevent or significantly relieve severe pain in 70–90% of patients with pancreatic cancer in randomized trials and should be considered for all patients whose tumors are believed to be incurable (49,50). Pain due to any tumor involving the celiac plexus will respond to this technique. In NCPB, neurolytic agents (50% ethanol, 6% phenol, or absolute alcohol) are injected on either side of the aorta at the level of the celiac plexus. In one randomized trial, pain relief was reported in 85% of patients postoperatively; although two third of patients had return of pain before death, pain scores remained lower when compared to patients who did not receive NCPB (50). NCPB also prevented the development of severe pancreatic pain in patients without pain at time of laparotomy. Interestingly, an increased survival time was also found for those who received NCPB. For patients not undergoing surgery, NCPB can be done percutaneously (51,52). In a meta-analysis of 989 patients who received NCPB percutaneously, pain was relieved in 89% of patients initially and in 70–90% until death (49). NCPB decreases narcotic requirements, adds little morbidity, and may increase survival.

Hypophysectomy

Hypophysectomy involves ablation or destruction of the pituitary gland through a stereotactic transsphenoidal approach and has been used to manage severe pain from diffuse bone metastases in patients with cancer. The mechanism of pain relief is not understood but may be due to stimulation of the hypothalamic pain-suppressing capability. Although not commonly performed, a recent study has demonstrated benefit in select patients (53).

Cordotomy

Cordotomy, where the anterolateral quadrant of the spinal cord containing the spinothalamic tract is divided, results in selective temperature loss and pain perception on the contralateral side several segments below the level of the division. Cordotomy may be useful to treat well-localized, unilateral, lower extremity, or perineal pain due to direct nerve plexus invasion by rectal or gynecologic cancers. The procedure may be done percutaneously or with an open technique (54).

SUPPORTIVE PROCEDURES

Biopsy

Increased or newly apparent pain may be the first sign that a tumor has recurred locally or has metastasized. New pain at follow-up should prompt a search for recurrence in a patient with cancer, including radiologic imaging, tumor marker measurements and physical examination. When recurrence is found, surgeons are occasionally called upon to perform incisional or excisional biopsies of newly discovered masses to help guide the palliative treatment of patients.

Vascular Access

Patients may require long-term or central vascular access for many reasons: chemotherapy, drugs, parenteral nutrition, blood sampling, or transfusions. Surgeons and interventional radiologists share the responsibility of inserting and maintaining permanent indwelling vascular access devices such as tunneled catheters and subcutaneous ports. Peripherally inserted central catheters (PICC lines) are a common and less-invasive option.

Enteral Feeding Tubes

While the ethical considerations regarding the insertion of feeding tubes to support patients with terminal illness is beyond the scope of this chapter, these tubes may be placed by a variety of percutaneous, laparoscopic, or open techniques (55).

SURGICAL DECISION-MAKING

The selection of the best palliative surgical procedure to recommend depends on the individual patient, the disease process, the risk-benefit ratio, and the available technical expertise (Table 51.3). Advances in laparoscopy and interventional radiology are of importance as these techniques may have lower morbidity compared to open procedures. It should be noted that abdominal laparoscopy still requires the use of a general and paralyzing anesthetic, which is a major contributor to morbidity. Generally, the most minimally invasive effective procedure is chosen so as to result in the least discomfort, morbidity, and time in hospital. However, this should not result in the withholding of more invasive procedures in appropriately selected patients when these procedures will be more effective for the relief of symptoms.

Palliative surgery must be carefully considered on an individual basis, with quality of life and symptom control being the main outcome measure, rather then the more frequently measured surgical endpoints of cure of disease and prolongation of life (56–58). Determining the benefits and optimal timing of a palliative surgical intervention requires an understanding of the patient's underlying disease, particularly, its natural history in that patient, and the treatment history. It may be reasonable to consider a palliative pelvic resection for pain in a patient with recurrent anal cancer, for example, if he or she has had a long disease-free interval, and metastases that have responded to chemotherapy; in contrast, such a decision may not be reasonable in a patient with local recurrence and widespread metastases several months after the initial potentially curative treatment. Knowledge of the disease may also allow the prevention of complications. Colonic resection in metastatic colorectal cancer, for example, is often offered to patients with obstructive symptoms to prevent acute obstruction, while recognizing that this will not alter the overall progression of disease. Operative morbidity and mortality is significantly higher after emergency rather than elective procedures.

An assessment of prognosis is essential to determine a risk/benefit ratio for the intervention. Studies of the ability of physicians to predict prognosis in patients with advanced cancer are mixed. One study found that clinicians estimated prognosis quite accurately when asked whether or not a patient with terminal cancer was expected to live 6 months (59). In another study, however, physicians tended to overestimate

TABLE 51.3

AN APPROACH TO THE SELECTION AND PREPARATION OF PATIENTS FOR PALLIATIVE SURGERY

INFORMATION GATHERING BEFORE MAKING A RECOMMENDATION
- Disease factors
  - Diagnosis, knowledge of natural history
  - Current status of tumor: local and staging imaging studies
- Patient factors
  - Prognosis
  - Health status
  - Patient goals and expectations
- Societal factors
  - Family and community resources
- Technical factors
  - Feasibility, choice of modality
  - Likelihood of successful palliation
  - Morbidity and mortality

DISCUSSION ABOUT GOALS OF CARE
- Review current status of disease with patient and family
- Make a recommendation based on likelihood of success
- Does this fit with the goals of care of the patient?

GENERAL PRINCIPLES
1. Anticipation and prevention of impending symptoms
2. Thorough preoperative evaluation to avoid intraoperative surprises
3. Avoid emergency situations
4. Communication with the patient and family about the goals of care
5. Commitment to continue to provide care despite outcome of surgery

patient survival and in particular failed to predict who would die within 2 months (60). Several clinical prognostic indices have been developed for patients with terminal cancer; these combine objective clinical criteria such as weight loss and performance status (patient function) with clinician estimates (61–64). Other less well-defined factors also impact on prognosis. In one study, extent of disease and quality of life together predicted survival better than each parameter alone in patients with breast cancer (65). In another study, symptom distress alone predicted survival in patients with lung cancer (66).

An exploration of alternatives to surgery may avoid an operation. Aggressive medical management of malignant bowel obstruction or the placement of a venting gastrostomy tube, for example, may allow patients with carcinomatosis to live without a nasogastric tube (55). Advances in medical therapy may also significantly alter the natural history of disease. The dramatic improvement in survival for patients with gastrointestinal stromal tumor with imatinib is a recent example (67). Palliative surgical procedures may now be contemplated where it was not rational to do so in the past.

As with any operation, the patient's overall physical status is an important consideration when assessing the patient's operative risk. Factors known to increase operative risk include increased age, the presence of underlying cardiac, renal, hepatic, or respiratory disease; poor performance status; and concurrent illness, such as sepsis, anemia, and uncontrolled metabolic abnormalities. Preoperative assessment using the American Society of Anesthesiologists Classification of Physical Status correlates well with postoperative mortality (68).

Asthenia, anorexia, and cachexia are common interrelated systemic symptoms that occur in many patients terminally ill with cancer, and contribute to the weakness and weight loss seen with advanced illness (69). Patients with these symptoms have significantly more complications and mortality after surgery (70). Decreased mobility from asthenia results in increased postoperative pulmonary complications. Anorexia leads to decreased oral intake, and the resultant malnutrition affects healing and immune function. If cachexia is present, the anabolism required for healing and immune function is further impaired. The presence of these symptoms preoperatively should caution against aggressive surgical intervention.

Because the goals of the procedure are the relief of suffering and improvement in quality of life, the patient's own perceptions and wishes are perhaps the most crucial determinants in procedure selection. Some time must be spent getting to know what is important to the patient. A few directed questions may be helpful, such as "Of all the symptoms that you have, which one bothers you the most?" and "If I were able to fix this symptom for you, would this significantly improve your life?" Because every procedure carries with it potential morbidity, only those procedures that will potentially improve symptoms that are important to the patient should be performed. Patient treatment choices are also determined by what the patient and family understand about the disease and prognosis. Weeks et al. found that the patient's decisions about whether to undergo aggressive therapy were related to their perception of their own survival (59). Patients with cancer tended to overestimate their life expectancy; those who believed that there was at least a 10% chance that they would die within 6 months were more likely to favor less aggressive therapies. Psychiatric conditions must also be kept in mind; Chochinov et al. found that patients who did not acknowledge their prognosis (9.5% of 200 patients with advanced cancer) were almost three times more likely to be clinically depressed (71).

The choice of procedure will be affected by the available community and personal resources available. These factors include the location where the patient is cared for after the procedure (hospital, hospice, or home), the expertise of the caregivers (nurse, family, palliative care physicians, or home health care aides), and the equipment available (e.g., portable pain pumps, or ostomy equipment). A procedure should make ongoing care as easy as possible for the patient and the caregivers. For example, an external drainage tube may be less invasive but will require management of a drainage bag; an internal stent placement may be more invasive but may require less care. Cost of the intervention may be a consideration for some families.

Pharmacologic Symptom Management in the Perioperative Setting

Patients with cancer undergoing palliative procedures are often taking a variety of medications for their symptoms, including appropriately high doses of narcotics. The high preoperative dosages of pain medication that patients require will complicate intra- and postoperative pain management, especially in hospitals that do not specialize in patients with cancer. The dosages of narcotics required for postoperative pain relief may be so high that physicians used to managing routine postoperative pain may become uncomfortable. For this reason, in our institutions, it is routine to ask the palliative care pain service to manage both the pre- and postoperative pain in patients with advanced cancer. In addition, patients who undergo an effective surgical intervention will require reassessment of their pain medications after the procedure. Dosages of long-acting medications may need to be titrated down and provisions made to allow for appropriate doses of breakthrough medications until a new threshold is attained. This is especially important after interventions that offer rapid relief, such as paracentesis for malignant ascites or biliary decompression by endoscopic or percutaneous stent placement.

CONCLUSION

The decision to offer any surgical procedure to a patient must balance the potential benefits of the intervention with the inevitable risks of postsurgical pain and complications. This is particularly important for the patient who is suffering from a terminal illness. For the surgeon, trained to intervene, a decision to operate is often the easiest one to make. The true skill of the surgeon as physician, however, lies in the careful selection and preparation of patients who will benefit from a surgical procedure, as well as a continued commitment to the care of patients for whom surgery is not selected. The question that must be answered is not "Can this operation be done?" but rather "Should this operation be done for this patient at this time?"

References

1. Friel JP, ed. *Dorland's illustrated medical dictionary*, 26th ed. Philadelphia, PA: WB Saunders, 1985.
2. Easson AM, Asch M, Swallow CJ. Palliative general surgical procedures. *Surg Oncol Clin N Am* 2001;10(1):161–184.
3. McCahill LE, Krouse RS, Chu DZ, et al. Decision making in palliative surgery. *J Am Coll Surg* 2002;195(3):411–422.
4. Ouchi K, Sugawara T, Ono H, et al. Palliative operation for cancer of the head of the pancreas: significance of pancreaticoduodenectomy and intraoperative radiation therapy for survival and quality of life. *World J Surg* 1998;22:413–417.
5. Finlayson CA, Eisenberg BL. Palliative pelvic exenteration: patient selection and results. *Oncology (Huntingt)* 1996;10(4):479–484.
6. Brophy PF, Hoffman JP, Eisenberg BL. The role of palliative pelvic exenteration. *Am J Surg* 1994;167(4):386–390.
7. Merimsky O, Kollender Y, Inbar M, et al. Is forequarter amputation justified for palliation of intractable cancer symptoms? *Oncology* 2001;60(1):55–59.
8. Krouse RS, McCahill LE, Easson AM, et al. When the sun can set on an unoperated bowel obstruction: management of malignant bowel obstruction. *J Am Coll Surg* 2002;195(1):117–128.
9. Miner TJ, Jaques DP, Karpeh MS, et al. Defining palliative surgery in patients receiving noncurative resections for gastric cancer. *J Am Coll Surg* 2004;198(6):1013–1021.
10. Ripamonti C. Management of bowel obstruction in advanced cancer patients. *J Pain Symptom Manage* 1994;9:193–200.
11. Parker MC, Baines MJ. Intestinal obstruction in patients with advanced malignant disease. *Br J Surg* 1996;83:1–2.
12. Gouma DJ, van Geenen R, van Gulik T, et al. Surgical palliative treatment in bilio-pancreatic malignancy. *Ann Oncol* 1999;10S4:269–272.
13. Shekarriz B, Shekarriz H, Upadhyay J, et al. Outcome of palliative urinary diversion in the treatment of advanced malignancies. *Cancer* 1999;85(4):998–1003.
14. Feng MI, Bellman GC, Shapiro CE. Management of ureteral obstruction secondary to pelvic malignancies. *J Endourol* 1999;13(7):521–524.
15. Christie N, Patel A, Landereneau R. Esophageal palliation-photodynamic therapy/stents/brachytherapy. *Surg Clin North Am* 2005;85(3):569–582.
16. Wood DE. Management of malignant tracheobronchial obstruction. *Surg Clin North Am* 2002;82(3):621–642.
17. Yamao T, Shimada Y, Shirao K, et al. Phase II study of sequential methotrexate and 5-fluorouracil chemotherapy against peritoneally disseminated gastric cancer with malignant ascites: a report from the Gastrointestinal Oncology Study Group of the Japan Clinical Oncology Group, JCOG 9603 Trial. *Jpn J Clin Oncol* 2004;34(6):316–322.
18. Chatzigeorgiou K, Economou S, Chrysafis G, et al. Treatment of recurrent epithelial ovarian cancer with secondary cytoreduction and continuous intraoperative intraperitoneal hyperthermic chemoperfusion (CIIPHCP). *Zentralbl Gynakol* 2003;125(10):424–429.
19. Lu C, Perez-Soler R, Piperdi B, et al. Phase II study of a liposome-entrapped cisplatin analog (L-NDDP) administered intrapleurally and pathologic response rates in patients with malignant pleural mesothelioma. *J Clin Oncol* 2005;23(15):3495–3501.
20. Sartori S, Tassinari D, Ceccotti P, et al. Prospective randomized trial of intrapleural bleomycin versus interferon alfa-2b via ultrasound-guided small-bore chest tube in the palliative treatment of malignant pleural effusions. *J Clin Oncol* 2004;22(7):1228–1233.
21. Mackey JR, Venner PM. Malignant ascites: demographics, therapeutic efficacy and predictors of survival. *Can J Oncol* 1996;6(2):474–480.
22. Doyle D, Hanks G, MacDonald N, eds. *Oxford textbook of palliative medicine*, 2nd ed. Oxford: Oxford University Press, 1999.
23. Aslam N, Marino CR. Malignant ascites: new concepts in pathophysiology, diagnosis, and management. *Arch Intern Med* 2001;161(22):2733–2737.
24. Schumacher DL, Saclarides TJ, Staren ED. Peritoneovenous shunts for palliation of the patient with malignant ascites. *Ann Surg Oncol* 1994;1(5):378–381.
25. Lee A, Lau TN, Yeong KY. Indwelling catheters for the management of malignant ascites. *Support Care Cancer* 2000;8(6):493–499.
26. Barnett TD, Rubins J. Placement of a permanent tunneled peritoneal drainage catheter for palliation of malignant ascites: a simplified percutaneous approach. *J Vasc Interv Radiol* 2002;13(4):379–383.
27. Sabatelli FW, Glassman ML, Kerns SR, et al. Permanent indwelling peritoneal access device for the management of malignant ascites. *Cardiovasc Intervent Radiol* 1994;17(5):292–294.
28. Murphy M, Rossi M. Managing ascites via the Tenckhoff catheter. *Medsurg Nurs* 1995;4(6):468–471.
29. Fletcher WS, Lakin PC, Pommier RF, et al. Results of treatment of inferior vena cava syndrome with expandable metallic stents. *Arch Surg* 1998;133(9):953–958.
30. Lee YCLR. Management of malignant pleural effusions. *Respirology* 2004;9(2):148–146.
31. Sahn SA. Malignancy metastatic to the pleura. *Clin Chest Med* 1998;19(2):351–361.
32. Dresler CM, Olak J, Herndon JE, et al. Phase III intergroup study of talc poudrage vs talc slurry sclerosis for malignant pleural effusion. *Chest* 2005;127(3):909–915.
33. Paschoalini MS, Vargas FS, Marchi E, et al. Prospective randomized trial of silver nitrate vs talc slurry in pleurodesis for symptomatic malignant pleural effusions. *Chest* 2005;128(2):684–689.
34. Pollak JS, Burdge CM, Rosenblatt M, et al. Treatment of malignant pleural effusions with tunneled long-term drainage catheters. *J Vasc Interv Radiol* 2001;12(2):201–208.
35. Robinson RD, Fullerton DA, Albert JD, et al. Use of pleural Tenckhoff catheter to palliate malignant pleural effusion. *Ann Thorac Surg* 1994;57:286–288.
36. Marrazzo A, Noto A, Casa L, et al. Video-thoracoscopic surgical pleurodesis in the management of malignant pleural effusion: the importance of an early intervention. *J Pain Symptom Manage* 2005;30(1):75–79.

37. DeCamp MM Jr, Mentzer SJ, Swanson SJ, et al. Malignant effusive disease of the pleura and pericardium. *Chest* 1997;112(4 Suppl):291S–295S.

38. Tsang TS, Seward JB, Barnes ME, et al. Outcomes of primary and secondary treatment of pericardial effusion in patients with malignancy. *Mayo Clin Proc* 2000;75(3):248–253.

39. Maher EA, Shepard FA, Todd TJR. Pericardial sclerosis as the primary management of malignant pericardial effusion and cardiac tamponade. *J Thorac Cardiovasc Surg* 1996;112:637–643.

40. Cady B, Easson A, Aboulafia AJ, et al. Part 1: Surgical palliation of advanced illness–what's new, what's helpful. *J Am Coll Surg* 2005;200(1):115–127.

41. Mirels H. Metastatic disease in long bones: a proposed scoring system for diagnosing impending pathologic fractures. *Clin Orthop Relat Res* 1989;249:256–264.

42. Damron TA, Morgan H, Prakash D, et al. Critical evaluation of Mirels' rating system for impending pathologic fractures. *Clin Orthop Relat Res* 2003;(415 Suppl):S201–S207.

43. van der Linden YM, Dijkstra PD, Kroon HM, et al. Comparative analysis of risk factors for pathological fracture with femoral metastases. *J Bone Joint Surg Br* 2004;86(4):566–573.

44. Wedin R, Bauer HC, Rutqvist LE. Surgical treatment for skeletal breast cancer metastases: a population-based study of 641 patients. *Cancer* 2001;92(2):257–262.

45. Wedin R, Bauer HC, Wersall P. Failures after operation for skeletal metastatic lesions of long bones. *Clin Orthop Relat Res* 1999;(358):128–139.

46. Patchell RA, Tibbs PA, Regine WF, et al. Direct decompressive surgical resection in the treatment of spinal cord compression caused by metastatic cancer: a randomised trial. *Lancet* 2005;366(9486):643–648.

47. Arbit E, Bilksy MH. Neurosurgical approaches in palliative care. In Doyle D, Hanks G, MacDonald N, eds. *Oxford textbook of palliative medicine*, Chapter 9.2.1. Oxford, England: Oxford University Press, 1999:414–419.

48. Rozen TD. Trigeminal neuralgia and glossopharyngeal neuralgia. *Neurol Clin* 2004;22(1):185–206.

49. Eisenberg E, Carr DB, Chalmers TC. Neurolytic celiac plexus block for treatment of cancer pain: a meta-analysis. *Anesth Analg* 1995;80(2):290–295.

50. Lillemoe KD, Cameron JL, Kaufman HS, et al. Chemical splanchnicectomy in patients with unresectable pancreatic cancer. A prospective randomized trial. *Ann Surg* 1993;217(5):447–455.

51. Le Pimpec Barthes F, Chapuis O, Riquet M, et al. Thoracoscopic splanchnicectomy for control of intractable pain in pancreatic cancer. *Ann Thorac Surg* 1998;65(3):810–813.

52. Saenz A, Kuriansky J, Salvador L, et al. Thoracoscopic splanchnicectomy for pain control in patients with unresectable carcinoma of the pancreas. *Surg Endosc* 2000;14(8):717–720.

53. Hayashi M, Taira T, Chernov M, et al. Role of pituitary radiosurgery for the management of intractable pain and potential future applications. *Stereotact Funct Neurosurg* 2003;81(1–4):75–83.

54. Jones B, Finlay I, Ray A, et al. Is there still a role for open cordotomy in cancer pain management? *J Pain Symptom Manage* 2003;25(2):179–184.

55. Easson AM, Hinshaw DB, Johnson DL. The role of tube feeding and total parenteral nutrition in advanced illness. *J Am Coll Surg* 2002;194(2):225–228.

56. Seely JF, Mount BM. Palliative medicine and modern technology. *Can Med Assoc J* 1999;161(9):1120–1121.

57. Easson AM, Lee KF, Brasel K, et al. Clinical research for surgeons in palliative care: challenges and opportunities. *J Am Coll Surg* 2003;196(1):141–151.

58. McLeod RS. Quality-of-life measurement in the assessment of surgical outcome. *Adv Surg* 1999;33:293–309.

59. Weeks JC, Cook EF, O'Day SJ. Relationship between cancer patients prediction of prognosis and their treatment preferences. *JAMA* 1998;279:1709–1714.

60. Vigano A, Bruera E, Jhangri GS, et al. Clinical survival predictors in patients with advanced cancer. *Arch Intern Med* 2000;160(6):861–868.

61. Sloan JA, Loprinzi CL, Laurine JA, et al. A simple stratification factor prognostic for survival in advanced cancer: the good/bad/uncertain index. *J Clin Oncol* 2001;19(15):3539–3546.

62. Morita T, Tsunoda J, Inoue S, et al. Improved accuracy of physicians' survival prediction for terminally ill cancer patients using the palliative prognostic index. *Palliat Med* 2001;15(5):419–424.

63. Maltoni M, Nanni O, Pirovano M, et al. Successful validation of the palliative prognostic score in terminally ill cancer patients. *J Pain Symptom Manage* 1999;17(4):240–247.

64. Knaus WA, Harrell FE Jr, Lynn J, et al. The SUPPORT prognostic model. Objective estimates of survival for seriously ill hospitalized adults. *Ann Intern Med* 1995;122(3):191–203.

65. Seidman AD, Portenoy R, Yao TJ, et al. Quality of life in phase II trials: a study of methodology and predictive value in patients with advanced breast cancer treated with paclitaxel plus granulocyte colony-stimulating factor. *J Natl Cancer Inst* 1995;87(17):1316–1322.

66. Degner LF, Sloan JA. Symptom distress in newly diagnosed ambulatory cancer patients and as a predictor of survival in lung cancer. *J Pain Symptom Manage* 1995;10(6):423–431.

67. Sawaki A, Yamao K. Imatinib mesylate acts in metastatic or unresectable gastrointestinal stromal tumor by targeting KIT receptors–a review. *Cancer Chemother Pharmacol* 2004;54(Suppl 1):S44–S49.

68. Dripps RD, Eckenhoff JE, Vandam LD. *Introduction to anesthesia: the principles of safe practice*, 6th ed. Philadelphia, PA: WB Saunders, 1988.

69. Bruera E. ABC of palliative care: anorexia, cachexia, and nutrition. *Br Med J* 1997;315:1219–1222.

70. Fearon KC, Barber MD, Moses AG. The cancer cachexia syndrome. *Surg Oncol Clin N Am* 2001;10(1):109–126.

71. Chochinov HM, Tataryn D, Wilson KG, et al. Prognostic awareness and the terminally ill. *Psychosomatics* 2000;41(6):500–504.

CHAPTER 52 ■ PALLIATIVE ORTHOPAEDIC SURGERY

JUAN SANTIAGO-PALMA AND JUAN C. JIMENEZ

Metastatic bone disease is the most common malignant bone lesion in adults. Seventy to 80% of all patients with cancer are likely to develop bone metastases (1) and approximately 9% will sustain a pathologic fracture (2). For many, a pathologic fracture is an indication of end-stage disease. It is estimated that only half these patients will survive beyond 1 year (3).

Bone metastases cause significant pain. Metastatic lesions produce inflammatory and osteolytic factors, which can activate nociceptors (4,5) and recruit osteoclasts (6,7). Patients experience pain as the tumor grows and increased tissue edema and intraosseous pressure develop. Osteoclastic activity erodes the cortex of the bone, which can eventually result in a pathologic fracture (6,7).

Over the past decade attention has been directed toward improving care for patients with bone metastases. Advancement in radiotherapy, surgical techniques, and the development of new drugs has improved the quality of life of patients with cancer and bone disease. Despite these advances, the management of painful bone metastases remains palliative.

In patients with metastatic bone disease the general objective of treatment shifts from curing the patient to providing symptom control and improving quality of life.

The cornerstone of treating symptomatic bone metastases is a combination of analgesics, external beam radiation therapy (EBRT), and bisphosphonates. Surgery, nerve blocks, chemotherapy, steroids, and hormones must be considered as adjunct therapies. In most patients, a combination of systemic modalities is required to keep the patient free of pain for extended periods of time. The key is to choose from different treatments to optimize pain, decrease treatment side effects, improve function, and quality of life.

EVALUATION

Pain is the most common symptom of bone metastases. Patients with skeletal disease present with pain over 75% of the time (8). Bone pain is the result of mechanical stress on the weakened bone, destruction of the bone, microfractures, periosteal distension, nerve compression, and tumor pressure on adjacent tissues. In addition several chemical factors, which mediate osteolytic, bone resorption, such as prostaglandins, bradykinin, substance P, interleukin-1 (IL-1), IL-6, and tumor necrosis factor activate the pain receptors of the periosteum (9).

Metastatic disease should be considered in any patient with limb or spine pain and a known history of cancer. Prostate and breast cancer are the most common tumors that cause bony metastases. Myeloma, lymphoma, and cancer of the lung and kidney are the most common malignancies with a lesion of bone as their first presentation (10).

The standard approach to evaluate a patient with metastatic bone disease is to follow an algorithm of clinical examination, laboratory tests, and imaging studies. A comprehensive evaluation must be made to determine the possibility of an impending pathologic fracture or neurologic compromise such as spinal cord compression.

Bone pain produces a well-localized dull ache that increases with weight bearing. Pain is usually aggravated with moving, standing, and walking. There is often focal tenderness. Bone pain is often associated with other pain syndromes. Metastases to the vertebrae may cause spinal cord compression, nerve root compression, or cauda equina syndrome. Metastases to the base of the skull can impinge on cranial nerves.

Initial diagnostic workup usually includes x-ray of the affected limb or spine. Plain radiographs are useful to assess for bony changes and fractures and can determine if the lesion is osteolytic or osteoblastic. Purely lytic lesions are prone to fracture, whereas purely blastic lesions seldom fracture (11). Bone metastases in patients with breast cancer and multiple myeloma are predominantly osteolytic in nature. By contrast, prostate bone lesions are mixed, containing both osteolytic and osteoblastic elements (12). Osteolytic lesions may not be apparent for several months, because, 30–75% of normal bone mineral content must be lost before the lesion becomes apparent on x-rays (13,14).

Bone scanning with technetium-99 is the most common diagnostic test used to detect bone metastasis (15,16). Bone scan detects increases in osteoblastic activity and skeletal vascularity (17,18). Sensitivity and specificity rates of technetium bone scanning range from 62–100% and specificity from 78–100% (19–23). Bone scan is considered sensitive for detecting osteolytic or osteoblastic bone metastases (24). False-negative findings can occasionally occur when osteolytic metastases grow rapidly, when bone turnover is slow, or when the tumor site is avascular (24).

Computed tomography (CT) scan offers excellent detail of the bone and bone marrow. CT scan is useful to distinguish structures of different densities. The sensitivity of CT scan for the diagnosis of bone metastases ranges from 71–100% (25,26).

Magnetic resonance imaging (MRI) provides detailed imaging of the bone and bone marrow. The diagnostic sensitivity of skeletal MRI ranges from 82–100%, and its specificity ranges from 73–100% (27–30). Bone marrow lesions are better visualized in MRI. MRI also has better resolution than CT scan for soft tissue and neurovascular structures. MRI is less accurate than CT scan to detect destruction of bone (17,31).

Positron emission tomography (PET) visualizes the uptake of positron-emitting radiopharmaceuticals by tissues. PET is used for whole-body scanning to detect metastases in either soft tissue or bone. Fluorodeoxyglucose (FDG) PET measures glucose metabolism in many types of cancer and can be useful for distinguishing benign from malignant bone lesions (32–34). Estimates of the sensitivity of FDG PET for detecting bone metastasis range from 62–100%, and specificity from 96–100% (35–37). The disadvantages of PET are its high cost and its relative lack of availability

Single photon emission computerized tomography (SPECT) uses the same radionuclide as bone scans. Like CT scan, SPECT uses a rotating camera to create tridimensional cross-sectional images. SPECT is useful to evaluate areas of increased uptake seen in bone scans due to its better resolution (38,39). Its sensitivity for the diagnosis of bone metastases is 87–92%, and its specificity is 91–93% (40,41). SPECT is useful to evaluate areas that are extensively surrounded by soft tissue such as the thoracolumbar spine and pelvis. In the spine SPECT useful for distinguishing benign from malignant lesions (42).

SURGICAL TREATMENT

The aim of surgery in metastatic bone disease is to stabilize the weakened bone and to eliminate the risk of pathologic fracture. Surgical treatment of a bone metastasis should be preceded by careful evaluation of the patient's needs, wishes, and prognosis. The goal of surgical treatment is to reduce pain, maintain function, and improve quality of life. A pathologic fracture is an obvious indication for surgery. Indications for surgical treatment without a fracture are less clear and must take into consideration the prognosis of the patient, failure of more conservative therapies and patients desire to proceed with surgery.

Studies indicate that the 1-year survival of patients with skeletal metastases who undergo surgical treatment is poor. Most studies have shown a 1-year survival of 0.30–0.54 (43–45). Various clinical features may help assess the survival in patients with metastatic bone disease. Patients with multiple myeloma, lymphoma, kidney and breast cancer have a better prognosis (38–40) and patients who suffer from lung cancer have a poorer prognosis. Complete pathologic fractures, and known visceral metastases are negative prognostic factors (41–43). Patients with poor Karnofsky scores, weight loss, and hemoglobin <7 mg per dL have a shorter survival (43,46,47).

There is no evidence that the surgical fixation of bone metastases influences long-term survival. Survival of patients who undergo surgery for bone complications is similar to that for patients with cancer who are treated by radiotherapy for bone pain. In a large randomized trial of radiotherapy for bone pain, the median survival was 6 months as compared with 6 months for patients who underwent surgery (45,48).

The decision to proceed with surgery in patients who are at risk of fracture is a complicated one. Although the avoidance of pathologic fracture is desirable, the principle of prophylactic surgery remains controversial. An attempt should be made to prevent fracture, by radiotherapy and the administration of bisphosphonates. Some studies have suggested that prophylactic fixation can result in decreased morbidity, shorter hospital stays, easier rehabilitation, and more pain relief when compared to fixation of pathologic fractures (49). However, survival curves have shown that if the bone does not fracture within 3 months, the chance of death occurring is 35%. Furthermore, pathologic fractures are relatively rare. In two trials for bone pain the rates for a long bone fracture were only 5 and 10% respectively (48,50). In a

population-based study of patients with cancer the risk of a long bone fracture was 12% (51).

Fracture Risk Assessment

Pathologic fractures of long bones such as the femur and the humerus can be quite debilitating. In the cancer population quantifying the risk of sustaining a pathologic fracture through a metastatic bone lesion is useful because early intervention with radiotherapy, surgery or agents such as bisphosphonates might aid in fracture prevention.

A number of systems have been proposed to assess fracture risk. The two systems most widely used are the Harrington and Mirels system. Harrington recommended prophylactic stabilization when a metastatic lesion was lytic in nature, more than half the diameter of the bone, >2.5 cm in diameter, or was associated with persistent pain or radiographic progression after radiation (1). However the Harrington's criteria have never been validated and their reliability and reproducibility has been questioned.

More recently, Mirels proposed a weighted scoring system to quantify the risk of sustaining a metastatic lesion in a long bone (50). This system objectively analyses and combines four radiologic and clinical risk factors into a single score. The four variables used in Mirels system are: degree of pain, lesional size, lytic versus blastic nature and anatomic location. Each of the four variables is given a score of 1–3 depending on the characteristics found and a total score is obtained by adding the individual scores. Scores range from 4–12 points (Table 52.1). Mirels recommends prophylactic stabilization with scores greater or equal to nine and suggest nonoperative care for patients with scores lower or equal to 7 (52). In an assessment of Mirels' system, reproducibility between observers was good and the sensitivity was 91%, but specificity was only 35%, In this study Mirels' system appear to be reproducible, valid, and more sensitive than clinical judgment (53).

Surgical Treatment of Upper Extremity Bone Lesions

The upper limb is the part of the skeleton least affected by bone metastases. Only 10–15% of bone metastases occur in this region (2). Most of these lesions occur in the humerus. The

TABLE 52.1

MIRELS' SCORING SYSTEM. EACH OF THE FOUR VARIABLES IS GIVEN A SCORE OF 1–3 DEPENDING ON THE CHARACTERISTICS FOUND AND A TOTAL SCORE IS OBTAINED BY ADDING THE INDIVIDUAL SCORES. MIRELS RECOMMENDS PROPHYLACTIC STABILIZATION WITH SCORES GREATER OR EQUAL TO NINE AND SUGGEST NONOPERATIVE CARE FOR PATIENTS WITH SCORES LOWER OR EQUAL TO 7

	Score		
Variable	1	2	3
Site	Upper limb	Lower limb	Peritrochanteric
Pain	Mild	Moderate	Functional
Lesion	Blastic	Mixed	Lytic
Size	<1/3	1/3–2/3	>2/3

proximal third and the diaphysis are the most frequent sites involved. The radius, ulna, and bones of the hand are rarely affected. Upper limb bone lesions present special difficulties as a result of their impact on patient function. Painful metastases in the humerus affect proximal range of motion of the upper extremity and the ability of positioning the hand to perform functional tasks and activities of daily living. The aim of treatment in these patients, as in patients with bone lesions in other regions of the body, is reduction of pain and maintenance or restoration of function. Most patients can be treated effectively with external beam radiation (11). In some cases a custom fitted brace device can be used to control pain.

Humeral Lesions

There are not absolute indications for surgical fixation of humeral lesions. In most cases intramedullary nailing is preferred. Intramedullary fixation has several advantages over plating including decrease surgical approach, decreased surgical operating time and superior biomechanics because fixation points are distant from the lesion (54). However, intramedullary nailing is commonly associated with decrease range of motion of the shoulder and rotator cuff tendinitis.

Intramedullary nailing can be performed by an open or closed technique. Closed nailing is usually selected for patients with minimal bone destruction and an intact segment proximal and distal to the fracture (11). Open nailing is used for fractures with large areas of bone destruction. However, open nailing requires extensive dissection to expose the humeral shaft and can be complicated by tumor bleeding and delayed wound healing (11).

The use of plating for prophylactic fixation has decreased. Plating requires a significant surgical approach because the plate requires a minimum number of cortical engagements to be stable (2). Plating also requires adequate cortical bone proximal and distal to the fracture. The advantages of plate fixation are that the rotator cuff is not subjected to the surgical trauma experienced with nailing.

In select cases when internal fixation cannot be achieved or when articular surfaces have been destroyed, a shoulder or elbow prosthetic device can be utilized. However, prosthetic devices require more surgical dissection and have higher incidence of complications (11).

Hand Lesions

Metastatic bone disease of the hand and wrist is rare. Only 0.1% of all metastatic skeletal lesions occur in this region (55–57). The phalanges are involved more frequently and the distal phalanx is the most common affected site. Metastases in the hand can mimic infections or inflammatory conditions. The median survival for patients with metastatic lesions of the hand is only 6 months. Radiation therapy is not frequently used because postradiation scarring and fibrosis can worsen hand function. Treatment options include simple curettage and cementation of the tumor and ray or a partial hand amputation (55,58).

Surgical Treatment of Lower Extremity Bone Lesions

Femoral and Acetabular Lesions

Patients with pathologic femoral fractures usually experience intense pain and are unable to ambulate. Surgical treatment of these fractures provides immediate reduction in pain and reestablishes walking. Pathologic fractures of the femoral neck are treated by hemiarthroplasty. Cementation of the femoral component is preferred because postoperative radiation may inhibit bone ingrowth. In addition cementation and appropriate soft tissue repair allow immediate full weight bearing. If the acetabulum is free of disease hemiarthroplasty is usually recommended, because of the lower risk of dislocation (56).

Fractures of the diaphysis may be treated with interlocking nails (59). With appropriately positioned interlocking screws placed into the femoral head and neck proximally and through the distal femur, the nail can protect the entire femur providing resistance to torsional and angular displacements. Trochanteric and subtrochanteric pathologic fractures can be fixated using reconstruction nails with locking screws into the femoral head or hemiarthroplasty. Reconstruction nails can potentially stabilize the whole femur and therefore offer some advantages over endoprosthesis.

Pelvic fractures rarely require surgical treatment. However, acetabular fractures cause intense pain and usually require surgical intervention. Acetabular lesions are treated with total hip arthroplasty with acetabular reinforcement by cement, rings, or pins (57).

Surgical Treatment of Spinal Lesions

Spinal metastases are the most common type of spinal tumor. Metastatic spinal cord compression is a medical emergency affecting 5–10% of patients with cancer. Spine metastases can lead to progressive pain and ultimately paralysis from spinal cord compression. Malignant spinal cord compression is most often associated with cancers of the breast, lung, prostate, and other tumors such as myeloma and lymphoma. Treatment does not prolong survival, but may reduce pain and improve quality of life.

Metastases spread to the spine directly or through the arterial or venous epidural plexus. Approximately two thirds of the patients have a single site of spinal cord compression at presentation while one third have multiple sites. Five to 10% of malignancies present initially with cord compression. The thoracic spine is the most commonly affected site.

Pain is the most common symptom in patients with spinal metastases. Movement or recumbency, particularly at night, exacerbates pain from metastatic spine disease. Pain usually increases with cervical spine extension and lateral rotation, straight leg raising, coughing, and local pressure. Cord compression can cause weakness, paresthesias, urinary and fecal incontinence, and autonomic dysfunction.

Patients with metastatic spine disease require judicious evaluation. Urgency for surgical intervention must be established. With severe neurologic deficits, an urgent decompression of the spinal cord combined with spinal stabilization will in many cases restore function. Plain films may show erosion of the pedicles and scalloping. An MRI of the affected area, if readily available and tolerated, should be obtained. A myelogram can be done if MRI is not available.

The goals of surgical treatment are pain control, preservation of spinal stability, maintenance of sphincter control and ability to ambulate. The extent of the disease as well as other medical comorbidities must be taken into consideration before considering surgery. The severity of the neurologic deficit must also be taken into account. If there is evidence of complete spinal cord injury, surgical intervention is unlikely to provide benefit and radiotherapy may be indicated. In patients without neurologic deficit EBRT is the treatment of choice. If survival is expected in the range of 3–6 months, it is reasonable to offer and pursue surgical decompression and stabilization. Recurrence after maximum doses of radiation is another indication for spinal surgery. If EBRT has been attempted and there is clinical deterioration or the tumor is radioresistant, surgical decompression and spinal stabilization should also be considered.

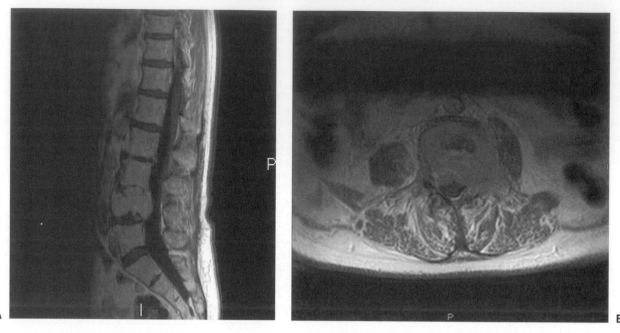

FIGURE 52.1. A and B: Eighty-year-old women with a 1-month history of intractable lower extremity radicular pain and weakness. MRI shows compression fracture of the L4 vertebral body and severe central canal stenosis.

The surgical treatment options can be tailored to the individual patient to allow for appropriate care. In cases of spinal cord compression and instability, simple laminectomy can further destabilize the spine and spinal reconstruction with a titanium cage or cadaveric bone graft is necessary. In these cases, the spine is further stabilized by spinal instrumentation such as pedicles, screws and rods (Fig. 52.1).

Surgical decompression of metastatic disease can also be obtained through minimally invasive spinal surgery technique. This technique involves the use of a tubular dilating system that spares the paraspinal musculature, minimizes disruption of the spine and decreases the chances of spinal instability.

Painful vertebral fractures without cord or root compression can be treated with kyphoplasty or vertebroplasty. In kyphoplasty and vertebroplasty a percutaneous cannula is inserted into the vertebral body through a transpedicular approach and methylmethacrylate is injected into the vertebral body to strengthen the bone and provide pain relief (Fig. 52.2). Kyphoplasty and vertebroplasty are minimally invasive techniques that can be performed under conscious

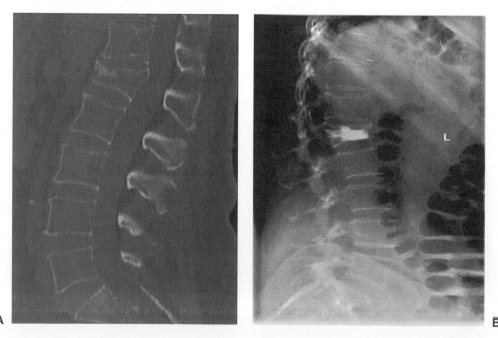

FIGURE 52.2. A and B: Sixty-one-year-old women with a 2-week history of severe upper lumbar pain. Almost complete pain relief was obtained immediately after kyphoplasty. Tissue obtained at the time of kyphoplasty provided diagnosis of carcinoma of the lung.

sedation and have infrequent and minor complications in experienced hands.

RADIATION THERAPY

EBRT provides effective symptomatic treatment for painful metastatic bone lesions. Local radiation therapy has been shown to be effective in relieving pain in 60–90% of patients (59–62). EBRT is also useful in preventing pathologic fractures and treating metastatic spinal cord compression.

It is speculated that EBRT provides pain relief by shrinking the tumor and inhibiting the release of chemical pain mediators. The rapid onset of pain relief is attributed to the decrease of chemical pain mediators whereas tumor shrinkage contributes to the long-lasting effect (5,63–65).

The clinical benefit of EBRT may be observed 24 hours after the initiation of therapy, but most often occurs 1–2 weeks after the first dose. Better responses are noted in patients with breast cancer, prostate cancer, and myeloma. Pain flare may occur in some patients at the beginning of EBRT. This flare usually lasts 2–3 days.

Radiation planning technique and fractionation schedules depend on the aim of therapy and the patient's status and prognosis. Single and multiple fractionated doses have been used with no significant difference in response. A single fraction is the treatment of choice for alleviating bone pain. A single fraction is used to treat both non–weight-bearing bones and weight-bearing bones without large lytic lesions. Terminally ill patients are usually treated with a single fraction. Patients who receive a single dose require further treatment more often than patients that receive multiple fractions (66,67).

Patients who have had surgical stabilization should be treated with EBRT. EBRT has been associated with an increase in functional status and a decrease in second procedures. Radiation is generally initiated 2–4 weeks after surgery. Disease progression occurs in 15–20% of patients treated with only surgery (68,69).

Painful, diffuse, metastatic disease may need hemibody radiation therapy. Most patients may be successfully treated with a single fraction to either the upper or the lower part of the body. A second fraction may be given 4–6 week later to the remaining portion of the body. Responses are usually observed within 24–48 hours (62,70).

Palliative radiotherapy for bone pain is well tolerated. Side effects are related to total dose and fraction size. Pelvic radiation may cause transient nausea and diarrhea. Treatment to the cervical or thoracic spine is associated with mucositis of the throat and esophagus. Radiation to neural structures can cause edema resulting in increase of pain and neurologic symptoms. Nausea, vomiting, and diarrhea frequently complicate large treatments. Radiation pneumonitis is commonly observed in upper body radiation therapy. Myelosuppression occurs in approximately 10% of patients treated with hemibody radiation (62).

Recurrent pain in a previously radiated area represents a significant problem. The tolerance of normal tissues may limit the use of additional radiation therapy. An alternative is to use systemic radiopharmaceuticals. The three approved radiopharmaceuticals used to treat metastatic bone pain are sodium phosphate (^{32}P), strontium chloride (^{89}Sr), and samarium (^{153}Sm) lexidronam. Radiopharmaceuticals are administered intravenously and target the painful bone metastases by accretion to the reactive bone sites with a high lesion-to-normal tissue ratio and a very low concentration in the underlying bone marrow and other structures (71). These agents target predominantly osteoblastic lesions. More than half of the patients who are treated obtain pain relief between 2 and 7 days. Pain relief may last several months after a single injection. Serial injections may be given after partial responses or if symptoms return after recovery of the bone marrow. Myelotoxicity is the major concern with the administration of radiopharmaceuticals to patients with bone metastases. The best results were seen in patients with carcinoma of the prostate (80% response) and breast cancer (89% response) (72). A less favorable response has been observed in patients with end-stage disease (73).

BISPHOSPHONATES

Bisphosphonates are efficacious in the treatment of symptomatic bone metastases and are an important therapeutic option in association with systemic treatments and EBRT. Bisphosphonates have been shown to decrease bone pain, as well as pathologic fractures. These agents are useful in the treatment of metastatic bone disease with marked osteolysis especially in patients with breast cancer and multiple myeloma. Pain relief is usually noted 2 weeks after the start of therapy but is more prominent after 4 months.

The two most commonly used bisphosphonates are pamidronate and zoledronic acid. These agents, like other bisphosphonates, directly inhibit osteoclast activity by cellular mechanisms that affect osteoclast attachment, differentiation, and survival. They also reduce osteoclast activity indirectly through effects on osteoblasts (74).

Bisphosphonates are generally well tolerated. The most common side effect are flu-like symptoms such as fever, arthralgias, and myalgias. These symptoms usually occur 24 hours after the start of therapy (75). Hypocalcemia is common but is rarely associated with symptoms. Supplemental calcium and vitamin D should be prescribed to reduce the risk of symptomatic hypocalcemia.

CORTICOSTEROIDS

Corticosteroids possess analgesic properties for a variety of cancer pain syndromes, including bone pain, neuropathic pain from infiltration or compression of neural structures. Corticosteroids are also effective in managing pain and symptoms from metastatic spinal cord compression (76,77).

Corticosteroids are thought to induce analgesia by decreasing peritumoral edema, inhibiting prostaglandin and leukotriene synthesis and decreasing ephaptic neural discharges.

The ideal corticosteroid, dose, and duration of therapy for bone pain is unknown. The current practice is derived from clinical experience. High doses of corticosteroids (e.g., dexamethasone, 100 mg, followed initially by 96 mg per day in divided doses) have been used for patients with spinal cord compression or an acute episode of severe pain that cannot be relieved with opioids (78). Low doses (e.g., dexamethasone at a dose of 2–4 mg once or twice daily) have been used for patients with advanced cancer who continue to have pain despite the use of opioids. Corticosteroids should be tapered to the lowest effective dose or discontinued to minimize the risk of adverse events.

References

1. Harrington KD. Impending pathologic fractures from metastatic malignancy: evaluation and management. *Instr Course Lect* 1986;35:357–338.
2. Sparkes J. Upper limb bone metastases. *Tech Orthop* 2004;19:9–14.
3. Bauer HCF. Controversies in the surgical management of skeletal metastases. *J Bone Joint Surg Br* 2005;87:608–617.
4. Mercadante S. Malignant bone pain: pathophysiology and treatment. *Pain* 1997;69:1–18.

5. Payne R. Mechanisms and management of bone pain. *Cancer* 1997;80(Suppl 8):1608–1613.
6. Guise TA, Chirgwin JM. Transforming growth factor-beta in osteolytic breast cancer bone metastases. *Clin Orthop* 2003;415(Suppl):S32–S38.
7. Kakonen SM, Mundy GR. Mechanisms of osteolytic bone metastases in breast carcinoma. *Cancer* 2003;97(Suppl 3):834–839.
8. Yazawa Y, Frassica FJ, Chao EYS, et al. Metastatic bone disease: a study of the surgical treatment of 166 pathologic humeral and femoral fractures. *Clin Orthop* 1990;251:213–219.
9. Poulsen HS, Nielsen OS, Klee M, et al. Palliative irradiation of bone metastases. *Cancer Trea Rev* 1989;16:41–44.
10. Wedin R, Bauer HCF, Skoog L, et al. Cytological diagnosis os skeletal lesions: fine-needle aspiration biopsy in 110 tumors. *J Bone Joint Surg Br* 2000;82:673–678.
11. Frassica FJ, Frassica DA. Evaluation and treatment of metastases of the humerus. *Clin Orthop* 2003;415(Suppl):212–218.
12. Solomayer EF, Diel IJ, Meyberg GC, et al. Metastatic breast cancer: clinical course, prognosis and therapy related to the first site of metastasis. *Breast Cancer Res Treat* 2000;59:271–278.
13. Coxon JP, Oades GM, Colston KW, et al. Advances in the use of bisphosphonates in the prostate cancer setting. *Prostate Cancer Prostatic Dis* 2004;7:99–104.
14. Edelstyn GA, Gillespie PJ, Grebbell FS. The radiological demonstration of osseous metastases: experimental observations. *Clin Radiol* 1967;18:158–162.
15. Krasnow AZ, Hellman RS, Timins ME, et al. Diagnostic bone scanning in oncology. *Semin Nucl Med* 1997;27:107–141.
16. Goris ML, Bretille J. Skeletal scintigraphy for the diagnosis of malignant metastatic disease to the bones. *Radiother Oncol* 1985;3:319–329.
17. Tryciecky EW, Gottschalk A, Ludema K. Oncologic imaging: interactions of nuclear medicine with CT and MRI using the bone scan as a model. *Semin Nucl Med* 1997;27:142–151.
18. Coleman RE. Monitoring of bone metastases. *Eur J Cancer* 1998;34:252–259.
19. Haubold-Reuter BG, Duewell S, Schilcher BR, et al. The value of bone scintigraphy, bone marrow scintigraphy and fast spin-echo magnetic resonance imaging in staging of patients with malignant solid tumours: a prospective study. *Eur J Nucl Med* 1999;20:1063–1069.
20. Crippa F, Seregni E, Agresti R, et al. Bone scintigraphy in breast cancer: a ten-year follow-up study. *J Nucl Biol Med* 1993;37:57–56.
21. Gosfield E, Alavi A, Kneeland B. Comparison of radionuclide bone scans and magnetic resonance imaging in detecting spinal metastases. *J Nucl Med* 1993;34:2191–2198.
22. Eustace S, Tello R, DeCarvalho V, et al. A comparison of whole-body turboSTIR MR imaging and planar 99mTc-methylene diphosphonate scintigraphy in the examination of patients with suspected skeletal metastases. *Am J Roentgenol* 1997;169:1655–1661.
23. Han LJ, Au-Yong TK, Tong WC, et al. Comparison of bone single-photon emission tomography and planar imaging in the detection of vertebral metastases in patients with back pain. *Eur J Nucl Med* 1998;25:635–638.
24. Cook GJ, Fogelman I. The role of positron emission tomography in the management of bone metastases. *Cancer* 2000;88:2927–2933.
25. Muindi J, Coombes RC, Golding S, et al. The role of computed tomography in the detection of bone metastases in breast cancer patients. *Br J Radiol* 1983;56:233–236.
26. Kido DK, Gould R, Taati F, et al. Comparative sensitivity of CT scans, radiographs and radionuclide bone scans in detecting metastatic calvarial lesions. *Radiology* 1978;128:371–375.
27. Kattapuram SV, Khurana JS, Scott JA, et al. Negative scintigraphy with positive magnetic resonance imaging in bone metastases. *Skeletal Radiol* 1990;19:113–116.
28. Algra PR, Bloem JL, Tissing H, et al. Detection of vertebral metastases: comparison between MR imaging and bone scintigraphy. *Radiographics* 1991;11:219–232.
29. Steinborn MM, Heuck AF, Tiling R, et al. Whole-body bone marrow MRI in patients with metastatic disease to the skeletal system. *J Comput Assist Tomogr* 1999;23:123–129.
30. Evans AJ, Robertson JF. Magnetic resonance imaging versus radionuclide scintigraphy for screening in bone metastases. *Clin Radiol* 2000;55:653.
31. Zimmer WD, Berquist TH, McLeod RA, et al. Bone tumors: magnetic resonance imaging versus computed tomography. *Radiology* 1985;115:709–718.
32. Dehdashti F, Siegel BA, Griffeth LK, et al. Benign versus malignant intraosseous lesions: discrimination by means of PET with 2-[F-18]fluoro-2-deoxy-D-glucose. *Radiology* 1996;200:243–247.
33. Aoki J, Inoue T, Tomiyoshi K, et al. Nuclear imaging of bone tumors: FDG-PET. *Semin Musculoskelet Radiol* 2001;5:183–187.
34. Malhotra P, Berman C. Evaluation of bone metastases in lung cancer: improved sensitivity and specificity of PET over bone scanning. *Cancer Control* 2002;9:259–260.
35. Shreve PD, Grossman HB, Gross MD, et al. Metastatic prostate cancer: initial findings of PET with 2-deoxy-2-[F-18]fluoro-D-glucose. *Radiology* 1996;199:751–756.
36. Bender H, Kirst J, Palmedo H, et al. Value of 18fluoro-deoxyglucose positron emission tomography in the staging of recurrent breast carcinoma. *Anticancer Res* 1997;17:1687–1692.
37. Bury T, Barreto A, Daenen F, et al. Fluorine-18 deoxyglucose positron emission tomography for the detection of bone metastases in patients with non-small cell lung cancer. *Eur J Nucl Med* 1998;25:1244–1247.
38. Gates GF. SPECT imaging of the lumbosacral spine and pelvis. *Clin Nucl Med* 1988;13:907–914.
39. Podoloff DA, Kim EE, Haynie TP. SPECT in the evaluation of cancer patients: not quo vadis; rather, ibi fere summus. *Radiology* 1992;183:305–317.
40. Savelli G, Chiti A, Grasselli G, et al. The role of bone SPECT study in diagnosis of single vertebral metastases. *Anticancer Res* 2000;20:1115–1120.
41. Kosuda S, Kaji T, Yokoyama H, et al. Does bone SPECT actually have lower sensitivity for detecting vertebral metastasis than MRI? *J Nucl Med* 1996;37:975–978.
42. Han LJ, Au-Yong TK, Tong WC, et al. Comparison of bone single-photon emission tomography and planar imaging in the detection of vertebral metastases in patients with back pain. *Eur J Nucl Med* 1998;25:635–663.
43. Hansen BH, Keller J, Laitinen M, et al. The Scandinavian sarcoma group skeletal metastasis register. Survival after surgery for bone metastases in the pelvis and extremities. *Acta Orthop Scand* 2004;75(Suppl 311):11–15.
44. Bono B, Cazzaniga P, Zurrida SM, et al. Palliative surgery of metastatic bone disease: a review of 83 cases. *Eur J Cancer* 1991;27:556–558.
45. Bauer HFC, Wedin R. Survival after surgery for spinal and extremity metastases. Prognostication in 241 patients. *Acta Orthop Scand* 1995;66:143–146.
46. Rex A, Marco W, Dhiren S, et al. Functional and oncological outcome of acetabular reconstruction for the treatment of metastatic disease. *J Bone Joint Surg* 2000;82:642.
47. Bohm P, Huber J. The surgical treatment of bony metastases of the spine and limbs. *J Bone Joint Surg Br* 2002;84:551–529.
48. Steenland E, Leer J, Van Houwelingen H, et al. The effect of a single fraction compared to multiple fractions on painful bone metastases: a global analysis of the Dutch bone metastases study. *Radiother Oncol* 1999;52:101–109.
49. Popken F, Schmidt J, Oegur H, et al. Treatment outcome after preventive stabilization vs management after pathological fracture. *Unfallchirurg* 2002;105:338–343.
50. Bone Trial Working Party. 8 Gy single fraction radiotherapy for the treatment of metastatic skeletal pain; randomized comparison with a multifraction schedule over 12 months of patient follow-up. *Radiother Oncol* 1999;52:111–121.
51. Wedin R, Bauer HCF, Rutqvist L. Incidence and outcome of surgical treatment for skeletal breast cancer metastases: a population based study of 641 patients. *Cancer* 2001;92:257–262.
52. Mirels H. Metastatic disease in long bones: a proposed scoring system for diagnosing impending pathologic fractures. *Clin Orthop* 1989;249:256–264.
53. Damron TA, Morgan H, Prakash D, et al. Critical evaluation of Mirel's rating system for impending pathologic fractures. *Clin Orthop* 2003;415(Suppl):201–207.
54. Damron TA, Rock MG, Choudhury SN, et al. Biomechanical analysis of prophylactic fixation form middle third humeral impending pathological fractures. *Clin Orthop* 1999;363:240–248.
55. Hayden RJ, Sullivan LG, Jebson PJ. The hand in metastatic disease and acral manifestations of paraneoplastic syndromes. *Hand Clin* 2004;20:335–343.
56. Weber KL, O'Connor MI. Operative treatment of long bone metastases: focus on the femur. *Clin Orthop* 2003;415(Suppl):276–278.
57. Hansen BH, Keller J, Laitinen M, et al. The Scandinavian sarcoma group skeletal metastasis register. Survival after surgery for bone metastases in the pelvis and extremities. *Acta Orthop Scand* 2004;75(Suppl 311):11–15.
58. Healey JH, Turnbull AD, Miedema B, et al. Acrometastases. A study of twenty-nine patients with osseous involvement of the hands and feet. *J Bone Joint Surg* 1986;68:743–746.
59. Blitzer PH. Reanalysis of the RTOG study of the palliation of symptomatic osseous metastases. *Cancer* 1985;55:1468–1472.
60. Friedland J. Local and systemic radiation for palliation of metastatic disease. *Urol Clin North Am* 1999;26:391–402.
61. Hoskin PJ. Radiotherapy in the management of bone pain. *Clin Orthop* 1995;312:105–119.
62. Salazar OM, Rubin P, Hendrickson FR, et al. Single dose half body irradiation for palliation of multiple bone metastases from solid tumors. *Cancer* 1986;58:29–36.
63. Hoskin PJ. Scientific and clinical aspects of radiotherapy in the relief of bone pain. *Cancer Surv* 1988;7:69–86.
64. Price P, Hoskin PJ, Easton D, et al. Prospective randomised trial of single and multifraction radiotherapy schedules in the treatment of painful bony metastases. *Radiother Oncol* 1986;6:247–255.
65. Mercadante S. Malignant bone pain: pathophysiology and treatment. *Pain* 1997;69:1–18.
66. Steenland E, Lee J, van Houwelingen H, et al. The effect of single fraction compared to multiple fractions in painful bone metastases: a global analysis of the Dutch Bone Metastasis Study. *Radiat Oncol* 1999;52:101–109.
67. Hoskin PJ, Ford HT, Harmer CL. Hemibody irradiation for metastatic bone pain in two histologically distinct groups of patients. *Clin Pathol* 1991;3:67–69.
68. Townsend PW, Smalley SR, Cozad SC, et al. Role of postoperative radiation therapy after stabilization of fractures caused by metastatic disease. *Int J Radiat Oncol Biol Phys* 1995;31:43–49.
69. Townsend PW, Rosenthal HG, Smalley SR, et al. Impact of postoperative radiation therapy and other perioperative factors on outcome after

orthopedic stabilization of impending or pathologic fractures. *J Clin Oncol* 1994;12:2345–2350.

70. Poulter CA, Cosmatos D, Rubin P, et al. A report of RTOG 8206: a phase III study of whether the addition of single dose hemibody irradiation to standard fractionated local field irradiation is more effective than local field irradiation alone in the treatment of symptomatic osseous metastases. *Int J Radiat Oncol Biol Phys* 1992;23:207–214.

71. Serafini AN. Therapy of metastatic bone pain. *J Nucl Med* 2001;42:895–906.

72. Robinson RG, Spicer JA, Preston DA, et al. Treatment of metastatic bone pain with strontium-89. *Int J Rad Appl Instrum B* 1987;14:219–222.

73. Rogers CL, Speiser BL, Ram PC, et al. Efficacy and toxicity of intravenous strontium-89 for symptomatic osseous metastasis. *Brachyther Int* 1998;4:133–142.

74. Michaelson MD, Smith MR. Bisphosphonates for treatment and prevention of bone metastases. *J Clin Oncol* 2005;23:8219–8224.

75. Zojer N, Keck AV, Pecherstorfer M. Comparative tolerability of drug therapies for hypercalcaemia of malignancy. *Drug Saf* 1999;21:389–406.

76. Greenberg HS, Kim JH, Posner JB. Epidural spinal cord compression from metastatic tumor: results with a new treatment protocol. *Ann Neurol* 1980;8:361–366.

77. Vecht CJ, Haaxma-Reiche H, van Putten WL, et al. Initial bolus of conventional versus high-dose dexamethasone in metastatic spinal cord compression. *Neurology* 1989;39:1255–1257.

78. Ettinger AB, Portenoy RK. The use of corticosteroids in the treatment of symptoms associated with cancer. *J Pain Symptom Manage* 1988;3:99–103.

CHAPTER 53 ■ PALLIATIVE ENDOSCOPIC AND INTERVENTIONAL RADIOLOGIC PROCEDURES

ANN MARIE JOYCE, ROSEMARY C. POLOMANO, MICHAEL C. SOULEN, AND MICHAEL L. KOCHMAN

Palliation of symptoms associated with advanced cancer can be accomplished through less invasive and more cost-efficient endoscopic and radiologic methods when compared with standard open surgical procedures. Specialization in oncologic procedures by gastroenterologists and interventional radiologists has spared many patients additional loss of time and postoperative pain associated with aggressive surgical interventions (1–3). Technologic advances and refinements in endoscopic and interventional radiologic procedures have eliminated the need for extensive surgeries and possibly lengthy recuperation in these patients, and have decreased the risks of associated complications. Patency of the gastrointestinal (GI) tract affected by cancerous tumor growth or strictures caused by radiotherapy can be restored with minimal discomfort and without significant threat to the patient's well-being. Internal and external drainage systems can be placed to relieve organ obstruction pain and inanition, and to prevent life-threatening end-organ dysfunction. Table 53.1 outlines palliative endoscopic and interventional procedures.

GASTROINTESTINAL TUBES FOR DECOMPRESSION AND NUTRITION

Nearly half of all patients undergoing gastrostomy and jejunostomy have cancer. Although most of them require GI tubes for enteral nutrition, gastrostomies and jejunostomies are inserted in a select group of patients for the purposes of decompression and drainage of intestinal obstructions. Approximately 40% of patients with ovarian cancer and as many as 28% of patients with colorectal cancer are at risk for developing bowel obstruction (4). Isolated malignant foci or widespread carcinomatosis of the abdomen causing external compression of GI structures are common causes of obstruction. Occlusion of the gastric outlet or intestine by tumor and adhesions from prior surgery, radiotherapy, and intraperitoneal chemotherapy are other mechanisms for gastric and intestinal blockages. Cramping and intestinal distention may be transiently relieved by vomiting, belching, flatus, and defecation; however, the unremitting cycle of these symptoms is often physically and emotionally intolerable. When initial management with aggressive pharmacotherapy, bowel rest, and temporary nasogastric decompression fails, GI decompression should be considered. Intolerable pain, fecal vomitus, intractable nausea or emesis,

and esophageal ulceration are clear indications for venting gastrostomies or jejunostomies (5–7).

Gastrostomy and jejunostomy, whether intended for venting purposes or for feeding, can be accomplished through surgical, radiologic, or endoscopic techniques (Table 53.2). In some instances endoscopic placement can be technically difficult because of carcinomatosis or ascites. A recent retrospective review of all patients with percutaneous endoscopic gastrostomy (PEG) placement for intestinal obstruction secondary to recurrent ovarian cancer demonstrated that it is possible to safely and effectively place a PEG in patients with diffuse carcinomatosis and ascites (8). Diffuse carcinomatosis was identified in 70 of the 77 patients who had a computed tomography (CT) scan before the procedure with ascites noted in 63% of the patients. Symptomatic relief was demonstrated in 86 (91%) of the 94 patients. The mean number of days to achieve relief was 1.7. There was a complication recognized in 17 of the 94 patients; the most common was leakage.

In a meta-analysis of the efficacy and safety of each technique (9), the 30-day mortality rate (8%) was the same for both radiologic and percutaneous endoscopic approaches. Statistical analyses revealed significantly fewer complications ($p < .001$) and decreased mortality ($p < .001$) with radiologic techniques compared to surgery and PEG. These data must be interpreted cautiously, as subset analyses were not performed. In some patients a gastrostomy or jejunostomy tube (J-tube) is not effective to relieve the obstruction or cannot be placed. An alternative type of decompressive tube, a cecostomy placed radiologically or endoscopically, has been tried in a few select patients with promising results (10).

Techniques for Gastrostomy and Jejunostomy Placement

Endoscopic Placement

Both percutaneous radiologic and endoscopic placement of gastrostomy tubes (G-tubes) and J-tubes for decompression and feeding provide an acceptable alternative to the uncomfortable presence of nasogastric tubes, and eliminate the need for operative procedures (6,11). Insertion of PEG involves a standard upper endoscopy with conscious sedation. After endoscopic examination of the stomach and duodenum to exclude significant ulcerations, the anterior gastric body

TABLE 53.1

COMMON ENDOSCOPIC AND INTERVENTIONAL PROCEDURES FOR ONCOLOGY PATIENTS

Type of procedure	Indication	Description of procedure	Considerations for oncology care (preprocedure/pain management/follow-up care)
Enteral tube placement for feeding percutaneous endoscopic gastrostomy/decompression	Enteral feedings in the absence of the ability to self-feed; decompression of gastrointestinal obstruction; nutritional support to prevent inanition and improve sense of well-being and functional status	The stomach or jejunum is punctured through the skin using x-ray guidance. The tract is dilated, and an 18- to 20-French tube is placed into the stomach and secured at the exit site of the skin	Preprocedure: antibiotics, coagulation and platelet determinations. Postprocedure: local wound care, possible need for temporary pain management
Tracheobronchial or esophageal stenting	Airway or esophageal intrinsic obstruction, extrinsic compression, or tracheoesophageal fistula; relief of obstruction or fistula closure to allow oral nutrition	Obstruction or fistula crossed with a guidewire under fluoroscopic/endoscopic guidance. Tumor is dilated if needed; expandable stent is placed under fluoroscopic/endoscopic guidance	Preprocedure: barium study, coagulation and platelet determinations, assurance of patient motivation. Postprocedure: barium study, possible need for temporary pain management, lifelong histamine type 2 receptor antagonist therapy, head of bed up to 30, aspiration precautions, modified diet
Percutaneous nephrostomy/stent	Ureteral obstruction; preserve renal function and prevent renal infection	Renal calyx is punctured with an 18- to 22-gauge needle through the skin under radiologic guidance. Tract is dilated, and the nephrostomy tube is placed. Stricture may be crossed, biopsied, or dilated, then stented	Preprocedure: coagulation, platelet, BUN, and creatinine determinations. Postprocedure: local wound care, possible need for temporary pain management, serial BUN and creatinine, monitoring of urine output
PTBD and ERBD with stent	Obstructive jaundice, cholangitis, and pruritus; relief of pruritus, prevention of systemic sepsis, and improvement in sense of well-being. Literature documents that ERBD is safer overall because of avoidance of puncture of liver capsule and placement of the catheters through hepatic parenchyma (3)	PTBD: bile duct is punctured with an 18- to 21-gauge needle under x-ray guidance. Tract is dilated and an 8- to 12-French tube is placed into the biliary tree-duodenum. Strictures are biopsied and dilated. Possible interval conversion to purely internal plastic or metal stent. ERBD: bile duct is cannulated at endoscopic retrograde cholangiopancreatography. Strictures are biopsied and dilated. Stricture may be stented with removable plastic or permanent metal stents. Nasobilary tube may be placed to facilitate/aid PTBD	Preprocedure: antibiotics, coagulation, platelet, and bilirubin determinations. Postprocedure: possible local wound care, possible need for temporary pain management, serial bilirubin to verify function
Embolization/chemoembolization	Treatment of unresectable, locally confined tumor; facilitate surgical resection; decrease tumor burden to improve sense of well-being and functional status	Hepatic artery providing blood supply to the tumor is identified and selectively catheterized. Embolic agents are injected into the vessel to occlude blood flow. Chemotherapeutic agents may be added to the embolic mixture for enhanced local effect	Preprocedure: coagulation, platelet, BUN, and creatinine, liver function test determinations. Postprocedure: local wound care, possible need for temporary pain management, evaluation for systemic effects. Management of postembolization syndrome (nausea and vomiting, fever, pain)

BUN, blood urea nitrogen; ERBD, endoscopic retrograde biliary drainage; PTBD, percutaneous transhepatic biliary drainage.
Adapted from Adelson MD, Kasowitz MH. Percutaneous endoscopic drainage gastrostomy in the treatment of gastrointestinal obstruction from intraperitoneal malignancy. *Obstet Gynecol* 1993;81:467, Table 53.2, with permission.

TABLE 53.2

GASTROSTOMY TUBE PLACEMENT

Technique	Advantage	Disadvantage
Endoscopic	Visualize upper gastrointestinal tract Least costly method	Technically difficult in patients with ascites, carcinomatosis, esophageal obstruction Risk of tumor seeding (not a concern for palliative use)
Radiologic	Preferred in patients with old tracts, even if closed Less risk of tumor seeding of ear, nose, and throat malignancies	Technically difficult in patients with esophageal obstruction
Surgery	Most successful	Longer recovery Most expensive

or antrum is transilluminated and the gastric body is fully insufflated. Using the endoscopic light source, a suitable area on the anterior abdominal wall is identified and the suitability of the site for a percutaneous tract is confirmed by gentle external compression at the potential entry site. These maneuvers allow for the determination of a safe site with the absence of any intervening viscera or major blood vessels. With some exceptions, dependent on the type of G-tube to be inserted and operator preference, a needle or trocar is passed into the gastric lumen and a guidewire is then threaded through the hollow needle and retrieved endoscopically. The guidewire is then pulled up to the patient's oropharynx and the G-tube is passed over the wire into the stomach and out of the anterior abdominal wall. Firm traction is applied to ensure passage of the internal bolster through the esophagus and to allow a traction seal and apposition of the gastric and abdominal walls to minimize leakage of gastric contents or feedings.

Recently, endoscopic ultrasound (EUS) has been used as an adjunct to aid in the endoscopic placement of G-tubes when the transillumination and indentation are not optimal (12). The advantage of this technique is that it may be performed in formerly complicated situations, including previously operated abdomens and in partial gastrectomy patients. The use of EUS imaging significantly improves visualization of the bowel and gastric viscera, which might otherwise be impeded by the formation of adhesions, presence of taut peritoneum or ascites, or diffuse intra-abdominal metastases. As a result, risks of inadvertent perforation of bowel, other organs, and metastatic foci are minimized. Studies show promising results over conventional procedures in facilitating ease of insertion and decreasing morbidity associated with the procedure (5).

Esophageal stents may be unsuccessful for palliation of patients with malignant dysphagia or in the management of tracheoesophageal (TE) fistulae. In some cases, the stent placement appears to be successful but the patient continues to have poor intake and may require enteral access. Placing a percutaneous gastrostomy was thought to be problematic in the setting of an esophageal stent but a small case series reviewed the success in eight patients (13). A PEG was placed in all nine patients but stent migration into the stomach was noted in one of the nine patients. This was managed endoscopically. Larger studies are needed to safety of this approach.

Radiologic Placement

Radiologic gastrostomy is performed using fluoroscopic guidance under local anesthetic, with conscious sedation if needed. If swallowing function is intact and there is no GI obstruction, the patient is given oral contrast the night before to opacify the transverse colon and splenic flexure the next day. A nasogastric tube is placed and the stomach insufflated with air. Ultrasound (US) is used to mark the left lobe of the liver if it crosses over the stomach. The anterior wall of the stomach is then punctured through the abdominal wall under fluoroscopy, avoiding both the colon and the liver. Aspiration of air and injection of contrast confirm that the needle tip is within the stomach. One or more "T-anchors" are placed for gastropexy, then the puncture tract is dilated over a guidewire and the tube placed. In patients with aspiration risk, the pylorus is crossed and a gastrojejunostomy catheter is placed with the tip beyond the ligament of Treitz. Single- or double-lumen catheters are available, with the second lumen allowing decompression of the stomach as well as jejunal feeding. The catheter is left to external drainage for 24 hours, and the patient is monitored for peritoneal signs. If the tube is to be used for feeding, an enteral cap is placed and feeds begun with water or dextrose solution at 30 mL per hour, which is advanced as tolerated. Peritoneal leakage, procedure-induced ileus, or bowel dysmotility may limit advancement of feeds.

Complications

Technical difficulties encountered during insertion tend to be relatively low, ranging from 4–8% (5,7,11,14,15). The inability to implant G-tubes has been attributed to tumor invasion of anterior gastric wall, anatomical anomalies, and massive ascites (11,16,17). Overall, such difficulties seem to be noted more frequently with endoscopic placement than for radiologic guidance (9). Complication rates for both procedures vary from study to study, and must be cautiously interpreted in view of different methods of placement, operator experience, and diversity of patients. Procedure-related deaths, typically defined as mortality within 30 days of the procedure, have been reported (9). However, mortality rates within 30 days of the procedure may reflect consequences of the underlying disease and the overall poor status of the patients rather than direct consequence of the procedure. Significant risks for complications include urinary tract infection, previous aspiration, and age >75 years (18).

Intestinal (colonic) perforation, peritonitis, and gastric hemorrhage are among the most serious complications. Isolated occurrences of mechanical intra-abdominal seeding of tumor (19) and stomal seeding (20) have been reported. Although the diameter of the lumen might be expected to increase adverse effects, Cannizzaro et al. found no appreciable differences in symptomatic relief and placement-related complications between patients who received 15- and 20-French lumen catheters (5). Prophylactic use of preprocedure and postprocedure antibiotic administration has been used to reduce the incidence of infection. The data are not clear, but it appears that the preprocedure use of antibiotics reduces the postprocedure incidence of tube site cellulitis and fasciitis. Meticulous cleansing of the tube site with an iodine prep or antibacterial soap and application of a sterile gauze dressing minimizes early wound infections. Once the sutures are removed (if used) and the subcutaneous tract has sealed (in approximately 3 weeks), no additional care to the site is generally required.

Jejunostomy Tube Placement

Radiologic and endoscopic placements of jejunostomies are valuable techniques associated with low risks while avoiding the need for surgery. Tubes can be placed into the jejunum indirectly through a gastric puncture site, such as a double-lumen gastrojejunostomy tube or a J-tube threaded through a G-tube (17,21). Alternatively, direct endoscopic jejunostomy is placed using methods similar to PEG placement with good success rates, low complication rates, and high patient satisfaction (22,23). The tubes are inserted distal to the ligament of Treitz under conscious sedation. The advantage of this technique is the relative stability of the direct J-tube placement in comparison with a J-tube threaded through a G-tube. In a study that compared the complications and the need for intervention with direct percutaneous endoscopic jejunostomy (D-PEJ) and percutaneous endoscopic gastrostomy with jejunostomy extension (PEG-J) revealed that 5 (13.5%) of 37 patients in the D-PEJ group required endoscopic reintervention compared with 19 (55.9%) of 34 patients in PEG-J group over a 6-month period (23). Eight of those 19 patients required the J-tube extension to be replaced at a mean of 33 days. Insertion of percutaneous jejunostomy catheters are more easily accomplished when a J-tube has previously been present because the small bowel is adherent to the abdominal wall, creating a secure tract. The bowel loop can be punctured under fluoroscopic or endoscopic guidance, the tract dilated, and a new tube placed. The absence of a well-established access site makes the initial percutaneous procedure technically more difficult because of bowel mobility. In these circumstances, a gastrojejunostomy catheter may be needed. Magnetic technology, which allows for transient fixation of otherwise mobile bowel segments against the anterior abdominal wall, may allow for easier endoscopic placement of J-tubes. This has been studied in a swine model, and holds promise for direct endoscopic enteral tube placement using minimally invasive techniques (24).

Considerations with Gastrointestinal Tube Placement

Several factors must be taken into account to select the best method and site of GI tube insertion. Both radiologic and endoscopic methods have similar procedural success rates, 30-day mortality rates, and types of complications (9,17). Local expertise and patient factors should be considered in selecting the appropriate method of placement. For instance, in patients with severe pharyngeal or esophageal strictures that prevent the passage of an endoscope, radiologic guidance may be preferred (17). It is also preferred to have radiologic placement in those who have old tracks that have healed. In other patients, who need visual investigation of the upper GI tract, endoscopic guidance is favored.

Other factors are considered in selecting the appropriate site of GI tube placement (gastric vs. jejunal). Feeding gastrostomies are preferred over jejunostomies for patients who may require skilled nursing placement, as J-tubes tend to fall out and clog more, frequently requiring more follow-up interventions.

Venting gastrostomies are indicated for patients with high upper intestinal or gastric outlet obstructions, whereas venting jejunostomies are more effective for decompression of intestinal obstructions that are more distal. Patients at risk for aspiration through emesis, as opposed to oropharyngeal dysphagia, are better candidates for jejunostomy feeding tubes. Through the use of a dual-lumen gastrojejunostomy tube, an artificial GI bypass can be constructed with a venting gastrostomy above the obstruction, enabling enteral feedings through a jejunostomy below the obstruction (25). Recently developed endoscopic techniques may mature allowing for endoscopic creation of gastrojejunostomies.

Lumen size appears to be more of an issue for patients who require intermittent or continuous decompression and wish to ingest soft food and fluids. Modifications in the contour of the tube and outflow portion, rather than lumen size, seem to be most critical in maximizing the flow of GI secretions mixed with semisolid foods and liquids (14). It is necessary to ensure that the tube selected for any patient is appropriate for its intended purpose. Some tubes now have one-way valves, which decrease the likelihood of patients expelling gastric contents if the end seal is loose, but these tubes are not suitable for gastric decompression. Most tubes are now designed in such a manner that they may be removed through firm traction and do not require repeat surgery or endoscopic procedure solely for removal. Replacement button devices and stomal tubes are available.

Above all, patient and family acceptance, motivation, and ability to care for the tube or administer feedings are critically important in the successful management of GI intubation. Patients and families are instructed to do the following:

1. Care for the tube exit site
2. Observe the site for any peristomal redness, ulceration, or drainage
3. Flush, cap, and connect the tube to the appropriate devices

The tube can be anchored to the abdomen with special securing devices. Arrangements for home health care are coordinated if patients are immediately discharged to home after tube placement, require nutritional support (enteral or total parenteral) or fluid replacement, or need additional teaching after hospitalization. This is necessary to assure proper monitoring as feeds are initiated and advanced, as well as to assist the patient and family with wound care and help them select an appropriate drainage container and operate suction devices for venting tubes.

Costs associated with the procedure must also be considered. Endoscopically and radiologically placed tubes can avoid the use of the operating room and general anesthesia, and their attendant costs and risks. Charges for PEG placement have been assessed around $2400 and radiologic placement at $4500 (9). Estimated reimbursement for professional fees remains similar, and for inpatients, the hospital reimbursement for the procedure is generally embedded into the fixed rate established for the diagnostic category.

PALLIATIVE MANAGEMENT OF GASTROINTESTINAL AND BILIARY OBSTRUCTION

Malignant intrinsic obstructions or extrinsic compressions of GI structures can be relieved through the placement of endoprostheses made from materials that restore both patency and function of the esophagus, colon, rectum, and biliary and pancreatic ducts. Over the past decade a dramatic improvement in the materials, design, and delivery systems has served to make these procedures both widely disseminated and less dangerous.

Esophageal Endoprosthetics

Indications

Esophageal endoprosthetic intubation is used to treat esophageal compression from locally advanced esophageal, mediastinal, or tracheobronchial malignancies, as well as strictures that may have resulted from prior radiotherapy. Endoprostheses (stents) also allow for the palliation and occlusion of TE fistula, permitting oral intake. The insertion of an artificial tube restores patency of the esophagus and can provide relief from dysphagia, pain, and the inability to swallow or effectively clear oral secretions.

Relative contraindications for the placement of esophageal stents include extensive circumferential tumor growth that occludes the lumen and interferes with passage of a guidewire and dilators, necrotic lesions that may hemorrhage, friable tissues that increase the chance for perforation, anticipated discomfort associated with the presence of the stent, and lack of patient acceptance or compliance with dietary modifications and follow-up care. The stents may leave a patient with a persistent globus sensation if placed within 2 cm of the upper esophageal sphincter. The placement of a stent into a fibrotic (post-therapy) stricture or one resistant to dilatation may result in mediastinal pain, as the pressure exerted by the stent in its attempt to deploy continues until full expansion.

Types of Stents

A variety of rigid and metal self-expandable stents are available as endoprosthetic devices. Selection of stents is dependent on several factors, including life expectancy, pattern of tumor growth (e.g., location, orientation of tumor invasion, extent of invasion, size), anticipated complications, and desired treatment outcomes (Table 53.3). Rigid stents have been manufactured from several materials, including polyvinyl tubing, silicone with metal reinforcements (Wilson-Cook, Wilson-Cook, Inc., Winston-Salem, NC), radiopaque silicone with metal reinforcements (Atkinson tube, Key-Med, Inc., Essex, UK). Promising results have been reported using cuffed

TABLE 53.3

RELATIVE INDICATIONS FOR RIGID AND EXPANDABLE METAL ENDOPROSTHESES

Situation	Rigid stents	Expandable metal stents
Cancer within 2 cm of upper esophageal sphincter	—	—
Airway compression by tube	—	–
Limited life expectancy	—	—
Lack of patient motivation	—	—
Luminal obstruction preventing passage of a guidewire	—	—
Noncircumferential tumors preventing anchoring of the stent	—	+
Soft or necrotic lesions with poor anchoring qualities	—	+
Profusely bleeding lesions	–	–
Horizontal orientation of the malignant lumen	–	+
Acutely angulated complex lesions	–	+

+, preferred; −, suboptimal; —, to be avoided if possible.

rigid stents in managing life-threatening sequelae associated with TE fistulas (26,27). Patients with TE fistulas tend to be poor surgical candidates because of respiratory distress, malnutrition, and debilitation from advanced stages of cancer. Mortality rates as high as 36% have been documented with attempts to surgically repair this type of fistula; however, peroral intubation using a cuffed rigid stent to seal off the fistula has reduced mortality to 24% (26). Expandable cuffs attached to rigid endoprostheses have been successful in occluding fistulas with less patient discomfort and reduced hospitalization compared to surgery, and without the risk of pressure necrosis (27).

The introduction of metal self-expanding esophageal stents, patterned after biliary and vascular stents, has minimized problems associated with the rigid polymeric stents and their fixed lumen diameters. Although self-expanding metal stents are approximately 10 times more expensive, their advantages of larger lumen size, ease of insertion, decreased complication rates, and greater success with more stenotic lesions often outweigh any cost expenditures. All of the metal stents share an ability to be placed into a narrow lumen on a small-bore delivery device and then allowed to expand once in correct anatomical position. Technical success rates for deployment are reported to be >95%, with significant improvement in dysphagia and tolerability of oral intake (28–31). A variety of self-expanding metallic stents are available that differ in design, elasticity, and resistance to angulation (32). Knowledge of their physical properties and tumor characteristics/anatomy can help in selecting the appropriate stent for a particular patient.

Some metallic self-expanding stents are covered with a polymeric sheet to inhibit tumor ingrowth and to facilitate occlusion of TE fistula tracts and have become the preferred design for most indications in the esophagus (31,33). A prospective, randomized study was performed to compare three covered metal stents: Gianturco-Z stent (Wilson-Cook, Bjaeverskov, Denmark), Flamingo Wallstent (Bulach, Switzerland), and Ultraflex stent (Microvasive Endoscopy/Boston Scientific, Natick, MA) (34). The study demonstrated that there were no differences in the technical success in placement, relief of dysphagia, mortality at 30 days and median survival among the three stents. There was a higher complication rate (36%) with the Gianturco-Z stent compared to the two other stents, but this result was not statistically significant ($p = .23$).

Antireflux stents have been developed to decrease reflux symptoms after placement for tumors near the gastroesophageal junction. Patients who have a stent placed across the gastroesophageal junction experience severe reflux, and this can result in aspiration pneumonia. Newer stents have been developed that have an artificial sleeve or valve to prevent reflux. Small studies have shown that these revised stents decrease reflux episodes (35,36).

Unlike rigid stents that can be taken out, metal self-expanding tubes are virtually impossible to remove short of an open surgical procedure, due to the expandable nature of the device and the design which favors an inflammatory tissue response which, while it decreases migration, causes difficulty with removal. One of the newer stents on the market is the Polyflex stent which is a silicone covered nonmetallic stent. Its major advantage is that it can be removed. The Polyflex stent (Boston Scientific, Natick, MA) is made of Trevira monofilaments with a silicone coat. The stent has a smooth inner surface and it a high expansive force. This stent was first introduced for the treatment of benign esophageal strictures but the indications are expanding to include patients with a malignant stricture who are undergoing chemoradiotherapy. Palliative radiation is effective in 60–80% of patients but it takes up to 4–6 weeks to see the improvement with dysphagia. Placement of a removable stent in this patient group is beneficial for reducing complications and related reintervention as demonstrated by Shin et al. (37).

In initial reports, Castamanga et al. showed a technical success rate of 75% of patients with inoperable esophageal strictures (38). In 4 of the 16 patients the stent placement was unsuccessful. In three of those patients, the delivery system could not be advanced across the stricture and in the one patient the stent did not open. In another similar study, the success rate was 100%. The disadvantages of the Polyflex stent include the bulky delivery system therefore resulting in the possible need for dilation and the resultant higher rate of stent migration (39).

Complications

Perforation, stent migration, pain, and hemorrhage are among the most common complications of esophageal stents. Perforation is the most serious complication and occurs with a frequency of approximately 6–8% with the rigid endoprostheses (40,41). The rate of perforation is <3% with the metallic self-expandable stents (28–31,42). Perforation may occur as a result of the endoscopy, esophageal dilatation, or the endoprosthetic placement itself. Factors associated with a higher incidence of perforation include prior radiotherapy and surgical intervention, sharp angulation from tortuous tumor involvement, and preexisting kyphoscoliosis. In most cases, perforations are identified at the time of stent placement by careful endoscopic inspection of the esophagus and pharynx, the physical examination findings of subcutaneous emphysema or crepitation of air, and radiographic detection of extraluminal air in the chest and neck areas. The exact location of a leak can be detected by the use of water-soluble contrast media.

Perforation always carries a risk for accompanying mediastinitis. Once identified, the use of acid-suppressive agents and intravenous antibiotics are the mainstays of therapy; the stent itself may seal off the site of the perforation. Consideration for the placement of an additional endoprosthetic or surgical repair may need to be entertained for open communicating tracts.

Stent migration and dislodgement may complicate metallic stent placement in up to 5% of patients (31). Some stents are designed to decrease migration (30), but further studies ascertaining their effectiveness for this complication are needed. Barium studies postprocedure documents location and function of the stent, and provides a baseline should migration be suspected in the future. Tumor ingrowth occludes stents in approximately 10–60% of cases, depending on the type of endoprosthesis used, the indication, and its length, and occurs a mean of 7 weeks postprocedure (28,31).

Bleeding related to expandable metallic stent placement occurs in <5% of cases (29,31). This is often insignificant, but more serious hemorrhage requiring transfusions has been reported (29). Aspiration may occur either during the placement of the endoprosthetic or subsequently, due to reflux of gastric contents. It is important to instruct patients that they should not lie supine or prone after placement; this is especially critical when the endoprosthetic bridges the gastroesophageal junction. A persistent globus sensation may occur if the stent is placed in the proximal esophagus, usually within 2 cm of the upper esophageal sphincter. Mediastinal pain may occur in 5–15% of patients, most often in those with preexisting pain or extraesophageal tumors (28,31,42).

It is useful to have a preprocedure barium study to assess for sharp angulation, unsuspected perforation, distance from the upper esophageal sphincter, and presence of fistula. Despite concern over complications of esophageal endoprosthetic placement, this procedure is relatively safe and offers considerable benefits for optimizing oral nutrition and improving quality of life. Patients are advised to gradually increase the consistency of their food but to avoid solid meats, breads, and baked products.

Colorectal Endoprostheses

Indications

The introduction of colorectal stents, designed similar to esophageal prostheses, has successfully relieved colorectal stenosis from obstructing tumors, particularly in patients with metastatic disease who are not potentially curable. Traditionally, a diverting colostomy was created as the standard for management of large bowel obstruction. If this surgery is done in the emergency setting, there is an increased mortality and morbidity rate. The tumors may involve the colon, rectum, bladder, ovary, or prostate. Most large bowel obstructions (70%) occur on the left side of the colon (43). In selected cases, endoprosthetic devices may be implanted for acute management of intestinal obstruction to allow for luminal decompression before palliative and definitive surgical resection (44,45). In other cases, colorectal stenting has been advocated as a primary palliative treatment (46). A review of the literature of 28 case series regarding colonic stenting revealed that stents were quite effective with low mortality and morbidity rates. Technical success was achieved in 92% of patients and clinical success was noted in 88% of patients. There was a mortality rate of 1% and perforation noted in 4% (47). De Gregorio et al. reported survival after colorectal stents ranging from 4–22 months (46), and others have determined that the time to reobstruction varies from 45–91 days (48). Three recent studies demonstrated that stent placement offered a better quality of life and was cost effective compared to surgical management (49–51).

Types of Colonic Endoprostheses

Endoprostheses used to restore and maintain colorectal patency are similar to the metal self-expanding tubes inserted to alleviate esophageal compression, but are not covered (to decrease the risk of migration). They may be placed under endoscopic or fluoroscopic guidance. The Wallstent (Boston Scientific, Natick, MA) is a popular stent, with models constructed with diameters of 18–22 mm and deployed lengths of 60–90 mm. Plastic stents have been used; however, one study comparing this technology to metal self-expanding stents found a higher incidence of placement failure due to iatrogenic perforation and temporary incontinence with plastic material (52).

Complications

Mild rectal bleeding may occur with colorectal stent procedures. More serious complications such as perforation seem to be more prevalent among patients with local tumor necrosis. Stent placement failures tend to be related to technical malfunctions or the inability to intubate the obstructed area due to extensive tumor involvement and luminal compromise. Stents placed within 3 cm of the anal verge may lead to the development of pain and tenesmus.

In a manner analogous to the placement of the esophageal endoprostheses, we have found it beneficial to obtain a preprocedure barium study, if possible, to rule out acute angulation and other unsuspected sites of obstruction. After colorectal stent placement, patients are advised to report signs and symptoms of increased pain, rectal bleeding, inability to defecate, abdominal distention, or stent protrusion through the anal opening. Consistent use of laxatives and stool softeners as well as dietary modifications may aid in maintaining bowel regularity.

Enteral Endoprostheses

Malignant gastric outlet, duodenal, and small bowel obstructions may be caused by occlusion of the lumen by intrinsic tumor mass or extrinsic compression. Until recently, surgical procedures were the only palliative option for these patients. Enteral stents can replace the need for palliative surgery by providing patients relief from symptoms and allowing maintenance of oral intake (53–55). A multicenter trial was performed that studied the outcomes of enteral stent placement in a total of 176 patients at four centers (56). Most of the obstructions were caused by pancreatic cancer, and the most common site of obstruction was the duodenum. Stent deployment was technically successful in 173 patients. Eight-four percent of the patients followed were able to tolerate oral intake. Complications were noted in 9% of the patients; stent migration was the most common complication. Similar results were demonstrated in another multicenter trial by Nassif et al. (57). A retrospective review of patients who had a duodenal stent placed versus patients who had a surgical gastrojejunostomy was performed (58). There were 20 patients in the stent group and 19 patients in the surgical group. Patients were able to tolerate oral intake earlier in the stent group (1 day vs. 9 days, $p < .0001$). The quality of life was also better in the stent group ($p < .05$). There were no differences noted in the technical or clinical success rates, patient survival or incidence of complications between the two modalities.

The types of endoprostheses are similar to the colorectal stents. One of the more popular models (Wallstent-Enteral, Boston Scientific, Natick, MA) is available in lengths of 60 and 90 mm, and in diameters of 18, 20, and 22 mm. They are usually placed under endoscopic and fluoroscopic guidance. Contrast studies and abdominal CT scans are helpful in defining anatomy and guiding appropriate placement. Types and rates of complications appear similar to those of esophageal and colorectal stenting, and include perforation and hemorrhage.

Biliary Stenting and Drainage Procedures

Indications

Palliative management of biliary obstruction or stenosis in patients with unresectable hepatic metastases, cholangiocarcinoma, and pancreatic carcinomas may improve quality of life (59–62). A measurable effect on psychosocial outcomes with placement of biliary stents has been observed (61).

Therapy for malignant biliary obstruction can be approached in a variety of ways. Surgical resection offers the possibility for cure, but is only possible in 10–15% of cases. Palliation can be achieved by surgical bypass or by endoscopic or percutaneous stenting combined with adjuvant radiation and chemotherapy. Comparative trials have shown no advantage between surgical and nonsurgical palliation of the obstruction in survival (63). Some surgeons prefer that all patients undergo preoperative biliary drainage, although a clear benefit from preoperative drainage has not been proved and the recent National Institutes of Health (NIH) Consensus Statement speaks against that as a routine practice (64).

Methods of Placement

Endoscopic therapy requires retrograde cannulation of the common bile duct, performance of a sphincterotomy in selected patients, and placement of a 7- to 11-French plastic endoprosthesis. A successful diagnostic endoscopic retrograde cholangiopancreatography was accomplished in 75–90% of patients, after which the technical success rate for performing a sphincterotomy was very high. For low strictures, such as pancreatic carcinoma, stent placement after successful cannulation of the duct was achieved in 95%, with a morbidity of 10% and a mortality of approximately 3% (65). Success rates for hilar strictures declined significantly to the 40–60% range, with an increase in morbidity and mortality to 18% and 8%, respectively (66,67). Higher success rates can be obtained using a rendezvous procedure, in which an interventional radiologist passes a guidewire percutaneously through the biliary tree into the duodenum, and is met by the endoscopist who pulls the guidewire out through the mouth. With this through-and-through approach, an endoprosthesis can be passed retrograde without creating a large transhepatic track. Use of the rendezvous technique increases the success rate for retrograde stenting of hilar strictures to almost 90% but also increases the complication rate (68).

Percutaneous biliary drainage is successful 95–100% of the time but suffers from an acute, serious complication rate of 15%. Once internal drainage has been achieved, conversion to an endoprosthesis is almost always possible with little added morbidity (69). Advantages of retrograde endoscopic stenting are its lower morbidity and the ability to change a clogged endoprosthesis. However, the endoscopic approach to the bile duct has a lower technical success rate than the percutaneous approach. Endoscopically placed plastic stents are usually smaller than those placed percutaneously, but metal stents are of the same size. Percutaneous internal–external drainage can almost always be accomplished regardless of the level of obstruction; this allows for larger tubes, which can be easily changed. Access is maintained for brachytherapy or for later interventions as the disease progresses.

Types of Stents

Technologic advancements in the perfection of metallic self-expanding implantable stents have maximized the efficiency of stents, but stent malfunction as a result of tumor ingrowth and overgrowth is a significant problem. Covered Wallstents (Microvasive Endoscopy, Boston Scientific, Natick, Mass), similar to those used in the esophagus, have been developed for the use in the biliary system to decrease the rate of tumor ingrowth and resultant occlusion. The diameter of the stent is 10 mm with lengths of 40, 60, and 80 mm. Recent studies demonstrate that there is less tumor ingrowth (0–14%) as compared with uncovered Wallstents. The major complication associated with the covered Wallstents is migration; this occurred in 6% of patients in Kahaleh et al. Cholecystitis may occur in 2.9–12% of patients with covered biliary endoprosthetics. Studies have not demonstrated a direct relationship between obstructing the cystic duct by the membranous portion of the covered Wallstent and the development of cholecystitis (70). Percutaneous or endoscopic deployment of metal stents has been associated with less pain during placement than plastic stents (67). The main advantage of metal stents appears to be a slightly longer duration of patency, 9–12 months.

Complications

Chronic internal–external drainage is associated with complications in up to 50% of patients, including cholangitis, skin infection, bleeding, leakage of bile and ascites, rib erosion, osteomyelitis, catheter fracture or dislodgement, and seeding of tumor cells along the track. The tubes require regular flushing and dressing. Even with optimal care, routine tube changes are necessary at 8- to 12-week intervals to avoid occlusion. For some, the distortion of their body image is psychologically distressing. Insertion of an endoprosthesis avoids many of the complications of having a chronic percutaneous catheter, but repeated drainage is required if the stent becomes obstructed.

Long-term patency rates are difficult to measure because of the high mortality in this population, but are in the range of 68–94% at a follow-up of 4–5 months (67,71–74). Occlusion of plastic stents occurs due to a sequence of bacterial adherence, glycoprotein deposition, and encrustation with bile salts. Newer series, employing longer stents made from smooth-surfaced polymers or antibacterial coatings, show patencies at the higher end of this range, with median patency of approximately 6.5 months (72,75). Long-term complications are common, with cholangitis in 20% and an average occlusion rate of 11%. Stents fractured or dislodged in 3–6% of cases. Average survival with malignant biliary obstruction is only 3–5 months. In the subset of patients with more indolent cholangiocarcinomas, stent placement can significantly increase survival.

Several studies have evaluated the efficacy of metal self-expanding stents in the treatment of neoplastic-related biliary obstruction by percutaneous insertion. Nicholson et al. who placed metal self-expanding stents percutaneously in 77 patients with inoperable biliary obstruction with no evidence of metastatic spread, found serum bilirubin levels returned to normal within 7 days of stent placement in 98.7% of patients (60). Use of metal stents may prove advantageous in patients with cholangiocarcinoma when intraductal radiation is administered through an iridium wire before stent placement, which can deliver 2000–3000 rads within a 1-cm radius. This can be supplemented by external beam therapy and chemotherapy with 5-fluorouracil. This combined modality approach can yield a mean survival of close to 2 years, with mean stent patency of 19.5 months (76). Intraductal brachytherapy does not appear to improve patency in patients with biliary obstruction from other types of tumors. In another series, successful placement and catheter longevity were noted for patients with cholangiocarcinoma ($n = 31$; mean survival 14 months), yet 77% of patients with sclerosing cholangitis from intra-arterial chemotherapy ($n = 11$) experienced catheter occlusions (59).

After catheter or stent placement, patients are followed with an anticipated reduction in serum bilirubin levels and resolution of pruritus over the first 7–10 days. Signs and symptoms of pain, fever, jaundice, or leakage at the tube site at any time may be a signal of stent occlusion or dislocation. Local care to the catheter exit site with a sterile dressing is done every day for the first few days, then every 3–4 days. Patients and family members are given instructions for catheter care and when to notify the physician or nurse regarding unusual findings. The site and dressing are continually observed for signs of bile leakage. The catheter is initially placed to straight drainage, with the output measured daily. Temperature is taken at least once a day for approximately 1 week after

insertion. Internal–external catheters can be capped after 24 hours to move the internal flow of bile into the duodenum. Biliary tubes require flushing thrice weekly whether capped or to external drainage. Patients with long-term external drainage systems are periodically monitored for electrolyte and bicarbonate depletion. Electrolyte loss can be avoided by reingestion of the bile.

TUMOR ABLATION TECHNIQUES

Endoscopic Ablative Palliation

Palliation of symptoms of GI malignancies may be achieved through the use of tumor ablative techniques (3). These methods may be applied endoscopically and include thermal debulking techniques (bipolar cautery, monopolar cautery, laser), tissue destruction (alcohol, chemotherapeutic agents, photodynamic therapy), and radiotherapy (afterloading techniques, seed implantation) (Table 53.4). The use of any of these methods is dependent on the local expertise and resources available, as well as a multidisciplinary approach to the overall care of the patient.

Esophagus

The maintenance of esophageal luminal patency is a goal for the palliation of nutritional support and the prevention of the aspiration of saliva, as well as for allowing the patient to obtain oral gratification. Many different techniques have been used. The technique most commonly applied in the past was bipolar cautery, but this has fallen out of favor due to concerns over full-thickness injury, stricture formation, the need for a circumferential tumor, and technical difficulties. This technique uses a rigid bipolar probe that is inserted into the tumor; serial applications of current are made as the probe is withdrawn under radiographic or direct visual guidance.

Neodymium:yttrium-aluminum-garnet (Nd:YAG) laser treatment has been the mainstay of the obliterative techniques used recently by gastroenterologists, but is being supplanted by PDT because of its overall lower significant complication rate. The technique is relatively fast and inexpensive if the cost of the laser power source is spread over several specialties. There is an 85% success rate with the use of Nd:YAG laser. The perforation rate may be as high as 6% and a TE fistula may occur in up to 9% of patients. Laser therapy appears to offer better palliation of dysphagia with low morbidity for tumors <5 cm in length compared to esophageal stents (77–79). Another technique is photodynamic therapy, a modality that

TABLE 53.4

ABLATIVE PROCEDURES

Procedure	Sites	Contraindications	Success	Complication
Nd:YAG	Esophagus, rectum	Fistula, coagulopathy	85%	Perforation, tracheoesophageal fistula
PDT	Esophagus	Fistula, respiratory compromise, severe cardiac disease	85%	Perforation, stricture, esophagitis, skin photosensitivity
Argon plasma coagulation	Esophagus	Fistula	89%	Perforation
Brachytherapy	Esophagus	Fistula, total obstruction	82%	Perforation, hemorrhage, stricture
Direct ethanol	Esophagus, liver	Fistula	67–80%	Intoxication, bleeding, vasovagal episodes, pleural effusion

Nd:YAG, neodymium:yttrium-aluminum-garnet; PDT, photodynamic therapy.

is currently approved by the U.S. Food and Drug Administration (FDA) for the palliation and restoration of luminal patency in esophageal cancer (80). Photodynamic therapy involves a two-stage process in which a photosensitizing agent is intravenously administered 1–3 days before endoscopic illumination. Several studies have shown significant improvement in dysphagia in patients with inoperable, obstructing esophageal cancer (81–83). Complications with this procedure may include perforation, stricture formation, esophagitis, and skin photosensitivity (82). PDT and laser appear to have similar efficacies. There is a lower rate of perforations with PDT which may be related to the limited depth of penetration. The main disadvantages with PDT are the photosensitivity and the cost of the equipment and repeated endoscopies (84). Further bench and clinical research will likely lead to better hematoporphyrin derivatives, better techniques, and additional applications.

Argon plasma coagulation (APC) is another form of ablative therapy that can be effective in the palliation of dysphagia in patients with esophageal tumors. It causes tissue coagulation and destruction through a noncontact probe that transfers energy through electrically charged argon gas. A retrospective study of 31 patients demonstrated that shrinkage of the tumor enabled passage of the endoscope in 89% of patients. Perforation was seen in 1.8% of treatments; procedure mortality was 1.2% (85). Further studies are needed to compare APC with established modalities of treatment.

Local radiotherapy (brachytherapy) may be directed and aided by endoscopic techniques, including EUS. Brachytherapy markers and delivery tubes may be placed endoscopically and location of the tumor precisely determined to allow for the accurate delivery of intraluminal and external beam therapy. Horns et al. compared single dose brachytherapy with metal stent placement. In this study, brachytherapy provided greater relief of dysphagia in the early stages of treatment with lower rate of complications compared with stent placement. Brachytherapy initially failed in 18% of patients and required stent placement (86). Stent placement usually provides immediate relief.

Direct ethanol injection into tumor masses has been used with success to debulk lesions, improve dysphagia, salvage endoprostheses when overgrowth has occurred, and maintain luminal patency. Scant data are available on which to base recommendations regarding its efficacy and safety. Pilot studies have shown that injection of cisplatin may be effective in palliation (87,88).

Rectum

The mainstay of endoscopic debulking of colorectal neoplasms has been the use of thermal ablation techniques. Large sessile or pedunculated lesions may be effectively debulked to allow for the passage of stool or for the preparation of the colon for a resection or stent placement. These techniques are relatively easily applied in the rectum below the peritoneal reflection, without much concern for the complication of free peritoneal perforation. The use of monopolar cautery snare resection coupled with saline injection is a technique that can be readily mastered and does not require a large investment in capital expenditures. Lesions that are commonly found in the rectum (and higher in the colon) tend to be circumferential and are not easily managed by application of cautery. Most of the lesions require the use of endoscopic laser therapy, most commonly performed with Nd:YAG. The potassium titanyl phosphate (KTP) laser (532 nm) is in clinical use in some centers, and we have found it to be quite effective. The laser energy may be applied through a free fiber and allowed to vaporize tissue to open the lumen, or it may be used with contact-type probes to allow for precise delivery of energy and, theoretically, a more controlled depth of penetration. There is a paucity of data

comparing this technique with others, although data that are published support its safety and efficacy when used by those experienced with the equipment and technique.

Percutaneous Ablation of Liver Tumors

In situ destruction of liver tumors has been performed with a variety of chemical and thermal techniques. Chemical ablation is most often performed with ethanol. Acetic acid has also been used. Thermal techniques include cryosurgery, hot saline injection, radiofrequency (RF), microwave, laser, and high-intensity focused US.

Patient Selection

The best candidates for percutaneous tumor ablation are those with small tumors, and with cancers that are confined to the liver but are nonetheless unresectable due to the distribution of disease, severity of underlying cirrhosis, or other comorbid diseases. Tumors must be accessible under imaging guidance. Patients with three or fewer lesions that are no more than 3 cm in diameter are excellent candidates for percutaneous treatment. Ablating lesions between 3 and 5 cm is more difficult, and above 5 cm the local failure rate increases dramatically.

Chemical Ablation

Chemical ablation with ethanol causes cell death due to cellular dehydration and protein denaturation. These processes, combined with small vessel thrombosis, lead to coagulative necrosis of tissue. Intravenous access is required for sedation and analgesia. Prophylactic antibiotics are not necessary. After localization of the tumor under CT scan guidance or US, the skin is prepped and draped and local anesthesia administered from the skin through the liver capsule. The lesion is then punctured with a 20–22 gauge (G) diamond-tip, multisidehole needle (e.g., Bernadino needle, Wilson-Cook, Inc., Winston-Salem, NC), passing the needle to the back wall of the tumor. Absolute alcohol is injected slowly while rotating the needle, preferably during real-time US monitoring. Alcohol is brilliantly echogenic on US, jet-black on CT scan. The needle is gradually withdrawn toward the proximal edge of the tumor. Injection is stopped and the needle repositioned if alcohol is observed to flow into a blood vessel, bile duct, or into the liver outside of the tumor. After completing the injection, the needle is left in place for 1–2 minutes to allow the alcohol to diffuse, then the needle is aspirated firmly during withdrawal to minimize leakage. Additional passes may be required to treat the entire tumor volume.

Lesions up to 3 cm are easily treated in a single session. Because the toxic dose of ethanol is 0.8–1.0 mL per kg, lesions 4 cm or larger usually require multiple treatment sessions. Patients can be brought back at weekly intervals for this simple outpatient procedure until the entire tumor has been treated. Pain and nausea are common during the procedure, and can be managed with medication. Patients will become intoxicated if sufficient alcohol is injected, particularly Asians with alcohol dehydrogenase deficiency. Fever and transient liver function test elevation typically occur in the days after the procedure, and do not require specific therapy. Patients can be discharged after a few hours of observation. Complications occur in 1–14% of procedures. Vasovagal episodes may occur; and intraperitoneal bleeding and pleural effusion are each reported after 0.5% of procedures. Rarer complications include pneumothorax, ascites, cholangitis, abscess, hepatic infarct, biliary stricture, and tumor seeding.

Successful chemical ablation causes an area of necrosis in the liver that is larger than the index lesion. Hence the apparent size of the lesion increases on follow-up imaging. It is essential to obtain "functional" imaging that is sensitive to cellular viability. At a minimum, CT scan or magnetic resonance imaging should be obtained using dynamic scanning during the arterial phase of contrast enhancement. Positron emission tomography and spectroscopy are more sophisticated techniques for assessing tumor viability. Serum tumor markers should be followed, if elevated at baseline. Fine-needle aspiration biopsy can be performed to evaluate regions suspicious for residual or recurrent tumor.

Over 1000 cases of hepatoma treated with percutaneous ethanol injection (PEI) have been reported (89–91). Among resected specimens, complete necrosis was observed in 67–80%. Local recurrence at the treated site occurred in up to 15%. Unfortunately, regional failure is high, with 64–98% of patients developing new liver tumors within 5 years. Survival rates at 5 years are reported to be 30–50%. Although these figures are remarkably high compared to most series reporting other therapies for hepatoma, it must be remembered that PEI patients are a highly selected group with very small tumor burden.

PEI does not work as well for metastatic lesions. Because metastases tend to be less vascular and are harder than the surrounding liver, the liquid alcohol tends to follow the path of least resistance back along the needle and on to infiltrate the liver, rather than diffusing through the tumor nodule. Complete necrosis is achieved in less than half of lesions, usually in tumors <2 cm in size.

PEI has been used extensively for treatment of focal hepatomas in patients with hepatic cirrhosis. However, it is being replaced by thermal ablation in many institutions. Livraghi et al. reported their comparative experience with the two techniques (92). These were not prospective or randomized trials. Among 84 patients/121 lesions treated with PEI and 96 patients/106 lesions treated with RF ablation, it took over four sessions of PEI on average to ablate the entire tumor, versus only 1.2 sessions for RF. Complete success as judged by imaging studies was similar for both modalities, but the local recurrence rate was 13% after PEI versus 2% for RF. There was one complication in the PEI group, five in the RF group. Lencioni et al. demonstrated that RF was superior to PEI in achieving complete tumor response and requiring fewer sessions in a prospective, randomized study of 102 patients (93). As in the Livraghi group, the recurrence rate was higher with PEI (92,93). The conclusion was that RF is more efficient and effective than ethanol in ablating hepatomas.

Acetic Acid

Acetic acid was first proposed as an ablation agent by Ohnishi et al. who reasoned that acetic acid, used in vitro to dissolve lipids and extract collagen from various tissues (including cirrhotic liver), may have applications in percutaneous ablation (94). Ohnishi initially demonstrated acetic acid to be superior to ethanol in cell kill in a rat model with a higher degree of necrosis and more homogenous diffusion. The cytotoxic mechanisms of acetic acid are similar to those of ethanol, including protein denaturation and dissolution of basement membrane and interstitial collagen resulting in coagulative necrosis of tumor cells. Dose–response studies in a rat model have shown the cytotoxic effects of acetic acid plateau at a concentration of 50% (approximately 8 mol per L). Acetic acid has an advantage of infiltrating the septae and capsule of tumors, whereas ethanol does not cross tumor septae. As a result, a smaller volume is required to achieve the same degree of cell kill with fewer treatment sessions.

These characteristics may account for the differences observed by Ohnishi et al. in the only prospective, randomized trial comparing ethanol ablation with acetic acid ablation for small (<3 cm) hepatocellular carcinomas (95). A total of 31 patients underwent acetic acid ablation and 29 patients

underwent ethanol ablation of one to four discrete tumors. The groups were well matched in terms of age, sex, underlying liver disease, Child-Pugh score, and tumor burden (size, number, and histologic grade). All patients underwent acetic acid or ethanol ablation by the same operator, using US guidance and a 22-G needle. The number of treatment sessions and total volume injected for all sessions was less with patients treated with acetic acid compared to those treated with ethanol. A significant and substantial difference was observed in cancer-free and overall survival. The 1- and 2-year cancer-free survival rates were 83% and 63% in the acetic acid group and 59% and 33% in the ethanol group. The 1- and 2-year overall survival rates were 100% and 92% in the acetic acid group and 83% and 63% in the ethanol group. No major complications occurred in either group; the minor postablation effects of pain and fever were seen in both groups.

Huo et al. performed a study to compare transarterial chemoembolization and percutaneous acetic acid injection in a total of 310 patients (96). There was no significant difference in the survival of the two groups but the transarterial chemoembolization seemed to be more effective in patients with larger tumors (3–6 cm). Therefore, in patients with small hepatocellular carcinoma (HCC) either treatment may be recommended.

Large-volume injections of acetic acid (>20 mL) should be avoided because of the potential for metabolic acidosis and direct renal toxicity of acetic acid. Preliminary observations indicate that acetic acid may be especially useful when treating hepatic metastases, which are notoriously difficult to treat with ethanol due to their hard, firm consistency. Acetic acid appears to infiltrate through firm lesions more homogenously than ethanol. Acetic acid may also hold promise in the treatment of nonhepatic neoplasms.

Thermal Ablation

Temperatures above 60°C cause cell death within minutes. This can be accomplished with various energy sources, including RF, microwave, laser, or high-intensity US. Of these, only RF electrocautery is commercially available in the United States. Heating has advantages over chemical ablation, in that it does not depend on direct contact with the cells. Energy is dispersed fairly evenly across the treatment volume, and is not limited by septations or areas of necrosis or fibrosis within the tumor. RF ablation works by inducing ionic agitation in the surrounding tissues. This results in localized frictional heating. Lesion size is proportional to the power of energy delivered (watts), time, and size of the probe. Reliable thermal lesions up to 3.5 cm can be created using a radial or multiprobe array.

The ablation technique is similar to PEI. Intravenous access is essential, as pain is a significant side effect of the procedure, and deep sedation or anesthesia may be required. Access to the lesion is obtained under imaging guidance, using local anesthesia. If necessary, multiple overlapping burns are performed to treat the entire tumor volume. Each burn takes 10–30 minutes, so the procedure is more time-consuming than PEI.

Immediate results of RF ablation based on follow-up imaging indicate absence of any enhancing tumor in 60–90% of tumors, with lesion size being the major determinant of success (97,98). Local recurrence rates have been reported to be from as low as 2% to as high as 40% within 1 year. As with any local approach, new lesions are the predominant mode of failure, occurring in up to 65% of patients within 1 year. Complications occur in approximately 2.4% of cases.

Combined Regional and Local Therapy

Chemoembolization (see section Chemoembolization), although treating a large volume, is limited in its ability to induce complete tumor necrosis. Conversely, RF ablation causes thorough tissue necrosis within a small volume, primarily limited by blood flow. Hence, combining the two techniques is an appealing approach to intermediate size lesions. Occlusion of the hepatic artery or portal vein during RF ablation results in substantially larger burn volumes. This is routinely done during intraoperative ablation, using the Pringle maneuver to temporarily reduce hepatic blood flow. Temporary balloon occlusion, embolization, or chemoembolization to devascularize the tumor allows effective RF ablation of tumors up to 8 cm in diameter. Blood flow to the surrounding liver is still preserved through the portal vein, so a "surgical" margin is not achieved. Experience with this combined modality therapy is still preliminary, so long-term follow-up for recurrence is not available (99). Given these findings, RF may be considered first-line therapy for HCC in patients who are not suitable for surgery.

Chemoembolization

Malignancies in the liver present one of the most challenging problems in clinical oncology. Other tumors that are less common but frequently develop fatal hepatic metastases despite a resectable primary include ocular melanoma, neuroendocrine tumors, and the rare GI sarcomas. Response rates of hepatoma and metastatic colorectal cancer to a variety of systemic chemotherapeutic agents are no better than 20–40%, and a significant survival benefit has not been demonstrated. Intra-arterial chemotherapy using continuous infusion of 5-fluorodeoxyuridine and steroids delivered by percutaneous catheters or by surgically implanted pumps has remained a popular regional approach to hepatic malignancies and colorectal metastases to the liver, although none of the phase III trials comparing intra-arterial to intravenous chemotherapy for metastatic colorectal cancer has shown a long-term survival benefit for intra-arterial infusions (100–103). Response rates of hepatoma to intra-arterial chemotherapy are 50–60%, with an increase in survival to 20–60% at 1 year (104,105).

Embolization of the hepatic artery has proved effective for palliation of liver metastases from neuroendocrine tumors, with response rates of 80–90% (106,107). Hepatoma has a more modest response to embolization (50–60%), with some increase in short-term survival (108,109). The efficacy of embolization is limited by the liver's ability to develop collateral blood supply when the hepatic artery is occluded. For this reason, benefits from hepatic artery embolization tend to be transient. Embolization has not been shown to extend survival for patients with colorectal metastases (110,111). Chemoembolization combines hepatic artery embolization with simultaneous infusion of a concentrated dose of chemotherapeutic drugs. Theoretical advantages of this technique include the following:

1. Embolization renders the tumor ischemic, depriving it of nutrients and oxygen and decreasing drug resistance.
2. Tumor drug concentrations are orders of magnitude higher than those achieved by infusion alone (112,113).
3. Blood flow is arrested, prolonging the dwelling time of the chemotherapy with measurable drug levels present as long as a month later (114,115).
4. Most of the drug is retained in the liver, minimizing systemic toxicity.

A variety of chemotherapeutic drugs and embolic agents are used around the world. Doxorubicin, in doses of 40–80 mg, is probably the most commonly used single agent. Often it is combined with *cis*-platinum (100–150 mg) or mitomycin-C (10–20 mg). These drugs can be dissolved in their powdered form directly in radiographic contrast. This solution can be injected directly, or emulsified with iodized oil (Ethiodol, Savage Laboratories, Melville, NY) before injection. Embolization is completed with small particles of gelatin sponge or polyvinyl alcohol sponge.

Critical to the selection of patients for regional therapy is tumor confinement to the liver. Patients with minimal or indolent extrahepatic disease may be candidates if the liver disease is considered to be the dominant source of morbidity and mortality. Tumors that typically meet these criteria include hepatoma, intrahepatic cholangiocarcinoma, and metastases from colorectal cancer, ocular melanoma, neuroendocrine tumors, and sarcomas. When the parenchyma is diseased, the liver becomes more dependent on the hepatic artery for its blood supply. Subgroups of patients have been identified who are at high risk of acute hepatic failure after hepatic artery embolization. They typically have >50% of the liver volume replaced by tumor, lactate dehydrogenase >425 IU per L, aspartate aminotransferase >100 IU per L, and total bilirubin >2 mg per dL (116). The presence of hepatic encephalopathy or jaundice is an absolute contraindication to embolization. Biliary obstruction is also a contraindication. Even with a normal serum bilirubin, the presence of dilated intrahepatic bile ducts places the patient at high risk for biliary necrosis in the obstructed segment(s) of the liver.

Evaluation for chemoembolization includes a tissue diagnosis, cross-sectional imaging of the liver, exclusion of extrahepatic disease, and laboratory studies. Given the significant discomforts, hazards, and expense of this treatment, its palliative role should be clearly understood. After hydration and premedication with antibiotics and antiemetics, diagnostic visceral arteriography is performed to determine the arterial supply to the liver and confirm patency of the portal vein. The origins of vessels supplying the gut, particularly the right gastric and supraduodenal arteries, are carefully noted to avoid embolization of the stomach or small bowel. Once the arterial anatomy is clearly understood, a catheter is advanced superselectively into the right or left hepatic artery, depending on which lobe holds the most tumor, and chemoembolization is performed. The patient receives intra-arterial lidocaine and intravenous fentanyl or morphine sulfate to alleviate pain during the embolization. After the procedure, vigorous hydration, intravenous antibiotics, and antiemetic therapy are continued. Opioids, prochlorperazine, and acetaminophen are liberally supplied for control of pain, nausea, and fever. The patient is discharged as soon as oral intake is adequate and parenteral narcotics are not required for pain control. Approximately one half of patients are discharged in 1 day, and most of the rest within 2 days. Oral antibiotics are continued for another 5 days, and antiemetics and opioids are continued as needed. Follow-up includes return for a second procedure directed at the other lobe of the liver 3–4 weeks later. Depending on the arterial anatomy, two to four procedures are required to treat the entire liver, after which response is assessed by repeat imaging studies and tumor markers. Eighty to 90% of patients suffer a postembolization syndrome, characterized by pain, fever, and nausea and vomiting. The severity of these symptoms varies tremendously from patient to patient, and they can last from a few hours to several days. Serious complications occur in up to 5% of procedures.

Major complications of hepatic embolization include hepatic insufficiency or infarction, hepatic abscess, biliary necrosis, and nontarget embolization to the gut. With careful patient selection and scrupulous technique, the incidence of these serious events collectively is 3–4%. Other complications include renal insufficiency and anemia requiring transfusion, with incidences of <1% each. Thirty-day mortality ranges from 1–4%.

Among combined series of 800 patients with unresectable HCC treated with chemoembolization in Asia, Europe, and the United States, response rates as measured by decreased tumor volume and decreased serum α-fetoprotein levels were 60–83% (114,117,118). Cumulative probability of survival ranged from 54–88% at 1 year, 33–64% at 2 years, and 18–51% at 3 years. Survival varies inversely with tumor volume, stage, and Childs class. Despite the large volume of single-institution experiences with chemoembolization of hepatoma published over the past decade, few controlled trials have been reported. A multicenter European trial comparing cisplatin/Lipiodol gelfoam chemoembolization to no therapy in 100 patients with relatively small tumor burdens (90% stage I) found 1-year survivals of 62% and 43%, respectively, and 2-year survivals of 38% and 26% (119). A French multicenter trial of 127 patients with more advanced disease (62% stage II or III) showed almost identical survival rates in the chemoembolization arm (64% and 38% at 1 and 2 years), with survival in the control arm of only 18% and 6%, respectively (p < .0001) (120). Several reports of chemoembolization for liver metastases from colon cancer have been reported (121,122). These consistently show a response in two thirds of patients, and median survivals on the order of 2 years, which is approximately double that seen with systemic chemotherapy alone. A phase III randomized trial is now under way to evaluate the benefit of chemoembolization in addition to standard chemotherapy in this disease.

CONSCIOUS SEDATION AND ANALGESIA

Interventional techniques for palliation are aimed at relieving pain and improving symptoms. However, in some circumstances these procedures may transiently worsen pain, exacerbate other symptoms, and sometimes, create new temporary sources for pain. The need for pain control before, during, and after procedures cannot be overestimated. Uncontrolled pain leads to a release of catecholamines that stimulates the sympathetic nervous system, which can stress the cardiovascular system, resulting in tachycardia, cardiac arrhythmias, or cardiac ischemia (123). It can also result in elevated blood pressure, which in turn may increase the risk of stroke and potential for hemorrhage at the procedural site (124). Nausea, vomiting, and bradycardia, which are parasympathetic responses, can accompany severe pain originating from the viscera or peritoneum as the result of an invasive procedure.

As areas of the body are manipulated, nociceptors (free nerve endings) are activated; giving rise to various painful sensations that may or may not be similar to the pain of cancer. A painful stimulus to viscera or organ structures, such as inflammation, that is sustained over time increases the vulnerability of visceral nociceptors to stimuli that would not normally evoke pain (125). The slightest manipulation of visceral structures affected by cancer pain can provoke significant pain. Moreover, ischemic pain caused by embolization procedures or damage to vasculature is so severe that adequate pain control during and after remains a clinical priority (126,127).

To some extent, the perception of pain can be diminished by percutaneous and intravascular local anesthetics, regional blocks, and liberal use of systemic opioid analgesics and sedating agents. Nonpharmacologic methods, such as relaxation techniques, can reduce the need for opioids and sedating agents, enhance amnesia, and improve the patient's overall well-being and outlook on the procedure (124). The level of complexity and duration of the procedure have warranted more liberal use of sedating agents and intensive monitoring in endoscopic and interventional radiology procedure units. Specific details are beyond the scope of this chapter and the following recommendations for the selection of sedating agents and opioids to manage procedural pain and anxiety that accompany interventional procedures for cancer (11,128–130).

CONCLUSION

Decisions for endoscopic and interventional radiologic techniques must be based on available data and sound clinical judgment, balancing potential risks and benefits. The ability to perform some palliative interventions is largely the result of local expertise and the availability of clinical resources. All possible comfort and supportive care measures should be considered or attempted before undertaking of invasive interventions. Moral, ethical, and social issues arise if patients are subjected to these procedures only to prolong intense pain and suffering when life expectancy is very limited. On the other hand, withholding therapeutic options for palliation of intolerable and unmanageable symptoms takes hope away from patients for a better quality of life for the remaining weeks or months of life.

Gastroenterologists and interventional radiologists may overlap in areas of expertise and perform similar procedures; however, each offers unique aspects to the technical performance of the procedure. Careful patient selection and knowledge of the local expertise and areas of interest of each specialist leads to a multidisciplinary effort and more options and opinions in regard to the therapy for the individual patient. Differences in how each specialty approaches an individual clinical situation may be readily evident, but despite these differences, the indications for treatment and the intended outcomes for treatment remain similar.

References

1. Jones SN. Interventional radiology in a palliative care setting. *Palliat Med* 1995;9:319.
2. Rossi P, Bezzi M. Interventional radiology in gastrointestinal neoplasms. *Curr Opin Oncol* 1995;7(4):367.
3. Botet JF. Interventional radiology. In: DeVita VT, Hellman S, Rosenberg SA, eds. *Cancer: principles and practice of oncology*, 5th ed. Philadelphia, PA: Lippincott-Raven, 1997:682.
4. Ripamonti C. Management of bowel obstruction in advanced cancer patients. *J Pain Symptom Manage* 1994;9:193.
5. Cannizzaro R, Bortoluzzi F, Valentino M, et al. Percutaneous endoscopic gastrostomy as a decompression technique in bowel obstruction due to abdominal carcinomatosis. *Endoscopy* 1995;27:317.
6. Cunningham MJ, Bromberg C, Kredentser DC, et al. Percutaneous gastrostomy for decompression in patients with advanced gynecologic malignancies. *Gynecol Oncol* 1995;59:273.
7. Campagnutta E, Cannizzaro R, Gallo A, et al. Palliative treatment of upper intestinal obstruction by gynecological malignancies: the usefulness of percutaneous endoscopic gastrostomy. *Gynecol Oncol* 1996;62:103.
8. Pothuri B, Montemarano M, Gerardi M, et al. Percutaneous endoscopic gastrostomy tube placement in patients with malignant bowel obstruction due to ovarian carcinoma. *Gynecol Oncol* 2005;96(2):330–334.
9. Wollman BD, Agostino HB, Walus-Wigle JR, et al. Radiologic, endoscopic, and surgical gastrostomy: an institutional evaluation and meta-analysis of the literature. *Radiology* 1995;197:699.
10. Howie SB, Amigo PH, O'Kelly K, et al. Palliation of malignant bowel obstruction using a percutaneous cecostomy. *J Pain Symptom Manage* 2004;27(3):282–285.
11. Adelson MD, Kasowitz MH. Percutaneous endoscopic drainage gastrostomy in the treatment of gastrointestinal obstruction from intraperitoneal malignancy. *Obstet Gynecol* 1993;81:467.
12. Panzer S, Harris M, Berg W, et al. Endoscopic ultrasound in the placement of a percutaneous endoscopic gastrostomy tube in the non-transilluminated abdominal wall. *Gastrointest Endosc* 1995;42(1):88–90.
13. Adler DG, Baron TH, Geels W, et al. Placement of PEG tubes through previously placed self-expanding esophageal metal stents. *Gastrointest Endosc* 2001;54(2):237–241.
14. Herman LL, Hoskins WJ, Shike M. Percutaneous endoscopic gastrostomy for decompression of the stomach and small bowel. *Gastrointest Endosc* 1992;38:314.
15. Marks WH, Perkal MF, Schwartz PE. Percutaneous endoscopic gastrostomy for gastric decompression in metastatic malignancy. *Surg Gynecol Obstet* 1993;177:573.
16. Bell SD, Carmody EA, Yeung EY, et al. Percutaneous gastrostomy and gastrojejunostomy: additional experience in 519 procedures. *Radiology* 1995;194:817.

17. de Baere T, Chapot R, Kuoch V, et al. Percutaneous gastrostomy with fluoroscopic guidance: single-center experience in 500 consecutive cancer patients. *Radiology* 1999;210:651–654.

18. Light VL, Slezak FA, Porter JA, et al. Predictive factors for early mortality after percutaneous endoscopic gastrostomy. *Gastrointest Endosc* 1995;42:330.

19. Becker G, Hess CF, Grund KE, et al. Abdominal wall metastasis following percutaneous endoscopic gastrostomy. *Support Care Cancer* 1995;3:313.

20. Lee DS, Mohit-Tabatabai MA, Rush BF, et al. Stomal seeding of head and neck cancer by percutaneous endoscopic gastrostomy. *Ann Surg Oncol* 1995;2:170.

21. Simon T, Fink AS. Recent experience with percutaneous endoscopic gastrostomy/jejunostomy (PEG/J) for enteral nutrition. *Surg Endosc* 2000;14:436–438.

22. Rumalla A, Baron TH. Results of direct percutaneous endoscopic jejunostomy, an alternative method for providing jejunal feeding. *Mayo Clin Proc* 2000;75:807–810.

23. Fan AC, Baron TH, Rumalla A, et al. Comparison of direct percutaneous endoscopic jejunostomy and PEG with jejunal extension. *Gastrointest Endosc* 2002;56(6):890–894.

24. Ginsberg GG, Scotiniotis I. Endoscopic magnetic-coupling for transient luminal fixation. *Gastrointest Endosc* 2000;51:AB3476.

25. Shike M. Percutaneous endoscopic stomas for enteral feeding and drainage. *Oncology* 1995;9:39.

26. Duranceau A, Jamieson GG. Malignant tracheoesophageal fistula: collective review. *Ann Thorac Surg* 1984;37:346.

27. Irving JD, Simson JNL. A new cuffed oesophageal prosthesis for the management of malignant oesophago-respiratory fistula. *Ann R Coll Surg Engl* 1988;70:13.

28. Grund KE, Storek D, Becker HD. Highly flexible self-expanding meshed metal stents for palliation of malignant esophagogastric obstruction. *Endoscopy* 1995;27:486–494.

29. Kozarek R, Raltz S, Brugge WR, et al. Prospective multicenter trial of esophageal Z-stent placement for malignant dysphagia and tracheoesophageal fistula. *Gastrointest Endosc* 1996;44:562–567.

30. Siersema PD, Hop WCJ, van Blankenstein M, et al. A new design metal stent (Flamingo stent) for palliation of malignant dysphagia: a prospective study. *Gastrointest Endosc* 2000;51:139–145.

31. Bartelsman JFW, Bruno MJ, Jensema AJ, et al. Palliation of patients with esophagogastric neoplasms by insertion of a covered expandable modified Gianturco-Z endoprosthesis: experience in 153 patients. *Gastrointest Endosc* 2000;51:134–138.

32. Chan ACW, Shin FG, Lam YH, et al. A comparison study on physical properties of self-expandable esophageal metal stents. *Gastrointest Endosc* 1999;49:462–465.

33. Vakil N, Morris AI, Marcon N, et al. A prospective, randomized, controlled trial of covered expandable metal stents in the palliation of malignant esophageal obstruction at the gastroesophageal junction. *Am J Gastroenterol* 2001;96(6):1791–1796.

34. Siersema PD, Hop WC, van Blankenstein M, et al. A comparison of 3 types of covered metal stents for the palliation of patients with dysphagia caused by esophagogastric carcinoma: a prospective, randomized study. *Gastrointest Endosc* 2001;54(2):145–153.

35. Shim CS. Esophageal stenting in unusual situations. *Endoscopy* 2003;35:14–18.

36. Laasch HU, Marriott A, Wilbraham L, et al. Effectiveness of open versus antireflux stents for palliation of distal esophageal carcinoma and prevention of symptomatic gastroesophageal reflux. *Radiology* 2002;225:359–365.

37. Shin JH, Song HY, Kim JH, et al. Comparison of temporary and permanent stent placement with concurrent radiation therapy in patients with esophageal carcinoma. *J Vasc Interv Radiol* 2005;16(1):67–74.

38. Costamagna G, Shah SK, Tringali A, et al. Prospective evaluation of a new self-expanding plastic stent for inoperable esophageal strictures. *Surg Endosc* 2003;17(6):891–895.

39. Radecke K, Gerken G, Treichel U. Impact of a self-expanding, plastic esophageal stent on various esophageal stenosis, fistulas, and leakages: a single-center experience in 39 patients. *Gastrointest Endosc* 2005;61:812–818.

40. Tytgat GNJ, Bartelsman JFWM, Vermeyden JR. Dilation and prosthesis for obstructing esophagogastric carcinoma. *Gastrointest Endosc Clin N Am* 1992;2(3):415.

41. Kadish S, Kochman M. Endoscopic diagnosis and management of gastrointestinal malignancies. *Oncology* 1995;9(10):967.

42. Ramirez FC, Dennert B, Zierer ST, et al. Esophageal self-expandable metallic stents—indications, practice techniques, and complications: results of a national survey. *Gastrointest Endosc* 1997;45:360–364.

43. Pothuri B, Guirguis A, Gerdes H, et al. The use of colorectal stents for palliation of large-bowel obstruction due to recurrent gynecologic cancer. *Gynecol Oncol* 2004;95(3):513–517.

44. Mainar A, Tejero E, Maynar M, et al. Colorectal obstruction: treatment with metallic stents. *Radiology* 1996;198:761.

45. Varda V, Daniljamo V, Hugao J, et al. Stent endoprosthesis for obstructing colorectal cancers. *Dis Colon Rectum* 1996;39:552.

46. De Gregorio MA, Mainar A, Tejero E, et al. Acute colorectal obstruction: stent placement for palliative treatment—results of a multicenter study. *Radiology* 1998;209:117–120.

47. Khot UP, Lang AW, Murali K, et al. Systematic review of the efficacy and safety of colorectal stents. *Br J Surg* 2002;89(9):1096–1102.

48. Rey JF, Romanczyk T, Greff M. Metal stents for palliation of rectal carcinoma: a preliminary report on 12 patients. *Endoscopy* 1995;327:501.

49. Xinopoulos D, Dimitroulopoulos D, Theodosopoulos T, et al. Stenting or stoma creation for patients with inoperable malignant colonic obstructions? Results of a study and cost-effectiveness analysis. *Surg Endosc* 2004;18(3):421–426.

50. Carne PW, Frye JN, Robertson GM, et al. Stents or open operation for palliation of colorectal cancer: a retrospective, cohort study of perioperative outcome and long-term survival. *Dis Colon Rectum* 2004;47(9):1455–1461.

51. Tomiki1 Y, Watanabe1 T, Ishibiki1 Y, et al. Comparison of stent placement and colostomy as palliative treatment for inoperable malignant colorectal obstruction. *Surg Endosc* 2004;18:1572–1577.

52. Rupp KD, Dohmoto R, Meffert R, et al. Cancer of the rectum: palliative endoscopic treatment. *Eur J Surg Oncol* 1995;21:644.

53. Feretis C, Benakis P, Dimopoulos C, et al. Palliation of malignant gastric outlet obstruction with self-expanding metal stents. *Endoscopy* 1996;28:225.

54. Kozarek RA, Brandabur JJ, Raltz SL, et al. Expandable stents: unusual locations. *Am J Gastroenterol* 1997;92:812.

55. Soetikno RM, Lichtenstein DR, Vandervoort J, et al. Palliation of malignant gastric outlet obstruction using an endoscopically placed Wallstent. *Gastrointest Endosc* 1998;47:267.

56. Telford JJ, Carr-Locke DL, Baron TH, et al. Palliation of patients with malignant gastric outlet obstruction with the enteral Wallstent: outcomes from a multicenter study. *Gastrointest Endosc* 2004;60(6):916–920.

57. Nassif T, Prat F, Meduri B, et al. Endoscopic palliation of malignant gastric outlet obstruction using self-expandable metallic stents: results of a multicenter study. *Endoscopy* 2003;35(6):483–489.

58. Maetani I, Tada T, Ukita T, et al. Comparison of duodenal stent placement with surgical gastrojejunostomy for palliation in patients with duodenal obstructions caused by pancreaticobiliary malignancies. *Endoscopy* 2004;36(1):73–78.

59. Coons H. Metallic stents for the treatment of biliary obstruction: a report of 100 cases. *Cardiovasc Intervent Radiol* 1992;15(6):367.

60. Nicholson AA, Royston CM. Palliation of inoperable biliary obstruction with self-expanding metal endoprostheses: a review of 77 patients. *Clin Radiol* 1993;47(4):245.

61. Ballinger AB, McHugh M, Catnach SM, et al. Symptom relief and quality of life after stenting for malignant biliary obstruction. *Gut* 1994;35(4):467.

62. Lichtenstein DR, Carr-Locke DL. Endoscopic palliation for unresectable pancreatic carcinoma. *Surg Clin North Am* 1995;75(5):969.

63. Smith AC, Dowsett JF, Russell RCG, et al. Randomised trial of endoscopic stenting versus surgical bypass in malignant low bile duct obstruction. *Lancet* 1994;344:1655–1660.

64. Cohen S, Bacon BR, Berlin JA, et al. NIH state-of-the-science statement on endoscopic retrograde cholangiopancreatography (ERCP) for diagnosis and therapy. *NIH Consens State Sci Statements* 2002;19(1):1–26.

65. Pereira-Lima JC, Jakobs R, Maier M, et al. Endoscopic biliary stenting for palliation of pancreatic cancer: results, survival predictive factor, and complication of 10-French with 11.5-French gauge stents. *Am J Gastroenterol* 1996;9:2179.

66. Magistrelli P, Masetti R, Coppola R, et al. Changing attitudes in the palliation of proximal malignant biliary obstruction. *J Clin Oncol* 1993;3:151.

67. Kauffman SL. Percutaneous palliation of unresectable pancreatic cancer. *Surg Clin North Am* 1995;75(5):989.

68. Tsang TK, Crampton AR, Bernstein JR, et al. Percutaneous-endoscopic biliary stenting in patients with occluded surgical bypass. *Am J Med* 1990;88:344–348.

69. Adam A, Chetty N, Roddie M, et al. Self-expandable stainless steel endoprosthesis for treatment of malignant bile duct obstruction. *AJR Am J Roentgenol* 1991;156:321–325.

70. Kahaleh M, Tokar J, Conaway MR, et al. Efficacy and complications of covered Wallstents in malignant distal biliary obstruction. *Gastrointest Endosc* 2005;61(4):528–533.

71. Huibregtse K, Carr-Locke DL, Cremer W, et al. Biliary obstruction—a problem with self-expanding metal stents. *Endoscopy* 1992;24:391.

72. Speer AG, Cotton PB, Rode J, et al. Biliary stent blockage with bacterial biofilm. *Ann Intern Med* 1988;108:546.

73. Cotton PB. Metallic mesh stents—is the expanse worth the expense? *Endoscopy* 1992;24:421.

74. Uflacker R. Percutaneous biliary procedures. *Gastrointest Endosc Clin N Am* 1996;6(1):177.

75. Seitz U, Vayeyar H, Soehendra N. Prolonged patency with a new design Teflon biliary prosthesis. *Endoscopy* 1994;26(5):478.

76. Eschelman DJ, Shapiro MJ, Bonn J, et al. Malignant biliary duct obstruction: long-term experience with Gianturco stents and combined-modality radiation therapy. *Radiology* 1996;220:717.

77. Lightdale CJ, Heier SK, Marcon NE, et al. Photodynamic therapy with porfimer sodium versus thermal ablation therapy with Nd:YAG laser for palliation of esophageal cancer: a multicenter randomized trial. *Gastrointest Endosc* 1995;42(6):507.

78. Cotton BP, Williams CP. *Practical gastrointestinal endoscopy*, 4th ed. London: Blackwell Science, 1996.

79. Carter R, Smith JS, Anderson JR. Laser recanalization versus endoscopic intubation in the palliation of malignant dysphagia: a randomized prospective study. *Br J Surg* 1992;79:1167–1170.

80. Overholt BF, Panjehpour M, DeNovo RC, et al. Balloon photodynamic therapy of esophageal cancer: effect of increasing balloon size. *Lasers Surg Med* 1996;18(3):248.

81. Maier A, Tomaselli F, Gebhard F, et al. Palliation of advanced esophageal carcinoma by photodynamic therapy and irradiation. *Ann Thorac Surg* 2000;69:1006–1009.

82. Luketich JD, Nguyen NT, Weigel TL, et al. Photodynamic therapy for treatment of malignant dysphagia. *Surg Laparosc Endosc Percutan Tech* 1999;9:171–175.

83. Moghissi K, Dixon K, Thorpe JA, et al. The role of photodynamic therapy (PDT) in inoperable oesophageal cancer. *Eur J Cardiothorac Surg* 2000;17:95–100.

84. Litle VR, Luketich JD, Christie NA, et al. Photodynamic therapy as palliation for esophageal cancer: experience in 215 patients. *Ann Thorac Surg* 2003;76(5):1687–1692; discussion 1692–1693.

85. Eriksen JR. Palliation of non-resectable carcinoma of the cardia and oesophagus by argon beam coagulation. *Dan Med Bull* 2002;49(4):346–349.

86. Homs MY, Steyerberg EW, Eijkenboom WM, et al. Single-dose brachytherapy versus metal stent placement for the palliation of dysphagia from oesophageal cancer: multicentre randomised trial. *Lancet* 2004;364(9444):1497–1504.

87. Harbord M, Dawes RF, Barr H, et al. Palliation of patients with dysphagia due to advanced esophageal cancer by endoscopic injection of cisplatin/epinephrine injectable gel. *Gastrointest Endosc* 2002;56(5):644–651.

88. Monga SP, Wadleigh R, Sharma A, et al. Intratumoral therapy of cisplatin/epinephrine injectable gel for palliation in patients with obstructive esophageal cancer. *Am J Clin Oncol* 2000;23(4):386–392.

89. Livraghi T, Solbiato L. Percutaneous ethanol injection in liver cancer: methods and results. *Semin Interv Radiol* 1996;10:69.

90. Shiina S, Niwa Y, Osmata M. Percutaneous ethanol injection therapy for liver neoplasms. *Semin Interv Radiol* 1996;10:57.

91. Livraghi T, Giorgio A, Marin G, et al. Hepatocellular carcinoma and cirrhosis in 746 patients: long-term results of percutaneous ethanol injection. *Radiology* 1995;197:101–108.

92. Livraghi T, Goldberg SN, Lazzaroni S, et al. Small hepatocellular carcinoma: treatment with radiofrequency ablation versus ethanol injection. *Radiology* 1999;210:655–661.

93. Lencioni RA, Allgaier HP, Cioni D, et al. Small hepatocellular carcinoma in cirrhosis: randomized comparison of radio-frequency thermal ablation versus percutaneous ethanol injection. *Radiology* 2003;228(1):235–240.

94. Ohnishi K, Ohyama N, Ito S, et al. Small hepatocellular carcinoma: treatment with U/S guided intratumoral injection of acetic acid. *Radiology* 1994;193:747–752.

95. Ohnishi K, Yoshioka H, Ito S, et al. Prospective randomized controlled trial comparing percutaneous acetic acid injection and percutaneous ethanol injection for small hepatocellular carcinoma. *Hepatology* 1998;27:67–72.

96. Huo T, Huang YH, Wu JC, et al. Comparison of transarterial chemoembolization and percutaneous acetic acid injection as the primary locoregional therapy for unresectable hepatocellular carcinoma: a prospective survcy. *Aliment Pharmacol Ther* 2004;19(12):1301–1308.

97. Curley SA, Izzo F, Ellis LM, et al. Radiofrequency ablation of hepatocellular cancer in 110 patients with cirrhosis. *Ann Surg* 2000;232:381–391.

98. de Baere T, Elias D, Dromain C, et al. Radiofrequency ablation of 100 hepatic metastases with a mean follow-up of more than 1 year. *AJR Am J Roentgenol* 2000;175:1619–1625.

99. Rossi S, Garbagnati F, Lencioni R, et al. Percutaneous radio-frequency thermal ablation of nonresectable hepatocellular carcinoma after occlusion of tumor blood supply. *Radiology* 2000;217:119–126.

100. Chang AE, Schneider PD, Sugarbaker PH, et al. A prospective randomized trial of regional vs. systemic continuous 5-FU chemotherapy in the treatment of colorectal metastases. *Ann Surg* 1987;206:685.

101. Hohn DC, Stagg RJ, Friedman MA, et al. A randomized trial of continuous intravenous versus hepatic intraarterial floxuridine in patients with colorectal cancer metastatic liver: The Northern California Oncology Group trial. *J Clin Oncol* 1989;7:1646.

102. Martin JK, O'Connell MJ, Wieand HS, et al. Intra-arterial floxuridine vs systemic fluorouracil for hepatic metastases from colorectal cancer. *Arch Surg* 1990;125:1022.

103. Kemeny N, Daly JM, Reichman B, et al. Intrahepatic or systemic infusion of fluorodeoxyuridine in patients with liver metastases from colorectal carcinoma: a randomized trial. *Ann Intern Med* 1987;107:459.

104. Onohara S, Kobayashi H, Itoh Y, et al. Intraarterial cisplatinum infusion with sodium thiosulfate protection and angiotensin II induced hypertension for treatment of hepatocellular carcinoma. *Acta Radiol* 1988;29:197.

105. Doci R, Bignami F, Bozzetti F, et al. Intrahepatic chemotherapy for unresectable hepatocellular carcinoma. *Cancer* 1988;61:1983.

106. Carrasco CH, Charnsangavej C, Ajani J, et al. The carcinoid syndrome: palliation by hepatic artery embolization. *Am J Radiol* 1986;147:149.

107. Ajani JA, Carrasco CH, Charnsangavej C, et al. Islet cell tumors metastatic to the liver: effective palliation by sequential hepatic artery embolization. *Ann Intern Med* 1988;108:340.

108. Lin DY, Liaw YF, Lee TU, et al. Hepatic arterial embolization in patients with unresectable hepatocellular carcinoma—a randomized controlled trial. *Gastroenterology* 1988;94:453.

109. Sato Y, Fujiwara K, Ogata I, et al. Transcatheter arterial embolization for hepatocellular carcinoma. *Cancer* 1985;955:2822.

110. Chuang VP, Wallace S. Hepatic artery embolization in the treatment of hepatic neoplasms. *Radiology* 1981;140:51.

111. Clouse ME, Lee RGL, Duszlak EJ. Peripheral hepatic artery embolization for primary and secondary hepatic neoplasms. *Radiology* 1983;147:407.

112. Konno T. Targeting cancer chemotherapeutic agents by use of Lipiodol contrast medium. *Cancer* 1990;66:1897.

113. Egawa H, Maki A, Mori K. Effects of intraarterial chemotherapy with a new lipophilic anticancer agent, estradiol-chlorambucil (KM2210), dissolved in Lipiodol on experimental liver tumor in rats. *J Surg Oncol* 1990;44:109.

114. Nakamura H, Hashimoto T, Oi H, et al. Transcatheter oily chemoembolization of hepatocellular carcinoma. *Radiology* 1989;170:783.

115. Sasaki Y, Imaoka S, Kasugai H, et al. A new approach to chemoembolization therapy for hepatoma using ethiodized oil, cisplatin, and gelatin sponge. *Cancer* 1987;60:1194.

116. Charnsangavej C. Chemoembolization of liver tumors. *Semin Invest Radiol* 1993;10:150.

117. Nakao N, Miura K, Takahashi H, et al. Hepatocellular carcinoma: combined hepatic arterial and portal venous embolization. *Radiology* 1986;161:303–307.

118. Van Beers B, Roche A, Cauquil P, et al. Transcatheter arterial chemotherapy using doxorubicin, iodized oil and gelfoam embolization in hepatocellular carcinoma. *Acta Radiol* 1989;30:415.

119. Groupe d'Etude de Traitment du Carcinome Hepatocellulaire. A comparison of lipiodol chemoembolization and conservative treatment for unresectable hepatocellular carcinoma. *N Engl J Med* 1995;332:1256.

120. Bronwicki JP, Vetter D, Dumas F, et al. Transcatheter oily chemoembolization for hepatocellular carcinoma. A 4-year study of 127 French patients. *Cancer* 1994;74:16.

121. Lang EK, Brown CL. Colorectal metastases to the liver: selective chemoembolization. *Radiology* 1993;189:417–422.

122. Sanz-Altamira PM, Spence LD, Huberman MS, et al. Selective chemoembolization in the management of hepatic metastases in refractory colorectal carcinoma. *Dis Colon Rectum* 1997;40:770–775.

123. Neuhaus C, Leppek R, Christ G, et al. Monitoring of vital functions in the course of interventional radiology procedures. In: Steinbrich W, Gross-Fengels W, eds. *Interventional radiology: adjunctive medication and monitoring.* New York: Springer-Verlag, 1993.

124. Lang EV, Chen F, Fick LJ, et al. Determinants of intravenous conscious sedation for arteriography. *J Vasc Interv Radiol* 1996;9(3):407–412.

125. Cervero E. Visceral pain: mechanisms of peripheral and central sensitization. *Ann Med* 1995;27:235.

126. Clark BA. A new approach to assessment and documentation of conscious sedation during endoscopy. *Gastroenterol Nurs* 1994;16:199.

127. Rospond RM, Mills W. Hepatic artery chemoembolization for hepatic tumors. *AORN J* 1995;61:573.

128. Molgaard CP, Teitelbaum GP, Pentecost MJ, et al. Intraarterial administration of lidocaine for analgesia in hepatic chemoembolization. *J Vasc Interv Radiol* 1990;1:81.

129. Hiew CY, Hart GK, Thomson KR, et al. Analgesia and sedation in interventional radiologic procedures. *Australas Radiol* 1995;39:128.

130. Polomano R, Soulen M, McDaniels C. Conscious sedation and analgesia with interventional radiologic procedures for oncology patients. *Crit Care Nurs Clin North Am* 1997;9(3):335–353.

CHAPTER 54 ■ PSYCHOSOCIAL CONSEQUENCES OF ADVANCED CANCER

JAMES R. ZABORA AND MATTHEW J. LOSCALZO

All psychosocial care is palliative in nature. Attention must be directed at the realities of one's life within their unique social context in order to maximize internal resources, activate external support systems, and focus on the dignity and quality of life (QOL). Psychosocial care within palliative care programs seeks ongoing evidence of effectiveness and clear benefit to patients, caregivers, and to the health care system. However, institutional support for these approaches always seems to be less than desirable.

Psychosocial concerns, to varying degrees, based on context and predisposition, are always at the core of the cancer experience. Life limiting illness and related demands are always stressful. However, there are also opportunities for the repairing and deepening of relationships and to make a meaningful contribution. In the absence of moderate to severe distress caused by physical symptoms, such as pain, nausea, or difficulty in breathing, the psychosocial and spiritual aspects of a person's identity and life become paramount. The psychosocial aspects of a person's life are what give them individuality and a context for living with a life-threatening illness.

Despite significant progress in research and treatments, the diagnosis of cancer creates fear and turmoil in the lives of every patient and family. In many respects cancer generates a greater sense of dread than other life-threatening illnesses with similar prognoses (1). Some studies have found that patients with cancer are sicker and have more symptoms than patients without cancer in the year before death, and most often, it is easier to predict the course of the illness (2).

Frequently, the greatest concern of patients with cancer is not death, pain, or physical symptoms, but rather the impact of the disease on their families (3). According to the World Health Organization (4), family refers to those individuals who are either relatives or other significant people as defined by the patient. Health care professionals must acknowledge the role of the family to maximize treatment outcomes. If the family is actively incorporated into patient care, the health care team gains valuable allies and resources. Families are the primary source of support and also fill in the caregiving roles for persons with cancer. Of note, women comprise most of the individuals who serve in these caregiving roles (5,6).

Although access to ongoing palliative care could potentially provide needed support for both patient and family, resources for palliative care are consistently limited. In the United States most palliative care is invested in hospice programs, but only one-third of all patients with cancer receive formal hospice care, often only in the final days of life (7,8). Furthermore, a discussion concerning a referral to hospice can seem quite sudden, and the patient and family can experience this transition as rejection. Despite the sobering survival statistics for many cancers, relatively few hospitals have developed a continuum of cancer care, which informs patients and families that most antineoplastic therapy is palliative and not curative. In particular, this is true for patients with cancer who enroll in Phase I and II clinical trials (9). This is significant given that most patients with cancer overestimate the probability of long-term survival (10). At present, patients and family members enter hospice care, which is the primary resource for comprehensive palliative care services, and attempt to accept that prolongation of life is no longer the goal of care. In addition to the shift in the focus from cure to care, the patient and family experience the loss of the health care team with whom trust has been imbued over months and sometimes many years. The loss occurs simultaneously at multiple levels. Although palliative care at the end of life should be a time of refocusing and resolution, the referral process may cause an iatrogenic crisis rather than comfort.

PSYCHOLOGICAL RESPONSES TO ADVANCED CANCER

The psychological impact of advanced cancer and its management is directly influenced by the interactions among the degree of physical disability, internal resources of the patient, the level of social support, the intensity of the treatment, side effects, and other adverse reactions, and the relationship with the health care team. The degree of physical distress placed on any individual and the inevitable drive to give meaning to the experience is the core from which the psychosocial concerns arise.

Adaptation to this phase of the illness begins with an appraisal of the extent of harm, loss, threat, and challenge that this experience generates. In many respects, this appraisal is linked to the intensity and quality of the patient's emotional response. Overall, this primary appraisal and definition of the meaning of advanced cancer results in an assessment of the extent of the potential harm, which then requires a secondary appraisal to be made. In this secondary level, patients must assess their personal (internal) and social (external) resources necessary to begin to address the demands and problems associated with advanced cancer (11).

In addition, two salient continuums related to patient and family adaptation must be considered. The level of psychological distress forms the first continuum and the second

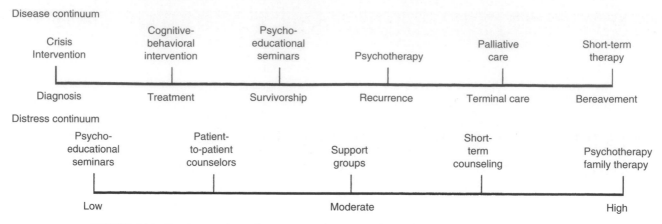

FIGURE 54.1. Continuum of care for patients with cancer and their families.

consists of the predictable and transitional phases of the disease process. Patients with a preexisting high level of psychological distress can experience significant difficulty with any attempt to adapt to the stressors associated with a cancer diagnosis. Although most patients experience significant distress at the time of their diagnosis, most patients gradually adjust during the following 6 months (12). Evidence indicates that the best predictor of positive adaptation is the psychological state of the patient with cancer before the initiation of any therapeutic regimens (13).

Figure 54.1 details potential interventions along the disease and distress continuums. The level of psychological vulnerability also falls along a continuum from low to high distress and should guide this selection of interventions (14). In addition, problem-solving interventions have been demonstrated to reduce distress among patients with cancer as well as among family members (15,16). Prevalence studies demonstrate that one of every three newly diagnosed patients (regardless of prognosis) needs psychosocial or psychiatric intervention (17–20). As disease advances, a positive relationship exists between the increase in the occurrence and severity of physiologic symptoms and the patient's level of emotional distress and overall QOL. For example, a study of 268 patients with cancer having recurrent disease observed that patients with higher symptomatology, greater financial concerns, and a pessimistic outlook experience higher levels of psychological distress and lower levels of general well-being (21).

In an effort to establish early identification of patients at high risk for poor adaptation, the National Comprehensive Cancer Network (NCCN) developed guidelines for the management of psychological distress among cancer patients across the disease continuum. These guidelines provide a framework for the development and implementation of psychosocial interventions based on the perspectives of psychiatry, social work, psychology, nursing, and pastoral care. Psychosocial screening serves as the mechanism to identify patients at higher levels of risk in order to provide interventions at a much earlier point in time. These guidelines can be accessed at www.nccs.org.

If distress levels can be identified through techniques such as psychosocial screening (22), patients can then be introduced into supportive care systems earlier in the treatment or palliative care process. Accordingly, any attempt to identify vulnerable patients and families in a prospective manner is worthwhile. Screening techniques are available through the use of standardized instruments which are able to prospectively identify patients and families that may be more vulnerable to the cancer experience (23). Preexisting psychosocial resources are critical in any predictive or screening process. In one approach, Weisman et al. (24) delineated key psychosocial variables in the format of a structured interview accompanied by a self-report measure (Table 54.1). However, in hospitals, clinics, or community agencies, which provide care to a high volume of patients and family members, a structured interview by a psychosocial provider is seldom feasible. Consequently,

TABLE 54.1

VARIABLES ASSOCIATED WITH PSYCHOSOCIAL ADAPTATION

Social support	History	Current concerns	Other variables
Marital status	Substance abuse	Health	Education
Living arrangements	Depression	Religion	Employment
Number of family members and relatives in vicinity	Mental health	Work-finance	Physical symptoms
Church attendance	Major illness	Family	Anatomic staging
	Past regrets	Friends	
	Optimism vs. pessimism	Existential	
		Self-appraisal	

From Weisman AD, Worden JW, Sobel HJ. *Psychosocial screening and interventions with patients with cancer: a research report.* Boston: Harvard Medical School and Massachusetts Hospital, 1980, with permission.

brief and rapid methods of screening are necessary. Brief screening techniques that examine components of distress, such as anxiety or depression, can be incorporated into the routine clinical care of the patient. Early psychosocial interventions may be less stigmatizing to the patient, and more readily accepted by patients, families, and staff if screening identifies the management of distress as one component of comprehensive care (25). Screening is also a cost-effective technique for case identification in comparison to an assessment of all new patients (26). Although screening for distress and problems have received much attention recently, there are extremely few screening programs in place, even in comprehensive cancer centers. The Moores University of California, San Diego (UCSD) Cancer Center is one of the few cancer programs that is screening all new patients with cancer for common problems and related distress. Although presently performed with pencil and paper, this screening and triage process is now being automated through touch-screen computers. For each of the problems listed, a triage plan is in place and can be accessed during the clinic visit by the physician, nurse or social worker. Not surprisingly, the 10 most common problems in rank order manifested by the first 300 patients with cancer were: fatigue (feeling tired), fear and worry about the future, finances, pain, feeling down, depressed or blue, being dependent on others, understanding my treatment options, sleeping, managing my emotions, and solving problems due to my illness. Of particular note, although pain was not the most frequently endorsed problem, it was the most emotionally distressing.

Standardized measures of psychological distress can differentiate patients into low, moderate, or high degree of vulnerability. Patients with a low or moderate level of distress may benefit from a psychoeducational program, which can enhance adaptive capabilities and problem-solving skills; high distress patients possess more complex psychosocial needs that require brief therapy or family therapy along with psychotropic drug therapy for the patient. For some patients ongoing mental health services are essential, whereas other patients may require assistance only at critical transition points. Clinical practice suggests that virtually all patients could benefit from some type of psychosocial intervention at some point along the disease continuum, especially at the end of life. Psychosocial interventions include educational programs, support groups, cognitive-behavioral techniques, problem-solving therapy or education, and psychotherapy (27). To further facilitate the process of screening, the Brief Symptom Inventory-18 was developed to create greater ease with administration and scoring and to develop gender-based norms (28,29).

The second continuum relates to the predictable phases of the disease process. This disease continuum extends from the point of diagnosis to cancer therapies and beyond. As patients move across this continuum, they may acquire experiences, knowledge, and skills that enable them to respond to the demands of their disease. The needs of a newly diagnosed patient with intractable symptoms differ significantly from a patient who has advanced disease and no further options for curative treatments.

The patient and family may be supported throughout the illness process and the family requires continuing support following the death of the patient. At times families are overwhelmed by the illness, and as a result are unable to effectively respond. For some families a death may represent a major loss of the family's identity and may paralyze the family's coping and problem-solving responses. Failure to respond and solve problems leads to a lack of control and may generate a significant potential for a chronic grief reaction (30). Although the disease continuum consists of specific points, Table 54.2 identifies a series of predictable and relevant crisis events and psychosocial challenges that occur as patients and families confront advanced disease.

FAMILY ADAPTABILITY AND COHESION

The Circumplex Model of Family Functioning, as developed by Olson et al. (31), categorizes families in a manner that explains the variation in their behavior. Although not specifically developed for cancer, this model conceptualizes families' responses to stressful events based on two constructs: adaptability, and cohesion. End-of-life care simultaneously generates significant stressors for both patients and families, especially in issues related to power, structure, and role assignments. Adaptability reflects the capability of a family to reorganize internal roles, rules, and power structure in response to a significant stressor. Given the impact of advancing cancer on the total family unit, families must frequently reassign roles, alter rules for daily living, and revise long-held methods for problem solving. Dysfunction in the family can relate to either low adaptability (rigidity) or excessively high adaptability (chaotic). A family characterized as rigid in its adaptability persists in the use of coping behaviors, such as frequent manifestations of anger, even when they are ineffective. Those that exhibit high adaptability create a chaotic response within the power structure, roles, and rules of the family; such families lack structure in their responses and attempt different coping strategies with every new stress. Although most families are in the more functional category of "structured adaptability," 30% are rigid or chaotic. These latter families are likely to exhibit problematic behaviors such as excessive demands of staff time or interference with the delivery of medical care that the health care team may find difficult to manage (32).

The second construct of Olson et al.—cohesion—is indicative of the family's ability to provide adequate support. Cohesion is the level of emotional bonding that exists among family members, and is also conceptualized on a continuum from low to high. Low cohesion (disengagement) suggests little or no connectedness among family members. A commitment to care for other family members is not evident and, as a result, these families are frequently unavailable to the medical staff for support of the patient or for participation in the decision-making process. At the other extreme, high cohesion (enmeshment) blurs the boundaries among family members. This results in the perception by health care providers that some family members seem to be just as affected by the diagnosis or treatment, or by each symptom, as the patient. Enmeshed families may demand excessive amounts of time from the health care team and be incapable of following simple medical directives. These families are not able to objectively receive and comprehend information which may be in the best interest of the patient. Also these families may assume a highly overprotective position in relation to the patient and may speak for the patient even when the patient's self-expression could be encouraged.

When engaging families, it is necessary to gain an appreciation for the rules and regulations within each particular family. Each family has its own rules, regulations, and communication styles. In gaining an understanding of the role of the patient in the family, it is helpful to ask the patient to describe the specific responsibilities he or she performs in the family, especially during a crisis. Generalities are less informative than descriptions of the specific experiences and duties of each family member during a crisis. These queries enable the patient to openly communicate and objectively evaluate his or her role and importance in the family system and provide a clinical opportunity to assess ongoing progress or deterioration. Patients and families can usually tolerate even the worst news or the most dire prognosis as long as it is framed within a context in which the patient and family know

TABLE 54.2

ADVANCING DISEASE AND PSYCHOSOCIAL TREATMENT

Crisis event	Personal meaning	Manifestation	Coping tasks	Survivor goals	Professional interventions
Recurrence/new primary	What did I do wrong? Was it my negative attitude? Was I foolish to hope this was over forever? God has failed me I beat this last time, I will beat it again	Anger Fear Depression Anxiety Shock Loss of hope Denial Guilt	Reestablish hope Accept the uncertainty about the future Understand information about new situation Regain a life focus and time perspective appropriate to the changed prognosis	Integrate reality with family functioning, maintain self-worth	Information Support Education Cognitive/behavioral skills training Physical availability Supportive psychotherapy Resource provision/referral
	Nothing ever works out good for me They said I was okay but I am not Do I have to start all over again?	Loss of trust Feelings of alienation Increased vulnerability Loss of control Confronting mortality Search for meaning	Communicate new status to others Make decisions about the new treatment course Integrate reality of ongoing nature of disease to probable death from cancer Tolerate changes in routine and roles again Adjust to increased dependency again Reinvest in treatment		
Advanced disease	I am out of control Will they offer new treatment? What am I doing wrong? Will it be as bad as the last time? Will I go broke?	Depression Anxiety Demoralization Fear Denial Anger Fear of intimacy	Maintain hope and direction Tolerate medical care Enhance coping skills Maintain open communication with family, friends, and health care professionals Assess treatment and care options Maintain relationships with medical team	Dignity Direction Role in work, family, and community	Support Cognitive/behavioral skills training Supportive psychotherapy Physical availability Resource provision/referral Information Education
Terminal	When am I going to die? Does dying hurt? What happens after you die? Why me? Why now? What did I do to deserve this? What will happen to my family? Will I be remembered by my family and friends? What if I start to die and I am all alone? Can't the doctors do something else, are they holding back on me, have they given up on me?	Depression Fear Anxiety Denial Demoralization Self-destructive behavior Loss of control Guilt Anger Fear of abandonment Fear of isolation Increased dependency Acceptance Withdrawal Search for meaning in past as well as present Pain/suffering Need to discuss afterlife	Maintain a meaningful quality of life Adjust to physical deterioration Plan for surviving family members Accept reality of prognosis Mourn actual losses Mourn the death of dreams Get things in order Maintain and end significant relationships Say good-bye to family and friends Accept impending death Confront the relevant existential and spiritual issues Talk about feelings Review one's life	Dignity Family support and bereavement	Physical availability Support Cognitive/behavioral skills training Therapeutic rituals Coordination of services Advocacy Information

how they are expected to respond and that the health care team will not abandon them.

IMPACT OF PHYSICAL AND PSYCHOLOGICAL SYMPTOMS

Patients with advanced illness experience pain, delirium, dyspnea, fatigue, nausea, anxiety, depression, sleeplessness, and many other symptoms that impair QOL. These noxious symptoms also compromise cognition, concentration, and memory (33), and override the underlying mental schema of patients. For the person in pain or acute physical distress, perception is confined to only the most immediate and essential elements of his or her sensory experience, and there is only a distant remnant of a past or future. The immediate need and goal is to stop or minimize the noxious experience. In some sense, pain, and other symptoms absorb the limited psychic energy of the patient, and valuable energy can only be made available if physical distress is effectively managed. The psychic life is subservient and dependent to the bodily experience. This is an important point for health care providers. Therefore, psychosocial interventions must simultaneously focus on physical symptoms in order to be effective. Furthermore, interventions that do not address the physical concerns of the patient may be unethical. The essence of psychosocial care is to raise the "bar" of what humanistic medical care means so that all of the concerns and needs of patients are effectively addressed and resolved. Unless physical and psychosocial distress are managed simultaneously, psychosocial interventions are less likely to be effective.

Moderate to severe pain is reported by 30–45% of patients undergoing (34) cancer treatments and 75–90% of patients with advanced disease (35). Pain seems to stand alone in its ability to gain the active attention of others although dramatically demonstrating a sense of being alone and vulnerable. This is especially true of patients with advanced disease, and their families. Although a patient is experiencing pain, another person only inches away is incapable of truly understanding what is so central and undeniable to the patient. This invisible and almost palpable boundary between the person in pain and his or her caregivers has significant implications for the quality and effectiveness of the therapeutic relationship (36).

Given that cancer pain can be adequately managed in almost all circumstances, its deleterious and at times life-threatening impact on the physical, psychological, and spiritual resources of both the patient and family are not only unnecessary but also evil. There is no known benefit to ongoing unrelieved pain. There are many known negative consequences. For example, O'Mahony et al. (37) found that the desire for death was correlated with ratings of pain and low family support but most significantly with depression. Given the relationship between pain and depression, the importance of adequate pain management can hardly be overstated. Recently Cobb et al. (38), in their comprehensive review of the delirium literature, found that poor pain control was identified as the number one cause or contributor for delirium. Given the obvious importance and prevalence of delirium as an indicator of QOL at the end of life, this is very important information.

Serlin et al. (39) were able to demonstrate that there is a positive correlation between pain intensity and function. As expected, low levels of pain intensity cause low levels of interference with life, whereas moderate to high levels of pain make it virtually impossible to have meaningful interactions with others and to feel part of a larger whole. Clinical experience consistently demonstrates that people with physical illness accompanied by high levels of pain intensity experience acute isolation, are unable to advocate for themselves and

are at very high risk to be badly cared for even in the best medical centers. Family and health care providers can be sensitive, caring, supportive, and concerned, but if pain is not adequately managed, the person confronting death has little possibility to think clearly, express his or her concerns, make a contribution and have anything resembling a peaceful death.

It is generally accepted that pain is poorly managed despite the availability of effective therapies (40–42). Of particular note, effective pain management may also be influenced by the race and ethnicity of the patient, but socioeconomic disadvantage is the more important predictor of disabling pain (43). Patients, families, and professional staff may share a reluctance to use opioid analgesics even when life expectancy is quite limited. Dysfunctional processes continue to exist which enable patients to accept suffering and to allow the health care team to permit unnecessary pain. This type of response represents an adaptive, but "dark side" of professional care. Although most patients with cancer are psychologically healthy (17,44), inadequately managed cancer pain and other symptoms can produce a variety of "pseudopsychiatric" syndromes, which are anxiety-provoking and confusing to patients, families, and clinicians. Patients with cancer and pain are also more likely to develop psychiatric disorders than patients with cancer without significant pain (42). In the short-term, pain provokes anxiety; over the long term, it generates depression and demoralization. Misguided priorities in the heath care system frequently result in needless pain and suffering in patients, and long-term guilt in family members and permanent mistrust of the intentions of health care providers.

The differences between depression and demoralization as clinical constructs have yet to be empirically explored. Depression is significantly related to higher levels of cancer pain and pain is likely to play a causal role related to depression. Overall depression rates for cancer patients are 20–25% (45) and estimates as high as 50–70% have been applied to populations with advanced disease (46). Patients who are demoralized are disheartened or discouraged by their circumstances but not in a pathologic sense. There is a significant correlation between affective disorders and pain and among the negative emotional states associated with pain (dysphoria, hopelessness, guilt, suicidal ideation, etc.). Anecdotal clinical experience consistently demonstrates that once pain and related distressing physical symptoms are relieved, and suffering, anxiety, depression, demoralization, and suicidal ideation are ameliorated, the impact on the family is equally significant (47).

Patients who are depressed distort reality and grossly minimize their perceived abilities in managing the demands of the illness and its treatment. Furthermore patients with cancer who are depressed and have inadequately controlled pain are at increased risk of suicide (37,48). For the patient who is depressed, acute sensitivity to physical sensations may lead to or exaggerate preexisting morbid or catastrophizing thoughts. The complex and interactive associations among physical sensations (neutral or noxious sensations), mentation (personal meaning given to the sensations), and behaviors (attempts to minimize threat and regain control) are all negatively influenced by depression. The destructive synergy of unrelieved pain and depression may lead to overwhelming suffering in patients and families and to a shared sense of helplessness and hopelessness (49). Consequently a patient or family may develop the faulty perception that suicide is their only remaining vestige of control. From this perspective, the value of a multimodality approach that combines pharmacology, supportive psychotherapy, and cognitive-behavioral skills training is clear (50). From a psychological perspective promotion of compliance with medical regimens, correction of distorted cognitive perceptions, acquisition of coping skills to manage physical tension, stress, and pain, and the effective use of valuable physical energy to maximize engagement of life become the focus of care.

SOCIOCULTURAL INFLUENCES ON PATIENT AND FAMILY ADAPTATION

Perceptions of illness and death can be conceptualized as experiences with both conscious and unconscious associations. These perceptions include concerns and fears that are beyond the limits of objective knowledge. Sociocultural beliefs may soothe anxiety or fear by providing comfort when a vacuum exists due to a lack of experience in the management of a chronic illness. Sociocultural attitudes also exert considerable influence as patients approach the end of their lives (51,52). These beliefs and attitudes are evident in direct observations of how the family cares for the patient, views of an afterlife, and rituals related to how the corpse is to be managed.

Koenig and Gates-Williams (53) offer a framework to assess cultural responses relevant to palliative care. This framework, which is consistent with a comprehensive psychosocial assessment, posits that "culture is only meaningful when interpreted in the context of a patient's unique history, family constellation, and socioeconomic status. Dangers exist in creating negative stereotypes—in simply supplying clinicians with an atlas or map of "cultural traits" common among particular ethnic groups."

Patients and their families can simply not be adequately understood without knowledge of their sociocultural backgrounds (54). Patients and families vary according to interests, beliefs, values, and attitudes. Individuals learn attitudes or values through family interactions and these patterns influence how patients respond to the health care team. Although the health care team represents expertise, safety, and authority, it is also an external and foreign force, which only through necessity has gained influence and power within the family system. In stressful situations the patient and family may project their own perceptions about themselves onto the health care team.

Although cultural characteristics are important these influences often diminish over time as families are assimilated into the predominant culture. Second-generation families are more similar to the host country than the country of origin. First-generation immigrants may possess old-world attitudes and values about authority and illness, whereas the perspectives of their offspring will be more consistent with the health care team.

Given the many and complex demands already made on health care professionals and the rapidly increasing diversity of institutions, is it reasonable to expect that staff be informed about the myriad cultures represented in such a pluralistic environment? For example, it is estimated that there are over 150 different languages spoken among the native Americans, with each tribe having its own rituals around end of life (55). One can only imagine trying to provide bereavement services to a group that demands that the name of the deceased never be mentioned again. Or that believes that even mentioning the word death will cause the event to happen. These barriers to effective and open communication, so respected by health care professionals in the United States, are not unique to native Americans (56). Furthermore, evidence exists that African Americans are far less likely to discuss end-of-life issues due to a belief that these discussions may result in less care being delivered (57).

Although there is no formula to making a connection with another person when he or she is ill, there are some areas that can be explored together that can be mutually enriching. The health care provider needs to specifically ask the patient and family about them as a system, patient, family, tribe, group, and so on. Some examples are:

- Because everyone is different, can you teach me how to help you get the information you need about your illness?
- How would you like me to share information with you about your illness?
- How much information, if any, would you like me to share with your family and others?
- Is there a particular person you would like me to include when you and I talk about serious matters?
- Would you like me to give you an overview of what is happening to you each time we meet or would you like me to simply answer your specific questions?
- What is your understanding of your health right now?
- What kinds of information would you like me to tell you?
- You have a very serious illness. Some people want to know what they have to prepare for in the near future. Is there anything that you would like to know now?
- Is there anything you think we need to share with your family and others that may be helpful to them and you?
- Is there anything we can do together to make this time meaningful for you and your family?
- Would you feel comfortable contacting me if you have any questions?

Ultimately, a relationship is always between two people at a time. Opening up one's self to be taught by the patient and family about who they are and how they want to manage the illness is the perfect counterpoint to the awesome power held by health care professionals.

PRINCIPLES OF EFFECTIVE PATIENT AND FAMILY MANAGEMENT

The family, as defined by the patient, is virtually always the primary supportive structure for the patient. The family serves as a supportive environment, which provides instrumental assistance, psychological support, and consistent encouragement, so that the patient seeks the best available medical care. Early in the diagnostic and treatment planning phases, a family's primary functions are to instill hope and facilitate communication. For the patient whose disease is beyond life-prolonging therapy, caregiving becomes the primary focus for the family. In the latter situation, families must prepare psychologically and financially for the experience of life without the patient (anticipatory grief). Cancer and its treatments is always a crisis and an assault on the family system. As an uninvited intruder, cancer challenges the viability of the family structure to tolerate and integrate a harsh and threatening reality, which cannot be overcome by force, denial, or even joint action. Joint action can be successful in terms of adaptation, and if the goals are clearly defined, there is an ongoing plan that promotes the optimal opportunity for successful goal attainment.

The health care team can guide the family in developing a problem-solving approach to the demands of the illness. Problem-solving therapy conceived by D'Zurilla, Nezu, and others, defines problem solving as a series of tasks rather than a single skill. According to the theoretical model, successful problem solving requires five component processes, each of which contributes directly to effective problem resolution (58). The five components are as follows:

1. Problem orientation, definition and formulation
2. Generation of alternatives

3. Decision making
4. Solution implementation and
5. Verification.

Problem orientation involves a motivational process; the other components consist of specific skills and abilities that enable a person to effectively solve a particular problem. Because problem solving is a set of skills, this approach has also been provided as an educational format.

The basic notion underlying the relevance of problem solving for cancer patients lies in the moderating role of coping through problem-solving serves in the general stress-distress relationship (59). The more effective people are in resolving or coping with stressful problems, the more probable it is that they will experience a higher QOL as compared with those persons facing similar problems who have difficulty in coping. Families also require guidance and support in managing the multiple problems associated with cancer, related treatments, adverse reactions, and rehabilitation. Following the diagnosis of cancer, families need to have honest, intelligible, and timely information whereas being reassured that competent health care professionals are genuinely caring for their family member.

Previous research indicates that problem-solving education for family caregivers improves their ability to manage care better, and cope more effectively with the stressors generated by caregiving. D'Zurilla, Nezu, and others (60,61) have developed conceptual frameworks for problem-solving therapy, and have conducted research that demonstrates that counseling caregivers, who are under stress, reduces their distress while increasing their problem-solving competence. This conceptual model has been applied successfully with a number of diverse health-related problems including cancer (62). Blanchard et al. (63) have shown that problem-solving counseling of family caregivers lessened caregiver distress and reduced long-term depression in the patients.

Therapeutic treatment plans must always be clearly communicated because it delineates each individual's responsibility so that the potential for goal attainment is maximized. For many families with histories of effective functioning, the cancer experience represents the first time that their joint action may not overcome an external threat. Consequently, the cancer experience must be reframed into more realistic terms so that the threat can be perceived as manageable rather than destructive. If this is not achieved, the family can manifest anger, avoidance, displacement, or other forms of regressive behavior. For the family with a history of multiple defeats and failures, the cancer experience may be perceived as more evidence that they are incapable of managing the demands of an overwhelming world. The cancer experience temporarily alters the family structure, but it also has the potential to inflict permanent change. The health care team can significantly influence how these changes are interpreted and integrated into family life.

Patients often identify the effect on the family as the most upsetting repercussion of the cancer (3). Therefore, any effective intervention must include the patient, the family, and other social support networks. When patients consider their families, they may experience guilt, shame, anger, frustration, and fear of abandonment. Family members may experience anger, fear, powerlessness, survivor guilt, and confusion as they attempt to care for the patient. Family members may demonstrate the defense mechanism of displacement, transferring emotion from one person or situation to another and potentially confusing health care professionals. This confusion can create tension for family members and providers at a time when clarity and effective interactions are essential.

With little exception, assessment of the primary players in the family system is a rather straightforward process. The patient can be asked the following directly:

- Who do you rely on most to assist you in relation to the practical needs of your illness (e.g., transportation, insurance company negotiations)?
- When you get scared or confused, with whom in your family are you most able to talk?
- Who in your family most concerns you?
- Is anyone in your family overwhelmed with your ongoing medical and practical needs?
- Who in your family is coping least well with your illness?
- Is anyone in your family openly angry with you because of your illness?
- Are you particularly worried about how a specific person in your family is coping?
- Who is most dependent on you in your family?
- For what are they dependent on you?
- What would happen to your family if you were unable to maintain your present level of functioning?
- Are you ever concerned that the demands of your illness will be too much for your family?

The answers to these questions communicate to the patient and family that it is appropriate and necessary to gauge the impact of the cancer and its treatment on their lives and also provide the groundwork for the coordination of patient and family functions. In addition, role modeling of open communication provides an environment of emotional support, flexibility in roles, trust, and the implied and spoken promise never to abandon each other. This cannot be achieved unless the patient and family accept that some treatment effects and life events are beyond their control and there are limits to what is possible. The medical team has the responsibility to manage the physical aspects of the disease whereas the patient and family actively strive to integrate change, maintain normalcy, and accept the reality of the illness. The course of the illness—including death—must be identified as one of the potentially uncontrollable issues so the patient and family can focus on areas that are amenable to their influence.

Financial resources are virtually always a major concern of patients and families. When discussions of money and resources occur within the family system, shame and guilt are common. These emotions are frequently alluded to but not openly discussed. This can be a barrier to open communication and can lead to patient fears and fantasies of abandonment. This is especially true for patients with advancing disease. Simultaneously the family may have concerns about life goals after the patient's acute need is past or death occurs. The expected range of emotional reactions within the family includes anger, fear, guilt, anxiety, frustration, powerlessness, and confusion. Cancer confronts people with the reality of limitations.

In addition to the increasing costs of health insurance and home care, there is a wide variety of nonreimbursable, illness-related costs that can be financially devastating to patients and families. Transportation, nutritional supplements, temporary housing, child care, and lost work days are but a few examples of costs borne almost totally by patients and families for which there is seldom any form of reimbursement (64). Schulz et al. (65) found that respondents spent more than $200 per month on health-related expenses and reported significant negative effects on amount of time worked. Other studies have confirmed the negative financial impact of advanced cancer (66,67).

Money is almost always a metaphor for value, control, and power (68). How patients and family members communicate about money can be an indication of their perceptions of whether treatment is progressing or not. Therefore interchanges about financial matters can actively represent latent communications about the perceived but unexpressed value of care and its potential outcome. For example, the patient and family may at the beginning of treatment state that money is no object and all resources must be expended so that the patient survives. When treatment becomes prolonged, however, a much more sober and realistic view concerning valuable and vanishing resources may become evident, and a greater discussion of investment and return may ensue. At this point in time, both patient and family may be actually talking about their ability to persevere. Concerns about money may then be an expression of exhaustion, diminishing hope, or anger. It is important that this metaphorical communication be seen as inadequate for open and direct communication. A metaphor is a signal and cue that indicate the need for open discussion. Openness is essential for the patient and family to discuss both their common and increasingly diverging needs. Patients and families must discuss their physical and spiritual fatigue, as well as specific financial concerns related to diminishing resources as a result of their struggle with cancer. The following clinical example illustrates a number of these points.

A 54-year-old married woman with three adolescent daughters expressed concern to the medical team about the ongoing cost of care for her terminally ill husband. The team felt that she was selfish and that it was unethical for them to consider the financial impact on the family in caring for the patient. Sensing their resistance to her plight, she felt rejected and became irate. A meeting with the patient, family, and relevant staff was organized by the social worker to openly address her financial concerns. The family had existing financial debts due to past medical treatments and consequently had ample reason for its concern related to the additional costs of care. Once this meeting resolved concerns over additional unneeded expenditures, the focus shifted to the much more emotionally laden issues related to the slow deterioration of the patient and the family's intense grief over the impending loss. It became evident that money for the family represented the loss of "everything."

In some cases, the family may begin to perceive the dying patient as already being deceased. Anticipatory grief and premature emotional withdrawal from the dying patient creates confusion and a sense of terror in the patient. As a result, the family experiences guilt and shame because they are prepared for the loss but the patient is still alive.

SPECIFIC PROBLEMATIC PATIENT AND FAMILY BEHAVIORS

Physicians almost always identify "difficult families" as one of the most challenging tasks as a medical provider. Within the context of the family milieu, conflicts with staff may be unavoidable. It is the management of these conflicts that will determine the quality of the relationship between the patient, family, and professional staff. Conflicts may result if a family cannot follow simple guidelines or is intolerant of any physical discomfort that the patient may experience. Families that frequently criticize staff may be held to more rigid standards of behavior. Unit guidelines become laws, and the struggle for control results in fear and mistrust. Conversely, patients and families who endear themselves to staff through verbal praise of the quality of care often receive warmth and flexibility, and, as a result, unit guidelines, such as visiting hours or number of visitors, may be relaxed.

The professional staff must be flexible in their communication styles or they may be perceived as violating family boundaries. This type of interaction can devolve into a battle for power and control. Conflicts that remain at the level of power and control make it virtually impossible to work with the patient and family to develop action-oriented, problem-solving strategies, which unite all in a common set of values and

goals. Effective symptom management is essential to engage the patient, family, and the staff toward a common goal. Poor management can lead to estrangement and abandonment (69). Open communication can establish goals within the context of the family and significantly reduce the strain. However health care providers must accept that at times any approach may be ineffective because the family structure cannot tolerate the influence of external forces. When this occurs continued attempts at open communication is the only alternative that can achieve some sense of mutual understanding and trust.

Families can exhibit a range of behaviors that the health care team defines as problematic and can potentially interfere with the delivery of medical care. Families can delay or prevent the completion of a procedure, verbally abuse the staff, or divide the team. Families may demand excessive amounts of staff time, repeatedly demanding sessions to review the same information. Confusion may reflect intense anxiety and the overwhelming nature of this experience for caregivers. Some families have unrealistic expectations and compare the responses of staff members searching for inconsistencies. Others fail to follow unit guidelines, consistently arriving well before visiting hours or delaying their departure from the hospital at the end of the day. Families may encourage patients to refuse medical recommendations or directives. Family members at times may speak for the patient and encourage the patient to withdraw and regress. Families may also possess unrealistic expectations of staff. Family members may perceive the staff as their own medical providers and seek personal care from the team (33).

Family functions include facilitation of medical decision making, reduction of stress, initiation of effective problem solving, and provision of comfort to the patient. If the family cannot provide these functions or is unavailable to the patient and staff, the staff may need to assume and fulfill these roles. At times, the staff may be resentful when families are unavailable or withdraw from participation. The burden on staff to care for these patients can be dramatically increased.

SPECIAL PATIENT AND FAMILY ISSUES

Children in the Home

Children of adult patients with cancer may be an unseen and forgotten population. In acute care settings, children are not observed due to the patients' daytime appointments or policies that prohibit visits to inpatient units. Within the palliative setting, however, children and grandchildren are often present and may play an active role in the caregiving process.

Although salient developmental differences exist among children of different ages, those 3 years or older are able to verbally communicate their concerns so that an ongoing dialogue can occur. Highly sensitive to emotional and physical changes, children benefit most from an environment where they are continually given information in a manner that they can understand and are then encouraged to ask questions. Adults should be prepared for questions to be rather concrete and egocentric, centered around the immediate needs of the child and any potential change in the immediate family. Children are specifically concerned about the continued presence of parents and their own safety. Questions from children usually come one or two at a time. Children often need time to interpret and integrate the adult responses before returning for additional information, which may occur days or weeks later.

Methods to deliver medical information or relieve distress must vary according to each child's developmental stage.

Children have fantasies about the etiology, meaning, and duration of a parent's illness. Young children need consistent information about the chronic nature of the disease so that they can anticipate changes and incorporate an understanding of these medical events into their world. Young children cannot fully appreciate the concept of permanence. The permanence of death or abstract terms, such as "forever," are beyond their ability to integrate on a cognitive level. Children need consistent support, measured doses of information, and an environment that can respond to their questions.

Developmentally, adolescence is the time for resolution of conflicts with parents as well as a quickened pace to individuation from the family. These processes can be delayed or significantly complicated by the family's focus on a loved one who is slowly deteriorating and dying. Competitiveness, sexuality, aggression, and peer relationships may compound and confuse attempts to cope with a loss and the end of a specific relationship.

Familial roles can be disrupted or confused during a parent's illness, and, as a result, adolescents may be required to assume adult responsibilities. There is a danger in treating an adolescent as an adult. The demands of adolescence under normal circumstances generate numerous stressors for the family, and a chronic illness at this point in the life cycle can significantly exacerbate the family's level of distress. Of particular concern, adolescents may be "parentified." Physical maturity should not be equated with emotional, intellectual, or spiritual development. Adolescents can easily be overwhelmed with guilt and shame when their normal sense of power and grandiosity cannot control symptoms or death. This may have a long-term negative effect on the ability to tolerate emotional relationships. If the death of a parent or grandparent is to occur in the home, children must be carefully assessed, and appropriate interventions and support should be offered.

Psychiatric Illness

Histories of psychiatric disorders present further challenges in the effective management of patients and families. Psychiatric symptoms must be assessed and appropriately managed if the patient is to truly benefit from supportive care interventions. For example, symptoms, such as severe depression, may dramatically influence a patient's perception of pain and the ability of the health care team to control it. Furthermore, psychiatric symptoms of a family member can also cause a significant concern given the health care team's expectations concerning caregiving in the home by family members. Frequently, expectations of family members as caregivers are relatively uniform despite the significant variation that exists in each family's level of functioning. Families must be assessed not only for their availability but also for their ability to provide adequate supportive care.

Patients or family members with a history of physical or sexual abuse may exhibit significant difficulty in the ability to develop a trusting relationship with the health care team and may require psychiatric management. Families with a history of abuse may try to withhold information related to the abuse and any attempt to assess the patient or family as an intrusion. Trust can only be developed over time as the health care team consistently verbalizes their concern for patient and family as well as their availability for support and intervention. Families with severe dysfunction isolate and protect themselves from the outside world with rigid outer boundaries. Health care providers may define such a family as problematic when initial offers of assistance are refused. The team may experience frustration and rejection, which is inevitably communicated directly to the patient and family. Consequently, the family is lost as an ally and resource and, as a result, their isolation is increased. Although few in number, timely psychiatric referrals for these patients and family members are essential.

Addictions

A current or past history of substance abuse or an active addiction within the patient or the family creates a sense of alarm within the health care team. For example, the patient with a history of substance abuse may simply not be trusted by health care providers. The patient's behavior may be viewed as manipulative and if pain is a problem, there may be reticence to prescribe higher opioid doses if the patient is in pain, or even when dying.

Patients should not needlessly suffer as a result of a prior history of opioid abuse or their current treatment in a methadone clinic. Patients with a history of opioid addiction that is remote or has been effectively managed in a drug treatment program may be at much greater risk for the undertreatment of cancer pain. Consultation with a drug treatment facility may be necessary to plan effective management strategies.

Family members of a substance abuser can negatively influence or reinforce the patient's drug-seeking behavior. These families frequently possess an extremely high level of cohesion, which can be characterized as enmeshed. Within this type of family, boundaries between family members are nebulous, and, as a result, family members may appear to be equally affected by the status of the patient. The care provided to the patient may be sporadic or inconsistent because the family may be overwhelmed by the severity of the illness. Careful medical and psychosocial coordination between patient, family, staff, and, when appropriate, a drug treatment center, is necessary to maximize cooperation and maintain quality care. Despite the level of frustration associated with this group of patients, dignified care is possible and attainable.

Intimacy and Sexuality

Advanced disease always affects sexuality and sexual functioning. Notwithstanding, the lack of libido and impaired sexual functioning are frequently overlooked or ignored as a concern of the patient. Open discussion of intimacy and sexuality with the team can actually result in enhancement of emotional vitality. In fact, an increase in intimacy can evolve as closeness is redefined and openly discussed. Patients' needs for intimacy and sexual activity must be examined and supported. A couple's expression of intimacy, even during terminal care, can create a sense of normalcy and relief in the midst of a highly traumatic course of medical events. As patients enter the terminal phase, these discussions require a high level of sensitivity. Most patients long to be touched and held, and it is not uncommon for spouses or children to lie in bed with a dying patient to provide comfort and experience closeness or intimacy.

Dying at Home

Although many patients and families describe a preference for death to occur in the comfort of their homes, this goal is not always attainable. Approximately 76–80% of patient deaths occur in medical institutions; only 10–14% of patients die in hospices, and the remaining 5–10% die in nursing homes or in patients' homes (70–72). The return to home, nursing homes, or hospices as the chosen places of death continues to increase, primarily as a result of the Medicare Hospice Benefit (73) and physician availability for home visits (74). A number of key psychosocial variables (Table 54.2) may inhibit or prevent the occurrence of death in the home even with the highest level of supportive care or hospice services. Families must be carefully assessed and prepared for the death event. Key family members can be specifically questioned concerning their level of comfort or toleration for stressful events within the home. Preparations, including advance directives, wills, and do-not-resuscitate orders, should begin as early as possible to resolve all questions and informational needs that the family may have. Typically, hospice services are only available in the home for a fraction of each day. Consequently, the patient's death will probably occur when the family is alone.

A family that wants to maintain a dying member at home despite complex needs may suddenly request that the patient die in the hospital. Reasons for rapid changes may be obvious and practical or may be irrational and unconscious. Either way, the resources and limitations of the family must be assessed and supported. Many patients who are terminally ill possess acute care needs (e.g., pain control, mental status changes, etc.), and admission may be warranted to provide brief respite for the family or to actually manage the death event.

When the Patient Dies

The final hours of the patient's life have significant meaning for the family and offer an opportunity for closure. The ritualistic need to be present at the exact moment of death can be very powerful for family members. The desire to be present for the death event is common, and for family members who are absent, significant regrets may result (75). Unexpected deaths occur in approximately 30% of patients; attempts to notify the family of the impending event is possible in 70% of cases (76).

Family members may require objective information concerning the cause of death, especially if the death was unexpected. Despite the terminal prognosis, many families need to understand why the patient died when he or she did. This information can mitigate a high level of mistrust and resulting distress, and address any irrational concerns and fears associated with the death as it is happening.

Interactions with staff that occur immediately following the death can have a long-term effect. Emotional reactions of family members are expected, and crying, sobbing, and wailing are common. The therapeutic demands associated with the provision of terminal care challenges the health care professional to communicate with empathy while facilitating the initiation of essential tasks such as removal of the body and funeral arrangements. Families vary in their ability to receive information and emotional support during this time. The relationship between the family and the health care team influences how much of these preparations can be made prior to the death event and how much clinical intervention the family requires and can tolerate. Generally, families elect a spokesperson to provide and receive information but care must be taken to assess other members of the family. A follow-up meeting with the family by a social worker or nurse in the home can be very helpful to identify any family member who may be at risk for an abnormal grief response (30).

CONCLUSIONS

All patients and families possess a personal meaning of disease, prolonged illness, and death. These meanings are influenced over time by numerous factors. A clear understanding of these meanings, associated emotions, and their antecedents enhances the health care team's ability to provide care and anticipate potential problems. Information and education must

be consistently available as the patient and family move across the disease continuum toward and post the death event (77).

Variables, such as cohesion, describe the quality and intensity of relationships within the family. High cohesion or enmeshed families lose more than a family member when the patient dies. For these families, part of their identity is also lost. Given their extreme level of dependence on one another, these families may experience the death as catastrophic, which prevents the effective resolution of the loss. Chronic grief can exacerbate current psychological symptoms and influence health care practices. Bereavement follow-up among high-risk families is essential as a means to develop psychosocial prevention programs. The psychosocial obligation to the family does not end with the patient's death, and some families may require follow-up beyond the customary 1-year period as the bereaved experience salient dates such as a birthday or anniversary for the first time without the loved one who has died. Most often, bereaved family members must experience the "four seasons of the year" as they attempt to celebrate holidays or experience a vacation following the death of their loved one (78). Given the intensity of the loss and the family's level of risk, grief must be monitored and resolved.

As with palliative care, despite data supporting effectiveness and benefits to patients, their caregivers and to the system, psychosocial services have been actively supported and demanded by consumers of these services. To its detriment, the health system has for too long resisted a wider view of the patient experience. Palliative care has actively promoted the importance of psychosocial services and has created an opportunity to give a strong voice to the humanistic agenda, where respect, dignity, identifying personal and social strengths are synergized into a health caring system where the needs of people are more wisely and appropriately balanced with the inquisitiveness and natural desire to defy the limits of what humans can presently accomplish while still maintaining our humanity.

Ultimately, the role of the health care team is to create an environment with exquisite symptom management and honest and open communication (79). If these components are present, the opportunity exists to provide meaning to the death event. If this occurs, a sense of growth is possible for patients who are dying and the surviving family.

ACKNOWLEDGMENTS

The authors wish to acknowledge the assistance of Karlynn BrintzenhofeSzoc, DSW, and the Department of Oncology Social Work of The Johns Hopkins Oncology Center in the development of the tables and figure.

References

1. Mishel MH. Reconceptualization of the uncertainty in illness theory. *Image J Nurs Sch* 1990;22:256.
2. Seale C, Cartwright A. *The year before death*. Brookfield, WI: Ashgate Publishing Company, 1994.
3. Levin DN, Cleeland CS, Dar R. Public attitudes toward cancer pain. *Cancer* 1985;56:2337.
4. World Health Organization. *Cancer pain and palliative care*, Technical Report 804. Geneva: World Health Organization, 1990.
5. Zarit SH, Todd PA, Zarit JM. Subjective burdens of husbands and wives as caregivers: a longitudinal study. *Gerontologist* 1986;26:260.
6. Brody EM. Women in the middle and family help to older people. *Gerontologist* 1981;21:471.
7. Iwashyna TJ, Christakis NA. Attitude and self-reported practice regarding hospice referral in a national sample. *J Palliat Med* 1998;1(3):241.
8. Bomba PA. Enabling the transition to hospice through effective palliative care. *Case Manager* 2005;16(1):48.
9. Zwerding T, Hamann K, Meyers F. Extending palliative care: is there a role for preventive medicine? *J Palliat Med* 2005;8(3):486.

10. Weeks JC, Cook EF, O'Day SJ, et al. Relationship between cancer patients' predictions of prognosis and their treatment preferences. *JAMA* 1998;279:1709.
11. Lazarus RS. *Emotion and adaptation.* New York: Oxford University Press, 1991.
12. Weisman AD, Worden JW. The existential plight in cancer: significance of the first 100 days. *Int J Psychiatry Med* 1976–1977;7:1.
13. Carlsson M, Mamrin E. Psychological and psychosocial aspects of breast cancer treatments. *Cancer Nurs* 1994;17:418.
14. Zabora JR, Loscalzo MJ, Weber J. Managing complications in cancer: identifying and responding to the patient's perspective. *Semin Oncol Nurs* 2003;19(4 Suppl 2):1.
15. Houts PS, Nezu AM, Nezu CM, et al. A problem-solving model of family caregiving for cancer patients. *Patient Educ Couns* 1996;27:63.
16. Bucher J, Loscalzo MJ, Zabora JR, et al. Problem-solving cancer care education for patients and caregivers. *Cancer Pract* 2001;9(2):66.
17. Derogatis LR, Morrow GR, Fetting J. The prevalence of psychiatric disorders among cancer patients. *JAMA* 1983;249(6):751.
18. Farber JM, Weinerman BH, Kuypers JA. Psychosocial distress in oncology outpatients. *J Psychosoc Oncol* 1984;2:109.
19. Stefanek M, Derogatis L, Shaw A. Psychological distress among oncology outpatients. *Psychosomatics* 1987;28:530.
20. Zabora J, BrintzenhofeSzoc K, Curbow B, et al. The prevalence of psychological distress by cancer site. *Psychooncology* 2001;10:19.
21. Schulz R, Williamson GM, Knapp JE, et al. The psychological, social, and economic impact of illness among patients with recurrent cancer. *J Psychosoc Oncol* 1995;13(3):21.
22. Zabora JR. Pragmatic approaches in the psychosocial screening of cancer patients. In: Holland J, Breitbart P, Loscalzo M, eds. *Handbook of psychooncology*, 2nd ed. London: Oxford Press, 1998.
23. Jacobsen PB, Donovan KA, Trask PC, et al. screening for distress in ambulatory cancer patients. *Cancer* 2005;103(7):1494.
24. Weisman AD, Worden JW, Sobel HJ. *Psychosocial screening and interventions with cancer patients: a research report.* Boston, MA: Harvard Medical School and Massachusetts Hospital, 1980.
25. Fawzy FI, Fawzy NW, Arndt LA, et al. Critical review of psychosocial interventions in cancer care. *Arch Gen Psychiatry* 1995;52:100.
26. Zabora JR, Smith-Wilson R, Fetting JH, et al. An efficient method for the psychosocial screening of cancer patients. *Psychosomatics* 1990;31(2):192.
27. Zabora JR, Loscalzo MJ, Smith ED. "Psychosocial Rehabilitation". In: Abeloff MD, Armitage JO, Lichter AS, et al. *Clinical oncology.* New York: Churchill Livingstone, 2002.
28. Derogatis LR. *BSI-18: administration, scoring and procedures manual.* Minneapolis, MN: National Computer Systems, 2000.
29. Zabora J, BrintzenhofeSzoc K, Jacobsen P, et al. Development of a new psychosocial screening instrument for use with cancer patients. *Psychosomatics* 2001;42(3):19.
30. BrintzenhofeSzoc K, Smith E, Zabora J. Development of a screening approach to predict complicated grief in surviving spouses of cancer patients. *Cancer Pract* 1999;7(5):233.
31. Olson DH, McCubbin HI, Barnes HL, et al. Predicting conflict with staff among families of cancer patients during prolonged hospitalizations. *J Psychosoc Oncol* 1989;7(3):103.
32. Zabora JR, Fetting JH, Shaley VB, et al. Predicting conflict with staff among families of cancer patients during prolonged hospitalization. *J Psychosoc Oncol* 1989;7(3):103.
33. Jamison RN, Sbrocco T, Parris W. The influence of problems in concentration and memory on emotional distress and daily activities in chronic pain patients. *Int J Psychiatry Med* 1988;18:183.
34. Daut RL, Cleeland CS. The prevalence and severity of pain in cancer. *Cancer* 1982;50(9):1913.
35. Bond MR, Pearson IB. Psychological aspects of pain in women with advanced cancer of the cervix. *J Psychosom Res* 1969;13:13.
36. Cleeland CS. The impact of pain on the patient with cancer. *Cancer* 1984;54:2635.
37. O'Mahony S, Goulet J, Kornblith A, et al. Desire for hastened death, cancer pain and depression: report of a longitudinal observational study. *J Pain Symptom Manage* 2005;29(5):446.
38. Cobb JL, Glantz MJ, Martin EW, et al. Delirium in patients with cancer at the end of life. *Cancer Pract* 2000;8(4):172.
39. Serlin RC, Mendoza TR, Nakamura Y, et al. When is cancer pain mild, moderate or severe? *Pain* 1995;61(2):277.
40. Von Roemn JH, Cleeland CS, Gonin R, et al. Physician attitudes and practice in cancer pain management. *Ann Intern Med* 1993;119:121.
41. Cleeland CS, Gonin R, Hatfield AK, et al. Pain and its treatment in outpatients with metastatic cancer. *N Engl J Med* 1994;330(9):592.
42. Grossman SA, Sheidler VR, Swedeen K, et al. Correlation of patient and caregiver ratings of cancer pain. *J Pain Symptom Manage* 1991;692:53.
43. Portenoy RK, Ugarte C, Fuller I, et al. population-based survey of pain in the United States: differences among white, African American, and Hispanic subjects. *J Pain* 2004;5(6):317.
44. Spiegel D, Sands SS, Koopman C. Pain and depression in patients with cancer. Cancer 1994;74:2570.
45. Razavi D, Delvaux N, Farvacques C, et al. Screening for adjustment disorders and major depressive disorders in cancer inpatients. *Br J Psychiatry* 1990;156:79.
46. Shacham S, Reinhart LC, Raubertas RF, et al. Emotional states and pain: intraindividual and interindividual measures of association. *J Behav Med* 1983;6:405.
47. Bucher JA, Trostle GB, Moore M. Family reports of cancer pain, pain relief, and prescription access. *Cancer Pract* 1999;792:71.
48. Bolund C. Suicide and cancer II: medical and care factors in suicide by cancer patients in Sweden, 1973–1976. *J Psychosoc Oncol* 1985;3:17.
49. Breitbart W, Rosenfeld B, Pessin H, et al. Depression, hopelessness, and desire for hastened death in terminally ill patients with cancer. *JAMA* 2000;284(22):2907.
50. Massie MJ, Holland JC. Depression and the cancer patient. *J Clin Psychiatry* 1990;51(Suppl 7):12.
51. Kagawa-Singer M. Diverse cultural beliefs and practices about death and dying in the elderly. In: Wieland D, ed. *Cultural diversity and geriatric care: challenges to the health professions.* New York: Haworth Press, 1994.
52. Hellman C. *Culture, health and illness,* 3rd ed. Newton, MA: Butterworth–Heinemann, 1995.
53. Koenig BA, Gates-Williams J. Understanding cultural difference in caring for dying patients. Caring for patients at the end of life. *West J Med* 1995;163(3):244.
54. Power PW, Dell Orto AE. Understanding the family. In: Power PW, Dell Orto AE, eds. *Role of the family in the rehabilitation of the physically disabled.* Baltimore, MD: University Park Press, 1980.
55. Van Winkle NM. End of life decision making in American Indian and Alaska Native cultures. In: *Cultural issues in end-of-life decision making.* Thousand Oaks, CA: Sage Publications Inc, 2000.
56. Parker SG. The challenge of bringing hospice to the Zuni Tribe. *Last Acts* 2001; 10.
57. Hopp F, Duffy SA. Racial variations in end-of-life care. *J Am Geriatr Soc* 2000;48(6):658.
58. Nezu AM, Nezu CM, Friedman SH, et al. *Helping cancer patients cope.* Washington, DC: American Psychological Associates, 1998.
59. Nezu AM, Nezu CM, Perri MG. *Problem-solving therapy for depression: theory, research, and clinical guidelines.* New York: Wiley, 1989.
60. D'Zurilla TJ, Nezu AM. *Social problem-solving in adults.* In: Kendall P, ed. *Cognitive-behavioral research and therapy.* New York: Academic Press, 1982.
61. Nezu AM, Nezu CM, Houts PS, et al. *Relevance of problem-solving therapy to psychosocial oncology. J Psychosoc Oncol* 1999;16(3–4).5–26.
62. Nezu AM, D'Zurilla TJ, *Social problem-solving and negative affective states.* In: Kendall P, Watson D, eds. *Anxiety and depression: distinctive and overlapping features.* New York: Academic Press, 1989.
63. Toseland RW, Blanchard CG, McCallion P. A problem solving intervention for caregivers of cancer patients. *Soc Sci Med* 1995;40(4):517.
64. Lansky SB, Cairns N, Lowman J, et al. Childhood cancer: non-medical costs of the illness. *Cancer* 1979;43(1):403.
65. Schulz R, Williamson GM, Knapp JE, et al. The psychological, social, and economic impact of illness among patients with recurrent cancer. *J Psychosoc Oncol* 1995;13(3):21.
66. Houts PS, Lipton A, Harvey HA, et al. Nonmedical costs to patients and their families associated with outpatient chemotherapy. *Cancer* 1984;53:2388.
67. Mor V, Guadagnoli E, Wool M. An examination of the concrete service needs of advanced cancer patients. *J Psychosoc Oncol* 1987;5(1):1.
68. Farkas C, Loscalzo M. Death without indignity. In: Kutscher AH, Carr AC, Kutscher LG, eds. *Principles of thanatology.* New York: Columbia University Press, 1987:133.
69. Loscalzo M, Amendola J. Psychosocial and behavioral management of cancer pain: the social work contribution. In: Foley KM, Bonica JJ, Ventafridda V, eds. *Advances in pain research and therapy,* Vol 16. New York: Raven Press, 1990:429.
70. Jordhoy MS, Saltvedt I, Fayers P, et al. Which cancer patients die in nursing homes? Quality of life, medical and sociodemographic characteristics. *Palliat Med* 2003;17(5):433.
71. Bruera E, Sweeney C, Russell N, et al. Place of death of Houston area residents with cancer over a two-year period. *J Pain Symptom Manage* 2003;26(1):637.
72. Sager M, Easterling D, Kindig D, et al. Changes in the location of death after passage of Medicare's prospective payment system. A national study. *N Engl J Med* 1989;320:433.
73. McMullan A, Mentnech R, Lubitz J, et al. Trends and patterns in place of death for medicare enrollees. *Health Care Financ Rev* 1990;12:1.
74. Leff B, Kaffenbarger KP, Remsburg RN. Prevalence, effectiveness, and predictors of planning the place of death among older persons followed in community-based long term care. *J Am Geriatr Soc* 2000;48(8):943.
75. Tolle SW, Bascom PB, Hickam DA, et al. Communication between physicians and surviving spouses following patient death. *J Gen Intern Med* 1986;1:309.
76. Tolle SW, Girard DW. The physician's role in the events surrounding patient death. *Arch Intern Med* 1982;143:1447.
77. Abbott KH, Sago JG, Breen CM, et al. Families looking back: one year after discussion of withdrawal or withholding of life-sustaining support. *Crit Care Med* 2001;25(1):197.
78. Worden JW. *Grief counseling and grief therapy: a handbook for the mental health practitioner,* 2nd ed. New York: Springer Publishing Company, 1991.
79. Steinhauser KE, Christakis NA, Clipp EC, et al. Factors considered important at the end of life by patients, families, physicians, and other care providers. *JAMA* 2000;284(19):2476.

CHAPTER 55 ■ DISORDERS OF SEXUALITY AND REPRODUCTION

URSULA S. OFMAN

As the effectiveness of medical treatment of cancer patients has improved a great deal during the past decades, quality of life outcomes have gained increasing attention of clinicians and researchers alike. Although nerve-sparing surgeries, conformal radiation, and new chemotherapies have greatly contributed to improved survivorship, the psychological realities post cancer treatment remain somewhat oblique. Sexuality is a complex area, in which biology and psychology intersect, and which is also strongly affected by interpersonal and behavioral factors. Even if oncology were able to successfully treat patients without creating any physical impairments to sexual function, sexual dysfunction would be part of many a patient's posttreatment life because of the severity of the psychological impact of cancer diagnosis and the experience of treatment on self image, confidence, attitude toward self and partner, and so on. After active treatment, survivors attempt to return to their previous daily routines. The challenge this represents for many cancer survivors is not trivial. Sexuality is one of the most complicated areas of functioning to regain. A diagnosis of cancer means having to face one's own mortality, possibly for the first time. The treatments are often painful, frightening, and intrusive and have the potential to erode one's sense of body integrity and body image. Memories of the illness and treatment together with their emotional aftereffects present a disruptive mix for sexual interest and functioning. These effects may continue long after active treatment is over and are "stirred up" again at every routine follow-up visit.

Many cancer treatments interfere physiologically with some aspect of physical functioning, which also may impede an easy return to pretreatment life. These disruptive, long-term effects are not only those that directly affect sexual organs or gonads but also include other aspects of functioning that may interfere with the patient's sexual self-image, such as scars, a change in physique as a result of hormone treatment, ostomies, disfiguring surgery, and so on. Any change in appearance or functioning and any long-term treatment side effect can be a reminder of the illness and its treatment and may interfere with a sensuous, virile, and confident sexual self-image.

Changes in gender-role behavior resulting from the physical and emotional side effects of cancer surgery or treatment may not only impair the patient's sexual interest, but also affect the partner's perception of the patient as a sexual object. For both the patient and the patient's partner, it may be difficult to view each other from the same perspective that had previously drawn them to each other sexually. The patient may have become physically and emotionally dependent on the partner, who in return may have had to assume a nurturing, parenting role. After treatment ends, it may be

impossible to return to the previous role distribution in the relationship. Both partners are also faced with the varying reactions of extended family, friends, and colleagues to the illness and subsequent difficulties. These reactions may range from affectionate support to angry withdrawal, adding to the psychosocial difficulty of the posttreatment period. Worries about the possibility of a recurrence, together with uncertainty about the future, heightened anxiety and depression, a sense of personal inadequacy, and diminished sense of control in either or both partners also can interfere seriously with the resumption of a sexual life (1–3).

Despite the consistently documented negative effects of cancer and cancer treatments on sexual functioning, most cancer survivors continue to maintain a sexual self-image, even if it is difficult to integrate physical and emotional changes over time. Little has been done to identify the richness of patients' attempts to integrate their cancer experiences into a new sexual self-concept. Research in this area has been hampered, among other factors, by methodological issues including the need for innovative approaches to solicit and measure responses (4,5). Few studies to date document the outcomes of structured interventions to ameliorate sexual difficulties posttreatment. Sexual recovery is usually just one among several goals of the studied interventions. The studies reviewed reported improved sexual outcomes for participants (6,7).

The psychosexual issues regarding the prospect of infertility in this population add to the overall experience of loss and mortality. To face death and at the same time to surrender one's chance of living on in one's offspring must present a depressing, noxious combination for many of the young, childless patients beginning treatment. On a marital level, the issue of possible infertility undoubtedly has a long-term negative effect on the stability of the relationship as well as the need to renegotiate aspects of the implicit relationship contract. Unattached patients may not worry about possible loss of fertility in the early stages of diagnoses and treatment but still may feel damaged and limited in their capacity as a potential mate. Efforts are being made to prevent or limit loss of fertility for some groups of patients. Further research in this area is urgently needed to alert the medical community to this issue and to develop strategies for helping these patients cope with this immense psychosocial stressor.

Although psychosocial causes are responsible for much of the sexual and procreative difficulty that survivors experience, physical causes are to some extent more easily researched and identified. Therefore, the vast majority of studies in this area focus on medically caused sexual and reproductive dysfunction. In the following sections, this literature is reviewed by disease site and treatment modality.

SEXUAL AND REPRODUCTIVE SIDE EFFECTS OF SURGERY

Breast Cancer

Breast cancer patients may be the best researched group in terms of the sexual impact of treatment on sexual functioning. Partly because radical mastectomy had been the treatment of choice for all breast cancer patients, the effects of breast loss on women's sexual experience and life were researched early. In recent years, it has been widely accepted that comparable survival rates may be obtained in early breast cancer patients treated either with traditional surgical procedures (modified radical mastectomy) or with breast-conserving techniques combined with radiation and, increasingly, chemotherapy. The psychological and psychosexual outcomes of these two approaches have been compared in a number of studies. Although some studies report a tendency toward better preservation of body image and higher level of enjoyment of breast caressing in patients with breast preservation or reconstruction (8,9), the groups do not show any differences in sexual frequency, ease of reaching orgasm and overall sexual satisfaction. It is also possible that age at the time of treatment plays a significant role in these patients' perception of quality of life. Wenzel et al. (10) found that immediately after treatment for breast cancer, younger women (50 years and younger) reported significantly worse overall quality of life than the older women in their study. No significant differences in sexual dysfunction or body image were noted in this study.

In an effort to clarify the nature of women's response to lumpectomy, McCormick et al. (11) studied 74 women following lumpectomy and radiation and reported that 39% of the sexually active patients avoided the treated breast, 20% stated that their partner avoided it, and 48% noted breast discomfort during sexual activity; still, 90% indicated a high level of satisfaction with the results of their treatment.

The implications of breast reconstruction for the psychological adjustment of the mastectomy population are also beginning to receive attention. Rowland et al. (12) studied 83 women who had undergone reconstruction after modified radical mastectomy for early stage breast cancer and reported that these patients generally returned to premorbid levels of sexual satisfaction and comfort. The timing of the reconstructive surgery may be a relevant factor for these women. In a retrospective study of women who had undergone immediate breast reconstruction after breast cancer surgery, and women who had delayed breast reconstruction, Al-Ghazal et al. (13) found significantly superior outcomes for women who had undergone breast reconstruction at the time of their initial surgery.

Although there is now a growing body of research dealing with the emotional and sexual consequences of surgery for early stage breast cancer, little is known about the effects of systemic regimens for breast cancer on sexual functioning. In a survey of 1098 women who had been diagnosed with breast cancer 1–5 years earlier and who had been treated with different adjuvant regimens, Ganz et al. (14) found that patients who had received chemotherapy seemed to experience a higher incidence of vaginal dryness and pain during intercourse, whereas women treated with tamoxifen reported a higher incidence of hot flashes, night sweats, and vaginal discharge. In another study of this population, Ganz (15) found that although rates of sexual activity did not decline, women taking tamoxifen reported slightly higher rates of difficulty with arousal and achieving orgasm. In a large survey of breast cancer survivors,

Meyerowitz et al. (16) found no significant differences between their subjects and age-matched healthy women on a standard measure of sexuality. However, women who were most likely to have reported negative impact on their sexuality from cancer treatment included women who had experienced changes in their hormonal status.

A further concern is posed by the large number of women now receiving hormonal treatment, especially tamoxifen, for long periods. The long-term side effects of these treatments are only now emerging slowly and require more research in the future. Research to date suggests that tamoxifen actually may produce estrogenic changes in the vaginal mucosa of postmenopausal women (17,18). However, its impact on symptomatic vaginal atrophy in these women is unknown (19).

Cancer of the Female Reproductive Organs

The incidence of sexual problems in women after gynecologic cancer treatment ranges in various reports from 0% to virtually 100% (20). This reflects both the many methodologic difficulties of assessment in this field and the varied treatments for gynecologic malignancies. These treatments range from laser surgery for cervical carcinoma *in situ* to total pelvic exenteration and vigorous chemotherapies for advanced gynecologic tumors. The gynecologic malignancies, with their obvious significance for sexual function, deserve comprehensive study to help women recover sexually as fully as possible. As Van de Wiel et al. (21) point out in their review of sexual function after cervical cancer treatment, many studies use frequency of intercourse as the sole indicator of the quality of sexual relations. This sheds little light on the true sexual status of the gynecologic cancer survivor. Further refinements in research instruments and methodology hopefully will benefit this population.

Cervical Cancer

Cervical cancer is the fourth most common neoplasm in women, with 13,000 new cases of invasive disease diagnosed annually in the United States. Excluding *in situ* lesions, treatment consists of radical hysterectomy, radiation therapy, or a combination of both approaches. Studies comparing sexual outcomes for radiation treatment and surgery indicate that at 6 months posttreatment, both surgery and radiation patients reported no significant changes in sexual functioning. At 1-year posttreatment, however, both populations reported decreased sexual interest and radiation patients reported significantly diminished sexual functioning with severe dyspareunia, postcoital bleeding, and pain on penetration. These studies highlight the difficulties posed for sexual recovery by pelvic irradiation for gynecologic cancer. The sequelae of fibrosis, vaginal stenosis, and decreased lubrication (22) are likely to interfere with sexual function unless treated appropriately, promptly, and continuously with vaginal dilators, effective vaginal lubricants (e.g., Astroglide and others) and, in some cases, a hormone-free vaginal moisturizer such as Replens.

Total pelvic exenteration is a surgical procedure occasionally performed to excise advanced pelvic tumors *en bloc* in the absence of distant metastases. The surgery entails removal of the bladder, urethra, vagina, uterus, ovaries, and rectum; two ostomies are created. The treatment is such a serious challenge to both physical and emotional recovery that early clinical reports explored whether postoperative quality of life justified the continued use of so radical an approach. Some researchers have reported that construction of a neovagina combined with special support and counseling efforts offers an improved chance for sexual rehabilitation after surgery (23).

At present, however, many questions remain regarding vaginal reconstruction. The long-term advantage to patient adjustment and satisfaction must be weighed against the risk of these procedures. The psychological and practical adjustments required by exenteration, which include body image, ostomy, and mortality concerns, also merit continued further study.

The impact of gynecologic cancer on a woman's sexual self-esteem or sense of worth as a sexual partner remains an intuitively powerful yet little studied factor in postcancer distress. Van de Wiel et al. (21) compared 11 women treated for cervical carcinoma with a group of nonpatient controls and found that although the frequency of sexual activity did not differ between the groups, the patients with cervical cancer valued sexual interactions significantly less and had a lower self-appraisal of themselves as sexual partners. Although the small populations studied and the retrospective nature of the work limit conclusions, this report marks a valuable effort to illuminate the subtler but far-reaching consequences of gynecologic cancer for sexual well-being.

Endometrial and Ovarian Cancer

Endometrial cancer presents most commonly in post-menopausal women. Treatment consists of surgery, radiation therapy, chemotherapy, or a combination of modalities. Ovarian cancer presents in premenopausal and postmenopausal women; surgical evaluation and debulking are ordinarily the first step in treatment, followed by a chemotherapeutic regimen with a combination of agents. Only with the advent of chemotherapy for ovarian cancer has the previously dismal prognosis for this tumor improved markedly. Studies of the long-term implications of this illness for the survivor's sexual function have begun to appear. Compared with healthy controls, women with these cancers report lower frequency of sexual behaviors, lower levels of arousal, increased incidence of dyspareunia, and problems with body image.

The ovarian cancer patient faces the serial trauma of a serious cancer diagnosis, major pelvic surgery with resultant changes to the vagina, a demanding chemotherapeutic regimen, treatment-related onset of menopause in the premenopausal patient, and complete loss of fertility. The psychological, physical, and hormonal impact on sexual function in this population merits further careful study.

The endometrial cancer patient must often contend with radiation changes to the vagina and pelvis. Vaginal changes include fibrosis with resultant shortening and narrowing; reduced elasticity of the vaginal wall; and diminished lubrication, creating high risk of dyspareunia. As mentioned earlier, the consequences of radiation to the vagina may be avoided or alleviated by the regular use of vaginal dilators and sexual comfort can be improved by the use of appropriate lubricants, vaginal moisturizers, and intercourse positions. An important area for future inquiry is the implementation of patient support and education plans for women facing pelvic radiation, which may increase contact with health care providers and encourage crucial patient compliance with these strategies during the demanding months of treatment, especially during the first year posttreatment, as radiation changes evolve and produce physical and relationship distress.

Vulvar Cancer

Vulvar carcinoma is a rare tumor arising primarily in older women. In early stage disease, treatment may consist of wide local excision (24). In more advanced disease, the lesions are often multicentric and radical vulvectomy is performed, which entails removal of clitoris, labia minora and majora,

and bilateral inguinal lymph node dissection. Postoperatively, patients may experience a high degree of complications, including wound infections and lymphedema of the lower extremities as well as introital stricture. Research attention has begun to focus on this population in recent years (25) and reports document that sexual dysfunction posttreatment for vulvar cancer is common and affects all phases of the sexual response cycle.

Sexual and Reproductive Implications of Systemic Cancer Treatments in Women

Sexual and reproductive consequences of surgery are obvious, occur at the time of treatment, and are usually permanent. In contrast, the side effects of radiation and chemotherapy may accumulate over time and may not be permanent. Premature menopause, which is a frequent long-term side effect of systemic cancer treatments, such as chemotherapy, hormone therapy, and pelvic irradiation, has implications for both sexual and reproductive functioning. Ovarian failure secondary to single agent and combination chemotherapy has been documented (26). Alkylating agents appear to be the most notorious cause of ovarian failure in older women (aged 40 and older). Resulting symptoms include amenorrhea and menopausal symptoms, such as hot flashes, irritability, vaginal dryness, and atrophy of the vaginal epithelium. The treatment increases the likelihood of vaginitis, dyspareunia, and decreased sexual interest. Although some women recover normal ovarian functioning after treatment, premature menopause is the long-term outcome for many women. Aside from the specific drug regimen used, age is an important variable in this context, with older women more prone to loss of fertility and early menopause, particularly after treatment with larger, cumulative drug doses. In a study of women who received high-dose chemotherapy for breast cancer with autologous bone marrow support, Winer et al. (27) found that although overall quality of life after treatment was relatively high in this population one or more years after completion of treatment, problems with sexual functioning were common.

Gonadal dysfunction and infertility after radiation therapy are difficult to predict. The central location of the ovaries within the pelvis, close to major nodal areas, makes damage from radiation scatter and leakage likely. As with chemotherapy, radiation damage is dose-related, cumulative, and age-dependent. Loescher et al. (28) found that permanent infertility after 25 treatments of 500 Gy occurred in 60% of women aged 15–40 years and in 100% in women aged over 40. Because pelvic radiation interferes with the vasocongestive processes of female sexual arousal, vaginal lubrication also may be impaired, and dyspareunia and vaginitis may develop. Therefore, pelvic radiation may result in long-term adverse effects on female sexual functioning.

Radiation treatment is often combined with chemotherapeutic regimens. In such cases, it is difficult to differentiate between toxicity incurred from radiation versus that due to the chemotherapeutic agent(s). Data from women who received combined radiation and chemotherapy for Hodgkin disease suggest that these combination treatments result in additive ovarian toxicity (29).

CANCER OF THE MALE REPRODUCTIVE ORGANS

Prostate Cancer

Prostate cancer is the most commonly diagnosed cancer in men. It affects mostly older men: 80% of all diagnoses are made in men aged 65 years and older. In recent years, partly due to improved screening and diagnostic methods, the proportion of younger men in the newly diagnosed population seems to increase. Older men and their partners in this age group are often at a developmental stage dominated by losses: retirement, death of peers, and separation from adult children who move away. These losses may include diminished sexual activity secondary to sexual dysfunction that precedes the cancer diagnosis. Changes in sexual functioning due to normal aging are often compounded by age-related chronic diseases and their treatments, such as hypertension and diabetes. Zinreich et al. (30) reported that 63% of 43 patients (mean age, 67.7 years) with varying stages of prostate cancer had erectile dysfunction before undergoing any cancer treatment. Of these, 44% were never able to obtain an erection and 56% reported difficulty maintaining erections during intercourse. For many elderly couples, the man's erectile difficulty results in a complete cessation of sexual activity.

Treatment for early stage disease commonly consists of surgery or radiation therapy. In early stage prostate cancer, the advances in medical technology have meant gains for sexual functioning posttreatment. Quinlan et al. (31), in a case series of 500 men, reported an incidence of erectile dysfunction of 32% with nerve-sparing surgery techniques, compared with 85% after radical prostatectomy. Recovery of erectile functioning is often slow, however, and may exceed 6 months in some patients.

Traditional radiation regimens for prostate cancer may also produce erectile dysfunction as a long-term side effect. Schover (32) found in a review of the literature that the generally estimated 50% of erectile dysfunction after definitive radiotherapy may be inflated. The actual incidence may lie between 14% and 46% of all cases. The mechanism believed to be responsible for the development of erectile dysfunction in radiation patients is vascular scarring, which may develop 6 months posttreatment or later. Helgason et al. (33) confirmed the general observation of increased incidence of erectile dysfunction in men treated with radical prostatectomy, compared to men treated with external beam radiation.

Advanced-stage prostate cancer is commonly treated with testosterone deprivation, accomplished by bilateral orchiectomy or the administration of estrogen, flutamide, or luteinizing hormone-releasing hormone analogues. All these interventions produce sexual side effects, including loss of desire for sexual activity and impaired erectile functioning. Men undergoing hormone treatments are also confronted with body image issues, reduced energy levels, and hot flashes, which may contribute to the development of sexual problems.

Testicular Cancer

Unlike prostate cancer, testicular cancer typically affects young men. It is the most common cancer in men aged 17 to 34 in the United States. These men are confronted with a life-threatening disease at a life stage in which they are supposed to separate from their families of origin and find their own identity as an adult. The demands of the illness interfere with the developmental goals of this population and interfere with the young man's concept of himself as an independent, strong, and virile person.

In the past, treatment routinely included unilateral orchiectomy, retroperitoneal lymphadenectomy, and either chemo-locoregional therapy for nonseminomatous tumors or radiation for seminomas. Men with metastatic seminomas may receive chemotherapy in addition to radiation. Despite the traumatic aspects of treatment for testicular cancer and the psychosocial issues faced by this group, survivors of the disease fare quite

well as far as their long-term sexual outcomes are concerned. Studies document levels of decreased levels of sexual desire and erectile difficulties that are not significantly different from age-matched controls. Fertility issues due to retrograde ejaculation as a result of surgical damage to paraaortic sympathetic nervous system pathways are a prominent concern for men after retroperitoneal lymphadenectomy (34). Rieker et al. (35) found in a retrospective study of 223 testicular cancer survivors who were more than 1-year postdiagnosis that 30% experienced overall performance distress, 10% had erectile difficulties, and 6% were anorgasmic. Fossa et al. (36) surveyed 31 men postbilateral orchiectomy and found that despite difficulties in dosing androgen replacement therapies, most patients were psychologically and sexually well adjusted to their situation. More evidence that sexual outcomes in this population are strongly influenced by psychosexual factors comes from Arai et al. (37), who found in a study that included patients who had been on a surveillance protocol postsurgery that these men reported the same extent and nature of sexual difficulty as men who had also been treated with chemotherapy or radiation.

Therefore, fertility concerns relating to retrograde ejaculation and chemotherapy appear to be the most common sexual side effects of testicular cancer and may impair sexual quality of life for these patients. Despite the relative low incidence of reported sexual dysfunction in this group, posttreatment sexual support seems to be warranted in this young population. They may experience problematic relationships because of persisting low-grade sexual dysfunction, which is treatable (38).

Sexual and Reproductive Implications of Systemic Cancer Treatments in Men

Testicular function in adult men is particularly susceptible to injury by chemotherapeutic agents. Affected are the germinal epithelium, the Leydig cells responsible for steroidogenesis, and the hypothalamic-pituitary-testicular axis (39). Dysfunction of the testis occurs shortly after initiation of treatment and can persist for months or years after function has returned to other tissues. Manifestations of toxicity are reduction in testicular volume, severe oligospermia or azoospermia, and infertility. The effects of the alkylating agents have been particularly well documented. For example, doses of chlorambucil below 400 mg cause reversible oligospermia, and cumulative doses in excess of 400 mg result in azoospermia and germinal aplasia (40). Low-sperm count and elevated follicle-stimulating hormone levels are physiologic indicators of germinal aplasia. The Sertoli cells are more resistant to chemotherapeutic agents and consequently, testosterone levels may remain within the normal range during and after treatment.

Combination chemotherapeutic regimens may have an even more disruptive effect on the germinal epithelium than treatment with a single agent. MOPP (nitrogen mustard, vincristine, procarbazine, and prednisone) results in irreversible germinal dysfunction in male lymphoma patients. However, other regimens that are equally effective seem to cause germ cell aplasia in fewer patients, many of whom experience the return of spermatogenesis with time. Chemotherapeutic agents are not known to affect the male sexual response cycle directly.

In contrast to the consequences of chemotherapeutic regimens on male reproductive capacity, which have been established for a number of antineoplastic agents, the effects of radiation therapy on sexual functioning and fertility have received little attention to date. The testis and both the germinal epithelium and the Leydig cells are very radiosensitive. Damage and recovery appear to be dose dependent. Doses as low as 150 cGy may result in a marked, if transient, suppression of sperm production. Disruption of sperm production increases with accelerating doses: at 2000 to 3000 cGy, recovery may take 3 years; at 4000 to 6000 cGy, approximately 5 years; and above 6000 cGy, sterility seems permanent (26). By affecting the vasocongestive mechanisms necessary for erectile functioning, pelvic radiation also may cause erectile dysfunction in men.

CANCER SITES IN BOTH SEXES

Bladder Cancer

Bladder cancer arises primarily in older men and women, who already may have experienced age-related changes in sexuality. Whereas treatment in the United States previously consisted of cystectomy for lesions of any stage, early bladder carcinoma *in situ* without infiltration may now be treated with local excision and bacille Calmette-Guérin.

In patients with invasive bladder cancer, cystectomy is still the treatment of choice. Recent advances in the development of nerve-sparing cystectomies in men and women promise improved sexual functioning outcomes in both sexes (41). A common sexual side effect for men after radical cystectomy is erectile dysfunction resulting from transection of the nerves governing erection and loss of ejaculation secondary to excision of the prostate at the time of surgery. Changes in the sensation of orgasm may ensue. Patient response to this loss is not well documented.

In women, cystectomy may result in a narrowed or shortened vagina, scarring, and numbness or loss of sensation, all of which may impair the excitement response. Furthermore, removal of both ovaries during surgery causes premature menopause in premenopausal patients, which may lead to reduced vaginal lubrication and desire. The simultaneous creation of a stoma and external diversion of urine generates concerns about body image, odor, leakage, and spills and therefore may contribute to sexual avoidance and other difficulties (42). In recent years, continent cutaneous urinary diversion and orthotopic bladder substitution have become clinically accepted alternatives to ileal conduit diversion. The *a priori* assumption had been that postoperative quality of life would be better following these types of continent cutaneous diversions. However, although studies on the validity of this assumption have been hampered by a lack of consensus regarding methodology, follow up studies do not seem to confirm any advantage in quality of life or sexual functioning in these patients.

Colorectal Cancer

Cancer of the colon and rectum is the second most common cancer in the United States; approximately 140,000 new cases are diagnosed annually, primarily in older men and women. Surgery remains the mainstay of treatment; resection of the tumor with pelvic lymphadenectomy may be followed by radiation, chemotherapy, or both. Pelvic lymphadenectomy may result in damage to the parasympathetic nervous system, causing erectile dysfunction, and to the sympathetic nervous system, causing retrograde or diminished ejaculation. Past studies have reported a varying incidence of these side effects after treatment. Havenga and Welvaart (43) studied 26 men with rectosigmoid carcinoma, nine of whom were treated with abdominoperineal resection and 17 of whom were treated with low anterior resection. Only two of the patients with abdominoperineal resection returned to sexual activity, five had erectile dysfunction, and seven were anorgasmic. Patients who had low anterior resection reported less sexual

dysfunction after surgery; 12 maintained sexual activity, and 4 reported either erectile dysfunction or anorgasmia. Further evidence that abdominoperineal resection produces significant sexual dysfunction was reported by Koukouras et al. (44), who studied 60 sexually active male patients with colorectal cancer who were treated with high anterior resection, low anterior resection, or abdominoperineal resection. Patients with the abdominoperineal resection had the highest incidence of sexual dysfunction; 65% became sexually inactive, 45% lost all erectile ability, and 50% reported absence of ejaculation. New surgery techniques to address primary rectal cancer promise to improve sexual outcomes for some of these patients (45). In a prospective study, Maas et al. (46) evaluated the sexual outcomes of operative procedures that combine pelvic nerve-preserving techniques with radical tumor resection to ensure optimal local tumor control with minimal bladder and sexual dysfunction. They found that the nerve-preserving technique results in low morbidity and good functional outcome. Impotence was related to sacrifice of the inferior hypogastric plexus and preservation of the superior hypogastric plexus was crucial for ejaculation.

Hojo et al. (47) described the use of a nerve-sparing approach to pelvic lymphadenectomy in 134 patients with advanced disease. They found that although bladder dysfunction was best prevented with a nerve-sparing procedure, preservation of sexual function in men is more difficult and requires a high degree of nerve preservation. This approach is therefore not advisable for patients with locally extensive disease.

In patients with early stage rectal cancer who are treated by amputation of the rectum alone, erectile dysfunction appears to be less prevalent, but problems with the orgasm phase persist. There is a glaring shortage of studies focusing on the sexual side effects of treatment for colorectal neoplasms in women.

After the creation of a colostomy, both men and women must contend with issues of changed body image and sensitivity about cleanliness, odor, and fear of accidents. Early studies by Sutherland et al. (48) have remained clinically on target; they found that the sexual impact of the ostomy far exceeds the extent of physical handicap. Depression, anger, and fear of being repugnant are common emotional reactions postoperatively and may contribute to a pattern of sexual avoidance. The medical staff must anticipate these issues and offer support to patients, whose challenges include self-care of the ostomy, overcoming fears concerning changed appearance, and regaining physical self-esteem. Other patients who are farther along in this process may provide invaluable help to the recovering colorectal patient in this regard. Overall adjustment to the colostomy may take more than 1 year, as documented by Hurny and Holland (49).

Sexual response after colorectal surgery remains an insufficiently understood area, particularly in view of the current high prevalence of this tumor. For women particularly, the issues of sexual recovery after colorectal and bladder cancer remain too little explored. Nonetheless the impact of pelvic surgeries on the female excitement and orgasm responses, as well as the impact of the ostomy issues on desire, may be surmised to be great. The value of treatment interventions for sexual dysfunction in this population, including both penile prosthesis implantation and sexual counseling for the patient or couple, is also an appropriate area of study.

Other Cancers

Patients with less common tumors and those with common tumors that do not directly affect the organs of sexual response have received little or no research attention with regard to the sexual sequelae of their treatment. The diagnosis and treatment of all cancers have far-reaching psychological implications for the patient and family that lie beyond the scope of this review. These matters are covered comprehensively elsewhere (50). Some cancer treatments pose a particularly severe challenge to the recovery of normal self-esteem and restored body image; treatments involving limb amputations, marked facial, and other appearance changes, or loss of normal phonation are examples. In a rare study of the sexual outcomes of patients with head and neck cancer, Monga et al. (51) found that although most of the patients studied continued to be interested in sex, only 49% were satisfied with their sexual functioning after treatment. Older patients (65 years and older) reported more satisfaction with their sexual partner and current sexual functioning than younger patients, who also tended to have more advanced disease and lower performance status, and significantly poorer sexual functioning.

The simple passage of time does not heal all wounds. In the area of sexuality, it is not uncommon for problems to become more severe with time. The adjustment to cancer and its elements of disfigurement is by nature a slow process, and problems with adjustment and recovery, including those in the sexual and relationship arena, may often be more accessible to counseling by oncology mental health professionals during the first and second posttreatment year than at a later stage in cancer survivorship.

Cancers that require systemic treatment with chemotherapy, whole body irradiation, or bone marrow transplant challenge the patient physically and emotionally more than most surgeries or radiation regimens. Treatments may be lengthy and arduous, depleting the patient of energy and causing severe side effects. Sexual functioning is clearly affected by many of these regimens (52). In recent years, the sexual concerns of women patients with bone marrow transplant have received some research attention. Ovarian failure secondary to conditioning treatment with melphalan or cyclophosphamide and total body irradiation is associated with profound effects on sexual functioning, most commonly vaginal dryness, loss of desire for sexual activity, and difficulties with sexual intercourse (53). Ostroff et al. (54) found that standard regimens of hormone replacement therapy did not alleviate all sexual impairment experienced by women with treatment-related ovarian failure. In a study comparing bone marrow transplant survivors and a matched sample undergoing maintenance chemotherapy, Altmaier et al. (55) found that bone marrow transplant patients reported a higher incidence of sexual difficulties. Ostroff and Lesko (52) confirmed the prevalence of sexual dysfunction in bone marrow transplant survivors. Clearly, this population is at increased risk for sexual dysfunction and would benefit from further research attention.

Patients with Hodgkin's disease are now often successfully treated with aggressive chemotherapy. Treatment is associated with a high degree of infertility in both men and in women. The interrelationship in young cancer survivors among cancer treatment, loss of desire and sexual dysfunction, lost or impaired fertility, and relationship distress remains clinically inescapable but very little studied.

A group that has also received very little attention concerning the sexual and fertility related sequelae of cancer and its treatment are survivors of childhood cancers. Relander et al. (56) surveyed 77 adult male survivors of childhood malignancies. One third of them had been treated for hematologic cancers, one third for central nervous system tumors, and one third for other malignancies. They found that patients treated for tumors in the hypothalamic pituitary region, with testicular irradiation, and those treated with high doses of alkylating agents suffered from severe gonadal and sexual dysfunction as adults. Puukko et al. (57) found in a survey of 31 female survivors of childhood leukemia

that although they did not differ from healthy, age-matched controls with regard to the frequency of sexual intercourse, their sexual identity was less well developed and they had more restrictive attitudes about sexuality and sexual pleasure. More research is needed to assess the long-term physical and emotional outcomes of these young patients with cancer.

PREVENTION AND MANAGEMENT OF SEXUAL AND REPRODUCTIVE DYSFUNCTION IN CANCER PATIENTS

Medical Strategies to Prevent and Manage Sexual and Reproductive Dysfunction

Efforts have been made to reduce sexual and reproductive morbidity by refining surgical and radiation therapies. Examples include the development of nerve-sparing surgical techniques to preserve erectile function after prostatectomy (58) and nerve-sparing retroperitoneal lymph node dissection (RPLND) for men with clinical stage I nonseminomatous testicular cancer to preserve emission and ejaculation. In some cases, the effort to preserve ejaculatory function and avoid other treatment side effects in men with nonseminomatous tumors who do not evidence metastatic spread led to the use of unilateral orchiectomy followed by careful observation. A further example of the attempt to preserve quality of life is the strategy of offering observation as a treatment for nonmetastatic seminomatous testicular cancer instead of immediately proceeding with chemotherapy post-RPLND, thereby preserving gonadal functioning. New, nerve-sparing techniques that involve preservation of the superior hypogastric plexus also may contribute to the preservation of ejaculatory functioning (59) in these men.

Similar attempts have been made to preserve sexual functioning in some treatments used for cancers in women. For example, wide local excision for vulvar cancer and lumpectomy of breast tumors mark efforts on the part of surgeons to preserve sexual function and body image as much as possible without compromising treatment efficacy.

In both men and women, efforts to keep pelvic radiation doses to a therapeutically efficacious minimum may reduce the incidence of radiation-induced sterility and allow recovery of gonadal function. Radiation damage to gonads in men may now be reduced drastically by employing a new testicular shield that reduces scatter to about 10% of the patient's prescription dose. In women, oophoropexy (the surgical transposition of the ovaries to a midline position behind the uterus) reduces the ovarian exposure of women receiving pelvic radiation in about 50% of patients (60). These developments reflect the growing willingness of the oncology world to try to preserve and maintain sexual and reproductive function while providing appropriately aggressive cancer therapy.

Medical treatments for iatrogenic sexual dysfunction and infertility also have begun to be developed. Loss of emission and ejaculation is a frequent side effect of RPLND in men. Because most men undergoing this procedure are young (17 to 34), this loss is a serious concern. For men with adequate sperm production before sterilizing cancer treatment, cryobanking is usually advised. However, many patients present with suboptimal sperm before treatment. To secure a postthaw sample adequate for spousal insemination, more than 20 million sperm per milliliter with at least 40% progressive motility is generally required (26). Multiple ejaculates, if time permits, can increase the total of viable sperm for storage.

For men after RPLND, antegrade ejaculation may return with time and, in some men, sympathomimetic drugs such as ephedrine or anticholinergic drugs, such as diphenhydramine or imipramine, may help to facilitate normal ejaculation. Electroejaculation is possible to harvest sperm in men who do not recover ejaculatory function (61). Recently, there have also been some encouraging medical developments to help patients overcome sexual difficulties. Since the introduction of injectable vasocongestive agents (Caverject), a whole arsenal of pharmacologic treatments for erectile dysfunction has been introduced and now includes a variety of oral medications that aid penile congestion in conjunction with physical stimulation. Although these medications are very effective for many, they may provide less relief for men with advanced collagenization of penile tissue and patients, postsurgery, who have compromised neurologic and/or vascular functioning. It must also be stated that these medications do not appear to help much in situations in which severe performance anxiety is present.

Sexual interest, which is governed by both hormonal and psychological factors in both men and women, is more difficult to address with pharmacologic means. Not much is understood about the interplay of hormonal environment and psychology that produces sexual interest in humans. One avenue to possibly ameliorate the problem of reduced sexual desire in patients with cancer could be androgen replacement in those with iatrogenic gonadal dysfunction. However, this strategy is contraindicated in patients who have hormone sensitive cancers. There are no medications to date that promise to effectively address diminished sexual interest in these patients. Few studies have focused on hormonal interventions to help cancer patients overcome iatrogenic gonadal dysfunction. Hall and others (62) treated nine women with acquired hypogonadotropic hypogonadism after therapy for cranial tumors using a physiologic replacement regimen of exogenous gonadotrophin-releasing hormone. This restored ovulation and fertility in 78% of the participants.

Women who undergo premature menopause after cancer treatment need medical intervention to alleviate menopausal symptoms and prevent atherosclerosis, hypertension, cardiovascular accidents, and osteoporosis. Unless an estrogen-sensitive tumor was involved, hormonal replacement should be considered to treat some of these symptoms (63). Wren (64) argued that hormone replacement may be feasible in most women after genital tract cancer. In his view, estrogen/progestogen regimens will not affect malignant cell growth in vulvar and vaginal cancer as well as squamous cell carcinoma of the cervix. Although the endometrium and the ovary contain hormone receptors that may respond to estrogen by increased growth factor production, a large number of women with these cancers were cured by the initial treatment and would benefit from hormone replacement without risk of stimulating cancer growth. Women who were not cured may benefit from treatment with progestogens alone or estrogen and progesterone in combination to relieve any discomfort caused by estrogen deficiency.

Aside from estrogen replacement therapy, nonhormonal medications, such as clonidine, methyldopa, and beta-blockers, may be used to control hot flashes (65). Emotional instability also may be addressed with serotonin selective reuptake inhibitors such as fluoxetine or sertraline. Topical solutions to counteract reduced lubrication, and changes of the vaginal lining include Replens, vitamin E oil, Chaste berry, 1–2% testosterone cream, and limited doses of estrogen cream or Vagifem (66). Androgen treatment may be indicated in women with reduced bioavailable androgen levels after chemotherapy (67) and may improve sexual interest.

Psychosocial Prevention and Intervention for Sexual Difficulties

Although efforts are under way to prevent and alleviate adverse sexual and reproductive side effects of cancer treatments medically, severe physical and emotional damage can occur nonetheless. Even patients whose treatments did not affect sexual end organs report being impaired in their sexual enjoyment after cancer treatment. Indeed, impaired sexual functioning during or after cancer treatment can occur regardless of the specific physiologic changes that have taken place. The sexual response cycle (desire, arousal, and orgasm) is a complex process that may be disrupted by a wide range of factors both physiologic and psychological.

Sexual response during and after cancer treatment is vulnerable to the impact of the cancer itself, medical treatment side effects, other medical problems, medications, pain, depression, anxiety, partner response, and subtler psychological effects, such as changed body image and belief in cancer myths. Patients with cancer must face their own mortality, undergo uncomfortable, sometimes lengthy, or disfiguring treatments, and deal with the effect of their illness on spouse, family, and work. An understandable consequence of this process can be loss of sexual desire and impaired sexual response. Von Eschenbach and Schover (68) found that the most frequent sexual side effect reported by men with cancer is erectile dysfunction, whereas women are more likely to lose interest in sex altogether. Loss or impairment of sexual desire may be triggered by the trauma of diagnosis and treatment, which interferes with the patient's perception of himself or herself as a sexual person. There may be concerns about one's attractiveness and the partner's reaction that contribute to an overall withdrawal from sexual activity. Concerns about sexual functioning may contribute to sexual avoidance even if sexual desire per se is not impaired.

Although inhibited sexual desire, sexual avoidance, and erectile dysfunction may be the most frequently observed sexual difficulties in this context, any sexual dysfunction may be caused by the patient's and the partner of the patient's reaction to the trauma of the experience. Little has been reported on how ethnic differences in sexual socialization and attitudes affect sexual outcomes of cancer treatments. Most populations studied at major cancer centers are predominantly white, and there often are not enough members of different backgrounds to enable researchers to compare subgroups along these lines. Wyatt et al. (69) compared 147 African American and white breast cancer survivors and found that although both groups in their study were from very similar sociodemographic backgrounds, African American women were significantly less likely to be comfortable with and practice oral sex and any self-touching/masturbation than their white counterparts. Also white women were much more likely to report that breast cancer had a negative impact on their sex lives. Ethnic differences in survivor groups deserve much more attention to enable treatment providers to deliver psychosexual support in an optimal fashion to all patient groups.

The medical team often fails to help prevent development of sexual dysfunction by not addressing the topic with the patient. This may be due to a number of factors such as discomfort with the topic or a concern about appearing intrusive or presumptuous. When the patients are elderly, young, single, widowed, or homosexual, sexual concerns appear to be particularly difficult to address (70). All too often, sexuality is viewed as being a concern only for men and women who are sexually active within a committed relationship. Every patient, regardless of current level of sexual activity, has a perception of himself or herself as a sexual being and is invested in knowing that he or she can function sexually even if not pursuing any sexual relationships at the moment. Often, the medical staff waits for the patient to open the topic and concludes that there is no interest in sexual issues if the patient remains silent. Vincent et al. (71) found that 80% of patients receiving cancer treatment were interested in more information about sex, although 75% said they would not initiate conversation about it with their doctor. Patients with cancer often feel they should be glad to be alive. Asking about sexual concerns may seem ungrateful and frivolous. If physicians and nurses initiate communication about sexual side effects of proposed treatments at the time of treatment decisions, they signal to the patient that sexual functioning is a legitimate concern that can be addressed.

Privacy and confidentiality are crucial prerequisites for discussing sexual concerns with patients. Sexual matters cannot be discussed productively during rounds, when several staff members are present or when a roommate is within earshot. Under such conditions, the clinician is likely to encounter vague responses and little enthusiasm for the topic. Assessment of the patient's sexual status and history at the time of treatment decision provides the crucial basis for members of the medical team to give appropriate support and information about the possible impact of treatment options on sexual functioning. It also signals to the patient that sexual concerns are understood to be an integral component of patients' quality of life. The time of diagnosis and treatment decision is a stressful one for the patient and his or her partner, and sexual concerns are not likely to be in the forefront of their minds. However, sexual functioning needs to be addressed from the start to support the patient in the struggle to adjust to the impact of cancer treatment on self-image and functioning. Clear and detailed information enables patients and their partners to anticipate problems and prepare for them. The nursing staff in particular can be instrumental in helping patients and their partners deal with both emotional and physical side effects by explaining the physiology involved, normalizing the experience, and giving pragmatic advice and coping with strategies. The timing of these interventions is determined by the situation. Certainly in emotional or medical crisis situations, such as when a relapse of the cancer is discovered, it is not helpful for the patient to be asked about sexual matters. Sexual advice is best received when it specifically addresses the problems with which the patient and his or her partner are currently struggling.

At the time of treatment decision, the patient needs to know about the sexual and reproductive issues that may arise as a result of the treatment. Patients also need reassurance that help is available should sexual difficulties occur. As treatment proceeds and patients are seen for follow-up visits, the sexual status should be assessed by asking open-ended questions such as, "How are things going in your relationship?" and "How are things sexually?" As patients express difficulty, it is easy for the caregiver to normalize the experience of the patient and to offer specific advice on how to improve matters sexually.

Because any change in appearance and functioning may have sexual consequences, the medical staff should consider the potential sexual implications of all treatments offered to the patient and address them with all patients. A good resource for both staff and patients is a pair of booklets published by the American Cancer Society that address sexual concerns of male and female patients after cancer treatment. The booklets are lucid, practical, and informative about both sexual side effects and strategies to deal with them (72). If patients continue to experience sexual difficulty after cancer treatment, referral to a sex therapist for careful evaluation and treatment may be indicated.

A short course of sexual counseling is often sufficient to facilitate better adaptation and functioning, particularly for patients who had a satisfactory sex life before the cancer

diagnosis. Sex therapy with cancer patients is geared to address the specific difficulty expressed by the patient and the patient's partner. Sexual attitudes and fears are explored, and frequently exercises are prescribed to do at home. These exercises are designed to reintroduce sexual activity slowly. Usually these exercises follow a graded approach, beginning with general physical pleasuring and gradually becoming more sexually focused. This approach is particularly helpful to patients who have a great deal of performance anxiety, who avoid sexual activity for fear of being unable to complete it, whose confidence in their ability to function is shaken, and who feel unattractive and shy about how their bodies were affected by cancer treatment. Similarly, partners are often just as reluctant to resume sexual activity as the patient, and may also benefit from the structure sex therapy provides.

SUMMARY

The focus of the available literature is primarily on the incidence of sexual and gonadal dysfunction after cancer treatment. Very few authors compare their population with normal age-matched controls. Considering the high incidence of sexual difficulty in the general population (73), such comparisons might reveal how, very successfully, many cancer survivors are able to integrate sexual side effects and continue some sexual life, despite the impairing physical and emotional side effects of their treatments. New medical strategies aim at prevention and amelioration of sexual side effects and infertility. Comprehensive psychosexual support during and after treatment promises to further aid patients and their partners in minimizing negative sexual outcomes. Sexual side effects in particular can be addressed in brief sexual counseling or therapy. Informing the patient of possible side effects before treatment makes early intervention in case of psychosexual difficulties possible. Psychosocial aspects of fertility concerns of the cancer patient during active treatment and as a survivor have received little attention so far, possibly because of previous experience, when long-term survival of young patients was rare. With advancing technology in cancer treatment, this cohort of long-term survivors is likely to grow and requires an adequate response to these medical and psychosocial needs.

References

1. Cella D, Tross S. Psychological adjustment to survival from Hodgkin's disease. *J Consult Clin Psychol* 1986;54:616.
2. Ostroff J, Smith K, Lesko L. Promotion of mental health among adolescents cancer survivors and their families. *Proceedings of the mental health services for children and adolescents in primary care settings: an NIMH Research Conference*, 1989.
3. Rieker P, Edbril S, Garnick M. Curative testis cancer therapy: psychosocial sequelae. *J Clin Oncol* 1985;3:1117.
4. van der Riet P. The sexual embodiment of the cancer patient. *Nurs Inq* 1998;5:248.
5. Andersen BL. Surviving cancer: the importance of sexual self-concept. *Med Pediatr Oncol* 1999;33:15.
6. Maguire P, Tait A, Brooke M, et al. Effects of counseling on the psychiatric morbidity associated with mastectomy. *Br Med J* 1980;281:1454–1456.
7. Christensen DN. Postmastectomy couple counseling: an outcome study of a structured treatment protocol. *J Sex Marital Ther* 1983;9:266–275.
8. Schover LR. Sexuality and body image in younger women with breast cancer. *J Natl Cancer Inst Monogr* 1994;(16):177–182.
9. Schover LR, Yetman RJ, Tuason LJ, et al. Partial mastectomy and breast reconstruction. A comparison of their effects on psychosocial adjustment, body image, and sexuality. *Cancer* 1995;75(1):54–64.
10. Wenzel LB, Fairclough DL, Brady MJ, et al. Age-related differences in the quality of life of breast carcinoma patients after treatment. *Cancer* 1999;86:1768.
11. McCormick B, Yahalom J, Cox L, et al. The patient's perception of her breast following radiation and limited surgery. *Int J Radiat Oncol Biol Phys* 1989;17:1299.

12. Rowland J, Holland JC, Chaglassian T, et al. Psychological response to breast reconstruction; expectation for and impact on post mastectomy functioning. *Psychosomatics* 1993;34(3):241–250.
13. Al-Ghazal SK, Sully L, Fallowfield L, et al. The psychological impact of immediate rather than delayed breast reconstruction. *Eur J Surg Oncol* 2000;26:17.
14. Ganz PA, Rowland JH, Meyerowitz BE, et al. Impact of different adjuvant therapy strategies on quality of life in breast cancer survivors. *Recent Results Cancer Res* 1998;152:396.
15. Ganz PA. Impact of tamoxifen adjuvant therapy on symptoms, functioning and quality of life. *J Natl Cancer Inst Monogr* 2001;(30):130–134.
16. Meyerowitz BE, Desmond KA, Rowland JH, et al. Sexuality following breast cancer. *J Sex Marital Ther* 1999;25:237.
17. Jordan VC. Long-term adjuvant tamoxifen therapy for breast cancer: the prelude to prevention. *Cancer Treat Rev* 1990;17:15.
18. Love RR. Antiestrogen chemoprevention of breast cancer: critical issues and research. *Prev Med* 1991;20:64.
19. Schover LR, Montague DK, Schain WS. Sexual problems. In: DeVita VT, Hellman S, Rosenberg SA, eds. *Cancer: principles and practice of oncology,* Vol. 2. Philadelphia, PA: JB Lippincott Co, 1993:2464.
20. Andersen BL, Jochimsen PR. Sexual functioning among breast cancer, gynecologic cancer, and healthy women. *J Consult Clin Psychol* 1985;53:25.
21. Van de Wiehl HBM, Weijmar Schultz WCM, Hallensleben A, et al. Sexual functioning following treatment of cervical carcinoma. *Eur J Gynaecol Oncol* 1988;9:275.
22. Seibel MM, Freeman MG, Graves WL. Carcinoma of the cervix and sexual function. *Obstet Gynecol* 1980;55:484.
23. Andersen BL, Hacker NF. Psychosexual adjustment following pelvic exenteration. *Obstet Gynecol* 1983;61:331.
24. Stehman FB, Bundy BN, Dvoretsky PM, et al. Early stage I carcinoma of the vulva treated with ipsilateral superficial inguinal lymphadenectomy and modified radical hemivulvectomy: a prospective study of the gynecologic oncology group. *Obstet Gynecol* 1992;79:490.
25. Andreasson B, Moth I, Jensen SB, et al. Sexual function and somatopsychic reactions in vulvectomy-operated women and their partners. *Acta Obstet Gynecol Scand* 1986;65:7.
26. Sherins RJ, Mulvihill JJ. Gonadal dysfunction. In: DeVita VT Jr, Hellman S, Rosenberg SA, eds. *Cancer: principles and practice of oncology.* Philadelphia, PA: JB Lippincott Co, 1989:2170.
27. Winer EP, Lindley C, Hardee M, et al. Quality of life in patients surviving at least 12 months following high dose chemotherapy with autologous bone marrow support. *Psychooncology* 1999;8:167.
28. Loescher L. Surviving adult cancers. Part 1: physiologic effects. *Ann Intern Med* 1989;3:411–432.
29. Horning SJ, Hoppe RT, Kaplan HS. Female reproductive potential after treatment for Hodgkin's disease. *N Engl J Med* 1981;304:1377.
30. Zinreich ES, Derogatis LR, Herpst J, et al. Pretreatment evaluation of sexual function in patients with adenocarcinoma of the prostate. *Int J Radiat Oncol Biol Phys* 1990;19:1001–1004.
31. Quinlan DM, Epstein JI, Carter BS, et al. Sexual function following radical prostatectomy: influence of preservation of neurovascular bundles. *J Urol* 1991;145:998.
32. Schover LR. Sexual rehabilitation after treatment for prostate cancer. *Cancer* 1993;71(Suppl 3):1024.
33. Helgason AR, Adolfsson J, Dickman P, et al. Factors associated with waning sexual function among elderly men and prostate cancer patients. *J Urol* 1997;158:155.
34. Caffo O, Amichetti M. Evaluation of sexual life after orchidectomy followed by radiotherapy for early-stage seminoma of the testis. *BJU Int* 1999;83:462.
35. Rieker PP, Fitzgerald EM, Kalish LA, et al. Psychosocial factors, curative therapies, and behavioral outcomes: a comparison of testis cancer survivors and a control group of healthy men. *Cancer* 1989;64:2399.
36. Fossa SD, Opjordsmoen S, Haug E. Androgen replacement and quality of life in patients treated for bilateral testicular cancer. *Eur J Cancer* 1999;35:1220.
37. Arai Y, Kawakita M, Okada Y, et al. Sexuality and fertility in long-term survivors of testicular cancer. *J Clin Oncol* 1997;15:1444.
38. Heidenreich A, Hofmann R. Quality-of-life issues in the treatment of testicular cancer. *World J Urol* 1999;17:230.
39. Constabile RA. The effects of cancer and cancer therapy on male reproductive function. *J Urol* 1993;149:1327.
40. Cheviakoff J, Calamera JC, Morgenfeld ML. Recovery of spermatogenesis in patients with lymphoma after treatment with chlorambucil. *J Reprod Fertil* 1973;33:155.
41. Venn SN, Popert RM, Mundy AR. 'Nerve-sparing' cystectomy and substitution cystoplasty in patients of either sex: limitations and techniques. *Br J Urol* 1998;82:361.
42. Schover LR, von Eschenbach AC. Sexual function and female radical cystectomy: a case series. *J Urol* 1985;134:465.
43. Havenga K, Welvaart K. Sexual dysfunction in men following surgical treatment for rectosigmoid carcinoma. *Ned Tijdschr Geneeskd* 1991;135:710.
44. Koukouras D, Spiliotis J, Scopa CD, et al. Radical consequence in the sexuality of male patients operated for colorectal carcinoma. *Eur J Surg Oncol* 1991;17:285.
45. Havenga K, Maas CP, DeRuiter MC, et al. Avoiding long-term disturbance to bladder and sexual function in pelvic surgery. *Semin Surg Oncol* 2000;18(3):235–243.
46. Maas CP, Moriya Y, Steup WH, et al. Radical and nerve preserving surgery for rectal cancer in The Netherlands: a prospective study on morbidity and functional outcome. *Br J Surg* 1998;85:92.
47. Hojo K, Vernava AM III, Sugihara K, et al. Preservation of urine voiding and sexual function after rectal cancer surgery. *Dis Colon Rectum* 1991;34:532.
48. Sutherland AM, Orbach CE, Dyk RB, et al. The psychological impact of cancer and cancer surgery: I. Adaptation to the dry colostomy: preliminary report and summary of findings. *Cancer* 1952;5:857.
49. Hurny C, Holland JC. Psychosocial sequelae of ostomies in cancer patients. *CA Cancer J Clin* 1985;36:170.
50. Holland JC, Rowland JH, eds. *Handbook of psychooncology: psychological care of the patient with cancer.* New York: Oxford University Press, 1989.
51. Monga U, Tan G, Ostermann HJ, et al. Sexuality in head and neck patients. *Arch Phys Med Rehabil* 2000;78:298.
52. Ostroff J, Lesko LM. Psychosexual adjustment of patients undergoing bone marrow transplantation: clinical/research issues and intervention programs. In: Whedon M, ed. *Bone marrow transplantation: principles, practice and nursing care.* Monterey, CA: Jones and Bartlett Publishers, 1991:312–333.
53. Cust MP, Whitehead MI, Powles R, et al. Consequences and treatment of ovarian failure after total body irradiation for leukaemia. *BMJ* 1989;299:1494.
54. Ostroff J, Stern V, Dukoff R, et al. The psychosocial adjustment of pre maturely menopausal cancer survivors treated with hormone replacement therapy. *American Psychosomatic Society Meeting,* 1991.
55. Altmaier EM, Gingrich RD, Fyfe MA. Two-year adjustment of bone marrow transplant survivors. *Bone Marrow Transplant* 1991;7:311.
56. Relander T, Cavallin-Stahl E, Garwicz S, et al. Gonadal and sexual function in men treated for childhood cancer. *Med Pediatr Oncol* 2000;35:52.
57. Puukko LR, Hirvonen E, Aalberg V, et al. Sexuality of young women surviving leukemia. *Arch Dis Child* 1997;76:197.
58. Walsh PC, Lepor H, Eggelston JC. Radical prostatectomy with preservation of sexual function. *Prostate* 1983;4:473.
59. Takasaki N, Okada S, Kawasaki T, et al. Studies on retroperitoneal lymph node dissection concerning postoperative ejaculatory function in patients with testicular cancer. *Hinyokika Kiyo* 1991;37:213.
60. Thomas PRM, Winstantly D, Peckham MJ. Reproductive and endocrine function in patients with Hodgkin's disease: effects of oophoropexy and irradiation. *Br J Cancer* 1976;33:226.
61. Bennett CJ, Seager SWJ, McGuire EJ. Electroejaculation for recovery of semen after retroperitoneal lymph node dissection. *J Urol* 1987;137:513.
62. Hall JE, Martin KA, Whitney HA, et al. Potential for fertility with replacement of hypothalamic gonadotrophin-releasing hormone in long term female survivors of cranial tumors. *J Clin Endocrinol Metab* 1994;79:1166.
63. Ettinger B. Overview of the efficacy of hormonal replacement therapy. *Am J Obstet Gynecol* 1987;156:1298.
64. Wren BG. Hormonal therapy following female genital tract cancer. *Int J Gynecol Cancer* 1994;4:217.
65. Laufer LR, Yohanan E, Meldrum DR. Effect of clonidine on hot flashes in postmenopausal women. *Obstet Gynecol* 1982;60:583.
66. Barbach L. *The pause: positive approaches to menopause.* New York: Plume Books, 1995.
67. Kaplan HS. A neglected issue: the sexual side effects of current treatments for breast cancer. *J Sex Marital Ther* 1992;18:1.
68. von Eschenbach AC, Schover LR. The role of sexual rehabilitation in the treatment of patients with cancer. *Cancer* 1984;54:2662.
69. Wyatt GE, Desmond KA, Ganz PA, et al. Sexual functioning and intimacy in African American and white breast cancer survivors: a descriptive study. *Womens Health* 1998;4:385.
70. Auchincloss SS. Sexual dysfunction in cancer patients: issues in evaluation and treatment. In: Holland JC, Rowland JH, eds. *Handbook of psychooncology.* New York: Oxford University Press, 1989:383–413.
71. Vincent CE, Vincent B, Greiss FC, et al. Some marital-sexual concomitants of carcinoma of the cervix. *South Med J* 1975;68:52.
72. Schover LR. *Sexuality and cancer; for the woman who has cancer, and her partner AND Sexuality and cancer; for the man who has cancer, and his partner.* New York: American Cancer Society, 2001.
73. Laumann EO, Paik A, Rosen RC. Sexual dysfunction in the United States. *JAMA* 1999;199:537.

CHAPTER 56 ■ HOME CARE AND CAREGIVERS

BETTY R. FERRELL AND BARBARA J. WHITLATCH

INTENSIVE CARE OF HOME CARE

Since the mid-1980s, there has been a major shift in home health care. In the United States this shift was caused originally by the prospective system; it has been sustained by current trends toward managed care. Long hospital stays have been replaced by early discharges and the shifting of the burden of care to the home. The intensity of care for these home care patients has also changed because of the demographics of both patients and caregivers. Home care nurses and family caregivers have been charged with managing patients with complex and highly technical treatment plans. Home care is characterized by intensive management of symptoms and the need for supportive care of both the patient and the family caregivers who assume the burdens of cancer and its treatment (1–3).

Complexities of Home Care

Until recently the study of symptom management has been largely confined to major symptoms, such as cancer pain, and acute care settings. Recent studies have focused on the special needs of patients in other settings, including the nursing home (4,5), the hospice (6,7), and the home (8,9). Several factors can influence palliative care in these settings. Heavy reliance on family members, access to diagnostic facilities, and, often, limited pharmacy services can influence the effectiveness of pain and symptom management at home.

It may be assumed that comfort is enhanced in home care, as the home environment has been considered preferable to institutional settings. Indeed, patients, families, and health care professionals often elect care at home because they assume that patients are more comfortable there. Research has not confirmed this perspective and has demonstrated that treatment may not be substantially better at home (10–12). As researchers have extended studies into the home care setting, barriers have been described that actually hinder pain management in the home, including patient's and family's fears of addiction, failure of the patient to report pain, and limited access to needed services. These facts emphasize that fulfilling the patient's preference to be at home may not necessarily result in effective symptom management.

Symptom management at home is different from that at the hospital or other institutional setting. Hospitals typically provide technical equipment and services for acutely ill patients. For patients with complex problems, inpatient care often includes a variety of aggressive or invasive strategies for diagnosis and definitive treatment of the underlying conditions. Home care, by contrast, relies heavily on low-tech strategies, concentrating mostly on symptom management. The overall effectiveness of these different strategies at home in comparison with hospitals remains difficult to analyze.

Cancer as a Family Experience

Cancer and other life-threatening illnesses, such as acquired immunodeficiency syndrome (AIDS), are generally recognized as affecting the entire family unit rather than a single individual. The recent shift in health care, with movement toward home care as the predominant setting, emphasizes the importance of family involvement in the total care needs of the patient. It is indeed remarkable that care which only a decade ago was reserved for intensive care units (ICUs) by specially trained registered nurses is now delegated to family caregivers in the home environment who have had little or no preparation to assume both the physical and emotional demands of illness. Home care has advanced from low-tech care, focused on follow-up for patients discharged from hospitals, into its current status as the setting for active treatments, including chemotherapy, intravenous fluid administration, blood transfusion, complex wound care, and many other technical procedures. Recent literature has acknowledged the intense demands of family caregiving at home largely in the areas of technical care, acquisition of skills, and provision of intense, 24-hour physical caregiving. Less emphasis has been placed on the emotional burdens of assuming responsibilities for the patient's well-being or peaceful death in the home. A study involving 28,777 patients with cancer published in 2004 revealed that care is in fact becoming more aggressive over time with increased use of chemotherapy, increased ICU stays and later referral to hospice (13).

The home environment can be viewed as a delicate balance. At one end of the spectrum are the many demands that the home care environment offers that, if out of balance, can result in intense burdens for family caregivers and compromised care for patients. At the other end are the many benefits of home care. The home care environment can potentially offer the patient improved physical comfort, the psychological comfort of familiar surroundings, an opportunity for healing of relationships, and the ability for patients and families to benefit from the compassion of giving and receiving comfort care and a shared transition from life to death (14–19).

Another significant trend has been the use of home as the setting of care. In the late 1970s and early 1980s, health care professionals generally made the decision whether to discharge a patient to the home or to offer an extended stay in an inpatient setting based on patient or family preferences. The decade of the 1990s transformed home care as the primary setting of active treatment as well as palliative care. Very important, however, has been the diminished choice on the part of patients and families primarily due to changes in the health care system. Although some patients and families have volitionally chosen home care, others have had care relegated to the home setting due to health care system or hospital determinants.

The outcomes of home care may often be best evaluated by the effects on family caregivers following the death of the patient and during bereavement. Hospice providers have long recognized that positive experiences with caregiving in the home result in positive bereavement and adaptation by family members after the patient's death. Feelings of inadequacy in providing home care, patient complications, and deaths that are less optimal than anticipated can result not only in the patient's diminished quality of life or quality of death, but also in long-term consequences for the family. Home care then is best viewed as not merely care provided to a single individual in the home environment but rather as a family experience in which every aspect of care provided to the patient or the provision of care by the family caregiver will impact the others (20–23).

Public Denial of Death and Influence on Care

Much literature has addressed the social need to deny death and the reluctance of individuals in society to accept death and dying amidst a health care system focused on cure. Efforts by the hospice movement, the social influences of AIDS, the prevalence of cancer, and other factors have in many ways made our society confront the reality of death in recent years. In an effort to diminish societal denial of death and heighten awareness of the growing end-of-life movement, the well-known documentary reporter Bill Moyers produced a four-part series for public television that aired in fall 2000. Through his years of work in preparing "On Our Own Terms: Dying in America," Moyers sought to address myriad aspects of how individuals, families, and the health care systems view and manage death in the United States. This was the first time in modern US history that such a well-known media personality devoted such substantial effort to examining the societal views toward the end of life. For professionals in the end-of-life movement, this represented a major coup in overcoming societal silence, denial, and aversion to such a critical stage in life.

In the 1990s, several other programs were developed in the United States to address the need for increased research, professional education, and advocacy in end-of-life care, including aspects of home care, hospice, and community involvement. The Project on Death in America was established by the Open Society Institute through a grant from the Soros Foundation, one of the wealthiest philanthropic foundations in the United States. Interestingly enough, the benefactor recognized the incredible dearth of resources and training in caring for those at the end of life. The Project on Death in America programs addressed aspects of end-of-life care in various professional fields, including medicine, nursing, social work, chaplaincy, and other social service fields.

These efforts at examining the end of life as a natural life stage have been balanced by intense media attention on new potentially curative therapies, such as gene therapy, biomedical engineering, and advanced technologies. This attention encourages continuation of the death-denying society. Health care providers should recognize that for many family caregivers and patients, the death that they are now witnessing is perhaps their first personal encounter with the termination of life. Family caregivers struggle with the sanctity of life and

denial of death just as do health care professionals and society at large. However, the profound experience of dying, or of caring for a loved one who is dying, transcends all aspects of home care. This experience has been described as an all-encompassing aspect of the clinical care of the terminally ill patient at home (24).

Physical and Psychosocial Issues

The needs of patients and family caregivers in home care span the domains of quality of life, as depicted in Figure 56.1. Home care needs most often involve physical needs, such as management of pain and other symptoms, and treatment of the side effects associated with treatment of the disease. Nutritional needs, sleep disturbance, fatigue, incontinence, and other physical aspects of disease and treatment are common priorities of home care. In fact the area of physical well-being and symptom management has been the focus of home care and is also the area with the greatest scientific basis for the practice of care in the home (25,26).

Psychological well-being is predicated on pharmacologic management of symptoms, such as anxiety and depression, as well as counseling to address issues such as fears, loss of control, and the many other psychological demands of life-threatening illness. Similar to psychological needs are the patient's social needs, such as the ability to maintain appearance and normal roles and relationships, and family issues such as financial concerns. The ability to meet psychological and social needs is more difficult outside palliative care programs, in which there is limited access to social workers, clinical psychologists, and other support personnel (27–29).

Spiritual well-being presents perhaps the greatest challenge in home care. In the institutional setting, such as the inpatient hospital, chaplaincy services may be more available. Yet it is during the advanced stages of illness, when care takes place in the home, that spiritual needs, like psychosocial needs, may become more prominent. This issue emphasizes the importance of psychosocial and spiritual assessment to determine unmet needs (30,31).

CHALLENGES TO SYMPTOM MANAGEMENT AT HOME

There are at present many uncertainties about the future of the health care system in the United States and in virtually all

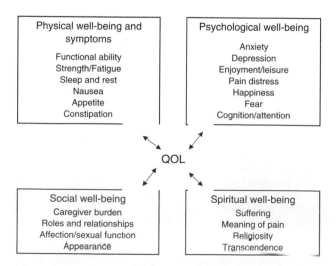

FIGURE 56.1. Dimensions of quality of life (QOL).

countries. A certainty, however, is that care continues to shift into the outpatient and home care environment. Therefore it is patients and families who will assume most of the care in the future. One of the greatest challenges in this area derives from demographical and social influences such as the impact of a steadily aging population of patients with multiple chronic illnesses. Care of the patient with cancer at home becomes far more difficult when the patient is 80 years old and also has concomitant illnesses such as cardiac disease, hypertension, and diabetes, with their associated medications and treatments (32,33). There is still limited attention focused on the special care needs of the geriatric population at home and that of their caregivers, who are often elderly children. Expanded efforts in attending to complex needs of the aging will need to be adopted, especially given the growing percentage of population over the age of 65 (34).

An equal challenge rests in the demographics of family caregivers in the home. Research has revealed that approximately 70% of caregiving is provided by elderly spouses in the home and an additional 20% is provided by daughters or daughters-in-law, who are often balancing full-time employment as well as the demands of their own families while providing intensive care to their loved ones.

One of the most challenging aspects of home care will be the future impact of managed care and similar factors influencing the types and extent of care to be provided in the home. Factors, such as limitations in the types of services available, the frequencies of visits, and the duration for which this care can continue, will make home care extremely challenging. In essence, as the intensity of needs is increasing, the available resources in home care are diminishing.

Involvement of Family Caregivers in Medications

A primary task of home care related to cancer and other terminal illness is management of medications. It is enlightening to realize that home care nurses and other professionals assume similar responsibilities in other settings only after formal courses in pharmacology and with support available from colleagues, pharmacists, and physicians reached by direct access. This is particularly true in oncology, where symptom management is often either accomplished on an as-needed basis for symptoms, such as nausea or anxiety, or with necessary titration of around-the-clock dosing of medication such as analgesics.

Management of medications is important not only to preserve the patient's comfort but also to diminish the burden on the family and avoid costly complications such as repeat hospitalizations when medications are not effectively used. Patients and family caregivers often do not have the necessary knowledge to judge indications for administration of medications or the delicate issues involved with titration or the side effects of medications. Health care providers can make a valuable contribution to the care of patients at home by insuring that medication schedules are made as simple as possible using single agents rather than multiple drugs, and maintaining the simplest possible routes of administration and dosage schedules. Patients require assistance with important decisions regarding the use and titration of medications and practical techniques such as written dosage schedules, use of self-care logs, and provision of guidelines to help in medication choices.

An additional burden of family caregiving, often neglected, is the costs assumed by patients and family caregivers themselves related to pain management and home care (35). Families incur significant expenses related to home care in advanced disease, much of which is not reimbursed. Costs include direct expenses, such as medications, as well as extensive indirect costs such as loss of wages. Most of the cost savings to third-party payors have resulted in increased costs assumed by patients and families.

Cultural Considerations of Home Care

The increase in multiculturalism in the United States has added another dimension to the complexity of health care provision as well as coverage. Language barriers, cultural traditions, and religious beliefs create the need for increased sensitivity and knowledge on the part of health care professionals. No longer is health care—or home care—merely for English-speaking, Anglo-Saxon, Judeo-Christian patients and families (36). These facts present additional challenges when considering assessment of pain and symptoms as well as issues related to beliefs about death in various cultures (37,38). Assessment and treatment are complicated by cultural factors, and health care providers along with researchers seek ways to understand and accomplish a nonbiased medium from which to practice. Likewise, health care providers may be caught by the demands for individualized care in the midst of a growing multicultural society (39).

Notably, in many non-Anglo communities, it is tacitly acknowledged as a "duty" in the culture that the burden of much health care automatically shifts to the extended family. In theory this increases the number of caregivers, but it does not increase the certainty of training, understanding, or efficacy of home care. In such environments, familiarity with one's ethnic, religious, or cultural beliefs—especially with respect to terminal care—is best appropriated within a person's respective community. Not only is this true for the patient but also for the surviving family and community. It may justify transcultural home care.

Home Care of Children

Most literature regarding home care has focused on the care of adults. The care of children is often perceived to be less demanding or even normal as families are usually expected to provide such pediatric home care. On the contrary such care is quite demanding because of the characteristics of the ill child, the parents, the siblings, and the extended family. Recent studies have explored the experience of parents in caring for a child with pain. These studies added a dimension to the previous research related to families and pain and also described the decisions and conflicts in pain management for children (40,41).

Parents of pediatric patients with cancer in pain often reported that their health care team did not take their child's pain seriously and did not provide adequate analgesia to relieve the pain. This is consistent with recent literature describing the inadequate assessment and management of pediatric pain and the overall deficiencies in pediatric palliative care (42). However, when specialized pain teams were involved, they were better able to relieve not only the child's pain but the parents' emotional suffering as well. The parents' role in decision making varied from allowing the child to have control whenever possible regarding his or her treatment to personally administering nondrug methods of pain relief that temporarily alleviated both the child's pain and the parents' feelings of helplessness.

SUPPORTING FAMILY CAREGIVERS IN HOME CARE

The literature consistently supports the importance of family members during advanced illness. The caregiver's own health, attitudes, and knowledge have a profound effect on the successful management of the patient's symptoms. This is especially important in the care of patients terminally ill with cancer at home (43–45).

The control of chronic pain remains a perplexing problem that may have important implications for stress experienced by the caregiver. Increased anxiety, depression, marital and family conflicts, embarrassment, guilt, resentment, low morale, and severe emotional and physical exhaustion are commonly reported by distressed caregivers (44–46). Studies have revealed an overall marked decrease in dimensions of caregiver quality of life, which are particularly prevalent when the patient has unmanaged pain and symptoms. Indeed pain management may present caregivers with unique kinds of stress. For example, pain management often requires drugs that must be monitored carefully to achieve maximum pain control safely with minimum side effects. Newer, high-tech pain strategies, such as infusion pumps and chronic spinal infusions, also require the caregivers to have special knowledge and skills. The areas of greatest burden for caregivers in the management of pain include demands on time, emotional adjustment, distressing symptoms, work adjustment, sleep adjustment, and family and relationship adjustments.

Jennings et al. (45,46) have discussed the ethical challenges the individual, family members, and society as a whole face as a result of the homebound chronically ill. Management of the chronically ill in the home results in social withdrawal and isolation, transformation of family relationships and roles, and the placing of new burdens on both the patient and family caregivers. Altilio and Rigoglioso (47) argued that payers and providers have moral and ethical responsibilities toward caregivers. Such responsibilities range from viewing the caregiver as a member of the health care team and involving them in all aspects of care planning to provide ongoing support, after-care, and bereavement care. Their plan includes the provision of improved insurance coverage for both the ill family member and the caregivers. Altilio and Rigoglioso noted that increased involvement in the care team may help caregivers feel more prepared to manage the huge challenge of home care. Conversely they also mention that there are dangers in incorporating caregivers as members of the treatment team because professionals may feel the right to abdicate their own responsibilities to the overburdened caregiver. Essentially, Altilio and Rigoglioso call for a paradigm shift in viewing caregivers. They assert that health care providers should be major advocates for caregivers in order to improve discharge planning to home care, provide ongoing education, skills training, and support, and simplify insurance coverage policies. This latter point is especially important because it would allow families to know exactly what to expect and how to safeguard against failure for lack of knowledge or understanding.

Assessment of Symptoms

Assessment of both acute and chronic symptoms can be difficult in the home. In the absence of diagnostic facilities and multidisciplinary specialists, care must be taken to avoid attributing symptoms to preexisting illness. Underreporting of symptoms may be common for a variety of reasons. Patients with cancer may not report pain because they fear the social implications of opioid analgesics. Elderly patients are often stoic and dread additional diagnostic tests, hospitalization, and new medications (17). Although home care nurses and family caregivers may be extremely helpful, most patients require careful evaluation of significant new complaints as well as continued assessment for the management of chronic or persistent symptoms.

Patients with chronic pain should be evaluated for psychological problems. Functional assessment, including ambulation and a broad variety of activities, may represent important indicators of overall physical well-being. Most patients with chronic pain also have significant anxiety or depression at some time. The need to identify and manage anxiety and depression cannot be overemphasized in the adjunctive management of chronic pain, because ongoing symptoms have been shown to significantly affect general emotional well-being, adjustment to illness, cognition, pain perception, and overall treatment outcome (48). Formal assessment screening instruments for functional and psychological impairments are helpful in this evaluation and minimize the possibility that detectable problems will be missed (18).

Nondrug Treatments

In addition to the extensive responsibilities related to the pharmacologic management of pain, patients and family caregivers use many nondrug strategies for pain relief at home. The home care environment offers the benefit of access to nondrug pain relief methods, and patients and families often feel more comfortable with these alternative methods at home. Previous research has demonstrated that patients and family caregivers infrequently receive formal information or guidance regarding nondrug strategies but rather rely on their own attempts to discover methods that may add to the patient's comfort (19).

Our experience has also demonstrated that patients and families are very eager to add nondrug interventions to their overall pain management (19). These provide great benefit to the patient by not only enhancing physical relief but also alleviating anxiety and giving the patient a better sense of control. We have also demonstrated that family caregivers have found nondrug comfort measures to be extremely valuable in reducing their sense of helplessness. Families are very eager to learn skills that will add to the patient's comfort. It is these family interventions that are often recalled during bereavement as positive memories of their ability to provide greater comfort during terminal illness. Other more structured interventions can also be incorporated by referral to health care professionals such as clinical psychologists, psychiatrists, social workers, and others who can offer many other treatments that might assist in the patient's comfort at home (49,50).

Other Efforts of Preparing Family Caregivers

In a review of literature from 1975–1999, Pasacreta and McCorkle (51) found a dearth of data-based literature and limited number of well-designed training programs for caregivers. The limited programs that were discovered represented three broad categories:

1. Educational
2. Counseling/psychotherapeutic
3. Hospice/palliative home care

Of those dimensions of training, most interventions were aimed at individuals or families, were typically located at one facility, and often represented selection bias in well-adjusted caregivers. Nonetheless the disparate and limited attempts at training caregivers further highlights the extent of the need. Pasacreta et al. discovered that a 6-hour psychoeducation program for cancer caregivers had a positive influence on several factors (51,52). For instance, caregivers displayed an improved sense of confidence in providing care as well as improved perception of their own health. The focus on skills and application of principles was particularly noteworthy as the training addressed symptom management, psychosocial support, and resource identification.

Resources for Caregivers

Since the middle 1990s, researchers and clinicians have recognized the need to develop resources specifically aimed at family caregivers. Stetz et al. (53) discovered five major categories of informational needs of family caregivers:

1. Preparing the caregiver
2. Managing the care
3. Facing challenges
4. Developing supportive strategies
5. Discovering unanticipated rewards and benefits

These researchers asserted that health care professionals have a responsibility to prepare family members with educational strategies that included skill development, access to and use of resources, home care management, decision-making, and self-care.

Just as the technology boom has advanced medical treatments, it has also allowed greater access to resources for caregivers. If a family is fortunate enough to own a computer and have access to the Internet, a wealth of information is available. Moreover, many treatment centers have created "information centers" that allow access to the World Wide Web. Although such an environment can offer volumes of material, caregivers will have to be cautious not to become further inundated and to find the time and energy to pursue such resources. The fact that such items are available within moments represents a step forward in trying to prepare caregivers for their "other full-time job" of managing the home treatment of their loved ones.

Public Policy Implications

To examine trends in end-of-life care across generations, Byock initiated a 10-year longitudinal study in Missoula, Montana. That project seemed to bring national attention to end-of-life care, and it seemed to propel new efforts in advocacy and public policy in that field. Despite the increase in advocacy efforts to enhance federal allocation of funding for home care efforts and the needs of caregivers, little has been done at the federal level to lessen the burden. At the outset of the 21st century, home care continues to face enormous and increasing challenges with decreased funding. The burden on health care professionals as well as on families has increased exponentially in the past decade. With the expanding aging populations, home care will likely take on a different look in the new millennium (54).

This is particularly relevant when considering the cost of caregiving. In 1997, the national economic value of informal caregiving—care provided by an untrained family member—was $196 billion, dwarfing the national expenditures of $32 billion for formal home health care and $83 billion for nursing home care. Notably the estimated economic value of informal caregiving represents approximately 18% of the total national health care expenditures (55). Although the outcome of the new $113 million caregiver program remains to be seen, at least there seems to be some recognition of the value and important role of family caregivers as well as the tremendous toll that providing such care takes on an individual and whole family system.

In addition to governmental factors, other policy experts have attempted to influence whole systems of care. In the late 1990s, Lynn, founder of the Center to Improve Care of the Dying as well as the advocacy group, Americans for Better Care of the Dying (ABCD), proposed a comprehensive system of managed care of end-of-life care. Her program, Medicaring, is based on the notion that capitated or salaried managed care systems offer important opportunities to provide high-quality, cost-effective care for seriously ill individuals nearing the end of life (56). Despite the fact that managed care systems for the most part have largely ignored the need for end-of-life care, Lynn argues that such systems inherently offer certain advantages that include coordinated care across delivery systems, interdisciplinary teams, integrated services, service arrays, utilization controls, and accountability for care standards. Capitated or salaried managed care systems may be well positioned to achieve marked change in end of life if they were to broaden their current focus to include end-of-life care and if payment reimbursements were revised to encourage such programming. The focus of managed care systems on prevention, patient education, cost efficiency, service coordination, integrated provider networks, and such organizational structures could potentially support real change in end-of-life care. Indeed some managed care organizations have expanded services to hospices, although with extensive limits. Lynn asserts that her "Medicaring" proposal encompasses the best components of palliative care within a structured managed care system. Such a program would be comprehensive and supportive and would offer community-based services to meet personal and medical needs with a focus on patient preferences, symptom management, family counseling, and support. Home care would be profoundly influenced if such a program became the standard of care in community-based managed care organizations. It is a larger system and societal change that needs to occur before such programs are institutionalized.

ENHANCING PROFESSIONAL TRAINING IN HOME CARE

Home Care Outreach for Palliative Care Education

Although palliative care principles are prevalent in hospice programs, such elements have not necessarily extended into other health care systems such as home care. This dearth of training exists despite the fact that home care agencies provide extensive care to patients and families facing physical and psychosocial demands at the end of life. Although nonhospice home care agencies are technically not intended for terminally ill, palliative care education is important to support home care providers given the challenges of the health care system in general and the greater demands on home care, essentially making it the primary setting of care (57).

Beginning in the middle 1990s, Ferrell et al. developed and implemented the Home Care Outreach for Palliative Care (HOPE) project for the following purposes:

1. Assess current practices within select nonhospice home care agencies regarding care of the dying
2. Design the HOPE educational program to include relevant content for realistic implementation in home care agencies
3. Implement the HOPE project in select home care agencies
4. Assess outcomes of the project and plan for future dissemination to home care agencies and organizations

The HOPE curriculum is organized into five modules. The first module presents a general overview of palliative care and end-of-life issues. The second and third modules address various aspects of pain and symptom management, respectively.

The fourth component focuses on communication, family caregivers, and spirituality. The last module, entitled "the good death," covers important elements of the last days of life. Key aspects of the modules are the attention given to psychosocial dimensions of care at home, cultural considerations, and the special care required at the time of death. In early 2001, the HOPE project was extended to a national training group with planned follow-up studies and additional programs scheduled. The first of its kind in a "train the trainers" format for palliative care education of home care providers, the HOPE project is aimed at changing the landscape of end-of-life care in the home care setting (57,58).

Communication Training

Of interest, the retrospective assessment provided by caregivers after the death of their family member is in large part influenced by how they viewed the relationship and communication with the health care professional (59). Missing components of "model" treatment programs can be overlooked if the caregiver feels sufficiently supported by the health care community (60). However in palliative care and home care studies, patients and their families are often dissatisfied with their interactions with health professionals. That may come as no surprise when one considers that ironically medical professionals spend up to 70% of their working time communicating but have virtually no education in that aspect of their work (59). Yet communication behaviors seem to play an important role in meeting the cognitive and affective needs of patients with cancer as well as the needs of their caregivers (61). Moreover, communication skills are particularly imperative in home care settings with its myriad of family dynamics, along with cultural, ethnic, and religious nuances of the home. Such issues have prompted researchers to develop training in communication skills for health care professionals. Adding another component of training to an already overburdened health care professional may not be a welcome endeavor. However some studies have demonstrated that such training has actually helped to reduce the intensity of the emotionally laden interactions and increase the professional's sense of confidence to adequately address the affective components of life-threatening illness and care (61).

Cultural Competency

Health care providers must be prepared to manage diverse, multicultural patient populations in various health care settings while working collaboratively with coworkers who also represent various cultural backgrounds (36). Home care presents a greater challenge in that the health care provider is essentially being immersed into the microculture of the family and the macrocosm of the community. Health care educators have recognized this changing demography of our culture, and some have developed programs in cultural competency for their workers (36). Of note, cultural competency does not necessitate that health care providers know and understand all the traditions and practices of the numerous ethnic groups. Rather the intent is to have managers, administrators, and front-line employees work collectively to increase their knowledge of cultural diversity, share that knowledge, and combine efforts to promote cultural awareness and sensitivity in practice settings.

Patient education efforts have also developed in the past few decades, and researchers advocate that health care professionals must consistently exercise heightened cultural sensitivity through their approach to patients as well as in information provided (36,62). Failing to do so runs the risk of necessitating more time and resources.

Davis (63) asserts that health care professionals traditionally have established a portrait of the "ideal dying patient," which implicitly places expectations on terminally ill patients with whom they come in contact. Such tacit anticipation runs the risk of causing a chasm between the health care provider and the patient and family. This may further heighten emotionally laden situations and make care and treatment even more complicated. In addition, lack of recognition of cultural factors may cause further difficulties in communication and understanding with regard to informed consent

TABLE 56.1

"FADING AWAY": FAMILY EXPERIENCES IN END-OF-LIFE CARE

Dimension	Description
Redefining	Redefining involves a shift from "what used to be" to "what is now." It demands adjustment in how individuals see themselves and each other.
Burdening	Feeling as if they are a burden for their family is common among patients. If patients see themselves as purposeless, dependent, and immobile, they have a greater sense of burdening their loved ones.
Struggling with paradox	Struggling with paradox stems from the fact that the patient is both living and dying. For patients, the struggle focuses on wanting to believe they will survive and knowing that they will not.
Contending with change	Those facing terminal illness in a family member experience changes in every realm of daily life—relationships, roles, socialization, and work patterns.
Searching for meaning	Searching for meaning has to do with seeking answers to help in understanding the situation. Patients tended to journey inward, reflect on spiritual aspects, deepen their most important connections, and become closer to nature.
Living day to day	If patients were able to find some meaning in their experience, then they were better able to adopt an attitude of living each day.
Preparing for death	Preparing for death involved concrete actions that would have benefit in the future, after the patient died. Patients had their family's needs uppermost in their minds and worked hard to teach or guide family members with regard to various tasks and activities that the patient would no longer be around to do.

Adapted from Davies B, Reimer JC, Brown P, et al. *Fading away: the experience of transition in families with terminal illness.* Amityville, New York: Baywood Publishing Company, Inc., 1995.

TABLE 56.2

INTERVENTIONS FOR ASSISTING FAMILIES IN HOME CARE

Acquisition of skills to perform treatments and procedures (e.g., care of decubitus ulcers, management of incontinence)
Knowledge regarding assessment of symptoms or disease status (e.g., signs of infection)
Scheduling of medical or laboratory appointments or coordination of home care services
Information regarding the disease, treatments, and expected prognosis
Emotional support in confronting the burdens of caregiving
Counseling to promote communication within the family and with the health care providers
Validation that the care they are providing is adequate to meet the patient's needs
Assessment and guidance regarding the physical strains of caregiving (e.g., lifting, turning, personal care)
Spiritual support for changing belief systems as a result of life-threatening illness
Assistance in maintaining a sense of normalcy in the household
Skills in assessing cognitive changes in the loved one and in dealing with the emotional burden associated with cognitive changes
Interventions to enhance the patient's and family's sense of control
Information and assistance to access community resources
Assistance in organizing the tasks of caregiving (e.g., teaching families to schedule assistance, establishing daily care schedules)
Coping skills to manage the uncertainty of illness
Immediate access to health care services for emergencies
Respite from emotional and physical exhaustion
Care that preserves hope, with attention to preservation of hope even in advanced disease
Respect for privacy in the home, and care that minimizes intrusions and preserves dignity

and truth-telling about diagnosis, prognosis, and treatment options.

As a result of the potential dangers associated with lack of recognition and training in multicultural care, Lister (64) presented a taxonomy for developing cultural competence among health care providers. Of interest, some policy advocates have argued for licensing boards to require cultural competency as a provision of licensure. Rather than adding more demands to the taxed home care system, De Savorgnani and Haring (65) assert that the impact of cultural issues on home care has the potential to serve as the impetus for development of "comprehensive diversity programs" that would enhance the lives of patients and staff in home care. Consistently in the past decade, researchers have demonstrated the benefits of a culturally sensitive staff as patients and their families have reported that they view their homes as the milieu that allows for continuity of lifestyle, family relationships, and cultural values. Many professional organizations now view transcultural training as a necessity given the changing demographics in the United States and in home care.

Fading Away

One of the most significant contributions in understanding family experiences in terminal illness has been the work by Betty Davies et al. titled "Fading Away" (66). This research describes the families' experiences as they coped with the terminal illness of a beloved family member. The research findings generated a theoretical scheme that conceptualized families' experiences as a transition that families themselves labeled as "fading away." The transition of fading away for families facing terminal illness began with the realization that the ill family member was no longer living with cancer but now dying from cancer.

The transition of fading away is characterized by seven dimensions: redefining, burdening, struggling with paradox, contending with change, searching for meaning, living day by day, and preparing for death. Davies et al. emphasized that the dimensions do not occur in linear fashion; but rather, they are interrelated and inextricably linked to one another. Table 56.1 summarizes these dimensions.

CONCLUSION

The home care environment can best be described as the ICU of the future. Home care is complex as a result of changing patient and family caregiver characteristics. The home environment is rich with benefits to enhance patient comfort, but it also provides challenges in providing optimum physical, psychosocial, and spiritual care. The literature has addressed many interventions that are helpful in assisting families in home care. These interventions include a range of suggestions about physical care, including the transferring of information about physical caregiving back to families, offering validation and support to families for their efforts at home care, and interventions to improve communication (Table 56.2).

There is a tremendous need for continuity of care as patients are increasingly cared for across many settings. It is essential that issues of care in the home are communicated to those involved in ambulatory care, inpatient care, and other areas of care. Expert care for patients at home, similar to all aspects of palliative care, begins with a thorough assessment of the patient's needs. Organized care based on a comprehensive perspective, which recognizes the physical, psychological, social, and spiritual needs during advanced illness, is best accomplished by empowering families to provide excellent care for patients at home.

References

1. Bentur N. Hospital at home: what is its place in the health system? *Health Policy* 2001;55(1):71–79.
2. Ferrell BR, Virani R, Grant M. Home care outreach for palliative care education. *Cancer Pract* 1998;6(2):79–85.
3. Franks PJ, Salisbury C, Bosanquet N, et al. The level of need for palliative care: a systematic review of the literature. *Palliat Med* 2000;14(2):93–104.
4. Baer WL, Hanson JC. Families' perception of the added value of hospice in the nursing home. *J Am Geriatr Soc* 2000;48(8):879–882.
5. Holzheimer A. The essentials of pain management for cancer patients receiving home care. *Home Care Provid* 1999;4(1):120–123.
6. Steinhauser KE, Christakis NA, Clipp EC, et al. Factors considered important at the end-of-life by patients, family, physicians, and other care providers. *JAMA* 2000;284(19):2476–2482.
7. Strang V, Koop PM. Factors which influence coping: home-based family caregiving of persons with advanced cancer. *J Palliative Care* 2003;19:107.

8. Krulish LH. Home care in the new millennium. *Home Health Nurse* 2000;18(2):144.

9. McCorkle R, Strumpf NE, Nuamah IF, et al. A specialized home care intervention improves survival among older post-surgical cancer patients. *J Am Geriatr Soc* 2000;48(12):1701–1713.

10. Bruera E, Sweeney C, Willey J, et al. Perception of discomfort by relatives and nurses in unresponsive terminally ill patients with cancer: a prospective study. *J Pain Symptom Manage* 2003;26:818–826.

11. Schumacher KL, Koresawa S, West C, et al. Putting cancer pain management regimens into practice at home. *J Pain Symptom Manage* 2002;23:369–382.

12. Mehta A, Ezer H. My love is hurting: the meaning spouses attribute to their loved ones' pain during palliative care. *J Palliative Care* 2003;19:87–94.

13. Earle CC, Neville BA, Landrum MB, et al. Trends in the aggressiveness of cancer care near the end-of-life. *J Clin Oncol* 2004;22:315–321.

14. Salmon JR, Kwak J, Acquaviva KD, et al. Transformative aspects of caregiving at life's end. *J Pain Symptom Manage* 2005;29(2):121–129.

15. Pierson CM. A good death: a qualitative study of patients with advanced AIDS. *AIDS Care* 2002;14(5):587–598.

16. Steinhauser KE, Clipp EC, McNeilly M, et al. In search of a good death: observations of patients, families, and providers. *Ann Intern Med* 2000; 132(10):825–832.

17. Clinical Practice Guidelines from the American Geriatrics Society. Guidelines at http://www.americangeriatrics.org/, 2006.

18. Zabora J. Screening procedures for psychological distress. In: Holland JC, ed. *Handbook of psycho-oncology*. New York: Oxford University Press, 1998.

19. Ferrell BR, Ferrell BA, Ahn C, et al. Pain management for elderly patients with cancer at home. *Cancer* 1994;74:2139–2146.

20. Panke JT, Ferrell BR. Emotional problems in the family. In: Doyle D, Hanks GWC, MacDonald N, eds. *Oxford textbook of palliative medicine*, 3rd ed.New York: Oxford University Press, 2004.

21. Koop PM, Strang VR. The bereavement experience following home-based family caregiving for persons with advanced cancer. *Clin Nurs Res* 2003; 23:127–144.

22. Strang V, Koop P, Peden J. The experience of respite during home-based family caregiving for persons with advanced cancer. *J Palliat Care* 2003; 18:97–104.

23. Teno Jm, Clarridge BR, Casey V, et al. Family perspectives on end-of-life care at the last place of death. *JAMA* 2004;291:88–93.

24. Cantor J, Blustein J, Carlson MJ, et al. Next-of-kin perceptions in physician responsiveness to symptoms of hospitalized patients near death. *J Palliat Med* 2003;6:531–539.

25. Perreault A, Fothergill-Bourbonnais F, Fiset V. The experience of family members caring for a dying loved one. *Int J Palliat Nurs* 2004;10:133–143.

26. Pooler J, McCrory F, Steadman Y, et al. Dying at home: a care pathway for the last days of life in a community setting. *Int J Palliat Nurs* 2003; 9:258–264.

27. Evers MM, Meier DE, Morrison RS. Assessing differences in care needs and service utilization in geriatric palliative care patients. *J Pain Symptom Manage* 2002;23:424–432.

28. Doyle D. Palliative medicine in the home: an overview. In: Doyle D, Hanks G, MacDonald N, eds. *Oxford textbook of palliative care*, 2nd ed. Oxford: Oxford University Press, 2004:1097–1114.

29. Beaver K, Luker K, Woods S. Primary care services received during terminal illness. *Int J Palliat Nurs* 2000;6:220–227.

30. Borneman T, Brown-Saltzman K. Meaning in illness. In: Ferrell B, Coyle N, eds. *Oxford textbook of palliative nursing*. Oxford: Oxford University Press, 2001:415–424.

31. Kemp C. Spiritual Care Interventions. In: Ferrell B, Coyle N, eds. *Oxford textbook of palliative nursing*. Oxford: Oxford University Press, 2001: 401–414.

32. Jaarsma T. End-of-life issues in cardiac patients and their families. *Eur J Cardiovasc Nurs* 2002;1:223–225.

33. Proot IM, Abu-Saad HH, Crebolder HF, et al. Vulnerability of family caregivers in terminal palliative care at home: balancing between burden and capacity. *Scand J Caring* 2003;17:113–121.

34. Carr D. A "good death" for whom? Quality of spouse's death and psychological distress among older widowed persons. *J Health Soc Behav* 2003;44:215–232.

35. Baker R, Wu AW, Teno JM, et al. Family satisfaction with end-of-life care in seriously ill hospitalized patients: findings of the SUPPORT program. *J Am Geriatr Soc* 2000;48:S61–S69.

36. Parsons LC, Reiss PL. Promoting collaborative practice with culturally diverse populations. *Semin Nurse Manag* 2000;7(4):160–165.

37. McDermott MA. Pain as a mutual experience for patients, nurses and families: international and theoretical perspectives from the four countries. *J Cult Divers* 2000;7(1):23–31.

38. Heineken J, McCoy N. Establishing a bond with clients of different cultures. *Home Health Nurse* 2000;18(1):45–51.

39. Gerrish K. Individualized care: its conceptualization and practice within a multiethnic society. *J Adv Nurs* 2000;32(1):91–99.

40. Vickers JL, Carlisle C. Choices and control: parental experiences in pediatric home care. *J Pediatr Oncol Nurs* 2000;17(1):12–21.

41. Wolfe J, Klar N, Greir HE, et al. Understanding prognosis among parents of children who died of cancer: impact on treatment goals and integration of palliative care. *JAMA* 2000;284(10):2469–2475.

42. Institute of Medicine. *When children die: improving palliative and end-of-life care for children and their families*. Washington, DC: The National Academies Press, 2003.

43. Kissane DW, McKenzie M, McKenzie DP, et al. Psychosocial morbidity associated with patterns of family functioning in palliative care: baseline data from the family focused grief therapy controlled trial. *Palliat Med* 2003; 17:527–537.

44. Stajduhar KI. Examining the perspectives of family members involved in the delivery of palliative care at home. *J Palliat Care* 2003;19:27–35.

45. Jennings B, Callahan D, Caplan AL. Ethical challenges of chronic illness. *Hastings Cent Rep* 1988;18(1):3–16.

46. Callahan D. Families as caregivers: the limits of morality. *Arch Phys Med Rehabil* 1988;69:323–328.

47. Altilio T, Rigoglioso RL. Payers' and providers' responsibilities towards caregivers. In: Levine C, ed. *Always on call: when illness turns families into caregivers*. New York: United Hospital Fund of New York, 2000.

48. Gatchel RJ, Turk DC, eds. *Psychosocial factors in pain: critical perspectives*. New York: Guilford Press, 1999.

49. Pan CX, Morrison RS, Ness J, et al. Complementary and alternative medicine in the management of pain, dyspnea, and nausea and vomiting near the end-of-life: a systematic review. *J Pain Symptom Manage* 2000;20(5): 374–387.

50. Ferrell BR, Grant M, Borneman T, et al. Family caregiving in cancer pain management. *J Palliat Med* 1999;2(2):185–195.

51. Pasacreta JV, McCorkle R. Cancer care: impact of interventions on caregiver outcomes. *Annu Rev Nurs Res* 2000;18(40):127–148.

52. Pasacreta JV, Barg F, Muamah I, et al. Participant characteristics before and after attendance at a family caregiver cancer education program. *Cancer Nurs* 2000;23(4):295–303.

53. Stetz KM, McDonald JC, Compton K. Needs and experiences of family caregivers during marrow transplantation. *Oncol Nurs Forum* 1996;23(9): 1422–1427.

54. Bowers G, Crisler K, Flammang M, et al. The future of home care. *Home Care Provid* 2000;5(1):18–24.

55. Levine C, ed. *Always on call: when illness turns families into caregivers*. New York: United Hospital Fund of New York, 2000.

56. Lynn J, O'Connor MA, Dular JD, et al. MediCaring: development and test marketing of a supportive care benefit for older people. *J Am Geriatr Soc* 1999;47(9):1058–1064.

57. Ferrell BR, Borneman T, Juarez G. Integration of pain education in home care. *J Palliat Care* 1998;14(3):62–68.

58. Ferrell BR, Virani R, Grant M. Improving end-of-life care education in home care. *J Palliat Med* 1998;1(1):11–19.

59. Hurny C. Communicating about cancer: patients' needs and caregivers' skills. *Support Care Cancer* 2000;8:437–448.

60. Friedrichsen MJ, Stang PM, Carlsson ME. Breaking bad news in the transition to palliative cancer care—patient's view of the doctor giving the information. *Support Care Cancer* 2000;8(6):472–478.

61. Kruijver IP, Kerkstra A, Bensing JM, et al. Nurse-patient communication in cancer care: a review of the literature. *Cancer Nurs* 2000;23(1): 20–31.

62. Douglas M. Pain as the fifth vital sign: will cultural variations be considered? *J Transcult Nurs* 1999;10(4):285.

63. Davis AJ. The bioethically constructed ideal dying patient in the USA. *Med Law* 2000;19(1):161–164.

64. Lister P. A taxonomy for developing cultural competence. *Nurse Educ Today* 1999;19(4):313–318.

65. DeSavorgnani AA, Haring RC. The impact of cultural issues on home care personnel and patients. *Caring* 1999;18(4):22–27.

66. Davies B, Reimer JC, Brown P, et al. *Fading away: the experience of transition in families with terminal illness*. Amityville, New York: Baywood Publishing Company, Inc., 1995.

CHAPTER 57 ■ MANAGEMENT OF SYMPTOMS IN THE ACTIVELY DYING PATIENT

PAUL ROUSSEAU

The obligation of physicians to relieve suffering is universal, particularly when death is imminent and the indignities of illness consume patients' final days and hours of life. This honored encumbrance transcends all other duties accorded by physicians and is fundamental to a death free of interminable symptoms and a satisfactory bereavement for surviving family members (1). Lamentably, the dying process can be a time of untold loss and suffering, and although spiritual and psychosocial concerns are basic domains in the inherent makeup of an individual, unrelieved physical suffering can detract the attention from important spiritual and psychosocial issues at the end of life. Accordingly, physicians must be competent in relieving physical distress and, in so doing, maintaining patient dignity and familial equanimity (2).

During the last days of life, there are characteristic symptoms that commonly occur, including dyspnea and noisy, gurgling respirations frequently referred to as the "death rattle," anxiety, restlessness, delirium, nausea and vomiting (NV), and pain (2–9). Although such symptoms are often multifactorial in etiology, treatment is usually empiric and palliative. Diagnostic evaluation is limited in recognition of the short life expectancy and impending death. Nevertheless, empiric treatment strategies do not suggest or encourage clinical indifference but rather mandate ongoing clinical assessment of therapeutic interventions in a continual effort to allay suffering. From time to time, terminal symptoms are refractory and unresponsive to aggressive and exhaustive interventions. In such cases, palliative sedation (PS) is an ethically and morally appropriate option that may be utilized to afford a more peaceful and tranquil death for the patient and a satisfactory grieving process for the remaining family members.

DYSPNEA AND THE DEATH RATTLE

Dyspnea

Dyspnea occurs in 29–90% of terminally ill patients and is the most common severe symptom as death approaches (9–13). Although it is more common in patients with pulmonary disorders, 23.9% of dyspneic patients in the National Hospice Study did not exhibit cardiac or pulmonary disease (11). Dyspnea is also reportedly more common in children dying from cancer, occurring in 80% of such patients (14,15). Dyspnea in terminally ill patients derives from five primary causes:

1. Existing disease [i.e., chronic obstructive pulmonary disease (COPD) and congestive heart failure]
2. Acute superimposed illness (i.e., pneumonia, pulmonary embolus)
3. Cancer-related complications (i.e., pleural effusion, lymphangitis carcinomatosis, tumor-induced bronchial obstruction, ascites)
4. Effects of cancer therapy (i.e., radiation and chemotherapy-induced pulmonary fibrosis), and
5. Miscellaneous causes (i.e., anemia, uremia, anxiety) (9,13,16).

As with any symptom, the treatment of dyspnea should address any easily correctable underlying cause, all the while recognizing and considering the limited life expectancy of the imminently dying patient and the invasiveness and discomfort of the proposed therapeutic interventions. Consequently, for most patients near death, opioids, benzodiazepines, phenothiazines, and corticosteroids are the mainstays of therapy (2,7–9,12,13,16,17).

Opioids purportedly relieve dyspnea by altering the perception of breathlessness (10,18), decreasing ventilatory response to hypoxia and hypercapnia (10,19), and reducing oxygen consumption at rest and with exercise (10,20). Controlled trials and anecdotal case reports on the use of systemic opioids in the treatment of malignant and COPD-associated dyspnea have generally demonstrated a reduction in dyspnea (10,17,21–25), including a recent Cochrane review that further confirmed the benefit of oral and parenteral opioids in improving dyspnea in patients with life-limiting disease (26–28). Although morphine preparations are generally utilized, any opioid should potentially alleviate dyspnea (Table 57.1). Opioids can be administered orally, rectally, sublingually, subcutaneously, intravenously, and by inhalation, but during the final hours of life when the ability to swallow declines and consciousness wanes, rectal, subcutaneous, and intravenous routes are more commonly used.

Inhalation of opioids is an unique and innovative approach to drug delivery. Controlled trials have revealed conflicting results (17,21,25,29–34), including a Cochrane review that showed no benefit of nebulized morphine over nebulized saline (26–28) but anecdotal reports have generally been favorable (13,35–37). In addition, a recent study by Bruera et al. noted that nebulized morphine was as good as

TABLE 57.1

PHARMACOLOGIC TREATMENT OF TERMINAL DYSPNEA

Drug	Dose[a]
Opioids	
Morphine	5–10 mg p.o., s.l., i.m., i.v., s.q., p.r. q1–4h; i.v. or s.q. doses should be adjusted accordingly using a 3:1 oral to parenteral ratio; titrate dose 30–50% daily or more frequently until symptoms improve or sedation becomes problematic; patients already on morphine may need to increase their regular dose by 25–50%; when dyspnea is severe and acute, 2–5 mg i.v. q15min or 5 mg s.q. q20min until dyspnea is relieved
Oxycodone	5–10 mg p.o., s.l., p.r. q1–4h
Hydromorphone	1–2 mg p.o., s.l., i.m., i.v., s.q., p.r. q1–4h; i.v. or s.q. doses should be adjusted accordingly using a 5:1 oral to parenteral ratio; titrate dose as per morphine recommendation
Nebulized morphine[b]	5 mg in 2 mL of normal saline q1–4h through nebulizer, may titrate to 20 mg q2–4h; hydromorphone may be substituted for morphine and started at 2 mg q1–4h
Corticosteroids	
Dexamethasone	4–8 mg p.o., s.l., i.m., i.v., s.q., p.r. daily
Prednisone	20–40 mg p.o., s.l. daily
Benzodiazepines	
Lorazepam	0.5–2 mg p.o., s.l., i.m., i.v., s.q., p.r. q1–4h
Diazepam	5–10 mg p.o., s.l., i.m., i.v., p.r. q1–4h
Midazolam	0.5 mg i.v. q15min until settled; 2.5–5 mg s.q., then 10–30 mg CSI q24h
Phenothiazine	
Chlorpromazine	12.5–25 mg i.v. q2–4h; 25 mg p.o., p.r. q2–4h

CSI, continuous subcutaneous infusion.
[a]Suggested starting doses may need to be clinically titrated; older frail patients may need doses adjusted appropriately.
[b]Nebulized morphine may cause histamine-mediated bronchospasm, particularly in opioid-naive patients or during the first nebulization; may be difficult for actively dying patients to take oral medications.

subcutaneous morphine in relieving dyspnea in patients with cancer; however, only 11 patients were included in the study, limiting its value (38). It is postulated that inhaled opioids exert their effect by means of opioid receptors that have been identified in the bronchial mucosa, as pharmacokinetic studies suggest that systemic bioavailability of nebulized morphine is extremely poor, varying from 4–8% (21,32,39). However, opioids may also stimulate histamine release from pulmonary mast cells and precipitate bronchospasm, worsening terminal dyspnea. Because this complication is usually a first-dose effect, careful observation is required during initial administration, and may warrant the prophylactic use of an antihistamine such as diphenhydramine. Although studies are generally nonsupportive and further research with randomized controlled trials is unquestionably warranted, in the dyspneic patient near death, nebulized opioids may be efficacious and worth a trial in an attempt to reduce breathlessness and assuage the horrific fear of suffocation when all other palliative measures have failed.

Benzodiazepines have been frequently utilized in dyspnea primarily when a component of anxiety is involved. However, studies and anecdotal reports are contradictory (17), with most well-designed randomized controlled trials failing to find significant benefit (40–42). Nevertheless, benzodiazepines are frequently beneficial in reducing dyspnea, particularly during the final days of life (43) and are increasingly used in hospice and palliative care programs. Buspirone, a popular nonbenzodiazepine anxiolytic and serotonin agonist, has been shown to relieve dyspnea in patients with anxiety and COPD at a dose of 15–45 mg daily (44). Because of its delayed onset of action, it may be of limited use in actively dying patients. Although not a benzodiazepine, the neuroleptic chlorpromazine has been used in dyspnea refractory to other medications. It appears to reduce air hunger and anxiety with minimal side effects (primarily sedation and hypotension) and has been efficacious in patients near death (9,45,46).

Although corticosteroids are useful when bronchospasm is associated with inflammation, most studies suggest that only 20–30% of patients with COPD improve with corticosteroid therapy. In the final days of life, corticosteroids are most useful when prescribed for dyspnea associated with airway obstruction, lymphangitis carcinomatosis, radiation pneumonitis, and superior vena cava syndrome (9,16). Corticosteroids can be administered orally, rectally, subcutaneously, intravenously, and by inhalation. Although side effects are of concern during chronic use, such concerns are negated by short-term use in dying patients.

Other medications are also available to attenuate dyspnea in the dying patient. These include diuretics, bronchodilators, and inhaled anesthetics. Oral and intravenous diuretics are useful when pulmonary edema and ascites contribute to dyspnea. The diuretic furosemide can also be administered through inhalation in a dose of 20 mg every 2–4 hours as needed, and appears to reduce dyspnea, irrespective of the underlying etiology (47–50). Although bronchodilators are best utilized in patients with a bronchospastic component to dyspnea (i.e., asthma, COPD with reactive airways), these drugs are frequently used when there is little-to-no evidence of bronchospasm and appear to provide subjective reduction of dyspnea in many patients. The use of adrenergic agonist bronchodilators, such as albuterol and metaproterenol, should be tempered by the possibility of resultant agitation, tremor, and heightened anxiety, potentially aggravating terminal dyspnea (9).

Nebulized anesthetics have been used infrequently for dyspnea in dying patients. In a study comparing nebulized saline and lidocaine, saline exerted a greater effect on the reduction of breathlessness (32,51). However, nebulized anesthetics have been useful for cough and may be considered when persistent coughing contributes to or aggravates dyspnea (17).

Nonpharmacologic interventions that are useful for terminal dyspnea include oxygen, a bedside fan, thoracentesis for pleural effusion, and paracentesis for ascites. The role of oxygen therapy in reducing dyspnea in patients near the end of life is somewhat controversial. In hypoxemic patients with disorders such as COPD, congestive heart failure, or pulmonary fibrosis, most studies suggest that there is significant symptomatic improvement (21,29,52). In patients without hypoxemia, however, its use is more contentious. Even so, the medical symbolism inherent in oxygen therapy may alleviate dyspnea by way of a placebo effect and should be considered in actively dying patients (a nasal cannula is better tolerated than a mask in most patients) (9,42). Moreover, oxygen therapy may provide many family members with the symbolic solace that "something is being done" to help their loved one, in spite of the fact that oxygen may actually provide only little therapeutic benefit.

A bedside fan may also be useful in alleviating dyspnea by reportedly stimulating thermal and mechanical receptors of the trigeminal nerve (V2 branch) in the cheek and nasopharynx, altering the central perception of breathlessness (9,45,53,54). The fan should be placed at the bedside, set on a low speed, and directed at the patient's face (9).

Thoracentesis and paracentesis may be useful when pleural effusion and ascites contribute to dyspnea (particularly if previous drainage has reduced dyspnea). In the final days of life, however, generally other strategies should be utilized unless noninterventional approaches have failed and breathlessness aggravates suffering. An indwelling thoracentesis or paracentesis catheter may obviate the need for repeated and painful intermittent thoracenteses and paracenteses, and should be considered in recurrent and disabling pleural effusions and ascites depending on estimated life expectancy.

Death Rattle

In the last 24–48 hours of life, most patients retain secretions in the back of the throat that produces a gurgling type of respiration frequently referred to as the death rattle (9,55). Fortunately, the patient is usually unaware of the noise. It can, however, be very disturbing to family members. Oropharyngeal suctioning is usually provided, but gagging and coughing may generate patient discomfort and further distress for relatives and caregivers. Instead, treatment with anticholinergic drugs is recommended to desiccate bronchial secretions and abolish the need for suctioning. Suggested medications include atropine, glycopyrrolate, scopolamine, and hyoscyamine (Table 57.2) (9,16). In one study, subcutaneous scopolamine

TABLE 57.2

PHARMACOLOGIC TREATMENT OF THE DEATH RATTLE

Drug	Dose
Scopolamine	0.4–0.6 mg s.q. q2–4h; 0.8–2.0 mg CSI q24h; 1–3 transdermal patches q3d
Hyoscyamine	0.125–0.250 mg s.l. q2–4h; 0.25–0.5 mg s.q. q2–4h; 1–2 mg CSI q24h
Glycopyrrolate	0.2 mg s.l., s.q. q2–4h
Atropine	0.4 mg s.q. q2–4h; may give 2 mg of atropine, 2.5–5.0 mg of morphine, and 2 mg of dexamethasone q2–4h through nebulizer

CSI, continuous subcutaneous infusion.

was more immediately efficacious when compared to subcutaneous glycopyrrolate; however, glycopyrrolate has a longer duration of action (26,33). Nevertheless, most anticholinergic medications work relatively well. These antisialagogues do not dry up secretions already present, and they should therefore be used at the first sign of noisy respirations (7). In addition, placing patients in a lateral recumbent position with the head slightly elevated may help reduce the pooling of secretions and diminish noisy respirations (2), as may discontinuing parenteral and enteral infusions whenever possible (14).

ANXIETY, RESTLESSNESS, AND DELIRIUM

Anxiety

Anxiety is one of the most common psychological problems in terminally ill patients and like most symptoms can have numerous etiologies (55–60). Anxiety can be a component of a preexisting anxiety disorder or, more commonly in actively dying patients, accompany medical disorders and complications of illness and medications (57,59). Medical disorders that can cause anxiety include hyperthyroidism, pheochromocytoma, and primary and metastatic brain tumors. Medical complications and medications that can precipitate anxiety include hypoxia, sepsis, unrelieved pain, dyspnea, and medications such as corticosteroids, bronchodilators, and antiemetics that cause akathisia (56–59). In addition, withdrawal states from benzodiazepines and opioids can result in anxiety and may occur inadvertently when medications are suddenly discontinued after admission to a hospital or long-term care facility (58).

The treatment of anxiety in the terminally ill often depends on etiology but generally involves nondrug maneuvers, specific interventions, and pharmacotherapy. Nondrug measures include meditation, biofeedback, progressive relaxation, and psychotherapy (58). In actively dying patients these nondrug methods are of little value. In some cases, specific interventions can be of benefit and include such measures as oxygen and opioids for dyspnea, opioids and other analgesics for pain, and discontinuing medications that cause akathisia, a movement disorder precipitated by neuroleptic medications (i.e., haloperidol, chlorpromazine, prochlorperazine), and characterized by motor restlessness, compulsive moving, and anxiety.

The principal therapy for anxiety includes the judicious use of benzodiazepines, neuroleptics, and antihistamines (56–59). Benzodiazepines are the mainstay of treatment in the terminally ill patient, with the shorter-acting agents, such as lorazepam and oxazepam, preferred in the patient with advanced disease (Table 57.3). These drugs are metabolized by conjugation in the liver and are safest when hepatic disease is present (56,57,59). This is in contrast to alprazolam and other benzodiazepines which are metabolized through oxidative pathways and may accumulate in debilitated patients (61). Midazolam, a water-soluble benzodiazepine, may be infused intravenously or subcutaneously and is very useful in controlling anxiety in the terminal phase of illness. The cost of midazolam may limit its use (56–59,62), particularly in managed care and capitated health systems, although a generic version is now available. Diazepam, an older but efficacious benzodiazepine, may be used rectally when no other route is available and the cost is of concern, with recommended dosages equivalent to oral regimens. Clonazepam, a long-acting benzodiazepine used for seizure disorders and myoclonus, is useful in patients who experience end-of-dose recurrence of anxiety on shorter-acting benzodiazepine medications (56–59).

TABLE 57.3

PHARMACOLOGIC TREATMENT OF ANXIETY

Drug	Dose[a]
Benzodiazepines	
Lorazepam	0.5–2.0 mg p.o., s.l., i.m., i.v., s.q. q1–4h
Midazolam	0.5–5.0 mg i.v., s.q. q1–4h; 10–30 mg CSI q24h
Diazepam	2.5–10.0 mg p.o., i.m., i.v., p.r. q1–4h
Clonazepam	0.5–2.0 mg p.o. b.i.d.–q.i.d.
Oxazepam	15 mg p.o. t.i.d.–q.i.d.
Neuroleptics	
Haloperidol	0.5–1.0 mg p.o., i.m., i.v., s.q. q1–6h
Chlorpro-mazine	10–25 mg p.o., i.m., i.v., p.r. q4–6h
Thioridazine	10–75 mg p.o. t.i.d.–q.i.d.
Antihistamines	
Hydroxyzine	10–50 mg p.o., i.m., i.v., s.q. q2–4h

CSI, continuous subcutaneous infusion.
[a]Suggested starting doses, may need to be clinically titrated; older frail patients may need doses adjusted appropriately, may be difficult for actively dying patients to take oral medications.

Other nonbenzodiazepine medications useful for anxiety include the neuroleptics chlorpromazine, thioridazine, and haloperidol, and the antihistamine hydroxyzine (Table 57.3). Neuroleptics may be used when benzodiazepines fail to relieve anxiety, when psychotic symptoms accompany anxiety, or when there is concern regarding the respiratory depressant effects of benzodiazepines (63). Hydroxyzine, an effective antihistaminic anxiolytic, may have coanalgesic effects (64) and may be a particularly useful alternative to benzodiazepines when pain accompanies or exacerbates anxiety, or when benzodiazepines and neuroleptics are contraindicated (i.e., allergy, respiratory depression, akathisia).

Restlessness

Restlessness is commonly observed during the last hours of life. Although it has multiple causes (and may overlap with delirium), specific treatment may not be possible (7). Restless patients may have diverse symptoms, including impaired consciousness, intermittent sleepiness, tossing and turning, moaning, grunting, crying out, and agitation, and muscle spasms or twitching (2). Restlessness may be caused by spiritual conflicts; by physical discomfort, such as a distended urinary bladder or bladder spasms, fecal impaction, unrelieved pain, and pressure ulcers; or by nausea, dyspnea, pruritus, hypoxia, extreme weakness, corticosteroids, and sudden withdrawal from benzodiazepines. Treatment involves identifying and managing the underlying cause or, if that is not possible, providing spiritual support, verbal and tactile reassurance, and utilizing a benzodiazepine such as midazolam, or a neuroleptic such as chlorpromazine (Table 57.3) (2,7).

Delirium

Delirium is a nonspecific global disorder of cognition and attention that occurs in 8–75% of hospitalized patients with cancer (58,59,65,66) and in 62–83% of patients just before death (67–70). It is a significant sign of physiologic disturbance and, analogous to anxiety, may be secondary to multiple etiologies, including primary or metastatic brain tumors, infection, organ failure, metabolic disturbances, vascular complications, nutritional deficiencies, medication side effects, radiotherapy, and paraneoplastic syndromes (67). In contrast to dementia, delirium is considered a reversible disorder with rapid onset; in the last 24–48 hours of life, however, it may be irreversible. According to the Diagnostic and Statistical Manual of the American Psychiatric Association (71), delirium is characterized by:

- Disturbance of consciousness (reduced awareness of the environment) with reduced ability to focus, sustain, or shift attention
- Change in cognition (memory deficit, disorientation, perceptual disturbances such as hallucinations, illusions, delusions) that is not related to a preexisting dementia
- Development over a short period of time, with usual fluctuation throughout the day
- Evidence from the history, physical examination, or laboratory tests of a general medical condition judged to be etiologically related to the causation of delirium

The assessment of delirium must take into consideration the life expectancy of the patient and the patient's goals for care. Most palliative care clinicians would undertake a diagnostic workup only when a clinically suspected cause can be easily identified and treated effectively with simple interventions that carry a minimal burden or risk of causing further distress (i.e., hypodermoclysis for dehydration). Most often, the cause of delirium in the actively dying patient is multifactorial and irreversible, and treatment is usually empiric (67). Similar to anxiety, nondrug supportive measures are of limited value (other than the presence of family members, a well-lit room, and familiar sounds and music). Consequently, pharmacologic interventions are the primary methods for treating delirium in patients near death.

Neuroleptic medications are the preferred pharmacologic agents and are particularly safe and efficacious in reducing disturbing cognitive symptoms in dying patients (Table 57.4) (16,56,58,59,65,67). Haloperidol is the usual

TABLE 57.4

PHARMACOLOGIC TREATMENT OF DELIRIUM

Drug	Dose[a]
Neuroleptics	
Haloperidol	0.5–1.0 mg p.o., i.m., i.v., s.q. q1–6h; 5–15 mg CSI q24h; in acute situations, 0.5–1.0 mg i.v., s.q. q45–60 min until symptoms controlled
Chlorpro-mazine	10–25 mg p.o., i.m., i.v., p.r. q4–6h
Risperidone	0.5–1.0 mg p.o. b.i.d.
Olanzapine	2.5–5 mg p.o. q.d.
Benzodiazepines	
Lorazepam	0.5–2.0 mg p.o., s.l., i.m., i.v., s.q. q1–4h
Midazolam	0.5–5.0 mg i.v., s.q. q1–4h; 10–30 mg CSI q24h

CSI, continuous subcutaneous infusion.
[a]Suggested starting doses, may need to be clinically titrated; older frail patients may need doses adjusted appropriately; may be difficult for actively dying patients to take oral medications if the patient is taking an opioid; rotating to another opioid with no active metabolites (i.e., hydromorphone) may help lessen delirium if the delirium is opioid induced; severe agitated delirium may require palliative sedation.

drug of choice and may be given orally, intravenously, and subcutaneously, with its use supported by three recent studies (72–75). However, clinicians should be aware that parenteral doses are approximately twice as potent as oral doses (65,67). It is the drug of choice because of its short half-life, lack of active metabolites, and minimal anticholinergic and cardiovascular side effects. It is also less likely to cause sedation or paradoxical delirium (76). The atypical antipsychotics such as olanzapine, risperidone, and quetiapine can also be considered in the management of delirium.

A short-acting benzodiazepine can be added if the patient is overly agitated, although (26) benzodiazepines alone are not indicated in the treatment of delirium. In fact, benzodiazepines may actually exacerbate the delirious state and should be used cautiously and discontinued if delirium worsens. When delirium is difficult to control in the last days of life, PS to the point of unconsciousness may be needed (6,77). In such situations a benzodiazepine, such as lorazepam or midazolam, is the drug of choice, either alone or in conjunction with a neuroleptic.

NAUSEA AND VOMITING

NV occur in 62% of patients with terminal cancer. Although the prevalence is 40–46% during the last 6 weeks of life (78), it rarely develops as a new symptom during the last days of life (8). NV is observed more frequently in women, individuals younger than 65 years, and patients with stomach and breast cancer (78).

The etiology of NV in terminal illness varies and is frequently multifactorial (9), particularly as death approaches. Although diagnostic evaluation can be done in the actively dying patient, treatment usually involves the empirical use of nonpharmacologic measures and antiemetics. However, if the clinician, patient, or family insists on an evaluation, simple tests, such as measurement of electrolytes, blood urea nitrogen, creatinine, calcium, albumin, glucose, and digoxin or anticonvulsant drug levels, are recommended and may readily disclose a reversible cause.

Nonpharmacologic measures used to treat NV include dietary manipulations (Table 57.5), elimination of emetogenic medications [i.e., nonsteroidal anti-inflammatories, digoxin, iron (79)], and the limited use of nasogastric suctioning, particularly for high gastrointestinal bowel obstruction. Nasogastric tubes can be uncomfortable and difficult to place, especially in the home environment, but intermittent use may be considered for severe and intractable vomiting refractory to antiemetic therapy. A percutaneous venting gastrostomy is

TABLE 57.5

DIETARY MANIPULATIONS FOR NAUSEA AND VOMITING

Minimize unpleasant odors
Sounds and smells of food preparation should be excluded
Avoid foods known to precipitate nausea and vomiting
Clear liquid diet may be best tolerated
Cold foods may be preferred
Sour foods, such as lemons, and rinsing of the mouth with weak lemon juice may reduce nausea
Utilize frequent small feedings if the patient wants to eat

Adapted from Lichter I. Nausea and vomiting in patients with cancer. *Hematol Oncol Clin North Am* 1996;10:207–220, with permission.

useful if placed prior to the active dying process. However, its placement in the patient near death is usually not practical.

Nine types of antiemetics are utilized in the treatment of terminal NV: dopamine antagonists, metoclopramide, anticholinergics, antihistamines, corticosteroids, serotonin antagonists, octreotide, cannabinoids, and benzodiazepines (Table 57.6) (9,79–81).

Dopamine antagonists include haloperidol and prochlorperazine and are the usual first-line antiemetics chosen by most clinicians. Haloperidol is an excellent antiemetic and is particularly useful in delirious patients with NV because both symptoms may be improved with a single medication. As mentioned earlier (see the section Delirium), parenteral doses are twice as potent as oral doses, and there is a reported ceiling effect at approximately 30 mg a day. Prochlorperazine is also efficacious and a favorite of many clinicians, and while promethazine and chlorpromazine are also prescribed, there is probably little advantage in using them over prochlorperazine (79). Although combination therapy for NV is common in the terminally ill, two or more dopamine antagonists should not be prescribed concurrently as the potential for adverse extrapyramidal reactions is increased without additional antiemetic benefit.

Metoclopramide is both a dopamine antagonist and a serotonin (5-HT4) agonist, but at doses greater than 120 mg a day it becomes a serotonin (5 HT3) antagonist (82). It is very useful as an antiemetic and a prokinetic agent for gastroparesis-induced vomiting but caution must be exercised with older patients as it may cause extrapyramidal reactions that may not be dose dependent (79).

Anticholinergic medications are most efficacious in NV related to colic and mechanical bowel obstruction (79,83). They include scopolamine, hyoscyamine, and glycopyrrolate. Antihistamines are effective in motion sickness, mechanical bowel obstruction, and increased intracranial pressure. These drugs comprise buclizine, meclizine, and diphenhydramine.

Corticosteroids have a synergistic effect with metoclopramide and the serotonin antagonists (79) but are rarely useful as single agents (however, they may reduce peritumor edema of gastrointestinal malignancies and brain metastases, and, in so doing, lessen emetic episodes). Dexamethasone is the favored agent due to the small pill size, minimal mineralocorticoid activity, and availability of intravenous and subcutaneous administration. Serotonin antagonists are relatively new and expensive agents. Although quite useful in chemotherapy- and radiation-induced emesis, their value in terminal NV is unknown. Nevertheless, they are frequently utilized in dying patients and are reportedly quite effective in reducing emesis, particularly NV associated with radiation, bowel obstruction, and renal failure (79,84).

Octreotide is a somatostatin analog that is useful in reducing NV associated with intestinal obstruction. This drug decreases gastrointestinal secretions, stimulates absorption of water and electrolytes, and inhibits intestinal peristalsis (85).

Dronabinol is the only commercially available cannabinoid available in the United States. It is rarely used in terminal NV. It exhibits antikinetic properties in the stomach and small bowel (79) and may be most useful in emesis related to small bowel obstruction. It may, however, potentially worsen gastroparetic conditions.

The benzodiazepines have little role as singular antiemetics in the actively dying patient unless anxiety is a dominant component. They are best utilized as adjuncts to other antiemetics through their amnesic, anxiolytic, and sedative properties (86).

Many hospice programs utilize compounding pharmacists to prepare diverse and innovative medications and delivery systems for symptom control in dying patients. A compounding pharmacist can prepare a topical gel and/or suppository

TABLE 57.6

PHARMACOLOGIC TREATMENT OF NAUSEA AND VOMITING

Drug	Dose[a]
Dopamine antagonists	
Haloperidol	0.5–2.0 mg p.o., i.m., i.v., s.q. q4–6h; 5–15 mg CSI q24h
Prochlorperazine	5–20 mg p.o., i.m., i.v. q4–6h; 25 mg p.r. q4h
Droperidol	2.5–5.0 mg i.v. q4–6h
Promethazine	25 mg p.o., p.r. q4–6h; 12.5–25.0 mg i.v. q4–6h
Substituted benzamide	
Metoclopramide[b]	5–20 mg p.o., i.m., i.v., s.q. q6h; 20–80 mg CSI q24h
Anticholinergics	
Scopolamine	0.3–0.8 mg p.o., s.q. q4–6h; 1–3 transdermal patches q3d; 0.8–2.0 mg CSI q24h
Hyoscyamine	0.125–0.250 mg p.o., s.l. q4h; 0.25–0.50 mg s.q. q4–6h; 1–2 mg CSI q24h
Antihistamines	
Buclizine	50 mg p.o. q4–6h
Meclizine	25–50 mg p.o. q4–6h
Diphenhydramine	25–50 mg p.o., i.m., i.v. q4–6h
Corticosteroids	
Dexamethasone	1–4 mg p.o., i.v., s.q. q6h; 2–12 mg CSI q24h
Serotonin antagonists	
Ondansetron	8 mg p.o., i.v., s.q. q8h; 8–24 mg CSI q24h
Granisetron	0.5–1.0 mg p.o., i.v., s.q. q12h
Somatostatin analogue	
Octreotide	150 µg s.q. t.i.d.; 0.2–0.9µg CSI q24h
Cannabinoid	
Dronabinol	2.5–7.5 mg p.o. b.i.d.–t.i.d.
Benzodiazepines	
Lorazepam	0.5–2.0 mg p.o., s.l., i.m., i.v., s.q. q4h
Compounded medication[c]	
ABHR, ABHRD, ABHRDC[d]	1 p.r. q4–6h

CSI, continuous subcutaneous infusion.

[a]Suggested starting doses, may need to be clinically titrated; older frail patients may need doses adjusted appropriately.

[b]Metoclopramide is a serotonin antagonist at high doses.

[c]Needs to be prepared by a compounding pharmacist.

[d]ABHR compounded medications have not been tested in a research setting and their use is not supported by well-designed trials.

variously known as *ABHR, ABHRD,* or *ABHRDC* that contain commercially available antiemetics, including Ativan (lorazepam), Benadryl or Dramamine (diphenhydramine), Haldol (haloperidol), Reglan (metoclopramide), Decadron (dexamethasone), or Cogentin (benztropine). These drugs are combined in various dosages (i.e., Ativan, 1.0 mg; Benadryl, 12.5–25.0 mg or Dramamine, 25–50 mg; Haldol, 0.5–1.0 mg; Reglan, 5–10 mg; Decadron, 10 mg; and Cogentin, 1 mg). The suppositories have been quite useful in refractory NV and may be very effective in patients near death. Although there have been no studies that assess the varied combinations, they appear to benefit some patients because of both antiemetic and sedative effects.

PAIN

As death approaches, pain may become less problematic because the patient becomes bedbound and experiences less movement-related pain. Nevertheless, opioids must not be stopped abruptly, and clinicians should be cognizant that patients may be disturbed by pain, even when comatose (7). Assessment of pain may become difficult and, in the final hours of life, patients may appear to show signs of pain when turned or repositioned, even when unconscious. Such pain may be due to an underlying medical disorder or due to joint stiffness secondary to bed rest and minimal body movement (87). Conversely, moaning and groaning is not uncommon in actively dying patients and may be interpreted as pain by family members. However, it is rare for uncontrolled pain to develop during the last hours of life, and in such patients, it is helpful to look for tension across the forehead, furrowing of the eyebrows, or facial grimacing, all evidence that the moaning and groaning may be secondary to pain (88,89).

Assessing pain in confused or demented patients may be problematic. Such patients frequently exhibit pain by facial grimacing, resistance to turning or repositioning, agitation, and a reduction in functional abilities. Conversely, signs of apparent discomfort may be noted when a patient who is hearing or visually impaired or confused is touched without forewarning. Such response may not in fact be pain but rather the result of a startled response from tactile stimulation without prior warning.

In the final hours of life, patients may be unable to swallow, and sublingual/buccal, transdermal, rectal, intravenous, or subcutaneous administration of analgesics may be necessary (Tables 57.7 and 57.8). Although rectal administration of sustained-release opioids is not approved by the U.S. Food and Drug Administration (FDA), studies suggest that rectal absorption is similar to oral administration. In addition, suppositories are available for nonsteroidal anti-inflammatory drugs, the tricyclic antidepressant doxepin, and the corticosteroid

TABLE 57.7

ALTERNATIVE ROUTES OF DELIVERY FOR PHARMACOLOGIC TREATMENT OF PAIN

Opioids that can be delivered subcutaneously
  Morphine
  Hydromorphone
  Methadone
  Fentanyl
Opioids that can be delivered topically
  Fentanyl[a]
  Morphine[b]
Oral opioids that can be delivered rectally
  Morphine[c]
  Oxycodone
Anesthetics that can be delivered subcutaneously
  Lidocaine[d]
Adjuvant medications and alternative routes of delivery

Dexamethasone	s.q., i.m., i.v., p.r.
Indomethacin	p.r.
Diclofenac	p.r.
Ketorolac[e]	s.q.
Carbamazepine[f]	p.r.
Valproic acid	p.r.
Doxepin	p.r.

[a]Available as a topical patch; to convert from an oral opioid, convert the opioid to a morphine equivalent dose, then divide the morphine dose by 2 to get the approximate strength of the fentanyl patch. From Storey P, Knight CF. *UNIPAC three: assessment and treatment of pain in the terminally ill.* Gainesville, FL: American Academy of Hospice and Palliative Medicine, 1996, with permission.
[b]Also available as a suppository; hydromorphone also available as a suppository.
[c]Morphine can be compounded into a gel for topical use, bioavailability is unknown.
[d]1–3 mg/kg (often 100 mg) i.v. over 20–30 min or s.q. over 30–60 min—if pain relieved, start an infusion either i.v. or s.q. at 0.5–2 mg/kg/h; serum levels may be monitored. See: Ferrini R. Parenteral lidocaine for severe intractable pain in six hospice patients continued at home. *J Palliat Med* 2000;3:193–200.
[e]Can be administered by a continuous subcutaneous infusion, 60 mg q24h.
[f]Crush the tablets, put in a gelatin capsule, and place rectally.

TABLE 57.8

ALTERNATIVE ROUTES OF MEDICATION ADMINISTRATION[a]

Route	Medication
Rectal	Valproic acid
	Carbamazepine
	Diazepam
	Indomethacin
	Doxepin
	Pentobarbital
	Phenobarbital
	Chlorpromazine
	Opioids
Inhalation	Furosemide
	Vasopressin
Sublingual	Liquid opioids[b]
	Hyoscyamine
	Atropine
	Lorazepam
Subcutaneous	Morphine
	Hydromorphone
	Midazolam
	Lorazepam
	Haloperidol
	Hyoscyamine
	Glycopyrrolate
	Metoclopramide
	Dexamethasone
	Lidocaine
	Ketorolac
Transdermal	Fentanyl
	Scopolamine

[a]List is not all inclusive.
[b]Methadone is lipophilic and therefore better absorbed across the buccal membrane than the other opioids.

dexamethasone. The antiepileptics carbamazepine and valproic acid are frequently administered rectally by placing them in gelatin capsules.

Unfortunately, many patients and family members are reluctant to utilize the rectal route for administration of medications, especially if pain is not controlled and frequent supplementary doses of analgesics are required. In such cases, subcutaneous infusions are appropriate and well tolerated. Opioids; the nonsteroidal anti-inflammatory ketorolac (90); the anticholinergics scopolamine, atropine, hyoscyamine, and glycopyrrolate; and the corticosteroid dexamethasone can all be given by means of the subcutaneous route in an effort to maintain or improve pain control. Epidural and other invasive analgesic interventions are rarely utilized when the patient is near death and should ideally be considered for use earlier in the disease process.

PALLIATIVE SEDATION

PS, also referred to as terminal sedation or controlled sedation, is the intentional use of pharmacologic agents to induce and maintain a deep sleep, but not deliberately cause death, in specific clinical circumstances complicated by refractory symptoms (91). The incidence of PS varies from 5–52% (92). This variation is attributable to diverse definitions of PS, the retrospective nature of studies, and cultural and ethnic diversity. A refractory symptom is at times subjective and nonspecific and includes physical as well as psychological symptoms (93). Cherny and Portenoy clarify the boundaries of a refractory symptom by offering three criteria that suggest a symptom is refractory:

1. It cannot be controlled adequately despite aggressive efforts to identify a tolerable therapy that does not compromise consciousness.
2. Additional invasive and noninvasive interventions are incapable of providing adequate relief.
3. The therapy directed at the symptom is associated with excessive and intolerable acute or chronic morbidity and is unlikely to provide relief within a tolerable time frame (91).

The ethical validity of PS derives from the doctrine of double effect, a doctrine that is applied to situations in which it is impossible for a person to avoid all harmful actions, and the precept of informed consent. The traditional formulations of the doctrine of double effect involves four basic conditions:

1. The nature of the act must be good or morally neutral and not in a category that is absolutely prohibited and intrinsically wrong.
2. The intent of the clinician must be good, and the good effect, not the bad effect, must be intended.
3. The demarcation between the means and effects must be acceptable, in other words, the bad effect must not be the means to the good effect.
4. Proportionality, whereby the good effect must exceed or balance the bad effect (94).

Contentious issues regarding PS revolve around the use of tube feedings and eventual dehydration, and the relationship of PS to physician-assisted suicide and euthanasia. Opponents of PS claim that the sedated patient dies of malnutrition and/or dehydration, not the underlying disease, although most patients have stopped eating and drinking before the initiation of PS, negating the argument of clinician-induced food and fluid deprivation. Nevertheless, if patients or surrogate family members wish to continue tube feedings, most clinicians discuss the futility of nutritional support but acquiesce to such requests, or more favorably suggest a time-limited use of enteral nutrition, and initiate PS.

Opponents of PS also contend that PS is nothing more than slow euthanasia. As proffered by the doctrine of double effect, however, the intent of the clinician must be considered. In the case of refractory symptoms, the intent is to alleviate suffering, not assist in suicide or euthanasia, although PS may undeniably hasten death. Auspiciously, the US Supreme Court fundamentally sanctioned PS in its decision opposing the constitutional right to physician-assisted suicide in 1997 (95,96), and in so doing, helped establish its value in the palliative armamentarium.

If PS is employed in a dying patient, guidelines should be followed (Table 57.9), including obtaining informed consent, as it is intimately integrated with autonomy and self-determination, and allows a reasonable person or surrogate to make independent and noncoerced treatment decisions (97). The reason for PS should be documented, as should the people present during the discussion, and if required by institutional or corporate policy, a completed consent form placed in the patient's chart. The choice of medications for PS is practitioner dependent; clinicians should choose the drugs they are most familiar with, considering efficacy, cost, and clinical circumstance. Drugs frequently used for

TABLE 57.9

GUIDELINES FOR PALLIATIVE SEDATION

Presence of a terminal illness with refractory symptom(s)
A do-not-resuscitate order
Exhaustion of all palliative treatments, including treatment for depression, delirium, anxiety, and familial discord
Consideration of ethical and psychiatric consultations
Consideration of assessment for spiritual issues by a skilled clinician or clergy member
Discussion regarding the discontinuation of parenteral or enteral nutrition or hydration
Obtaining informed consent
Consideration of respite sedation, particularly in patients with refractory existential distress

Adapted from Rousseau P. Palliative sedation in the management of refractory symptoms. *J Support Oncol* 2004;2:181–186.

TABLE 57.10

MEDICATIONS FOR PALLIATIVE SEDATION

Drug	Dose
Benzodiazepines	
Midazolam	5 mg s.q. bolus, then 1 mg/h s.q., titrate as needed
Lorazepam	2–5 mg s.q. bolus, then 0.5–1.0 mg/h s.q., titrate as needed; 1–4 mg q1–4h s.l., p.r.
Barbiturates	
Thiopental	5–7 mg/kg/h i.v. bolus, then 20–80 mg/h i.v., titrate as needed
Pentobarbital[a]	2–3 mg/kg i.v. bolus, then 1 mg/h i.v., titrate as needed; 60–120 mg p.r. q4h
Phenobarbital	200 mg i.v., s.q. bolus, then 25 mg/h i.v., s.q., titrate as needed
Neuroleptics	
Haloperidol	2–10 mg i.v., s.q. bolus, then 5–15 mg/d, titrate as needed
Chlorpromazine[a]	25–100 mg p.r. q4h
Anesthetic	
Propofol	10 mg/h i.v., titrate as needed; boluses of 20–50 mg may be administered for urgent sedation

[a]Available as a suppository.

PS include benzodiazepines, barbiturates, neuroleptics, and propofol (Table 57.10).

FAMILY VIGIL

As death nears, family members tend to gather for comfort, solace, and support of themselves and their dying loved one. Emotions may become capricious and volatile, and aggressive treatments may be requested in an attempt to delay or preclude death. A "long-lost" family member may also suddenly appear and precipitate dissension among family members. Such disruption can distract health care providers as well as family members from providing the care and sustenance the dying patient needs. The clinician must keep in mind that such actions are often a manifestation of grief and fear, a desire to control an uncontrollable situation, or apprehension regarding one's own predestined death. It is important to maintain open communication with family members and reaffirm the goal of comfort care. Social work, nursing, and chaplain involvement can help direct family members in accepting the inevitable death of their loved one and provide reassurance that they will be there during this final journey.

Involving family members in the plan of care for the patient will enhance cooperation and a sense of contribution, as will frequent interaction with and discussion of their loved ones decline. They should be encouraged to assist in care by swabbing the oral mucosa, applying cool compresses to the eyes, performing gentle range of motion, and holding the hand of their loved one. The signs and events of the dying process should be reinforced, and personal, cultural, and religious beliefs and rituals honored (98,99). Family members may also be encouraged to convey the five affirmations recommended by Ira Byock: I forgive you, forgive me, I love you, thank you, and good-bye (100). Facilitating and supporting the opportunity for resolution and closure, personal and spiritual growth, and emotional healing is cardinal to a constructive death and bereavement, and should be provided for and encouraged.

To preclude confusion and turmoil during a home death, family members should be advised not to call "911." Specific instructions should be given about whom to call (i.e., hospice nurse, social worker, chaplain, or physician). Family members should also be instructed about the physiologic events that occur as the patient dies [e.g., the heart stops beating, breathing stops, pupils may dilate, eyes may remain open, urine and stool may be released, jaw may drop open (98)] and offered sufficient time to ask questions. Once death occurs, there is no immediacy to deliver the body to the morgue or funeral home, and family members should be allowed private time with their deceased loved one. Intravenous lines and catheters should be removed and, if desired by the spouse or children, the deceased bathed by family members; the latter can facilitate closure and allow expressions of immediate grief in a supportive setting (99). Finally, if the clinician is present to pronounce the patient, forthright and candid respect should be shown to the patient and family. Words such as, "I'm sorry, he/she has died," and "My deepest condolences" are appropriate. However, silence, touch, and mere presence can be the greatest forms of communication and compassion at the time of death.

TIME OF DEATH

No matter how well family members and health care professionals are prepared, the time of death can be challenging and difficult (88). If the patient is at home, family members should have been instructed to call the hospice program or their family physician if hospice was not involved. Rarely is it necessary to involve the coroner, unless the death was unexpected or surrounded by suspicious circumstances. If the death occurs in an institution, a medical student or resident may be called to certify or pronounce death; in nonteaching institutions, the responsibility may fall on the nurse (89). However, one issue that may arise before and after death is what are the signs of death, especially if the patient is dying at home away from professional caregivers. Family members should be counseled on the signs of death, particularly in homebound patients (88,89). Basic signs of death include absence of heart sounds, pulses, and respiration, fixed pupils, pale and waxen color as blood settles, and release of urine and stool with relaxation of sphincter tone (88).

Once death has occurred, the focus of care should immediately shift from the patient to the family and caregivers; although death had been expected, no one understands the emotions and depth of loss until it actually occurs. Families should be allowed to spend time with their deceased loved one before the body is moved; time spent with the body immediately after death reportedly helps family members assimilate and deal with acute grief (88,89). Moreover, moving the body is a direct confrontation with the reality of death, so providing ample time with the body and asking whether family members wish to witness the removal is suggested (88). Finally, professional caregivers should offer to assist the family in notifying other family members and friends, and provide a telephone number where they can be reached should unforeseen issues or questions arise.

References

1. Rousseau PC. The losses and suffering of terminal illness. *Mayo Clin Proc* 2000;75:197–198.
2. Abrahm JL. *A physician's guide to pain and symptom management in cancer patients.* Baltimore, MD: The Johns Hopkins University Press, 2000.
3. Nelson KA, Walsh D, Behrens C, et al. The dying cancer patient. *Semin Oncol* 2000;27:84–89.
4. Conill C, Verger E, Henriquez I, et al. Symptom prevalence in the last week of life. *J Pain Symptom Manage* 1997;14:328–331.
5. Fainsinger R, Miller M, Bruera E, et al. Symptom control during the last week of life on a palliative care unit. *J Palliat Care* 1991;7:5–11.
6. Ventafridda V, Ripamonti C, DeConno F, et al. Symptom prevalence and control during cancer patients' last days of life. *J Palliat Care* 1990;6:7–11.
7. Twycross R, Lichter I. The terminal phase. In: Doyle D, Hanks GWC, MacDonald N, eds. *Oxford textbook of palliative medicine*, 2nd ed. Oxford: Oxford University Press, 1998:977–992.
8. Adam J. ABC of palliative care. The last 48 hours. *BMJ* 1997;315:1600–1603.
9. Rousseau PC. Nonpain symptom management in terminal care. *Clin Geriatr Med* 1996;12:313–327.
10. Bruera E, MacMillan K, Pither J, et al. The effects of morphine on the dyspnea of terminal cancer patients. *J Pain Symptom Manage* 1990;5:341–344.
11. Reuben DB, Mor V. Dyspnea in terminally ill cancer patients. *Chest* 1986;89:234–236.
12. Sykes NP. Advances in symptom control for dysphagia and dyspnea. *J Cancer Care* 1992;1:47–52.
13. Hsu DHS. Dyspnea in dying patients. *Can Fam Physician* 1993;39:1635–1638.
14. Von Roenn JH, Paice JA. Control of common, non-pain cancer symptoms. *J Support Oncol* 2005;32:200–210.
15. Wolfe J, Grier HE, Klar N, et al. Symptoms and suffering at the end of life in children with cancer. *N Engl J Med* 2000;342:326–333.
16. Rousseau PC. Hospice and palliative care. *Dis Mon* 1995;41:769–844.
17. Manning HL. Dyspnea treatment. *Respir Care* 2000;45:1342–1351.
18. Light RW, Muro JR, Sato RI, et al. Effects of oral morphine on breathlessness and exercise tolerance in patients with chronic obstructive pulmonary disease. *Am Rev Respir Dis* 1989;139:126–133.
19. Weil JV, McCullough RE, Kline JS, et al. Diminished ventilatory response to hypoxia and hypercapnia after morphine in normal man. *N Engl J Med* 1975;292:1103–1106.
20. Woodcock AA, Gross ER, Gellert A, et al. Effects of dihydrocodeine, alcohol, and caffeine on breathlessness and exercise tolerance in patients with chronic obstructive lung disease and normal blood gases. *N Engl J Med* 1981;305:1611–1616.
21. Ripamonti C. Management of dyspnea in advanced cancer patients. *Support Care Cancer* 1999;7:233–243.
22. Allard P, Lamontagne C, Bernard P, et al. How effective are supplementary doses of opioids for dyspnea in terminally ill cancer patients? A randomized continuous sequential clinical trial. *J Pain Symptom Manage* 1999;17:256–265.
23. Boyd KJ, Kelly M. Oral morphine as symptomatic treatment of dyspnea in patients with advanced cancer. *Palliat Med* 1997;11:277–281.
24. Bruera E, MacEachern T, Ripamonti C, et al. Subcutaneous morphine for dyspnea in cancer patients. *Ann Intern Med* 1993;119:906–907.
25. LeGrand SB, Walsh D. Palliative management of dyspnea in advanced cancer. *Curr Opin Oncol* 1999;11:250–254.
26. Plonk WM, Arnold RM. Terminal care: the last weeks of life. *J Palliat Med* 2005;8:1042–1054.
27. Jennings AL, Davies AN, Higgins JP, et al. Opioids for the palliation of breathlessness in terminal illness. *Cochrane Database Syst Rev* 2001;(4):CD002066, www.cochranc.org.
28. Abernethy AP, Currow DC, Frith P, et al. Randomised double blind placebo controlled trial of sustained release morphine in the management of refractory dyspnea. *BMJ* 2003;327:523–528.
29. Ripamonti C, Fulfaro F, Bruera E. Dyspnoea in patients with advanced cancer: incidence, causes, and treatments. *Cancer Treat Rev* 1998;24:69–80.
30. Chrubasik J, Wust H, Friedrich G, et al. Absorption and bioavailability of nebulized morphine. *Br J Anaesth* 1988;61:228–230.
31. Ripamonti C, Bruera E. Transdermal and inhalatory routes of opioid administration: the potential application in cancer pain. *Palliat Med* 1992;6:98.
32. Davis C. The role of nebulised drugs in palliating respiratory symptoms of malignant disease. *Eur J Palliat Care* 1995;2:9–15.
33. Zeppetella G. Nebulized morphine in the palliation of dyspnea. *Palliat Med* 1997;11:267.
34. Coyne P, Viswanathan R, Smith TJ. Fentanyl by nebulizer reduces dyspnea (Abstract). *Proc Am Soc Clin Oncol* 2001;20:402A.
35. Farncombe M, Chater S. Case studies outlining use of nebulized morphine for patients with end-stage chronic lung and cardiac disease. *J Pain Symptom Manage* 1993;8:221–225.
36. Quelch PC, Faulkner DE, Yun JWS. Nebulized opioids in the treatment of dyspnea. *J Palliat Care* 1997;13:48–52.
37. Farncombe M, Chater S. Clinical application of nebulized opioids for treatment of dyspnea in patients with malignant disease. *Support Care Cancer* 1994;2:184–187.
38. Bruera E, Sala R, Spruyt O, et al. Nebulized versus subcutaneous morphine for patients with cancer dyspnea: a preliminary study. *J Pain Symptom Manage* 2005;29:613–618.
39. Masood AR, Thomas SHL. Systemic absorption of nebulized morphine compared with oral morphine in healthy subjects. *Br J Clin Pharmacol* 1996;41:250–252.
40. Zeppetella G. The palliation of dyspnea in terminal disease. *Am J Hosp Palliat Care* 1998;15:322–330.

41. Booth S, Wade R. Johnson M, et al. For the Expert Working Group of the Scientific Community of the Association of Palliative Medicine. The use of oxygen in the palliation of breathlessness. *Respir Med* 2004;98:66–77

42. Bruera E. *Symptom control in the terminally ill cancer patient. UpToDate*[R] (www.uptodateonline.com), Accessed April 19, 2005.

43. Storey P. Symptom control in advanced cancer. *Semin Oncol* 1994;21:748–753.

44. Craven J, Sutherland A. Buspirone for anxiety disorders in patients with severe lung disease. *Lancet* 1991;338:249.

45. McIver B, Walsh D, Nelson K. The use of chlorpromazine for symptom control in dying cancer patients. *J Pain Symptom Manage* 1994;9:341–345.

46. Walsh D. Dyspnoea in advanced cancer. *Lancet* 1993;324:450–451.

47. Ong KC, Kor AC, Chong WF, et al. Effects of in haled furosemide on exertional dyspnea in chronic obstructive lung disease. *Am J Respir Crit Care Med* 2004;169:1029–1033.

48. Stone P, Kurowska A, Tookman A. Nebulized furosemide for dyspnea. *Palliat Med* 1994;8:256.

49. Shimoyama N, Shimoyama M. Nebulized furosemide as a novel treatment for dyspnea in terminal cancer patients. *J Pain Symptom Manage* 2002;23:73–76.

50. Kohara H, Ueoka H, Aoe K, et al. Effect of nebulized furosemide in terminally ill cancer patients with dyspnea. *J Pain Symptom Manage* 2003;26:962–967.

51. Wilcock A, Corcoran R, Tattersfield AE. Safety and efficacy of nebulised lignocaine in patients with cancer and breathlessness. *Palliat Med* 1994;8:35–38.

52. Bruera E, de Stoutz ND, Velasco-Leiva A, et al. Effects of oxygen on dyspnoea in hypoxaemic terminal cancer patients. *Lancet* 1993;342:13–14.

53. Enck RE. *The medical care of terminally ill patients.* Baltimore, MD: The Johns Hopkins University Press, 1994.

54. Dudgeon DJ, Rosenthal S. Management of dyspnea and cough in patients with cancer. *Hematol Oncol Clin North Am* 1996;10:157–171.

55. Sorenson HM. Managing secretions in dying persons. *Respir Care* 2000;45:1355–1362.

56. Breitbart W, Chochinov HM, Passik S. Psychiatric aspects of palliative care. In: Doyle D, Hanks GWC, MacDonald N, eds. *Oxford textbook of palliative medicine,* 2nd ed. Oxford: Oxford University Press, 1998: 933–954.

57. Breitbart W, Jacobsen PB. Psychiatric symptom management in terminal care. *Clin Geriatr Med* 1996;12:329–347.

58. Roth AJ, Breitbart W. Psychiatric emergencies in terminally ill cancer patients. *Hematol Oncol Clin North Am* 1996;10:235–259.

59. Breitbart W. Psycho-oncology: depression, anxiety, delirium. *Semin Oncol* 1994;21:754–769.

60. Holland JC. Anxiety and cancer: the patient and family. *J Clin Psychiatry* 1989;50:20–25.

61. Hollister LE. Pharmacotherapeutic considerations in anxiety disorders. *J Clin Psychiatry* 1986;47:33–36.

62. Bottomley DM, Hanks GW. Subcutaneous midazolam infusion in palliative care. *J Pain Symptom Manage* 1990;5:259–261.

63. Massie MJ, Holland JC. Depression and the cancer patient. *J Clin Psychiatry* 1990;51:12–17.

64. Beaver WT, Feise G. Comparison of the analgesic effects of morphine, hydroxyzine and their combination in patients with post-operative pain. In: Bonica JJ, Albe Fessard D, eds. *Advances in pain research and therapy.* New York: Raven Press, 1976:553–557.

65. Ingham J, Breitbart W. Epidemiology and clinical features of delirium. In: Portenoy RK, Bruera E, eds. *Topics in palliative care,* Vol. 1. New York: Oxford University Press, 1997:7–19.

66. Massie MJ, Holland JC, Glass E. Delirium in terminally ill cancer patients. *Am J Psychiatry* 1983;140:1048–1050.

67. Breitbart W, Strout D. Delirium in the terminally ill. *Clin Geriatr Med* 2000;16:357–372.

68. Pereira J, Hanson J, Bruera E. The frequency and clinical course of cognitive impairment in patients with terminal cancer. *Cancer* 1997;79:835–842.

69. Back IN, Jenkins K, Blower A, et al. A study comparing hyoscine hydrobromide and glycopyrrolate in the treatment of death rattle. *Palliat Med* 2001;15:329–336.

70. Casarett DJ, Inouye SK. Diagnosis and management of delirium near the end of life. *Ann Intern Med* 2001;135:32–40.

71. American Psychiatric Association. *Diagnostic and statistical manual of mental disorders,* 4th ed. Washington, DC: American Psychiatric Association, 1994.

72. Jackson KC, Lipman AG. Drug therapy for delirium in terminally ill patients. *Cochrane Database Syst Rev* 2004;(2):CD004770; www.cochrane.org.

73. Kehl KA. Treatment of terminal restlessness: a review of evidence. *J Pain Palliat Care Pharmacother* 2004;18:5–30.

74. Breitbart W, Marotta R, Platt NM, et al. A double blind trial of haloperidol, chlorpromazine, and lorazepam in the treatment of delirium in hospitalized AIDS patients. *Am J Psychiatry* 1996;153:231–237.

75. Finucane TE. Delirium at the end of life. *Ann Intern Med* 2002;137:295.

76. Stiefel F, Fainsinger R, Bruera E. Acute confusional states in patients with advanced cancer. *J Pain Symptom Manage* 1992;7:94–98.

77. Fainsinger R, Bruera E. Treatment of delirium in a terminally ill patient. *J Pain Symptom Manage* 1992;7:54–56.

78. Reuben DB, Mor V. Nausea and vomiting in terminal cancer patients. *Arch Intern Med* 1986;146:2021–2023.

79. Davis MP, Walsh D. Treatment of nausea and vomiting in advanced cancer. *Support Care Cancer* 2000;8:444–452.

80. Lichter I. Nausea and vomiting in patients with cancer. *Hematol Oncol Clin North Am* 1996;10:207–220.

81. Baines M. Nausea and vomiting in the patient with advanced cancer. *J Pain Symptom Manage* 1988;3:81–85.

82. Axelrod R. Antiemetic therapy. *Compr Ther* 1997;23:539–545.

83. Rousseau PC. Management of malignant bowel obstruction in advanced cancer: a brief review. *J Palliat Med* 1998;1:65–72.

84. Currow D, Coughlan M, Fardell B, et al. Use of ondansetron in palliative medicine. *J Pain Symptom Manage* 1997;13:302–307.

85. Riley J, Fallon MT. Octreotide in terminal malignant obstruction of the gastrointestinal tract. *Eur J Palliat Care* 1994;1:23–25.

86. Rousseau P. Antiemetic therapy in adults with terminal disease: a brief review. *Am J Hosp Palliat Care* 1995;12:13–18.

87. Saunders C. Pain and impending death. In: Wall PD, Melzack E, eds. *Textbook of pain.* London: Churchill Livingstone, 1989:624–631.

88. Ferris FD. Last hours of living. *Clin Geriatr Med* 2004;20:641–667.

89. Ferris FD, von Gunten CF, Emanuel LL. Competency in end-of-life care: last hours of life. *J Palliat Med* 2003;4:605–613.

90. Trotman IF, Myers KG. Use of ketorolac by continuous subcutaneous infusion for control of cancer-related pain. *Postgrad Med J* 1994;70:359–362.

91. Cherny NI, Portenoy RK. Sedation in the management of refractory symptoms: guidelines for evaluation and treatment. *J Palliat Care* 1994;10:31–38.

92. Rousseau PC. Terminal sedation in the care of dying patients. *Arch Intern Med* 1996;156:1785–1786.

93. Rousseau PC. The ethical validity and clinical experience with palliative sedation. *Mayo Clin Proc* 2000;75:1064–1069.

94. Quill TE, Dresser R, Brock DW. The role of double effect—a critique of its role in end-of-life decision making. *N Engl J Med* 1997;337:1768–1771.

95. *Vacco v Quill,* 117 SCt 2293 1997.

96. *Washington v Glucksberg,* 117 SCt 2258 1997.

97. Rousseau P. Palliative sedation in the management of refractory symptoms. *J Support Oncol* 2004;2:181–186.

98. American Medical Association. *Education for physicians on end-of-life care, module 12.* Chicago: American Medical Association, 1999:M12–1–M12–37.

99. Twaddle M. The process of dying and managing the death event. *Prim Care* 2001;28(2):329–338.

100. Byock I. *Dying well: peace and possibilities at the end of life.* New York: Riverhead Books, 1997.

CHAPTER 58 ■ SPIRITUALITY

CHRISTINA M. PUCHALSKI

Dying is a normal part of life. In today's society, however, dying is still treated as an illness. All too often, people die in hospitals or nursing homes, alone and burdened with unnecessary treatment. In many cases, treatments would be refused if patients were given the chance to talk about their choices with their physicians long before the deathbed scene. Dying people are not always listened to . . . their wishes, their dreams, their fears go unheeded. They want to share those with us.

At the turn of the century, an average American's life expectancy was 50 years (1). Now, 73% of deaths are among people at least 65 years old, and 24% of deaths are among those at least 85 years old. The leading causes of deaths in 1900 were influenza, tuberculosis, diphtheria, heart disease, cancer, and stroke. Today, heart disease is the number one cause of death, followed by cancer and stroke. Modern medicine has granted more people an old age, but it also slows the process of dying. The end of life can last several years.

Because the end of life can last so long, the question arises as to how to live with dying. Some people choose to live fighting their illness to the end, with much of their focus on the fight. Others focus their attention on other aspects of their lives, such as work, family, and hobbies. Still others pursue a mix of these approaches. Each person's way of handling his or her dying is reflective of who that person is, what is important to him or her, and how he/she faces crisis. One needs to remember that there is no set map for living with dying. Each individual patient creates his or her own path and approach.

MEANING AND PURPOSE

Illness and the prospect of dying can call into question the very meaning and purpose of a person's life. Illness can also cause people to suffer deeply. Victor Frankl wrote that man is not destroyed by suffering; he is destroyed by suffering without meaning (2). Writing about concentration camp victims, he noted that survival itself might depend on seeking and finding meaning. Harold Kushner also noted that pain may be the reason, and out of pain and suffering may come the answer (3). In my own clinical experience, I have found that people may cope with their suffering by finding meaning in it. Illness can present people with the opportunity to find new meaning in their lives. Many patients say that out of their despair they were able to realize an entirely new and more fulfilling meaning in their lives. Rabbi Cohen wrote:

> When my mother died, I inherited her needlepoint tapestries. When I was a little boy, I used to sit at her feet as she worked on them. Have you ever seen needlepoint from underneath? All I could see was chaos; strands of thread all over with no seeming purpose. As I grew, I was able to see her work from above. I came to appreciate the patterns, the need for the dark threads as well as the light and gaily colored ones. Life is like that. From our human perspective, we cannot see the whole picture, but we should not despair or feel that there is no purpose. There is meaning and purpose even for the dark threads, but we cannot see that right away. (4)

Spirituality helps people find hope in the midst of despair. As caregivers, we need to engage our patients on that spiritual level. This is where spirituality plays such a critical role—the relationship with a transcendent being or concept can give meaning and purpose to people's lives, to their joys and to their sufferings. Spirituality is concerned with a transcendental or existential way to live one's life at a deeper level, "with the person as human being" (5). All people seek meaning and purpose in life; this search may be intensified when someone is facing death.

There are many different ways people can derive meaning from their lives:

- Work
- Relationships
- Hobbies
- Art, music, dance
- Reflective writing
- Sports
- Relationship with God/sacred/Divine
- Religious, spiritual, philosophical, or existential beliefs
- Religious, spiritual, or cultural rituals

Some of these activities or practices provide an important but perhaps transient meaning (meaning with a small m); others provide a more transcendent and spiritual meaning (meaning with a large M). For example, work may provide an immense amount of meaning to a person. But when that person is ill or dying and unable to work, what then will provide meaning? Therefore there are activities, relationships, and values that are meaningful but do not define the ultimate purpose of one's life. Illness, aging, and dying strip away all those things that were meaningful but that do not ultimately sustain us. When we confront ourselves in the nakedness of our dying, it is then that we have the opportunity to find deep and transcendent meaning—that is, values, beliefs, practices, relationships—expressions that lead one to the awareness of transcendence/God/Divine and to a sense of ultimate value and purpose in life. Everyone's sense of meaning evolves over their life in response to experiences and life in general. People can fluctuate between "meaning" and "Meaning."

Downey defined spirituality as "an awareness that there are levels of reality not immediately apparent and that there is a quest for personal integration in the face of forces of fragmentation and depersonalization" (6). Spirituality is that aspect of human beings that seeks to heal or be whole. Foglio and Brody wrote:

> For many people religion [spirituality] forms a basis of meaning and purpose in life. The profoundly disturbing effects of illness can call into question a person's purpose in life and work; responsibilities to spouse, children, and parents . . . Healing, the restoration of wholeness (as opposed to merely technical healing) requires answers to these questions (7).

Healing, then, is not synonymous with recovery. Indeed, healing may occur at any time, independent of recovery from illness. In dying, for example, restoration of wholeness may be manifested by a transcendent set of meaningful experiences while very ill. It may be reflected by a peaceful death. In chronic illness, healing may be experienced as the acceptance of limitations (5). A person may look to medical care to alleviate his or her suffering, and when the medical system fails to do so, begin to look toward spirituality for meaning, purpose, and understanding. As people are faced with serious illness or the prospect of dying, questions often arise:

- Why did this happen to me?
- What will happen to me after I die?
- Why would God allow me to suffer this way?
- Will I be remembered?
- Will I be missed?

These questions can cause people to undergo a life review whereby they analyze their lives, accomplishments, relationships, and perceived failings (8). This questioning can result in fears, anxieties, and unresolved feelings, which in turn can result in despair and suffering as people face themselves and their eventual mortality. Cassell wrote, "Since in suffering, disruption of the whole person is the dominant theme, we know of the losses and their meaning by what we know of others out of compassion for their suffering" (9). Compassion is essential in the care of all patients, particularly those who are dealing with chronic and serious illnesses and are dying. Two Latin words form the root of the word compassion: "cum," meaning "with," and "passio," meaning "suffering with" (10). What compassionate care asks us to do is to suffer with our patients, that is, to be present to them fully as they suffer and to partner with them in the midst of their pain.

HUMANIZING HEALTH CARE

Medicine has enjoyed tremendous technologic advances that have helped treat illness and prolong lives. These advances have shaped medical care in the Western world. Although this is very positive, it has tended to focus care on the technologic and curative aspects, diminishing the importance of the humanitarian and compassionate aspects of care. As Doka wrote, "Efforts to humanize patient care are essential if the integrity of the human being is not to be obscured by the system" (5).

Dying is a natural occurrence in life. However, the western medical and social culture still treats dying as if it were just a biological occurrence. Dying should be as natural an experience as birth. It should be a meaningful experience for dying persons, a time in which they find meaning in their suffering and have all the dimensions of their experience addressed by their caregiver. These dimensions are the physical, psychological, social, and spiritual (Table 58.1).

Patients encounter all types of suffering—spiritual as well as physical. Cecily Saunders, the founder of St. Christopher's Hospice in London and of the Hospice movement, stated that one of the aims of hospice is that there be relief of "total pain," including the physical, emotional, psychological, social, and spiritual (11). It should be the obligation of all physicians and

TABLE 58.1

THE DIMENSIONS OF THE DYING EXPERIENCE

Physical	Pain and other symptom management
Psychological	Anxiety and depression
Social	Social isolation, economic issues
Spiritual	Purpose and meaning, relationships with the transcendent, search for ultimate meaning, hope, reconciliation, despair

other caregivers to respond to, as well as attempt to relieve, all suffering if possible. Because people may cope with suffering using their spiritual resources, physicians should be able to communicate with their patients about spiritual issues. They should recognize the spiritual as well as physical dimensions of suffering and make resources available for those patients who wish them. Physicians have the responsibility to listen to people as they struggle with their dying. We *need* to be willing to listen to their anxieties, their fears, their unresolved conflicts, their hopes, and their despairs. If people are stuck in despair, they will suffer deeply. It is through their spirituality that people become unstuck from despair.

SPIRITUALITY IN CLINICAL PRACTICE

Medical professionals are recognizing that there are inadequacies in the health care system in terms of care of the dying. The American College of Physicians convened an end-of-life consensus panel, which concluded that physicians should extend their care for those with serious medical illness by attentiveness to psychosocial, existential, or spiritual suffering (12). Other national organizations have also supported the inclusion of spirituality in the clinical setting. The Joint Commission on Accreditation of Healthcare Organizations has a policy that states: pastoral counseling and other spiritual services are often an integral part of the patient's daily life. When requested, the hospital provides, or provides for, pastoral counseling services (13).

The interest in spirituality in medicine among medical educators has been growing exponentially. Medical schools are now teaching courses in end-of-life care and in spirituality and medicine. Only one school had a formal course in spirituality and medicine in 1992. Now, over 100 medical schools are teaching such courses (14). The key elements of these courses have to do with listening to what is important to patients, respecting their spiritual beliefs, and being able to communicate effectively with them about these spiritual beliefs, as well about their preferences at the end of life.

In 1998, the Association of American Medical Colleges (AAMC), responding to concerns by the medical professional community that young doctors lacked these humanitarian skills, undertook a major initiative—The Medical School Objectives Project (MSOP)—to assist medical schools in their efforts to respond to these concerns. The report notes that "Physicians must be compassionate and empathetic in caring for patients. . . they must act with integrity, honesty, respect for patients' privacy and respect for the dignity of patients as persons. In all of their interactions with patients they must seek to understand the meaning of the patients' stories in the context of the patients', and family and cultural values" (15). In recognition of the importance of teaching students how to respect patients' beliefs, AAMC has supported the development of courses in spirituality and medicine.

In 1999, a consensus conference with AAMC was convened to determine learning objectives and methods of teaching courses on spirituality, cultural issues, and end-of-life care. The findings of the conference were published as Report III of the MSOP. This report included a clinically relevant definition of spirituality: spirituality is recognized as a factor that contributes to health in many persons. The concept of spirituality is found in all cultures and societies. It is expressed in an individual's search for ultimate meaning through participation in religion and/or belief in God, family, naturalism, rationalism, humanism, and the arts. All of these factors can influence how patients and health care professionals perceive health and illness and how they interact with one another (16).

Spirituality, that which gives us meaning, can be expressed in many ways. When approaching patients' spiritual issues, it is important to recognize that the definition of spirituality is broad and all-encompassing. It is critical to allow the patient to inform the physician and other care providers what spirituality means to that patient. The outcome goals stated in MSOP III are that students will:

- Be aware that spirituality, as well as cultural beliefs and practices, are important elements of the health and well-being of many patients
- Be aware of the need to incorporate awareness of spirituality, and cultural beliefs and practices, into the care of patients in a variety of clinical contexts
- Recognize that their own spirituality, and cultural beliefs and practices, might affect the ways they relate to, and provide care to, patients
- Be aware of the range of end-of-life care issues and when such issues have or should become a focus for the patient, the patient's family, and members of the health care team involved in the care of the patient
- Be aware of the need to respond not only to the physical needs that occur at the end of life, but also to the emotional, sociocultural, and spiritual needs that occur (16)

DATA DEMONSTRATING PATIENT NEED

The need for attentiveness to the spiritual concerns of dying patients has been well recognized by many researchers (17,18). A survey conducted in 1997 by the George H. Gallup International Institute showed that people overwhelmingly want their spiritual needs addressed when they are close to death. In the preface to the survey report, George H. Gallup, Jr., wrote: "The overarching message that emerges from this study is that the American people want to reclaim and reassert the spiritual dimensions in dying" (19). In the study, survey respondents said they wanted warm relationships with their providers, to be listened to, to have someone to share their fears and concerns with, to have someone with them when they are dying, to be able to pray and have others pray for them, and to have a chance to say goodbye to loved ones. When asked what would worry them, they said not being forgiven by God or others, or having continued emotional and spiritual suffering. When asked about what would bring them comfort, they said they wanted to believe that death is a normal part of the life cycle and that they would live on, either through their relationships, their accomplishments, or their good works. They also wanted to believe that they had done their best in their life and that they will be in the presence of a loving God or higher power. It is as important for health care providers and other caretakers to talk with patients about these issues as it is to address the medical-technical side of care.

In a recent study, most of the people surveyed said that their second highest concern, if they were facing death, was being at peace in general and at peace with God specifically (12).

The 1990 Gallup survey found that 75% of Americans say religion is central to their lives; a majority feels that their spiritual faith can help them recover from illness (20). Additionally, it was found that 63% of patients surveyed believe it is good for doctors to talk to patients about spiritual beliefs. Lehman et al. found that 94% of patients with religious beliefs agreed that physicians should ask them about their spiritual beliefs if they become gravely ill; 45% of patients who denied having any religious beliefs still agreed that physicians should ask their patients about their spiritual beliefs (21). In this survey, 68% of patients said they would welcome a spiritual question in a medical history; only 15% said they actually recalled being asked by their physicians whether spiritual or religious beliefs would influence their decisions. A study surveying more than 200 hospital inpatients found that 77% believed physicians should consider patients' spiritual needs. Furthermore, 37% wanted their physician to discuss spiritual beliefs with them more frequently and 48% wanted their physicians to pray with them (22).

In a more recent study, McCord et al. asked patients in a family practice setting when those patients would welcome spiritual discussions with their clinicians (23). The following responded positively: 94% responded yes if they were seriously ill, with the possibility of dying; 91% said yes if they were suffering from an ongoing serious illness; 87% said yes if suffering from a loss; 83% said yes if admitted to a hospital; and 60% responded positively during a history or initial visit. This has important implications for palliative care as palliative care clinicians work with patients in all these categories (23).

RELATIONSHIP BETWEEN SPIRITUALITY AND COPING

The beneficial effects of spirituality in helping people cope with serious illness and dying are well documented (24). Furthermore, researchers have noted that most patients with cancer in a palliative care setting experience spiritual pain, which is expressed as an internal conflict, a loss or interpersonal conflict, or in relation to God/Divine. Fitchett and others have shown that spiritual struggles are associated with poor physical outcome and higher rates of morbidity (25). Spiritual pain is also related to psychological distress so that patients presenting with depression or anxiety may actually be suffering from spiritual conflict (26).

Quality of life instruments used in end-of-life care try to measure an existential domain, which addresses purpose, meaning in life, and capacity for self-transcendence. In studies of one such instrument, three items have been found to correlate with good quality of life for patients with advanced disease: if the patient's personal existence is meaningful; if the patient finds fulfillment in achieving life goals; and if life to this point has been meaningful (27). This supports the importance of addressing meaning and purpose in a dying person's life. Spirituality and nonorganized religion have also been associated positively with the will to live in patients with HIV (28).

The observations noted in patient stories (5) and in the writings of Foglio and Brody (7)—that illness can cause people to question their lives, their identities, and what gives their life meaning—is supported by research. For example, in a study of 108 women undergoing treatment for gynecologic cancer, 49% noted becoming more spiritual after their diagnosis (29). In a study of parents with a child who had died of cancer, 40% of those parents reported a strengthening of their own spiritual commitment over the course of the year before their child's death (30). Illness, facing one's mortality, is an opportunity for new experience, self-awareness, and meaning in life.

Religion and religious beliefs can play an important role in how patients understand their illness. In a study asking older adults about God's role in health and illness, many respondents saw health and illness as being partly attributable to God and, to some extent, God's interventions (31). Pargament et al. have studied both positive and negative coping, and have found that religious experiences and practices, such as seeking God's help or having a vision of God, extends the individual's coping resources and are associated with improvement in health care outcomes (32). Patients showed less psychological distress if they sought control through a partnership with God or a higher power in a problem-solving way, if they asked God's forgiveness or were able to forgive others, if they reported finding strength and comfort from their spiritual beliefs, and if they found support in a spiritual community. Patients had more depression, poorer quality of life, and callousness toward others if they saw the crisis as a punishment from God, if they had excessive guilt, or if they had an absolute belief in prayer and cure and an inability to resolve their anger if cure did not occur. Pargament et al. have also noted that sometimes patients refuse medical treatment based on religious beliefs (33).

There are a number of studies on meditation, as well as other spiritual and religious practices that demonstrate a positive physical response, especially in relation to levels of stress hormones and modulation of the stress response (34). Although more solid evidence is needed, there appears to be an association between meditation and some spiritual or religious practices and certain physiologic processes, including cardiovascular, neuroendocrine, and immune function.

SPIRITUAL COPING

How does spirituality work to help people cope with their dying (Table 58.2)? One mechanism might be through hope. Hope is a powerful inner strength that helps one transcend the present situation and helps foster a positive belief or outlook. Spirituality and religion offer people hope, and help people find hope in the midst of the despair that often occurs in the course of serious illness and dying. Hope can change during a course of an illness. Early on, the person may hope for a cure; later, when a cure becomes unlikely, the person may hope for time to finish important projects or goals, travel, make peace with loved ones or with God, and have a peaceful death. This can result in a healing, which can be manifested as a restoration of one's relationships or sense of self. Often our society thinks in terms of cures. Whereas cures may not always be possible, healing—the restoration of wholeness—may be possible to the very end of life. Hope has also been shown to be an effective coping mechanism. Patients who are more hopeful tend to less depressed.

Religious beliefs offer a sense of hope. For example, in Catholicism, hope in Jesus' promise of victory over death

through resurrection and salvation gives Catholics hope in a life beyond death. In the funeral rites, it is stated: "I believe in the resurrection of the dead and the life of the world to come" (35). In the Protestant view, the concept of salvation in death gives hope. Jesus' dying and rising from the dead means that those who participate in His death no longer participate in the sinful human nature (36). In Eastern traditions such as Buddhism and Hinduism, the hope of rebirth and a belief in karma offer people hope in the face of mortality (37). In Judaism, there are many diverse ways of viewing death. For some, hope is found in living on through one's children. In the orthodox and conservative views, there is a belief in a resurrection in which the body arises to be united with the soul (38). For patients with and without specific religious beliefs, there is a need to transcend death, which also may be manifested through living on through one's relationships or one's accomplishments and deeds (39). Irion suggests that humans may create abstractions by portraying a life after death (40). For the religious, this may take the form of concepts found in their religious traditions. For others, life after death might be in terms of one's descendants. For some, it might be being immortalized in the memory of others or in the contributions one makes in life. Cultural beliefs and traditions can also contribute to how people find meaning and hope in the midst of despair (41).

Finding meaning in the midst of suffering and uncertainty is critical to effective coping. Spiritual beliefs in general and religious, in particular, can help people find this meaning and purpose. Religion provides a system of beliefs, ritual, and community that can help people find meaning in the context of their illness and dying (42). One very powerful intervention that addresses meaning with patients with advanced cancer has had positive outcomes in these patients. It involved a brief meaning-centered group psychotherapy intervention that is centered on helping patients find meaning in the midst of their suffering (43).

Spirituality can offer people a sense of control. Illness can disrupt life completely. Some people find a sense of control by turning worries or a situation over to a higher power or to God (44). Similarly, people can use their beliefs to help them accept their illness and find strength to deal with their situation (45). Reconciliation may be an important aspect of a dying person's spiritual journey. Often people seek to forgive others or themselves as they review their lives and their relationships.

SPIRITUAL CARE

Framework of Care

An approach to the care of a patient is to recognize that spirituality is an essential part of being human. It is the part of a person that seeks transcendent meaning and purpose in life. It is that part of each individual from which each person can heal by becoming whole again in the midst of suffering, loss, and stress. Therefore, in caring for patients, health care professionals must not only attend to the physical, emotional, and social domains of a patient's life as is supported by the biopsychosocial model of care, but also the spiritual domain, therefore a biopsychosocialspiritual model of care. In a recent Ethics Conference with the George Washington Institute of Spirituality and Health, as well as the AAMC, spiritual care was described as an essential element of health care and not an amenity (46).

During the time a person experiences illness, suffering, loss or stress, he/she will engage actively in the health care system. Health care professionals will often meet people during profoundly difficult times in their patients' lives. During these

---

TABLE 58.2

SPIRITUAL COPING

Hope: for a cure, for healing, for finishing important goals, for a peaceful death
Sense of control
Acceptance of the situation
Strength to deal with the situation
Meaning and purpose: in life, in midst of suffering

times, patients are vulnerable and often afraid, lonely, and confused. Spiritual care offers a framework for health care professionals to connect with their patients, listen to their fears, dreams, and pain, collaborate with their patients as partners in their care, and provide through the therapeutic relationship an opportunity for healing. Healing is distinguished from cure in this context. It refers to the ability of a person to find solace, comfort, connection, meaning and purpose in the midst of suffering, disarray, and pain. The care the clinician provides is rooted in spirituality through compassion, hopefulness, and the recognition that, although a person's life may be limited or no longer socially productive, it remains full of possibility (47).

There are studies that document the importance of the doctor-patient relationship (48). Dr. Francis Peabody wrote in his 1927 medical classic, *The Care of the Patient*, "One of the essential qualities of the clinician is interest in humanity, for the secret care of the patient is in caring for the patient" (49). This relationship can have potential positive impact on health care outcomes, compliance, and patient satisfaction (48). Because healing springs from the therapeutic relationship, spiritual care is grounded in relationship-centered care. Spiritual care begins from the moment the health care professional enters the patient's room.

Practice with Intention

The health care practitioner intentionally opens himself/herself to the possibility of openness, connection, and mystery. *Intention to openness* refers to the willingness to listen to the patient without a preconceived agenda, with full respect of the patient as an individual with a unique story (cultural, personal, spiritual), and a commitment to be fully present in the encounter with the patient. *Intention to connection* refers to the willingness and ability to actively and appropriately form a connection with the patient on a spiritual and emotional level thereby affording the patient the opportunity to experience a sense of belonging, care, and love. By relating from our humanness, we can help to form deeper and more meaningful connections with our patients. *Intention to mystery* refers to the acceptance that none of us controls another, ourselves, life, or outcome. Life is full of mysteries—being open to mystery allows the health care practitioner to let go of a need to be in control and fully responsible for outcome. It implies a humbleness as one accepts that both the health care practitioner and the patient are walking a journey together which may have many unplanned and unexpected turns. This reframes the commitment from fixing or solving to a commitment of presence, persistence, partnership, and a willingness to walk with the unknown and handle situations as they arise together. It removes the illusion of expert and client and offers the reality of spiritually equal partners.

Training Requirements for Spiritual Care

In order to be able to engage in spiritual care, health care professionals need training on how to be intentionally open, willing, and accepting of mystery. This means that the clinician brings his or her whole being to the encounter and places full attention on the patient, not allowing distractions to interfere with that attention. Integral to this is the ability to listen and to be attentive to all dimensions of patients' and their family's lives. Some clinicians suggest that current medical practices do not allow enough time for this. However, being wholly present to the patient is not time dependent. It simply requires the intention on the part of the physician to be fully present for their patients. One becomes fully present when one approaches the patient with deep respect, respect

stemming from a commitment to honoring of the whole person. Mohamad Reaz Abdullah Asian Institute for Development Communication said: "When we say 'I respect you,' what exactly are we saying? We are really respecting a quality that has been expressed by the person, and we are forming a symbiotic relationship with a quality that we admire. However, when the divinity in the individual that is common to all beings is respected, then the meaning of respect is taken on golden wings to a new height." This is the essence of a spiritually based relationship with others.

Spiritual Self-care

Because this work is intense and personal it opens up to the possibility of emotional and spiritual reaction on the part of both patient and health care professional. This requires an awareness of the physician's own values, beliefs, and attitudes, particularly toward the physician's own mortality. By confronting one's own mortality, one can better understand what the patient is facing. Many physicians speak of their own spiritual practices and how those practices help them in their ability to deliver good spiritual care and, in fact, good medical care (5,50). Therefore, in order to practice spiritual care effectively, the health care professional needs to be aware of and supported in their spiritual needs and journey. It is also critical to train and support the health care professional in how to practice relationship-centered care in a way that respects the power differential of the contextual relationship—doctor–patient, nurse–patient, and so on.

Intrinsic and Extrinsic Spiritual Care

All medical care has intrinsic (the behavior, attitudes, and values the health care professionals bring to the encounter) and extrinsic aspects (the knowledge and skills applied in the encounter). The relationship-centered aspect of medical care is the intrinsic essential aspect of all care from which extrinsic care emanates, including physical, emotional, and social care. That is, spiritual intrinsic care refers to the intention of presence; physical extrinsic care refers to taking vital signs, for example, and spiritual extrinsic care refers to the ability to reorganize spiritual issues and problems as they present in relationship to the presenting health care problem or situation. It also refers to recognizing patients' inner resources of strength or a lack of those resources. Once these are recognized, clinicians then incorporate patients' spirituality into the care plan if appropriate to the clinical situation. Everyone on the interdisciplinary health care team practices spiritual care, but the specifics of how the spiritual care is delivered is dependent on the context which it is given. A chaplain provides spiritual care in the context of his/her training as a spiritual counselor in health care setting; clergy provides spiritual care in the context of a religious setting, a nurse, and physician practice spiritual care in the context of caring for patients in a spiritual health care situation (hospital, clinic, patient visits, education). Although the relationship-centered and caring aspects are similar in how each profession deals with the patient, how patient spiritual issues and problems are dealt with depend on the health care professional's level of training and context. Chaplains and clergy work primarily with spiritual issues and spiritual problems in-depth and not necessarily in relation to health and illness. They may be secondarily aware of and interface with social, emotional, and physical issues but deal with them more in a supportive way. Nurses and doctors are trained primarily to address the physical issues with which patients present. However, emotional, social, and spiritual issues may affect or be related to the physical issue. Therefore, nurses and

TABLE 58.3

SPIRITUAL CARE

Compassionate presence
   Intention to openness
   Intention to connection
   Intention to mystery
Relationship-centered care
   Partnership
   Not agenda driven
   Listening to patients' fears, hopes dreams, meaning
Spirituality of health care professional
   Awareness of one's own spirituality
   Awareness of one's own mortality
   Having a spiritual practice
Extrinsic spiritual care
   Taking a spiritual history
   Recognizing patients' spiritual issues
   Recognizing patients' spiritual problems or spiritual pain
   Recognizing patients' resources of inner strength or lack of resources
   Incorporating patients' spirituality into treatment or care plans (presence, referral, rituals, meditation, etc.)

doctors recognize, support and/or triage those spiritual issues appropriately to the spiritual care professionals (Table 58.3).

Taking a Spiritual History and Formulating a Spiritual Care Plan

Obtaining a spiritual history is one way to listen to what is deeply important to the patient (51). When one gets involved in a discussion with a patient about his or her spirituality, one enters the domain of what gives the person meaning and purpose in life and how that person copes with stress, illness, and dying. The spiritual history affords the patient the space and opportunity to address his or her suffering and hopes. A spiritual history validates the importance of a patient's spirituality and gives the patient permission to discuss their spirituality, if they desire to. Having the physician or other clinician inquire about the patient's spiritual beliefs gives the patient an opening and an invitation to discuss spiritual beliefs, if that is what the patient would like to do. It also enables the physician to connect with the patient on a deep, caring level. In fact, many physicians who obtain spiritual histories remark that the nature of the doctor-patient relationship changes. As soon as they bring up these questions, they feel that it establishes a level of intimacy, an understanding of who the person is at a much deeper level than is typical. The relationship feels less superficial (51). Patients note that they feel more trusting of a physician who addresses and respects their spiritual beliefs. In one survey, 65% of patients in a pulmonary outpatient clinic noted that a physician's inquiry about spiritual beliefs would strengthen their trust in the physician (21).

SPIRITUAL ISSUES

Some of the spiritual issues that patients present with in the clinical setting are as follows:

- Lack of meaning and purpose
- Hopelessness
- Despair
- Not being remembered
- Guilt/shame

- Anger at God/others
- Abandonment by God/others
- Feeling out of control
- Existential suffering
- Trust
- Reconciliation
- Grief/loss
- Loneliness
- Lack of love or connection to others or to God
- Fear

Personal and professional caregivers also have similar spiritual issues, as well as spiritual issues that relate to the caregiving role:

- Loss of meaning (no time for activities, relationships)
- Guilt/shame (not being able to be present 100% to patient
- Questions of faith/God
- Anger at God
- Sense of abandonment
- Powerlessness
- Loneliness
- Fear

In addition to identifying and addressing the spiritual issues discussed in the preceding text, it is important to assess the spiritual resources of strength for patients—hope, sense of meaning and purpose, ability to transcend suffering, as well as support from spiritual or religious community, family, or friends.

Communities, such as churches, temples, mosques, spiritual, or other support groups or a group of like-minded friends, can serve as strong support systems for some patients. The absence of these resources could impact in an adverse way how patients cope with illness and/or dying.

Once the clinician finds out about the patient's spiritual beliefs, their issues, and their resources for coping, he or she can then address any spiritual practices that are important to the patient. These might be prayer, meditation, listening to certain music, enjoying solitude, or writing poetry, or journeying. One can then incorporate these practices as appropriate. Possible options for a spiritual care plan, then are as follows:

- Referrals to:
  - A meaning-centered psychotherapy group or to counseling
  - Appropriate spiritual care professionals, such as chaplains, to help with spiritual distress or lack of spiritual resources or resources of strength. Chaplains should be integrated into interdisciplinary health care teams. Hospice teams often have chaplains as part of the care team
  - Spiritual directors
  - Pastoral or other counselors
  - Music thanatologists
  - Art therapy
  - Meditation
  - Yoga, tai chi
  - Specific spiritual support groups
  - Religious or sacred spiritual reading or rituals (based on what the patient has identified as appropriate for them)
- Incorporating spiritual practices or rituals as appropriate
- Presence to patient as he/she works on spiritual issues with the health care professional

Spiritual History

The main elements of a spiritual history, which have been developed for physicians and other health care providers, can be recalled by using the acronym "FICA" (51) (Table 58.4).

TABLE 58.4

FICA

F—Faith and belief
"Do you consider yourself spiritual or religious?" or "Do you have spiritual beliefs that help you cope with stress or difficult times?" If the patient asks what is meant by the word spiritual, reflect back to the patient to define that for themselves. If a patient relates to the question as only religious, suggest that spiritual can be broader than religion and often refers to what gives a deep meaning to a person's life. Also ask what gives deep meaning to the patients' life.
I—Importance
"What importance does your belief system or faith have in your life? Have your beliefs influenced how you take care of yourself in this illness? What role do your beliefs play in coping with your illness or in healing?" Do your beliefs affect your health care decision making?
C—Community
"Are you a part of a spiritual or religious community? Is this of support to you and how? Is there a group of people you really love or who are important to you?"
A—Address/action in care
The physician and other health care providers can think about what needs to be done with the information the patient shared—referral to chaplain, other spiritual care provider, or other resource. This is the part of the history that is used for formulating a treatment plan.

This acronym helps clinicians structure questions that help elicit patients' spiritual beliefs and values. This tool was developed with a focus group of primary care physicians. The goal was to identify the basic information clinicians need to know in order to determine how a patient's spirituality might impact their care. The tool is primarily used as a way to invite the patient to share their spiritual beliefs and values with their clinician, if they would like to. Anecdotal evidence suggests that patients experienced increased trust in their clinician once these conversations are initiated. Patients also express feeling respected and that the clinician is interested in who they are as people. Clinicians also find that the information obtained from the spiritual history allows the clinician to come up with a more comprehensive treatment plan.

The initial question of FICA affords the patient the opportunity to talk about spiritual matters. These spiritual issues can be religious, spiritual, or other sources of deep meaning and purpose in life. In this first question, it is important to assess what the patient's belief system is and also if that belief system or something else gives meaning to the person's life. The second question allows the clinician to determine if these belief systems are important to the patient. For some people, identified spiritual beliefs may not be important to them but there may be other philosophies or activities that give deeper meaning or purpose. This is also the place where patients might reveal if they have any spiritual issues that need attending to. For example, patients might reveal spiritual distress, such as meaninglessness or guilt. It is also important to know if there is anything else about the belief system that might impact health care decision making. This is particularly important with advanced directives: wishes for how a patient would like to be treated and who should be involved in the decision-making process. Many patients would like their clergy or culturally based healers involved. The fourth question has to do with the extrinsic aspect of the patient's belief system—is there a community that the patient identifies as their spiritual or main support community. This could be church, temple, or mosque or could be like-minded friends, family, or other spiritual support group (e.g., a cancer support group could be thought of by some as a spiritual support group). Finally, the "A" (assessment or action) section is not a specific question one has to ask, but rather it is one to be considered in terms of what specific aspects of the treatment plan might be affected. So, if the patient is in spiritual distress, a referral to a chaplain might be appropriate. Or if a patient would like to learn to meditate, then a referral to a teacher or class might be beneficial.

FICA is not meant to be used as a checklist, but rather as a guide as to how to start the spiritual history and what to listen for as the patient talks about his or her beliefs. Mostly, FICA is a tool to help physicians and other health care providers know how to open a conversation to spiritual issues and issues of meaning and value. In the context of the spiritual history, patients may relate those fears, dreams, and hopes to their care provider. The spiritual history can be done in the context of a routine history or at any time in the patient interview, usually as a part of the social history. In addition to religious or spiritual beliefs and values and other aspects of the spiritual history, the social history should address lifestyle, home situation, and primary relationships; other important relationships and social environment; work situation and employment; social interests/avocation; life stresses; and lifestyle risk factors (e.g., tobacco, alcohol, or illicit drugs).

The spiritual history is patient-centered. One should always respect patients' wishes and understand appropriate boundaries. Physicians and other health care providers must respect patients' privacy regarding matters of spirituality and religion and should avoid imposing their own beliefs on the patient (52).

The following case illustrates how FICA can be used. A patient who died of metastatic malignant melanoma was an Episcopalian. Her religious beliefs were central to her life, and in fact, were the means through which she came to be at peace with dying. During her last hospitalization, the house officers caring for her were apprehensive about discussing advance directives and dying. However, during the spiritual history, the patient told them how her religious beliefs helped her come to terms with dying and how she was ready to die naturally. She handed them her living will. She also asked that her church members be allowed to visit her often. She later told me that being asked about her beliefs helped her feel respected and valued by the physicians and that she felt that she could trust them more. The physicians stated that once they asked a spiritual history, the nature of the interaction between themselves and this patient changed. It felt "more natural, more comfortable, warmer, and more honest."

Another case illustrates the variability encountered in practice. When asked "if you have any spiritual beliefs that help you with stress," a patient undergoing a routine examination answered that she found meaning and purpose while sitting in the woods near her house—that nature brought her peace. This was very important to her, as she noted that on days when she did not meditate there in the morning, she would become scattered and tense. Her community consisted of a group of like-minded friends who shared her beliefs. She asked that her medical record indicate that when she became seriously ill or dying, she wanted a room in her hospice overlooking the trees. She also asked to learn basic meditation techniques. In a subsequent visit many months later, she reported that she had stopped meditating, with negative results; resuming meditation helped her cope better with her stress.

ETHICAL ISSUES: ROLE OF SPIRITUALITY IN THE CLINICAL SETTING

It is critical for physicians and other health care providers to address spiritual issues with their patients because spirituality affects patients' clinical care in a direct manner. Spiritual issues can impact clinical care in various ways, which are illustrated by the following cases.

Case 1

Spiritual beliefs may be a dynamic in patients' understanding of their illness. Julie was a 28-year-old woman whose husband left her recently. She learned through the family grapevine that he has acquired immunodeficiency syndrome. She came into a clinic and saw a physician for the first time to get tested for HIV. When she returned to the clinic for her test results, she found out that she was HIV positive. The physician attempted to present an optimistic picture by relaying all the newest information on treatment for HIV. The patient, however, continued to cry out about "God doing this to me." The physician persisted in discussion of the medical and technical aspects of the diagnosis while the patient continued to make references to God. After some time, the physician asked the patient why she thought her illness was coming from God. She told the physician that she was raped as a teenager, got pregnant, and had an abortion. She said, "I have been waiting for the punishment for 15 years, and this is it." The patient refused all medications and treatment.

Patients come to understand their health, illness, and dying through their beliefs, cultural backgrounds, past experience, and values. In this case, Julie had been carrying guilt for an event that happened many years before. The temptation for the physician was to alleviate this guilt by talking about how understandable the abortion was in the context of the rape. However, this is not what the patient felt, and by trying to erase her guilt, it actually precluded the patient from talking about her feelings. The physician instead listened to the patient and did not force the issue of medications and preventive care. The physician continued to see the patient regularly, listening to her issues around the diagnosis. She also referred Julie to a chaplain who worked further with Julie on these issues. It took approximately a year before Julie was able to see God as forgiving and was able to forgive herself. It was then that she could focus on the treatment of her HIV disease. Issues like these can be complicated. What part of Julie's beliefs came from strongly held religious dogma and what part from low self-esteem or depression? Chaplains are trained to understand the difference in the roots of these beliefs, and they are trained to help patients resolve these types of conflicts. In addition, physicians can be helpful by listening to patients, giving patients the time to resolve conflicts, and respecting patients' rights to their own beliefs.

Case 2

Religious convictions/beliefs may affect health care decision making. Frank was an 88-year-old man dying of pancreatic cancer in the intensive care unit. He was on pressors and a ventilator. The team approached the family about withdrawing support. The family was very religious and believed that their father's life was in God's hands; they believed there would be a miracle and that their father would survive.

These types of cases are very common and are often handled poorly. Physicians and intensive care unit teams get frustrated that patients' families cannot see that their loved one is dying, and the family feels hurt and angry that the medical teams do not understand their beliefs. The discussion often gets polarized and difficult to resolve. It is critical that the medical teams, even if they do not agree with the family, respect family beliefs. Often, simply listening to the family about what they mean by a "miracle" can open up the conversation to many feelings that the family is experiencing. For example, the physician could simply say, "I can understand that a miracle would be wonderful," and then wait to see what the family says. Or the physician could ask, "What does a miracle mean to you?" If families feel respected, they are not as likely to feel threatened and that the medical team opposes them. The medical team, in turn, can get to know the values and beliefs of the family. Referral to a chaplain would be critical in this case. The chaplain, someone who is not perceived as being a part of the medical team per se, can explore the issues of miracles in a very nonthreatening way.

In Frank's case, the chaplain worked with the family. Over time, they began to see the possibility of a miracle independent of whether their father was on a ventilator. The family was then at peace with withdrawing ventilator support. The family was invited to bring their minister in during the whole process, and there were prayers and rituals at the bedside. Their father lived for several days and then died at peace.

Case 3

Spirituality may be a patient need. Rebecca was a 60-year-old woman who had a stroke and had had diabetes and hypertension for many years. She was very debilitated, being wheelchair bound with a speech impediment. Her major coping strategy was prayer. She was Catholic. Her church group and family were her major social supports. It was very important for her to discuss her spiritual beliefs with her physician.

Rebecca's faith was central to her life and was the basis of all her decisions. It was the way she coped with the effects of her chronic illnesses and with her dying. It was important for her to talk about her faith at every visit. She had an inner strength that was rooted in her religious beliefs and enabled her to withstand numerous physical and emotional challenges. In the end, it was her faith that probably gave her the will to live beyond what medical statistics would have predicted for someone as ill as she was. Daily prayer was so important to her that it also became an indicator for her well-being. At one point in her illness, she became very depressed. Although she denied symptoms of depression, she related that she was too tired to pray. She was then able to recognize symptoms of depression. Her church group was also a strong support. In fact, they were so present to her that they were clearly part of her extended family.

Case 4

Spirituality may be important in patient coping. Ronda was a 54-year-old woman with advanced ovarian cancer. Her husband, who was her major support, died unexpectedly. Ronda, who was Jewish, dealt with her suffering and depression through her faith in God. She also joined Jewish Healing Services for support and guidance.

Ronda was raised Jewish but was not observant throughout her adult life. She described herself as an optimist and saw that attitude as an inner strength. Her will to live was strong, and her fight to survive her cancer in the face of dismal odds gave her meaning in life. She spoke of her cancer as a gift in that it gave her a new perspective of life. She came to understand her life in a different, deeper way. She expressed a sense of gratitude for being alive each moment of the day and did not take anything, or anyone, for granted. During times of stress and loss, she relied on her inner strength as a resource. She reached out to support networks, such as the Jewish Healing Services. When her cancer metastasized, she looked at her religious roots for an understanding of death and of suffering. It was important for her to talk with her physicians about these issues and for her to be respected. For a physician to dismiss her will to live and try new therapies simply because of a statistical understanding of her disease would be to dismiss who she is as a person, a "statistic of one," as she said. It was important for her to be able to talk with her physician about her will to live and also about her search for meaning in the midst of suffering. She made a "dream list" as to what was important for her to accomplish before her death. Therapy was adjusted around her ability to complete her dream list.

Case 5

Spirituality may be integral to whole patient care. Joe was a 42-year-old man with irritable bowel syndrome. He had major stressors in his life, including a failed marriage and dissatisfaction at work. He had signs of depression, including insomnia, excessive worrying, decreased appetite, and anhedonia. Overall, he felt that he had no meaning and purpose in life.

Joe did not respond to medication and diet changes alone. However, with the addition of meditation and counseling, Joe improved. In this case, the physical, emotional, social, and spiritual issues all interplayed and affected how he coped with illness.

ETHICAL ISSUES: PROFESSIONAL AND PERSONAL BOUNDARIES

Performing a spiritual history has been included in coursework on spirituality and medicine (51). The spiritual history emphasizes the practice of compassion with one's patients, and helps the clinician learn to integrate patients' spiritual concerns into the therapeutic plans. Given the data suggesting that spirituality may be beneficial for patients who are coping with illness, health care institutions should have written policies stating that the patient has a right to express his or her spirituality and religiosity in a respectful and supportive clinical environment.

Physicians should strive to discuss patients' spiritual concerns in a respectful manner and as directed by the patient. The spiritual history is patient-centered, not physician-centered (Table 58.5). A physician should always respect patients' privacy regarding matters of spirituality and religion, and must be vigilant in avoiding imposing his or her beliefs on the patients. The relationship between physician and patient is not an equal one. There is an intimacy in the relationship, but it is intimacy with formality. The patient comes to the physician in a vulnerable time of his or her life, often looking to the physician as a person of authority. The physician should not abuse

TABLE 58.5

ETHICAL AND PROFESSIONAL BOUNDARIES

Spiritual history: patient-centered
Recognition of pastoral care professionals as experts
Proselytizing is not acceptable in professional settings
More in-depth spiritual counseling should be under the
  direction of chaplains and other spiritual leaders
Praying with patients:
  Not initiated by physicians unless there is no pastoral care
    available and the patient requests it
  Physician can stand in silence as patient prays in his/her
    tradition
  Referral to pastoral care for chaplain-led prayer

that authority by imposing his or her own beliefs, or lack of beliefs, onto patients. A vulnerable patient may adopt a physician's belief simply because the patient is fearful and assumes the physician knows more. In terms of spiritual intervention, physicians can recommend a variety of interventions, such as chaplain referral, meditation, yoga, prayer, or other spiritual practice. But the decision to recommend these comes from the patient. For example, physicians could recommend religious and spiritual practices to a patient if these practices are already part of that patient's belief system. However, an agnostic patient should not be told to engage in worship any more than a highly religious patient should be criticized for frequent church attendance. Therefore, if a patient states that prayer helps with stress, the physician could suggest that prayer might help in dealing with a serious diagnosis. Or, if a patient finds meaning and purpose in nature, a physician might suggest meditation techniques focused on nature.

Patients sometimes ask their physician about the physician's beliefs. Given the unequal relationship between patient and physician, it is important that the question be handled carefully and with the same guidelines that are used when addressing other sensitive issues such as sexual history or domestic violence. Patients sometimes ask personal questions of their physicians to take the attention off themselves. Sometimes, it is to see if they can connect with the physician by reassuring themselves that the physician has the same beliefs as they. In general, if asked about his or her own beliefs, the physician could ask the patient why it is important for him or her to know that information. The physician can reassure the patient that the focus of the encounter is on the patient's needs and issues, not the doctor's. In some cases, patients still feel the need to know. A patient of a certain religious belief may want to work only with a doctor of that same religion. In some cases, it may not be possible to accommodate the patient, but at least the physician can explore with the patient the reasons for the request. Some patients want to know that their beliefs will not be ridiculed. A response from the physician that he or she respects and supports a patient's beliefs might serve to reassure the patient. In general, it is best to avoid sharing one's personal beliefs unless one already knows the patient and is comfortable that this sharing would not coerce the patient into adopting the physician's beliefs or intimidate the patient from sharing more about his or her own beliefs. A physician should not do anything that violates his or her own comfort level as well. Many physicians prefer to keep their private lives private in the professional context of the doctor-patient relationship.

Patients often ask physicians to pray with them. A physician need not worry that it is somehow inappropriate to allow a moment of silence or a prayer if the patient requests this. In fact, walking away and not showing respect for the request may leave the patient with a sense of abandonment by the physician. If the physician feels conflicted about praying with patients, he or she need only stand by quietly as the patient prays in his or her own tradition. Alternatively, the physician could suggest calling in the chaplain or the patient's clergyperson to lead a prayer. Physician-led prayer is generally not recommended, as that is usually the role of the clergy or chaplain. In addition, having the physician lead a prayer opens the possibility of having the prayer be of the physician's belief, not of the patient's. Furthermore, clergy and chaplains are trained specifically in techniques of leading prayer in ecumenical and health care contexts.

Appropriate referrals to chaplains are important to good health care practice and are as appropriate as referrals to other specialists. Chaplains are clergy or laypersons certified in a pastoral training program designed to train them as chaplains. Chaplains work in hospital settings, outpatient clinics, businesses, schools, and prisons. They are trained to be spiritual care providers working with people to explore meaning in life, cope with suffering, and use their beliefs to help them cope with illness or stress. Chaplains work with people of all faiths, as well as with nonreligious people. Clergy are trained to provide religious care usually only to people of their specific denomination.

Where are the boundaries between what chaplains do and what physicians do? Some would argue that discussions with patients about spiritual matters should be initiated solely by chaplains (53). Physicians can use spiritual histories as a screening tool. By inquiring about a patient's beliefs, the physician can evaluate whether the beliefs are helpful or harmful to the patient's health and medical care. If a patient has beliefs that support him or her and give meaning and peace of mind, the physician can encourage those beliefs. In cases in which spiritual beliefs interfere with a patient's getting needed therapy—for example, a patient who thinks an illness is a punishment caused by God and therefore refuses medicine or treatment because of a feeling that the punishment is deserved—a referral to a chaplain would be very helpful. Patients have the right to refuse medical treatment. However, it is important that the choice be made with full informed consent. Therefore, if a patient refuses treatment based on a religious or spiritual belief, it may be appropriate to refer the patient to a chaplain so that the chaplain can explore these beliefs with the patient.

Sometimes, refusal of treatment is based on accepted religious tenets. Other times, the patient may attribute the reasons for refusal to religious beliefs when it actually stems from other concerns, such as lack of self-esteem or depression. The chaplain is trained to explore the beliefs with the patient further and help the patient differentiate between the two. The physician should be respectful of the patient's beliefs, but still explain the consequences of refusal of treatment without being coercive. This way the patient can have enough medical and spiritual information to make a fully informed decision. Physicians in general are not trained to explore the theological aspects of belief, although they can listen and learn about belief from patients. However, physicians can listen to and support patients as they make decisions for themselves. Sometimes, simply listening to a patient in a nonjudgmental fashion and asking a few open-ended questions, such as "tell me more about your belief," can help patients resolve issues of belief and treatment for themselves.

Although many studies suggest that spirituality can be helpful, there are also circumstances in which spirituality can have a negative effect on health. It is important for health care providers to recognize this dynamic. For example, a person who interprets his or her illness as a punishment from God might attempt to refuse treatment. In such a scenario, a chaplain or other religious advisor could perhaps work with the patient's beliefs to help him or her work through the guilt

issues. The patient might accept treatment or refuse it, but at least the decision wouldn't be motivated solely by guilt, and would be more of an informed decision. Some people who feel guilt in their relationships with God might also relate to others in their lives in a similar way. Counseling may also be helpful. Some religious beliefs forbid certain medical practices, such as Jehovah's Witnesses' refusal to accept blood transfusions. It is important to recognize the difference between refusing treatment based on an established religious principle versus refusal of treatment stemming from depression, unwarranted guilt, or a misperceived sense of punishment from God. Some patients may have complicated ethical and spiritual issues. Physicians need not feel that they must solve these dilemmas on their own. Chaplains, members of ethics committees, and counselors often work with physicians in the care of patients.

It is important to recognize that spirituality in the health care setting is not in any one person's domain. Physicians, nurses, social workers, and chaplains all can deal with patient spirituality. It also is true, however, that most physicians are not trained to deal with complex spiritual crises and conflicts. Chaplains and other spiritual caregivers are. Therefore, it is important that physicians obtain a spiritual history as a way of inquiry about spiritual issues that might impact a patient but that physicians also recognize when to make a referral to these specialists.

NEUROTHEOLOGY

Patients may talk about spiritual or mystical experiences, which might manifest as visions, feeling God's or a deceased loved one's presence, altered states of consciousness, locutions, or sensory experiences (unusual smells, sights, or sounds). From the clinical standpoint, there is a debate as to the difference between spiritual experience and psychopathology. Many patients close to death talk of seeing loved ones or angels in the room. Some physicians medicate patients if these experiences cause distress or agitation. This assumes that spiritual experiences are comforting versus psychopathologic ones, which may cause agitation. Theologians would argue that, in fact, not all spiritual experiences are comforting, and that medicating people in the midst of a spiritual experience might be in conflict with patients' beliefs and religious traditions.

There are no clear-cut answers to this dilemma. But there is a new area of research and study called *neurotheology*, the study of the neurobiology of religion and spirituality. By using brain-imaging studies, scientists are attempting to identify the brain's spirituality circuit. Results indicate that certain spiritual experiences, such as deep meditation or intense religious moments in prayer, can be associated with distinct neural activity in the brain. However, this does not mean that such experiences are mere neurologic illusions, nor do these studies establish cause and effect. Andrew Newberg, a physician who does this research at the University of Pennsylvania, notes that "there is no way to determine whether the neurologic changes associated with spiritual experience mean that the brain is causing those experiences or is instead perceiving a spiritual reality" (54).

Theologians suggest that neurotheologians identify religion with specific experiences and feelings. Spiritual or mystical experiences may be part of a person's life, but those experiences have nothing to do with how well people communicate with God nor with the spiritual practices inherent in religions, such as prayer or virtue. Neurotheologians suggest that we may be "wired for God" (55) or that evolution has programmed the brain to find pleasure in transcending the self. But most mystics and spiritual leaders write not so much of pleasure from spiritual practice as of the perseverance of a spiritual practice, which at times can be difficult and seemingly empty. Most mystics, such as Teresa of Avila, have seen spiritual practices as leading them beyond themselves to the practice of charity and love of neighbors (56). Teresa of Avila and other mystics regarded spiritual or mystical experiences as special gifts of God but not essential to spiritual growth. Furthermore, spiritual experiences do not indicate the level of charity or love present in the heart of the person—only external acts of charity do.

Neurobiologists can correlate certain experience with certain brain activity, but it would be reductionistic to conclude that the brain is the only source of the experience. For example, science cannot measure the influence of spiritual grace. Therefore, in the clinical setting, it is important to recognize the limits of science and to relinquish the need for reductionistic explanatory models for spiritual beliefs and experiences. Much of what happens to our patients may have no answers. Illness causes us to ask questions that are deeply spiritual and unanswerable scientifically: who am I? Why am I suffering? What is the meaning of my illness and suffering? Illness, in and of itself, is a spiritual journey, which may include emptiness, joy, despair, hope, and mystical experiences. As physicians and caregivers, our job is to support our patients as they go through this journey.

Although it is critical to respect professional boundaries and not try to do the chaplain's job, there is a spectrum along which most physicians can operate. Some physicians elect to pursue issues of religion or spirituality with a patient in greater depth than would others. Consider as an analogy the treatment of depression by an internist. Some internists treat simple cases of depression, referring only the more complex ones to psychiatrists. Others refer a patient to a psychiatrist immediately on diagnosis of depression. Each physician must be honest in recognizing his or her own professional and personal limitations. Ultimately, the goal is to do what is best for the patient. If early referral to a chaplain or other support person is in the best interest of the patient, then that is the appropriate course of action.

CARING FOR OUR PATIENTS

Beyond the data, writings, and courses are personal stories from physicians and their patients. In the experience of many physicians who care for patients with chronic and terminal illnesses, there is a feeling of being privileged and honored to care for people who are facing death. Their strength and courage in the midst of suffering is inspiring. Our patients are greater teachers to us and to our students on the meaning of life than any philosophical text. The stories they share are ones of personal transcendence, courage, and dignity. Our patients continually live with dying and, in the midst of that, are often able to face their losses, their fears, and their pain, and transcend to a place where they see their lives as rich and fulfilling. They reprioritize and thereby are able to find a place of deep meaning and purpose in their lives. It is often humbling for us to recognize that what we now place importance on in life, may have little or no importance in the end when facing our own mortality. Annoyance at rush hour traffic when late or our emphasis on academic success pale in comparison to our patients' descriptions of a glowing sunrise or the deep love they feel for another. We would encourage all students reading this text to look on your patients as teachers and to approach dying patients not with trepidation and fear but with openness to all the joy and wisdom you can experience with them.

We should have systems of care that allow for people to die in peace, to die the way they want to, and to be able to engage in those activities that bring peace to them: prayer, meditation, listening to music, art, journaling, sacred ritual, and relationships with others. Our systems of care should be interdisciplinary, with physicians, nurses, social workers, chaplains, and other spiritual care providers all working together to provide spiritual and holistic care for our patients. It is then that health care systems will become caring communities rather than impersonal, technologically driven ones.

Our culture and our profession as a whole must look at dying very differently from the way it currently does. We need to see dying not as a medical problem but as a natural part of life that can be meaningful and peaceful. We can broaden and perhaps even enhance our lives now by knowing that one day we will die. By thinking about our mortality early in life, we will not be caught off guard and pressured by the dilemmas of choices at the end of life. We will have had a chance to think about some of those choices sooner and to come to peace with our mortality. This is where religious organizations can be particularly helpful. They can facilitate our discussions of dying and what that means to us. They can educate their members about the importance of preparing themselves for the choices, both spiritual and medical, that need to be made near the end of life. We, the interdisciplinary care team, can jointly assist the dying person come to peace in life's last moments.

All of us, whether actively dying or helping care for the dying, have one thing in common: we all will die. The personal transformation that is often seen in patients as they face death can occur in all of our lives. By facing our inevitable dying, we can ask ourselves the same questions that dying patients face—what gives meaning and purpose to our lives, who are we at our deepest core, and what are the important things we want to do in our lives. By attending to the spiritual dimensions of our personal and professional lives, however, we express that, we can better provide care to our patients (57).

Wayne Muller has written:

There are times in all of our lives when we are forced to reach deep into ourselves to feel the truth of our real nature. For each of us there comes a moment when we can no longer live our lives by accident. Life throws us into questions that some of us refuse to ask until we are confronted by death or some tragedy in our lives. What do I know to be most deeply true? What do I love, and have I loved well? Who do I believe myself to be and what have I placed on the center of the altar of my life? Where do I belong? What will people find in the ashes of my incarnation when it is over? How shall I live my life knowing that I will die? And what is my gift to the family of earth (58)?

Of all life's difficult yet important experiences, dying may be the most difficult one we will ever have. The moment of death, and the dying that precedes it, brings to a close the journey that each one of us has been on. We are the privileged persons who attend people while they are dying, be they our patients or our loved ones and friends. We are the persons who can bring hope and comfort to dying patients as they complete their lives. We need to ensure that our society and our systems of care preserve and enhance the dignity of all people, especially when they are made vulnerable by illness and suffering. We need to listen to the dying and to all our patients, and be with them, for them. The process of dying can be a meaningful one, one that we can all embrace and celebrate rather than fear and dread.

References

1. Field MJ, Cassel CK, eds. Committee on Care at the End of Life, Division of Health Care Services, Institute of Medicine. *Approaching death: improving care at the end of life.* Washington, DC: National Academy Press, 1997.
2. Frankl V. *Man's search for meaning.* New York: Simon & Schuster, 1984.
3. Kushner HS. *When bad things happen to good people.* New York: Schocken Books, 1981.
4. Cohen KL. In: Lynn J, Harrold J, eds. *Handbook for mortals.* New York: Oxford University Press, 1999:31.
5. Doka KJ, Morgan JD, eds. *Death and spirituality.* Amityville, NY: Baywood Publishing Company, 1993.

6. Downey M. *Understanding Christian spirituality*. New York: Paulist Press, 1997.
7. Foglio JP, Brody H. Religion, faith and family medicine. *J Fam Pract* 1988; 27:473–474.
8. Kubler-Ross E. *On death and dying*. New York: Collier Books/Macmillan Publishing Co., 1997.
9. Cassell EJ. *The nature of suffering and goals of medicine*. New York: Oxford University Press, 1991.
10. *Webster's 7th new collegiate dictionary*. Springfield, MA: Meriam-Webster, 1965.
11. Wald FS. The emergence of hospice care in the United States. In: Spiro HM, McCrea-Curnen MG, Wandel LP, eds. *Facing death*. New Haven, CT: Yale University Press, 1996.
12. Lo B, Quill T, Tulsky J. Discussing palliative care with patients. ACP-ASIM end-of-life care consensus panel. *Ann Intern Med* 1999;130:744–749; See also: Karlawish J, Quill T, Meier D. A consensus-based approach to providing palliative care to patients who lack decision-making capacity. ACP-ASIM end-of-life care consensus panel. *Ann Intern Med* 1999;130: 835–840.
13. Joint Commission on Accreditation of Healthcare Organizations (JCAHO). *Implementation section of the 1996 standards for hospitals by JCAHO*. Oakbrook Terrace, IL: Joint Commission on Accreditation of Healthcare Organizations, 1996.
14. Puchalski CM, Larson DB. Developing curricula in spirituality and medicine. *Acad Med* 1998;73(9):970.
15. Association of American Medical Colleges. *Learning objectives for medical student education: guidelines for medical schools. Medical School Objectives Project (MSOP)*. Washington, DC: American Association of Medical Colleges, 1998.
16. Association of American Medical Colleges. *Report III—Contemporary issues in medicine: communication in medicine. Medical School Objectives Project (MSOP III)*. Washington, DC: Association of American Medical Colleges, 1999:25.
17. Conrad NL. Spiritual support for the dying. *Nurs Clin North Am* 1985;20:415–426.
18. Moberg DO. Spiritual well-being of the dying. In: Lesnoff-Caravaglia G, ed. *Aging and the human condition*. New York: Human Sciences Press, 1982:139–155.
19. The George H. Gallup International Institute. *Spiritual beliefs and the dying process: a report on a national survey*. Conducted for the Nathan Cummings Foundation and the Fetzer Institute, 1997. Available at http://www.ncf.org/reports/program/reports_health.html.
20. Corbett JM. *Religion in America*. Englewood Cliffs, NJ: Prentice Hall, 1990.
21. Ehman JW, Ott BB, Short TH, et al. Do patients want physicians to inquire about their spiritual or religious beliefs if they become gravely ill? *Arch Intern Med* 1999;159:1803–1806.
22. King DE, Bushwick B. Beliefs and attitudes of hospital inpatients about faith, healing, and prayer. *J Fam Pract* 1994;39:349–352.
23. McCord G, Gilchrist VJ, Grossman SD, et al. Discussing spirituality with patients: a rational and ethical approach. *Ann Fam Med* 2004;2(4): 356–361.
24. Cohen SR, Boston P, Mount BM, et al. Changes in quality of life following admission to palliative care units. *Palliat Med* 2001;15(5):363–371.
25. Fitchett G, Rybarczyk BD, DeMarco GA, et al. The role of religion in medical rehabilitation outcomes: a longitudinal study. *Rehabil Psychol* 1999;44(4):333–353.
26. Fitchett G, Murphy PE, Kim J, et al. Religious struggle: prevalence correlates and mental health risks in diabetic, congestive heart failure, and oncology patients. *Int J Psychiatry Med* 2004;34(2):179–196.
27. Cohen SR, Mount BM, Strobel MG, et al. The McGill quality of life questionnaire: a measure of quality of life appropriate for people with advanced disease. A preliminary study of validity and acceptability. *Palliat Med* 1995;9:207–219.
28. Tsevat J, Puchalski CM, et al. *Spirituality and religion in patients with HIV/AIDS*, in preparation 2005.
29. Roberts JA, Brown D, Elkins T, et al. Factors influencing views of patients with gynecologic cancer about end-of-life decisions. *Am J Obstet Gynecol* 1997;176(1):166–172.
30. Cook JA, Wimberly DW. If I should die before I wake: religious commitment and adjustment to death of a child. *J Sci Study Relig* 1983;22:222–238.
31. Bearon LB, Koenig RG. Religious cognitions and use of prayer in health and illness. *Gerontologist* 1990;30:249–253.
32. Pargament KI, David SE, Kathryn F, et al. God help me: I, religious coping efforts as predictors of the outcomes to significant negative life events. *Am J Community Psychol* 1990;18:793–824.
33. Pargament KI, Smith BW, Koenig HG, et al. Patterns of positive and negative religious coping with major life stresses. *J Sci Study Relig* 1998;37(4):710–724.
34. Seeman TE, Aubin LF, Seema M. Religiosity/spirituality and health: a critical review of the evidence for biological pathways. *Am Psychol* 2003;58(1):53–63.
35. Rutherford R. *The death of a Christian: the rite of funerals*. New York: Pueblo, 1980.
36. Klass D. Spirituality, Protestantism and death. In: Doka KJ, Morgan JD, eds. *Death and spirituality*. Amityville, NY: Baywood Publishing Company, 1993:61.
37. Ryan D. Death: eastern perspectives. In: Doka KJ, Morgan JD, eds. *Death and spirituality*. Amityville, NY: Baywood Publishing Company, 1993:81.
38. Grollman EA. Death in Jewish thought. In: Doka KJ, Morgan JD, eds. *Death and spirituality*. Amityville, NY: Baywood Publishing Company, 1993:25–27.
39. VandeCreek L, Land Nye C. Trying to live forever: correlates to the belief in life after death. *J Pastoral Care* 1994;48(3): 273–280.
40. Irion PE. Spiritual issues in death and dying for those who do not have conventional religious beliefs. In: Doka KJ, Morgan JD, eds. *Death and spirituality*. Amityville, NY: Baywood Publishing Company, 1993.
41. Meagher D, Bell CP. Perspectives on death in the African American community. In: Doka KJ, Morgan JD, eds. *Death and spirituality*. Amityville, NY: Baywood Publishing Company, 1993:113–130.
42. Puchalski CM, O'Donnell E. *Religious and spiritual beliefs in end-of-life care: how major religions view death and dying. Techniques in Regional Anesthesia and Pain Management*, 2005;9(3):114–121.
43. Breithart W. Spirituality and meaning in supportive care. Spirituality and meaning-centered group psychotherapy interventions in advanced cancer. *Supportive Care Center* 2002;10:272–280.
44. *44 Questions: Questions and answers about Alcoholics Anonymous*. AA World Services, Inc., 1952.
45. Strachan JG. *Alcoholism, treatable illness: an honorable approach to man's alcoholism problem*. Center City, MN: Hazelden, 1982.
46. Puchalski CM, Anderson BM, Lo B, et al. *Ethical guidelines for spiritual care*. AAMC Report, in press, 2006.
47. O'Connor P. The role of spiritual care in hospice. Are we meeting patients' needs? *Am J Hosp Care* 1988;5:31–37.
48. DiBlasi Z, Harkness E, Ernst E, et al. Influence of context effects on health outcomes: a systematic review. *Lancet* 2001;357(9258):757–762.
49. Peabody FW. *The care of the patient*. Cambridge, MA: Harvard University Press, 1927.
50. Sulmasy DP. *The healer's calling: a spirituality for physicians and other health care professionals*. New York: Paulist Press, 1997.
51. Puchalski CM, Romer AL. Taking a spiritual history allows clinicians to understand patients more fully. *J Palliat Med* 2000;3:129–137; See also: Puchalski CM. Spiritual assessment tool. *J Palliat Med* 2000;3(1):131.
52. Post SG, Puchalski CM, Larson DB. Physicians and patient spiritual- ity: professional boundaries, competency, and ethics. *Ann Intern Med* 2000;132(7):578–583.
53. Sloan RP, Bagiella E, VandeCreek L, et al. Should physicians prescribe religious activities? *N Engl J Med* 2000;342(25):1913–1916.
54. Begley S, Underwood A. God and the brain: how we're wired for spirituality. *Newsweek* 2001;69:50–57.
55. Benson H. *Timeless healing: the power and biology of belief*. New York: Simon & Schuster, 1996.
56. St. Teresa of Avila. *Interior castle*. Washington, DC: ICS Publications, 1997.
57. Newman LF, Epstein L. Doctor-patient relationships: know thy patient, know thyself. *Med Health R I* 1996;79(8):308–310.
58. Muller W. *Touching the divine: teachings, meditations and contemplations to awaken your true nature [Audiocassettes]*. Louisville, CO: Sounds True, Inc., 1994.

CHAPTER 59 ■ BEREAVEMENT CARE

AREEJ RAED EL-JAWAHRI AND HOLLY G. PRIGERSON

BEREAVEMENT

Bereavement refers to the situation of losing to death a person to whom one is attached. Grief refers to the emotional response to that loss. Bereavement and grief are universal experiences that almost all adults must confront at some point in their lifetime. Nearly 2.5 million US citizens died in 2003 each leaving behind many to grieve their loss (1). Approximately 9.7% of women and 2.5% of men in the United States are widows and widowers, respectively (2). Most of those experiencing widowhood are older than 64, when their health is likely to be already compromised, and bereavement may compound their health difficulties.

Bereavement has been considered as one of the most stressful events experienced in one's life (3,4). It has been associated with an increased risk of cardiac events, hypertension, cancer, and suicidal ideation (5–10). It has also been associated with reduced quality of life, disability, functional impairments (social, family, and occupational), adverse health behaviors such as alcohol and cigarette consumption, hospitalizations, and increased risk for morbidity and mortality (11–15). Bereavement is a well-established risk factor for elevated depressive symptomatology and an increased likelihood of major depressive episodes (16–20), and anxiety-related symptoms and disorders (21–23). In light of these health risks, clinicians need to strive to minimize the potential negative health consequences of bereavement. Additionally, bereavement care should be the final phase of any comprehensive palliative care plan. One must look at the family as the unit of care when providing palliative services and hence bereavement care becomes an essential aspect to complete and facilitate the family's healing process.

NORMAL, UNCOMPLICATED, GRIEF

Normal, or uncomplicated, grief reactions are those that, though painful, move the survivor toward an acceptance of the loss and an ability to carry on with his or her life. Approximately, 80–90% of bereaved individuals experience normal or uncomplicated grief (24). It is important to recognize that most people are able to adjust to the loss over time in a fairly satisfactory way.

One of the main myths concerning uncomplicated grief is that it follows a direct stage-by-stage pathway from denial to anger, separation distress, depression, and finally recovery (25). In fact, data suggest that there are no clear stages of grief resolution. In contrast to the hypothesized grief resolution graph [Figure 59.1 (25)], the data reveal a gradual reduction in distress over time from loss. Contrary to the stage theory of the course of grief, disbelief was not found to be the most frequently endorsed initial reaction to loss. The predominant symptom throughout the first 6 months post-loss was yearning. Depressed mood did not peak after disbelief, yearning and anger had subsided; rather, disbelief, yearning, and depressed mood all declined significantly from 2 to 20 months post-loss. As shown in Figure 59.1, levels of anger remained stably low and did not peak after disbelief had faded. Additionally, acceptance of death increased significantly over time and revealed a pattern inverse to disbelief and yearning. Figure 59.1 suggests a parallel shift downward in all the grief indicators over time from loss. These data are inconsistent with the phases of grief resolution model.

While uncomplicated grief can be an extremely painful and sad experience, by 6 months the bereaved individuals develop some sense of acceptance and are capable of finding some meaning or purpose in their lives. They see the future holding potential enjoyment for them and are capable of engaging in productive activities. They are also able to maintain connections with others and their sense of competence and self-esteem are not markedly changed by their loss. They are capable of functioning without substantial impairment (24). Survivors may initially exhibit many symptoms of complicated grief, but by 6 months post-loss there is usually improvement in their ability to focus on other things and move beyond the loss. Those who have elevated levels of a specific set of symptoms [Table 59.1 (24)] for more than 6 months after the death may cause concern.

DIAGNOSTIC CRITERIA FOR COMPLICATED GRIEF: EVIDENCE OF DISTINCTIVE SYMPTOMS, COURSE, AND OUTCOMES

Studies have found that complicated grief symptoms form a coherent cluster of symptoms distinct from bereavement-related depressive and anxiety symptom clusters (7,8,10,12, 26). Bereaved individuals with complicated grief, experience disruptive and distressing yearning, pining, and longing for the deceased that endures for longer than 6 months. They also report extreme difficulty "moving on" with their life (feeling "stuck" in their grief) as well as feelings of numbness and detachment, bitterness, and a lack of meaning in life without the deceased. They have trouble accepting the death and see no potential for future happiness. Bereaved individuals experiencing complicated grief report having these symptoms

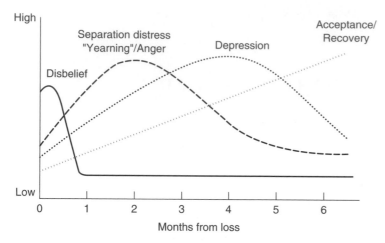

Hypothesized grief resolution [1-5]

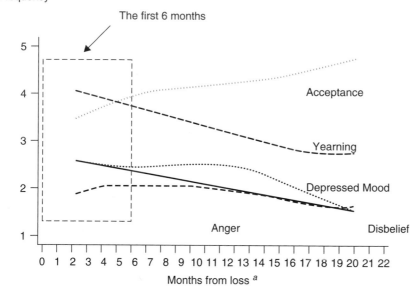

Unadjusted mean grief resolution scores over time

a: All of the lines start from 2 months after loss and end at 20 months
b: 1 = Less than once a month; 2 = Monthly; 3 = Weekly; 4 = Daily;
   5 = Several times a day except for indicator of "depressed mood"

FIGURE 59.1. Hypothesized resolution of grief model and observed changes in grief symptomatology over time from loss. From: Zhang B, Maciejewski PK, Vanderwerker LC, et al. A Preliminary Empirical Examination of the State Theory of Grief Resolution (25).

several times a day and find these symptoms impair their ability to function normally (7,12,27–37) [Table 59.1 (24)].

It is important to note that this conceptualization of complicated grief specifies that these particular distress symptoms persist for at least 6 months, regardless of when those 6 months occur. Hence, delayed and chronic subtypes of grief may both come under the complicated grief diagnosis as long as, whatever the delay in onset, symptoms continue for 6 months. Typically, however, the overwhelming feelings of those who are diagnosed with complicated grief are not delayed; it is much more often the case that their grief has been intense and unrelenting since the death (24).

Recent research demonstrates that bereaved individuals with high levels of complicated grief symptoms have substantially greater dysfunction than those with lower levels of these symptoms. Complicated grief symptoms may endure for several years and predict substantial morbidity and adverse health behaviors beyond depressive symptoms (5–15). Complicated grief has been shown to be a substantial risk for suicidal thoughts and behaviors, with incidence of cardiac events, high blood pressure, and even cancer, in studies that took into account the effect of major depression and generalized anxiety disorder (5–10,24). It is a risk factor for quality of life impairments such as poor social interactions and role functioning, loss of energy, and self perception of illness, disability and functional impairments, loss of work days, and adverse health behaviors such as changes in patterns of consumption of alcohol, food, and tobacco (5–10,24). It has also been shown that complicated grief increases the risk for ulcerative colitis (11). Table 59.2 provides a summary of the several negative health consequences associated with complicated grief.

TABLE 59.1

CRITERIA FOR DIAGNOSING COMPLICATED GRIEF

Criterion A: chronic and persistent yearning, pining, longing for the deceased
Yearning and longing—"Do you feel yourself yearning and longing for the person who is gone?"
Criteria B: the person must have four of the following eight remaining symptoms at least several times a day or to a degree intense enough to be distressing and disruptive:

1. **Trouble accepting the death**—"Do you have trouble accepting the loss of ____?"
2. **Inability to trust others**—"To what extent has it been hard for you to trust others because of the loss of ____?
3. **Excessive bitterness or anger related to the death**—"Do you feel angry about the loss of ____?"
4. **Uneasy about moving on**—"Sometimes people who lose a loved one feel uneasy about moving on with their life. To what extent do you feel that moving on (for example, making new friends, pursuing new interests) would be difficult for you?"
5. **Numbness/detachment**—"Do you feel emotionally numb or have trouble feeling connected with others ____ since died?"
6. **Feeling life is empty or meaningless without deceased**—"To what extent do you feel that life is empty or meaningless without ____?"
7. **Bleak future**—"Do you feel that the future holds no meaning or prospect for fulfillment without____?"
8. **Agitated**—"Do you feel on edge or jumpy since ____ died?"

Criterion C: the above symptom disturbance causes marked and persistent dysfunction in social, occupational, or other important domains
Criterion D: the above symptom disturbance must last at least 6 months
Complicated grief diagnosis—criteria A, B, C, and D must be met

From: Prigerson HG, Maciejewski PK. A call for sound empirical testing and evaluation of criteria for complicated grief proposed for DSM-V. Omega. *J Death Dying* 2005–2006;52(1):9–19.

Research suggests that complicated grief at 6 months predicts impairment and complications at 13–23 months post-loss (6–8,10). Hence, recognizing the signs and symptoms of complicated grief at 6 months would be a good way for health care professionals to identify survivors who may experience further adjustment difficulties in the future.

WHY DO PHYSICIANS NEED TO CARE FOR BEREAVED PERSONS?

When looking at the outcomes of complicated grief, one is able to see why physicians should play a role in all aspects of bereavement care. There remains little doubt about the excess morbidity associated with bereavement, and with complicated grief, specifically. Additionally, bereavement tends to occur most often in later life, when health and adaptive capacities may already be compromised and hence physicians need to play an integral role in caring for bereaved patients and in preventing the unchecked progression of complicated grief.

TABLE 59.2

OUTCOMES OF COMPLICATED GRIEF

Increased risk of suicidal thoughts and behaviors
Increased risk of major depressive disorder
Increased risk of anxiety disorders (generalized anxiety disorder, posttraumatic stress disorder, and panic disorder)
Increased incidence of cardiac events
Increased incidence of high blood pressure
Significant changes in consumption of food, alcohol, and tobacco
Increased risk of impairment in social and occupational functioning
Impaired quality of life

There are several compelling reasons for physicians to actively engage themselves in bereavement care. First, they are already involved in caring for bereaved patients and will become increasingly so as the population ages. Empathic "aftercare" for bereaved patients demonstrates the physicians' respect for the deceased and concern for the surviving family members. It may reduce the family's sense of abandonment by the health care system and soften the psychological blow of losing a loved one. Enhanced discussion between bereaved family members and physicians may help both in attaining a sense of closure. Finally, engaging in the active care of bereaved individuals may reduce the negative health consequences and complications associated with the bereavement process in the surviving family members.

WHAT SHOULD CLINICIANS DO TO ASSIST BEREAVED PATIENTS?

Health care professionals can use the algorithm in Table 59.1 to diagnose complicated grief. Although many of these signs and symptoms are similar to the manifestation of uncomplicated grief during the first 6 months following the loss, it is the persistence of these symptoms and their overall effects on the functioning of the bereaved individuals that are the hallmarks of complicated grief (Figure 59.2). Figure 59.2 shows the mean grief resolution scores (a summation of the nine symptoms presented in Table 59.1) over time from loss for those with and without complicated grief (diagnosed at 6 months post-loss). In contrast to the significant average decline in grief and associated distress over time displayed in Figure 59.1, Figure 59.2 illustrates how the mean grief score remains stably high from 2 to 20 months post-loss for the group diagnosed with complicated grief. These results indicate that bereaved persons diagnosed with complicated grief at 6 months post-loss are unlikely to resolve their grief naturally and may benefit from interventions aimed at reducing their chronically high levels of grief (see following section on Treatment of Complicated Grief).

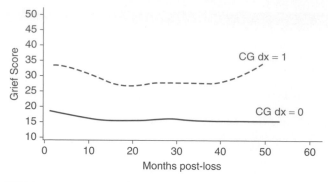

FIGURE 59.2. Mean grief score over time, stratified by complicated grief diagnosis. dx, diagnosis.

DISTINCTIONS BETWEEN COMPLICATED GRIEF AND OTHER PSYCHIATRIC DISORDERS SECONDARY TO BEREAVEMENT

Complicated grief distinguishes itself from other psychiatric disorders. Research has found the symptoms of complicated grief to be distinct from symptoms of major depressive disorder, generalized anxiety disorder and post-traumatic stress disorder (PTSD) (5,6,8–13). Data have shown that symptoms of complicated grief form a cluster that hold together cohesively and that they are distinct from depression and anxiety symptoms (6,8–10,14).

Distinguishing Complicated Grief from Post-traumatic Stress Disorder

There are many symptomatic differences that can be perceived when distinguishing between PTSD and complicated grief (38). Traumatized individuals are typically anxious about the threat related to the traumatic event, whereas for persons bereaved from nontraumatic deaths separation anxiety is the more salient response (38). In general, fears of violent harm to self or significant others play a less significant role for the bereaved than it does among trauma victims. Additionally, grieving individuals uniquely experience yearning and pining. Efforts to cope with complicated grief should involve reorienting oneself in the world without the deceased rather than processing the events of the death, as might occur following a traumatic event (38). Furthermore, one's personal sense of safety is frequently challenged after a trauma, but not necessarily following bereavement. Although there appear to be similarities in the phenomenology of PTSD and complicated grief such as reexperiencing (intrusive thoughts), and agitation, the core meaning behind the symptoms of these two disorders is quite dissimilar (38). PTSD intrusive thoughts and reexperiencing involve memories of the traumatic event that are negative and distressing. Intrusions experienced by individuals with complicated grief, on the other hand, are often positive and comforting (38). In fact, PTSD and complicated grief are further distinguished because of the tendency of some grieving individuals to treasure and permit these positive memories to remain in their consciousness, often to the extent that they are maladaptive and prohibit themselves from moving forward (38). When looking at avoidance, traumatized individuals more frequently avoid reminders of the event, whereas the bereaved might seek reminders of the deceased (38). Individuals with complicated

grief do not appear to avoid reminders of threat as individuals with PTSD often do, but rather avoid reminders of the absence of the deceased through denial (38). In fact, they tend to seek out reminders of the deceased's presence. They are more likely to speak with others about the loss including the deceased, whereas individuals with PTSD try to avoid discussions that will entail a painful return to the traumatic experience (38).

Distinguishing Complicated Grief from Bereavement-Related Depression

Distinguishing complicated grief from the major depressive disorder has been difficult because these disorders may co-exist following bereavement (8,10). Despite their potential co-occurrence, their symptom profiles are distinct (8,10). Symptoms of yearning, intrusive thoughts, preoccupation with thoughts of the deceased, disbelief regarding the death, and feeling that a part of oneself died with the deceased are all specific to complicated grief and are distinct from depressive symptoms (8,10). Symptoms of depressed mood, psychomotor retardation, and damaged self-esteem are indicators of depression (8,10). It is important, however, for health care professionals to realize that complicated grief and bereavement-related depression are often seen together following bereavement and being able to recognize the differences between and the distinctiveness of these disorders may be essential in guiding decisions for effective intervention. Later in this chapter, we will discuss the treatments of complicated grief and bereavement-related psychiatric complications such as depression.

RISK FACTORS FOR COMPLICATED GRIEF

There are many risk factors that may predispose certain individuals to experiencing complicated grief. Understanding these risk factors and their implications will help health care providers in identifying individuals at risk for complicated grief and in providing the necessary support to help survivors through their grieving process. Complicated grief appears to be associated with attachment disturbance and a high degree of insecurity and unstable sense of self and one's relationship with others (29,39,40). Survivors who were in a dependent, close, and confiding relationship with the deceased are more likely to experience complicated grief (29,39,41,42). Interestingly, individuals who have experienced childhood abuse and serious neglect have also been shown to have a higher risk for complicated grief (43). Individuals who are generally averse to lifestyle changes are also more likely to experience complications (44). Complicated grief is less likely to be seen in survivors with a good social support network and with some advance preparation for the death (45,46).

Table 59.3 shows a list of risk factors that health care professionals can keep an eye on when dealing with bereaved individuals. Monitoring these risk factors can be a clue to identify bereaved individuals who may be at risk for deteriorating social and psychological illness and associated impairment. For example, individuals lacking a good social support structure should be encouraged to participate in support groups and in bereavement organizations such as the AARP Widowed Persons Service to reduce isolation, normalize the challenges that they face, and obtain useful practical advice and empathy, as well as companionship.

TABLE 59.3

RISK FACTORS OF COMPLICATED GRIEF

Close, dependent relationship to the deceased
Relationship—parents and spouses are most adversely affected
Abuse or serious neglect in childhood
Separation anxiety in childhood
Preference for lifestyle regularity—averse to
   change/disruptions
Lack of preparation for the death

COMPLICATED GRIEF AND USE OF HEALTH SERVICES

It is important to note that bereaved people with complicated grief are less likely to seek medical care than those without grief complications (47). This suggests a need for greater outreach by making an extra effort to identify appropriate services and encourage those with complicated grief to use them.

MANAGEMENT OF BEREAVED INDIVIDUALS

Health care professionals can make the grieving process a more tolerable experience for the survivors. If health care professionals approach taking care of bereaved individuals as part of their duty and as an integral part of end-of-life care, some incidents of complicated grief might be prevented, detected early, and/or brought under control before causing significant damage to the health and quality of life of bereaved individuals.

As noted earlier, preparedness for the death tends to decrease the risks of developing complicated grief and hence the first task for health care professionals who may have a chance to make family members more prepared for their loss, is to facilitate a peaceful and dignified loss, encourage them to say goodbye to their loved ones, and to deal with any guilt or regrets they might have. Following the death, health care professionals should provide an opportunity for survivors to spend some time with the body of the deceased, when possible. This will facilitate acceptance of the death and help in overcoming the denial and shock due to the loss.

In the first couple of months post-loss, the physician might make telephone calls to offer condolences and also to recommend a visit to evaluate and then monitor the survivors' health care needs. The content of office visits between the physician and the bereaved individual might shift from ordinary practice to a discussion about the course of grief, the ways the bereaved individual have attempted to cope with the loss, their daily practices, their feelings, emotions, and thoughts, their worries, and hopes for the future. During these consultations, physicians can closely monitor the grieving process, its natural progression, and watch out for signs and indicators of complicated grief. Physicians should expect bereaved individuals to exhibit some signs and symptoms that may be associated with complicated grief during the first few months following the loss, but they should see a gradual decline in these symptoms and a progression toward acceptance of the death and ability to move on by 6 months post-loss.

Physicians sometimes feel reluctant to approach the deceased patient's surviving family because of a common perception that the family is angry with them, and perhaps due to a sense of guilt and/or helplessness about being unable to prevent the death. In a study of reactions to terminal care, 30% of surviving family members reported dissatisfaction with the information provided about the cause of death (11). Physicians who contact bereaved patients and express sorrow and concern may minimize the anger directed toward them.

The physician's discomfort or uncertainty about what to say or do when taking care of bereaved patients must be overcome in favor of taking active steps to help them. Tables 59.4 and 59.5 show a list of comments and practices in communicating with and caring for grieving patients, which has been derived from a synthesis of discussions with widowed persons, and participation in grief support groups (11). Physicians should acknowledge the loss and let the bereaved person know that they feel for him/her. Furthermore, they should acknowledge their inability to fully comprehend the magnitude of their loss and the feelings that the bereaved individuals may be experiencing. Physicians should encourage conversations about the deceased, remembering him/her, and allowing the bereaved individual to talk freely about their thoughts of the deceased. Additionally, physicians should provide an opportunity for the bereaved individuals to ask any of their unanswered questions, to address their concerns about the final moments in the deceased's life, and to provide a sense of closure for the family. Physicians should always express concern for the bereaved individuals and provide them with an opportunity to talk about their loss and its effect on their lives.

In managing bereaved individuals, health care professionals can facilitate healing and minimize the risk of complicated grief by encouraging certain behaviors and providing some helpful advice for bereaved individuals. Physicians can encourage bereaved individuals to be involved in social practices, develop new routines and skills, and maintain an active lifestyle. Furthermore, health care professionals can serve as advocates for good health behaviors such as discouraging bereaved persons from excessive drinking, smoking, or eating.

TREATMENT OF COMPLICATED GRIEF

While managing bereaved individuals, being able to recognize risk factors and symptoms of complicated grief will help health professionals in identifying individuals who are having a really difficult time coping with the loss and in recommending further counseling and support. Treatment and counseling that get at the meaning of the loss to the survivor's sense of self and attitudes toward their surrounding environment, and interventions that enhance the survivor's sense of their prospects for future fulfillment would target the core attachment issues that lay at the root of complicated grief (11). Treatments that foster a sense of competence and independence in the survivor, that promote development of new, meaningful relationships, and encourage new routines and skills would be beneficial (52,53). When dealing with patients suffering from complicated grief, health care providers should recommend maintaining an active daily routine, monitoring caloric intake, getting adequate sleep (6.5–9 hours/night), and exercising several times each week just as they would with any bereaved individual. Bereaved individuals experiencing difficulties, adjusting to the loss as predicted, should also be encouraged to participate in support groups that will help them find empathic support, feel less isolated or abnormal, and potentially learn ways to enhance their sense of independence and "survival" skills, and generally assist them in coping with their loss (11,48–55).

It is important for health care professionals to be able to distinguish between complicated grief and bereavement related psychiatric complications such as bereavement-related depression because they might call for different treatment protocols and different therapies.

TABLE 59.4

COMMUNICATION STRATEGIES FOR PHYSICIAN INTERACTIONS WITH BEREAVED INDIVIDUALS

Things to say . . .	Things not to say . . .
I am sorry, or I am sorry she/he's gone. This acknowledges the loss and shows a genuine concern for the bereaved	*Call me.* This puts the burden on the bereaved. Make the effort to contact the bereaved and demonstrate an interest
I can't imagine what you are going through; I can't imagine how you feel. Bereaved people are often angered by comments that minimize the way they are feeling or assume that others know how they are feeling; acknowledgement of your inability to imagine fully how they feel is often appreciated	*I know how you feel.* Nobody can fully know how anyone else feels even when dealing with a very similar situation. Bereaved individuals may resent you for assuming you know what they are going through
Say the deceased's name. Mentioning the name of the deceased can be a reminder that you have not forgotten the deceased, which can be comforting to the bereaved who worry about the deceased being forgotten	*How are you* (casually)*?* This appears insincere because they are probably not feeling well but are disinclined to discuss this in a brief, passing conversation
What are you remembering about the deceased today? Do not worry about bringing up sad memories for the bereaved, they are often thinking and remembering the deceased. Help them to express their thoughts and show that you care by asking them what they are thinking and feeling	*It was probably for the best.* Bereaved people may not feel that this is totally, or even partly, true
Talk about the deceased. Depending on your relationship with the deceased, you may want to say it was an honor to know him/her and that you will miss him/her	*He/she is happy now.* You have no way of knowing this and the patient might resent your assumption
How are you feeling since the deceased's death? How has the deceased's death affected you? Bereaved patients appreciate the concern and this will allow doctors to know how bereaved patients are adapting to the loss, potentially revealing problematic adjustment	*It is God's will.* This can confuse the religious and offend the nonreligious people
There are things that are not within our control. This is often a good thing to say to bereaved patients who are questioning the reasons behind their tragedy. This may help patients to accept that they have no control over what happened	*The world is so unsettled right now, you should be happy that he/she is in heaven and at peace.* Do not make religious references that may not fit with the patient's belief system
I hope you find the strength to bear your loss. This is good. Mourning is about the loss, not the strength of the bereaved. Do not say "you are strong enough to deal with this". Focus on the mourning itself	*It was his/her time to go.* Bereaved patients often do not feel this way and they protest their loved one's departure regardless of how long or how happily they had lived their life
I know you'll miss him/her. This acknowledges that you feel for the patient and appreciate their loss	*I am sorry I brought it up.* Do not apologize for talking about an upsetting topic that is very much on the minds of the bereaved. Bereaved people want to talk about their loss
How are you sleeping or ("eating")? This may be a window into coping difficulties. This provides a segue into discussing other health behaviors that may be adversely affected by the loss and provides you with an opportunity to encourage healthy eating, drinking, and sleeping habits	*Let's change the subject.* Try not to avoid the topic because it is uncomfortable for you. Aiding the bereaved person is about attending to their needs and not about your discomfort or awkwardness
You are entitled to these feelings. This is a natural part of the grieving process. It is often comforting for bereaved patients to know that their pain and feelings are natural and that the pain they are experiencing is normal	*You should work toward getting over this by now.* Physicians should reassure patients that the intense emotions they are experiencing frequently endure for many months if not longer and should not put pressure on the bereaved to move on before they feel they are able

Adapted from Prigerson HG, et al. Caring for bereaved patients "all doctors just suddenly go". *JAMA* 2001;286:1369–1376.

Prospect for Pharmacotherapy and Psychotherapy

Initial studies indicated that interpersonal psychotherapy (IPT) and tricyclic antidepressants are not effective in ameliorating symptoms of complicated grief (56,57). Recent trials suggest that selective serotonin reuptake inhibitors may be effective in treating symptoms of both major depressive disorder and complicated grief, though results await confirmation from randomized control trials (58,59).

William Piper's interpretative and supportive therapies (60), and Mardi Horowitz's eclectic integrated cognitive-dynamic approach to case formulation and treatment (61) are all promising psychotherapeutic techniques for complicated grief, although again, conclusive results await publication of randomized controlled trials. Katherine Shear's complicated grief therapy (CGT) (62) is the first randomized controlled trial for complicated grief with proven efficacy for the reduction of complicated grief symptomatology. Because complicated grief includes depressive symptoms such as sadness, guilt, and social withdrawal, Shear used a framework for the treatment based on previous research with IPT for grief-related depression (62). Because of the presence of PTSD like symptoms of disbelief, as well as unique symptoms related to the death, Shear modified

TABLE 59.5

PRACTICES IN COMMUNICATING WITH AND CARING FOR GRIEVING PATIENTS

Practices to implement	Practices to avoid
Death notification. Establish a system whereby you are notified of patient deaths, recent losses, and deaths within patient's families	**Passivity.** Avoid being passive, vague, or insincere. Do not place the burden on the bereaved patient to approach you, because they probably will not. Take an initiative to help them cope with their loss
Outreach. Express your sorrow for the loss, invite bereaved patients to talk about their loss, and monitor their coping and lifestyle changes throughout their grieving process	**Avoidance.** Do not avoid talking about their loss to the bereaved patients. They often want to talk about their loss, want you to know how they are feeling, and desire your help and advice in making them feel normal
Have useful information available. Provide a list of resources for bereaved patients: support groups, brochures and educational material about bereavement, clergy, mental health professionals, lawyers, and financial planners	**Making comparisons with other losses.** Do not attempt to minimize the bereaved patient's loss or compare it to other losses. Each loss is different, as are bereaved person's reactions to the loss
Follow-up. Remember that bereavement is a process, and that you cannot monitor bereaved patients with just a one-time visit. Do not hesitate to call bereaved patients if you have not heard from them; monitor their symptoms and adjustment. Evaluate those whom you believe to be at risk of complicated grief	**Pressure and inappropriate positivity.** Try not to imply that they should be moving forward with their life and that they should be feeling better by now. Do not try to place them on a stage of grief, or suggest that their outlook should be more positive

Adapted from Prigerson HG, et al. Caring for bereaved patients "all doctors just suddenly go". *JAMA* 2001;286:1369–1376.

IPT techniques to include cognitive-behavioral therapy-based techniques for addressing death trauma (62). The cognitive strategies were used when working with loss-specific distress. Shear reports that her new integrated approach, her targeted CGT is an improved treatment over IPT that shows higher response rates and faster time to response for symptoms of complicated grief, specifically (62).

TREATMENT OF BEREAVEMENT-RELATED PSYCHIATRIC COMPLICATIONS

The results of research on bereavement interventions suggest that treatment selection should be based on the patient's specific psychiatric diagnosis or diagnoses (11). For patients diagnosed with bereavement-related depression, the treatment should follow the guidelines for treating major depressive disorder including the prescription of selective serotonin reuptake inhibitors or tricyclic antidepressant (11). Similarly, if the bereaved individuals show distinct signs and symptoms of any other major psychiatric disorder, treatment should follow the guidelines for treating that specific disorder independent of the complicated grief treatment.

Here, once again, one can see the importance of an accurate understanding of the distinct differences between the clinical presentation of complicated grief and other psychiatric disorders in the bereavement setting. The success of treating the patient's symptoms will depend on the ability to accurately diagnose their symptoms and the progression of their illness throughout their bereavement process.

IMPLICATIONS FOR PALLIATIVE CARE

Barry et al. evaluated the association between the bereaved persons' perceptions of death (e.g., extent of suffering, violent vs. peaceful death) and preparedness for the death and psychiatric disorders (45). Barry et al. showed that the perception of death as more violent was associated with major depressive disorder at 4 months post-loss. More importantly, this work indicated that the perception of lack of preparedness for the death was associated with complicated grief at 4 and 9 months post-loss.

Recent work (63) suggests that earlier hospice enrollment may reduce the risk for major depressive disorder during the first 6–8 months of bereavement. This is consistent with Barry's work because earlier hospice enrollment might indicate more preparedness for the death. Additionally, another study in the Netherlands indicated that the bereaved family and friends of cancer patients who died by euthanasia coped better with respect to grief symptoms and posttraumatic stress reactions than the bereaved of comparable cancer patients who died a natural death (64). These data strongly suggest that preparation in advance for the loss may help reduce the risk of developing complicated grief and make the grieving process less painful for the survivors.

This information can have tremendous implications for palliative care services and hospices by allowing them to play a key role in reducing the risks of developing complications in bereaved individuals during their grieving process. Palliative care services as well as hospices can help families orient to their loss and provide them with a chance to accept and deal with that loss. Furthermore, this information should also be used by health care professionals when dealing with patients suffering from terminal illnesses. Health care professionals should be encouraged to recommend hospice and palliative care services to their patients when it is appropriate to do so to prevent prolongation of suffering in them, allow them a peaceful ending, and also help their families prepare for their loss, which may lower their risk of developing complicated grief.

CONCLUSION

Bereavement is a natural and nearly universal experience that causes a great deal of distress and sorrow for those who experience the loss of an intimate person. However, an individual's experience with grief and bereavement may vary depending on many factors including social elements, relationship (e.g., parents, spouses) and closeness to the deceased, and, particularly, emotional dependency on the deceased. Past experiences with loss, intrapersonal factors, as well as interpersonal factors are all influential in determining bereavement adjustment.

Because of the many negative health care consequences associated with bereavement and complicated grief, bereavement care should be a responsibility assumed by health care providers and an integral part of any comprehensive palliative care plan that focuses on providing good quality end-of-life care for the dying patient as well as support for the survivors. Health care professionals need to recognize the symptoms associated with complicated grief and identify the persons having difficulties in coping with their loss. Additionally, having a good understanding of the various risk factors that predispose certain individuals to complicated grief will help health care providers in closely monitoring individuals at risk and also in recommending proper treatment and support options.

Bereavement care currently does not get the proper attention in the education and the development of tomorrow's physicians. Medical and psychiatric training often devotes little time to the recognition of complicated grief. Without the proper education, physicians might not be able to recognize the signs and symptoms of complicated grief, comprehend their duty to take care of the family and survivors who are left behind, and provide adequate help and encouragement for bereaved individuals attempting to cope with their loss. Furthermore, all health care professionals will probably be exposed to grieving individuals, and survivors will probably be greatly helped by having a doctor who is comfortable in addressing their grief, capable of helping them cope with their loss, and supporting their efforts to bring closure to the loss, and to move on with their lives. Hence, it is essential that bereavement care becomes an integral part of current educational programs directed at developing better physicians who are capable of managing all aspects of their patient's struggles, including their grieving process.

In this chapter, we have also tried to outline the importance of preparing families for their loss, for experiencing a peaceful resolution and a nonviolent death when possible, and for the advantages of early hospice enrollment in lowering the risk of developing complicated grief. This provides yet another reason for health care professionals to reassess their priorities and their efforts when providing quality end-of-life care for their patients and their families. Aggressive therapies and prolongation of life above all else might not be the best strategy to implement when taking care of patients and their families. Instead, preparing the families for the loss, and accepting death as part of the natural life cycle rather than a failure in the medical care provided may prove extremely helpful for the bereaved individuals and their grieving process. Finally, we hope that the research findings outlined in this chapter will help in shaping palliative care programs and shaping hospices' roles in the bereavement process as well as in physicians' attitudes, perceptions, and actions when providing end-of-life and bereavement care for their patients and for those who are left behind.

References

1. Hoyert DL, Kung HC, Smith BL. *Deaths: preliminary data for 2003.* National Vital Statistics Reports Vol 33, # 15, Center for Disease Control, Feb. 28, 2005, http://www.cdc.gov/nchs/data/nvsr/nvsr53/nvsr53_15.pdf.
2. America's Families and living Arrangement 2003 March Current Population Survey Report, U.S. Census Bureau, March 2003, http://www.census.gov/prod/2004pubs/p20-553.pdf.
3. Holmes TH, Rahe RH. The social readjustment rating scale. *J Psychosom Res* 1967;11:213–218.
4. Osterweis M, Solomon F, Green M, eds. *Bereavement: reactions, consequences and care.* Washington, DC: National Academy Press, 1984.
5. Prigerson HG, Bridge J, Maciejewski PK, et al. Influence of traumatic grief on suicidal ideation among young adults. *Am J Psychiatry* 1999;156:1994–1995.
6. Chen JH, Bierhals AJ, Prigerson HG, et al. Gender differences in the effects of bereavement-related psychological distress in health outcomes. *Psychol Med* 1999;29:367–380.
7. Prigerson HG, Bierhals AJ, Kasl SV, et al. Traumatic grief as a risk factor for mental and physical morbidity. *Am J Psychiatry* 1997;154:616–623.
8. Prigerson HG, Bierhals AJ, Kasl SV, et al. Complicated Grief as a disorder distinct from bereavement-related depression and anxiety: a replication study. *Am J Psychiatry* 1996;153:1484–1486.
9. Prigerson HG, Maciejewski PK, Reynolds CF III, et al. Inventory of Complicated Grief: a scale to measure maladaptive symptoms of loss. *Psychiatry Res* 1995;59:65–79.
10. Prigerson HG, Frank E, Kasl SV, et al. Complicated Grief and bereavement-related depression as distinct disorders: preliminary empirical validation in elderly bereaved spouses. *Am J Psychiatry* 1995;152:22–30.
11. Prigerson HG, Jacobs Sc. Perspectives on care at the close of life. Caring for bereaved patients: "all the doctors just suddenly go. *JAMA* 2001;286:1369–1376.
12. Silverman GK, Jacobs SC, Kasl SV, et al. Quality of life impairments associated with diagnostic criteria for traumatic grief. *Psychol Med* 2000;30:857–862.
13. Prigerson HG, Shear MK, Jacobs SC, et al. Consensus criteria for traumatic grief. A preliminary empirical test. *Br J Psychiatry* 1999;174:67–73.
14. Boelen PA, van den Bout J, de Keijser J. Traumatic grief as a disorder distinct from bereavement-related depression and anxiety: a replication study with bereaved mental health care patients. *Am J Psychiatry* 2003;160:1229–1241.
15. Ott CH. The impact of Complicated Grief on mental and physical health at various points in the bereavement process. *Death Stud* 2003;27:249–272.
16. Brown GW, Harris TO. Depression. In: Brown GW, Harris TO. *Life events and illness.* New York, Guilford Press, 1989:49–94.
17. Bruce ML, Kim K, Leaf PJ, et al. Depressive episodes and dysphoria resulting from conjugal bereavement in a prospective community sample. *Am J Psychiatry* 1990;147:608–611.
18. Clayton PJ. Bereavement and depression. *J Clin Psychiatry* 1990;51:34–38.
19. Lund D, Dimond M, Caserta MS. Identifying elderly with coping difficulties two years after bereavement. *Omega* 1985;16:213–224.
20. Zisook S, Shuchter S. Uncomplicated bereavement. *J Clin Psychiatry* 1993;54:365–372.
21. Bornstein PE, Clayton PJ, Halikas JA, et al. The depression of widowhood after 13 months. *Br J Psychiatry* 1973;122:561–566.
22. Parkes CM, Wiss RS. *Recovery of bereavement.* New York: Basic Books, 1983.
23. Jacobs S, Hansen F, Kasl S, et al. Anxiety disorders during acute bereavement: risk and risk factors. *J Clin Psychiatry* 1990;51:269–274.
24. Prigerson HG. Complicated Grief: when the path of adjustment leads to a dead-end. *Bereavement Care* 2004;23:38–40.
25. Zhang B, Maciejewski PK, Vanderwerker LC, et al. A preliminary empirical examination of the state theory of grief resolution. (Submitted manuscript).
26. Prigerson HG, Bridge J, Maciejewski PK, et al. Traumatic grief as a risk factor for suicidal ideation among young adults. *Am J Psychiatry* 1997;156:1994–1995.
27. Bowlby J. *Loss: sadness and depression.* New York: Basic Books, 1980.
28. Lindemann E. Symptomatology and management of acute grief. *Am J Psychiatry* 1944;101:141–148.
29. Prigerson HG, Shear MK, Frank E, et al. Traumatic grief: a case of loss-induced distress. *Am J Psychiatry* 1997;154:1003–1009.
30. Schut HA, De Keijser J, Van den Bout J, et al. Post-traumatic stress symptoms in the first years of conjugal bereavement. *Anxiety Res* 1991;4:225–234.
31. Zisook S, Chentsova-Dutton Y, Shuchter SR. PTSD following bereavement. *Ann Clin Psychiatry* 1998;10:157–163.
32. Lewis CS. *A Grief Observed.* New York: Bantam Seabury Press, 1963.
33. Middleton W, Burnett P, Paphael B, et al. The bereavement response: a cluster analysis. *Br J Psychiatry* 1996;169:167–171.
34. Horowitz MJ, Siegel B, Holen A, et al. Criteria for Complicated Grief disorder. *Am J Psychiatry* 1997;154:905–910.
35. Jacobs S, Kasl S, Schaefer C, et al. Conscious and unconscious coping with loss. *Psychosom Med* 1994;56:557–563.
36. Bonanno GA, Keltner D, Holen A, et al. When avoiding unpleasant emotions might not be such a bad thing: verbal-autonomic response dissociation and midlife conjugal bereavement. *J Pers Soc Psychol* 1995;69:975–989.
37. Stroebe MS, Stroebe W. Does "grief work" work? *J Consult Clin Psychol* 1991;59:479–482.
38. Lichtenthal WG, Cruess DG, Prigerson HG. A case for establishing Complicated Grief as a distinct mental disorder in DSM-V. *Clin Psychol Rev* 2004;24:637–662.
39. van Doorn C, Kasl SV, Beery LC, et al. The influence of marital quality and attachment styles on traumatic grief and depressive symptoms. *J Nerv Ment Dis* 1998;186:566–573.

40. Carr D, House JS, Wortman C, et al. Psychological adjustments to sudden and anticipated spousal loss among older widowed persons. *J Gerontol Psychol Soc Sci* 2001;56:S237–S248.

41. Prigerson HG, Maciejewski PK, Rosenheck R. The interactive effects of marital harmony and widowhood on Health, health service utilization and costs. *Gerontologist* 2000;40:349–357.

42. Johnson JG, Vanderwerker LC, Bornstein RF, et al. Development and validation of an instrument for the assessment of dependency among bereaved persons. *J Psychopathol Behav Assess (in press)*.

43. Silverman GK, Johnson JG, Prigerson HG. Preliminary explorations of the effects of prior trauma and loss on risk of psychiatric disorders in recently widowed people. *Isr J Psychiatry Relat Sci* 2001;38:202–215.

44. Beery LC, Prigerson HG. Lifestyle regularity as a unique risk factor for Complicated Grief. *Submitted manuscript*.

45. Barry LC, Kasl SV, Prigerson HG. Psychiatric disorders among bereaved persons: the role of perceived circumstances of death and preparedness for death. *Am J Geriatr Psychiatry* 2001;10:447–457.

46. Vanderwerker LC, Prigerson HG. Social support, technological connectedness and periodical readings as protective factors in bereavement. *J Loss Trauma* 2004;9:45–57.

47. Prigerson HG, Silverman GK, Jacobs SC, et al. Disability, traumatic grief, and the underutilization of health services. *Prim Psychiatry* 2001;8:61–69.

48. Main J. Improving management of bereavement in general practice based on a survey of recently bereaved subjects in a single general practice. *Br J Gen Pract* 2000;50:863–866.

49. Morgan DL. Adjusting to widowhood: do social networks really make it easier? *Gerontologist* 1989;29:101–107.

50. Schneider DS, Sledge PA, Shuchter SR, et al. Dating and remarriage over the first two years of widowhood. *Ann Clin Psychiatry* 1996;8:51–57.

51. Marmar CR, Horowitz MJ, Wess DS, et al. A controlled trail of brief psychotherapy and mutual help group treatment of conjugal bereavement. *Am J Psychiatry* 1988;145:203–309.

52. Brown LF, Reynolds CF, Monk TH, et al. Social rhythm stability following late-life spousal bereavement: associations with depression and sleep impairment. *Psychiatry Res* 1996;62:161–169.

53. Prigerson HG, Reynolds CF III, Frank E, et al. Stressful life events, social rhythms, and depressive symptoms among the elderly: an examination of hypothesized causal linkages. *Psychiatry Res* 1991;51:33–49.

54. Pennebaker JW, Zech E, Rime B. Disclosing and sharing emotion: psychological, social and health consequences. In: Stroebe MS, Hansson RO, Stroebe W, et al. *Handbook of bereavement research: consequences, coping and care*. Washington, DC: American Psychological Association, 2001:517–544.

55. Esterling BA, Antoni MH, Fletcher MA, et al. Emotional disclosure through writing or speaking modulates latent Epstein-Barr virus antibody titers. *J Consult Clin Psychol* 1994;62:130–140.

56. Rosenzweig AS, Pasternak RE, Prigerson HG, et al. Bereavement-related depression in the elderly. Is drug treatment justified? *Drugs Aging* 1996;8:323–328.

57. Reynolds CF III, Miller MD, Pasternak RE, et al. Treatment of bereavement-related major depressive episodes interpersonal psychotherapy. *Am J Psychiatry* 1999;156:202–208.

58. Zygmont M, Prigerson HG, Houck PR, et al. A post hoc comparison of paroxetine and nortriptyline for symptoms of traumatic grief. *J Clin Psychiatry* 1998;59:241–245.

59. Zisook S, Shuchter SR, Pedrelli P, et al. Bupropion sustained release for bereavement: results of an open trial. *J Clin Psychiatry* 2001;62:227–230.

60. Piper WE, McCallum M, Joyce AS, et al. Patients personality and time-limited group psychotherapy for Complicated Grief. *Int J Group Psychother* 2001;51:525–555.

61. Marmar CR, Horowitz MJ, Weiss DS, et al. A controlled trial of brief psychotherapy and mutual-help group treatment of conjugal bereavement. *Am J Psychiatry* 1988;145:203–209.

62. Shear MK, Frank E, Houck P, et al. Treatment of Complicated Grief: a randomized controlled trial. *JAMA* 2005;293:2601–2659.

63. Bradley EH, Prigerson HG, Carlson MD. Depression among surviving caregivers: does length of hospice enrollment matter? *Am J Psychiatry* 2004;161:2257–2262.

64. Swarte NB, Van der Lee ML, Van der Born JG, et al. Effects of euthanasia on the bereaved family and friends: a cross sectional study. *Br Med J* 2003;327:189–194.

CHAPTER 60 ■ STARTING A PALLIATIVE CARE PROGRAM

HANNAH I. LIPMAN AND DIANE E. MEIER

INTRODUCTION: WHY PALLIATIVE CARE?

The Case for Palliative Care

Palliative care is comprehensive medical care focused on relieving the suffering of patients facing serious or life-threatening illness and that of their families. It is provided across the continuum of illness from first diagnosis until death, should it occur, and bereavement. Curative or life-prolonging treatment may be provided concurrently with palliative care, as appropriate. An interdisciplinary team may provide palliative care in all medical settings: inpatient, outpatient, in the home, in long-term care, and in the emergency department.

The field of palliative care has expanded rapidly over the last two decades. This has been in response to the challenge to our health care system to provide high-quality care to increasing numbers of older patients with multiple chronic illnesses in recognition of the fact that symptom control, advance care planning and shared decision making, coordination of care across settings, and care of the dying patients are integral to the care of all seriously ill patients.

Clinical Imperative for Palliative Care

There is a high burden of pain and other symptoms among hospitalized patients (1), chronically ill patients in the community (2), and dying patients in all care settings (3). Most deaths occur in the hospital (50%) and nursing home (25%), despite most people's stated preference for dying at home (4). As the population ages and the burden of chronic illness increases, the number of seriously ill patients who are in the oldest old age group increases. The use of nonbeneficial life-sustaining treatments for these patients is high despite preferences for care focused on quality and quantity of life (5).

Interviews with chronically ill patients show that the factors they value most are relief from physical symptoms, shared decision making with clinicians, avoiding a prolonged dying process, lessening the burden on caregivers, and strengthening personal relationships (6–9). However, caregivers of dying patients report dissatisfaction with the quality of care in these areas at end of life (3,10).

Most people with serious or chronic illness require assistance with care at home. This burden falls on their families (11). Caregivers are more likely to be depressed, face significant economic stress, and have a higher morbidity and mortality rate than age-matched controls (12). Physicians and policy makers, as well as the general public, express concern about the ability of the medical system to address the care needs of the chronically ill (13). Taken together, these factors have driven the rapid growth in palliative care programs in recent years.

Financial Imperative for Palliative Care

A striking 68% of all Medicare dollars are spent on 23% of all beneficiaries who have five or more chronic medical conditions (14). One fourths of all Medicare dollars are spent in the last year of life (15). Medical spending on those who die in any given year is not significantly different from spending on patients with similar illness burden who do not die in that year (15). This emphasizes the difficulty in prognosticating life expectancy accurately. Therefore, palliative care should be delivered throughout the continuum of illness on the basis of need and independent of prognosis, addressing the high utilization and the need for care for all patients with multiple chronic illnesses.

Educational Imperative for Palliative Care

To meet the challenges detailed in the preceding text, current and future generations of medical students and house staff must be educated in palliative care, the quality management of complex chronic illness. At present, medical education takes place primarily in acute care hospitals. The growth of palliative care programs in teaching hospitals aims to ensure that medical students and house staff are taught the core skills of palliative care: pain and symptom management, expert communication about care alternatives and decision support, and a sophisticated ability to help patients and families manage a complex and fragmented health care system. In 2000, 26% of a random sample of 100 teaching hospitals had a palliative care consultation service or inpatient unit (16). By 2003, according to data from the American Hospital Association survey, 68% of hospitals belonging to the American Association of Medical Colleges Council of Teaching Hospitals reported a palliative care program (17). The number of physicians trained to provide specialist-level palliative care is also increasing. As of 2005, there are currently over 50 palliative medicine fellowship programs and 1891 physicians are certified in the subspecialty in the United States (18). Progress is being made toward recognition of the specialty by the American Board of Medical Specialties (19).

HOW TO APPROACH STARTING A PALLIATIVE CARE PROGRAM

Starting a new palliative care program in a health care institution is a challenging but rewarding task. The recommendations contained in this chapter are drawn from the data and experience of the Center to Advance Palliative Care (CAPC), an organization committed to increasing the number and quality of palliative care programs in the United States through the provision of technical assistance. Further details, links to relevant resources, and *A Guide to Building a Hospital-Based Palliative Care Program* (20), a publication of the CAPC may be found at www.capc.org (21).

Leadership

An effective leader to act as program champion throughout the planning and implementation process is critical to success. In addition to commitment to the mission of palliative care to relieve suffering, improve communication and care across settings, and meet the system-wide challenges of an aging population with chronic illness, the ideal program champion should be an experienced leader, an effective communicator, command respect throughout the institution, and have credibility with key institutional decision makers. The professional discipline of the program champion is less important than these personal leadership qualities. Whether the champion is a physician, a nursing leader, an administrator, or some other professional will depend on local institutional factors.

BUILDING THE CASE AT YOUR INSTITUTION

Securing Support

A successful program must be aligned with the mission, priorities, needs, and culture of the home institution. Taking the time to thoroughly understand these institutional characteristics before planning the program will pay off later. The institution's mission statement and annual report are good sources of information about the hospital's goals and clinical and financial strengths. Informal interviews with leaders of other recently implemented new programs may be informative about how to negotiate the approval and funding processes in the institution.

The new palliative care program will have an impact on the care provided by and work environment of clinicians from other medical services with similar goals, skills, and patient base, such as anesthesia pain, oncology, critical care, and geriatrics, as well various other hospital staff, including social work services, pharmacy, and nutrition. Meeting informally with representatives from these areas, as well as with key institution decision makers, provides an early opportunity to assess their needs, knowledge, and misconceptions about palliative care, as well as to educate them about what palliative care is and how it can successfully integrate with their work. Barriers to smooth implementation of the new service are therefore identified and may be overcome early in the planning process through this informal interviewing process.

These informal meetings may also identify candidates for the planning team, which will need to continue to build support within the hospital. Team members should have some of the same leadership qualities as the program champion, be committed to a collaborative effort, and represent the range of disciplines that provide palliative care. The team should also include at least one community representative invested in the success of the new program, such as a leader from an established and respected local hospice or a member of the institution's Board of Trustees. The planning team will be responsible for conducting the system and needs assessment (see next section) that will yield quantitative and qualitative data about clinical care at and financial status of the hospital, including both strengths and opportunities for improvement, and will help recruit palliative care providers when the program is to be implemented. This core planning team projects an attitude of enthusiasm for seizing opportunities for positive change, advocates for the program in their spheres of influence, and works to overcome the inevitable barriers that face any new clinical service.

System and Needs Assessment

The purpose of the system and needs assessment is to thoroughly review and document the existing strengths and opportunities for improvement specific to the home institution before the design and implementation of the new program. A structured system assessment yields information about current institutional strengths and resources, which the palliative care program will build on. Examples of such resources are physicians, nurses, social workers, chaplains, and other providers who have expertise or interest in palliative care, elements of clinical infrastructure such as an electronic medical record or billing system, a strong anesthesia pain service, an efficient discharge planning or case management team, and productive relationships with local hospice leaders and community philanthropic leaders.

A structured needs assessment answers the question: does this institution need a palliative care program and, if yes, on what services and which patient populations can the new program have a biggest positive impact? Baseline data on the number of annual deaths, their mean and median length of stay, and their Diagnosis Related Group (DRG) categories will be the basis for comparison to data collected after program implementation to demonstrate success. Examples of institutional needs identified with system assessment are the prevalence of untreated or undertreated pain and other symptoms, patient and family satisfaction, nursing and staff satisfaction and turnover, number of patients exceeding national benchmark length of stay for DRG, costs per day for such outliers, discharge delays, and pharmacy costs.

Adequate access to hospital data is necessary to conduct thorough system and needs assessments. Sources of data include the hospital information technology and financial records departments, results of ongoing quality-improvement initiatives, and patient and family satisfaction surveys mandated by the Joint Commission on Accreditation of Healthcare Organizations. The planning team may design and conduct its own surveys and informal interviews to supplement existing data. See Table 60.1 for a list of data to be gathered for the system and needs assessment.

Making the Financial Case

Palliative care improves the financial health of the institution primarily by cost avoidance, as opposed to revenue generation. Under Medicare, the major insurer of the chronically ill, hospitals are reimbursed for an inpatient stay according the DRG. The average length of stay and costs for the admission

TABLE 60.1

USEFUL DATA FOR PALLIATIVE CARE PROGRAMS

Statistics describing the hospital

Total number staffed acute inpatient beds
Overall hospital occupancy rate
ICU occupancy rate
Average LOS for all admissions
Average LOS for Medicare admissions
Average LOS in ICU
Number of admissions with an LOS of >20 d
Number of admissions who die in the hospital
List of top 20 DRGs by case frequency for patients who die as inpatients
Mean and median LOS for an admission within top 20 DRGs
Mean and median LOS for top 20 DRG patients who died in the hospital vs. those in same DRG discharged alive
Mean and median LOS for DRG 483 (tracheostomy with mechanical ventilation 96+ hours) for those who died in the
  hospital vs. those discharged alive
Payer mix for patients in the top 20 DRGs for those discharged alive and for those who died in the hospital
Presence or absence of a dedicated hospice unit, number of hospice beds, hospital–hospice contracts
Number of hospice referrals per year

Description of hospital patient population

Annual number of admissions for patients younger than 21, 22–62, and older than 65
Total number of admissions per year
Total number of Medicare admissions per year
Total number of Medicaid admissions per year
Total number of commercially insured patients per year
Total number of "self-pay" (uninsured) patients per year

Data on clinical outcomes

Assessments of pain and other symptoms
JCAHO pain scores
Prevalence of advance care planning
Prevalence of documented goals of care
Chart review of clinical assessments and interventions

Patient and family satisfaction data

Pain and symptom control
Treatment quality
Attitudes of providers
Timeliness of provider response
Provider communication
Customer service

Measures of staff satisfaction

Retention rate of staff
Staff stress due to time pressures
Staff perceptions of understaffing for care of patients with life-threatening conditions

ICU, intensive care unit; LOS, length of stay; DRG, diagnosis related group; JCAHO, joint commission on accreditation of healthcare organizations.
Reprinted with permission from The Center to Advance Palliative Care. *A Guide to Building a Hospital-based Palliative Care Program*. Available at www.capc.org.

diagnosis determine the appropriate DRG. Given this system, it is in the financial interest of the hospital, assuming that enough care has been provided to justify the designated DRG, to limit both length of stay and costs per day (22–24). The palliative care team facilitates timely clarification of goals of care, which often allows discharge to a less acute level of care, thereby shortening length of stay (25), and avoidance of nonbeneficial procedures, tests, and medications, thereby reducing daily hospital pharmacy, imaging, and ancillary costs.

Clinical research data support these claims. One case–control study showed that daily hospital charges were reduced by 66% after transfer to a palliative care unit compared to the charges before transfer and by 59% compared to matched controls, without increasing mortality (26). Another study of palliative care for patients with cancer showed a decrease in proportion of patients dying in the hospital from 39% to 21% (27).

Interventions designed to identify patients in the intensive care unit (ICU) unlikely to benefit from critical care, improve physician–patient communication, and decrease delay in clarification of goals of care (28–31) have been shown to decrease ICU length of stay, decrease overall hospital days, and limit use of nonbeneficial life-sustaining treatment in critically ill patients without increasing mortality when compared to a control group. Over 80% of patients/surrogate, nurse, and physician participants in one study (30) found the intervention helpful. A detailed financial analysis (32) conducted by Gilmer et al. of their study (30) on ethics consultation (decision support similar to that provided by palliative care consultants) in the ICU showed reduced total costs through a reduction in length of stay among patients who did not survive to hospital discharge and a decrease in the number of patients with hospital stays of 10 or more days.

Studies of comprehensive outpatient palliative care also show a decrease in system-wide costs driven by a decrease in the use of acute care services including emergency department visits, hospital days (33), and outpatient primary care and urgent visits (34).

To make this financial case clear to the hospital administration, the planning team must show how these findings apply to the home institution. The needs assessment has identified specific opportunities for cost saving. Study data from the CAPC provide estimates of the probable financial impact of palliative care. The following example illustrates how these data can be integrated to show how the new program will impact the institution in a real way.

First, estimate referral volume to show how many patients the new palliative care team will impact. Applying the national inpatient average death rate of 2.5% to the total annual hospital admissions will yield the approximate number of expected inpatient deaths in the institution per year. Approximately half of all referrals to inpatient palliative care consultation programs die in the hospital. Therefore, the potential number of referrals to the program annually can be estimated at 5% of all hospital admissions. This estimate should be compared to the institution's actual inpatient mortality rate and adjusted accordingly if it deviates significantly from the national average of 2.5%. It is reasonable to assume that perhaps 20% of these potentially appropriate patients will be referred in the first year of the program. For example, 5% of a hypothetical 16,000 annual admissions yields 800 possible palliative care referrals. Assuming that only 20% of appropriate referrals will actually come to the service in the first year, the service can anticipate 160 referrals in this period (Table 60.2). This is only one method of estimating referral volume. Please refer to the CAPC Web site at www.capc.org for a detailed alternative and downloadable spread sheets for these financial projections and other interactive tools (21).

The next step is to estimate, on the basis of hospital-specific data, how much costs can be reduced per patient. The greatest impact can be made for patients with the longest lengths of stay. By comparing hospital-specific length of stay data to national benchmarks for each of the DRGs that is most likely to be referred to palliative care, estimate dollars that would have been saved by meeting the national benchmark. Exactly why the hospital exceeds the benchmark, and, therefore, how the team can effect the greatest improvement, can be elucidated from chart review and informal interviews with care providers. The deviation of the hospital length of stay from the benchmark is the potential number of days saved. By calculating potential days saved for each DRG with long length of stay and multiplying by the cost per day for that DRG, the cost savings per hospitalization is determined. For example, if hospital length of stay for a given DRG exceeds national benchmark by 1.7 days and cost per day is $1200, then $2040 can be saved per case by bringing length of stay in line with the national benchmark (Table 60.2). The total potential annual cost reduction is estimated by multiplying potential savings per patient by annual referral volume.

Similarly, savings by reduction in daily costs will have the greatest impact when appropriate patients are transferred from the very costly ICU setting to a medical surgical unit. Examine case histories of patients with long ICU cases in detail to determine how to have the greatest impact. Estimate how many ICU days are saved by timely discussion of prognosis and goals of care, first with all involved physicians and then with the patient (if possible) and family. The difference in cost between ICU and acute care beds can then be used to determine costs saved per case simply by transferring patients out of the critical care setting. Similarly, potential savings from avoidance of nonbeneficial tests and treatments can be estimated by examining the case histories of a sample of patients dying in the ICU or after a prolonged ICU stay. Estimate annual number of ICU referrals to palliative care by examining length of stay data and by having informal discussions with ICU staff.

Going through this process using hospital-specific data is crucial because it yields concrete estimates of the program's real potential financial impact. Only hospital-specific data will demonstrate the program's likely worth to administrators and decision makers.

For institutions without opportunities to lower length of stay to national benchmarks, the financial case should focus on other relevant priorities (e.g., reduction in costs per day or strong customer satisfaction and community reputation), as determined by the needs assessment. For example, if increasing bed occupancy is a priority, show how a palliative care program will improve the institution's competitive position in the local market.

Making the Clinical Case

Palliative care improves control of pain and other physical symptoms (25,34–37); attends to spiritual, emotional, and social suffering of the patient and family (34); improves patient–physician communication; facilitates shared decision making; and increases patient and family/caregiver satisfaction (25,33). Mortality is not increased in patients receiving palliative care (26,30,34,38). Recommendations made by palliative care consultation services are implemented at a rate of 84–91% (39,40), indicating need for and utilization of the service provided.

Concrete patient narratives and examples are critical to making the clinical case in a meaningful and powerful way. The needs assessment will reveal areas of opportunity for clinical improvement. Use case presentations, real or hypothetical, to demonstrate concrete opportunities for positive change. Demonstrate who the palliative care patient is, what the needs of that patient and family and caregivers are, and at what points in the hospital stay the care of the patient and family can be improved with good palliative care.

Presenting the Case for Palliative Care

The presentation to administration synthesizes both the existing strengths and the opportunities for improvement at the institution and summarizes how the new palliative care program will leverage existing hospital resources to address the challenges to improve clinical care; patient, family, and staff satisfaction; and the hospitals' financial health. The case is presented positively and enthusiastically. The goal is to demonstrate why the program should be approved and funded. Stakeholders need to see that the program is aligned with the mission and priorities of the hospital, integrates and leverages existing services, improves compliance with national standards such as those of the Joint Commission on Accreditation

TABLE 60.2

EXAMPLES OF FINANCIAL CALCULATIONS

Estimating year 1 referrals	
Total hospital admissions per year	16,000 patients
Percentage of total admissions palliative care appropriate	× 5%
Potential annual volume of patients who could benefit	800 patients
Referral rate for year 1	× 20%
Estimated year 1 program referrals	160 patients
Estimating dollars saved by reducing LOS	
Average hospital LOS for a given DRG	6.7 d
National benchmark LOS for that DRG	−5 d
Potential days saved by meeting national benchmark	1.7 d
Hospital costs per day for that DRG	× $1200
Total dollars saved per case	$2040
Estimating number of beds for an inpatient palliative care unit	
Estimated annual program referrals	584 patients
One half transferred to palliative care unit	292 patients
Average LOS on palliative care unit	× 8 d
Total annual inpatient days on palliative care unit	2336 patient d
	Divide by 365 d
Average daily census	6.4 patients
Ideally, beds are filled to at least 80% of capacity	× 1.25
Number of beds supported by referral volume	8 beds
Estimating average daily census for consultation service	
Estimated year 1 program referrals	160 patients
Average hospital LOS	6 d
Average palliative care patient LOS	8 d
Average LOS on palliative care consultation service	5 d
Total inpatient days (160 × 5)	800 patient d
	Divide by 365 d
Average daily census	2.19 patients

LOS, length of stay; DRG, diagnosis related group.
Adapted with permission from The Center to Advance Palliative Care. *A Guide to Building a Hospital-based Palliative Care Program.* Available at www.capc.org.

of Healthcare Organizations, and improves clinical and financial outcomes. Stakeholders also need to know that the team, and especially its leader, is fully committed to shepherding the program to success, planning and prepared for growth, such that their short-term investment will be realized in long-term gain.

DESIGNING A PROGRAM

Characteristics to Consider

The size and time commitment of the new palliative care team is determined by the size of the institution and estimated referral volume. Small teams with an advance practice nurse providing daily clinical care and a part-time physician may meet the needs of a small community hospital. Small teams draw on the services of the available interdisciplinary team members, such as social work and chaplaincy, on a part-time, shared basis. Large tertiary hospitals will need to support a full team with dedicated full-time interdisciplinary members. The process by which referrals are made and which patients who will make up the target population will also depend on local factors. During the design process, determine in detail how each resource will be utilized and how resources will be brought together into a smoothly functioning whole. The long-term goal is to offer full continuity of palliative care including inpatient consultation, a dedicated inpatient unit, and an outpatient and long-term care practice. Plan ahead for how the program will grow to meet this goal.

Choice of Clinical Palliative Care Delivery Models

Palliative Care Consult Team

Introducing the new program with a palliative care consultation team has several advantages. Start-up costs are low because only salaries of team members, office space, and supplies are required. Existing programs and services (e.g., social work, chaplaincy) can be tapped for part-time, shared use by the consult team.

The consultation model is familiar to referring physicians. Physicians' concerns about losing control over the care of their patients, with whom they have long-established relationships, are allayed. *The client of the palliative care consult team is the referring physician.* Therefore, if the palliative care team is asked to provide help with pain management and not goals of care, the consultation advice should be limited to that requested by the referring physician.

However, if requested by the referring physician, the palliative care consult team may assume primary responsibility for patients with complex and time-consuming needs. Primary patients need not be geographically separated in a dedicated palliative care unit but may be scattered throughout the hospital. Consultation teams are highly visible throughout the hospital, with frequent opportunities to teach palliative care principles and basic symptom management techniques. Referral volume can increase rapidly as informal curbside questions become opportunities for formal consultations.

The main disadvantage of the consultation model is lesser degree of control over patient clinical outcomes and costs than may be achieved on a dedicated inpatient care unit.

Inpatient Palliative Care Unit

A palliative care inpatient unit is a set of beds reserved specifically for palliative care patients, either within another medical unit or separate and freestanding. Palliative care providers are usually the primary physicians for these patients, but an open unit is also possible. Dedicated palliative care units are appropriate for patients with complex symptom management needs or complex family dynamics, or for those who are imminently dying. Approximately ten beds at high occupancy are necessary for economies of scale to make a palliative care unit financially feasible (41). Space, 24/7 nurse and ancillary staff, and supplies may or may not be shared with other units. The initial financial investment of staff and space and, therefore, risk of starting an inpatient palliative care unit may be greater than those associated with starting a consultation service.

There are advantages to having a dedicated palliative care unit. It can be decorated to have a more peaceful and home-like feel, building on the model of the in-hospital hospice unit. The staff of the palliative care unit, such as nursing assistants, registered nurses (RNs), and housekeeping will be trained and made experts in palliative care delivery. In a palliative care unit, the palliative care team has greater control over the care and the clinical and financial outcomes for patients than is possible on the palliative care consult team. These units can also serve as centers of excellence in clinical care, teaching (41), and research.

Disadvantages of the inpatient palliative care unit may include lost opportunities to interface with and teach referring clinicians, house staff, and students throughout the hospital. Segregation of dying patients may reinforce out-of-date ideas that palliative care is only appropriate for patients with a terminal prognosis. It is also undesirable to convey the message that the unit is someplace patients go to die, thereby perpetuating the idea that care of the dying is someone else's responsibility.

Because starting a palliative care program with a dedicated inpatient unit may convey an unintended message that palliative care is only for the imminently dying, it is preferable to begin with a consultation service and expand to include an inpatient unit only when the consultation model is widely accepted and utilized.

Outpatient Practice

Starting an outpatient palliative care practice usually follows from the growth of an inpatient service. Patients discharged from the inpatient service who are well enough to travel may be followed up in the outpatient practice. Additionally, it is an access point for patients who have received a diagnosis of serious or life-threatening illness but do not yet require inpatient or home care. Outpatient practices may be autonomous or housed within other primary care or appropriate specialty practices. Preliminary reports of two outpatient palliative care programs suggest that there exist a sufficient number of appropriate patients to sustain a referral base (34,42).

Administrative Home

The appropriate administrative home for the new program will depend on local organizational structure, institutional culture, and the home department of the team leadership. Established programs in the United States reside in a variety of homes, such as oncology, geriatrics, general internal medicine, nursing, and case management. Once the administrative home is determined, understanding the consequences of its location is important. Consider how the organizational structure affects visibility and respect throughout the institution. The goal is to offer palliative care services to all seriously ill patients regardless of specific diagnosis or prognosis. Plan how to outreach to physicians and nurses in departments other than the administrative home.

Estimating Costs and Revenues

It is important to take time to estimate a budget with details about how much revenue the program will bring in (e.g., clinical income, philanthropy, grants, cost avoidance dollars) relative to how much it will cost to operate (e.g., staff salaries, space). Staff salary will make up most of the operational costs for a consultation service or inpatient unit. On the basis of estimated referral volume (see section Making the Financial Case), determine staffing needs.

Staffing an Inpatient Palliative Care Unit

In planning an inpatient palliative care unit, first determine what size unit can be supported by the estimated referral volume. A dedicated unit is only financially feasible if its beds are filled. To balance costs of overhead and the minimum staff necessary to keep the unit running 24 hours each day, a minimum of six beds is recommended. The optimal number of beds from a staffing ratio standpoint, however, is 15. Assuming that half of all consultation referrals will be transferred to the palliative care unit (adjust this on the basis of local referral patterns and expectations), average daily palliative care unit census can be calculated from the expected total consult referral volume and the estimated average length of stay in the unit. An 80% occupancy rate is the minimum recommended for financial feasibility. Therefore, number of inpatient unit beds needed should be calculated as the estimated average daily census multiplied by 1.25 (Table 60.2).

Some assumptions about ideal staffing ratios are necessary to make concrete estimates of staffing needs. On an inpatient unit, an adequate ratio of nurses to patients is necessary not only for patient care but also to avoid staff burnout. An RN to patient ratio of 1:4 on the day shift and 1:5 at night has been recommended (22) because of the high physical and emotional care needs and the serious illness burden of hospitalized palliative care patients. Similarly, estimate how many patient care assistants and licensed practical nurses will be needed on the unit on the basis of how such staff operate in the local institution. Budget for other professionals, such as social work and chaplain, on the basis of whether they will be shared with other units or on the unit full time. A typical 12–15-bed palliative care unit will require one full-time physician or an advance practice nurse and a part-time physician.

Staffing a Palliative Care Consult Service

Budgeting for a palliative care consult service requires making an assumption about how many physicians and nurses are required to meet the needs of the estimated volume of patients.

On the basis of the expected referral volume and average length of stay in the palliative care service, average daily census can be estimated. Start with the institution's average length of stay for patients in DRGs who are likely to be referred for palliative care. Add 2 days because patients referred for palliative care are more complex and usually have longer length of stay. However, actual referral to palliative care is not likely before the third day of hospitalization. Starting with a hypothetical 6 days average length of stay for the institution will yield an average length of stay on the palliative care service of 5 days. For example, if estimated annual referrals is 160, total annual inpatient days is calculated to be 800. The average daily census is then estimated at 2.19 patients per day (Table 60.2).

From the average daily census, determine staff needs on the basis of optimal patient to staff member ratios. For example, if it is assumed that one physician can see 12 patients per day and the average daily census is 2, approximately 0.2 physician full-time equivalents are needed.

On the basis of total staff needs and salary, benefits, and overhead, add up to total staff expenses.

Billing Fee for Service

Direct revenue for the program will come from two sources: hospital reimbursement (the DRG or other insurance payment to the hospital) and physician or nurse practitioner billing. Hospital reimbursement can be estimated on the basis of service volume and projected DRG mix of the patients served. Estimates depend on the primary insurance and payer mix that covers the target patient population. Financial professionals from the home institution can help determine this.

Revenue from physician billing can be estimated on the basis of patient volume, types of services billed for, and the insurance coverage of the target patient population. Two billing codes are required for each patient encounter. The procedure/service codes are listed in the *Current Procedural Terminology* (CPT) manual. Palliative care specialists commonly use the evaluation and management codes. The appropriate code is determined by the complexity of the patient's encounter *or* by the time spent caring for the patient. Determining the CPT code on the basis of time is allowed when >50% of the time spent with the patient is used for care coordination or counseling, as is often the case in palliative care interactions. Other CPT codes are appropriate when procedures are performed. See the CAPC Web site's published documentation guidelines for more guidance.

The second code identifies the diagnoses and/or symptoms that justify the palliative care services. These are chosen from the International Classification of Disease-Clinical Modification (ICD-9-CM) codes (24). Palliative care consultation teams typically bill using symptom and condition codes (e.g., pain or debility), not the primary disease codes, to avoid conflict with the billing diagnoses of the primary physician and other consultants. Advance practice nurses, who are certified by the American Nursing Credentialing Center, are eligible for reimbursement for services provided under Medicare. However, because individual states regulate the practice of advance practice nurses, their ability to bill for services provided, and their ability to prescribe, each team will need to identify state-specific requirements. Where allowed, the process of billing by an advance practice nurse is similar to that described in the preceding text for physicians (43).

PRESENTING THE BUSINESS PLAN

The purpose of the business plan is to state clearly, positively, and concisely why the proposed palliative care program is necessary, how it will run in detail, and what it will take to ensure a successful program. A member of the planning team with experience and skill at writing should be responsible for putting together the business plan. It may be helpful to consult a business or marketing specialist or work closely with an administrator or board member with relevant expertise (44). The executive summary introduces the reader briefly (in one page) to the components within the full business plan.

The full business plan first summarizes the results of the system and needs assessments, describing current clinical and financial conditions at the institution and highlighting where there are opportunities for improvement, as well as areas that are functioning well (45). Next, these institutional conditions are set in national and local context. Include national standards of care and guidelines, such as the Joint Commission on Accreditation of Healthcare Organizations standard, the National Consensus Project Guidelines for Quality Palliative Care (46), recommendations of the American Pain Society for management of cancer pain (47), and the palliative care services provided by competitor institutions in the local market.

The business plan should then summarize data showing the effectiveness of palliative care in improving symptom management and patient and family satisfaction, and reducing costs. Describe exactly how the new program will function, how resources will be used, who will staff the service, how the service will be delivered, who the target patient population is, and how the program will integrate with existing hospital resources and services. Use clinical case examples to illustrate concretely how the new palliative care service will operate and serve the needs of the institution and its patients. Show the calculations of costs and revenues of the program compared with the potential for cost avoidance.

The business plan should convince administrators that the proposed new services will improve the quality of care for patients, be financially feasible or advantageous for the institution, provide a competitive advantage in the market, and represent a strategic investment of scarce resources and that the proposed team is committed and is therefore the optimal group to bring these goals to fruition.

IMPLEMENTING THE SERVICE

Despite the careful detailed planning that has been invested in the new service to this point, unforeseen barriers and challenges will inevitably arise as the program is implemented. Overcoming unforeseen barriers requires flexibility. Success of the program is dependent on producing highest quality service for the program's primary clients, the referring physicians. This means responding to consultation requests in a timely manner and being responsive to feedback from referring physicians, as well as patients and families, hospital staff, and institution administrators.

Growth of the program depends on meeting the clinical and financial projections laid out in the planning stage. Decreasing length of stay requires family meetings and discussions of the pros and cons of the various treatment alternatives early in the hospital stay (23). A good working relationship with hospital case management and local nursing home, home care, and hospice providers facilitates timely transfer of care to more appropriate community settings (48,49). Realizing projected revenue requires meticulous attention to documentation and a systematized billing process (Fig. 60.1).

MEASURING QUALITY AND IMPACT

Growth and sustainability of the program depends critically on documentation of outcomes. Prospectively gathered data about symptom management, patient and family satisfaction, and cost savings will have the greatest impact (50). What variables to measure and how to collect data on a daily basis should be planned before implementation of the new program. There are many available tools for gathering clinical data and evaluating patient satisfaction (Table 60.3). Build on the data gathered in the needs assessment to show concrete improvement as compared to baseline measures. Qualitative data including the perspective of patients and families will also have an impact on convincing leadership of the benefit of the program (51). In addition to showing positive impact of the new program, the goal of measurement is to identify opportunities for further quality improvement. Focus on measurable outcomes that can be improved upon by changing processes of care (52).

Palliative Care Consult Record

Name plate

Consultant_____ MD # _____
Consult request date _____
Patient location _____
Primary service _____
Date of hospital admission _____
Attending MD _____
Attending MD contact # _____
Referring clinician _____
Referring clinician contact # _____

Palliative care Dx:	Secondary Dx:		Underlying Dx:		
Initial Consult (enter dates)					
99251 Consult Focused/Straightforward (20 min)					
99252 Consult Expanded/Straightforward (40 min)					
99253 Consult Detail/ Low Complexity (55 min)					
99254 Consult High/Moderate Complexity (80 min)					
99255 Consult High/High Complexity (110 min)					
Subsequent Hospital Care					
99231 Focused/Low (15 min)					
99232 Expanded/Moderate (25 min)					
99233 Detail/High (35 min)					
99356 Prolonged Services Face to Face 1st hour					
99357 Face to face each additional 30 minutes					

Rate: None [0] Mild [1] Moderate[2] Severe[3]

Family mem/Patient/MD reporting? Please circle	F P MD	F P MD	F P MD	F P MD	F P MD
Pain					
Dyspnea					
Anxiety					
Other_____					
MSO$_4$ Levels					
Vitals					

FIGURE 60.1. Consult Record/Billing Card, 63/8″ × 57/8″, which can be folded in half to fit in pocket. **A:** Side one. **B:** Side two. (Adapted with permission from the online tools from The Center to Advance Palliative Care. Available at www.capc.org.)

Code status	Full	Advance directive? Y / N	If yes:	Living will	DPOA
DNR DNI					

Estimated life expectancy	24 hours	1 week	1 month	6 months	>6 months
	Pt aware of prognosis & plan ? Y / N		Family aware of prognosis & plan ? Y / N		

Current interventions   ET Tube   BiPap   FT/PEG   TPN   Drains   IV   Other_____

Symptoms/Issues	Interventions	Symptoms/Issues	Interventions
pain		death rattle	
dyspnea		GI symptoms	
fever/chills		agitation	
cough		other	

Family issues/interactions with patient and staff   Contact

person_____ # _____
                                        Address:

Transfers Admit to PCU _____   PCU Wait List _____   Pall. Care on Floor _____
                         (date)   (date)   Room_____   (date)

Person writing PCU admit orders _____ beeper _____

Clinical History
VRE? MRSA?
Active TB ?
Ventriculostomy ?
Endotracheal Tubes ?
Active c. difficile ?

© UCSF 2002

Bereavement follow-up	Discharge Date/Disposition

FIGURE 60.1. (*continued*).

MARKETING THE PROGRAM

A good marketing plan ensures that referring physicians, patients, families, and administrators are aware of the services the program provides, how the service can help them, how they can access the service, and what it will cost them (in terms of time, effort, complexity, and cost) to access the service. Match the message and the method of delivery to the audience. Patients and families want to know how palliative care will address their symptoms, improve communication with their physician, and lessen the burden on family caregivers. Informational brochures (see the CAPC Web site for examples), Web sites, and presentations at disease-specific societies, such as the Leukemia and Lymphoma Society and Alzheimer's Association, are effective means of reaching patients and families.

Referring physicians want to know how to quickly and easily reach the palliative care team for a consultation request and how the team will communicate with them to assist with patient care. Word of mouth, grand rounds, and other presentations are among the approaches used to reach referring physicians. Administrators want to know how the program improves the financial health and market position of the institution and how best to invest in the program's future. Present updates with financial and clinical outcome data to administrators at key time points in the budget cycle. In all cases, investigate and use existing channels of communication, such as the hospital Web site and local advertising venues.

SUSTAIN AND GROW

Successful demonstration of quality improvement through the word of mouth of satisfied referring physicians and their patients, in addition to continuous marketing, will ensure program growth. Plan ahead for growth by negotiating early how the administration will support expansion of the clinical team and services provided as volume rises. Prospectively collect the data that the stakeholders will need to determine whether to fund an expanded clinical team. Hiring additional staff usually lags behind the growth in referral volume. A busy

TABLE 60.3

DATA NEEDED TO MEASURE QUALITY OF CARE

Data element(s)	Source	Where stored?	Importance
Patient characteristics (date of consult, religion, ethnicity, education)	PPI	PCD	Required
Patient characteristics (Age; sex; medical record number; DRG; primary, secondary, tertiary diagnoses [ICD-9 code]; insurance; procedure codes)	HD	HD	Required
Functional status (e.g., Karnofsky score)	PPI	PCD	Required
Advance directive status	PPI	PCD	Important
Surrogate/NOK contact information	PPI	PCD	Required
Pain and symptom assessment	PPI	PCD	Required
Palliative care interventions	PCR	PCD	Nice to have
Postdischarge/death satisfaction	PPI	PCD	Important
Site of discharge	MR	PCD	Required
Documentation of advance directives[a]	MR/HD[b]	PCD/HD	Nice to have
Length of stay (hospital and ICU)	HD	HD	Required
Pharmacy information[b]	MR/HD	PCD/HD	Important/Nice to have
Cost measures	HD	HD	Required
Reimbursement rates by payer category for nonreimbursed services	HD	HD	Important
Philanthropy and grant funding	PCR	HD/PCD	Required

PPI, patient/proxy interview; PCR, palliative care records or palliative care team interview; MR, medical record; HD, hospital database; PCD, palliative care database; HD, hospital database; ICD-9, international classification of disease-9; NOK, next of kin.

[a]Some hospital database systems store this information.

[b]If pharmacy information is readily accessible from a hospital database, it can become a very powerful data element. If it is only available by chart review, it may not be worth the labor required to gather it.

Reprinted with permission from the center to advance palliative care. *A Guide to Building a Hospital-based Palliative Care Program.* Available at www.capc.org.

palliative care service is emotionally and physically demanding for staff and can pose a risk of burnout and staff turnover. Create a plan to support staff through the busiest times. Failing to plan for growth and professional self care (53) poses the single largest threat to the sustainability of hospital palliative care programs.

SUMMARY AND TAKE HOME POINTS

1. Document the hospital's need for a palliative care team through a system assessment process.
2. Understand and align the mission and priorities of the hospital with those of the palliative care program.
3. Thoroughly investigate the institution's strengths and needs before designing the new program.
4. Draw on existing institutional strengths and resources to leverage opportunities for positive change.
5. Using hospital-specific data, calculate how the new program will contribute to the financial health of the hospital through cost avoidance by decreasing length of stay and daily hospital costs.
6. Use clinical case examples to show how the new program will improve pain and symptom management; facilitate timely decision making; address the psychological, spiritual, and social needs of seriously ill patients and their families; and improve patient and family satisfaction.
7. Present the case for palliative care positively and, often, using opportunities to dispel myths.
8. Design a program that fits the institution's resources and needs.

9. Remember that the client is the referring physician and provide high-quality service to the client. Answer the question asked. Be timely and communicate personally.
10. Document success.
11. Plan for growth.

CONCLUSION

The recent rapid growth in the number of hospital palliative care services is testimony to their added quality and utility in the acute care setting. Hundreds of programs have successfully used the steps outlined here to initiate and sustain a palliative care program. More detail is available from the CAPC (www.capc.org) and the *Journal of Palliative Medicine.*

RESOURCES

- CAPC: technical assistance for clinicians and hospitals seeking to establish or strengthen a palliative care program—www.capc.org
- Palliative Care Leadership Centers: six exemplary palliative care programs providing site visits, hands-on training, and technical assistance to support new palliative care clinicians and programs nationwide—www.capc.org/pclc
- Promoting Excellence in End-of-Life Care: organization and Web site supporting innovative approaches to delivery of palliative care, plus comprehensive web-based tools and other resources—www.promotingexcellence.org

References

1. Desbiens NA, Mueller-Rizner N, Connors AF Jr, et al. The symptom burden of seriously ill hospitalized patients. SUPPORT Investigators. Study to Understand Prognoses and Preferences for Outcome and Risks of Treatment. *J Pain Symptom Manage* 1999;17(4):248–255.

2. Walke LM, Gallo WT, Tinetti ME, et al. The burden of symptoms among community-dwelling older persons with advanced chronic disease. *Arch Intern Med* 2004;164(21):2321–2324.

3. Teno JM, Clarridge BR, Casey V, et al. Family perspectives on end-of-life care at the last place of care. *JAMA* 2004;291(1):88–93.

4. Pritchard RS, Fisher ES, Teno JM, et al. Influence of patient preferences and local health system characteristics on the place of death. SUPPORT Investigators. Study to Understand Prognoses and Preferences for Risks and Outcomes of Treatment. *J Am Geriatr Soc* 1998;46(10):1242–1250.

5. Somogyi-Zalud E, Zhong Z, Hamel MB, et al. The use of life-sustaining treatments in hospitalized persons aged 80 and older. *J Am Geriatr Soc* 2002;50(5):930–934.

6. Singer PA, Martin DK, Kelner M. Quality end-of-life care: patients' perspectives. *JAMA* 1999;281(2):163–168.

7. Steinhauser KE, Christakis NA, Clipp EC, et al. Preparing for the end of life: preferences of patients, families, physicians, and other care providers. *J Pain Symptom Manage* 2001;22(3):727–737.

8. Steinhauser KE, Christakis NA, Clipp EC, et al. Factors considered important at the end of life by patients, family, physicians, and other care providers. *JAMA* 2000;284(19):2476–2482.

9. Steinhauser KE, Clipp EC, McNeilly M, et al. In search of a good death: observations of patients, families, and providers. *Ann Intern Med* 2000;132(10):825–832.

10. Baker R, Wu AW, Teno JM, et al. Family satisfaction with end-of-life care in seriously ill hospitalized adults. *J Am Geriatr Soc* 2000;48(5 Suppl):S61–S69.

11. Emanuel EJ, Fairclough DL, Slutsman J, et al. Assistance from family members, friends, paid care givers, and volunteers in the care of terminally ill patients. *N Engl J Med* 1999;341(13):956–963.

12. Emanuel EJ, Fairclough DL, Slutsman J, et al. Understanding economic and other burdens of terminal illness: the experience of patients and their caregivers. *Ann Intern Med* 2000;132(6):451–459.

13. Anderson GF. Physician, public, and policymaker perspectives on chronic conditions. *Arch Intern Med* 2003;163(4):437–442.

14. Anderson GF. Medicare and chronic conditions. *N Engl J Med* 2005;353(3):305–309.

15. Hogan C, Lunney J, Gabel J, et al. Medicare beneficiaries' costs of care in the last year of life. *Health Aff (Millwood)* 2001;20(4):188–195.

16. Billings JA, Pantilat S. Survey of palliative care programs in United States teaching hospitals. *J Palliat Med* 2001;4(3):309–314.

17. Morrison RS, Maroney-Galin, Kralovec PD, et al. The growth of palliative care programs in us hospitals. *J Palliat Med* 2005;8(6):1127–1134.

18. American Academy of Hospice and Palliative Medicine. Available at www.aahpm.org. Accessed on November 21, 2005.

19. von Gunten CF, Sloan PA, Portenoy RK, et al. Physician board certification in hospice and palliative medicine. *J Palliat Med* 2000;3(4):441–447.

20. CAPC. A guide to building a hospital-based palliative care program. New York: Center to Advance Palliative Care, 2004:www.capc.org.

21. Center to Advance Palliative Care. www.capc.org. Accessed November 22, 2005.

22. Davis MP, Walsh D, Nelson K, et al. The business of palliative medicine: management metrics for an acute-care inpatient unit. *Am J Hosp Palliat Care* 2001;18(1):26–29.

23. Davis MP, Walsh D, Nelson KA, et al. The business of palliative medicine–Part 2: the economics of acute inpatient palliative medicine. *Am J Hosp Palliat Care* 2002;19(2):89–95.

24. von Gunten CF. Financing palliative care. *Clin Geriatr Med* 2004;20(4):767–781, viii.

25. Finlay IG, Higginson IJ, Goodwin DM, et al. Palliative care in hospital, hospice, at home: results from a systematic review. *Ann Oncol* 2002;13(Suppl 4):257–264.

26. Smith TJ, Coyne P, Cassel B, et al. A high-volume specialist palliative care unit and team may reduce in-hospital end-of-life care costs. *J Palliat Med* 2003;6(5):699–705.

27. Back AL, Li YF, Sales AE. Impact of palliative care case management on resource use by patients dying of cancer at a veterans Affairs medical center. *J Palliat Med* 2005;8(1):26–35.

28. Dowdy MD, Robertson C, Bander JA. A study of proactive ethics consultation for critically and terminally ill patients with extended lengths of stay. *Crit Care Med* 1998;26(2):252–259.

29. Lilly CM, De Meo DL, Sonna LA, et al. An intensive communication intervention for the critically ill. *Am J Med* 2000;109(6):469–475.

30. Schneiderman LJ, Gilmer T, Teetzel HD, et al. Effect of ethics consultations on nonbeneficial life-sustaining treatments in the intensive care setting: a randomized controlled trial. *JAMA* 2003;290(9):1166–1172.

31. Campbell ML, Guzman JA. Impact of a proactive approach to improve end-of-life care in a medical ICU. *Chest* 2003;123(1):266–271.

32. Gilmer T, Schneiderman LJ, Teetzel H, et al. The costs of nonbeneficial treatment in the intensive care setting. *Health Aff (Millwood)* 2005;24(4):961–971.

33. Brumley RD, Enguidanos S, Cherin DA. Effectiveness of a home-based palliative care program for end-of-life. *J Palliat Med* 2003;6(5):715–724.

34. Rabow MW, Dibble SL, Pantilat SZ, et al. The comprehensive care team: a controlled trial of outpatient palliative medicine consultation. *Arch Intern Med* 2004;164(1):83–91.

35. Higginson IJ, Finlay IG, Goodwin DM, et al. Is there evidence that palliative care teams alter end-of-life experiences of patients and their caregivers? *J Pain Symptom Manage* 2003;25(2):150–168.

36. Du Pen SL, Du Pen AR, Polissar N, et al. Implementing guidelines for cancer pain management: results of a randomized controlled clinical trial. *J Clin Oncol* 1999;17(1):361–370.

37. Jack B, Hillier V, Williams A, et al. Hospital based palliative care teams improve the symptoms of cancer patients. *Palliat Med* 2003;17(6):498–502.

38. Ringdal GI, Jordhoy MS, Kaasa S. Family satisfaction with end-of-life care for cancer patients in a cluster randomized trial. *J Pain Symptom Manage* 2002;24(1):53–63.

39. Chong K, Olson EM, Banc TE, et al. Types and rate of implementation of palliative care team recommendations for care of hospitalized veterans. *J Palliat Med* 2004;7(6):784–790.

40. Manfredi PL, Morrison RS, Morris J, et al. Palliative care consultations: how do they impact the care of hospitalized patients? *J Pain Symptom Manage* 2000;20(3):166–173.

41. Fischberg D, Meier DE. Palliative care in hospitals. *Clin Geriatr Med* 2004;20(4):735–751, vii.

42. Casarett DJ, Hirschman KB, Coffey JF, et al. Does a palliative care clinic have a role in improving end-of-life care? Results of a pilot program. *J Palliat Med* 2002;5(3):387–396.

43. Kuebler KK. The palliative care advanced practice nurse. *J Palliat Med* 2003;6(5):707–714.

44. Walsh D, Gombeski WR Jr, Goldstein P, et al. Managing a palliative oncology program: the role of a business plan. *J Pain Symptom Manage* 1994;9(2):109–118.

45. Cohn KH, Schwartz RW. Business plan writing for physicians. *Am J Surg* 2002;184(2):114–120.

46. National Consensus Project. *Clinical Practice Guidelines for Quality Palliative Care.* Available at www.nationalconsensusproject.org. Accessed on November 21, 2005.

47. Gordon DB, Dahl JL, Miaskowski C, et al. American pain society recommendations for improving the quality of acute and cancer pain management: American Pain Society Quality of Care Task Force. *Arch Intern Med* 2005;165(14):1574–1580.

48. Meier DE. When pain and suffering do not require a prognosis: working toward meaningful hospital-hospice partnership. *J Palliat Med* 2003;6(1):109–115.

49. Meier DE, Thar W, Jordan A, et al. Integrating case management and palliative care. *J Palliat Med* 2004;7(1):119–134.

50. Nelson KA, Walsh D. The business of palliative medicine–Part 3: the development of a palliative medicine program in an academic medical center. *Am J Hosp Palliat Care* 2003;20(5):345–352.

51. Gysels M, Hughes R, Aspinal F, et al. What methods do stakeholders prefer for feeding back performance data: a qualitative study in palliative care. *Int J Qual Health Care* 2004;16(5):375–381.

52. Morrison RS, Siu AL, Leipzig RM, et al. The hard task of improving the quality of care at the end of life. *Arch Intern Med* 2000;160(6):743–747.

53. Meier DE. Planning for the mixed blessing of unexpected growth. *J Palliat Med* 2005;8(5):906–908.

CHAPTER 61 ■ STAFF STRESS AND BURNOUT

MARY L.S. VACHON AND CHRISTOPHER SHERWOOD

Stress in the care of the dying has been being studied for more than 30 years (1,2). Recent research (3,4) indicates that little seems to have changed in the last four decades. Some improvements have been made. However, at times, organizations for a variety of reasons, including economic concerns, may go through phases when they are more or less open and able to make the changes that might decrease staff stress. Caregivers need to take responsibility for dealing with some of their own issues and incorporating proven stress management techniques into their lives, making sure that the job of dealing with issues related to staff stress is not totally the responsibility of the organizations.

This chapter will provide a selective review of the literature showing that many of the stressors appear not to have changed in the last four decades and will then look at current research to do both, better understand the process of what is happening and attempt to remedy the situation, changing what can be changed. Research shows that younger caregivers have more stress (5,6) and fewer coping mechanisms (5), so it is not surprising that there continues to be stress as new people come into the field. Issues inherent in responding to increasing number of patients with cancer, new treatment methods, "demanding consumers", dealing with cancer as a chronic illness, overwork, coping with life and death issues, communicating with people who are at a critical and vulnerable point in their lives, and dealing with colleagues who can be both a major source of support as well as a major stressor in our lives (5) will not be easy to deal with. Both personal and organizational approaches will be required to prepare new caregivers for the field; to support those in the middle of their career as they are juggling many family and career issues; and to provide the senior members of our disciplines with an opportunity of their lives in which their rich experiences can be valued and used to provide wisdom for those who will follow in their footsteps and develop their own paths, from which we can all benefit. It is to the benefit of many of us that there will be sufficient resources and resilient staff to deal with our families and us when it is our time to avail ourselves of the skill of those in supportive oncology and palliative care.

OVERVIEW

This chapter will review a variety of models that caregivers might consciously or unconsciously follow in their practice of supportive oncology and palliative care; will review recent concepts of burnout (7,8) and compassion fatigue (9,10) differentiating burnout from depression (11,12); will discuss the concepts of job engagement (7) and compassion satisfaction (CS) (13) and utilize a framework developed by Maslach et al. (7) to understand the general factors contributing to burnout, showing that many of the sources of stress and burnout in supportive oncology and palliative care have not changed in the last 30 years. Finally, works on job satisfaction in the areas of supportive oncology and palliative care will be reviewed and recent research on improving both organizational and personal coping will be discussed. In general, the focus in this chapter will be on recent literature; the history of the field and the literature have been reviewed elsewhere (14,15).

MODELS OF CARING

In their powerful book, *Crossing Over: Narratives of Palliative Care*, which describes the experience of palliative care in two settings in the United States and Canada, Barnard, Towers, Boston, and Lambrinidou (16) state, "palliative care is whole-person care not only in the sense that the whole person of the patient (body, mind, spirit) is the object of care, but also in that the whole person of the caregiver is involved. Palliative care is, par excellence, care that is given through the medium of a human relationship" (16, p. 5). The authors document the experiences of patients, families, and caregivers during some of their finest and not so fine moments. The reader comes to understand the humanity of all involved.

A more recent study of nurses in a Netherlands academic palliative care setting (17) was undertaken by Georges et al. to gain insight into the fact that many nurses were leaving, frustrated by the far-reaching medical orientation on the ward and feeling unable to provide the care they wanted to give. These nurses were not neophytes. They were generally oncology nurses aged 35–55 years and had been working on this unit from 6 months to more than 4 years. They raised questions about the benefits and burdens of the medical treatment with which they collaborated. This study challenges whether the assumptions of Barnard are completely generalizable at this point in time and may shed some light on some of the conflicts in supportive oncology and palliative care in the early 21st century. This study will be compared with that of Bernice Catherine Harper (18). Dr. Harper is a social worker, whose initial work involved supervising other social workers at the City of Hope Hospital in California. Her initial work was in the 1970s, drawing from much earlier work done in the 1950s, and was updated in 1994. Harper carefully supervised social workers and developed a Schematic Comfort-Ability Growth and Development Scale in coping with professional anxieties in death and dying. Her model proposes "learning to be comfortable in working with the dying patient and his family must be preceded by a growth and developmental process or sequence including cycles of productive change, observable behavior, and feeling" (18, p. 124).

Comfort-Ability Growth and Development in Coping with Professional Anxieties in Death and Dying

Harper has a six-stage model, taking the caregiver from being a neophyte in the first month of working in the oncology field to a stage of 10 years or more of practice. The process involves careful supervision with a focus on the care of the dying and implies that the caregiver wishes to become more involved at an emotional level with clients.

Stage I Intellectualization 1–3 months.
- Provides practical help. Generally, the clinician relates on an intellectual basis, rejecting any emotional involvement.
- Marked by periods of brisk activities as the worker tries to manage latent anxiety by completely understanding the hospital setting, policies, and procedures, but at the same time familiarizing oneself with the disease and the physical aspects of death and dying. Ineffective coping and managing of anxiety results in withdrawing and not being able to speak with the patient and the family about death and dying.
- At this point in the professional career caregivers might be seen as experiencing empathic failure, the failure of one part of a system to understand the meaning and experience of another (19).

Stage II Emotional Survival 3–6 months.
- The caregiver experiences trauma, often accompanied by guilt and anxiety.
- As one confronts the reality of the patient's impending death, one must confront simultaneously one's own eventual death. The caregiver comes face to face with the reality that "but by the grace of God go I."
- Feelings of self-pity exist along with feelings of pity for the patient. These feelings often lead to feelings of guilt and frustration. "This traumatized state of awareness often fosters extreme hostility within the worker as one tries to 'fight back'. With this emotional experience, stage I passes into stage II, thereby jolting the worker out of the inertia of intellectualization into the activity of emotional involvement. Without this, the emotional growth could not transpire" (18, p. 45).

Stage III Depression 6–9 months.
- The most crucial in the schematic growth and development scale–the "Grow or Go" stage.
- Mastery of self is a real challenge in this stage and this requires a growing acceptance of death and an orientation to the reality of death and dying.
- Some workers experience extreme anxiety, grief, and depression. They question their usefulness, and real ability to contribute and be helpful; and express anger, hurt, and inability to come to terms with the situation. The pain, mourning and grieving are a part of the regression of not accepting the loss and then a moving forward to accept death and dying.
- Depending on how caregivers handle their feelings of depression, they may quit the job or learn to live with it.

Stage IV Emotional Arrival 9–12 months.
- Marked by a sense of freedom—freedom from the debilitating effects, which are inhered in the previous stages of the experiential growth process. The caregiver is now largely free from identifying with the patient's symptoms, free from the preoccupation with one's own death and dying, free from guilt feelings about one's own good health, and free from incapacitating periods of depression.
- The caregiver is not insensitive, rather the caregiver's sensitivities have sharpened. Although one is not free from pain, one is typically free from its incapacitating effects. At this stage the caregiver has "appropriate" emotions and has the sensitivity to grieve and the resilience to recover. "In other words one has reached the stage at which one has the control to practice the art of one's science" (18, p. 71).

Stage V Deep Compassion 12–24 months.
- Involves self-realization, self-awareness, and self-actualization. The developmental process involves the caregiver 'doing for himself'. This growth process contains all the elements of stages I–IV plus personal values, self-reliance, and the realistic acceptance of life and death.
- At this point caregivers have seen all the physical aspects of the illness and have come to know and understand that in some cases living can be more painful for the patient and family than dying.
- "Stage V is the culminating point of all the growth and development that has previously transpired. The learning process was anxious, traumatic, painful, and depressing, but the product of the process in terms of professional growth and development is rewarding" (18, p. 83).
- The caregiver's behavior and performance are enhanced by the dignity and self-respect one feels toward the self, thus enabling one to give dignity and respect to the dying person.
- The deep compassion felt by the caregiver toward the dying person is translated into constructive and appropriate activities on the basis of human and professional assessment of the needs of the dying person and the family.

Stage VI The Doer 8–10 years beyond stage V.
- Demonstrates inner knowledge and wisdom, inner power, and inner strength. "… there is reinforcement, enhanced wisdom and knowledge to the understanding of death and dying. There is less and less misunderstanding of death. The professional and caregiver see, understand and accept death as a part of life's transitions" (18, p. 122). "In order to use what you know, you must know what you use" (18, p. 99).
- This stage is the flowering of the health professional. It is characterized by "the mature seasoned professional who operates, acts, and reacts on the basis of maturity. Mature adults are well aware of self. They know where they have been, where they want to go and what they need to do to get there"

(18, p. 99). This person is able to work well with the sick, terminally ill, and their families.

- "The Burned-Out Syndrome is not a point at issue. Professional growth and development of the seasoned health professionals prevent burnout because these professionals take each stage and each phase of growth and development in their stride and grow in the process. They are able to identify with the terrible events and diseases of the patients without letting these events destroy them, without getting 'burned out'".
- Acceptance, competence, and trust are exhibited in stage VI.
- To some extent, doers have learned how to gather from the universe what they need, to do their work. Their clients recognize something in them and give feedback information that can then be used to help others.

For some, "gathering from the universe" might mean plugging into an intuitive wisdom, which comes over time. Dr. David Cumes is a urologic surgeon, originally from South Africa where he learned about traditional ways of healing before coming to the United States and specializing at Stanford Medical Center, where he also taught. Cumes (20) writes about getting in touch with the Inner Healer and one's intuitive wisdom, in part through wilderness trekking and connecting with what he calls the 'Field'. He quotes The Bhagavad Gita "*Whatever being comes to be, be it motionless or moving, derives its being from the 'field' and 'knower of the field'. Know this.*" Cumes speaks of us all being "knowers" of the Field.

> "Not only are we in the Field, but the Field is in us. The cosmic Field seems to extend from us as an energy reservoir in space through which signals pass back and forth. We could divide the messages that traverse the Field simply into Knowable and Unknowable. Light, sound, radio, TV, electromagnetic pulses and chemicals as subtle as pheromones are some of the Knowable signals that travel through the Field.
> Many Knowable "mini" Fields are encountered in nature. We see the marvel of a termite colony, where the Field of intelligence of the colony far exceeds the capacity of the nervous system of any singular termite...However, there are also Unknowable forces transmitted through the Field such as telepathic and healing energies, which science has been unable to define or measure" (20, p. 114).

Cumes writes of returning from a wilderness trek in Peru to a busy schedule of patients, one of whom was a young man requiring a lymph node dissection for a cancerous tumor Dr. Cumes had removed before going on his trip. He did the surgery. The next morning he woke up at 5:00 AM

> "... with an unusual degree of clarity. In this wide-awake state I was unable to get back to sleep and lay restlessly in bed. I felt uneasy about something, but could not put my finger on it. I decided to go to the hospital to make rounds early. It was dark when I arrived at the hospital to visit Jim. The nurse wondered what I was doing at the hospital so early and accompanied me to his bed. As we entered his room, it was obvious that Jim had stopped breathing. The nurse had seen him shortly before I arrived and everything had been fine. We began to ventilate him immediately because his reaction might have been due to an oversensitivity to morphine, gave him a drug called Narcan, which reverses the effect of morphine. There was a dramatic response and Jim began to breathe immediately. He came to, confused and wanting to know what had happened, but none the worse for the experience.
> When I left the hospital after the incident, I gave a sigh of relief and realized how different the outcome could have been if something had not awakened me that morning. I wondered if my sensitivity to messages from the Field had been increased after the past two weeks in the pristine wilderness of the Andes" (20, p. 120).

Cumes states that "All healing involves four factors: the healer, the patient, the place where the healing occurs and the presence of a universal Field that embraces both healer and patient" (20, p. 11).

Michael Kearney, a hospice physician, also tries to elucidate these concepts (21). He uses concepts in the new physics to describe the integration between the traditional medical model and the healing model, which can be applied in palliative care and its relevance to the relationship between the caregiver and the patient. "The quantum idea that ours is a participatory universe has implications for carers. Although there are still subjects and objects within the healing model, the boundaries may not be as clear as they are within the medical model. Caring now becomes a dynamic event. While the roles of 'carer' and 'patient' remain, there is also an interweaving of the two. The term 'clinical objectivity' is joined by that of 'clinical subjectivity', acknowledging a shared dimension to the healing encounter".

Striving to Adopt a Well-Organized and Purposeful Approach versus Striving to Increase the Well-being of the Patient

A very different approach to caring comes from the work of Georges et al. (17). They reported that "the academic character of the ward, focus on palliative treatment of symptoms, and need to achieve a high turnover rate of patients because of high demand and reduced bed capacity seem to encourage nurses to adopt an attitude promoting a more rational approach to care". The authors quoted an earlier study on an intervention on that unit by Van Staa et al. (22) as noting that, "Although the mission of the unit has been stated as: 'to put the patient and his or her loved ones first in mind, heart and soul', little attention had been given to substantial deepening of the philosophy of palliative care. Paying attention to emotions and questions of meaning and developing a therapeutic and relational approach were seen by the management committee as typical of the hospice movement. Therefore, it was thought that efforts must be directed essentially to the development of an instrumental approach involving developing care protocols and increasing outreach activities (22,23). Therefore, nurses were much more preoccupied with issues of competence and other practical matters and developed task-oriented attitudes".

The unit was having trouble retaining nursing staff. Two methods of practice described the nurses' actual activity: the first was the more prominent, 'striving to adopt a well-organized and purposeful approach as a nurse on an academic ward' (n = 12); the second is 'striving to increase the well-being of the patient' (n = 2). Although the sample size is small, the issues presented may shed some very important light on some of the issues in palliative care and supportive oncology. The following section is adapted from reference 24.

The Striving of Nurses to Adopt a Well-Organized and Purposeful Approach in an Academic Setting

Several of the nurses adopted an academic attitude, underpinning their nursing practices with a scientific and professional rationale. They felt that it was important to use a 'scientific' classification system of nursing diagnosis, to formulate nursing interventions in relation to the diagnosis, and to work within the limits set by the policy of the ward and the hospital. They were concerned with appropriate bed utilization and attempted to make discharge arrangements at an early stage to avoid unnecessary occupation of beds. Carrying out the nursing process in a professional manner was more important than investing in their relationships with patients.

Developing a Professional Attitude

The nurses took a rational approach principally directed at gaining information about patients' symptoms and gaining insight into their problems. These nurses had a more detached attitude and tended to focus on identified tasks and problems. For example, when giving information to patients, nurses may pay much attention to clarity and completeness while failing to consider the emotional impact of the message.

Striving to Remain Objective

Patients' health problems were described in a formal language. The nurses avoided speaking about problems that could not be labeled well because they were not sure members of the multidisciplinary team could understand them. They argued that being objective was more in accordance with current professional developments in the field of nursing. They used diagnostic instruments to establish their observations. This allowed them to feel more comfortable when speaking with physicians, to feel they were seen as being more trustworthy, and hence to be involved in the decision-making process. These nurses consciously strive to avoid allowing their feelings to have an impact on their response to situations.

Being Task Oriented

These nurses are mostly committed to improving the situation of patients by solving or reducing their problems. They find it important to see that their interventions actually do improve the situation. When it is not possible to find a solution for patients' problems, for example, to achieve sufficient symptom control, especially pain, nurses feel powerless and feel that they have not been able to achieve something meaningful for patients.

Avoiding Emotional Stress

Coping with the emotional aspects of palliative care was a leading theme in the interviews with these nurses. The stress they experienced seemed to be related mainly to their appraisal of, and approach to, palliative care. Some said that the gravity of caring for dying patients would inevitably lead to burnout, so they did not plan to work too long in palliative care. They tended to distance themselves from patients by focusing on tasks and the treatment of symptoms. Some nurses explain that their experience has taught them to remain more professional and detached, while others decided consciously not to invest too much in their relationship with patients because it would be too demanding.

Embracing a Practitioner-Focused Perspective

Nurses found it difficult to distance themselves from their own beliefs and to learn to be available to discern the perspective of patients and the meaning of the situation for them. Working in accordance with rules, they emphasized the need to respect important rules of the ward. When, for example, patients mention that they are considering euthanasia, some nurses explain that patients first have to follow the procedures in the organization and then go on to explain them to the patient. "These nurses, by being mainly directed to using a rational and 'scientific' approach to their tasks, could fail to meet the real needs of patients and to pay sufficient attention to the development of a compassionate attitude. This perception, which was very much present on the ward, is mainly characterized by a distant approach towards patients and a well-developed self-awareness to work on one's own development as a professional."

Striving to Increase the Well-being of the Patient

Nurses who practiced under the second model striving to increase the well-being of the patient felt that it was important to use their individual capabilities, such as being sensitive to patients' concerns, and adapted their approach to individual patients. They found that, when fully aware of the needs of patients, it was not difficult to explain them to other caregivers.

Care appeared to be a central concern for these nurses and a main source of satisfaction. They were aware that, thanks to their caring attitude, they could mean something to patients, even if only for a short time, and they felt this to be rewarding. The characteristics of these nurses are discussed in the following sections.

Adopting a Humble Attitude

To act in accordance with the needs of patients, these nurses put their own considerations aside and found a way to cope with their own emotions. They strove to adopt an unobtrusive approach and to show their availability to patients without forcing anything, even without expecting patients to answer their 'invitation'. This concept is similar to that described by Roshi Joan Halifax and Barbara Dossey (25) "An unknown territory, death often produces unpredictable responses that challenge all of us. The 'trouble spots' are the ground for learning to open our hearts. As we open our hearts we learn to let go of our conceptions, and letting go is the basis of equanimity. It provides the deepest opportunity to practice the three tenets of not-knowing, bearing witness, and healing. Maybe we find ourselves a little more humble and wiser for it all" (25, p. 157).

Giving Attention to Patients and Their Experiences

This approach was shaped by sensitivity to the feelings of patients, trying to discover and understand what patients experience and why they react as they do. To be conscious of patients' experiences requires being really present. Some nurses, for example, are concerned that giving inadequate or incomplete information to patients could badly affect the direction of their decision about further treatment. By their sensitivity to the experiences of patients they become more connected with them and try to really help them, even if they have to 'break the rules'.

Being Available

Being available, truly present, appears to be a major virtue of nurses so they can perceive the troubles and needs of a patient. They speak about being sensitive to unspoken messages and about trusting their intuition. Being receptive to what is going on helps them see how they can contribute to the well-being of patients.

Valuing a Caring Attitude

The meaning that nurses assign to their work is mainly based on their experience as nurses and on their daily encounters with patient care. They developed a caring attitude on the basis of authentic relationships with patients.

Remaining Attentive and Thoughtful

To find solutions to the problems they are confronted with, these nurses used self-reflection, striving to adopt a patient-centered attitude and to improve their caring attitude. They were also attentive to the context of their work, particularly to what should be changed to make it easier to express a caring perspective.

Trying to Accept and Cope with Emotional Strain

Nurses recognized that by caring for patients whose life is limited they are exposed to painful moments. However, they tried to accept emotionally difficult situations as a part of their own reality and did not attempt to avoid them. They strove to remain 'authentic' and stay close to patients even if they could not alleviate their problems.

Reflections on a Comparison of the Two Models

A comparison of Harper's (18) work with that of Georges et al. (17) shows that, while Harper's model is very useful to describe the career path of some staff in supportive oncology and palliative care, there may be others who do not progress in the manner which Harper describes. From her perspective, these staff members may never have evolved beyond the first stage of comfortability. They are still involved in an intellectual approach to their role and are defending against allowing emotions to intrude. However, the nurses in the category striving to increase the well-being of the patient could be seen to be in Harper's stage IV or higher in which they have "the control to practice the art of one's science" (18, p. 71).

Part of the reason for the split between the two approaches to nursing may be due to the bureaucratization of hospice palliative care. Byock (26) notes that Max Weber, the renowned German sociologist, observed that while social movements evolve to meet the needs of the time, they continue only through the process of bureaucratization. "Routinization is part and parcel of a social movement's success; with it comes stability, confidence and bureaucracy" (27). Some of the issues being confronted by the nurses in the Georges et al. study (17) can be seen as related to the bureaucratization and standardization of palliative care. Doyle (28) and Kearney (29) warned earlier that palliative care specialists needed to avoid becoming merely symptomatologists. The field needed to recognize that "We are, in the presence of death, working toward health-that balance of body, mind and spirit that is so much more than freedom from disease. For that reason I believe we have no choice but to be alert to and responsive to human spiritual needs" (28).

> "..(I)t as though the dragon (that is the patient's distress) also guards a treasure-something essential for that particular individual's healing at that moment in time. It is suggested that if we in palliative medicine fail to accept this view, a view which allows that there may also be a potential in the suffering of the dying process, if we sell out completely to the literalism of the medical model with its view that such suffering is only a problem, we will be in danger of following a pattern which could lead to our becoming 'symptomatologists', within just another specialty" (29).

STRESS, BURNOUT, AND COMPASSION FATIGUE

Response to stress in oncology and palliative care has been measured in a number of ways including measuring various aspects of stress, psychological distress, and burnout.

More recently there has been interest in the concept of compassion fatigue (9,10). Compassion fatigue (9) has been used to describe a syndrome that shares some characteristics with burnout: depression, anxiety, hypochondria, combativeness, the sensation of being on "fast forward," and an inability to concentrate. Garfield et al. (30) state, however, that in contrast to one who has burned out, the caregiver with compassion fatigue can still care and be involved. Wright (31), a clinical nurse specialist and trauma/bereavement counselor

working in an Accident and Emergency Department in the United Kingdom, gives the following signs of compassion fatigue: 'no energy for it anymore'; 'emptied, nothing left to give'; 'not wanting to go there again'; 'feeling depleted in every dimension'; 'too many questions and no answers'; 'why am I doing this?'.

Table 61.1 gives the definition of terms related to burnout and compassion fatigue and their more positive aspects of job engagement and CS. Table 61.2 gives a list of symptoms reflective of compassion fatigue and burnout. Stamm (13) suggests that if compassion fatigue and burnout are combined there may be no energy available to sustain the vision of a better world, in which one could find satisfaction. Burnout, characterized by exhaustion, seems to make it impossible to envision a world in which one is not overwhelmed by an ability to be efficacious (39,40). The lack of efficacy (individual or corporate) likely colors negatively a person's view of his or her fit with a personal belief system (13).

Burnout and Depression

Brenninkmeyer et al. (41) differentiated burnout from depression. Given that the clinical picture of depression seems to reflect a general sense of self defeat, they hypothesized that individuals high in burnout and low in superiority (how individuals see themselves in comparison to others) would experience depressive symptoms. Depressive symptomatology was highest among individuals high in burnout who experienced a decline in superiority. "Depression was more strongly related to superiority than emotional exhaustion and depersonalization. In fact, emotional exhaustion, which constitutes the core symptom of burnout, did not have a significant association with superiority" (41, p. 879).

They concluded "reduced sense of superiority and a perceived loss of status are more characteristic of depressed individuals than for individuals who are burnt out. It seems that burnt-out individuals are still 'in the battle' for obtaining status and consider themselves as potential winners, while depressed individuals have given up" (41, p. 879).

Two recent large European studies have assessed the overlap between depression and burnout. In a Finnish study (11), burnout and depressive disorders were clearly related. The risk of depressive disorders, especially major depressive disorder (12-month prevalence), was greater when burnout was severe. Half of the participants with severe burnout had some depressive disorder. Those with a current major depressive episode suffered from serious burnout more often than those who had suffered a major depressive episode earlier.

The Dutch study (12) involved 3385 employees in a variety of work settings; after controlling for background variables, the strongest predictor of all three burnout facets was current depressive symptomatology. Hospital personnel (mostly female with a high level of interpersonal contact) reported the most depressive symptoms. Independent of the effects of background variables and current depressive symptoms, having ever experienced a depressive episode further predicted current symptoms of two burnout facets: emotional exhaustion and cynicism. In addition, a history of depression in close family members independently predicted current symptoms of emotional exhaustion. The authors concluded that a predisposition to depression, as reflected by a personal and family history of depression, may increase the risk for burnout.

In a southern European study of oncologists (42), low psychosocial orientation and burnout symptoms (i.e., emotional exhaustion, depersonalization, and poor personal accomplishment in their job) were associated with lower confidence in

TABLE 61.1

DEFINITION OF TERMS

Stress	■ The strain that remains "in response to the failure to manage tensions well and to overcome stressors" (32) ■ Observed at the physiologic, psychological, and behavioral levels of analysis (33,34) ■ An ongoing process affected by individual personality factors and environmental variables. The individual constantly responds to and interacts with the environment ■ Whether the stress is a benefit or a harm to the individual depends greatly on the individual's cognitive appraisal of the stress and subsequent coping process ■ "There is increasing consensus around defining work-related stress in terms of the 'interactions' between employee and (exposure to hazards in) their work environment. Within this model stress can be said to be experienced when the demands from the work environment exceed the employee's ability to cope with (or control) them" (35)
Burnout	■ "The progressive loss of idealism, energy and purpose experienced by people in the helping professions as a result of the conditions of their work" (36) ■ A syndrome of responses involving increased feelings of emotional exhaustion, negative attitudes toward the recipients of one's service (depersonalization), a tendency to evaluate oneself negatively with regard to one's work, and a feeling of dissatisfaction with accomplishments on the job (8) ■ The root cause of burnout lies in people's need to believe that their life is meaningful, and that the things they do—and consequently they themselves—are important and significant (37)
Job engagement	■ The opposite of burnout ■ Engagement is defined as a persistent, positive-affective-motivational state of fulfillment in employees that is characterized by vigor, dedication, and absorption ■ Involves energy, involvement, and efficacy ■ The individual's relationship with work, involving: a sustainable workload, feelings of choice and control, appropriate recognition and reward, a supportive work community, fairness and justice, and meaningful and valued work ■ Engagement is also characterized by high levels of activation and pleasure (7)
Compassion fatigue	■ Compassion fatigue is a more user-friendly term for secondary traumatic stress disorder which is almost identical to Post-traumatic Stress Disorder (PTSD), except that it applies to those emotionally affected by the trauma of another (usually a client or family member) (10) ■ Most often this concept is associated with the "cost of caring" for others in emotional pain (38) ■ Also known as *secondary or vicarious traumatization* ■ One form of burnout (37) ■ On the Compassion Satisfaction and Fatigue (CSF) Test a higher score on compassion fatigue reflects symptoms of work-related PTSD, rapid onset as a result of exposure to highly stressful caregiving (13)
Compassion satisfaction	■ The satisfaction derived from the work of helping others ■ Compassion satisfaction plays a vital role in the equation of human services ■ May be the portrayal of efficacy ■ Compassion satisfaction may be happiness with what one can do to make the world in which one lives a reflection of what one thinks it should be ■ On the CSF Test a higher score on compassion satisfaction reflects better satisfaction with ability to caregive (e.g., derives pleasure from helping, likes colleagues, feels good about ability to help, makes contribution (13)

communication skills and higher expectation of a negative outcome following physician–patient communication.

A MODEL FOR UNDERSTANDING OCCUPATIONAL STRESS

Maslach et al. (7) reviewed the research on burnout over the last three decades. Previous research focused on the Person-Environment Fit model (43). More recent research has focused on the degree of match or mismatch between the person and the six domains of the job environment. The greater the gap or mismatch between the person and the environment, the greater the likelihood of burnout. The greater the match or the fit, the greater the likelihood of engagement with work. Mismatches arise when the process of establishing a

psychological contact leaves critical issues unresolved, or when the working relationship changes to something that the person finds unacceptable. Mismatches lead to burnout. Six areas of work life come together in a framework that encompasses the major organizational antecedents of burnout. These include: workload, control, reward, community, fairness, and values.

Burnout arises from severe mismatches between people and their work settings in some or all of these areas. Preliminary evidence suggests that the area of values may play a central mediating role for the other areas. Alternatively, people may vary in the extent to which each of the six areas is important to them, as can be hypothesized from the earlier section Models Of Caring. Some people may place a higher weight on rewards than on values, or people may be prepared to tolerate a mismatch regarding workload if they receive praise, good pay, and have good relationships with colleagues.

TABLE 61.2

EXAMPLES OF COMPASSION FATIGUE BURNOUT SYNDROMES

Cognitive	Emotional	Behavioral	Spiritual	Personal relations	Somatic	Work performance
Lowered concentration	Powerlessness	Impatient	Questioning the meaning of life	Withdrawal	Shock	Low morale
Decreased self-esteem	Anxiety	Irritable	Loss of purpose	Decreased interest in intimacy or sex	Sweating	Low motivation
Apathy	Guilt	Withdrawn	Lack of self satisfaction	Mistrust	Rapid heartbeat	Avoiding tasks
Rigidity	Anger/rage	Moody	Pervasive hopelessness	Isolation from others	Breathing difficulties	Obsession about details
Disorientation	Survivor guilt	Regression	Anger at God	Overprotection as a parent	Aches and pains	Apathy
Perfectionism	Shutdown	Sleep disturbances	Questioning prior religious beliefs	Protection of anger or blame	Dizziness	Negativity
Minimization	Numbness	Nightmares	Loss of faith in a higher power	Intolerance	Increased number and intensity of medical maladies	Lack of appreciation
Preoccupation with trauma	Fear	Appetite changes	Greater skepticism about religion	Loneliness	Other somatic complaints	Detachment
Thoughts of self harm or harm to others	Helplessness	Hypervigilance		Increased interpersonal conflicts	Impaired immune system	Poor work commitments
	Sadness	Elevated startle response				Staff conflicts
	Depression	Accident proneness				Absenteeism
	Emotional roller coaster	Losing things				Exhaustion
	Depleted					Irritability
	Overly sensitive					Withdrawal from colleagues

Table used with permission from Figley CR, ed. *Treating compassion fatigue*. New York: Brunner-Routledge, 2002.

While the literature has been somewhat divided as to whether the care of the dying is a major stressor in hospice palliative care (5,15), recent research in the burnout area has focused explicitly on emotion–work variables (e.g., requirement to display or suppress emotions on the job, requirements to be emotionally empathic) and has found that these emotional factors do account for additional variance in burnout scores over and above job stressors (7). Table 61.3 uses this model to review select studies in stress and burnout from the last four decades involving research in Canada (2–4,44,45), the United States (46), the United Kingdom (6,47,48), France (49), and Turkey (50) and an international study of close to 600 caregivers who came from many countries and were interviewed individually or in small groups in Canada, the United States, Australia, and Europe (5). In Table 61.3 the column on values has been omitted because this area has not been explicitly studied in the cited research. This section will apply the framework to the studies in Table 61.3 as well as refer to some other relevant recent studies.

Workload

Excessive workload exhausts the individual to the extent that recovery becomes impossible. Emotional work is especially draining when the job requires people to display emotions inconsistent with their feelings. Workload relates to the exhaustion component of burnout. In Table 61.3, it can be seen from the early 1970s that there were perceived difficulties with workload, and insufficient staff to do the job at hand. From the 1970s, through the ensuing decades to the 21st century, staffs report being overwhelmed with the workload imposed by the increase in cancer and the chronic nature of the illness. Sometimes different terms are used to describe the same phenomenon. Vachon (5) uses the term role overload to describe what Grunfeld (4) describes as feeling under pressure to meet deadlines and the term role conflict to describe "having conflicting demands on time". In the original research by Vachon (5), job–home interaction was seen as a manifestation of

stress; in more recent work, the problem continues to exist but is labeled as a stressor.

Van Staa et al. (22) studied the staff in a hospice in the Netherlands and found that direct patient care activities have an impact on stress through a heavy workload of complex care, a shortage of staff, and an experienced lack of competence. Palliative care workers in rural Australia spoke of the difficulty involved in being expected to work beyond normal working hours and of the lack of anonymity in a small rural community (51).

Control

Control is related to inefficacy or reduced personal accomplishment. Mismatches often indicate that individuals have insufficient control over the resources necessary to do their work or insufficient authority to pursue the work in what they believe is the most effective manner. From the 1970s, stress has resulted from a lack of knowledge in interpersonal skills and a lack of communication and/or management skills (6,44,47–49). Issues arise when patients become more demanding consumers (3,4,44). Consistently, caregivers report having difficulty performing in their jobs because of a lack of organizational resources (3,4,6,47). In addition, they report feeling disenfranchised (46) and having an imbalance between their job and their authority (50).

Recent practices in hospice led by fiscal constraints have raised increasing concern. Nurses are sometimes expected to perform procedures without adequate supervision and training, in the community. When people are expected to assume responsibility with inadequate training, they have difficulty functioning. Nurses report being in situations both in the hospital and in the community where they feel responsible for alleviating the pain of a palliative care patient, yet do not have a physician willing to order the medication they feel will be sufficient to control pain. In addition, with earlier discharge of very sick patients, nurses with limited experience may be expected to care for seriously ill palliative care patients in

TABLE 61.3

FACTORS ASSOCIATED WITH STRESS AND BURNOUT IN ONCOLOGY AND PALLIATIVE CARE OVER THE LAST 30 YEARS

Description of study	Workload	Control	Reward	Community	Fairness	Emotion–work variables
Vachon et al. (44) Research begun in 1971—all nurses in a cancer hospital. Author-constructed questionnaire, specific stressors, and major difficulty in nursing	Lack of resource personnel	Lack of knowledge and skills in interpersonal relationships Lack of communication skills		Problems with staff communication	Pressure to discharge dying patients because of being an active treatment hospital	Natural fear of illness and death Difficulty dealing with the emotional needs of patients and families Watching patients suffer and die Feelings of personal inadequacy Dealing with patients' feelings about illness, prognosis, and death Grief, especially with the death of younger patients
Vachon et al. (44) Conversations and observations made about oncologists and oncology residents in the 1970s in travels throughout North America	Tremendous workload imposed by the prevalence of cancer, the increased life expectancy, and chronic nature of the disease	Rotating interns and residents fearing prescribing narcotics because of risk of addiction Patients demanding more active involvement to arrange treatment around their schedules and to stop treatment when they feel that it is doing no good				Ever increasing demands to be sensitive to and deal with the psychosocial needs of patients, families, and staff Role strain, dealing with research and clinical issues when patients are dying Residents trying to decide for themselves which model of care to follow
Vachon (5,45) International sample of oncology staff in 1980s (n = 110). Qualitative individual and group interviews with caregivers from around the world	Role overload Role ambiguity Role conflict Inadequate resources	Unrealistic expectations of organization Lack of control		Team communication problems Communication problems with others in the system		Patient/family difficulties with coping or personality problems Patient/family difficulties in communication Identification with patient/family

Vactor (5,15) International sample of 100 palliative care staff Qualitative individual and group interviews with caregivers from around the world	Role ambiguity Role conflict Inadequate resources	Communication problems with administration The nature of the system	Communication problems with others in the system Team communication problems	Unrealistic expectations of the organization	Patient and family communication problems Dealing with patients and families with coping and personality problems
Ramirez et al. (6) 393 oncologists, radiotherapists, and palliative care specialists in the United Kingdom Instruments—12 item General Health Questionnaire, Maslach Burnout Inventory, author-developed stressful and satisfying aspects of work questionnaire	Being overloaded and its effect on home life—this problem was more for medical and radiation oncologists than for palliative care specialists Insufficiently trained in communication and management skills Low levels of satisfaction from not having adequate resources to perform one's role	Deriving little satisfaction from professional status/esteem High stress and low satisfaction from dealing with patients	Medical oncologists—stress from organizational responsibilities/conflicts		Clinical (radiation) oncologists reported most of their stress from treatment toxicity and errors, and dealing with patient suffering Dealing with patients suffering
Graham et al. (47) 214 clinical radiologists in the United Kingdom. Instruments—stressful situations and satisfactions measured by author-constructed instruments	Work overload the most stressful aspect of work Having conflicting demands on one's time Feeling under pressure to meet deadlines Inadequacies in current staffing and facilities Insufficiently trained in communication and management skills	Uncertainty over future funding of your unit or institution Feeling that your accumulated skills and experience are not being used to the full Feeling poorly paid for the work that you do	Impositions made on radiologists by other clinicians Stress in relationships with consultant colleagues	Concerns about funding	

(continued)

TABLE 61.3

(CONTINUED)

Description of study	Workload	Control	Reward	Community	Fairness	Emotion–work variables
Kash et al. (46) 261 house staff, nurses, and medical oncologists at a US cancer research hospital. Instruments—Maslach Burnout Inventory, Psychiatric Epidemiology Research Interview, Hopkins Symptom Checklist, Hardy Personality, Work Environment Scales, The Stress Questionnaire	Nurses feel more overwhelmed by the enormity of the tasks of patient care. Feel overworked	Nurses and house staff complain about doing "chores" and not having information about the bigger, more interesting picture. Feel disenfranchised		Oncologists perceived significantly less support from others than did nurses or house staff	Nurses may feel less supported by hospital structure to meet patients' needs, especially psychological needs	Nurses and house staff see the patient when they are most ill with symptoms, or in the terminal stage of disease. Stressor contributing most to burnout and demoralization was dealing with a high number of deaths, or struggling over a do-not-resuscitate (DNR) decision with another colleague or family member. Dealing with ethical issues
Payne (48) 72 female hospice nurses and 17 female nursing assistants from nine UK hospices. Instruments—Maslach Burnout Inventory, Nursing Stress Scale, Ways of Coping Scale, demographic information	Workload was a frequently reported stressor but was not related to burnout as were the other items mentioned in the table	Inadequate preparation		Conflict with staff		Death and dying
Escot et al. (49) 37 members of nursing staff in a French oncology hospital. Instruments—Nursing Stress Scale, Maslach Burnout Inventory, General Health Questionnaire	Problems of time pressure which leave staff with inadequate opportunity to deal with the psychological components of caregiving and to face suffering and death	Inadequate training to deal with psychologic aspects of caregiving and suffering leading to the feeling that one's interventions are inadequate. A lack of information at the time of diagnosis. Persistent fear of developing cancer		Absence of doctor at time of death. Associated with distress lasting for a week after death		Over one third report disgust with preparing dead bodies for the mortuary, especially with stuffing orifices. Feelings of impotence in the face of lack of improvement in a patient

Source and instruments						
Grunfeld et al. Cancer care Ontario staff (n = 681), (3) Focus groups at six cancer centers (n = 108) (4) Instruments—Maslach Burnout Inventory, 12 item General Health Questionnaire, Sources of stress and satisfaction from Ramirez et al. (6)	Increased incidence of cancer Increase in the complexity of cases Heavy workloads Inadequate staffing Available treatment options (new agents to treat previously untreatable cancers to new palliative options for advanced cancer) Feeling under pressure to meet deadlines Having conflicting demands on time Having home life disrupted because of long working hours	Better-informed patients Health service restructuring and reduced spending has led to downsizing of acute and chronic care services in the hospital Fewer health care professionals Changing roles and responsibilities for health care workers The increasing demand for oncology care has not been consistently matched with a commensurate increase in human and material resources, or improvements in systems of care delivery			Heavy workloads—leading to a perceived decrease in the quality of patient care and staff morale Having inadequate staffing to do the job properly	Being involved with the emotional distress of patients
Isikhan et al. Staff from five cancer hospitals in Turkey 50) (n = 109)	Responsibilities of their role Long and tiring work hours Not having enough time for family and social life Scarcity of health care professionals Rapid increase in the population of patients with cancer	Imbalance between job and authority	Lack of appreciation of effort by supervisors	Conflict with colleagues	Imbalance between jobs and responsibilities Unfairness in job promotion opportunities Inadequacy of equipment High cost of drugs	Problems with patients and their relatives

their homes, without access to physicians skilled in effective palliative care and symptom management (52).

Reward

Lack of reward may be financial when one does not receive a salary or benefits commensurate with achievements, or lack of social rewards when one's hard work is ignored and not appreciated by others. The lack of intrinsic rewards (e.g., doing something of importance and doing it well) can also be a critical part of this mismatch. The studies chosen for review have not found difficulties in the area of financial rewards with the exception of the Graham et al. (47) study of clinical radiologists in the United Kingdom.

From the 1980s, there are reports of communication problems with administration, often reflecting a lack of social rewards (5,50). In the study by Ramirez et al. (6) deriving little satisfaction from work was associated with burnout for oncologists. There are concerns about the future funding of units and feeling that skills are being underutilized (47). Participants in an Australian study of hospice providers reported that economic pressures resulted in less staff support, competition between services for funding, inadequate funding to provide services in areas of need, lack of support for psychosocial needs including bereavement care, and experienced staff leaving palliative care (53).

Community

This mismatch arises when people lose a sense of personal connection with others in the workplace. Social support from people with whom one shares praise, comfort, happiness and humor affirms membership in a group with a shared sense of values. Problems with colleagues have been reported in most of the studies in Table 61.3 (5,6,15,44,45,47–49). In the Kash et al. study (46), oncologists were found to have less support from their colleagues than nurses or fellows. In the European Union, recognition of communication problems between palliative care mobile teams (PCMTs) and hospital staff led to a program of intervention, to be discussed subsequently (54).

Fairness

This mismatch arises when there is not perceived fairness in the workplace. Fairness communicates respect and confirms people's self worth. Mutual respect among people is central to a shared sense of community. A lack of fairness was perceived in discharging dying patients from an active treatment hospital (44) and in the unrealistic expectations of the organization (5). There are concerns about funding (47), nurses not feeling supported in meeting patients' emotional needs (46), and having inadequate resources to do the job properly (3,4). In Turkey, oncology nurses and oncologists experienced an imbalance between their jobs and responsibilities, unfairness in job promotion, inadequacy of equipment, and high cost of drugs (50).

Values

People might feel constrained by their job to do something unethical and not in accord with their own values. Alternatively, there may be a mismatch between their personal career goals and the values of the organization. People can also be caught in conflicting values of the organization, such as when there is a discrepancy between a lofty mission statement and actual practice, or when the values are in conflict (e.g., high quality service and cost containment do not always coexist). The values of caregivers were not specifically mentioned in the research in Table 61.3 but can be seen to reflect through many of their other stressors such as inadequate staffing and resources. Staffing problems can lead to not being able to do the job properly, a decrease in quality patient care, and decreased staff morale (3,4). Nurses working with critically ill and dying children in Hong Kong and Greece experienced stress when they felt unable to provide quality care because of the shortage in nursing personnel (55).

In contrast, Webster and Kristjanson's (53) Australian study of caregivers in palliative care found that the work allowed caregivers to bring personal values to the workplace and encouraged personal growth.

Emotion–Work Variables

Table 61.3 shows that staff consistently report difficulty in various aspects of communicating with sick, suffering, and dying patients. Forty-three percent of United Kingdom general practitioner (GP) respondents needed more time to give to dying patients, around one third had trouble coping with their own emotional responses to dying patients. These GPs seemed most likely to have difficulty communicating with patients who were dying and their relatives (56). Oncologists in Portugal, Spain, and Italy felt they were quite confident in eliciting patients' worries, favoring their patient's openness, breaking bad news, and summarizing. However, they were less confident in evaluating anxiety and depression, helping with uncertainty, dealing with denial, and promoting family communication. The authors concluded that low psychosocial orientation of these oncologists negatively affected their communication skills and was associated with higher levels of burnout (42).

Personal Variables Associated with Stress and Burnout

Other variables associated with stress and burnout include younger age (5,50); being younger than 55 (6); being older (49); female gender (46,47); being a single physician in the United Kingdom (57) or a married physician or oncology nurse in Turkey (50); being house staff (46); and experiencing job–home interaction (3,6).

Factors associated with less stress and burnout included: being an experienced oncologist (11 or more years of experience) (50), being religious, and having a 'hardy personality' (46).

COPING

Personal Coping Mechanisms

Table 61.4 shows personal coping mechanisms that have been suggested in the literature.

Job Engagement and Compassion Satisfaction

Job engagement (7) and CS (13) are two ways of providing a framework to understand what keeps workers functioning and enjoying their work in difficult situations.

Job engagement is conceptualized as being the opposite of burnout. It involves energy, involvement, and efficacy.

TABLE 61.4

LIFESTYLE MANAGEMENT TECHNIQUES

- Recognize and monitor symptoms
- Good nutrition
- Meditation
- Spiritual life
- Grieving losses, personally and as a team
- Decrease overtime work
- Exercise—aerobics, yoga, qi gong, tai chi
- Time in nature—walking, gardening
- Music—singing, listening to music, playing an instrument
- Energy work—reiki, healing touch, therapeutic touch
- Maintain sense of humor
- Balance work and home lives to allow sufficient "time off"
- Have a good social support system—personally and professionally
- Seek consultation if symptoms are severe
- Discuss work-related stresses with others who share the same problems
- Visit counterparts in other institutions; look for new solutions to problems
- Remember the Serenity Prayer at work: God grant me the serenity to accept the things I cannot change, the wisdom to change the things I can, and the wisdom to know the difference. Sometimes work-related problems can be solved, other times, leaving the work environment and taking the wisdom gained with one is a good solution (24)

Engagement involves the individual's relationship with work. It involves a sustainable workload, feelings of choice and control, appropriate recognition and reward, a supportive work community, fairness and justice, and meaningful and valued work. Engagement is also characterized by high levels of activation and pleasure (7). Engagement is defined as a persistent, positive-affective-motivational state of fulfillment in employees, which is characterized by vigor, dedication, and absorption (7).

CS (13) is satisfaction derived from the work of helping others. It may be the portrayal of efficacy. CS may be happiness with what one can do to make the world in which one lives a reflection of what one thinks it should be. Caregivers with CS derive pleasure from helping others, like their colleagues, feel good about their ability to help and make a contribution. Stamm (13) describes a balancing act between compassion fatigue and CS. She notes that caregivers in humanitarian settings may be experiencing compassion fatigue, yet they like their work because they derive positive benefits from it. They believe what they are doing is helping others and may even be redemptive. When a person's belief system is well maintained with positive material, a person's resiliency may be enhanced (58). What seems to count most for resilience is the opportunity to encounter pain within a context of meaning and to find that one's compassion (one's suffering with) has power. These sustain an underlying belief that the world is good and in order (59).

The compassion of caregivers often catches the attention of others, even at the most difficult times of their lives. Dr. Peter Frost was professor of organizational behavior at the University of British Columbia. When he was being treated for metastatic melanoma he observed the nurses of the British Columbia Cancer Agency "whose highly professional and empathic behavior caught my attention when I was in their care. They sparked my initial interest in exploring the meaning and practice of compassion" (60, p. 9). Observing and reflecting on the compassion of these nurses led to his book *Toxic Emotions at Work: How Compassionate Managers Handle Pain and Conflict*, which is hailed as one of the top management books of 2003. "My illness—a trigger for changes, obviously in my personal life—also set in motion my thinking about the kinds of hidden forces that determine our well-being, even to the point of acquiring disease. And in particular, how the behavior of organizations and the people in them can affect the health of certain individuals ... a few months after my surgery I found myself at a week-long seminar on health and healing. That is where my ideas about emotional pain in organizations, and its effects on people who try to manage that pain for organizations began to crystallize" (60, p. 2).

How do Professionals Cope and Find Meaning in Their Work?

When caregivers to the critically ill, dying, and bereaved were interviewed and asked what enabled them to continue working in the field, the top five coping mechanisms identified were: a sense of competence, control, or pleasure in one's work (13%); team philosophy, building, and support (11%); control over aspects of practice (10%); lifestyle management (9%); and a personal philosophy of illness, death, and one's role in life (9%) (5).

More recent studies have looked at sources of satisfaction in the work of palliative care and oncology staff. These include: dealing well with patients and relatives (6); patient care or patient contact was the major source of satisfaction in oncologists, allied health personnel, and support staff, even if their job did not involve much patient contact (4); having professional status and esteem, deriving intellectual satisfaction, and having adequate resources to perform one's role (6); and having good relationships with colleagues (61). Oncology was felt to be a special environment, often because of longstanding relationships with patients; having good relationships with patients, families, and colleagues were the three top sources of satisfaction; being perceived to do the job well was fourth highest for all groups; and having variety in one's job was amongst the top for all groups (4).

Palliative care has been described as a way of living. Vitality—the capacity to live and develop which is associated with energy, life, animation, and importance—is the core meaning of palliative care. The way of living involves unity with self, being touched to the heart, and personal meaning. Crucial to the experience of palliative care was the patient and family, holistic care, and the interdisciplinary team (53). Helping patients find meaning in suffering was rewarding (16,21); as was having a deep sense of satisfaction from contributing to the care of dying children, feeling they were doing a difficult but meaningful job, feeling they had a unique role, and being appreciated by the family of dying children for their involvement and intimate relationships (55).

Studies of Intervention

Despite a variety of articles describing intervention with palliative care staff, there have been few studies documenting the efficacy of intervention in this or other groups. Van Staa et al. (22) describe an intervention in a new palliative care unit in the Netherlands, which is the same one referred to in the

Georges et al. article (17) cited earlier. A carefully designed training program and staff support activities were meant to enhance personal growth, to give emotional support, and to deal with death and bereavement issues. The interventions did not involve mutual collaboration, practical problems, managerial and communication skills, and the skills needed to deliver complex palliative care. There was a cultural difference between the external consultants who embraced a relational therapeutic worldview and the hospice staff who came from a rational technical hospital environment. The former approach involves complete trust and openness in order to work. Not all staff members were convinced of the value of the nondirective approach. In addition, a therapeutic group is fundamentally different from a group that has to work together after the session. The authors suggest that future leaders should focus on content as well as process issues. They also suggest that adequate resources, a supportive management structure, an extensive educational training program, and attention to individual needs should accompany support groups.

DiMeglio et al. (62) report on an intervention on a nursing unit of one of the American Magnet hospitals. These are hospitals that the American Nurses Credentialing Center recognizes as consistently demonstrating higher satisfaction for nurses, lower turnover and vacancy rates, and they build magnetism into the organization. The hospital where the research was conducted has organizational development that incorporates a focus on systems, teams, and change. In the intervention, their main objective was to identify those elements that create high-performing teams. Other objectives included: identifying barriers to effective teamwork, distinguishing traits of staff, dealing with change and conflict, and using learned communication techniques to improve group cohesion. Data was gathered using the instrument *How Well Are We Working Together?* This provided a baseline assessment of each particular unit's cultures including expectations, decision making, and areas of conflict. There was a minimum of three 1-hour meetings on each unit in which participants were asked to describe what this unit is like and what makes a high-performing team here. A modified Myers-Briggs Type indicator (MBTI) inventory was used, allowing a safe atmosphere in which to speak of styles and personal characteristics that could account for various team differences and shift conflicts. Personality types were identified and discussed including: introvert/extrovert, intuitive/sensing, thinking/feeling, judging/perceiving. The intervention improved group cohesion, nurse satisfaction and retention, and teamwork. The team came to the insight that there was a group of nurses who articulated high levels of professional autonomy and perceived themselves as expert clinicians. They presented themselves as the "ultimate" team-cohesive, highly skilled nurses, and expert at training newer nurses. However, the newer nurses did not agree and saw them as an insider group. This led to a discussion about orientation, mentorship, and integration of new team members into existing teams.

Another study by Cohen-Katz et al. (63) was done on a unit where there was already work to improve employee satisfaction and retention; a nursing advisory council had been set up; there was work to enhance the model of self-governance and increased opportunity for education and professional development. An 8-week Mindfulness-Based Stress Reduction (MBSR) program was held based on the work of Jon Kabat Zinn (64). Mindfulness is defined as being fully present to one's experience without judgment or resistance. Its emphasis on self care, compassion, and healing makes it relevant as an intervention for helping nurses. The results of the study showed that the treatment group had decreased scores on the Maslach Burnout Inventory and these changes lasted for 3 months. Specifically, there was significantly decreased emotional exhaustion and depersonalization and a trend towards significance in personal accomplishment.

Examples of Other Intervention

In an intervention experienced by Christopher Sherwood, a residential hospice program developed a staff support system that anecdotally has demonstrated great effectiveness at being able to assist its health care provider staff to cope with the day-to-day burdens that result from life, both in and out of their work. This system relies on the consistency of the nursing staff to "check-in" with one another at the start of each shift prior to attending to the needs of the inpatients and their families.

This idea was borrowed from the hospice's bereavement program after significant benefits were found for people who as facilitators with the program's bereavement groups, check-in with each other prior to each group session. This occurs with the bereavement coordinator leading a premeeting that focuses a portion of time on *how* each cofacilitator is doing at that moment. Each person is provided the opportunity to share with his/her cofacilitators what he/she is thinking and feeling at the time, and to reciprocate to others by listening to them in return. The rationale behind this approach is based on the principle that the emotional depth achieved by facilitators with the families they support is mirrored by the depth they achieve amongst themselves.

Transferring the idea of check-in sessions to the staff who work on the inpatient unit was initially facilitated by a fellow staff member who was very skilled in providing psychosocial care. A session, which usually takes no more than 5–10 minutes, allows each person the opportunity to both give and receive support from fellow staff members, as in the bereavement group. It was noted by many staff, shortly after this program was started, that the check-in times were extremely valuable for promoting interdependency among team members, which in turn has been very helpful for the interdisciplinary team in being able to provide care to patients and families.

Table 61.5 shows the model of collaborative coping developed by the Emotional Safety Committee of St. Joseph's Hospice in Auckland New Zealand.

Communication Training

Given that burnout has been associated with difficulty in communication skills (42), a number of authors have developed communication skills interventions. Fallowfield et al. (65) showed improvement in the communication skills of oncologists, which the authors hypothesize that leads to personally and professionally more rewarding consultations, which can have a significant impact on clinical care and patients' and physicians' well-being. Gysels et al. (66) reviewed studies that assessed communication skills training in oncology. All the interventions demonstrated modest improvements (effect sizes ranged from 0.15–2.0) and deterioration in the outcomes measured was found. They concluded that training improved basic communication skills. In clinical practice, positive attitudes and beliefs are needed to maintain skills over time and to effectively handle emotional situations.

Meier et al. (67) recently proposed an approach to physician awareness that involves identifying and working with emotions that may affect patient care. This involves looking at physician, situational, and patient risk factors that can affect physician feelings and thus influence patient care.

The steps include the following:

- Identifying the factors that predispose to emotions that might affect patient care

TABLE 61.5

EMOTIONAL SAFETY: AN ORGANIZATIONAL AND PERSONAL RESPONSIBILITY

How do we keep ourselves, our colleagues, and our team SAFE at St. Joseph's?

There are several structures and opportunities, which are currently in place.

The maintenance of personal safety and integrity as a partnership. There are expectations you should have of the organization, and expectations we should have of each other as individuals.

Some of the organizational responsibilities include:
- Appropriate recruitment
- Appropriate orientation
- Ongoing and regular opportunities for supervision and support
- Exposure to timely critical incident debriefing
- Regular and appropriate feedback
- Acknowledgment on sadness and burden of work
- Celebration of successes
- Healthy rostering
- Time for reflection and ritual
- Noncritical acknowledgment of personal pressures
- Regular forums for communication

Some personal responsibilities include:
- Making sure you derole at the end of the day
- Using ritual to acknowledge your own losses
- Giving and receiving support—from peers and management
- Admitting and acknowledging helplessness and painful experiences
- Giving prompt feedback to peers and management—as opposed to harboring resentment and blame
- Not expecting too much of yourself, especially in light of all the suffering that you see. Set limits
- Using the supervisory process regularly—even when you feel that you do not need it
- Maintaining careful boundaries and limiting your work to professional connections
- Taking regular holidays and time out
- Making sensible roster requests
- Exercising regularly
- Eating a healthy diet
- Enjoying and having fun with the team, and outside work
- Spoil yourself rotten—YOU DESERVE IT

- Monitoring for signs (behavioral) and symptoms (feelings) of emotions
- Naming and accepting the emotion
- Identifying possible sources of the emotion
- Responding constructively to the emotion
  - Step back from the situation to gain perspective
  - Identify behaviors resulting from the feeling
  - Consider implications and consequences of behaviors
  - Thinking through alternative outcomes for patients, according to different behaviors
  - Consulting a trusted professional colleague

Studies in Process

Medland et al. (61) describe an intervention with 150 members of the multidisciplinary team in the oncology department at Northwestern Memorial Hospital. The program aims to decrease absenteeism and enhance a sense of community to create a meaningful and rewarding work environment. The program targets both individual and organizational issues. Research has not yet been conducted but staff retention has improved. Plans are under way to measure the effectiveness of the program through increased overall patient satisfaction, psychosocial patient satisfaction, and spiritual patient satisfaction scores. The level of staff psychosocial wellness, as evidenced by follow-up human services surveys, is planned for the future. Most importantly,

staff will be monitored for changes in behavior reflecting use of positive coping strategies and constructive self-care behaviors.

Another model for shifting established patterns is being developed in the European Union with a goal of improving the interaction between PCMTs and the hospital staff with whom they interact (54). In this model, recognizing the full range of convictions held by persons in a hospital setting, the concept of palliative care/terminal care has been bolstered by the concept of **Continuous Care**. Continuous care tends to **articulate** curative and palliative procedures focusing on the holistic care of patients and their family. "'Promoting the integration of continuous care in the hospital' intends to identify the challenges in integrating continuous care through an inventory and analysis of the activity of PCMT in several countries of Europe. Competencies for PCMTs have been derived, and based on these, a pilot three phase educational programme with PCMTs undertaken and evaluated" (54, p. 4).

CONCLUSIONS

While many of the stressors in palliative care appear not to have changed in the last four decades, important work that has been recently completed or is underway is available to help understand the differences in vulnerability to burnout, stress, and compassion fatigue and the overlap between depression and burnout, and to develop programs of intervention to target various stressors such as communication issues, team building, organizational development, and self care. Some concern must be expressed, however, about the future of supportive oncology and palliative care from the study by Georges et al. (17). Will the field become primarily a specialty of symptomatologists as Kearney (29) and Doyle (28) warned, or will it be able to meet the challenge of Dr. Ira Byock to devise a palliative care system that is "cutting edge, medically crisp, but tender and loving" (26)? In such a system it is to be hoped that caregivers will have compassion for themselves and their colleagues, as well as the patients and families whom they serve.

References

1. Rochester SR, Vachon MLS, Lyall WAL. Immediacy in language: a channel to care of the dying patient. *J Comm Psychol* 1974;2:75–76.
2. Lyall WAL, Vachon MLS, Rogers J. A study of the degree of stress experienced by professionals caring for dying patients. In: Ajemian I, Mount BM, eds. *The RVH manual on hospice/palliative care*. New York: ARNO Press, 1980:498–508.
3. Grunfeld E, Whelan TJ, Zitzelsberger L, et al. Cancer care workers in Ontario: prevalence of burnout, job stress and job satisfaction. *Can Med Assoc J* 2000;163:166–169.
4. Grunfeld E, Zitzelsberger L, Coristine M, et al. Job stress and job satisfaction of cancer care workers. *Psychooncology* 2005;14:61–69.
5. Vachon MLS. *Occupational stress in the care of the critically ill, dying and bereaved*. Washington, DC: Hemisphere Publishing, 1987.
6. Ramirez AJ, Graham J, Richards MA, et al. Burnout and psychiatric disorder among cancer clinicians. *Br J Cancer* 1995;71:1263–1269.
7. Maslach C, Schaufeli WB, Leiter MP. Job burnout. *Annl Rev Psychol* 2001;52:397–422.
8. Maslach M. *Burnout, the cost of caring*. New York: Prentice-Hall, 1982.
9. Figley CR, ed. *Compassion fatigue: coping with secondary traumatic stress disorder in those who treat the traumatized*. New York: Brunner/Mazel, 1995.
10. Figley CR, ed. *Treating compassion fatigue*. New York: Brunner-Routledge, 2002.
11. Ahola K, Honkonen T, Isometsä E, et al. The relationship between job-related burnout and depressive disorders-results from the Finnish Health 2000 Study. *J Affect Disord* 2005;88(1):55–62.
12. Nyklícek I, Pop VJ. Past and familial depression predict current symptoms of professional burnout. *J Affect Disord* 2005;88(1):63–68.
13. Stamm BH. Measuring compassion satisfaction as well as fatigue: developmental history of the compassion satisfaction and fatigue test. In: Figley CF, ed. *Treating compassion fatigue*. New York: Brunner-Routledge, 2002:107–119.
14. Vachon MLS. Reflections on the history of occupational stress in hospice/palliative care. In: Corless IB, Foster Z, eds. *The hospice heritage: celebrating our future*. New York: The Hayworth Press, Inc, 1999:229–246; Published simultaneously as *Hosp J* 1999;14:3–4.
15. Vachon MLS. Staff stress in palliative/hospice care: a review. *Palliat Med* 1995;9:91–122.
16. Barnard D, Towers A, Boston P, et al. *Crossing over: narratives of palliative care*. New York: Oxford, 2000.
17. Georges JJ, Grypdonck M, De Casterle BD. Being a palliative care nurse in an academic hospital: a qualitative study about nurses' perceptions of palliative care nursing. *J Clin Nurs* 2002;11(6):785–793.
18. Harper BC. *Death: the coping mechanism of the health professional*, Rev ed. Greenville, SC: Southeastern University Press, Inc, 1994.
19. Neimeyer RA, Jordan j. Disenfranchisement as empathic failure. In: Doka K, ed. *Disenfranchised grief*, 2nd ed. Champaign, Ill: Research Press, 2002.
20. Cumes D. *The spirit of healing*. St. Paul, MN: Llewellyn, 1999.
21. Kearney M. *A place of healing: working with suffering in living and dying*. Oxford: Oxford University Press, 2000.
22. van Staa AL, Visser A. van der Zouwe Caring for caregivers: experiences and evaluation of interventions for a palliative care team. *Patient Edu Couns* 2000;41:93–105.
23. van Staa AL, van der Zouwe N, Visser A. Pionieren met palliatieve zorg. *Tijdschrift Voor Gezondheidswetenschappen* 1999;77:472–478.
24. Vachon MLS. The experience of the nurse in end-of-life care in the 21st century. In: Ferrell B, Coyle N, eds. *Oxford textbook of palliative nursing*, 2nd ed. Oxford University Press, 2005:1011–1029.
25. Halifax J, Dossey B. *Compassionate care of the dying: manual and standards for practice*. Santa Fe, New Mexico: Upaya Zen Center, 2005.
26. Byock I. Dying in America: past, present and future. Paper presented at The Great Journey, Death, Dying and Bereavement, Tucson, AZ, 27 March 2004.
27. Byock I. From innocence to audit: transatlantic lessons on the routinization of hospice. *Am J Hosp Palliat Care* 1994;11(1):4–7.
28. Doyle D. Have we looked beyond the physical and psychosocial? *J Pain Symptom Manage* 1992;7:302–311.
29. Kearney M. Palliative medicine-just another specialty? *Palliat Med* 1992;6:41.
30. Garfield C, Spring C, Ober D. *Sometimes my heart goes numb: love and caring in a time of AIDS*. San Francisco: Jossey-Bass, 1995.
31. Wright B. Compassion fatigue: how to avoid it. *Palliat Med* 2004;18(3):4–5.
32. Antonovsky A. *Health, stress and coping*. San Francisco: Jossey-Bass, 1979.
33. Lazarus RS, Cohen J. Psychological stress and adaptation: some unresolved issues. In: Selye H, ed. *Selye's guide to stress research*, Vol. 1. New York: Von Nostrand Reinhold, 1980:90–117.
34. Lazarus R, Launier R. Stress related transactions between person and environment. In: Pervin L, Lewis M, eds. *Perspectives in international psychology*. New York: Plenum Publishing, 1978:287–327.
35. European Agency for Safety and Health at Work. *Safety at work*. http://agency.osha.eu.int/publications/factsheets/8/en/facts8_en.pdf, 2000.
36. Edelwich J, Brodsky A. *Burn-out: stages of disillusionment in the helping professions*. New York: Springer-Verlag New York, 1980.
37. Pines AM. Burnout: an existential perspective. In: Schaufeli W, Maslach C, Marek T, eds. *Professional burnout*. Washington, DC: Taylor and Francis, 1993.
38. Figley CR. Traumatization and comfort: close relationships may hazardous to your health. Keynote presentation at the *Conference on Families and Close Relationships: Individuals in Social Interaction*. Lubbock, TX: Texas Tech University, 1982.
39. Demerouti E, Bakker AB, Nachreiner f, et al. The job demands-resources model of burnout. *J Appl Psychol* 2001;86:499–512.
40. Lee RT, Ashforth BE. On the meaning of Maslach's three dimensions of burnout. *J Appl Psychol* 1990;75:743–747.
41. Brenninkmeyer V, Van Yperen NW, Buunk BP. Burnout and depression are not identical twins: is decline of superiority a distinguishing feature? *Pers Individ Dif* 2001;30:873–880.
42. Travado L, Grassi L, Gil F, et al. Physician-patient communication among Southern European cancer physicians: the influence of psychosocial orientation and burnout. *Psychooncology* 2005;14:661–670.
43. French JRP, Rodgers W, Cobb S. Adjustment as person-environment fit. In: Coelho GV, Hamburg DA, Adams E, eds. *Coping and adaptation*. New York: Basic Books, 1974:316–333.
44. Vachon MLS, Lyall WAL, Freeman SJJ. Measurement and management of stress in health care professionals working with advanced cancer patients. *Death Educ* 1978;1:365–375.
45. Vachon MLS. Stress and coping in cancer professionals. In: Godden J, ed. *Cancer care searching for balance*. Toronto: The Ontario Cancer Treatment and Research Foundation, 1991:87–92.
46. Kash KM, Holland JC, Breitbart W, et al. Stress and burnout in oncology. *Oncology* 2000;14:1621–1637.
47. Graham J, Ramirez AJ, Field S, et al. Job stress and satisfaction among clinical radiologists. *Clin Radiol* 2000;55:182–185.
48. Payne N. Occupational stressors and coping as determinants of burnout in female hospice nurses. *J Adv Nurs* 2001;33:396–405.
49. Escot C, Artero S, Gandubert C, et al. Stress levels in nursing staff working in oncology. *Stress Health* 2001;17:273–279.
50. Isikhan V, Comezb T, Zafer D. Job stress and coping strategies in health care professionals working with cancer patients. *Eur J Oncol Nurs* 2004;8(3):234–244.
51. McConigley R, Kristjanson LJ, Morgan A. Palliative care nursing in Western Australia. *Intl J Pal Care Nurs* 2000;6(2):80–90.
52. Coyle N. Focus on the nurse: ethical dilemmas with highly symptomatic patients dying at home. *Hosp J* 1997;12(2):33–41.
53. Webster J, Kristjanson LJ. "But isn't it depressing?" The vitality of palliative care. *J Palliat Care* 2002;18(1):15–24.
54. European Commission. *Promoting the development and integration of palliative care mobile support teams in the hospital*. Brussels: Directorate-General for Research Food Quality and Safety, 2004.
55. Papadatou D, Martinson IM, Chung P, et al. Caring for dying children: a comparative study of nurses' experiences in Greece and Hong Kong. *Cancer Nurs* 2001;24(5):402–412.
56. Seale C, Cartwright A. *The year before death*. Aldershot: Avebury, 1994.
57. Ramirez AJ, Graham J, Richards MA, et al. Mental health of hospital consultants: the effect of stress and satisfaction at work. *Lancet* 1996;347:724–728.
58. Pearlman L, Saakvitne K. *Trauma and the therapist: countertransference and vicarious traumatization in psychotherapy with incest survivors*. New York: Norton, 1995.
59. Young-Eisendrath P. *The Resilient Spirit* Reading, MA: Perseus Books 1996.
60. Frost PJ. *Toxic Emotions at Work*. Boston, MA: Harvard Business School Press, 2003.
61. Medland J, Howard-Ruben J, Whitaker E. Fostering psychosocial wellness in oncology nurses: addressing burnout and social support in the workplace. *Oncol Nurs Forum* 2004;31(1):47–54.

62. DiMeglio K, Padula C, Piatek C, et al. Group cohesion and nurse satisfaction: examination of a team-building approach. *J Nurs Adm* 2005;35(3):110–120.
63. Cohen-Katz J, Wiley SD, Capuano T, et al. The effects of mindfulness-based stress reduction on nurse stress and burnout: a quantitative and qualitative study. *Holist Nurs Pract* 2004;18(6):302–308.
64. Kabat-Zinn J. *Full catastrophe living: using the wisdom of your body and mind to face stress, pain, and illness.* New York: Delta, 1990.
65. Fallowfield L, Jenkins V, Farewell V, et al. Efficacy of a cancer research UK communication skills training model for oncologists: a randomized controlled trial. *Lancet* 2002;359:650–656.
66. Gysels M, Richardson A, Higginson IJ. Communication training for health professionals who care for patients with cancer: a systematic review of effectiveness. *Support Care Cancer* 2004;12:692–700.
67. Meier DE, Back AL, Morrison RS. The inner life of physicians and the care of the seriously ill. *JAMA* 2002;286(23):3007–3014.

ETHICAL CONSIDERATIONS IN PALLIATIVE CARE

CHAPTER 62 ■ ADVANCE DIRECTIVES AND ASSESSMENT OF DECISION-MAKING CAPACITY

LINDA L. EMANUEL

Many oncology patients would like to have some control over their medical care, not only when they are alert but also when they are too sick to participate in making decisions. Similarly, those who have to make decisions for patients who are unable to participate would like to be guided by the patient's wishes. Advance care planning evolved in response to these needs. Having discussions about goals in different types of scenarios and including both the family and the physician in that discourse are the key issues. For effective discussions, it helps to have the patient and the family go through validated worksheets that walk them through the various considerations resulting in expressions of preference that are clinically meaningful. This should usually be done on the patient's and the family's own time, with opportunities to check in with the physician and the team to ensure coordination and agreement. Ideally, this can happen over time, integrated into the course of care.

TERMS, HISTORY, AND LAW

Two main modalities exist by which a person can make preparations in anticipation of future incapacity (1). One is to appoint a proxy to speak in the place of the principal person. The other is to write down wishes in a directive. These two modalities are usually complementary, because written statements cannot provide for all eventualities, and proxy decision makers cannot speak accurately on behalf of patients without the patient's guidance.

Proxy Designation

Physicians should be aware of three key issues on which to advise patients and proxies. First, patients, professionals, and the proxies themselves should understand the proxy's role. Speaking in place of the patient can take two distinctly different forms. In one form, the patient asks the proxy to represent the patient's prior wishes and to hold steadfast to these known prior preferences, extrapolating them if necessary to the situation at hand. In the other form, the proxy speaks according to the proxy's own judgment (2). In this alternative role, the proxy remains more independent of the patient's stated prior wishes and tries instead to imagine what the patient would have wanted in the circumstances, judge the

best interests of the patient, and balance other issues as he or she sees fit. These two modalities can be merged. For instance, a patient may tell a proxy to apply his or her prior wishes, albeit with latitude and taking particular types of unpredictable family issues into consideration (3).

Second, patients and proxies should know that studies have found that proxies often guess the prior wishes of patients inaccurately and, furthermore, that proxies often imagine that the patients' prior wishes are for more intervention than patients actually select (4). Even a proxy who has had a close relationship with the patient may not be able to make accurate judgments. It is possible that close relationships do not often include discussions about medical aspects of dying, or that patients do not even know their own preferences until they have discussed or faced a relevant matter. It is also possible that proxies face significant emotional issues that may hinder their ability to imagine the patients' wishes. Regardless, physicians must counsel patients to discuss relevant perspectives explicitly and well in advance of a deteriorating medical situation that may result in incompetence (5).

Third, patients should be aware that friends and family members have their own interests and issues, which may conflict with their role as proxy. Common examples include the difficulty of letting go of the loved patient, the great emotional burden of making life-and-death decisions, the difficulty of finding the extensive time it takes to perform the proxy role well, and the difficulty of choosing how to allocate limited family resources (e.g., to the patient's medical care vs. the children's education) (4). Conflicting motivations are inevitable and need not prohibit the proxy role. Nonetheless, the proxy may need help distinguishing different motivations and abiding by those that are most suited to the proxy role.

Instructional Directives

The history of the development of instructional directives reflects the search for the most valid form of expressing prior wishes. The earliest commonly used instructional directive was the Do Not Resuscitate (DNR) order, written by the physician after discussion with the patient and the family (6). After its proposal in 1976, a set of studies and a culture evolved around the DNR discussion. It is still relevant and can be included in comprehensive advance planning discussions (7). A hazard of isolated DNR discussions is that they occur too late, either missing the patients who need them or occurring in such "out of the blue" conversations that alarmed patients make decisions without the benefit of settled reflection (8–10). A more recent approach involves a cluster of doctors' orders concerning life-sustaining intervention, such as through the Physicians' Orders for Life-Sustaining Treatment or POLST form (11). This approach can prompt more optimal discussions with patients and families.

An earlier modality for making instructional directives was the living will. This was introduced in 1968 by a lawyer, Louis Kutner. The living will attempted to express the widespread view that heroic levels of technological intervention should be avoided if the patient's prognosis was hopeless. The statements made in living wills were true enough to the sentiment, but in practice they were insufficient to guide the specific decision making needed in real clinical circumstances. Different interpretations of what constitutes a heroic intervention and what constitutes a hopeless prognosis meant that this early type of living will was liable to bring as much confusion as clarity to the decisions.

Efforts to increase the specificity of living wills began, starting most notably with Sissela Bok's and Michigan's living will (12,13). Thereafter, developments began along two lines: one to better describe the general health-related values of the patient (values histories) and one to formulate ways in which patients could make very specific treatment preference statements (treatment-specific directives) (14,15). Empirical evidence that general statements cannot predict specific wishes has supported the more balanced view that these two modalities work best together (16–18). Some patients are inclined to write a free-prose letter encapsulating their wishes. Such letters can be worthwhile, but many patients do not have the writing skills or the specialized expertise that ensures coverage of relevant matters. In such cases, the concurrent use of predrafted documents is to be encouraged. More recently, efforts have been focused on the need to validate predrafted instructional directives, just as any other instrument that seeks to record subjective matters needs to be validated (19). A few forms have been validated, and at least one validated form that is tailored to cancer exists (20–22). One of the more studied forms, which is generic and adaptable and has been validated in several studies, is the Medical Directive (17,23–26). Physicians should provide and advise patients to use validated forms, because using nonvalidated forms risks misrepresentation of patients' true wishes and can confuse decision making. Validated forms also provide a succinct method of ensuring that patients have considered the major areas that most people need to cover. The use of a validated form as a worksheet for thought and discussion can be as important as its use as a recorded document.

Statutory versus Advisory Documents

All states and the District of Columbia have statutes that endorse advance directives in one way or another. Some endorse the use of proxies, others endorse the use of instructional directives, and most now endorse both (27). Most state statutes have a corresponding document, which is often available from local health care facilities or state medical organizations. The fundamental purpose of state statutes is to allow the physicians to follow the patient's wishes without fear of liability. The interests of the patient are served indirectly by protecting physicians who follow patients' wishes and rendering physicians vulnerable if they do not. Many states specifically honor the statutory documents of other states, although some differences exist, and frequent travellers may wish to have documents from their frequented state bound together with those from their home state.

It is part of common law that competent patients have the right to accept or refuse medical intervention, even life-sustaining intervention. Even casual statements have been honored as sufficient evidence, and this has held true even in the face of national political campaigns (28). Written statements have been explicitly identified as desirable evidence of patients' preferences (29,30). Physicians can therefore be assured that patients' statements carry legal authority whether or not they are recorded in a manner not specifically designed for local state statutes. Statements made in a nonstatutory form can be considered as advisory documents. In this sense, distinctions between legal and "nonlegal" or "illegal" forms in this context are erroneous. A statutory form is legally binding, and a nonstatutory advisory document is also binding if it provides clear evidence of the patient's wishes. Because statutory forms are written to comply with legal criteria, they are often far less informative than advisory documents, which can address personal values and clinical issues.

The Patient Self-Determination Act, and Recommendations of the Joint Commission on Accreditation of Health Care Organizations

The United States' Patient Self-Determination Act of 1990 requires that patients be asked about the existence of an advance directive at the time of enrollment or admission to a health care facility. The intent of the law was to increase awareness and documentation of advance directives. In addition, the Joint Commission on Accreditation of Health Care Organizations recommends that facilities have arrangements for counseling patients who wish to complete advance directives. Completion of advance directives is best done in the more stable setting of continuing outpatient care, but occasionally their completion in the inpatient setting is unavoidable. Therefore, although minimal compliance with the Patient Self-Determination Act and the recommendations of the Joint Commission require relatively little from physicians, the spirit of both requirements involves thoughtful, longitudinal involvement of the physician and the other members of the interdisciplinary team in discussion with the patient.

CONCEPTUAL FOUNDATIONS, EMPIRICAL BACKGROUND

Honoring Patients' Wishes

The notion that autonomy can be extended into times of incompetence by recording wishes ahead of time is not straightforward. How can anyone know whether the wishes of an incompetent person are represented by previously recorded wishes? What about patients who are incompetent for decision making but are awake and appear to be capable of feelings and wishes, and these apparent wishes differ from the prior wishes? Responding to these two questions, which motivated considerable debate in the advance directive movement, depends on two points. First, the justifying principle for advance directives is surviving interests, rather than the broader principle of autonomy. Second, the condition of the patient in which advance directives pertain unequivocally is wishlessness; equivocal situations can occur when the patient is incompetent but has discernable wishes (31).

Surviving Interests

Ordinarily, autonomy involves the application of real-time wishes. But because it is impossible to create real-time wishes when there are none, autonomy can be extended only by applying prior wishes. A surviving interest constitutes a distinct form of autonomy and should not be confused with the more general autonomy. *Surviving interest*, ordinarily a legal term, refers to the right of the individual to determine decisions on matters in which he or she has an overriding interest even after losing the direct ability to act on these matters. The most common example is the estate will, in which individuals exercise their right to determine disposal of their property after death. A related arrangement that relies on a surviving interest concerns the funeral directions by the principal planning for his or her own death. Another example is the organ donor card. The important point is that arrangements predicated on surviving interests do not rely on real-time wishes; they rely on prior wishes. Advance directives rely on prior wishes in just the same way as these more traditional applications of surviving interests. Even when a proxy is instructed to make decisions without reference to the patient's prior wishes, the proxy's authority relies on the patient's prior wishes to designate him or her, and although proxies may make use of their own real-time judgments, there is no application of the patients' (nonexistent) real-time wishes. The question "How can anyone know if the wishes of the patient who is incompetent are represented by the recorded wishes?" can be answered as follows, When there are no reliable real-time wishes, it is prior wishes that must be represented.

The Zone between Incompetence and Wishlessness

Patients who are in a state in which it is not possible to have wishes, such as occurs when there is complete absence of neo-cortical function, clearly meet the criteria by which advance directives can be activated. A problem arises when a patient is not wishless but is decisionally incapacitated, as can occur in advanced stages of cancer. Many such circumstances involve such a significant change in the patients' personality or states of being that they are very different from the former selves who made out the directive. There is limited ethical imperative to apply the wishes of the former person to the current person if the latter is a significantly altered or a truncated version of the former (32). Under these circumstances, advance directives may be said to represent a weak version of the surviving interests of the patients, and other factors must therefore be considered. Technical and legal statements as to when advance directives can be activated often fail to make this distinction. Nonetheless, physicians should be particularly careful to meet ethical standards as well as legal ones under these circumstances. The question "How should one represent patients who are decisionally incapacitated who seem to have wishes that differ from the recorded wishes?" can be answered as follows: a combination of guidance by the advance directive and substituted or best interests judgment should determine the physicians' and the proxies' decisions for patients in this circumstance.

Substituted Judgment and Best Interests Judgment

Whenever patients' surviving interests are unknown, decisions must be made by using standards of substituted judgment or best interests judgment. The application of prior wishes is not the same thing as using substituted judgment. Even when prior wishes are inferred from stated wishes to fit unpredicted decisions, this is a form of prior-preference–guided judgment that is justified by surviving interests.

Substituted judgment usually refers to attempts to judge as the patient would have if he or she could have. In the words of Justice Hughes, who wrote the opinion for Karen Quinlan's case, "if Karen were herself miraculously lucid for an interval (not altering the existing prognosis of the condition to which she would soon return) and perceptive of her ... condition, she [would] decide upon ... [the decision of the court offered on her behalf]" (33). Substituted judgment is an intrinsically difficult concept and is just as difficult to implement in reality. Understanding what a person would want is hard enough in ordinary circumstances. Understanding what a person would want when the person is in a state that neither the patient nor the proxy have ever been in is even harder. When that state is such that the individual is incapable of having wishes, it is impossible. This last key difficulty centers on the fact that real-time wishes are being created when there are none. Commentators have noted that substituted judgment usually ends up being a version of best interest judgment. It may also end up being a version of prior-preference–guided judgment in that attempts are made to guess what the prior healthy person would have wanted if he or she could have anticipated the eventual condition.

Best interests judgment is somewhat easier conceptually, but is still difficult to implement. The idea is to judge according to the best interests of the patient. It has this advantage: not only is real time used, but also there need be no reliance on notions of the patient's wishes. The difficulty of this concept is determining what the best interests of the patient are, because this involves highly subjective value assessments. It may also be the case that the patient is so debilitated and "absent" that ordinary real-time interests do not exist. Despite these difficulties, it is the best guiding standard available when prior preferences cannot be used.

AUTHENTICITY OF WISHES

Cultural Differences

Advance care planning has evolved in the contexts of western cultures and is often thought of in terms suited to social contexts in which individual's rights have some priority. However, the idea of planning is not predicated on individualism and is readily accomplished in cultures that emphasize extended families and community responsibility.

Other cultural differences also invite special consideration, and similarly can usually be accommodated. When the role of deciding for others traditionally falls to a particular role or person in a culture it may seem that advance planning threatens that role. Or if there is distrust of those who seek to plan by those who will be affected, then planning may be omitted or counterproductive unless trustworthiness is established (34). Delegated decision making to family heads has been identified in families of Asian origins; trust concerns have been identified in African American patients and families; and concerns over precipitating undesired outcomes if they are discussed has been identified among Navajo families (35–37). Perhaps the most problematic cultural issues have to do with cultural inhibitions against discussing dying. This taboo has been as strong in modern western cultures as elsewhere.

Although cultural issues are powerful, generalizations are also problematic. Every case must be engaged on its own issues. The clinician who approaches people with genuine respect and, with an open mind, who inquires about and honors cultural differences should be able to accomplish advance care planning when it is appropriate in forms that suit each case and setting.

Three practical tips can help with many situations: if extended family decision making may be desired, ask the patient how he or she would like the decision managed and include the relevant people in the process, perhaps suggesting designation of the decision maker in the family as the proxy. If trust may be insufficient, spend longer time establishing trustworthiness by explaining the nature of your thinking as a clinician, by including other members of the family or community and by avoiding arrogation of decision making and instead sharing information fully and carefully. If death is difficult to talk about, be extra sure that you are comfortable with the topic and that you approach it with simplicity and a listening disposition. Ask if there are methods of talking about dying that might be easier and try to accommodate any requests.

Informed Consent and Competence Standards for Advance Directives

Patients' prior wishes are articulated in real time and must be held to the same standards as any other real-time decisions, namely, to ordinary standards of informed consent. Informed consent has received considerable attention, and its standards can be read about elsewhere (38–40). Although standards may evolve, for the present physicians should ensure that patients understand the nature of the decision, the alternatives, and the risks (common or serious) and benefits. Patients should be over 18 years of age, have decision-making capacity in the relevant areas, and give evidence of having made actual active decisions. Informed consent specifically for advance directives can be considered in two parts. First, patients must consent to making out an advance directive. Patients must know what the basic procedures are (to discuss the issues and record preferences) and understand that traditional decision making (having physicians and legal next of kin use their best judgment) is the alternative. They must know that there are risks either way (e.g., careless advance directives can lead to unintended actions, but traditional decision making is known to correspond poorly to patients' wishes). To be competent in the use of instructional directives, patients have to be competent using imagined scenarios. Otherwise, they will not be able to understand the intervention choices they are making for future potential situations. This is not as dissimilar as it may initially seem from real-time decisions, because real-time decisions are also based on how people think they will feel in the future while living with the consequences of the immediate decision.

Second, discussions of advance directives need to ensure adequate information and decision making for any specific treatment decisions made. This can be difficult because of the large number of decisions included in some instructional directives and because of the sketchy nature of delineated scenarios in the advance directive. Many instructional directives specifically state that they are to be used as a guide to the patient's wishes rather than as a series of treatment decisions. For this reason, standards of informed consent can be relaxed to some degree. Nonetheless, the standards must be sufficient to provide an accurate picture of the patient's wishes. The use of well-designed brochures or other information packets that describe key interventions can help ensure informed consent standards. The key interventions should include mechanical respiration, resuscitation, chemotherapy or radiation therapy, dialysis, simple diagnostic tests, and pain control (including the potential side effects of dulled cognition and respiratory depression). Whether or not information aides are used, physicians must ensure evidence of patients' comprehension.

Valid Expressions

An efficient means for physicians to assist patients in making valid expressions and recordings of prior preferences is to provide them with a validated predrafted instructional directive and to go through it. If patients have been able to complete such a directive, meeting standards of informed consent for the wishes they express, then the statements recorded must be considered valid. The validation of predrafted instruments for the articulation of subjective matters is a well-developed discipline in itself. Generally speaking, instruments must meet standards of content validity, construct validity, criterion-related validity, and test–retest reliability. The first requires that the instrument cover the relevant content matter, the second that items in the instrument be constructed to fit the concepts of the subject matter, the third that the items bear sensible relationships to existing relevant scales and to one another, and the fourth that if the same items were used again at a different time a reasonably similar set of responses would be obtained (19). Predrafted advance directives should meet these standards, as adapted to the needs of advance directives; unfortunately, few directives are available that meet such standards (31,41).

HOW TO DO IT

Five Steps in a Continuing Process

The creation of recorded advance directives is one step in a longitudinal process that should be integrated into the totality of clinical care. Although five steps can be identified, they will rarely be so distinct in actual practice. First is raising the topic. Second, and most important, is structuring a core discussion to cover the main issues and to start the patient thinking about his or her views. Third is reviewing the final document and putting it in the medical record. Fourth is updating the directive from time to time. Fifth is ensuring its availability and use, applying it to decisions that arise after the patient has become wishless (42).

Raising the Topic, Providing Background Information, and Advising on Proxy Choice

First, the topic must be raised. This may be the hardest part, although once expected and routinized, it is a surprisingly easy matter.

With whom should the topic be raised? Among oncology patients, everyone should have the opportunity for advance care planning, whether the prognosis for cure is excellent or poor. Sometimes, patients would have discussed advance care planning with their primary care or other physician. The oncologist can build on this foundation. The topic should not be avoided on the assumption that it has been dealt with. Patients who have completed advance care planning before receiving their oncologic diagnosis may have since changed their perspective. The extent and structure of the planning may not have been as good as what the oncologist can offer. Most important of all, the oncologist needs to know the substance of the patient's current health advance care planning.

In an oncology or a palliative care practice, the topic can be raised by the fourth or fifth visit, depending on the emotional and medical circumstances. Time should be allowed before advance care planning for confirmation of the diagnosis, exploration of treatment options, establishment of a solid therapeutic relationship, and adjustment by the patient to his or her diagnosis (9,43). Earlier mention, say at the second or third visit, that advance planning will be a component of the routine care that should occur for all patients with or without cancer can facilitate the process.

One manner in which the topic can be raised is as follows:

"Ms/r. X, I want to talk with you about planning for future medical care. Many now recommend that people make plans whether or not they have an illness, and that doctors discuss these issues routinely with patients. There is even a federal law that aims to let people know that advance planning is available to all people. We should go through these issues together. It is part of getting to know your values and helping to ensure that you are cared for the way you would want to be even in times of life-threatening illness when communication may be impossible. There is nothing new about your health, and I am not hiding bad news that we have not already discussed; planning for the future simply is prudent. Is this something you have explored before?"

It is helpful to be able to add, as is true for many oncologists:

"I myself have done this as a routine matter, despite being in good health."

Some issues for the patient to consider in selecting a proxy can be included at this point, in particular that being a proxy is a complex and burdensome task, and that family members and close friends may have interests that conflict with the patient's. Most people prefer to select someone close to them as a proxy nonetheless, and usually for good reason, but the possibilities of appointing a more distant friend or a professional such as a social worker or lawyer are worth considering. Some patients suggest appointing the physician as proxy. Because the idea of a proxy is to have someone to talk with the physician, this is usually not the best idea. The patient should be reassured that the physician will in any case be working to make the best decision for the patient and that additional proxy powers are usually unnecessary; participation by the physician in creating a written directive, perhaps without a designated proxy can be a helpful alternative.

Nonphysician health care providers can assist in the first step of raising the topic and providing background information. Reports of interventions to improve advance care planning have included physician-led, nurse-led, social worker-led, and multifaceted interventions (44–50). Brochures and predrafted forms and videos or closed-circuit television programs can also be made available in patient information libraries and patient rooms.

Structured Discussion: Discerning Personal Thresholds and Goals for Care

Second, the topic must be discussed. This is usually done best by the patient and the family on their own time, once they have been oriented to key features of the task. The proxy should be present at this discussion whenever possible. He or she can be advised to listen and ask for any needed clarification, in preparation for the potential role of speaking for the patient, and may even act as a scribe, penciling down the patient's statements. An efficient way of structuring a discussion is to go through a validated blank directive, using it as a worksheet (31). Using a pencil rather than a pen to fill in the patient's wishes, and having the pencil in the patient's or the proxy's hand, can help emphasize explicitly that in this discussion the directive is being used as a worksheet and not as a final document. Start the discussion in the following manner:

"Let's look at these standardized circumstances. You will go through one or two and then perhaps another one or two more. You can then do the rest later. Imagine this first case in the worksheet. Say you are in a coma with no awareness. Assume there is a chance that you might wake up, but it isn't likely, and recovery may involve serious disability. Some people would want us to withdraw treatment and let them die, others would want us to attempt everything possible, and yet others would want us to try

to restore quality of life but stop treatment if it was not working. What do you think your goals for medical care would be?"

Useful scenarios to have the patient and the family go through include the following:

1. A coma with a small chance of recovery (see preceding text)
2. A persistent vegetative state and
3. A moribund state with waxing and waning consciousness

The first three or so scenarios should be standard scenarios designed to cover the major situations commonly encountered when advance directives pertain. Then two or three additional scenarios can be used that are tailored to the patient. One may be created by the physician, based on the patient's illness and expectable circumstances (20). Another may be created by the patient if he or she wishes, based on what the patient considers to be a state worse than death that has not already been covered in previous scenarios (22). It may also be important to consider a scenario in which the patient is in his or her current health and acquires a new life-threatening illness involving incompetence.

In each scenario, the patient's goals for care are selected and then illustrated with some selected intervention preferences. The commonly considered intervention preferences are as follows:

1. Resuscitation
2. Mechanical respiration
3. Chemo- or radiation therapy
4. Renal dialysis
5. Major surgery, and
6. Artificial nutrition/hydration

In addition, preferences regarding simple diagnostic tests and antibiotics provide useful information.

When scenario-based documents with intervention choices are used, it is possible to derive a patient's personal thresholds for intervention. These can be particularly helpful when inferring from scenarios in a prior statement to real situations. For instance, when using the Medical Directive, scenarios are arrayed in a sequence that approximates a gradient of prognosis severity (41). For each scenario, potential interventions are arranged approximately by the level of burdensomeness. An individual tends to have a threshold regarding burdensomeness and regarding prognosis that can be seen when all the options are filled in. Table 62.1 illustrates schematically how this can occur; the dark line represents one patient's, personal thresholds for prognosis and for burdensomeness. This approach is supported by the finding that most patients are concerned about prognosis and treatment burden when they engage in advance care planning (51–53).

Another threshold can often be seen by looking at a patient's goals for care across the scenarios. A wide range of goals is possible; far from being a dichotomous choice between intervention versus comfort, care can be a unique blend of both for every scenario. A patient's thresholds for goals can serve as a combination of prognosis and intervention thresholds, that is, as an overall guide. Table 62.2 illustrates the same hypothetical patient's thresholds for goals. Because research indicates that extrapolating from a person's goals for care to specific interventions is reasonably accurate, it may be best to focus primarily on goals for care in an advance care planning discussion, especially if time is short (18).

Some sensitive issues should be specifically addressed, not least because they may not fit the rest of the person's pattern of preferences (26). One of these has to do with comfort measures because pain control may blunt alertness. Most people can also say whether pain control or being alert and unconfused to the last possible moment is more important to them.

TABLE 62.1

DISCERNING PERSONAL THRESHOLDS FOR INTERVENTION WITH MEDICAL DIRECTIVES

Scenario ▶	Best prognosis	Less good prognosis	Worse prognosis	Worst prognosis
▼ Intervention				
Least burdensome	Consent	Consent	Decline	Decline
Less burdensome	Consent	Consent	Decline	Decline
More burdensome	Decline	Decline	Decline	Decline
Most burdensome	Decline	Decline	Decline	Decline

After these scenarios, patients can be asked what they would consider to be the best to be hoped for from the dying process. Most can say, for instance, that they want enough time to settle things with people they are involved with, that they want to have done one particular thing, or that they want to be in a particular place. Elicitation of these images of a good dying should not be construed as promises to fulfill them; rather, the physician should tell the patient that the images may help in orchestrating care that fits as much as possible with the patient's wishes.

There are certain key positions that patients should be encouraged to articulate during or after their consideration of the scenarios. One is their position on withholding versus withdrawing life-sustaining therapy, because some people have strong positions on the distinction or lack thereof between the two, and it is well to have a specific indication whether an unwanted intervention, if in place already, should be withdrawn. Another topic that can be included in the scenarios is the place of pain control. Use of pain medications intended to control pain but with a known side effect of hastening death is generally considered morally acceptable. Physician-assisted suicide, although not generally accepted, is receiving wide attention, and it may be helpful to clearly articulate preferences and positions on this matter. Physicians who have patients requesting actions they cannot condone should advise the patients of this fact at this early stage. Similarly, the proxy should raise objections at this stage if necessary.

Even if the physician is involved in structuring most of the discussion, the entire process need take no more than 15 minutes once the physician has gained experience with it. The intent is not to reach final resolution or to elicit extended narratives. Rather, it is to identify the key issues that patients should think about and to provide them with a good method for recording their preferences. Nonetheless, during these steps patients commonly communicate deeply held values. Witnessing such expressions can give physicians a strong sense of the privilege of caring for patients, and the knowledge that ensues about how health issues fit with the individual patient's sense of meaning in life can be of great practical importance. Involvement of other members of the interdisciplinary team can make matters more efficient and can assist the team in having a care plan that is well understood. Reciprocally, patients can feel clearer, more understood, and confident.

Patients should be encouraged to absorb the informational materials and to talk over all the issues with their family, friends, pastor, lawyer, counselor, or whomever they consider to be relevant, until they have reached a settled view for themselves (9). The patient can then prepare a statement, preferably in a fashion that includes a validated advisory form and a statutory form that can then be stapled together if they are not already combined.

Recording the Document

Once the patient has completed the essential personal discussions outside the physician's office, he or she can bring the document in for a final review by the physician. At this point, the physician can check for medical misconceptions and major changes that may need inquiry. This should take only a few moments in most cases. It is useful to have a space where the physician can cosign the document (54). This signature should not be a requirement, but its presence fosters the physician's involvement and carries an important implicit message of partnership between the patient and the physician.

Updating the Document

Documents should be reviewed at routine intervals. For a patient who has undergone a cure or for whom the prognosis

TABLE 62.2

DISCERNING PERSONAL THRESHOLDS FOR GOALS USING MEDICAL DIRECTIVES

Scenario ▶	Best prognosis	Less good prognosis	Worse prognosis	Worst prognosis
▼ Goal				
Comfort and quality of life are the primary goals				√
Treat readily curable conditions and also emphasize comfort and quality of life			√	
Treat everything but reconsider often		√		
Treat everything; longevity is the primary goal	√			

is good, this review should occur every 1 to 5 years and after major life changes such as childbirth, marriage, divorce, significant health status changes, bereavement, and important experiences of others' ill health. Most reviews will be rapid. Specific treatment decisions are about as durable as other major life decisions, such as marriage (23,55–57). When a patient shows a particularly high level of instability, this may indicate incompetence for advance decision making, and the physician should review the matter, perhaps advising simple designation of a proxy instead of instructional directives.

Applying the Document to Real Decisions

Occasionally, prior preferences fit the eventual circumstances and application of the prior preferences requires little interpretation or extrapolation. More often, the fit is not perfect and prior preferences can guide but not precisely direct the decisions. Interpretation and extrapolation is necessary. In doing so, it is important to know that certain patterns of decisions have high degrees of predictability. If a patient's prior directives do not cover the decision at hand, it may well be possible to extrapolate from the preferences that are provided in the directive. Such predictions can be far more accurate than unguided judgments. Decline of less-invasive interventions predicts decline of more-invasive interventions, and acceptance of more-invasive interventions predicts acceptance of less-invasive interventions. Acceptance of intervention in poor-prognosis scenarios predicts acceptance in better-prognosis scenarios, and decline in better-prognosis scenarios predicts decline in poorer prognoses. The use of simple calculations can even provide probability estimates of specific decisions, which, when very high or very low, can be a comforting guide to proxy decision makers (24).

Pitfalls and Preventive Measures

A common pitfall is to omit advance care planning discussions altogether (58). Another variation on this theme is to mistakenly suppose that a "DNR discussion" is sufficient advance care planning. Discussing cardiopulmonary resuscitation and use of a DNR order in the absence of considering a range of scenarios and goals for care is often needlessly frightening for patients, considering as it does only the moment of death, and often yields unstable decisions and poor guidance to providers (23,24). If a clinician cares for a patient for whom a DNR order is written without comprehensive orders, such as are outlined in a POLST form, this should prompt a review of advance care planning with that patient (11).

As advance directives gradually come into more general use, common pitfalls are emerging (59). Assessment of a patient's competence to undertake advance care planning can be difficult if profound psychological issues or psychiatric diagnoses are involved. Occasionally, for instance, a patient will show major inconsistency in treatment plans or will ask for extremes of no treatment or undue intervention. These may be indications of ineffective emotional adjustment to medical circumstance. Although not strictly incompetent for completing advance directives, these patients may do better using proxy designation rather than instructional directives to preserve flexible decision making. Alternatively, advance care planning can be deferred or updated frequently until psychotherapy or other assistance has secured better emotional adjustment.

A further problem is the noninclusion of relevant parties at the early stages of planning. The noninclusion of the proxy or of the family members or close friends who have divergent opinions can lead to fractured decision making. The noninclusion of the physician can lead to inadequate sensitization of the physician to the patient's thinking. For

instance, a recent major study showed that when a nurse is the main communicator in advance planning, the physician's understanding of the patient's wishes is not improved (60).

Poor informed consent and documentation constitute another pair of pitfalls. For example, a patient may express a strong desire to avoid perpetual dependence on a respirator, but the wording of the advance directive may indicate that a respirator should never be used. In the event of reversible pneumonia, the patient may well want temporary use of a respirator. A properly validated directive should require this kind of distinction, and physicians should ensure this minimum level of patients' understanding. Physicians should check the document for improbable statements and ask patients to briefly state their wishes in free words, checking for correspondence with medical possibilities.

Perhaps the most common pitfall of all is the activation of advance directives before patients have reached a wishless state, and sometimes even before they have reached an incompetent state for making the decision(s) at hand. A widespread tendency to avoid direct communication with patients appears to exacerbate this problem. Advance directives, as distinct from their predecessor, the DNR order, have no authority when they are first written and must not be activated until the patient is decisionally incapacitated and wishless.

A final crucial pitfall is the poor application of wishes to eventual decisions. Some studies have indicated that physicians rather commonly override advance directives (61). Whether this is because patients are decisionally incapacitated but not wishless, or because proxy opinions persuade physicians more than the patient's advance directives, or for other reasons is not well studied. Nonetheless, if a patient has a validated advance directive that uses scenarios and specific intervention choices, extrapolation to unstated decisions can be accomplished with considerable accuracy in many cases.

BROADER USES

Structured Deliberation

An unforeseen benefit brought about by the idea of advance directives was a general increase in attention to the questions of how patients' health care values can be elicited, understood, documented, and used as the driving force behind therapeutic decision making. In a sense, the field emerged from a desire to move the medical question from "What is the right decision?" to "Who should make the decision?" with the intended answer being "the patient." However, as the desirability of multilateral decision making became more accepted, the question has become "What is the right kind of deliberative process for the decision?" This latter question is potentially relevant to a wide range of decisions and circumstances. In delineating a set of validated worksheets and structured deliberations for advance directives, the concept of structured deliberation for a wide range of medical decisions and approaches has emerged (62,63). Clinicians who engage in structured deliberation will find that advance care planning fits seamlessly into their routines of care.

Structuring Other Care Plans

The use of care plans need not be limited to scenarios involving incompetence and wishlessness. Plans can usefully be made for situations involving no loss of competence as well. Nursing home and hospice facilities often make use of such plans. A common example is prior decision making regarding transfer to a hospital facility in case of medical deterioration. Those who decline may have a written "Do Not Hospitalize" order. Similar decisions about levels of medical care within the facility can also be made. For instance, some patients may elect comfort care only, whereas others may elect simple diagnostic maneuvers but no invasive ones, and others may elect full aggressive care. Corresponding orders and/or notes can be written in patients' records. Such decisions must always be subject to change if the patient wishes, just as advance directives are adjustable while the patient is competent. Nonetheless, such planning provides important communication and often streamlines decision making in the event of otherwise difficult decisions.

Intervention for Turbulent Thought Processes

Patients in difficult medical circumstances often face existential decisions. Turbulent emotions and turbulent thinking are common. For instance, a patient may understand that he or she has incurable cancer and therefore decline chemotherapy, but when faced with the need to make a decision about resuscitation may be precipitated into an emotional crisis by the sense of imminent death or impending abandonment and may decline a "Do Not Resuscitate" order. Such decisions are often perplexing to providers, and discord between parties readily ensues. Discord over goals or treatment decisions should alert physicians to the likelihood that patients are facing emotional and moral turbulence. A structured dialogue can be very helpful. The preset scenarios in a validated generic advance directive provide an excellent structure. By going back over preset scenarios that the patient knows were designed independently and that cover questions likely to be relevant (because the document is validated), the physician may be able to discern the structure of the patient's nonturbulent moral thought. With the more stable structure returned, it is possible to reapproach a scenario that is tailored to the patient and, finally, the patient's current situation. Often, the patient no longer feels threatened by the sense of imminent mortality, and coherent thought processes and decisions can occur again. If these discussions are conducted in the presence of the proxy and other relevant care providers, there can be a refocusing of the entire group of providers on the retrieved coherent plan. Difficult personal interactions and time-consuming confusions can be put aside, allowing people to get on with the business of reaching a state of existential maturity, and when relevant, preparing for death on a personally meaningful level (64).

Structured deliberations such as these can also provide an approach to patients who request euthanasia or physician-assisted suicide. Some patients may have firm and persuasive reasons for requesting such actions, but many patients are in fact seeking something else. Some seek control, some attempt to avoid pain, and some try to address concerns about being a burden or being abandoned. A structured path through scenarios allows patients to assert control and gain assurances that pain can be controlled in most cases, that there are ways of planning for burden and nonabandonment, and that there are ways to exit this world without active euthanasia or assisted suicide. Some physicians find active euthanasia morally defensible in some instances, and others do not. But all must agree that patients who request it erroneously, actually seeking care, should be identified and guided toward the actions they really desire. Structured deliberations can provide a sensitive, professional, and efficient method to help patients understand their own desires. Importantly, they also provide physicians with a chance to communicate explicitly what their moral position is; physicians who do not find active euthanasia or physician-assisted suicide acceptable can make this clear in the supportive setting while simultaneously making clear what comfort care they can offer.

LIMITATIONS AND FUTURE DIRECTIONS

As important as advance directives may be, they have clear limitations and should not be construed as a panacea for decision making about life-sustaining interventions. Especially in the case of patients who are moderately demented or otherwise decisionally incapacitated but not wishless, advance directives offer no more than tangible evidence of one among other perspectives to be weighed in the decision. Even for patients who are wishless, advance directives provide a way to augment the honoring of surviving interests, but they do not offer perfect evidence of all relevant wishes.

No Evidence for Direct Cost Savings

Some advocates have suggested that the use of advance directives can effect considerable cost savings. This perspective has been motivated by the assumption that their use would help avoid unwanted and costly interventions and therefore help reduce the costs of medical care. Although end-of-life care is very costly, there is evidence that patients tend to opt for more treatment than physicians and nurses, and that proxies opt for even more intervention (65,66). In addition, although hospice and palliative care have traditionally been less costly than hospital care for dying patients, these populations are self-selecting. A randomized controlled trial found no cost savings, perhaps indicating that patients, taken in the aggregate, may be getting more or less the degree of intervention that they want (67,68). Studies have not calculated the indirect or nonmedical costs as well as the direct, medical costs. Because the costs of care and of opportunities lost to the families appear to be high (69), studies that examine comprehensive costs are still necessary. In the meantime, however, individual matches with patients' wishes are found to be poor in many studies, and advance planning should continue with the goal of closing this gap. These motivations for advance planning have overwhelming independent merit and should not be confused with false economic incentives.

When Patients Have No Advance Directive

About half of all patients have an estate will. If even this form of well-accepted planning for death is not used by more patients, it is likely that advance directives will also have a similar "ceiling." To meet the objective of attempting to match decisions with patients' prior preferences, it may be helpful to have supplementary approaches (70). In circumstances when the patient comes from a population of patients whose preferences have been studied and documented, it is possible to refer to those data to help guide their decisions. Therefore, if it is known that the patients registered at the hospital in question declined resuscitation for the situation at hand in 85% of instances, the proxy may find this to be useful guiding information. In cases when the proxy has no idea how to speak on behalf of the patient, the physician may indicate that the greatest likelihood of matching the patient's prior wishes, if only the patient had had a chance to articulate them, will be by following the majority preferences of others. Naturally, these default guidelines should not be coercive or replace valid personal directives.

References

1. President's Commission for the Study of Ethical Problems in Medicine and Biomedical Research. *Deciding to forego life-sustaining treatment: a report on the ethical, medical, and legal issues in treatment decisions.* Washington, DC: Government Printing Office, 1983.

2. Lynn J. Why I don t have a living will. *Law Med Health Care* 1991;19:101–104.

3. Seghal A, Galbraith A, Chesney M, et al. How strictly do dialysis patients want their advance directives followed? *JAMA* 1992;267:59–63.

4. Emanuel EJ, Emanuel LL. Proxy decision making. *JAMA* 1992;267:2221–2226.

5. Hines SC, Glover JJ, Babrow AS, et al. Improving advance care planning by accommodating family preferences. *J Palliat Med* 2001;4(4):481–489.

6. Rabkin MT, Gillerman G, Rice NR. Orders not to resuscitate. *N Engl J Med* 1976;295:364–366.

7. Emanuel LL. Does the do-not-resuscitate order need life sustaining intervention? Time for advance care directives. *Am J Med* 1989;86:87–90.

8. Ratner E, Norlander L, McSteen K. Death at home following a targeted advance-care planning process art home: the kitchen table discussion. *J Am Geriatr Soc* 2001;49(6):778–781.

9. Voogt E, van der Heide A, Rietjens JA, et al. Attitudes of patients with incurable cancer toward medical treatment in the last phase of life. *J Clin Oncol* 2005;23(9):2012–2019.

10. Bedell SE, Delbanco TL. Choices about cardiopulmonary resuscitation in the hospital: when do physicians talk with patients? *N Engl J Med* 1984;310:1089–1093.

11. Cantor MD. Improving advance care planning: lessons form POLST. Physician orders for life-sustaining yes. *J Am Geriatr Soc* 2000;48(10):1343.

12. Bok S. Personal directions for care at the end of life. *N Engl J Med* 1976;295:367–369.

13. Relman AS. Michigan's sensible living will. *N Engl J Med* 1979;300:1270–1272.

14. Doukas DJ, McCullough LB. The values history: the evaluation of the patient's values and advance directives. *J Fam Pract* 1991;32:145–153.

15. Emanuel LL, Emanuel EJ. The medical directive: a new comprehensive advance care document. *JAMA* 1989;261:3288–3293.

16. Schneiderman LJ, Pearlman RA, Kaplan RM, et al. Relationship of general advance directive instructions to specific life-sustaining treatment preferences in patients with serious illness. *Arch Intern Med* 1992;152:2114–2122.

17. Fischer G, Alpert H, Stoeckle JD, et al. Relationship between goals and treatment preferences in advance directives. *J Gen Intern Med* 1994;9:93.

18. Doukas DJ, Gorenflo DW. Analyzing the values history: an evaluation of patient medical values and advance directives. *J Clin Ethics* 1993;4:41–45.

19. Nunally JC. *Psychometric theory*, 2nd ed. New York: McGraw-Hill, 1978:265–270.

20. Singer PA. Disease-specific advance directives. *Lancet* 1994;344:594–596.

21. Berry SR, Singer PA. The cancer-specific advance directive. *Cancer* 1998;82(8):1570–1577.

22. Patrick DO, Starks HE, Cain KC, et al. Measuring preferences for health states worse than death. *Med Decis Making* 1994;14:9–18.

23. Emanuel LL, Emanuel EJ, Stoeckle JD, et al. Advance directives: stability of patients treatment choices. *Arch Intern Med* 1994;154:209–217.

24. Emanuel LL, Barry MJ, Emanuel EJ, et al. Advance directive: can patients stated treatment choices be used to infer unstated choices? *Med Care* 1994;32:95–105.

25. Alpert H, Hoijtink R, Fischer G, et al. Psychometric analysis of an advance directive. *Med Care* 1996;34:1055–1063.

26. Schwartz CE, Merriman MP, Reed GW, et al. Measuring patient treatment preferences in end-of-life care research: applications for advance care planning interventions and response shift research. *J Palliat Med* 2004;7(2):233–245.

27. *Right to life legislation*. New York: Choice in Dying, 1994.

28. Gostin LO. Ethics, the constitution, and the dying process: the case of Theresa Marie Schiavo. *JAMA* 2005;293:2403–2407.

29. Weir RF, Gostin L. Decisions to abate life-sustaining treatment for non-autonomous patients: ethical standards and legal liability for physicians after Cruzan. *JAMA* 1990;264:1846–1853.

30. Emanuel EJ. A review of the ethical and legal aspects of terminating medical care. *Am J Med* 1988;84:291–301.

31. Emanuel LL. What makes a directive valid? *Hastings Cent Rep* 1994;24 (6 Suppl):S27–S29.

32. Dresser RS. Advance directives, self-determination, and personal identity. In: Hackler C, Moseley R, Vawter DE, eds. *Advance directives in medicine.* New York: Praeger Publishers, 1989:155–170.

33. *In re Karen Ann Quinlan* 70 N.J. 10, 355 A.2d 647 1976.

34. Perkins HS, Geppert CM, Gonzales A, et al. Cross-cultural similarities and differences in attitudes about advance care planning. *J Gen Intern Med* 2002;17(1):48–57.

35. Blackhall LJ, Murphy ST, Frank G, et al. Ethnicity and attitudes toward patient autonomy. *JAMA* 1995;274:820–825.

36. McKinley ED, Garrett JM, Evans AT, et al. Differences in end-of-life decision making among black and white ambulatory cancer patients. *J Gen Intern Med* 1996;11:651–656.

37. Carrese JA, Rhodes LA. Western bioethics on the Navajo reservation: benefit or harm? *JAMA* 1995;274:826–829.

38. Appelbaum PS, Lidz CW, Meisel A. *Informed consent: legal theory and clinical practice.* New York: Oxford University Press, 1987.

39. Faden RR, Beauchamp TL. Decision-making and informed consent: a study of the impact of disclosed information. *Soc Indic Res* 1980;7:313–336.

40. Shapiro R. Informed consent. In: Berger A, Levy MH, Portenoy RK et al. eds. *Principles and practice of supportive oncology.* Philadelphia, PA: JB Lippincott Co, 1996.

41. www.medicaldirective.org.

42. Emanuel LL, Danis M, Pearlman RA, et al. Advance care planning as a process. *Am Geriatr Soc* 1995;43:440–446.

43. Knight S, Emanuel L. *Creative adaptation to loss: a conceptual model J Palliative Medicine* 2006;(In press).

44. Wenger NS, Kanouse DE, Collins RL, et al. End-of-life discussions and preferences among persons with HIV. *JAMA* 2001;285(22):2880–2887.

45. Grimaldo DA, Wiener-Kronish JP, Jurson T, et al. A randomized, controlled trial of advanced care planning discussions during preoperative evaluations. *Anesthesiology* 2001;95(1):43–50.

46. Lorenz KA, Lynn J. Oregon's lessons for improving advance care planning. *J Am Geriatr Soc* 2004;52(4):233–237.

47. Henderson ML. Gerontological advance practice nurses: an end-of-life care facilitators. *Geriatr Nurs* 2004;25(4):247–254.

48. Morrison RS, Chichin E, Carter J, et al. The effect of a social work intervention to enhance advance care planning documentation in the nursing home. *J Am Geriatr Soc* 2005;53(2):290–294.

49. Briggs LA, Kirchhoff KT, Hammes BJ, et al. Patient-centered advance care planning in special patient populations: a pilot study. *J Prof Nurs* 2004;20(1):47–58.

50. Pearlman RA, Starkes H, Cain KC, et al. Improvements in advance care planning in the Veterans Affairs System: results of a multifaceted intervention. *Arch Intern Med* 2005;165(6):667–674.

51. Weeks JC, Cook EF, O'Day SJ, et al. Relationship between cancer patient's predictions of prognosis and their treatment preferences. *JAMA* 1998;279:1709–1714.

52. Fried TR, Bradley EH, Towle VR, et al. Understanding the treatment preferences of seriously ill patients. *N Engl J Med* 2002;346:1061–1066.

53. Fried TR, Bradley EH. What matters to seriously ill older persons making end-of-life treatment decisions?: a qualitative study. *J Palliat Med* 2003;6(2):237–244.

54. Orentlicher D. Advance medical directives. *JAMA* 1990;263:2365–2367.

55. Silverstein MD, Stocking CB, Antel JP, et al. Amyotrophic lateral sclerosis and life-sustaining therapy: patient s desires for information, participation in decision making, and life-sustaining therapy. *Mayo Clin Proc* 1991;66:906–913.

56. Everhart MA, Pearlman RA. Stability of patient preferences regarding life-sustaining treatments. *Chest* 1990;97:159–164.

57. Danis M, Patrick DL, Garrett J, et al. Stability of choices about life-sustaining treatments. *Ann Intern Med* 1994;120:567–573.

58. Lynn J, Goldstein NE. Advance care planning for fatal chronic illness: avoiding commonplace errors and unwarranted suffering. *Ann Intern Med* 2003;138(10):812–818.

59. Emanuel LL. Appropriate and inappropriate use of advance directives. *Clin Ethics* 1994;5(4):357–359.

60. The SUPPORT investigators. A controlled trial to improve decision-making for seriously ill hospitalized patients: the struggle to understand prognoses and preferences for outcomes and risks of treatments (SUPPORT). *JAMA* 1995;274(20):1591–1598.

61. Danis M, Southerland LI, Garrett JM, et al. A prospective study of advance directives for life-sustaining care. *N Engl J Med* 1991;324:882–888.

62. Emanuel LL. Structured deliberation for medical decision making for the seriously ill. *Hastings Cent Rep* 1995;25(6):514–518.

63. Kasper JF, Mulley AG Jr, Wennberg JE. Developing shared decision-making programs to improve the quality of health care. *Qual Rev Bull* 1992;18(6):183–190.

64. Schwartz C, Lennes I, Hammes B, et al. Honing and advance care planning intervention using qualitative analysis: the Living Well interview. *J Palliat Med* 2003;6(4):593–603.

65. Steiber SR. Right to die: public balks at deciding for others. *Hospitals* 1987;61:72.

66. Gillick MR, Hesse K, Massapica N. Medical technology at the end of life. What would physicians and nurses want for themselves? *Arch Intern Med* 1993;153:2542–2547.

67. Kane RL, Wales J, Bernstein L, et al. A randomized controlled trial of hospice care. *Lancet* 1984;1:890–894.

68. Emanuel EJ, Emanuel LL. The economics of dying–the illusion of cost savings at the end of life. *N Engl J Med* 1994;330:540–544,

69. Covinsky K, Goldman L, Cook EF, et al. The impact of serious illness on patient's families. *JAMA* 1994;272:1841–1844

70. Emanuel LL, Emanuel EJ. When patients have no advance directives: institutional default guidelines defined by communities of patients. *Hastings Cent Rep* 1993;23:6–14.

CHAPTER 63 ■ WITHHOLDING AND WITHDRAWING POTENTIALLY LIFE-SUSTAINING TREATMENT

RICHARD J. ACKERMANN

> "I will define what I conceive medicine to be: In general terms, it is to do away with the suffering of the sick, to lessen the violence of their disease, and to refuse to treat those who are overmastered by their disease, realizing that in such cases medicine is powerless."
> Hippocrates of Cos, 460-380 B.C.

More than 500,000 patients die of cancer in the United States every year. A couple of generations ago, these patients died rather speedily, from cardiopulmonary failure, sepsis, or other causes. Now, a substantial number of patients with cancer find themselves dying over a prolonged period in highly technologic and sometimes impersonal environments, such as the intensive care unit. By the time patients are dying in the intensive care unit, fewer than 10% can participate in the decision-making process, except through advance directives or surrogates. More and more, we are faced with decisions to forego cardiopulmonary resuscitation (CPR) or other forms of life-sustaining treatments. At least 65% of patients with cancer prefer to die at home, but only 30% are successful in doing so (1–3).

Helping patients and families make decisions about potential life-sustaining treatments is an essential skill for cancer specialists. The oncologist needs to understand the legal and ethical issues, as well as practical issues of implementation. All 50 states have laws and regulations on informed consent and the withdrawal of life-sustaining treatments. In hospitals and other institutions, the general policy is that physicians should provide all available treatment, unless there are specific decisions to the contrary (4). Over 70% of deaths in US intensive care units now occur as a withdrawal of life-sustaining treatments. The General Medical Council of the United Kingdom has produced a practice guideline on the subject (5).

There are at least three reasons why a physician might agree to withhold or withdraw a potentially life-sustaining treatment. First and by far the most important, we do so to comply with the wish of an autonomous patient or their surrogate, assuming that fully informed consent has been obtained. Second, we do so because the therapy cannot meet the overall treatment goal, even if it would have some short-term physiologic effect. And third, we do so because the therapy has failed and is prolonging the dying process (6).

The central issue for patients suffering from advanced malignancy is not *when* to switch from curative to comfort measures. Appropriate palliation of symptoms is always a goal, from the first diagnosis of cancer through terminal care. Rather, the primary issue is whether continued aggressive care has a realistic chance of working, or whether it is more appropriate to concentrate on comfort, letting the disease take its natural course, and allowing the patient to die (6). Withdrawal of life support should occur when the burdens of treatment outweigh the benefits, as determined by the overall goals of the patient. This is vague but reflects clinical reality. Table 63.1 addresses common concerns oncologists have regarding withholding and withdrawing potentially life-sustaining treatments.

The overall legal and ethical consensus behind withholding and withdrawal is based on patient autonomy. Every competent adult has the right to decide which medical interventions she wants, including the right to refuse treatment, even if that would lead to death. If the patient lacks decision-making capacity, then in all 50 states there is arrangement for a surrogate to be named, who has full legal authority to act. All medical interventions are included, including the decision to use or not use artificial nutrition and hydration (ANH). Patients who die as a result of withdrawal of life-sustaining treatments die of their underlying disease process, not from assisted suicide or euthanasia (8).

There is no moral or legal distinction between withholding and withdrawing a treatment. However, from an emotional and clinical perspective, it is nearly always easier not to begin a treatment rather than to stop it (9).

It is not useful to make a distinction between "ordinary" and "extraordinary" treatments, because these terms can only be defined by each individual. A much better method is to look at the benefits and burdens of the proposed intervention. The "ordinary" treatment of intravenous hydration in a healthy patient with pneumonia may be considered burdensome by another patient who is suffering from end-stage malignancy. Further, the "extraordinary" treatment of hemodialysis and vasopressors can certainly be justified in patients with cancer who experience a complication of cancer or its treatment. Ask this question: what are the benefits and the burdens of the intervention in this particular patient? (1).

Physicians can ensure appropriate care in the hospital, outpatient clinics, and across care settings, even if patients desire not to use certain medical interventions. Unfortunately, studies have documented that too many patients die without attention to these issues. For example, the Study to Understand Prognoses and Preferences for Outcomes and Risks of Treatment (SUPPORT) documented that despite advance directives, many patients underwent invasive medical treatments against previously stated wishes (10).

TABLE 63.1

TYPICAL LEGAL AND ETHICAL CONCERNS CANCER SPECIALISTS MAY HAVE REGARDING THE WITHHOLDING OR WITHDRAWING OF POTENTIALLY LIFE-SUSTAINING TREATMENTS

Are physicians legally required to provide all life-sustaining measures possible?
No. To the contrary, patients have a right to refuse any medical treatment, including life-sustaining treatments such as mechanical ventilation, or even artificial hydration and nutrition.

Is withdrawal or withholding of treatment equivalent to euthanasia?
No. There is a strong general consensus that withdrawal or withholding of treatment is a decision that allows the disease to progress on its natural course. It is not a decision to seek death and end life. Euthanasia actively seeks to end the patient's life.

Are you killing the patient when you remove the ventilator and treat the pain?
No. The intent and sequence of actions are important, as are the means chosen. If the intent is to secure comfort, not death, if the medications are chosen for and titrated to the patient's symptoms, if the medications are not administered with the primary intent to cause death, then ventilator withdrawal and pain medication are not euthanasia.

Can the treatment of symptoms constitute euthanasia?
No. For patients who have been on opiates for pain, it is very difficult to give such high doses that death is caused or even hastened in the absence of a disease process that is leading to imminent death. Patients tend to sleep off the effect if they receive too much medication. However, in the rare circumstance when opiates might contribute to death, provided the intent was to treat the symptoms, then opiate use is not euthanasia.

Is it illegal to prescribe large doses of opiates to relieve pain, breathlessness, or other symptoms?
No. Even very large doses of opiates (thousands of milligrams per day) are permitted and appropriate, if the doses are titrated to the patient's needs.

Adapted with permission from Emanuel LL, von Gunten CJ, Ferris FD. *Education on end-of-life care trainer's guide*, Module 11, withholding, withdrawing therapy. Chicago, IL: Institute for Institute for Ethics at the American Medical Association, EPEC Project, The Robert Wood Johnson Foundation, 1999 (7).

In the SUPPORT, 316 patients with colon cancer metastatic to liver and 747 patients with stage IV non–small cell lung cancer who died within one year of an index hospitalization were studied. During the last 3–6 months of life, more than 50% of both groups preferred treatment that focused on comfort care, even if this shortened their lives. Despite this preference, >25% were in severe pain in the last 3–6 months and >40% were in severe pain the last three days of life (11).

In some circumstances, oncologists have a long-term relationship with patients in community settings, which may facilitate communication at the end of life. In these settings, end-of-life discussions may occur in small pieces over several months or years. In other circumstances, the cancer specialist may be serving as a consultant and may not have the luxury of a long-term relationship. Consultation with palliative care specialists may improve end-of-life care and reduce use of nonbeneficial resources (12).

Patients with cancer may consider many life-sustaining treatments, either related to cancer (chemotherapy, radiation, surgery) or not, such as CPR. There are many other choices patients can make, including elective intubation, mechanical ventilation, dialysis, blood transfusion, artificial nutrition and hydration, diagnostic tests, antibiotics, other medications and treatments, as well as admissions to the hospital or to an intensive care unit. The patient's treatment choices and complexities often increase as the patient becomes overmastered by aggressive malignancy. Many patients who initially want to cure the cancer will have no care restrictions at the beginning of the physician–patient relationship. Patients in whom cancer does not respond to treatment may opt for a do-not-resuscitate status, with progressively more restrictions as the disease progresses. As patients approach the end of life, physicians tend to withdraw life-sustaining treatments in a logical sequence, starting with restricting blood products and progressing through restrictions on dialysis, vasopressors, mechanical ventilation, parenteral nutrition, antibiotics, intravenous fluids, and enteral tube feeding (13).

One reason that physicians (and also patients) may not consider palliative approaches until too late is uncritical acceptance of new technology. Physicians may by seduced by authority—you do something because someone you really respect advocates the procedure, although there is little evidence of its merit. Not only do we accept new technology uncritically, but we also become almost reverent about it. Part of this is that procedures and technology are usually reimbursed well. We also tend to accept unproved dogmas of decades or centuries; some of these turn out to be useless or even harmful. Finally, we sometimes practice medicine based on our last wonderful success or disaster, or ones we have heard about—anecdotal medicine—rather than practicing evidence-based medicine (14).

Generally, medicines such as chemotherapy must have rigorous proof of both efficacy and safety before they are approved for clinical use. However, tests and procedures have no FDA approval. Demand rigorous proof of technologies before incorporating them into practice. Just because a new cancer operation has been invented does not mean it should replace the standard—well-crafted randomized clinical trials should compare the new operation with the old (14).

Oncologists should not only provide general guidelines but also feel free to provide specific advice to patients with cancer and families who are struggling with these difficult decisions. The thoughtful clinician can provide frank advice based on science but also on personal experience. For example, it might be appropriate in one setting to say:

> "You have advanced lung cancer. We can't change that awful fact, but there is much we can still control. Inserting a feeding tube into your stomach may increase the number of days you would live, but the cost may be that the quality of your remaining days would be worse."

The Education for Physicians on End-of-life Care curriculum, supported by the AMA, suggests a workable 8-step process when deciding whether to withhold or withdraw therapy (Table 63.2). Ideally, these steps occur during routine

TABLE 63.2

EIGHT-STEP PROTOCOL TO DISCUSS WITHHOLDING OR WITHDRAWING THERAPY

1. Be thoroughly familiar with your institutional policies and state laws.
2. Choose an appropriate, private setting for the discussion, such as your private office or a counseling room in the hospital.
3. Ask the patient and family what they understand. Make sure everyone is on the same page and understands the medical issues, treatment options, and prognosis. If there is uncertainty or disagreement among physicians, express that uncertainty.
4. Discuss the patient's values and general goals of care. That is, find out what the guiding principle should be—for example, squeezing every possible minute or day from life, living until a daughter's wedding, staying out of the hospital, or relief of symptoms.
5. Establish a context for the discussion. For example:

   "We need to decide now if we should go with more transfusions and bone marrow stimulants," or "Your father's cancer has blocked both of his kidneys, causing kidney failure, and we need to decide if we should proceed to dialysis."

6. Discuss specific treatment preferences. Review the realistic options and make a recommendation on which one(s) seem most reasonable, given the general goals of care.
7. Respond to emotions.
8. Establish and implement the plan. Sometimes, all that will be accomplished is the discussion, and no decision will be made except to continue talking.

Adapted with permission from Emanuel LL, von Gunten CJ, Ferris FD. *Education on end-of-life care trainer's guide*, Module 11, withholding, withdrawing therapy. Chicago, IL: Institute for Institute for Ethics at the American Medical Association, EPEC Project, The Robert Wood Johnson Foundation, 1999 (7).

office follow-ups, although in many cases, they won't happen until a crisis such as febrile neutropenia or a mechanical complication of advanced malignancy has occurred (7).

Patients have different preferences, or styles, in medical decision making. For example, some want all the possible information and then make the decision themselves, while others may want the physician to decide. In a study of 999 women with breast cancer, 18% of women preferred a paternalistic model where the physician makes decisions, 15% wanted the physician to make the decision after hearing her input, 44% wanted a joint physician–patient decision, 14% wanted to make the decision herself after getting the physician's input, and 9% wanted to make all decisions herself (15).

Physicians should find out what the patient or family knows about the current medical situation. There are often tragic misconceptions or misunderstandings, and patients often seek to blame something in their past or medical treatment for their current predicament. Avoid medical jargon, and judge just how much detail is helpful. Some patients want to know everything, while others simply want an overview such as "your kidney function is stable." Provide an honest opinion, express doubt if you have it or if physician consultants disagree. Ask if the patient or family want more information or a second (or third) opinion.

The key to the discussion is determining the general goals of care. For example, the physician may summarize like this:

"Let me tell you what I hear you saying."

If the patient no longer has decision-making capacity, ask the appointed decision maker to articulate the patient's values and goals of care. Encourage the family to use substituted judgment, where they transmit what they believe their loved one would say, rather than what will reduce their guilt. If family disagreements occur, spend more time on the overall goals of care before proceeding to specific treatment options.

Some patients may ask you to "do everything." This "everything" is very broad and easily misinterpreted. It implies that the choice is between everything and nothing, which is almost never true. Further, it assumes that the physician has power over the disease, which is also not true. For example, never ask a family:

"Do you want us to do everything?"

because the obvious answer is:

"Yes, of course we want everything for our mother, whom we love dearly."

If the patient is terminally ill, establish context by a statement such as:

"Your father is dying from the lung cancer, despite everything we have done to try and treat it. His death will probably occur in the next few days or weeks."

After establishing the overall goal of care and a context for decision making, talk about specific treatment options. Provide this information in small pieces. For example, if this is the visit when you tell the patient she has cancer, it is likely that nothing else you say at the visit will be heard. Simply say:

"I have some really bad news. The biopsy came back positive for cancer of the pancreas,"

and wait, sitting silently. Stop to assess for reactions and clarify misunderstandings. Most importantly, allow time for emotion. Patients and their families may be profoundly disturbed, especially at key times such as diagnosis, first metastasis, complications, or failure of standard therapies. You made need other colleagues, such as counselors, to assist. Patients are nearly always grateful for the advice and continued presence of the physician, even if the advice is withdrawing an ineffective treatment (7).

Patients deserve a full and clear understanding of proposed therapies. With advanced cancer, especially when the prognosis is doubtful, always include a discussion of palliative options, even if initial curative/remittive therapy has not yet been offered. Patients may wish comfort-based care to take center stage at some point.

Finally, try to establish a plan. If the patient or her decision maker simply can't do this, then agree to meet again or perhaps convene a family meeting. Ask if a chaplain, social worker, or out-of-town family member should be consulted (7).

HOPE FOR THE BEST, AND PREPARE FOR THE WORST

Patients and oncologists often feel they must choose between fighting the disease and preparing for death. The physician may be reluctant to discuss palliative care or withdrawal of ongoing treatment, because the patient will "lose hope." But hoping for cure and preparing for eventual death need not be exclusive. A recent editorial calls this tension "Hope for the best, and prepare for the worst" (16). These authors give concrete advice on how to talk about chemotherapy and palliative care. Conversations such as these should occur early and often, not just when facing the final weeks of life.

Give time to both hoping and preparing.

> Doctor: "I will do everything I can to put your cancer into remission. We are hoping for the best. Still, I think we should prepare for the worst in case the treatment does not work."

Align the hopes of the patient and physician.

> Doctor: "Tell me more about your hopes for your treatment."

Encourage, but do not impose, the dual agenda of hoping and preparing.

> Patient: "When you talk about preparing for the worst, it feels like you're ready to give up on me."
> Doctor: "The way I think about it, preparing for the worst helps me give you the best medical care, no matter what happens. I want to be your doctor and take care of you. I'm not giving up on you."

Support this dual agenda of hope and preparation over time, as you develop a trusting relationship with the patient and family.

> Patient: "I don't want to think about preparing for the worst."
> Doctor: "It sounds like this is hard for you to consider. Can you describe what makes it hard to consider?"
> Patient: "What if my wife can't handle the worst?"

Respect hopes and fears, and respond to emotions.

> Doctor: "I can see that caring for your family is very important to you. I have some ideas that may help in case the treatment doesn't go the way you and I want it to" (16).

Many patients with cancer are facing a chronic, progressive disease, in which death is approaching at some pace. There are at least two reasons for this. First, the cancer itself may be incurable or relatively so. But second, many patients with cancer also have organ failure, dementia, or other life-limiting illnesses, and the cancer is one more layer of complexity on an already complex set of medical problems.

Ideally, patients and their families are fully informed throughout the trajectory of their illnesses, and palliative care is part of the plan from the beginning. At diagnosis, some patients with cancer have already experienced a brush with death, and some will have had relatives or friends who died from malignancy. Many patients with cancer can be cured. On the other hand, patients with aggressive, incurable diseases expect active care, but they also want it in the context of comfort, dignity, and some level of control.

Avoid prognostic paralysis—if the patient is clearly declining, failing multiple courses of active cancer therapy, do not avoid the obvious. Ask yourself "Would I be surprised if my patient were to die in the next 12 months?" If the answer is no, you would not be surprised, then allow the patient and their family to plan for a better death, rather than simply measuring tumor load and biochemical markers until the moment of death (17). While there is usually no exact answer, there is a good literature to help the physician offer realistic information to patients and families. A recent systematic review showed that experienced clinicians routinely over-estimate survival, although the predictions remain highly correlated, even if miscalibrated (18).

The most important predictive factor in advanced cancer is functional ability, that is, a measure of what the patients can do for himself (16). Commonly used indices are the Karnofsky score (0 is dead, and 100 is normal) and the ECOG (Eastern Cooperative Oncology Group) scale (just the reverse—0 is normal, and 5 is dead). In patients with advanced malignancy, a medical survival of 3 months correlates with a Karnofsky score <50 or ECOG >3 (19). Ask the patient this question:

> "How much time do you spend in bed or lying down?"

If the answer is >50% of the time and is progressively increasing, this correlates with a medical survival of 3 months. Survival would be less if there were substantial symptoms related to the cancer, especially if dyspnea is present.

Several well-recognized cancer syndromes have very short median survival times (19):

- Malignant hypercalcemia—8 weeks (except for newly diagnosed breast cancer or myeloma)
- Malignant pericardial effusion—8 weeks
- Carcinomatous meningitis—8–12 weeks
- Multiple brain metastases—1–2 months without radiation, 3–6 months with radiation

VOLUNTARILY STOPPING EATING AND DRINKING

Sometimes, patients who are perfectly capable of taking in nutrition make a conscious decision to stop all oral intake. The physician is asked to accept this decision, and the patient gradually loses consciousness, usually dying of dehydration or another complication. If all oral intake is stopped, patients usually live 1–3 weeks. If some oral or parenteral fluids are continued, patients may live much longer.

Voluntarily stopping eating and drinking (VSED) does not actually require the participation of the physician, although the physician may be able to support the patient's independence and decision making. Most patients lose appetite and thirst in end-stage malignancy, but not all do. For a few patients, increases in hunger or thirst may actually increase suffering. It can also be difficult for family or the medical team to allow VSED to occur, because some individuals may find the decision immoral. Almost all patients will lose their ability to direct actions at the end, and it may be difficult for the treatment team to continue withholding hydration and nutrition (20).

CARDIOPULMONARY RESUSCITATION

Decisions about resuscitation should take place in the context of the overall goal of care. For example, you might start the conversation with:

> "Let me see if I have this right. You want us to do all we can to fight the tumor, but when your time comes, you want to die peacefully. Is that right?"

A decision *not* to use CPR in the event of death (DNR, do not resuscitate), can also be framed in a more positive, natural way: Allow Natural Death (AND) (21).

"We will do everything we can to keep your father comfortable. Should his heart or lungs give out, we will allow him to die naturally and peacefully."

Following this, you can ask the patient to explain the values that underlie that decision—for example:

"Tell me why you feel that way."

Do not imply the impossible or use the word "everything":

"Do you want us do everything?" or
"Do you want us to put mom on a breathing machine or start her heart?"

Rather, ask the same question in this way:

"If your heart should stop beating or your breathing should stop, would you want us to use 'heroic' measures?"
"Would you want us to compress your chest and put a tube in your lungs to try to get your heart and breathing started again?"

If a patient has indicated he does not want CPR, you could summarize like this:

"It looks like we're agreed that we need to concentrate on your comfort and get you back home. With that in mind, I would recommend against the use of artificial or heroic means to keep you alive. If that's correct, I will write an order in the chart that if your heart stops or you stop breathing, we will not attempt to revive you."

In other cases, the situation may be more ambiguous, or the patient's goals of care may be unclear. Try something like this:

"If you begin to die in spite of all of our aggressive treatment, do you want us to use heroic measures to try and bring you back, or shall we allow a natural death?"

Another suggestion is:

"How do you want things to be when you die?"

After confirming a DNR (or AND) order, always reassure the patient that this restriction does not address any other aspect of care except preventing CPR. A DNR/AND order is not a proxy for any other life sustaining treatment. For example,

"I will write the DNR/AND order in the chart. I want you to know that we are still going to use maximal medical therapy to meet your goals."

Affirm that all other aspects of medical care will still be continued. But if you think other restrictions might be appropriate, either address that or ask for consultation from hospice or palliative care colleagues (22).

Sometimes, patients and families continue to want CPR, even when the physician does not think this therapy is in the patient's best interest. This "unreasonable" request may come from several different areas.

First, patients may have an inflated perception of the success of CPR. While the general public believes that CPR is usually successful, in fact, the actual survival of hospital-based CPR is 10–15% for all patients. For those older than age 70 years, survival to hospital discharge is <15%, and for patients with metastatic cancer or renal failure, survival is much lower (23). Ask the patient,

"What do you know about CPR?"

Guilt can play a powerful role in clinging to aggressive treatment, including CPR. A son may be guilty because he lives 2000 miles away and has not been there to care for his dying mother. You may be able to give an explicit recommendation, or even permission, that it is OK to stop fighting. Open the door with a comment like:

"Deciding on these issues seems very hard for you. I want your mother to have the best care possible. I know that you still want

her to have CPR, and I am hesitant about that. Can you tell me more about your decision?"

For some patients, agreeing to a DNR (AND) order may be equivalent to choosing to die. Acceptance of death in terminal illness does not occur at the same rate for all patients, and for some, it never occurs. The patient/family may view CPR as the "last chance" for continued life. Use a gentle probe such as:

"What do you think we would do differently, after CPR, that we aren't doing now?"

If, after discussion, the patient chooses CPR, their wishes should be accepted, but the discussion can be approached again. Do not forget to talk about other important end-of-life decisions, such as whether to keep up transfusions, bone marrow support, or antibiotic treatment.

Some patients and families have a deep distrust of the medical system, particularly cultures that have traditionally been denied access to first-rate medical care. Or the patient may have had an abrupt experience with a previous physician, or a situation where a dire prognosis was given to a family member, who outlived the prognosis. In some cases, withdrawal of life support may be interpreted as active euthanasia. Address this openly:

"Your decision makes me wonder if you fully trust in the doctors and nurses who are caring for you. Do you have any concerns like that?" (6)

If you believe that CPR cannot work—that it simply will not restore physiologic function, then you have several choices. You can accede to the wish for CPR, continuing to gently counsel against its use. You can also discuss what happens after, if CPR does "work"—would they want to continue on life support measures? If the patient doesn't have a legal surrogate, encourage him to name one while he still has decision-making capacity. However, you are not legally or ethically obligated to do something that you think is wrong. Other options include transfer of care to another physician or facility, but this is often not practical or possible (24,25).

Disagreements between physician and patient/family are best handled through continued conversation and negotiation. Appealing to medical futility is rarely appropriate or practical. The main reason for this is lack of a clear definition of futility. If a patient or family demands care that the physician thinks is futile, Table 63.3 provides several options (26).

A DNR (AND) order may not be valid or respected if a patient dies at home. Remain the patient's advocate and insist that the DNR/AND request be honored. Advise the families of patients who wish to avoid CPR at home to call you or the Hospice in the event of death, not 911, to avoid tragic misunderstandings (27).

MECHANICAL VENTILATION

There are two main options for ventilator withdrawal: immediate extubation and terminal weaning. In immediate extubation, the patient is suctioned and the endotracheal tube is removed. Humified oxygen may be given to keep the airway moist. This is the preferred method if the patient is conscious, secretions are minimal, and the airway is unlikely to be compromised post-extubation. A physician should supervise the extubation—decide if you will do that, or would prefer a palliative care consultant to manage this procedure.

In terminal weaning, ventilator parameters such as tidal volume, FiO_2, PEEP, and rate are progressive decreased, with the endotracheal tube still in place. Terminal weaning can be done over several days or over 30–60 minutes. If the patient survives the terminal wean, the physician may opt to leave

TABLE 63.3

SUGGESTIONS WHEN PATIENTS OR FAMILY DEMAND "FUTILE" TREATMENT

Obtain a second (or third) opinion.
Ask the patient the meaning of the intervention and why they want it.
Get the support of someone who shares the patient's belief system.
Give the patient and family space and time to digest your advice.
Talk about hoping for the best, but planning for the worst.
Ask for consultation from the hospital ethics committee or palliative care team.
Utilize the chaplain service to address spiritual issues.
Ask social workers or other counselors to facilitate communication.
Agree to a time trial of the proposed intervention, agreeing to stop if it is ineffective.
If no progress is made, consider transfer of the patient to another physician or institution.

From Cohen RA. A tale of two conversations. *Hastings Cent Rep* 2004;34(3):49 (21)

the ET tube in place, providing oxygen through a T-piece. Terminal weaning may be preferred for patients are on high-level ventilatory support and for those who have trouble clearing and protecting their airway, to avoid struggling and gasping (8).

Before proceeding to extubation or terminal weaning, the physician needs to counsel the patient/family about likely outcomes of the withdrawal. Some patients will die within minutes, particularly those who are septic or on maximal pressure support. Most patients will die within hours to days, depending on their underlying condition and the details of other medical support. In some cases, there is a small possibility that the patient may regain cardiorespiratory stability, perhaps even enough to resume other treatments and consider hospital discharge. Have an honest discussion of the prognostic uncertainty (28).

Assume that the family knows nothing about the procedure of ventilator withdrawal. Explain what will happen in simple terms, and answer questions. Decide with the family if the endotracheal tube will be removed. Review how you will use oxygen and other medications to manage symptoms. Especially emphasize that you can manage the patient's breathlessness and tachypnea. Let the family know that their loved one will likely need to be asleep to control symptoms. Counsel the family that involuntary gasping or moving does not indicate suffering, if the patient is properly sedated.

Encourage the family to gather and arrange for any special music, rituals, or religious observations. Ask if anyone else should be present, such as friends or clergy. Write a note in the chart, describing the clinical conditions, discussion with the surrogate or family, and the plan. Turn off all monitors and alarms—it is very distressing to watch the oxygen saturation drop point by point or hear ventilator alarms going off.

Turn off any paralytic agents well before the withdrawal. Patients rarely survive ventilator withdrawal, so paralysis is almost always inappropriate.

Remove any restraints and other unnecessary medical equipment, such as nasogastric tubes, telemetry, and venous compression devices. Maintain an i.v. line. Discontinue inotropes, blood pressure support medications, antibiotics, and dialysis. In most cases, turn off the artificial hydration; but if the family cannot accept it, maintain that support.

Clear plenty of space around the bedside for the family to gather. It is important to allow the family to be present, if they wish, throughout the whole process of withdrawal. Offer chairs for the family. One or more family members may wish to hold their loved one's hand. You may have to break hospital rules and allow multiple family members at the bedside, for prolonged times outside regular visiting hours.

Ensure that symptoms such as pain and dyspnea are well managed before extubation. Have a syringe or i.v. drip of an opiate and a benzodiazepine such as midazolam or lorazepam immediately accessible, in case tachypnea, dyspnea, or pain becomes apparent.

If extubation is to occur, it is helpful to have a respiratory therapist or nurse take that function, so you can stand at the foot of the bed for supervision and support of the family. The therapist should have suction and a washcloth at the ready. In general, reduce ventilatory support in the following order: eliminate PEEP, reduce the FiO_2, reduce IMV, reduce pressure support, eliminate IMV breaths, and use a T-piece (in many cases, some of these steps are not needed). Deflate the ET tube and remove it into a waiting towel. Deal with any secretions. Someone should be assigned to silence the ventilator and move it out of the way. Use suction for heavy oropharyngeal secretions, but not routinely. If the patient is awake at all, ask if they would like to be suctioned. If possible, raise the head of the bed to 30°. For the patient who can support his own ventilation, extubation allows closer contact with the family.

Provide tissues for crying. Stay there for a few minutes, if possible. Some patients die immediately, but it is more likely that a patient will live for hours or even days. Spend a few minutes to answer any questions and to ensure that distressing symptoms are managed. The family is often very anxious, wondering if they have done the right thing, and they will need support from their physician. When the patient dies, allow the family to spend as much as time as they want at the bedside (29,30).

The two most common distressing symptoms seen with ventilator withdrawal are dyspnea and anxiety. Be prepared to pretreat and treat both symptoms. Opiates and benzodiazepines are the mainstays of therapy, often at doses that will cause some sedation. There is no medical, legal, or ethical justification for withholding sedation, when death after ventilator withdrawal is the expected outcome, out of fear that death will be hastened. On the other hand, increasing doses beyond those required to effect sedation, with the intention of hastening death, is unacceptable (31).

Provide sedation to all patients undergoing ventilator withdrawal, even those who are deeply comatose. Patients who are fully awake or who have been taking substantial doses of opiates or benzodiazepines will require higher doses to achieve symptom control. The physician should be at the bedside just before and after extubation, to assure symptom management.

For medication-naive patients, give a bolus of morphine 2–10 mg i.v., followed by a morphine infusion of 50% of the bolus dose/hour. Alternatively, fentanyl at 100–250 µg i.v. every 3–5 minutes is appropriate. At the same time, give 1–2 mg i.v. bolus of midazolam, followed by 1 mg/hour intravenously (or diazepam 5–10 mg i.v. every 10 minutes). Get expert help with children. Titrate these medications to achieve excellent control of anxiety and dyspnea prior to extubation (30).

After extubation, if distress is severe, give an immediate intravenous bolus of 5–10 mg morphine and/or 2–4 mg midazolam, every 10 minutes, until symptoms are controlled. Adjust infusion rates to match. The overall goal is not a specific dose but rather relief of symptoms. In general, keep the respiratory rate <30/minute, heart rate <100/minute, and eliminate grimacing and agitation. If titrated morphine or midazolam are ineffective, consider the use of a short-acting barbiturate like pentobarbital, haloperidol, propofol, or consultation with an expert in palliative medicine (30).

ARTIFICIAL NUTRITION AND HYDRATION

Physicians as well as patients have particular problems with withholding or withdrawing artificial nutrition and hydration (ANH). Food and water are powerful social and religious symbols of caring, so withholding ANH may be perceived as callous or neglectful. Some physicians may personally find it unethical to withhold or withdraw these interventions; however strong legal and ethical support is in place for a thoughtful discussion of these issues. Table 63.4 lists situations when withdrawing/withholding ANH may be appropriate.

There are no randomized trials of tube feeding in patients with advanced malignancy. However, there is anecdotal evidence that tube feeding may be life prolonging in very special circumstances, such as patients with proximal GI obstruction and a high functional status, and patients receiving chemotherapy or radiation therapy involving the proximal GI tract. Observational studies have shown no improvement in quality of life in dying patients who receive enteral tube nutrition. Tube feeding may clearly have negative effects on the quality of life, such as the need for physical or chemical restraints, infection, pain, loss of dignity, and loss of the pleasure of eating (32).

Several clinical trials have examined the effect of total parenteral nutrition in patients with advanced malignancy. For example, 128 patients with small cell lung carcinoma who were beginning chemotherapy were randomized to 28 days of total parenteral nutrition (TPN) or no parenteral nutrition. Patients receiving TPN had no benefit in survival, response to chemotherapy, or tolerance to chemotherapy. However, there was a four-fold increased risk of febrile episodes among those receiving TPN, consistent with an increased risk of infection (33). A review of over 70 clinical trials of nutritional support in patients with advanced malignancies

---

TABLE 63.4

CLINICAL CONSIDERATIONS IN STARTING, STOPPING, OR WITHHOLDING ARTIFICIAL NUTRITION AND HYDRATION

Indications to consider starting ANH
The patient or decision maker, after being provided appropriate counseling and options, chooses this intervention to reflect personal values.

  When the primary goal of the patient is to maximize the quantity of life
  When the patient is stable or improving, and the intervention has a reasonable chance of reaching the patient's goals
  When the risk/benefit ratio is unclear, or the evolution of the disease is uncertain. In this case, consider a trial of the intervention, with withdrawal if little or no benefit occurs
  As short-term interventions in healthy patients or those with mild or moderately severe illness (acute neutropenic infections, perioperative use)
  In selected chronic conditions (e.g., patients with esophageal obstruction or massive bowel resection, where oral intake is not possible or inadequate)
  When a patient is unable to swallow and remains hungry or thirsty
  When delirium may be due to dehydration
  To maintain life for a period, while the decision maker/family struggles with end-of-life decisions
  When there is no clear decision-maker, or the family cannot reach a consensus
  When the quality of life is good, as defined by the patient

Potential reasons to consider withholding or withdrawing ANH
The patient or decision maker, after being provided appropriate counseling and options, decides against this intervention to reflect personal values.

  When the primary goal of the patient is palliation of symptoms
  When the intervention is bound to fail (e.g., in widely metastatic small cell lung carcinoma)
  When the patient is dying, and the intervention is merely prolonging the dying process or causing suffering
  When a patient has moderate or severe, irreversible cognitive impairment (e.g., multiple strokes or Alzheimer's dementia)
  When the intervention causes complications (e.g., agitation requiring sedation or physical restraints, infection, multiple tube obstructions or withdrawals, aspiration pneumonia)
  To help relieve symptoms of fluid overload (e.g., dyspnea, diarrhea, urinary frequency or bowel obstruction) in terminally ill patients
  When the patient has end-stage organ failure (e.g., respiratory, cardiac, renal)
  When other end-stage diseases, such as advanced acquired immunodeficiency syndrome, are present
  When a patient has had a stroke, brain metastasis, or cerebral edema, is profoundly impaired and does not recover useful swallowing function
  When the risks exceed the benefits

Adapted with permission from Emanuel LL, von Gunten CJ, Ferris FD. *Education on end-of-life care trainer's guide*, Module 11, withholding, withdrawing therapy. Chicago, IL: Institute for Institute for Ethics at the American Medical Association, EPEC Project, The Robert Wood Johnson Foundation, 1999 (7).

showed no benefit on survival, morbidity, or duration of hospitalization (34).

Similarly, placing a feeding tube in a patient with advanced dementia does not prevent aspiration, has little effect on malnutrition, does not improve survival or function, does not prevent or treat pressure sores, and may cause discomfort and other effects (35,36).

The first step in helping patients and families decide about feeding tubes is to evaluate the patient's overall values and goals of care. Review the medical conditions, and then assess the potential for ANH to help achieve these goals. For example, if the patient has advanced cancer, what is the expected course of the cancer? Is anything reversible? How will intravenous or enteral tube fluids and nutrition improve the situation? In the best of all worlds, these decisions are made before a crisis, at which time the decision maker often becomes overwhelmed by the number and complexity of decisions that must be made.

Address common misperceptions. Many patients believe that a lack of appetite and poor oral intake is the cause of the debility, assuming that "if Mom would just get some nutrition in, she could get stronger and fight the cancer better." Use clear, simple language, focusing on the true cause of the problem:

> "The advanced cancer is taking all of the calories and strength away," or
> "Your heart is so weak and it causes you to lose your appetite and feel so drained."

In some equivocal cases, it may be appropriate to advocate for a monitored clinical trial of hydration. However, in terminally ill patients, ANH often worsens physical symptoms like dyspnea, ascites, diarrhea, vomiting, incontinence, or edema. Sometimes a family may feel more comfortable withdrawing intravenous fluids after a trial has shown no benefit.

Providing food and water to loved ones meets powerful emotional and social needs. For patients who have decided against ANH, give family members specific tasks to accomplish in the nonmedical care of dying patients, such as taking turns holding vigil, holding the patient's hand, singing or reading poetry or scripture, or stroking the forehead.

As patients lie dying, families are often worried that the lack of fluids and nutrition will cause suffering. While there are of course no randomized clinical trials that answer this question, there is a large body of observational data that suggests that dehydration is a normal part of the dying process (37). Reversing a normal, natural process often leads to discomfort, without affecting the eventual outcome. If the patient is not experiencing hunger or thirst, which is typical in patients with end-stage malignancy, then providing ANH will not relieve a symptom. Some patients with no cognitive impairment may even make a conscious decision to stop eating and drinking at the end.

Several Supreme Court cases, culminating in the Nancy Cruzan case, have established that Americans have a constitutional right to decline ANH, and that surrogates can make these choices for patients who lack decision-making capacity (38). The recent Terry Schiavo case broke no new legal or ethical ground; all the judges involved in this convoluted case agreed that her decision maker had the right to withdraw her feeding tube (39,40).

Like all procedures, tube feeding is not inevitable; it is a choice.

There are many complications of nutritional support, whether enteral or parenteral. IV-catheter associated complications include pneumo- and hydrothorax, sepsis, infection, and venous thrombosis. Enteral tubes may cause epistaxis, nasal alar necrosis, aspiration, airway obstruction, nasopharyngosinusitis, esophagitis and stricture, intestinal obstruction, nausea, vomiting, and diarrhea. Both modalities may cause serious electrolyte disturbances, hyperosmolarity, refeeding

syndrome, and hepatic steatosis. Probably the most serious complication is the need for physical and chemical restraints in most patients (41).

In the fasting state, glycogen is broken down to produce glucose, which is essential for brain metabolism, while peripheral tissues are able to utilize fatty acids as fuel. When glycogen is depleted, amino acids from muscle may be utilized to produce glucose, using hepatic gluconeogenesis. What is not widely appreciated is that with prolonged (more than a week) fasting, the brain becomes able to use ketones as an energy source. Ketonemia markedly suppresses gluconeogenesis, thereby preserving skeletal muscle (42).

Ketonemia also causes a euphoric state, provides pain relief (probably through release of endogenous opiate-like substances), and most importantly, markedly suppresses hunger. If the ketonemia is reversed, even by as few as 400 calories per day, pain increases and hunger returns. Therefore, there is a strong physiologic reason for not reversing the ketonemia of the dying patient, unless there is some reversible process at play (42).

Further, terminal dehydration is relatively benign. Several observational studies have shown little problem except for dry mouth and lips, which can be managed by nursing interventions. A minority of dehydrated patients at the end of life may become delirious; if this is possible, a limited trial of hydration may be indicated. Fluid depletion in the dying patient makes many fluid-related symptoms better—for example, dyspnea, edema, diarrhea, and frequent urination. If artificial nutrition has been withheld, it makes little sense to provide intravenous fluids, especially fluids containing glucose (43).

The large majority of dying patients will experience some delirium, which is often reversible. Common causes of reversible delirium include hypoxia, fever, medications, opiate or benzodiazepine withdrawal, or even dehydration. Dehydration generally causes no symptoms in dying patients. Hydration can be an option if the patient wishes to be more alert. A trial of hydration may be warranted in dehydrated patients who are delirious, but more research is needed in this area (44).

Does withholding food cause suffering? There obviously are no randomized trials to answer this question. In one prospective study, 32 mentally aware, competent, and terminally ill patients were admitted to a palliative care unit. All patients were offered whatever food and drink they desired; symptoms such as pain and dyspnea were managed, avoiding sedation. Patients were followed up until their deaths. Twenty (63%) never had any hunger, and an additional 11 (34%) had only mild hunger at the beginning of the study (45).

References

1. Pawlik TM, Curley SA. Ethical issues in surgical palliative care: am i killing the patient by "letting him go"? *Surg Clin North Am* 2005;85:273–286.
2. Murray SA, Boyd K, Sheikh A, et al. Developing primary palliative care. People with terminal conditions should be able to die at home with dignity. *BMJ* 2004;329:1056–1057.
3. Lynn J. Serving patients who may die soon and their families. The role of hospice and other services. *JAMA* 2001;285:925–932.
4. Ackermann RJ. Withholding and withdrawing life-sustaining treatment. *Am Fam Physician* 2000;62:1555–1560, 62,64.
5. Withholding and withdrawing life-prolonging treatments: good practice in decision-making. General Medical Council—United Kingdom, at www.gmc-uk.org, 2006.
6. Prendergast TJ, Puntillo KA. Withdrawal of life support. Intensive caring at the end of life. *JAMA* 2002;288:2732–2740.
7. Emanuel LL, von Gunten CJ, Ferris FD. *Education for physicians on end-of-life care trainer's guide*. Module 11, withholding, withdrawing therapy. Chicago, IL: Institute for Ethics at the American Medical Association, 1999.
8. Prendergast TJ. Withholding or withdrawal of life-sustaining therapy. *Hosp Pract* 2000;35:91–92, 95–100, 102.
9. Melltorp G, Nilstun T. The difference between withholding and withdrawing life-sustaining treatment. *Intensive Care Med* 1997;23:1264–1267.

10. The SUPPORT Principal Investigators. A controlled trial to improve care for seriously ill hospitalized patients. The study to understand prognoses and preferences for outcomes and risks of treatments (SUPPORT). *JAMA* 1995;273:1591–1598 [Published erratum appears in *JAMA* 1996;275:1232.

11. McCarthy EP, Phillips RS, Zhong Z, et al. Dying with cancer: patients' function, symptoms, and care preferences as death approaches. *J Am Geriatr Soc* 2000;48:S110–S121.

12. Campbell ML, Guzman JA. A proactive approach to improve end-of-life care in a medical intensive care unit for patients with terminal dementia. *Crit Care Med* 2004;32:1839–1843.

13. Asch DA, Faber-Langendoen K, Shea JA, et al. The sequence of withdrawing life-sustaining treatment from patients. *Am J Med* 1999;107:153–156.

14. Grimes DA. Technology follies. The uncritical acceptance of medical innovation. *JAMA* 1993;268:3030–3033.

15. Lee SJ, Back AL, Block SD, et al. Enhancing physician-patient communication. *Hematology Am Soc Hematol Ed Program* 2002;1:464–483.

16. Back AL, Arnold RM, Quill TE. Hope for the best, and prepare for the worst. *Ann Intern Med* 2003;138:439–443.

17. Murray SA, Boyd K, Sheikh A. Palliative care in chronic illness. We need to move from prognostic paralysis to active total care. *BMJ* 2005;330:611–612.

18. Glare P, Virik K, Jones M, et al. A systematic review of physicians' survival predictions in terminally ill cancer patients. *BMJ* 2003;327:195–198.

19. Weissman D. Fast fact and concept #13: determining prognosis in advanced cancer. At www.eperc.mcw.edu, May 2000.

20. Quill TE, Lo B, Brock DW. Palliative options of last resort. A comparison of voluntarily stopping eating and drinking, terminal sedation, physician-assisted suicide, and voluntary active euthanasia. *JAMA* 1997;278:2099–2104.

21. Cohen RA. A tale of two conversations. *Hastings Cent Rep* 2004;34(3):49.

22. Weissman D, von Gunten C. Fast fact and concept #23: DNR orders in the hospital—Part 1. At www.eperc.mcw.edu, September 2000.

23. Saklayen M, Liss H, Markert R. In-hospital cardiopulmonary resuscitation: survival in 1 hospital and literature review. *Medicine* 1995;74:163–175.

24. Weissman D, von Gunten C. Fast fact and concept #24: DNR orders in the hospital setting—Part 2. At www.eperc.mcw.edu, September 2000.

25. Cantor MD, Braddock CH, Derse AR, et al. Do-not-resuscitate orders and medical futility. *Arch Intern Med* 2003;163:2689–2694.

26. Stagno SJ, Zhukovsky DS, Walsh D. Bioethics: communication and decision-making in advanced disease. *Semin Oncol* 2000;27:94–100.

27. Muller D. Do not resuscitate. *Health Aff* 2005;24(5):1317–1322.

28. O'Mahony S, McHugh M, Zallman L, et al. Ventilator withdrawal: procedure and outcomes. Report of a collaboration between a critical care division and a palliative care service. *J Pain Symptom Manage* 2003;26:954–961.

29. von Gunten C, Weissman DE. Fast fact and concept #33: ventilator withdrawal (Part I). At www.eperc.mcw.edu, January 2001.

30. von Gunten C, Weissman DE. Fast fact and concept 334: symptom control for ventilator withdrawal in the dying patient (Part II). At www.eperc.mcw.edu, Feb 2001.

31. Alpers A, Lo B. The supreme court addresses physician-assisted suicide. Can its rulings improve palliative care? *Arch Fam Med* 1999;8:200–205.

32. Hallenbeck J, Weissman D. Fast fact and concept #10: tube feed or not tube feed? At www.eperc.mcw.edu, April, 2000.

33. Clamon GH, Feld R, Evans WK, et al. Effect of adjuvant central IV hyperalimentation on the survival and response to treatment of patients with small cell lung cancer; a randomized trial. *Cancer Treat Rep* 1985;9:167–177.

34. Klein S, Koretz RL. Nutrition support in patients with cancer: what do the data really show? *Nutr Clin Pract* 1994;9:91–100.

35. Finucane TE, Christmas C, Travis K. Tube feeding in patients with advanced dementia: a review of the evidence. *JAMA* 1999;282:1365–1370.

36. Gillick MR. Rethinking the role of tube feeding in patients with advanced dementia. *N Engl J Med* 2000;342:206–210.

37. Ashby M, Stoffell B. Artificial hydration and nutrition and alimentation at the end of life: a reply to craig. *J Med Ethics* 1995;21:135–140.

38. *Cruzan v. Director.* Missouri Department of Health. 1990;497 US 261.

39. Annas GJ. "Culture of life" policies at the bedside—the case of Terri Schiavo. *New Engl Med* 2005;352:1710–1715.

40. Goston LO. Ethics, the constitution, and the dying process. The case of Theresa Marie Schiavo. *JAMA* 2005;293:2403–2407.

41. Mitchell SL, Kiely DK, Hamel MB. Dying with advanced dementia in the nursing home. *Arch Intern Med* 2004;164:321–326.

42. Winter SM. Terminal nutrition: framing the debate for withdrawal of nutritional support in terminally ill patients. *Am J Med* 2000;109:723–726.

43. Pasman HR, Onwuteaka-Philipsen BD, Kriegsman DMW, et al. Discomfort in nursing home patients with severe dementia in whom artificial nutrition and hydration is forgone. *Arch Intern Med* 2005;165:1729–1735.

44. Bruera E, Sala R, Rico MA, et al. Effects of parenteral hydration in terminally ill cancer patients: a preliminary study. *J Clin Oncol* 2005;23:2366–2371.

45. McCann RM, Hall WJ, Groth-Juncker A. Comfort care for terminally ill patients. The appropriate use of nutrition and hydration. *JAMA* 1994;272:1263–1266.

CHAPTER 64 ■ PALLIATIVE CARE AND PHYSICIAN-ASSISTED DEATH

BARBARA A. SUPANICH

Many events have occurred since 2001 that have stimulated many sectors of the United States society to ponder, reflect, and debate the issues regarding physician-assisted death. Recently, in the United States, the debate has involved the US Supreme Court; (1) the US Congress and US President George W. Bush (in the Teri Schiavo debate), and multiple discussions in state legislatures, local communities, and multiple physician, nurse, patient, and public surveys (2–7). Recently, the issues have focused on personal choice at the end-of-life, ethical treatment and decision issues at the end of life, and the State's responsibility for "preserving life."

Although the US Supreme Court in 1997, made a unanimous decision to uphold the right of states to prohibit physician-assisted death, this decision also allows states to permit it (8,9). In late 2001, then US Attorney General John Ashcroft made an unsuccessful attempt to halt the practice of physician-assisted death in Oregon; (7) by focusing on prescriber rights to prescribe opiates to terminally ill patients.

The recent heated public discussion and debates regarding the withdrawal of artificial nutrition and hydration from Teri Schiavo highlight the need for better education of health professionals, legislators, patients and their families and the general public on end of life treatment choices for themselves, and their loved ones. For professionals involved in palliative care and hospice care, our current US social milieu provides many unique challenges to our provision of excellent and compassionate palliative care to our patients and their families.

This chapter will review some of the major ethical arguments, look more specifically at the challenges posed for the palliative care professional, and propose ethically sound clinical strategies for responding to the challenges of a patient's or family member's request for physician-assisted death.

DEFINITIONS

Discussions regarding physician-assisted death are often complicated by the participants not properly understanding the ethical terms regarding end of life care treatment options.

Withdrawing or withholding life-sustaining treatment refers to decisions to stop or not initiate certain medical therapies, with the anticipated outcome that the patient will die from the underlying disease. Common examples include withdrawing of a ventilator from a patient in end-stage emphysema; forgoing the use of anti biotics in a patient with terminal cancer and suspected pneumonia; and refusal of tube feeding by a patient with an end-stage neuromuscular disease.

Voluntary active euthanasia refers to the direct administration of a lethal agent to the patient by another party, with a merciful intent. This chapter considers only *voluntary active euthanasia* because that is the only form being seriously advocated in the United States today.

Assisted suicide refers to the patient intentionally and willfully ending his or her own life, with the assistance of another party. This assistance may include different levels of involvement—merely providing information about how to commit suicide; providing the means to commit suicide, such as a lethal quantity of pills; or actively participating in the suicide, such as being present at the scene and inserting an intravenous line through which the patient may then administer a lethal dose (9). The widely publicized actions of Dr. Timothy Quill (10) and Dr. Jack Kevorkian (11,12) provide examples of the second and third levels of involvement, respectively. In the State of Oregon, physician-assisted suicide involves a discussion with the patient regarding the diagnosis, prognosis, capacity for healthcare decision making, and the voluntary nature of the request. After appropriate consultation, the attending or consulting physician can then write a prescription for a lethal dose of medication (8).

For this chapter, *assisted death* refers jointly to the practices of voluntary euthanasia or assisted suicide. Most of the literature on ethics has focused on the special problems of the physician's role that is, the practice of *physician-assisted death*. In the context of hospice, the roles of other health professionals and the family are extremely important, and in some cases, the patient may request assistance in dying from one or more of them as well as (or instead of) from the physician.

It is important to be clear about what is *not* assisted death. As noted, it is *not* an assisted death if a competent person decides not to initiate a specific therapy (e.g., further chemotherapy, antibiotics for a pneumonia or another septic process, renal dialysis or artificial nutrition, or hydration). The use of high doses of opioids, when the intent is to relieve pain and not to hasten death, is *not* physician-assisted death. Although many still believe that high-dose opioids pose a serious risk of fatal respiratory depression, palliative specialists know that this very seldom occurs with proper titration of analgesic doses, even when very large doses of opioids are administered in terminal illness (13). Even if respiratory depression is a foreseen (but unintended) consequence of adequate analgesia, administering the analgesics is not considered to be physician-assisted death.

Withholding and withdrawing life-sustaining treatment is widely accepted today, both in ethics and law, as appropriate and compassionate care. When the adult competent patient is fully informed and freely chooses these options or has clearly documented these choices in an advance care plan document, all 50 states accept these decisions as legally and ethically binding. As a matter of fact, there have been no successful lawsuits against physicians or others for following a patient's written choices in an advance directive. Physicians are at more risk of a wrongful life suit for *not* following the directive than they are of a wrongful death suit. Some, notably Dixon (14), have argued that there is no morally relevant difference between this practice and the practice of assisted death. Dixon argues that fairness requires that if we legalize physician-assisted suicide that we should also make active euthanasia legally available (14). In this chapter, without giving detailed arguments, I have prepared a review of ethical arguments on both sides of the question. I will assume that if assisted death can be justified, it must be justified on its own merits and not merely because it shares some moral features with the relatively uncontroversial practice of withdrawing or withholding life-sustaining treatment (15–18).

ETHICAL ARGUMENTS

Patient Integrity

Patients who are living with a life-limiting illness want their personal values and goals maintained and respected. For many patients, the most important personal values are autonomy and personal integrity. From the patient's perspective, this means that one's belief system, personal values, and life goals will be honored and respected, and that they will play a vital role in treatment plans and palliative care planning. Most patients have the expectation that their suffering will be moderated, their pain will be controlled and they will have the opportunity to have meaningful conversations with their physicians and family concerning the type and extent of their treatments (5,6,19–21). A recent report of the Oregon Health Division (22) confirms that 67% of the 26 persons who experienced a physician-assisted death in 1999 identified loss of autonomy, an inability to participate in activities that would make life meaningful, and loss of bodily functions as reasons for seeking an assisted death.

Proponents of assisted death would argue that they are honoring the personal integrity and the personal autonomy of the person by being willing to discuss and assist the patient with *all* treatment/care options for the patient, including assisted death. Proponents also claim that physician-assisted death minimizes harm to the patient and others. They argue that the patient would determine what counts as a harm and may legitimately decide that ongoing life with severe suffering is a greater harm than a painless death (22,23).

Opponents claim that, however important the moral value of patient autonomy is, it is insufficient to justify the practice of assisted death (6,14,15,24–26). Autonomy may justify withdrawing or withholding treatment because that constitutes a negative right of noninterference, which is strongly grounded in the concept of respecting personal bodily integrity. But it cannot justify a positive right to demand that others take specific actions to promote one's own idea of one's welfare—especially when those actions cause death. Some opponents also make the claim that causing a death is one of the greatest harms that a clinician could inflict on a patient. The basic principle of "Do no harm" should be understood as requiring a healing relationship between the physician and the patient and, therefore it is in direct conflict with respect to patient autonomy when assistance in dying is requested.

Compassionate Response to Suffering

For some physicians, a request by a patient for death assistance is viewed as a plea to release the patient from intolerable suffering. From this perspective, such assistance is understood as an act of compassion. Quill and others (10,27–30) have argued that a willingness to discuss this option with the patient often may act as a suicide deterrent since once the patient's concerns and fears have been fully discussed, the physician may be able to propose alternative means of relieving suffering short of death (5,6,22,30–32). By contrast, if physicians refuse to offer assistance, suffering patients may avoid these searching conversations and instead commit suicide in a manner that actually increases their own and the family's suffering.

It is a serious mistake to equate suffering narrowly with pain and other unpleasant physical symptoms. Suffering is defined through the experiences of the individual, which includes a personal sense of impaired quality of life, and is understood as a fundamental threat to one's wholeness as a person. Suffering is ultimately tied to one's personal belief system. It reflects how those beliefs define the reality of the human person, and how one experiences an illness in the overall context of one's life journey and personal expectations for the future. Two patients may report similar symptoms but have vastly different experiences of suffering (30,32–35).

Proponents of assisted death point to the multifaceted and complex nature of suffering as a defense for the individual's right to choose a quicker death because no one can really comprehend the severity of anyone's suffering. Palliative care may be able to relieve unpleasant symptoms very well but it may be much less capable of restoring meaning and function to a life that has irreversibly lost both. Whereas excellent palliative care and hospice care should greatly reduce the number of patients who may request death assistance, it would not negate the need for this option in some cases.

By contrast, opponents claim that proponents have a short-sighted and simplistic approach to the relief of suffering. Precisely because suffering is multifaceted and intimately tied to personal meaning, there are numerous options to offer the suffering individual to assist them in restoring a sense of meaning in her life. To relieve suffering by eliminating the sufferer must always be viewed as an inadequate response. Attending adequately to loneliness, fear of death, depression, unresolved conflicts, and lack of forgiveness, anger, and hopelessness is harder, but ultimately will allow a better personal resolution. This is especially important work for the physician, nurses, and family members since they may tend to project their own suffering onto the patient and, therefore, conclude that a premature death is actually the merciful choice from the patient's perspective (5,6,30,36).

Safeguards

Both proponents and opponents of physician-assisted death agree that safeguards are needed to protect the patient's safety and integrity and to protect society from physicians who might abuse the end of life choice (6,26,27,37–39). Table 64.1 lists some commonly proposed safeguards and guidelines for discussing the choice of assisted death (27,38).

As previously discussed, proponents believe that patients are the best judge of their own suffering and should have the option of discussing their situation with their personal physicians and developing a mutually agreeable plan for control of their pain and suffering. Proponents also believe that multiple compassionate and appropriately timed conversations between the patient and the primary physician over time will build the trust and rapport necessary for honest and uncoerced

TABLE 64.1

SAFEGUARDS AND GUIDELINES FOR THE DISCUSSION OF ASSISTED DEATH

(1) The patient must have a condition that is incurable (not necessarily terminal) and is associated with severe suffering without hope of relief.

(2) All reasonable comfort-oriented measures must have been considered or tried.

(3) The patient must express a clear and repeated request to die that is not coerced (e.g., emotionally or financially).

(4) The physician must ensure that the patient's judgment is not distorted, i.e., the patient is competent to make a rational treatment choice.

(5) Physician-assisted death must be carried out only in the context of a meaningful physician-patient relationship.

(6) Consultation must be obtained from another physician to ensure that the patient's request is rational and voluntary.

From Quill T, Cassel C, Meier D. Care of the hopelessly ill—proposed clinical criteria for physician-assisted suicide. *N Engl J Med* (Sounding Board) 1992;327:1380 (27); Miller F, Quill T, Brody H, et al. Regulating physician-assisted death. *N Engl J Med* 1994;31:119 (38).

conversations among the patient, the physician, and the family members. Many proponents also believe that consultation with at least one other physician is a vital safeguard. A parallel safeguard is the assurance of accurate and clear documentation that all appropriate guidelines have been followed.

Most opponents would agree that suffering is both personal and unique and that all reasonable comfort measures should be discussed with the patient and tried. They would agree that more open and frank discussions between the physician and the patient should occur on topics such as pain and symptom control, and the patient's perception and experiences of suffering. In their opinion, these types of discussions and the subsequent individualized plan of care for the patient would negate the need for the option of assisted death. Opponents see the potential for coercion as very real and often quite difficult to ascertain, so that the proposed guidelines would be inadequate in practice. Opponents are also concerned about the erosion of the patient-physician relationship occurring when physicians start providing the means of death for their patients. They also would point out flaws in the consultation and documentation guidelines, for example, choosing a like minded consultant, and question the ability of the guidelines to protect patient safety (6).

Professional Integrity

Opponents of physician-assisted death often argue that causing death is inconsistent with the moral integrity of the physician as a healer and never an agent of death. In this view, even if society deemed it appropriate to permit assistance in dying, ethical physicians would be obligated to refuse to provide such assistance. Another group of professionals would have to be appointed by society for that role (40). Similar arguments have been made on behalf of nurses, pharmacists, and other health care professionals (7,25,41,42).

Another key argument for proponents lies in their interpretation of the nature of healing and the moral goals of medicine, and the physician's professional integrity. For them, the goals of medicine include relief of suffering, respect for the patient's voluntary and thoughtful choices and aiding patients to achieve the most peaceful and dignified death possible. Suffering that has been unrelieved by excellent palliative care in a patient who has made repeated voluntary requests for death assistance would constitute an exception to the general prohibition. In such narrowly defined cases, a physician could assist death although maintaining ethical integrity (so long as assisting death did not violate any of that physician's moral or religious values) (43).

Slippery Slope

Concern about a "slippery slope" is one of the main arguments raised by opponents. They argue that once the legal barriers to physician-assisted death are broken there will be little justification for limiting the practice to only the terminally ill. What is today an *option,* to choose assisted death, might become an *obligation,* to choose it, especially under pressures of cost containment, family financial pressures, and biases toward vulnerable populations such as the nursing home population, minorities, the disabled, and those living with HIV/AIDS (44).

Proponents respond that proper attention to safeguards will prevent many problems and concerns raised by the slippery slope argument. Typical of the dispute between proponents and opponents of assisted death are sharply divergent interpretations of the current Oregon experience. One side argues that this is the manifestation of our worst fears regarding physician-assisted death (6,26,32). The other side suggests that the published reports from the public health department in Oregon confirms that the safeguards are working, palliative care and hospice care have markedly increased and in reality, very few patients over the past 6 years have requested and carried out an assisted death (22).

Substituted Judgment

Opponents worry that society will extend physician-assisted death to incompetent patients. Most proposals for physician-assisted death in the United States today specifically exclude the option of choosing physician-assisted death by an advance care directive. This topic is still being debated in multiple arenas in United States society, including the Congress and several state referenda (45–47).

IMPLICATIONS FOR PALLIATIVE CARE AND HOSPICE

Official Policies

Both the National Hospice and Palliative Care Organization (NHPCO) and the American Academy of Hospice and Palliative Medicine (AAHPM) have position statements opposing the legalization of assisted death (48,49). The AAHPM statement is brief and states that competent palliative care usually relieves the pain and suffering of patients and their families. This statement calls for reforms to ensure comprehensive palliative care for all. The NHPCO position paper (Table 64.2) is considerably more detailed and reviews all of

TABLE 64.2

MAJOR POINTS OF THE NATIONAL HOSPICE AND PALLIATIVE CARE
ORGANIZATION'S POSITION STATEMENT ON ASSISTED DEATH

In November 1990, a resolution was adopted rejecting the practice of voluntary euthanasia
and assisted suicide:
(1) These practices are counter to the organization's core principles of relief of suffering,
coordination of palliative and support services for the patient and family, a focus in
maintaining the quality of remaining life, and a commitment to affirm life that neither
hastens nor postpones death.
(2) Hospice offers competent, appropriate, and compassionate palliative care to patients
and their families as an effective choice for the care of dying patients and their families.
(3) Aggressive palliative care can improve the quality and quantity of remaining life, as
defined by the patient's life goals and choices.
(4) Patients and their families need to be given the opportunity to discuss the accuracy of
the diagnosis, prognosis, and range of palliative treatment options appropriate for their
personal situation and lifestyle.
(5) The administrative and financial requirements of developing and maintaining assisted
death as a component of the health care delivery system could competitively diminish
the support needed to increase assets to appropriate health care and palliative care.

Board of Directors. *Statement opposing the legalization of euthanasia and assisted suicide.* Arlington, VA:
National Hospice and Palliative Care Organization (49).

the major points discussed previously. In summary, NHPCO
statement maintains that allowing unpreventable death to occur with dignity and comfort is quite different from accepting
death as an expeditious way out of difficult situations for an
individual or society.

Both organizations see hospice as an ethically sound model
of compassionate, cost-effective, patient-and-family–oriented
care. They also would argue that hospice care should be
available to all and affordable for all who would opt
for palliative care, and that all health care professionals
should possess basic knowledge of hospice and palliative care
management principles.

Attitudes

As one might expect from official policy statements, there
is a marked difference in attitudes toward physician-assisted
death among hospice professionals compared to United States
health care workers, in general. A slight majority of physicians
in the states of Washington and Michigan favor a policy
that would permit the option of physician-assisted death;
other surveys have shown that from 33–40% of physicians
favor such a policy (8,50,51). By contrast, surveys of hospice
physicians, nurses, and volunteers show only a minority in
favor of allowing physician-assisted death and about two-
thirds strongly opposed (25).

It is understandable that those who devote so much of
their energy to relief of symptoms, and who see the vast
majority or their patients "living well until they die," might
view the occasional patient who chooses physician-assisted
death as either a failure or a threat. Some of these patients
may have had prior exposure to hospice, and their decision
for assisted death can be experienced as a rejection of the
hospice philosophy. Even patients who had never experienced
organized palliative care may seem to be saying, by choosing
assisted death, that they do not value what is offered by
palliative care. So, there are understandable philosophical and
emotional reasons for hospice caregivers to react negatively to
physician-assisted death.

The hospice professional's approach to care of the terminally ill and dying emphasizes that each person will be
supported through a variety of personal and professional

resources in order to live well and be well supported in
their death experience. At first glance, physician-assisted death
would seem to be inappropriate, unnecessary, or both in every
case (44). The philosophy of some hospice professionals is inconsistent with the views of proponents of assisted death. Both
have in common a rejection of the dominant mode of dying
that seems to characterize the American hospital setting—a
death prolonged by excessive use of technology, inadequately
attended by concern for amelioration of symptoms, and a
depersonalized and deindividualized death; as patients' true
choices are routinely ignored and human relationships and human caring are given short shrift in the environment of technology. Both hospice professionals and assisted death advocates
agree that the death experience in America can be improved
through a greater understanding and appreciation of human
needs, individual values, and choices. Most hospice professionals would disagree with assisted death advocates, however, by
choosing improvements in the approach to caring for the dying
in contrast to advocating for assisted death methods.

Success of Palliative Care

Advocates of physician-assisted death assume that palliative
care modalities, although normally highly successful, do not
have a 100% success rate for all patients. There will of necessity be a few patients whose unpleasant symptoms, personal
suffering, or inability to achieve personal goals will not be
ameliorated by even the most highly skilled palliative interventions. Many advocates of physician-assisted death would
favor restricting the option of death to that small percentage
of patients who cannot be assisted effectively by palliative care
treatments. Palliative care specialists would counter this observation by stating that their modalities are much more effective
than physician-assisted death advocates (or the general public)
appreciate. It is well known to palliative care specialists that
the average United States health professional underestimates
the effectiveness of palliative care approaches and mislabels
undertreatment or suboptimal treatments as "failures" of palliative care. As previously stated, palliative care specialists
would argue that excellent, high quality palliative care offered
to all persons living with a life-limiting illness would bring the
demand for physician-assisted death to almost zero.

But both well-designed studies and common sense would lead to the conclusion that no medical therapy, however marvelous, can always succeed (29,52). Although challenged, palliative care specialists admit that they cannot effectively treat 100% of all patients' symptoms. The 3–5% of patients whose physical suffering does not respond well to current treatment modalities (traditional and complementary) can be offered palliative sedation (52). Since the intent is to relieve the symptoms and not to shorten life, pharmacologically induced coma does not constitute physician-assisted death but is an acceptable, if extreme, use of palliative treatment (53).

Defenders of physician-assisted death have offered two rebuttals to this argument. First, they have argued that in many instances in which pharmacologically induced coma might be used, death follows so surely and within so short a span of time that it is a semantic quibble not to view this as physician-assisted death *from a moral point of view* (although recognizing from a *legal point of view*, sedation to the point of coma is quite acceptable even in jurisdictions where physician-assisted death would be a crime).

To understand these moral and legal nuances, it is important to discuss the application of the ethical principle of double effect to high-dose opioids for analgesia and to pharmacologically induced coma. To opponents of physician-assisted death, the two instances are quite analogous. In both cases, one intends the relief of symptoms, not death. One foresees the risk that the means used to relieve the symptoms could cause a hastened death, but hastening death is not one's true intent. Therefore, death is a foreseen but unintended consequence of an action that is morally defensible, and so the use of that means is morally justified.

To proponents of physician-assisted death, however, the two cases raise difficult issues regarding issues of personal control of symptoms and the controversies regarding the ability to relieve spiritual or existential suffering with palliative sedation. Palliative care professionals are well aware that very few patients actually have significant respiratory depression from properly administered opioids in terminal illness.

Palliative sedation can be another treatment choice for patients with refractory symptoms such as terminal delirium, pain, or myoclonus (54–59). Administration of pharmacologic agents to relieve these refractory terminal symptoms and/or suffering may be an acceptable treatment option for a patient's consideration. There are three common characteristics of cases in which palliative sedation might be considered:

(1) Alternative means of relieving the symptoms have been ineffective or have intolerable side effects

(2) The goal or intention of sedation is to relieve symptoms and not to shorten the patient's life and

(3) The patient is usually near death or in the actively dying process (59)

Currently, the careful titration of one of several pharmacologic agents used for palliative sedation includes midazolam, propofol, or a barbiturate in combination with an opioid (59). Of these three agents, many physicians are most comfortable with midazolam IV infusions.

It is also important for the palliative physician to have an explicit discussion of the goals and the outcomes of palliative sedation for the patient, with the patient, family members, and palliative team members. The discussion should include an explicit and compassionate discussion of the goals and expected outcomes, a discussion of the common concerns and misunderstandings of palliative sedation, answer questions regarding concerns about the dying process, and allow the family and friends time for engaging in final conversations, cultural death rituals, and religious rituals.

A second rebuttal is that some terminally ill persons who have demanded the right to physician-assisted death have claimed that a palliative sedation typifies the loss of control and dignity that is their overriding goal to avoid. For at least this group of patients, palliative care experts might relieve unpleasant symptoms, but only at the cost of violating the patient's own deeply held values regarding quality of life.

Pain versus Suffering

Suffering is experienced as a personal experience by each individual, including a personal sense of impaired quality of life as well as a threat to one's personal integrity and wholeness. Suffering is ultimately tied to one's personal belief system and how the person experiences an illness in the overall context of the person's life and expectations for the future. The best available study of patient attitudes in a setting where physician-assisted death is openly practiced and legally tolerated reveals that approximately 10% of patients requesting euthanasia suffer principally from pain and approximately 50% suffer from physical symptoms of the sort that can easily be relieved by palliative medical interventions. A significant number of requests to die arise from those who state that they are merely tired of life or whose general level of functioning has deteriorated below their personally acceptable minimum (53). Reports from Oregon identified the most common reasons for asking for assisted death include loss of autonomy, loss of control of bodily functions, an inability to participate in activities that make life enjoyable, and a determination to control the manner of death (22). A recent study which examined physician attitudes regarding physician-assisted death and AIDS patients revealed that 48% of the physicians would assist the patient in the survey's case scenario and 53% had positively responded to a patient request in their own practices (5).

Possibly many or even most patients could be aided by emotional and/or spiritual counseling to the point where they would no longer request assisted death. A more sensitive and patient-centered approach requires understanding the meaning the patient attaches to the individual circumstances and not merely the assumption that palliative care treatments have been underutilized (19,21,53).

Funding for Palliative Care

One recurring argument against allowing physician-assisted death is that hospice and palliative care have been chronically underfunded in the United States. According to this argument, as soon as physician-assisted death is a legal option, patients will be steered toward a quick, painless, cheap death and will be discouraged from seeking potentially expensive hospice care. The net result will be the serious underfunding of all types of palliative care programs, and the option to choose palliative care will be an option on paper only for most United States patients. Many United States hospice professionals charge that palliative care has been very slow to develop in the Netherlands and that country's euthanasia policy is directly to blame. Hospice professionals have experienced the problems and challenges of chronic underfunding and of working with physicians, administrators and legislators who were often ill informed about hospice care. Understandably, they are skeptical of any proposal that assumes that palliative care has arrived and that adequate funding is on the horizon (54).

Defenders of the assisted death option have argued in reply that a properly regulated and legalized option for physician-assisted death could actually support the expansion of hospice. The most recent report on the Oregon experience with physician-assisted death would support this argument (8).

Many such proposals include the stipulation that no patient will be granted the request to die until palliative care experts have concluded that the patient cannot be effectively helped by appropriate treatments. In effect, the proposals would require that every patient requesting physician-assisted death undergo a trial of palliative care (27,38). Proponents further assume that in most cases, the patients would be so impressed with the success of the treatments that they would elect to remain in the hospice program rather than be put to death. The result, they argue, will be additional political support for hospice programs and for palliative care training and research.

It is possible that health care professionals might merely rubber-stamp requests for assisted death rather than engaging in detailed conversations with their patients. Ironically, this outcome would be more likely if the nation moves toward legalizing physician-assisted death and if (as opinion polls now suggest) the best trained palliative care specialists refuse as a matter of conscience to have anything to do with the assisted death program, even to the extent of screening patients and consulting on palliative care alternatives (25,54).

CLINICAL MANAGEMENT OF REQUESTS FOR ASSISTED DEATH

Although the debate between opponents and proponents of assisted death is complex and apparently intractable, many aspects of the practical management of patients who request direct assistance in dying will be the same, regardless of the clinician's moral stance. These are clinical approaches that should fit both moral positions comfortably. A few areas of practice will differ, however, to remain consistent with the clinician's own moral commitments (Table 64.3).

Reactions to Patient Request

As noted in the preceding text, a hospice patient who requests physician-assisted death may well trigger intensely negative emotional reactions among members of the care team. It is very important that those emotional reactions be validated by other team members but not be allowed to derail the necessary conversations with the patient that will support the patient's values and choices, as well as assess future care needs. Ideally, the patient's request should be received both respectfully and sympathetically. The patient may be told that she is hardly alone among patients facing death in making such a request and that the clinician very much appreciates the trust shown by the patient in honestly sharing her request. The clinician would then engage in dialogue with the patient regarding her underlying reasons for the request and come to a mutual agreement that this request will be discussed at her next care meeting.

Alternatively, a patient may confide this request, or the fact that she is seriously considering assisted death, to only one member of the palliative care team with whom she may experience a deeper personal trust. In that event, the team member ought initially to respect the confidence but state clearly that she feels a very strong obligation to share that information with all other team members, so that as a team they can discuss how best to offer assistance to the patient. The clinician should persist in seeking the patient's permission to share the disclosure with the rest of the team members. If the selective disclosure indicates that there are unresolved issues of distrust between the patient and other team members, the most therapeutic approach may be to address those issues head-on as part of the negotiations about the disclosure. If the patient continues to refuse permission to share this information, then the clinician is faced with the very difficult conflict about when it is justifiable to violate a patient's confidence. One must balance the goal of preventing harm to the patient against the possibility that violating a confidence (or threatening to do so) may lead to even less disclosure of key information and, therefore, a lessened opportunity to help the patient in the future.

If the clinician, on balance, thinks that the secret ought to be revealed to colleagues, the justification would be that the clinician is at the patient's bedside not as a solo practitioner but as a representative of the team; and not to allow the team to function cohesively is in a sense to reject the clinician's care. This justification will be most plausible when the team aspects of care, and the sharing of information in the team, have been fully disclosed to the patient as a part of the admission process. In order to minimize further loss of trust, the clinician who feels obligated to reveal secret information should frankly inform the patient of this and the reasons for the disclosure.

Some requests for death assistance are transparently a result of a temporary stress or mood change and are very unlikely to represent the considered, enduring posture of the patient. The clinician may deal with such requests by validating the emotional state of the patient and responding with appropriate brief counseling techniques.

All patients should be informed at this stage that it is the practice of the team to take all requests for death assistance very seriously. The patient should be informed that it is the experience of the team that the concerns and problems that prompt such requests can usually be ameliorated once the team has carefully assessed the patient's situation and further care options. The clinician should provide speedy attention to these concerns and full communication of the team's planning process.

TABLE 64.3

SUGGESTED STEPS FOR THE CLINICAL MANAGEMENT OF A REQUEST FOR ASSISTED DEATH

(1) The clinician should listen to the request for assisted death in an open and empathetic manner and evaluate the issues underlying the request.

(2) The clinician should share her personal stance with the patient in an open and professional manner, always assuring the patient that he will be supported throughout the process of his personal decision making process.

(3) All clinicians should take appropriate steps to process their personal emotional reactions to the patient's request, e.g., hospice team meetings.

(4) The clinician should have a continuing dialogue with the patient and appropriate family members or support persons concerning the development and implementation of the therapeutic treatment plans, including a request for assisted death, in a manner consistent with both the law and the clinician's moral values and belief system.

Miller F, Quill T, Brody H, et al. Regulating physician-assisted death. *N Engl J Med* 1994;31:119 (38).

At this point in the inquiry, the clinician, or the organization will take different approaches depending on their moral position on physician-assisted death. A clinician (or team) who is morally opposed to this practice in all cases should share this information with the patient, lest the patient entertain unrealistic hopes of later assistance. The statement of refusal to consider the option of assisted death should be coupled with the promise to stand by the patient until the moment of death and to continue to search exhaustively for any means other than death assistance to ameliorate the patient's suffering. The clinician may wish to add that a moral distaste for the action of assisting death does not equate with a moral condemnation of the suffering individual who is making the request.

In jurisdictions where assisted dying is legal, the clinician (or team) who is morally willing to consider the permissibility of assisting a patient's death (in carefully selected cases) may share that stance with the patient. (Assisted suicide is currently legal only in the State of Oregon.) The clinician would next share the procedure the team will follow in order to be sure that the patient is making a voluntary, considered choice and is suffering in ways that cannot be relieved by any other measures. The estimated amount of time needed for this determination, and to consider and suggest alternatives, should be shared with the patient. In any event, the patient needs to be informed that no quick and easy acquiescence is contemplated. The clinician may wish to inform the patient of the statistical chances that the patient will select an alternative means of addressing her suffering and will, in that event, no longer request a quick death.

Possible Scenarios

After this initial discussion around the patient's first request for assisted death, the palliative care team should engage in a careful inquiry to determine the nature and origin of the patient's suffering, taking at face value that if the patient was prompted to ask to die the suffering must be more severe than the team had previously appreciated. The inquiry will be aided by understanding some common scenarios observed among patients making such requests (55). The categories developed by Quill are very useful; (29,31) the following six scenarios illustrate situations in which all observers should agree that the best option lies not in assisting death but in providing alternate forms of care.

Inadequately Treated Physical Symptoms

The easiest category to deal with is the patient who seeks death because of suffering caused by inadequately treated physical symptoms. The palliative care team may have missed the onset, duration, or severity of a symptom. The patient may have felt compelled for a variety of emotional reasons to deny or minimize the symptoms. Or a previously prescribed treatment may be producing unpleasant or intolerable side effects that the patient similarly feels obligated to deny or minimize, possibly to avoid hurting the feelings of the clinicians. In any case, a searching discussion in which physical symptoms and treatment side effects are explicitly explained should reveal the source(s) of the problem, or other family members may be able to enlighten the hospice team on the nature of the complaint. A trial of an improved treatment strategy, to show the patient that the troublesome symptom can be relieved to tolerable levels, will also be successful in helping the patient experience and believe that their symptoms are able to be relieved.

Depression

Untreated depression can cause a patient to experience intense hopelessness, despair, and to have strong desires for death. A team member skilled in the differential diagnosis of depression should interview the patient with this possibility in mind. In an elderly patient, special expertise in geropsychiatry may be required, both to distinguish the signs of depression from the effects of aging or chronic illness, and to determine a type and dose of antidepressant medication which is appropriate for this particular patient (56). As always in palliative care, the treatment of depression in the terminal patient should be aimed at relief of troublesome symptoms rather than the cure of a disease. This may require flexibility and creativity in combining medication with emotional supports.

Family Dysfunction or Conflict

A patient's wish to die may grow out of conflicts within a troubled family relationship. A patient may wish to die because of a fear that painful and dissatisfying family relationships are not going to improve. In other cases, a request may be a manipulative counteroffensive aimed at punishing other family members. Most hospice teams have social workers and chaplains, as well as other team members, who are capable of evaluating family dysfunction and developing an appropriate management plan.

Spiritual Crisis

A request for assisted death may signal the fact that the belief system that previously provided the patient with a sense of meaning in her life is no longer experienced as supportive or meaningful, and the patient now feels that further existence would be without meaning for her. It may also suggest that this patient had been able to cope with previous life stressors without invoking any spiritual belief system and is now belatedly confronting the fact that she has no such resource to draw upon in looking at her own impending death.

Spiritual counseling may help to resolve the crisis and to restore a sense of meaning to the patient's life in the context of her illness and impending death. To be effective, the counseling needs to be tailored to the patient's spiritual beliefs or values and current needs. A careful assessment of the patient's sense of the nature of the current conflict and the reasons why previously helpful spiritual or emotional supports no longer seem to be working is essential for identifying the most helpful spiritual counselor for each patient. Human beings often assign meanings to events through the construction of narrative. Engaging patients in telling or writing stories about their past lives or present illness, or about their hopes for their survivors, may facilitate the process of restoring personal hope and meaning (36,48,53,57).

Unremitting Suffering Despite Adequate Support

It is the expectation of all palliative care specialists that this category would include relatively few patients. Clinicians who accept the permissibility of physician-assisted death would regard a patient in this extreme clinical and human condition a candidate for this assistance if she met the following criteria:

(1) Failed to achieve adequate relief of suffering through appropriate trials of palliative treatments
(2) Received appropriate emotional, social, and spiritual supports without adequate relief of suffering and
(3) The patient has retained her capacity for decision making and persists in voluntary request for death assistance

It is important for clinicians to recall that it is much harder to make the case that assistance in dying is the *right* of the terminally ill patient than that such death assistance is *permissible* in rare, selected circumstances. If patients have no moral right to death assistance, then physicians can refuse to assist death in all dubious cases. This effectively places the burden of proof on the patient rather than the physician—a negative situation if one adopts a strongly libertarian posture but a positive one if one is concerned about the ease with which any policy of assisted death may be abused to the detriment of vulnerable persons.

When faced with a patient who has unremitting suffering, those morally opposed to death assistance will again wish to affirm their commitment not to abandon the patient and to always stand by her in her suffering, although continuing to try new approaches and new combinations of treatments despite the waning likelihood of success. Spiritual counseling becomes critically important at this juncture—for the clinician to understand the patient's philosophy/spirituality regarding suffering as well as her coping strategies to ascertain meaning in the midst of the suffering, and for the patient to have the opportunity to utilize the expertise of chaplains or her own spiritual/religious advisors.

Hastening Death by Withdrawing Nutrition and Hydration

A policy proposal (56) and a case report (58) awakened interest in a legally permissible strategy allowing patients to hasten death, even in jurisdictions prohibiting physician-assisted suicide. A challenging case scenario for the palliative physician is one in which the patient chooses to voluntarily stop artificial nutrition and hydration because she has determined that life is not worth living and that an early death is preferable. The clinician wants to continue the support to prevent any discomfort of dehydration since the patient is not actively dying. For some, it will seem a clear-cut case of providing compassionate symptom relief although a patient exercises her legal and moral right to refuse medical interventions, including artificial nutrition and hydration. For others, it will seem an obvious subterfuge in which one stays on the "right" side of the law although engaging in an act, which is morally indistinguishable from physician-assisted suicide. After all, the patient refuses artificial nutrition and hydration not because of an inability to eat or drink, and not because artificial administration is excessively painful or burdensome, but because the patient has determined that future life is not worth living and that an early death is preferable. This case situation will be very challenging for the palliative care specialist and her team. It is paramount in these situations that the clinician have repeated conversations with the patient to ascertain her reasons for the decision to assure that this decision is consistent with the patient's values and life goals, her sense of how burdensome this treatment is, as well as the reality of her current clinical condition. Those who favor physician-assisted death will regard a prolonged death from dehydration, even if symptoms are well controlled, as an undignified travesty of what could otherwise have been a quick and painless death had more direct means been used. Those who advocate physician-assisted death but fear legal repercussions may find this an acceptable temporary solution. Some who oppose physician-assisted death would only support such a decision if the patient was actively dying and the artificial nutrition and hydration were no longer effective as treatments for the patient. They would ethically evaluate this treatment in the same manner as they would treatments such as ventilators, renal dialysis, or antibiotic treatments. If the burden of the treatment for the patient far outweighs the benefits,

then it is morally acceptable to withdraw or not choose such a treatment within this value system.

Considerable patient-and-family education is beneficial and necessary because most laypersons and some healthcare professionals are unaware that such a death can be relatively painless and comfortable with proper palliative support (19,57,58). Some patients or families may still find the prospect unacceptable even after several conversations. For those patients who might elect to use this method, it will be important to allow for shared conversations with family and providers to articulate the patient's goals, values, and her sense of the balance of benefits and burdens regarding this treatment and adequate symptom relief.

CONCLUSIONS

The foregoing sections have explored the ethical issues, the professional implications for hospice professionals, and the clinical management of requests for assisted death from hospice patients. Commentators on these issues (6,19,27,28,50) emphasize that there needs to be a stepwise approach to requests for assisted death which should include assessment of decision making capacity and lack of depression, excellent discussions regarding advance care planning, evaluation for treatable causes of symptoms and treatment if possible, proper utilization of professional resources (including spiritual), a network of caring (both professional and family), conversations with the patient and family which balance the patient's stated values with the known beneficial and non-beneficial aspects of treatment choices, and a death that expresses personal values and dignity (6).

References

1. *Vacco v Quill.* US Citation: 521 US 793, 1997;Docket:95–1858.
2. Saurez-Almazor ME, Belzile M, Bruera E. Euthanasia and physician-assisted suicide: a comparative survey of physicians, terminally ill cancer patients, and the general population. *J Clin Oncol* 1997;15:418–427.
3. Young A, Volker D. Oncology nurses attitudes regarding voluntary, physician-assisted dying for competent, terminally ill patients. *Oncol Nurse Forum* 1993;20(3):445.
4. Doukas DJ, Waterhouse D, Gorenflo DW, et al. Attitudes and behaviors on physician-assisted death: a study of Michigan oncologists. *J Clin Oncol* 1995;13:1055.
5. Slome LR, Mitchell TF, Charlebois E, et al. Physician-assisted suicide and patients with human immunodeficiency virus disease. *N Engl J Med* 1997;336:417–421.
6. Emanuel LL. Facing requests for physician-assisted suicide: toward a practical and principled clinical skill set. *JAMA* 1998;280:643–647.
7. Ersek M. The continuing challenge of assisted death. *J Hosp Palliat Nurs* 2004;6(1):46–59.
8. *The Oregon death with Dignity Act: a guide for health care providers,* 2nd ed., 2005 (Website: www.ohsu.edu/ethics).
9. Watts DT, Howell T. Assisted suicide is not voluntary active euthanasia. *J Am Geriatr Soc* 1992;40:1043.
10. Quill T. Death and dignity: a case of individualized decision making. *N Engl J Med* 1991;324:691.
11. Kevorkian J. *Prescription: medicine—the goodness of planned death.* Buffalo, New York: Prometheus Books, 1991.
12. Annas G. Physician-assisted suicide—Michigan's temporary solution. *N Engl J Med* 1993;328:1573.
13. Wilson WC, Smedira NG, Fink C, et al. Ordering and administration of sedatives and analgesics during the withholding of life support from critically ill patients. *JAMA* 1992;267:949.
14. Dixon N. On the difference between physician-assisted suicide and active euthanasia. *Hastings Cent Rep* 1998;28(3):25–29.
15. Annas G. Death by prescription—the oregon initiative. *N Engl J Med* 1994;331:1240.
16. Callahan D. Pursuing a peaceful death. *Hastings Cent Rep* 1992;22(4):33–38.
17. Kass L. Why doctors must not kill. Euthanasia: California proposition 161. *Commonweal* 1991;118(14):473.
18. Emanuel EJ. The history of euthanasia debates in the United States and Britain. *Ann Intern Med* 1994;121(10):793.
19. Peteet J. Treating patients who request assisted suicide. *Arch Fam Med* 1994;3:723.

20. Ferrel B, Rhiner M. High-tech comfort: ethical issues in cancer pain management for the 1990's. *J Clin Ethics* 1991;Summer:108.
21. Steinmetz D, Walsh MGabel LL, et al. Family physician's involvement with dying patients and their families. *Arch Fam Med* 1993;2:753.
22. Sullivan AD, Hedberg K, Fleming DW. Legalized physician-assisted suicide in Oregon—the second year. *N Engl J Med* 2000;342:598–604.
23. Davies J. Altruism towards the end of life. *J Med Ethics* 1993;19(2):111.
24. Clark PA. Pain management—theological and ethical principles governing the use of pain relief for dying patients. *Health Prog* 1993:30.
25. Campbell CS, Hare J, Matthews P. Conflicts of conscience: hospice and assisted suicide. *Hastings Cent Rep* 1995;25(3):36.
26. Emanuel EJ, Daniels ER, Fairclough DL, et al. The practice of euthanasia and physician-assisted suicide in the United States: adherence to proposed safeguards and effects on physicians. *JAMA* 1998;280:507–513.
27. Quill T, Cassel C, Meier D. Care of the hopelessly ill—proposed clinical criteria for physician-assisted suicide. *N Engl J Med* (Sounding Board) 1992; 327:1380.
28. Brody H. Assisted death—a compassionate response to a medical failure. *N Engl J Med* 1992;327:1384.
29. Quill T. *Death and dignity: making choices and taking charge.* New York: WW Norton, 1993.
30. Quill TE, Lo B, Brock DW. Palliative care options of last resort: a comparison of voluntarily stopping eating and drinking, terminal sedation, physician-assisted suicide and voluntary active euthanasia. *JAMA* 1997; 278:2099–2104.
31. Quill T. Doctor, I want to die, will you help me? *JAMA* 1993;270:870.
32. Drane JF. Physician-assisted suicide and voluntary active euthanasia: social ethics and the role of hospice. *Am J Hosp Palliat Care* 1995; 3–10.
33. Cassel EJ. The nature of suffering and the goals of medicine. *N Engl J Med* 1982;306:639.
34. Cassel EJ. *The nature of suffering and the goals of medicine.* New York: Oxford University Press, 1991.
35. Gunderson M, Mayo DJ. Restricting physician-assisted death to the terminally ill. *Hastings Cent Rep* 2000;30(6):17–23.
36. Miles S. Physicians and their patients' suicides. *JAMA* 1994;271:1786.
37. Battin M. Voluntary euthanasia and the risks of abuse: can we learn anything from the Netherlands? *Law Med Health Care* 1992;20(1–2):133.
38. Miller F, Quill T, Brody H, et al. Regulating physician-assisted death. *N Engl J Med* 1994;31:119.
39. Weir RF. The morality of physician-assisted suicide. *Law Med Health Care* 1992;20(1–2):116.
40. Kass LR. Neither for love nor money: why doctors must not kill. *Public Interest* 1989;94:25.
41. Haddad A. Physician-assisted suicide: the impact on nursing and pharmacy of value. *SHHV Newsletter* December, 1994.
42. Rupp MT, Isenhower HL. Pharmacist's attitudes toward physician-assisted suicide. *Am J Hosp Pharm* 1994;51(1):69.
43. Miller FG, Brody H. Professional integrity and physician-assisted death. *Hastings Cent Rep* 1995;25(3):8.
44. Campbell CS. Aid-in-dying and the taking of human life. *J Med Ethics* 1992;18(3):128.
45. *Harvard Law Review.* Physician-assisted suicide and the right to die with assistance. *Harv Law Rev* 1992;105:2021.
46. Kamisar Y. Are laws against assisted suicide constitutional? *Hastings Cent Rep* 1993;23(3):32.
47. Sedler RA. The constitution and hastening inevitable death. *Hastings Cent Rep* 1993;23(5):20.
48. Board of Directors. *Position Statement.* Gainesville, FL: American Academy of Hospice and Palliative Medicine, 1998.
49. Board of Directors. *Statement opposing the legalization of euthanasia and assisted suicide.* Arlington, VA: National Hospice and Palliative Care Organization.
50. Doukas DJ, Gorenflo DW, Supanich BA. Primary care physician attitudes and values toward end-of-life care and physician-assisted death. *Ethics Behav* 1999;9(3):210–230.
51. Cohen J, Fihn S, Boyko EJ, et al. Attitudes toward assisted suicide and euthanasia among physicians in Washington state. *N Engl J Med* 1994;331:89–94.
52. Emanuel EJ, Fairclough DL, Emanuel LL. Attitudes and desires related to euthanasia and physician-assisted suicide among terminally ill patients and their caregivers. *JAMA* 2000;284:2460–2468.
53. Freeman J, Pellegrino E. Management at the end of life. *Arch Fam Med* 1993;2:1078.
54. Miller RJ. Hospice care as an alternative to euthanasia. *Law Med Health Care* 1992;20(1–2):127.
55. Foley KM. The relationship of pain and symptom management to patient requests for physician-assisted suicide. *J Pain Symptom Manage* 1991;6:289.
56. Block SD, Billings JA. Patient requests to hasten death: evaluation and management in terminal care. *Arch Intern Med* 1994;154(18):2039.
57. Frank AW. *The wounded storyteller: body, illness, and ethics.* Chicago, IL: University of Chicago Press, 1995.
58. Bernat JL, Gert B, Mogielnicki RP. Patient refusal of hydration and nutrition: an alternative to physician-assisted suicide or voluntary active euthanasia. *Arch Intern Med* 1993;153:2723.
59. Lo B, Rubenfeld G. Palliative sedation in dying patients: "We turn to it when everything else hasn't worked". *JAMA* 2005;294(14):1810–1816.

CHAPTER 65 ■ PALLIATIVE CARE: ETHICS AND THE LAW

ROBERT A. BURT AND MICHAEL K. GOTTLIEB

During the past 30 years, a dramatic change has occurred in the legal and ethical principles governing provision of care for terminally ill patients. Withholding or discontinuing life-prolonging treatment has now received widespread approval in judicial opinions, state statutes, and the intraprofessional norms of medical practice. The first significant judicial opinion was rendered in 1976 by the New Jersey Supreme Court in the *Karen Quinlan* case, which authorized the removal of a ventilator from a patient in a persistent vegetative state (1). Numerous state legislatures and courts subsequently endorsed the proposition that where patients or their surrogates requested this course, physicians could withhold or withdraw life-prolonging treatment with no fear of criminal or civil liability (2). In 1990, the United States Supreme Court bestowed ultimate legitimacy on this changed norm of medical practice by ruling, in effect, that mentally competent patients had a constitutional right to refuse life-prolonging treatment (3). Seven years later, the Justices unanimously declined to extend this ruling beyond a "right of refusal;" the court rejected any constitutional right to active acceleration of death by physician-assisted suicide even if requested by a mentally competent patient (4). The court did clearly indicate that state legislatures were free to authorize this practice; to date, only Oregon has done so (5).

From its very beginning in the *Quinlan* case, however, the "right to refuse treatment" has been afflicted by a disconnect between conception and reality. In authorizing ventilator removal, the New Jersey Supreme Court relied on the principle of respect for autonomous choice. The court gave no weight to the wishes of Karen's parents or to those of her physicians; the only person with any legally recognizable claim was Karen herself. But Karen, of course, was in no position to make any choice about the continuation of the respirator. She was then incompetent, with no prospect of ever regaining competence; and before her cerebrovascular accident, when she had been competent; she had never expressed any opinion about her wishes in the event she might become ventilator-dependent. The court quickly bypassed the central problem in applying the autonomy ideal to her by positing that

1. If she had been competent, she would have had a right to choose withdrawal
2. She should not lose this right "merely" because she was now incompetent and
3. Her father could exercise this right for her, so long as he acted on the basis of what he believed to be her wishes rather than his own view of her best interests

From its modern origins in the *Quinlan* case, the autonomy framework for conceptualizing end-of-life decision making has therefore had a distinctly artificial cast of mind. It is only 30 years after *Quinlan*, however, that we can now clearly see what should have been evident from the beginning: the autonomy framework in the context of end-of-life decision making simply does not fit the facts.

This is not to deny that protecting patient autonomy in end-of-life care, as in all medical treatment and research, is an important principle. Nor does this deny that disregard for patient choice has been a longstanding and unjustifiable feature of medical treatment and research. But in reality, applying the autonomy framework in end-of-life decision making has had little practical effect and much fictitious posturing. Efforts to persuade people to execute advance directives to protect their autonomy if they should become incompetent have essentially failed. Where incompetent patients have previously completed advance directives and treating physicians disregard their clear import, however, courts have been willing to award civil damages (6). The fictive character of these directives is revealed with special clarity in the laws of some 33 states providing that where an incompetent person has not specified a health care proxy in advance, the state will make that choice itself on the premise that most people would want what the state wants for them—that is, spouse first, adult children second, and so forth (7). Most state surrogacy laws require that the surrogate follow a "substituted judgment" standard—that is, the surrogate is obliged somehow to discern what the incompetent patient would have wanted based on prior statements or general values (8). A few states provide that, where the patient's prior wishes are unclear, the surrogate is permitted to act on the basis of the patient's "best interests" (9).

The explanation for the failure of the advance directive movement emerged with considerable force in the empirical findings of the study to understand prognoses and preferences for outcomes and risks of treatments (SUPPORT) (10). Carried out in the 1990s, the study tested the most extensive, rigorous effort that had ever been tried to assist critically ill patients and their families in making informed choices about end-of-life care. Notwithstanding the magnitude of this effort toward promoting choice, it produced no effective results. The SUPPORT data instead revealed—in findings that have been subsequently confirmed in other settings—that most patients and their families simply did not want to make decisions about their end-of-life care. Although most patients in the study were persuaded to fill out advance directives, a substantial portion of these patients and their families ignored their prior directives as death drew near. They simply did not want to talk about the imminently looming reality that they were facing death; and most medical professionals returned the favor with equal reluctance to speak about this inevitability.

There are two ways to respond to the consistently confirmed insufficiency of advance directives and end-of-life planning. One way—the dominant way during the past 30 years—has been to redouble efforts to promote patient and family choice making. The second way is to turn our focus of attention away from the autonomous choice framework in thinking about end-of-life decision making. This alternative is preferable—not to override autonomous choice but to remove this value from the center of attention and to recast our thinking about end-of-life care to promote different, although not necessarily inconsistent, goals.

Our preference for this alternative arises from more than the practical failure of efforts to promote individual end-of-life care choice making. More fundamentally, the pursuit in itself carries substantial social dangers that are likely to yield abuses as bad as, and even directly similar to, the abuses of physician authoritarianism that the autonomy framework was intended to correct. The crucial impetus for the modern embrace of the autonomy framework for terminally ill patients was mistrust of physicians, based on a belief that they regularly disregarded both the wishes and interests of their dying patients by pursuing aggressive, painful therapies with no realistic possibility of success, by withholding effective pain relief generally, and by abandoning their patients when death became patently unavoidable. The equivalent dangers in the autonomy framework arise from the practical reluctance of most people to exercise choice.

That reluctance, we believe, comes from cognitive difficulties that inescapably afflict everyone in contemplating the reality of his or her own death. Proponents of the autonomy framework during the past thirty years have not ignored these difficulties but instead have inveighed against them. From their perspective, the cognitive obstacles to rationalizing death are not insurmountable. According to their view, we should—individually and collectively—end our "denial of death" and reconceive death (as some say it once was conceived in western civilization, or in some other contemporary cultures) as a "natural part of life" to be accepted in the same way that we accept any inevitable biological givens. We suggest, however, that there is more at play in the avoidance of death's biological inevitability than the simple fear of it. There is, more importantly, a cognitive drag on our ability to comprehend death. We may parrot the language of rational choice in comparing our fears about death with our fears about continued life. We may enact a convincing appearance of autonomous choice in contemplating death. But it is very difficult, at the core of our thinking, to convince ourselves that death is rationally comprehensible. Death is more than a future condition fraught with uncertainties about benefits and detriments. It is more than the absence of life. It is the absence, the intrinsic contradiction, of meaningfulness. The very concept of the choice-making self, the construct on which the autonomy principle depends for its coherence, is radically unsettled—even made incomprehensible—by the actual, imminent approach of death.

The more conventional view is that some people may be afflicted with this difficulty but some—perhaps many or even most—are not; and the task for application of the autonomy principle is to devise guidelines for distinguishing those who are and are not "competent" to exercise rational choice. But the difficulties of drawing this distinction are so profound and the consequences of our inevitable failures to make convincing distinctions are so grave that we should not put this differentiating enterprise at the center of our practices about end-of-life care.

We believe that the most convincing explanation for the medical abuses inflicted by physicians on dying patients is the physicians' own sense of the "wrongness" of death. The incomprehensibility of death readily translates into a conviction that death is a kind of grammatical error, a misfit in a world that can be rationally comprehended. In the medical lexicon, death is therefore understood as an error to be corrected, opposed, and negated. Displacing physicians and blaming their commitment to rational mastery over death does not, however, cure the problem posed by the incomprehensibility of death. Its conceptual status as a grammatical error leads to medical triumphalism and the abuses of dying patients that follow from this relentless warfare against error. Its incomprehensibility translates with equal ease in lay terms to a conviction that death is "wrong" as a moral proposition. Even if one's rational intellect can comprehend that there are worse things than death, and that it is nonsensical to imbue a biological inevitability with moral condemnation, nonetheless a persistent undertow pulls continuously in the opposite direction. This moral ambivalence toward death might be consciously denied. And some people may be more capable than others of rigidly maintaining this denial into the maw of death itself. But for most people, successful resistance to this moralized understanding is akin to success in refusing to think about elephants in response to a command that you must not—whatever you do, *you must not*— think about elephants.

The actual consequences of thinking forbidden thoughts about elephants are much less fraught with danger than thinking forbidden thoughts about the moral wrongness of death. If actual death is a moral wrong and you cannot avoid dying—indeed, if you actively embrace dying—then it follows that some wrong has been committed and someone must be punished for this wrongdoing. Physicians might, of course, punish their dying patients for this transgression. But when physicians are removed from their previously central choice-making role, the impulse to blame does not vanish; it simply moves to a new target. The ironic consequence of the autonomy principle—that decisions about death are the legitimate prerogative of no one but the dying person—is that blame too will be attached only to the dying person. As the choice belongs to the individual, the punishment will be individually self-inflicted. The precise content of this punishment would vary—perhaps patients' insistence on aggressive and painful, although patently futile treatments, perhaps their refusal to request effective pain relief, perhaps their embrace of premature death. But in all such cases, the abuse previously inflicted by physicians on dying patients will reappear, for the same underlying reasons, as abuse inflicted by dying patients on themselves.

Abuse of dying patients—either self-inflicted or iatrogenic—is not, however, inevitable. It is only ambivalence about death—some lurking, ineradicable sense of its wrongfulness juxtaposed against all rational arguments for its inevitability and even preferability—that is inevitable. The impetus for turning this ambivalence toward abuse is denial—not "denial of death," in the conventional sense of that cultural construct, but denial of the negative valences in the ambivalence toward death. Like trying not to think about elephants, the negative valences cannot be entirely repressed; and if they are banished from consciousness by a single-minded insistence that death is "good" or "dignified" or "accepted," the unconsciously buried sense of wrongness and guilt accompanying death will push toward expression in action. This is the dynamics by which an unacknowledged sense of wrongdoing and guilt expresses itself by wrongful action that implicitly invites condemnation whereas, at the same time, the action is explicitly enshrined in protestations of righteous conduct.

The challenge for social regulation of end-of-life care is to identify the circumstances in which this malign dynamic is likely to take hold and to design countervailing schemes. Reliance on patient autonomy is not an effective countervailing scheme, any more than the now-discredited reliance on physician autonomy for deciding whether and when death should occur. We believe, however, that the following three principles are alternatives responsive to the current overinvestment in patient autonomy:

1. No one should be socially authorized to engage in conduct that directly, purposefully, and unambiguously inflicts death, whether on another person or on oneself.
2. Decisions that indirectly lead to death should be acted upon only after a consensus is reached among many people; no single individual should be socially authorized to exercise exclusive control over decisions that might lead to death, whether that individual is the dying person, the attending physician, or a single family member acting as health care proxy.
3. As much as possible, end-of-life care should not depend on explicit decisions made at the bedside of a specific dying person but rather should be implicitly dictated by systems-wide decisions about available resources, personnel, and institutional settings—that is, by setting up default pathways that implicitly guide and even control caretaking decisions in individual cases.

PRINCIPLE 1: NO INFLICTION OF DEATH

The rationale for the first principle is that the direct, purposeful, and unambiguous infliction of death leaves no psychological space for acknowledged ambivalence. Whether the infliction is carried out on oneself or on others, it demands an unambivalent claim of rightness and righteousness that is psychologically impossible and therefore invites self-contradictory expressive actions. (The clearest model for this demand is in the administration of the death penalty, where the possibility of executing an innocent person must be entirely excluded and yet the difficulties of obtaining this ironclad assurance lead to a lingering sense of guilt and abusive inflictions in the enterprise.)

Our current regulations for end-of-life decision making do offer psychological space for acknowledged ambivalence in various ways. The rules that permit withholding or withdrawing life-sustaining care provide some comforting assurance that these actions do not in themselves inflict death because the underlying illness is the cause of death. At the same time, the logical tenuousness of this reasoning promotes conscious acknowledgment of ambivalence—that is, of the close proximity of these actions to wrongful conduct. (This protective dynamic is compellingly revealed in a case presentation by Miles Edwards and Susan Tolle, describing their actions and reactions in removing a competent, conscious postpolio patient from a ventilator, in response to his insistent request. Although rationally convinced of the moral correctness of this course, Drs. Edwards and Tolle report the sense of wrongdoing—of "purposeful killing" that nonetheless attended their actions and that powerfully troubled them (11).

The logical tenuousness of the distinction between relieving pain and hastening death in the high-dosage administration of opioids to dying patients—the so-called "double effect" principle—has the same psychologically protective function, serving simultaneously as permission and a warning sign about dealing with death. According to the double effect principle, consequences that would be wrong if caused intentionally become acceptable, even when foreseen or indeed expected, if the actions creating those consequences were intended for a morally permissible purpose (12). Typically, reliance on the principle of double effect requires the presence of the following four conditions:

1. The act creating the risk of adverse consequences must be beneficial, or at least morally neutral
2. The actor must intend the beneficial effect and not the harmful effect, although the harmful effect may be foreseen
3. The harmful effect must not be a means to the beneficial effect and
4. The beneficial effect must outweigh the harmful effect (13)

In the context of palliative care, under this principle, a physician may administer pain medication to a patient, knowing that medication may hasten the patient's death, so long as the intent of the physician is solely to relieve the patient's pain. In this scenario, the "beneficial" effect of pain relief is intended, whereas the "harmful" effect of death is merely foreseen.

The protective function of logically tenuous rules tends to erode over time, as their routine application dulls everyone's sense of the close correspondence between permitted and forbidden conduct authorized by these rules. The clearest indication of this erosion is in the arguments put forward with increasing social acceptance by advocates for physician-assisted suicide and euthanasia. These advocates insist that withholding or withdrawing life-sustaining treatment or application of the "double effect" principle is logically identical to purposeful, unambiguous infliction of death, and that this logical identity means that all these steps are morally equivalent and morally correct. These contemporary advocates fail to see that, far from justifying this "next step" toward purposeful killing, the plausibility of their logical claims about existing practices should raise concerns that these practices have themselves lost their function as protective expressions of ambivalence toward death. Our guiding principle for social regulation should be that the more comfortable clinicians and patients are with actions implicating death, the more socially dangerous these actions become. Preserving these "illogical" lines between accepting and hastening death—between physician-assisted suicide and withholding or withdrawing treatment or administering high-dosage opioids—is in the service of promoting conscious awareness of moral discomfort. Eliminating this discomfort, as urged by advocates for physician-assisted suicide and euthanasia, is logical but terribly wrong—and socially dangerous because the unconsciously buried conviction of wrongdoing ultimately will express itself in eruptions of blameworthy conduct.

PRINCIPLE 2: CONSENSUS DECISION MAKING FOR DEATH

Our second principle, that social regulations should not designate any single individual to exercise exclusive control over decisions that might lead to death, would require a more radical departure from existing arrangements. Forged on the anvil of autonomous individual choice, existing arrangements search relentlessly for a single designated decision-maker based on a clear-cut hierarchy of authority. The desperate intensity of this search is revealed by the state laws, noted in the preceding text, that denominate proxy decision makers even where an incompetent patient has made no prior selection. In particular, this intense search is apparent in the provision of those laws regarding multimember proxies, such as parents or children or siblings; the laws typically specify that for this class of proxies, majority vote shall prevail and, in the event of tie votes, the class is disqualified from decision-making authority. The implicit goal in these laws is not simply to find some single decision maker but to find an unambiguous choice about life-sustaining treatment.

There is a practical imperative behind this goal because of the binary character of the decision to treat or not to treat. But, honoring this imperative means suppressing the ambivalence that is likely to accompany this decision. If, as we believe, it is more socially and psychologically protective to acknowledge and address this ambivalence in the course of decision making, the better course would be to amplify the opportunities for expression of differing views—therefore forcing everyone's ambivalence about death-dispensing decisions toward visible acknowledgment. To accomplish this goal, provision of life-sustaining treatment must be the default option unless and until all of the affected participants have come to a consensus about withholding or withdrawing.

When the patient is competent and prepared to make a decisive choice, the autonomy principle does properly bestow hierarchically superior authority with the patient. But even in this clear-cut case, there are other, importantly affected participants who should have some voice in the patient's ultimate decision—not a veto but a voice in talking to the patient and thereby potentially addressing and amplifying the ambivalence that the decisive patient himself is likely to feel but also likely to deny.

Beyond—or perhaps one should say, above—this psychological benefit of consultation, there is an ethical principle that demands this consultative process. The competent patient may have the ethically highest priority in decision making; but his or her decision to continue or discontinue treatment has powerful and lasting impact on family members and on health care clinicians. The current ethical fixation on the patient's autonomous choice ignores the legitimacy of these others' stake in this decision. That stake may ultimately deserve less weight than the competent patient's choice; but some weight nonetheless is appropriate and can be respected by rules providing for some consultative processes.

Perhaps these consultations should be mandatory in all cases; perhaps some exception should be made where the patient adamantly resists any consultation, but even here the patient should be required to explain his refusal to some third party (although not necessarily to convince this party about the intrinsic correctness of his willful isolation in decision making). In this required explanation, some degree of respect at least would be paid by the patient both to the possibility that he is suppressing his own ambivalence about his decision and that others will be powerfully affected by his decision and therefore have some ethically mandated stake in it.

Where there is no competent patient or clear-cut advance directive from the now-incompetent patient, the autonomy principle provides no ethical basis for giving priority to any one among many plausibly affected parties. The practical imperative of making some unambiguous choice among binary alternatives could justify some ultimate arbitrarily imposed hierarchy among potential decision makers. But, unlike existing arrangements, this ultimate imposition should be postponed for some considerable time while the parties are forced by their explicitly shared decision-making authority to collaborate with one another and to explore the possibilities of a genuine consensus.

This extended consultative process cuts against the grain of current medical practice for at least two reasons. The process is time consuming and it is emotionally draining. Clinicians are not adequately compensated financially or psychologically for these costs. They are, moreover, typically not trained to engage in these consultative processes. Extended consultation with distressed family members in conflict with one another about treatment alternatives requires considerable emotional investment and resilience among clinicians. It requires, among other things, that clinicians confront their own discomfort, their own ambivalence, about the death-dispensing decisions that are a required part of their daily routine. The automatic, instantaneous designation of a single decision-maker—whether it is the competent patient or one family member among many to speak for the incompetent patient—permits clinicians to avoid these arduous, complicated confrontations with conflicting family members and with conflicts within themselves. This is the path of least resistance—and the path of greatest individual and social danger toward routinized, unacknowledged impositions of abuse.

Some clinicians may be tempted to avoid difficult consultation with patients or their families by invoking a principle of "medical futility." In certain circumstances, this principle is clearly well-founded. To use an extreme example, if a patient suffering from lung cancer requests that his physicians amputate a limb, the requested treatment has no relevance to the presenting illness and a physician is not only justified but is professionally obligated to refuse the request. In this sense, the principle of "medical futility" continuously guides proper medical practice (14). But some have argued for a broader application of this principle, and invoke it to justify physician refusals of treatments that have very low (but not demonstrably zero) probabilities of success (15). If, however, the patient or his surrogate believes it worthwhile to pursue such therapy, the ethical basis for the physician's refusal is not clear.

The physician may have a personal moral objection to providing some requested treatments—for example, abortions or discontinuance of life-prolonging treatment. State statutes typically provide conscientious exemptions regarding such procedures for health care professionals (although also requiring that physicians or hospitals assist patients in finding facilities where the requested procedures will be provided) (16). In other circumstances, apparently futile treatment may involve health care professionals in such assaultive interventions—for example, the administration of cardiopulmonary resuscitation (CPR) to a hopelessly terminal patient—that the professionally hallowed principle of "primum non nocere" could justify refusals. But refusal of treatments based simply on physicians' generalized conviction of "futility" too readily undermines the physicians' primary obligation to consult with and attempt to persuade rather than unilaterally override the wishes of patients or their families (17).

PRINCIPLE 3: SYSTEMIC PATHWAYS FOR DECISION MAKING ABOUT DEATH

Our third principle that systems-wide default pathways should self-consciously be constructed to implicitly guide and even dictate caretaking decisions in individual cases, derives from the same psychological premises as the other principles. Systems-wide decisions establish the context and frequently dictate the content of individual bedside decisions on such matters as allocation of resources, locus of care (home vs. hospital vs. nursing home), and roles of professional and nonprofessional caretakers (reliance on family, consistent vs. multiple, episodic involvement of health care professionals, respective and/or collaborative roles of physicians, nurses, social workers, clergy).

This is the lesson, for example, of the SUPPORT finding that whether patients died at home or in institutional settings did not depend on the individual preferences of patients or families, but correlated directly with the availability of institutional beds—the more beds in any region, the more likely that terminally ill patients in those regions would die in those beds. Notwithstanding the clarity and persuasiveness of these data, however, it is highly unlikely that anyone involved in the systems-wide decision making that produced more or fewer hospital beds in any given locale acknowledged, even to themselves, that their decisions would have direct impact on dying patients and virtually dictate whether these patients would die at home or in hospital. The impact of these systems-wide choices on actual dying people was, in an important sense, invisible to everyone—although a moment's clear thought would have made this impact visible.

We can see this same phenomenon in the familiar example of the psychological difference between systems-wide decisions to withhold resources for improving coal mine safety and particularized decisions to withhold rescue resources from workers trapped in coal mine accidents. In both contexts, it is clear that lives will be lost by withholding safety and rescue resources, and the numbers of lost lives are precisely calculable. But in withholding expenditures for coal mine safety, the lives lost are statistical projections. For trapped coal miners, these impending deaths have names, faces, and specifically identifiable families. The ethical costs and psychological dangers of withholding resources from rescue are therefore much greater than for withholding preventive expenditures. Withholding rescue resources feels like inflicting death on people and is inevitably guilt provoking, whereas withholding preventive safety resources feels more like impersonal policy decisions.

In the terms we have been using, the preventive expenditure context permits easy dominance of the rational perspective that death may be socially desirable because of the costs of preventing it. But when this logical rationing calculus is applied to trapped coal miners or at the bedside of an identifiable person, then the negative valence regarding the intrinsic evil of death—and the blameworthy status of those involved in choosing death—insistently asserts itself (18). In making decisions about the care of dying people, we should take advantage of the psychological protective implications of systems-wide decision making. As much as possible, we should make systems-wide decisions in which, at the moment when the decisions are made, no specific dying person is an acknowledged target.

Provision of pain control is one clear context in which reliance on individual decision making has historically failed to yield even minimally adequate results. The SUPPORT study, for example, revealed that more than half of all dying patients suffered considerable, although treatable and therefore unnecessary, pain during the last 3 days of life. Reliance on initiatives from individual physicians or demands for better pain relief from individual patients or their families offers very little prospect for needed changes in practice. In part this is because the barriers to provision of adequate pain relief are, to an important degree, systemically created; and therefore the remedy must be systemic. And in part this is because individual initiatives, like those born out of the proautonomy movement, are too haphazard to effect significant change. The decisions of individual patients in this environment are too often subject to the influence or perceived influence of physicians, of families, and of institutions. Often physicians, themselves, continue to view certain conservative methods of pain treatment as medically appropriate, even when the medical literature indicates the opposite view. Fortunately, many of the significant systemic barriers to the provision of adequate pain control in the United States have recently become the focus of changing regulatory and institutional policies. Such change is evident not only in emerging federal and state laws, which have traditionally provided for such a high degree of regulatory scrutiny that some physicians have felt reluctant to prescribe controlled substances to patients for whom such prescriptions were medically appropriate, but also in federal and state enforcement policy and practice.

Federal enforcement of the Controlled Substances Act (CSA), for instance, continues to evolve toward more appropriate standards. The CSA establishes a range of administrative, civil, and criminal penalties for the inappropriate prescription or distribution of controlled substances. Many of these penalties are substantial and go beyond the attorney general's authority [through the Drug Enforcement Agency (DEA)] to suspend or revoke a physician's registration to distribute prescription drugs if he or she has acted in a manner "inconsistent with the public interest."

Historically, enforcement of the CSA exacerbated practitioners' fears of investigation (thereby reducing overall appropriate pain management). But more recently, and despite the prosecutorial power afforded by the CSA, and the few highly publicized cases in which physicians have misused or overprescribed pain medication, actual federal prosecution for abusive prescription of controlled substances is relatively rare. Although there are more than 1,100,000 practitioners registered with the DEA to prescribe controlled substances (19), an average of 25 registrations have been revoked in each of the past 5 years (20).

In fact, the DEA has revised its policies over the last 15 years to encourage effective pain management. In its 1990 *Physician's Manual*, for instance, the DEA indicated that the use of controlled substances to manage pain is a legitimate medical use and encouraged physicians to prescribe, dispense or administer narcotics when used for a legitimate medical purpose.

More recently, in 2001, the DEA joined with 21 pain and health organizations to issue a joint statement on the use and abuse of pain medication and physician reluctance to manage pain with controlled substances. The statement was noteworthy, not only because it affirmed government support for the legitimate use of prescription drugs for patients in pain, but also because it was the first ever public collaboration between the DEA and organizations supporting pain management. The statement recognized that the undertreatment of pain is a serious problem in the United States that affects both chronic pain sufferers and the terminally ill. Most importantly, perhaps, the statement emphasized that although the prevention of drug abuse is an important societal goal, it should not thwart pain management efforts. In November of 2004, the DEA released an Interim Policy Statement titled "Dispensing of Controlled Substances for the Treatment of Pain," that recognized the crucial importance of not discouraging medical practitioners engaged in legitimate pain treatment from providing proper medication to patients.

Regulatory progress has been achieved in fits and starts, but federal policy now specifically reflects the appropriateness of using narcotics to treat pain. This should be viewed by health care providers as encouragement to prescribe pain medication without fear of reprisals. It is also clear from the language of the CSA that Congress intended it to *not* unduly restrict practitioners from prescribing narcotics. Section 801 of the CSA recognizes that controlled substances "have a useful and legitimate medical purpose and are necessary to maintain the health and general welfare of the American people" (21).

The CSA further provides that psychotropic substances should be controlled in accordance with established drug schedules to ensure that these substances are available for legitimate medical and scientific purposes. This is significant given the frequent use of psychotropic drugs with opioids to treat pain caused by nervous system damage. Congressional support for legitimate medical use of psychotropics, including for medical pain management, suggests concomitant support for the legitimate medical use of opioids to treat pain.

Moreover, during the past 10 years, several states have attempted to improve patient access to pain management and address physician reluctance to prescribe opioids for fear of disciplinary action by enacting Intractable Pain Treatment Acts ("IPTAs"). These laws immunize physicians from disciplinary action by state medical boards provided that the physicians comply with certain requirements. For example, Texas's IPTA prohibits a medical board from subjecting a physician to disciplinary actions where, in the course of the physician's treatment of a person for intractable pain, the physician prescribed or administered dangerous drugs or controlled substances. The Texas IPTA defines "intractable pain" as a "pain state in which the cause of the pain cannot be removed or otherwise treated and which in the generally accepted course of medical practice no relief or cure of the cause of the pain is possible or none has been found after reasonable efforts" (22). Despite the changing trend in federal and state policies governing certain types of prescriptions for pain medications, however, undertreatment of chronic pain remains a problem. This may be due to the historical fear among physicians of high regulatory scrutiny and potential penalties (despite extremely rare prosecutions), or a continued and widespread lack of understanding among physicians about the relative risks of prescribing opioids. Notwithstanding extensive research evidence to the contrary, many physicians continue to believe that the use of opioids will sedate a patient into irreversible unconsciousness or death. Whereas depressed respirations, sedation, and confusion are potential side effects of opioid therapy, research has demonstrated that opioids do not hasten death when titrated appropriately (23). A systemic approach to encouraging appropriate pain management is necessary, therefore, to undo the historical and persistent bias against appropriate treatment—for whatever reasons.

The threat of civil liability is also emerging as an additional systemic incentive for providers to treat pain. There are only a few cases alleging the undertreatment of pain as the basis for a medical malpractice claim, but recent court decisions indicate that these actions are likely to increase. In one of the first cases that held a physician liable for undertreatment of pain medication, the state licensing board made it clear that overestimating the relative risk of pain medication is no defense to liability for undertreatment. In 1999, the Oregon Board of Medical Examiners cited a pulmonary specialist for unprofessional or dishonorable conduct and gross or repeated acts of negligence for failing to adequately treat six seriously ill or dying patients with pain medication from 1993 to 1998 (24). In at least three of the cases, the physician purportedly failed to prescribe controlled substances for pain relief for fear that pain medication would suppress the respiratory drive of his patients despite medical research demonstrating that appropriate titration of controlled substances does not depress patient respirations. The Oregon Board's disciplinary actions came just 18 months after a national nonprofit patient advocacy group, Compassion in Dying, called on all fifty states' medical boards and the Federation of State Medical Boards to penalize physicians who failed to give adequate pain control to terminally ill patients (25).

In a recent line of California cases, claims for pain and suffering due to inadequate pain management have been successfully brought under the state's "elder abuse statute." In *Bergman v. Chin* (2001) (26), a California jury found that a physician's failure to adequately manage the pain of a terminally ill patient was a form of elder abuse. Although it was not the first case to base a claim on poor pain management (27), it was the first time that undertreatment was framed as the cause of action under an "elder abuse statute" in a civil trial. The jury awarded the survivors of an 85-year-old lung cancer patient $1.5 million for unnecessary pain and suffering caused by the inadequate treatment of pain.

The case involved a patient diagnosed with multiple spinal compression fractures and a strong possibility of lung cancer.

Although the emergency room physician initially prescribed morphine, the attending physician at the hospital changed the prescription to meperidine, with instructions to administer the pain medication as needed. During the 5 days the patient remained hospitalized, he complained of severe pain (reporting a range from seven to 10), but remained on meperidine as needed. At discharge, when the patient reported pain at level 10, he was prescribed an oral form of hydrocodone, but was known to have difficulties swallowing. He was eventually prescribed meperidine by injection and a fentanyl patch. In hospice, the patient's regular physician re-prescribed liquid morphine and two additional patches, which effectively relieved the pain. The patient died 3 days after his hospital discharge.

Because California's malpractice law did not provide for survival of an action for pain and suffering, the plaintiffs in *Bergman* asserted a cause of action under the state's Elder Abuse and Dependent Adult Civil Protection Act. The basis for their claim was that the defendant's failure to establish an adequate pain management plan was reckless, resulted in severe injury (excruciating pain), and was therefore a violation of the state's statute prohibiting elder abuse. This meant, however, that the plaintiffs needed to meet a higher burden of proof. California's malpractice laws requires proof of negligence by a preponderance of the evidence, but the elder abuse statute requires proof that conduct rose to the level of recklessness through clear and convincing evidence. Bergman's estate successfully showed that the defendant physician acted with "deliberate disregard of the high probability that an injury [would] occur [,]" and that the conduct constituted "a conscious choice of a course of action... with knowledge of the serious danger to others involved in it" (28).

Two years after the *Bergman* verdict, California's second pain case was successfully brought under the state's elder abuse statute. In *Tomlinson v. Bayberry Care Center* (29), an 85-year-old patient who suffered from mesothelioma was admitted to a hospital where records indicated that the patient experienced pain "all the time," often reaching a reported level of 10. Pain relief was only sporadically provided. After being transferred to a nursing home, Tomlinson frequently reported pain. Round-the-clock pain control was never provided, however, and medication was only administered after Tomlinson's family requested it based on their own research into various pain medications. Despite the fact that Tomlinson had an advance directive expressly stating his wishes for aggressive pain treatment, the days prior to his death were characterized as "twenty days of unremitting agony" (30). The hospital, the attending physician at the hospital, the nursing care facility, and the physician at the facility, all settled for undisclosed amounts and agreed to participate in continuing education classes.

Whereas the settlements by all of the defendants were caused in part by the *Bergman* verdict, the overriding cause was a shift in perspective in the medical and health care communities. As a result of these cases, a standard of care for pain management is being established, and much of the ambiguity surrounding pain medication prescription effectively removed. Clinical practice guidelines and standards are closer to offering authoritative, legally enforceable statements on adequate pain management, and are presumptive evidence of due care. Consequently, health care providers can no longer escape liability by offering evidence of inadequate treatment as the "usual or customary" practice in the community, and California physicians are now required to receive continuing medical education instruction in pain management (31).

Illustrative of this shift are the disciplinary actions taken by the California Medical Board, and the pursuance of fraud charges by the federal Center for Medicare and Medicaid Services (CMS). In *Bergman*, the California Medical Board refused to pursue disciplinary action despite finding inadequate care on the part of the defendant. In *Tomlinson*, however, not only did the board file an accusation with the state attorney general, but it also issued a public reprimand of the physician involved. Of equal significance, CMS launched an investigation and is considering pursuing federal fraud charges. The premises of the charges would be that adequate pain management is the standard of care, and billing for treatment that falls short of the standard constitutes fraud.

This emerging line of case law will likely grow in California and (in time) elsewhere, and will continue to reinforce the existing systemic approaches to improving pain management through the delivery of appropriate pain medication.

The three principles we have advanced have one common theme: That the focus of attention should shift away from individual choice-making autonomy in the social arrangements regarding end-of-life care. Because it has no substantive content—because it is ostentatiously silent about whether death is desirable or undesirable, but insists only that each individual should make this value choice for himself—the autonomy focus has served the same psychological purpose that we are criticizing. This psychological purpose is to deny ambivalence about death—to deny that death can be both attractive and repulsive at the same time, and to deny that decisions either to accept or to resist death are more fraught with possibilities of abuse when this core ambivalence is suppressed rather than acknowledged in an open and sustained way. Acknowledging this ambivalence is difficult. These difficulties have given impetus to the relentless search for a single decision-maker regarding end-of-life care—whether that decision-maker was the attending physician, under the old ethos of physician paternalism, or the individual patient, under the new ethos of individual autonomy (32). We have seen enough by now to know that the new path is not a reliable improvement over the old.

References

1. In re Quinlan, 355 A.2d 647 (N.J. 1976), *cert den* 429 US 922.
2. *See, for example*, Ala Code § 22-8A-7; Alaska Stat § 18.12.060; Ariz Rev Stat Ann §§ 36–3205, 36–3261.C; Ark Code Ann § 20-17-208; Cal Health & Safety Code § 7190.5; Cal Probate Code § 4750; Colo Rev Stat §§ 15-14-508, 15-18-110; Conn Gen Stat Ann § 19a-571; Del Code Ann tit 16 § 2510; DC Code Ann § 6–2427(a); Ga Code Ann §§ 31-32-7,31-36-2(c), 31-36-8; Haw Rev Stat § 327D 18; Idaho Code § 39–4508; Ill Comp Stat tit 755 § 35/4, 7; Ind Code Ann §§ 16-36-4-7(c), 16-36-4-13(d), 30-5-9-10; Iowa Code Ann §§ 144A.9, 144B.9; Kan Stat Ann § 65-28, 106; Ky Rev Stat Ann § 311.635; La Rev Stat Ann § 40:1299.58.8; Me Rev Stat Ann tit 18A § 5–809; Md Health-Gen Code Ann § 5–609; Mass Ann Laws ch 201D § 8; Minn Code Ann § 145C.11; Miss Code Ann §§ 41-41-117(1), 41-41-173; Mo Ann Stat §§ 404.855, 459.040; Mont Code Ann § 50-9-204; Neb Rev Stat §§ 20–410, 30–3423(2); Nev Stat Ann § 449.630; NH Rev Stat Ann §§ 137-H:9, 137J:11 II; NJ Stat Ann § 26:2H-73;"NM Stat Ann § 24-7A-9; NY Pub Health Law § 2986; NC Gen Stat § 32A-24(c), 90–321(h); ND Cent Code §§ 23-06.4-09, 23-06.5.12; Ohio Rev Code Ann §§ 1337.15, 2133.11; Okla Stat Ann tit 63 § 3101.10; Or Rev Stat §§ 127.560,. 620; Pa Cons Stat Ann § 5407(a); RI Gen Laws §§ 23-4.10-7, 23-4.11-8; SC Code Ann § 62-5-504(J); SD Codified Laws Ann §§ 34-12D-13, 59-7-8; Tenn Code Ann § 32-11-110(h), 34-6-208; Tex Health & Safety Code Ann § 672.015, Tex Civ Prac & Rem Code § 135.010; Utah Code Ann § 75-2-1114; Vt Stat Ann tit 14 § 3462, tit 18 § 5259; Va Code Ann § 54.1–2988; Wash Rev Code Ann § 70.122.051; W Va Code Ann 16-30-7(a), 16-30A-10(a); Wis Stat Ann §§ 154.07, 155.50; Wyo Stat Ann §§ 3-5-208, 35-22-106, 35- 22-108.
3. *See* Cruzan v. Director, Missouri Dep't of Health, 497 U.S. 261 (1990).
4. *See* Washington v. Glucksberg, 521 US 702 (1997); Vacco v. Quill, 521 US 793 (1997).
5. *See* The Oregon Death with Dignity Act, Or. Rev. Stat. 127.800 (2003); In 1997, an injunction against operation of the Act was vacated by Lee v. Oregon, 107 F.3d 1382, 1392 (9th Cir. 1997).
6. *See* Bartling v. Glendale Adventist Medical Center, 184 Cal. App. 3d 961, 229 Cal. Rptr. 360, 363 (2d Dist. 1986); Ficke v. Evangelical Health Systems, 285 Ill. App. 3d 886, 221 Ill. Dec. 95, 674 N.E.2d 888, 892 (1st Dist. 1996); Anderson v. St. Francis-St. George Hosp., Inc., 77 Ohio St. 3d 82, 671 N.E.2d 225, 227 (1996); Stolle v. Baylor College of Medicine, 981 S.W.2d 709, 712 (Tex. App. Houston 1st Dist. 1998), reh'g overruled, (Oct. 14, 1998) and review denied, (Feb. 25, 1999).
7. *See* Alabama: Ala. Code 1975 § 22-8A-11 and -6; Alaska: Alaska Stat. § 13.52.030; Arizona: Ariz. Rev. Stat. Ann. § 36–3231; Arkansas: Ark. Code Ann. § 20-17-214; California: Cal. Health & Safety Code § 24178; Delaware: Del. Code Ann. tit. 16, §§ 2507; Washington, D. C.: D.C. Code 1981 § 21–2210; Florida : Fla. Stat Ann. § 765.401; Georgia: Ga. Code Ann. § 31-9-2 (informed consent statute) and Ga. Code Ann. § 31-36A-1 to -7; Illinois: 755 ILCS 40/1 to 40/65, specifically 40/25; Iowa: Iowa Code Ann. § 144A.7; Kentucky: Ky. Rev. Stat. § 311.631; Louisiana: La. Rev. Stat. Ann. § 40:1299.58.1 to. 10; Maine: Me. Rev. Stat. Ann tit. 18-A, § 5–801 to § 5–817, specifically § 5–805; Maryland: Md. Health-Gen. Code Ann., § 5–605; Mississippi : Miss. Code Ann. §§ 41-41-201 to -229, particularly §§ 41-41-203(s), -211, and -215(9); Montana: Mont. Code Ann. § 50-9-106; Nevada: Nev. Rev. Stat. § 449.626; New Mexico: N.M. Stat. Ann. 1978 § 24-7A-5; New York: N.Y. Pub. Health Law § 2965; North Carolina: N.C. Gen. Stat. § 90–322 (assigning priority first to patient's spouse, then to "relatives of the first degree"); North Dakota: N.D. Cent. Code § 23-12-13; Ohio: Ohio Rev. Code Ann. § 2133.08; Oregon: Or. Rev. Stat. § 127.635 and § 127.505(12) and 127.535(4); South Carolina: S.C. Code 1976 Ann. § 44-66-10 to -80; South Dakota: S.D. Codified Laws § 34-12C-1 to -8; Tennessee: Tenn. Code Ann § 68-11-1801 to -1815, particularly § 68-11-1806; Texas: Tex. [Health & Safety] Code Ann. § 166.039 (providing for joint surrogacy between supervising physician and family member, according to priority); Utah: Utah Code Ann. § 75-2-1105, -1105.5, -1107; Virginia: Va. Code § 54.1–2986; Washington: Wash. Rev. Code Ann. § 7.70.065; West Virginia: W. VA. Code Ann. § 16-30-8; Wisconsin: Wisc. Stat. Ann. § 50.06 (applicable only for certain facility admissions): States that list "interested parties "who must decide among themselves which shall act as surrogate include the following: Colorado : Colo. Rev. Stat. Ann. § 15–18.5-101 to -1003; Idaho: Idaho Code § 39–4303; Indiana: Ind. Code Ann. § 16-36-1-1 to -14 (West 2005); Michigan: Mich. Comp. Laws Ann. § 333.5651 to 5661, particularly § 333.5653(g) and. 5655(b); Wyoming: Wyo. Stat. § 3-5-209 and § 35-22 105.
8. States that do have legislation directing the selection of surrogate decision-makers in the absence of an advance directive, but do not provide any standard for decision making include the following: Arkansas, Colorado (Colorado's "Separate Surrogate Consent Act" requires that the patient's surrogate be an individual with whom the patient has a close relationship and who is likely to be aware of the patient's wishes with regard to medical treatment; *see* Colo. Rev. Stat. Ann. § 15–19.5-103(4)(a)), Idaho, Indiana, Louisiana, Michigan, North Carolina, Oklahoma, Utah, and Wisconsin.
9. *See, e.g.,* the Uniform Health Care Decisions Act (adopted with modification by several states, and without substantial revision by California: Cal. Probate Code §§ 4600 to -4948; Delaware: Del. Code Ann. tit. 16, §§ 2501 to 2518; Hawaii: Hawaii Rev. Stat. §§ 327E-1 to - 16; Maine: Me. Rev. Stat. Ann. tit. 18A, § 5–801 to § 5–817; Mississippi: Miss. Code Ann. §§ 41-41-201 to -229; New Mexico: N.M. Stat. Ann. §§ 24-7A-1 to -18; and Tennessee: Tenn. Code Ann § 68-11-1801 to - 1815). Some states have combined the "substituted judgment" and "best interests" standards. *See e.g.* Virginia: Va. Code Ann. § 54.1–2981.
10. Lynn J. Unexpected returns: insights from SUPPORT. In: Isaacs S, Knickman J, eds. *To improve health and health care.* San Francisco: Jossey-Bass, 1997:165; The SUPPORT project was carried out in two stages, with a first stage of description (1989–1991) and the second stage of intervention (1992–1994).
11. Edwards MJ, Tolle SW. Disconnecting a ventilator at the request of a patient who knows he will then die: the doctor's anguish. *Ann Intern Med* 1992;117:254–256.
12. *See* Vacco v. Quill, 521 U.S. 793, 801-02 & n.11 (1997); *See also* Quill TE, Lo B, Brock DW. Palliative options of last resort: a comparison of voluntarily stopping eating and drinking, physician-assisted suicide, and voluntary active euthanasia. *JAMA* 1997;278:2099.
13. Quill TE, Dresser R, Brock DW. The rule of double effect - a critique of its role in end-of-life decision making. *N Engl J Med* 1997;337:1768.
14. See Menikoff J. Demanded medical care. *Ariz State Law J* 1998;30:1091, 1095.
15. For example, Texas law provides that physicians may refuse to provide "non-beneficial" treatment, notwithstanding the request of the patient or surrogate, so long as a hospital ethics committee agrees. The hospital is obliged to assist in finding a facility that will provide the treatment, but after ten days, the disputed treatment may be discontinued. *See* chapter 166 of the Texas Health and Safety Code. As enacted in 1999, this provision applied only to adult patients, but in 2003 was extended to treatment disputes involving children.
16. *See, e.g.,* Ala Code § 22-8A-8; Alaska Stat § 18.12.050; Ark Code Ann §§ 20-17-202(d), 20-17-207; Cal Health & Safety Code § 7190; Colo Rev Stat § 15-18-113(5); Conn Gen Stat Ann § 19a-580a; Del Code Ann tit 16 § 2508(e),(g); DC Code Ann § 6–2427(b); Fla Stat Ann § 765.308; Ga Code Ann § 31-32-8(b); Haw Rev Stat § 327D-11; Idaho Code § 39–4508; Ill Comp Stat tit 755 § 35/3(d), 6, 45/4-7, 4–8; Ind Code Ann § 16-36-4-13(e), (f) (if transfer not possible, physician's decision controls over patient's); Iowa Code Ann § 144A.8; Kan Stat Ann § 65-28, 107(a); Ky Rev Stat Ann § 311.633; La Rev Stat Ann § 40:1299.58.7; Me Rev Stat Ann tit 18A § 5–807(E), (F), (G); Md Health-Gen Code Ann § 5–613; Mass Ann Laws ch 201D §§ 14, 15; Minn Stat Ann § 145B.06.subd.1; Miss Code Ann § 41-41-115(2); Mo Ann Stat §§ 404.830, 404.872 (prohibition of retaliatory discharge against one who refuses to withdraw treatment

because of conscience), 459.030; Mont Code Ann § 50-9-203; Neb Rev Stat §§ 20–409, 30–3428; Nev Rev Stat Ann § 449.628; NH Rev Stat Ann §§ 137-H:6, 137-J:8 II; NJ Stat Ann §§ 26:2H-62 (individuals), 26:2H-65 (private, religious institutions); NM Stat Ann § 24-7A-7E; NY Pub Health Law §§ 2984.3 (private hospitals), .4 (individuals); ND Cent Code §§ 23-06.4-08, 23.06.5–09; Ohio Rev Code Ann §§ 2133.02(D), .10; Okla Stat Ann tit 63 § 3101.9; Or Rev Stat §§ 127.555, .625; Pa Cons Stat Ann § 5409 (if transfer not possible, health care provider's wishes prevail); RI Gen Laws §§ 23-4.10-6, 23-4.11-7; SC Code Ann § 44-77-100, 62-5-504(R); SD Codified Laws Ann §§ 34-12D-11, 34-12D-12; Tenn Code Ann §§ 32-11-108, 34-6-214; Utah Code Ann § 75-2-1112; Vt Stat Ann tit 14 § 3459, tit 18 § 5256; Va Code Ann § 54.1–2987; Wash Rev Code Ann § 70.122.060 (no transfer requirement, but health care providers must try to reach agreement with patient); W Va Code Ann §§ 16-30-7(b), 16-30A-10(b); Wis Stat Ann § 155.50(b); Wyo Stat Ann § 35-22-104.

17. *See* Burt Robert. The medical futility debate: patient choice, physician obligation, and end-of-life care. *J Palliat Med* 2002;5:249–254; Burt Robert, Randall Curtis J. Why are critical care clinicians so powerfully distressed by family demands for futile care? *J Crit Care* 2003;18:22–24.

18. For an extended, illuminating discussion of this proposition, *see* Calabresi Guido, Bobbitt Philip. *Tragic choices.* New York: W. W. Norton, 1978.

19. U.S Department of Justice, Drug Enforcement Agency, Office of Diversion Control, Registrant Population Summary as of August 2, 2005, available at http://www.deadiversion.usdoj.gov/drugreg/pop/summary.htm

20. Approximately half of these revocations were issued because the practitioner was no longer licensed to practice medicine. The remaining causes for revocation are represented by the revocations issued as of October, 2005, and include the following: no doctor-patient relationship existed (3 revocations issued), fraud (3 revocations issued), personal recreational use (1 revocation issued), improper "gray market" distribution (e.g., through gas stations) (2 revocations issued), and improper distribution through the internet (3 revocations issued). *See* U.S. Department of Justice, Drug Enforcement Agency, Office of Diversion Control, Federal Register Notices, Registrant Actions, available at http://www.deadiversion.usdoj.gov/fed_regs/index.html.

21. 21 U.S.C. § 801(1) (2000).

22. Tex. Rev. Civ. Stat. Ann. art. 4495c, § 2(3)

23. *See* Fohr SA. The double effect of pain medication: separating myth from reality. *J Palliat Med* 1998;1:315, 320. ("The literature contains little data to support the belief that appropriate use of opioids hastens death in patients dying from cancer and other chronic diseases"); Another prevalent, but erroneous belief is that patients prescribed opioids are subjected to a high risk of addiction, *See* Joranson DE, Ryan KM, Gilson AM, et al., Trends in medical use and abuse of opioid analgesics. *JAMA* 2000;283:1710, 1712 (noting that the incidence of drug addiction for patients taking opioids is less than one percent); *see also* Tanabe Paula, Buschmann Mary Beth. Emergency nurses' knowledge of pain management principles. *J Emerg Nurs* 2000;26:299,299.

24. *See* Or. Bd. of Med. Examiners, Guide to Licensing Action Report (Apr. 22, 2005), available at www.bme.state.or.us/licensactionrpt.html; *See also* Barnett EH. Case marks big shift in pain policy. *Oregonian* September 2, 1999.

25. Medical boards urged to penalize docs who give little pain relief to dying. *Med Health* January 19, 1998. WL 10321284.

26. No. H205732-1 (Cal. Super. Ct. June 13, 2001); *See also* Okie Susan. California jury finds doctor negligent in managing pain. *Washington Post* June 15, 2001:A02.

27. *See e.g.*, Estate of Henry James v. Hillhaven Corp., Super. Ct. Div. 89CVS64, Hertford County, NC (1990) (in which the estate was awarded $15 million for failure to adequately treat patient's cancer pain); Gaddis v. U.S., 7 F. Supp. 2d 709 (D.S.C. 1997) (in which patient's daughter was awarded $125,000, nurses failed to administer prescribed pain medication; and additional $953,526 was awarded in compensatory damages).

28. Bergman v. Chin, No. A091386 at 3 (Cal. Super. Ct. June 13, 2001) (citing Delaney v. Baker, 20 Cal.4th 23, 31–32 (1999)).

29. No. C 02–00120 (Cal. Super. Ct. Contra Costa County, 2003).

30. Pls. ' Mediation Br., Tomlinson v. Bayberry Care Ctr., No. C 02–00120 (Cal. Super. Ct. Contra Costa County, 2003), *available at* http://www.compassionindying.org/tomlinson/tomlinson_brief.pdf.

31. Albert Tanya. California requires doctors take CME in pain management. *Am Med News* 2001.

32. *See generally* Burt RA. *Death is that man taking names: intersections of American medicine, law, and culture.* Berkeley: University of California Press, 2002.

SPECIAL INTERVENTIONS IN SUPPORTIVE AND PALLIATIVE CARE

CHAPTER 66 ■ HEMATOLOGIC SUPPORT OF THE CANCER PATIENT

DAVEY B. DANIEL AND JEFFREY CRAWFORD

No one thinks of how much blood it costs.—Dante Alighieri

Anemia, neutropenia, and thrombocytopenia are common complications of cancer and its treatment. Physicians caring for oncology patients must recognize the high frequency of myelosuppression, the significant impact on quality of life (QoL), and the risks inherent in severe myelosuppression. Originally armed only with transfusion products, antibiotics, and time, oncologists now have powerful, yet expensive tools to deal with cytopenia. The annual cost of recombinant erythropoietin agents is >1% of overall drug costs in the United States and European Union (1) and approximately 10% of overall direct costs for cancer care (2). Granulocyte growth factors add to the costs and are increasingly used in both hematologic and solid malignancies. On the other hand, the impact of hospitalization for fever and neutropenia are substantial in economic terms and may result in adverse patient outcomes. Therefore, it is critically important that a rationale approach be taken to growth factor use and transfusion support. This requires both an understanding of the literature and clinical judgment. This chapter will review much of this data as well as the current clinical treatment guidelines for anemia, neutropenia, and thrombocytopenia caused by cancer and its treatment.

Chemotherapy can cause both transient and sustained cytopenia. The storage compartment of the marrow contains enough maturing cells to maintain peripheral counts for approximately 8–10 days after stem cell production ceases. Therefore, the effect of cell cycle–specific chemotherapy will be notable by the tenth day after treatment, nadir counts are manifest between days 14 and 18, and recovery generally occurs between days 21 and 28. In contrast, G_0 active agents are characterized by delayed nadir counts (4 weeks) and prolonged recovery time (6 weeks) owing to the preferential effect on resting stem cells. Scheduling of chemotherapy is also important as repeated dosing of chemotherapy, especially during early marrow recovery, may result in sustained toxicity and persistent pancytopenia. Likewise, radiation therapy further contributes to myelosuppression, particularly when the marrow is already suppressed from chemotherapy or malignant involvement. Recent trends in medical oncology have focused on providing therapy in more dose intense (autologous stem cell transplantation) and dense fashions (adjuvant breast cancer given every 2 weeks). These regimens along with more myelotoxic agents such as the taxanes have increased the incidence of myelosuppression in commonly treated tumors.

ANEMIA

Anemia is a frequent finding and a major cause of morbidity in oncology patients. Rates of anemia depend on the tumor type, the myelotoxic treatment given, and the patient's comorbidities. Anemia is almost universal in patients with hematologic malignancies even prior to treatment. A retrospective study of over 500 patients with lymphoma, lung, breast, colon, or ovarian cancer showed high rates of anemia, from 44 to 95%, depending on tumor type (Table 66.1), but severe anemia was infrequent (<10%). In this study, age, gender, and disease stage were all important predictors of anemia. Although estimates of anemia rates are imprecise, it is obvious that anemia occurs more frequently as medical oncologists adopt more aggressive regimens. Rates vary by regimen but combinations regimens such as CHOP (cyclophosphamide, doxorubicin, vincristine, and prednisone) have rates of grade III anemia (Hb <8.0 g per dL) as high as 70% (3). It is difficult to estimate the actual rates of chemotherapy-induced anemia (CIA) based on newer regimens as many studies only report profound, grade III anemia, and study populations are often healthier and less prone to anemia than the typical patient in the community setting. (See Table 66.2 for explanations of the common toxicity criteria for cytopenias.) Despite the difficulty in pinpointing precise rates, anemia is recognized as a common and treatable side effect of cancer and continues to require treatment. A large retrospective audit of cancer centers in the United Kingdom in the late 1990s found that more than a third of patients required at least one transfusion during the course of their treatment for cancer with high rates in those with lung or ovarian cancer (40%) (4).

The etiology of anemia in patients with cancer is multifactorial, often arising from both the cancer itself and its treatment. Tumor cells can invade the bone marrow or can suppress marrow and erythropoietin production by cytokine production. Blood loss, shortened red cell survival, nutritional deficits, and underlying infection (again causing cytokine-related suppression of the marrow) can be sources of anemia. Less common causes include acute hemorrhage from the malignancy itself, hemolytic states such as disseminated intravascular coagulation associated with promyelocytic leukemia and sepsis, and immune hemolytic anemia from chronic lymphocytic leukemia and lymphomas. Anemia of chronic disease occurs frequently in patients with cancer and is characterized by normocytic and normochromic morphology on peripheral and bone marrow examination, low serum iron and iron binding capacity,

TABLE 66.1

RATES OF ANEMIA IN A RETROSPECTIVE STUDY OF PATIENTS UNDERGOING
CHEMOTHERAPY. PRE- AND POST-TREATMENT INCIDENCE OF ANEMIA

Cancer type	Chemotherapy treatments	Pretreatment anemia incidence (%)	Anemia incidence during treatment (%)
Breast ($n = 165$)	FAC, CMF	44	60
Lung ($n = 128$)	EP	70	95.0
Colon ($n = 75$)	CPT-11, FUFA	71	71
Ovarian ($n = 84$)	PT, PC	68	91.5
Lymphoma ($n = 100$)	CEOP, ABVD	82	82

FAC, 5-fluorouracil, adriamycin, and cyclophosphamide; CMF, cyclophosphamide, methotrexate and
5 fluorouracil; EP, etoposide and cisplatin (platinum); CPT-11, Irinotecan; FUFA, fluorouracil and folinic
acid; CEOP, cyclophosphamide, epirubicin, vincristine; ABVD, doxorubicin, bleomycin, vinblastine, and
dacarbazine; PT, cisplatin and paclitaxel; PC, carboplatin and paclitaxel.
Tas F, Eralp Y, Basaran M, et al. Anemia in oncology practice: relation to diseases and their therapies. *Am J
Clin Oncol* 2002;25:371–379 (5).

normal or increased marrow iron stores, and blunted erythropoietin levels and response. CIA is common in patients with cancer and the focus of much research and treatment. The continued bombardment of the marrow by myelotoxic regimens can cause significant and prolonged anemia with repeated cycles causing a cumulative injury to production.

Symptoms and Signs

Fatigue is an all too frequent symptom of cancer, and anemia is often the only treatable cause of cancer-related fatigue. In a survey of 1171 patients, fatigue was identified as the leading complaint of patients with cancer—greater than pain, nausea, or emesis (6). Although the physicians' major focus is often on treating pain, patients often note that fatigue is a greater concern. In addition to fatigue, anemia may be associated with other symptoms: shortness of breath, tachycardia, chest pain, dizziness, headache, claudication pain, angina, and even depression. The pattern of symptoms and the individual's ability to tolerate them is significantly dependent on the rapidity of onset of the anemia, the patient's baseline functional status, and comorbid conditions. Although patients with anemia may show pallor, orthostasis, and hypoxia, these are usually present in patients with large acute hemorrhages who have not had sufficient time for volume expansion. It is the gradual onset of anemia that is much more characteristic of oncology patients and is more often associated with the insidious symptoms of fatigue, decreased exercise tolerance, and sometimes confusion, particularly in the elderly. Indeed, elderly patients have a lower

reserve capacity and may display any of these symptoms even at higher hemoglobin levels. With laboratory testing, the diagnosis of anemia is rarely difficult. The history and examination clarifies how well a patient is tolerating the anemia. Physical examination findings are highly variable. Pallor can be difficult to recognize and is very dependent on pigmentation but mucosal membranes, nail beds, and palmar creases are often areas where pallor is more consistently noted. The decreased blood volume due to anemia may cause widened pulse pressure, a hyperdynamic precordium, and systolic flow murmurs loudest at the apex with radiation along the sternum to the neck. Finally, patients with severe anemia can show signs of high output cardiac failure with peripheral edema and an S_3 gallop.

Thresholds for Treatment

Oxygen delivery is maximized at hematocrits between 30 and 40%, but observational studies have shown no difference in mortality in patients with hematocrits as low as 10%—provided sufficient intravascular volume is maintained. In the intensive care medicine literature, there remains a debate over what transfusion threshold should be used. A multicenter randomized trial of 838 intensive care unit patients showed that a restrictive transfusion strategy, using 7 g per dL of hemoglobin versus 10 g per dL in the control, yielded similar 30-day mortality rates and had statistically significant lower in-hospital mortality and transfusion rates (7). Although the higher threshold did not increase mortality in this acute

TABLE 66.2

NATIONAL CANCER INSTITUTE COMMON TERMINOLOGY CRITERIA FOR
ADVERSE EVENTS

	Neutrophils/granulocytes	Hemoglobin	Platelets
Grade 1	<LLN–1500 mm^3	<LLN–10.0 g/dL	<LLN–75,000/ mm^3
Grade 2	<1500–1000 mm^3	<10.0–7.9 g/dL	<75,000–50,000/ mm^3
Grade 3	<1000–500 mm^3	<8.0–6.5 g/dL	<50,000–25,000/ mm^3
Grade 4	<500 mm^3	<6.5 g/dL	<25,000/ mm^3

LLN, lower limit of normal.

setting, we do not know long-term effects including mortality and QoL.

This intensive care population is also very different from the patients usually seen in oncology. The patient with cancer often has a chronic anemia, and the focus is generally not on short-term mortality but rather on QoL and symptom management. It had been thought that chronically anemic patients fare better than others through compensatory mechanisms of maintenance of plasma volume, increased cardiac output, and shifts in the oxygen–hemoglobin dissociation curve from 2,3-diphosphoglycerate production. However, there is now mounting evidence that oncology patients with chronic anemia may benefit significantly from hemoglobin levels near normal, which are far greater than that we have sought to maintain in oncology patients in the past or currently in other patient populations. The decision to transfuse a patient with blood products must take into consideration the degree of physiologic stress from the anemia, comorbid illness, the potential of recovery without transfusion, and finally, transfusion risks. Transfusion thresholds vary but are often carried out only when hemoglobin levels dropped substantially, sometimes below 8 g per dL. New data arising from the use of erythropoietin agents suggest that QoL may be better maintained at much higher hemoglobin levels (near 12 g per dL), suggesting that many patients may be undertreated. With the availability of recombinant erythropoietin, there is now an alternative to transfusion, allowing for these higher treatment goals.

Role of Erythropoietin

Erythropoietin plays a key role in red blood cell (RBC) production and in the anemia due to cancer. An obligatory growth factor and regulatory molecule, erythropoietin affects RBC production by stimulating the burst forming units–erythroid (BFU-E) and the colony forming units–erythroid (CFU-E). The BFU-E cells are early cells within erythropoiesis, which proliferate rapidly and have a low number of erythropoietin receptors. Therefore, a higher level of erythropoietin is necessary to stimulate entry into the cell cycle for BFU-E cells. The later CFU-E cells have a high number of erythropoietin receptors and require a constitutive level of erythropoietin for continued survival, growth, and production. Erythropoietin therefore shows a keen regulatory mechanism for red cell production. In the adult, approximately 90% of erythropoietin is produced within the peritubular fibroblastoid cells of the inner cortex of the kidney, and the remainder is produced in the liver. Within the peritubular interstitial cells, erythropoietin production is constitutive and inducible with baseline levels produced from each cell and additional cells recruited to increase production for hypoxic states. As arterial Po_2 levels decrease and tissue hypoxia increases, erythropoietin levels increase, acting as a key regulatory mechanism. Erythropoietin has been shown to be responsive to hypoxic states, and as seen in the setting of anemia, it increases committed red cell progenitors and the rate of maturation of the reticulocytes. The erythropoietin level is fairly constant for an individual with stable hemoglobin level, does not vary significantly with gender or age, and has no biologically inactive precursor or stores.

Cancer can affect erythropoietin by decreasing the marrow responsiveness to erythropoietin or by decreasing erythropoietin production, as tumor necrosis factor and some nephrotoxic agents can. In both a rat model and in a group of patients with lung cancer, cisplatin was shown to cause depressed erythropoietin levels from the expected compared to controls with similar levels of anemia (8). These patients did not mount the usual increased erythropoietin response levels to anemia after receiving cisplatin but were capable of producing increased levels once cisplatin treatment had been completed

and renal function improved. Although this study suggests that some patients have insufficient erythropoietin production, others show that marrow of patients with cancer may be unable to respond to the physiologically increased levels in response to cancer (9).

Epoetin α and β

There has been rapid progress during the last two decades as biotechnology has changed our treatment of anemia. It was only in 1985 that recombinant human erythropoietin (rHuEPO) was purified and cloned. In 1987, it was approved for treatment of anemia related to renal disease and then, in 1990, it was approved for human immunodeficiency virus (HIV)–related anemia. A number of small phase I and II trials in the early 1990s proved efficacy in the treatment of anemia related to cancer or chemotherapy. In a phase I and II trial of 21 patients receiving cisplatin with hemoglobin levels <11 g per dL, patients were randomized to 100 units per kg or 200 units per kg five times per week and the overall response rate was >50%, with a mean rise in hemoglobin of 2.5 g per dL (10). A number of nonrandomized phase II trials confirmed these findings. Suddenly, mild to moderate anemia (hemoglobin of 8–11 g per dL) was now treatable. Recombinant erythropoietin in the form of epoetin α was approved for treatment of CIA in 1993. However, it had not yet been shown to be effective in large trials with a variety of tumor types. Three large community-based, observational studies of epoetin α were completed during the late 1990s. Each prospectively examined the open-label use of erythropoietin in anemic patients with cancer undergoing chemotherapy and evaluated changes in hemoglobin, transfusion requirements, and QoL measurements. All three studies reached similar conclusions regarding the effectiveness of erythropoietin in increasing both hemoglobin levels and QoL scores (Fig. 66.1).

Demetri et al. (11) examined 2370 patients with nonmyeloid malignancies, the majority (78%) of whom had solid tumors (24% lung, 17% breast, and 13% gynecologic). Roughly one-fourth of these patients received a platinum-based therapy—a drug that causes significant anemia. Each had a hemoglobin

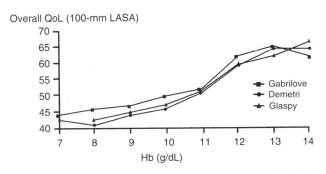

FIGURE 66.1. Community-based trials. Overall quality of life (QoL) associated with hemoglobin (Hb) levels (cross-sectional). LASA, Linear Analog Scale Assessment, also known as *Cancer Linear Analog Scale* (CLAS). (From references: Littlewood TJ, Bajetta E, Nortier JWR, et al. Effects of epoetin alfa on hematologic parameters and quality of life in cancer patients receiving nonplatinum chemotherapy: results of a randomized, double-blind, placebo-controlled trial. *J Clin Oncol* 2001;19(11):2865–2874; Macdougall IC, Gray SJ, Elston O, et al. Pharmacokinetics of novel erythropoiesis stimulating protein compared with epoetin alfa in dialysis patients. *J Am Soc Nephrol* 1999,10.2392–2395; Quirt I, Robeson C, Lau CY, et al. Epoetin alfa therapy increases hemoglobin levels and improves quality of life in patients with cancer-related anemia who are not receiving chemotherapy and patients with anemia who are not receiving chemotherapy. *J Clin Oncol* 2001;19:4126–4134; with permission.)

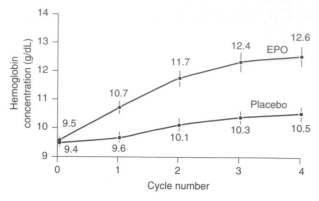

FIGURE 66.2. Change in mean hemoglobin values in patients with advanced cancer with chemotherapy induced anemia who were randomly assigned epoetin α (40,000 units per week) or placebo. EPO, erythropoietin. (Witzig TE, Silberstein PT, et al. Phase III, randomized, double-blind study of epoetin alfa compared with placebo in anemic patients receiving chemotherapy. *J Clin Oncol* 2005;23(12):2606–2617.)

level <11 g per dL, with an overall mean hemoglobin of 9.3 g per dL, and were given 10,000 units of epoetin α three times weekly with increased doses to 20,000 units if unresponsive at week four. Sixty-three percent of patients responded by an increase of at least 1 g per dL after 4 weeks of treatment. After 16 weeks, the mean hemoglobin had risen by 2 g per dL, and 61% of patients had achieved either a 2-g per dL response or a hemoglobin >12 g per dL. The transfusion rate had decreased from 29% the month before treatment to 5% at week 16. These results were consistent with a similar study by Glaspy et al. (12) of 2352 patients and a third study by Gabrilove et al. with 3012 patients (13). The main difference in these trials was the dosing schedule— weight-based dosing three times weekly (Glaspy), flat dosing at 10,000 units three times per week (Demetri), and weekly dosing with 40,000 units per week (Gabrilove). Each had hemoglobin response rates from 53.4–68%, mean hemoglobin rise of 1.8 g per dL to 2.0 g per dL, and significant decreases in transfusion requirements. The use of three times weekly dosing schedule is somewhat inconvenient, but a recent randomized, blinded, placebo-controlled study confirmed that weekly epoetin α as studied in Gabrilove et al. is a reasonable treatment choice for patients with CIA (14) and resulted in a significant difference in mean hemoglobin and RBC transfusions compared to placebo (Fig. 66.2). A recent observational study of community use of epoetin α showed that >72% of those examined used epoetin α dosed weekly at 40,000 units with more frequent dosing now uncommon in the community setting (15).

A number of randomized trials using various dosing regimens have now been performed. A 2005 meta-analysis of 27 randomized trials (3287 patients) examining treatment with epoetin α or epoetin β from 1985 to present showed that patients treated with erythropoietin had lower transfusion rates and increased hematologic responses. Those treated with erythropoietin had transfusion rates 33% lower than untreated patients [RR = 0.67 (0.62, 0.73)] (1). In a sub analysis of 14 trials in this meta-analysis, 48% of patients receiving erythropoietin had a hemoglobin response [RR = 3.60 (3.07, 4.23)].

Quality of Life

Although clinical parameters such as hemoglobin level and transfusion requirements are important, much of the drive to treat CIA lies in the effects on QoL. Each of the community-based trials examined patient self reported QoL

parameters; all three used a linear analog scale assessment (LASA), a 100-mm visual analog scale with questions on energy, activity, and overall QoL. The Demetri and Gabrilove studies also used a 20-item questionnaire that examines well being associated with fatigue and anemia (FACT-An). Each trial confirmed a correlation between increase in hemoglobin levels and improvement in QoL (Fig. 66.1). In the Demetri trial, the difference between those treated and those untreated was statistically different ($p < .001$) with those with the greatest increase in hemoglobin showing the most improvement. Those with a <2 g per dL response also had improvement in QoL measurements if the disease was stable or responsive to chemotherapy. As might be expected, patients did not have an improvement in QoL if hemoglobin level did not increase or the QoL effect was blunted if they had disease progression. Each of these large trials was open labeled; so, self reported QoL changes could be suspect due to patient bias. However, a blinded, randomized trial of thrice weekly epoetin α in patients receiving nonplatinum based chemotherapy showed QoL benefits in three primary QoL scales (FACT-General, FACT-An, and CLAS subscales) with trends in two other scales (SF-36 Physical Component Summary and Mental Component Summary). This confirmed in a blinded study the QoL benefits of treating CIA with epoetin α (16). In addition, there are additional studies that support the use of erythropoietin agents in patients who have anemia secondary to cancer, but not resulting from chemotherapy. These included epoetin α, epoetin β, and darbepoetin treatments.

Darbepoetin

Darbepoetin α is an analog of erythropoietin with two additional oligosaccharide chains; it is a larger molecule (38,500 vs. 30,400 d) with a slightly different amino acid structure (five amino acid substitutions). With the increased glycosylation, its half-life is far greater. Intravenously administered darbepoetin's half-life measures 25.4 hours, and the subcutaneous half-life is even longer at >48 hours (17). Although its affinity for the erythropoietin receptor is somewhat less than rHuEPO's affinity, this does not seem to impact its effectiveness. In 1999, darbepoetin was approved for patient with renal failure. In July 2002, the U.S. Food and Drug Administration (FDA) approved darbepoetin for treatment of CIA. Five randomized clinical trials have shown that treatment with darbepoetin reduces transfusions requirements and increases hemoglobin levels in patients with CIA, anemia caused by lymphoproliferative disease, and patients with anemia caused by solid tumors (18–22). Hemoglobin response rates of 40–70% were seen. Darbepoetin therapy has also been shown to improve QoL with FACT-F scores showing significant improvement at 4 weeks and continuing through treatment (20). Two large head to head trials comparing darbepoetin to epoetin α have now been completed and show few differences in clinical response between the two agents (23,24). Both were industry-sponsored trials that have differences in structure and analysis that make decisions regarding differences in efficacy difficult. Waltzman et al. (23) examined 352 patients randomized to epoetin α or darbepoetin; this study reported higher mean hemoglobin levels (1.2 vs. 0.8), higher rates of hemoglobin response (>2 g per dL) (57 vs. 41%), and shorter median time to 1 g increase in hemoglobin for epoetin α treated patients compared to darbepoetin (35 vs. 48 days). The trial by Glaspy et al. had a noninferiority design with similar dose adjustment rules between the two drugs (24). This showed no statistically significant differences between the two drugs in regard to transfusion requirements and percentage of patients achieving the hemoglobin target. At this point, much of the decision of which erythropoietic agent is driven by patient

TABLE 66.3

COMMON DOSING OPTIONS FOR EPOETIN ALPHA AND DARBEPOETIN ALPHA

Epoetin α (Procrit, Ortho Biotech)	Initial approval 150 U/kg^2 t.i.w.
	Common usage 40,000 U^2 q wk
	Investigational front loading:
	   60,000 U^2 qwk $\times$ 4; then
	   120,000 U q3wk
		Increase to 300 U/kg t.i.w. in 4 wk if <1 g/dL increase
		Increase to 60,000 U^2 qwk in 4 wk if <1 g/dL increase

Darbepoetin α (Aranesp, Amgen)	Initial approval 2.25 μg/kg q1wk
	Common usage
	  200 μg q2wk
	  300 μg q3wk
	Investigational front loading:
	  325 μg or 4.5 μg/kg qwk until
	  HB >12 g/dL, then q3wk
		Increase to 4.5 μg/kg^2 q1wk in 6 wk if <1 g/dL increase
		Increase to 300 μg^2 q2wk in 6 wk if <1 g/dL increase

convenience and economics which are specific to the patient and clinical setting.

Recent and ongoing trials continue to examine alternative dosing regimens including the use of so-called front loading regimens. The front loading studies have looked at higher initial doses of epoetin α and darbepoetin followed by either lower or less frequent dosing as maintenance. Pilot studies of epoetin α have shown increased response rates of 86% (Hb increases of 2 g per dL by week 8) (25); this is far superior to those results seen in the standard 40,000 units per week community-based trials. Darbepoetin dosed weekly initially, then on an every 3-week maintenance schedule has also been studied and also shown to have similarly high rates of response, 84–86% (26). However, it is important to note that these dosing strategies have not been studied in a large community setting and that response rates are generally higher in pilot trials than in larger phase III trials or in actual practice.

Erythropoietin and Myelodysplasia

The most common morbidity of myelodysplastic syndrome is anemia, and it is often difficult to manage. Repeated transfusions are often necessary and eventually lead to iron overload. For those with symptomatic cytopenias, the use of growth factors [epoetin α, darbepoetin, and sometimes, granulocyte colony-stimulating factor (G-CSF)] has improved management of anemia in myelodysplastic syndromes (MDS). However, response rates remain low. Other causes of anemia such as concurrent iron or B$_{12}$ deficiencies or hemolytic anemia should be been ruled out or treated prior to considering the use of recombinant factors. In general, patients with myelodysplastic syndrome lack normal marrow response to erythropoietin and are less responsive to elevations in native erythropoietin often seen in these patients. However, the use of erythropoietin (40,000 units per week or 150 units per kg three times weekly) (27) or darbepoetin (150 μg per wk) (28) has been shown to have responses in up to 45% of patients. Those with lower levels of native serum erythropoietin (<100 mU per mL) often have higher response rates. National Comprehensive Cancer Network (NCCN) guidelines, however, call for consideration of Erythropoietic agents in patients with serum erythropoietin levels <500 mU per mL. Responses may be delayed, so 2–3 months of treatment are often recommended. For patients unresponsive to erythropoietin, the addition of G-CSF can be considered, particularly in those with sideroblastic anemia and relatively low levels of baseline erythropoietin. In patients who fail to respond after 2 to 3 months, it may be time to consider more aggressive therapy such as the DNA methylation inhibitors.

Treatment Guidelines

The 2005 NCCN guidelines (29) call first for a determination of whether immediate correction is required. If so, then transfusion is recommended. For those with mild anemia (Hb 10–11 g per dL) and who are symptomatic, the panel recommended consideration of erythropoietin therapy. Consideration of treatment was strongly recommended for those with hemoglobin <10 g per dL. All patients should be evaluated for other causes of anemia, including reviewing the peripheral blood film, and when appropriate, iron studies, B$_{12}$, folate, and other anemia evaluations. Measuring erythropoietin levels is generally not of value in treating CIA because levels do not correlate with response as they do when treating patients with anemia due to myelodysplasia. It is also important to remember that many patients require dose titration, usually performed after 4 weeks of treatment with epoetin α and 6 weeks after treatment of darbepoetin with subsequent assessment of response between 8 and 12 weeks. The 2005 NCCN guidelines recommend discontinuing erythropoietin therapy if there is no response after 8–12 weeks. Table 66.3 has various dosing strategies and titration recommendations.

Although all of the studies discussed thus far have focused on the treatment of CIA, several trials shifted toward early treatment and prevention of anemia. Several small trials

TABLE 66.4

MULTINATIONAL ASSOCIATION OF SUPPORTIVE CARE IN CANCER SCORING SYSTEM

Risk factor	Points
Burden of illness: no or mild symptoms	5
No hypotension	5
No chronic obstructive pulmonary disease	4
Solid tumor and no previous fungal infection	4
No dehydration	3
Burden of illness: moderate symptoms	3
Outpatient status	3
Age <60 years	2

Maximum score: 26 Threshold for low risk patients $\geq$ 21
Tanneberger S, Melilli G, Strocchi E, et al. Use of red blood cell transfusion in palliative care services: is it still up to date or is cancer-related anaemia controlled better with erythropoietic agents? *Ann Oncol* 2004;15:839–840 (30).

have shown that treating prior to development of anemia results in less anemia. However, larger trials examining this strategy have met some difficulty. Two of these trials [the Beta-Blocker Evaluation in Survival Trial (BEST) in breast cancer and the Henke trial in head and neck cancer] have been closed at interim analysis because of adverse events (31,32), whereas three others were closed because of concerns arising out of the first two trials. These two prevention trials will be discussed with the adverse events discussion to follow. Although it is likely that anemia can be prevented by early use of erythropoietic agents, this use has not yet been shown to be clinically beneficial or safe. Both the NCCN 2005 Guidelines and the 2004 European Organisation for Research and Treatment of Cancer (EORTC) Guidelines for use of Erythropoietic Proteins (33) do not recommend the treatment of patients prophylactically before the development of anemia unless done in the context of a well designed clinical trial.

Thirty to 50% of patients do not respond initially to erythropoietin treatment for CIA using traditional dosing regimens. Recent data suggest intravenous iron may be useful in unresponsive oncology patients with CIA and in increasing the proportion of patients with an initial response. Previous studies in dialysis population report improvement in response to erythropoietin agents when iron supplementation is added because of the large amounts of iron required to meet the demands of erythropoiesis, suggesting that many may suffer from a functional iron deficiency despite adequate stores. A multicenter open-label study randomized 157 patients to no-iron, oral iron, bolus iron dextran, or iron dextran total dose infusion (34). All patients had hemoglobin of <10.5 g per dL, serum ferritin of <450 pmol per L or <= 675 with transferrin saturation of <19% and had other causes of anemia excluded. Those receiving intravenous iron dextran had higher mean increases in hemoglobin and higher hematologic responses (Hb rise of 2 g per dL or hemoglobin of 12 g per dL or greater) than those with no-iron or oral iron. 68% responded to iron dextran, 25% to no-iron, and 36% to oral iron. There were also significant differences in QoL as measured by LASA scores. Only one acute hypersensitivity reaction occurred with a test dose of iron dextran. The reported incidence of severe reactions to iron dextran is approximately 0.7% but may be important clinically if intravenous iron dextran supplementation becomes more common.

Anemia and Treatment Response

A number of studies have shown that tumor hypoxia reduces the tumor responsiveness to radiation therapy. It is thought that oxygen is required to prevent cellular repair of DNA damage from hydroxyl ions produced from radiation. These oxygen molecules fix the damaged areas, preventing repair of sublethal damage from radiation. Not surprisingly, the radiation dose required to kill cells in a hypoxic environment is significantly higher than those with an adequate oxygen supply. Brizel et al. have shown that patients with head and neck tumors treated with radiation therapy have lower 2-year survival (70 vs. 31%) and 2-year local tumor control (82 vs. 41%) if the Po_2 within the tumor site is <10 mm Hg (35). Likewise, differences in survival based on hemoglobin level have been shown in non–small cell lung cancer (Hb >13), and in bladder, prostate, head and neck, and anal cancer. Although no current trials have been published showing that using epoetin α to increase hemoglobin levels will increase tumor responsiveness to radiation therapy, the studies mentioned in the preceding text suggest that it is fertile ground for further investigation. The Littlewood trial of erythropoietin in the treatment of chemotherapy-related anemia included survival as a secondary end point (16). Although it confirmed other studies

showing correlation between improvement in hemoglobin levels and QoL scales, it also showed a trend toward improved survival. Although not reaching statistical significance, mean survival in the epoetin α group was 17 months, compared to 11 months in those patients treated with placebo ($p = .13$). However, both the Henke and BEST trials had adverse survival outcomes in patients who were treated with erythropoietin agents to prevent anemia. Therefore, there is currently no conclusion of whether epoetin α and β have beneficial or adverse effects on survival. The BEST trial examined the use of epoetin α (Eprex) to prevent the development of anemia in patients receiving front-line therapy for metastatic breast cancer. Based on predetermined stopping rules, the trial was halted after a 12-month survival analysis showed a significant decrease in survival at 1 year (76 vs. 70%) among those patients receiving erythropoietin ($p = .0117$). Although the survival curves converged at 19 months, it was apparent that during the first 4 months of therapy, patients receiving erythropoietin had higher rates of disease progression (6 vs. 3%) and higher rates of thrombotic events (1 vs. 0.2%). A similar trial in patients with head and neck cancer evaluated 351 patients at multiple centers looking at patients with very mild anemia (Hb <12 g per dL or 13 g per dL), assigning patients to treatment with epoetin β three times weekly or. placebo. Although 82% of patients randomized to epoetin β had correction of their anemia to levels >14 mg per dL (women) or 15 mg per dL (men), this increase did not correlate with an improvement in survival. On the contrary, patients in the treatment arm actually had lower progression-free survival rates. There are several possible biologic explanations for why erythropoietin could lead to tumor growth or resistance to therapy. One of which is the presence of erythropoietin receptors identified in a number of cancer cell lines and tumors including breast and lung cancer, although no clinical data has been demonstrated that these receptors are functional. Furthermore, an Oncology Drug Advisory Committee reviewed all trials of epoetin α, epoetin β, and darbepoetin α. They found no evidence to change current recommendations. The results of several additional prospective trials of anemia prevention are ongoing and eagerly awaited.

Adverse Effects of Erythropoietin Therapy

Just as transfusions can have rare but significant side effects, erythropoietin therapy is not without risks. Hypertension develops in 20–30% of renal patients receiving erythropoietin (4–9%). This has been a rare event in the cancer population. Likewise, although a number of cases of pure red cell aplasia have been reported in renal patients, no clinical trials in oncology patients have reported any cases of pure red cell aplasia or antierythropoietic antibodies. However, risk of venous thrombosis and other thrombovascular events are likely increased in treated patients. Pooled results from 12 trials showed 43 thrombotic events in 1019 patients compared to 14 in 719 placebo patients [RR 1.58 (0.94–2.66)] (1). These translate to a 4% rate of thromboembolic events in treated patients compared to 2% in untreated patients. However, given the overlapping confidence interval, the meta-analysis did not show a definitive increase in thrombotic risk. Some trials have suggested that higher levels of hemoglobin, 14–16 g per dL, are associated with higher rates of thrombovascular events (31,32). In a clinical trial in which a number of patients had hemoglobin levels in the normal range, rates of vascular events were 11% compared with 5% in untreated patients (32). Therefore, current clinical guidelines call for holding dose if hemoglobin exceeds 12 g per dL or reducing dose if hemoglobin climbs by >1 g per dL in a 2-week period.

Hematologic Support in the Hospice Setting

A focus on symptom management is the hallmark of palliative care, and erythropoietic agents are important treatments for anemia related fatigue. Treatment of anemia is entirely appropriate and often the mainstay of palliative treatment for some patients such as those with myelodysplasia. Likewise, minimizing adverse treatment side effects in those receiving palliative chemotherapy is an important aspect of their care. However, use of these agents in many patients, particularly those enrolled in a hospice care program has not been well studied. Substantial responses to growth factors (increase in hemoglobin of 2 g per dL) often take from 4 to 6 weeks, and many patients (up to 40%) have smaller responses or no response. With delayed responses, patients who are deteriorating rapidly may never benefit from such interventions. Furthermore, economic considerations may be prohibitive as erythropoietin and darbepoetin could consume a lion's share of the limited financial resources available in the hospice setting. However, the use of erythropoietic agents may be appropriate and consistent with palliative care in patients who are likely to live long enough to benefit and have an improvement in functional status.

The use of blood transfusions in the hospice and palliative setting is also controversial. Unfortunately, there are little data to guide this decision. One study of 112 patients with advanced cancer in a hospital at home care program examined responses to home transfusions (30). This study showed that two thirds of patients transfused had improvements in their self-rated QoL with most reporting improvements in sleep disturbances and fatigue. Responses in symptom control were maintained for a mean of 18.5 days after transfusion. A second prospective study of 246 patients with cancer in an inpatient hospice unit showed that 51.4% reported subjective benefit in well-being the day following transfusions (36). However, these were self reported assessments in unblinded studies; it is unclear that the improvements seen were clinically meaningful. Pretransfusion hemoglobin levels, degree of fatigue, and severity of dyspnea did not predict which of the patients would benefit from transfusion, adding little to determine which of the patients clinicians should consider for transfusion. Ultimately, the decision to transfuse a patient in the palliative or hospice setting is driven by the individual patient's symptoms, functional status, and prognosis. Transfusion in ambulatory patients who will obtain functional improvements is a reasonable and recognized indication for a RBC transfusion. Likewise, platelet transfusions in those with active bleeding and thrombocytopenia are usually consistent with the individual patient's plan of care. Just as in the use of erythropoietin agents, a careful examination of the likelihood of the individual patient receiving a substantial benefit can often avoid costly, ineffective treatment.

NEUTROPENIA

Neutropenia and its associated complications remains the major dose-limiting toxicities of most chemotherapeutic regimens. Febrile neutropenia (FN) is an oncologic emergency and requires close observation. Mortality as a consequence of neutropenia may still be as high as 8% in hospitalized patients with solid tumors (37). Mortality rates in patients with hematologic conditions are even higher at 13%. Although this is substantially lower than decades ago when odds of living through neutropenic fever were about even, we often underestimate the risks that remain for neutropenic patients. Supportive care for neutropenia continues to be aggressive with broad-spectrum antibiotics and hospitalization for those at moderate to high risk; oral antibiotic regimens have been

shown to be appropriate in certain low-risk populations (38). The risk of developing fever while neutropenic is roughly 10% per day of neutropenia. In addition to the infectious risk, neutropenia often further complicates treatment by requiring dose reductions and delays, the consequences of which are difficult to discern. In this section we will discuss treatment of FN and the prophylactic use of granulocyte growth factors to prevent neutropenia (Table 66.5).

Growth Factor Use—Primary and Secondary Prophylaxis

G-CSF (filgrastim [Neupogen], Amgen) is a lineage-specific growth factor that hastens maturation and release of the committed progenitor pool and prolongs circulation of released granulocytes. The growth factor also enhances neutrophil efficacy through increases in chemotaxis and phagocytosis and primes granulocytes for respiratory burst. With stimulation by growth factors, progenitor cell production and maturation of neutrophils may occur within a single day, compared with the usual 5-day maturation process. Pegfilgrastim, a conjugate with a 20 kDa polyethylene glycol attached to the N-terminus of the standard recombinant human G-CSF molecule, has a prolonged serum half-life, while maintaining all other biologic effects of G-CSF. Because it is not renally cleared, pegfilgrastim (Neulasta, Amgen) levels at the neutrophil remain elevated until absolute neutrophil count levels begin to rise and are then cleared by receptors on the neutrophil itself. This self-regulation allows dosing once per chemotherapy cycle, reducing inconvenience and overall health care costs. Toxicity related to G-CSF is generally mild. Up to 40% of patients complain of medullary bone pain. Infrequent reactions include allergic reactions, Sweet's syndrome, infection site reaction, and reduction in platelet counts.

Granulocyte macrophage colony stimulating factor (GM-CSF) [sagramostim (Leukine, Prokine)] is a lineage-nonspecific factor that acts synergistically with other cytokines to enhance erythroid and multipotent colonies, with resulting broader hematologic effects. Clinical effects include expansion of the myeloid, eosinophil, and monocyte/macrophage pools as well as increased neutrophil activity similar to G-CSF's effects. GM-CSF has a broader range of side effects; patients may note fever, nausea, headache, bone pain, diarrhea, thrombosis, and anorexia.

The use of growth factors in cancer treatment must be considered in two individual circumstances—primary and secondary prophylaxis of neutropenia. Data have shown that the recombinant colony-stimulating factors filgrastim, pegfilgrastim, and sargramostim are effective at reducing the nadir and duration of neutropenia. A meta-analysis of eight studies examining filgrastim prophylaxis showed approximately a 50% decrease in FN episodes. Filgrastim has been shown to decrease the risk of FN (OR = 0.38), documented infection (OR = 0.51), and infection-related mortality (OR = 0.60) when given prior to the development of neutropenia (39). Pegylated G-CSF (pegfilgrastim) has similar efficacy with reductions in the risk of FN of approximately 50% when used with highly myelosuppressive chemotherapy. A recent study in patients with metastatic breast cancer receiving weekly docetaxel (100 mg per m^2) showed a dramatic reduction in the rate of FN from 17 to 1% (40) and showing even more significant reductions with moderately myelosuppressive regimens.

Because of the difficulty in identifying high-risk patients for primary prophylaxis, the most common current clinical practice is secondary prophylaxis. This is a population of patients who have already proved themselves to be at high risk for neutropenic fever and its adverse effects by a first episode of FN. In a study of patients receiving cyclophosphamide,

TABLE 66.5

NATIONAL COMPREHENSIVE CANCER NETWORK GUIDELINES FOR INITIAL ANTIBIOTIC TREATMENT IN FEBRILE NEUTROPENIA

Oral antibiotic combination therapy (low-risk patients only):
- Ciprofloxacin + amoxicillin/clavulanate (for penicillin-allergic patients, may use ciprofloxacin + clindamycin)

Intravenous monotherapy (choose one):
- Cefepime
- Ceftazidime
- Imipenem/cilastatin
- Meropenem

Intravenous antibiotic dual therapy:
- Aminoglycoside + antipseudomonal penicillin ± β-lactamase inhibitor or extended-spectrum cephalosporin (cefepime, ceftazidime)
- Ciprofloxacin + antipseudomonal penicillin
- Double β-lactam (extended-spectrum cephalosporin + antipseudomonal penicillin or monobactam)

Intravenous vancomycin, if appropriate, added to monotherapy or dual therapy

---

doxorubicin, and etoposide for advanced small cell lung cancer, Crawford et al. showed that in patients with previous FN, the use of G-CSF reduced the duration of FN in subsequent cycles (from 6 to 2.5 days) and the rate of FN (from 100 to 23%) even when maintained on the same dose (41). A phase IV open-label study conducted by Epstein et al. (42) showed that primary prophylaxis with filgrastim in more than 780 pediatric and adult patients with various cancers and regimens allowed at least 90% of the planned chemotherapy to be given at full dose and on schedule. Therefore, it appears that growth factor use can increase the ability to maintain full dose intensity of chemotherapy. However, there is still a paucity of data to guide CSF use in maintaining dose intensity in most cancers. Although the concept that maintaining dose intensity and schedule leads to improved survival seems reasonable, is suggested by retrospective studies, and is consistent with current strategies, there have been no definitive studies that prove this.

Two major guideline groups have generated recommendations for the primary use of growth factors. The American Society of Clinical Oncology (ASCO) CSF committee reviews the literature and updates its evidence-based recommendations for clinical practice (43), with the last published guidelines in 2000. The 2005 National Comprehensive Cancer Center Guidelines for use of growth factor have been able to incorporate more recent data and differ substantially from the 2000 ASCO guidelines. The primary distinction between the two guidelines is the threshold for individual chemotherapeutic regimens that should prompt the primary prophylactic use of growth factors. The 2000 ASCO guidelines were based to some extent on earlier cost minimization data from Lyman et al. that recommends primary prophylaxis for regimens that have high rates of FN be restricted. Based on an estimated 50% decrease in FN rates and economic costs from the early 1990s, previous cost minimization analyses determined that primary prophylaxis with growth factor in regimens with a risk of FN of 40% or greater would result in cost savings compared to no prophylaxis (44). Very few regimens commonly used cause this rate of FN. However, costs of hospitalization have significantly increased in the past decade, whereas the cost of prophylactic growth factor use has remained stable. More recent data suggests that a lower threshold may be appropriate when all costs of care are considered (45).

The 2005 NCCN guidelines lower the threshold to include regimens that have FN rates of 20% or greater (46). This was based not on cost analysis, but on more recent clinical efficacy data. A recent study in patients with metastatic breast cancer receiving weekly docetaxel (100 mg per m^2) has now shown a dramatic reduction in the rate of FN with primary prophylaxis in moderately myelosuppressive regimens (40). Nine hundred twenty-eight patients with metastatic breast cancer were given docetaxel 100 mg per m^2 every 21 days and randomized 1:1 to placebo or day 2 pegfilgrastim. The rate of FN was significantly lower in treated patients than those receiving placebo (1 vs. 17%); hospitalizations were also lower in the group receiving pegfilgrastim (1 vs. 14%). This showed the utility of using pegfilgrastim in moderately suppressive regimens in the 10–20% range. This was part of the data supporting a lower threshold of 20% for beginning primary prophylaxis. This lower threshold now would include a number of commonly used regimens such as carboplatin/docetaxel, TAC (docetaxel, doxorubicin, cyclophosphamide), and ESHAP (etoposide, methylprednisolone, cisplatin, cytarabine). The NCCN guidelines also call for consideration of prophylactic growth factors for those with lower risk chemotherapy (10–20%) who have additional FN risk factors such as age, nutritional status, and comorbidities. Rates of neutropenia in treatment regimens for non-Hodgkin's lymphoma varied between 21 and 47% in a number of studies of elderly patients. Even more important, risk for infectious death can be up to 30% in these patients with the majority occurring following the first cycle of chemotherapy. Therefore, a less stringent standard may need to be considered for older and sicker patients. Other populations recognized by the ASCO committee that may benefit from prophylaxis are those with extensive previous chemotherapy or radiation and those in whom there may be significantly increased risk of infection. Indeed, the ASCO guidelines recommend that clinical discretion prevail in cases in which the clinical risk of neutropenia is judged to be substantial. An important consideration for the NCCN guidelines is the inclusion of treatment intent (curative, life-extending, palliative) in the decision for prophylactic growth factor versus use of a less myelosuppressive regimen or dosage schedule, if of comparable benefit to the patient.

THROMBOCYTOPENIA

Platelet Transfusions

Decreased platelet counts are common in the patients with cancer; the causes include invasion of the marrow by tumor, nutritional deficiencies, myelosuppression due to cytokines from the tumor, and myelosuppression/myeloablation from intensive chemotherapeutic regimens. Thrombocytopenia was originally a common complication of acute leukemias and their treatment, but it is now an increasing complication of solid tumor treatment as multiagent chemotherapy is adopted in a variety of malignancies, including lung and lymphoma.

Although mortality from major hemorrhages in an oncology patient is increasingly rare, thrombocytopenia is a frequent concern. Complications vary from harmless ecchymoses and petechiae to disruptive epistaxis and gingival bleeds, to life-threatening gastrointestinal and intracranial hemorrhages. Whether the patient has simple petechiae or a major hemorrhage, the treatment for thrombocytopenia is still the same: prevent or treat the hemorrhage by supplementing the platelet level. More than 9 million platelet units were transfused in 1997, and oncology patients and transplant patients consumed as much as half of these transfused platelets. Although most platelets transfused in the surgical patient are one-time transfusions in direct response to bleeding episodes and increased consumption of platelets, much of that used in the oncology patient is given for prophylaxis, with multiple transfusions required over longer periods of time. Prophylactic platelet transfusions are common, frequent, and are now considered the standard in the care of oncology patients. However, the standard at which one should transfuse has shifted over the last decade. As late as 1992, 80% of physicians sampled were using a standard threshold for prophylaxis of 20,000 per μL (47).

On the basis of recent studies, the last ASCO committee on platelet transfusions now recommends the new threshold of 10,000 per μL at which to transfuse oncology patients (Table 66.6). There has been one retrospective and two prospective trials of prophylactic transfusions comparing 20 K to 10 K as the threshold for transfusion. The largest was a multicenter trial by Rebulla et al. (48) Transfusion thresholds of 10,000 per μL and 20,000 per μL were compared in 255 adolescent and adult patients with AML (excluded acute promyelocytic leukemia). During episodes of fever to 38° C, active bleeding, or invasive procedures, the higher threshold was used (this occurred 22.6% of the time). Major bleeding episodes were similar in the two groups with 21.5% (10,000 per μL group) and 20% (20,000 per μL) of patients having episodes greater than petechiae, mucosal, or retinal bleeding ($p = .41$). One fatal bleed, a cerebral hemorrhage, did occur in the lower threshold group, but this event occurred when the platelet count was 32,000. Platelet transfusions were 21.5% lower in the 10,000 per μL threshold group ($p = .001$). Gastrointestinal bleeding did occur twice as often (12 vs. 5 episodes) at the more restrictive threshold, but there were no differences in the number of red cell transfusions required due to this.

Bishop et al. (49) showed that the thrombocytopenic patient can undergo major surgery provided adequate transfusion support is given. The retrospective analysis of 95 patients with acute leukemia requiring a variety of surgeries showed that, provided counts exceed 50,000, blood loss is usually minimal. On the basis of this study, the ASCO committee recommended a threshold of 50,000 per μL before major invasive procedures (50). There is little guidance in the literature regarding the appropriate levels before lumbar puncture or bone marrow aspiration. Several retrospective studies of no more than 20 adult patients have recommended transfusions before lumbar puncture for levels of <20,000, but this has not been examined in larger trials.

Refractoriness

Refractoriness to platelet transfusion is a common and significant effect of repeated transfusions and may be as high as 35% in patients with AML (50). Refractoriness to platelet transfusion is thought to be because of platelet-reactive alloantibodies against histocompatibility antigens. These antibodies consume large numbers of transfused platelets and leave little to show for the transfusions.

It is now recognized that leukocytes contaminating the platelet transfusion play a role in immunization (51). Because platelets lack class II histocompatibility antigens, another agent must serve as a costimulant along with its class I antigens. Several methods are used to reduce leukocytes within a transfusion. Filtration is the older process but varies in its ability to filter leukocytes; it usually results in a three log

---

TABLE 66.6

AMERICAN SOCIETY OF CLINICAL ONCOLOGY CLINICAL PRACTICE GUIDELINES FOR PLATELET TRANSFUSIONS

10,000/μL should be the prophylactic threshold for adult patients with adult leukemia and most solid tumors

20,000/μL should be considered for some tumors that, due to tumor necrosis, are particularly at risk for bleeding. Examples include melanoma, bladder, gynecologic, and colorectal tumors

Platelet counts >50,000/μL should be reached before surgery

To reduce alloimmunization, leukoreduced blood products should be used in patients who will require continued platelet transfusions

Patients refractory to platelet transfusions should be treated with HLA-matched platelets

From Schiffer CA, Anderson KC, Bennett CL, et al. Platelet transfusion for patients with cancer: clinical practice guidelines of the American Society of Clinical Oncology. *J Clin Oncol* 2001;19(5):1519–1538, with permission.

TABLE 66.7

TRANSFUSION REACTIONS AND INFECTIONS

TRANSFUSION REACTIONS	
Febrile (FNHTR)	1–4:100
Allergic	1–4:100
Delayed hemolytic	1:1000
TRALI	1:5000
Acute hemolytic	1:12,000
Anaphylactic	1:150,000
INFECTIONS	
Bacterial contamination of products	1:3000
Risk of septic reaction (platelets)	1:50,000
Risk of septic reaction (PRBC)	1:500,000
Serious viral pathogen	1:300,000
Hepatitis B	1:60,000
Hepatitis C	1:1,600,000
HIV-1	1:2,000,000

FNHTR, febrile nonhemolytic transfusion reaction; TRALI, transfusion related acute lung injury; PRBC, packed red blood cells; HIV, human immunodeficiency virus.

reduction in the volume of leukocytes. Newer methods have used ultraviolet light to reduce antigenicity of transfusions. In the Trial to Reduce Alloimmunization to Platelets, over 600 patients were randomized to receive either pooled, filtered, single-donor filtered, or pooled irradiated platelets. Each of the methods to reduce the number of viable leukocytes transfused led to a reduction in the production of antibody formation compared with simple transfusion with pooled platelets (17 vs. 45%). Leukocyte-depleted transfusion products (both RBCs and platelets), therefore, should be used in leukemic patients receiving induction and consolidation. The data behind those with solid tumors who require platelet transfusions are not as clear, mostly because these patients rarely require the prolonged transfusions common in the treatment of patients with leukemia. Leukodepleted transfusions are also less likely to cause transfusion reactions (Table 66.7), which are thought to be mediated by cytokines from leukocytes. However, both methods of leukocyte reduction are inefficient, costing a loss of up to 25% of platelets and driving up the costs of transfusions.

Although patients who received repeated transfusion often develop antibodies, other factors also play a role in a poor response to an individual platelet transfusion. Fever, infection, and an active bleeding source all consume additional platelets and may be reflected in a less than expected response to a transfusion. The ASCO committee has recommended that following transfusions, platelet counts be measured again to determine an adequate increase in platelet counts. If a patient fails to have adequate increases in post-transfusion platelet counts in at least two ABO-compatible transfusions, the clinician should consider alloimmunization and other causes of platelet destruction such as disseminated intravascular coagulation, sepsis, and immune thrombocytopenia purpura. Often patients with alloimmunization can be transfused with HLA-matched platelets with good response (up to 50%), but it is critical that further transfusion be coordinated with blood bank personnel. If HLA-matched platelets fail to produce adequate responses, cross-matched or family-member donated platelets may then be considered.

Thrombopoietic Agents

Platelet transfusions are costly, at times ineffective, and place the recipient at risk for transfusion reactions and infectious exposures. Given the promising responses of anemia and neutropenia to growth factors, it is hoped that a pharmacologic alternative to platelet transfusion will soon be found. Early efforts using cytokines to stimulate platelet production showed significant toxicities, including fevers and hypotension interleukin IL-1 and headaches, fatigue, and fevers (IL-6), but little clinical benefit. However, IL-11 has been approved as a thrombopoietic agent based on promising data in patients with breast cancer. IL-11 was originally derived from stromal cells and was found to stimulate proliferation of a murine plasmacytoma cell line. It has multiple effects on both hematopoietic cells and other organ systems such as intestinal and bronchial epithelial cells. IL-11 either alone or in concert with other cytokines has been shown to increase megakaryocyte maturation markers, megakaryocyte polyploidy, and platelet size. *In vitro* studies showed little activity alone, but *in vivo*, it has been shown to promote megakaryocytopoiesis and increase platelet production. In a study of 93 breast cancer patients, platelet transfusions were reduced in 30% of patients (52). However, side effects are significant and include edema, fatigue, myalgias, and cardiovascular events. This has limited use in general clinical practice and fueled the drive to find other agents to stimulate platelet production.

It has been less than a decade since the c-MPL ligand was identified and cloned. From this development, two variants of the c-MPL ligand have been produced and studied, showing mixed results in clinical trials. RhTPO, an intact recombinant thrombopoietin, and PEG-rHuMGDF, a truncated and pegylated human recombinant megakaryocyte growth and development factor, showed early promise in phase I trials. Studies in leukemic and stem cell transplant patients failed to show clinical benefit. Furthermore, there was concerning evidence of antibody production to the pegylated MGDF when injected subcutaneously causing prolonged thrombocytopenia. For this reason, the manufacturer halted further US clinical trials of PEG-rHuMGDF in September 1998. Current approaches involve the development of thrombopoietin-mimetic peptides that have now entered early phase clinical trials.

BLOOD TRANSFUSION PRODUCTS

Transfusions of blood products are necessary at times to support the oncology patient. The choice of transfusion product should be driven by the underlying deficit. Fresh whole blood transfusions consist of RBCs, plasma with coagulation factors, and fresh platelets and is rarely used except to treat severe hypovolemia in patients with large, acute blood loss. In fact, packed red blood cells (PRBC), fresh frozen plasma (FFP), and platelet concentrates are more appropriate in most patients requiring large volume replacement. PRBC products typically have a hematocrit of 60–90% and are the most frequent transfusion products given to oncology patients. One 300-mL unit typically raises the recipient's hemoglobin by 3–4%. Platelet transfusion preparations can be random donor pooled platelet concentrates or single-donor apheresis platelet concentrates (which in turn can be used to provide either random or HLA-matched platelets). FFP contains both plasma proteins and all coagulation factors (1 unit ~7% of coagulation factors). FFP (180–300 mL per unit) is used for correcting congenital or acquired coagulation factor deficiencies and is usually sufficient for hemostasis once coagulation factor levels reach roughly 25% of normal and fibrinogen levels are >75 mg per dL. For correction of a prolonged prothrombin time, doses of roughly 10–15 mL per kg body weight are necessary. For patients with larger deficits in fibrinogen and on von Willebrand factor (vWF), cryoprecipitate may be necessary. Each unit of cryoprecipitate (1 unit ~15 mL) contains fibrinogen (~150 mg), factor VIII (~80 units), and large amounts of vWF. More purified coagulation products are also available but are rarely needed in patients without congenital or acquired coagulopathies.

Complications of Blood Product Transfusions

Transfusions of blood products are frequently necessary in the oncology patient, but they are not without consequence. Six hundred ninety-four patient deaths resulting from blood transfusions were reported from 1985 to 1999 (52). There were likely many more transfusion deaths that went unreported or unrecognized. Hemolytic transfusion reactions occur infrequently but may be responsible for as many as 1.0–1.2 deaths per 100,000 patients transfused.

Alloimmunization is the most frequent complication of blood transfusions with estimates of rates varying from 7 to 30% (53). In a retrospective analysis of 564 patients with myeloproliferative or lymphoproliferative disorders from 1987 to 1996, Schonewille et al. found an overall immunization rate of 9% of patients receiving long-term transfusion support, with the risk of immunization of 0.5% per each RBC unit transfused. As seen in the previous section, platelet alloimmunization is a major problem in the treatment of oncology patients. However, there is some suggestion that those undergoing chemotherapy may not produce as active a response to incompatible transfusions as others requiring transfusions, thereby lowering actual alloimmunization rates in oncology patients.

Hemolytic Transfusion Reactions

Acute reactions occur during and immediately after transfusion and vary from the discomfort of an allergic reaction with urticaria to life-threatening hemolysis and multiorgan system dysfunction associated with acute hemolytic reactions. Due to strict and thorough crossmatching, acute hemolytic reactions are infrequent, <1 per 200,000 units transfused (54), but up to 16 deaths per year may be attributable to this immunologic response to an incompatible blood product. Symptoms occur early in transfusion, often within the first 5 minutes of beginning the transfusion, but reactions can occur several hours after transfusion. Fever, chills, and hypotension typically dominate the presentation, but reactions can include such nonspecific complaints as flushing, low back pain, dyspnea, nausea, chest pain, or abdominal pain.

Laboratory evidence of acute hemolytic transfusion reaction (AHTR) includes early and rapid decrease in serum haptoglobin levels and increases in serum bilirubin, plasma hemoglobin, and urine hemoglobin peaking approximately 6 hours after initiation of reaction. With prompt attention and discontinuation of the instigating transfusion, AHTR need not be fatal. The transfusion must be stopped immediately, intravenous saline continued, and both the transfusion sample and the patient's serum sent for investigation. Intravenous furosemide and fluid can diminish some of the effects of the intrarenal shunting. Hemolysis can also occur because of nonimmunologic mechanisms including mechanical forces, osmotic pressure (e.g., contact with nonisotonic fluid or in G6PD-deficient transfusions in patients receiving reducing agents).

Delayed hemolytic transfusion reactions tend to be less fulminant and manifest by falling hematocrits with elevated bilirubin, fever, hemoglobinuria, and a positive Coombs test seen 5–10 days following transfusion. Usually asymptomatic and undetected, some prospective work has shown that the actual incidence may be as high as 0.5%. More significant reactions may lead to renal failure, jaundice, and further deterioration of an already ill patient. The likely precipitating event of the reaction is an amnestic response to RBC antigens or de novo development of non–ABO antigens. Anti-Kidd and Duffy antibodies may play a role in those clinically significant reactions, but these are difficult to detect. Management is symptomatic support.

Transfusion-Related Acute Lung Injury

Transfusion-related acute lung injury (TRALI) is a rare but life-threatening acute noncardiogenic pulmonary edema with symptoms similar to adult respiratory distress syndrome. Patients experience tachypnea and dyspnea and exhibit bilateral pulmonary edema. Differing from cardiogenic edema and cases of fluid overload, the etiology is thought to be donor HLA antibodies reacting with recipient neutrophils. These activated granulocytes are sequestered in the pulmonary vasculature, where they wreak havoc, releasing proteolytic enzymes that damage the microvasculature. Pulmonary leak then occurs, allowing fluid and protein to fill the alveoli. TRALI often occurs early in transfusion, within 2 hours but has also been reported much later. Respiratory compromise typically lasts several days, and most recover without lasting sequelae. However, some patients require short-term ventilator support. Mortality rates have been reported as high as 6%. There is no method of predicting which transfusions will result in TRALI, although multiparous women may have an increased frequency of antibodies due to exposures during pregnancy and delivery.

Febrile Nonhemolytic Transfusion Reactions

Febrile nonhemolytic transfusion reactions, the most frequently seen of transfusion reactions, is a cluster of symptoms similar to AHTR but without the specter of fatality. Patients complain of fever, chills, nausea, emesis, and/or malaise and often have a rapid increase in body temperature of 1–2° C. Although originally attributed to antileukocyte antibodies, it is now recognized that recipient's immunologic system may also contain antiplatelet or antigranulocyte antibodies that create these symptoms. In some cases, no precipitating antibody is found at all, and cytokines are thought to play the key role. As the number of leukocyte-depleted blood products transfusions have increased, the frequency of these reactions has declined. Patients can be treated with antipyretics, usually acetaminophen, for symptomatic relief. Platelet transfusions much more frequently cause febrile reactions than other blood products. Although some are attributable to antibodies, cytokines likely play a role. Transfusions of stored platelets more frequently cause reactions perhaps because of the production of cytokines during storage. If donor-end, leukodepleted platelet transfusions are used, the incidence of febrile nonhemolytic transfusion reactions is dramatically reduced.

Anaphylaxis and Allergic Reactions

Anaphylactic reactions are infrequent, but rapid death can occur as laryngeal edema, bronchospasms, and hypotension develop from mast cell degranulation. Most of these reactions are seen in immunoglobulin A (IgA)-deficient patients who have anti-IgA antibodies and are then transfused with products from an IgA donor. Patients can be treated with corticosteroids, antihistamines, and support measures. Future reactions can be prevented by transfusing components from IgA-deficient donors or by washing packed RBCs and platelet products to reduce the possibility of transfusing IgA. Benign allergic reactions are fairly common with any transfusion product. Antigens present in the transfused products can cause urticaria. Treatment is again antihistamines, but routine prophylactic treatment is not recommended. Patients who have had previous reactions, however, are commonly treated prophylactically with each transfusion and the use of washed RBCs and platelets should be considered.

Infectious Risks and Complications

As improved record keeping and crossmatching eliminate hemolytic reactions and improved surveillance decrease viral infections, bacterial contamination has become a significant proportion of transfusion-related morbidity and mortality. Seventy-seven of 694 transfusion-related deaths from 1985 to 1999 were attributable to bacterial infections (53). Contamination generally occurs at the time of collection from skin flora of inadequately prepared donors or from asymptomatic bacteremia from the donor. Platelets have a higher incidence of contamination because storage and increased exposure from the multiple donors of pooled platelets. These units are frequently contaminated with skin flora, which then replicates with storage at room temperature. For this reason, platelet storage is limited to 5 days. Because RBCs are stored at cooler temperatures, contaminants in these products are frequently *Yersinia, Serratia, Pseudomonas,* and *Enterobacter* species, which can survive cooler temperatures. Patients frequently present with symptoms of sepsis at the time of transfusion. Hypotension and shock can develop rapidly as accumulated endotoxin is released into the recipient. Symptoms may later develop as bacteremia occurs within the host. Efforts at prevention are largely focused on improved sterile collection techniques.

The safety of the US blood supply has improved over recent years such that the risk of transmission of a serious viral pathogen is approximately 29 per million units (55). Yet fear of this iatrogenic complication is often the greatest concern of blood product recipients. Failure to detect the presence of virus in the contaminated units is largely the result of donation and testing during the "window period" shortly after the donor has acquired the infection and before serologic conversion. Nevertheless, viral infection is rare and seldom a significant event for the adult oncology patient.

Many other clinical infections have been related to blood transfusion, including common pathogens such as Epstein-Barr virus and parvovirus, as well as rarer illnesses such as Chagas' disease, Creutzfeldt-Jakob disease, leishmaniasis, malaria, babesiosis, and syphilis. Fortunately the transfusion-related incidence of these diseases is uncommon. Cytomegalovirus (CMV) deserves special note because of the high seroprevalence in the United States (35–80% varying by region) and the potentially devastating effects on the immunosuppressed host who acquires the infection. CMV is a leukocyte-associated virus; therefore any blood product contaminated with white blood cells is capable of transmitting infection. Several studies have shown decreased rates of CMV infection in patients receiving leukodepleted blood products, but prospective trials comparing leukocyte reduced versus CMV seronegative transfusions are limited. Therefore CMV-negative donors are still used as the standard of care for those patients in whom CMV infection could be devastating, including seronegative bone marrow transplant patients.

CONCLUSION

The discovery of the hematopoietic growth factors and their introduction into clinical practice has dramatically changed our understanding of hematopoiesis. In addition, the clinical consequences of anemia, neutropenia, and thrombocytopenia in the patient with cancer have become much better characterized. Clinical practice guidelines have been developed

and are continually being revised as our knowledge base increases. Meanwhile, the areas of transfusion medicine and infectious diseases have clarified the appropriate settings for transfusion support and antibiotics and the risks and benefits of these approaches (56). In addition, economic studies and outcome research have focused on this critical area of supportive care to help us understand the best approaches to be used for our patients. With the advent of second-generation hematopoietic growth factors, further benefits are anticipated, including trials that may shift emphasis from treatment of cytopenias to more preventive strategies. In this rapidly changing area, readers are encouraged to follow the results of ongoing randomized clinical trials as well as the updates of evidence-based, clinical practice guidelines to best incorporate the use of hematopoietic growth factors, transfusions, transfusion support, and antibiotics in the clinical care of their patients.

References

1. Bohlius J, Langensiepen S, Schwarzer G, et al. Recombinant human erythropoietin and overall survival in cancer patients: results of a comprehensive meta-analysis. *J Natl Cancer Inst* 2005;97(7):489–498.
2. Marchetti M, Barosi G. Clinical and economic impact of epoetins in cancer care. *Pharmacoeconomics* 2004;22(16):1029–1045.
3. Meyer RM, Browman GP, Samosh ML, et al. Randomized phase II comparison of standard CHOP with weekly CHOP in elderly patients with non-Hodgkin's lymphoma. *J Clin Oncol* 1995;13(9):2386–2393.
4. Barrett-Lee PJ, Bailey NP, O'Brien MER, et al. Large-scale UK audit of blood transfusion requirements and anaemia in patients receiving cytotoxic chemotherapy. *Br J Cancer* 2000;82:93–97.
5. Tas F, Eralp Y, Basaran M, et al. Anemia in oncology practice: relation to diseases and their therapies. *Am J Clin Oncol* 2002;25:371–379.
6. Cella D. Factors influencing quality of life in cancer patients: anemia and fatigue. *Semin Oncol* 1998;25:43–46.
7. Hebert PC, Wells G, Blajchman MA, et al. A multicenter, randomized, controlled clinical trial of transfusion requirements in critical care. *N Engl J Med* 1999;340:409–417.
8. Wood PA, Hrushesky WJ. Cisplatin-associated anemia: an erythropoietin deficiency syndrome. *J Clin Invest* 1995;95(4):1650–1659.
9. Dowlati A, R'Zik S, Fillet G, et al. Anaemia of lung cancer is due to impaired erythroid marrow response to erythropoietin stimulation as well as relative inadequacy of erythropoietin production. *Br J Haematol* 1997;97(2):297–299.
10. Miller CB, Platanias LC, Mills SR, et al. Phase I-II Trial of erythropoietin in the treatment of cisplatin-associated anemia. *J Natl Cancer Inst* 1992;82:98–103.
11. Demetri GD, Kris M, Wade J, et al. Quality-of life benefit in chemotherapy patients treated with epoetin alfa is independent of disease response or tumor type: results from a prospective community oncology study. Procrit Study Group. *J Clin Oncol* 1998;16(10):3412–3425.
12. Glaspy J, Bukowski R, Steinberg D, et al. Impact of therapy with epoetin alfa on clinical outcomes in patients with nonmyeloid malignancies during cancer chemotherapy in community oncology practice. Procrit Study Group. *J Clin Oncol* 1997;15(3):1218–1234.
13. Gabrilove JL, Cleeland CS, Livingston RB, et al. Clinical evaluation of once-weekly dosing of epoetin alfa in chemotherapy patients: Improvements in hemoglobin and quality of life are similar to three-times-weekly dosing. *J Clin Oncol* 2001;19(11):2875–2882.
14. Witzig TE, Silberstein PT, Loprinzi CL, et al. Phase III, randomized, double-blind study of epoetin alfa compared with placebo in anemic patients receiving chemotherapy. *J Clin Oncol* 2005;23(12):2606–2617.
15. Herrington JD, Davidson SL, Tomita DK, et al. Utilization of darbepoetin alfa and epoetin alfa for chemotherapy-induced anemia. *Am J Health Syst Pharm* 2005;62(1):54–62.
16. Littlewood TJ, Bajetta E, Nortier JWR, et al. Effects of epoetin alfa on hematologic parameters and quality of life in cancer patients receiving nonplatinum chemotherapy: results of a randomized, double-blind, placebo-controlled trial. *J Clin Oncol* 2001;19(11):2865–2874.
17. Macdougall IC, Gray SJ, Elston O, et al. Pharmacokinetics of novel erythropoiesis stimulating protein compared with epoetin alfa in dialysis patients. *J Am Soc Nephrol* 1999;10:2392–2395.
18. Glaspy JA, Jadeja JS, Justice G, et al. Darbepoetin alfa given every 1 or 2 weeks alleviates anaemia associated with cancer chemotherapy. *Br J Cancer* 2002;87:268–276.
19. Hedenus M, Adriansson M, Miguel JS, et al. Efficacy and safety of darbepoetin alfa in anaemic patients with lymphoproliferative malignancies: a randomized, double-blind, placebo-controlled study. *Br J Haematol* 2003;122:394–403.

20. Quirt I, Robeson C, Lau CY, et al. Epoetin alfa therapy increases hemoglobin levels and improves quality of life in patients with cancer-related anemia who are not receiving chemotherapy and patients with anemia who are not receiving chemotherapy. *J Clin Oncol* 2001;19:4126–4134.

21. Vansteenkiste J, Pirker R, Massuti B, et al. Double-blind, placebo-controlled, randomized phase trial of darbepoetin alfa in lung cancer patients receiving chemotherapy. *J Natl Cancer Inst* 2002;94:1211–1220.

22. Glaspy J, Jadeja J, Justice G, et al. A randomized, active-control, pilot trial of front-loaded dosing regimens of darbepoetin-alfa for the treatment of patients with anemia during chemotherapy for malignant disease. *Cancer* 2003;97:1312–1320.

23. Waltzman RJ, Croot C, Williams D. Final hematologic results: epoetin alfa (EPO) 40,000 U qW vs darbepoetin alfa (DARB 200mcg q 2 w in anemic cancer patients (pts) receiving chemotherapy. *ASCO Annual Meeting (Abs no 8030)*. 2005.

24. Glaspy J, Berg R, Tomita D, et al. Final results of a phase 3, randomized, open-label study of darbepoetin alfa 200 mcg every 2 weeks (Q2W) versus epoetin alfa 40,000 U weekly (QW) in patients with chemotherapy-induced anemia (CIA). *ASCO Annual Meeting (Abs no 8125)*. 2005.

25. Patton J, Kuzur M, Liggett W, et al. Epoetin alfa 60,000 u once weekly followed by 120,000 u every 3 weeks increases and maintains hemoglobin levels in anemic cancer patients undergoing chemotherapy. *Oncologist* 2004;9:90–96.

26. Hesketh PJ, Arena F, Patel D, et al. Front-loaded darbepoetin alfa with q3w maintenance administered as a fixed or weight-based dose in anemic cancer patients results in similar efficacy profiles (Abs 2941). *Proc Am Soc Clin Oncol* 2003;22:731.

27. Musto P, Falcone A, Sanpaolo G, et al. Efficacy of a single, weekly dose of recombinant erythropoietin in myelodysplastic syndromes. *Br J Haematol* 2003;122(2):269–271.

28. Musto P, Lanza F, Balleari E, et al. Darbepoetin alpha for the treatment of anaemia in low-intermediate risk myelodysplastic syndromes. *Br J Haematol* 2005;128(2):204–209.

29. NCCN Guidelines Cancer and Treatment Related Anemia. http://www.nccn.org/professionals/physician_gls/PDF/anemia.pdf, 2004.

30. Tanneberger S, Melilli G, Strocchi E, et al. Use of red blood cell transfusion in palliative care services: is it still up to date or is cancer-related anaemia controlled better with erythropoietic agents? *Ann Oncol* 2004;15:839–840.

31. Henke M, Laszig R, Rube C, et al. Erythropoietin to treat head and neck cancer patients with anaemia undergoing radiotherapy: randomised, double-blind, placebo-controlled trial. *Lancet* 2003;362(9392):1255.

32. Leyland-Jones B. Breast cancer trial with erythropoietin terminated unexpectedly. *Lancet Oncol* 2003;4:459–460.

33. Bokemeyer C, Aapro MS, Courdi A, et al. EORTC guidelines for the use of erythropoietic proteins in anaemic patients with cancer. *Eur J Cancer* 2004;40(15):2201.

34. Auerbach M, Ballard H, Trout JR, et al. Intravenous iron optimizes the response to recombinant human erythropoietin in cancer patients with chemotherapy-related anemia: a multicenter, open-label, randomized trial. *J Clin Oncol* 2004;22(7):1301–1307.

35. Brizel DM, Dodge RK, Clough RW, et al. Oxygenation of head and neck cancer: changes during radiotherapy and impact on treatment outcome. *Radiother Oncol* 1999;53(2):113–117.

36. Massimo M, Castellani L, Berlusconi A, et al. Use of red blood cell transfusions in terminally ill cancer patients admitted to a palliative care unit. *J Pain Symptom Manage* 1996;12(1):18–22.

37. Lyman GH, Kuderer NM, Agboola O, et al. The epidemiology and economics of neutropenia in hospitalized cancer patients: data from the University Health System Consortium. Poster presented at the *43rd Annual Meeting of the American Society of Hematology*. December 7–11, 2001, (Abstr no 1813).

38. Maher DW, Graham JL, Green M, et al. Filgrastim in patients with chemotherapy induced febrile neutropenia: a double blind, placebo-controlled trial. *Ann Intern Med* 1994;121:492–501.

39. Lyman GH, Kuderer NM, Djulbegovic B. A meta-analysis of granulocyte colon-stimulating factor (rH-G-CSF) to prevent febrile neutropenia in patients receiving cancer chemotherapy. *Am J Med* 2002;112:406–411.

40. Vogel CL, Wojtukiewicz MZ, Carroll RR, et al. First and subsequent cycle use of pegfilgrastim prevents febrile neutropenia in patients with breast cancer: a multicenter, double-blind, placebo-controlled phase III study. *J Clin Oncol* 2005;23:1178–1184.

41. Crawford J, Ozer H, Stoller R, et al. Reduction by granulocyte colony-stimulating factor of fever and neutropenia induced by chemotherapy in patients with small-cell lung cancer. *N Engl J Med* 1991;325(3):164–170.

42. Epstein JM, Donnelly SM, O'Byrne JM, et al. Community experience with filgrastim in diverse nonmyeloid malignancies: an open-label phase 4 study. *J Support Oncol* 2004;2(Suppl 2):54–55.

43. Ozer H, Armitage JO, Bennett CL, et al. American Society of Clinical Oncology. 2000 update of recommendations for the use of hematopoietic colony-stimulating factors: evidence-based, clinical practice guidelines. American Society of Clinical Oncology Growth Factors Expert Panel. *J Clin Oncol* 2000;18(20):3558–3585.

44. Lyman GH, Lyman CG, Sanderson RA, et al. Decision analysis of hematopoietic growth factor use in patients receiving cancer chemotherapy. *J Natl Cancer Inst* 1993;85:488–493.

45. Cosler LE, Calhoun EA, Agboola O, et al. Effects of indirect and additional direct costs on the risk threshold for prophylaxis with colony-stimulating factors in patients at risk for severe neutropenia from cancer chemotherapy. *Pharmacotherapy* 2002;24:488–489.

46. Crawford J, Althaus B, Armitage J, et al. National Comprehensive Cancer Network. Myeloid growth factors clinical practice guidelines in oncology. [Guideline. Journal Article. Practice Guideline]. *J Natl Compr Cancer Netw* 2005;3(4):540–555. Jul.

47. Pisciotto PT, Benson K, Hume H, et al. Prophylactic versus therapeutic platelet transfusion practices in hematology and/or oncology patients. *Transfusion* 1995;35(6):498–502.

48. Rebulla P, Finazzi G, Marangoni F, et al. The Gruppo Italiano Malattie Ematologiche Maligne dell'Adulto: the threshold for prophylactic platelet transfusions in adults with acute myeloid leukemia. *N Engl J Med* 1997;337:1870–1875.

49. Bishop JF, Schiffer CA, Aisner J, et al. Surgery in acute leukemia: a review of 167 operations in thrombocytopenic patients. *Am J Hematol* 1987;26:147–155.

50. Schiffer CA, Anderson KC, Bennett CL, et al. Platelet transfusion for patients with cancer: clinical practice guidelines of the American Society of Clinical Oncology. *J Clin Oncol* 2001;19(5):1519–1538.

51. Group TTS. Leukocyte reduction and UV-B irradiation of platelets to prevent alloimmunization and refractoriness to platelet transfusion. *N Engl J Med* 1997;337:1861–1869.

52. Tepler I, Elias L, Smith JW II, et al. A randomized placebo-controlled trial of recombinant human interleukin-11 in cancer patients with severe thrombocytopenia due to chemotherapy. *Blood* 1996;87:3607–3614.

53. Brecher ME, Hay SN. Bacterial contamination of blood components. *Clin Microbiol Rev* 2005;18(1):195–204.

54. Schonewille H, Haak HL, van Zijl AM. Alloimmunization after blood transfusion in patients with hematologic and oncologic diseases. *Transfusion* 1999;39(7):763–771.

55. Sazama K. Reports of 355 transfusion-associated deaths: 1976–1985. *Transfusion* 1990;30:583–590.

56. Goodnough LT, Brecher ME, Kanter MH, et al. Transfusion Medicine—Blood Transfusion-First of Two Parts. *N Engl J Med* 1999;340:438–447.

CHAPTER 67 ■ NUTRITION SUPPORT

WILLIAM A. MOURAD, CAROLINE M. APOVIAN, AND CHRISTOPHER D. STILL

Malignant disease is frequently accompanied by profound weight loss and malnutrition. In fact, cancer patients have the highest prevalence of malnutrition of any hospitalized group of patients (1). In its most severe form, weight loss due to malignancy is termed the *anorexia-cachexia syndrome* and is characterized by anorexia, skeletal muscle atrophy, tissue wasting, and organ dysfunction (2). Malnutrition associated with malignancy is an indicator of a poor prognosis. It is associated with a higher mortality rate (3) and higher perioperative morbidity in severely malnourished patients (4–6). However, it is unclear if the routine use of nutritional support in cancer patients can mitigate those consequences. A great deal of research has attempted to answer this question and guidelines for use of nutrition support have been set up by the American Society for Parenteral and Enteral Nutrition, the American Gastroenterological Association, and the American College of Physicians (7–9).

Choosing the appropriate route of nutrition support for a malnourished patient is an important decision predicated on the patient's clinical situation. Although enteral feeding is the preferred route for patients with a functional gastrointestinal (GI) tract, many patients have relative or absolute contraindications to and are unable to tolerate enteral feedings (5,7–9). Patients with severe diarrhea, abdominal distention, high nasogastric tube output, or unobtainable safe access to the GI tract are poor candidates for enteral nutrition. The complications of enteral nutrition include pulmonary aspiration, diarrhea, and intestinal ischemia or infection. The risks of parenteral nutrition include infection, electrolyte imbalances, and a failure of large controlled studies showing an improvement except in selected patient populations (the severely malnourished surgical patient and bone marrow transplant patients) (4–10).

This chapter will address the following questions: what is the effect of nutrition support on the outcomes of patients with cancer undergoing various treatment modalities? What is the role of nutrition support in the treatment of cytokine-mediated cancer anorexia and altered host metabolism? Are there specific nutritional supplements that take on a pharmacologic role by modulating tumor cell growth? Finally, is preservation of quality of life, by reduction of fatigue and other effects of malnutrition, an adequate outcome of adjuvant nutritional therapy? Because of the ongoing controversies associated with these issues and ethical issues regarding nonvolitional feeding guidelines, nutrition support of the patient with cancer should be emphasized in the clinical setting. Nonetheless, nutrition support is an integral component of comprehensive cancer care in patients who are carefully selected through the use of nutritional screening tools and for whom appropriate goals of treatment have been established.

MALNUTRITION IN THE CANCER PATIENT

Malnutrition in the patient with cancer results from several mechanical and metabolic processes. The cachexia of malignancy is a complex metabolic disorder characterized by involuntary weight loss which, if not treated, often leads to death (3). Certain tumors predispose individuals to cancer cachexia. Table 67.1 depicts the frequency of weight loss among approximately 3000 patients with cancer studied by the Eastern Cooperative Oncology Group. Breast cancer and sarcomas rarely resulted in significant host weight loss compared with cancers involving digestive organs such as stomach and pancreas. Patients with lung cancer or prostate cancer also demonstrated significant weight loss and malnutrition. The Eastern Cooperative Oncology Group survey demonstrated a lower morbidity and longer survival in patients without weight loss, except in cases of pancreatic or gastric cancer. The role, however, of nutritional support preventing weight loss remains unclear.

Causes of Malnutrition

Table 67.2 lists the potential etiologic factors in the development of malnutrition and cancer anorexia. The development of malnutrition in the individual patient is usually the result of a combination of these mechanisms (11).

Anorexia of Malignancy

Several factors, including changes in the central nervous system, changes in taste perception due to tumor, depression, and its associated reduced physical activity, have been implicated as causes of cancer anorexia. The regulation of appetite is complex and is mediated by blood nutrient levels, host nutrient resources, liver function, GI capacity or toxicity, medications, and environmental cues (7,8,11,12). When weight loss is encountered despite adequate caloric intake, it is termed the *anorexia-cachexia syndrome*. Recently, considerable attention has been directed to the role of various cytokines and tumor byproducts as mediators of this syndrome which are discussed in detail later in this chapter under mediators of cancer cachexia.

From DeWys WD, Begg C, Lavin PT, et al. Prognostic effect of weight loss prior to chemotherapy in cancer patients. *Am J Med* 1980;69:491–497, with permission.

TABLE 67.1

FREQUENCY OF WEIGHT LOSS IN CANCER PATIENTS

Tumor type	Number of patients	Weight loss in the previous 6 mo (%)			
		0	0–5	5–10	>10
Favorable non-Hodgkin's lymphoma	290	69	14	8	10
Breast	289	64	22	8	6
Sarcoma	189	60	21	11	7
Unfavorable non-Hodgkin's lymphoma	311	52	20	13	15
Colon	307	46	26	14	14
Prostate	78	44	27	18	10
Lung, small cell	436	43	23	20	14
Lung, non–small cell	590	39	25	21	15
Pancreas	111	17	29	28	26
Nonmeasurable gastric	179	17	21	32	30
Measurable gastric	138	13	20	29	38
Total	2918	42	22	18	16

NUTRITIONAL EFFECTS OF CANCER TREATMENTS

Radiation

The site, magnitude, and duration of radiation therapy all influence the severity of nutritional compromise. This injury may be associated with both acute and long-term effects of radiation therapy (13,14).

After radiotherapy of the oral cavity and pharynx, patients can experience either heightened or suppressed taste sensation. Loss of taste is severe and rapid after oropharyngeal irradiation, as measured by quantitative tests of sensitivity to sour, sweet, and bitter substances. Fortunately, patients often regain preradiation taste sensitivity 60 to 120 days after therapy is completed.

Radiation to the head and neck may inhibit adequate salivation, leading to changes in eating habits. Also, patients may experience increased sensitivity of their teeth to extreme temperature and sweetness. In a study of weight loss during a 6- to 8-week course of external beam radiation therapy to the head and neck regions, 93% of 114 patients lost an average of 3.7 kg. In addition, approximately 9% of individuals lost more than one tenth of their body weight during their 6- to 8-week course of radiation (14).

Radiation to the gastric area and small and large intestine is associated with various complications that may influence nutritional status. Low doses of gastric irradiation reduce gastric acidity whereas higher doses may induce ulcer formation. Nausea, vomiting, and diarrhea are common in individuals undergoing radiation to the small and large bowel. In addition, chronic diarrhea or bowel obstruction may develop due to radiation-induced enteritis following high-dose GI irradiation.

Upper abdominal radiation may produce radiation-induced hepatitis, characterized by anorexia, nausea, vomiting, and abdominal distention. This disorder is usually temporary. Radiation to the pancreas may similarly result in acute anorexia, nausea, and vomiting.

TABLE 67.2

ETIOLOGY OF THE ANOREXIA-CACHEXIA SYNDROME

Direct and indirect tumor effects
    Change in taste
    Dysphagia
    Pain
    Gastrointestinal tract obstruction
    Early satiety
    Anorectic factors (cytokines) produced by tumor or host
Antineoplastic therapy
    Chemotherapy
    Radiotherapy
    Anorexia/anosmia
    Nausea
    Mucosal/ulcerations/infections

Chemotherapy

Chemotherapy can affect host tissue in addition to the targeted neoplasm and thereby cause short-term nutritional defects. Many chemotherapies and immunotherapy products can produce nausea, vomiting, and diarrhea. This can lead to anorexia, electrolyte imbalance, and malnutrition.

Mucosal toxicity, manifested as oral ulcerations, cheilosis, glossitis, and pharyngitis, may be inevitable with the use of some chemotherapeutic agents. This often leads to odynophagia and anorexia. Specific agents, such as actinomycin D, cytarabine, 5-fluorouracil, hydroxyurea, and methotrexate, can produce ulcerations of the entire GI epithelium (15). Therapy itself does not induce malabsorption but, because of its side effects, can aggravate the effect of tumor-related malabsorption syndromes (15). With either a single agent or combination chemotherapy, small intestinal absorptive function remains well preserved in most instances. Nutrition support is usually unnecessary in the initially well nourished patient if the ill effects of chemotherapy are significantly limited in time and intensity.

Multiple major organ systems are affected by chemotherapeutic agents which results in decreased efficiency of metabolism. The liver is especially vulnerable, and hepatic injury is commonly associated with anorexia. Diffuse hepatocellular damage often results in hypoalbuminemia. Several additional agents affect other organ systems. Hydroxyurea may cause renal impairment. Doxorubicin may cause cardiac toxicity leading to congestive heart failure, water retention, and electrolyte imbalance. Carter (16) provides extensive discussions of the nutritional consequences of chemotherapy and immunotherapy.

Surgery

Nutritional depletion can be attributed to surgical intervention in many cancer patients. Nutrition support can be a beneficial tool, as a patient with good nutritional status develops fewer postoperative complications. Poor nutritional status can affect wound healing immune function and several studies have shown that when patients with severe malnutrition receive nutritional support the complication rate improves (4–6).

Certain surgical procedures may require nutritional intervention. Surgery of the upper GI tract can compromise a patient's ability to take oral feedings. Conditions associated with esophagectomy and esophageal reconstruction may include delayed gastric emptying secondary to vagotomy, malabsorption, and the development of a fistula or stenosis. Gastric surgery may result in dumping syndrome, malabsorption, and/or hypoglycemia.

The site and extent of intestinal resection can result in a variety of nutritional complications. Jejunal resection can decrease the efficiency of absorption of carbohydrates, protein, fat, water, and electrolytes. Ileum resection commonly results in vitamin B_{12} deficiency and bile salt losses. With extensive small bowel resection, malabsorption can result. Abnormalities in sodium and water balance are commonly associated with ileostomy and colostomy formation. In addition, gastric and intestinal bypass surgery to relieve obstruction can result in a blind loop syndrome with specific nutritional deficiencies.

Individuals with pancreatic cancer should be nutritionally assessed because they frequently lose weight before their diagnosis and surgical intervention. After pancreatectomy, malabsorption as well as endocrine and exocrine insufficiency are common problems that may require insulin and pancreatic enzyme replacement. Patients with cancer undergoing uretero-sigmoidostomy may experience hyperchloremic acidosis and hypokalemia in addition to other more common postoperative problems.

If it is anticipated that nutritional intervention will be required postoperatively, a nasoenteric feeding tube can be placed intraoperatively. With patients in whom a longer recuperative course is anticipated, surgical placement of a gastrostomy tube or jejunostomy tube may be more appropriate.

Carbohydrate Metabolism

Abnormal glucose metabolism, a major source of caloric wasting, is a hallmark of cancer cachexia (17). Both, increased glucose production and utilization as well as insulin resistance are characteristic. Glucose intolerance may be attributable to a reduced tissue sensitivity to insulin (17). There may be decreased pancreatic β-cell receptor sensitivity in patients with cancer as well, leading to inadequate insulin release in response to a glucose load. Such abnormalities in peripheral glucose metabolism simulate a type II diabetic state and also share elements similar to the stress state (17).

An increase in gluconeogenesis in the liver of the patient with cancer is a common finding. This can be the result of an increased release of glucogenic fuel substrates, such as lactate and alanine, as well as an increased induction of hepatic gluconeogenetic enzymes (17–19). The energy drain created by increased hepatic gluconeogenesis leads to host depletion of protein and calories. Elevation level of hepatic glucose production in a tumor-bearing host requires energy; three moles of adenosine triphosphate are necessary to convert each mole of lactate to glucose. Therefore, abnormal glucose kinetics can result in calorie-consuming futile metabolic cycles, with a drain on host energy. Patients with cancer who lose weight may exhibit increases in glucose flux and glucose oxidation rates. This mechanism is central in the development of host depletion in cachexia, although the energy expenditure involved in these processes suggests that they are more likely associative than causative (20,21).

Protein Metabolism

Cancer anorexia is accompanied by wasting of host protein mass, leading to fatigue, weakness, and altered host cell-mediated immune response. Clinical signs include skeletal muscle and visceral organ atrophy, hypoalbuminemia, and anergy. Host protein wasting results from alterations in total body protein turnover, muscle protein synthesis and catabolism, hepatic protein metabolism, and plasma secretory protein levels. Several studies have shown that cachectic cancer patients have elevated rates of protein turnover and that the normal adaptation of reduced protein metabolism (i.e., protein sparing) in the setting of starvation does not occur (22). With nutritional depletion, patients with cancer anorexia continue to manifest elevated rates of skeletal protein mobilization rather than the normal response of decreased protein turnover and protein sparing. Protein turnover rates in cachectic patients with cancer are significantly higher compared with similarly malnourished control patients without cancer. A loss of less than 100 g of protein nitrogen or 625 g of body protein equal to 2.5 kg of lean body mass can produce mild protein malnutrition, fatigue, weakness, and altered immune response (23). Explanations for this phenomenon of increased nitrogen turnover remain controversial. However, the findings suggest an injury response to cancer with the tumor acting as a "nitrogen sink."

Lipid Metabolism

The most common impairments in lipid metabolism seen in patients with cancer are hyperlipidemia and depletion of fat stores (24–26). Abnormal lipoprotein lipase activity alters the ability of fatty acids to be utilized as protein-sparing energy fuels and is a major cause of protein malnutrition. The hyperlipidemia seen in patients with cancer is significant and may play a role in disease outcome. Elevated lipid levels may have an inhibitory effect on monocytes and macrophages. The combination of increased lipolysis, fatty acid recycling through very low density lipoprotein, and the impairment of lipoprotein lipase enzyme activity leading to decreased lipid clearance can be immunosuppressive.

Suppression of lipoprotein lipase occurs in patients with cancer, but the mechanism is different from that which occurs in starvation. In the latter, lipid mobilization occurs despite a decrease in lipoprotein lipase activity because of a 50% decrease in plasma insulin levels. Vlassara et al. (27) have shown that cancer-associated reductions in plasma lipoprotein lipase are accompanied by normal or even increased insulin levels. This represents a maladaptive host response, since insulin promotes lipid storage, not fat oxidation. Impaired glucose and fat oxidation provide a sink for loss of gluconeogenic amino acids, therefore producing an energy deficit and malnutrition.

Biochemical Mediators of the Anorexia-Cachexia Syndrome

The anorexia-cachexia syndrome incorporates a group of symptoms and signs such as inanition, severe anorexia, weakness, skeletal muscle wasting, organ dysfunction, and progressive weight loss. Physiologically it is characterized by dramatic loss of triglycerides from adipose tissue and loss of visceral and skeletal protein mass (28). Potential etiologies of cancer anorexia are listed in Table 67.2. Cachexia was previously thought to be the result of increased energy demanded by the growing tumor mass. Recent research has demonstrated that it is primarily due to immune mediators [e.g., tumor necrosis factor (TNF), interluekin-6, and eicosanoids], and tumor byproducts (e.g., proteolysis—inducing factor, lipolytic hormone) causing abnormalities in carbohydrate, protein, and lipid metabolism (11). This means that anorexia, an almost universal characteristic of cachexia, should be interpreted as the result of metabolic abnormalities rather than the main cause of cachexia, and that the weight loss seen is not simply a result of decreased caloric intake. In addition to risks that worsening nutritional status has on complication rates of surgery, radiation therapy, and chemotherapy, the cachexia and anorexia are also a source of psychological distress for patients and their families (12).

There has been much interest in the possible role of cytokines in cancer anorexia. Prominent cytokines include TNF, interleukin-1α, and β (IL-1), interleukin-6 (IL-6), interferon-α (IFN-α), and differentiation factor, also known as *leukemia inhibitory factor* (29,30). The peptides are pyrogens, and their administration, with the exception of IL-6, can produce many of the systemic vascular effects seen in sepsis and shock. For example, IL-1 and TNF-α share the capacity to up-regulate gene transcription of endothelial cell adhesion molecules, increase procoagulant activity, promote the transendothelial migration of leukocytes out of the vascular component into the pulmonary epithelium, and activate the release of toxic superoxide and other enzyme products from neutrophils (31).

Features of cancer cachexia can also be reproduced by cytokine administration. For example, IL-1 (32) and, to a lesser extent, TNF-α (33) and IFN-α (34) are potent anorexia-producing agents. Some cytokine effects are mediated through the hypothalamus (32), and others act directly on the GI tract, causing decreased gastric emptying (33). Other cytokines may promote cachexia by increasing resting energy expenditure. Warren et al. (35). reported that patients with cancer receiving cytokines as antineoplastic therapy had a dose-dependent increase in resting energy expenditure.

A mechanism proposed by Kern and Norton (2) to explain the anorexia and metabolic derangements of the anorexia-cachexia syndrome is shown in Figure 67.1. Some cancers incite a paracrine-induced systemic host response with production of cytokines such as interleukins or cachectin/TNF. These are secreted by immune cells and may be part of the host defense in an attempt to destroy the tumor. However, cytokines have negative secondary effects on host organs, resulting in anorexia and abnormalities in carbohydrate, protein, and lipid metabolism. Mobilization of nutrients from fat and skeletal muscle during the acute phase of sepsis or in patients with trauma rapidly provides a physiologic source of nutrients to the liver so that it can synthesize acute injury proteins. In a patient with cancer, the low-grade release of cytokines persists because of the metabolic activity of the tumor and eventually causes severe depletion of host cell mass, skeletal muscle wasting, and abnormal lipolysis. The anorexia of chemotherapy, radiotherapy, or surgery only exacerbates this process, adding to the net effect of host depletion. The "at-risk" patient with cancer can be identified by a rapid weight loss of greater than 10% of usual body weight.

There are other prominent mediators aside from cytokines that appear to play a prominent role in skeletal muscle wasting. A 24-kilodalton proteoglycan, called *proteolysis-inducing factor* (PIF), was identified in the murine MAC16 colonic adenocarcinoma model of anorexia. This factor was subsequently identified in the urine of weight-losing patients with cancer but not in the urine of weight-stable patients with cancer or weight-losing controls with benign disease (29,36,37). There is also some evidence that eicosanoids play a role in the metabolic affects PIF and affect protein and fat metabolism (38,39).

Although the murine MAC16 model demonstrates muscle wasting to PIF and not to certain cytokines, there are other models that show similar metabolic activity with cytokine production but do not demonstrate activity of PIF. One final pathway of these multiple mediators of skeletal muscle

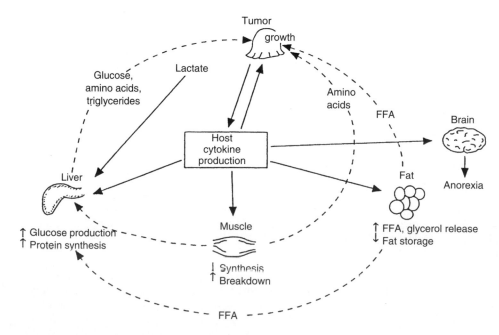

FIGURE 67.1. Proposed mechanism of the cancer anorexia syndrome. Tumor–host interaction results in production of metabolically active cytokines that cause anorexia and abnormalities in host intermediary metabolism. FFA, free fatty acids. (From Kern KA, Norton JA. Cancer cachexia. *JPEN J Parenter Enteral Nutr* 1988;12:286–298, with permission.)

catabolism could be the ATP-ubiquitin-proteasome pathway. In fact, animal studies have shown that both TNF and PIF can increase proteasome activity (38,40,41). This suggests that these multiple mediators may share a common downstream affect on catabolism (11).

Fordy et al. reported that patients with significant weight loss from colorectal liver metastases required a large tumor volume (42). This weight loss was not explained by changes in diet, quality of life, or hormones, but activation of the innate immune systems and incomplete activation of the acquired immune systems were likely to be involved. Agents that attenuate either the acute-phase inflammatory response or T lymphocyte IL-2 receptor up-regulation might reduce weight loss in patients with metastatic disease (42). Some studies have looked at targeting other inflammatory mediators like eicosanoids with NSAIDs or COX2 inhibitors as a means of preventing weight loss (43). The final role anticatabolic medications will play in reversing the weight loss seen in cancer cachexia has yet to be determined.

Preventing malnutrition is easier than reversing it. Reversing malnutrition in a patient with advanced cancer is nearly impossible. Patients with cancer often lose weight and become malnourished at a time when they most need nutrition support (44). Current pharmacologic therapies as well as complementary and alternative methods are recommended for patients with cancer cachexia (45). In recent years, anabolic medications, such as corticosteroids and progestational drugs, have proven effective in relieving symptoms of cancer cachexia. Corticosteroids have a limited effect (lasting up to 4 weeks) on symptoms such as appetite, food intake, sense of well-being and performance status, but none of the studies proved that patients had weight gain (12). Recent studies involving terminally ill patients have shown that progestational drugs improved the symptoms of fatigue and anorexia even in the absence of weight gain. If abruptly discontinued, both megestrol and medroxyprogesterone could induce thromboembolic phenomena, breakthrough vaginal bleeding, peripheral edema, hyperglycemia, hypertension, Cushing's syndrome, alopecia, adrenal suppression, and adrenal insufficiency. However, in most clinical trials, the adverse effects rarely led patients to discontinue these drugs. There has also been much interest in appetite stimulants (Cannaboids) and anticatabolic medications (eicosapentaenoic acid, pentoxifylline), but the most consistent data so far has been for megestrol and medroxyprogesterone (12,46).

ADJUNCTIVE NUTRITION SUPPORT DURING ANTINEOPLASTIC TREATMENT

The goal of nutritional care in the cancer patient should always be considered supportive whether the aim of primary therapy is cure or palliation. Nutritional therapy should be aimed at improving metabolic status, body composition, functional status, and, ultimately, quality of life. Nutrition support can prevent further deterioration in all of these parameters. However, because of the metabolic derangements of cancer cachexia, attempts to reverse severe nutritional depletion are almost universally unsuccessful.

A concern also exists about the possibility of disproportionately stimulating tumor growth while trying to replete the malnourished cancer patient, but recent work has not supported this theory (47,48). Undoubtedly in a cachectic noncancer patient receiving either total parenteral nutrition (TPN) or enteral feeding, nitrogen balance, wound healing, and outcome are improved. However, controversy continues about the role of nutrition support in patients with cancer. In the setting of chemotherapy, the risk of providing nutrition

support inappropriately must be foremost in clinical decision making. TPN is not indicated for patients with advanced metastatic cancer who are not receiving antineoplastic treatment, and the routine use of TPN in patients with cancer who can tolerate enteral nutrition is unjustified. The potential adverse consequences of nutrition support in the setting of cancer make it important to establish the therapeutic benefits before the initiation.

"If the gut works, use it" has become the motto of most nutrition support teams around the country. The use of the GI tract is encouraged whenever possible because it is safe, physiologic, and cost effective. There is also evidence that enteral nutrition may improve visceral protein synthesis. In addition, enteral feeding is superior to TPN in supporting GI mucosal growth and function. This may be important for critically ill patients in whom the gut mucosal barrier may become compromised.

Nutrition Support in Patients Treated with Chemotherapy and Radiotherapy

Currently, in the patient with advanced cancer the literature does not support routine use of TPN or enteral feeding (49). Two older metaanalytic reviews (50,51) concluded that TPN provided no added benefits in terms of survival, tumor response, or chemotherapy toxicity. Also, the American College of Physicians recommended against using TPN routinely in patients undergoing chemotherapy. The studies examining TPN in radiation therapy similarly show lack of benefit. TPN unfortunately was found to have more infectious complications. Studies evaluating enteral feeding in patients receiving chemotherapy or radiation therapy also could not show a consistent benefit. However, there is some data in patients with bone marrow transplants (see in the following text) or cancers of the head and neck that suggest that nutritional therapy either improves outcome or quality of life. For patients with advanced head and neck cancer who are usually underweight at the start of therapy, chemoradiation therapy is associated with significant mucosal toxicity and there has been interest in prophylactic nutritional support. Data in these patients suggest that enteral feedings can improve quality of life, reduce hospitalizations, and reduce interruptions in treatment (13), although there is still some debate as to which is the best mode of delivery (52,53). So, although routine use of nutritional support is not recommended for all patients undergoing chemo or radiation therapy, nutritional therapy should be considered for those patients who have severe malnourishment, a prolonged treatment related anorexia, or for patients whose malnutrition is a major obstacle to a continued reasonable quality of life (54).

Nutrition Support in Patients Treated with Bone Marrow Transplantation

Bone marrow transplantation (BMT) requires intensive chemotherapy and often radiation. This can lead to mucositis, esophagitis, nausea, diarrhea, and graft versus host disease, all of which may compromise a patient's ability to maintain adequate oral intake. Many patients undergoing BMT are routinely started on parenteral nutrition. In a 1987 study, Weisdorf et al. (55). reported increased survival in patients undergoing BMT who received TPN as compared with controls who received maintenance intravenous fluids. Other studies suggested that TPN was associated with a higher rate of infections (56). A study by Iestra et al. (57) attempted to identify subsets of patients that would benefit from TPN and found that when using the indications of severe malnutrition on admission, a prolonged period of minimal oral intake, and clinical weight loss of over 10%, TPN was required in about one third of autologous BMT recipients conditioned without total body irradiation (for lymphoma) compared with 92% of recipients of a mismatched graft. In another recent study on autologous BMT, TPN was associated with a significant preservation of weight compared with controls on oral diets and showed trends toward better quality of life and infections. The authors concluded that in autologous BMT, TPN was better suited for patients with malnutrition or unable to take an oral diet (58).

There has also been several studies looking at the effect of specialized nutrition support in patients undergoing BMT. Glutamine is an amino acid that helps attenuate mucosal damage in the GI tract caused by chemotherapy and radiation, thereby decreasing bacterial translocation and bacteremia. Glutamine-enriched TPN is hypothesized to decrease the occurrence of systemic infection in predisposed patients. In one study (59) Ziegler et al. reported similar survival but decreased infection rates and shortened length of stay in patients receiving glutamine-TPN versus those receiving standard TPN. However, Schloerb et al. (60) performed a recent randomized double-blind trial with oral and parenteral glutamine in patients with both hematologic and solid tumors. Although there is a suggestion of improved long-term survival, similar rates of survival, infections, and length of hospitalization were seen in both hematologic and solid tumors.

In conclusion, most clinical trials failed to demonstrate the clinical efficacy of providing routine nutritional support to most patients with cancer. However, there are some selected cases where nutritional support seems to be beneficial. These would include patients who are severely malnourished or who are at risk of becoming so, severely malnourished patients with cancer needing to undergo major surgery, and patients undergoing bone marrow transplant.

Nutrition Support in the Perioperative Setting

Presurgical and postsurgical nutritional therapy has been investigated extensively in the literature for both, patients with and without cancer. Malnourished patients have increased morbidity and mortality postoperatively. The question remains if perioperative nutrition, either enteral or parenteral, can change this outcome. Many of the older studies differ in terms of study size, patient population, methods, and end points and the conclusions are not consistent. Two older meta-analytic reviews found that the combined morbidity or mortality of perioperative TPN was one half to two thirds that of the control group (50,61). A large multicenter Veterans Affairs study (10) examined preoperative and postoperative TPN in patients receiving abdominal and thoracic surgeries against control groups who received enteral nutrition or no nutrition. Mildly or moderately malnourished patients treated with TPN actually experienced more infectious complications than controls, but the severely malnourished patients experienced a significant comparative decrease in noninfectious complications. The benefit in severely malnourished patients was also observed in a study on patients with gastric or colorectal cancer who had lost over 10% of their body weight (4). TPN given 10 days before and 9 days after surgery was associated with fewer postoperative complications compared with controls who received only postoperative supplementation, with the bulk of the improvement seen from a reduction in infectious complications. In contrast, a study on postoperative TPN given to patients undergoing major pancreatic resection for malignancy noted a higher major complication rate, mostly infections relating to abscess formation rather than catheter-related complications (62). A more recent meta-analysis also found that perioperative TPN had a trend toward fewer complications, although the mortality rates did not differ (6).

However, this trend was seen in studies done before 1988 with less rigorous methodology and the authors concluded that the benefit of TPN was more likely to occur in severely malnourished patients.

The literature supporting perioperative enteral feedings is less ambiguous. Many trials initially showed similar lengths of hospital stay and perioperative mortality in enterally fed patients compared with control groups. An older study looking at the effect of postoperative jejunostomy tube feeding with a formula enriched with arginine, ribonucleic acids, and omega-3 fatty acids in patients with cancer reported fewer complications and shortened length of stay compared with patients receiving a standard formula (63). And in a recent large prospective randomized Italian study, enteral feeding was compared to parenteral nutrition in malnourished patients with GI malignancy (5). The authors found that in the enterally fed group, postoperative complications were reduced and hospital stay decreased from 15.0 to 13.6 days and they felt that the differences were not due to an increase in complications from TPN.

GUIDELINES AND RISK FACTOR ASSESSMENT FOR NUTRITION SUPPORT

Global Assessment Tools

All critically ill patients require a thorough nutritional assessment to determine who is likely to benefit from nutrition support and whether nutrition is to be provided through an enteral route, parenteral route, or a combination. The implementation of nutrition support teams as well as proper guidelines and protocols for surveillance are the first steps

TABLE 67.3

NUTRITIONAL ASSESSMENT PARAMETERS

Parameters	Standards
Initial evaluation	
Body mass index (kg/m^2)	
Rate weight loss (% weight loss/time)	(see Table 67.5)
Serum albumin (g/dL)	>3.5 g/dL
Comprehensive evaluation	
Anthropometrics	
Triceps skinfold (mm)	
Arm muscle circumference	
Biochemical indices	
Urine	
Creatine height index	
Urine urea nitrogen	6–7 g/24 h
Nitrogen balance	0–1 g/24 h
Catabolic index	(see text)
Serum	
Transferrin (g/dL)	>170 g/dL
Total lymphocyte count	>1500 cells/mm^3
Prealbumin	18–45 mg/dL
Immune function: delayed hypersensitivity	
Skin tests	
Candida	>5-mm induration
Mumps	>5-mm erythema/induration
Tetanus toxoid	>5-mm induration

in ensuring that malnourished patients are identified through nutritional screening (Table 67.3). The principal factors that determine who will need nutrition support include current nutritional status, recent weight loss, the anticipated duration of inadequate nutrient intake, and the presence and degree of the stress response. A nutritional assessment begins with a thorough history and physical examination. Other simple assessment measures which can be used initially to screen for protein calorie malnutrition include height and weight to determine body mass index (BMI) (64), percent of regular weight lost, serum protein levels (albumin, prealbumin, transferrin), and anthropomorphics. Although each of these measures have their drawbacks, they are sensitive enough to identify most patients with protein calorie malnutrition. Other indicators from the Nutrition Screening Initiative level II screen (65) include midarm muscle circumference, triceps skinfold, and serum cholesterol. In addition, clinical history, drug use, eating habits, living environment and income, and functional status, as well as mental and cognitive functioning, need to be assessed.

Among the many indices that have been proposed, perhaps the most beneficial tool for nutritional screening in the patient with cancer is the Subjective Global Assessment (SGA) (Table 67.4) modified by Ottery (66,67) for the practicing oncologist and other health care providers. The original SGA (68) estimates nutritional status on the basis of medical history (i.e., weight and weight history, dietary intake, GI symptoms with >2 weeks duration, functional status, and metabolic demands) and physical examination (five determinations of muscle, fat, and fluid status) (69). On the basis of these features, the patient is categorized as (a) well nourished, (b) having moderate or suspected malnutrition, or (c) having severe malnutrition (70). Two modifications of the SGA have been developed specifically for use in patients with cancer (66,67). Figure 67.2 demonstrates an algorithm for optimal nutritional oncology intervention based on the SGA (71).

Individual Screening Tools

Body Mass Index

The BMI may be a useful tool to identify individuals at risk for protein calorie malnutrition as it normalizes body weight for height and is independent of sex.

$$BMI = weight\ (kg)/height\ (m^2)$$

A BMI of less than 22 may be indicative of possible protein calorie malnutrition, especially among patients with cancer and a value less than 18 is consistent with significant malnutrition.

TABLE 67.4

PATIENT-GENERATED SUBJECTIVE GLOBAL ASSESSMENT OF NUTRITIONAL STATUS

History	Functional capacity
Weight change: I weigh about ____ pounds I am about __ feet and __ inches tall A year ago I weighed about ____ pounds Six months ago I weighed about ____ pounds During the past 2 weeks my weight has: ____ decreased ____ not changed ____ increased I would rate my food intake during the past month (compared to my normal) as: ____ no change ____ changed ____ more than usual ____ much less than usual ____ taking little solid food ____ taking only liquids ____ taking only nutritional supplements ____ really taking in very little of anything Over the past 2 weeks I have had the following problems that keep me from eating enough (check all that apply): ____ no problems eating ____ no appetite, just did not feel like eating ____ nausea ____ vomiting ____ diarrhea ____ constipation ____ mouth sores ____ dry mouth ____ pain ____ things taste funny or have no taste ____ smells bother me __ other	Over the past month I would rate my activity as generally: ____ 0 = normal, no limitations ____ 1 = not my normal self but able to be up and about with fairly normal activities ____ 2 = not feeling up to most things but in bed less than half the day ____ 3 = able to do little activity and I spend most of the day in bed or chair ____ 4 = pretty much bedridden (rarely out of bed) The remainder of this form will be filled in by your doctor, nurse, or therapist. Thank you. Disease and its relation to nutrition requirements: Primary diagnosis _____ (stage, if known _____)[a] Metabolic demand (stress): ____ no stress ____ low stress ____ moderate stress ____ high stress Physical (for each trait specify: 0 = normal, 1 + = mild, 2 + = moderate, 3 + = severe) ____ loss of subcutaneous fat (triceps, chest) ____ muscle wasting (quadriceps, deltoid) ____ ankle edema ____ sacral edema ____ ascites Selective global assessment rating (select one) ____ A = well nourished ____ B = moderately (or suspected of being) malnourished ____ C = severely malnourished

[a]Modification of the original selective global assessment for oncology patients (69).

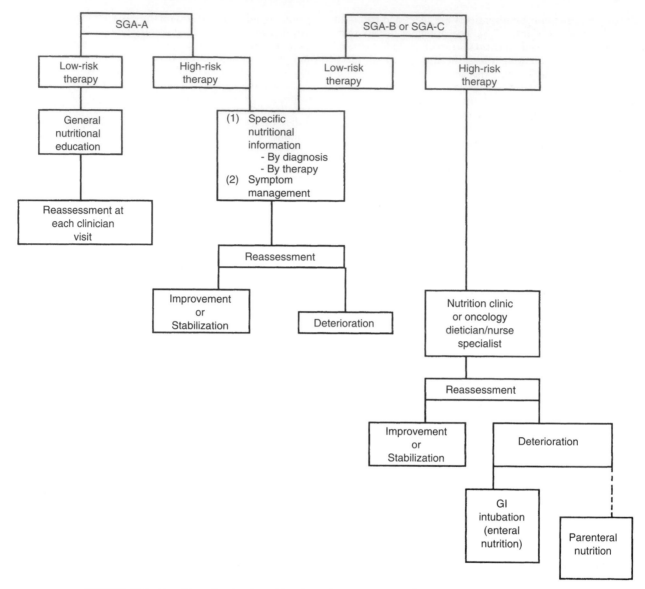

FIGURE 67.2. Algorithm of optimal nutritional oncology intervention: baseline nutritional status (SGA). "Risk" refers to nutritional risk. *GI*, gastrointestinal; *SGA*, subjective global assessment; *SGA-A*, well nourished; *SGA-B*, moderately malnourished; *SGA-C*, severely malnourished. (From Kern KA, Norton JA. Cancer cachexia. *JPEN J Parenter Enteral Nutr* 1988;12:286–298, with permission.)

Weight Loss

Documentation of the patient's weight history is an important and easily obtainable index for the suspected presence or progression of malignancy. Weight alone may be a poor indicator of short-term nutritional status as fluctuations in total body water may cause significant weight changes. There are several parameters available to interpret weight measurements including the weight/height index and the percentage of weight lost. Because the patient's height remains essentially constant, the weight/height index remains a reliable tool for estimating nutritional status. An index less than 90% of standard would suggest moderate nutritional risk whereas a weight/height index less than 75% of standard suggests severe malnutrition.

Table 67.5 focuses on the percentage of regular weight lost. This too can be a good indication of the severity of nutritional deficiency. For example, "severe" weight loss should be considered with a 5% loss of body weight in 1 month or a 10% loss within 6 months (72).

Serum Albumin and Prealbumin

Serum albumin concentration is a commonly used index of nutritional status. Albumin, synthesized in the liver, has a half-life of approximately 20 days with normal serum concentrations of greater than 3.5 g/dL (Table 67.3).

As a nutritional marker, serum albumin concentrations may be beneficial for detecting malnutrition. Table 67.6 demonstrates that, in hospitalized patients, hypoalbuminemia is associated not only with anergic immune status but with increased morbidity and mortality, and is a poor prognostic indicator (73).

There are limitations to the use of serum albumin concentration as a nutritional index for stressed and critically ill patients. During an acute illness or stress, such as injury, infection, or surgery, serum albumin synthesis decreases. Albumin concentrations can also be affected by fluid status, volume repletion, heart disease, renal disease, and liver disease. In addition, due to the long half-life, serum albumin does not respond on a daily or weekly basis to nutrition support. This has

TABLE 67.5

EVALUATION OF WEIGHT CHANGE

	Significant weight loss (%)	Severe weight loss (%)
1 wk	1–2[a]	>2
1 mo	5	>50
3 mo	7.5	>7.5
6 mo	10	>10

[a]Percent weight change, usual weight—actual weight divided by 100 ∞ usual weight.
From Blackburn GL, Harvey KB. Nutritional assessment as a routine in clinical medicine. *Postgrad Med* 1982;71:46, with permission.

led to use of measuring prealbumin for short-term assessment of nutrition. Although concentrations can be decreased for the same reasons as serum albumin, the half-life of prealbumin is on the order of 1 to 2 days.

Transferrin

Transferrin is a 90-kd globulin that binds and transports iron. The half-life of transferrin, which is primarily synthesized in the liver, is 8 to 10 days. Visceral protein depletion is reflected with transferrin levels less than 170 g/dL. This makes it more sensitive than albumin as an index of improvement in nutritional status. There are, however, two instances when transferrin levels are unreliable for nutritional status: in iron-deficient or iron-overloaded patients who tend to show high and low transferrin levels, respectively, and in patients who have had multiple transfusions (74).

Anthropometrics

Anthropometric techniques are tools that may be beneficial in defining fat stores in the patient with cancer. One of the major sites of fat deposition in the human body is the subcutaneous space (75). Subcutaneous fat represents approximately 30% and 33% of total body fat in men and women, respectively; these numbers vary according to age, level of obesity, and measurement techniques (76).

A useful anthropometric assessment of body fat mass is the triceps skinfold (TSF) measurement. This measurement is performed by using large calipers at the upper left arm. Knowing the TSF, one can derive the more valuable arm muscle circumference (AMC):

$$AMC = \text{arm circumference} - TSF$$

The AMC is compared with standard tables and values less than 60% of standard are consistent with protein depletion (75). As with all anthropometric techniques, interobserver

TABLE 67.6

PROBABILITY ESTIMATES USING SERUM ALBUMIN

	<10%	<25%	50%	>75%	>90%
Anergy	5.2	4.2	3.2	2.2	1.2
Sepsis	4.3	3.7	3.1	2.5	1.9
Death	4.9	4.0	3.2	2.3	1.5

From Langstein HN, Norton JA. Mechanisms of cancer cachexia. *Hematol Oncol Clin North Am* 1991;5:103–123, with permission.

and intraobserver variation ranges from 15% to 20%, and the exact correlation between upper arm circumference and total body protein stores is unknown.

Delayed Hypersensitivity

Assessment of the function of the cellular immune system through delayed hypersensitivity testing to common skin antigens can be a marker of nutritional status. Anergy has been correlated with an increased incidence of postoperative morbidity and mortality in older studies (77). The common recall antigens used are *Candida*, mumps, dermatophytes, or tetanus toxoid. After 24 to 48 hours, 5 mm or greater of induration is considered a positive response. Cellular immunity is most sensitive to malnutrition, but protein deficiency also reflects leukocyte function, particularly immune cell activation and cytokine release.

Evaluation of Ongoing Nutrition Support

Patients undergoing administration of nutrition support require assessment of several parameters to tailor daily requirements of specific nutrients. Many of these parameters, notably serum albumin, AMC, and BMI, are not sensitive enough to detect the short-term effects of nutrition support. In addition to daily electrolyte determinations, physical examination, and accurate body weights, other parameters, such as nitrogen balance, may be more beneficial in assessing the impact of nutritional therapy on a short-term basis.

Health care providers must, however, differentiate an increase in weight caused by fluid retention from lean body mass. Malnourished patients who are suddenly overfed can develop an increase in intravascular volume, congestive heart failure, and electrolyte abnormalities, which can be fatal (78).

Nitrogen Balance

The nitrogen balance determination is a dependable measure that can reflect the influence of nutrition support on lean body mass. Nitrogen balance reflects the difference between nitrogen intake versus output over a 24-hour period. With 1 g of nitrogen representing 6.25 g of protein, the nitrogen balance is calculated as

$$\text{Nitrogen balance} = \text{Nitrogen intake} - \text{Nitrogen loss}$$
$$= [\text{protein intake}/6.25] - (\text{Urine urea nitrogen} + 4)$$

The principal form of urine nitrogen is called *urine urea nitrogen*, which can be easily measured. Urea excreted in the urine reflects protein degradation. In addition to urea, other forms of nitrogen are excreted, including nonurea urine nitrogen, fecal nitrogen, and integumental nitrogen. These are lost at a fairly constant rate except when diarrhea is present. In calculating nitrogen loss, 4 g is added to the nitrogen output as an estimate of fecal and integumental losses.

NUTRITION SUPPORT

Parenteral Nutritional Requirements

Caloric Requirements

The primary goal of parenteral and enteral nutrition support is to supply adequate protein and nonprotein calories to prevent further catabolism and to promote the accrual of protein. The goals of parenteral and enteral nutrition remain supportive:

1. Improving wound healing
2. Bolstering immune function
3. Influencing acid-base and mineral homeostasis and
4. Minimizing obligate nitrogen loss in the catabolic postinjury state

These goals are achieved by

1. Providing substrate (protein, carbohydrate, lipid, electrolytes, minerals, and vitamins) for ongoing metabolic functions
2. Improving cardiac and respiratory function by restoring glycogen stores in cardiac and diaphragmatic muscle and
3. Potentially modifying the systemic inflammatory response (72,78,79)

The "gold standard" for estimating basal energy requirements was derived by Harris and Benedict around the turn of the century (80). Basal metabolic requirements (BMRs) can be calculated using the following Harris-Benedict equations:

$$\text{BMR for males} = 66.4730 + (13.7516W)$$
$$+ (5.0033H) - (6.7550A)$$
$$\text{BMR for females} = 65.5095 + (9.563W)$$
$$+ (1.8496H) - (4.6756A)$$

where W is weight in kilograms, H is height in centimeters, and A is age in years.

The mild to moderately stressed patient usually requires 25 to 35 kcal/kg and 1.5 g of protein/kg of ideal body weight in order to maintain positive nitrogen balance. Nonprotein calories are supplied by both carbohydrates and lipids, with glucose being the major energy source for the central nervous system, red blood cells, and renal medulla. These organ systems require a minimum of 100 to 150 g/day (75). The maximal infusion of dextrose given should be 5 mg/kg/minute. Exceeding this rate may lead to hepatic steatosis and excess fat synthesis and carbon dioxide production (75). The caloric density of glucose is 3.4 kcal/g; approximately 60 to 70% of nonprotein calories should be provided as dextrose (79).

Lipid Requirements

Fat emulsions, derived from soybean or safflower oil, provide 2.0 kcal/mL in standard 20% solutions. The usual dose of lipid is 0.5 to 1.0 g/kg/day, with the maximum of 2.5 g/kg/day (81). Lipid emulsions are usually formulated to provide approximately 30% of total nonprotein calories. However, a minimum of 0.5 mg/kg/day is sufficient to prevent essential fatty acid deficiency.

Protein Requirements

The protein requirements for a mild to moderately stressed patient may be estimated at 1.5 to 2.0 g protein/kg based on ideal body weight. Although nonprotein calories may spare nitrogen in the nonstressed state, patients with cancer usually require an infusion of 0.2 to 0.3 g nitrogen/kg/day to maintain a positive nitrogen balance (82).

Fluid Requirements

Fluid requirements depend on baseline requirements, losses, and fluid deficits. Fluid status is dynamic and should be monitored on a constant basis by physical examination and accurate daily weights. The average fluid requirement varies from 1250 to 3000 mL/day, depending on body habitus. The average semistressed patient requires approximately 35 mL/kg/day. A wide array of fluid abnormalities can be seen in patients with cancer due to the disease process and therapies such as surgery, radiation therapy, and chemotherapy.

Electrolytes

Electrolytes are included in all parenteral nutrition solutions. Electrolyte requirements for patients with cancer are essentially the same as for patients with nonmalignant forms of disease.

The electrolyte composition of TPN will be dependent on the hormonal milieu, GI, and pulmonary losses, disease state, and renal and hepatic function (75). In addition, treatment modalities (i.e., amphotericin B administration) can alter electrolyte requirements. Daily serum electrolyte measurements are important to customize the patient's daily nutritional prescription. Limitations exist for calcium, phosphorus, and magnesium in parenteral nutritional solutions. Calcium and phosphorus can form a precipitate if they are not compounded properly or if excessive amounts are added to the solution (83). The pH, temperature, and type of amino acid solution will also affect the compatibility of calcium and phosphorus (84). Hypophosphatemia may result from hyperalimentation without adequate supplementation. A minimum of 20 meq of potassium phosphate per 1000 kcal will usually prevent hypophosphatemia (85).

Enteral Feedings

If the GI tract is intact and functioning, liquid formula diets are preferred. Oral supplements provide an excellent source of calories and protein to bolster a modest oral intake or as an adjunct to hyperalimentation. Unfortunately, patients with cancer often suffer from anorexia, nausea, oropharyngeal obstruction, or central nervous system pathology and cannot meet their caloric needs despite a functioning intestinal tract. These individuals can benefit from tube feeding. Small pliable nasogastric tubes are available and well tolerated by most patients. Delivery methods can be by either bolus feeding, gravity, or mechanical pump systems. In the critically ill patient, the literature supports the use of continuous rather than intermittent tube feeding. In this population, continuous tube feedings have been associated with positive nitrogen balance and weight gain as compared to intermittent tube feedings (86). Continuous tube feedings require less energy expenditure because of diet-induced thermogenesis and have been shown to be effective in the prevention of stress ulceration (87,88).

Although most patients' needs can be met with one or two enteral formulations, there are a myriad of disease-specific products available. Slow rates should be initiated at 10–20 mL/hour and then increased 10 mL every 8 to 12 hours until full flow rates are obtained. There is usually no reason to dilute low-fat, well-tolerated formulas such as Peptamen, Vital, or Vivonex. The patient's head should be maintained at a 30° elevation with nasogastric and nasoduodenal feedings to avoid aspiration. For patients needing chronic enteral feedings, surgical or endoscopically placed gastrostomy or jejunostomy tubes may be beneficial.

Nutritional Adjuncts and Immunonutrition in Cancer Patients

Over the past several decades, our appreciation of the importance of feeding patients who are unable to take in calories adequate for metabolic requirements has increased extensively. As discussed earlier, there have been many studies showing improved outcomes in malnourished patients. In patients with cancer, however, in addition to malnutrition there may also be the affects of altered immune status from cachexia, compromised GI mucosal barriers, bone marrow transplants, and effects of chemotherapy. There has been interest in using adjuncts to enteral or parenteral nutrition to either support immune function or to help curb the catabolic state of the cachexia-anorexia syndrome. Initially, growth hormone showed some promise, but more recent studies have not been as favorable. Takala et al. actually found an increased mortality in critically ill patients given growth hormone (89).

Because of this, growth hormone is not recommended at this time. Special enteral diets have been formulated to contain high amounts of arginine together with omega-3 fatty acids, nucleic acids, and sometimes glutamine. All these substances have been shown to enhance or preserve host immune responses and/or to reduce harmful and exaggerated inflammatory responses. This therapeutic approach has been termed *immunonutrition* (90).

Since 1990, standard enteral and parenteral preparations have been modified by adding immunonutrients. This new category of dietary compounds has peculiar properties. Among the most interesting and carefully investigated immunonutrients are the following:

1. Arginine, which improves macrophage tumor cytotoxic effects, bactericidal activity, and vasodilation through production of nitric oxide; stimulates T-cell proliferation, natural killer cell cytotoxic effects, and generation of lymphokine-activated killer cells; and modulates nitrogen balance and protein synthesis (91)
2. Omega-3 polysaturated fatty acids, derived from fish oil, which are potent anti-inflammatory agents through pathway of coagulation, and upregulate the immune response and
3. Glutamine, which is known to facilitate the transport of nitrogen between organs, reduce the skeletal and intestinal protein waste during stress, enhance macrophage, and neutrophil phagocytosis, and preserve the intestinal permeability by being the major fuel for different cell types (92,93)

Prebiotic bacteria, such as *Lactobacillus plantarum,* seem not only to preserve key nutrients, such as omega-3 fatty acids, but also increase its content during storage conditions. *L. plantarum* competes with gram-negative potential pathogens for receptor sites at the mucosal cell surfaces, eliminates nitrate, and produces nitric oxide; this may help recondition the GI mucosa. To produce a *L. plantarum*–containing formula, a treatment policy is regarded as an extension of the immunonutrition program, and is called *ecoimmunonutrition*. Patients with radiation therapy or cancer are candidates for ecoimmunonutrition (94).

The conception of immunonutrition has gained a great deal of clinical attention, and multiple studies have been performed in a wide variety of settings in an attempt to demonstrate clinical outcome benefits (59,95–99).

Glutamine is a nonessential amino acid that has been noted to be depleted in patients with cancer. Standard TPN solutions do not contain glutamine because of instability issues. Addition of glutamine to TPN formulations has been shown to improve nitrogen balance and promote protein synthesis without stimulating tumor growth (100). There have been multiple studies of glutamine in different patient populations. Ziegler and et al. in a double-blind prospective trial found that patients undergoing bone marrow transplant who received glutamine-enriched TPN had an improved nitrogen balance, fewer infections, and shortened length of hospitalization compared with controls (59). In a small randomized double-blinded study, Morlion and et al. showed that patients undergoing surgery for colorectal cancer had quicker onset of immune recovery and had shorter hospital stays (6.2 days less) if they received glutamine-enriched TPN when compared to patients receiving standard TPN (101). Gianotti and Bragna et al. randomized 305 malnourished patients (<10% weight loss) with GI cancer and compared those receiving enteral feedings with arginine, omega-3 fatty acids, and RNA given preoperatively or pre- and postoperatively, against those receiving no perioperative nutrition. The patients given the perioperative immunonutrition showed improvements in postoperative infections and in length of hospital stay when compared with the control group (96).

It is unlikely that there are adverse effects of immunoenhancing nutrients given the modest amounts of the nutrients that are in the enteral formulas and the relatively short period (e.g., a few weeks) patients are fed formulas with immunoenhancing nutrients. However, any nutrient that can alter immune function needs to be critically evaluated for potential adverse effects. Certain lines of breast cancer cells, for example, may also be stimulated to replicate when large doses of either L-arginine or L-glutamine are administered (102,103). It has been hypothesized that nitric oxide synthesized from L-arginine triggers vascular smooth muscle dilation and could potentially promote septic shock (104). A sheep model of sepsis has demonstrated administration of excessively high amounts (e.g., 200 mg/kg/h) of L-arginine parenterally had adverse outcomes (105). However, this dose of arginine would be equivalent to over 300 g/day for a 70-kg man, which would not occur with the levels found in immunoenhancing formulas.

However, meta-analysis provides the best estimate of overall treatment effect. In two published meta-analyses of immunonutrition, different investigators came up with different estimates of the overall effect on mortality. Heys et al. combined 11 randomized trials of immunonutrition in critically ill and surgical patients (97). However, this meta-analyses did not include several key papers in non-English journals published subsequent to 1998. Subsequently, Beale and et al. aggregated the results of 12 randomized trials of immunonutrition in surgical and critically ill patients. Although there was some overlap between the two meta-analyses, the study by Beale et al. included recently published studies but was limited to studies of Impact (Novartis Nutrition Corp., Bern, Switzerland) and Immun-Aid (McGaw Inc., Irvine, CA) (98). Moreover, Impact and Immun-Aid, the two enteral feeding preparations enriched with these "immunonutrients" that have been developed commercially for critically ill patients, are slightly different in composition. Both of these meta-analyses demonstrated reductions in infectious complications and hospital length of stay, but did not find a mortality benefit. Heyland et al. performed another meta-analysis to include newer studies and to cover the topics the above meta-analysis did not include. He also found a decrease in infections without an overall mortality benefit, but noted that the treatment effect varied depending on patient population (surgical patients had better outcomes than critically ill patients), intervention, and methodologic quality of the study (99).

Home Parenteral and Enteral Nutrition

Oral or tube feedings in the home setting are both financially and physiologically preferred over parenteral nutrition. However, patients who cannot tolerate oral or tube feedings may benefit from home TPN. The technology and science of nutrition support has flourished in the last 20 years but not without a significant increase in costs. It has been estimated that nutrition support accounts for approximately 1% of all health care dollars (106,107). As expected, most of these dollars are spent on hospitalized patients, but approximately 20% are spent on patients living outside the hospital (106). Half of these patients are nursing home residents and half reside at home. Twenty percent of home patients receive parenteral nutrition support and 80% receive enteral nutrition support (106). The cost for enteral feeding is estimated at $15,000/year with home parenteral nutrition support being at least 10 times as costly (107).

Patients with a curable malignancy, who require aggressive primary treatment causing anorexia, nausea, and/or ileus, may benefit from home nutrition support. Other indications for home nutrition support are patients who are "cured" from their primary cancer but are left with bowel dysfunction from irradiation or resection.

A voluntary patient registry, the North American Home Parenteral and Enteral Patient Registry, was formed in 1984 to follow clinical outcomes of home patients receiving home parenteral or enteral nutrition. There are approximately 204 programs with more than 10,000 home nutrition patients registered. The Oley Foundation has published outcomes information on patients registered to date.

For the individual deemed a candidate for home nutrition support, techniques used at home and in the hospital are essentially similar. In the home setting, the patient and the patient's family may take responsibility for solutions administered (108). For parenteral nutrition, central catheter administration is the preferred route for hyperalimentation. This allows provision of adequate calories and protein without large fluid volumes. If possible, a Hickman catheter is preferred because it has two Dacron cuffs that help secure placement and reduce the risk of ascending bacterial infection. Strict sterile technique is essential to reduce the risk of catheter infection and sepsis. Even with precautionary measures, the incidence of catheter-related sepsis is 4.5 to 11.0% (109). In addition to the traditional subclavian or internal jugular central venous access, peripherally inserted central catheters (110,111) can be inserted into the basilic or cephalic vein in the antecubital fossa and threaded into the superior vena cava. Peripherally inserted central catheter lines are safe and reliable central venous access routes for patients receiving parenteral nutrition, long-term antibiotics, and chemotherapy without the complications of pneumothorax or hemopneumothorax. For all patients with intravenous lines, close follow-up with a nutrition support team is important to monitor fever, fluid status, and electrolyte abnormalities. To improve quality of life, patients can have enteral or parenteral feeding cycled at night to allow mobility during the day.

CONCLUSIONS

It is well known that patients with malignancy have a high incidence of malnutrition and cachexia resulting from decreased intake as well as metabolic alterations due to the influence of the tumor. The clinician must not only identify those patients at risk for malnutrition but must also identify those select few who will benefit from nutrition support.

Routine use of TPN in patients with cancer has not been substantiated in the literature (112). The clinician must carefully assess the severity of malnutrition, treatment options, and potential quality of life in a patient with cancer before opting to use nutrition support as an adjunctive therapy. Decisions regarding methods and aggressiveness of the nutritional intervention should be based on these issues as well. The enteral route is always preferable to TPN in terms of physiologic response, immune competence, quality of life, and cost (113).

References

1. Bistrian BR, Blackburn GL, Vitale J, et al. Prevalence of malnutrition in general medical patients. *JAMA* 1976;235:1567–1570.
2. Kern KA, Norton JA. Cancer cachexia. *JPEN J Parenter Enteral Nutr* 1988;12:286–298.
3. DeWys WD, Begg C, Lavin PT, et al. Prognostic effect of weight loss prior to chemotherapy in cancer patients. *Am J Med* 1980;69:491–497.
4. Bozzetti F, Gavazzi C, Miceli R, et al. Perioperative total parenteral nutrition in malnourished, gastrointestinal cancer patients: a randomized, clinical trial. *JPEN J Parenter Enteral Nutr* 2000;24:7.
5. Bozzetti F, Braga M, Gianotti L. Postoperative enteral versus parenteral nutrition in malnourished patients with gastrointestinal cancer: a randomised multicentre trial. *Lancet* 2001;358:1487.
6. Heyland DK, Montalvo M, MacDonald S, et al. Total parenteral nutrition in the surgical patient: a meta-analysis. *Can J Surg* 2001;44:102.
7. Russell MK, Andrews MR, Brewer CK, et al. American Society for Parenteral and Enteral Nutrition Board of Directors Guidelines for the use of parenteral and enteral nutrition in adult and pediatric patients. *JPEN J Parenter Enteral Nutr* 2002;26:SA1–S138.
8. American Gastroenterological Association Medical position statement: parenteral nutrition. *Gastroenterology* 2001;121:966–969.
9. Mcgeer AJ, Detsky AS, O'rourke K. Parenteral nutrition in patients receiving cancer chemotherapy. American College of Physicians. *Ann Intern Med* 1989;110:734.
10. Perioperative total parenteral nutrition in surgical patients. The Veterans Affairs Total Parenteral Nutrition Cooperative Study Group. *N Engl J Med* 1991;325:525.
11. MacDonald N, Easson AM, Mazurak VC. Understanding and managing cancer cachexia. *J Am Coll Surg* 2003;197:143–161.
12. Bruera E. ABC of palliative care, anorexia, cachexia and nutrition. *BMJ* 1997;315:1219–1222.
13. Lee JH, Machtay M, Unger LD, et al. Prophylactic gastrostomy tubes in patients undergoing intensive irradiation for cancer of the head and neck. *Arch Otolaryngol Head Neck Surg* 1998;124:871.
14. Donaldson SS. Nutritional problems associated with radiotherapy. In: Newell GR, Ellison NM, eds. *Nutrition and cancer: etiology and treatment.* New York: Raven Press, 1981.
15. Mitchell EP, Schein PS. Gastrointestinal toxicity of chemotherapeutic agents. *Semin Oncol* 1982;9:52–64.
16. Carter SK. Nutritional problems associated with cancer chemotherapy. In: Newell GR, Ellison NM, eds. *Nutrition and cancer: etiology and treatment.* New York: Raven Press, 1981.
17. Heber D, Byerly LO, Chlebowski RT. Medical abnormalities in the cancer patient. *Cancer* 1985;55:225–229.
18. Lundholm K, Edstrom S, Karlberg I, et al. Glucose turnover, gluconeogenesis from glycerol in estimation of net glucose cycline in cancer patients. *Cancer* 1982;50:1142–1142.
19. Waterhouse C. Lactate metabolism in patients with cancer. *Cancer* 1974; 33:66–71.
20. Norton JA, Burt ME, Brennan MF. *In Vivo* utilization of substrate by human sarcoma-bearing limbs. *Cancer* 1980;45:2934–2939.
21. Warnold I, Lundholm K, Schersten T. Energy balance and body composition in cancer patients. *Cancer Res* 1978;38:1801–1807.
22. Shaw JHF, Humberstone DM, Douglas RG, et al. Leucine kinetics in patients with benign disease, non-weight losing cancer, and cancer cachexia: studies at the whole body and tissue level and the response to nutritional support. *Surgery* 1991;109:37–50.
23. Blackburn GL, Wolfe RR. Clinical biochemistry in intravenous hyperalimentation. In: Alberti KGM, Price CP, eds. *Recent advances in biochemistry.* Edinburgh: Churchill Livingstone, 1981:217–223.
24. Kralovic RC, Zepp A, Canedella RJ. Studies of the mechanism of carcass fat depletion in experimental cancer. *Eur J Cancer* 1977;13:1071–1079.
25. Legaspi A, Jevanandam M, Staves HF, et al. Whole body lipid and energy metabolism in the cancer patient. *Metabolism* 1987;36:958–963.
26. Beck SA, Tisdale MJ. Production of lipolytic and proteolytic factors by a Murine tumor producing cachexia in the host. *Cancer Res* 1987;47: S919–S923.
27. Vlassara H, Spiegel RJ, Doval DS, et al. Reduced plasma lipoprotein lipase activity in patients with malignancy-associated weight loss. *Horm Metab Res* 1986;18:698–703.
28. Tisdale MJ. Protein loss in cancer cachexia. *Science* 2000;289:2293–2294.
29. Todorov P, Cariuk P, McDevitt T, et al. Characterization of a cancer cachectic factor. *Nature* 1996;379:739–742.
30. Guttridge DC, Mayo MW, Madrid LV, et al. NF-[kappa]-induced loss of MyoD messenger RNA: possible role in muscle decay and cachexia. *Science* 2000;289:2363–2366.
31. Moldawer LL, Rogy MA, Flowery SF. The role of cytokines in cancer cachexia. *JPEN J Parenter Enteral Nutr* 1992;16:43S–49S.
32. Uehara A, Sekya C, Takasugi Y, et al. Anorexia induced by interleukin-1: involvement of corticotropin-releasing factor. *Am J Physiol* 1989;257: R613–R617.
33. Bodnar RJ, Pasternak GW, Mann PE, et al. Mediation of anorexia by human recombinant tumor necrosis factor through a peripheral action in the rat. *Cancer Res* 1989;49:6280–6284.
34. Langstein HN, Doherty GM, Frajer DL, et al. The role of alpha interferon and tumor necrosis factor in an experimental rat model of cancer cachexia. *Cancer Res* 1991;51:2302–2306.
35. Warren RS, Starnes HF, Gabrilove JL, et al. The acute metabolic effects of tumor necrosis factor administration in humans. *Arch Surg* 1987;122: 1396–1400.
36. Wigmore SJ, Todorov PT, Barber MD, et al. Characteristics of patients with pancreatic cancer expressing a novel cancer cachectic factor. *Br J Surg* 2000;87:53–58.
37. Cabal-Manzano R, Bhargava P, Torres-Duarte A, et al. Proteolysis-inducing factor is expressed in tumours of patients with gastrointestinal cancers and correlates with weight loss. *Br J Cancer* 2001;84:1599.
38. Lorite MJ, Smith HJ, Arnold JA, et al. Activation of ATP-ubiquitin-dependent proteolysis in skeletal muscle *in vivo* and murine myoblasts *in vitro* by a proteolysis-inducing factor (PIF). *Br J Cancer* 2001;85:297.

39. Ross JA, Fearon KC. Eicosanoid-dependent cancer cachexia and wasting. *Curr Opin Clin Nutr Metab Care* 2002;5:241–248.

40. Baracos VE. Regulation of skeletal-muscle-protein turnover in cancer-associated cachexia. *Nutrition* 2000;16:1015–1018.

41. Llovera M, Garcia-Martinez C, Agell N, et al. TNF can directly induce the expression of ubiquitin-dependent proteolytic system in rat soleus muscles. *Biochem Biophys Res Commun* 1997;230:238.

42. Fordy C, Glover C, Henderson D, et al. Contribution of diet, tumour volume and patient-related factors to weight loss in patients with colorectal liver metastases. *Br J Surg* 1999;86:639–644.

43. Lundholm Ke, Daneryd P, Bosaeus I, et al. Palliative nutritional intervention in addition to cyclooxygenase and erythropoietin treatment for patients with malignant disease: effects on survival, metabolism, and function. *Cancer* 2004;100(9):1967–1977.

44. Wilkes G. Nutrition: the forgotten ingredient in cancer care. *Am J Nurs* 2000;100:46–51.

45. Finley JP. Management of cancer cachexia. *AACN* 2000;11:590–603.

46. Desport JD, Gory-Delabaere G, Blanc-Vincent MP, et al. Standards, options and recommendations for the use of appetite stimulants in oncology (2000). *Br J Cancer* 2003;89(suppl 1):S98–S100.

47. Torosian MH. Stimulation of tumor growth by nutrition support. *JPEN J Parenter Enteral Nutr* 1992;16:72S–75S.

48. Bozzetti F, Gavazzi C, Mariani L, et al. Glucose-based total parenteral nutrition does not stimulate glucose uptake by human tumours. *Clin Nutr* 2004;23:417–421.

49. Klein S, Koretz RL. Nutrition support in patients with cancer: what do the data really show? *Nutr Clin Pract* 1994;9:91–100.

50. Klein S, Simes J, Blackburn G. Total parenteral nutrition and cancer clinical trials. *Cancer* 1986;58:1378–1386.

51. McGeer AJ, Detsky AS, O'Rourke KO. Parenteral nutrition in cancer patients undergoing chemotherapy: a meta-analysis. *Nutrition* 1990;6:233–240.

52. Magne N, Marcy PY, Foa C, et al. Comparison between nasogastric tube feeding and percutaneous fluoroscopic gastrostomy in advanced head and neck cancer patients. *Eur Arch Otorhinolaryngol* 2001;258:89.

53. Mekhail TM, Adelstein DJ, Rybicki LA, et al. Enteral nutrition during the treatment of head and neck carcinoma: is a percutaneous endoscopic gastrostomy tube preferable to a nasogastric tube? *Cancer* 2001;91:1785.

54. Souba WW. Nutritional support. *N Engl J Med* 1997;336(1):41–48.

55. Weisdorf SA, Lysne J, Wind D, et al. Positive effect of prophylactic total parenteral nutrition on long-term outcome of bone marrow transplantation. *Transplantation* 1987;43:833–838.

56. Szeluga DJ, Stuart RK, Brookmeyer R, et al. Nutritional support of bone marrow transplant recipients: a prospective randomized clinical trial comparing total parenteral nutrition to an enteral feeding program. *Cancer Res* 1987;47:3309–3316.

57. Iestra JA, Fibbe WE, Zwinderman AH, et al. Parenteral nutrition following intensive cytotoxic therapy: an exploratory study on the need for parenteral nutrition after various treatment approaches for haematological malignancies. *Bone Marrow Transplant* 1999;23:933.

58. Roberts S, Miller J, Pineiro L, et al. Total parenteral nutrition *vs* oral diet in autologous hematopoietic cell transplant recipients. *Bone Marrow Transplant* 2003;32:715–721.

59. Ziegler TR, Young LS, Benfell K, et al. Clinical and metabolic efficacy of glutamine-supplemented parenteral nutrition after bone marrow transplantation. *Ann Intern Med* 1992;116:821–828.

60. Schloerb PR, Skikne BS. Oral and parenteral glutamine in bone marrow transplantation: a randomized, double-blind study. *JPEN J Parenter Enteral Nutr* 1999;23(3):117–122.

61. Detsky AS, Baker JP, O'Rourke K, et al. Perioperative parenteral nutrition: a meta-analysis. *Ann Intern Med* 1987;107:195–203.

62. Brennan MF, Pisters PW, Posner M, et al. A prospective randomized trial of total parenteral nutrition after major pancreatic resection for malignancy. *Ann Surg* 1994;220:436.

63. Foschi D, Cavagna G, Callioni F, et al. Hyperalimentation of jaundiced patients on percutaneous transhepatic biliary drainage. *Br J Surg* 1986;73:716–719.

64. Ferro-Luzzi A, Sette S, Franklin M, et al. A simplified approach of assessing adult chronic energy deficiency. *Eur J Clin Nutr* 1992;46(3):173–186.

65. Nutrition Screening Initiative. *Nutrition intervention manual for professionals caring for older Americans*. Washington, DC: Nutrition Screening Initiative (2626 Pennsylvania Avenue NW, Suite 301, Washington, DC 20037), 1992.

66. Ottery FD. Rethinking nutritional support of the cancer patient: a new field of nutritional oncology. *Semin Oncol* 1994;21:770–778.

67. Ottery FD. Modification of subjective global assessment (SGA) of nutritional status (NS) for oncology patients. In: *19th Clinical Congress*, American Society for Parenteral and Enteral Nutrition, Miami, FL, January 15–18, 1995, Abstract 119.

68. Detsky AF, McLaughlin JR, Baker JP, et al. What is subjective global assessment of nutritional status? *JPEN J Parenter Enteral Nutr* 1987;11:8–13.

69. Ottery FD. Supportive nutrition to prevent cachexia and improve quality of life. *Semin Oncol* 1995;22:98–111.

70. Sluys TE, van de Ende ME, Swart GR, et al. Body composition in patients with acquired immunodeficiency syndrome: a validation study of bioelectrical impedance analysis. *JPEN J Parenter Enteral Nutr* 1993;17:404–406.

71. Ottery FD. Cancer cachexia: prevention, early diagnosis, and management. *Cancer Pract* 1994;2:123–131.

72. Blackburn GL, Harvey KB. Nutritional assessment as a routine in clinical medicine. *Postgrad Med* 1982;71:46–63.

73. Herrmann FR, Safran C, Levkoff SE, et al. Serum albumin level on admission as a predictor of death, length of stay, and readmission. *Arch Intern Med* 1992;152:125–130.

74. McGeer AJ, Detsky AS, O'Rourke K. Parenteral nutrition in patients undergoing cancer chemotherapy: a meta-analysis. *Nutrition* 1990;6:233–240.

75. Harrison LE, Brennan MF. The role of total parenteral nutrition in the patient with cancer. *Curr Probl Surg* 1995;32(10):833–924.

76. Brennan MF. Total parenteral nutrition in the cancer patient. *N Engl J Med* 1981;305:375–382.

77. Pietsch JB, Meakins JL, MacLean LD. The delayed hypersensitivity response: application in clinical surgery. *Surgery* 1977;82:349–355.

78. Apovian CM, McMahon MM, Bistrian BR. Guidelines for refeeding the marasmic patient. *Crit Care Med* 1990;18:1030–1033.

79. Grant JP. *Handbook of total parenteral nutrition*, 2nd ed. Philadelphia, PA: WB Saunders, 1992:208–209.

80. Harris JA, Benedict FG. *A biometric study of basal metabolism in man*. Washington, DC: Carnegie Institute of Washington, 1919.

81. Aspen Board of Directors. Guidelines for the use of total parenteral nutrition in the hospitalized patient. *JPEN J Parenter Enteral Nutr* 1986;10:441–444.

82. Lowry SF, Brennan MS. Intravenous feeding in the cancer patient. In: Rombeau JL, Caldwell MD, eds. *Parenteral nutrition*. Philadelphia, PA: WB Saunders, 1986;445–470.

83. American Medical Association, Department of Food and Nutrition. Multivitamin preparations for parenteral use: a statement by the nutrition advisory group. *JPEN J Parenter Enteral Nutr* 1986;10:441–445.

84. Brown R, Querchia RA, Sigman R. Total nutrient admixture: a review. *JPEN J Parenter Enteral Nutr* 1986;10:650–658.

85. Rombeau JL, Rolandelli RH, Wilmore DW. Nutritional support. In: Wilmore DW, Brennan MF, Harken AH et al., eds. American College of Surgeons. *Care of the surgical patient*. New York: Scientific American, 1994;1–40.

86. Parker P, Stroop S, Greene H. A controlled comparison of continuous versus intermittent feeding in the treating of infants with intestinal disease. *J Pediatr* 1981;99:360–364.

87. Heymsfield S, Casper K, Grossman G. Bioenergetic and metabolic response to continuous versus intermittent nasogastric feeding. *Metabolism* 1987;36:570–575.

88. Zarling EJ, Parmar JR, Mobarhan S, et al. Effective enteral formula infusion rate, osmolality and chemical composition upon clinical tolerance and carbohydrate absorption in normal subjects. *JPEN J Parenter Enteral Nutr* 1986;10:588–590.

89. Takala J, Ruokonen E, Webster NR, et al. Increased mortality associated with growth hormone treatment in critically ill adults. *N Engl J Med* 1999;341:785.

90. Barbul A. Immunonutrition comes of age [editorial]. *Crit Care Med* 2000;28:884–885.

91. Moncada S, Higgs A. The L-arginine-nitric oxide pathway. *N Engl J Med* 1993;329:2002–2012.

92. Hall JC, Heel K, McCauley R. Glutamine. *Br J Surg* 1996;83:305–312.

93. Calder PC. More good news about glutamine. *Nutrition* 2000;16:71–72.

94. Bengmark S. Immunonutrition: role of biosurfactants, fiber, and probiotic bacteria. *Nutrition* 1998;14:585–594.

95. Novak F, Heyland DK, Avenell A, et al. Glutamine supplementation in serious illness: a systematic review of the evidence. *Crit Care Med* 2002;30:2022.

96. Gianotti L, Braga M, Nespoli L, et al. A randomized controlled trial of preoperative oral supplementation with a specialized diet in patients with gastrointestinal cancer. *Gastroenterology* 2002;122(7):1763–1770.

97. Heys SD, Walker LG, Smith I, et al. Enteral nutritional supplementation with key nutrients in patients with critical illness and cancer: a meta-analysis of randomized controlled clinical trials. *Ann Surg* 1999;229:467.

98. Beale RJ, Bryg DJ, Bihari DJ. Immunonutrition in the critically ill: a systematic review of clinical outcome. *Crit Care Med* 1999;27:2799.

99. Heyland DK, Novak F, Drover JW, et al. Should immunonutrition become routine in critically ill patients? A systematic review of the evidence. *JAMA* 2001;286:944.

100. Klimberg VS, Souba WW, Salloum RM, et al. Glutamine enriched diets support muscle glutamine metabolism without stimulating tumor growth. *J Surg Res* 1990;48:319–323.

101. Morlion BJ, Stehle P, Wachtler P, et al. Total parenteral nutrition with glutamine dipeptide after major abdominal surgery: a randomized, double-blind, controlled study. *Ann Surg* 1998;227:302.

102. Parks KGM, Heys SD, Blessing K, et al. Stimulation of human breast cancers by dietary L-arginine. *Clin Sci* 1992,82.413–417.

103. Souba WW. Glutamine and cancer. *Ann Surg* 1993;218:715–728.

104. Lorente JA, Landin L, De Pablo R, et al. L-arginine pathway in the sepsis syndrome. *Crit Care Med* 1999;27:2474–2479.

105. Lorente JA, Delgado MA, Tejedor C, et al. Modulation of systemic hemodynamics by exogenous L-arginine in normal and bacteremic sheep. *Crit Care Med* 1999;27:2474–2479.

106. Howard L. Parenteral and enteral nutrition therapy. In: Wilson JD, Braunwald E, Isselbacher KJ, et al. eds. *Harrison's principles of internal medicine*, 12th ed. New York: McGraw-Hill, 1990;434.
107. North American Home Parenteral and Enteral Nutrition Patient Registry. *Annual Report 1985–1990*. Albany, New York: Oley Foundation, 1987–1992;1228.
108. Flowers JF, Ryan JA, Gough JA. Catheter-related complications of total parenteral nutrition. In: Fischer JE, ed. *Total parenteral nutrition*. Boston, MA: Little Brown, 1991:25–45.
109. Rogers JZ, McKee K, McDermott E. Peripherally inserted central venous catheters. *Support line*. 1995;17(5):5–10.
110. Loughran SC, Borzatta M. Peripherally inserted central catheters: a report of 2506 catheter days. *JPEN J Parenter Enteral Nutr* 1995;19:133–136.
111. Harvey KB, Moldawer LL, Bistrian BR, et al. Biological measures for the formulation of a hospital prognostic index. *Am J Clin Nutr* 1981;34:2013–2022.
112. Chan S, Blackburn GL. Total parenteral nutrition in cancer patients. In: Heber D, Blackburn GL, Go VLW, eds. *Nutrition oncology*. San Diego, CA: Academic Press, 1999;573–578.
113. Chlebowski RT. Enteral nutrition in cancer patients. In: Heber D, Blackburn GL, Go VLW, eds. *Nutrition oncology*. San Diego, CA: Academic Press, 1999;581–584.

CHAPTER 68 ■ ISSUES IN NUTRITION AND HYDRATION

CHRISTINE S. RITCHIE AND ELIZABETH KVALE

The issues surrounding artificial nutrition and hydration (ANH) pose challenges for clinicians, patients, families, and society. Legal precedent and ethical principles guide medical practice; yet with regard to critical questions in this area our scientific base for establishing benefit or harm is so primitive and methodologically inadequate that evidence-based decisions are illusory. Decisions regarding the use of hydration and nutrition in palliative care often boil down to an honest if imperfect discussion of the potential harm and benefit of nutrition and hydration in a particular setting, filtered through the values of each patient and their family.

WHAT IS NUTRITION AND HYDRATION?

Definitions

Artificial hydration is the provision of water or electrolyte solutions by any nonoral route. *Artificial nutrition* includes total parenteral nutrition (TPN), enteral nutrition (EN) by nasogastric tube (NGT), percutaneous endoscopic gastrostomy (PEG) tube, percutaneous endoscopic gastrostomy jejunostomy (PEG-J) tube, gastrostomy tube, or gastrojejunostomy tube.

History

In the 1920s, continuous infusion of i.v. glucose was introduced in humans. It was not until the 1960s that parenteral nutrition was used, first in seriously ill adult surgical patients and then in children and adults with short bowel syndrome (1). These children, who before these therapies died of starvation, were able to live for years, sustained with artificial nutrition. Parenteral nutrition use then expanded to many other patient populations, often without clear or well-established indications. Only in the past decade has some light been shed in critical care settings as to when TPN is beneficial and when it may be more harmful (2,3).

In the late 1970s, gastrostomies began to be performed and were often used for swallowing problems in children (4). Their use became widely generalized to adults such that EN is now commonly used among patients with stroke, neurologic disease, and cancer (5). Between 1988 and 1995 the number of tubes placed in the United States doubled; in 2000, more than 216,000 tubes were placed. Recent data from Veterans Administration and Medicare database reviews suggest a stabilization of this trend in some settings (Fig. 68.1).

Whereas i.v. hydration is a well-established part of medical practice, its role in end-of-life care remains less clear. IV hydration is often used for treatment of terminal delirium and agitation. Whether it is beneficial, and if so, at what rate of infusion, remains an area of controversy.

ETHICAL AND LEGAL FRAMEWORK

Nutrition and hydration decisions may be more difficult for some families than ventilator support or cardiac resuscitation. Families may equate foregoing of artificial nutrition with starvation. The potential harms associated with artificial nutrition (such as restraint use, immobility, and decreased social contact) are often not considered. Because of the dearth of good scientific data to assist clinicians in addressing whether or not artificial nutrition has meaningful benefit, it is often difficult to provide guidance to patients' families.

In medicine, ethical principles guide how a patient should be treated or how a treatment dilemma should be handled. The ethical principle of *autonomy* states that a person should have the ability to govern oneself. This principle was applied in the court decisions of Barber in 1983, Bouvia in 1986, and Cruzan in 1990, all of which stated that competent adults should be the final arbiters of decisions regarding their own health care. If nutritional support is unwanted, then providing artificial nutrition does not adhere to the principle of *autonomy* and lessens patient dignity. *Beneficence* is the ethical principle that states that physicians should always provide care that benefits the patient. In the case of artificial nutrition, the physician needs to ask if the artificial nutrition is actually "doing good" for their patient. The principle of *nonmaleficence* addresses the complimentary principle that one should "do no harm"—*primum non nocere*. In the case of ANH, physicians must weigh the potential for this medical treatment to harm their patient in any way. If this treatment was contributing to more harm than benefit, than the principle of *nonmaleficence* would support its discontinuation (Fig. 68.2).

The argument for the discontinuation of nutritional support states that ANH are indistinguishable from other medical treatments. In the 1990 Cruzan decision, the U.S. Supreme Court stated that "the law does not distinguish artificial feeding from other forms of medical treatment" (6). The right of patients to refuse this treatment is supported, and within this framework artificial nutrition is considered medical intervention

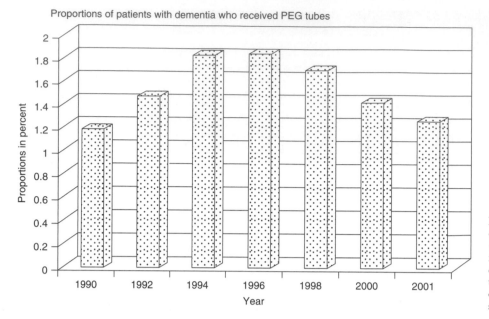

Proportions of patients with dementia who received PEG tubes

FIGURE 68.1. Time trends in the use of percutaneous endoscopic gastrostomy (PEG) tube feeding: proportion of demented patients in the administrative database of the Veterans Health Administration shown as percent of total number of demented patients. A decreasing trend since 1996 is identified.

and not basic care. Withdrawing artificial nutritional support and allowing a patient to die is not considered equivalent to euthanasia. In the former instance, the goal of discontinuing therapy is to remove burdensome interventions; in the latter, the intended result is the death of the patient. Nevertheless, as demonstrated by the Schiavo case, public acceptance of these distinguishing features in nutritional support varies greatly. Furthermore, some faith communities take issue with the distinction between artificial and basic nutrition.

In addition, much legal confusion persists because advance directive statutes may make it more difficult for a person capable of making decisions to prospectively forego ANH, and many state statutes are poorly written and confusing (7).

INDICATIONS

No clear palliative indications exist for artificial nutrition. The American Gastroenterological Association (AGA) endorses PEG tube placement for prolonged tube feeding (specifically more than 30 days), and nasogastric feeding when enteral

feeding is required for shorter periods (Table 68.1). In practice, PEG tubes are placed for a variety of different clinical conditions, including dysphagia, prolonged illness, anorexia, neurologic/psychiatric disorders, oropharyngeal or esophageal disorders or cancers, or increased nutritional needs that the patient is unable to meet with oral intake. Studies show that neurologic illnesses (e.g., dysphagia following stroke, dementia), cancer (obstruction secondary to tumor, postradiation, postchemotherapy, or postresection), and the prevention of aspiration account for most placements (8–10).

Indications for artificial hydration are relatively straightforward in critical care settings or when an otherwise healthy patient presents with volume depletion. Indications for hydration at the end of life have not been established. In the acute care setting, parenteral hydration is routinely given. In the hospice setting, parenteral hydration is not routine, but may be considered in instances where the patient is experiencing neuropsychiatric symptoms such as delirium, myoclonus, and agitation.

With regards to ANH, the scientific literature lacks high quality randomized trials that might yield clear indications

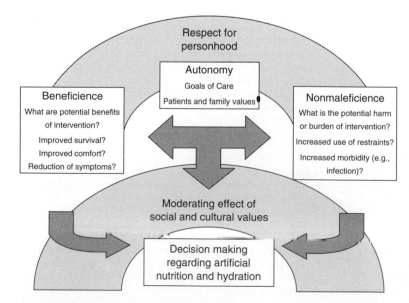

FIGURE 68.2. Integration of ethical principles into decisionmaking regarding artificial nutrition and hydration.

TABLE 68.1

AMERICAN GASTROENTEROLOGICAL ASSOCIATION
GUIDELINES ON ENTERAL FEEDING

- The patient cannot or will not eat
- The gut is functional
- The patient can tolerate the placement of the device[a]

[a]American Gastroenterological Association. American
Gastroenterological Association medical position statement: guidelines
for the use of enteral nutrition. *Gastroenterology* 1995;108:1280–
1301.

to guide practice. Benefits and harms are often gleaned from
imperfect evidence from heterogeneous populations.

POTENTIAL BENEFIT OF ARTIFICIAL NUTRITION

Common rationale for use of artificial nutrition includes improved survival, comfort, reduction in pressure ulcers, and
reduction in aspiration. Although most of the studies performed to date are compromised by substantial methodological
problems, none have consistently demonstrated improved outcomes in these arenas with the exceptions of improved survival
for short bowel syndrome, decreased hepatic encephalopathy
in alcoholic cirrhosis, decreased length of hospital stay in hip
fracture patients, and decreased postoperative complications
of patients with gastric cancer given artificial nutrition preoperatively (11,12). Although no controlled trials exist, follow-up
studies suggest increased survival of patients in persistent
vegetative state who are likely to die within weeks without
artificial nutrition, but may live for many years with artificial
nutrition (13). There is also moderately strong evidence that
artificial nutrition can prolong life when it is used in short-
term critical care (14). A summary of the levels of evidence

for benefit from artificial nutrition is given in Tables 68.2 and
68.3.

Survival

A number of retrospective studies and a few prospective
studies have been performed in patients to ascertain survival
benefit in patients receiving artificial nutrition. The largest
study to date was a retrospective review by Grant et al. of
81,105 medicare beneficiaries who received gastrostomies in
1991. No comparison group was identified for this study.
Cerebrovascular disease, neoplasms, fluid and electrolyte
disorders, and aspiration pneumonia were the most common
primary diagnoses. The mortality rate at 1 and 3 years
was 63.0–81.3%. The median survival for was 28.9 weeks
for women and 17.6 weeks for men. At 30 days, primary
diagnoses of malnutrition and fluid and electrolyte disorders,
and secondary diagnoses of swallowing disorders, dementia,
or cerebrovascular disease were characterized by the *lowest*
mortality rates. Thirty-day mortality rates were *highest* among
those with primary diagnoses of nonaspiration pneumonia
or influenza, and secondary diagnoses of congestive heart
failure, or any neoplasm (8). Rabeneck et al. studied 7369
patients receiving PEG tubes at VA facilities between 1990
and 1992. In this retrospective cohort study, 23.5% died
during their index hospitalization. The median survival of the
full cohort was 7.5 months from the time of tube placement.
The overall mortality rates at 1, 2, and 3 years were 59,
71, and 77%, respectively. The highest mortality rates were
observed for patients with lung or pleural cancer (46.4%),
followed by esophageal cancer (20.8%) and head and neck
cancer (18.8%) (15). Survival decreased with increasing age.
The median survival across clinical diagnostic categories was
13.9 months for cerebrovascular disease, 13.4 months for
other organic neurologic diseases, 9.6 months for nutritional
deficiency, 8.0 months for head and neck cancer, and 4 or
fewer months for all other cancers. Among 674 older (age
>50) adults referred to a community gastroenterology group
for PEG insertion over a 10-year period, mortality rates at 1, 2,
and 3 years were 54.3, 73.2, and 84.5%, respectively. Like

TABLE 68.2

LEVELS OF EVIDENCE FOR ARTIFICIAL NUTRITION

Population/type of artificial nutrition	Outcome	Classification	Level of evidence
Stroke			
PEG vs. NG tube	Improved albumin/weight	IIa	B1
PEG vs. NG tube/oral feeding	Survival	IIb	B1
Acquired immunodeficiency syndrome			
TPN in advanced disease	Increased weight	IIa	B1
TPN in advanced disease	Survival	IIb	B1
Cancer			
TPN	During chemotherapy	III	B1
Prophylactic enteral nutrition[a] before treatment in head and neck cancer	Weight stabilization	IIa	B2
Enteral nutrition before surgery	Gastrointestinal cancer	IIa	A
Dementia			
Enteral nutrition	Survival	III	B2
Enteral nutrition	Aspiration	III	B2
Enteral nutrition	Pressure sores	IIb	C

PEG, percutaneous endoscopic gastrostomy; NG, nasogastric; TPN, total parenteral nutrition.
[a]Enteral nutrition includes NG, gastrostomy and PEG tube feeding.

TABLE 68.3

RECOMMENDATION CLASSIFICATIONS AND LEVELS
OF EVIDENCE

Classification
  Class I: Intervention is useful and effective
  Class IIa: Weight of evidence/opinion is in favor of
    usefulness/efficacy
  Class IIb: Usefulness/efficacy less well-established by
    evidence/opinion
  Class III: Intervention is not useful/effective and may be
    harmful
Level of Evidence
  A: Sufficient evidence from multiple randomized trials
  B: Limited evidence from
    1. Single, randomized trial or
    2. Other nonrandomized studies
  C: Based on expert opinion, case studies, or standard of care

Rabeneck's study, the overall median survival was between 6 months and 1 year; however, those receiving tube feeding in this cohort were much more likely to be patients with stroke or other neurologic conditions. Very few of the PEGs were placed in patients with cancer. Risk factors for mortality in this cohort were being male, having feeding difficulty, having diabetes, being referred from a hospital and being 80 years of age or greater (16). Similar to Grant's cohort, dementia was *not* an independent risk factor for decreased survival. Because these studies used large databases, identification of truly comparable control groups would have been challenging. Nevertheless, because there was no comparable control group, the impact of gastrostomies on survival could not be ascertained.

Comfort

The small body of literature evaluating patient symptoms at the end of life suggests a relatively low prevalence of hunger (17). In McCann's study of 32 patients in a comfort care unit, 63% denied hunger entirely, while 34% reported hunger during the first quarter of their course in the unit. In all patients reporting either hunger or thirst, these symptoms were consistently and completely relieved by oral care or the ingestion of small amounts of food and fluid. In a case study of a patient refusing nutrition and hydration, the patient experienced no discomfort and died peacefully (18). A survey of Oregon hospice nurses found that among those who had cared for patients who declined nutrition and hydration, the majority reported the ensuing death to be peaceful (19).

Studies of healthy volunteers engaged in fasting report resolution of hunger in less than 24 hours. The resulting ketosis is associated with relief of hunger and a mild euphoria. Animal studies suggest that ketosis may also have a mild analgesic effect. When ketosis is minimized by small feedings, hunger may persist (20).

Reduction in Pressure Ulcers

There is some evidence that malnutrition is positively correlated with pressure ulcer incidence and severity (21,22). However, only two nutrition intervention studies for pressure ulcer prevention or treatment included artificial nutrition.

Hartgrink et al. performed a randomized controlled trial (RCT) with 140 patients with fracture of the hip and an increased pressure ulcer risk. The intervention group was treated with standard hospital diet and additional NGT feeding administered overnight. The comparison group received the standard hospital diet alone (23). No significant difference was found between the groups. Chernoff et al. utilized artificial nutrition in an RCT of 12 tube-fed patients with pressure ulcers. The treatment comparison, however, was amount of protein intake, not tube feeding (24). Thus, it is not possible to draw any firm conclusions on the effect of enteral and parenteral nutrition on the prevention and treatment of pressure ulcers.

Reduction in Aspiration Rates

In prospective studies of EN, aspiration pneumonia is not demonstrably decreased. Progression of aspiration to pneumonia is difficult to predict and is influenced by a number of factors, including decreased level of alertness, prolonged supine position, and colonization of the oropharynx (25). Tube feeding is in fact a risk factor for development of aspiration pneumonia among nursing home residents (odds ratio 3.0) (26). A recent meta-analysis suggests that small bowel feeding reduces the frequency of aspiration pneumonia compared with intragastric feeding (27).

POTENTIAL HARM

Complications

Complications from nasal intubation can include pharyngeal or esophageal perforation, and accidental bronchial insertion. Approximately 25% of NGTs "fall out" or are pulled out by patients soon after insertion; fine bore tubes can be displaced by coughing or vomiting. Immediate complications of percutaneous gastrostomy and jejunostomy tubes include abdominal wall or intraperitoneal bleeding and bowel perforation (28). Significant surgical intervention is needed in fewer than 5%. Postinsertion tube related complications from percutaneous gastrostomy and jejunostomy tubes include infection at the insertion site, peristomal leaks, accidental tube removal, peritonitis, sepsis, and necrotizing fasciitis.

Restraints

Families are often unaware that patients with PEG tubes may require restraints (29). In Peck's study of nursing home residents with dementia, those receiving EN were more likely to be restrained (71%) than those who were not (56%) (30). When a select cohort of nursing home residents were asked, a third stated that they would prefer tube feeds if they were unable to eat. But 25% then declined when they were informed that restraints are sometimes applied during the feeding process.

Social Isolation

Patients fed enterally may be given fewer opportunities to taste food or experience the social interaction that can occur at mealtimes. They may experience sensory deprivation and social isolation if feeding comprises simply hanging a bag of nutrients on a pole for delivery through a tube. Hand feeding, though more labor intensive than EN, enhances the dietary impact of feeding through touch, social engagement, and nurturing interactions.

CONDITIONS FOR WHICH ARTIFICIAL NUTRITION IS OFTEN CONSIDERED

Stroke

Two randomized studies of stroke patients with dysphagia who received PEG tube feeds showed improvement in albumin and weight gain at 6 weeks follow-up (31,32). Norton et al. performed a prospective randomized comparison of PEG versus NGT feeding after acute dysphagic stroke. Thirty patients with persisting dysphagia 14 days after acute stroke were randomly assigned to PEG (16 patients) versus NGT feeding (14 patients). Mortality at 6 weeks was significantly lower in the PEG group, with two deaths compared with eight deaths in the NGT group. Patients with PEG were more likely to have received the total amount of prescribed feeding and showed statistically greater improvement in nutritional state as well as discharge rate at 6 weeks. The comparison groups for both of these studies were patients receiving NGT feeding, not oral feeding. A meta-analysis of the three completed trials comparing PEG and NGTs estimated that the odds ratio for death is 0.88 (95% confidence interval [CI], 0.59–1.33) in favor of PEG. This value is not significant; CIs were wide and included the possibility of a large advantage or disadvantage with respect to survival for PEG over nasogastric feeding.

More recently, Iizuka and Reding performed a case-matched control of PEG versus no-PEG for 193 PEG patients. Controls were matched to the greatest extent possible on (from highest to lowest priority):

1. Sex
2. Duration from onset to stroke unit admission (interval poststroke)
3. Functional status on admission
4. Age
5. Diagnosis (ischemic vs. hemorrhagic)
6. Year of admission

No significant differences were found between the 2 groups except for functional status, which was significantly lower for the PEG group. There was a 4.7-fold greater frequency of death in the PEG group. Medical complications (pneumonia, cardiac events, stroke progression) were also greater in this group. Both groups, however, showed a similar frequency of home discharge for survivors (33).

The largest controlled trial in stroke patients is the FOOD trials, which consisted of two trials for dysphagic stroke patients. In one trial, patients enrolled within 7 days of admission were randomly allocated to early enteral tube feeding or no tube feeding for more than 7 days (early vs. avoid). In the other, patients were assigned to PEG or nasogastric feeding. In the early versus avoid trial, early tube feeding was associated with a nonsignificant reduction in absolute risk of death of 5.8% (95% CI, 0.8–12.5, $p = .09$). There was no increase in pneumonia associated with early tube feeding; however, the improved survival was offset by a 4.7% excess of survivors with a poor outcome with a worse quality of life. Thus, early feeding might have kept patients alive in a severely disabled state when they would otherwise have died. In the PEG versus nasogastric trial, PEG feeding was associated with a nonsignificant increase in the absolute risk of death of 1.0% (34).

End-Stage Acquired Immunodeficiency Syndrome

Retrospective and prospective observational studies have reported conflicting results regarding the impact of TPN or EN on body weight and body composition in patients with human immunodeficiency virus (HIV) infections. In a 2-month RCT of 31 malnourished and severely immunodepressed acquired immunodeficiency syndrome (AIDS) patients, subjects were assigned to receive either dietary counseling ($n = 15$) or home TPN ($n = 16$) Bodyweight increased by 8 kg in the TPN group and decreased by 3 kg in the control group ($p < .0006$). Lean body mass increased in the TPN group and decreased in the control group $p < .004$). However, no difference in survival rate was noted. Quality of life in this trial was measured with a self-assessed "subjective health feeling" that demonstrated improvement in 83% of participants in the intervention arm, while 91% of participants in the control group reported feeling worse. Karnofsky scores stabilized in the intervention group and decreased in the control group (-12%), though this change was only statistically significant at one-time point (35). Other studies of TPN have also demonstrated increases in lean body mass and body weight, but only in patients who do not have a systemic infection (12).

Cancer

TPN and EN cancer-randomized studies in patients with a variety of tumors and therapies have generated inconsistent results. In a meta-analysis of 28 prospective RCTs evaluating the use of TPN in patients with cancer, TPN was found to be possibly useful when used preoperatively in patients with gastrointestinal tract cancer. It appeared to be beneficial in reducing major surgical complications and operative mortality but increased risk of infection. No statistically significant benefit from TPN could be demonstrated in survival, treatment tolerance, treatment toxicity, or tumor response in patients receiving chemotherapy or radiotherapy (36). A meta-analysis of patients receiving TPN during chemotherapy failed to demonstrate any clinical benefits (37). The poor outcomes observed in these trials culminated in a consensus statement from the American College of Physicians. This statement advised that the routine use of parenteral nutrition should be discouraged in patients undergoing chemotherapy and that when it is used in patients with cancer with malnutrition, physicians should consider the possibility of increased risk (38). This statement and the clinical trials that led to its issuance have curbed the use of TPN in the United States in patients with metastatic, incurable disease. However, subsequent studies evaluating TPN and EN remain mixed. In other countries, TPN continues to be used regularly for patients with advanced cancer.

Like TPN, EN in patients with cancer has not been shown to improve survival, improve tumor response, decrease toxicity, or decrease surgical complications. The only exception is in patients with cancer in head and neck, and esophagus (39). In a retrospective case–control study of 88 patients treated for locally advanced head and neck cancer with accelerated radiation or concurrent chemoradiotherapy, prophylactic gastrostomy tubes (PGTs) were associated with half of the weight loss compared to the control group. There were significantly fewer hospitalizations for nutritional or dehydration issues in those with PGTs than in the control group; the use of PGTs had no influence on overall survival or local control. Although in animal studies nutritional support has been shown to increase rates of tumor growth, this has not been demonstrated consistently in humans (40).

Both TPN and EN have been able to improve some nutritional indices, such as body weight, fat mass, nitrogen balance, and whole-body potassium. Thyroxine-binding pre-albumin and retinol-binding protein levels increase only with TPN, whereas some immune response indices (complement factors and lymphocyte number) improve only with EN. EN appears to be more available for use in protein synthesis than TPN (41). The results of randomized studies comparing TPN and EN have been conflicting, but demonstrated a potential marginal advantage to TPN with regard to weight gain, and nitrogen balance (42,43). Taken as a whole, TPN and EN both appear able to prevent further deterioration of the nutritional state and sometimes improve some metabolic indices in patients with cancer. However, no real demonstrable benefit has been shown on quality of life, and no large randomized trials have been performed in patients with advanced cancer.

Dementia

Dementia is a progressive disease that worsens in recognizable stages. In the Functional Assessment Staging System (FAST), one system used to follow the course of Alzheimer's disease; it is at the final stage seven when Alzheimer's disease patients may stop eating spontaneously. At stage seven, patients usually die within a year. They lose the ability to speak, ambulate, eat, control their muscles, and smile. When patients reach this stage it is very difficult to maintain nutrition because encouragement to eat becomes less successful. In this instance, difficulty eating is a marker for the terminal phase of Alzheimer's dementia.

The same is not true in other forms of dementia. For example, patients with Parkinson's disease often lose the ability to maintain adequate caloric intake at an earlier stage of their disease; in this setting, a feeding tube may be required. PEG tube placement does not prevent aspiration; aspiration rates may continue to range between 25 and 40% (44). PEG tubes in patients with advanced dementia do not prevent aspiration pneumonia, reduce the risk of infection or pressure sores, or improve function. Based on Rimon's findings and those of others not showing dementia to be a risk factor for increased mortality, the impact of EN on survival remains unclear.

Amyotrophic Lateral Sclerosis

Some studies suggest that the benefits of a PEG in amyotrophic lateral sclerosis (ALS) are adequate nutritional intake and weight stabilization (45–47). Whether PEG increases survival time remains unclear (48). PEG placement may be associated with increased pulmonary risks and shorter survival time when done in patients with reduced vital capacity, defined as forced vital capacity <50% of predicted. Recent studies, however, call this into question (49,50).

POTENTIAL BENEFIT FROM ARTIFICIAL HYDRATION

Comfort

A common argument for providing artificial hydration in palliative care is to alleviate thirst. Healthy volunteers who undergo experimentally induced dehydration, often report thirst, yet this sensation is relieved by ad lib sips of fluid in cumulative volumes insufficient to restore physiologic fluid balance. The few studies evaluating patient symptoms at the end of life suggest a high prevalence of dry mouth and thirst that is not correlated with hydration status but can be alleviated with ice chips and sips of water (17). In several studies of palliative care patients, no statistically significant association was found between thirst and fluid intake, serum sodium, urea, or osmolality (51,52).

Reduction of Delirium or Opioid Toxicity

Retrospective studies have suggested that hydration might be able to reduce neuropsychiatric symptoms such as sedation, hallucinations, myoclonus, and agitation (53). In the first RCT of hydration versus placebo in patients with cancer, Bruera et al. compared the effects of hydration with either 1000 or 100 mL of normal saline on target symptoms of sedation, fatigue, hallucinations, and myoclonus. Although the study did not meet its accrual goals, 53 (73%) of 73 target symptoms experienced by the treatment group improved, compared with 33 (49%) of 67 target symptoms in the placebo group ($p = .006$), suggesting a potential benefit of hydration in this population. This study was underpowered and characterized by many subjective measures, and was not performed in hospice patients. Nevertheless, it highlights the importance of further study in this controversial area.

POTENTIAL HARM FROM ARTIFICIAL HYDRATION

Commonly cited side effects of artificial hydration in palliative care include fluid overload and increased respiratory secretions. Because no controlled trials exist, the association between these adverse effects and artificial hydration are hard to measure.

Fluid Overload

Concerns regarding hydration often center on the potential impact such hydration might have on edema, ascites, and respiratory distress. A comparison of two different health care settings (a palliative care unit and an acute care unit) demonstrated marked differences in volume of hydration ordered. The acute care group ordered higher volumes of hydration, but also prescribed a higher number of diuretics, suggesting that increased hydration could be associated with greater likelihood for fluid overload (54). Morita's study of terminally ill patients also noted an association between hydration and symptom scores for edema, ascites, and pleural effusion (55).

Increased Respiratory Secretions

Many palliative care providers believe hydration may worsen retained respiratory secretions at the very end of life. However, the effect of hydration on respiratory secretions at the end of life is unclear. Neither Ellershaw nor Morita found a correlation between hydration status and bronchial secretions.

METHODOLOGICAL ISSUES IN EVALUATING EFFECTIVENESS OF NUTRITION INTERVENTIONS

In reviewing the current ANH literature, one is struck by the dearth of methodologically rigorous studies available to inform practice. With the exception of several large retrospective cohort studies, most studies had small sample sizes and heterogeneous patient populations. These cohort studies did not include meaningful comparison groups, so evaluating the true impact of ANH is problematic.

Very little attention has been given to the nature of the nutritional intervention being provided through artificial nutrition. PEG placement or tube feeding might or might not lead to adequate caloric intake. Evaluating differences in outcome between those receiving adequate nutrients and those that did not would elucidate whether or not outcomes varied by actual caloric intake. In most studies, the composition of the nutrition or fluid formulations in these studies was rarely addressed or identified.

In almost all instances, RCTs either do not exist or are underpowered to evaluate the main outcomes. Most studies had difficulty with recruitment and high dropout rates. Furthermore, the follow-up time was often very short (days to weeks). Hence these trials are not likely to detect true effects of the intervention.

For the preponderance of observational studies influencing this field, confounding is not adequately addressed. For example, in observational studies of patients with dementia receiving EN, it is possible that tubes are placed primarily in a subgroup of patients whose oral intake has become insufficient to sustain life, thus prolonging their survival from 0 to 1 month to 6 to 7 months (confounding by indication). On the other hand, it is likely that tubes were not placed in the subgroup of patients who retained some capacity to eat; those patients also survived a median of roughly 6–7 months. The ability to eat could then be a confounding factor that explains the similar survival between groups receiving and not receiving artificial nutrition. Measuring the ability to eat and controlling for this risk factor in the analysis could help to ascertain the true association between tube placement and survival. Because many patients have multiple conditions, the nature and severity of these conditions (especially in Medicare databases) may be difficult to capture and therefore adequately control for in analyses.

Many of the outcomes chosen in these studies provide inadequate information for clinicians to guide patients. Most studies have evaluated survival and nutritional or medical indicators. Most have not addressed quality of life outcomes or quality-adjusted life years.

WHAT ARE CULTURAL AND RELIGIOUS DIMENSIONS TO THESE FORMS OF TREATMENT?

Ethnicity

Among NH residents with severe cognitive impairment, African Americans were almost four times more likely than whites to have a feeding tube (56). Despite a recent trend toward decreased PEG tube placement in dementia patients, racial discrepancies persist. In a review of the Veterans Health Administration database, Braun et al. found that although only 18.4% of dementia patients were African American,

they accounted for 28.8% of all PEG tube recipients with dementia (57). Reasons cited for this discrepancy include mistrust of the health care system, a greater desire for more aggressive medical treatment near the end of life, and differences in underlying religious beliefs and values. The possibility remains that African Americans are receiving a different standard of care with regard to ANH at end of life.

Religious Background

Jewish, Islamic, and Catholic traditions place a priority on "sanctity of life," often preferring greater life-sustaining treatments over "quality of life." Jewish and Islamic traditions do not distinguish tube feeding from other forms of basic nutrition (58). According to most Jewish religious authorities, "nutrition in any form is a basic human need and should be provided to all patients" (59). How cognitively impaired the patient is, is not relevant, because human life of any quality is of supreme value. Jewish tradition, however, does not argue for *any* treatment that is not of benefit to the patient and relies on scientific evidence in making an ethical judgment on a particular treatment modality.

GUIDELINES FOR ENTERAL/PARENTERAL NUTRITION IN PALLIATIVE CARE

Improve the Scientific Literature Base

Because all the current data regarding ANH have significant methodological weaknesses, providers should be circumspect about the true benefits and harm of nutrition support, especially in the enteral form. Improvements in the overall quality could be made by:

1. Collaboration with epidemiologists/biostatisticians from the beginning stages of the study
2. Agreement on appropriate outcome measures
3. Use of the highest quality design for the clinical question at hand

More rigorous studies are needed to increase the confidence that current clinical practice is based on the higher levels of evidence.

Improve the Assessment Process

Before initiating artificial nutrition, it is worth asking the following questions:

1. Is the patient able to swallow properly? If so, oral nutrition is preferable and safer than tube feeding.
2. If the patient can swallow properly, is the patient maintaining adequate nutritional intake to meet nutritional needs? If not, dietary supplementation is preferable and safer than tube feeding.
3. If the patient can swallow but cannot maintain adequate nutritional intake, is it due to a specific modifiable cause? If so, addressing the underlying cause is preferable and safer than tube feeding. For example:
   - Does the patient have a psychological condition such as depression that affects nutritional intake?
   - Does the patient have mouth pain, poorly fitted dentures or loss of teeth?

- Is the food or the eating environment unappealing?
- Does the patient have the physical dexterity needed to eat without assistance?
- Does the patient need to be reminded how to chew and swallow?
- Is the patient receiving the help he or she needs to eat?
- Are language barriers, ethnic or cultural dietary restrictions, or religious beliefs keeping the patient from taking an adequate amount of nutrition?

4. If the patient is unable to eat or does not have adequate nutritional intake, address the following questions before considering tube feeding:
   - Does the clinical decision to employ tube feeding respect the autonomy of the patient and family to decline the intervention?
   - Is conservative treatment a better option? Has it been tried? If not, why?
   - Is there scientific evidence that supports tube feeding as a better option than oral intake in this situation?
   - Are there any contraindications to artificial feeding in this patient?
   - When and how will the effectiveness of and continued need for tube feeding be reassessed (i.e., reaching a specific therapeutic goal or a prespecified time period)?

Improve the Informed Consent Process

The current quality of informed consent for EN and, in particular, placement of gastrostomy tubes is poor. In a review of 154 consecutive hospitalized adults undergoing placement of gastrostomy tubes, only 1 medical record documented a procedure-specific discussion of benefits and burdens of and alternatives to tube feeding (60).

Specific information that should be provided

The informed consent process should include discussion of median, 1- and 3-year survival rates. It should also identify both physical (restraints) and potential psychosocial (social isolation and sensory deprivation) adverse effects associated with artificial nutrition. In patients who are not imminently dying, alternatives such as carefully monitored hand feeding should be discussed, including the observation that there is no difference in survival for PEG tubes versus hand feeding for demented and nondemented patients (61). In patients who are in the terminal phase of their illness, findings regarding the common lack of hunger experienced by patients, should be communicated to patients' families to allay concerns regarding potential patient distress associated with minimal oral intake.

Poor prognostic factors consistently noted in the literature should be described, including increased age (>80), chewing and swallowing disorders, and the presence of underlying malignancies (62).

GUIDELINES FOR HYDRATION IN PALLIATIVE CARE

Hydration may be of benefit in patients with potential opioid toxicity, confusion, or nausea. Patients and families, should be informed regarding the lack of correlation between hydration and thirst and the finding that sips of water, ice chips, lip moisteners, salivary substitutes, mouth swabs, hard candy, and routine mouth care are more effective at addressing the sense of dry mouth and thirst than is artificial hydration.

CONCLUSION

Evidence regarding the potential benefit or harm associated with ANH in palliative care continues to be limited by underpowered or poorly designed studies. Decisions regarding ANH should be informed by treatment goals and patient preference (autonomy) and the application of the principles of nonmaleficence and beneficence where potential harm or benefits can be determined. While case law regards artificial nutrition as medical treatment, in the absence of a developed literature to provide a scientific basis for decision making, social values may continue to guide decisions in some instances. Many religious traditions do not distinguish artificial nutrition from basic food and water, a point which renders moot discussion of harm and benefits for some decision makers. Physicians should inform the patient or their family as fully as possible regarding the potential benefit and harm associated with ANH and assist them to make the best decision possible based on the patient's values and available information about risks and benefits.

References

1. Dudrick SJ. A 45-year obsession and passionate pursuit of optimal nutrition support: puppies, pediatrics, surgery, geriatrics, home TPN, ASPEN, etc. *J Parenter Enteral Nutr* 2005;29:272–287.
2. Heyland DK, MacDonald S, Keefe L, et al. Total parenteral nutrition in the critically ill patient: a meta-analysis. *JAMA* 1998;280:2013–2019.
3. Heyland DK, Montalvo M, MacDonald S, et al. Total parenteral nutrition in the surgical patient: a meta-analysis. *Can J Surg* 2001;44:102–111.
4. Gauderer MW. Percutaneous endoscopic gastrostomy-20 years later: a historical perspective. *J Pediatr Surg* 2001;36:217–219.
5. Callahan CM, Haag KM, Weinberger M, et al. Decision-making for percutaneous endoscopic gastrostomy among older adults in a community setting. *J Am Geriatr Soc* 1999;47:1105–1109.
6. Missouri Department of Health. Cruzan v Director, Missouri Department of Health, 110 S. Ct. 2841 1990.
7. Kapp MB. Regulating the foregoing of artificial nutrition and hydration: first, do some harm. *J Am Geriatr Soc* 2002;50:586–588.
8. Grant MD, Rudberg MA, Brody JA. Gastrostomy placement and mortality among hospitalized Medicare beneficiaries. *JAMA* 1998;279:1973–1976.
9. Light VL, Siezak FA, Porter JA, et al. Predictive factors for early mortality after percutaneous endoscopic gastrostomy. *Gastrointest Endosc* 1995;42:330–335.
10. Taylor CA, Larson DE, Ballard DJ, et al. Predictors of outcome after percutaneous endoscopic gastrostomy: a community-based study. *Mayo Clin Proc* 1992;67:1042–1049.
11. Wasa M, Takagi Y, Sando K, et al. Long-term outcome of short bowel syndrome in adult and pediatric patients. *J Parenter Enteral Nutr* 1999;23 (Suppl 5):S110–S112.
12. Klein S, Kinney J, Jeejeebhoy K, et al. Nutrition support in clinical practice: review of published data and recommendations for future research directions. *Am J Clin Nutr* 1997;66:683–706.
13. Tresch DD, Sims FH, Duthie EH, et al. Clinical characteristics of patients in the persistent vegetative state. *Arch Intern Med* 1991;151:930–932.
14. Heyland DK, Dhaliwal R, Drover JW, et al. Canadian clinical practice guidelines for nutrition support in mechanically ventilated, critically ill adult patients. *J Parenter Enteral Nutr* 2003;27:355–373.
15. Rabeneck L, Wray NP, Petersen NJ. Long-term outcomes of patients receiving percutaneous endoscopic gastrostomy tubes. *J Gen Intern Med* 1996;11:287–293.
16. Rimon E, Kagansky N, Levy S. Percutaneous endoscopic gastrostomy; evidence of different prognosis in various patient subgroups. *Age Ageing* 2005;34:353–357.
17. McCann RM, Hall WJ, Groth-Juncker A. Comfort care for terminally ill patients. The appropriate use of nutrition and hydration. *JAMA* 1994;272:1263–1266.
18. Eddy D. A conversation with my mother. *JAMA* 1994;272:179–181.
19. Ganzini L, Goy ER, Miller LL, et al. Nurses' experiences with hospice patients who refuse food and fluids to hasten death. *N Engl J Med* 2003;349:359–365.
20. Byock IR. Patient refusal of nutrition and hydration; walking the ever-finer line. *Am J Hosp Palliat Care* 1995;12:9–13.
21. Berlowitz DR, Wilking SV. Risk factors for pressure sores. A comparison of cross-sectional and cohort-derived data. *J Am Geriatr Soc* 1989;37:1043–1050.

22. Bergstrom N, Braden MJ, Laguzza A, et al. Prospective study of pressure sore risk among institutionalized elderly. *J Am Geriatr Soc* 1992;40:747–758.

23. Hartgrink HH, Wille J, Konig P, et al. Pressure sores and tube feeding in patients with a fracture of the hip: a randomized clinical trial. *Clin Nutr* 1998;17:287–292.

24. Chernoff RS, Milton KY, Lipschitz DA. The effect of a very high-protein liquid formula on decubitus ulcers healing in long-term tube-fed institutionalized patients. *J Am Diet Assoc* 1990;90:A–130.

25. McClave SA, DeMeo MT, DeLegge MH, et al. North American summit on aspiration in the critically ill patient: consensus statement. *J Parenter Enteral Nutr* 2002;26:S80–S85.

26. Langmore SE, Terpenning MS, Schork A, et al. Predictors of aspiration pneumonia: how important is dysphagia? *Dysphagia* 1998;13:69–81.

27. Heyland DK, Drover JW, MacDonald S, et al. Effect of postpyloric feeding on gastroesophageal regurgitation and pulmonary microaspiration: results of a randomized controlled trial. *Crit Care Med* 2001;29:1495–1501.

28. Stroud M, Duncan H, Nightingale J. Guidelines for enteral feeding in adult hospital patients. *Gut* 2003;52:1–12.

29. Sullivan-Marx EM, Strumpf NE, Eans LK, et al. Predictors of continued physical restraint use in nursing home residents following restraint reduction efforts. *J Am Geriatr Soc* 1999;47:342–348.

30. Peck A, Cohen CE, Mulvihill MN. Long-term enteral feeding of aged demented nursing home patients. *J Amer Geriatr Soc* 1990;38:1195–1198.

31. Norton B, Homer-Ward M, Donnelly MT, et al. A randomized prospective comparison of percutaneous endoscopic gastrostomy and nasogastric tube feeding after acute dysphagic stroke. *Br Med J* 1996;312:13–16.

32. Park RH, Allison MC, Lang J, et al. Randomised comparison of percutaneous endoscopic gastrostomy and nasogastric tube feeding in patients with persisting neurological dysphagia. *Br Med J* 1992;304:1406–1409.

33. Iizuka M, Reding M. Use of percutaneous endoscopic gastrostomy feeding tubes and functional recovery in stroke rehabilitation: a case-matched controlled study. *Arch Phys Med Rehabil* 2005;86:1049–1052.

34. Dennis MS, Lewis SC, Warlow C. FOOD Trial Collaboration. Effect of timing and method of enteral tube feeding for dysphagic stroke patients (FOOD): a multicenter randomized controlled trial. *Lancet* 2005;26:764–772.

35. Melchior JC, Chastang C, Gelas P, et al. Efficacy of 2-month total parenteral nutrition in AIDS patients: a controlled randomized prospective trial. The French Multicenter Total Parenteral Nutrition Cooperative Group Study. *AIDS* 1996;10:379–384.

36. Klein S, Simes J, Blackburn GL. Total parenteral nutrition and cancer clinical trials. *Cancer* 1986;58:1378–1386.

37. McGeer AJ, Detsky AS, O'Rourke K. Parenteral nutrition in cancer patients undergoing chemotherapy: a meta-analysis. *Nutrition* 1990;6:233–240.

38. American College of Physicians. Parenteral nutrition in patients receiving cancer chemotherapy. *Ann Intern Med* 1989;110:734–736.

39. Lee JH, Machtay M, Unger LD, et al. Prophylactic gastrostomy tubes in patients undergoing intensive irradiation for cancer of the head and neck. *Arch Otolaryngol Head Neck Surg* 1998;124:871–875.

40. Bozzetti F, Gavazzi C, Mariani L, et al. Artificial nutrition in cancer patients: which route, what composition? *World J Surg* 1999;23:577–583.

41. Dresler CM, Jeevanandam M, Brennan MF. Metabolic efficacy of enteral feeding in malnourished cancer and non-cancer patients. *Metabolism* 1987;36:82.

42. Burt ME, Gorschboth CM, Brennan MF. A controlled, prospective, randomized trial evaluating the metabolic effects of enteral and parenteral nutrition in the cancer patient. *Cancer* 1982;49:1092–1095.

43. Lim STK, Choa RG, Lam KH, et al. Total parenteral nutrition versus gastrostomy in the preoperative preparation of patients with carcinoma of the esophagus. *Br J Surg* 1981;68:69–72.

44. McClave SA, Chang WK. Complications of enteral access. *Gastrointest Endosc* 2003;58:739–751.

45. Klor BM, Milianti FJ. Rehabilitation of neurogenic dysphagia with percutaneous endoscopic gastrostomy. *Dysphagia* 1999;14:162–164.

46. Mazzini L, Corra T, Zaccala M, et al. Percutaneous endoscopic gastrostomy and enteral nutrition in amyotrophic lateral sclerosis. *J Neurol* 1995;242:695–698.

47. Kasarskis EJ, Scarlata D, Hill R, et al. A retrospective study of percutaneous endoscopic gastrostomy in ALS patients during the BDNF and CNTF trials. *J Neurol Sci* 1999;169:118–125.

48. Desport JC, Preux PM, Truong CT, et al. Nutritional assessment and survival in ALS patients. *Amyotroph Lateral Scler Other Motor Neuron Disord* 2000;1:91–96.

49. Gregory S, Siderowf A, Golaszewski AL, et al. Gastrostomy insertion in ALS patients with low vital capacity: respiratory support and survival. *Neurology* 2002;58:485–487.

50. Boitano J, Jordan T, Benditt JO. Noninvasive ventilation allows gastrostomy tube placement in patients with advanced ALS. *Neurology* 2001;56:413–414.

51. Burge F. Dehydration symptoms of palliative care cancer patients. *J Pain Symptom Manag* 1993;8:454–464.

52. Ellershaw JE, Sutcliffe JM, Saunders CM. Dehydration and the dying patient. *J Pain Symptom Manag* 1995;10:192–197.

53. Bruera E, Franco JJ, Maltoni M, et al. Changing pattern of agitated impaired mental status in patients with advanced cancer: association with cognitive monitoring, hydration and opioid rotation. *J Pain Symptom Manag* 1995;10:287–291.

54. Lanuke K, Fainsinger RL, De Moissac D. Hydration management at the end of life. *J Palliat Med* 2004;7:257–263.

55. Morita T, Hyodo I, Yoshimi T, et al. Association between hydration volume and symptoms in terminally ill cancer patients with abdominal malignancies. *Ann Oncol* 2005;16:640–647.

56. Gessert CE, Curry NM, Robinson A. Ethnicity and end-of-life care: the use of feeding tubes. *Ethn Dis* 2001;11:97–106.

57. Braun UK, Rabeneck L, McCullough LB, et al. Decreasing use of percutaneous endoscopic gastrostomy tube feeding for veterans with dementia—racial differences remain. *J Am Geriatr Soc* 2005;53:242–248.

58. Gordon M, Alibhai SMH. Ethics of PEG tubes—Jewish and Islamic perspectives. *Am J Gastroenterol* 2004;99:1194.

59. Jotkowitz AB, Clarfield AM, Glick S. The care of patients with dementia: a modern Jewish ethical perspective. *J Am Geriatr Soc* 2005;53:881–884.

60. Brett AS, Rosenberg JC. The adequacy of informed consent for placement of gastrostomy tubes. *Arch Intern Med* 2001;161:745–748.

61. Franzoni S, Frisoni GB, Boffelli S, et al. Good nutritional oral intake is associated with equal survival in demented and nondemented very old patients. *J Am Geriatr Soc* 1996;44:1366–1370.

62. Mitchell SL, Buchanan JL, Littlehale S, et al. Tube-feeding versus hand-feeding nursing home residents with advanced dementia: a cost comparison. *JAMA* 2003;4:27–33.

CHAPTER 69 ■ REHABILITATIVE MEDICINE

REBECCA G. SMITH AND MARY M. VARGO

Because the effects of cancer and its treatment are so varied, the individual with cancer can present with rehabilitation needs of virtually any sort (1). The key concept in rehabilitation is the need for definable goals. For cancer rehabilitation, Dietz (2) has outlined four types of goals: preventative, restorative, supportive, and palliative. According to the World Health Organization International Classification of Functioning, Disability, and Health (WHO/ICF) (3), illness can act at a number of levels. Terminology was revised in 2002 to incorporate a "health" rather than "disease" perspective. Most basic is the effect of disease on the body itself (in most recent terminology "body structures" and "body functions", formerly "impairment"). The next rung considers one's ability to perform basic daily living functions ("activity limitations", formerly known as "disability"), followed by the broader concept of impact on one's societal role ("participation restrictions", formerly known as "handicap"). Environmental influences on the person are also considered. Rehabilitation goals are highly individualized and may be set at any one or more of these levels.

Another important concept is measurement of rehabilitation outcomes. While at the body structure or body function level this may be straightforward (i.e., joint range of motion, limb girth, manual muscle testing), quantifying activity limitations or participation restrictions can be more complicated. Traditional functional scales applied to the cancer population, such as Karnofsky or East Cooperative Oncology Group (ECOG) scores, do not afford a level of detail that is useful in monitoring gradual increments in progress. In recent years, quantitative functional outcome tools, such as the Functional Independence Measure (FIM) (4), have been successfully used for measuring outcomes in patients with cancer, mainly in the inpatient rehabilitation setting. Other tests or scales measuring parameters such as quality of life, fatigue, pain, psychological tests, and specific functions (timed walk; swallowing studies; cognitive or language batteries) may also be of use in specific contexts.

SPECTRUM OF FUNCTIONAL IMPAIRMENTS

The range of impairments caused by cancer is not only broad, but also dynamic. Problems seen may be attributable to the tumor itself, to treatment effects, or to other comorbidities. The issues may be immediately evident, or they may occur in a delayed manner. While some types of problems have excellent potential for improvement with rehabilitation (restorative goal), other impairments are permanent (maintenance goal,

to prevent progression or secondary complications). The kind of rehabilitation problems, and the goals of treatment, will also vary with the stage of disease (Table 69.1).

Common issues across many types of cancer include pain, fatigue, and deconditioning. Pain and fatigue management are discussed in more detail in other chapters. Attention to differential diagnosis for these issues is critical. Rehabilitation interventions for pain include nonpharmacologic treatments such as heat, cold, and electricity-based modalities, injections, manual therapies, targeted exercise, and psychological strategies. Adjunctive pain medications may also be of benefit depending on the nature of the pain. Complementary and alternative medicine strategies such as acupuncture have gained increasing acceptance. Rehabilitation interventions for fatigue include exercise, energy conservation techniques, and pharmacologic adjustments. This may include use of stimulants or antidepressants, attention to sleep–wake cycle, and general care in minimizing the sedating or fatiguing side effects of medicines (5,6).

Other problems are less universally seen, but need significant rehabilitation services when they do occur. Neurologic deficits can result from peripheral neuropathies; nerve root, spinal cord, or brain involvement; as well as from myopathies or conditions affecting the myoneural junction. Musculoskeletal issues can include major amputation or deformity (such as might present after a limb-sparing procedure), contracture, and muscle strain. Orthopaedic stability needs to be considered when bony metastatic disease presents. Communication and swallowing problems may occur, especially with conditions involving brain or head and neck structures. Cognitive deficits also can result from brain tumor or therapies. Limb edema, especially lymphedema, is a common problem often caused by tumor invasion of lymph nodes, and especially, by surgical and radiation treatment across lymph structures.

DECONDITIONING

Deconditioning, or debility, is a multisystem complication of prolonged immobility (7,8). While not specific to cancer, individuals with cancer are at risk due to the lack of physical activity that can result from the cancer itself, as well as from treatment. Deconditioning may also coexist with other forms of weakness, such as corticosteroid myopathy, critical illness polyneuropathy, myoneural junction disorders, or other neurologic insult. Of note, deconditioning is different from cachexia, and strategies to combat deconditioning (primarily restorative exercise programs) will probably not be tolerated

TABLE 69.1

CANCER REHABILITATION: A DYNAMIC LANDSCAPE

Core concepts	Individualized, patient-centered goals; team approach; interdisciplinary communication
Goals	Preventative, restorative, supportive, palliative
Phases	Pretreatment, primary treatment, posttreatment/survivor/ intercurrent, recurrence, end of life
Types of need	Systemic (i.e., fitness; fatigue management); tumor specific (including localized, metastatic, paraneoplastic effects)
Reasons for rehabilitation need	Cancer; treatment effect; comorbidity
Time course	Immediate/early effects; late effects (includes early effects that are permanent, and effects that have delayed onset)

in the patient who is cachectic. Strategies to prevent and treat deconditioning are presented in Table 69.2. Many of the figures cited in the following text apply to individuals on complete bedrest. However, any limited activity status can also produce some degree of deconditioning.

Weakness is the best-known effect of deconditioning. Various studies have found a loss of 10–20% strength per week of bedrest (1–1.5% per day), plateauing at 25–50% of strength at 3–5 weeks, and 50% loss of muscle bulk at 2 months (8,9). The muscles develop increased fat and fibrous tissue, reduced concentration of oxidative enzymes, and increased jitter in neuromuscular transmission. Antigravity muscles show the most pronounced loss of muscle bulk, and large muscles lose strength twice as quickly as smaller ones (10). Stretching may delay muscle atrophy, and, conversely, limb positioning in a muscle-shortened configuration results in quicker atrophy (7). Daily isometric contractions at 10–20% maximum, held for 10 seconds, have been shown in one study to maintain isometric muscle strength, but it is unclear whether this is enough in all cases (9). With submaximal exercise, strength rebuilds at 6% per week, therefore it takes about twice as long to reverse the deconditioning process as it takes to develop (7–9). Generally isotonic (nonresistive) exercise is favored over isometric, because of its favorable effects on both musculoskeletal and cardiovascular systems (8).

Contracture formation occurs because of increased collagen cross-links and turnover in loose areolar tissue, and eventual joint capsule tightness (7). Aggravating factors include local trauma, edema, hemorrhage, poor circulation, and joint degeneration, and accelerating factors include pain, poor positioning, weakness, and spasticity. Contractures result in increased work of physical activity (most notably walking), abnormal joint forces during weight bearing, impaired self-care, and in severe cases, more difficult nursing care. Stretching for 10–15 minutes daily prevents contractures, but in the setting of mild contractures, passive range-of-motion exercises for 20–30 minutes twice daily, with sustained terminal stretch, is required. For more severe contractures even more aggressive stretching is required, often in combination with other modalities, such as heat or dynamic splinting. Serial casting can also be done (8).

Osteopenia primarily affects weight-bearing bone, with mineral content falling nearly 1% per week, plateauing at approximately 50% of the original mass (7). Hypercalcemia may occur, typically approximately 4 weeks after starting bedrest, with symptoms including nausea, vomiting, abdominal pain, lethargy, weakness, and anorexia (7). In the setting of cancer, alternative reasons for bone loss should be weighed, such as tumor invasion or paraneoplastic phenomena.

Cardiovascular effects include loss of plasma volume, decreased stroke volume and cardiac output, increased resting heart rate (half a beat per day during the first 2 months of bedrest), decreased VO_2 max, increased blood viscosity, and decreased plasma proteins (7). With reconditioning, attention must be paid to heart rate and blood pressure responses to activity, and in particular to postural hypotension, which can be treated with compression stockings, use of a tilt table, adequate salt and fluid intake, and in refractory cases sympathetic or mineralocorticoid medications (8). For the patient with co-morbid coronary artery disease, additional precautions may be needed when approaching reconditioning. Pulmonary effects include reduced tidal volume, increased respiratory rate, ciliary dryness, ineffective cough (especially with recumbency), and ventilation/perfusion mismatches. The patient should have frequent position changes, perform deep breathing exercises including incentive spirometry, and undergo appropriate chest physical therapy to facilitate clearing of secretions (8). Genitourinary effects include impaired emptying, bladder infection, and stones. Gastrointestinal effects include reduced peristalsis and poor appetite. Attention should be paid to adequate fluid and fiber intake, pharmacologic measures to address constipation (stool softeners, suppositories, laxatives), and, if urinary retention is suspected, checking of post-void residual volumes (8). Medications with anticholinergic or otherwise constipating side effects should be avoided, if possible. Cognitive and psychologic effects of deconditioning also occur, such as confusion, depressed mood, and anxiety. Attending to the patient's comfort (including, to the extent possible, enjoyable activities), maintaining familiar people and environments, a regular daily routine, and adequate sleep are probably important in minimizing these effects.

REHABILITATION INTERVENTIONS

Therapeutic Exercise

While much remains to be delineated, especially regarding the extent to which precautions are needed, exercise has been one of the best-studied areas of cancer rehabilitation in recent years. In addition to benefits relating to physical conditioning, improvements have been found in quality of life, psychological factors, and fatigue, even duration of neutropenia and of hospital stay (11–15). Beneficial effects have been seen in populations ranging from inpatients in the midst of intensive antineoplastic treatment, to outpatients recovering from breast cancer treatment (16), to long-term survivors (17). The goals of exercise vary with the stage of disease and the patient's place in the treatment trajectory. For example, for an acutely ill hospitalized patient, the main goal of exercise might be to slow down the loss of strength, whereas posttreatment the goals will be genuinely restorative. Exercise can be conceptualized both in terms of maximizing general fitness (strength, cardiopulmonary conditioning), as well as targeting specific issues that the individual with cancer might need to address (such as lymphedema, amputation, hemiparesis, contracture). While formal conditioning programs do not

TABLE 69.2

DECONDITIONING EFFECTS AND TREATMENT STRATEGIES

Effect	Prevention	Treatment
Muscle weakness/reduced muscle mass	Isometric muscle contraction at least 20–30% maximal for a few seconds daily; positioning to avoid pressure palsies (fibular head, ulnar groove, spiral groove of humerus)	Strengthening exercise; consider/address comorbid etiologies of weakness
Contracture	Range-of-motion exercise (especially large muscle groups and muscles crossing two joints; attention to hips, knees, ankles, shoulders, elbows, neck, back); splinting, positioning	Manual stretches (20–30 minutes twice daily with sustained terminal stretch), with pain-control measures if needed; deep heat (contraindicated if area is insensate or if tumor in affected part); dynamic splinting; serial casting; blocks; surgical releases
Osteopenia	Weight-bearing exercise as feasible; adequate calcium and vitamin D intake	Same as for prevention; however, avoid high-impact weight bearing if severe osteopenia or metastatic disease
Cardiovascular	Adequate hydration; conditioning (aerobic) exercise as feasible (can use supine ergometer if patient in bed); thromboembolic prophylaxis	Conditioning (aerobic) exercise to training effect; include warm-up and cool-down; if postural hypotension—compression stockings, fall prevention strategies, possible sympathetic or mineralocorticoid agents; initially check pulse and blood pressure pre- and postexertion (rule out inotropic insufficiency or exaggerated heart rate response to activity)
Pulmonary	Deep breathing exercise control/mobilize secretions (hydration, bronchodilators, cough, suctioning)	Conditioning (aerobic) exercise; supplemental oxygen if needed to maintain saturation during physical activity
Gastrointestinal	Stool softener; high fiber diet; avoid constipating medications as feasible; nutritional strategies to for optimal intake, possible appetite stimulant	Same; laxatives, bulk-forming agents, suppository program or use of enemas if necessary
Urinary	Adequate hydration; remove catheter as soon as feasible; void upright if possible; monitor for retention	Same; treat bladder infections (especially once catheter removed, or if symptomatic with the catheter); catheterization program if failure to void or retention present, until resolved
Psychological/central nervous system	Maintain familiar people, environment and routine as feasible; monitor for signs of depression and anxiety; regulate sleep–wake; adequate pain control and other symptom management; avoid medications with cognitive side effects as feasible	Same; treat psychologic/psychiatric sequelae with pharmacologic and/or nonpharmacologic strategies; safety precautions (such as supervision, fall prevention strategies, possible restraints) for confusion

generally have a role in end-stage cachexia, rehabilitation therapies such as physical or occupational therapies may still be of benefit to help address the patient's functional needs and overall independence level (18,19). On the other end of the spectrum, for obese individuals, exercise is an important component of meeting weight loss goals, and shows promise in preventing weight gain in patients with breast cancer receiving chemotherapy (20). Special considerations regarding obesity in the cancer population are its association with reduced survival (and increased risk of malignancy in the first place) for at least some tumor types (21), and its association with lymphedema (22). A number of studies have shown benefits of exercise in cancer-related immune parameters (23). Physical activity has been associated with reduced overall and site-specific (breast, colon) cancer risk (24).

Many exercise precautions have been cited for individuals with cancer, on a commonsense basis, but the evidence basis is very limited (Table 69.3). Factors to consider include blood counts (especially platelet count), bony integrity, and cardiovascular status. Generally, exercise can be unlimited with platelet count greater than 30–50 K, should be limited to low-impact, nonresistive activities when the platelets are under that level, and totally restricted (except perhaps brief

walking) when platelets are under 10–20 K. The concern is that bleeding will result from the physical impact or from blood pressure response to activity. If there is a concern of bony stability, orthopaedic assessment is indicated for possible surgical fixation, bracing, or use of an assistive device before initiating the exercise program (25). Cardiovascular problems are common in the general population, and given the demographics of cancer they must be considered. A cancer-specific concern is cardiotoxicity of anthracycline chemotherapy. In this setting, warm-up and cool-down phases are essential, and the patient might not mount a predictable heart rate response to activity (26). Improved physical performance results from exercise, but is considered to be due to peripheral adaptation rather than intrinsic cardiac factors (27). Weight-lifting restrictions have sometimes been recommended for individuals with lymphedema, but, in the authors' opinion, there is no one-size-fits-all cut-off as to how much may be lifted. Rather, patients should be counseled to build their activity gradually, avoiding sudden exposure to heavy weights.

A perennial difficulty with exercise programs, as with many therapies, is long-term compliance, and, of course, quality of life is always a consideration. Therefore, to the extent possible the patient's enjoyment of the activity and

TABLE 69.3

EXERCISE PRECAUTIONS IN CANCER REHABILITATION (EMPIRIC)

Thrombocytopenia

\>50000: no restrictions
30000–50000: aerobic (nonresistive) exercise permissible
20000–30000: gentle nonresistive exercise (active or passive) only
<10,000–20000: essential activity only

Anemia[a]

Hematocrit >35%: activity as tolerated
Hematocrit 25–35%: light aerobic activity and light weights permissible
Hematocrit <25%: essential activity, light isometric activity; avoid progressive aerobic programs

Bony metastasis

Lesion >2.5 cm (in femur), or >50% cortex involved; non–weight bearing (i.e., walker, crutches) until stability reestablished; avoid twisting/torques
25–50% Cortex involved—avoid high bony impact, torques; consider assistive device for pain control and partial assist with weight bearing
<25% Cortex involved—no restrictions

Lymphedema

Avoid over-strenuous use of the affected limb (sudden unaccustomed activity)

[a]Must be interpreted in light of overall health status.

access concerns, must be considered and incorporated into the exercise recommendations. Courneya has outlined exercise programs for early stage patients and long-term healthy survivors (28).

Generally, when cardiovascular conditioning is desired, an aerobic program is favored. Data is lacking as to when the exercise program needs to be supervised versus self-directed (16). Ideally, there should be a method of monitoring exercise intensity, to assure that a training effect is being reached. Over time, the individual will be able to increase his or her exercise intensity, with progressively greater physical work being performed before the anaerobic threshold is reached. Possible parameters include target heart rate based on exercise stress test data (the ideal, especially in the setting of known cardiac problems, but not always feasible) or calculated values (220 less age in years as a rough gauge of maximum heart rate in a healthy individual). Target exercise heart rate is typically 60–85% of maximum, with those in poor physical condition aiming for the lower end of this spectrum. Alternatively, for the frail individual, one might aim empirically for an approximately 20 beats per minute increase from resting heart rate, or use the Borg Rating of Perceived Exertion, a self-administered rating scale which has been shown to correlate with heart rate and other physiologic training effect parameters (26). While adjunctive pharmacologic strategies, such as use of stimulants, anabolic steroids, or red blood cell promoting agents, have been considered to improve exercise tolerance and/or muscle mass in the patient with cancer, data as to effectiveness and specific indications is pending. One study of weight losing cancer patients did exhibit improved exercise tolerance with erythropoietin (29).

Strengthening is initially best tolerated with isotonic (non-resistive, high-repetition) activities, gradually incorporating more intensity into the program. However, when one desires to minimize forces across a joint (e.g., in the presence of bony invasion, pain, or arthritis), isometric exercise may be best tolerated. Isometric exercise consists of muscle contraction in the absence of joint excursion. Isometric strength is important for some aspects of functional activity, such as transfers, and maintaining a wheelchair push-up.

Flexibility on the part of the therapist is needed, and tolerance may be limited by medical complications and fatigue. Even if, while acutely ill, the level of participation is minimal,

the patient benefits from the "habit" and trust that is built with the therapist, which may translate into quicker transition to physical activity when the patient is ready (30,31).

For individuals with focal weakness, the activity program will include strengthening of the affected parts, and compensatory strategies. The prognosis for improvement will vary with the etiology and severity of the lesion (see section Mobility and Gait Training). For those with contracture, a stretching program is important (see section Deconditioning). Stretches are also an important preventative strategy, especially for patients who have received radiation therapy across a joint, amputation (contractures will impede prosthetic use), or with a weakness pattern resulting in imbalance in the strength of agonist/antagonist muscles surrounding a joint.

Exercise is an important part of complex decongestive therapy (CDT) for lymphedema (see section Lymphedema), although it has not been well studied as an isolated modality for this condition.

Mobility and Gait Training

Mobility refers to the ability to move and explore one's environment. It includes the ability to move in bed (bed mobility) including changing positions from supine to sitting, rolling on one's side, sitting on the side of the bed, and transferring from one surface to another. It may be at the wheelchair or ambulatory level. Impaired mobility may be caused by a number of conditions (see section Spectrum of Functional Impairment). Cognitive and visual perception factors imposed by central nervous system lesions may also limit mobility and pose additional challenges in rehabilitation.

For the severely impaired person having difficulty moving in bed, poor sitting tolerance, and inability to transfer, physical therapy is needed. Physical therapy may also be indicated to attain a higher functional level (reconditioning), or to help the patient regain deficient skills. The therapy may begin at the bedside to promote independent mobility in bed, balance and sitting tolerance, and transfers out of bed to a standing position or to another chair. The use of a tilt table may allow the person with autonomic dysfunction to gradually tolerate changes in position from supine to sitting and eventually to standing. Locomotion may be achieved with a wheelchair, or

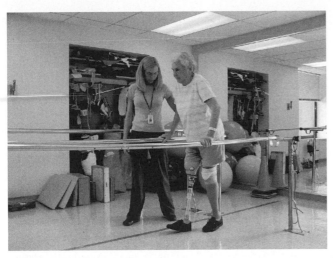

FIGURE 69.1. Gait training: patient with right transfemoral amputation and a left transtibial amputation.

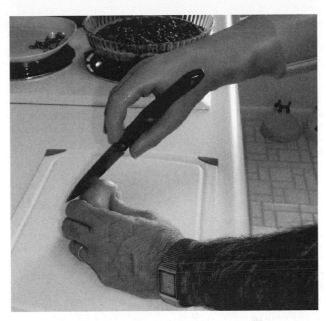

FIGURE 69.2. Patient with a transradial amputation learning to perform kitchen activities in occupational therapy. (Photograph courtesy of Albert Esquenazi, MD.)

walking with an assistive device such as a walker or cane. The prescription of an orthosis or prosthesis may be necessary to promote functional independence. Additional physical therapy goals may include strengthening affected muscles, stretching contractures, reducing spasticity, improving proprioception and balance, and helping develop compensatory strategies for those with visual–spatial deficits or communication disorders.

Gait disturbances due to weakness, spasticity, proprioceptive deficits, and leg-length discrepancies may be corrected with a combination of orthoses, specially adapted assistive devices and gait training. Physical therapists also provide gait training to those who have had lower limb amputations. This may include teaching them to ambulate using assistive devises such as crutches or a walker, as well as providing prosthesis (artificial limb) training. Gait abnormalities associated with poorly fitting or incorrectly fitted prostheses can also be identified and corrected by a team including the physical therapist, physiatrist, and prosthetist (Figure 69.1).

Functional abnormalities due to spasticity including ambulation and gait may be addressed with a combination of physical therapy, medications, and other interventions if necessary. Pharmacologic management of spasticity may be initiated if the conventional therapeutic techniques of stretching and bracing are not effective and if the condition limits ambulation, activities of daily living (ADL), and hygiene and/or causes pain. These agents include baclofen, tizanidine, and dantrolene. Interventional techniques such as botulinum toxin injections, neurolysis with phenol and intrathecal baclofen pumps are additional strategies that physiatrists may use to reduce the complications of spasticity that often limit ambulation, as well as other ADL.

Activities of Daily Living

Functional ADL include activities of self-care including bathing, grooming, personal hygiene, toileting, eating, and dressing. Additional instrumental ADL include meal preparation, shopping, paying bills, and household duties. The inability to perform ADL may be due to the same factors that limit mobility including cognitive and visual perception deficits.

Occupational therapists are trained to help people regain their ability to perform their ADL. They help the patient develop compensatory strategies to perform self-care activities including functional transfers to the commode and bath or shower, based on the individual's impairments. Assistive

devices such as a reacher or shochorn may help a person regain the ability to dress. Modified eating utensils and upper extremity orthoses may assist in self-feeding. Additional devices including a raised toilet seat and tub or shower chair may help compensate for orthopaedic or neurologic impairments and allow a person to perform toileting and bathing activities.

Occupational therapists are also trained to provide focused therapies to improve generalized upper extremity weakness and range of motion, and implement techniques such as constraint-induced therapy for those with long-standing upper extremity hemiparesis. They, along with physical therapists, are trained to provide education and training to patients and their families, as well as, teach safety techniques and energy conservation strategies (such as pacing, prioritization, planning, and attention to posture with activities) and perform a home checkout. Home therapies may be effective in establishing independence and compensatory strategies in the home environment, as well as in developing home modifications to improve safety and accommodate specific limitations and equipment (Figure 69.2).

Cognitive and Communication Disorders

Cancer and/or treatment sequelae may interfere with one's cognition and ability to communicate. Impaired cognition may be related to brain pathology, but also to depression, medications, or endocrine/electrolyte disturbances. An acute change in mental status should prompt a thorough evaluation of treatable causes.

Aphasia refers to an impaired ability to comprehend or express verbal or written language. It may occur as a consequence of a central nervous system lesion in the language area of the dominant cerebral hemisphere. Its classification includes evaluation of fluency of speech, as well as one's ability to comprehend, repeat, and name objects (32,33). Speech and cognitive therapies can help improve comprehension and expression by various facilitation, compensation, and education strategies (33,34).

Facilitative strategies emphasize restoring normal speech patterns including silent rehearsals, self-cueing, self-monitoring of comprehension, and feedback generation to verify comprehension. Compensation strategies develop alternative forms of communication. These may include gesturing or drawing, emphasizing key words, using a communication board, the speaker slowing their rate of speech to improve comprehension and speaker gesturing (33). Patient and family education promotes understanding of the underlying disorder and enables family members to use the strategies mentioned earlier to improve communication at home and in the community.

Unilateral spatial neglect refers to a deficit in attention to one side of the body. It may result from a lesion involving specific brainstem nuclei, thalamus, striatum, cingulate gyrus, frontal lobe, or posterior parietal cortex. Unilateral spatial neglect may create significant barriers to safe ambulation and ability to perform ADL including dressing and eating. Rehabilitation strategies to improve attention to the neglected side include cueing, visual stimulation of the affected side, prism adaptation, eye patching, and electric stimulation (33,35).

Dysarthria refers to impaired communication due to oral-motor weakness. It may be due to central nervous system lesions in the cerebral hemisphere or brainstem. It may also be a complication of peripheral nerve or muscle injury following head and neck surgery. Speech therapies can help improve communication skills with oral-motor strengthening exercises, communication boards and other compensatory strategies.

The ability to communicate may also be compromised following tumor invasion and/or subsequent resection of lesions in the head and neck, including the palate, tongue, mandible, pharynx, vocal cords, and larynx. Speech therapies can be individualized to promote and improve ability to communicate by a number of techniques. These include vocal cord adduction and oral-motor/labial strengthening exercises, communication boards, and adaptive, nonverbal gestures, and writing equipment (34,35). Voice restoration following laryngectomies may be facilitated using several techniques that include esophageal speech and tracheoesophageal puncture (TEP) speech. Sophisticated voice restoration devices include voice and telephone amplifiers for whispered or dysphonic speech, artificial speaking devices (electrolarynxes), body-powered tone generators, and speech synthesizers. Text telephones and fax machines may help improve communication in the work setting (34). See Chapter 12 of this book for a more detailed discussion.

Swallowing Dysfunction

Impaired swallowing is referred to as dysphagia. It may result from unilateral or bilateral cerebral hemispheric or brainstem lesions (32,33). It may also result as a consequence of tumor invasion or resection in the head and neck, as well as, a complication of radiation and chemotherapy. Dysphagia has many associated complications including aspiration, fear of choking, loss of appetite, weight loss, and malnutrition (34).

An initial bedside swallow study can be performed to evaluate swallowing dysfunction and risks of aspiration. Predictors of aspiration on bedside examination include dysphonia, dysarthria, abnormal cough, cough after swallowing, abnormal gag reflex, and change in voice after swallowing (33). A video fluoroscopy study is then performed to visualize the swallowing mechanism. Aspiration is defined by video fluoroscopy as penetration of contrast material below the level of the true vocal cords (33). Speech therapies promote improved swallowing by facilitatory and compensatory swallowing techniques such as oral-motor exercises, thermal stimulation, postural modifications such as tucking one's chin and tilting one's head, and dietary modifications. In the case of severe dysphagia or malnutrition, supplemental or alternative feeding strategies should be considered. These include temporary use of a small bore nasogastric tube, or a gastrostomy or jejunostomy

tube if long-term enteric feeding is required (33,34). Refer to Chapter 12 (in this book) for a detailed description of the phases of swallowing, as well as for further evaluation and rehabilitation interventions.

Physical Modalities for Pain Relief

Physical modalities are physical agents used to produce a therapeutic effect in tissues. They include heat, cold, and electrotherapy. They are frequently used to reduce pain, facilitate stretch, aid in wound care, and introduce medications such as corticosteroids. Heat includes superficial and deep heating modalities. Superficial heat is applied to the surface of the skin to achieve maximum tissue temperatures in skin and subcutaneous fat. It is applied using heating pads, moist compresses, hydrocollator packs, paraffin baths, and whirlpool baths. Deep heat is directed to the heat muscle, tendons, ligaments or bone. It is most commonly applied using ultrasound waves. Medication such as 1% lidocaine or corticosteroids may be applied using ultrasound. This technique is known as *phonophoresis*. The ultrasound waves facilitate the diffusion of the medication into the deeper tissue zones. Phonophoresis is often used to treat tendinitis, bursitis, scar tissue, neuromas, and adhesions that may be complications associated with cancer or its treatments (36).

Cold modalities, also known as *cryotherapy*, are often used to treat acute pain and inflammation associated with musculoskeletal disorders, as well as, myofascial pain, spasticity, and emergent care of minor burns. Cryotherapy should not be used in cold intolerant patients or in those with cryopathies such as cold hypersensitivity and Raynaud's disease (36).

Transelectrocutaneous electrical nerve stimulation (TENS) is the most common form of electroanalgesia. It has been used to help reduce both neuropathic and nociceptive pain conditions, depending on the type of TENS unit and parameters chosen. It is applied by placing 1–4 electrode pads surrounding the area of pain. A small stimulating unit is connected and a specific frequency, pulse width, and amplitude are selected on the basis of the type of pain and the patient's response. The analgesic affect of TENS may be due to a combination of mechanisms including acting as a counterirritant in the central nervous system to inhibit activity of dorsal horn nociceptive neurons, activating the production of endogenous opioids and possibly activating other neurotransmitter systems including the serotonergic and substance P systems (37). The TENS unit should not be applied over or near malignancy, unless it is being used in terminally ill patient with cancer (36).

There are precautions that should be considered when prescribing modalities. Heat should not be applied to an area of acute trauma and inflammation, and in patients with bleeding diatheses, edema, peripheral vascular disease, large scars, impaired sensation, and cognitive or communication deficits that impair their ability to report pain. The use of all heat forms and electricity are contraindicated directly over malignancies because of their potential for increasing the rate of tumor growth or hyperemia necessary for hematogenous spread. This precaution may be overlooked in the terminally ill patient if modalities are to be used as adjuvants to improve pain relief or reduce inflammation (36). Cryotherapy is the treatment of choice for acute trauma and inflammation. It may also be used in patients with bleeding diathesis and large scars.

Orthotics

Orthoses are fabricated devices used to provide support or improve function of a moveable body part (38). They are commonly prescribed for individuals with neurologic sequelae of cancer or its treatment, including those with hemiparesis from cerebral lesions, quadriparesis or paraparesis from spinal cord involvement, as well as weakness from plexopathies, peripheral neuropathies, and myopathies. They include upper and lower extremity devices. The upper extremity devices, such as the balanced arm orthosis, may permit gravity-eliminated movements of the arms to aid in eating and grooming functions in an individual with a C5 level of spinal cord injury. The static wrist splints protect the joint and facilitate the use of a weakened grasp in those with no or weak wrist extension. Dynamic wrist splints, including the tenodesis splint, are used to enhance or create a functional grip. They may also be used to reduce spasticity or prevent contractures (38). Environmental control units provide those with severe upper and lower extremity weakness the ability to mobilize and perform ADL through controls such as their mouth.

Lower extremity orthoses are used to stabilize and protect the lower limb joints, as well as aid in therapeutic standing and therapeutic and functional ambulation. It can be modified to provide varying degrees of ankle support, as well as reduce spasticity and clonus. The type of the lower extremity orthosis is influenced by the severity and location of weakness. Persons with thoracic or high lumbar spinal cord lesions, or those with significant lower extremity weakness including hip flexion, will require hip-knee-ankle-foot orthoses (HKAFO) to promote more hip support and control. A reciprocating gait orthosis is a type of bilateral HKAFO that enables people with these levels of spinal cord injury to ambulate. The knee-ankle-foot orthosis (KAFO) is used in people with weak quadriceps but intact thigh flexors. The KAFO locks the knee in extension while ambulating. An ankle-foot orthosis (AFO) is often prescribed for those with good hip and thigh strength, but varying degree of leg and foot weakness. It is commonly used in those with weak ankle dorsiflexion and/or plantar flexion due to isolated peripheral nerve injuries, peripheral neuropathies, or distal lower limb weakness following a cerebral or spinal cord lesion. The AFO provides support and assistance with dorsiflexion and/or plantar flexion of the ankle (38) (Figure 69.3).

Spinal orthoses include those that provide stability to the cervical, thoracic, and lumbosacral regions of the vertebral column. There are a number of types of spinal orthoses that provide varying degrees of stability and motion. Prescription depends on the goals of the orthoses, for example stabilization status post–tumor resection and/or pain relief due to compression fractures. See Chapter 6 for a detailed description of the types of spinal orthoses.

Prosthetic and Limb Salvage Issues

Compared with other populations who have had amputation (traumatic, dysvascular), those with cancer tend to have a more proximal level of amputation (39), which makes prosthetic management more challenging; however, they also tend to be younger individuals, which is a favorable prognostic characteristic for prosthetic use. In appropriate cases, limb-sparing procedures can be performed and do not compromise life expectancy (40). Limb-sparing options are quite varied and include wide local incision, autologous tissue transfers, intercalary amputation and reconstruction (e.g., the Van Nes procedure in the lower limb), allografts, endoprostheses, and composite techniques (39). While quality of life outcomes have been found to be comparable between patients undergoing amputation and those receiving a limb-sparing intervention, the latter has been associated with more long-term complications, such as endoprosthetic loosening or infection, or need for future procedures to accommodate growth. Generally, however, patient satisfaction with limb-sparing procedure results

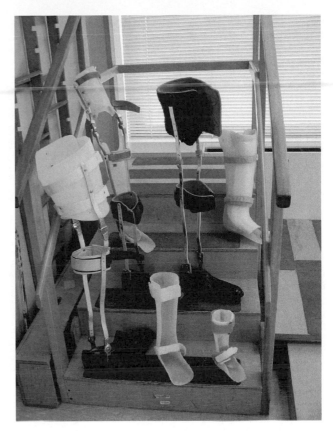

FIGURE 69.3. Collection of knee- and ankle-foot orthoses including plastic molded and double metal upright models.

is high, except when there have been complications, in which case satisfaction is often greater after amputation is (eventually) performed (41). For those who have had amputation, important aspects of preprosthetic care include edema control, exercise for flexibility and strengthening of the residual limb, general conditioning, and education as to functional expectations with a prosthesis.

For those with very proximal upper limb (such as forequarter level) amputation, functional prosthetic use is not likely to be a viable goal. Fabrication of a molded shoulder prosthesis allows a better fit of clothing. Ideally, mold of the shoulder should be made prior to the amputation. For upper and lower limb amputations above the elbow or knee, immediate postoperative casting is often employed, and the patient is fitted with a permanent prosthesis at approximately 6 weeks, if adequate healing has occurred and no further chemotherapy is planned (due to concern of fluid shifts affecting limb size). Numerous prosthetic options are available, depending on the patient's general condition (active versus limited use anticipated) and priorities (cosmesis versus durability) (25) (Figure 69.4).

Rehabilitation after limb-sparing procedure will depend on the nature of the intervention. Functional goals will be similar, or sometimes higher than with amputees; however, postsurgical considerations such as weight bearing, soft tissue healing, or compromise of neural or articular structures may be factors in pacing, strategies, and expectations for rehabilitation.

Lymphedema

Various effective therapies have been developed for lymphedema (42,43), however, an ongoing daily routine is needed

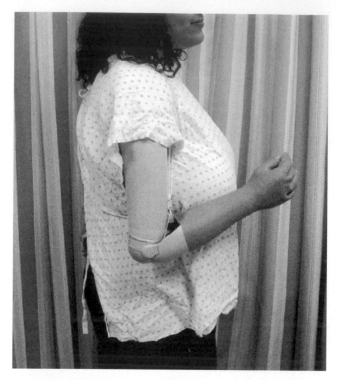

FIGURE 69.4. Patient with a transfemoral amputation demonstrating an upper limb prosthesis. (Photograph courtesy of Albert Esquenazi, MD.)

in most cases. In general, posttreatment lymphedema has a better prognosis than lymphedema due to active malignancy (42). Lymphedema is also more responsive to therapy in the early stages, but improvement can occur later as well. Surgery and radiation to lymph structures present additive risk, and obesity is associated with a higher risk of lymphedema (44). Sentinel lymph node biopsy appears to be dramatically reducing, but not eliminating, the risk in patients with breast cancer.

Many commonsense precautions have been developed for lymphedema prevention, such as avoiding sudden constriction or pressure changes to the limb (blood pressure cuff, hot tubs, air travel, purse straps) or cuts to the skin (due to concern of infection and aggravation of lymphedema from the inflammatory process); however, these precautions have not been rigorously studied. Of greatest concern, among the precautions sometimes stated are activity limitations, such as being told not to lift more than 10 pounds with the affected arm. The concern is that such a limitation will affect quality of life and also subject the contralateral limb to strain. The authors prefer not to set an absolute limit on physical activity, for the reasons given earlier and also because muscle actions may be beneficial in promoting lymph flow. Rather, patients should be advised to build their activity level gradually, avoiding sudden exertions, and to be attentive for any possible aggravating or relieving effects of activity.

Among treatment methods, CDT—a combination of multi-layer wraps, a specialized massage technique called *manual lymphatic drainage* (MLD), exercises, and skin care—has been best studied (45). In a controlled trial, a wrapping program followed by long-term use of compression garments was more effective in reducing swelling than garments alone (46). Compression garments are considered the mainstay for maintenance care, although many patients use other aspects of CDT long term. Various garment strengths (commonly 40/30 or 30/20 mm Hg, with the higher pressures distally) and designs are available, and customized garments can be made for those

with unusual limb contour. Compression pumps and other specialized devices are available, but data on their effectiveness is limited (47,48). Although often helpful for other causes of edema, diuretics are not helpful for lymphedema. Coumarins have also been studied, with some benefit found in European studies, however, not in a large US trial (49).

Because lymphedema management involves a daily routine, lifestyle implications and compliance must be considered. It is best to educate patients in a wide array of strategies, allowing them to incorporate those that align best with their preferences, abilities, and routine. When gauging improvement, one should consider not just the limb size, but also soft tissue status, the patient's perception of effectiveness, and status of any comorbid issues, such as skin infections or muscle/tendon strains.

Pulmonary Rehabilitation

Pulmonary compromise in the oncology patient may be related to lung cancer or the sequelae of lung resection, radiation and/or chemotherapy. It also occurs in patients with spinal cord injuries to the cervical through midthoracic spine due to weakened or paralyzed muscles of respiration. Additionally, immobilized patients are at an increased risk of developing atelectasis and pneumonia.

Chest physical therapy to mobilize pulmonary secretions is an important approach. This reduces the work of breathing and limits infection and atelectasis. Respiratory therapists and some physical therapists are trained to mobilize secretions using a number of techniques including chest percussion and vibration, postural drainage, incentive spirometry, and facilitation of a cough using manual and mechanical techniques (50). Additional rehabilitative strategies include teaching energy conservation techniques and pursed lip breathing.

Lung cancer and its sequelae lead to significant morbidity and mortality. The most common symptoms associated with lung cancer and its surgical, chemotherapy, and radiation treatments include fatigue, pain, dyspnea, cough, and insomnia (51). The results of a recent study indicate that the impact of dyspnea, pain, and fatigue on daily life activities in ambulatory patients with advanced lung cancer is significant (52).

Lung cancer rehabilitation has classically been described in two phases, a preoperative or pretreatment phase and a postoperative phase. The preoperative phase includes a thorough medical, social, and functional assessment. Patients are given breathing exercises to perform before their surgery to improve air entry, increase efficiency of respiratory muscles, increase chest mobility, and decrease risk of pneumonia. Patients are instructed to perform these exercises before and after surgery (34). The use of nonpharmacologic interventions including special breathing and relaxation techniques, activity pacing, counseling, and/or positive thinking can help reduce the sense of dyspnea in patients with lung cancer (51,53). Additional exercises, including daily stretches, walking, and stair climbing, as tolerated, should be encouraged. These activities may improve cardiopulmonary status, and reduce symptoms. They may also improve a patient's sense of well-being and generate a restored sense of hope and power (51,54).

The initial postoperative phase involves relieving postoperative pain, and preventing the complications of immobility by initiating passive range-of-motion exercises, skin care including pressure relief techniques, and prevention of thromboemboli. The patient is instructed to perform breathing exercises and use incentive spirometry following extubation. The patient should be mobilized and encouraged to ambulate with appropriate assistive devices as soon as possible. Patients with lung cancer also suffer from sequelae imposed by metastatic disease. These commonly affect the central nervous, peripheral nervous, and musculoskeletal systems (34). Symptoms or signs of involvement of these organ systems should prompt the clinician to further investigate the etiology, as well as, refer for an evaluation by rehabilitation specialists to maximize function and quality of life.

The patient's postoperative treatment plan and functional potential should be considered to facilitate appropriate referral for inpatient or outpatient rehabilitation, skilled nursing care, or a home rehabilitation program. Counseling regarding the patient's prognosis, functional limitations, and changing functional and social roles will help facilitate the patient's and family's adjustment and understanding of his or her condition. Palliative care issues may also need to be addressed.

Rehabilitation Strategies for Bladder and Bowel Dysfunction

Patients with cancer often experience bowel and/or bladder dysfunction. Bowel complications include diarrhea, often a side effect of chemotherapy or a result of pseudomembranous colitis, gastroenteritis, or viral infection (34). Dehydration and electrolyte disturbances may also develop. Therefore, appropriate identification of the cause by stool culture and white blood cell count when indicated, rehydration, and appropriate antibiotics and antimotility medications should be initiated.

Constipation is another common complication of medications such as opioids, immobility, obstruction from tumors or abdominal adhesions, or neurologic sequelae. The neurogenic causes of bowel dysfunction include lesions in the brain, spinal cord, peripheral nerves, or enteric nervous system. The complications associated with the neurogenic bowel are related to the site of injury and often classified as either upper motor neuron (UMN) or lower motor neuron (LMN) syndromes (55,56). Both slow bowel transit time and lead to constipation. The LMN bowel dysfunction has an associated weak external anal sphincter and therefore is also associated with fecal incontinence (55,56). A bowel program should be prescribed for both neurogenic causes. The patient with LMN bowel dysfunction should take stool bulking agents and perform a bowel program once or more times daily to reduce the risk of fecal incontinence.

All patients with constipation should be counseled on the need for a diet that is high in fluids and fiber, as well as, the need for regular exercise. Often a stool softener such as ducosate sodium and daily laxative such senna can be prescribed. A bowel program includes a series of daily rituals that promote regular bowel movements. It includes scheduling a bowel movement daily, usually after a meal to facilitate the gastrocolic reflex. The patient should be encouraged to sit upright on a commode and not use a bedpan. Rectal digital stimulation and the use of a suppository laxative such as glycerol or bisacodyl will facilitate the rectoanal reflex and promote an effective bowel movement. In patients with cognitive and/or communication deficits that limit one's ability to recognize the urge to defecate or are unable to communicate this need, timed voiding for both bowel and bladder functions should be performed.

Complaints of constipation associated with nausea, vomiting, abdominal bloating and discomfort, loss of appetite, and inability to tolerate oral intake of foods should prompt the clinician to further evaluate for a paralytic ileus or bowel obstruction. Fecal impaction may present with symptoms of severe constipation and associated diarrhea. Treatment by fecal disimpaction and an enema should relieve the symptoms.

Bladder dysfunction may present as either urinary incontinence or urinary retention. Common causes of bladder dysfunction in patients with cancer, in addition to tumor invasion causing obstruction of urinary outflow, are related to side effects of radiation, medication such as opioid or tricyclic antidepressants, infection, cognitive limitations, mobility and ADL dysfunction, and neurogenic bladder. Additional premorbid factors such as benign prostatic hypertrophy and stress incontinence may be present to complicate the symptoms (34,56,57). All these conditions should be considered when evaluating a patient with cancer and urinary complaints because the cause of the symptoms may be multifactorial and require a multidisciplinary approach to optimize treatment goals.

Patients with cancer who have voiding dysfunction as a result of neurologic injury are described as having a neurogenic bladder. The dysfunction may be due to lesions in the cerebral cortex, brainstem, spinal cord, lumbosacral plexus, or peripheral nerves. The neurogenic bladder may be classified according to a number of systems. The anatomic system classifies the dysfunction according to the site of injury. This includes suprapontine, suprasacral, and infrasacral lesions (56,57). A second system of classification is based on the type of physiologic dysfunction and includes the areflexic bladder, hyperreflexic bladder, and detrusor sphincter dysynergy (DSD). A urologic evaluation that includes urodynamic study will help in objectively determining the physiologic mechanism(s) of the dysfunction (56,57). Management depends of the type of urologic dysfunction and may include a combination of interventional, behavioral, and pharmacologic strategies.

Normal voluntary control of micturition is a well-coordinated interaction between the somatic central and peripheral nervous systems, the autonomic nervous system and peripheral nerves. The cortex provides descending inhibitory regulation of the micturition reflex. The pontine region of the mesocephalic reticular formation has been identified as the micturition reflex center (58). Lesions above the pons may cause loss of voluntary control of micturition and subsequent incontinence. However, the spinal reflexes remain intact. Sympathetic afferent and efferent reflex activation at the spinal cord levels T10-L3 functions to store urine in the bladder primarily by its α-adrenergic stimulation of the internal urethral sphincter. Parasympathetic afferent and efferent reflex activation at spinal cord levels S2-4 leads to the emptying of urine from the bladder by causing detrusor muscle contraction through muscarinic acetylcholine receptor stimulation. The somatic pudendal nerve formed from spinal roots S2-4 controls the voluntary striated urethral sphincter (56,57).

Classically, the suprapontine lesions clinically demonstrate urinary incontinence due to detrusor hyperreflexia (57). The supraspinal lesions demonstrate urinary retention with overflow incontinence secondary to DSD where both detrusor muscle and internal urethral sphincter are overactive and uncoordinated. The infraspinal lesions demonstrate urinary retention due to detrusor areflexia (57).

Pharmacologic interventions include anticholinergic medications to relax the detrusor muscle in detrusor hyperreflexia and α-adrenergic blockade to relax an overactive internal urethral sphincter as in DSD (56,57). In those patients with urinary retention as with an areflexic bladder, often a Valsalva's maneuver or Crede voiding technique that applies manual pressure in the suprapubic region over a distended bladder will initiate emptying of the bladder. Catheterization techniques may also be necessary and include a number of variations depending on the type of bladder dysfunction, and the underlying functional and cognitive levels of the patient. The variations in catheterizations include the clean intermittent catheterization technique that must be performed at least every 6 hours by the patient or caregiver, condom catheterization for men with urinary incontinence and no retention, an indwelling Foley catheterization, suprapubic catheterization, and an iliovesicular conduit (56,57). Each of these catheterization techniques has its benefits and associated risks. An individualized bladder management plan should be initiated to optimize bladder function, hygiene, and convenience, as well as, minimize social embarrassment, barriers, and risks associated with bladder dysfunction and catheterizations. Behavioral strategies include timed voiding and limiting the amount of fluids especially at night. Rehabilitation interventions include initiating treatment, and patient and caregiver education and instruction regarding the individualized bladder management program.

A special consideration must be made for those with spinal cord lesions at the T6 level or higher. Patients with injuries at and above the T6 level are at risk of developing autonomic dysreflexia (AD). AD is defined as an increase in blood pressure of greater that 20 mm Hg above baseline. It results from stimulation of the splanchnic division of the sympathetic nervous system by a noxious stimulus below the level of the lesion and causes the sympathetic responses of vasoconstriction and hypertension. The body's autoregulation mechanisms are interrupted due to the spinal cord lesion and the uncontrolled blood pressure. Classically, the patient's heart rate will decrease because of the intact response of the parasympathetic nervous system through the vagus nerve. The patients may develop a severe headache, experience an increase in spasticity, and describe a vague discomfort. This is a medical emergency and immediate treatment must be initiated. This includes making the person sit upright, loosening tight fitting clothing, checking for bladder distension, and either checking an indwelling catheter for kinks or initiating urinary catheterization. A urine sample should be sent for analysis and culture. A rectal examination should be performed to evaluate for and treat fecal impaction, and an inspection for ingrown toenails and infected decubiti should be made. If the source of the autonomic stimulation is not found and/or the blood pressure continues to be elevated, nitroglycerin paste can be applied (34,59). If the source of the stimulus is not found and/or the blood pressure continues to be elevated, the patient should be transferred to the intensive care unit for treatment with intravenous nitroprusside.

REHABILITATION SETTINGS

Acute Care

Acute care physical therapy will maintain the range of motion of joints, help prevent pressure ulcers by mobilization and pressure relief, promote independence with bed mobility and transfers, maintain cardiopulmonary function, and prevent other complications of immobility. Prescription of acute care occupational therapy will help maintain the range of motion and strength of upper limb joints and muscles and promote maintenance or functional restoration of ADL. Referral for speech therapy will help promote improved swallowing, communication, and/or cognitive skills. These therapeutic interventions will allow for the determination of safety and need for assistive devices. Physiatrists should be consulted to provide a comprehensive functional evaluation to assist with current care and predicted future rehabilitation needs.

Inpatient Rehabilitation

In recent years, progress of patients with cancer in acute rehabilitation units has been studied, with generally comparable findings in functional gains and discharge to community as non–cancer patients at rehabilitation units. Patients with cancers involving the brain or spinal cord have been particularly well studied (60–65). All patients in acute rehabilitation units are expected to tolerate 3 hours of active rehabilitation therapy

per day, and therefore the studies discussed here involve a preselected population. Typically, patients admitted to rehabilitation units will have Karnofsky scores between 30 and 70 (66). One study that monitored progress in rehabilitation units stratified cancer rehabilitation according to Dietz goal (see introductory text) (67). Patients with restorative goals made greater motor gains than those with supportive or palliative goals, however, patients in each Dietz classification made significant motor gains, including palliative cases. Cognitive gains were seen in patients with restorative and supportive goals, but not in those with palliative goals. When considered according to impairment group (asthenia, central nervous system dysfunction, orthopaedic, and postoperative), all exhibited gains, although less in those with central nervous system dysfunction than the other groups. In another study, patients in various subgroups (primary intracranial neoplasm, spinal cord, breast cancer, and other) made similar gains (68). Among patients with brain tumor, there is no significant difference in improvement between those with primary or metastatic brain involvement. Individuals tend to make better progress in their first rehabilitation hospitalization than during a repeat admission (69). Findings regarding impact of ongoing brain radiation therapy on rehabilitation progress have been variable (68–70). Patients on corticosteroids should not be fully tapered until after the radiation therapy is completed. Management of deep venous thrombosis, a common complication, can be problematic, as inferior vena cava filters may have a high complication rate in this population (71), and therefore systemic anticoagulation should be given consideration. The role of temporary filters in patients with cancer has not been studied to our knowledge.

A matched study of neoplastic spinal cord patients (compared to traumatic spinal cord injury) found shorter length of stay in the cancer group, lower total functional gains, but comparable efficiency of functional gains (improvement in function per day) and comparable discharge to community rate (72).

Rehabilitation progress in subacute units has not been as rigorously examined, but this level of care may be appropriate for those unable to tolerate more intensive rehabilitation, or, on the other end of the spectrum, for those with less functional debility that does not need the intensity of acute rehabilitation.

Outpatient Rehabilitation

Outpatient rehabilitation systems for the cancer population have not been as systematically developed and studied as inpatient rehabilitation. Many lymphedema clinics exist, and studies of exercise regimens for those with cancer are showing promising results (11,16,17). Issues such as pain and contracture, as well as other ongoing functional impairments are often best addressed in an outpatient setting.

Home Therapies and Hospice Settings

Home-based rehabilitation, including physical, occupational, and speech therapies may be effective in establishing independence in ADL and mobility through development of compensatory strategies in the home environment. Home therapies may also be initiated to develop home modifications for improved safety and to accommodate specific limitations and equipment. They are usually initiated at the time of discharge from an acute care or rehabilitation setting and are necessary if the patient is unable to tolerate outpatient services or community activities.

When the terminally ill patients reach the stage where the life expectancy is less than 6 months, hospice care should be considered. Although rehabilitation of the terminally ill patient sounds counter-intuitive, the goals of both palliative care in the hospice setting and rehabilitation are very similar. The two share a common multidisciplinary approach to maximize function, reduce caregiver burden, and maintain psychological and spiritual well-being.

The most common symptoms in patients with advanced cancer include fatigue, pain, and generalized weakness (73). These factors, among others, lead to significant functional decline and loss of independence. At this stage, the burden on the caretaker increases and the patient may experience significant psychological distress. A number of epidemiologic studies have reported an association between functional decline and psychological distress in the patient with cancer (18,74–76). The "loss of ability to do what one wants" was rated as the highest among end-of-life concerns (74). Additionally, 88% of 301 terminally ill patients expressed a strong desire for mobility (18). Depression and loss of quality of life has been associated with compromised self-care behaviors and dependence on others for ADL (75,76). Patients' perception of increasing dependency predicts interest in physician-assisted suicide (77). Finally, the fear of becoming a burden was among the most frequently cited reasons for euthanasia requests in Holland where physician-assisted suicide is legal (78).

Although, research evaluating the outcomes of rehabilitative intervention in the terminally ill patient is limited, epidemiologic studies support the utility of rehabilitative interventions in the palliative care setting. One noteworthy study investigated 301 patients in a hospice facility receiving physical therapy. At the outset of therapy, 80% of the 301 patients had difficulty performing their ADL. Following rehabilitation, a mean 27% improvement was measured in the Barthel mobility index. Forty-nine patients achieved sufficient functional autonomy to be discharged home. In the same study, a questionnaire was completed by 169 families of the deceased patients. These families indicated that 88% of the patients had indicated a desire for ambulation or mobility and 63% considered the terminal rehabilitation procedures to be effective. The author concluded that rehabilitation could make a significant contribution to the care of the terminally ill patient with cancer (18).

The rehabilitation strategy for the terminally ill patient with cancer is individualized to heighten quality of life and maximize function with the intervention of physical, occupational, and speech therapies. The use of assistive devices, orthoses, and mobility aids are utilized as needed. Family members are trained to provide care in transfers, ADL, and communication. Future research is needed to help establish outcome-supported appropriate interventions for terminally ill patients with cancer. This will maximize the benefits of rehabilitation, including functional independence and quality of life.

CONCLUSION

Individuals with cancer may exhibit a wide spectrum of functional impairments, which rehabilitation can effectively address. The needs of patients with cancer vary by tumor type, treatment type, and stage of disease. Rehabilitation in the setting of palliative or end-of-life concerns remains a relatively under-studied area; the limited data available is promising.

References

1. Lehmann J, DeLisa JA, Warren CG, et al. Cancer rehabilitation: assessment of need, development, and evaluation of a model of care. *Arch Phys Med Rehabil* 1978;59:410.
2. Dietz JH. Rehabilitation of the cancer patient. *Med Clin North Am* 1969;53(3):607–624.
3. *Towards a common language for functioning, disability and health*. World Health Organization. Geneva, 2002 (http://www.who.who.int/classifications/icf/en/).
4. Granger CV, Hamilton BB, Sherwin FS. *Guide for the use of uniform data set for medical rehabilitation*. Buffalo, New York: Uniform Data System for Medical Rehabilitation, 1986.
5. Dimeo F, Schmittel A, Fietz T, et al. Physical performance, depression, immune status and fatigue in patients with hematological malignancies after treatment. *Ann Oncol* 2004;15:1237–1242.
6. Escalante CP, Grover T, Johnson BA, et al. A fatigue clinic in a comprehensive cancer center. *Cancer* 2001;92:1708–1713.
7. Buschbacher RM, Porter CD. Deconditioning, conditioning and the benefits of exercise. In: Braddom RL, ed. *Physical medicine and rehabilitation*, 2nd ed. Philadelphia, PA: WB Saunders, 2000:702–726.
8. Halar EM, Bell KR. Immobility and inactivity: physiological and functional changes, prevention and treatment. In: DeLisa JA, ed. *Physical medicine and rehabilitation: principles and practice*, Philadelphia, PA: Lippincott Williams & Wilkins, 2005:1447–1467.
9. Mueller EA. Influence of training and of inactivity on muscle strength. *Arch Phys Med Rehabil* 1970;51:449–462.
10. Dietrick JE, Whedon GD, Shorr E. Effects of immobilization upon various metabolic and physiologic functions of normal men. *Am J Med* 1948;4:3–32.
11. Courneya KS. Exercise in cancer survivors: an overview of research. *Med Sci Sports Exerc* 2003;35(11):1846–1852.
12. Dimeo FC. Effects of exercise on cancer-related fatigue. *Cancer Suppl* 2001;92(6):1689–1693.
13. Dimeo F, Fetscher S, Lange W, et al. Effects of aerobic exercise on the physical performance and incidence of treatment-related complications after high dose chemotherapy. *Blood* 1997;90:3390–3394.
14. Dimeo FC, Stieglitz R-D, Novelli-Fischer U. Effects of physical activity on the fatigue and psychologic status of cancer patients during chemotherapy. *Cancer* 1999;85(10):2273–2277.
15. Courneya KS, Keats MR, Turner AR. Physical exercise and quality of life in cancer patients following high dose chemotherapy and autologous bone marrow transplantation. *Psychooncology* 2000;9:127–136.
16. Segal R, Evans W, Johnson D, et al. Structured exercise improves physical functioning in women with stages I and II breast cancer: results of a randomized controlled trial. *J Clin Oncol* 2001;19:657–665.
17. Courneya KS, Mackey JR, Bell GJ, et al. Randomized controlled trial of exercise training in postmenopausal breast cancer survivors: cardiopulmonary and quality of life outcomes. *J Clin Oncol* 2003;21:1660–1668.
18. Yoshioka H. Rehabilitation for the terminal cancer patient. *Am J Phys Med Rehabil* 1994;73:199.
19. Porock D, Kristjanson LJ, Tinnelly K, et al. An exercise intervention for advanced cancer patients experiencing fatigue: a pilot study. *J Palliat Care* 2000;16(3):30–36.
20. Schwartz A. Exercise and weight gain in breast cancer patients receiving chemotherapy. *Cancer Pract* 2000;8(5):231–237.
21. Curry SJ, Byers T, Hewitt M, eds. *Fulfilling the potential of cancer prevention and early detection*, Institute of Medicine Report. Washington, DC: National Academies Press, 2003.
22. Johansson K, Ohlsson K, Ingvar M, et al. Factors associated with the development of arm lymphedema following breast cancer treatment: a match pair case control study. *Lymphology* 2002;35:59–71.
23. Fairey AS, Courneya KS, Field CJ, et al. Physical exercise and immune system function in cancer survivors. *Cancer* 2002;94:539–551.
24. Thune I, Furberg A. Physical activity and cancer risk: dose-response and cancer, all sites and site-specific. *Med Sci Sports Exerc* 2001;33(Suppl 6):S530–S550.
25. Vargo MM, Gerber LH. Rehabilitation for patients with cancer diagnoses. In: DeLisa JA, ed. *Physical medicine and rehabilitation: principles and practice*. Philadelphia, PA: Lippincott Williams & Wilkins, 2005:1771–1791.
26. Shah SK. Cardiac rehabilitation. In: DeLisa JA, ed. *Physical medicine and rehabilitation: principles and practice*. Philadelphia, PA: Lippincott Williams & Wilkins, 2005:1811–1838.
27. Sharkey AM, Carey AB, Heise CT, et al. Cardiac rehabilitation after cancer therapy in children and young adults. *Am J Cardiol* 1993;71:1488–1490.
28. Courneya KS, Mackey JR, McKenzie DC. Exercise for breast cancer survivors: research evidence and clinical guidelines. *Phys Sportsmed* 2002; 30(8):(http://www.physsportsmed.com/issues/2002/08_02/courneya.htm).
29. Daneryd P, Svanberg E, Korner U, et al. Protection of metabolic and exercise capacity in unselected weight-losing cancer patients following treatment with recombinant erythropoietin: a randomized prospective study. *Cancer Res* 1998;58:5374–5379.
30. James MC. Physical therapy for patients after bone marrow transplantation. *Phys Ther* 1987;67:946–952.
31. Gillis TA, Donovan ES. Rehabilitation following bone marrow transplantation. *Cancer* 2001;92(Suppl 4):998–1007.
32. Roth ElliotJ, Harvey RichardL. Rehabilitation of stroke syndromes. In: Braddom Randall, ed. *Physical medicine and rehabilitation*, 1st ed. Philadelphia, PA: WB Saunders, 1996:1053–1087.
33. Black-Schaffer RM, Kirsteins AE, Harvey RL. Stroke rehabilitation: comorbidities and complications. *Arch Phys Med Rehabil* 1999;80:S8–S15.
34. Gerber Lynn, Vargo Mary, Smith RebeccaG. Rehabilitation of the cancer patient. In: Devita Vincent, ed. *Cancer principles and practice of oncology*, 7th ed. Philadelphia, PA: Lippincott Williams & Wilkins, 2005:2719–2746.

35. Bogey RossA, Geis CarolyC, Bryant Philip, et al. Stroke and neurodegenerative disorders. Stroke: rehabilitation medicine. *Arch Phys Med Rehabil* 2004;85(Suppl 1):S15–SS19.

36. Weber DC, Brown AW. Physica agent modalities. In: Braddom RL, ed. *Physical medicine and rehabilitation,*. 1st ed. Saunders WB, Philadelphia. 1996:449–463.

37. Mysiw JW, Jackson RD. Electrical Stimulation. In: Braddom RL, ed.*Physical medicine and rehabilitation*. 1st ed. Saunders WB, Philadelphia. 1996:464–492.

38. Dietz Mark A, Mindy A. Spinal cord injury. *Orthotics in neurological rehabilitation*. New York: Demos Publications, 1992:97–103.

39. King JC, Williams RP, McAnelly RD, et al. Rehabilitation of tumor amputees and limb salvage patients. *Phys Med Rehabil* 1994;8(2): 297–319.

40. Nagarajan R, Neglia JP, Clohisy DR, et al. Limb salvage and amputation in survivors of pediatric lower extremity bone tumors: what are the long term implications? *J Clin Oncol* 2002;20:4493–4501.

41. Lane JM, Christ GH, Khan SN, et al. Rehabilitation for limb salvage patients: kinesiologic parameters and psychologic assessment. *Cancer* 2001; 92:1013–1019.

42. Foldi E, Foldi M, Clodius L. The lymphedema chaos: a lancet. *Ann Plast Surg* 1989;22:505–515.

43. Casley-Smith JR, Casley-Smith JR. Modern treatment of lymphoedema I. Complex physical therapy: the first 200 Australian limbs. *Australas J Dermatol* 1992;33:61–68.

44. Erickson VS, Pearson ML, Ganz PA, et al. Arm edema in breast cancer patients. *J Natl Cancer Inst* 2001;93(2):96–111.

45. Megens A, Harris SR. Physical therapist management of lymphedema following treatment for breast cancer: a critical review of its effectiveness. *Phys Ther* 1998;78(12):1302–1311.

46. Badger CMA, Peacock JL, Mortimer PS. A randomized, controlled, parallel group clinical trial comparing multilayer bandaging followed by hosiery versus hosiery alone in the treatment of patients with lymphedema of the limb. *Cancer* 2000;88(12):2832–2837.

47. Dini D, Del Mastro L, Gozza A, et al. The role of pneumatic compression in the treatment of postmastectomy lymphedema. A randomized phase III study. *Ann Oncol* 1998;9:187–190.

48. Richmond DM, O'Donnell TF, Jr, Zelikovski A. Sequential pneumatic compression for lymphedema: a controlled trial. *Arch Surg* 1985;120:1116–1119.

49. Loprinzi CL, Kugler JW, Sloan JA, et al. Lack of effect of coumarin in women with lymphedema after treatment for breast cancer. *N Engl J Med* 1999;340:346–350.

50. Alba AS. Concepts in pulmonary rehabilitation. In: Braddom RL, ed. *Physical medicine and rehabilitation*, 1st ed. 1996:671–672.

51. Fialka-Moser Veronika, Crevenna Richard, Korpan Marta, et al. Cancer rehabilitation. particularly with aspects of physical impairments. *J Rehabil Med* 2003;35:153–162.

52. Tanaka Keiko, Tatsuo Akechi, Okuyama Toru, et al. Impact of dyspnea, pain, fatigue on daily life activities in ambulatory patients with advanced lung cancer. *J Pain Symptom Manage* 2002;23(5):417–423.

53. Hately Juliet, Laurence Virginia, Scott Ann, et al. Breathlessness clinics within specialist palliative care settings can improve the quality of life and functional capacity of patients with lung cancer. *Palliat Med* 2003;17: 410–417.

54. Wall LM. Changes in hope and power in lung cancer patients who exercise. *Nurs Sci Q* 2000;13(3):234–242.

55. Steins StevenA, Bergman SusanBiener, Goetz LanceL. Neurogenic bowel dysfunction after spinal cord injury: clinical evaluation and rehabilitation management. *Arch Phys Med Rehabil* 1997;78:S86–S102.

56. Cardenas DD, Mayo ME, King JC. Braddom RL, ed. Urinary tract and bowel management in the rehabilitation setting. *Physical medicine and rehabilitation*, 1st ed. Saunders WB, Philadelphia. 1996:555–579.

57. Linsenmeyer TA, Stone JM. Neurogenic bladder and bowel. In: DeLisa JA, ed. *Rehabilitation medicine: principles and practice*, 3rd ed. Philadelphia, PA: Lippincott Williams & Wilkins, 1998:1073–1106.

58. Kaynan AM, Perkash I. Neurogenic bladder. In: Frontera WR, Silver JK, eds. *Essentials of physical medicine and rehabilitation*. Philadelphia, PA: Hanley & Belfus, 2002:626–637.

59. McKinley WO, Gittler MS, Kirshblum SC, et al. Spinal cord medicine. Medical complications after spinal cord injury: identification and management. *Arch Phys Med Rehabil* 2002;83(3S-1):S58, S90.

60. Kirshblum S, O'Dell MW, Ho C, et al. Rehabilitation of persons with central nervous system tumors. *Cancer Suppl* 2001;92(4):1029–1037.

61. Huang ME, Cifu DX, Keyser-Marcus L. Functional outcome after brain tumor and acute stroke: a comparative analysis. *Arch Phys Med Rehabil* 1998;79:1386–1390.

62. Huang ME, Wartella JE, Kreutzer JS. Functional outcomes and quality of life in patients with brain tumors: a preliminary report. *Arch Phys Med Rehabil* 2001;82:1540–1546.

63. Mukand JA, Blackinton DD, Crincoli MG, et al. Incidence of neurologic deficits and rehabilitation of patients with brain tumors. *Am J Phys Med Rehabil* 2001;80:346–350.

64. Murray PK. Functional outcome and survival in spinal cord injury secondary to neoplasia. *Cancer* 1985;55:197–201.

65. Philip PA, Ayyanger R, Vanderbilt J, et al. Rehabilitation outcome in children after treatment of primary brain tumor. *Arch Phys Med Rehabil* 1994;75:36–39.

66. O'Toole DM, Golden AM. Evaluating cancer patients for rehabilitation potential. *West J Med* 1991;155:384–387.

67. Cole RP, Scialla SJ, Bednarz L. Functional recovery in cancer rehabilitation. *Arch Phys Med Rehabil* 2000;81:623–627.

68. Marciniak CM, Sliwa JA, Spill G, et al. Functional outcome following rehabilitation of the cancer patient. *Arch Phys Med Rehabil* 1996;77:54–57.

69. Marciniak CM, Sliwa JA, Heinemann AW. Functional outcomes of persons with brain tumors after inpatient rehabilitation. *Arch Phys Med Rehabil* 2001;82:457–463.

70. O'Dell MW, Barr K, Spanier D, et al. Functional outcome of inpatient rehabilitation in persons with brain tumors. *Arch Phys Med Rehabil* 1998;79:1530–1534.

71. Levin JM, Schiff D, Loeffler JS, et al. Complications of therapy for venous thromboembolic disease in patients with brain tumors. *Neurology* 1993;43:1111–1114.

72. McKinley WO, Huang ME, Brunsvold KT. Neoplastic versus traumatic spinal cord injury: an outcome comparison after inpatient rehabilitation. *Arch Phys Med Rehabil* 1999;80:1253–1257.

73. Coyle N, Adelhart J, Foley KM, et al. Character of terminal illness in the advanced cancer patient: pain and other symptoms during the last four weeks of life. *J Pain Symptom Manage* 1991;6:408–410.

74. Axelsson B, Sjoden PO. *Urinary tract and bowel management in the rehabilitation setting. Palliat Med* 1998;12(1):29–39.

75. Longman AJ, Braden CJ, Michel MH. Side effects burden in women with breast cancer. *Cancer Pract* 1996;4(5):274–280.

76. Ulander K, Jeppsson B, Grahn G. Quality of life and independence in activities of daily living preoperatively and at follow-up in patients with colorectal cancer.. *Support Care Cancer* 1997;5(5):402–409.

77. Fairclough DL. Quality of life, cancer investigation, and clinical practice. *Cancer Invest* 1998;16(7):478–484.

78. Van der Maas PJ, Pijnenborg L, van Delden JJ. Changes in Dutch opinions on active euthanasia, 1966 through 1991. *JAMA* 1995;273(18):1411–1414.

CHAPTER 70 ■ COMPLEMENTARY AND ALTERNATIVE APPROACHES

BARRIE R. CASSILETH AND GARY DENG

A vast collection of disparate approaches, from unproven cancer cures to soothing, adjunctive regimens, is subsumed under the single umbrella term *complementary and alternative medicine*, known commonly by the acronym "CAM." Although they are typically discussed in the aggregate, it is clinically and conceptually necessary to distinguish between the two categories because they comprise profoundly different modalities.

Alternative therapies may generally be perceived literally as such; they are promoted as cancer treatments and sometimes as cancer cures, and are often sold for use instead of mainstream therapy. By definition, alternative therapies are unproven. If they were backed by solid data, they would not be "alternative." Rather, they would be found in every oncology program and used as viable treatments. Alternative regimens, which are typically invasive and biologically active, are usually very expensive and potentially harmful. They may harm directly through physiologic activity, or indirectly when patients postpone receipt of mainstream care. Late-stage patients are especially vulnerable to these therapies, as they often promise cure of even advanced disease.

Complementary therapies, in contrast, are used for symptom management and to enhance well-being. They serve as adjuncts to mainstream care; promoted not as cancer cures, but as means of enhancing patients' quality of life. Complementary therapies are supportive, palliative care in every respect. They address body, mind, and spirit, aiming to control pain and other symptoms and to optimize quality of life for patients and families. This definition is essentially identical to that proposed by the World Health Organization for palliative care (1).

In CAM, therefore, we must work with two poles of a continuum. Patients need the knowledge and support to forego the siren calls to seek metabolic therapies in Tijuana; to buy shark cartilage; to self-treat with high-dose vitamins and other products sold over the counter or delivered intravenously in alternative clinics; and to seek remission of disease through self-proclaimed healers, electromagnetic cures, and many other products and approaches.

At the same time, patients need access to the comfort of supportive complementary modalities. These therapies are becoming increasingly available not only directly to patients on a private basis, but also in hospitals, clinics, and homes as part of symptom control and the general effort to ease the physical, psychosocial, and spiritual distresses associated with cancer and especially with end-stage disease.

This chapter addresses the state of CAM in the larger health care system, and reviews the alternative therapies that are so widely and temptingly available to patients and families. Physicians and other caregivers need to know about these pervasive alternatives. Helpful complementary therapies are reviewed as the conclusion to this chapter.

IMPACT OF COMPLEMENTARY AND ALTERNATIVE MEDICINE ON THE HEALTH CARE SYSTEM

The acceptance of unconventional therapies, along with the advent of managed care, advances in biotechnology, and other significant medical and societal events, marked health care in the 1990s and were among the significant changes that occurred during that time. The popularity of CAM has affected every component of the health care system and all specialties of medicine, including palliative oncologic care. It has left its mark on the thinking and practice of physicians and other health professionals, and broadened patients' involvement and influence in their own care.

Unconventional cancer medicine today, no longer a collection of covert practices (2), is highly visible, and information about it is widely available to the general public thanks to the advent of the Internet. It is a multibillion dollar business in the United States, and of equivalent impact and importance throughout the developed world.

Internationally, as well as in North America, the use of CAM for cancer is widespread. A systematic review (3) located 26 surveys of patients with cancer from 13 countries, including 5 from the United States. The average prevalence of CAM use across all studies was 31%. Therapies most commonly adopted around the world included dietary treatments, herbs, homeopathy, hypnotherapy, imagery or visualization, meditation, megavitamins, relaxation, and spiritual healing. All, but one of the US surveys, obtained information about specific therapies employed. Patients used Laetrile, metabolic therapies, diets, spiritual healing, megavitamins, imagery, and "immune system stimulants" (3). Across samples, the prevalence of CAM use in the United States ranged from 7 to 50%.

A recent report presented the most comprehensive and reliable findings to date on Americans' use of CAM in general. The National Center for Health Statistics 2002 National Health Interview Survey involved 31,044 adults and found that 75% used some form of CAM (4). When prayer specifically for health reasons was excluded, the percentage was 50%. As found in virtually all previous surveys, CAM use was most common among women, better educated people, those hospitalized in the previous year and former smokers, indicating a more health conscious segment of the population.

Prevalence rates from all CAM studies conducted in the United States and internationally vary from less than 10% to more than 70%. This broad range with its apparent discrepancies is attributable primarily to variable understandings and definitions of CAM. Surveys often do not define CAM, or more typically, define it extremely broadly, resulting in the inclusion of lifestyle activities such as weight loss efforts, exercise, church attendance, and support activities such as group counseling, thus resulting in bloated figures for CAM use. Moreover, few studies distinguish between the use of alternative therapies (in lieu of mainstream cancer treatment) versus adjunctive use of complementary modalities.

Although research evidence is scanty (2), it appears that approximately 8–10% of patients diagnosed with tissue-biopsy cancer eschew mainstream therapy and immediately seek alternative care. Most CAM users, however, seek complementary, not alternative, therapies for cancer-related problems.

In 1994, legislation was passed allowing herbal medicines and other "food supplements" to be sold over the counter without U.S. Food and Drug Administration (FDA) review. This resulted in an estimated doubling of dietary supplement sales in the following 6 years. According to National Nutritional Food Association, annual sale of dietary supplements reached $19.8 billion in 2003, among them $4.2 billion in herbs. Although the sale of most supplements increases each year, the sale of herbs declined by 3% in 2002 and 1.8% in 2003 (5). The decline is presumed due to unrealistically high public expectations, media reports about safety concerns and questionable effectiveness, and public confusion about the vast array of products.

Despite the drop in sales of herbal remedies, CAM use by patients with cancer has grown in recent years (3); a secondary analysis of close to 3000 patients with cancer estimates a 64% increase after 1987 (6). It is likely that this reflects expanded variety of over-the-counter remedies and broader availability of complementary therapies in mainstream cancer programs and centers.

Complementary and Alternative Medicine Use Among Pediatric Patients with Cancer

The use of CAM methods among pediatric patients with cancer represents a special and understudied issue. Surveys in Australia and Finland, in British Columbia, and in the Netherlands indicate substantial interest in CAM, especially in more recent years, with 40–50% of pediatric patients with cancer in those countries receiving alternative or complementary therapies (3).

Few studies of CAM use among US pediatric patients with cancer have been published in the past 10 years. A 1998 article reported that 65% of 81 US patients with cancer used CAM, whereas 51% of 80 control-group children receiving routine checkups did so. Of particular interest is the type of CAM received. Prayer, exercise, and spiritual healing accounted for more than 96% of CAM used. Excluded from this sample by definition, however, were the pediatric patients brought for alternative treatment to clinics in the United States, Mexico, Germany, or elsewhere. Patients who received only alternative cancer therapies did not appear in CAM surveys, because all but one such survey was conducted in mainstream clinics or hospitals.

Public Access to Information

CAM today is very much an open and public issue, discussed widely in the media and readily found on the Internet.

Magazines and television specials provide the general public with details about new CAM therapies. The yellow pages of telephone books in most cities and towns typically list various types of CAM practitioners. Information available to the public varies widely in accuracy. Many Web sites and publications that appear to be objective actually are sponsored by commercial enterprises that promote and sell the products they report. Misinformation about health issues is widespread. In 1999, the U.S. Federal Trade Commission (FTC) announced that it had identified hundreds of Web sites promoting and selling phony cures for cancer and other serious ailments among the estimated 15,000–17,000 health-related Web sites. Because today there are approximately 874,000,000 such sites, it is likely that those selling bogus treatments have increased accordingly.

Recognition by Mainstream Journals and Physicians

A survey of 295 family physicians in the Maryland-Virginia region (7) revealed that up to 90% view complementary therapies such as diet and exercise, behavioral medicine, and hypnotherapy as legitimate medical practices. A majority refers patients to nonphysicians for these therapies or provides the services themselves. Homeopathy, Native American medicine, and traditional Oriental medicine were not seen as legitimate practices.

Two hundred Canadian general practitioners held similar views, noting their patients' interest especially in chiropractic. These physicians perceive chiropractic care, hypnosis, and acupuncture for chronic pain as the most effective CAM therapies, and homeopathy and reflexology as less efficacious (8). A meta-analysis of 12 studies in Great Britain suggests that British physicians view complementary medicine as only moderately effective (9), a level of enthusiasm that contrasts with the fervent efforts of the British Royal Family to promote homeopathy and other complementary therapies, and to merge them with mainstream care.

In addition to increasing coverage of CAM services by health insurers, a final marker of mainstream interest noted here is the publication of CAM research articles in major mainstream medical journals. Articles about CAM in major journals shifted from commentaries through the 1970s expressing realistic concern about quackery, to surveys of patients' knowledge and use of unproven methods in the 1980s, to reports of actual research results starting primarily in the mid-1990s.

The *Journal of the American Medical Association*, the *New England Journal of Medicine*, the *Lancet*, the *British Medical Journal*, and specialty journals such as *Cancer* and the *Journal of Clinical Oncology* have published reports of CAM research in recent years. In 1996–1997, the National Library of Medicine added many new CAM search terms to its medical subject headings, and began to cover alternative medicine journals previously not reviewed for inclusion in Medline. In large part, mainstream science opposition is being replaced by emphasis on the importance of methodologically sound research, which now increasingly occurs in numerous respectable institutions around the world.

COMPLEMENTARY AND ALTERNATIVE MEDICINE THERAPIES AND PRACTITIONERS

While recognizing overlap, the National Center for Complementary and Alternative Medicine (NCCAM) groups CAM therapies into four domains: biologically based practices;

mind–body medicine; manipulative and body-based practices; and energy medicine. In addition, whole medical systems cut across all domains. Traditional Chinese medicine, for example, includes biologically active botanicals, mind–body practices, manipulative techniques, and acupuncture. Therapies commonly sought by patients with cancer are discussed in the following sections. Many of these approaches are unproven methods promoted as alternatives to mainstream cancer treatment. Helpful complementary or adjunctive therapies are discussed separately at the end of this chapter.

Diet and Nutrition

Advocates of dietary cancer treatments typically extend mainstream assumptions about the protective effects of fruits, vegetables, fiber, and avoidance of excessive dietary fat in reducing cancer risk, to the idea that food or vitamins can cure cancer. Proponents of this belief make their claims in books with titles such as *The Food Pharmacy: Dramatic New Evidence that Food is your Best Medicine, Prescription for Nutritional Healing*, and *New Choices in Natural Healing*.

The macrobiotic diet is a persistently popular example of such dietary approaches. As currently constructed, it is similar to recent U.S. Department of Agriculture dietary pyramid recommendations for healthful eating, except that the macrobiotic diet omits dairy products and meat. This diet derives 50–60% of its calories from whole grains, 25–30% from vegetables, and the remainder from beans, seaweed, and soups. All animal meat and certain vegetables and processed foods are to be avoided, and soybean consumption is promoted. Despite claims in publications and Web sites, there is no evidence that this or any other diet can cure cancer.

Metabolic Therapies and Detoxification

Metabolic therapies continue to draw patients from North America to the many clinics in Tijuana, Mexico. These therapies involve practitioner-specific combinations of diet plus vitamins, minerals, enzymes, and "detoxification." One of the best known sites for metabolic therapy is the Gerson clinic, where treatment is based on the belief that toxic products of cancer cells accumulate in the liver, leading to liver failure and death. The Gerson treatment aims to counteract liver damage with a low-salt, high-potassium diet, coffee enemas, and a gallon of fruit and vegetable juice daily (10). The clinic's use of liquefied raw calf liver injections was suspended in 1997 following sepsis in a number of patients.

Other Tijuana clinics and practitioners provide their own versions of metabolic therapy, each applying an individualized dietary and "detoxification" regimen. Additional components of treatment are included according to practitioners' preferences. Metabolic regimens are based on belief in the importance of "detoxification," which is thought necessary for the body to heal itself. Practitioners view cancer and other illnesses as symptoms of the accumulation of toxins. This is a nonphysiologic but venerable concept that originated in ancient Egyptian, Ayurvedic, and other early efforts to understand illness and death, both of which were believed caused by the putrefaction of food in the colon. Decay and purging were major themes in early cultures' therapeutic regimens. Neither the existence of toxins nor the benefit of colonic cleansing has been documented.

Modern variations on the older approach to internal cleansing are drinkable cleansing formulas, said to detoxify and rejuvenate the body. Many variations are available in health food stores, books, and on the Internet. A shake of liquid clay, psyllium seed husks, and fruit juice, for example, is said to remove harmful food chemicals and air pollutants. These products tend to function as major laxatives, potentially dangerous when taken over days or weeks or on a regular basis as recommended by promoters, and of special concern for patients with cancer.

Megavitamin and Orthomolecular Therapy

Some patients and alternative practitioners believe that large dosages of vitamins—typically hundreds of pills a day—or intravenous infusions of high-dose vitamin C can cure disease. In 1968, Nobel Laureate Linus Pauling coined the term *orthomolecular* to describe the treatment of disease with large quantities of nutrients. His claims that massive doses of vitamin C could cure cancer were disproved in clinical trials (11), but megavitamin and orthomolecular therapy—the latter adds minerals and other nutrients—remain popular among patients with cancer. There is no evidence that megavitamin or orthomolecular therapy is effective in treating any disorder.

Mind–Body Techniques

The potential to influence health with our minds is an extremely appealing concept in the United States. It affirms the power of the individual, a belief intrinsic to U.S. culture. Some mind–body interventions have moved from the category of alternative, unconventional therapies into mainstream complementary or supportive care. Good documentation exists, for example, for the effectiveness of meditation, biofeedback, and yoga in stress reduction and the control of some physiologic reactions (12).

The argument that patients can use mental attributes or mind–body work to cure cancer is not tenable (13,14). Attending to the psychological health of patients with cancer is a fundamental component of good cancer care. Support groups, good doctor–patient relationships, and the emotional and instrumental help of family and friends are vital. However, the idea that patients can influence the course of their disease through mental or emotional work is not substantiated and can evoke feelings of guilt and inadequacy when disease continues to advance despite patients' best spiritual or mental efforts (15).

Bioelectromagnetics

Bioelectromagnetics is the study of interactions between living organisms and their electromagnetic fields. According to proponents, magnetic fields penetrate the body and heal damaged tissues, including cancers. No peer-reviewed publications could be located for this work, or for any clinical cancer-related claims regarding bioelectromagnetics. Despite the lack of data and the patent absurdity of these claims, proponents continue to sell electromagnetic therapy as a cure for cancer and other major illnesses.

Electromagnetic therapy and the related group of energy therapies, discussed in the section Manual Healing Methods, illustrate a striking difference between previous and currently popular alternative practices. Whereas many earlier alternatives reflected concepts important to scientific study of the time, many of today's popular alternatives are mystical and explicitly contrary to contemporary scientific and medical thought. It is as though the new millennium encouraged deeper adoption of explanatory notions applied in millennia past.

Alternative Medical Systems

This category includes ancient systems of healing typically based on concepts of human physiology that differ from those accepted by modern western science. Two of the most popular healing systems are traditional Chinese medicine and India's Ayurvedic medicine, popularized by best-selling author Deepak Chopra, MD (16).

"Ayurveda" comes from the Sanskrit words "ayur" (life) and "veda" (knowledge). Ayurveda's ancient healing techniques are based on the classification of people into one of three predominant body types. There are specific remedies for disease, and regimens to promote health, for each body type. This medical system has a strong mind–body component, stressing the need to keep consciousness in balance. It uses techniques such as yoga and meditation to do so. Ayurveda also emphasizes regular detoxification and cleansing through all bodily orifices.

Traditional Chinese medicine explains the body in terms of its relationship to the environment and the cosmos. Concepts of human physiology and disease are interwoven with geographic features of ancient China and with the forces of nature. Chi, the life force said to run through all of nature, flows in the human body through vertical energy channels known as *meridians*.

The 12 main meridians are believed to be dotted with acupoints. Each acupoint corresponds to a specific body organ or system, so that needling (acupuncture) or pressing an acupoint (acupressure) can redress the life-force imbalance causing the problem in that particular organ. To determine the source of the blockage, the practitioner relies on pulse diagnosis, a technique applied by doctors of traditional Chinese medicine today as it was millennia ago. It involves concentration on several body pulses by the practitioner for approximately 45 minutes.

Although the very existence of chi or a "vital energy force" remains unproven, acupuncture has been shown to induce measurable neurophysiologic change. It also helps reduce certain symptoms experienced by patients with cancer. Tai chi, a gentle exercise technique with a mind–body component to foster the smooth flow of Chi, is useful in preventing falls among the frail or elderly (17). Traditional Chinese medicine also includes a full herbal pharmacopoeia with remedies for most ailments, including cancer (18). The potential anticancer and immunomodulatory benefits of many Chinese herbs and other botanicals are under investigation in the United States and elsewhere.

Pharmacologic and Biologic Treatments

Because pharmacologic and biologic alternative treatments are invasive and biologically active, they tend to be highly controversial. An example is antineoplastons, developed by Stanislaw Burzynski, MD, PhD, and available in his clinic in Houston, Texas. Laboratory analysis conducted by a respected scientist concluded that antineoplastons did not normalize tumor cells (19). Promising anecdotal reports encouraged a clinical trial for pediatric patients with brain tumors, but a National Cancer Institute research effort failed to accrue patients. Further research at the Burzynski Institute was permitted under an investigational new drug (IND), but preliminary data were criticized as uninterpretable, and the therapy as useless and toxic, by respected mainstream scientists. Burzynski and his patients continue the antineoplaston therapy and remain vocal advocates of its efficacy.

Immunoaugmentive therapy (IAT) was developed by the late Lawrence Burton, PhD, and offered in his clinic in the Bahamas. Injected IAT is said to balance four protein components in the blood and to strengthen the patient's immune system. Burton claimed that IAT was particularly effective in treating mesothelioma. Documentation of IAT's efficacy remains anecdotal. The clinic has continued to operate after Burton's death, but its popularity seems to have waned.

Interest in shark cartilage as a cancer therapy was activated by a 1992 book by I. William Lane, PhD, *Sharks Don't Get Cancer*, and by a television special that displayed apparent remissions in patients treated with shark cartilage in Cuba. The televised outcome was strongly disputed by oncologists in the United States. Advocates base their therapy on its putative antiangiogenic properties. A recent randomized controlled trial found neither survival benefit nor improved quality of life in patients with advanced cancer (20). The product was poorly tolerated due to its unpleasant taste.

Cancell is another biological remedy that appears to be especially popular in Florida and the midwestern United States. Proponents claim that it returns cancer cells to a "primitive state" from which they can be digested and rendered inert. FDA laboratory studies, which showed Cancell to be composed of common chemicals, including nitric acid, sodium sulfite, potassium hydroxide, sulfuric acid, and catechol, found no basis for proponent claims of Cancell's effectiveness against cancer (21).

Manual Healing Methods

Osteopathic and chiropractic doctors were among the earliest groups to use manual methods. Today, there are numerous approaches involving touch and manipulation techniques, including hands-on massage. The benefit of chiropractic treatment of low back pain was supported by a National Institutes of Health (NIH) consensus conference (22), but its value is widely disputed by mainstream physicians.

One of the most popular manual healing methods is therapeutic touch (TT), which, despite its name, involves no direct contact. In TT, healers move their hands a few inches above a patient's body and sweep away "blockages" to the patient's energy field. Although a study in the *Journal of the American Medical Association* showed that experienced TT practitioners were unable to detect the investigator's "energy field" (23) and despite mainstream scientists' unwillingness to accept its fundamental premises, TT is taught in North American nursing schools and practiced by nurses in the United States and other countries. Reiki, which can involve light touch, is defined as spiritually guided life force, the manipulation of energy surrounding the patient. This energy is called "ki" in Japanese lore or "qi or Chi" in Chinese tradition. A small study reported better pain control in advanced cancer patients receiving Reiki when compared to usual care (24). Reduction of heart rate and diastolic blood pressure has been reported in a randomized controlled trial of 45 subjects (25). However, the existence of the bioenergy field and its subjection to a practitioner's manipulation has never been convincingly demonstrated.

Several other therapies also involve manipulation of a putative human energy field, or use of an individual's special gift for energy healing. Healing of this type, which has remained popular over the centuries in less developed areas of the world (26), has gained increasing public interest and acceptance in the United States. Healers in many areas of the United States claim the ability to cure people of cancer. Although they may cause only minor difficulties when patients also receive mainstream care, many patients are firmly convinced of healers' abilities and decline even to have tumors removed surgically in favor of healers' ministrations.

Herbal Treatments for Cancer

Herbal remedies typically are part of traditional and folk healing methods with long histories of use. Herbal medicine is found is most areas of the world and across all cultures historically. Although many herbal remedies are claimed to have anticancer effects, only a few have gained substantial popularity as alternative cancer therapies.

For decades, Essiac has remained a popular herbal cancer alternative in North America. Developed initially by a Native healer from Southwestern Canada, it was popularized by a Canadian nurse, Rene Caisse (Essiac is Caisse spelled backwards). Essiac is comprised of four herbs: burdock, turkey rhubarb, sorrel, and slippery elm. Researchers at the National Cancer Institute and elsewhere found that it has no anticancer effect.

Iscador, a derivative of mistletoe, is a popular cancer remedy in Europe, where it is said to have been in continuous use as folk treatment since the Druids. It is used in many mainstream European cancer clinics, typically in conjunction with chemotherapy. Despite many studies, definitive data in support of the usefulness of Iscador have not emerged.

Patients with cancer use many over-the-counter herbal products in addition to or instead of those promoted specifically as cancer treatments. It is therefore important to recognize herbal remedies that are toxic or tend to interact with other medications as well as those that may help patients with cancer. Because neither the FDA nor any other agency examines herbal remedies for safety and effectiveness, few products have been formally tested for side effects or quality control, but information is beginning to emerge on the basis of public experience with over-the-counter supplements.

Reports in the literature describe severe liver and kidney damage from some herbal remedies. These reports underscore the fact that "natural" products, contrary to apparent consumer belief, are not necessarily safe or harmless (21). Most members of the public apparently are not aware that herbs are essentially dilute natural drugs that contain scores of different chemicals, most of which have not been documented. Effects are not always predictable.

Moreover, the potential for herb–drug interaction is sufficiently problematic that patients on chemotherapy or other major medications should not use herbal remedies. Similar cautions are necessary for patients receiving radiation, as some herbs photosensitize the skin and cause severe reactions. Some herbs interfere with coagulation and produce dangerous blood pressure swings and other unwanted interactions with anesthetics (21). Herbs such as feverfew, garlic, ginger, and ginkgo have anticoagulant effects and should be avoided by patients on warfarin sodium (Coumadin), heparin sodium, aspirin, and related agents. The risk of herb–drug interactions appears to be greatest for patients with kidney or liver problems. Herbs can alter metabolism of prescription medicine through the cytochrome P-450 system, possibly worsening side effects or compromising efficacy (21).

The California Department of Health found unsafe levels of mercury and other toxic metals in more than a third of Asian patent medicines studied. Several instances of heart problems resulting from digitalis-contaminated supplements have been reported (27). Prostate cancer (PC)-SPES, an herbal mixture popular in 2002 as a treatment for prostate cancer, was found to be contaminated with prescription medicine (28). Concerns have been raised even about dietary antioxidants, which may interact with certain groups of chemotherapeutic agents (29).

Regulatory and Safety Issues

Dietary supplements, which include vitamins and minerals, homeopathic remedies, herbal treatments, antioxidants, and other over-the-counter products, are probably the most popular unconventional remedies used today by patients with cancer, as well as by the public in general. Legal standards for the processing and packaging of herbs as well as quality-control standards and overseeing are very much needed. Because they are not yet mandatory, few food supplement companies voluntarily self-impose quality evaluation and control. Consumer protection and enforcement agencies cannot provide protection against contaminated or falsely advertised products. Current federal regulations do not permit such overseeing, and regulatory capability would prohibit full analysis and ongoing overseeing of the estimated 20,000 food supplement items now sold over the counter.

The magnitude and seriousness of the problem hopefully will result in the establishment of government overseeing programs of some kind, despite anticipated efforts on the part of the food supplement industry to block efforts that could lead to regulation. Information provided by manufacturers and marketers are not without bias and conflict of interest. Reputable sources of information are listed in Table 70.1.

COMPLEMENTARY THERAPIES

Complementary therapies are safe, nontoxic, noninvasive, easy to use, and inexpensive. Many may be self managed, meaning that practitioners are often unnecessary, which gives patients the rare and important opportunity to maintain a measure of control over their well-being. Supportive or complementary modalities also are soothing, comforting, and distracting, and are backed by good efficacy data.

Some complementary therapies, such as relaxing in a warm bath or painting soothing mental pictures, are intuitively comforting and helpful. Major supportive therapies have been singled out here for more detailed review. These

TABLE 70.1

REPUTABLE SOURCES OF ON-LINE INFORMATION ON COMPLEMENTARY AND ALTERNATIVE MEDICINE

National Center for Complementary and Alternative Medicine: http://nccam.nih.gov
National Cancer Institute: http://www.cancer.gov/cam/index.html
American Cancer Society: http://www.cancer.org/docroot/ETO/ETO_5.asp?sitearea=ETO
USDA Food and Nutrition Information Center: http://www.nal.usda.gov/fnic
NIH Office of Dietary Supplements: http://dietary-supplements.info.nih.gov
U.S. Pharmacopeia: http://www.usp.org/dietarySupplements
http://www.cancer.org/docroot/ETO/ETO_5.asp?sitearea=ETO
Memorial Sloan-Kettering Cancer Center: http://www.mskcc.org/aboutherbs
M. D. Anderson Cancer Center: http://www.mdanderson.org/departments/CIMER
Institute of Medicine: http://www.iom.edu/board.asp?id=3788

therapies—music therapy, therapeutic massage, acupuncture, and mind–body modalities—address some of the most pervasive and difficult problems faced by patients under palliative care. Although data do not always come from the patient population of concern to us here, research shows that these minimally invasive, side effect–free therapies effectively reduce anxiety, depression, pain, dyspnea, nausea, and fatigue (30).

Music Therapy

Music therapy is provided by professional musicians who are also trained music therapists. They often hold professional degrees in music therapy, and are adept in dealing with the psychosocial as well as clinical issues faced by patients and family members.

Music therapy is particularly effective in the palliative care setting. Formal music therapy programs in palliative medicine exist in many major institutions. Although music therapy extends back to folklore and Greek mythology (Apollo was the god of both music and medicine), it has been studied scientifically only in recent years.

Controlled trials indicate that music therapy produces emotional and physiologic benefits, reducing anxiety, stress, depression, and pain. Music intervention significantly reduced heart rate, respiratory rate, and anxiety scores among inpatients after myocardial infarction, ventilatory assistance, and patients undergoing flexible sigmoidoscopy (31). Live versus recorded music more effectively reduced anxiety.

In the preoperative setting, randomized trials found that music reduced anxiety and its physiologic correlates such as blood pressure and salivary cortisol, a biochemical marker of stress and anxiety. Music lowered blood pressure and anxiety scores during and after eye surgery (32) and among women undergoing hysterectomies in a randomized, controlled trial (33).

Music therapy was shown to be effective against laboratory-induced pain, among patients with cancer (34) and among cancer patients with chronic pain (35). Music reduced intraoperative analgesic requirements compared to controls, and patients randomized to a music intervention reported significantly less pain and required less pain medication. In what was possibly the largest trial of its type, 500 surgical patients were randomized to control, recorded music, jaw relaxation, or a music/jaw relaxation combination. Music led to significant decreases in both pain intensity and related distress associated with pain (36). Music also can help reduce depression (37).

In a randomized controlled trial of patients with cancer undergoing autologous stem cell transplantation, anxiety, depression, and total mood disturbance scores were significantly lower in music therapy group when compared with standard care controls (38).

Massage Therapy

The benefits of massage therapy are documented for the terminally ill (39), and the pain-reducing effects of this intervention are well documented for patients with cancer at various stages of illness (40). In the largest study to date, 87 hospitalized patients with cancer were randomized to foot massage (also called *reflexology*) or to control on a crossover basis. Pain and anxiety scores fell with massage, with differences between groups achieving substantial significance ($p = .001$) (34). Pain scores fell by two thirds immediately after the first massage of patients with postburn itching and pain and improvements appeared to be cumulative. No similar changes were seen in controls. Other studies found similar results for patients with postoperative pain. In an analysis of 1290 patient reports of symptom severity pre- and postmassage therapy, 0–10 ratings of pain, fatigue, stress/anxiety, nausea, depression, and "other" were reduced by approximately 50%, even for patients reporting high baseline scores. Benefits persisted with no return toward baseline scores throughout 48-hour follow-up (41).

Acupuncture

Pain is the most common and the best studied indication for acupuncture. It relieves both acute (e.g., postoperative dental pain) and chronic (e.g., headache) pain (42,43). A recent randomized controlled trial of 570 patients with osteoarthritis of the knee found that a 26-week course of acupuncture significantly improved pain and dysfunction when compared with sham-acupuncture control. In this study all patients received other usual care for osteoarthritis. At week 8, improvement in function but not in pain was observed, indicating that long-term treatment maybe required to achieve full effect (44).

Acupuncture appears effective against cancer-related pain. A randomized placebo-controlled trial tested auricular acupuncture for patients with pain despite stable medication. A total of 90 patients were randomized to needles placed at correct acupuncture points (treatment group), versus acupuncture or pressure at nonacupuncture points. Pain intensity decreased by 36% at 2 months from baseline in the treatment group, a statistically significant difference compared with the two control groups, for whom little pain reduction was seen (45). Skin penetration *per se* showed no significant analgesic effect. The authors selected acupuncture points by measuring electrodermal signals. These results are especially important because most of the patients had neuropathic pain, which is often refractory to conventional treatment.

Acupuncture helps lessen chemotherapy-induced nausea and vomiting. In one study, 104 patients with breast cancer receiving highly emetogenic chemotherapy were randomized to receive electroacupuncture at the PC6 acupuncture point, minimal needling at nonacupuncture points, or pharmacotherapy alone. Electroacupuncture significantly reduced the number of episodes of total emesis when compared with pharmacotherapy only. Most patients did not know the group to which they had been assigned (46). The effects of acupuncture do not appear entirely due to attention, clinician–patient interaction, or placebo.

Acupuncture has been reported to reduce xerostomia (severe dry mouth). Radiotherapy for head and neck cancer causes acute and chronic xerostomia, which may persist despite the use of pilocarpine (Salagen) and amifostine (Ethyol). Acupuncture improved Xerostomia Inventory scores in 18 patients with head and neck cancer and pilocarpine-resistant xerostomia in uncontrolled trials. Patients with breast or prostate cancer may experience vasomotor symptoms (hot flashes) during estrogen or androgen ablation therapy. A few uncontrolled studies investigated acupuncture to treat these symptoms. Self-stimulation of implanted miniature acupuncture needles attenuated tamoxifen-related hot flashes in 8 of 12 patients with breast cancer (47), and similar results were found in a case series of patients with breast (48) and prostate cancer (49). Controlled trials are under way at several centers.

Fatigue following chemotherapy or irradiation, another major and common problem, has few reliable treatments in patients without a correctable cause such as anemia. In an uncontrolled trial of fatigue after chemotherapy, acupuncture reduced fatigue 31% after 6 weeks of treatment. Among those with severe fatigue at baseline, 79% had nonsevere fatigue scores at follow-up (50), whereas fatigue was reduced only in 24% of patients receiving usual care in another center (51).

Mind–Body Therapies

The varied group of mind–body therapies is geared to decrease stress and promote relaxation in different ways. Hypnotherapy has been shown to reduce chemotherapy-related nausea and vomiting in children, and possibly to control anxiety and nausea. Hypnosis for pain is well supported (52). Other techniques, including visualization and progressive relaxation, also decrease pain and promote well-being (53).

Meditation can help stress reduction. In a randomized wait-list control study of 109 patients with cancer, participation in a 7-week Mindfulness-Based Stress Reduction Program was associated with significant improvement in mood disturbance and symptoms of stress (54). A single arm study of patients with breast and prostate cancer showed significant improvement in overall quality of life, stress, and sleep quality, but symptom improvement was not significantly correlated with program attendance or minutes of home practice (55).

Yoga, which combines physical movement, breath control, and meditation, improved sleep quality in a controlled trial of 39 patients with lymphoma. Practicing a form of yoga that incorporates controlled breathing and visualization significantly decreased sleep disturbance when compared to wait-list controls (56). Mindfulness-Based Stress Reduction techniques must be practiced to produce beneficial effects (57).

Other Therapies

The use of pet animals (pet therapy) is thought to help reduce loneliness and improve quality of life, especially for those who are elderly, alone or demented. Most pet therapy research has been conducted in psychiatric settings. A randomized clinical trial with pain and palliative care cancer patients, conducted at the NIH Clinical Center, began enrollment in 2005. This study will examine how animal-assisted therapy affects pain in patients with cancer receiving pain and palliative care at the NIH Clinical Center.

Art therapy is a behavioral modality that uses creative expression to help develop coping skills. Many cancer centers provide access to artistic expression on a recreational basis or guided by professional art therapists. A few reports showed better association of art therapy with children with leukemia undergoing painful procedures or with reduced stress and lowered anxiety in family caregivers of patients with cancer. Although scientific study of art therapy is minimal, it is clear that many patients enjoy creative activity, and the enjoyment per se is an important end in and of itself.

Other complementary therapies, such as spiritual care, counseling, and group support, have been part of supportive and palliative care in cancer for decades. The complementary therapies discussed here represent an extension of those efforts to decrease symptoms and enhance patients' quality of life. Our challenge is to help patients avoid the pitfalls of useless unproven therapies, while ensuring their access to the safe, noninvasive, beneficial complementary modalities reviewed here (58).

SUMMARY

Alternative therapies are unproven or disproved, and potentially harmful. Patients should be advised to avoid them. Complementary therapies, on the other hand, can reduce many symptoms experienced by patients with cancer. An increasing body of evidence supports the use of acupuncture, massage, music and mind–body therapies for symptom control. These therapies should be considered particularly when conventional treatment produces unwarranted side effects or fails to bring satisfactory symptom relief. It is important to tailor the use of complementary therapies to the needs and preferences of each patient.

Other factors, such as economic concerns, patients' belief systems and cultural backgrounds, may also play a role in applying complementary therapies in palliative care. In the light of product quality-control issues and potential interactions with prescription medications, it is helpful to be familiar with supplements commonly used by patients with cancer or refer patients to reliable sources of information (21).

There have been concerted efforts to raise awareness and encourage the use of evidence-based complementary therapies in palliative care and supportive oncology (www.IntegrativeOnc.com). Integrating complementary therapies into cancer care is likely to provide a sense of patient empowerment, reduce troubling symptoms, improve patient satisfaction, and enhance the physician–patient relationship.

References

1. WHO. *Cancer pain and relief*. Technical Report Series 804. Geneva: World Health Organization, 1990.
2. Cassileth BR, Lusk EJ, Strouse TB, et al. Contemporary unorthodox treatments in cancer medicine. A study of patients, treatments, and practitioners. *Ann Intern Med* 1984;101(1):105–112.
3. Ernst E, Cassileth BR. The prevalence of complementary/alternative medicine in cancer: a systematic review. *Cancer* 1998;83(4):777–782.
4. Barnes PM, Powell-Griner E, McFann K, et al. Complementary and alternative medicine use among adults: United States, 2002. *Adv Data* 2004;343: 1–19.
5. http://www.nnfa.org/facts/index.htm Accessed June 10, 2005.
6. Abu-Realh MH, Magwood G, Narayan MC, et al. The use of complementary therapies by cancer patients. *Nursingconnections* 1996;9(4):3–12.
7. Berman BM, Singh BK, Lao L, et al. Physicians' attitudes toward complementary or alternative medicine: a regional survey. *J Am Board Fam Pract* 1995;8(5):361–366.
8. Verhoef MJ, Sutherland LR. General practitioners' assessment of and interest in alternative medicine in Canada. *Soc Sci Med* 1995;41(4):511–515.
9. Ernst E, Resch KL, White AR. Complementary medicine. What physicians think of it: a meta-analysis. *Arch Intern Med* 1995;155(22):2405–2408.
10. Green S. A critique of the rationale for cancer treatment with coffee enemas and diet. *JAMA* 1992;268(22):3224–3227.
11. Moertel CG, Fleming TR, Creagan ET, et al. High-dose vitamin C versus placebo in the treatment of patients with advanced cancer who have had no prior chemotherapy. A randomized double-blind comparison. *N Engl J Med* 1985;312(3):137–141.
12. Integration of behavioral and relaxation approaches into the treatment of chronic pain and insomnia. NIH technology assessment panel on integration of behavioral and relaxation approaches into the treatment of chronic pain and insomnia. *JAMA* 1996;276(4):313–318.
13. Cunningham AJ, Edmonds CV, Jenkins GP, et al. A randomized controlled trial of the effects of group psychological therapy on survival in women with metastatic breast cancer. *Psychooncology* 1998;7(6):508–517.
14. Gellert GA, Maxwell RM, Siegel BS. Survival of breast cancer patients receiving adjunctive psychosocial support therapy: a 10-year follow-up study. *J Clin Oncol* 1993;11(1):66–69.
15. Cassileth BR. The social implications of mind-body cancer research. *Cancer Invest* 1989;7(4):361–364.
16. Chopra D. *Ageless body, timeless mind*. New York: Harmony Books, 1993.
17. Henderson NK, White CP, Eisman JA. The roles of exercise and fall risk reduction in the prevention of osteoporosis. *Endocrinol Metab Clin North Am* 1998;27(2):369–387.
18. Cai Y, Luo Q, Sun M, et al. Antioxidant activity and phenolic compounds of 112 traditional Chinese medicinal plants associated with anticancer. *Life Sci* 2004;74(17):2157–2184.
19. Green S. 'Antineoplastons'. An unproved cancer therapy. *JAMA* 1992;267 (21):2924–2928.
20. Loprinzi CL, Levitt R, Barton DL, et al. Evaluation of shark cartilage in patients with advanced cancer. *Cancer* 2005;104:176–182.
21. About herbs http://www.mskcc.org/aboutherbs Accessed June 10, 2005.
22. Lawrence DJ. Report from the consensus conference on the validation of chiropractic methods. *J Manipulative Physiol Ther* 1990;13(6):295–296.
23. Rosa L, Rosa E, Sarner L, et al. A close look at therapeutic touch. *JAMA* 1998;279(13):1005–1010.

24. Olson K, Hanson J, Michaud M. A phase II trial of Reiki for the management of pain in advanced cancer patients. *J Pain Symptom Manage* 2003; 26(5):990–997.

25. Mackay N, Hansen S, McFarlane O. Autonomic nervous system changes during Reiki treatment: a preliminary study. *J Altern Complement Med* 2004;10(6):1077–1081.

26. Cassileth BR, Vlassov VV, Chapman CC. Health care, medical practice, and medical ethics in Russia today. *JAMA* 1995;273(20):1569–1573.

27. Slifman NR, Obermeyer WR, Aloi BK, et al. Contamination of botanical dietary supplements by digitalis lanata. *N Engl J Med* 1998;339(12):806–811.

28. Walsh PC. Prospective, multicenter, randomized phase II trial of the herbal supplement, PC-SPES, and diethylstilbestrol in patients with androgen-independent prostate cancer. *J Urol* 2005;173(6):1966–1967.

29. Labriola D, Livingston R. Possible interactions between dietary antioxidants and chemotherapy. *Oncology (Huntingt)* 1999;13(7):1003–1008; discussion 1008, 1011–2.

30. Deng G, Cassileth BR, Yeung KS. Complementary therapies for cancer-related symptoms. *J Support Oncol* 2004;2(5):419–426; discussion 427–9.

31. Chlan L, Evans D, Greenleaf M, et al. Effects of a single music therapy intervention on anxiety, discomfort, satisfaction, and compliance with screening guidelines in outpatients undergoing flexible sigmoidoscopy. *Gastroenterol Nurs* 2000;23(4):148–156.

32. Allen K, Golden LH, Izzo JL Jr, et al. Normalization of hypertensive responses during ambulatory surgical stress by perioperative music. *Psychosom Med* 2001;63(3):487–492.

33. Mullooly VM, Levin RF, Feldman HR. Music for postoperative pain and anxiety. *J N Y State Nurses Assoc* 1988;19(3):4–7.

34. Beck SL. The therapeutic use of music for cancer-related pain. *Oncol Nurs Forum* 1991;18(8):1327–1337.

35. Zimmerman L, Pozehl B, Duncan K, et al. Effects of music in patients who had chronic cancer pain. *West J Nurs Res* 1989;11(3):298–309.

36. Good M, Stanton-Hicks M, Grass JA, et al. Relaxation and music to reduce postsurgical pain. *J Adv Nurs* 2001;33(2):208–215.

37. Hanser SB, Thompson LW. Effects of a music therapy strategy on depressed older adults. *J Gerontol* 1994;49(6):P265–P269.

38. Cassileth BR, Vickers AJ, Magill LA. Music therapy for mood disturbance during hospitalization for autologous stem cell transplantation: a randomized controlled trial. *Cancer* 2003;98(12):2723–2729.

39. Wilkinson S, Aldridge J, Salmon I, et al. An evaluation of aromatherapy massage in palliative care. *Palliat Med* 1999;13(5):409–417.

40. Ferrell-Torry AT, Glick OJ. The use of therapeutic massage as a nursing intervention to modify anxiety and the perception of cancer pain. *Cancer Nurs* 1993;16(2):93–101.

41. Cassileth BR, Vickers AJ. Massage therapy for symptom control: outcome study at a major cancer center. *J Pain Symptom Manage* 2004;28(3): 244–249.

42. NIH Consensus Conference. Acupuncture. *JAMA* 1998;280(17):1518–1524.

43. Melchart D, Linde K, Fischer P, et al. Acupuncture for recurrent headaches: a systematic review of randomized controlled trials. *Cephalalgia* 1999;19(9):779–786; discussion 765.

44. Berman BM, Lao L, Langenberg P, et al. Effectiveness of acupuncture as adjunctive therapy in osteoarthritis of the knee: a randomized, controlled trial. *Ann Intern Med* 2004;141(12):901–910.

45. Alimi D, Rubino C, Pichard-Leandri E, et al. Analgesic effect of auricular acupuncture for cancer pain: a randomized, blinded, controlled trial. *J Clin Oncol* 2003;21(22):4120–4126.

46. Shen J, Wenger N, Glaspy J, et al. Electroacupuncture for control of myeloablative chemotherapy-induced emesis: a randomized controlled trial. *JAMA* 2000;284(21):2755–2761.

47. Towlerton G, Filshie J, O'Brien M, et al. Acupuncture in the control of vasomotor symptoms caused by tamoxifen. *Palliat Med* 1999;13(5):445.

48. Porzio G, Trapasso T, Martelli S, et al. Acupuncture in the treatment of menopause-related symptoms in women taking tamoxifen. *Tumori* 2002; 88(2):128–130.

49. Hammar M, Frisk J, Grimas O, et al. Acupuncture treatment of vasomotor symptoms in men with prostatic carcinoma: a pilot study. *J Urol* 1999; 161(3):853–856.

50. Vickers AJ, Straus DJ, Fearon B, et al. Acupuncture for postchemotherapy fatigue: a phase II study. *J Clin Oncol* 2004;22(9):1731–1735.

51. Escalante CP, Grover T, Johnson BA, et al. A fatigue clinic in a comprehensive cancer center: design and experiences. *Cancer* 2001;92(6 Suppl): 1708–1713.

52. Sellick SM, Zaza C. Critical review of 5 nonpharmacologic strategies for managing cancer pain. *Cancer Prev Control* 1998;2(1):7–14.

53. Walker LG, Walker MB, Ogston K, et al. Psychological, clinical and pathological effects of relaxation training and guided imagery during primary chemotherapy. *Br J Cancer* 1999;80(1–2):262–268.

54. Speca M, Carlson LE, Goodey E, et al. A randomized, wait-list controlled clinical trial: the effect of a mindfulness meditation-based stress reduction program on mood and symptoms of stress in cancer outpatients. *Psychosom Med* 2000;62(5):613–622.

55. Carlson LE, Speca M, Patel KD, et al. Mindfulness-based stress reduction in relation to quality of life, mood, symptoms of stress and levels of cortisol, dehydroepiandrosterone sulfate (DHEAS) and melatonin in breast and prostate cancer outpatients. *Psychoneuroendocrinology* 2004;29(4): 448–474.

56. Cohen L, Warneke C, Fouladi RT, et al. Psychological adjustment and sleep quality in a randomized trial of the effects of a Tibetan yoga intervention in patients with lymphoma. *Cancer* 2004;100(10):2253–2260.

57. Shapiro SL, Bootzin RR, Figueredo AJ, et al. The efficacy of mindfulness-based stress reduction in the treatment of sleep disturbance in women with breast cancer: an exploratory study. *J Psychosom Res* 2003;54(1):85–91.

58. Cassileth B. *The alternative medicine handbook: the complete reference guide to alternative and complementary therapies.* New York: WW Norton, 1998.

SPECIAL POPULATIONS

CHAPTER 71 ■ LONG-TERM SURVIVORSHIP: LATE EFFECTS

NOREEN M. AZIZ

BACKGROUND AND SIGNIFICANCE

With continued advances in strategies to detect cancer early and treat it effectively along with the aging of the population, the number of individuals living years beyond a cancer diagnosis can be expected to continue to increase. Statistical trends show that, in the absence of other competing causes of death, 64% of adults diagnosed with cancer today can expect to be alive in 5 years (1–4). Relative 5-year survival rates for those diagnosed as children (age <19 years) are even higher, with almost 79% of childhood cancer survivors estimated to be alive at 5 years and 75% at 10 years (5).

Survival from cancer has seen dramatic improvements over the past three decades, mainly as a result of advances in early detection, therapeutic strategies, and the widespread use of combined modality therapy (surgery, chemotherapy, and radiotherapy) (6–10). Medical and sociocultural factors such as psychosocial and behavioral interventions, active screening behaviors, and healthier lifestyles may also play an integral role in the length and quality of that survival (11).

Although beneficial and often lifesaving against the diagnosed malignancy, most therapeutic modalities for cancer are associated with a spectrum of late complications ranging from minor and treatable to serious or, occasionally, potentially lethal (2,6,12–15). Although living for extended periods of time beyond their initial diagnosis, many cancer survivors often face various chronic and late physical and psychosocial sequelae of their disease or its treatment. Additionally, as the number of survivors and their length of survival expand, long-term health issues specific to cancer survival are also fast emerging as a public health concern. Questions of particular importance to cancer survivors include surveillance for the adverse sequelae, or late and long-term effects, of treatment; the development of new (second) cancers; and recurrence of their original cancer. One fourth of *late deaths* occurring among survivors of childhood cancer during the extended survivorship period, when the chances of primary disease recurrence are negligible, can be attributed to a treatment-related effect such as a second cancer or cardiac dysfunction (16). The most *frequently observed* medical sequelae among pediatric cancer survivors include endocrine complications, growth hormone deficiency, primary hypothyroidism, and primary ovarian failure. Also included within the rubric of late effects are second cancers arising as a result of genetic predisposition (e.g., familial cancer syndromes) or the mutagenic effects of therapy. These factors may act independently or synergistically. Synergistic effects of

mutagenic agents such as cigarette smoke or toxins such as alcohol are largely unknown (2,6,12).

Therefore, there is today a greater recognition of symptoms that persist after the completion of treatment and which arise years after primary therapy. Both acute organ toxicities such as radiation pneumonitis and chronic toxicities such as congestive cardiac failure, neurocognitive deficits, infertility, and second malignancies are being described as the price of cure or prolonged survival (2,6,12). The study of late effects, originally within the realm of pediatric cancer, is now germane to cancer survivors at all ages because concerns may continue to surface throughout the life cycle (2,6). These concerns underscore the need to follow-up and screen survivors of cancer for toxicities such as those mentioned and also to develop and provide effective interventions that carry the potential to prevent or ameliorate adverse outcomes.

The goal of survivorship research is to focus on the *health and life* of a person with a history of cancer *beyond* the acute diagnosis and treatment phase. Survivorship research seeks to examine the causes of, and to prevent and control the adverse effects associated with, cancer and its treatment, and to optimize the physiologic, psychosocial, and functional outcomes for cancer survivors and their families. A hallmark of survivorship research is its emphasis on understanding the integration/interaction of multidisciplinary domains.

This chapter presents definitional issues relevant to cancer survivorship; examines late effects of cancer treatment among survivors of pediatric and adult cancer; and articulates gaps in knowledge and emerging research priorities in cancer survivorship research relevant to late effects of cancer treatment. It draws heavily from pediatric cancer survivorship research because a paucity of data continues to exist for medical late effects of treatment for survivors of cancer diagnosed as adults. Research on late effects of cancer treatment began in the realm of pediatric cancer and continues to yield important insights for the impact of cancer therapies among adults.

DEFINITIONAL ISSUES

Fitzhugh Mullan, a physician diagnosed with and treated for cancer himself, first described cancer survivorship as a concept (17). Definitional issues for cancer survivorship encompass three related aspects (2,6):

1. *Who is a cancer survivor?* Philosophically, anyone who has been diagnosed with cancer is a survivor, from the

time of diagnosis to the end of life.* Caregivers and family members are also included within this definition as secondary survivors.

2. *What is cancer survivorship?* Mullan described the survivorship experience as similar to the seasons of the year. Mullan recognized three seasons or phases of survival: acute (extending from diagnosis to the completion of initial treatment, encompassing issues dominated by treatment and its side effects); extended (beginning with the completion of initial treatment for the primary disease, remission of disease, or both, dominated by watchful waiting, regular follow-up examinations, and, perhaps, intermittent therapy); and permanent survival (not a single moment; evolves from extended disease-free survival when the likelihood of recurrence is sufficiently low). An understanding of these phases of survival is important for facilitating an optimal transition into and management of survivorship.

3. *What is cancer survivorship research?* Cancer survivorship research seeks to identify, examine, prevent, and control adverse cancer diagnosis and treatment-related outcomes (such as late effects of treatment, second cancers, and quality of life); to provide a knowledge base regarding optimal follow-up care and surveillance of cancer survivors; and to optimize health after cancer treatment (2,6).

Other important definitions include those for long-term cancer survivorship and late versus long-term effects of cancer treatment. Generally, *long-term cancer survivors* are defined as those individuals who are 5 or more years beyond the diagnosis of their primary disease and embody the concept of permanent survival described by Mullan. *Late effects* refer specifically to unrecognized toxicities that are absent or subclinical at the end of therapy and become manifest later with the unmasking of hitherto unseen injury caused by any of the following factors: developmental processes, the failure of compensatory mechanisms with the passage of time, or organ senescence. *Long-term effects* refer to any side effects or complications of treatment for which a patient with cancer must compensate; also known as persistent effects, they begin during treatment and continue beyond the end of treatment. Late effects, in contrast, appear months to years after the completion of treatment. Some researchers classify cognitive problems, fatigue, lymphedema, and peripheral neuropathy as long-term effects whereas others classify them as late effects (18–21). Chemotherapeutic drugs for which late effects have been reported most frequently include adriamycin, bleomycin, vincristine, methotrexate, cytoxan, and many others (Table 71.1) (22–46).

This chapter focuses largely on the *physiologic* or *medical* long-term and late effects of cancer treatment. Physiologic sequelae of cancer treatment can also be further classified as follows:

1. System specific (e.g., organ damage, failure, or premature aging, immunosuppression, or issues related to compromised immune systems, and endocrine damage)
2. Second malignant neoplasms (such as an increased risk of recurrent malignancy, increased risk of a certain cancer associated with the primary malignancy, and/or increased risk of secondary malignancies associated with cytotoxic or radiologic cancer therapies (this topic is not covered in detail in this chapter as it is reviewed comprehensively elsewhere in this book) and
3. Functional changes such as lymphedema, incontinence, pain syndromes, neuropathies, fatigue; cosmetic changes such as amputations, ostomies, and skin/hair alterations;

and comorbidities such as osteoporosis, arthritis, and hypertension

REVIEW OF LATE AND LONG-TERM EFFECTS BY ORGAN SYSTEM OR TISSUES AFFECTED†

System-Specific Physiologic Sequelae‡

Cardiac Sequelae

The heart may be damaged by both therapeutic irradiation and chemotherapeutic agents commonly used in the treatment for cancer. Several types of damage have been reported, including pericardial, myocardial, and vascular. Cardiac damage is most pronounced after treatment with the anthracycline drugs doxorubicin and daunorubicin, used widely in the treatment of most childhood cancers and adjuvant chemotherapy for breast and many other adult cancers. An additive effect has also been reported when anthracyclines are used in conjunction with cyclophosphamide and radiation therapy. Anthracyclines cause myocardial cell death, leading to a diminished number of myocytes and compensatory hypertrophy of residual myocytes (47). Major clinical manifestations include reduced cardiac function, arrhythmia, and heart failure. Chronic cardiotoxicity usually manifests itself as cardiomyopathy, pericarditis, and congestive heart failure.

Cardiac injury that becomes clinically manifest during or shortly after completion of chemotherapy may progress, stabilize, or improve after the first year of treatment. This improvement may either be of a transient nature or last for a considerable length of time. There is also evidence of a continuum of injury that will manifest itself throughout the lives of these patients (48). From a risk factor perspective, patients who exhibit reduced cardiac function within 6 months of completing chemotherapy are at increased risk for the development of late cardiac failure (49). However, a significant incidence of late cardiac decompensation manifested by cardiac failure or lethal arrhythmia occurring 10–20 years after the administration of these drugs has also been reported (50).

In a recent study of Hodgkin's disease (HD) survivors, investigators reported finding cardiac abnormalities in most of the participants (51). This is an important finding especially because the sample consisted of individuals who did not manifest symptomatic heart disease at screening and described their health as "good." Manifestations of cardiac abnormalities include the following:

1. Restrictive cardiomyopathy (suggested by reduced average left ventricular dimension and mass without increased left ventricular wall thickness)
2. Significant valvular defects
3. Conduction defects
4. Complete heart block
5. Autonomic dysfunction (suggested by a monotonous heart rate in 57%)
6. Persistent tachycardia and
7. Blunted hemodynamic responses to exercise

The peak oxygen uptake (VO_{2max}) during exercise, a predictor of mortality in heart failure, was significantly reduced

---

*From the National Coalition for Cancer Survivorship.

†Common to both children and adults depending on cancer site and treatment(s) received.

‡These include organ damage, failure, or premature aging resulting from chemotherapy, hormone therapy, radiation, surgery, or any combination thereof.

TABLE 71.1

POSSIBLE LATE EFFECTS OF RADIOTHERAPY AND CHEMOTHERAPY

Organ system	Late effects/sequelae of radiotherapy	Late effects/sequelae of chemotherapy	Chemotherapeutic drugs responsible
Bone and soft tissues	Short stature, atrophy, fibrosis, osteonecrosis	Avascular necrosis	Steroids
Cardiovascular	Pericardial effusion, pericarditis; coronary arterial disease	Cardiomyopathy, congestive cardiac failure	Anthracyclines Cyclophosphamide
Pulmonary	Pulmonary fibrosis, decreased lung volumes	Pulmonary fibrosis Interstitial pneumonitis	Bleomycin, BCNU Methotrexate, adriamycin
Central nervous system	Neuropsychological deficits, structural changes, hemorrhage	Neuropsychological deficits, structural changes Hemiplegia, seizure	Methotrexate
Peripheral nervous system		Peripheral neuropathy, hearing loss	Cisplatin, vinca alkaloids
Hematologic	Cytopenia, myelodysplasia	Myelodysplastic syndromes	Alkylating agents
Renal	Decreased creatinine clearance Hypertension	Decreased creatinine clearance Increased creatinine, renal filtration Delayed renal filtration	Cisplatin Methotrexate Nitrosoureas
Genitourinary	Bladder fibrosis, contractures	Bladder fibrosis, hemorrhagic cystitis	Cyclophosphamide
Gastrointestinal	Malabsorption, stricture, abnormal LFT	Abnormal LFT, hepatic fibrosis, cirrhosis	Methotrexate, BCNU
Pituitary	Growth hormone deficiency, pituitary deficiency		
Thyroid	Hypothyroidism, nodules		
Gonadal	Men: risk of sterility, Leydig cell dysfunction	Men: sterility	Alkylating agents
	Women: ovarian failure, early menopause	Women: sterility, premature menopause	Procarbazine
Dental/oral health	Poor enamel and root formation, dry mouth		
Ophthalmologic	Cataracts, retinopathy	Cataracts	Steroids

BCNU, carmustine; LFT, liver function test.
Data from Ganz (1998, 2001) (12,13) and Aziz (2002, 2003) (2,6).

(<20 mL/kg/m^2) in 30% of survivors and was correlated with increasing fatigue, increasing shortness of breath, and a decreasing physical component score on the SF-36. Given the presence of these clinically significant cardiovascular abnormalities, investigators recommend serial, comprehensive cardiac screening of HD survivors who fit the profile of having received mediastinal irradiation at a young age.

Congestive cardiomyopathy is directly related to the total dose of the agent administered; the higher the dose, the greater the chance of cardiotoxicity. Subclinical abnormalities have also been noted at lower doses. The anthracyclines doxorubicin and daunorubicin are well-known causes of cardiomyopathy that can occur many years after completion of therapy. The incidence of anthracycline-induced cardiomyopathy, which is dose dependent, may exceed 30% among patients receiving cumulative doses in excess of 600 mg per m^2. A cumulative dose of anthracyclines >300 mg per m^2 has been associated with an 11-fold-increased risk of clinical heart failure, compared with a cumulative dose of <300 mg per m^2, the estimated risk of clinical heart failure increasing with time from exposure and approaching 5% after 15 years.

A reduced incidence and severity of cardiac abnormalities was reported in a study of 120 long-term survivors of acute lymphoblastic leukemia (ALL) who had been treated with lower anthracycline doses (90–270 mg per m^2), compared

with previous reports in which subjects had received moderate anthracycline doses (300–550 mg per m^2) (52,53). Twenty-three percent of the patients were found to have cardiac abnormalities, 21% had increased end-systolic stress, and only 2% had reduced contractility. The cumulative anthracycline dose within the 90–270 mg per m^2 range did not relate to cardiac abnormalities. The authors concluded that there may be no safe anthracycline dose to completely avoid late cardiotoxicity. A recent review of 30 published studies in childhood cancer survivors found that the frequency of clinically detected anthracycline cardiac heart failure ranged from 0 to 16% (54). In an analysis of reported studies, the type of anthracycline (e.g., doxorubicin) and the maximum dose given in a 1-week period (e.g., >45 mg per m^2) was found to explain a large portion of the variation in the reported frequency of anthracycline-induced heart failure.

Cyclophosphamide has been associated with the development of congestive cardiomyopathy, especially when administered at the high doses used in transplant regimens. Cardiac toxicity may occur at lower doses when mediastinal radiation is combined with the chemotherapeutic drugs mentioned above. Late onset of congestive heart failure has been reported during pregnancy, rapid growth, or after the initiation of vigorous exercise programs in adults previously treated for cancer during childhood or young adulthood as a result of increased afterload and the impact of the additional stress of such events on marginal cardiac reserves. Initial improvement in cardiac function after completion of therapy appears to result, at least in part, from compensatory changes. Compensation may diminish in the presence of stressors such as those mentioned earlier and myocardial depressants such as alcohol.

The incidence of subclinical anthracycline myocardial damage has been the subject of considerable interest. Steinherz et al. found 23% of 201 patients who had received a median cumulative dose of doxorubicin of 450 mg per m^2 had echocardiographic abnormalities at a median of 7 years after therapy (55). In a group of survivors of childhood cancer received a median doxorubicin dose of 334 mg per m^2, it was found that progressive elevation of afterload or depression of left ventricular contractility was present in approximately 75% of patients (47). A recent review of the literature on subclinical cardiotoxicity among children treated with an anthracycline found that the reported frequency of subclinical cardiotoxicity varied considerably across the 25 studies reviewed (frequency ranging from 0 to 57%) (56). Because of marked differences in the definition of outcomes for subclinical cardiotoxicity and the heterogeneity of the patient populations investigated, it is difficult to accurately evaluate the potential long-term outcomes within anthracycline-exposed patient populations or the potential impact of the subclinical findings.

Effects of radiation on the heart may be profound, and include valvular damage, pericardial thickening, and ischemic heart disease. Patients with radiation-related cardiac damage have a markedly increased relative risk (RR) of both angina and myocardial infarction [RR, 2.56] years after mediastinal radiation for HD in adult patients, whereas the risk of cardiac death is 3.1 (57). This risk was greatest among patients receiving >30 Gy of mantle irradiation and those treated before 20–21 years of age. Blocking the heart reduced the risk of cardiac death due to causes other than myocardial infarction (58).

In general, among anthracycline-exposed patients, the risk of cardiotoxicity can be increased by mediastinal radiation (59), uncontrolled hypertension (60,61), underlying cardiac abnormalities (62), exposure to nonanthracycline chemotherapeutic agents (especially cyclophosphamide, dactinomycin, mitomycin C, dacarbazine, vincristine, bleomycin, and methotrexate) (63,64), female gender (65), younger age (66), and electrolyte imbalances such as hypokalaemia and hypomagnesaemia (67). Previous reports have suggested that doxorubicin-induced cardiotoxicity can be prevented by continuous infusion of the drug (68). However, Lipshultz et al. compared cardiac outcomes in children receiving either bolus or continuous infusion of doxorubicin, and reported that continuous doxorubicin infusion over 48 hours for childhood leukemia did not offer a cardioprotective advantage over bolus infusion (69). Both regimens were associated with progressive subclinical cardiotoxicity, therefore suggesting that there is no benefit from continuous infusion of anthracyclines.

Chronic cardiotoxicity associated with radiation alone most commonly involves pericardial effusions or constrictive pericarditis, sometimes in association with pancarditis. Although a dose of 40 Gy of total heart irradiation appears to be the usual threshold, pericarditis has been reported after as little as 15 Gy, even in the absence of radiomimetic chemotherapy (70,71). Symptomatic pericarditis, which usually develops 10–30 years after irradiation, is found in 2–10% of patients (72). Subclinical pericardial and myocardial damage, as well as valvular thickening, may be common in this population (73,74). Coronary artery disease has been reported after radiation to the mediastinum, although mortality rates have not been significantly higher in patients who receive mediastinal radiation than in the general population (58).

Given the known acute and long-term cardiac complications of therapy, prevention of cardiotoxicity is a focus of active investigation. Several attempts have been made to minimize the cardiotoxicity of anthracyclines, such as the use of liposomal-formulated anthracyclines, less-cardiotoxic analogs, and the additional administration of cardioprotective agents. The advantages of these approaches are still controversial, but there are ongoing clinical trials to evaluate the long-term effects. Certain analogs of doxorubicin and daunorubicin, with decreased cardiotoxicity but equivalent antitumor activity, are being explored. Agents such as dexrazoxane, which are able to remove iron from anthracyclines, have been investigated as cardioprotectants. Clinical trials of dexrazoxane have been conducted in children, with encouraging evidence of short-term cardioprotection (75); however, the long-term avoidance of cardiotoxicity with the use of this agent has yet to be sufficiently determined. The most recent study by Lipshultz et al. reported that dexrazoxane prevents or reduces cardiac injury, as reflected by elevations in troponin T, which is associated with the use of doxorubicin for childhood ALL without compromising the antileukemic efficacy of doxorubicin. Longer follow-up will be necessary to determine the influence of dexrazoxane on echocardiographic findings at 4 years and on event-free survival (76).

Another key emerging issue is the interaction of taxanes with doxorubicin. Epirubicin-taxane combinations are active in treating metastatic breast cancer, and ongoing research is focusing on combining anthracyclines with taxanes in an effort to continue to improve outcomes following adjuvant therapy (77). Clinically significant drug interactions have been reported to occur when paclitaxel is administered with doxorubicin, cisplatin, or anticonvulsants (phenytoin, carbamazepine, and phenobarbital), and pharmacodynamic interactions have been reported to occur with these agents that are sequence- or schedule dependent (78). Because the taxanes undergo hepatic oxidation through the cytochrome P-450 system, pharmacokinetic interactions from enzyme induction or inhibition can also occur. A higher than expected myelotoxicity has been reported. However, there is no enhanced doxorubicinol formation in human myocardium, a finding consistent with the cardiac safety of the regimen (79). Investigators have suggested that doxorubicin and epirubicin should be administered 24 hours before paclitaxel and the cumulative anthracycline dose be limited to 360 mg per m^2, thereby preventing the enhanced toxicities caused by sequence- and schedule-dependent interactions between anthracyclines and paclitaxel (78). Conversely, they also suggest that paclitaxel should be administered at least 24 hours before cisplatin to avoid a decrease in clearance and increase in myelosuppression. With concurrent anticonvulsant therapy, cytochrome P-450 enzyme induction results in decreased paclitaxel plasma steady-state concentrations, possibly requiring an increased dose of paclitaxel. A number of other drug interactions have been reported in preliminary studies for which clinical significance has yet to be established (78).

The human epidermal growth factor receptor (HER) 2 is overexpressed in approximately 20–25% of human breast cancers and is an independent adverse prognostic factor. Targeted therapy directed against this receptor has been developed in the form of a humanized monoclonal antibody, trastuzumab. Unexpectedly, cardiac toxicity has developed in some patients treated with trastuzumab, and this has a higher incidence in those treated in combination with an anthracycline (80,81). Both clinical and in vitro data suggest that cardiomyocyte HER2/erbB2 is uniquely susceptible to trastuzumab (82). Trastuzumab has shown activity as a single agent in metastatic breast cancer both before chemotherapy and in heavily pretreated patients, and its use in combination with an anthracycline or paclitaxel results in a significant improvement in survival, time to progression, and response (80). The HER2 status of a tumor is a critical determinant of response to trastuzumab-based treatment; those expressing HER2 at the highest level on immunohistochemistry, 3+, derive more benefit from treatment with trastuzumab than those with overexpression at the 2+ level. Interactions between the estrogen receptor and HER2 pathway have stimulated interest in using trastuzumab in combination with endocrine therapy.

Neurocognitive Sequelae

Long-term survivors of cancer may be at risk of neurocognitive and neuropsychological sequelae. Among survivors of childhood leukemia, neurocognitive late effects represent one of the more intensively studied topics. Adverse outcomes are generally associated with whole-brain radiation and/or therapy with high-dose systemic or intrathecal methotrexate or cytarabine (83–85). High-risk characteristics, including higher dose of central nervous system (CNS) radiation, younger age at treatment, and female sex, have been well documented. Results from studies of neurocognitive outcomes are directly responsible for the marked reduction (particularly in younger children) in the use of cranial radiation, which is currently reserved for treatment of very high-risk subgroups or patients with CNS involvement (86).

A spectrum of clinical syndromes may occur, including radionecrosis, necrotizing leukoencephalopathy, mineralizing microangiopathy, and dystrophic calcification, cerebellar sclerosis, and spinal cord dysfunction (87). Leukoencephalopathy has been primarily associated with methotrexate-induced injury of white matter. However, cranial radiation may play an additive role through the disruption of the blood–brain barrier, therefore allowing greater exposure of the brain to systemic therapy.

Although abnormalities have been detected by diagnostic imaging studies, the abnormalities observed have not been well demonstrated to correlate with clinical findings and neurocognitive status (88,89). Chemotherapy- or radiation-induced destruction in normal white matter partially explains intellectual and academic achievement deficits (90). Evidence suggests that direct effects of chemotherapy and radiation on intracranial endothelial cells and brain white matter as well as immunologic mechanisms could be involved in the pathogenesis of CNS damage.

Neurocognitive deficits, as a general rule, usually become evident within several years of CNS radiation and tend to be progressive in nature. Survivors of leukemia treated at a younger age (e.g., <6 years of age) may experience significant declines in intelligence quotient (IQ) scores (91). However, reductions in IQ scores are typically not global, but rather reflect specific areas of impairment, such as attention and other nonverbal cognitive processing skills (92). Affected children may experience information-processing deficits, resulting in academic difficulties. These children are particularly prone to problems with receptive and expressive language, attention span, and visual and perceptual motor skills, most often manifested in academic difficulties in the areas of reading, language, and mathematics. Accordingly, children treated with CNS radiation or systemic or intrathecal therapy with the potential to cause neurocognitive deficits should receive close monitoring of academic performance. Referral for neuropsychological evaluation with appropriate intervention strategies, such as modifications in curriculum, speech and language therapy, or social skills training, implemented in a program tailored for the individual needs and deficits of the survivor should be taken into consideration (93). Assessment of educational needs and subsequent educational attainment have found that survivors of childhood leukemia are significantly more likely to require special educational assistance, but have a high likelihood of successfully completing high school (37,94). However, when compared with siblings, survivors of leukemia and non-Hodgkin's lymphoma (NHL) are at greater risk of not completing high school. As would be anticipated from the results of neurocognitive studies, it has been shown that survivors, particularly those under 6 years of age at treatment, who received cranial radiation and/or intrathecal chemotherapy were significantly more likely to require special education services and least likely to complete a formal education (86,95,96).

Progressive dementia and dysfunction have been reported in some long-term cancer survivors as a result of whole-brain radiation with or without chemotherapy, and occur most often in patients with brain tumor and patients with small cell lung cancer who have received prophylactic therapy. Neuropsychological abnormalities have also been reported after CNS prophylaxis utilizing whole-brain radiation for leukemia in childhood survivors. In fact, cognitive changes in children began to be recognized as treatments for childhood cancer, especially ALL, became increasingly effective. These observations have resulted in changes in treatment protocols for childhood ALL (97,98).

Several recent studies have reported cognitive dysfunction in women treated with adjuvant therapy for breast cancer (99,100). In one study (101), investigators compared the neuropsychological performance of long-term survivors of breast cancer and lymphoma treated with standard-dose chemotherapy who carried the epsilon 4 allele of the apolipoprotein E (APOE) gene to those who carry other APOE alleles. Survivors with at least one epsilon 4 allele scored significantly lower in the visual memory (p <.03) and the spatial ability (p <.05) domains and tended to score lower in the psychomotor functioning (p <.08) domain as compared with survivors who did not carry an epsilon 4 allele. No group differences were found on depression, anxiety, or fatigue. The results of this study provide preliminary support for the hypothesis that the epsilon 4 allele of APOE may be a potential genetic marker for increased vulnerability to chemotherapy-induced cognitive decline.

Although cranial irradiation is the most frequently identified causal factor in both adults and children, current work in adults indicates that cognitive problems may also occur with surgery, chemotherapy, and biologic response modifiers (102–104). These findings need to be validated in prospective studies along with the interaction among treatment with chemotherapeutic agents, menopausal status, and hormonal treatments. Emotional distress has also been related to cognitive issues in studies of patients beginning cancer treatment.

Patients have attributed problems in cognition to fatigue, and others have reported problems with concentration, short-term memory, problem-solving, and concerns about "chemo-brain" or "mental pause" (105). Comparisons across studies are difficult because of different batteries of neuropsychological tests used, and differences among patient samples by diagnosis, age, gender, or type of treatment received, and, finally, inconsistency in the timing of measures in relation to treatment landmarks. Despite these methodological issues, studies have shown impairments in verbal information processing, complex information processing, concentration, and visual memory (106–109).

Current studies indicate that cognitive deficits are often subtle but a observed consistently in a proportion of patients, may be durable, and can be disabling (110). Deficits have been observed in a range of cognitive functions. Although underlying mechanisms are unknown, preliminary studies suggest a genetic predisposition. Cognitive impairment may be accompanied by changes in the brain, detectable by neuroimaging. Priorities for future research include the following:

1. Large-scale clinical studies that use both a longitudinal design and concurrent evaluation of patients with cancer who do not receive chemotherapy. Such studies should address the probability and magnitude of cognitive deficits, factors that predict them, and underlying mechanisms
2. Exploration of discrepancies between subjective reports of cognitive dysfunction and the objective results of cognitive testing
3. Studies of cognitive function in patients receiving treatment for diseases other than breast cancer, and in both men and women, to address the hypothesis that underlying mechanisms relate to changes in serum levels of sex hormones and/or to chemotherapy-induced menopause
4. Development of interventions to alleviate these problems and
5. Development of animal models and the use of imaging techniques to address mechanisms that might cause cognitive impairment

Endocrinologic Sequelae

Thyroid. Radiation exposure to the head and neck is a known risk factor for subsequent abnormalities of the thyroid. Among survivors of HD and, to a lesser extent, survivors of leukemia, abnormalities of the thyroid gland, including hypothyroidism, hyperthyroidism, and thyroid neoplasms, have been reported to occur at rates significantly higher than those found in the general population (111–114). Hypothyroidism is the most common nonmalignant late effect involving the thyroid gland. Following radiation doses above 15 Gy, laboratory evidence of primary hypothyroidism is evident in 40–90% of patients with HD, NHL, or head and neck malignancies (113,115,116). In a recent analysis of 1791 5-year survivors of pediatric HD (median age at follow-up, 30 years), Sklar et al. reported the occurrence of at least one thyroid abnormality in 34% of subjects (114). The risk of hypothyroidism was increased 17-fold compared with sibling control subjects, with increasing dose of radiation, older age at diagnosis of HD, and female sex as significant independent predictors of an increased risk. The actuarial risk of hypothyroidism for subjects treated with 45 Gy or more was 50% at 20 years following diagnosis of their HD. Hyperthyroidism was reported to occur in only 5%. Finally, it is important to note that the risk of hypothyroidism in adult patients treated with mantle irradiation for HD is significant. Most of the adult cases occur in the first 5 years but the risk is lifelong. These issues are of key importance for survivors of adult cancer with a history of RT for head and neck cancer.

Hormones affecting growth. Poor linear growth and short adult stature are common complications after successful treatment of childhood cancers (117). The adverse effect of CNS radiation on final height as an adult among patients with childhood leukemia has been well documented, with final heights below the fifth percentile occurring in 10–15% of survivors (43,118,119). The effects of cranial radiation appear to be related to age and gender, with children younger than 5 years at the time of therapy and female patients being more susceptible. The precise mechanisms by which cranial radiation induces short stature are not clear. Disturbances in growth hormone production have not been found to correlate well with observed growth patterns in these patients (31,120). The phenomenon of early onset of puberty in girls receiving cranial radiation may also play some role in the reduction of final height (33,121). In survivors of childhood leukemia, not treated with cranial radiation, there are conflicting results regarding the impact of chemotherapy on final height (122).

Hormonal rationale for obesity. An increased prevalence of obesity has been reported among survivors of childhood ALL (123–125). Craig et al. investigated the relationship between cranial irradiation received during treatment for childhood leukemia and obesity (126). Two hundred thirteen (86 boys and 127 girls) irradiated patients and 85 (37 boys and 48 girls) nonirradiated patients were enrolled. For cranially irradiated patients, an increase in the body mass index (BMI) Z score at the final height was associated with female sex and lower radiation dose but not with age at diagnosis. Severe obesity, defined as a BMI Z score >3 at final height, was present only in girls, who received 18–20 Gy irradiation, at a prevalence rate of 8%. Both male and female nonirradiated patients had raised BMI Z scores at latest follow-up, and there was no association with age at diagnosis. The authors concluded that these data demonstrated a sexually dimorphic and dose-dependent effect of cranial irradiation on BMI. In a recent analysis from the Childhood Cancer Survivor Study, Oeffinger et al. compared the distribution of BMI of 1765 adult survivors of childhood ALL with that of 2565 adult siblings of survivors of childhood cancer (127). Survivors were significantly more likely to be overweight (BMI, 25–30) or obese (BMI, 30 or more). Risk factors for obesity were cranial radiation, female gender, and age from 0 to 4 years at diagnosis of leukemia. Girls diagnosed under the age of 4 who received a cranial radiation dose >20 Gy were found to have a 3.8-fold-increased risk of obesity.

Gonadal dysfunction. Treatment-related gonadal dysfunction has been well documented in both men and women following childhood malignancies (128). However, survivors of leukemia and T-cell NHL treated with modern conventional therapy are at a relatively low risk of infertility and delayed or impaired puberty. Treatment-related gonadal failure or dysfunction, expressed as amenorrhea or azoospermia, can lead to infertility in both male and female survivors of cancer, and may have its onset during therapy (129). Infertility can be transient, especially in men, and may recover over time after therapy. Reversibility is dependent on the dose of gonadal radiation or alkylating agents. Ovarian function is unlikely to recover long after the immediate treatment period because long-term amenorrhea commonly results from loss of ova. Cryopreservation of sperm before treatment is an option for men (130), but limited means are available to preserve ova or protect against treatment-related ovarian failure for women (131–133). A successful live birth after orthotopic autotransplantation of cryopreserved ovarian tissue has been recently reported (134–137). A reasonable body of research on topics relating to the long-term gonadal effects of radiation and chemotherapy exists (138–161) and provides a basis for counseling patients and parents of the anticipated outcomes on pubertal development and fertility. A detailed review of this topic is beyond the scope of this chapter.

Among survivors of adult cancer, the risk of premature onset of menopause in women treated with chemotherapeutic agents such as alkylating agents and procarbazine or with abdominal radiation therapy is age related, with women older than age 30 at the time of treatment having the greatest risk of treatment-induced amenorrhea and menopause, and sharply increased rates with chemotherapy around the age of 40. Tamoxifen has not been associated with the development of amenorrhea so far (162). Cyclophosphamide at doses of 5 g per m^2 is likely to cause amenorrhea in women over 40, whereas many adolescents will continue to menstruate even after >20 g per m^2 (163). Although young women may not become amenorrheic after cytotoxic therapy, the risk of early menopause is significant. Female disease-free survivors of cancer diagnosed at ages 13–19 who were menstruating at age 21 were at fourfold-higher risk of menopause compared with controls (140).

Fertility and Pregnancy Outcomes

Fertility. The fertility of survivors of childhood cancer, evaluated in the aggregate, is impaired. In one study, the adjusted relative fertility of survivors compared with that of their siblings was 0.85 [95% confidence interval (CI), 0.78, 0.92]. The adjusted relative fertility of male survivors (0.76; 95% CI, 0.68, 0.86) was slightly lower than that of female survivors (0.93; 95% CI, 0.83, 1.04). The most significant differences in the relative fertility rates were demonstrated in male survivors who had been treated with alkylating agents with or without infradiaphragmatic irradiation (164).

Fertility can be impaired by factors other than the absence of sperm and ova. Conception requires delivery of sperm to the uterine cervix and patency of the fallopian tubes for fertilization to occur and appropriate conditions in the uterus for implantation. Retrograde ejaculation occurs with a significant frequency in men who undergo bilateral retroperitoneal lymph node dissection. Uterine structure may be affected by abdominal irradiation. Uterine length was significantly reduced in 10 women with ovarian failure who had been treated with whole-abdomen irradiation. Endometrial thickness did not increase in response to hormone replacement therapy in three women who underwent weekly ultrasound examination. No flow was detectable with Doppler ultrasound through either uterine artery of five women and through one uterine artery in 3 additional women (165,166). Similarly, four of eight women who received 1440 cGy total-body irradiation had reduced uterine volume and undetectable uterine artery blood flow (167). These data are pertinent when considering the feasibility of assisted reproduction for these survivors.

Pregnancy. Most chemotherapeutic agents are mutagenic, with the potential to cause germ cell chromosomal injury. Possible results of such injury include an increase in the frequency of genetic diseases and congenital anomalies in the offspring of successfully treated childhood and adolescent cancer patients. Several early studies of the offspring of patients treated for diverse types of childhood cancer identified no effect of previous treatment on pregnancy outcome and no increase in the frequency of congenital anomalies in the offspring (168–170). However, a study of offspring of patients treated for Wilms' tumor demonstrated that the birth weight of children born to women who had received abdominal irradiation was significantly lower than that of children born to women who had not received such irradiation (171), a finding that was confirmed in several subsequent studies (172–174). The abnormalities of uterine structure and blood flow reported after abdominal irradiation might explain this clinical finding.

Prior studies of offspring of childhood cancer survivors were limited by the size of the population of offspring and the number of former patients who had been exposed to mutagenic therapy. Several recent studies that attempted to address some of these limitations did not identify an increased frequency of major congenital malformations (175–180), genetic disease, or childhood cancer (181,182) in the offspring of former pediatric cancer patients, including those conceived after bone marrow transplant (183). However, there are data suggesting a deficit of males in the offspring of the partners of male survivors in the Childhood Cancer Survivor Study cohort (184), as well as an effect of prior treatment with doxorubicin or daunorubicin on the percentage of offspring with a birth weight <2500 g born to female survivors in the Childhood Cancer Survivor Study who were treated with pelvic irradiation (185).

Pulmonary Sequelae

The *acute* effects of chemotherapy on the lungs may be lethal, may subside over time, may progress insidiously to a level of clinical pulmonary dysfunction, or may be manifested by abnormal pulmonary function tests. Classically, high doses of bleomycin have been associated with pulmonary toxicity. However, drugs such as alkylating agents, methotrexate, and nitrosoureas may also lead to pulmonary fibrosis, especially when combined with radiation therapy. Radiation is thus an important contributor to pulmonary sequelae of chemotherapy (186). Alkylating agents can injure the lung parenchyma, cause restrictive lung disease by inhibiting chest wall growth, and lead to thin anteroposterior chest diameters even 7 years after completion of therapy. Bleomycin may cause pulmonary insufficiency and interstitial pneumonitis (187).

Pulmonary fibrosis can cause late death in the survivorship period. Among children treated for brain tumors with high doses of nitrosurea and radiotherapy, 35% died of pulmonary fibrosis, 12% within 3 years and 24% after a symptom-free period of 7–12 years (188). The risk for overt decompensation continues for at least 1 year after cessation of therapy and can be precipitated by infection or exposure to intraoperative oxygen. In terms of long-term outcomes, a recent study noted that 22% of HD patients with normal pulmonary function tests at the end of therapy (three cycles each of Mustargen, Vincristine (Oncovin), Procarbazine, Prednisone (MOPP) and Adriamycin, Bleomycin, Vinblastine, Dacarbazine (ABVD) or two cycles of each plus 2550 cGy of involved-field radiotherapy) developed abnormalities with follow-up of 1 7 years.

The long-term outcome of pulmonary toxicity is determined by factors such as the severity of the acute injury, the degree of tissue repair, and the level of compensation possible. Pulmonary dysfunction is usually subclinical and may be manifested by subconscious avoidance of exercise owing to symptoms. Premature respiratory insufficiency, especially with exertion, may also become evident with aging. Recent aggressive lung cancer treatment regimens consisting of surgery, radiation, and chemotherapy may well put patients at high risk for decreased pulmonary function and respiratory symptoms.

Genitourinary Tract

Several drugs such as cisplatin, methotrexate, and nitrosoureas have been associated with both acute and chronic toxicities such as glomerular and tubular injury (189). Glomerular injury may recover over time, whereas tubular injury generally persists. Hemodialysis to counteract the effects of chronic renal toxicity may be warranted for some patients. Ifosfamide may cause Fanconi's syndrome with glycosuria, phosphaturia, and aminoaciduria, and may affect glomerular filtration. Hypophosphatemia may result in slow growth with possible bone deformity if untreated.

Radiation therapy may cause tubular damage and hypertension as a result of renal artery stenosis, especially in doses >20 Gy, especially among children (190). Radiation and chemotherapy may act synergistically, the dysfunction occurring with only 10–15 Gy.

The bladder is particularly susceptible to certain cytotoxic agents. Acrolein, a metabolic by-product of cyclophosphamide and ifosfamide, may cause hemorrhagic cystitis, fibrosis, and occasionally diminished bladder volume. An increased risk of developing bladder cancer also exists. Radiation may lead to bladder fibrosis, diminished capacity, and decreased contractility, the severity of which is proportional to dose and area irradiated. The resultant scarring may diminish urethral and ureteric function.

Gastrointestinal/Hepatic

There are few studies describing long-term effects to this system, either due to underdetection or to a longer latency period than for other organs. Hepatic effects may result from the deleterious effects of many chemotherapeutic agents and radiotherapy. Transfusions may increase the risk of viral hepatitis. Hepatitis C has also been identified in increasing numbers of survivors, 119 of the 2620 tested. Of these patients, 24 of 56 who agreed to participate in a longitudinal study underwent liver biopsy. Chronic hepatitis was noted in 83%, fibrosis in 67%, and cirrhosis in 13%. Fibrosis and adhesions are known to occur after radiotherapy to the bowel.

Compromised Immune System

Hematologic and immunologic impairments can occur after either chemotherapy or radiation and are usually acute in nature. They are temporally related to the cancer treatment. Occasionally, persistent cytopenias may persist after pelvic radiation or in patients who have received extensive therapy with alkylating agents. Alkylating agents may cause myelodysplastic syndrome or leukemia as a late sequela. Immunologic impairment is seen as a long-term problem in HD, relating to both the underlying disease and the treatments used. HD patients are also at risk for serious bacterial infections if they have undergone splenectomy.

Peripheral Neuropathies

These effects are particularly common after taxol, vincristine, and cisplatin. However, despite the frequent use of such chemotherapeutic agents, few studies have characterized the nature and course of neuropathies associated with these drug regimens or dose levels (191,192). Peripheral neuropathy may or may not resolve over time, and potential residual deficits are possible. Clinical manifestations include numbness and tingling in the hands and feet years after completion of cancer treatment.

Second Malignant Neoplasms and Recurrence

Second malignant neoplasms occur as result of an increased risk of second primary cancers associated with the following:

1. Primary malignancy
2. Iatrogenic effect of certain cancer therapies (193–196)

Examples include the development of breast cancer after HD, ovarian cancer after primary breast cancer, and cancers associated with the *HNPCC* gene. Survivors of cancer in childhood have an 8–10% risk of developing a second malignant neoplasm within 20 years of the primary diagnosis (197,198); this is attributable to the mutagenic risk of both radiotherapy and chemotherapy (199–212). This increased risk may be further potentiated in patients with genetic predispositions to malignancy (213–219). The risk of secondary malignancy induced by cytotoxic agents is related to the cumulative dose of drug or radiotherapy (dose dependence).

The risk of malignancy with normal aging results from the risk of cumulative cellular mutations. Compounding the normal aging process by exposure to mutagenic cytotoxic therapies results in an increased risk of secondary malignancy, particularly after radiotherapy, alkylating agents, and podophyllotoxins. Commonly cited secondary malignancies include the following:

1. Leukemia after alkylating agents and podophyllotoxins (220)
2. Solid tumors such as breast, bone, and thyroid cancer in the radiation fields in patients treated with radiotherapy (221)
3. Bladder cancer after cyclophosphamide
4. A higher risk of contralateral breast cancer after primary breast cancer and
5. Ovarian cancer after breast cancer

A detailed discussion of this significant topic is beyond the scope of this chapter. However, the importance of the risk of breast cancer in women treated with chest irradiation and the importance of second primaries in patients with a prior head and neck cancer cannot be overemphasized.

Ancillary Sequelae

Lymphedema. Lymphedema can occur as a persistent or late effect of surgery and/or radiation treatment, and has been reported most commonly after breast cancer treatment, incidence rates ranging between 6 and 30% (222). Lymphedema can occur in anyone with lymph node damage or obstruction to lymphatic drainage. Women undergoing axillary lymph node dissection and high-dose radiotherapy to the axilla for breast cancer are regarded as the highest risk group. Clinically, lymphedema symptoms may range from a feeling of fullness or heaviness in the affected limb to massive swelling and major functional impairment. Recommendations from the American Cancer Society conference on lymphedema in 1998 emphasize the need for additional research on prevention, monitoring, early intervention, and long-term treatment. Treatments suggested encompass multiple treatment modalities including skin care, massage, bandaging for compression, and exercise. Intermittent compression pumps were recommended only when used as an adjunct to manual approaches within a multidisciplinary treatment program, and routine use of medications such as diuretics, prophylactic antibiotics, bioflavinoids, and benzopyrones was discouraged in the absence of additional research. The impact of sentinel node biopsy in lieu of extensive axillary node dissection procedures for breast cancer on the incidence of lymphedema is not known at this time. A recent review by Erickson et al. found that arm edema was a common complication of breast cancer therapy, particularly when axillary dissection and axillary radiation therapy were used, and could result in substantial functional impairment and psychological morbidity (223). The authors note that although recommendations for "preventive" measures (e.g., avoidance of trauma) are anecdotally available, these measures have not been well studied. They found that nonpharmacologic treatments, such as massage and exercise, have been shown to be effective therapies for lymphedema, but the effect of pharmacologic interventions remains uncertain.

Fatigue. Fatigue has been reported as a persistent side effect of treatment in many studies (95,224–226). This is especially true among patients who have undergone bone marrow transplantation (227). Treatment-related fatigue may be associated with various factors such as anemia, infection, changes in hormonal levels, lack of physical activity, cytokine release, and sleep disorders (228). The impact of exercise interventions on fatigue is a promising area of research. Fatigue is an important influence on quality of life for both the patient and the family and needs to be managed effectively.

Sexuality and intimacy. Sexuality encompasses a spectrum of issues ranging from how one feels about one's body to the actual ability to function as a sexual being and has been reported as a persistent effect of treatment. In a recent study on breast, colon, lung, and prostate cancer survivors, issues related to sexual functioning were among the most persistent and severe problems reported. Preexisting sexual dysfunction may also be exacerbated by cancer and its treatment (229). A detailed discussion of this topic is beyond the scope of this chapter.

Surgical and radiation-induced toxicities. *Surgical* effects include increased risk of infections and physiologic comprise associated with nephrectomy (lifestyle changes to prevent trauma to remaining kidney), splenectomy (increased risk for sepsis resulting from encapsulated bacteria), and limb amputation.

Radiation therapy may especially exert effects on the musculoskeletal system and soft tissues among children and young adults, causing injury to the growth plates of long bones and muscle atrophy, osteonecrosis, and fractures (2,5). Short stature can occur as a result of direct bone injury or pituitary radiation and resultant growth hormone deficiency. Chronic pain, the result of scarring and fibrosis in soft tissues surrounding the joints and large peripheral nerves, is a particularly distressing problem among patients who have received moderately high doses of radiation. Soft tissue sarcomas, skin cancers at previously irradiated sites, and pregnancy loss due to decreased uterine capacity in young girls after abdominal radiation are also possible.

CANCER SURVIVORS, HEALTH CARE UTILIZATION, AND COMORBID CONDITIONS

Cancer survivors are high health care utilizers affecting distinct health care domains (230,231). Data clearly show that cancer survivors are at greater risk for developing secondary cancers, late effects of cancer treatment, and chronic comorbid conditions. Exposures leading to these risks include cancer treatment, genetic predisposition, and/or common lifestyle factors (232–234). Although the threat of progressive or recurrent disease is at the forefront of health concerns for a cancer survivor, increased morbidity, and decreased functional status and disability that result from cancer, its treatment, or health-related sequelae are also significant concerns. The impact of chronic comorbid conditions on cancer and its treatment is heightened more so among those diagnosed as adults and those who are elderly at the time of diagnosis.

Presented next is a brief overview of some factors potentiating the risk for chronic comorbid conditions among cancer survivors. A brief discussion of the major comorbid illnesses observed among survivors is also presented.

Metabolic Syndrome-Associated Diseases: Obesity, Diabetes, and Cardiovascular Disease

Obesity is a well-established risk factor for cancers of the breast (postmenopausal), colon, kidney (renal cell), esophagus (adenocarcinoma), and endometrium; therefore, a large proportion of patients with cancer are overweight or obese at the time of diagnosis (235,236). Additional weight gain can also occur during or after active cancer treatment, an occurrence that has been frequently documented among individuals with breast cancer, but recently has been reported among patients with testicular and gastrointestinal cancers as well (228,237). Given data that obesity is associated with cancer recurrence in both breast and prostate cancer, and reduced quality of life among survivors, there is compelling evidence to support weight control efforts in this population (14,15,238,239). Also, gradual weight loss has proven benefits in controlling hypertension, hyperinsulinemia, pain, and dyslipidemia and in improving levels of physical functioning, conditions that are reportedly significant problems in the survivor population (14,15,21,240). Accordingly, the ACS Recommendations for Cancer Survivors list the "achievement of a healthy weight" as a primary goal (14).

Obesity represents one of several metabolic disorders that are frequently manifest among cancer survivors, disorders that are grouped under the umbrella of "the metabolic syndrome" include diabetes and cardiovascular disease (CVD). Insulin resistance is the underlying event associated with the metabolic

syndrome, and insulin resistance, co-occurring hyperinsulinemia, or diabetes has been reported as health concerns among cancer survivors (241–243). As Brown et al. observe (232), diabetes may play a significant role in the increased number of noncancer-related deaths among survivors; however, its role in progressive cancer is still speculative.

Although there is one study that suggests that older breast cancer patients derive a cardioprotective benefit from their diagnosis and/or associated treatments (most likely tamoxifen) (244), most reports indicate that CVD is a major health issue among survivors, evidenced by mortality data that show that half of noncancer-related deaths are attributed to CVD (10). Risk is especially high among men with prostate cancer who receive hormone ablation therapy, as well as with patients who receive adriamycin and radiation treatment to fields surrounding the heart (245). Although more research is needed to explore the potential benefits of lifestyle interventions specifically within survivor populations, the promotion of a healthy weight through a low saturated fat diet with ample amounts of fruits and vegetables and moderate levels of physical activity is recommended (14,15).

Osteoporosis

Osteoporosis and osteopenia are prevalent conditions in the general population, especially among women. Despite epidemiologic findings that increased bone density and low fracture risk are associated with increased risk for breast cancer (246–254), clinical studies suggest that osteoporosis is still a prevalent health problem among survivors (255–258). Data of Twiss et al. indicate that 80% of older breast cancer patients have T-scores <-1 and therefore had been clinically confirmed with osteopenia at the time of their initial appointment. Other cancer populations, such as premenopausal breast and prostate cancer patients, may possess good skeletal integrity at the onset of their disease, but are at risk of developing osteopenia that may ensue with treatment-induced ovarian failure or androgen ablation.

Decreased Functional Status

Previous studies indicate that functional status is lowest immediately after treatment and tends to improve over time; however, the presence of pain and co-occurring diseases may affect this relationship (259). In the older cancer survivor, regardless of duration following diagnosis, the presence of comorbidity, rather than the history of cancer per se, correlates with impaired functional status (260). Cancer survivors have almost a twofold increase in having at least one functional limitation; however, in the presence of another comorbid condition, the odds ratio increases to 5.06 (95% CI, 4.47–5.72) (261). These findings have been confirmed by other studies in diverse populations of cancer survivors (262–264). A cost analysis by Chirikos et al. (264) indicates that "the economic consequence of functional impairment exacts an enormous toll each year on cancer survivors, their families, and the American economy at large."

GRADING OF LATE EFFECTS

The assessment and reporting of toxicity, based on the toxicity criteria system, plays a central role in oncology. Grading of late effects can provide valuable information for systematically monitoring the development and/or progression of late effects (265). Although multiple systems have been developed for grading the adverse effects[§] of cancer treatment, there is, to date, no universally accepted grading system (3). In contrast to the progress made in standardizing acute effects, the use of multiple late effects grading systems by different groups hinders the comparability of clinical trials, impedes the development of toxicity interventions, and encumbers the proper recognition and reporting of late effects. The wide adoption of a standardized criteria system can facilitate comparisons between institutions and across clinical trials.

Multiple systems have been developed and have evolved substantially since being first introduced more than 20 years ago (266). Garre et al. developed a set of criteria to grade late effects by degree of toxicity as follows: grade 0 (no late effect), grade 1 (asymptomatic changes not requiring any corrective measures, and not influencing general physical activity), grade 2 (moderate symptomatic changes interfering with activity), grade 3 (severe symptomatic changes that require major corrective measures and strict and prolonged surveillance), and grade 4 (life-threatening sequelae) (267). The SPOG (Swiss Pediatric Oncology Group) grading system has not been validated so far. It also ranges from 0 to 4: grade 0, no late effect; grade 1, asymptomatic patient requiring no therapy; grade 2, asymptomatic patient, requires continuous therapy, continuous medical follow-up, or symptomatic late effects resulting in reduced school, job, or psychosocial adjustment while remaining fully independent; grade 3, physical or mental sequelae not likely to be improved by therapy but able to work partially; and grade 4, severely handicapped, unable to work independently) (268).

The National Cancer Institute Common Toxicity Criteria (CTC) system was first developed in 1983. The most recent version, CTCAE v3.0 (Common Terminology Criteria for Adverse Events version 3.0) represents the first comprehensive, multimodality grading system for reporting *both* acute and late effects of cancer treatment. This new version requires changes in the following two areas:

1. Application of adverse event criteria (e.g., new guidelines regarding late effects, surgical and pediatric effects, and issues relevant to the impact of multimodal therapies) and
2. Reporting of the *duration* of an effect

This instrument carries the potential to facilitate the standardized reporting of adverse events and a comparison of outcomes between trials and institutions.

It is important to be aware that tools for grading late effects of cancer treatment are available, to validate them in larger populations, and to examine their utility in survivors of adult cancers. Oncologists, primary care physicians, and ancillary providers should be educated and trained to effectively monitor, evaluate, and optimize the health and well-being of a patient who has been treated for cancer. Additional research is needed to provide adequate knowledge about symptoms that persist following cancer treatment or those that arise as late effects, especially among survivors diagnosed as adults. Prospective studies that collect data on late effects will provide much needed information regarding the temporal sequence and timing of symptoms related to cancer treatment. It may be clinically relevant to differentiate between onset of symptoms during treatment, immediately posttreatment, or months later. Continued, systematic follow-up of survivors will result in information about the full spectrum of damage caused by

cytotoxic and/or radiation therapy and possible interventions that may mitigate these adverse effects. We also need to examine the role of comorbidities on the risk for, and development of, late effects of cancer treatment among, especially, adult cancer survivors. Guidelines for the practice of follow-up care of survivors of cancer and evaluation and management of late effects need to be developed so that effects can be mitigated when possible. Clearly, survivors can benefit from guidelines established for the primary prevention of secondary cancers as well as for continued surveillance (269,270).

FOLLOW-UP CARE FOR LATE AND LONG-TERM EFFECTS

Optimal follow-up of survivors includes both ongoing monitoring and assessment of persistent and late effects of cancer treatment and the successful introduction of appropriate interventions to ameliorate these sequelae. The achievement of this goal is challenging and inherent in that challenge is the recognition of the importance of preventing premature mortality from the disease and/or its treatment and the prevention or early detection of both the physiologic and psychological sources of morbidity. The prevention of late effects, second cancers, and recurrences of the primary disease requires watchful follow-up and optimal utilization of early detection screening techniques. Physical symptom management is as important in survivorship as it is during treatment, and effective symptom management during treatment may prevent or lessen lasting effects.

Regular monitoring of health status after cancer treatment is recommended, because this should:

1. Permit the timely diagnosis and treatment of long-term complications of cancer treatment
2. Provide the opportunity to institute preventive strategies such as diet modification, tobacco cessation, and other lifestyle changes
3. Facilitate screening for, and early detection of, a second cancer
4. Ensure timely diagnosis and treatment of recurrent cancer and
5. Permit the detection of functional or physical or psychological disability

There has been no consensus on overall recommendations for routine follow-up after cancer therapy for *all* cancer survivors. A recent review by Kattlove and Winn can help guide oncologists in providing continuing quality care for their patients—care that spans a broad spectrum of medical areas ranging from surveillance to genetic susceptibility (271). Health promotion is a key concern of patients once acute management of their disease is complete. Increasingly, cancer survivors are looking to their oncology care providers for counsel and guidance with respect to change in lifestyle that will improve their prospects of a healthier life and possibly a longer one as well. Although complete data regarding change in lifestyle among cancer survivors have yet to be determined, and there remains an unmet need for behavioral interventions with proven efficacy in various cancer populations (272), the oncologist can nonetheless make use of extant data and also should be attentive to new developments in the field.

Follow-up care and monitoring for late effects is usually done more systematically and rigorously for survivors of childhood cancer while they continue to be part of the program or clinic where they were treated. The monitoring of adult cancer sites for the development of late effects, particularly outside the oncology practice, is neither thorough nor systematic. It is important that survivors of both adult and childhood cancers be monitored for the late and long-term effects or treatment, as discussed in preceding sections, at regular intervals.

[§]Any new finding or undesirable event that may or may not be attributed to treatment. Some adverse events are clinical changes or health problems unrelated to the cancer diagnosis or its treatment. A definitive assignment of attribution cannot always be rendered at the time of grading.

It is now recognized that cancer survivors may experience various late physical and psychological sequelae of treatment and that many health care providers may be unaware of actual or potential survivor problems (273). Until recently, there were no clearly defined, easily accessible risk-based guidelines for cancer survivor follow-up care. Such clinical practice guidelines can serve as a guide for doctors, outline appropriate methods of treatment and care, and address specific clinical situations (disease-oriented) or use of approved medical products, procedures, or tests (modality-oriented). In response to this growing mandate, the Children's Oncology Group has now developed and published its guidelines for long-term follow-up for Survivors of Childhood, Adolescence, and Young Adults Cancer (274). These risk-based, exposure-related clinical practice guidelines are intended to promote earlier detection of and intervention for complications that may potentially arise as a result of treatment for pediatric malignancies, and are both evidence based (utilizing established associations between therapeutic exposures and late effects to identify high-risk categories) and grounded in the collective clinical experience of experts (matching the magnitude of risk with the intensity of screening recommendations). Importantly, they are intended for use beginning 2 or more years following the completion of cancer therapy and are not intended to provide guidance for follow-up of the survivor's primary disease.

Of great significance to survivors of adult cancer, using the best available evidence, the American Society of Clinical Oncology (ASCO) expert panels have also identified and developed recommendations for practice for posttreatment follow-up of specific cancer sites (breast and colorectal; source: www.asco.org). In addition, ASCO has also created an expert panel tasked with the development of follow-up care guidelines geared toward the prevention or early detection of late effects among survivors diagnosed and treated as adults.

To facilitate optimal follow-up during the posttreatment phase, the patient's age at diagnosis, side effects of treatment reported or observed during treatment, calculated cumulative doses of drugs or radiation, and an overview of late effects most likely for a given patient given the treatment history should be summarized and kept on file. A copy of this summary should be provided to the patient or to the parent of a child who has undergone treatment for cancer. The importance of conveying this detailed treatment history to primary care providers should be clearly communicated, especially if follow-up will occur in the primary/family care setting. Finally, screening tests that may help detect subclinical effects that could become clinically relevant in the future should be listed.

Recommendations for regular, ongoing follow-up of cancer survivors are summarized in Table 71.2. For the prevention or early detection of second malignant neoplasms occurring as a late effect of treatment, providers should remain ever vigilant for the possibility. A detailed history and physical examination is always appropriate, in conjunction with screening at age-appropriate intervals or as outlined by panel recommendations arrived through consensus.

Physicians, caregivers, and the family must be able to hear and observe what the patient is trying to communicate, reduce fear and anxiety, counter feelings of isolation, correct misconceptions, and obtain appropriate symptom relief. Practitioners inheriting care for child or adult survivors need to understand the effects of cytotoxic therapies on the growing child or the adult at varying stages/ages of life and be knowledgeable about interventions that may mitigate the effects of these treatments.

Patient education should guide lifestyle and choices for follow-up care, promote adaptation to the disease or relevant sequelae, and help the patient reach an optimal level of wellness and functioning, both physical and psychological, within the context of the disease and treatment effects.

REVIEW AND CONCLUSIONS

Our knowledge about the late effects of cancer treatment, in large part, comes from studies conducted among survivors of pediatric cancer. We need to explore further the impact of cancer treatment on late effects in survivors who were adults when diagnosed. We also need to examine the role of comorbidities on the risk for, and development of, late effects of cancer treatment among these adult cancer survivors. Future research must be directed toward identification of risks associated with more-recent treatment regimens, as well as the very late occurring outcomes resulting from treatment protocols utilized three or more decades ago. As treatment- and patient-related factors impact the subsequent risk of late occurring adverse outcomes, clear delineation of those survivors who are at high risk of specific adverse outcomes is essential for the rational design of follow-up guidelines, prevention, and intervention strategies.

Each person with cancer has unique needs based on the extent of the disease, effects of treatment, prior health, functional level, coping skills, support systems, and many other influences. This complexity requires an interdisciplinary approach, by all health professionals, that is organized, systematic, and geared toward the provision of high-quality care. This ambience may facilitate the adaptation of cancer survivors to temporary or permanent sequelae of the disease and its treatment.

The sizeable population of cancer survivors presents many important questions related to treatment decisions, the impact of medical effects of cancer treatment on health, and long-term follow-up care needs related to cancer as well as other chronic comorbid conditions. It is critical, if we are to develop effective research priorities and recommendations for clinical care, education, and policy related to care for survivors of cancer, that we note the two following key points:

1. The population of cancer survivors consists of individuals with varying needs and issues—those cured of their disease and no longer undergoing active treatment, as well as patients with recurrences or resistant disease requiring ongoing treatment.
2. Regardless of disease status, any survivor may experience lasting adverse effects of treatment (275).

Research conducted with cancer survivors indicates that long-term adverse outcomes are more prevalent, serious, and persistent than expected. However, the late effects of cancer and its treatment in survivors, especially among those who were adults when diagnosed, and/or those belonging to ethnoculturally diverse or medically underserved groups, remain poorly documented (275). In addition, survivors of cancer have significantly poorer health outcomes on multiple burden of illness measures than do people without a history of cancer. These health decrements may occur or continue many years after diagnosis. Comorbid conditions are another major issue for many diagnosed with cancer, yet little is known about the quality of the noncancer-related care received by these survivors (276). It has been reported that it is more likely that survivors would not receive recommended care across a broad range of chronic medical conditions (e.g., angina, congestive heart failure, and diabetes). Quality of life issues in long-term survivors of cancer differ from the problems they face at the time of diagnosis and treatment (274). Interventions with the potential to treat or ameliorate these many and varied late and chronic effects of cancer and its treatment must be developed, evaluated for efficacy, and disseminated.

The larger scientific community has begun to champion the need for cancer survivorship research, and to call for solutions that will lead to both increased length and quality of life for all survivors of cancer (277). This demand is reflected in

TABLE 71.2

FOLLOW-UP CARE AND SURVEILLANCE FOR LATE EFFECTS

Follow-up visit	Content of clinic visit	Suggested evaluative procedures and ancillary actions
Chemotherapy/treatment cessation visit	1. Review complete treatment history 2. Calculate cumulative dosages of drugs 3. Document regimen(s) administered 4. Radiation ports, dosage, machine 5. Document patient age at diagnosis/treatment 6. Side effects during treatment 7. Identify likely late effects 8. Baseline "grading" of late effects (Garre or Swiss Pediatric Oncology Group)	Develop late effect risk profile Summarize all information in previous column Provide copy to patient (or parent if minor child) Instruct that this summary should be provided to primary care or other health care providers Keep copy of summary in patient chart
General measures at every visit	1. Detailed history 2. Complete physical examination 3. Review systems 4. Medication, maintenance, prophylactic antibiotics 5. Education: grade point average, school performance 6. Employment history 7. Menstrual status/cycle 8. Libido, sexual activity 9. Pregnancy and outcome	Evaluate symptomatology, patient reports of issues Review any intercurrent illnesses Evaluate for disease recurrence, second neoplasms Systematic evaluation of long term (persistent) and late effects (see specific measures) Grade long-term and late effects: Garre or SPOG criteria Complete blood cell, urinalysis; other tests depending on exposure history and late effect risk profile
Specific measures to evaluate late effects Relevance differs by: 1. Age at diagnosis/treatment 2. Specific drugs, regimens 3. Combinations of treatment modalities 4. Dosages administered 5. Expected toxicities (based on mechanics of action of cytotoxic drugs; cell-cycle–dependent; proliferation kinetics) 6. Exceptions occur to the theoretical assumption that least susceptible organs/tissues are those that replicate slowly or not at all (vinca, methotrexate, adriamycin) 7. Combinations of radiation/chemotherapy more often associated with late effects	Growth: includes issues such as short stature, scoliosis, hypoplasia	Monitor growth (growth curve); sitting height, parental heights, nutritional status/diet, evaluate scoliosis, bone age, growth hormone assays, thyroid function, endocrinologist consult; orthopaedic consult
	Cardiac	Electrocardiogram, echo, afterload reduction, cardiologist consult Counsel against isometric exercises if high risk, advise ob/gyn risk of cardiac failure in pregnancy
	Neurocognitive	History and examination Communicate: school, family, special education Compensatory remediation techniques Neuropsychology consult; computed tomography or magnetic resonance imaging; cerebral spinal fluid; basic myelin protein Written instructions, appointment cards
	Neuropathy	History/examination: neurologic examination, sensory changes hands/feet, paresthesias, bladder, gait, vision, muscle strength Neurologist consult
	Gonadal toxicity	History for primary vs. secondary dysfunction, gonadal function (menstrual cycle, pubertal development/delay, libido); hormone therapy; interventions (bromocriptine) Premature menopause: hormone replacement unless contraindicated; dual energy x-ray absorptiometry scans for osteoporosis; calcium Endocrinologist consult Reproductive technologies
	Pulmonary	Chest x-ray; pulmonary function tests; pulmonologist consultation
	Urinary	Urinalysis; blood urea nitrogen/creatinine; urologist if hematuria
	Thyroid	Annual thyroid stimulating hormone; thyroid hormone replacement; endocrinologist

TABLE 71.2

(CONTINUED)

Follow-up visit	Content of clinic visit	Suggested evaluative procedures and ancillary actions
	Weight history	Evaluate dietary intake (food diary)/physical activity
		Nutritionist and/or endocrinologist consult
	Lymphedema	History/exam: swelling, sensations of heaviness/fullness
	Fatigue	Rule out hypothyroidism; anemia, cardiac/pulmonary sequelae; evaluate sleep habits
		Evaluate physical fitness and activity levels
		Regular physical activity unless contraindicated
	Surgical toxicity	Antibiotic prophylaxis (splenectomy)
	Gastrointestinal/hepatic	Liver function, hepatitis screen, gastroenterologist consult
Screening for second malignant neoplasms	Screening guidelines differ by age	Follow guidelines for age-appropriate cancer screening (mammogram, Pap smear, fecal occult blood test/flexible sigmoidoscopy)
	Oncologist consult	Mammogram at age 30 if history of mantle radiation for Hodgkin's disease
		Screen for associated cancers in hereditary nonpolyposis colorectal cancer family syndrome
		Screen for ovarian cancer if history of breast cancer and BRCA I and II.
Assess/manage comorbidities	Osteoporosis; heart disease; arthritis, and so on	History/examination; be cognizant of risk; appropriate consult

Evaluations are suggestions only. Relevance will differ by treatment history and late effect risk profile.
Data from Aziz (2002, 2003). (2,6)

the language of several Institute of Medicine (IOM) reports, PRG documents, and National Cancer Institute (NCI) bypass budgets. The IOM report on cancer survivors who were adults when diagnosed articulates key areas for research and care delivery, especially with respect to the development of a formal care plan for survivors that integrates, within one document, key treatment relevant variables, exposures, late effect risks, and management/follow-up care needs (278). The recent IOM report on childhood survivorship cites the need to create and evaluate standards and alternative models of care delivery, including collaborative practices between pediatric oncologists and primary care physicians as well as hospital-based long-term follow-up clinics (279). Another IOM report, Ensuring Quality Cancer Care, recognized that attributes of high-quality care could be linked to optimal outcomes such as enhanced length and quality of survival, and that continued medical follow-up of survivors should include basic standards of care that address the specific needs of long-term survivors.

Survivors of cancer who have completed initial therapy generally require significant amounts of follow-up care during the first 2 years of diagnosis. The frequency and intensity of monitoring diminishes each year thereafter, a dramatic decrease occurring 2–5 years posttreatment. Conversely, the risk of late effects and the impact of long-term effects increases with time. This progressive fall-off in cancer and noncancer related medical visits may reflect either a failure of the medical system to convey the risk for adverse, treatment-related sequelae, or a manifestation of system driven barriers (unequal access, disparities in receipt of quality care). Patient-driven factors (fear of recurrence or of findings) are also critical. Not all survivors may be aware of the late effects they may be at risk for. Therefore, physicians and institutions treating them must provide survivors with a discharge summary detailing

key treatment/exposure and baseline health information that may be relevant if or when late effects become manifest.

Most of the cancer survivors return to their primary care providers for medical follow-up once treatment ends, many of whom may be unaware of the additional health risks of cancer treatment. Providing education and training is therefore necessary. Extant published international long-term follow-up care guidelines provide a logical basis for informed practice, but are not truly evidence based and must be updated regularly and communicated optimally to providers and survivors to be truly effective and useful (280,281).

Cancer survivors are a vulnerable population due to the impact of cancer and its treatment on various health outcomes, and also because of the potential impact of their cancer history on comorbid conditions. Attention may shift away from important health problems not related to cancer, or, surveillance may become over vigilant. The lack of evidence base that can help tailor optimal care strategies needs to be addressed. The relative roles of primary care providers and specialists in the care of cancer survivors are not clear. Developing and testing interventions that examine outcomes among groups of survivors managed under different follow-up care settings is a critical need.

It is imperative that we achieve an evidence-based understanding of the frequency, content, setting and experiences of follow-up care received by the broader population of cancer survivors in order to develop standards for such care with a view toward preventing, detecting early, or ameliorating long term or late effects of cancer and its treatment. Findings from methodologically rigorous studies will improve our understanding of the nature and extent of the burden of illness carried by cancer survivors, yield key information regarding follow-up care, and facilitate future efforts focusing on the development of standards or best practices for such care, especially when notable health disparities might exist.

References

1. American Cancer Society. *Cancer facts and figures, 2003.* Atlanta, GA: American Cancer Society, 2004.
2. Aziz N, Rowland J. Trends and advances in cancer survivorship research: challenge and opportunity. *Semin Radiat Oncol* 2003;13:248–266.
3. Jemal A, Clegg LX, Ward E, et al. Annual report to the nation on the status of cancer, 1875–2001, with a special feature regarding survival. *Cancer* 2004;101:3–27.
4. Rowland J, Mariotto A, Aziz N, et al. Cancer survivorship—United States, 1971–2001. *MMWR Morb Mortal Wkly Rep* 2004;53:526–529.
5. Ries LAG, Smith MA, Gurney JG, et al., eds. *Cancer incidence and survival among children and adolescents: United States SEER program 1975–1995.* NIH Publication 99-4649. Bethesda, MD: National Cancer Institute, 1999.
6. Aziz NM. Long-term survivorship: late effects. In: Berger AM, Portenoy RK, Weissman DE, eds. *Principles and practice of palliative care and supportive oncology,* 2nd ed. Philadelphia, PA: Lippincott Williams & Wilkins, 2002:1019–1033.
7. Chu KC, Tarone RE, Kessler LG. Recent trends in U.S. breast cancer incidence, survival, and mortality rates. *J Natl Cancer Inst* 1996;88: 1571–1579.
8. McKean RC, Feigelson HS, Ross RK. Declining cancer rates in the 1990s. *J Clin Oncol* 2000;18:2258–2268.
9. Ries LAG, Wing PA, Miller DS. The annual report to the nation on the status of cancer, 1973–1997, with a special section on colorectal cancer. *Cancer* 2000;88:2398–2424.
10. Shusterman S, Meadows AT. Long term survivors of childhood leukemia. *Curr Opin Hematol* 2000;7:217–220.
11. Demark-Wahnefried W, Peterson B, McBride C. Current health behaviors and readiness to pursue life-style changes among men and women diagnosed with early stage prostate and breast carcinomas. *Cancer* 2000;88: 674–684.
12. Ganz PA. Late effects of cancer and its treatment. *Semin Oncol Nurs* 2001; 17(4):241–248.
13. Ganz PA. *Cancer survivors: physiologic and psychosocial outcomes.* Alexandria, VA: American Society of Clinical Oncology, 1998:118–123.
14. Schwartz CL. Long-term survivors of childhood cancer: the late effects of therapy. *Oncologist* 1999;4:45–54.
15. Brown ML, Fintor L. The economic burden of cancer. In: Greenwald P, Kramer BS, Weed DL, eds. *Cancer prevention and control.* New York: Marcel Dekker, 1995:69–81.
16. Sklar CA. Overview of the effects of cancer therapies: the nature, scale and breadth of the problem. *Acta Paediatr Suppl* 1999;88:1–4.
17. Mullan F. Seasons of survival: reflections of a physician with cancer. *N Engl J Med* 1995;313:270–273.
18. Loescher LJ, Welch-McCaffrey D, Leigh SA. Surviving adult cancers. Part 1: physiologic effects. *Ann Intern Med* 1989;111:411–432.
19. Welch-McCaffrey D, Hoffman B, Leigh SA. Surviving adult cancers. Part 2: psychosocial implications. *Ann Intern Med* 1989;111:517–524.
20. Herold AH, Roetzheim RG. Cancer survivors. *Prim care* 1992;19:779–791.
21. Marina N. Long-term survivors of childhood cancer. The medical consequences of cure. *Pediatr Clin North Am* 1997;44:1021–1041.
22. Green DM. Late effects of treatment for cancer during childhood and adolescence. *Curr Probl Cancer* 2003;27(3):127–142.
23. Mertens AC, Yasui Y, Neglia JP, et al. Late mortality experience in five-year survivors of childhood and adolescent cancer: The Childhood Cancer Survivor Study. *J Clin Oncol* 2001;19:3163–3172.
24. Robison LL, Bhatia S. Review: late-effects among survivors of leukaemia and lymphoma during childhood and adolescence. *Br J Haematol* 2003; 122:345–356.
25. Boulad F, Sands S, Sklar C. Late complications after bone marrow transplantation in children and adolescents. *Curr Probl Pediatr* 1998;28: 273–304.
26. Bhatia S, Landier W, Robison LL. Late effects of childhood cancer therapy. In: DeVita VT, Hellman S, Rosenberg SA, eds. *Progress in oncology.* Sudbury: Jones and Bartlett, 2002:171–213.
27. Dreyer ZE, Blatt J, Bleyer A. Late effects of childhood cancer and its treatment. In: Pizzo PA, Poplack DG, eds. *Principles and practice of pediatric oncology,* 4th ed. Philadelphia, PA: Lippincott Williams & Wilkins, 2002:1431–1461.
28. Hudson M. Late complications after leukemia therapy. In: Pui CG, ed. *Childhood leukemias.* Cambridge, MA: Cambridge University Press, 1991: 463–481.
29. Blatt J, Copeland DR, Bleyer WA. Late effects of childhood cancer and its treatment. In: Pizzo PA, Poplack DG, eds. *Principles and practice of pediatric oncology,* revised ed. Philadelphia, PA: Lippincott-Raven, 1997: 1091–1114.
30. Kirk JA, Raghupathy P, Stevens MM, et al. Growth failure and growth-hormone deficiency after treatment for acute lymphoblastic leukemia. *Lancet* 1987;1:190–193.

31. Blatt J, Bercu BB, Gillin JC, et al. Reduced pulsatile growth hormone secretion in children after therapy for acute lymphoblastic leukemia. *J Pediatr* 1984;104:182–186.
32. Silber JH, Littman PS, Meadows AT. Stature loss following skeletal irradiation for childhood cancer. *J Clin Oncol* 1990;8:304–312.
33. Leiper AD, Stanhope R, Preese MA, et al. Precocious or early puberty and growth failure in girls treated for acute lymphoblastic leukemia. *Horm Res* 1988;30:72–76.
34. Ogilvy-Stuart AL, Clayton PE, Shalet SM. Cranial irradiation and early puberty. *J Clin Endocrinol Metab* 1994;78:1282–1286.
35. Furst CJ, Lundell M, Ahlback SO. Breast hypoplasia following irradiation of the female breast in infancy and early childhood. *Acta Oncol* 1989; 28(4):519–523.
36. Meyers CA, Weitzner MA. Neurobehavioral functioning and quality of life in patients treated for cancer of the central nervous system. *Curr Opin Oncol* 1995;7:197–200.
37. Haupt R, Fears TR, Robeson LL, et al. Educational attainment in long-term survivors of childhood acute lymphoblastic leukemia. *JAMA* 1994;272:1427–1432.
38. Stehbens JA, Kaleih TA, Noll RB, et al. CNS prophylaxis of childhood leukemia: what are the long-term neurological, neuropsychological and behavioral effects? *Neuropsychol Rev* 1991;2:147–176.
39. Ochs J, Mulhern RK, Faircough D, et al. Comparison of neuropsychologic function and clinical indicators of neurotoxicity in long-term survivors of childhood leukemia given cranial irradiation or parenteral methotrexate: a prospective study. *J Clin Oncol* 1991;9:145–151.
40. Ash P. The influence of radiation on fertility in man. *Br J Radiol* 1990; 53:155–158.
41. Didi M, Didcock E, Davies HA, et al. High incidence of obesity in young adults after treatment of acute lymphoblastic leukemia in childhood. *J Pediatr* 1995;127:63–67.
42. Oberfield SE, Soranno D, Nirenberg A, et al. Age at onset of puberty following high-dose central nervous system radiation therapy. *Arch Pediatr Adolesc Med* 1996;150:589–592.
43. Sklar C, Mertens A, Walter A, et al. Final height after treatment for childhood acute lymphoblastic leukemia: comparison of no cranial irradiation with 1,800 and 2,400 centigrays of cranial irradiation. *J Pediatr* 1993; 123:59–64.
44. Greendale GA, Petersen L, Zibecchi L, et al. Factors related to sexual function in postmenopausal women with a history of breast cancer. *Menopause* 2001;8:111–119.
45. Ganz PA, Greendale GA, Petersen L, et al. Managing menopausal symptoms in breast cancer survivors: results of a randomized controlled trial. *J Natl Cancer Inst* 2000;5:1054–1064.
46. Yancik R, Ganz PA, Varricchio CG, et al. Perspectives on comorbidity and cancer in older patients: approaches to expand the knowledge base. *J Clin Oncol* 2001;19:1147–1151.
47. Lipshultz SE, Colan SD, Gelber RD, et al. Late cardiac effects of doxorubicin therapy for acute lymphoblastic leukemia in childhood. *N Engl J Med* 1991;324:808–814.
48. Bu'Lock FA, Mott MG, Oakhill A, et al. Left ventricular diastolic function after anthracycline chemotherapy in childhood: relation with systolic function, symptoms and pathophysiology. *Br Heart J* 1995;73:340–350.
49. Goorin AM, Borow KM, Goldman A, et al. Congestive heart failure due to adriamycin cardiotoxicity: its natural history in children. *Cancer* 1981;47:2810–2816.
50. Steinherz LJ, Steinherz PG. Cardiac failure and dysrhythmias 6–19 years after anthracycline therapy: a series of 15 patients. *Med Pediatr Oncol* 1995;24:352–361.
51. Adams MJ, Lipsitz SR, Colan SD, et al. Cardiovascular status in long-term survivors of Hodgkin's disease treated with chest radiotherapy. *J Clin Oncol* 2004;22(15):3139–3148.
52. Kremer LCM, van Dalen EC, Offringa M, et al. Anthracycline-induced clinical heart failure in a cohort of 607 children: long-term follow-up study. *J Clin Oncol* 2001;19:191–196.
53. Sorensen K, Levitt G, Chessells J, et al. Anthracycline dose in childhood acute lymphoblastic leukemia: issues of early survival versus late cardiotoxicity. *J Clin Oncol* 1997;15:61–68.
54. Kremer LCM, van Dalen EC, Offringa M, et al. Frequency and risk factors of anthracycline-induced clinical heart failure in children: a systematic review. *Ann Oncol* 2002;13:503–512.
55. Steinherz LJ, Steinherz PG, Tan CT, et al. Cardiac toxicity 4–20 years after completing anthracycline therapy. *JAMA* 1991;266:1672–1677.
56. Kremer LCM, van der Pal HJH, Offringa M, et al. Frequency and risk factors of subclinical cardiotoxicity after anthracycline therapy in children: a systematic review. *Ann Oncol* 2002;13:819–829.
57. Hancock SL, Tucker MA, Hoppe RT. Factors affecting late mortality from heart disease after treatment of Hodgkin's disease. *JAMA* 1993; 270:1949–1955.
58. Hancock SL, Donaldson SS, Hoppe RT. Cardiac disease following treatment of Hodgkin's disease in children and adolescents. *J Clin Oncol* 1993; 11:1199–1203.
59. Fajardo L, Stewart J, Cohn K. Morphology of radiation-induced heart disease. *Arch Pathol* 1968;86:512–519.
60. Minow RA, Benjamin RS, Gottlieb JA. Adriamycin (NSC-123127) cardiomyopathy: an overview with determination of risk factors. *Cancer Chemother Rep* 1975;6:195–201.

61. Prout MN, Richards MJ, Chung KJ, et al. Adriamycin cardiotoxicity in children: case reports, literature review, and risk factors. *Cancer* 1977;39:62–65.
62. Von Hoff DD, Layard MW, Basa P, et al. Risk factors for doxorubicin-induced congestive heart failure. *Ann Intern Med* 1979;91:710–717.
63. Kushner JP, Hansen VL, Hammar SP. Cardiomyopathy after widely separated courses of adriamycin exacerbated by actinomycin-D and mithramycin. *Cancer* 1975;36:1577–1584.
64. Von Hoff DD, Rozencweig M, Piccart M. The cardiotoxicity of anticancer agents. *Semin Oncol* 1982;9:23–33.
65. Lipshultz SE, Lipsitz SR, Mone SM, et al. Female sex and drug dose as risk factors for late cardiotoxic effects of doxorubicin therapy for childhood cancer. *N Engl J Med* 1995;332:1738–1743.
66. Pratt CB, Ransom JL, Evans WE. Age-related adriamycin cardiotoxicity in children. *Cancer Treat Rep* 1978;62:1381–1385.
67. Pai VB, Nahata MC. Cardiotoxicity of chemotherapeutic agents: incidence, treatment and prevention. *Drug Saf* 2000;22:263–302.
68. Legha SS, Benjamin RS, Mackay B, et al. Reduction of doxorubicin cardiotoxicity by prolonged continuous intravenous infusion. *Ann Intern Med* 1982;96:133–139.
69. Lipshultz SE, Giantris AL, Lipsitz SR, et al. Doxorubicin administration by continuous infusion is not cardioprotective: the Dana-Farber 91-01 acute lymphoblastic leukemia protocol. *J Clin Oncol* 2002;20:1677–1682.
70. Marks RD Jr, Agarwal SK, Constable WC. Radiation induced pericarditis in Hodgkin's disease. *Acta Radiol Ther Phys Biol* 1973;12:305–312.
71. Martin RG, Ruckdeschel JC, Chang P, et al. Radiation-related pericarditis. *Am J Cardiol* 1975;35:216–220.
72. Ruckdeschel JC, Chang P, Martin RG, et al. Radiation-related pericardial effusions in patients with Hodgkin's disease. *Medicine* 1975;54:245–259.
73. Perrault DJ, Levy M, Herman JD, et al. Echocardiographic abnormalities following cardiac radiation. *J Clin Oncol* 1985;3:546–551.
74. Kadota RP, Burgert EO Jr, Driscoll DJ, et al. Cardiopulmonary function in long-term survivors of childhood Hodgkin's lymphoma: a pilot study. *Mayo Clin Proc* 1988;63:362–367.
75. Wexler LH. Ameliorating anthracycline cardiotoxicity in children with cancer: clinical trials with dexrazoxane. *Semin Oncol* 1998;25:86–92.
76. Lipshultz SE, Rifai N, Dalton VM, et al. The effect of dexrazoxane on myocardial injury in doxorubicin-treated children with acute lymphoblastic leukemia. *N Engl J Med* 2004;351(2):145–153.
77. Gluck S. The expanding role of epirubicin in the treatment of breast cancer. *Cancer Control* 2002;9(suppl 2):16–27.
78. Baker AF, Dorr RT. Drug interactions with the taxanes: clinical implications. *Cancer Treat Rev* 2001;27(4):221–233.
79. Sessa C, Perotti A, Salvatorelli E, et al. Phase IB and pharmacological study of the novel taxane BMS-184476 in combination with doxorubicin. *Eur J Cancer* 2004;40(4):563–570.
80. Jones RL, Smith IE. Efficacy and safety of trastuzumab. *Expert Opin Drug Saf* 2004;3(4):317–327.
81. Schneider JW, Chang AY, Garratt A. Trastuzumab cardiotoxicity: speculations regarding pathophysiology and targets for further study. *Semin Oncol* 2002;293(Suppl 11):22–28.
82. Schneider JW, Chang AY, Rocco TP. Cardiotoxicity in signal transduction therapeutics: erbB2 antibodies and the heart. *Semin Oncol* 2001;28:18–26.
83. Meadows AT, Gordon J, Massari DJ, et al. Declines in IQ scores and cognitive dysfunctions in children with acute lymphocytic leukaemia treated with cranial irradiation. *Lancet* 1981;2:1015–1018.
84. Jankovic M, Brouwers P, Valsecchi MG, et al. Association of 1800 cGy cranial irradiation with intellectual function in children with acute lymphoblastic leukaemia. ISPACC. International Study Group on Psychosocial Aspects of Childhood Cancer. *Lancet* 1994;344:224–227.
85. Hertzberg H, Huk WJ, Ueberall MA, et al. The German Late Effects Working Group. CNS late effects after ALL therapy in childhood. Part I. Neuroradiological findings in long-term survivors of childhood ALL: an evaluation of the interferences between morphology and neuropsychological performance. *Med Pediatr Oncol* 1997;28:387–400.
86. Green DM, Zevon MA, Rock KM, et al. Fatigue after treatment for Hodgkin's disease during childhood or adolescence. *Proc Am Soc Clin Oncol* 2002;21:396a.
87. Price R. Therapy-related central nervous system diseases in children with acute lymphocytic leukemia. In: Mastrangelo R, Poplack DG, Riccardi R, eds. *Central nervous system leukemia: prevention and treatment.* Boston, MA: Martinus Nijhoff, 1983:71–83.
88. Peylan-Ramu N, Poplack DG, Pizzo PA, et al. Abnormal CT scans of the brain in asymptomatic children with acute lymphocytic leukemia after prophylactic treatment of the central nervous system with radiation and intrathecal chemotherapy. *N Engl J Med* 1978;298:815–818.
89. Riccardi R, Brouwers P, Di Chiro G, et al. Abnormal computed tomography brain scans in children with acute lymphoblastic leukemia: serial long-term follow-up. *J Clin Oncol* 1985;3:12–18.
90. Mulhern RK, Reddick WE, Palmer SL, et al. Neurocognitive deficits in medulloblastoma survivors and white matter loss. *Ann Neurol* 1999;46:834–841.
91. Packer RJ, Sutton LN, Atkins TE, et al. A prospective study of cognitive function in children receiving whole-brain radiotherapy and chemotherapy: 2-year results. *J Neurosurg* 1989;70:707–713.
92. Peckham VC, Meadows AT, Bartel N, et al. Educational late effects in long-term survivors of childhood acute lymphocytic leukemia. *Pediatrics* 1988;81:127–133.
93. Moore IM, Packer RJ, Karl D, et al. Adverse effects of cancer treatment on the central nervous system. In: Schwarta CL, Hobbie WL, Constine WL, et al., eds. *Survivors of childhood cancer: assessment and management.* St. Louis, MO: Mosby, 1994:81–95.
94. Mitby PA, Robison LL, Whitton JA, et al. Utilization of special education services among long-term survivors of childhood cancer: a report from the Childhood Cancer Survivor Study. *Cancer* 2003;97:1115–1126.
95. Loge JH, Abrahamsen AF, Ekeberg O, et al. Hodgkin's disease survivors more fatigued than the general population. *J Clin Oncol* 1999;17:253–261.
96. Knobel H, Loge JH, Lund MB, et al. Late medical complications and fatigue in Hodgkin's disease survivors. *J Clin Oncol* 2001;19:3226–3233.
97. Chessells JM. Recent advances in the management of acute leukaemia. *Arch Dis Child* 2000;82:438–442.
98. Pui CH. Acute lymphoblastic leukemia in children. *Curr Opin Oncol* 2000;12:2–12.
99. van Dam FS, Schagen SB, Muller MJ, et al. Impairment of cognitive function in women receiving adjuvant treatment for high-risk breast cancer: high-dose versus standard-dose chemotherapy. *J Natl Cancer Inst* 1998;90:210–218.
100. Brezden CB, Phillips KA, Abdolell M, et al. Cognitive function in breast cancer patients receiving adjuvant chemotherapy. *J Clin Oncol* 2000;18:2695–2701.
101. Ahles TA, Saykin AJ, Noll WW, et al. The relationship of APOE genotype to neuropsychological performance in long-term cancer survivors treated with standard dose chemotherapy. *Psychooncology* 2003;12(6):612–619.
102. Ganz PA. Cognitive dysfunction following adjuvant treatment of breast cancer: a new dose-limiting toxic effect? *J Natl Cancer Inst* 1998;90:182–183.
103. Hjermstad M, Holte H, Evensen S, et al. Do patients who are treated with stem cell transplantation have a health-related quality of life comparable to the general population after 1 year? *Bone Marrow Transplant* 1999;24:911–918.
104. Walker LG, Wesnes KP, Heys SD, et al. The cognitive effects of recombinant interleukin-2 therapy: a controlled clinical trial using computerised assessments. *Eur J Cancer* 1996;32A:2275–2283.
105. Curt GA, Breitbart W, Cella D, et al. Impact of cancer related fatigue on the lives of patients: new findings from the fatigue coalition. *Oncologist* 2000;5:353–360.
106. Ahles TA, Tope DM, Furstenberg C, et al. Psychologic and neuropsychologic impact of autologous bone marrow transplantation. *J Clin Oncol* 1996;14:1457–1462.
107. Ahles TA, Silberfarb PM, Maurer LH, et al. Psychologic and neuropsychologic functioning of patients with limited small-cell lung cancer treated with chemotherapy and radiation therapy with or without warfarin: a study by the Cancer and Leukemia Group B. *J Clin Oncol* 1998;16:1954–1960.
108. Mulhern RK, Kepner JL, Thomas PR, et al. Neuropsychologic functioning of survivors of childhood medulloblastoma randomized to receive conventional or reduced-dose craniospinal irradiation: A Pediatric Oncology Group study. *Clin Oncol* 1998;16:1723–1728.
109. Raymond-Speden E, Tripp G, Lawrence B, et al. Intellectual, neuropsychological, and academic functioning in long-term survivors of leukemia. *J Pediatr Psychol* 2000;25:59–68.
110. Tannock IF, Ahles TA, Ganz PA, et al. Cognitive impairment associated with chemotherapy for cancer: report of a workshop. *J Clin Oncol* 2004;22(11):2233–2239.
111. Shalet SM, Beardwell CG, Twomey JA, et al. Endocrine function following the treatment of acute leukemia in childhood. *J Pediatr* 1977;90:920–923.
112. Robison LL, Nesbit ME Jr, Sather HN, et al. Height of children successfully treated for acute lymphoblastic leukemia: a report from the Late Effects Study Committee of Childrens Cancer Study Group. *Med Pediatr Oncol* 1985;13:14–21.
113. Hancock SL, Cox RS, McDougall IR. Thyroid diseases after treatment of Hodgkin's disease. *N Engl J Med* 1991;325:599–605.
114. Sklar C, Whitton J, Mertens A, et al. Abnormalities of the thyroid in survivors of Hodgkin's disease: data from the Childhood Cancer Survivor Study. *J Clin Endocrinol Metab* 2000;85:3227–3232.
115. Glatstein E, McHardy-Young S, Brast N, et al. Alterations in serum thyrotropin (TSH) and thyroid function following radiotherapy in patients with malignant lymphoma. *J Clin Endocrinol Metab* 1971;32:833–841.
116. Rosenthal MB, Goldfine ID. Primary and secondary hypothyroidism in nasopharyngeal carcinoma. *JAMA* 1976;236:1591–1593.
117. Sklar CA. Growth and neuroendocrine dysfunction following therapy for childhood cancer. *Pediatr Clin North Am* 1997;44:489–503.
118. Berry DH, Elders MJ, Crist W, et al. Growth in children with acute lymphocytic leukemia: A Pediatric Oncology Group study. *Med Pediatr Oncol* 1983;11:39–45.
119. Papadakis V, Tan C, Heller G, et al. Growth and final height after treatment for childhood Hodgkin disease. *J Pediatr Hematol Oncol* 1996;18:272–276.
120. Shalet SM, Price DA, Beardwell CG, et al. Normal growth despite abnormalities of growth hormone secretion in children treated for acute leukemia. *J Pediatr* 1979;94:719–722.
121. Didcock E, Davies HA, Didi M, et al. Pubertal growth in young adult survivors of childhood leukemia. *J Clin Oncol* 1995;13:2503–2507.

122. Katz JA, Pollock BH, Jacaruso D, et al. Final attained height in patients successfully treated for childhood acute lymphoblastic leukemia. *J Pediatr* 1993;123:546–552.
123. Odame I, Reilly JJ, Gibson BE, et al. Patterns of obesity in boys and girls after treatment for acute lymphoblastic leukaemia. *Arch Dis Child* 1994;71:147–149.
124. Van Dongen-Melman JE, Hokken-Koelega AC, Hahlen K, et al. Obesity after successful treatment of acute lymphoblastic leukemia in childhood. *Pediatr Res* 1995;38:86–90.
125. Sklar CA, Mertens AC, Walter A, et al. Changes in body mass index and prevalence of overweight in survivors of childhood acute lymphoblastic leukemia: role of cranial irradiation. *Med Pediatr Oncol* 2000;35:91–95.
126. Craig F, Leiper AD, Stanhope R, et al. Sexually dimorphic and radiation dose dependent effect of cranial irradiation on body mass index. *Arch Dis Child* 1999;81:500–510.
127. Oeffinger KC, Mertens AC, Sklar CA, et al. Obesity in adult survivors of childhood acute lymphoblastic leukemia: a report from the Childhood Cancer Survivor Study. *J Clin Oncol* 2003;21:1359–1365.
128. Thomson AB, Critchley HOD, Wallace WHB. Fertility and progeny. *Eur J Cancer* 2002;38:1634–1644.
129. Lamb MA. Effects of cancer on the sexuality and fertility of women. *Semin Oncol Nurs* 1995;11:120–127.
130. Brougham MF, Kelnar CJ, Sharpe RM, et al. Male fertility following childhood cancer: current concepts and future therapies. *Asian J Androl* 2003;5(4):325–337.
131. Wallace WH, Anderson R, Baird D. Preservation of fertility in young women treated for cancer. *Lancet Oncol* 2004;5(5):269–270.
132. Opsahl MS, Fugger EF, Sherins RJ. Preservation of reproductive function before therapy for cancer: new options involving sperm and ovary cryopreservation. *Cancer J* 1997;3:189–191.
133. Oktay K, Newton H, Aubard Y, et al. Cryopreservation of immature human oocytes and ovarian tissue: an emerging technology? *Fertil Steril* 1998;69:1–7.
134. Donnez J, Dolmans MM, Demylle D, et al. Livebirth after orthotic transplantation of cryopreserved ovarian tissue. *Lancet* 2004;364(9443):1405–1410.
135. Wallace WH, Pritchard J. Livebirth after cryopreserved ovarian tissue autotransplantation. *Lancet* 2004;364(9451):2093–2094.
136. Bath LE, Tydeman G, Critchley HO, et al. Spontaneous conception in a young woman who had ovarian cortical tissue cryopreserved before chemotherapy and radiotherapy for a Ewing's sarcoma of the pelvis: case report. *Hum Reprod* 2004;19(11):2569–2572.
137. Wallace WH, Kelsey TW. Ovarian reserve and reproductive age may be determined from measurement of ovarian volume by transvaginal sonography. *Hum Reprod* 2004;19(7):1612–1617.
138. Chapman RM, Sutcliffe SB, Malpas JS. Cytotoxic-induced ovarian failure in Hodgkin's disease. II. Effects on sexual function. *JAMA* 1979;242:1882–1884.
139. Waxman JHX, Terry YA, Wrigley PFM, et al. Gonadal function in Hodgkin's disease: long-term follow-up of chemotherapy. *Br Med J* 1982;285:1612–1613.
140. Byrne J, Fears TR, Gail MH, et al. Early menopause in long-term survivors of cancer during adolescence. *Am J Obstet Gynecol* 1992;166:788–793.
141. Madsen BL, Giudice L, Donaldson SS. Radiation-induced premature menopause: a misconception. *Int J Radiat Oncol Biol Phys* 1995;32:1461–1464.
142. Li FP, Gimbreke K, Gelber RD, et al. Outcome of pregnancy in survivors of Wilms' tumor. *JAMA* 1987;257:216–219.
143. Constine LS, Rubin P, Woolf PD, et al. Hyperprolactinemia and hypothyroidism following cytotoxic therapy for central nervous system malignancies. *J Clin Oncol* 1987;5:1841–1851.
144. Lushbaugh CC, Casarett GW. The effects of gonadal irradiation in clinical radiation therapy: a review. *Cancer* 1976;37:1111–1125.
145. Stillman RJ, Schinfeld JS, Schiff I, et al. Ovarian failure in long-term survivors of childhood malignancy. *Am J Obstet Gynecol* 1981;139:62–66.
146. Wallace WHB, Thomson AB, Kelsey TW. The radiosensitivity of the human oocyte. *Hum Reprod* 2003;18:117–121.
147. DaCunha MF, Meistrich ML, Fuller LM, et al. Recovery of spermatogenesis after treatment for hodgkin's disease: limiting dose of MOPP chemotherapy. *J Clin Oncol* 1984;2:571–577.
148. Narayan P, Lange PH, Fraley EE. Ejaculation and fertility after extended retroperitoneal lymph node dissection for testicular cancer. *J Urol* 1982;127:685–688.
149. Schlegel PN, Walsh PC. Neuroanatomical approach to radical cystoprostatectomy with preservation of sexual function. *J Urol* 1987;138:1402–1406.
150. Rowley MJ, Leach DR, Warner GA, et al. Effect of graded doses of ionizing radiation on the human testis. *Radiat Res* 1974;59:665–678.
151. Speiser B, Rubin P, Casarett G. Aspermia following lower truncal irradiation in Hodgkin's disease. *Cancer* 1973;32:692–698.
152. Shamberger RC, Sherins RJ, Rosenberg SA. The effects of postoperative adjuvant chemotherapy and radiotherapy on testicular function in men undergoing treatment for soft tissue sarcoma. *Cancer* 1981;47:2368–2374.
153. Green DM, Brecher ML, Lindsay AN, et al. Gonadal function in pediatric patients following treatment for Hodgkin disease. *Med Pediatr Oncol* 1981;9:235–244.
154. Sklar C. Reproductive physiology and treatment-related loss of sex hormone production. *Med Pediatr Oncol* 1999;33:2–8.

155. Shalet SM, Horner A, Ahmed SR, et al. Leydig cell damage after testicular irradiation for lymphoblastic leukaemia. *Med Pediatr Oncol* 1985;13:65–68.
156. Leiper AD, Grant DB, Chessells JM. Gonadal function after testicular radiation for acute lymphoblastic leukaemia. *Arch Dis Child* 1986;61:53–56.
157. Sklar CA, Robison LL, Nesbit ME, et al. Effects of radiation on testicular function in long-term survivors of childhood acute lymphoblastic leukemia: a report from the Children Cancer Study Group. *J Clin Oncol* 1990;8:1981–1987.
158. Chapman RM, Sutcliffe SB, Malpas JS. Cytotoxic-induced ovarian failure in women with Hodgkin's disease. I. Hormone function. *JAMA* 1979;242:1877–1881.
159. Whitehead E, Shalet SM, Jones PH, et al. Gonadal function after combination chemotherapy for Hodgkin's disease in childhood. *Arch Dis Child* 1982;57:287–291.
160. Ortin TT, Shostak CA, Donaldson SS. Gonadal status and reproductive function following treatment for Hodgkin's disease in childhood: the Stanford experience. *Int J Radiat Oncol Biol Phys* 1990;19:873–880.
161. Mackie EJ, Radford M, Shalet SM. Gonadal function following chemotherapy for childhood Hodgkin's disease. *Med Pediatr Oncol* 1996;27:74–78.
162. Goodwin PJ, Ennis M, Pritchard KI, et al. Risk of menopause during the first year after breast cancer diagnosis. *J Clin Oncol* 1999;17:2365–2370.
163. Koyama H, Wada T, Nishzawa Y, et al. Cyclophosphamide induced ovarian failure and its therapeutic significance in patients with breast cancer. *Cancer* 1977;39:1403–1409.
164. Byrne J, Mulvihill JJ, Myers MH, et al. Effects of treatment on fertility in long-term survivors of childhood or adolescent cancer. *N Engl J Med* 1987;317:1315–1321.
165. Critchley HOD, Wallace WHB, Shalet SM, et al. Abdominal irradiation in childhood: the potential for pregnancy. *Br J Obstet Gynaecol* 1992;99:392–394.
166. Critchley HOD. Factors of importance for implantation and problems after treatment for childhood cancer. *Med Pediatr Oncol* 1999;33:9–14.
167. Bath LE, Critchley HO, Chambers SE, et al. Ovarian and uterine characteristics after total body irradiation in childhood and adolescence: response to sex steroid replacement. *Br J Obstet Gynaecol* 1999;106:1265–1272.
168. Li FP, Fine W, Jaffe N, et al. Offspring of patients treated for cancer in childhood. *J Natl Cancer Inst* 1979;62:1193–1197.
169. Hawkins MM, Smith RA, Curtice LJ. Childhood cancer survivors and their offspring studied through a postal survey of general practitioners: preliminary results. *J R Coll Gen Pract* 1988;38:102–105.
170. Byrne J, Rasmussen SA, Steinhorn SC, et al. Genetic disease in offspring of long-term survivors of childhood and adolescent cancer. *Am J Hum Genet* 1998;62:45–52.
171. Green DM, Fine WE, Li FP. Offspring of patients treated for unilateral Wilms' tumor in childhood. *Cancer* 1982;49:2285–2288.
172. Byrne L, Mulvihill JJ, Connelly RR, et al. Reproductive problems and birth defects in survivors of Wilms' tumor and their relatives. *Med Pediatr Oncol* 1988;16:233–240.
173. Li FP, Gimbreke K, Gelber RD, et al. Outcome of pregnancy in survivors of Wilms' tumor. *JAMA* 1987;257:216–219.
174. Hawkins MM, Smith RA. Pregnancy outcomes in childhood cancer survivors: probable effects of abdominal irradiation. *Int J Cancer* 1989;43:399–402.
175. Hawkins MM. Is there evidence of a therapy-related increase in germ cell mutation among childhood cancer survivors? *J Natl Cancer Inst* 1991;83:1643–1650.
176. Green DM, Zevon MA, Lowrie G, et al. Pregnancy outcome following treatment with chemotherapy for cancer in childhood and adolescence. *N Engl J Med* 1991;325:141–146.
177. Nygaard R, Clausen N, Siimes MA, et al. Reproduction following treatment for childhood leukemia: a population-based prospective cohort study of fertility and offspring. *Med Pediatr Oncol* 1991;19:459–466.
178. Dodds I, Marrett LD, Tomkins DJ, et al. Case-control study of congenital anomalies in children of cancer patients. *Br Med J* 1993;307:164–168.
179. Kenny LB, Nicholson HS, Brasseux C, et al. Birth defects in offspring of adult survivors of childhood acute lymphoblastic leukemia. *Cancer* 1996;78:169–176.
180. Green DM, Fiorello A, Zevon MA, et al. Birth defects and childhood cancer in offspring of survivors of childhood cancer. *Arch Pediatr Adolesc Med* 1997;151:379–383.
181. Mulvihill JJ, Myers MH, Connelly RR, et al. Cancer in offspring of long-term survivors of childhood and adolescent cancer. *Lancet* 1987;2:813–817.
182. Hawkins JJ, Draper GJ, Smith RA. Cancer among 1,348 offspring of survivors of childhood cancer. *Int J Cancer* 1989;43:975–978.
183. Sanders JE, Hawley J, Levy W, et al. Pregnancies following high-dose cyclophosphamide with or without high-dose busulfan or total-body irradiation and bone marrow transplantation. *Blood* 1996;87:3045–3052.
184. Green DM, Whitton JA, Stovall M, et al. Pregnancy outcome of partners of male survivors of childhood cancer. A report from the Childhood Cancer Survivor Study. *J Clin Oncol* 2003;21:716–721.
185. Green DM, Whitton JA, Stovall M, et al. Pregnancy outcome of female survivors of childhood cancer. A report from the Childhood Cancer Survivor Study. *Am J Obstet Gynecol* 2002;187:1070–1080.

186. Horning SJ, Adhikari A, Rizk N. Effect of treatment for Hodgkin's disease on pulmonary function: results of a prospective study. *J Clin Oncol* 1994; 12:297–305.

187. Samuels ML, Douglas EJ, Holoye PV, et al. Large dose bleomycin therapy and pulmonary toxicity. *JAMA* 1976;235:1117–1120.

188. O'Driscoll BR, Hasleton PS, Taylor PM, et al. Active lung fibrosis up to 17 years after chemotherapy with carmustine (BCNU) in childhood. *N Engl J Med* 1990;323:378–382.

189. Vogelzang NJ. Nephrotoxicity from chemotherapy: prevention and management. *Oncology* 1991;5:97–112.

190. Dewit L, Anninga JK, Hoefnagel CA, et al. Radiation injury in the human kidney: a prospective analysis using specific scintigraphic and biochemical endpoints. *Int J Radiat Oncol Biol Phys* 1990;19:977–983.

191. Hilkens PHE, Verweij J, Vecht CJ, et al. Clinical characteristics of severe peripheral neuropathy induced by docetaxel, taxotere. *Ann Oncol* 1997;8:187–190.

192. Tuxen MK, Hansen SW. Complications of treatment: neurotoxicity secondary to antineoplastic drugs. *Cancer Treat Rev* 1994;20:191–214.

193. Bhatia S, Robison LL, Meadows AT, LESG Investigators. High risk of second malignant neoplasms (SMN) continues with extended follow-up of childhood Hodgkin's disease (HD) cohort: report from the Late Effects Study Group. *Blood* 2001;98:768a.

194. van Leeuwen FE, Klokman WJ, Stovall M, et al. Roles of radiotherapy and smoking in lung cancer following Hodgkin's disease. *J Natl Cancer Inst* 1995;87:1530–1537.

195. Kreiker J, Kattan J. Second colon cancer following Hodgkin's disease. A case report. *J Med Liban* 1996;44:107–108.

196. Deutsch M, Wollman MR, Ramanathan R, et al. Rectal cancer twenty-one years after treatment of childhood Hodgkin disease. *Med Pediatr Oncol* 2002;38:280–281.

197. Hawkins MM, Draper GJ, Kingston JE. Incidence of second primary tumors among childhood cancer survivors. *Br J Cancer* 1984;56:339–347.

198. Meadows AT, Baum E, Fossati-Bellani F, et al. Second malignant neoplasms in children: an update from the Late Effects Study Group. *J Clin Oncol* 1985;3:532–538.

199. Bhatia S, Robison LL, Oberlin O, et al. Breast cancer and other second neoplasms after childhood Hodgkin's disease. *N Engl J Med* 1996; 334:745–751.

200. Malkin D, Li FP, Strong LC, et al. Germline p53 mutations in a familial syndrome of breast cancer, sarcomas, and other neoplasms. *Science* 1990; 250:1333–1338.

201. Neglia JP, Friedman DL, Yasui Y, et al. Second malignant neoplasms in five-year survivors of childhood cancer: childhood cancer survivor study. *J Natl Cancer Inst* 2001;93:618–629.

202. Bhatia S, Sather HN, Pabustan OB, et al. Low incidence of second neoplasms among children diagnosed with acute lymphoblastic leukemia after 1983. *Blood* 2002;99:4257–4264.

203. Neglia JP, Meadows AT, Robison LL, et al. Second neoplasms after acute lymphoblastic leukemia in childhood. *N Engl J Med* 1991;325:1330–1336.

204. Relling MV, Rubnitz JE, Rivera GK, et al. High incidence of secondary brain tumours after radiotherapy and antimetabolites. *Lancet* 1999; 354:34–39.

205. Hawkins MM, Wilson LM, Stovall MA, et al. Epipodophyllotoxins, alkylating agents, and radiation and risk of secondary leukaemia after childhood cancer. *Br Med J* 1992;304:951–958.

206. Tucker MA. Solid second cancers following Hodgkin's disease. *Hematol-Oncol Clin North Am* 1993;7:389–400.

207. Beatty O III, Hudson MM, Greenwald C, et al. Subsequent malignancies in children and adolescents after treatment for Hodgkin's disease. *J Clin Oncol* 1995;13:603–609.

208. Jenkin D, Greenberg M, Fitzgerald A. Second malignant tumours in childhood Hodgkin's disease. *Med Pediatr Oncol* 1996;26:373–379.

209. Sankila R, Garwicz S, Olsen JH, et al. Risk of subsequent malignant neoplasms among 1,641 Hodgkin's disease patients diagnosed in childhood and adolescence: a population-based cohort study in the five Nordic countries. Association of the Nordic Cancer Registries and the Nordic Society of Pediatric Hematology and Oncology. *J Clin Oncol* 1996;14:1442–1446.

210. Wolden SL, Lamborn KR, Cleary SF, et al. Second cancers following pediatric Hodgkin's disease. *J Clin Oncol* 1998;16:536–544.

211. Green DM, Hyland A, Barcos MP, et al. Second malignant neoplasms after treatment for Hodgkin's disease in childhood or adolescence. *J Clin Oncol* 2000;18:1492–1499.

212. Metayer C, Lynch CF, Clarke EA, et al. Second cancers among long-term survivors of Hodgkin's disease diagnosed in childhood and adolescence. *J Clin Oncol* 2000;18:2435–2443.

213. Wrighton SA, Stevens JC. The human hepatic cytochromes P450 involved in drug metabolism. *Crit Rev Toxicol* 1992;22:1–21.

214. Hayes JD, Pulford DJ. The glutathione S-transferase supergene family: regulation of GST and the contribution of the isoenzymes to cancer chemoprotection and drug resistance. *Crit Rev Biochem Mol Biol* 1995;30: 445–600.

215. Raunio H, Husgafvel-Pursiainen K, Anttila S, et al. Diagnosis of polymorphisms in carcinogen-activating and inactivating enzymes and cancer susceptibility: a review. *Gene* 1995;159:113–121.

216. Smith G, Stanley LA, Sim E, et al. Metabolic polymorphisms and cancer susceptibility. *Cancer Surv* 1995;25:27–65.

217. Felix CA, Walker AH, Lange BJ, et al. Association of CYP3A4 genotype with treatment-related leukemia. *Proc Natl Acad Sci U S A* 1998;95: 13176–13181.

218. Naoe T, Takeyama K, Yokozawa T, et al. Analysis of genetic polymorphism in NQO1, GST-M1, GST-T1, and CYP3A4 in 469 Japanese patients with therapy-related leukemia/myelodysplastic syndrome and de novo acute myeloid leukemia. *Clin Cancer Res* 2000;6:4091–4095.

219. Blanco JG, Edick MJ, Hancock ML, et al. Genetic polymorphisms in CYP3A5, CYP3A4 and NQO1 in children who developed therapy-related myeloid malignancies. *Pharmacogenetics* 2002;12:605–611.

220. Zim S, Collins JM, O'Neill D, et al. Inhibition of first-pass metabolism in cancer chemotherapy: interaction of 6-mercaptopurine and allopurinol. *Clin Pharmacol Ther* 1983;34:810–817.

221. Hildreth NG, Shore RE, Dvoretsky PM. The risk of breast cancer after irradiation of the thymus in infancy. *N Engl J Med* 1989;321:1281–1284.

222. Petrek JA, Heelan MC. Incidence of breast carcinoma-related lymphedema. *Cancer* 1998;83(Suppl 12):2776–2781.

223. Erickson VS, Pearson ML, Ganz PA, et al. Arm edema in breast cancer patients. *J Natl Cancer Inst* 2004;93:96–111.

224. Andrykowski MA, Curran SL, Lightner R. Off-treatment fatigue in breast cancer survivors: a controlled comparison. *J Behav Med* 1998;21:1–18.

225. Broeckel JA, Jacobsen PB, Horton J, et al. Characteristics and correlates of fatigue after adjuvant chemotherapy for breast cancer. *J Clin Oncol* 1998;16:1689–1696.

226. Greenberg DB, Kornblith AB, Herndon JE, et al. Quality of life for adult leukemia survivors treated on clinical trials of cancer and Leukemia Group B during the period 1971–1988. *Cancer* 1997;80:1936–1944.

227. Bush NE, Haberman M, Donaldson G, et al. Quality of life of 125 adults surviving 6–18 years after bone marrow transplant. *Soc Sci Med* 1995; 40:479–490.

228. Mock V, Piper B, Escalante C, et al. National comprehensive cancer network. NCCN practice guidelines for cancer-related fatigue. *Oncology* (Williston Park). 2000;14(11A):151–161.

229. Ganz PA, Schag CAC, Lee JJ, et al. The CARES: a generic measure of health-related quality of life for cancer patients. *Qual Life Res* 1992; 1:19–29.

230. Demark-Wahnefried W, Aziz NM, Rowland JH, et al. Riding the Crest of the Teachable Moment. *J Clin Oncol* 2005;23(24):5814–5830.

231. Day RW. Future need for more cancer research. *J Am Diet Assoc* 1998;98:523.

232. Brown BW, Brauner C, Minnotte MC. Noncancer deaths in white adult cancer patients. *J Natl Cancer Inst* 1993;85:979–997.

233. Meadows AT, Varricchio C, Crosson K, et al. Research issues in cancer survivorship. *Cancer Epidemiol Biomarkers Prev* 1998;7:1145–1151.

234. Travis LB. Therapy-associated solid tumors. *Acta Oncol* 2002;41:323–333.

235. Bergstrom A, Pisani P, Tenet V, et al. Overweight as an avoidable cause of cancer in Europe. *Int J Cancer* 2001;91:421–430.

236. World Health Organization. *IARC handbook of cancer prevention*, vol 6. Geneva: World Health Organization, 2002.

237. Nuver J, Smit AJ, Postma A, et al. The metabolic syndrome in long-term cancer survivors, an important target for secondary measures. *Cancer Treat Rev* 2002;28:195–214.

238. Freedland SJ, Aronson WJ, Kane CJ, et al. Impact of obesity on biochemical control after radical prostatectomy for clinically localized prostate cancer: a report by the shared equal access regional cancer hospital database study group. *J Clin Oncol* 2004;22:446–453.

239. Chlebowski RT, Aiello E, McTiernan A. Weight loss in breast cancer patient management. *J Clin Oncol* 2002;20:1128–1143.

240. Argiles JM, Lopez-Soriano FJ. Insulin and cancer. *Int J Oncol* 2001; 18:683–687.

241. Bines J, Gradishar WJ. Primary care issues for the breast cancer survivor. *Compr Ther* 1997;23:605–611.

242. Yoshikawa T, Noguchi Y, Doi C, et al. Insulin resistance in patients with cancer: relationships with tumor site, tumor stage, body-weight loss, acute-phase response, and energy expenditure. *Nutrition* 2001;17:590–593.

243. Balkau B, Kahn HS, Courbon D, et al. Paris Prospective Study. Hyperinsulinemia predicts fatal liver cancer but is inversely associated with fatal cancer at some other sites: the Paris Prospective Study. *Diabetes Care* 2001;24:843–849.

244. Lamont EB, Christakis NA, Lauderdale DS. Favorable cardiac risk among elderly breast carcinoma survivors. *Cancer* 2003;98:2–10.

245. Hull MC, Morris CG, Pepine CJ, et al. Valvular dysfunction and carotid, subclavian, and coronary artery disease in survivors of Hodgkin lymphoma treated with radiation therapy. *JAMA* 2003;290:2831–2837.

246. Buist DS, LaCroix AZ, Barlow WE, et al. Bone mineral density and endogenous hormones and risk of breast cancer in postmenopausal women (United States). *Cancer Causes Control* 2001;12:213–222.

247. Buist DS, LaCroix AZ, Barlow WE, et al. Bone mineral density and breast cancer risk in postmenopausal women. *J Clin Epidemiol* 2001;54:417–422.

248. Cauley JA, Lucas FL, Kuller LH, et al. Bone mineral density and risk of breast cancer in older women: the study of osteoporotic fractures. Study of Osteoporotic Fractures Research Group. *JAMA* 1996;276:1404–1408.

249. Lamont EB, Lauderdale DS. Low risk of hip fracture among elderly breast cancer survivors. *Ann Epidemiol* 2003;13:698–703.

250. Lucas FL, Cauley JA, Stone RA, et al. Bone mineral density and risk of breast cancer: differences by family history of breast cancer. Study of Osteoporotic Fractures Research Group. *Am J Epidemiol* 1998;148:22–29.

251. Newcomb PA, Trentham-Dietz A, Egan KM, et al. Fracture history and risk of breast and endometrial cancer. *Am J Epidemiol* 2001;153:1071–1078.

252. van der Klift M, de Laet CE, Coebergh JW, et al. Bone mineral density and the risk of breast cancer: the Rotterdam Study. *Bone* 2003;32:211–216.

253. Zhang Y, Kiel DP, Kreger BE, et al. Bone mass and the risk of breast cancer among postmenopausal women. *N Engl J Med* 1997;336:611–617.

254. Zmuda JM, Cauley JA, Ljung BM, et al. Study of Osteoporotic Fractures Research Group. Bone mass and breast cancer risk in older women: differences by stage at diagnosis. *J Natl Cancer Inst* 2001;93:930–936.

255. Schultz PN, Beck ML, Stava C, et al. Health profiles in 5836 long-term cancer survivors. *Int J Cancer* 2003;104:488–495.

256. Twiss JJ, Waltman N, Ott CD, et al. Bone mineral density in postmenopausal breast cancer survivors. *J Am Acad Nurse Pract* 2001;13:276–284.

257. Ramaswamy B, Shapiro CL. Osteopenia and osteoporosis in women with breast cancer. *Semin Oncol* 2003;30:763–775.

258. Diamond TH, Higano CS, Smith MR, et al. Osteoporosis in men with prostate carcinoma receiving androgen-deprivation therapy: recommendations for diagnosis and therapies. *Cancer* 2004;100:892–899.

259. Ko CY, Maggard M, Livingston EH. Evaluating health utility in patients with melanoma, breast cancer, colon cancer, and lung cancer: a nationwide, population-based assessment. *J Surg Res* 2003;114:1–5.

260. Garman KS, Pieper CF, Seo P, et al. Function in elderly cancer survivors depends on comorbidities. *J Gerontol A Biol Sci Med Sci* 2003;58:M1119–M1124.

261. Hewitt M, Rowland JH, Yancik R. Cancer survivors in the U.S.: age, health and disability. *J Gerontol A Biol Sci Med Sci* 2003;58:82–91.

262. Ashing-Giwa K, Ganz PA, Petersen L. Quality of life of African-American and white long term breast carcinoma survivors. *Cancer* 1999;85:418–426.

263. Baker F, Haffer S, Denniston M. Health-related quality of life of cancer and noncancer patients in medicare managed care. *Cancer* 2003;97:674–681.

264. Chirikos TN, Russell-Jacobs A, Jacobsen PB. Functional impairment and the economic consequences of female breast cancer. *Womens Health* 2002;36:1–20.

265. Trotti A. The evolution and application of toxicity criteria. *Semin Radiat Oncol* 2002;121(Suppl 1):1–3.

266. Hoeller U, Tribius S, Kuhlmey A, et al. Increasing the rate of late toxicity by changing the score? A comparison of RTOG/EORTC and LENT/SOMA scores. *Int J Radiat Oncol Biol Phys* 2003;55(4):1013–1018.

267. Garre ML, Gandus S, Cesana B, et al. Health status of long term survivors after cancer in childhood. *Am J Pediatr Hematol Oncol* 1994;16:143–152.

268. Von der Weid N, Beck D, Caflisch U, et al. Standardized assessment of late effects in long term survivors of childhood cancer in Switzerland: results of a Swiss Pediatrics Oncology Group (SPOG) study. *Int J Pediatr Hematol Oncol* 1996;3:483–490.

269. Brown JK, Byers T, Doyle C, et al. Nutrition and physical activity during and after cancer treatment: an American Cancer Society guide for informed choices. *CA Cancer J Clin* 2003;53:268–291.

270. Rock CL, Demark-Wahnefried W. Nutrition and survival after the diagnosis of breast cancer: a review of the evidence. *J Clin Oncol* 2002;20:3302–3316.

271. Kattlove H, Winn RJ. Ongoing care of patients after primary treatment for their cancer. *CA Cancer J Clin* 2003;53:172–196.

272. Robison LL. Cancer survivorship: unique opportunities for research. *Cancer Epidemiol Biomarkers Prev* 2004;13:1093.

273. Eshelman D, Landier W, Sweeney T, et al. Facilitating care for childhood cancer survivors: integrating children's oncology group long-term follow-up guidelines and health links in clinical practice. *J Pediatr Oncol Nurs* 2004;21:271–280.

274. Deimling GT, Kahana B, Bowman KF, et al. Cancer survivorship and psychological distress in later life. *Psychooncology* 2002;11(6):479–494.

275. Yabroff KR, Lawrence WF, Clauser S, et al. Burden of illness in cancer survivors: findings from a population-based national sample. *J Natl Cancer Inst* 2004;96(17):1322–1330.

276. Earle CC, Neville BA. Under use of necessary care among cancer survivors. *Cancer* 2004;101(8):1712–1719.

277. Ferrell BR, Hassey Dow K. Quality of life among long-term cancer survivors. *Oncology (Williston Park)* 1997;11(4):565–568, 71; discussion 72, 75–6.

278. Hewitt M, Greenfield S, Stovall E, eds. *From cancer patient to cancer survivor: lost in transition.* Washington, DC: National Academies Press, 2005.

279. Hewitt M, Weiner S, Simone J, eds. *Childhood cancer survivorship: improving care and quality of life.* Washington, DC: National Academies Press, 2003.

280. Taylor A, Blacklay A, Davies H, et al. Long-term follow-up of survivors of childhood cancer in the UK. *Pediatr Blood Cancer* 2004;42(2):161–168.

281. Wallace WH, Blacklay A, Eiser C, et al. Developing strategies for long-term follow-up of survivors of childhood cancer. *BMJ* 2001;323:271–274.

CHAPTER 72 ■ PSYCHOSOCIAL ASPECTS OF CANCER SURVIVORSHIP

SUSAN A. LEIGH AND ELIZABETH J. CLARK

What happens when my body breaks down happens not just to that body but also to my life, which is lived in that body. When the body breaks down, so does the life. Even when medicine can fix the body, that doesn't always put the life back together again (1).
—Arthur Frank

Survivorship is not just about long-term survival but about quality of life from the moment of diagnosis onward. To better understand this issue from the consumer's perspective, it is helpful to understand the difference between curing and healing. The concept of cure has become a medical reality for many types of cancer; yet, the concept of healing after cancer and its treatment is a completely different story. Although curing resides within a disease-repair system and is defined biomedically, healing focuses on health and wellness and can be explained both physically and psychosocially. *Disease* is what is seen, treated, and measured and is the tangible focus for cure. *Illness* is what is felt and experienced and is a more intangible focus for healing. Lerner notes that, "Although the capacity to heal physically is necessary to any successful cure, healing can also take place on deeper levels whether or not physical recovery occurs" (2). By understanding the difference between the treatment of an external disease and the personal, lived experience of illness, physicians can more readily acknowledge and appreciate the psychosocial sequelae, which may include spiritual or existential influences, that often accompany or follow a diagnosis of cancer. This chapter will attempt to redefine the cancer experience, especially from the consumer's perspective, review psychosocial aspects of survival along an expanded continuum, and offer strategies to enhance survivorship.

CANCER MYTHS

Cancer continues to instill dread and to masquerade as a ruthless, secretive assailant. During the first half of the last century, it was believed that, "If it was not fatal, it was not cancer" (3). In *Illness as Metaphor*, Sontag (3) writes that a diagnosis of cancer will remain an automatic death sentence until its causes are known and effective treatments are discovered. Although recent advances in science and medical technology have increased the chances for survival, the often-paralyzing fear of eventual death from the disease still lingers today. This fear will obviously continue to invade our lives as long as certain types of cancer are untreatable or incurable.

Along with the myth of imminent death, cancer evokes other misunderstandings, especially concerning causation. Decades ago, many individuals theorized that cancer was caused by emotional resignation and hopelessness (3). Although attempts to identify "cancer personalities" became a popular trend in the 1970s, there were suggestions that patients unfortunate enough to be diagnosed with cancer must have done, thought, or repressed something to allow this disease to happen. Current pop psychology that often oversimplifies causation and blames the sick individual for having done something wrong may be rooted in this myth. Although the paranoia surrounding cancer is gradually diminishing, the disease continues to harbor elements of fear, stigma, shunning, discrimination, and withdrawal of support (4). Fortunately, the growth of advocacy organizations is helping to raise awareness about the new realities of life with and beyond cancer and is helping to dispel this paranoia.

When the biology of a disease is not understood, mythological speculation, and oversimplification are apt to define the sickness. Of major importance in defining cancer is that it continues to be identified as a homogeneous disease. Cancer is less often seen as many diseases with multiple causes and treatments and more frequently seen as a single entity with simple causation. Therefore, many individuals look for the "magic bullet" that will cure cancer, meaning all cancers! Also, a popular theory that stress causes cancer often overrules other causative factors, such as genetic predisposition, decreased or damaged immune competence, dangerous health habits, and environmental carcinogens. But not all myths are rooted in the individual. The health care system itself is also full of myths and misunderstandings.

HEALTH CARE MYTHS

As medical researchers and clinicians focus on extending and saving lives, patients become acutely aware of issues affecting the quality of their lives. Two current myths involved with quality of life concerns are the all-powerful role of the physician and the healing environment within our hospitals (4).

The power and control in the management of patients was historically held by doctors. In this current age of increased bureaucracy, expensive delivery of care, and cost containment, decision-making powers have shifted to financing and regulatory agencies (5). Physicians are required to spend increasing amounts of time on administrative matters, and have daily patient quotas along with time limitations spent per case. These restrictions can have a major impact on the quality of the patient/physician interaction and care. Patients also wait longer for appointments and have a more limited choice of doctors. Meanwhile, owing to the rapidly increasing population of *baby boomers*, we have seen the emergence of a new type of health care consumer. Out of necessity these consumers are more assertive in asking questions and requesting information, and are more inclined toward partnership *with* rather than paternalism *from* their providers of care. As the decision-making powers shift, this attitude can either enhance or strain the already challenged physician–patient relationship.

The second area of misunderstanding is the type of environment in which healing is fostered. The delivery of care is now complicated by diagnosis-related groups, gatekeepers, cost containment, utilization reviews, managed care, and mountains of paperwork. Although the old system allowed unlimited stays in the hospital and actually encouraged passivity and invalidism, the new system has gone to the other extreme. The so-called *healing environment* in the hospital is now hurried, understaffed, and overflowing with critically ill patients. Consequently, discharging patients from the hospital as soon as possible has become fiscally prudent, and patients return home sooner and sicker. The healing environment, then, becomes the home rather than the hospital, and greater responsibility is placed on the patient and family members or other caregivers. These changing social trends are actually forcing a shift from passive patienthood to a more proactive survivorship.

SEMANTICS OF SURVIVORSHIP

The concept of survivorship was initially introduced to the field of oncology in 1986 with the founding of the National Coalition for Cancer Survivorship. The events preceding this organizational meeting included medical advances and social trends that provoked exploration of new issues related to cancer. As new therapies became available to treat cancer, the hopes and expectations of surviving this disease were elevated. Access to information about scientific breakthroughs became readily available to the general public; awareness about cancer prevention, early detection, second opinions, and treatment options increased; many types of cancers shifted from acute to chronic diseases; and some patients were actually cured. Oncologists were finally able to rejoice, along with their patients, because not everyone would die of this feared disease. Yet, as patients and family members savored the sweetness of survival, they also realized that life would never be the same and that it would always be full of uncertainty. In *Of Dragons and Garden Peas*, wherein a patient talks to doctors, Trillin sums up this dilemma: "So, once we have recognized the limitations of the magic of doctors and medicine, where are we? We have to turn to our own magic, to our ability to 'control' our bodies" (6).

Control comes in many forms. It was not too long ago that the cancer patient's agenda was more often than not set by health care providers, especially physicians. Eventually, patients decided to take more control, either directly or indirectly, over all aspects of cancer care that affected their lives. Therefore, support groups, hotlines, resource materials, and patient networks proliferated. As the shift to recognize the consumer voice began, the concept of *survivorship* emerged.

Mullan describes survivorship as "the act of living on ... a dynamic concept with no artificial boundaries" (7). Carter further describes this theme as a process of *going through*, suggesting movement through phases (8). From these models, the concept of survivorship is viewed as a continual, ongoing process rather than a specific time frame, stage, or outcome of survival (9). Survivorship is not just about long-term survival, which is how the medical profession generally defines it. Rather, it is the experience of living with, through, or beyond cancer (10,11). From this point of view, survivorship begins at

the moment of diagnosis and continues for the remainder of life (7,10).

Although this philosophic definition of survivorship as a continual *process* is accepted by many advocates, it is not necessarily the case within the medical community. Physicians tend to define survivorship as a phase of cancer care, specifically the time right after initial treatment is completed and there is no evidence of disease. It will end if the disease recurs, if a secondary malignancy is diagnosed, or the survivor enters the phase of palliative care or dies. This difference in viewing survivorship as a stage versus a process exemplifies differences between medical or quantitative models of health care delivery and psychosocial models that are more qualitative in nature. Neither model is right or wrong. But because there is still no consensus on what survivorship actually means, it becomes imperative that the term is defined within the context it is used.

Other discrepancies in semantics revolve around who is or is not a cancer survivor. When cancer was considered incurable, the term *survivor* applied to the family members whose loved one had died of the disease. This terminology was used for years by the medical profession and insurance companies. But when potentially curative therapy became a reality, physicians selected a 5-year parameter to measure survival. Freedom from disease and biomedical longevity became the standards of success where the outcome was measurable and quantifiable.

As treatment successes improved over the years, this limited definition failed to consider patients who are not cured of their disease, require maintenance therapy, or periodically change treatment modalities, yet remain alive for more than 5 years. Others experience late recurrences, are diagnosed with second malignancies, or develop delayed effects of treatment. Even as the 5-year landmark has been modified as a parameter for describing survival, medical professionals seem inclined to categorize anyone receiving therapy or not completely free of disease as a "patient" and everyone who is not under treatment or with no evidence of disease as a "survivor."

Many individuals who have histories of cancer feel that survivorship extends far beyond the restrictions of time and treatment. Yet, while many individuals with a history of cancer love the term *survivor*, just as many abhor it. Labels such as victors, graduates, triumphers, veterans, and thrivers are now part of the survivorship lexicon. Others express a greater sense of power as activists, advocates, conquerors, and warriors. More recently, an African-American group considered survivorship a spiritual journey and asked to be called *the blessed*. Although all these labels can confuse providers and consumers alike, Gray (12) notes in *Persons With Cancer Speak Out* that, "The act of defining is an act of power." This is all about the individuals—the survivors—identifying their own issues and defining themselves rather than relying on the agendas and descriptives of the health care community (9). Again, any or all of these labels can be considered correct and simply need to be defined when clarification is needed. Therefore, the term *survivor* in this chapter reflects the National Coalition for Cancer Survivorship definition: "from the time of its discovery and for the balance of life, an individual diagnosed with cancer is a survivor" (7,10).

STAGES OF SURVIVAL

Obviously, cancer survivors have different issues, depending on their circumstances along the survival continuum. In the classic article, "Seasons of Survival: Reflections of a Physician with Cancer," Mullan (13) was the first to propose a model of survival that includes acute, extended, and permanent stages.

Acute Stage

The acute (or immediate) stage begins at the time of the diagnostic workup and continues through the initial courses of medical treatment. The survivor is commonly called a *patient* during this stage, and the primary focus is on treating the disease and physical survival. Usually, without any prior training, individuals diagnosed with cancer are required to make sophisticated medical decisions at a time of intense vulnerability, fear, and pressure. Inexperienced in navigating the complicated culture of medicine, many survivors continue to rely solely on their physicians to make treatment-related decisions. Others, though, ask for information, explanations, and more effective communication in an attempt to understand their choices.

Although supportive care services are most available at the time of diagnosis and treatment, their availability is at risk due to current cost constraints. If clinics and hospitals are unable to meet the increasing demands for supportive care at this stage, community-based models of support often fill in some of these gaps. Access to the health care team, counselors, patient support networks, resource libraries, hotlines, advocacy organizations, and family support systems helps survivors navigate this initial stage of survival. But the picture changes, sometimes dramatically, once treatment ends.

Extended Stage

If the disease responds during the initial course of therapy, the survivor moves into the extended (or intermediate) stage of survival. This stage is often described as one of watchful waiting, limbo, or remission, as survivors monitor their bodies for symptoms of disease recurrence. Uncertainty about the future prevails, as medical-based support systems are no longer readily available. Recovery entails dealing with the physical and emotional effects of treatment, and reentry into social roles is often challenged by ignorance and discrimination.

Although no longer a patient, the individual may not feel entirely healthy and may have difficulty feeling like a survivor. Ambiguity defines this stage, as survivors find themselves afloat in a mixture of joy and fear, happy to be alive and finished with treatments, yet afraid of what the future may hold.

The need for continued supportive care during this transitional stage began to receive attention in the mid-1980s as community and peer networks started augmenting or replacing institutional support (7–11). Because recovery from most types of cancer treatments entails regaining both physical and psychological stamina, rehabilitation programs might include physical and occupational therapies, exercise programs, nutrition classes, support groups, individual counseling, family therapy, or vocational training. There is no particular timetable for this type of rehabilitation or reentry to happen.

Permanent Stage

For many survivors, a certain level of trust and comfort gradually returns, and the permanent (or long-term) stage of survival just seems to happen. This is roughly equivalent to cure or sustained remission. Although most survivors experience a gradual evolution from a state of "surviving to thriving," as described by Hassey-Dow (14), others must deal with the chronic, debilitating, or delayed effects of therapy. Although many of these long-term survivors have no physical evidence of disease and appear to have fully recovered, the life-threatening experience of having survived cancer is never forgotten. The metaphor of the Damocles syndrome illustrates the apprehension or fear of living under the sword, never knowing whether or when it might drop (15,16).

For many cancer survivors, long-term follow-up tends to be as unpredictable as today's health care system. Generally, there are scant, if any, guidelines for specific follow-up, nor are there wellness-focused programs tailored to the altered health care needs of this population. One exception is pediatric oncology, which is far beyond adult oncology in the systematic follow-up of long-term survivors. Standardized assessments in specialized clinics help identify problems, such as disease recurrence, second malignancies, or late effects of treatment, and interventions can be initiated as soon as possible.

Adults, on the other hand, often feel burdened by a "glorification of recovery" (17), whereby they are praised for overcoming adversity and encouraged to minimize their complaints. The appearance of health can actually hamper the identification of real problems, as no one wants to believe that something might still be wrong (17,18). But symptoms of distress, both biomedical and psychosocial, must be taken seriously. And, in this age of cost containment and managed care, survivors need continued access to appropriate specialists who understand the consequences of survival and can treat accordingly.

As the population of cancer survivors increases, attention to survival issues are finally receiving much-needed attention. Yet, even if the disease is eradicated, the psychosocial sequelae of surviving a life-threatening experience must be recognized as barriers to a full recovery. Although the National Comprehensive Cancer Network (NCCN) has a number of current guidelines available on its website (www.NCCN.org), there is little information that focuses specifically on long-term survival. Yet it is does list topics under the supportive care heading that deal with quality of life and can be considered survivorship-related.

Following the development of the NCCN guidelines and recent reports focusing on adult survivorship issues, the American Society of Clinical Oncology (ASCO) created a new Survivorship Task Force. Under this initiative, it also convened an expert panel in January 2005, to begin the process of developing clinical practice guidelines for the long-term care of adult cancer survivors. As these guidelines are to be evidence-based, this is simply the beginning of a lengthy and time-consuming process as little systematic follow-up has occurred in this population. But it is a "beginning" that will encourage physicians to begin serious work identifying topics such as late physiologic effects of disease and treatment, secondary malignancies, and psychological and social fallout surrounding survival.

PSYCHOSOCIAL ASPECTS

How well an individual adapts psychologically and socially to living with cancer depends on a wide variety of factors. First are the physical factors, including the age and sex of the individual, the type and stage of disease, the kinds and duration of recommended treatments, the outcomes of treatment, disease progression, and residual side effects. Added to these are permanent disabilities, physical limitations, and possible disfigurement and altered body image. Next are the psychological variables. Where is the individual in life-stage development? What previous experiences has the individual had with illness in general and with cancer in particular? What individual psychological strengths and weaknesses are brought to the cancer experience? What kinds of coping mechanisms usually are employed by the individual in crisis situations? Does the individual have a history of emotional problems such as depression, anxiety, or other mental health concerns? Self esteem, independence and motivation, as well as interactional skills, also play a part.

When aspects of social functioning are added to the equation, many other variables need to be considered. These include the sociodemographic factors such as marital status, race, ethnicity, religious orientation, educational level, employment history, and financial stability. Next are the social roles ascribed to the individual such as spouse, partner, parent, employee, and friend. In addition to the sociodemographic variables, other social factors include the type of social support available to the individual. What kinds of changes will a history of cancer bring for the individual and the family? Will the individual be able to fulfill existing job requirements, or will joblessness or employment discrimination become a factor? Despite this wide range of individual variability, there are numerous shared experiences that occur along the continuum of cancer survivorship. Also shared are the most common problems and needs faced by individuals with cancer.

Needs of Cancer Survivors

At last, the needs of cancer survivors have caught the attention of the oncology community and governmental agencies. Although a myriad of oncology researchers and clinicians have identified survivor needs over the past 20 years, recognition of this special population has recently become a focus of multiple agencies dedicated to national health. Examples of these recent reports include:

- 2001 *Voices of a Broken System: Real People, Real Problems.* A report published by the National Cancer Institute (NCI) summarizing information gathered from the President's Cancer Panel (PCP). It focuses on the delivery of care in our health care system; who is served and not served; barriers to access and delivery of quality cancer care; and the impacts on minorities and the underserved (19).
- 2003 *Childhood Cancer Survivorship: Improving Care and Quality of Life.* A report by the Institute of Medicine (IOM), National Research Council of the National Academies. This extensive report, solicited by the National Cancer Advisory Board (NCAB), recommends developing guidelines for follow-up care of childhood cancer survivors; developing standards for comprehensive systems to deliver survivorship care; raising awareness of late effects; improving professional education and training in the area of long-term survival; and increasing research in this area (20).
- 2003 *Living Beyond Cancer: Finding a New Balance.* This is another PCP report from NCI and differentiates survivor issues across the lifespan. As with all other PCP reports, this one too goes directly to the President. It includes long-term health issues and follow-up care, legal and regulatory protections, problems with privacy and insurance portability provisions, access to education and information, availability of psychosocial and supportive care needs, health insurance, and surveillance and research (21).
- 2004 *A National Action Plan for Cancer Survivorship: Advancing Public Health Strategies.* This report is jointly sponsored by the Centers for Disease Control (CDC) and the Lance Armstrong Foundation (LAF) and identifies cancer survivorship as a new challenge to public health. Owing to increasing numbers of individuals surviving cancer and living with lingering or delayed effects of the disease or treatment, it becomes imperative to assist in preventing and controlling existing or potential health problems. The proposed National Action Plan will hopefully be used as a guide to help decrease the burden of cancer, improve the quality of life of all Americans affected by this disease, and increase funding for survivorship research and delivery of culturally appropriate care (22).
- 2005 Published in November 2005 is the much anticipated report from the IOM entitled *Cancer Survivorship: Charting the Course to Improve Care and Quality of Life.* This report will focus on adult survivors just as the 2003 IOM report focused on pediatrics.

Multiple categories of unmet needs are identified within this assortment of reports. Collectively they encompass different combinations of categories that include physical, psychological, social, spiritual, economic, financial, legal, vocational, and cultural needs.

One of the most utilized and replicated models to categorize dimensions of quality of life in long-term cancer survivors is one by Ferrell et al. entitled Quality of Life Model Applied to Cancer Survivors. It is now available on-line through the City of Hope website (23). This model incorporates four domains that apply to cancer survivors, and includes physical, social, psychological, and spiritual well-being. Multiple topics are included under each domain. For example, economic, vocational, and financial needs would all fall under the social domain.

Earlier work that utilized a Quality of Life–Cancer Survivors Tool found that the psychological well-being subscale had the lowest score. The authors conclude that although distress related to the cancer experience abates over time, the psychological impact of the distress lingers (24).

Addressing the wide variety of psychosocial needs and concerns of patients with cancer mentioned in the preceding text is beyond the scope of this chapter. However, several salient themes have been selected to receive expanded coverage and to indicate some psychosocial sequelae that perhaps are specific to the cancer experience.

Normlessness (Lack of Societal Norms) of the Cancer Experience

Many of the psychological problems associated with cancer are related to a lack of knowledge and requisite skills needed for negotiating the cancer experience. Cancer survivors experience a sequence of crises for which habitual problem-solving activities are not adequate and that do not lead to the previously achieved balanced state (25). Therefore, cancer may be a normless or anomic situation for a significant number of individuals.

Anomia can be defined as "a temporary state of mind occasioned by a sudden alteration in one's life situation, and characterized by confusion and anxiety, uncertainty, loss of purpose, and a sense of separateness from one's usual social support system" (26). Individuals newly diagnosed with cancer may not know how to think or talk about their situation. They need information, but because of the shock and unfamiliarity of the situation, they may be unable to understand the broad significance or assimilate what information they do receive.

Added to this is the stigma that accompanies a cancer diagnosis. Despite treatment advances and extended survival rates for various cancers, cancer remains a stigmatized disease, and individuals with cancer must contend with the consequent societal attitudes, prejudices, and discrimination (1,3).

Eventually, most individuals with cancer become experts about their own illness and treatment. They know more or less what to expect medically, and they learn how best to navigate the health care system. They develop the requisite language and needed coping skills to manage the crisis periods. They often interact with other patients with cancer, perhaps by attending support groups or online chat rooms, or they seek extra care from their health care team and counselors. These interactions may help survivors see that while the disease of cancer is a personal experience, there are numerous commonalities among individuals regarding the illness process and its consequences. In short, they learn how to live with cancer. There may be recurrent crisis situations, both physical and psychosocial, but gradually the normlessness first experienced after the cancer diagnosis subsides, and life takes on a somewhat normal, a "new normal," cadence that incorporates the physical, emotional, and spiritual changes catalyzed by the cancer experience (25).

Problems with Reentry

For many patients, active cancer therapy eventually ends, but the successful end of cancer treatment does not necessarily signal an end to the difficulties and stresses faced by individuals with cancer and their family members. The period of waiting to see whether the treatment abated the disease process, and worry about not receiving any active intervention, may create new anxiety and fear (27). The survivor enters what Hurt et al. (28) refer to as "neutral time": a period of remission characterized by uncertainty and lacking in "safety signals" indicating that the disease will not return. At this time, some individuals face an illness-related identity crisis. They may no longer be perceived as cancer "patients" because they are not in active treatment, yet they may have difficulty thinking about themselves as cancer "survivors" or achieving reentry into a "well-role" (11). Another anomic situation, what Maher (26) refers to as "the anomia of good fortune," may occur.

When the concept of anomia is applied to cancer recovery, the positive experience of doing well, perhaps even of being cured, may be mixed with negative elements. These elements might include the following:

1. The withdrawal of the intensified social support that accompanied diagnosis and treatment
2. Ambivalence about the discontinuation of treatment
3. Anxiety about recurrence of disease
4. Adjustment to permanent disabilities resulting from the disease or its treatment
5. The need to resume life-oriented modes of thought after a successful adjustment to the idea of death
6. Anger at perceived inadequacies or
7. Confusion about feelings of depression when the objective situation has improved (26)

Reentry also entails problems with assuming previous roles and responsibilities, and with readjustment and readaptation to daily life (25). The stress of a diagnosis of cancer and its subsequent treatment disrupts the patterns of a lifetime and requires adaptation to personal and interpersonal changes. While active treatment is ongoing, family members frequently assume some of the instrumental, and even emotional, duties of the individual with cancer. This redistribution of tasks can have a marked impact on the family unit. When cancer treatment ends, interpersonal relationships may be further strained because the new patterns of interaction and functionality need to be negotiated once again. Another area of reentry that may be of concern for some cancer survivors is rejoining the workforce. Most individuals with cancer remain actively employed during the treatment phase, but some experience brief or extended absences from work. Returning to work can entail various psychological stresses. There may be a difference in the way the employee is treated by others. Some coworkers may still believe that cancer carries an automatic death sentence and may stigmatize and isolate the returning employee. There may be changes in physical appearance, such as permanent disfigurement from cancer surgery, or temporary changes in appearance, such as hair loss, that initially make the cancer survivor feel insecure and awkward. An added concern may be reduced physical stamina, which makes it difficult to meet the previous work demands and can have an impact on relationships with coworkers.

Employment Discrimination

Of paramount importance to most survivors is financial stability and the opportunity to retain their jobs during or after therapy. Yet, many who are able and willing to work encounter discrimination by being dismissed or demoted, by having benefits reduced or eliminated, or by experiencing conflict with coworkers because of a lack of understanding, ignorance, or fear about cancer (29,30). Hoffman (30) reports that approximately 7% (or 1 in 7) survivors report being fired because of their cancer experience, and that survivors are laid off five times more often than other workers. Health care professionals, as well as cancer survivors, must take action on three levels to combat cancer-based discrimination: individual and group advocacy, public and professional education, and appropriate use of legal remedies (30).

Advocates hoped for legal protection against employment discrimination for qualified survivors with the passage of the Americans With Disabilities Act, but this has recently been challenged in court. Also, the Federal Rehabilitation Act of 1973 affords limited protection to those survivors whose employers receive federal funds. Most states have laws against discrimination in general, while a few states protect cancer survivors specifically. A major challenge is to test the system and file suit when discrimination is suspected.

Living with Uncertainty

Reentry may require some compromises on both the personal and the interpersonal levels. The cancer survivor may have to learn to live with physical compromises related to the disease or to the effects of the cancer therapy. Adverse late effects of treatment may not appear for years after the completion of therapy, and the individual with a history of cancer has to live with an awareness of the vulnerability associated with delayed treatment effects, recurrence of disease, or susceptibility to a second cancer. Family members also must live with these fears, and their overprotectiveness may be an issue after the completion of treatment. Even when there are no obvious physical limitations, many survivors and their loved ones continue to be concerned about the survivors' activity level, and the general consensus has been "to take it easy." For most survivors, a lack of exercise most likely does more harm than good. Researchers are now finding that exercise helps to decrease the fatigue and depression that is often associated with cancer and its treatment (31). While reports show that moderate exercise can help survivors by decreasing muscle atrophy, maintaining heart and lung function, and preserving strength and endurance, translation of this information into practical programs is now available (31).

Maintaining a Positive Future Orientation

For a while after a cancer diagnosis, the future is foreshortened, reduced to the span of time between treatments or between episodes of active disease (26), and frustration and disappointment may occur as a result of the nonlinear quality of healing (7). Cancer in the family can have a profound negative impact, and yet hopefulness and a positive future orientation are important components for quality of life in cancer survivorship. Hope is a complex concept and often is misunderstood by health care professionals. Much of the reason for this confusion is that health care professionals generally think only in terms of therapeutic hope—that is, hope that refers to a cure or remission of disease (32). Many other kinds of hope, generalized and particular, are described in the literature (33).

Hope constitutes an essential experience of the human condition. It functions as a way of feeling, a way of thinking, a way of behaving, and a way of relating to oneself and one's world (34). Hope has the ability to be fluid in its expectations, and in the event that the desired object or outcome does not occur, hope can still be present (32). It is also a cognitive-affective resource that is a psychological asset. The purpose of hope is to guard against despair, and, as a coping strategy, it can reduce ongoing stress and discomfort quickly and for prolonged periods.

Hope is individualistic, and individuals have various capacities for hoping and different approaches for maintaining hope. Individual hope is generally influenced by the patterns of hoping within the family (33,34).

There is a temporal aspect to hope that involves a consideration of the future, and hope changes as situations and circumstances change. Even when hope for survival is dim, individuals will find other things to hope for: pain control, mending strained relationships, or even a dignified death. Disconfirmation of one's hope usually leads to a reformulation of hope, not to its destruction.

Cancer survivors need and desire accurate and honest information about their disease, its treatment, and the potential side effects. They need to be aware of problems that they may have to face in the future. If these issues and concerns are presented with compassion and with assurance for continuing support, they can accept even bad news, and new, more realistic goals can be assimilated into the hoping process.

Cancer survivors are challenged to find ways to cope with uncertainty and with maintaining a positive future orientation. The fear of recurrence of cancer and heightened vulnerability may diminish over time, but the consensus is that it never completely goes away (35).

Survivor Guilt

One additional, related aspect of long-term cancer survival deserves special mention. Numerous long-term survivors express guilt over the fact that they have survived when many others have not (36). This may be a particularly salient issue for individuals who have been well integrated into a support group and who have watched other members of that group succumb to their disease.

Arthur Frank, in his book *At the Will of the Body*, gives an excellent example of the concept of survivor guilt: "At the same time I was diagnosed as having cancer, a good friend my age also was diagnosed, and my mother-in-law came out of remission again. They both have died. I can make no sense of their deaths and my survival" (1).

Many survivors search for meaning and purpose in their survival and make a renewed commitment to life (37). They also may decide to try to "give something back" in practical and tangible ways. This often includes advocacy efforts on behalf of other survivors.

Living with Loss

Nothing ever prepares us for the really bad things in life, and loss is an encompassing life theme. Losses are a part of life—we lose loved ones, we lose jobs, we lose chances, and we lose dreams. There are many necessary losses when one has cancer. Some of these losses, such as hair loss and loss of fertility, are physical, but emotional losses are associated with cancer as well. For example, cancer survivors may have to learn to live with some limitations, and they may have to alter goals, expectations, and hopes to fit the current, after-cancer reality.

Every loss requires a concomitant grief response or some type of mourning, but American society is uncomfortable with grief. Therefore, individuals tend to hide their feelings and emotions. A secondary factor is that the individual who appears to be coping well relieves others of the burden of support, so hidden grief is reinforced.

Grief, however, cannot be postponed indefinitely. It must reach expression in some way, and hidden grief may be transformed into a variety of emotional responses such as anger, guilt, anxiety, helplessness, or sadness.

The literature on the tasks of mourning is well developed (38,39). These tasks can be summarized as the following:

1. Accepting the reality of the loss
2. Experiencing the pain of the grief
3. Adjusting to a changed environment and
4. Emotionally relocating the loss in one's life and moving on

Perhaps the most important way of helping individuals experiencing loss is to "enfranchise" their grief (40). This includes recognizing their right to express emotions and encouraging them to verbalize their feelings and sadness. A basic step in helping individuals live with loss is educating them about the grief process and encouraging them to openly discuss loss issues. Through expression can come emotional healing.

REDEFINING THE CANCER EXPERIENCE

With an increasing sense of empowerment, survivors are redefining the cancer experience for themselves. They are requesting—and sometimes demanding—that nonmedical supportive services be an integral part of cancer care and recovery. Many are working on their own to provide support, resources, and education for fellow survivors, while others are working in conjunction with health care institutions and communities to provide these services. Survivors are joining support groups, producing publications, staffing telephone hotlines, and sharing information through Internet services. Others are developing community-based educational and mutual aid networks, are testifying before Congress, and are forming national organizations and coalitions. Advocacy—on personal, community, national, and public policy levels—has become a major component of the cancer care equation and is increasingly important to assure access to quality cancer care.

The Cancer Survivor's Bill of Rights (see Appendix) is one of the earliest examples of a consumer commentary documenting quality of life issues from a nonmedical perspective. Survivors themselves identify individual, interpersonal, and social rights to greater care and satisfaction throughout the cancer experience.

FINDING MEANING

Weil (41) suggests that there is no meaning to cancer—it is simply cancer. The meaning attached to the experience is different for everyone and reflects individual interpretations of the disease, treatments, and circumstances. While formulas or guidelines are needed to improve the continuity of quality cancer care, they are not enough to assess and care for individuals who are distressed and suffering. Ferrell fears that the concept of quality of life is an endangered species in today's medical and political climate and "may be lost during health care reform and amidst what [she has] termed the 'dehumanization' of cancer" (42). Therefore, the increasing needs, both biomedical and psychosocial, of this burgeoning population of survivors call for cooperative efforts among the recipients and providers of care, the payors who finance care, the scientists who develop better methods of care, and the politicians who set public policy as to what kind of care will be available and to whom. To ensure the integrity of our health care system, the mythology of cancer must be dispelled, caring must expand into long-term survival, and attention must be paid to the psychosocial aspects of living with, through, and beyond cancer.

References

1. Frank AW. *At the will of the body*, Vol. 8 Boston, MA: Houghton Mifflin, 1991:137.
2. Lerner M. *Choices in healing*. Cambridge, MA: MIT Press, 1994:14.
3. Sontag S. *Illness as metaphor and AIDS and its metaphors*. New York: Anchor, 1988:19.
4. Leigh S. Myths, monsters, and magic: personal perspectives and professional challenges of survival. *Oncol Nurs Forum* 1992;19:1475.
5. Anderson JG. The deprofessionalization of American medicine. In: Miller G, ed. *Current research on occupations and professions*, Vol. 7 Greenwich, CT: JAI Press, 1992;241.
6. Trillin AS. Of dragons and garden peas. *N Engl J Med* 1981;304:699–700.
7. Mullan F. Survivorship: an idea for everyone. In: Mullan F, Hoffman B, eds. *Charting the journey: an almanac of practical resources for cancer survivors*. Mount Vernon, NY: Consumers Union, 1990:1.
8. Carter B. Going through: a critical theme in surviving breast cancer. *Innov Oncol Nurs* 1989;5:2.
9. Leigh S. Cancer survivorship: a consumer movement. *Semin Oncol* 1994; 21:783.
10. Leigh S. Defining our destiny. In: Hoffman B, ed. *A cancer survivor's almanac: charting your journey*. Hoboken, NJ: John Wiley and Sons, 2004: 292–300.
11. Welch-McCaffrey D, Loescher LJ, Leigh SA, et al. Surviving adult cancer. Part 2: psychosocial implications. *Ann Intern Med* 1989;3:517.
12. Gray RE. Persons with cancer speak out: reflections on an important trend in Canadian health care. *J Palliat Care* 1992;8:30.
13. Mullan F. Seasons of survival: reflections of a physician with cancer. *N Engl J Med* 1985;313:270.
14. Hassey-Dow K. The enduring seasons in survival. *Oncol Nurs Forum* 1990;17:511.
15. Koocher G, O'Malley J, eds. *The damocles syndrome: psychosocial consequences of surviving childhood cancer*. New York: McGraw Hill, 1981.
16. Smith D, Lesko LM. Psychosocial problems in cancer survivors. *Oncology* 1988;2:33.
17. Siegal K, Christ GH. Hodgkins disease survivorship: psychosocial consequences. In: Lacher MJ, Redman JR, eds. *Hodgkins disease: consequences of survival*. Philadelphia, PA: Lea & Febiger, 1990:383.
18. Smith DW. *Survival of illness*. New York: Springer-Verlag, 1981.
19. National Cancer Institute (NCI). *Voices of a broken system: real people, real problems*. NIH Publication No. 03–5301: Available at http://pcp.cancer.gov; 2002.
20. Institute of Medicine (IOM). *Childhood cancer survivorship :improving care and quality of life*. Washington, DC: National Academies Press; 2003.
21. National Cancer Institute (NCI). *Living beyond cancer: finding a new balance*. Available at http://pcp.cancer.gov; 2004.
22. Centers for Disease Control and Prevention (CDC) and the Lance Armstrong Foundation (LAF). *A National Action Plan for Cancer Survivorship: Advancing Public Health Strategies*. Available at http://www.cdc.gov/cancer; 2004.
23. City of Hope Beckman Research Institute. *Quality of Life*. Available at http://www.cityofhope.org/prc/pain_qual_life.asp; 2005.
24. Ferrell BR, Dow KH, Leigh S. Quality of life in long-term cancer survivors. *Oncol Nurs Forum* 1995;22:915.
25. Clark E. Family challenges: communication and teamwork. In: Hoffman B, ed. *A cancer survivor's almanac: charting your journey*. Hoboken, NJ: John Wiley and Sons, 2004:133–146.
26. Maher EL. Anomic aspects of recovery from cancer. *Soc Sci Med* 1982; 16:907–911.
27. Tross S, Holland JC. Psychological sequelae in cancer survivors. In: Holland JC, Rowland JH, eds. *Handbook of psychooncology*. New York: Oxford University Press, 1990:101.
28. Hurt GJ, McQuellon RP, Darrett RJ. After treatment ends. *Cancer Pract* 1994;2:417.
29. Leigh S, Welch-McCaffrey D, Loescher LJ, et al. Psychosocial issues of long-term survival from adult cancer. In: Groenwald SL, Frogge MH, Goodman M, et al. eds. *Cancer nursing: principles and practice*, 3rd ed. Boston, MA: Jones and Bartlett, 1993:484.
30. Hoffman B. Working it out: your employment rights. In: Hoffman B, ed. *A cancer survivor's almanac: charting your journey*. Hoboken, NJ: John Wiley and Sons, 2004:241–269.
31. Schwartz AL. *Cancer fitness: exercise programs for patients and survivors*. New York: Simon & Schuster, 2004.
32. Clark E. *You have the right to be hopeful*. Silver Spring, MD: National Coalition for Cancer Survivorship, 2003.
33. Groopman JE. *The anatomy of hope: how people prevail in the face of illness*. New York: Random House, 2004.
34. Clark EJ. Confronting the end of life. In: Hoffman B, ed. *A cancer survivor's almanac: charting your journey*. Hoboken, NJ: John Wiley and Sons, 2004:191–200.
35. Wells NL, Turney ME. Common issues facing adults with cancer. In: Lauria MM, Clark EJ, Herman JF, Stearns NM, eds. *Social work in oncology: supporting survivors, families, and caregivers*. Atlanta, GA: American Cancer Society, 2001:38.
36. Shanfield SB. On surviving cancer: psychological considerations. *Compr Psychol* 1980;21(2):128.
37. Maxwell T, Aldredge-Clanton J. Survivor guilt in cancer patients: a pastoral perspective. *J Pastoral Care* 1994;48(1):25.
38. Hedlund SC, Clark EF. End of life issues. In: Lauria MM, Clark EJ, Hermann JF, Stearns NM, eds. *Social work in oncology: supporting survivors, families, and caregivers*. Atlanta, GA: American Cancer Society, 2001.
39. Worden JW. *Grief counseling and grief therapy: a handbook for the mental health practitioner*, 3rd ed. New York: Springer Publishing Co, 2001.
40. Doka KJ. *Disenfranchised grief: recognizing hidden sorrow*. New York: Lexington Books, 1989.
41. Weil A. *Health and healing*. Boston, MA: Houghton Mifflin, 1988.
42. Ferrell BR. To know suffering. *Oncol Nurs Forum* 1993;20:1471.

APPENDIX

Cancer Survivors' Bill of Rights

The American Cancer Society presents this Survivors' Bill of Rights to call public attention to survivor needs, to enhance cancer care, and to bring greater satisfaction to cancer survivors, as well as to their physicians, employers, families, and friends:

1. Survivors have the right to assurance of lifelong medical care, as needed. The physicians and other professionals involved in their care should continue their constant efforts to be
   - sensitive to the cancer survivors' lifestyle choices and their need for self-esteem and dignity;
   - careful, no matter how long they have survived, to have symptoms taken seriously, and not have aches and pains dismissed, for fear of recurrence is a normal part of survivorship;
   - informative and open, providing survivors with as much or as little candid medical information as they wish, and encouraging their informed participation in their own care;
   - knowledgeable about counseling resources, and willing to refer survivors and their families as appropriate for emotional support and therapy which will improve the quality of individual lives.

2. In their personal lives, survivors, such as other Americans, have the right to the pursuit of happiness. This means they have the right:
   - to talk with their families and friends about their cancer experience if they wish, but to refuse to discuss it, if that is their choice and not to be expected to be more upbeat or less blue than anyone else;
   - to be free of the stigma of cancer as a "dread disease" in all social relations;

   - to be free of blame for having gotten the disease and of guilt for having survived it.

3. In the workplace, survivors have the right to equal job opportunities. This means they have the right:
   - to aspire to jobs worthy of their skills, and for which they are trained and experienced, and, therefore, not to have to accept jobs they would not have considered before the cancer experience;
   - to be hired, promoted, and accepted on return to work, according to their individual abilities and qualifications, and not according to "cancer" or "disability" stereotypes;
   - to privacy about their medical histories.

4. Because health insurance coverage is an overriding survivorship concern, every effort should be made to assure all survivors adequate health insurance, whether public or private. This means:
   - for employers, that survivors have the right to be included in group health coverage, which is usually less expensive, provides better benefits, and covers the employee regardless of health history;
   - for physicians, counselors, and other professionals concerned, that they keep themselves and their survivor-clients informed and up-to-date on available group or individual health policy options, noting, for example, what major expenses, such as hospital costs and medical tests outside the hospital are covered and what amount must be paid before coverage (deductibles);
   - for social policy makers, both in government and in the private sector, that they seek to broaden insurance programs, such as Medicare to include diagnostic procedures and treatment which help prevent recurrence and ease survivor anxiety and pain.

Adapted from Spingarn ND. *The cancer survivors' bill of rights*. Atlanta, GA: American Cancer Society, 1988, with permission.

CHAPTER 73 ■ PALLIATIVE CARE IN PEDIATRICS

JAVIER R. KANE AND BRUCE P. HIMELSTEIN

Palliative medicine for children is the art and science of family centered care aimed at enhancing quality of life and minimizing suffering. Inherent in this definition is the possibility of delivering palliative care in partnership with curative care for children with life-limiting illness or for children who may not die. Many principles already reviewed in other sections of this book are universally applicable across the age spectrum of the dying, so this chapter provides an overview of issues specific to the care of the life-threatened child.

Each year in the United States, approximately 50,000 children die, compared with approximately 2.3 million adults. National Vital Statistics for 2003, the last year published to date, demonstrate that accidents remain the number one cause of death in the age 1–19 child (1). The second leading cause of death for children for ages 1–4 is congenital malformations, deformations, and chromosomal abnormalities; ages 5–14 is malignancy; and for ages 15–19 is homicide. For infants, the leading causes of death are congenital malformations, deformations, and chromosomal abnormalities, disorders related to short gestation and low birth weight, sudden infant death syndrome, and newborns affected by maternal complications of pregnancy such as uterine rupture. Hundreds of thousands more children are living with life-threatening conditions. Goldman et al. estimated that 50/100,000 children were living with life-threatening illness (2). Feudtner et al. have done extensive research characterizing the epidemiology of childhood death (3). They have defined a group of complex chronic conditions (CCCs) "that can be reasonably expected to last at least 12 months (unless death intervenes) and to involve either several different organ systems or one organ system severely enough to require specialty pediatric care and probably some period of hospitalization in a tertiary care center." National data demonstrated that of 1.75 million deaths occurring in the 0–24-year old population from 1979 to 1997, 5% were attributable to cancer CCCs, 16% to non–cancer CCCs, 43% to injuries, and 37% to all other death causes. Non–cancer CCCs accounted for approximately 25% of infant deaths, 20% of childhood deaths, and 7% of adolescent deaths. Death rates from CCCs are declining slowly. Feudtner estimates that each year approximately 15,000 infants, children, adolescents, young adults might benefit from supportive care services delivered both at home and in the hospital, and that on any given day, approximately 5000 are living in the last 6 months of their lives, many of whom die in hospitals after prolonged periods of inpatient care and artificial life-sustaining therapies (4,5).

The diseases of childhood which might be appropriate for palliative care might include:

1. Conditions for which curative or life prolonging treatment is possible but may fail, such as advanced or progressive malignancy or malignancy with a poor prognosis, or complex and severe congenital or acquired heart disease;
2. Conditions requiring long periods of intensive treatment aimed at prolonging quality of life such as human immunodeficiency virus (HIV), cystic fibrosis, severe gastrointestinal disorders or malformations such as gastroschisis, severe epidermolysis bullosa, severe immunodeficiencies, renal failure when dialysis and/or transplantation are not available or indicated, chronic or severe respiratory failure, or muscular dystrophy;
3. Progressive conditions in which treatment is exclusively palliative from diagnosis such as mucopolysaccharidoses or other storage disorders, progressive metabolic disorders, certain chromosomal abnormalities such as Trisomy 13 or Trisomy 18, or severe forms of osteogenesis imperfecta; and
4. Conditions with severe, non-progressive disability, causing extreme vulnerability to health complications such as severe cerebral palsy with recurrent infection or difficult symptoms, extreme prematurity, severe neurologic sequelae of infectious disease, hypoxic/anoxic brain injury, or holoprosencephaly or other severe brain malformations. Given the uncertainty of prognosis, many children with these conditions will not fit eligibility criteria for hospice care in the United States (6).

EPIDEMIOLOGY OF SUFFERING

Despite best efforts, children living with chronic, life-threatening, and terminal illnesses experience substantial suffering. This experience of serious disease is multidimensional. It has broad-ranging implications in the child's life as a whole and in the family as a functional unit. Suffering results from a threat to one's physical and psychological self, from a threat to one's relationships with others, and from a threat to one's relationship with a transcendent source of meaning (7). Suffering is a profoundly personal experience and is endurable, and at times even fulfilling, when it becomes meaningful (8). Serious illness threatens children's sense of personal integrity and shatters all aspects of their lives. Physical pain and other symptoms cause fear, depression, and isolation. Illness affects their daily activities, sense of well-being, physical strength and agility, and the motives and quality of their relationships. Disease crushes their sense of security, and brings fears of the unknown, rejection, and punishment. Children also become confused by the experience of a mixed variety of emotions of anger, anxiety, sadness, loneliness, and isolation in the presence of a threatening situation (9). Children are highly vulnerable to the stress inherent to the experience of severe illness. They have an egocentric view of the world and lack a fully developed repertoire of coping mechanisms, such as problem solving or decision making, which are influenced by age-dependent behavior and cognitive abilities.

Within the physical realm, the published experience speaks best to those with malignant diseases. Recent studies by Wolfe (10) and Collins et al. (11,12) point to the wide variety and high prevalence of symptoms from which children with life-threatening illness suffer. There appears to be significant discrepancies between the reports of parents and physicians regarding the children's symptoms in the last month of life, with parents reporting each symptom more than the physicians. Furthermore, currently available treatments may not be successful in easing suffering associated with these symptoms that can cause significant distress. For children with nonmalignant diseases, some of the more troublesome symptoms might include gastroesophageal reflux, neuroirritability, immobility, incontinence, seizures, muscle spasms, pressure ulcers, contractures, recurrent infections, increased secretions, restlessness, sleep disturbance, and edema. There are few valid and reliable tools available to assess these symptoms and little data to substantiate the use of many of the interventions currently prescribed.

Suffering, for the parents of a child with a life-threatening illness, can also be a multidimensional experience of pain, fear, failure, despair, powerlessness, hopelessness, purposelessness, and vulnerability. Parental anxiety is due in part to the changing parent-child structure, the need to understand the illness experience, become familiar with the hospital environment, adapt to the changing relationships with their child and other family members, and negotiate with professionals about their care (13,14). Parents must also deal not only with the immediate threat of disease on their child's life, but also with important additional family stressors during treatment such as lifestyle changes, marital tension, financial strain, loss of self-esteem, and even loss of sleep (15). Furthermore, when confronted with the suffering and possible death of their child, parents frequently recognize their own limitations and mortality. Their perception of life, death, and the world around them is changed dramatically by the reality of the loss of their child. In addition, parents must also satisfy the emotional needs of other children in the family which many times parallel those of the seriously ill child (16). Finally, children and their families may also suffer spiritually. This may be manifested as a sense of isolation and abandonment, a sense of hopelessness and uncertainty about the meaning and ultimate purpose of life.

The American Academy of Pediatrics supports an integrated model of palliative care in which the components of palliative care are offered at diagnosis and continued throughout the course of illness, whether the outcome ends in cure or death (17). Basic principles of pediatric palliative care include the following:

1. Care is child-focused, family oriented and relationship-centered
2. Care focuses on relief of suffering and enhancing quality of life for the child and family
3. All children suffering from chronic, life-threatening and terminal illnesses are eligible
4. Care is provided for the child as a unique individual and the family as a functional unit
5. Palliative care is incorporated into the mainstream of medical care regardless of the curative intent of therapy
6. Care is not directed at shortening life
7. Care is coordinated across all sites of care delivery

8. Care is goal directed and is consistent with the beliefs and values of the child and his or her caregivers
9. An interdisciplinary team is always available to families to provide continuity
10. Advocacy for participation of the child and caregivers in decision making is paramount
11. Facilitation and documentation of communication are critical tasks of the team
12. Respite care and support are essential for families and caregivers
13. Bereavement care should be provided for as long as needed
14. "Do Not Resuscitate" orders should not be required and
15. Prognosis for short-term survival is not required

These essentials do not mandate a particular structure for care delivery other than to suggest the function of an interdisciplinary team of health care and allied health care professionals to provide care coordination and to facilitate the delivery of services with the goal to minimize suffering and improve quality of life.

ADVANCED CARE COORDINATION

Much of the fragmentation of services that occurs in modern health care systems results from the lack of a coordinating entity. The loss of continuity may be addressed by providing a medical home for these children along with the services of an advanced-illness care coordinator. This may be a registered nurse whose primary responsibilities are to enhance communication across settings, facilitate the participation of the patient and family in the decision-making process, ensure that health care providers adhere to the goals and principles of palliative care, and honor the patient and family's wishes. The coordinator may also be responsible for ensuring access to proper management of pain, and psychosocial and spiritual support. The advanced-illness care coordinator may advocate for change in the nature of the palliative care interventions according to the stage of disease and the patient and family's expectations, values, and beliefs. In our experience, provision of a trained advanced-illness care coordinator to facilitate end-of-life communication also increases utilization of and length of stay in end-of-life services and completion of advance directives. The roles provided by a physician advocate and the integration of services facilitated by the advanced care coordinator are essential for maintaining a patient-focused, relationship-centered approach and promotion of palliative care goals (18).

ETHICAL ISSUES

Shared decision making in pediatrics, driven by communication between child, parent, and physician, defines the standard in medical ethics. Clinicians must establish an effective process to ensure that all treatment decisions are made in the best interest of the child. Understanding the illness experience from the perspective of the child and family, establishing accurate prognosis and communicating it effectively, setting reasonable goals and establishing a comprehensive advanced-illness care plan are indispensable steps in this process. Judgments that relate to withholding and/or withdrawing certain therapies, as well as judgments concerning medically inappropriate interventions, are essentially subjective but realistically indispensable (19). There is marked variability among physicians regarding the use of artificial life support, but in general, these decisions must be goal directed and in consonance with the child's and family's beliefs and values (20).

Withholding and withdrawing artificial life-sustaining interventions in children, particularly medically provided artificial hydration and nutrition, is often controversial. However, in patients with no hope of regaining some potentiality for function, clinicians may find insufficient justification for continued treatment if the burden of therapy is greater than the benefits to the patient and family (21,22). Discontinuation of nonbeneficial interventions is squarely within the scope of parental decision-making authority for their child and is not inconsistent with the child's best interests. Although children are allowed to assent rather than to consent to plans regarding their care, parents and health care providers must recognize the subjective personal nature of suffering and respect the child's autonomy and capacity to make decisions, particularly for emancipated and mature minors (23). Whenever possible, caregivers must make an effort to invite children to participate in medical decision making and honor their end-of-life care wishes. This is particularly important for any child, regardless of age, who can understand his or her medical condition, who can communicate his or her preferences, and who is able to reach a reasonable decision and can understand its consequences (24). In addition, the principles that guide the rule of double effect and sedation of highly symptomatic patients with pain or dyspnea in adults also apply in the care of children (25). In difficult cases, institutional ethics committees can help resolve conflicts about treatment decisions, provide a forum for discussion of hospital policies, and educate the health care community about ethical concepts (26). Of note, although some alternative medicine practices in the care of seriously ill children may be justified; there are no published guidelines for the use of these practices in children (27). Parents of seriously ill children may be willing to try a variety of approaches, some of which may be potentially harmful, hoping for benefit in a desperate situation, particularly when the condition imposes a heavy burden for which mainstream therapies are insufficient (28). To best serve the interest of children, physicians must maintain a scientific perspective, provide balanced advice about therapeutic options, and establish and maintain a trusting relationship with families (29).

SYMPTOM CONTROL

Pain Assessment and Management

Pain is "an unpleasant sensory and emotional experience associated with actual or potential tissue damage, or described in terms of such damage" (30). Several outstanding and more comprehensive resources are available for pain management in children (31–34). It is subjective in nature. The experience of pain can be modulated by environmental, developmental, behavioral, psychological, familial, and cultural factors. Unrelieved pain for the child can produce fear, mistrust, irritability, impaired coping, and posttraumatic stress symptoms. Parents feel guilt and anger when pain is undertreated. Many children have pain at some time during their course with life-threatening illness; it can be disease related, treatment related, and/or related to psychological distress. Incidental, or traumatic pain, can still occur in a life-threatened child as well.

Pain assessment must be age-appropriate and requires a careful history and physical examination, determination of the primary cause(s) of pain, and evaluation of secondary causes and modulating features. Pain complaints should always be taken seriously; severe pain for a child is a medical emergency.

Elements of the pain assessment should include the quality of the pain, region and radiation, severity, temporal factors, and provocative and palliative factors. Additional historical elements include disease stage and context, fear of pain, ability to take medication, prior analgesic use, potential role of disease-specific treatment, reactions of parents and family context, and other nonpain symptoms, including depression and/or anxiety, sleep disturbance, and most important, interference with activities of daily life, including play.

Methods of pain assessment must be appropriate to the child's age, situation, emotional resources, developmental level and context, and wishes of the child and family. Ideally, pain assessment, being subjective, should be by self-report. For children >7 years of age, visual analogue or verbal response scales are appropriate. For children ages 3–7, several validated, self-report tools are available, including Faces Scale (35), Oucher (36), poker chip tool (37), body maps, and pain thermometers (38). The Bieri modification of the Faces Scale has improved morphometrics and score distribution (39,40).

For infants, toddlers, and preverbal children, several behavioral assessment scales exist, including CRIES (41), the Neonatal Infant Pain Scale (42), and Children's Hospital of Eastern Ontario Pain Scale (CHEOPS) (43) among others (44). Tools for the assessment of pain in the cognitively impaired child have also been described (45). In general, pain management for children should follow the World Health Organization analgesic ladder (46). Table 73.1 lists some of the more commonly used and available medications for mild, moderate, and severe pain. Particularly for children who cannot swallow pills, the long half-life, low cost, and availability in concentrated liquid formulation make methadone a good choice for long-term analgesia and for preventing opioid withdrawal symptoms (47,48). A short initial and long terminal half-life requires judicious titration to prevent oversedation. Given toxic metabolite accumulation and the availability of several alternatives, meperidine cannot be recommended and is excluded from the table. Medications for pain should be administered according to a regular schedule. Rescue doses should be provided for intermittent or more severe breakthrough pain. Effective management of procedural pain is as critical as expert anticipation, prevention, and treatment of medication side effects. (49,50). Depending on the etiology of the pain being treated, there are many nonopiate adjunct therapies available. Table 73.2 lists some of the more commonly used medications and their indications.

For children, in particular, choose the simplest, most effective, least painful route which for most will be oral or sublingual, or for those with central venous access, parenteral. Intramuscular injections should be avoided if possible. Rectal administration is possible, and many medications, including nonopiates and opiates as well as medication for nonpain symptoms, can be absorbed rectally. Subcutaneous infusion, popular in adult hospice and palliative medicine, is possible in children but may be inadvisable for needle-phobic children. Transdermal and inhalational routes may also be used in children, but little pharmacokinetic data is available regarding their use; anecdotally, absorption and/or metabolism of transdermal fentanyl may be faster in children, requiring patch changes every 2 days if breakthrough pain occurs. Promotion of good psychosocial and spiritual care must be partnered with appropriate pharmacology (51). Children should be given choices as often as possible. Behavioral methods, such as deep breathing (blowing bubbles), progressive relaxation, and biofeedback, have a role in pain management for children. Physical methods, such as touch therapies, including massage, transcutaneous electrical nerve stimulation, physical therapy, heat/cold, and acupuncture and/or acupressure, for example, are helpful adjuncts. Cognitive modalities, including distraction, music, art, play, imagery, and hypnosis, are also effective in children. Studies have demonstrated efficacy of many of these modalities alone or in combination with pharmacologic therapies (52). These therapies should be approached from a family centered perspective; parents can

TABLE 73.1

OPIOID AND NONOPIOID ANALGESICS

Drug	Initial dose (mg/kg/dose)	Route	Interval	Maximum dose	Formulation
Acetaminophen	10–15	p.o./p.r.	q4h	1 g/dose; 4 g/d	T, CT, L, D, S
Ibuprofen	5–10	p.o.	q6h	2.4 g/d; 3.4 g/d (adults)	T, CT, L, D
Choline magnesium trisalicylate	7.5–20	p.o.	b.i.d.–t.i.d.	1.5 g/dose	T, L
Naproxen	5–7	p.o.	q8–12 h	1 g/d	T, L
Ketorolac	0.5	p.o., i.v., i.m.	q6h	30 mg/dose i.v., 10 mg/dose p.o.	I, T
Codeine	0.5–1	p.o., s.q., i.m.	q3–4 h	60 mg/dose	T, L, I
Tramadol	1–2	p.o.	q6h	100 mg/dose, 400 mg/d	T
Morphine	0.2–0.5	p.o., s.l., p.r.	q3–4 h	Titrate	T, L, D, S
	0.1	i.v., s.q., i.m.	q2–4 h	Titrate	I
	0.3–0.6 (long-acting)	p.o.	q8–12 h	Titrate	SRT
Hydromorphone	0.03–0.08	p.o., p.r.	q3–4 h	Titrate	T, L, S
	0.015	i.v., s.q., i.m.	q2–4 h	Titrate	I
Methadone	0.2	p.o.	q8–12 h	Titrate	T, L
	0.1	i.v., s.q., i.m.	q8–12 h	Titrate	I
Fentanyl	0.5–1 µg/kg/h	Transdermal	q48–72 h	Titrate	P
	5–15 µg/kg (sedative)	t.m.	q4–6 h	Titrate	LO
	1–2 µg/kg	i.v., s.q.	q1–2 h	Titrate	I
Oxycodone	0.05–0.15	p.o.	q6h	Titrate	T, L
	0.1–0.3 (long-acting)	p.o.	q12h	Titrate	SRT

CT, chewable tablet; D, drops; I, injection; L, liquid; LO, lozenge; P, patch; S, suppository; SRT, sustained release tablet; T, tablet or capsule.

easily be taught many of these techniques. Providing effective tools for parental involvement in symptom management should increase feelings of control in an often uncontrollable situation.

Respiratory Symptoms

Dyspnea is a distressing symptom for children. Possible causes include tumor metastases, pneumonia, effusions, or neuromuscular problems that impair breathing. Measurement of dyspnea is difficult as it is subjective and does not correlate well with respiratory rate, work of breathing, or oxygen level. In older children, the modified Borg scale or 15-count breathlessness score may be useful (53). Treatment typically involves treatment of the underlying cause, if possible, oxygen, oral and/or parenteral opiates and/or benzodiazepines. There are no clear randomized clinical trials supporting the use of nebulized opiates in children despite widespread use in practice. There are anecdotal reports available (54).

Gastrointestinal Symptoms

Nausea and vomiting are among the most common gastrointestinal symptoms seen in children and cause significant distress and diminish function and quality of life. In young children, nausea may manifest as inactivity, weakness, irritability, and poor appetite. In older children, self-report is the preferred method of assessment. Nausea and vomiting may be secondary to gastrointestinal illness such as gastroenteritis, constipation, gastric stasis, ileus, peritoneal irritation, pancreatitis, obstruction, appendicitis, food poisoning, or overfeeding. Neurologic causes of nausea and vomiting include increased intracranial pressure secondary to brain tumor, subdural hemorrhage, or obstructive hydrocephalus. Middle ear disease or some brain tumors may cause nausea and vomiting from stimulation of the vestibular pathway. Certain medications, including chemotherapy, opioids, antibiotics, nonsteroidal anti-inflammatory agents, and anticholinergics can cause severe nausea and vomiting. Systemic infections as well as other illnesses, such as congenital adrenal hyperplasia, inborn errors of metabolism, and Reye's syndrome, among others, can also present with emesis. Anticipatory nausea and vomiting may reflect the presence of anxiety and stress. Postoperative nausea and vomiting is also a common occurrence in children. Identification of the source of these symptoms is important in order to select the appropriate therapy. Table 73.3 lists some of the antiemetics used in the treatment of children. Prokinetic agents, such as metoclopramide, are useful in the treatment of ileus and intestinal hypomotility. Antihistamines (e.g., diphenhydramine, dimenhydrinate, meclizine), phenothiazines (e.g., promethazine, chlorpromazine), and butyrophenones (e.g., haloperidol) are useful in the treatment of centrally mediated nausea and vomiting. Ondansetron and granisetron, which are 5-HT3 antagonists, are the treatment of choice in chemotherapy and radiation therapy–induced and postoperative nausea and vomiting. Corticosteroids have intrinsic antiemetic properties and potentiate effect of other antiemetics. Cannabinoids have antiemetic properties, as well, but its use in pediatrics is limited. Benzodiazepines may reduce anxiety and the likelihood of anticipatory nausea. Nondrug measures for palliation of nausea and vomiting that may enhance the effect of antiemetic drugs include acupuncture, psychological techniques, and transcutaneous electrical nerve stimulation (55).

Constipation, defined as the passage of small hard feces infrequently and with difficulty, is a common complaint among pediatric patients. In the child with severe constipation, encopresis may be mistaken by diarrhea. On physical examination, clay-like masses may be palpated in a partially distended

TABLE 73.2

ADJUVANT DRUGS USEFUL IN PEDIATRIC PAIN MANAGEMENT

Drug	Initial dose (mg/kg/dose)	Route	Interval	Maximum dose	Formulation	Indication
Amitriptyline	0.1	p.o.	q.h.s.	2 mg/kg/d	T, I	Neuropathic pain, depression, sleep disturbance
Nortriptyline	0.2–0.5	p.o.	q.h.s.	3 mg/kg/d	T, L	Neuropathic pain, depression, sleep disturbance
Paroxetine	10 mg/dose	p.o.	q.a.m.	60 mg/d	T, L, SRT	Neuropathic pain, depression
Fluoxetine	0.2	p.o.	q.a.m.	80 mg/d	T, L, SRT, 90 mg/q/wk	Neuropathic pain, depression
Carbamazepine	2.5–5	p.o., p.r.	b.i.d.–q.i.d.	2400 mg/d	T, L, SRT, CT	Neuropathic pain
Valproic acid	5	p.o.	q.d.–t.i.d.	60 mg/kg/d	T, L, SRT	Neuropathic pain
	5	i.v.	q6–8 h		I	
	10–15	p.r.	q8h		L	
Clonazepam	0.003–0.01	p.o.	t.i.d.–q.i.d.	0.2 mg/kg/d	T	Neuropathic pain
Gabapentin	5	p.o.	b.i.d.–t.i.d.	2400 mg/d	T, L	Neuropathic pain
Methylphenidate	0.1	p.o.	q4h–q24	60 mg/d	T, SRT	Coanalgesia, decreased sedation with opiates
Dextroamphetamine	0.1	p.o.	q4h–q24	40 mg/d	T, SRT	Co-analgesia, decreased sedation with opiates
Diazepam	0.1–0.2	i.v., i.m.	q2–4 h	10 mg/dose	T, L, I	Anxiety, muscle spasm
	0.2–0.3	p.o.	q4–6 h	10 mg/dose	T, L	
	0.3–0.5	p.r.	q2–4 h	20 mg/dose	I, S	
Midazolam	0.05–0.1	i.v., s.q., i.m.	q2–4 h	2.5 mg/dose	I	Anxiety, muscle spasm
	0.2–0.3	Intranasal			I	
	0.25–0.5	p.o.			L	
Lorazepam	0.05	p.o., s.l., p.r., i.v., i.m.	q4–6 h	2 mg/dose	T, L, I	Anxiety, muscle spasm
Dexamethasone	Varies by indication	p.o., i.v., i.m., s.q.	q6–12 h	10 mg/dose	T, L, I	Bone pain, increased intracranial pressure

CT, chewable tablet; I, injection; L, liquid; S, suppository; SRT, sustained release tablet or capsule; T, tablet or capsule.

abdomen and hard stools may be palpated on rectal examination. Opioids, vincristine, and drugs with anticholinergic effects, such as phenothiazines and tricyclic antidepressants, may cause constipation. Other causes include malignant intestinal obstruction and metabolic conditions such as dehydration, cystic fibrosis, hypothyroidism, and hypercalcemia. Spinal cord injuries or other neuromuscular illnesses may be associated with constipation as well. As in adults, prophylactic measures are the first line of intervention (56). Mobility, adequate fluid intake and increased fiber in the diet are helpful. Also, children must be encouraged to attempt defecation after meals to take advantage of the gastrocolic reflex. Hospital staff must allow children privacy for defecation and, whenever possible, the use of a commode or lavatory rather than a bedpan should be encouraged. Treatment of constipation in children includes a variety of oral laxatives and/or enemas. Patients with hard stools can receive laxatives with predominately softening action such as mineral oil, lactulose, or docusate sodium. If on physical examination the rectum is full of soft feces, a predominantly peristalsis-stimulating agent such as senna or bisacodyl may be indicated. Osmotic laxatives, such as polyethylene glycol or magnesium citrate, and rectal laxatives, such as glycerin suppositories, sodium docusate, or sodium phosphate enemas, can also be used in symptomatic children with severe constipation (57). Maintenance therapy may be necessary for patients with chronic constipation. The

use of laxatives in these patients does not lead to dependence. Mineral oil does not cause malabsorption of fat-soluble vitamins and may be used in children as part of a maintenance regimen but should be avoided in neurologically impaired children at risk of bronchoaspiration. The use of biofeedback in the treatment of constipation has not been clearly defined (58).

Diarrhea, one of the most common problems encountered by pediatricians, is defined as the passage of frequent, loose stools. Viral, bacterial, and parasitic infections are among the most common causes of acute diarrhea. Most patients with acute diarrhea have viral gastroenteritis, especially if stools are watery and do not contain either blood or mucus (59). Patients with fever, abdominal cramps, and/or bloody stools most likely have dysentery syndrome and should be treated empirically with trimethoprim/sulfamethoxazole while awaiting results of culture and bacterial susceptibility (60). Diarrhea persisting for longer than 3 weeks is said to be chronic and may be linked to serious organic noninfectious diseases such as anatomic defects, malabsorption syndromes, endocrinopathies, and neoplasms. Dehydration is particularly common in young children with diarrhea and vomiting. Aggressive, prophylactic treatment with hydration solutions (e.g., Pedialyte) and careful follow-up are paramount to prevent serious complications. Products containing salicylates (e.g., bismuth subsalicylate) should be avoided in children. The use

TABLE 73.3

ANTIEMETICS

Drug	Initial dose (mg/kg/dose)	Route	Interval	Maximum dose	Formulation
Butyrophenones					
Droperidol	0.05–0.06	i.m., i.v.	q4–6 h	2.5–5 mg/dose	I
Haloperidol	0.01–0.05	p.o., i.m., i.v., s.q.	q8–12 h	0.15 mg/kg/d	T, L, I
Prokinetic agents					
Metoclopramide	0.1–0.2 (postoperative)	p.o., i.m., i.v., s.q.	q6–8 h	10 mg/dose	T, L, I
	1–2 (chemo-induced)	p.o., i.v.	q2–4 h		
Phenothiazines					
Promethazine	0.25–1.0	p.o., i.m., i.v., p.r.	q4–6 h	25 mg/dose	T, L, I, S
Chlorpromazine	0.5–1.0	p.o., p.r.	q4–6 h	200 mg/d	T, L, I, S
	0.5–1.0	i.m., i.v.	q6–8 h	75 mg/d	
Prochlorperazine	0.1–0.15	p.o., i.m.	q6–8 h	2.5 mg/dose	T, L, I, S
Thiethylperazine	10 mg/dose (>12 y)	p.o., i.m., p.r.	q8–24 h	10 mg/dose	T, I, S
Antihistamines					
Diphenhydramine	0.5–1.0	p.o., i.m., i.v.	q6–8 h	300 mg/d	T, L, I
Dimenhydrinate	0.5–1.0	p.o., i.m., i.v.	q6–8 h	150 mg/d	T, CT, L, I
Hydroxyzine	2 mg/kg/d	p.o., i.m.	q6–8 h	100 mg/dose	T, L, I
Meclizine	25 mg/dose (>12 y)	p.o.	q12–24 h	100 mg/d	T, CT
Trimethobenzamide	5.0	p.o., i.m., p.r.	q6–8 h	200 mg/dose	T, I, S
Serotonin antagonists					
Ondansetron	0.1–0.15	p.o., i.v.	t.i.d.	8 mg/dose	T, L, I
Granisetron	0.01–0.02	p.o., i.v.	q.d., b.i.d.	2 mg/d	T, I
Steroids					
Dexamethasone	0.1–0.2	p.o., i.v., s.q.	q4–6 h	20 mg/dose	T, L, I
Cannabinoids					
Dronabinol	5 mg/m^2	p.o.	q4–6 h	20 mg/d	T

CT, chewable tablet; I, injection; L, liquid; S, suppository; T, tablet or capsule.

of kaolin/pectin and probiotics appear to be a useful adjunct to rehydration solutions (61).

Gastroesophageal reflux is particularly common in children with neurologic impairment, some of whom may require surgical fundoplication to reduce symptoms and decrease the risk of aspiration pneumonia. Useful medications include aluminum hydroxide with or without magnesium hydroxide, calcium carbonate, and H_2-receptor blockers (e.g., ranitidine) and proton pump inhibitors (e.g., omeprazole or lansoprazole) (62).

For patients experiencing cachexia as a result of prolonged, chronic childhood diseases, megestrol acetate, a synthetic progesterone derivative, appears promising as an agent to reverse the growth failure observed in these patients but may cause symptomatic adrenal suppression requiring treatment with hydrocortisone (63). Cyproheptadine can be used as an appetite stimulant in children. Corticosteroids and cannabinoids may also have a therapeutic role.

Pruritus

Pruritus may be multifactorial in children but is most commonly related to dry skin or to medication side effects, in particular, opiates. There are no standardized assessment tools for pruritus. Physical signs include excoriation, lichenification, and/or erythema. Patients may show behavioral clues such as rubbing of eyes, nose, and/or other skin surfaces. Treatment depends upon the cause; topical therapy with moisturizers and emollients may ameliorate itching associated with dry skin. Systemic corticosteroids may be effective for the severe pruritus associated with progressive lymphomas. For drug-induced

pruritus, modification of the drug regimen is the best therapy. If children must be maintained on a medication associated with pruritus, appropriate pharmacotherapy should be instituted, including antihistamines or opiate antagonists such as nalbuphine or low-dose naloxone (64).

Bone Marrow Failure

Bone marrow failure is most often associated with progressive leukemias or solid tumor with marrow involvement. It may lead to fatigue from progressive anemia, infection related to leukopenia, and bleeding as a result of thrombocytopenia. These may diminish the child's ability, and often the parent's willingness, to allow the child to fully participate in the activities of daily living. Decisions regarding interventions must be made based on quality of life goals; parents and providers alike often must be weaned from their adherence to following blood counts. Palliative transfusions may be a part of an overall care plan for a child with end-stage leukemia. Packed red blood cell and platelet infusions may be indicated, for example, for a leukemic child who is still able to go to school, whereas they may not be indicated for an unresponsive, bedbound child. For neutropenic patients proactive decisions may be made regarding the level of intervention for infection, be it comfort measures only, oral broad-spectrum antibiotics, or parental antibiotics, depending upon parent and child preferences in care. The presence of bone marrow failure impacts the way in which the child receives medical care. Children with leukemia, for example, are less likely than patients with solid tumors to receive hospice care and less likely to have support withdrawn (65).

Urinary Symptoms

Urinary retention is often a side effect of medications with anticholinergic properties, with urinary infection, or in children with metastasizing tumors or spinal cord involvement. Treatments may include medication changes, catheterization, physical measures such as compresses or gentle pressure to the bladder, cholinergic medications such as bethanechol, or opiate antagonists for opiate induced retention (66).

Fatigue

Fatigue is one of the most prevalent symptoms in children dying with cancer (67). It is a nonspecific symptom that is difficult to measure and describe due to its subjective nature and the lack of confirmed physiologic and laboratory indicators. Symptoms of fatigue may include physical weakness, mental exhaustion, disruption of sleep, reduced energy, emotional withdrawal, decreased play, or participation in usual activities. Fatigue may be observed in a wide variety of childhood illnesses, including infectious, inflammatory, malignant, and chronic processes, or psychological conditions such as stress, anxiety, and depression. Some medications, including chemotherapeutic regimens used in the treatment of cancer, can cause fatigue and generalized weakness (68).

Fatigue measurement instruments have been developed and tested (69). Common causes of prolonged fatigue such as anemia, hypothyroidism, sleep disturbances, anxiety, and depression, among others should be excluded. A good history and physical examination may point to other potential causes that may respond to therapy. If available, treatment should be directed at the medical or psychiatric condition most likely associated with fatigue. In addition, a graded and gradual increase in exercise and rehabilitation may be helpful. Cognitive-behavioral approaches may also be an effective counseling technique to assist the child in switching to a more adaptive coping strategy. Whenever possible, graded reintegration with peer and school activities is recommended. The use of drugs has not been explored well in children. Steroids, transfusion of blood products, thyroxine, recombinant erythropoietin, and methylphenidate have been used in the treatment of fatigue with varying results (70).

Neurologic Symptoms

Some of the more common and distressing neurologic symptoms in children with malignant disease may include seizures, headaches, and sleep disturbances. Children with neurodegenerative disorders or static encephalopathies may suffer from muscle weakness, muscle spasms, contractures, progressive immobility, and loss or nongain of developmental milestones and communication difficulties. An interdisciplinary and proactive approach to these complex symptoms coupled with patient-family education, is paramount.

Seizures in children with malignancy are often due to primary or metastatic brain lesions, metabolic disturbances, or as a side effect of chemoradiotherapy or medications. For children with known seizures, maintenance medications are appropriate; for children at risk for seizures, availability of at least one anticonvulsant in the home should be planned. For children unable to take medications orally, as most would be during a generalized seizure, administration of several agents by alternative routes is possible, including valproic acid, phenytoin,

pentobarbital, lorazepam, and diazepam rectally, lorazepam sublingually, midazolam and phenobarbital subcutaneously, and fosphenytoin, phenobarbital, and lorazepam intramuscularly. Rectal diazepam gel provides premeasured medication in a convenient dose delivery device: its efficacy and safety in childhood have been demonstrated in randomized clinical trials (71).

Headache, like seizures, is often multifactorial. A careful history and examination of the child will often suggest the cause. Increased intracranial pressure may result in symptoms associated with headache, such as nausea, vomiting, photophobia, lethargy, transient neurologic deficits, or severe irritability, in the preverbal child. Depending on the cause, increased intracranial pressure may be treated with surgery, chemotherapy, radiotherapy, steroids, or expectant management only. Immediate and aggressive use of analgesics, antiemetics, and, often, benzodiazepines, is critical for management of rapidly escalating headache.

For children oversedated from opiates, the addition of adjuvant medications may permit dose reductions. Psychostimulants such as methylphenidate or dexamphetamine have been used empirically to improve quality of life. The use of long-acting oral preparations or continuous parenteral infusions may reduce periods of increased sedation due to large bolus doses.

Sleep disturbance and insomnia in children are often undetected unless specifically elicited in the history. Problem sleeplessness in children may result from behavioral, circadian, biological, or medical abnormalities. In chronically ill children, the presence of other symptoms, such as pain, dyspnea, or wheezing, and emotional symptoms, such as anxiety, may be contributing factors and should be treated aggressively. Hypnotics are the mainstay of therapy for inadequate sleep; low-dose tricyclic antidepressants, such as amitriptyline, may also be appropriate, particularly for children also presenting with neuropathic pain (72).

PSYCHOSOCIAL SUPPORT

The death of a child is the most catastrophic loss a human being can face, and is inherently difficult to prepare for. Psychosocial support in palliative care calls for attention to effective communication and informed decision making to assure optimum quality of life and to decrease suffering in all of its dimensions (73). Open communication helps the sick child deal with uncertainty (74). Good psychosocial care encompasses listening empathically and asking questions, providing honest information, talking about feelings and fears, and identifying hopes and realistic goals of care. The beliefs, attitudes, and functional dynamics of individual family members, the family unit, as well as of the extended community, have a significant influence on the child's experience of severe disease and death. Families with low cohesion, high conflict, and poor conflict resolution report higher intensity of grief and psychosocial morbidity (75). Palliative care teams must include services to provide care and support for the siblings of seriously ill children, and extend their educational activities to school classmates (76,77).

Sick children and their parents need to feel in control of some aspects of their lives. Central to the existence of the dying person, adult and child alike, are the needs to have meaningful relationships, a sense of completion in one's life, a sense of meaning, and a sense of unconditional love. Maintaining a sense of normalcy in the child's life is equally important. Table 73.4 describes the illness experience according to the child's stage of cognitive development. The psychological adaptation of the primary caregivers to the challenges of serious illness is important for the mental health of the children (78). Generally speaking, families must be supported

TABLE 73.4

ILLNESS EXPERIENCE

Infant
Developmental task	Achievement of awareness of being separate from significant other
Impact of illness	Potential distortion of differentiation of self from parent/significant others
Cognitive age/stage	Sensorimotor (birth through 2 years)
Major fears	Separation, strangers
Concept of death	Unable to differentiate death from temporary separation or abandonment
Spiritual interventions	Provide consistent caretakers. Minimize separation from parents and significant others. Decrease parental anxiety, which is projected to infant. Maintain crib/nursery as "safe place" where no invasive procedures are performed. Actively listen to parents, reassure parents of the adequacy of their parenting skills, encourage parental presence. Encourage/facilitate use of spiritual support system for the family

Toddler
Developmental task	Initiation of autonomy
Impact of illness	Interference with development of sense of control, loss of independence
Cognitive age/stage	Preoperational thought (2–7 y): egocentric, magical, little concept of body integrity
Major fears	Separation, loss of control
Concept of illness	Phenomenism (2–7 years): perceives external, unrelated, concrete phenomena as cause of illness, e.g., "being sick because you don't feel well." Contagion: perceives cause of illness as proximity between two events that occurs by "magic," e.g., "getting a cold because you are near someone who has a cold"
Concept of death	Recognizes death in terms of immobility. Often viewed as reversible, temporary, or foreign
Spiritual interventions	Minimize separation from parents/significant others. Keep security objects at hand. Provide simple, brief explanations. Explain and maintain consistent limits. Encourage participation in daily care, etc. Provide opportunities for play and play therapy. Set limits. Reassure the child that disease is not punishment (by God, Higher Power, or other authority figure)

Preschooler
Developmental task	Creation of sense of initiative
Impact of illness	Interference/loss of accomplishments such as walking, talking, controlling basic bodily functions
Cognitive age/stage	Preoperational thought (3–7 y): egocentric, magical, tendency to use and repeat words the child does not understand, providing own explanations and definitions. Literal translation of words. Inability to abstract
Major fears	Bodily injury and mutilation; loss of control; the unknown; the dark; being left alone
Concept of illness	Phenomenism; contagion (3–7 y)
Concept of death	Recognizes death in terms of immobility. Often viewed as reversible, temporary, or foreign. Begins to question and develop a mature concept
Spiritual interventions	Do not underestimate level of comprehension. Provide simple, concrete explanations. Advance preparation is important; days for major events, hours for minor events. Verbal explanations are usually insufficient, so use pictures, models, actual equipment, medical play. When appropriate, initiate discussion of love and caring from Higher Power to relieve anxiety and loneliness. Show behavioral qualities of love, trust, respect, caring, and setting of firm limits and disciplining without anger

School-age child
Developmental task	Development of a sense of industry
Impact of illness	Potential feelings of inadequacy/inferiority if autonomy and independence are compromised
Cognitive age/stage	Concrete operational thought (7–10+ y): beginning of logical thought but tendency to be literal
Major fears	Loss of control; bodily injury, and mutilation; failure to live up to expectations of important others; death
Concept of illness	Contamination: perceives cause as person, object, or action external to the child that is "bad" or "harmful" to the body, e.g., "getting a cold because you didn't wear a hat." Internalization: perceives illness as having an external cause but being located inside the body, e.g., "getting a cold by breathing in air and bacteria"
Concept of death	Recognizes all the components of irreversibility, universality, nonfunctionality, and causality
Spiritual interventions	Provide choices whenever possible. Stress contact with school or organized religious peer group. Use diagrams, pictures, and models for explanations. Emphasize the "normal" things the child can do. Reassure child he/she has done nothing wrong; hospitalization, etc., is not "punishment." Be alert to anxiety about being punished by deity. Provide appropriate concrete explanations in response to questions regarding spiritual beliefs. Continue spiritual rituals; if appropriate promote prayer and relationship with child's concept of God. Model behaviors that show forgiveness and acceptance

Adolescent
Developmental task	Achievement of a sense of identity
Impact of illness	Potential alteration/relinquishment of newly acquired roles and responsibilities
Cognitive age/stage	Formal operational thought (11+ y): beginning of ability to think abstractly. Existence of some magical thinking (e.g., feeling guilty for illness) and egocentrism
Major fears	Loss of control; altered body image; separation from peer group

TABLE 73.4

(CONTINUED)

Concept of illness	Physiologic: perceives cause as malfunctioning or nonfunctioning organ or process; can explain illness in a sequence of events. Psychophysiological: realizes that psychologic actions and attitudes affect health and illness
Concept of death	Speculates on the implications and ramifications of death. Understands effect of death on other people and society as a whole. Future oriented, has difficulty in understanding reality of death as a present possibility
Spiritual interventions	Allow adolescent to be an integral part of decision making regarding care. Give information sensitively, because this age-group reacts to content of information as well as the manner in which it is delivered. Allow as many choices and as much control as possible. Be honest about treatment and consequences. Stress what the adolescent can do for him- or herself and the importance of cooperation and compliance. Assist in maintaining contact with peer group. Provide answers without bias and enable participation in discussions of illness in terms of philosophical or spiritual beliefs. Encourage contact with friends and use of spiritual rituals if adolescent continues to use them. Observe and document verbalizations of patient's values and beliefs

Modified from Gibbons MB. Psychosocial aspects of serious illness in childhood and adolescence. In: Armstrong-Dailey A, Zarbock Goltzer S, eds. *Hospice care for children.* New York: Oxford University Press, 1993:62–63. Concept of death from Faulkner KW. Children's understanding of death. In: Armstrong-Dailey A, Zarbock Goltzer S, eds. *Hospice care for children.* New York: Oxford University Press, 1993:9–21. Spiritual interventions from Hart D, Schneider D. Spiritual care for children with cancer. *Semin Oncol Nurs* 1997;13:263–270.

in the "letting go" process of anticipatory grieving and in their quest to fulfill the universal needs of meaning, purpose, value, self-worth, and a sense of competence in the care of their child (79). Psychosocial interventions in palliative care can also be directed to encourage honest communication between children, their families, and health care professionals, and strengthen interpersonal relationships so that they may feel connected and part of each other (80). The palliative care team can gently encourage the patient and the family to act on the opportunities for reconciliation, to express their love for each other, their forgiveness of past transgressions, and their gratitude. Interventions also aim to help patients understand their condition, to participate in the decision-making process, and to restore their sense of personal integrity, dignity, autonomy, self-mastery, and self-control. Overall, there is evidence of effectiveness for interventions incorporating cognitive-behavioral techniques on variables such as self-efficacy, self-management of disease, family functioning, psychosocial well-being, reduced isolation, social competence, hope, and pain (81). Family support and family therapy are important means of intervention for seriously ill children and their families to improve family function, particularly cohesiveness, conflict resolution, and expression of thoughts and feelings (82). Parental grief after the death of the child may be overwhelming (83). Except for the pharmacologic treatment of depression, however, no rigorous evidence-based recommendation regarding the treatment of bereaved persons is currently possible (84). Emphasis on parents holding on to their relationship with their dead children, rather than letting go of their emotional bonds has been suggested (85).

Children's Understanding of Death

Most children suffering from a life-limiting illness understand death better than other children their age. From birth to 3 years, children grasp events at the level of feeling and action which corresponds to Piaget's sensorimotor stage of cognitive development. Children at this age may interpret death as a temporary separation or abandonment. Children of ages 3–6 years, preoperational stage of cognitive development according to Piaget, view death as a state of immobility, which may be temporary and reversible. Between 6 and 12 years of age,

Piaget's stage of concrete operations, children begin to realize that people who die are not able to function. By the age of 7, most children recognize the four major concepts regarding death: irreversibility, finality, inevitability, and causality (86). As children enter what Piaget calls the stage of formal operations, which usually spans from 12 years of age onward, they develop the ability for abstract reasoning, and their thoughts about death are similar to those of a mature adult. It is again important to note that chronically ill and dying children, given the appropriate explanations, may come to understand concepts of death and dying well beyond that expected for their chronologic age. Stories, games, play, art, or music are among many tools that caregivers have to stimulate communication and help children freely express their thoughts and emotions.

Adjustment Disorder

Chronically ill children who have difficulty coping with the challenges imposed on their lives are often diagnosed as having an adjustment disorder. Children with serious and chronic illness are at increased risk for adjustment disorders (87). When present, these may occur with depressed mood, anxiety, disturbance of conduct, or a combination of these. Identification of children who may have difficulty adjusting is important as most of these children may benefit from appropriate behavioral and cognitive-behavioral therapies.

Anxiety

Anxiety disorders are one of the most prevalent categories of childhood and adolescent psychopathology (88). One of the dilemmas in clinical practice is to define what constitutes an anxiety disorder in comparison with normal anxiety in the presence of stressful life circumstances. Seriously ill children are under considerable personal and family strain and may experience symptoms of anxiety as a manifestation of psychological distress without meeting the criteria for diagnosis of an anxiety disorder. Children who experience difficulty functioning as a result of their anxiety symptoms may have an adaptive disorder. Some of the most common subclinical anxiety symptoms in children include over-concern about competence, excessive need for reassurance, fear of the dark, fear of harm to self or an attachment figure, and somatic complaints. Teenagers may also manifest unrealistic fears, excessive worry about past behavior, and self-consciousness as signs of increased anxiety. Working with the family system is the key way to decrease the anxiety symptoms experienced by the child (89). The aim of the therapy is to disrupt the dysfunctional patterns of interaction that promote family insecurity and to support areas of family competence. Attention to the child–parent relationship is vital to preventing and treating anxiety symptoms. Behavioral therapy, cognitive-behavioral therapy, and psychodynamic psychotherapy are useful therapeutic techniques to help the child and family in the process of coping with the challenges of a life-limiting illness. Commonly selected medications for treating anxiety symptoms include tricyclic antidepressants and selective serotonin reuptake inhibitors. Selection of the medication depends on the presence of comorbidities (90).

Depression

Major depression and dysthymia are common disorders occurring in children and adolescents. Fortunately, although children with medical problems appear to be at slightly elevated risk for depression and have higher rates of maladjustment, most children with chronic disease are not depressed. The clinical picture of depression in children and adolescents varies considerably across different developmental stages. Younger children may show more somatic complaints, auditory hallucinations, temper tantrums, and other behavioral problems. Older children may report low self-esteem, guilt, and hopelessness. The family relationships of youth with depressive symptomatology are frequently characterized by conflict, maltreatment, rejection, and problems with communication, with little expression of positive affect and support (91,92). For children at the end of life, depressive symptoms may occur as a normal reaction to grief and could suggest the need to explore their fears and concerns, and find support in their search for meaning and understanding of their disease, suffering, and imminent death.

The most important tool in diagnosis of depression in children is the comprehensive psychiatric evaluation that should be conducted by a trained clinician. Standardized interviews, however, are long and may not be appropriate for children with chronic illness in whom "depressive" symptoms may be related to the illness. Psychiatric symptom checklists derived from these standardized interviews have been developed and can be useful screening tools. The treatment of depressive youth should be provided in the least restrictive treatment setting that is safe and effective for a given patient. Given the developmental and psychosocial context in which depression unfolds, pharmacotherapy alone usually is not sufficient. Treatment may include a combination of cognitive-behavioral therapy, interpersonal therapy, psychodynamic psychotherapy, and other psychotherapies. For patients requiring pharmacotherapy, selective serotonin reuptake inhibitors are the initial treatment of choice (93).

SPIRITUAL SUPPORT

Patients and their families are especially concerned with spirituality in the contexts of suffering, debilitation, and dying. Spirituality is that part of our human nature that enables us to find a sense of meaning in our experiences. Many agree that the key to emotional coping with serious illness and disability is frequently found within the matrix of spirituality. Spirituality gives us meaning and direction, and brings a sense of order into our lives. This is equally true for children. Children, as well as adults, ask questions, search for a deeper understanding of their experiences, and express their emotions in response to their own interpretation of reality (94). Children are likely to base their spirituality on the relationship with their parents or other primary caregivers. Children's spirituality matures and evolves out of these important relationships, which suggests that spiritual care should be offered to the patient as well as his or her family (95). In addition, children often take religious teachings literally and require explanations beyond these literal meanings to assist them in the process of understanding and interpreting their life experiences.

The developmental stages may assist in the determination of appropriate interventions for spiritual care for the seriously ill child (96). Spiritual interventions introduced into the mainstream of medical therapy are directed to help children articulate their questions, express their emotions, and search for creative answers (97). These activities may allow patients and their families to discover meaning and purpose in their experiences, a sense of oneness with life, of belonging to something beyond themselves, of being part of something greater. This spiritual experience of transcendence beyond the self may facilitate coping by providing a sense of order despite the experience of serious illness and death. Many times at this stage, patients and families manifest a deep yearning for life but also a willingness to accept death, and to live their lives in harmony, giving and receiving love. Inadequate staffing, inadequate training of health care providers to detect patients' spiritual needs, and being called to visit with patients and families too late to provide all the care that could have been provided have been identified as barriers for effective spiritual care (98). Suggested spiritual interventions are included in Table 73.4.

References

1. Martin JA, Kochanek KD, Strobino DM, et al. Annual summary of vital statistics. *Pediatrics* 2005;115(3):619–634.
2. Goldman A. *Care of the dying child.* Oxford: Oxford University Press, 1999.
3. Feudtner C, Hays RM, Haynes G, et al. Deaths attributed to pediatric complex chronic conditions: national trends and implications for supportive care services. *Pediatrics* 2001;107(6):E99.
4. Feudtner C, DiGiuseppe DL, Neff JM. Hospital care for children and young adults in the last year of life: a population-based study. *BMC Med* 2003;1(1):3.
5. Feudtner C, Christakis DA, Zimmerman FJ, et al. Characteristics of deaths occurring in children's hospitals: implications for supportive care services. *Pediatrics* 2002;109(5):887–893.
6. Himelstein BP, Hilden JM, Boldt AM, et al. Pediatric palliative care. *N Engl J Med* 2004;350(17):1752–1762.
7. Brenneis JM. Spirituality and suffering. In: Parris WC, ed. *Cancer pain management.* Boston, MA: Butterworth–Heinemann, 1997:507–515.
8. Byock IR. The nature of suffering and the nature of the opportunity at the end of life. *Clin Geriatr Med* 1996;12:237–252.
9. Attig T. Beyond pain: the existential suffering of children. *J Palliat Care* 1996;12:20–23.
10. Wolfe JW, Grier HE, Klar N, et al. Symptoms and suffering at the end of life in children with cancer. *N Engl J Med* 2000;342:326–333.
11. Collins JJ, Devine TD, Dick GS, et al. The measurement of symptoms in young children with cancer: the validation of the memorial symptom assessment scale in children aged 7–12. *J Pain Symptom Manage* 2002;23(1): 10–16.
12. Drake R, Frost J, Collins JJ. The symptoms of dying children. *J Pain Symptom Manage* 2003;26(1):594–603.
13. Contro N, Larson J, Scofield S, et al. Family perspectives on the quality of pediatric palliative care. *Arch Pediatr Adolesc Med* 2002;156(1):14–19.
14. Meyer EC, Burns JP, Griffith JL, et al. Parental perspectives on end-of-life care in the pediatric intensive care unit. *Crit Care Med* 2002;30(1):226–231.
15. Durbin M. From both sides now: a parent-physician's view of parent-doctor relationships during pediatric cancer treatment. *Pediatrics* 1997; 100.263 267.
16. Sharpe D, Rossiter L. Siblings of children with a chronic illness: a meta-analysis. *J Pediatr Psychol* 2002;27(8):699–710.
17. American Academy of Pediatrics. Committee on bioethics and committee on hospital care. Palliative care for children. *Pediatrics* 2000;106:351–357.

18. http://www.ippcweb.org/modules.asp#mod6, 2006.

19. American Medical Association. Medical futility in end-of-life care. Report of the council on ethical and judicial affairs. *JAMA* 1999;281:937–941.

20. Randolph AG, Zollo MB, Egger MJ, et al. Variability in physician opinion on limiting pediatric life support. *Pediatrics* 1999;103(4):e46.

21. American Medical Association. Medical futility in end-of-life care. Report of the council on ethical and judicial affairs. *JAMA* 1999;281:937–941.

22. Nelson LJ, Rushton CH, Cranford RE, et al. Forgoing medically provided nutrition and hydration in pediatric patients. *J Law Med Ethics* 1995; 23:33–46.

23. Freyer DR. Care of the dying adolescent: special considerations. *Pediatrics* 2004;113:381–388.

24. American Academy of Pediatrics. Committee on bioethics. Guidelines on forgoing life-sustaining medical treatment. *Pediatrics* 1994;93:532–536.

25. Fleischman A. Commentary: ethical issues in pediatric pain management and terminal sedation. *J Pain Symptom Manage* 1998;15(4):260–261.

26. American Academy of Pediatrics. Committee on bioethics. Institutional ethics committees. *Pediatrics* 2001;107:205–209.

27. Kemper K, Cassileth B, Ferris T. Holistic pediatrics: a research agenda. *Pediatrics* 1999;103:902–909.

28. Angell M, Kassirer JP. Alternative medicine—the risks of untested and unregulated remedies. *N Engl J Med* 1998;339:839–841.

29. American Academy of Pediatrics. Counseling families who choose complementary and alternative medicine for their child with chronic illness or disability. *Pediatrics* 2001;107:598–601.

30. Pain terms: a list with definitions and notes on usage. Recommended by the IASP Subcommittee on Taxonomy. PMID: 460932. *Pain* 1979;6(3):249–252.

31. Yaster M, Krane EJ, Kaplan RF, et al., eds. *Pediatric pain management and sedation handbook.* St. Louis, MO: Mosby, 1997.

32. American Pain Society. *Guideline for the management of acute and chronic pain in sickle cell disease.* Glenview, IL: American Pain Society, 1999.

33. *Cancer pain relief and palliative care in children.* Geneva QZ 275 CAN (97731): World Health Organization, 1998:76.

34. Berde CB, Sethna NF. Analgesics for the treatment of pain in children. *N Engl J Med* 2002;347(14):1094–1103.

35. Wong DL. *Whaley and Wong's essentials of pediatric nursing,* 5th ed. St. Louis, MO: Mosby, 1997.

36. Beyer JE. *The Oucher: a user's manual and technical report.* Evanston, IL: Hospital Play Equipment, 1984.

37. Hester NO, Foster R, Kristensen K. Measurement of pain in children. Generalizability and validity of the pain ladder and the poker chip tool. In: Tyler DC, Krane EJ, eds. *Pediatric pain: advances in pain research and therapy,* Vol. 15. New York: Raven Press, 1990:79–84.

38. Finley GA, McGrath PJ. *Measurement of pain in infants and children.* Seattle, WA: IASP Press, 1998.

39. Goodenough B, Addicoat L, Champion GD, et al. Pain in 4- to 6-year-old children receiving intramuscular injections: a comparison of the faces pain scale with other self-report and behavioral measures. *Clin J Pain* 1997; 13(1):60–73.

40. Hicks CL, von Baeyer CL, Spafford PA, et al. The faces pain scale-revised: toward a common metric in pediatric pain measurement. *Pain* 2001;93(2):173–183.

41. Krechel SW, Bildner J. CRIES: a new neonatal postoperative pain measurement score. Initial testing of validity and reliability. *Pediatr Anaesth* 1995;5:53–61.

42. Lawrence J, Alcock D, McGrath P, et al. The development of a tool to assess neonatal pain. *Neonatal Netw* 1993;12:59–66.

43. McGrath PJ, Johnson G, Goodman JT. CHEOPS: a behavioral scale for rating postoperative pain in children. In: Fields HL, Dubner R, Cervero F, et al., eds. *Advances in pain research and therapy. Proceedings of the fourth world congress on pain.* New York: Raven Press, 1985:395–402.

44. Mathew PJ, Mathew JL. Assessment and management of pain in infants. [Review] [47 refs] [Journal Article. Review. Review, Tutorial]. *Postgrad Med J* 2003;79(934):438–443.

45. Solodiuk J, Curley MA. Pain assessment in nonverbal children with severe cognitive impairments: the Individualized Numeric Rating Scale (INRS). *J Pediatr Nurs* 2003;18(4):295–299.

46. Zech DF, Grond S, Lynch J, et al. Validation of World Health Organization guidelines for cancer pain relief: a 10 year prospective study. *Pain* 1995; 63:65–76.

47. Shir Y, Rosen G, Zeldin A, et al. Methadone is safe for treating hospitalized patients with severe pain. *Can J Anaesth* 2001;48(11):1109–1113.

48. Siddappa R, Fletcher JE, Heard AM, et al. Methadone dosage for prevention of opioid withdrawal in children. *Paediatr Anaesth* 2003;13(9):805–810.

49. Young KD. Pediatric procedural pain. *Ann Emerg Med* 2005;45(2):160–171.

50. Murat I, Gall O, Tourniaire B. Procedural pain in children: evidence-based best practice and guidelines. *Reg Anesth Pain Med* 2003;28(6):561–572.

51. Howard RF. Current status of pain management in children. *JAMA* 2003;290(18):2464–2469.

52. Mercadante S. Cancer pain management in children. *Palliat Med* 2004; 18(7):654–662.

53. Prasad SA, Randall SD, Balfour-Lynn IM. Fifteen-count breathlessness score: an objective measure for children. *Pediatr Pulmonol* 2000;30(1):56–62.

54. Cohen S, Dawson T. Nebulized morphine as a treatment for dyspnea in a child with cystic fibrosis. *Pediatrics* 2002;110:e38.

55. Burish TG, Tope DM. Psychological techniques for controlling the adverse side effects of cancer chemotherapy. Finding from a decade of research. *J Pain Symptom Manage* 1992;7:287–301.

56. Roma E, Adamidis D, Nikolara R, et al. Diet and chronic constipation in children: the role of fiber. *J Pediatr Gastroenterol Nutr* 1999;28:169–174.

57. Bell EA, Wall GC. Pediatric constipation therapy using guidelines and polyethylene glycol 3350. *Ann Pharmacother* 2004;38(4):686–693.

58. Heymen S, Jones KR, Scarlett Y, et al. Biofeedback treatment of constipation: a critical review. *Dis Colon Rectum* 2003;46(9):1208–1217.

59. Clark B, McKendrick M. A review of viral gastroenteritis. [Review] [104 refs] [Journal Article. Review. Review, Tutorial]. *Curr Opin Infect Dis* 2004;17(5):461–469.

60. Nataro J. Treatment of bacterial enteritis. *Pediatr Infect Dis J* 1998;17:420–421.

61. Allen SJ, Okoko B, Martinez E, Gregorio G, Dans LF. Probiotics for treating infectious diarrhea. *Cochrane Database Syst Rev.* 2006;(2):CD003048.

62. Israel DM, Hassel E. Omeprazole and other proton pump inhibitors: pharmacology, efficacy, and safety, with special reference to use in children. *J Pediatr Gastroenterol Nutr* 1998;27:568–577.

63. Orme LM, Bond JD, Humphrey MS, et al. Megestrol acetate in pediatric oncology patients may lead to severe, symptomatic adrenal suppression. *Cancer* 2003;98(2):397–405.

64. Maxwell LG, Kaufmann SC, Bitzer S, et al. The effects of a small-dose naloxone infusion on opioid-induced side effects and analgesia in children and adolescents treated with intravenous patient-controlled analgesia: a double-blind, prospective, randomized, controlled study. *Anesth Analg* 2005;100(4):953–958.

65. Klopfenstein KJ, Hutchison C, Clark C, et al. Variables influencing end-of-life care in children and adolescents with cancer. *J Pediatr Hematol Oncol* 2001;23(8):481–486.

66. Yamanishi T, Yasuda K, Kamai T, et al. Combination of a cholinergic drug and an alpha-blocker is more effective than monotherapy for the treatment of voiding difficulty in patients with underactive detrusor. [Clinical Trial. Journal Article. Randomized Controlled Trial]. *Int J Urol* 2004; 11(2):88–96.

67. Hockenberry M. Symptom management research in children with cancer. [Review] [38 refs] [Journal Article. Review. Review, Tutorial]. *J Pediatr Oncol Nurs* 2004;21(3):132–136.

68. Viner R, Christie D. Fatigue and somatic symptoms. *BMJ* 2005;330(7498):1012–1015.

69. Hockenberry MJ, Hinds PS, Barrera P, et al. Three instruments to assess fatigue in children with cancer: the child, parent and staff perspectives. *J Pain Symptom Manage* 2005;25(4):319–328.

70. Mock V, Atkinson A, Barsevick A, et al. National Comprehensive Cancer Network. NCCN Practice Guidelines for Cancer-Related Fatigue. *Oncology* 2000;14(11A):151–161.

71. Dreifuss FE, Rosman NP, Cloyd JC, et al. A comparison of rectal diazepam gel and placebo for acute repetitive seizures. *N Engl J Med* 1998;338(26):1869–1875.

72. Sheldon SH. Insomnia in children. *Curr Treat Options Neurol* 2001;3:37–50.

73. Chesson RA, Chisholm D, Zaw W. Counseling children with chronic physical illness. *Patient Educ Couns* 2004;55(3):331–338.

74. Beale EA, Baile WF, Aaron J. Silence is not golden: communicating with children dying from cancer. *J Clin Oncol* 2005;23(15):3629–3631.

75. Kissane DW, Bloch SB, Onghena P, et al. The Melbourne family grief study I: psychosocial morbidity and grief in bereaved families. *Am J Psychiatry* 1996;153:659–666.

76. Doka KJ, ed. *Living with grief: children, adolescents and loss.* Washington, DC: Hospice Foundation of America, 2000.

77. Sharpe D, Rossiter L. Siblings of children with a chronic illness: a meta-analysis. [Review] [21 refs] [Journal Article. Meta-Analysis. Review]. *J Pediatr Psychol* 2002;27(8):699–710.

78. Johnson G, Kent G, Leather J. Strengthening the parent-child relationship: a review of family interventions and their use in medical settings. *Child Care Health Dev* 2005;31(1):25–32.

79. Byock I. *Dying well.* New York: Riverhead, 1997.

80. Kane JR, Hellsten MB, Coldsmith A. Human suffering: the need for relationship-based research in pediatric end-of-life care. *J Pediatr Oncol Nurs* 2004;21(3):180–185.

81. Barlow JH, Ellard DR. Psycho-educational interventions for children with chronic disease, parents and siblings: an overview of the research evidence base. *Child Care Health Dev* 2004;30(6):637–645.

82. Kissane DW, Bloch SB, Onghena P, et al. The Melbourne family grief study I: perceptions of family functioning in bereavement. *Am J Psychiatry* 1996;153:650–658.

83. American Academy of Pediatrics. Committee on psychosocial aspects of child and family health. The pediatrician and childhood bereavement. *Pediatrics* 2000;105:445–447.

84. Amanda LForte, Malinda Hill, Rachel Pazder, et al. Bereavement care interventions: a systematic review. *BMC Palliat Care* 2004;3:3.

85. Davies R. New understandings of parental grief: literature review. *J Adv Nurs* 2004;46(5):506–513.

86. Wass H. Concepts of death: a developmental perspective. In: Wass H, ed. *Childhood and death*. Washington, DC: Hospice Foundation of America, 1995.
87. Wallander JL, Thompson RJ. Psychosocial adjustment of children with chronic physical conditions. In: Roberts MC, ed. *Handbook of pediatric psychology*. New York: Guilford Press, 1995:124–141.
88. Bernstein GA, Borchardt CM, Perwien AR. Anxiety disorders in children and adolescents: a review of the past 10 years. *J Am Acad Child Adolesc Psychiatry* 1996;35:1110–1119.
89. Norberg AL, Lindblad F, Boman KK. Coping strategies in parents of children with cancer. *Soc Sci Med* 2005;60(5):965–975.
90. American Academy of Child and Adolescent Psychiatry. Work group on quality issues. Practice parameters for the assessment and treatment of children and adolescents with anxiety disorders. *J Am Acad Child Adolesc Psychiatry* 1997;36:69S–84S.
91. Birmaher B, Ryan ND, Williamson DE, et al. Childhood and adolescent depression: a review of the past 10 years. Part I. *J Am Acad Child Adolesc Psychiatry* 1996;35:1427–1439.
92. Birmaher B, Ryan ND, Williamson DE, et al. Childhood and adolescent depression: a review of the past 10 years. Part II. *J Am Acad Child Adolesc Psychiatry* 1996;35:1575z–11583.
93. American Academy of Child and Adolescent Psychiatry. Practice parameters for the assessment and treatment of children and adolescents with depressive disorders. *J Am Acad Child Adolesc Psychiatry* 1998;37:63S–83S.
94. Sommer DR. Exploring the spirituality of children in the midst of illness and suffering. *ACCH Advocate* 1994;1:7–12.
95. Houskamp BM, Fisher LA, Stuber ML. Spirituality in children and adolescents: research findings and implications for clinicians and researchers. *Child Adolesc Psychiatr Clin N Am* 2004;13(1):221–230.
96. Heilferty CM. Spiritual development and the dying child: the pediatric nurse practitioner's role. *J Pediatr Health Care* 2004;18(6):271–275.
97. Stuber ML, Houskamp BM. Spirituality in children confronting death. *Child Adolesc Psychiatr Clin N Am* 2004;13(1):127–136, viii.
98. Feudtner C, Haney J, Dimmers MA. Spiritual care needs of hospitalized children and their families: a national survey of pastoral care providers' perceptions. *Pediatrics* 2003;111(1):e67–e72.

CHAPTER 74 ■ GERIATRIC PALLIATIVE CARE

JESSICA ISRAEL AND R. SEAN MORRISON

In our society, the overwhelming majority of people who die are elderly. They typically die slowly of chronic diseases, over long periods of time, with multiple coexisting problems, progressive dependency on others, and heavy care needs met mostly by family members. They spend most of their final months and years at home but, in most parts of the country, actually die surrounded by strangers in the hospital or nursing home. Abundant evidence suggests that the quality of life during the dying process is often poor, characterized by inadequately treated physical distress, fragmented care systems, poor to absent communication between doctors and patients and families, and enormous strains on family caregiver and support systems. In this chapter, we focus on the palliative care needs of older adults.

BIOLOGY OF AGING

Body Composition

Aging is a process that converts healthy adults into frail ones with diminished reserves in most physiologic systems and with an exponentially increasing vulnerability to most diseases and death (1). Aging is the most significant and common risk factor for disease in general. The process itself is a mystery, still poorly understood even in this age of advanced biotechnologic capability. Normal aging appears to be a fairly benign process. The body's organ system reserves and homeostatic control mechanisms steadily decline. Commonly, this slow erosion only becomes obvious in times of maximum body stress or serious illness. However, as the process continues, it takes less and less insult for the underlying physiologic weakness to become apparent. It is difficult to differentiate the effects of aging alone from those of concurrent disease or environmental factors. Eventually, a critical point is reached, when the body's systems are overwhelmed, and death ultimately results. Morbidity is often compressed into the last period of life (2).

Substantial changes occur in body composition with aging. These changes become important when related to nutritional needs, pharmacokinetics, and metabolic activity. As adults age, the proportion of bodily lipid doubles and lean body mass decreases. Bones and viscera shrink and the basal metabolic rate declines. Although specific age-associated changes occur in each organ system, changes in body composition

and metabolism are highly variable from individual to individual.

Renal Function

The aging kidney loses functioning nephrons. Cross-sectional and longitudinal studies have also demonstrated a decline in creatinine clearance. There is also evidence to show decreased renal plasma flow, decreased tubular secretion and reabsorption, decreased hydrogen secretion and decreased water absorption and excretion (3). When kidney disease complicates this aging process, the outcome can be highly deleterious.

Underlying renal function is an important issue in geriatric pharmacology. Many medications rely on the kidneys' mechanisms for excretion and their metabolites may accumulate and lead to side effects or toxic injury in an impaired system. For example, the renally cleared metabolite of meperidine, normeperidine, can accumulate in the elderly and predispose to delirium, central nervous system excitement, and seizure activity. Commonly used medications are more likely to damage older kidneys, including nonsteroidal anti-inflammatory drugs (NSAIDs), aminoglycosides, and intravenous contrast dye (4).

Gastrointestinal and Hepatic Function

The gastrointestinal tract changes less with aging than normal systems, but there are still some deficiencies that may affect medication delivery and breakdown, as well as nutritional status and metabolism. The esophagus may show delayed transit time. The stomach may atrophy and produce less acid. Colonic transit is greatly slowed, whereas small intestinal transit appears unaffected. Pancreatic function is usually well maintained, although trypsin secretion may be decreased.

The liver usually retains adequate function, although there are variable changes seen in its metabolic pathways. The cytochrome P-450 system may decline in efficiency and liver enzymes may be less inducible. The most significant change is the sharp decline in demethylization, the process that metabolizes medications such as benzodiazepines in the liver. This change may necessitate dosage adjustments. In addition, drugs that undergo hepatic first pass metabolism by extraction from the blood may have altered clearance with increasing age because of decreased hepatic blood flow.

Brain and Central Nervous System Changes

The brain and central nervous system slowly atrophy with age. Neurons stop proliferating and are not replaced when they die, resulting in neuronal loss as well as loss of dendritic arborization. These are also some degree of neurotransmitter and receptor loss. The extent of this loss is not well understood.

Age-related changes in pain perception may exist, but their clinical importance is uncertain. Although degenerative changes occur in areas of the central and autonomic nervous system that mediate pain, the relevance of these changes has yet to be determined (5). Clinical observations from elderly patients who report minimal pain and discomfort despite the presence of cardiac ischemia or intraabdominal catastrophe suggest that pain perception may be altered in the elderly. However, experimental data suggest that significant, age-related changes in pain perception probably do not occur (6). Until further studies conclusively demonstrate that the perception of pain decreases with age, stereotyping of most elderly patients as experiencing less pain may lead to inaccurate clinical assessments and needless suffering (5).

DEMOGRAPHY OF DYING AND DEATH IN THE UNITED STATES

The median age at death in the United States is now 77 years and has been associated with a steady and linear decline in age-adjusted death rates since 1940. In 1900, life expectancy at birth was <50 years; a girl born today may expect to live to age 79 and a boy to age 73. Those reaching 65 years can expect to live another 18 years on average and those reaching age 80 can expect to live an additional 8 years. These unprecedented increases in life expectancy (equivalent to that occurring between the Stone Age and 1900) are due primarily to decreases in maternal and infant mortality, resulting from improved sanitation, nutrition, and effective control of infectious diseases. As a result, there has been an enormous growth in the number and health of the elderly. By the year 2030, 20% of the United States' population will be over age 65, as compared to fewer than 5% at the turn of the twentieth century (7).

Although death at the turn of the twentieth century was largely attributable to acute infectious diseases or accidents, the leading causes of death today are chronic illness such as heart disease, cancer, stroke, and dementia. With advances in the treatment of atherosclerotic vascular disease and cancer, many patients with these diseases now survive for years. Many diseases that were rapidly fatal in the past have now become chronic illnesses.

In parallel, deaths that occurred at home in the early part of the twentieth century now occur primarily in institutions (57% in hospitals and 17% in nursing homes) (8). The reasons for this shift in location of death are complex, but appear to be related to health system and reimbursement structures that promote hospital-based care and provide relatively little support for home care and custodial care services despite the significant care burdens and functional dependency that accompany life-threatening chronic disease in the elderly. The older the patient, the higher the likelihood of death in a nursing home or hospital, with an estimated 58% of persons over 85 spending at least some time in a nursing home during the last year of their life (8). These statistics, however, hide the fact that most of an older person's last months and years is still spent at home in the care of family members, with hospitalization and/or nursing home placement occurring only near the very end of life. National statistics also obscure the

variability in the experience of dying. For example, the need for institutionalization or paid formal caregivers in the last months of life is much higher among the poor and women. Similarly, persons suffering from cognitive impairment and dementia are much more likely to spend their last days in a nursing home compared with cognitively intact, elderly persons dying from nondementing illnesses.

CARE SYSTEMS FOR OLDER ADULTS WITH SERIOUS AND LIFE-THREATENING ILLNESS

The incentives promoting an institutional—as opposed to home—death persist despite evidence that patients prefer to die at home. These incentives persist in the United States despite the existence of the Medicare Hospice Benefit (9), which was designed to provide substantial professional and material support (medications, equipment, skilled nursing visits) to families caring for the dying at home for their last 6 months of life. Reasons for the low rate of utilization of the Medicare Hospice Benefit vary by community but include the inhibiting requirements that patients acknowledge that they are dying in order to access the services, that physicians certify a prognosis of 6 months or less, and that very few hours (usually 4 or less) of personal care home attendants are covered under the benefit. In addition, the fiscal structure of the Medicare Hospice Benefit lends itself well to the predictable trajectory of late-stage cancers or acquired immunodeficiency syndrome (AIDS), but not so well to the unpredictable chronic course of other common causes of death in the elderly such as congestive heart failure, chronic lung disease, stroke, and dementing illnesses.

Traditional Medicare coverage in the United States also fails to meet the needs of the seriously ill, older adult. Neither paid personal care services at home nor nursing home costs for the functionally dependent elderly are covered by Medicare, but instead are paid for approximately equally from out-of-pocket and Medicaid budgetary sources that were originally developed to provide care for the indigent.

In nursing homes, standards of care focus on improvement of function, and maintenance of weight and nutritional status. Evidence of the decline that accompanies the dying process is typically regarded as a measure of substandard care (10). Therefore, a death in a nursing home is often viewed as evidence particularly by state regulators; of poor care rather than an expected outcome for a frail, chronically ill, older person. The financial and regulatory incentives and quality measures that currently exist in long-term care promote tube feeding over spoon feeding and transfer to hospital or emergency department in the setting of acute illness or impending death. They fail to either assess or reward appropriate attention to palliative measures, including relief of symptoms, spiritual care, and promotion of continuity with concomitant avoidance of brink-of-death emergency room and hospital transfers (11) (Table 74.1).

PALLIATIVE CARE NEEDS OF OLDER ADULTS

Although death occurs far more commonly in older adults than in any other age group, remarkably little is known about how death occurs in the oldest old, those over age 75. Most research on the experience of dying has been done in younger populations, and most studies examining pain and symptom management have focused on younger populations with cancer or AIDS. Studies in older adults have focused

TABLE 74.1

BENEFITS AND RISKS OF TUBE FEEDING IN OLDER ADULTS/NURSING HOME RESIDENTS

Benefits of tube feeding in older adults/Nursing home patients	Risks of tube feeding in older adults/Nursing home patients
Improved survival for patients in persistent vegetative state	Dementia patients more likely to be physically restrained
Improved survival for patients with extreme short bowel syndrome or proximal bowel obstruction	Increased risk of aspiration pneumonia, diarrhea, gastrointestinal discomfort, and problems associated with accidental feeding tube removal by the patient
Improved survival **AND** quality of life for patients with bulbar amyotrophic lateral sclerosis	With impaired renal function or in last days of life patient may have choking, increased pulmonary secretions, dyspnea, pulmonary edema, ascites
Improved survival for patients in acute phase of stroke or head injury	
Improved survival in patients receiving short-term critical care	
Improved nutritional status of patients with advanced cancer undergoing intensive radiation therapy	
No Survival Benefit in patients with dementia	

Table adapted from data summarized in Casarett D, Kapo J, Caplan A. Appropriate use of artificial nutrition and hydration-fundamental principles and recommendations. *N Engl J Med* 2005;353:2607–2612.

primarily on patients' preferences for care rather than the actual care received. Indeed, the largest study to date of the dying experience in the United States [study to understand prognoses and preferences for outcomes and risks of treatments (SUPPORT)] studied the hospital experience of patients with a median age of 66 (9). The median age of death in the United States is 77 years, and many of the oldest old die in nursing homes or at home rather than in hospital. Data from Medicare and state Medicaid registries suggest that expensive and high technology interventions are less frequently applied to the oldest patients, independent of functional status and projected life expectancy. Whereas these discrepancies may reflect patient preferences and indicate appropriate utilization of resources and patient preferences, it is more likely that they represent a form of implicit rationing of resources based on age. The implication is disturbing, considering that half of the highest-cost, Medicare enrollees survive at least 1 year (12).

Aside from pain and other sources of physical distress [discussed in the subsequent text (see the section Symptom Management: The Challenge of Pain)], the key characteristic that distinguishes the dying process in the elderly from that experienced by younger groups is the nearly universal occurrence of long periods of functional dependency and need for family caregivers in the last months to years of life. In SUPPORT, the median age of participants was 66 years and 55% of patients had persistent and serious family caregiving needs during the course of their terminal illness (13), and in another study of 988 terminally ill patients, 35% of families had substantial care needs (14). This percentage rises exponentially with increasing age. Although paid care supplements provides the sole source of care in 15–20% of patients (transportation, homemaker services, personal care, and more skilled nursing care), the remaining 80–85% of patients receive most of their care from unpaid family members (14). Furthermore, most family caregiving is provided by women (spouses and adult daughters and daughters-in-law), placing significant strains on the physical, emotional, and socioeconomic status of the caregivers. Those ill and dependent patients without family caregivers, or those whose caregivers can no longer provide nor afford needed services, are placed in nursing homes. In the United States, this typically occurs after patients exhaust all of their financial savings in order to become eligible for Medicaid. At present, 20% of the over age 85 population reside in a skilled nursing facility, and this number is expected to increase dramatically in the next 50 years (15). Present estimates suggest the current number of skilled nursing facility beds in the United States will be woefully inadequate for the needs of our aging population.

SYMPTOM MANAGEMENT: THE CHALLENGE OF PAIN

The constellation of symptoms seen in dying, older, adult patients is different from that of young adults. Delirium, sensory impairment, incontinence, dizziness, cough, and constipation are more prevalent in older adults (16). The elderly, on average, have 1.5 more symptoms than younger persons in the year prior to death, and 69% of the symptoms reported for people aged 85 or more lasted more than a year as compared with 39% of those for younger adults (<55 years) (16).

Studies focusing specifically on the prevalence of pain have shown consistently high levels of untreated or undertreated pain in older adults. In one study of elderly cancer patients in nursing homes, 26% of patients with daily pain received no analgesic at all and 16% received only acetaminophen, a percentage that rose with increasing age and minority status (17). A subsequent study revealed that 41% of patients who were assessed having pain on their first assessment continued to have moderate or excruciating daily pain on their second assessment 60–180 days later (18). Studies comparing pain management in cognitively intact versus demented elderly with acute hip fracture also found a high rate of undertreatment of pain in both groups, a phenomenon that worsened with increasing age and cognitive impairment (19,20). Similarly, a study of outpatients with cancer found that age and female sex were predictors of undertreatment, a disturbing observation given the dramatic rise in cancer prevalence with increasing age (21,22). Chronic pain due to arthritis, other bone and joint disorders, and low back pain syndrome is probably the most common cause of distress and disability in the elderly, affecting 25–50% of community-dwelling, older adults. It is likely that these symptoms also are consistently undertreated (23). These data suggest that the time before death among elderly persons is often characterized by significant physical distress that is neither identified nor properly treated.

Despite the high prevalence of pain and other symptoms in the elderly, most studies focusing on the assessment and treatment of pain and other symptoms have enrolled young patients with cancer. It is unclear whether these results can be generalized to a geriatric population. Pain assessment in the elderly is often complicated by the coexistence of cognitive impairment. The assessment and management of pain in the cognitively impaired patient present special challenges to the health care professional. The cognitively impaired patient is often unable to express pain adequately, request analgesics, or operate patient-controlled, analgesia devices. This increases the risk of undertreatment. The fear of precipitating or exacerbating a delirious episode by employing opioids in the management of pain may also lead to inadequate pain management.

As with the cognitively intact patient, the initial step in the assessment of pain in the demented individual is to ask the patient. Although patients with severe dementia may be incapable of communicating, many patients with moderate degrees of impairment can accurately localize and grade the severity of their pain (24,25). In the noncommunicative patient, alternative means of assessment must be identified. The need for careful pain assessment in this population of patients is underscored by evidence that suggests that medical professionals undertreat pain in the presence of cognitive impairment (19,20,26) and that pain may be aggravated in the presence of cognitive deficits (24). Untreated pain can result in agitation, disruptive behavior, and may worsen or precipitate a delirious episode (27–29).

Pain assessment in the noncommunicative patient should begin with observation of both nonverbal cues, such as facial expressions (grimacing, frowning) and motor behavior (bracing, restlessness, agitation), and verbal cues, such as groaning, screaming, or moaning. Data from cognitively intact individuals suggest that nonverbal behaviors correlate with self-reported pain in nondemented patients recovering from surgery (30,31). Pharmacologic therapy should be titrated upward in small, incremental doses until the nonverbal/verbal behavior disappears or side effects become apparent. This approach is particularly useful in the agitated patient whose behavior may well stem from untreated or undertreated pain. The risk of undertreating severe pain is generally more concerning, both medically and ethically, than the risk of worsening delirium with medications.

Pharmacologic therapy for pain must be modified in older adults. The World Health Organization's analgesic ladder approach may not be appropriate for the elderly. For example, the increased risk of side effects, including renal failure and gastrointestinal bleeding, mandates great caution in the use of NSAIDs. This caution extends to currently available parenteral NSAIDs because of the significantly increased risk of gastrointestinal bleeding, particularly with higher doses and with duration of use >5 days (32–34). Selective COX-2 antagonists have been associated with a decreased incidence of gastrointestinal events and are probably preferred for use in older adults over traditional NSAIDs (35–37). A recent systematic review, however, suggest that there may be an increase in adverse cardiovascular events associated with the use of COX-2 inhibitors although the magnitude of this risk has yet to be determined (38). The American Geriatrics Society has recently recommended that opioids be considered as a first step treatment rather than NSAIDs (23). If NSAIDs are used, careful monitoring of renal function and close observation for the development of gastrointestinal bleeding must be undertaken.

Opioid therapy remains the cornerstone of pain management in palliative care and this is also true for older adults. Some aspects of opioid therapy require special consideration in the elderly. Older adults will have a more pronounced pharmacologic effect after any weight-adjusted opioid dose than younger patients. The analgesia is more intense, and cognitive and respiratory effects, and perhaps constipation, are more severe. This enhanced effect is likely due to a lesser volume of distribution (approximately half that of younger patients), a decreased clearance, and diminished target organ reserve (central nervous system, pulmonary function, and bowel function). Age is the single most important predictor of initial opioid dose requirements for postoperative pain (39). The following formula, based on a review of records of >1000 adults between age 20 and 70 years undergoing major surgery, provides a rough estimate of the appropriate starting dose in parenteral morphine sulfate equivalents for adult opioid naive patients (with the exception of the oldest old): average first 24-hour morphine (mg) requirement for patients over 20 years of age = 100—age (39). Other factors that will influence opioid effects, but to a lesser degree than that of age, are body weight, severity of pain, abnormal renal function, nausea/vomiting, and cardiopulmonary insufficiency. After the initial dose determination, drugs should be titrated on the basis of analgesic effect.

There are no data as to appropriate starting doses for analgesia in older adults. A reasonable starting dose may be 30–50% of that recommended for a younger adult.

Practically speaking, however, the best advice is almost obvious. In opioid naive older adults one should start with the smallest dose available for the product. The key to prescribing a correct regimen is not in the first order you write, but rather, in what happens when this dose becomes effective. In an acute pain syndrome, the reassessment of the patient's level of pain at the right follow up interval will lead to the appropriate dose titration. An intravenous medication should be effective within 6 to 15 minutes, oral medications within an hour. Reassessing effective analgesia needs to occur frequently in an acute pain crisis.

Several opioids are best avoided in older adults. Meperidine is particularly hazardous as a result of the accumulation of its toxic metabolite, normeperidine, in patients with impaired renal function. Indeed, toxic levels can accumulate in older adults with "normal kidneys" due to age-related changes in creatinine clearance. There are almost no circumstances in which meperidine should be used on older adults. Similarly, pentazocine should also be avoided in older adults because of the increased incidence of delirium and agitation associated with its use. Finally, opioids with long half-lives (e.g., methadone, levorphanol) or opioids with sustained release preparations (e.g., sustained release morphine and oxycodone, and transdermal fentanyl) should be used with caution, rarely be used in opioid naive geriatric patients, and should probably only be used following steady state accumulation of shorter acting opioids.

With respect to adjuvant agents, amitriptyline, and the other tricyclic antidepressants, although efficacious in some neuropathic pain syndromes, are poorly tolerated in older adults due to their anticholinergic properties. Bowel and bladder dysfunction, orthostatic hypotension resulting in falls, delirium, movement disorders, and dry mouth are very common with these medications. If tricyclics are to be used, then nortriptyline or desipramine are the agents of choice and initial dosages should be very low and dose titration should be undertaken very slowly.

ALZHEIMER'S DISEASE AND RELATED DEMENTIAS

Irreversible dementia is a frightening and difficult diagnosis for geriatric patients and their families. A diagnosis of dementia means a certain and progressive decline in cognitive abilities over time and an eventual loss of independence. Dementia is a progressive, incurable illness, and all treatments are palliative. The average survival after a diagnosis of Alzheimer disease ranges from 7–10 years. Patients with dementia require medical care that focuses on preserving dignity and quality of life. Physicians should seek to aggressively manage the symptoms that endanger these goals. This must be done in early stages of the disease, the more moderate stages, and finally the advanced stages. The needs of patients in each stage are different, but the focus is always to preserve dignity and quality of life.

In early dementia, perhaps the most important job for the physician is to recognize and diagnose the disease and then to educate patients and their families about what they can expect. At this stage, patients can still make decisions for themselves. Physicians should ask patients about their preferences for medical treatments in the later stages of their disease and facilitate these important conversations between their patients and caregivers. Specific discussions about life-prolonging treatments, such as artificial nutrition and hydration, should take place. Physicians should ask patients to designate one or more primary decision makers to speak for them in preparation for later stages of disease when they are no longer able to make decisions for themselves. Patients should be encouraged to talk with their designated caregivers and loved ones about their views about advanced medical therapies such as feeding tubes, mechanical ventilation, and cardiopulmonary resuscitation (CPR). Although it is important to explore patients' specific preferences with regard to medical technology, it is equally important to explore the patients' values and goals of medical care: what is most important in their lives? What makes their lives worth living? What religious or spiritual values may be important? There is evidence that early conversations about advance directives help to prepare families for future decision making and may reduce the difficulty that comes with later surrogate decision making (40).

The early stages of Alzheimer's disease may be amenable to pharmacologic therapy with cholinesterase inhibitors. Treatment with these medications may improve performance in activities of daily living, modestly improve cognitive function, or slow the progression of the disease process. Aggressive control of vascular risk factors and the use of aspirin and cholesterol-lowering agents may slow the progress of vascular dementia. The goals of both types of therapies are to preserve independence for as long as possible.

Many patients with early-stage disease have concurrent psychiatric issues. Depression is especially common, affecting approximately 50% of the early Alzheimer's disease population (41). The symptoms of depression in early disease may be atypical and include indifference, difficulties with emotional engagement, and decreased motivation. Antidepressant therapies are often indicated, and cholinesterase inhibitors may be beneficial. Support groups may also be helpful at this stage of disease, both for patients and their caregivers.

Moderate-stage dementia is the longest stage of the disease. The physician's focus should be keeping the patient's environment safe, treating psychiatric symptoms, and supporting the patient's caregivers. As patients move to this more middle stage of disease, their need for supervision at home and help with performing activities of daily living become greater. Behavioral disturbances, agitation, and paranoia often occur in concert with increased dependence. These changes may become significant sources of caregiver stress. Palliative measures in moderate-level dementia include recognition and attention to caregiver stress, treatment of behavioral and psychiatric disturbance, and instituting environmental safety modifications. Additionally, patients with a moderate degree of cognitive impairment often exhibit impaired eating behaviors, and physicians must work with patients and their caregivers to meet nutritional demands, as well as modifying food products for easier mealtimes.

Caregiver stress is common, as relatives take on a more active and demanding role in the everyday routines of patients with progressive dementia. Many have never been in the role of primary caregiver for anyone other than their own children. Some primary caregivers may be geriatric patients themselves. Most families will face a high level of financial stress. Unless a patient has access to social services (Medicaid in the United States), out-of-pocket costs for additional help at home, pharmaceutical products, and durable medical equipment are high. Adult day programs may be hard to find, and respite programs are typically expensive. Patients with this degree of cognitive compromise may be difficult to place in nursing homes because often they do not carry other comorbid diagnoses, and the reimbursement rate for pure custodial care is low. Many caregivers leave their jobs or families behind to care for their loved ones. Some need to take on a second job to keep up with the financial burdens.

Caregivers may feel underappreciated because their loved ones fail to acknowledge how hard they are working or the sacrifices they are making. Eventually, patients fail to be able to even recognize who their caregivers are. These very real stresses need to be recognized, acknowledged, and supported. Physicians should question caregivers about fatigue, social isolation, depression, and physical symptoms. They should remind caregivers to take breaks and encourage other family members to help out. Caregiver support groups may also be helpful.

Behavioral disturbances become more frequent as dementia progresses. Although they may occur at any stage of disease, they are associated with increasing cognitive and functional decline. Symptoms include anxiety, depression, paranoia, delusions, hallucinations, sleep disorders, agitation, and combativeness. The presence of behavioral disturbance, especially paranoia and aggression, can increase the likelihood of nursing home placement. Treatment should be aimed at improving the quality of life of the patient and caregiver and should include both pharmacologic and nonpharmacologic considerations. Careful attention should be given to alternative causes of behavioral disturbance, such as uncontrolled pain, untreated infection, or suboptimal management of concurrent disease. Treatment of underlying medical illness may lead to sustained improvement in both cognitive status and behavior. In addition, the etiology of agitation may be based on basic human needs—hunger, thirst, or the need to change wet or soiled clothing. Identifying the root of the problem may be difficult, as patients with moderate degrees of dementia cannot tell their caregivers what exactly is bothering them. Nevertheless, the presence of a new behavioral disturbance should precipitate a medical evaluation and should not simply be considered a consequence of the underlying dementing illness.

Treating obvious etiologies as well as addressing possible modifications in the patient's care environment can be useful ways to address behavioral disturbances. For example, a careful history may demonstrate that agitated and paranoid behavior occurs at bath time. In this case, perhaps changing the water temperature or moving from a tub to a sponge bath may be less threatening for patients and lead to decreased agitation (42). Evidence suggests that involving patients actively in grooming routines may also decrease agitation. Calm environments, the use of usual routines, favorite pieces of music, and visits from children or pets may all be soothing. Attention to a patient's sleeping patterns is also important. Increasing daytime activities and decreasing daytime napping may help patients sleep better at night.

In addition to these behavioral interventions, low-dose standing or as-needed major tranquilizers, such as haloperidol, risperidone, or olanzapine, may be required to successfully manage behavioral disturbances and prevent hospital admissions. Bedtime dosing with major tranquilizers or with trazodone may help with sleep disturbances. Benzodiazepines may be associated with paradoxical agitation, excessive somnolence, and falls, and should be avoided in most patients.

Advanced dementia is the final stage of this terminal disease. Patients with end-stage dementia are dying. Research has demonstrated a median 6-month survival rate for patients with end-stage dementia, with or without tube feeding, although the range of survival times is wide (42–45). Most patients in this stage of disease are bedbound and nonverbal. Many patients in this stage of disease are placed in a nursing home because of their increasing care demands. Although comfort care and palliation of suffering should be the paramount focus of care, patients with advanced dementia often receive nonpalliative interventions at the end of life, such as tube feedings, CPR, mechanical ventilation, and systemic antibiotics in their final days of life (20,43,46,47).

Surrogate decision making in end-stage disease is inevitable. The process is made easier for all involved if, in the early stages of disease, the aforementioned critical discussions of treatment goals and end-of-life preferences have occurred. Caregivers may face multiple, difficult decisions, including emergency surgery, intubation, feeding tubes, and CPR. Even if the advance wishes were well communicated, it may still be difficult for family members to carry them out. Nonetheless, decisions should always be based on previously expressed wishes (if known) and the best interest of the patient with respect to the potential benefits or burdens of the proposed treatment. Physicians should offer caregivers continued support and offer them regular and repeated reviews of the goals of treatment and the expectations that follow interventions.

Comfort measures and the relief of suffering should be the primary palliative goals. Careful attention to potential sources of discomfort, such as pain and concurrent illness, is important. Pain is very commonly overlooked and undertreated in this population. Analgesic therapy should be empiric and preventive if an underlying source exists or the patient faces potentially uncomfortable procedures such as dressing changes or position changes. Physicians should also recognize that patients with advanced dementia may experience more discomfort from routine procedures, such as vital signs monitoring, phlebotomy, finger sticks, and bladder catheterizations, because they cannot understand what is being done to them and why. Unnecessary procedures should be discontinued. Topical anesthetic preparations may make the necessary procedures more bearable.

CONCLUSION

As a result of the unprecedented improvements in maternal and infant mortality and successes in the control, if not cure, of common chronic diseases, most people who die in the United States are old and frail. Conservative projections suggest that in the next 30 years, we will see a dramatic shift in demographics, with over 20% of the United States population being over age 65 in the year 2030. The elderly die of chronic, progressive illnesses (such as end-stage heart and lung disease, cancer, stroke, and dementia). These diseases have unpredictable clinical courses and prognoses, and current care systems are not well adapted to the trajectory of illness or the clinical needs of this group of patients. In contrast to younger adults, older adults often have unrecognized and untreated symptoms, cognitive impairment, and an extremely high prevalence of functional dependency and associated family caregiver burden. It is clear that our current systems of reimbursement are ill equipped to provide primary care with continuity, support for family caregivers, and home care and nursing home services. Because care for a frail, older adult typically includes preventive, life-prolonging rehabilitation and

palliative measures in varying proportions and intensity based on the individual patient's needs and preferences, any new models of care will have to be responsive to this range of service requirements. Several "mixed management" models of care have recently been proposed to address the needs of the frail elderly. They include the program of all-inclusive care for the elderly (PACE) Demonstration Program (48), a capitated Medicare and Medicaid waiver program, and the *MediCaring* model (49,50), a program targeted at patients with advanced heart and lung disease. But these programs have to date targeted only a small percentage of the growing number of older adults. Future research needs to be targeted at understanding the palliative care needs of older adults, developing medical interventions that address these needs, and developing models and systems of care that will meet the global needs of these patients and their families.

References

1. Miller RA. The biology of aging and longevity. In: Hazzard WR, Blass JP, Ettinger WH, et al., eds. *Principles of geriatric medicine and gerontology.* New York: McGraw-Hill, 1999:1–19.
2. Fries J. Aging, natural death and the compression of morbidity. *N Engl J Med* 1990;303:130.
3. Avorn J, Gurwitz J. Principles of pharmacology. In: Cassell C, Cohen H, Larson E, et al., eds. *Geriatric medicine,* 3rd ed. New York: Springer-Verlag, 1997.
4. Perneger TV, Whelton PK, Klag MJ. Risk of kidney failure associated with the use of acetaminophen, aspirin, and nonsteroidal antiinflammatory drugs. *N Engl J Med* 1994;331:1675–1679.
5. Ferrell B. Pain management in elderly people. *J Am Geriatr Soc* 1991; 39:64–73.
6. Harkins S. Pain perceptions in the old. *Clin Geriatr Med* 1996;12:435–459.
7. Olshansky SJ. Demography of aging. In: Cassel CK, Cohen HJ, Larson EB, et al., eds. *Geriatric medicine,* 3rd ed. New York: Springer-Verlag, 1997.
8. Meier D, Morrison R. Old age and care near the end of life. *Generations* 1999;23:6–11.
9. The SUPPORT Principal Investigators. A controlled trial to improve care for seriously ill hospitalized patients. The study to understand prognoses and preferences for outcomes and risks of treatments (SUPPORT). *JAMA* 1995;274:1591–1598.
10. Keay TJ, Fredman L, Taler GA, et al. Indicators of quality medical care for the terminally ill in nursing homes. *J Am Geriatr Soc* 1994;42:853–860.
11. Engle VF. Care of the living, care of the dying: reconceptualizing nursing home care. *J Am Geriatr Soc* 1998;46:1172–1174.
12. Lubitz JD, Riley FF. Trends in medicare payments in the last year of life. *N Engl J Med* 1993;328:1092–1096.
13. Covinsky KE, Landefeld CS, Teno J, et al. Is economic hardship on the families of the seriously ill associated with patient and surrogate care preferences? SUPPORT investigators. *Arch Intern Med* 1996;156:1737–1741.
14. Emanuel EJ, Fairclough DL, Slutsman J, et al. Assistance from family members, friends, paid caregivers, and volunteers in the care of terminally ill patients. *N Engl J Med* 1999;341:956–963.
15. Ferrell B. Overview of aging and pain. In: Ferrell BR, Ferrell BA, eds. *Pain in the elderly: a report of the task force on pain in the Elderly of the International Association for the study of pain.* Seattle,WA: IASP Press, 1996.
16. Seale C, Cartwright A. *The year before death.* Brookfield, WI: Ashgate Publishing Co, 1994.
17. Bernabei R, Gambassi G, Lapane K, et al. Management of pain in elderly patients with cancer. *JAMA* 1998;279:1877–1882.
18. Teno JM, Weitzen S, Wetle T, et al. Persistent pain in nursing home residents. *JAMA* 2001;285:2081.
19. Feldt KS, Ryden MB, Miles S. Treatment of pain in cognitively impaired compared with cognitively intact older patients with hip-fracture. *J Am Geriatr Soc* 1998;46:1079–1085.
20. Morrison RS, Siu AL. A comparison of pain and its treatment in advanced dementia and cognitively intact patients with hip fracture. *J Pain Symptom Manage* 2000;19:240–248.
21. Cleeland CS, Gonin R, Hatfield AK, et al. Pain and its treatment in outpatients with metastatic cancer. *N Engl J Med* 1994;330:592–596.
22. Stein W. Cancer pain in the elderly. In: Ferrell BR, Ferrell BA, eds. *Pain in the elderly: a report of the task force on pain in the Elderly of the International Association for the study of pain.* Seattle, WA: IASP Press, 1996.
23. American Geriatrics Society. The management of chronic pain in older persons: AGS panel on chronic pain in older persons. *J Am Geriatr Soc* 1998;46:635–651.
24. Parmelee P. Pain in cognitively impaired older persons. *Clin Geriatr Med* 1996;12:473–487.

25. Ferrell BA, Ferrell BR, Rivera LSO. Pain in cognitively impaired nursing home patients. *J Pain Symptom Manage* 1995;10:591–598.
26. Sengstaken E, King S. The problem of pain and its detection among geriatric nursing home residents. *J Am Geriatr Soc* 1993;41:541–544.
27. Duggleby W, Lander J. Cognitive status and postoperative pain: older adults. *J Pain Symptom Manage* 1994;9:19–27.
28. Lynch EP, Lazor MA, Gellis JE, et al. The impact of postoperative pain on the development of postoperative delirium. *Anesth Analg* 1998;86:781–785.
29. Morrison RS, Magaziner J, Gilbert M, et al. Relationship between pain and opioid analgesics on the development of delirium following hip fracture. *J Gerontol A Biol Sci Med Sci* 2003;58:76–81.
30. Mateo OM, Krenzischek DA. A pilot study to assess the relationship between behavioral manifestations and self-report of pain in postanesthesia care unit patients. *J Post Anesth Nurs* 1992;7:15–21.
31. Le Resche L, Dworkin S. Facial expressions of pain and emotions in chronic TMD patients. *Pain* 1988;35:71–78.
32. Strom BL, Berlin JA, Kinman JL, et al. Parenteral ketorolac and risk of gastrointestinal and operative site bleeding. A postmarketing surveillance study. *JAMA* 1996;275:376–382.
33. Camu F, Lauwers MH, Vanlersberghe C. Side effects of NSAIDs and dosing recommendations for ketorolac. *Acta Anaesthesiol Belg* 1996;47:143–149.
34. Maliekal J, Elboim CM. Gastrointestinal complications associated with intramuscular ketorolac tromethamine therapy in the elderly. *Ann Pharmacother* 1995;29:698–701.
35. Watson DJ, Harper SE, Zhao PL, et al. Gastrointestinal tolerability of the selective cyclooxygenase-2 (COX-2) inhibitor rofecoxib compared with nonselective COX-1 and COX-2 inhibitors in osteoarthritis. *Arch Intern Med* 2000;160:2998–3003.
36. Langman MJ, Jensen DM, Watson DJ, et al. Adverse upper gastrointestinal effects of rofecoxib compared with NSAIDs. *JAMA* 1999;282:1929–1933.
37. Silverstein FE, Faich G, Goldstein JL, et al. Gastrointestinal toxicity with celecoxib vs nonsteroidal anti-inflammatory drugs for osteoarthritis and rheumatoid arthritis: the CLASS study: a randomized controlled trial. Celecoxib Long-term Arthritis Safety Study. *JAMA* 2000;284:1247–1255.
38. Mukherjee D, Nissen SE, Topol EJ. Risk of cardiovascular events associated with selective COX-2 inhibitors. *JAMA* 2001;286:954–959.
39. Macintyre PE, Jarvis DA. Age is the best predictor of postoperative morphine requirements. *Pain* 1996;64:357–364.
40. Tilden VP, Tolle SW, Nelson CA, et al. Family decision-making to withdraw life-sustaining treatments from hospitalized patients. *Nurs Res* 2001;50:105–115.
41. Wells DL, Dawson P, Sidani S, et al. Effects of an abilities-focused program of morning care on residents who have dementia and on caregivers. *J Am Geriatr Soc* 2000;48:442–449.
42. Meier DE, Ahronheim JC, Morris J, et al. High short-term mortality in hospitalized patients with advanced dementia: lack of benefit of tube feeding. *Arch Intern Med* 2001;161:594–599.
43. Morrison RS, Siu AL. Survival in end-stage dementia following acute illness. *JAMA* 2000;284:47–52.
44. Fabiszewski KJ, Volicer B, Volicer L. Effect of antibiotic treatment on outcome of fevers in institutionalized Alzheimer patients. *JAMA* 1990;263:3168–3172.
45. Luchins DJ, Hanrahan P, Murphy K. Criteria for enrolling dementia patients in hospice [See comments]. *J Am Geriatr Soc* 1997;45:1054–1059.
46. Ahronheim J, Morrison R, Morris J, et al. Palliative care in advanced dementia: a randomized controlled trial and descriptive analysis. *J Palliat Med* 2000;3:265–273.
47. Ahronheim JC, Morrison RS, Baskin SA, et al. Treatment of the dying in the acute care hospital. Advanced dementia and metastatic cancer. *Arch Intern Med* 1996;156:2094–2100.
48. Eng C, Pedulla J, Eleazer GP, et al. Program of all-inclusive care for the elderly (PACE): an innovative model of integrated geriatric care and financing [See comments]. *J Am Geriatr Soc* 1997;45:223–232.
49. Lynn J. Caring at the end of our lives [Editorial; Comment]. *N Engl J Med* 1996;335:201–202.
50. Field MJ, Cassel CK, Institute of Medicine. *Approaching death: improving care at the end of life*. Washington, DC: National Academy Press, 1997.

CHAPTER 75 ■ PALLIATIVE CARE IN HIV/AIDS

PETER A. SELWYN

In its beginning phases in the United States in the 1980s, acquired immunodeficiency syndrome (AIDS) care was understood almost fully within the context of palliative care, and many hospice and palliative care clinicians became expert at managing the complex medical, psychological, spiritual, and broader societal issues that were routinely generated by the care of patients with advanced human immunodeficiency virus (HIV)/AIDS. However in a relatively rapid timeframe—beginning in the late 1980s and accelerating dramatically with the advent of the protease inhibitor class of antiretroviral therapy agents in 1996—AIDS became a "manageable" disease and quickly resulted in a growing medicalization and subspecialization of care which defines the current paradigm of HIV treatment. Although these rapid therapeutic advances,—collectively referred to as highly active antiretroviral therapy, or highly active antiretroviral therapy (HAART)—have provided great benefit to people living with AIDS, an unintended consequence of the HAART era has been the further separation of HIV/AIDS care from palliative care, and an increasing tendency to dismiss the importance of comprehensive palliative as well as disease-specific therapy for patients with AIDS and their families. The intent of this review is to highlight the many ways in which palliative and disease-specific therapy for HIV can and should coexist in an integrated model in order to meet the complex needs of patients now living with AIDS. Palliative care interventions remain important in the routine care of patients with HIV/AIDS across the continuum of care, not only in order to improve quality of life and address the wide range of medical and psychosocial issues related to chronic, progressive illness, but also to help enhance adherence with HIV-specific therapies, and as a consequence, potentially improve morbidity and mortality as well.

EPIDEMIOLOGY

Improvements in antiretroviral therapy, especially with the advent of the protease inhibitor class of antiretroviral agents in the mid 1990s, resulted in dramatic decreases in HIV-related mortality in the developed world, with declines in AIDS death rates of 50–60% in the United States and Europe occurring between 1996 and 2000 (1–5) (Fig. 75.1). However, several points must be noted:

1. The rate of decline in death rates has leveled off since 2000, and there remain approximately 15,000 deaths per year in the United States in patients with AIDS (3)

2. An increasing number of these deaths have resulted not necessarily from end-stage HIV disease but rather from other important and often untreatable comorbidities, such as cirrhosis and liver failure because of chronic hepatic C, hepatitis B, and/or alcohol-related liver disease, as well as non–AIDS-defining cancers which occur in greater than expected frequency in patients with AIDS, such as lung, gastrointestinal, and head and neck cancers. Indeed, in several series, mortality from these non–AIDS-defining comorbidities have accounted for up to 50% of all deaths among patients with AIDS in the past few years (6–11). Of these, hepatitis C is perhaps the most significant, given the high prevalence of hepatitis C among HIV-infected drug users generally 75% or higher in most series—as well as recent data suggesting more rapid progression to cirrhosis and death in coinfected patients, and the likelihood that drug users as a group may be less likely to receive therapy with interferon and ribavirin than other patient groups (12,13). In some respects, ironically, it is the prolonged survival with HIV/AIDS in the HAART era that has left patients vulnerable to growing mortality risks from end-organ failure, malignancies, and other chronic, progressive diseases that previously had not posed major risks because patients died before having had the time to develop them (7,14,15)

3. Disparities in access and adherence with HIV-specific antiretroviral therapy have also resulted in differential mortality risk in subpopulations of people with AIDS, such that AIDS-related mortality has diminished less among women, racial-ethnic minorities, and injection drug users than it has among caucasian men, and HIV/AIDS remains a leading cause of death for young African American and Hispanic men and women in the 20–50 year age range (3,16)

4. Toxicities from antiretroviral therapies (17,18), and other challenges to adherence and maintenance of effective treatment regimens over time, have resulted in patients for whom there are few therapeutic options, and in whom antiretroviral therapy may no longer be effective in preventing disease progression and decreasing mortality risk

5. Overall decreases in AIDS deaths, together with no decrease in the incidence of new HIV infections, have resulted in an increased prevalence of HIV infection, including a larger number of people living with symptomatic HIV disease for longer periods of time (3,16);

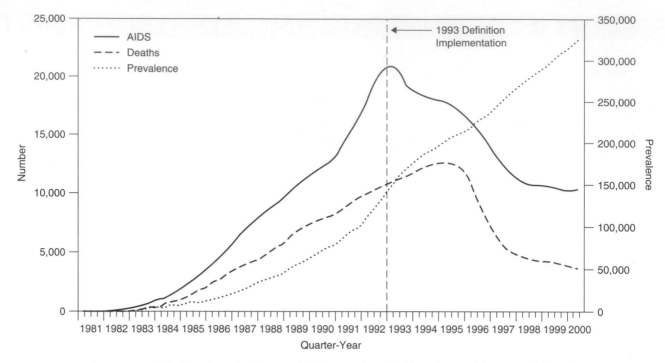

FIGURE 75.1. Estimated acquired immunodeficiency syndrome incidence (adjusted for reported delays), deaths, and prevalence, by quarter-year of diagnosis/death—United States, 1981–2000. (CDC. MMWR 2001;50:430–434).

6. With the bulk of antiretroviral therapy still regrettably limited to the developed world, palliative care for HIV/AIDS remains an important element of AIDS care worldwide, and will continue to be relevant even as the benefits of therapy are extended to the millions of people worldwide who urgently need it

All of these trends lead to the conclusion that there is an important and ongoing need for effective and expert palliative care interventions for the care of patients with HIV/AIDS in both the developed and developing world, and that the goal of comprehensive AIDS care must be to integrate palliative and disease-specific therapy on both individual and programmatic levels, across the continuum of disease, including but by no means limited to the end-of-life and late-stage disease (19). In many ways, in fact, AIDS in the HAART era has become less of a rapidly and uniformly fatal disease (similar to an aggressive and untreatable cancer), and more of a chronic, progressive illnesses [similar to congestive heart failure, chronic obstructive pulmonary disease (COPD), etc.], with all of the challenges that are posed in palliative care practice for conditions for which the prognosis and clinical course can be quite variable (19,20).

PAIN AND SYMPTOM MANAGEMENT

Since early in the epidemic, patients with AIDS have been documented to have a high prevalence of pain and other symptoms (21–35). Pain in AIDS has been believed to be a result of one or more of the following major categories:

1. AIDS-related opportunistic infections (e.g., cryptococcal meningitis, invasive herpes or measles virus (MV) infections, esophageal candidiasis)
2. HIV-related neurotoxicity (e.g., distal symmetric polyneuropathy (DSP), mononeuritis multiplex)

3. Medication toxicity (e.g., dideoxynucleoside peripheral neuropathy, didanosine-induced pancreatitis, zidovudine-induced headache)
4. Coexisting painful conditions (e.g., musculoskeletal pain, trauma, and other sequelae of injection drug use) and
5. Other nonspecific entities (e.g., the observed association between HIV infection and headache)

(See Table 75.1 for a summary of common pain-producing infections and neoplasms in patients with AIDS, and Table 75.2 for a summary of the types of pain that may be associated with the use of antiretroviral and other HIV-related therapies.) As is true in other conditions in addition to AIDS, the most effective treatment for AIDS-related pain may sometimes be disease specific [e.g., anti-CMV therapy for cytomegalovirus (CMV) esophagitis or colitis], sometimes more nonspecific (e.g., opioids and adjuvants for the neuropathic pain of DSP), and sometimes both (e.g., fluconazole plus a mucositis "cocktail" for odynophagia caused by esophageal candidiasis).

Pain management in patients with HIV/AIDS should follow the same basic principles as in other patient populations, with several important qualifications:

1. Pain in patients with AIDS tends to be underdiagnosed and undertreated (23,36,37), and most HIV care tends to be provided within a disease-specific framework (i.e., identifying a specific opportunistic infection and treating it), in which the focus on pain *per se* is minimal or secondary to the emphasis on diagnosing and treating specific HIV-related complications. As a result, patients are at risk for undertreatment of pain unless this is specifically addressed by clinicians capable of responding effectively.
2. Frequently, there is also a reluctance among physicians to prescribe opioid analgesics to drug-using patients, which is problematic given the high prevalence of current or prior substance use among injecting drug-using patients with HIV/AIDS (38,39). In effect, this means in practice

TABLE 75.1

PAIN-PRODUCING INFECTIONS AND NEOPLASMS

Infectious etiology

Pain site/Type	Oropharynx	Esophagus	Abdomen	HA	Chest	Biliary	Cutaneous	Anorectal	Peripheral neuropathy	Arthritis/ Arthralgia	Myopathy/ Polymyositis
HBV	—	—	X	—	—	—	—	—	—	X	—
HSV	X	X	—	—	—	—	X	X	—	—	—
HCV	—	—	X	—	—	—	—	—	—	X	—
CMV	X	X	X	—	—	X	—	—	X	—	—
HIV	—	—	—	X	—	—	—	—	X	X	X
EBV	X	—	—	—	—	—	—	—	—	—	—
Toxoplasmosis	—	—	—	X	—	—	—	—	—	—	—
Fungi, e.g. Candida	X	X	—	—	—	—	—	—	—	—	—
Microsporidiosis	—	—	X	—	—	X	—	—	—	—	—
MAC	—	—	X	—	—	X	—	—	—	—	—
Cryptococosis	—	—	—	X	—	—	—	—	—	—	—
Cryptosporidiosis	—	—	X	—	—	X	—	—	—	—	—
VZV	—	X	—	—	—	—	X	—	—	—	—
Salmonella Shigella Campylo-bacter	—	—	X	—	—	X	—	—	—	—	—
Neoplastic Etiology											
Kaposi's sarcoma	—	X	X	X	X	—	—	—	—	—	—
Lymphoma	—	X	X	X	X	—	—	—	—	—	—

HA, headache; HBV, hepatitis B virus; HSV, herpes simplex virus; HCV, herpes C virus; CMV, cytomegalovirus; HIV, human immunodeficiency virus; EBV, Epstein Barr virus; MAC, *mycobacterium avium* complex; VZV, varicella zoster virus.
Rainone F, Selwyn PA. Pain in Human Immunodeficiency Virus (HIV) and Acquired Immune Deficiency Syndrome (AIDS). In Schmidt RF, Willis WD, eds. *Encyclopedic reference of pain*. New York: Springer-Verlag, 2005.

TABLE 75.2

HUMAN IMMUNODEFICIENCY VIRUS–RELATED THERAPEUTIC AGENTS THAT MAY CAUSE PAIN[a]

Class/Agent	Headache	Peripheral neuropathy	Pancreatitis	Abdominal pain	Hepatitis	Nephrolithiasis
NRTIs						
Zidovudine	X	—	—	X	X	—
Lamivudine	—	—	X	—	X	—
Emtricitabine	X	—	—	—	X	—
Didanosine	—	X	X	X	X	—
Stavudine	—	X	X	—	X	—
Abacavir	—	—	—	X	—	—
Zalcitabine	—	X	X	X	X	—
NTRTI						
Tenofovir	X	—	—	—	—	—
NNRTI						
Nevirapine	—	—	—	—	X	—
Efavirenz	X	—	—	—	—	—
Delavirdine	X	—	—	—	—	—
PI						
Ritonavir	—	—	—	X	X	—
Indinavir	—	—	—	X	X	X
Saquinavir	—	—	—	X	X	—
Atazanavir	—	—	—	X	X	—
(Fos) amprenavir	—	—	—	X	X	—
Lopinavir	—	—	—	X	X	—
Nelfinavir	—	—	—	X	X	—
Tipranavir	—	—	—	X	X	—

NRTI, nucleoside reverse transcriptase inhibitor; NTRTI, nucleotide reverse transcriptase inhibitor; NNRTI, non-nucleoside reverse transcriptase inhibitor; PI, protease inhibitor.
[a]'Xs' indicate most commonly reported pain syndromes in association with different HIV-related therapeutic agents, although this may be seen with lesser frequency with agents not so indicated here.
Rainone F, Selwyn PA. Pain in Human Immunodeficiency Virus (HIV) and Acquired Immune Deficiency Syndrome (AIDS). In Schmidt RF, Willis WD, eds. *Encyclopedic reference of pain*. New York: Springer-Verlag, 2005.

that a history of substance use is also a risk factor for untreated or undertreated pain. Physicians have a professional obligation to diagnose and treat pain in patients with AIDS and substance use disorders, although this will require attention to their need for substance abuse treatment as well, if necessary, in collaboration with addiction medicine specialists. Palliative care physicians are also particularly well situated to help manage the complex interplay of pain, psychosocial issues, and concerns about addiction in patients with advanced diseases.

3. There is a wide range of common neuropathic pain syndromes in patients with AIDS (40–44), and these have increased in prevalence with longer survival because of HAART—another example of the ways in which the benefits of antiretroviral therapy have sometimes led inadvertently to new clinical challenges in palliative care and pain management (45). Moreover, some of the same medications which have helped prolong life as part of basic antiretroviral regimens (e.g., didanosine, stavudine, zalcitabine) can themselves cause peripheral neuropathy, which can further complicate regimen choice and the balance between disease-modifying and palliative agendas.

4. Some of the medications used in treating HIV/AIDS and related conditions (e.g., non-nucleoside reverse transcriptase inhibitors, protease inhibitors, rifamycins) can potentially be involved in pharmacokinetic interactions with opioids, anticonvulsants, benzodiazepines, and other medications used in pain management and palliative care, given their metabolism through the hepatic cytochrome P-450 enzyme system (46,47).

As a result of these and other related issues which pertain to the balance and coordination of palliative and disease-specific care, the management of pain in patients with AIDS is perhaps even more challenging and complex than in the pre-HAART era, which highlights the importance of expert palliative care input into the total care of this patient population.

PAIN IN SUBSTANCE USERS

Studies have suggested that chronic opioid addicts, including patients on chronic methadone maintenance, may have a lower threshold for painful stimuli than comparison groups (48,49). In addition, the phenomenon of pharmacologic tolerance suggests that when narcotic analgesics are used in opioid dependent patients, they may need *higher* doses, which may sometimes need to be given at even *more frequent* intervals, than in non–opioid-dependent individuals (50). (Unfortunately, this is not the first response of most clinicians outside of palliative care settings, and indeed many clinicians' ambivalence or discomfort about prescribing opioids to substance abusers often leads predictably to underdosing, which may lead to acting out or drug-seeking behavior by the patient, which reinforces the negative stereotypes harbored by the provider, etc.) Lastly, there remains the possibility that these patients may in fact be more likely to misuse or manipulate their prescriptions of controlled drugs than other patient populations, so particular safeguards and systems need to be implemented to minimize the risk of abuse. Indeed, one study which compared prescription drug misuse among patients with cancer and AIDS found that the latter group was far more likely to have misused prescribed analgesics, obtained analgesic medication from friends or on the street, and so on, demonstrating that one cannot treat pain effectively without also addressing the underlying drug use behaviors in this population (51). Another study has suggested a framework for assessing the likelihood of drug abuse–related behaviors concerning the use of narcotic analgesics in patients at risk for substance abuse, which can assist clinicians in identifying

---

TABLE 75.3

SPECTRUM OF ABERRANT DRUG-RELATED BEHAVIORS OCCURRING DURING TREATMENT WITH NARCOTIC ANALGESICS

LESS SUGGESTIVE OF ADDICTION

Aggressive complaining about the need for more drugs
Drug hoarding during periods of reduced symptoms
Requesting specific drugs
Openly acquiring similar drugs from other medical sources
Occasional unsanctioned does escalation or other noncompliance
Unapproved use of the drug to treat another symptom
Reporting psychic effects not intended by the clinician
Resistance to change in therapy associated with tolerable adverse effects
Intense expressions of anxiety about recurrent symptoms
Concept of "pseudo addiction"

MORE SUGGESTIVE OF ADDICTION

Reports of "lost" or "stolen" prescriptions
Selling prescription drugs
Prescription forgery
Stealing drugs from others
Injecting oral formulations
Obtaining prescription drugs from nonmedical sources
Concurrent abuse of alcohol or illicit drugs
Repeated dose escalations or similar noncompliance despite multiple warnings
Repeated visits to other clinicians or emergency rooms without informing the prescriber
Drug-related deterioration in function at work, in the family, or socially
Repeated resistance to changes in therapy despite evidence of adverse drug effects

Passik SD, Portenoy RK. Substance abuse issues in palliative care. In: Berger A, ed. *Principles and practice of supportive oncology.* Philadelphia, PA: Lippincott Williams & Wilkins, 1998:513–529.

high risk patients (Table 75.3) (52). Another study suggests a screening tool to help identify patients at risk for opioid prescription misuse (53).

Commonly effective safeguards to help prevent prescription drug misuse include the following (54–56):

1. Setting clear limits on the amount and frequency of controlled drug prescriptions
2. Limiting the prescribing clinician to one person whenever possible
3. Establishing a clear and consistent policy that "lost" or "stolen" prescriptions will not be replaced
4. Dispensing only small amounts of medication in cases when abuse is suspected to be a risk
5. Enlisting responsible family members or other caregivers to help manage controlled drug supplies
6. Using less "tempting" alternatives whenever possible (e.g., high-dose nonsteroidal anti-inflammatory drug (NSAID)s, liberal use of adjuvants for neuropathic pain, weak opioids, or tramadol when feasible, etc.) and
7. Having clear contingency planning or contracting for the consequences of patients' misuse of prescribed medications, which may be stipulated in advance with the patient, and which may include the possibility that the prescriber will decline to continue to prescribe this medication if the patient shows evidence of abusing the agreement between them (57). [See Ref. (57)] for discussion of opioid contracts.)
8. Making full use of the multi-disciplinary team, facilitate communication and information sharing about problematic patient behaviors to prevent staff "splitting," and provide mutual support in working with these sometimes challenging patients
9. Consulting effectively with addictionologists and other substance abuse treatment professionals as part of the palliative care/pain management team. It should also be recognized that for patients on methadone maintenance, their single daily dose of methadone provides no analgesic effect, and they require additional short- or long-acting narcotics in the event that strong analgesia is needed. Their underlying tolerance to opioids also requires that they receive higher and more frequent dosing than would normally be initiated in opioid-naive patients. Theoretically, one could argue from a pharmacotherapeutic standpoint that such patients might be treated both for their opioid dependence and their chronic pain needs by the use of increasing methadone

dosing given on a thrice daily schedule as opposed to maintaining their ongoing daily methadone dose and supplementing this with additional short or long-acting narcotics (58). Although this option may be available in some settings, the regulatory and programmatic guidelines which govern the operation of methadone maintenance treatment programs frequently preclude this possibility (54,59). (One exception or special circumstance may occur at the end of life, when patients are largely home- or bedbound, and if their pain requirements are such that they need a continuous subcutaneous opioid infusion, the total daily opioid requirement including the underlying standing daily methadone dose can be converted to a single opioid for continuous infusion, which can then be managed like any other such system in patients with severe pain and advanced disease.)

In addition to pain management and drug interactions (the latter is discussed in more detail in the following text), it should be noted that there are important ways in which methadone maintenance and HIV treatment overlap in the clinical context. Given the high prevalence of HIV infection among drug users, methadone maintenance programs have long been identified as important sites for providing care to drug users with or at risk for HIV. Successful examples exist of different models for combining HIV care and drug abuse treatment within methadone maintenance programs (60–64), as well as coordination with palliative care services for patients with late-stage disease or complicated pain management (65). Lastly, recent studies also suggest the potential importance of buprenorphine maintenance as a comparable substitution therapy to methadone, with the advantage that buprenorphine may be prescribed in primary care settings outside of drug treatment programs (66,67), and with the added benefit that it may be less likely to cause significant drug–drug interactions through the cytochrome P-450 system (68). Regardless of the drug treatment modality, palliative care clinicians need to work closely with HIV specialists and addictionologists in order to provide effective care to HIV-infected drug users with multiple medical and psychosocial comorbidities.

NEUROPATHIC PAIN SYNDROMES

Patients with AIDS have been found to be at risk for a wide range of neuropathic pain syndromes, occurring at different stages of HIV disease progression (40–44,69–73). Table 75.4

TABLE 75.4

HUMAN IMMUNODEFICIENCY VIRUS (HIV)-ASSOCIATED NEUROPATHIES

Type	Stage of disease	Course/Frequency	Symptoms
DSP	Mid to late	Indolent, protracted Common	Distal pain, paresthesias, and numbness especially in feet
Toxic	All	Common	Same
IDP			
Acute	Any stage	Rare	Global limb weakness
Chronic	Mid to late stages	Rare	Global limb weakness
PP	Advanced	Rare, may show rapid progression	Cauda equina syndrome. Saddle anesthesia
		May be associated with CMV infection	May respond to anti-CMV therapy if infection present
MM	Early, late	Infrequent	Self-limited multifocal motor
			sensory, or mixed somatic or cranial neuropathy
AN	All	Common (subclinical)	Varied

DSP, distal sensory polyneuropathy; IDP, inflammatory demyelinating polyneuropathy; PP, progressive polyradiculopathy; CMV, cytomegalovirus; MM, mononeuropathy multiplex: AN, autonomic neuropathy.

summarizes the major disease entities along with some of their clinical characteristics. The most common HIV-related neuropathic syndrome is the DSP, which primarily involves the distal lower extremities, particularly the soles of the feet but sometimes more extensive, and is associated with allodynia, burning or tingling pain, decreased vibratory sensation, and relative preservation of motor function. Reflexes may be diminished as well. Pain can be aching, most severe on the bottoms of the feet; patients may find it difficult to wear shoes and have antalgic gait. This syndrome is clinically difficult to distinguish from the distal bilateral peripheral neuropathy associated with the use of the reverse transcriptate inhibitors didanosine and stavudine (as well as the less commonly use agent zalcita zalcitabine), however, in the case of medication-induced peripheral neuropathy the symptoms often subside within weeks of stopping the medication, although pain may persist in up to one third of patients. [See Ref. (96) and http://aidsinfo.nih.gov for more information about specific agents.] The occurrence of DSP has been associated with elevated HIV viral loads in serum, suggesting that effective HAART may in fact help prevent this condition, although its incidence has steadily increased in the HAART era because of prolonged survival, and it may occur or persist even in patients with good virologic control. Treatment has been attempted with a variety of agents (41,74–78); some have been found to have no benefit (e.g., peptide T, topical capsaicin cream), and others have had demonstrated efficacy in clinical trials (e.g., lamotrigine). Many adjuvant medications exist for the treatment of neuropathic pain in conjunction with NSAID's and/or opioids. A combination of a weak or strong opioid together with an anti-convulsant such as lamotrigine, gabapentin, carbamazepine, or less commonly one of the tricyclic antidepressants, can usually be used with moderate to good results. Experimental studies with recombinant nerve growth factor suggested possible efficacy, but this product is not available, not being in commercial development at this time. More recent preliminary studies have suggested possible benefit from a transdermal capsaicin patch, and smoked marijuana (which is also available as oral dronabinol), in the treatment of chronic neuropathic pain in AIDS (79,80). Treatment of the other HIV-related neuropathies in addition to DSP is supportive and symptom-based, with the exception of the progressive polyradiculopathy syndrome, which may be caused by CMV infection, in which case specific antiviral therapy with valganciclovir, foscarnet, or cidofovir may be of benefit.

In addition to peripheral neuropathy syndromes, and aside from the well-known central nervous system (CNS) opportunistic infections seen in AIDS (e.g., cryptococcal meningitis, cerebral toxoplasmosis, progressive multifocal leukoencephalopathy), patients with AIDS are also at risk for a range of myelopathy syndromes, including the vacuolar myelopathy which was described early in the epidemic, and which continues to occur even in the HAART era. The etiology of AIDS-related myelopathy is not well understood, and although uncommon, may represent another condition such as DSP which may increase in frequency with longer survival because of HAART. Myelopathy generally involves the cervical and/or thoracic cord, and often results in spastic paraparesis or paraplegia, with loss of bowel and bladder function. Apart from causing symptomatic neurologic deficits, patients with myelopathy syndromes and AIDS may also experience painful muscle spasms, and be at risk from infectious complications caused by skin breakdown because of immobility, and urinary tract infections and sepsis caused by bladder dysfunction. All of these potential complications suggest the need for excellent palliative care and nursing practice to help minimize these adverse outcomes.

SYMPTOM MANAGEMENT IN ACQUIRED IMMUNODEFICIENCY SYNDROME

In addition to pain, patients with AIDS have been found to have a high prevalence of other symptoms, in studies both prior to and including the HAART era (Table 75.5). A number of studies have demonstrated a remarkable consistency in the prevalence of common symptoms, primarily in but not limited to patients with advanced disease (81). These symptoms include a mixture of medical and mental health symptoms (e.g., anorexia, fatigue, anxiety, nausea/vomiting, diarrhea, depression); like with pain, sometimes the best symptom management intervention may be disease-specific (e.g., antiretroviral therapy for fatigue and weight loss), and sometimes nonspecific and supportive (e.g., dronabinol for nausea and anorexia).

Consistent with the basic principles of palliative care, the decision whether and how to treat specific symptoms should be made within the context of the intended goals of care, and an assessment of the risks-benefits of specific types of interventions in relation to patient and family wishes. For example, in some patients for whom recovery of function and improvement in immunologic status is a viable and desired option, treating disseminated *mycobacterium avium* complex (MAC) infection is probably best done with combination antimycobacterial therapy (i.e., azithromycin, ethambutol), whereas in others with late-stage disease who are primarily receiving supportive care, a combination of prednisone and nonsteroidal anti-inflammatory drugs might provide enhanced symptom relief without undesirable medication toxicity. A listing of common symptoms in AIDS and potential disease-specific and supportive interventions is presented in Table 75.6.

In addition to the treatment interventions commonly used in other palliative care patient populations, it is important to highlight two areas in the realm of constitutional symptoms where symptom management in AIDS can have a profound impact on quality of life, patient functioning, and even the stigma and psychological burden which continue to be important for patients living with AIDS and their families. For anorexia and wasting, successful palliative interventions can include

TABLE 75.5

PREVALENCE OF SYMPTOMS IN PATIENTS WITH ACQUIRED IMMUNODEFICIENCY SYNDROME (AIDS)[a]

Symptoms	Percentage range
Fatigue or lack of energy	48–45
Weight loss	37–91
Pain	29–76
Anorexia	26–51
Anxiety	25–40
Insomnia	21–50
Cough	19–60
Nausea or vomiting	17–43
Dyspnea or respiratory symptoms	15–48
Depression or sadness	15–40
Diarrhea	11–32
Constipation	10–29

[a]Based on available descriptive studies of patients with AIDS, predominantly in patient with late-stage disease, 1990–2002.

TABLE 75.6

COMMON SYMPTOMS IN PATIENTS WITH ACQUIRED IMMUNODEFICIENCY SYNDROME (AIDS) AND POSSIBLE DISEASE-SPECIFIC AND SYMPTOM-SPECIFIC INTERVENTIONS

		Possible causes	Disease-specific Rx	Symptom-specific Rx
Constitutional	Fatigue, weakness	AIDS Opportunistic infections Anemia	HAART Treat specific infections, erythropoietin, transfusion	Corticosteroids (prednisone, dexamethasone) Psychostimulants (methylphenidine, pemoline, dextroamphetamine, modafinil)
	Weight loss/anorexia	HIV Malignancy	HAART Chemotherapy Nutritional support/ enteral feedings	Corticosteroids Testosterone/androgens Oxandrolone Megestrol acetate Dronabinol Recombinant growth hormone
	Fevers/sweats	Disseminated *mycobacterium avium* complex CMV HIV Lymphoma, malignancy	Azithromycin, ethambutol ganciclovir, foscarnet HAART Chemotherapy	NSAIDs (ibuprofen, indomethacin, cox-2 inhibitors) Corticosteriods Anticholinergics (hyoscine, thioridazine) H2-antagonists (cimetidine)
Pain	Nociceptive –Somatic –Visceral	Opportunistic infections, HIV-related malignancies, nonspecific	Treat specific disease entities	NSAIDs Opioids Corticosteroids
	Neuropathic	HIV-related peripheral neuropathy CMV Varicella zoster virus Dideoxynucleosides (didanosine, zalcitabine, stavudine) Other medications (isoniazid)	HAART Ganciclovir, foscarnet acyclovir, famciclovir Change antiretroviral or other regimen	NSAIDs Opioids (especially methadone) and adjuvants –Tricyclic antidepressants (amitriptyline, imipramine) –Benzodiazepines (clonazepam) –Anticonvulsants (gabapentin) Corticosteroids Acupuncture
Gastrointestinal	Nausea/vomiting	Esophageal candidiasis CMV HAART	Fluconazole, amphotericin-B, ganciclovir, foscarnet Change antiretroviral regimen	Dopamine antagonists (haloperidol, prochlorperazine) prokinetic agents (metoclopramide) Antihistamines (diphenhydramine, promethazine) Anticholinergics (hyoscine, scopolamine) Serotonin antagonists (granisetron, ondansetron, dolasetron) H2-blockers (cimetidine) Proton pump inhibitors (omeprazole) Somatostatin analogues (octreotide) Benzodiazepines (lorazepam) Corticosteroids
	Diarrhea	Mycobacterium avium-intracellulare Cryptosporidiosis CMV Microsporidiosis Other intestinal parasites Bacterial gastroenteritis Malabsorption	Azithromycin, ethambutol Paromomycin Ganciclovir, foscarnet Albendazole Other antiparasitic agents Other antibiotics	Bismuth, methylcellulose, kaolin Diphenoxylate + atropine Loperamide Octreotide Tincture of opium

(continued)

TABLE 75.6

(CONTINUED)

		Possible causes	Disease-specific Rx	Symptom-specific Rx
	Constipation	Dehydration	Hydration	Activity/diet
		Malignancy	Radiation/chemotherapy	Prophylaxis on opioids
		Anticholinergics, opioids	Medication adjustment	Softening agents
				—surfactant laxatives (docusate)
				—bulk-forming agents (bran, methylcellulose)
				—osmotic laxatives (lactulose, sorbitol)
				—saline laxatives (magnesium hydroxide)
				Peristalsis-stimulating agents
				—anthracenes (senna)
				—polyphenolics (bisacodyl)
Respiratory	Dyspnea	PCP	Trimethoprim/sulfameth-oxazole, pentamidine, atovaquone etc.	Use of fan, open windows, oxygen
				Opioids
		Bacterial pneumonia	Other antibiotics	Bronchodilators
		Anemia	Crythropocitin, transfusion	Methyl xanthines
		Pleural effusion/mass/obstruction	Drainage/radiation/surgery	Benzodiazepines (lorazepam)
		Decreased respiratory muscle function		
	Cough	*Pneumocystis Carinii* pneumonia, bacterial pneumonia	Anti-infective therapy (as earlier)	Cough suppressants (dextromethorphan, codeine, other opioids)
		Tuberculosis	Anti-tuberculous Chemotherapy	Decongestants, expectorants (various)
	Increased secretions ("death rattle")	Fluid shifts, ineffective cough, sepsis, pneumonia	Antibiotics as indicated	Atropine, hyoscine, transdermal or subcutaneous scopolamine, glycopyrrolate, fluid restriction, discontinue intervenous fluids
Dermatologic	Dry skin	Dehydration	Hydration	Emollients ± salicylates
		End-stage renal disease	Dialysis	Lubricating ointments
		End-stage liver disease malnutrition	Nutritional support	
	Pruritus	Fungal infection	Antifungals	Topical agents (menthol, phenol, calamine, doxepin, capsaicin)
		End-stage renal disease	Dialysis	Antihistamines (diphenhydramine)
		End-stage liver disease dehydration	Hydration, steroids, antifungals	Corticosteroids
		Eosinophilic folliculitis		Serotonin antagonists (ondansetron)
				Opioid antagonists (naloxone, naltrexone)
				Antidepressants
				Anxiolytics
				Neuroleptics
				Thalidomide (?)
	Decubiti/pressure Sores	Poor nutrition	Nutrition, increase mobility	Prevention (nutrition, mobility, skin integrity)
		Decreased mobility, Prolonged bed rest		Wound protection (semipermeable film/hydrocolloid dressing)
				Debridement (normal saline, enzymatic agents, alginates)
Neuropsychiatric	Delirium/agitation	Electrolyte imbalances, Dehydration	Correct imbalances hydration Sulfadiazine/	Neuroleptics (haloperidol, risperidone, chlorpromazine)
		Toxoplasmosis, Cryptococcal meningitis	pyrimethamine antifungals	Benzodiazepines (lorazepam, midazolam)
		Sepsis	Antibiotics	

TABLE 75.6

(CONTINUED)

	Possible causes	Disease-specific Rx	Symptom-specific Rx
Dementia	AIDS-related dementia	HAART	Psychostimulants (methylphenidate, dextroamphetamine) low-dose neuroleptics (haloperidol)
Depression	Chronic illness, reactive depression, major depression	Antidepressants (tricyclics, SSRIs, MAO inhibitors, other)	Psychostimulants (methylphenidate, pemoline, dextroamphetamine, modafinil) Corticosteroids (prednisone, dexamethasone)

HAART, highly active antiretroviral therapy; HIV, human immunodeficiency virus; CMV, cytomegalovirus; NSAIDs, nonsteroidal anti-inflammatory drugs; SSRI, selective serotinin reuptake inhibitor; MAO, monoamine oxidase.
Selwyn PA, Forstein M. Comprehensive care for late-stage HIV/AIDS: overcoming the false dichotomy of "curative" vs. "palliative" care. *JAMA* 2003;290:806–814.

corticosteroids, dronabinol, megestrol acetate, oxandrolone, testosterone, other anabolic steroids, and recombinant growth hormone, and thalidomide. To varying degrees, these therapies have been associated with increased weight gain, appetite, sense of well-being, energy, lean muscle mass, and even survival (especially correlated with increased lean muscle mass) (82,83). The anabolic agents and growth hormone have been associated with greater increases in lean muscle mass than the other classes of agents, but may be associated with hepatotoxicity (oxandrolone, anabolic steroids) and the possibility of insulin resistance (growth hormone) (82–86). For fatigue and the psychomotor retardation which can accompany HIV-related dementia or encephalopathy, psychostimulants such as methylphenidate or dextroamphetamine (87), in addition to HAART, can result in improved functioning and increased energy. Most patients tolerate these medications well, without significant risk of misuse even in substance users; sympathomimetic side effects can generally be avoided by using low doses and titrating upward gradually. Modafinil is another nonamphetamine-like agent which has not been widely used in AIDS but may be of potential benefit as well (88). Table 75.7 summarizes common medications and dosing schedules for the treatment of constitutional symptoms in AIDS.

In addition to relief from suffering and improvements in quality of life, it must be stressed that effective symptom management can help improve adherence with HAART, and therefore contribute to improved clinical outcomes and potentially, survival. Many of the medications used in HIV treatment can cause symptoms such as anorexia, nausea/vomiting, diarrhea, and certain types of pain, and in fact recent data suggest that the occurrence of these medication-related symptoms may be an important risk factor for nonadherence with HAART (89–91). Therefore, the appropriate and evidence-based use of palliative care medications can help facilitate patients' long-term adherence with HAART by controlling some of the symptoms which can otherwise adversely affect patient compliance, and therefore palliative interventions may indirectly have an important survival benefit.

DRUG INTERACTIONS

The growing pharmacopeia of AIDS-related medications has resulted in the growing awareness of potential drug–drug

interactions involving different commonly used therapeutic agents (46,47). Most of the drug interactions are mediated by the cytochrome P-450 enzyme system in the liver, which includes the pathways through which many of the AIDS-related medications are metabolized, as inducers, inhibitors, and/or substrates. Most importantly among them, the two main non-nucleoside reverse transcriptase inhibitors (nevirapine and efavirenz), together with the rifamycins used to treat mycobacterial diseases (rifampin, rifapentine, and rifabutin), are P-450 inducers, and the protease inhibitors (especially ritonavir, but also indinavir, saquinavir, and others) are P-450 inhibitors. Some of these known metabolic effects are used to advantage in HIV therapy, for example, the combined or "boosted" use of one protease inhibitor plus low-dose ritonavir to help increase blood levels of the primary drug, and others are used to help calculate dosage adjustments to ensure therapeutic levels (e.g., an increased dose of lopinavir/ritonavir when used with nevirapine) (92).

With the addition of palliative care medications to chronic HIV-related therapies, the potential complexity of drug interactions increases. Certain medications which might be used for palliative indications are contraindicated with ritonavir (e.g., midazolam, triazolam, terfenadine, astemizole), and the metabolism of certain opioids may also be affected by some of these AIDS-specific medications as well. One of the most important examples is methadone: methadone blood levels are predictably *decreased* by certain non-nucleocide reverse transcriptase inhibitors [nevirapine, efavirenz (93)], requiring methadone dosage increases to maintain blood levels, and may have important but less predictable responses to protease inhibitors such as ritonavir coadministration—although ritonavir is a P-450 inhibitor, the continued effect of all the metabolic pathways seems to result in mild decreases in methadone levels in some patients—requiring close clinical follow-up and possibly therapeutic drug level monitoring (92,94). Table 75.8 lists some of the classes of medications and their potential for drug–drug interactions; in individual cases, it is important to anticipate possible interactions, and as appropriate consult with pharmacist colleagues to help ensure the best choice of therapeutic combinations. Readers are also referred to more detailed resources on pharmacokinetic drug interactions in HIV/AIDS and their implications for palliative care (46,47,94–96).

TABLE 75.7

MANAGEMENT OF CONSTITUTIONAL SYMPTOMS IN HUMAN IMMUNODEFICIENCY VIRUS (HIV)/ACQUIRED IMMUNODEFICIENCY DEFICIENCY (AIDS)[a]

Symptom	Therapeutic intervention	Comments
HIV wasting	**Appetite stimulants** Megestrol acetate 400–800 mg p.o. q.d.	Can increase both appetite and body weight (primarily fat). Potential side effects include diabetes, Cushing's, hypogonadism, adrenal insufficiency (upon withdrawal)
	Prednisone 20–80 mg p.o. q.d.	Use lowest effective dose. Best reserved for patients with short prognosis and severe symptoms
	Dexamethasone 4–16 mg p.o./i.v./d in one dose or two divided doses Dronabinol 2.5–5 mg p.o. b.i.d.–t.i.d. **Testosterone** Testoderm TTS patch 5 mg/d Androderm patch 2.5–5 mg/d AndroGel topical 5 g/d Testosterone enanthate or testosterone cypionate 200 mg i.m. q2wk	Can increase weight, lean body mass, and quality of life score in men with concomitant hypogonadism. Investigational in women
	Other anabolic agents Oxandrolone 10–20 mg/d in two to four divided doses	Can promote weight gain in eugonadal men. May cause severe liver toxicity. Additional risk of virilization in women
	Growth hormone 0.1 mg/kg/day s.c.	Long-term effects unknown. Should not be considered first line. Extremely expensive
Fatigue	**Psychostimulants** Methylphenidate 2.5–5 mg p.o. q.a.m. or b.i.d. in a.m. and at noon; Maximum 60 mg/d in two divided doses Dextroamphetamine Same doses as methylphenidate Pemoline 18.75 mg p.o. q.a.m. or b.i.d. at a.m. and noon	Do not give after noon. Also good for depression and for sedation due to opioids. Avoid if anxiety, agitation As for methylphenidate Severe hepatotoxicity possible. Not first line
	Corticosteroids Dexamethasone 4–16 mg p.o./i.v. q.d in one dose or two divided doses	Studied only in patients with progressive, disseminated MAC
Fever and sweats	**Antipyretics** Acetaminophen 650–1000 mg p.o./p.r. q.6.h Choline magnesium trisalicylate 500–1000 mg po bid–t.i.d. Ibuprofen 200–600 mg p.o. q.6.h Indomethacin 25–50 mg p.o./p.r. t.i.d.	Nonsteroidal anti-inflammatory drugs may be particularly useful in patients with underlying malignancies. Less gastrointestinal toxicity with choline magnesium trisalicylate or rofecoxib than with ibuprofen
	Corticosteroids Dexamethasone 4–16 mg p.o./i.v. q.d. in one dose or two divided doses	Studied only in patients with progressive, disseminated MAC
	Anticholinergics (for sweats) Hyoscyamine 0.125–0.25 mg p.o. q.h.s–q4h Glycopyrrolate 1–2 mg p.o. q.h.s.–t.i.d. or 0.1–0.2 mg s.c./i.v. q.h.s.–q.i.d.	May cause dry mouth, constipation, tachycardia Hyoscyamine may cause confusion
	H2-antagonists (for sweats) Cimetidine 400–800 mg p.o. b.i.d.	

MAC, *mycobacterium avium* complex.
[a]Hurtado R, Krakauer EL. Constitutional symptoms. In O'Neill J, Selwyn PA, Schietinger H, eds. A clinical guide to supportive and palliative care for HIV/AIDS. Rockville, MD: Health Resources and Services Administration, 2003.

TABLE 75.8

POTENTIAL DRUG INTERACTIONS BETWEEN COMMON HUMAN IMMUNODEFICIENCY VIRUS AND PALLIATIVE CARE MEDICATIONS[a]

HIV medications	Palliative care medications

CYTOCHROME P-450 INHIBITORS

Protease inhibitors	Antifungals
Ritonavir[b]	Ketoconazole
Indinavir	Fluconazole
Nelfinavir	Itraconazole
Saquinavir	
Amprenavir	

Non-nucleoside reverse transcriptase inhibitors
Delavirdine

CYTOCHROME P-450 INDUCERS

Non-nucleoside reverse transcriptase inhibitors
Efavirenz
Nevirapine

Antimycobacterials
Rifampin
Rifabutin

CYTOCHROME P-450 INHIBITORS

Antidepressants
Fluoxetine
Paroxetine
Sertraline

CYTOCHROME P-450 INDUCERS

Anticonvulsants
Carbamazepine
Phenytoin
Phenobarbital

CYTOCHROME P-450 SUBSTRATES

Opioids	Benzodiazepines
Meperidine[c]	Clonazepam
Methadone	Diazepam
Codeine	Triazolam[c]
Morphine	Midazolam[c]
Fentanyl	
Antidepressants	**Hypnotics**
Nefazodone	Zolpidem
Sertraline	
Desipramine	
Appetite stimulants/antiemetics	**Antihistamines**
Dronabinol	Terfenadine[c]
	Astemizole[c]

[a]The palliative care medications listed may require careful monitoring due to potential drug interactions with certain HIV medications. Multiple pathways and feedback loops may exist, especially when multiple P-450–active medications are combined, and net effects are not always predictable. Most agents are active through the CYP3A4 isoform of the P-450 system, but other isoforms are involved to a lesser degree (CYP206, CYP2D19).
[b]The most potent P-450 inhibitor among the protease inhibitors.
[c]Not recommended for use with ritonavir or indinavir.
The reader is referred to more complete references and on-line resources to assess the importance of any potential drug interactions in clinical practice. See Refs. 47,94–96.
Selwyn PA, Forstein M. Comprehensive care for late-stage HIV/AIDS: overcoming the false dichotomy of "curative" vs. "palliative" care. *JAMA* 2003;290:806–814.

PROGNOSIS AND ADVANCE CARE PLANNING

The dramatic impact of HAART on survival has made it difficult to use the traditional prognostic markers to predict mortality in current patients with AIDS. In patients who have not experienced the benefit of an effective HAART regimen, even the most important mortality predictors from the pre-HAART era—for example, CD4+ T-lymphocyte count, prior opportunistic infections, wasting syndrome, certain laboratory markers—may be over-ridden by the introduction of effective antiretroviral therapy. The National Hospice Organization's proposed criteria suggesting less than 6 months prognosis in patients with AIDS (Table 75.9) (97) will not be meaningful in current patients unless one incorporates a variable related to HAART, that is, if patients have the opportunity to benefit from an appropriate and effective HAART regimen, in which case the poor prognostic variables may need to be revised. In addition to accounting for the possible benefits of HAART, recent studies have suggested that functional status

(e.g., Karnofsky score, or deficits in activities of daily living) may be important in predicting mortality in late-stage patients, for whom the traditional markers may no longer be useful because of their advanced disease stage (e.g., CD4 count). These factors are important in the consideration of palliative care treatment plans, because planning for goals of care needs to be informed whenever possible by an understanding of the possibility for survival given disease-specific therapy. Recent recommendations stress the need for current evidence-based guidelines to help uniform prognosis and assessment in late-stage patients in the HAART era (98).

The difficulty of prognostication in AIDS in the HAART era further compounds earlier observations that patients with AIDS are less likely than other patient populations to discuss advance directives with their physicians, particularly patients who are nonwhite and have histories of injection drug use (99–102). Moreover, given the known history and documentation of important cultural differences between different racial-ethnic groups regarding advance directives and end-of-life care planning, it is critical that discussion of goals of care and advance care planning in AIDS be attentive to these

TABLE 75.9

NATIONAL HOSPICE ORGANIZATION CRITERIA[a] FOR SUGGESTING ≤6 MONTHS PROGNOSIS IN PATIENTS WITH ACQUIRED IMMUNODEFICIENCY SYNDROME

CD4[+] T-lymphocyte count <25 cells/mm^3
HIV RNA>100,000 copies/mL
Persistent serum albumin <2.5 g/dL
CNS lymphoma
PML
Cryptosporidiosis
Severe wasting
Disseminated MAC (untreated)
Visceral Kaposi's sarcoma
Advanced HIV-related dementia
Toxoplasmosis
Severe cardiomyopathy
Chronic severe diarrhea

and

Documented failure to respond to or tolerate an
adequate trial of antiretroviral therapy
Additional criteria suggestive of short-term mortality:[b]
Impairments in greater than or equal to two activities of daily living
Clinically significant cognitive impairment
Serious medical comorbidity (Life-threatening malignancy, end-stage cirrhosis/liver failure, renal failure not on dialysis, and/or other organ system failure)

HIV, human immunodeficiency virus; CNS, central nervous system; PML, progressive multifocal leukoencephalopathy; MAC, *mycobacterium avium* complex.
[a]Adapted from National Hospice Organization. *Guidelines for determining prognosis for selected non-cancer diagnoses*. Alexandria, VA: National Hospital Organization, 1996. Suggested criteria are not weighted and have not been validated prospectively.
[b]See Ref. (65).

important psychosocial issues for patients and families. This is one of many examples in which the availability of a multidisciplinary (and multicultural) palliative care team can provide invaluable help for patients and families in addressing the complex issues involved in end-of-life decision making and goals of care for advanced HIV/AIDS. Other research suggests that different patient groups (e.g., cancer vs. AIDS) may have different primary concerns in end-of-life decision making (e.g., maintenance of hope, relief of pain), suggesting that clinicians need to be attuned to the disease-specific issues that may emerge (103). In addition, the special concerns of same-sex partners pertaining to heath care agent designation, legacy, and survivorship, all need to be effectively addressed (104). Lastly other researchers have documented that "disease-specific" advance directives may be very important in helping to achieve a "patient centered" approach to end-of-life decision making and goals of care (105–109). This has been found to be true for patients with AIDS, in which the use of an "HIV-specific advance directive," which described scenarios and medical conditions relevant to HIV/AIDS as part of a discussion of treatment choices, was preferred over a more generic advanced directive document by 77 versus 23% of patients surveyed (105–109).

WITHDRAWAL OF DISEASE-SPECIFIC THERAPY

With the advent of HAART, there have been numerous, frequently revised guidelines issued regarding the appropriate time to initiate antiretroviral therapy. Interestingly, however, there are no published guidelines which address the appropriate time to withdraw antiretroviral therapy in a patient who has exhausted all possibility of benefit. This perhaps reflects the important therapeutic and increasingly "curative" treatment paradigm that has accompanied the growth of effective therapy for HIV/AIDS, and indeed these advances are welcome and need to be extended to all people in need on a global basis. Nevertheless, despite all available medications and the best efforts of expert clinicians, sometimes there is little if any demonstrable benefit from continued HAART regimens, when the toxicity and negative quality-of-life impact of continued medication dosing may outweigh any realistic clinical benefit. Clearly the decision to stop therapy—which is often emotionally laden and not taken lightly by patients or families—needs to be individualized and should ultimately rest with the patient, but at times can cause unnecessary therapeutic confusion, and serve as a distraction from the end-of-life issues that need to be addressed, when patients continue to focus on future-directed therapy such as HAART without ever having had the possibility of stopping therapy be broached by their clinicians. In addition, although this is unproved, there is a theoretical and empiric basis for the concept of "viral fitness." This suggests that even in the face of high-level resistance to all antiretroviral agents, a less "fit" virus such as will be promoted by the continued exposure to antiretroviral medications, may be less pathogenic or likely to cause CD4 cell destruction than what would happen in the absence of such selective pressure (110,111).

Although these considerations are important, a thoughtful discussion about actual risks and benefits of continued HAART—instead of the uncritical continuation of therapy simply because the patient has been maintained on it in the past, despite ongoing disease progression—should ideally be undertaken between patients, families, and their physicians as part of routine care planning (Table 75.10). Similarly,

TABLE 75.10

POTENTIAL BENEFITS AND RISKS OF HIGHLY ACTIVE ANTIRETROVIRAL THERAPY IN LATE-STAGE HUMAN IMMUNODEFICIENCY VIRUS DISEASE

POTENTIAL BENEFITS[a]

Selection for "less fit" virus (i.e., less pathogenic than wild type), even in the presence of elevated viral loads
Protection against human immunodeficiency virus encephalopathy/dementia[a]
Relief/easing of symptoms possibly associated with high viral loads (e.g., constitutional symptoms)[a]
Continued therapeutic effect, albeit attenuated
Psychological and emotional benefits of continued "disease combating" therapy

POTENTIAL RISKS

Cumulative and multiple drug toxicities in the setting of therapeutic futility
Diminished quality of life from demands of treatment regimen
Therapeutic confusion (i.e., use of future-directed, disease-modifying therapy in a dying patient)
Distraction from end-of-life and advance care planning issues, with narrow focus on medication adherence and monitoring

[a]Evidence is lacking for some of these potential benefits, although they are commonly considered in clinical decision-making.
Selwyn PA, Forstein M. Comprehensive care for late-stage HIV/AIDS: overcoming the false dichotomy of "curative" vs. "palliative" care. *JAMA* 2003;290:806–814.

with opportunistic infection prophylaxis or suppression, there may be instances when continued disease-specific therapy may be important for quality of life, even in a patient with irreversibly advanced disease (e.g., anti-CMV therapy to preserve sight in CMV retinitis), and others when palliative interaction may be important as patients approach the end of life (e.g., analgesics and antipyretics instead of multidrug antimycobacterial therapy in patients with disseminated *m. avium* complex disease). Like with HAART, the decision to continue or discontinue disease-specific therapy should be dictated by a consideration of the goals of care, and the anticipated risks-benefits of treatment, rather than simply on the more medically narrow approach which dictates more reflexively that specific diagnoses "require" treatment.

In addition, there are other psychosocial issues for both patients and clinicians regarding the acceptance of death in the HAART era, a time in which the current biomedical paradigm seems to suggest that patients are not "supposed" to die. This new context has made thinking and talking about death in AIDS less common and less predictable—at least in the developed world—than it had been during the long and difficult time in which no treatment was available. It is important to recognize some of these psychological and cultural factors in order to help inform and clarify current decision making and discussions about goals of care in patients with late-stage disease for whom dying—despite our new more curative model of care—remains an important possibility (Table 75.11).

In addition to the psychosocial and contextual issues relevant to palliative care for HIV/AIDS in the HAART era, there are a number of particular treatment decisions regarding end-of-life care—both HIV-specific and more generic—that need to be anticipated and addressed by clinicians, patients, and families. Some of these are listed in Table 75.12.

INTEGRATION OF HUMAN IMMUNODEFICIENCY VIRUS CARE AND PALLIATIVE CARE

We have seen a remarkable evolution in AIDS care in the past 10 years, in which AIDS has changed from a rapidly and uniformly fatal illness to a complex but manageable chronic disease, with a whole new range of challenges and needs. Whereas care of patients with AIDS initially—and by necessity— included both palliative and disease-specific care,

TABLE 75.11

PSYCHOSOCIAL ISSUES FOR PALLIATIVE CARE IN THE ERA OF HIGHLY ACTIVE ANTIRETROVIRAL THERAPY

From "fate" to "tragedy": the universal becomes selective (i.e., uniform, fatal course vs. variability in outcome)
Renewed isolation/ostracism of the dying: death as reminder of the fallibility of HAART
Acceptance of death in the therapeutic era
Empowerment, guilt, and blame
New hope for success/greater possibility for failure
"Provider guilt"
    Pitfalls of sequential monotherapy
    Previously "complaint" patients at virologic disadvantage
    "Iatrogenic therapeutic failure"
    Emotional withdrawal/inappropriate overtreatment
Medicalization of acquired immunodeficiency syndrome
    Challenge to patient-provider communication
Bereavement needs of survivors

HAART, highly active antiretroviral therapy.

TABLE 75.12

TREATMENT DECISIONS AT THE END OF LIFE IN PATIENTS WITH HUMAN IMMUNODEFICIENCY VIRUS/ACQUIRED IMMUNODEFICIENCY SYNDROME IN THE HIGHLY ACTIVE ANTIRETROVIRAL THERAPY ERA

NON-HIV SPECIFIC

Laboratory/diagnostic testing
  discontinue "routine testing"
  Tests dictated by goals of therapy
Nutrition/hydration
  Emotional vs. medical decisions
  Sociocultural meaning of food and water
  Risks of parenteral/enteral feeding
Family and cultural issues involving young patients at end of life
Social and historical context of HIV/AIDS

HIV-SPECIFIC

Withdrawal of antiretroviral therapy?
  Symbolic meaning of HAART
  Patient preference
  Patient/family guilt (withdrawal = "giving up")
  Therapeutic confusion
  Toxicity vs. benefit
  Prognostic uncertainty
  "Lazarus syndrome" (i.e., near-death patients experiencing dramatic recoveries after
    initiation of HAART)
Withdrawal of prophylactic/suppressive therapy?
  Anticipated life expectancy
  Past history of osteogenesis imperfectas
  Symptom severity
  Toxicity vs. benefit
  Effectiveness of symptomatic/supportive therapy
Goals of expected therapy/outcomes?

HIV, human immunodeficiency virus; AIDS, acquired immunodeficiency syndrome; HAART, highly active antiretroviral therapy.

at a time when the options for disease-specific therapy were so limited, the emergence of the HAART era has now resulted in a growing separation between AIDS care and palliative care providers. Regrettably, this has resulted in a fragmentation of care for patients with AIDS and their caregivers, and arguably a loss of therapeutic effectiveness within a largely medical model of care. Rather than reproduce the false dichotomies of curative *versus* palliative care which have adversely impacted on the care of patients with cancer and other life-threatening conditions, it is important for AIDS care to reaffirm the important basis for coordinated disease-specific and supportive care which will optimize outcomes for patients and families. This is true both for the developed world, where perhaps the need for palliative care in AIDS has been too much overlooked by AIDS care providers in recent years, and in the developing world, where the appropriate and desperately needed focus on increasing access to antiretroviral therapy to the millions who need it should not obscure the need to treat pain and suffering with timely and important palliative care interventions as well. The science of palliative medicine has much to offer to the care of patients with AIDS in the HAART era; the challenge is to incorporate the best of palliative care with the best of disease-specific therapy on both for individual patients and in the development and implementation of clinical programs and services.

References

1. Center for Disease Control. Update: trends in AIDS incidence, deaths, and prevalence-United States, 1996. *MMWR Morb Mortal Wkly Rep* 1997; 46(8):165–173.

2. Palella FA Jr, Delaney KM, Moorman AC, et al. Declining morbidity and mortality among patients with advanced human immunodeficiency virus infection. *N Engl J Med* 1998;338:853–860.

3. Centers for Disease Control and Prevention. HIV/AIDS Surveillance Report. Atlanta: US Department of Health and Human Services. Centers for Disease Control and Prevention. 2004;15:1–44. http://www.cdc.gov/hiv/stats/hasrlink.htm.

4. Chiasson MA, Berenson L, Li W, et al. Declining HIV/AIDS mortality in New York City. *J Acquir Immune Defic Syndr* 1999;21:59–64.

5. Egger M, Hirschel B, Francioli P, et al. Impact of new antiretroviral combination therapies on HIV infected patients in Switzerland: prospective multicentre study. *BMJ* 1997;315:1194–1199.

6. Sansone RG, Frengley JD. Impact of HAART on causes of death of persons with late-stage AIDS. *J Urban Health* 2000;77:165–175.

7. Selwyn PA, Goulet JL, Molde S, et al. HIV as a chronic disease: long-term care for patients with HIV at a dedicated skilled nursing facility. *J Urban Health* 2000;77:187–203.

8. Puoti M, Spinetti A, Ghezzi A, et al. Mortality from liver disease in patients with HIV infection: a cohort study. *J Acquir Immune Defic Syndr* 2001; 24:211–217.

9. Centers for Disease Control and Prevention. HIV and AIDS - United States, 1981–2000, *MMWR Morb Mortal Wkly Rep* 2001;50:430–434.

10. Kravcik S, Hawley-Foss N, Victor G, et al. Causes of death in HIV-infected persons in Ottowa, Ontario, 1984–1995. *Arch Intern Med* 1997; 157:2069–2073.

11. Valdez H, Chowdhry TK, Asaad R, et al. Changing spectrum of mortality due to HIV: analysis of 260 deaths during 1995–1999. *Clin Infect Dis* 2001;32(1487):1493.

12. Tedaldi EM, Baker RK, Moorman AC, et al. Influence of coinfection with hepatitis C virus on morbidity and mortality due to human immunodeficiency virus infection in the era of highly active antiretroviral therapy. *Clin Infect Dis* 2003;36(3):363–367.

13. Powderly WG. Antiretroviral therapy in patients with hepatitis and HIV: weighing risks and benefits. *Clin Infect Dis* 2004;38(Suppl 2):S109–S113.

14. Lee L, Karon J, Selik R, et al. Survival after AIDS diagnosis in adolescents and adults during the treatment era, United States, 1984–1997. *JAMA* 2001;285:1308–1315.

15. Lynn L. An 88-Year-Old woman facing the end of life. *JAMA* 1997; 277:1633–1640.
16. Center for Disease Control. HIV and AIDS—United States, 1981–2000. *MMWR Morb Mortal Wkly Rep* 2001;50:430–434.
17. Powderly WG. Long-term exposure to lifelong therapies. *J Acquir Immune Defic Syndr* 2002;29(Suppl 1):S28–S40.
18. Montessori V, Press N, Harris M, et al. Adverse effects of antiretroviral therapy for HIV infection. *CMAJ* 2004;170(2):229–238.
19. O'Neill JF, Selwyn PA, Schietinger H, eds. *Clinical guide for supportive and palliative care for HIV/AIDS*. Rockville, MD: Health Resources and Services Administration, 2003.
20. Selwyn PA, Arnold R. From fate to tragedy: the changing meanings of life, death, and IDS. *Ann Intern Med* 1998;129:899–902.
21. LaRue FFA, Colleau SM. Underestimation and undertreatment of pain in HIV disease: multicentre study. *BMJ* 1997;314:23–28.
22. Singer JE, Fahy-Chandon B, Chi S, et al. Painful symptoms reported by ambulatory HIV-infected men in a longitudinal study. *Pain* 1993;54:15–19.
23. Breitbart W, Rosenfeld B, Passik SD, et al. The undertreatment of pain in ambulatory AIDS patients. *Pain* 1996;65:243–249.
24. O'Neill W, Sherrard J. Pain in human immunodeficiency virus disease: a review. *Pain* 1993;54:3–14.
25. Breitbart W, McDonald MV, Rosenfeld B, et al. Fatigue in ambulatory AIDS patients. *J Pain Symptom Manage* 1998;15:159–167.
26. Wood CGA, Whittet S, Bradbeer CS. ABC of palliative care: HIV infection and AIDS. *BMJ* 1997;315:1433–1436.
27. LaRue F, Brasseur L, Musseault P, et al. Pain and symptoms in HIV disease: a national survey in France. Abstract: Third Congress of the European Association for palliative care. *J Palliat Care* 1994;10:95.
28. Foley F. AIDS palliative care. Abstract: 10th International Congress on the Care of the Terminally Ill. *J Palliat Care* 1994;10:132.
29. Moss V. Palliative care in advanced HIV disease: presentation, problems, and palliation. *AIDS* 1990;4(Suppl 1):S235–S242.
30. Fontaine A, LaRue F, Lassauniere JM. Physicians; recognition of the symptoms experienced by HIV patients: how reliable? *J Pain Symptom Manage* 1999;18:263–270.
31. Filbet M, Marceron V, HGVA Alix F. A retrospective study of symptoms in 193 terminal inpatients with AIDS Abstract: Third Congress of the European Association for palliative care. *J Palliat Care* 1994;10:92.
32. Fantoni M, Ricci F, Del Borgo C, et al. Multicentre study on the prevalence of symptoms and symptomatic treatment in HIV infection. *J Palliat Care* 1997;13(2):9–13.
33. Vogl D, Rosenfeld B, Breitbart W, et al. Symptom prevalence, characteristics, and distress in AIDS outpatients. *J Pain Symptom Manage* 1998; 18:253–262.
34. Mathews W, McCutcheon JA, Asch S, et al. National estimates of HIV-related symptom prevalence from the HIV Cost and Services Utilization Study. *Med Care* 2000;38(750):762.
35. Kelleher P, Cox S, McKeogh M. HIV infection: the spectrum of symptoms and disease in male and female patients attending a London hospice. *Palliat Med* 1997;11(2):152–158.
36. Breitbart W, Kaim M, Rosenfeld B. Clinicians' perceptions of barriers to pain management in AIDS. *J Pain Symptom Manage* 1999;18:203–212.
37. Breitbart W, Passik S, McDonald MV, et al. Patient-related barriers to pain management in ambulatory AIDS patients. *Pain* 1998;76(1–2):9–16.
38. Todd KH, Samaroo N, Hoffman JR. Ethnicity as a risk factor for inadequate emergency department analgesia. *JAMA* 1993;269(12):1537–1539.
39. Morrison RS, Wallenstein S, Natale DK, et al. "We don't carry that" - failure of pharmacies in predominantly nonwhite neighborhoods to stock opioid analgesics. *N Engl J Med* 2000;342:1023–1026.
40. Sacktor N. The epidemiology of human immunodeficiency virus-associated neurological disease in the era of highly active antiretroviral therapy. *J Neurovirol* 2002;8(Suppl 2):115–121.
41. Wulff EA, Wang AK, Simpson DM. HIV-associated peripheral neuropathy: epidemiology, pathophysiology and treatment. *Drugs* 2000;59(6):1251–1260.
42. Tan SV, Guiloff RJ. Hypothesis on the pathogenesis of vacuolar myelopathy, dementia, and peripheral neuropathy in AIDS. *J Neurol Neurosurg Psychiatry* 1998;65(1):23–28.
43. Rachlis AR. Neurologic manifestations of HIV infection. Using imaging studies and antiviral therapy effectively. *Postgrad Med* 1998;103(3):147–161.
44. Simpson DM. Selected peripheral neuropathies associated with human immunodeficiency virus infection and antiretroviral therapy. *J Neurovirol* 2002;8(Suppl 2):33–41.
45. Bacellar H, Munoz A, Miller E, et al. Temporal trends in the incidence of HIV-1-related neurologic disease: Multicenter AIDS Cohort Study, 1985–1992. *Neurol* 1994;44:1892–1900.
46. Piscitelli SC, Gallicano KD. Drug therapy: interactions among drugs for HIV and opportunistic infections. *N Engl J Med* 2001;344:984–996.
47. Ogbuokiri J. Pharmacologic interactions of HIV and palliative medications. In: O'Neill J, Selwyn PA, eds. *A clinical guide to supportive and palliative care for HIV/AIDS*. Rockville, MD: Health Resources and Services Administration, 2003.
48. Compton P, Charuvastra VC, Ling W. Pain intolerance in opioid-maintained former opiate addicts: effect of long-acting maintenance agent. *Drug Alcohol Depend* 2001;63:139–146.
49. Compton P, Charuvastra C, Kintaudi K, et al. Pain responses in methadone-maintained opioid abusers. *J Pain Symptom Manage* 2000;20(4):237–245.
50. Kreek MJ. Medical safety and side effects of methadone in tolerant individuals. *JAMA* 1973;223:665–668.
51. Passik SD, Kirsh KL, McDonald MV, et al. A pilot survey of aberrant drug-taking attitudes and behaviors in samples of cancer and AIDS patients. *J Pain Symptom Manage* 2000;19(4):274–286.
52. Passik SD, Portenoy RK. Substance Abuse Issues in Palliative Care. In: Berger A, ed. *Principles adn practice of supportive oncology*. Philadelphia, PA: Lippincott Williams & Wilkins, 1998:513–529.
53. Compton P, Darakjian J, Miotto K. Screening for addiction in patients with chronic pain and "problematic" substance use: evaluation of a pilot assessment tool. *J Pain Symptom Manage* 1998;16(6):355–363.
54. Passik SD, Kirsh KL. Opioid therapy in patients with a history of substance abuse. *CNS Drugs* 2004;18(1):13–25.
55. Weaver M, Schnoll S. Abuse liability in opioid therapy for pain treatment in patients with an addiction history. *Clin J Pain* 2002;18(4 Suppl):S61–S69.
56. Currie SR, Hodgins DC, Crabtree A, et al. Outcome from integrated pain management treatment for recovering substance abusers. *J Pain* 2003; 4(2):91–100.
57. Fishman SM, Kreis PG. The opioid contract. *Clin J Pain* 2002;18(4 Suppl): S70–S75.
58. Manfredi PL, Gonzales GR, Cheville AL, et al. Methadone analgesia in cancer pain patients on chronic methadone maintenance therapy. *J Pain Symptom Manage* 2001;21(2):169–174.
59. Collins ED, Streltzer J. Should opioid analgesics be used in the management of chronic pain in opiate addicts? *Am J Addict* 2003;12:93–100.
60. Selwyn PA, Feingold AR, Iezza A, et al. Primary care for patients with human immunodeficiency virus (HIV) infection in a methadone maintenance treatment program. *Ann Intern Med* 1989;111:761–763.
61. Selwyn PA, Budner NS, Wasserman WC, et al. Utilization of on-site primary care services by HIV-seropositive and seronegative drug users in a methadone maintenance program. *Public Health Rep* 1993;108:492–500.
62. Lucas GM, Weidle PJ, Hader S, et al. Directly administered antiretroviral therapy in an urban methadone maintenance clinic: a nonrandomized comparative study. *Clin Infect Dis* 2004;38(Suppl 5):S409–S413.
63. De Castro S, Sabate E. Adherence to heroin dependence therapies and human immunodeficiency virus/acquired immunodeficiency syndrome infection rates among drug abusers. *Clin Infect Dis* 2003;37(Suppl 5): S464–S467.
64. Conway B, Prasad J, Reynolds R, et al. Directly observed therapy for the management of HIV-infected patients in a methadone program. *Clin Infect Dis* 2004;38(Suppl 5):S402–S408.
65. Selwyn PA, Rivard M, Kapell D, et al. Palliative care for AIDS at a large urban teaching hospital: program description and preliminary outcomes. *Innov End-of-Life Care* www2 edc org/lastacts 2002;4(3).
66. Umbricht A, Hoover DR, Tucker MJ, et al. Opioid detoxification with buprenorphine, clonidine, or methadone in hospitalized heroin-dependent patients with HIV infection. *Drug Alcohol Depend* 2003;69(3):263–272.
67. Mattick RP, Kimber J, Breen C, et al. Buprenorphine maintenance versus placebo or methadone maintenance for opioid dependence. *Cochrane Database Syst Rev* 2003;(2): Art No.:CD002207. DOI: 10. 1002/14651858. CD002207.
68. McCance-Katz EF, Pade P, Friedland G, et al. Efavirenz decreases buprenorphine exposure, but is not associated with opiate withdrawal in opioid dependent individuals, *12th conference on retroviruses and opportunistic infections*. Boston, MA: 2005, Abstract No. 653.
69. Gray F, Chretien F, Vallat-Decouvelaere AV, et al. The changing pattern of HIV neuropathology in the HAART era. *J Neuropathol Exp Neurol* 2003;62(5):429–440.
70. Aboulafia DM, Taylor L. Vacuolar myelopathy and vacuolar cerebellar leukoencephalopathy: a late complication of AIDS after highly active antiretroviral therapy-induced immune reconstitution. *AIDS Patient Care STDS* 2002;16(12):579–584.
71. Maschke M, Kastrup O, Esser S, et al. Incidence and prevalence of neurological disorders associated with HIV since the introduction of highly active antiretroviral therapy (HAART). *J Neurol Neurosurg Psychiatry* 2000;69(3):376–380.
72. Di Rocco A. Diseases of the spinal cord in human immunodeficiency virus infection. *Semin Neurol* 1999;19(2):151–155.
73. Di Rocco A, Simpson DM. AIDS-associated vacuolar myelopathy. *AIDS Patient Care STDS* 1998;12(6):457–461.
74. Berger JR, Nath A. Remedies for HIV-associated peripheral neuropathy. *Neurol* 2000;54(11):2037–2038.
75. Simpson DM, Olney R, McArthur JC, et al. A placebo-controlled trial of lamotrigine for painful HIV-associated neuropathy. *Neurol* 2000; 54(11):2115–2119.
76. Simpson DM, McArthur JC, Olney R, et al. Lamotrigine for HIV-associated painful sensory neuropathies: a placebo-controlled trial. *Neurol* 2003;60(9):1508–1514.
77. Simpson DM, Dorfman D, Olney RK, et al. The Peptide T Neuropathy Study Group. Peptide T in the treatment of painful distal neuropathy associated with AIDS: results of a placebo-controlled trial. *Neurol* 1996;47(5):1254–1259.
78. Paice JA, Ferrans CE, Lashley FR, et al. Topical capsaicin in the management of HIV-associated peripheral neuropathy. *J Pain Symptom Manage* 2000;19(1):45–52.

79. Nelson KE, Vlahov D, Cohn S. Sexually transmitted diseases in a population of intravenous drug users; associated with seropositivity in the human immunodeficiency virus (HIV). *J Infect Dis* 1991;164:456–463.

80. Nelson K, Walsh D, Sheehan F. The cancer anorexia-cachexia syndrome. *J Clin Oncol* 1994;12(1):213–225.

81. Selwyn P, Rivard M. Palliative care for AIDS: challenges and opportunities in the era of highly active anti-retroviral therapy. *J Palliat Med* 2003;6:475–487. [Originally in Innovations in End-of-Life Care 2002; (2002;4(3), www.edc.org/lastacts)].

82. Polsky B, Kotler D, Steinhart C. HIV-associated wasting in the HAART era: guidelines for assessment, diagnosis, and treatment. *AIDS Patient Care STDS* 2001;15(8):411–423.

83. Grinspoon S, Mulligan K. Weight loss and wasting in patients infected with human immunodeficiency virus. *Clin Infect Dis* 2003;36(Suppl 2):S69–S78.

84. Windisch PA, Papatheofanis FJ, Matuszewski KA. Recombinant human growth hormone for AIDS-associated wasting. *Ann Pharmacother* 1998; 32:437–445.

85. Wagner GJ, Rabkin R. Effects of dextroamphetamine on depression and fatigue in men with HIV: a double-blind, placebo-controlled trial. *J Clin Psychiatry* 2000;61(6):436–440.

86. Weinroth SE, Parenti DM, Simon GL. Wasting syndrome in AIDS: pathophysiologic mechanisms and therapeutic approaches. *Infect Agents Dis* 1995;4(2):76–94.

87. Brietbart W, Rosenfeld B, Kaim M, et al. A randomized, double-blind, placebo-controlled trial of psychostimulants for the treatment of fatigue in ambulatory patients with human immunodeficiency virus disease. *Arch Intern Med* 2001;161:411–420.

88. Fishbain DA, Cutler RB, Lewis J, et al. Modafinil for the treatment of pain-associated fatigue: review and case report. *J Pain Palliat Care Pharmacother* 2004;18(2):39–47.

89. Voss JG, Corless IB, Nicolas PK, et al. Impact of fatigue on daily activities and adherence to ARV medications. *XV International AIDS Conference*, Bangkok, Thailand: 2004.

90. Spire B, Bouhnik AD, Carrieri MP, et al. Depression, non-adherence and clinical progression in HIV infected drug users treated with highly active antiretroviral therapy, *XV international AIDS conference*, Bangkok, Thailand: 2004.

91. Reynolds NR, Kirksey KM, Bunch EH, et al. Type, frequency, and effectiveness of nausea self-care management strategies: an international, multi-site study. *XV international AIDS conference*, Bangkok, Thailand: 2004.

92. www.AIDSinfo.nih.gov. Antiretroviral Treatment Guidelines, Guidelines for the Use of Antiretroviral Agents in HIV-Infected Adults and Adolescents - April 07, 2005. Viewed, 9/13/05.

93. Calvo R, Lukas JC, Rodriguez M, et al. Pharmacokinetics of methadone in HIV-positive patients receiving the non-nucleoside reverse transcriptase efavirenz. *Br J Clin Pharmacol* 2002;53(2):212–214.

94. Gourevitch MN, Friedland GH. Interactions between methadone and medications used to treat HIV infection: a review. *Mt Sinai J Med* 2000; 67:429–436.

95. Faragon JJ, Piliero PJ. Drug interactions associated with HAART: focus on treatments for addiction and recreational drugs. *AIDS Read* 2003;13(9):433–41–446.

96. www.hiv-druginteractions.org. Viewed, 9/13/05.

97. National Hospice Organization. *Guidelines for determining prognosis for selected non-cancer diagnoses.* Alexandria, VA: National Hospital Organization, 1996.

98. Alexander C, Back A. Workgroup on Palliative and EndofLife Care in HIV/AIDS. Integrating Palliative Care into the Continuum of HIV Care.

99. Wenger NS, Kanouse DE, Collins RL, et al. End-of-life discussions and preferences among persons with HIV. *JAMA* 2001;22:2880–2887.

100. Randall Curtis J, Patrick DL, Caldwell E, et al. The quality of patient-doctor communication about end-of-life care: a study of patients with advanced AIDS and their primary care clinicians. *AIDS* 1999;13(9):1123–1131.

101. Randall Curtis J, Patrick DL, Caldwell ES, et al. Why don't patients and physicians talk about end-of-life care? *Arch Intern Med* 2000;160:1690–1696.

102. Randall Curtis J, Patrick DL. Barriers to communication about end-of-life care in AIDS patients. *J Gen Intern Med* 1997;12(12):736–741.

103. Randall Curtis J, Wenrich MD, Carline JD, et al. Patients' perspectives on physician skill in end-of-life care: differences between patients with COPD, cancer, and AIDS. *Chest* 2002;122:356–362.

104. Stein GL, Bonuck KA. Attitudes on end-of-life care and advance care planning in the lesbian and gay community. *J Palliat Med* 2001;4(2):173–190.

105. Singer PA, Martin DK, Lavery JV, et al. Reconceptualizing advance care planning from the patient's perspective. *Arch Intern Med* 1998; 158:879–884.

106. Martin DK, Thiel EC, Singer PA. A new model of advance care planning. *Arch Intern Med* 1999;159:86–92.

107. Singer PA, Martin DK, Kelner M. Quality end-of-life care. *JAMA* 1999; 281(2):163–168.

108. Aikman PJ, Thiel EC, Martin DK, et al. Proxy, health, and personal care preferences: implications for end-of-life care. *Camb Q Healthc Ethics* 1999;8:200–210.

109. Singer PA, Thiel EC, Salit I, et al. The HIV-specific advance directive. *J Gen Intern Med* 1997;12(12):729–735.

110. Deeks S, Wrin T, Liegler T, et al. Virologic and immunologic consequences of discontinuing combination antiretroviral-drug therapy in HIV-infected patients with detectable viremia. *N Engl J Med* 2001;344:472–480.

111. Frenkel L, Mullins J. Should patients with drug-resistant HIV-1 continue to receive antiretroviral therapy? *N Engl J Med* 2001;344:520–522.

CHAPTER 76 ■ PALLIATIVE CARE IN THE INTENSIVE CARE UNIT SETTING

THOMAS J. PRENDERGAST

Intensive care units (ICUs) combine, in one physical location, the most desperately ill patients with the intensive care physicians and nursing staff who are trained to use the latest in medical technology. The result is an approach to patient care that has been characterized as "rescue medicine." (1) This term correctly suggests that a primary goal of critical care medicine is to save the lives of patients who would have died without their aggressive interventions. The term also carries a negative connotation: in their zeal to save lives, critical care practitioners (intensivists) may undervalue the wishes of the patient, the needs of the family, pain and suffering caused by the treatment, and the potential for functional recovery, as opposed to mere survival. Because these concerns form the very core of palliative medicine, there is a widespread assumption that critical care medicine is at best indifferent and at worst antithetical to palliative care. For example, one of the major (negative) outcome measures of the Study to Understand Prognoses and Preferences for Outcomes and Risks of Treatments (SUPPORT) study was the presence of a patient in an ICU before death (2).

Accusations of a rescue mentality are anecdotal and difficult to assess (3). We might infer a mindset of rescue medicine when all dying patients receive all therapies, including ineffective cardiopulmonary resuscitation (CPR). From the inception of ICUs in the 1960s till the 1980s, this was the approach to patients dying in ICUs. Since then there has been an astonishing evolution in critical care practice (Table 76.1). In 2001, most ICU deaths followed a considered decision to either withhold or to withdraw life-sustaining therapy (10). In the past decade, intensivists have acquired a new responsibility to manage the death of patients who do not survive. This is not yet palliative care, but it opens the door to palliative care because it raises the question: how is this newly appreciated responsibility to the dying patient handled, and how well (11)?

APPROACHES TO PALLIATIVE CARE IN THE INTENSIVE CARE UNIT

Some patients are referred to the ICU for symptom control that cannot easily be provided elsewhere in the hospital. Palliation of symptoms may require intensity of nursing care that is not available in the ward. It may require interventions that can be comfortably managed in the ICU [e.g., treatment of intractable distress with barbiturate or propofol coma (12)]. The therapeutic goal may be to initiate ICU-specific interventions (e.g., vasopressor support or assisted ventilation) allowing time for the family to arrive to say good-bye. Instances of specific, circumscribed palliative care are a legitimate, although uncommon, use of critical care resources. For such patients, the ICU is not only an appropriate location but also quite likely, the best place to die.

Patients admitted for symptom control represent a small minority of ICU admissions. Most patients are admitted to the ICU emergently, under the presumption of treatment until more information is available, or because the clinician and patient/surrogate have made a decision to pursue a trial of curative therapy. There is an expectation of recovery or, at least, uncertainty about prognosis. Most patients improve and are discharged. Mortality rates vary from <5% of admissions to some surgical ICUs, to 15% of admissions to general medical ICUs, to >40% of admissions to ICUs that primarily treat oncology patients (10,13,14). Age alone does not appear to be an independent predictor of mortality (15). Certain diagnoses place patients at higher risk for death (16,17). Critically ill patients with cancer have a particularly poor prognosis, with multiple studies documenting in-hospital mortality rates from 50% to >90% in patients who develop critical illness following bone marrow transplant (18). A recent attempt to develop a mortality prediction model, specifically for patients with cancer identified three variables associated with higher mortality: allogeneic bone marrow transplant, progression of underlying disease, and poor performance status (13).

Patients admitted to the ICU for curative therapy also may benefit from palliative care. It is uncertain, however, which patients will benefit and when palliation should be emphasized in their course of intensive care. One approach emphasizes symptom control in patients known to be dying. Therefore, intensivists may arrive at palliative care through a natural extension of the ICU's core mission to rescue the grievously ill: treat aggressively for cure until death appears inevitable, then redirect the goals of care to control the patient's symptoms. This model and the accompanying language of transitioning from curative to comfort care have become commonplace in critical care medicine (19,20). The transition approach demonstrates a willingness to acknowledge the dying and to attend to the details of patients' deaths. In this sense, it is a significant advance beyond the relentless drive to treat, that sometimes has characterized critical care medicine. There are drawbacks to a transition approach, however. To state the obvious, there is more to palliative care than symptom control of the imminently dying. Another problem, one that remains underappreciated outside critical care medicine, is that it is surprisingly difficult to predict who is going to die (21,22).

849

TABLE 76.1

CHANGING MANAGEMENT OF DEATH WITHIN AMERICAN INTENSIVE CARE UNITS

Year	Case	Description
1968	*Ad Hoc* Committee on Brain Death[a]	Harvard Medical School committee proposes new criteria for death that use impairment of brain function. Reasons to redefine death include: need for organs for transplantation and to preclude inappropriate prolongation of critical care. Withdrawal of intensive care not considered possible without first declaring the patient dead
1976	Karen Quinlan[b]	Family of 21-year-old woman who is in a persistent vegetative state requests removal of mechanical ventilation. Hospital and physicians refuse. Family appeals to New Jersey State Supreme Court. In a landmark decision, the Court grants permission to withdraw the ventilator
1983	Clarence Herbert[c]	Two physicians in Los Angeles withdraw artificial nutrition and hydration from a terminally ill patient at the request of his family and in accordance with the patient's expressed wishes. The physicians are charged in criminal court with homicide. Ultimately, they are acquitted of all charges
1990	Nancy Cruzan[d]	U.S. Supreme Court rules that individual states may set evidentiary standards for the withdrawal of life support from incompetent patients but affirms the right of all patients to refuse unwanted therapies even when such refusal may result in death
1990	Helga Wanglie[e,f]	Physicians at University of Minnesota petition the local court to have the husband of an 88-year-old woman who is in a persistent vegetative state, removed as surrogate decision maker because he wishes to continue her intensive care. The court rejects their petition. Mrs. Wanglie dies on a ventilator without attempted resuscitation
1998	National Survey of ICU practice[g]	Data from 131 ICUs in 37 states collected in 1994–95 shows that 76% of deaths were preceded by withholding or withdrawal of life-support

[a]From JAMA. A definition of irreversible coma. Report of the *Ad Hoc* Committee of the Harvard Medical School to Examine the Definition of Brain Death. *JAMA* 1968;205:337–340, (4) with permission.
[b]From *In re Quinlan*, 70 NJ 10, 1976, (5) with permission.
[c]From Lo B. The death of Clarence Herbert: withdrawing care is not murder. *Ann Intern Med* 1984;101:248–251, (6) with permission.
[d]From *Cruzan v Director*, Missouri Department of Health, 497 U.S. 261, 1990, (7) with permission.
[e]From Miles SH. Informed demand for "non-beneficial" medical treatment. *N Engl J Med* 1991;325:512–515, (8) with permission.
[f]From Angell M. The case of Helga Wanglie. A new kind of "right to die" case. *N Engl J Med* 1991; 325:511–512, (9) with permission.
[g]From Prendergast TJ, Claessens MT, Luce JM. A national survey of end-of-life care for critically ill patients. *Am J Respir Crit Care Med* 1998; 158:1163–1167, with permission.

A transition model of palliative care in the ICU depends on the intensivist's ability to identify a clinical change in individual patients that redirects the goals of care away from curative therapy toward symptom control. Experienced intensivists can accurately predict the short-term mortality of groups of patients; many computer-based mortality prediction models do the same (23). Neither computer-aided decision systems nor expert clinical opinion allows specific identification of the individual patient who will die (22). Data from the SUPPORT study (21) demonstrate that, in most patients, there are no identifiable points when death becomes imminent that allows for a change in direction of care (Table 76.2). These data challenge the assumption that we have advance notice of death. The uncomfortable reality is that a high percentage of ICU patients die but individual ICU patients are difficult to identify as dying. Therefore, if the criterion for palliative care in ICU patients is that the providers first recognize that the patient is imminently dying, ICU practice will be deficient in two ways. Many patients will die without the benefit of palliative medicine because they will die unexpectedly. Those

TABLE 76.2

MEDIAN PREDICTED 2-MONTH MORTALITY STUDY TO UNDERSTAND PROGNOSES AND PREFERENCES FOR OUTCOMES AND RISKS OF TREATMENTS

Patient population	One day before death (%)	One week before death (%)
All deaths	17	51
Coma	5	27
Congestive heart failure	42	62
Chronic obstructive pulmonary disease	21	41

From Lynn J, Harrell F Jr, Cohn F, et al. Prognoses of seriously ill hospitalized patients on the days before death: implications for patient care and public policy. *New Horiz* 1997;5:56–61, with permission.

who do receive palliative care will receive it very late in their disease course.

Despite an emerging consensus that palliative care can coexist in parallel with aggressive critical care, many clinicians in and out of ICUs strongly support the concept of a transition to palliative care. There are many reasons for the persistence of this approach. A few patients do have an abrupt change in their clinical course that significantly changes their prognosis (e.g., the elderly patient with lung cancer who has a myocardial infarction that precipitates cardiogenic shock). Predicted survival may drop precipitously with additional organ dysfunction, and appreciation of this change may facilitate a decision to limit therapy. In other patients, the decision to change the direction of therapy is based on nonprognostic factors, such as suffering, quality of life, or comorbid illnesses, that suggest a high likelihood of recurrent hospitalization or death despite the possibility of short-term recovery (24). The same patient, although hemodynamically stable but with severe permanent left ventricular dysfunction, may face a degree of debilitation that he and his family may find to be unacceptable. Sometimes, clinicians and families frame the facts to suit their need for explanations in a way that creates transitions (25). Perhaps the patient's quality of life will be no different after the myocardial infarction but the event reshaped the patient and family's thinking toward acceptance of his mortality.

Finally, the transition model permits separation of the curative and palliative roles. To the extent that this separation allows the intensivist to withdraw from involvement as death approaches, it may represent a strategy to cope with feelings of helplessness, failure, and grief (26). The alternative, to assert that all patients at high risk of dying need palliative care, asks the intensivist simultaneously to be an advocate of rescue and palliative medicine (21,27). To assume both these roles is to move far beyond the transition model.

ADAPTING PALLIATIVE CARE TO THE INTENSIVE CARE UNIT

Palliative care in or out of the ICU starts with adequate symptom control. Symptom control is essential because pain and suffering without purpose are destructive, because untreated pain may adversely affect outcomes (28,29), and because unrelieved pain and suffering interfere with the patient's ability to address important life issues that may be brought to closure before death. Palliative medicine promises more than symptom control, however. It emphasizes the possibility of growth at the end of life. Palliative care means acknowledging and addressing psychological suffering (depression, anxiety), existential suffering (estrangement, alienation, lost opportunities, and the meaning of one's life), and spiritual suffering (Why am I dying?) (30). This ideal of palliative care depends upon a predictable disease course that allows time to plan and a patient who is alert enough to speak for himself and to participate in discussions of both medical planning and personal growth with a provider who has a relationship with the patient and, preferably, has known the patient and the family over time. Critical care medicine violates this model in almost every respect (Table 76.3) (31).

Some of the barriers to palliative care listed in Table 76.3 actually contribute to the success of critical care medicine. An emphasis on technology, and expert providers willing to push its limits, are desirable if they help the desperately ill and injured. Other barriers seem inevitable if less desirable. In an environment dedicated to treating the sickest patients, prognostic uncertainty dictates that some patients will die under aggressive therapy to successfully treat those who survive. This is neither a mistake nor necessarily a failure but an expected consequence of not knowing who will respond to treatment (27). The nature of critical illness is that clinical situations change rapidly and decisions must be made quickly. Pervasive prognostic uncertainty, pressure to make decisions, and significant mortality seem an inescapable part of the ICU environment. Some barriers shown in Table 76.3 are cultural and, therefore, subject to change. Struggling to save lives is fully consistent with acknowledging that the quality of death can be as important as the quality of life (32). To teach the importance of interpersonal relations and communications skills, need not devalue the technical and scientific accomplishments that distinguish modern critical care. Technology does not imply dehumanization; intensivists can be full participants in the human stories being played out under their care.

There are key elements of palliative care that are adaptable to the ICU in a way that improves the care of patients while respecting the critical care provider's appropriate role as advocate for the desperately ill. These features of palliative medicine are not inconsistent with good ICU practice. They are increasingly seen to define good ICU practice (19,27,33–35). The internist or oncologist whose patient is admitted to the

---

TABLE 76.3

SOME OBSTACLES TO PALLIATIVE CARE IN THE INTENSIVE CARE UNIT

The *raison d'être* of critical care medicine is to push the limits of what medicine can accomplish. Success is measured in lives saved. Lives lost may be accounted as failure. The importance of the quality of death is not part of the culture[a]

ICUs are different from other hospital locations in that the organizing principle is the acuity of illness. Geographically and organizationally, the focus of care is on technology and interventions rather than on interpersonal relations[b]

The ICU environment is characterized by acute illnesses with unpredictable outcomes.[c] Clinical status may change rapidly, necessitating rapid decision-making about life and death issues

Patients rarely have a preexisting relationship with their providers. Most patients who die are too ill to participate in discussions of their needs and wishes. Communications with family and surrogates are strained by lack of prior relationships, time-pressured decision-making, and uncertainty of prognosis[d]

Critical care education has emphasized the core mission of aggressive treatment of the acutely ill or injured, with little attention to palliative medicine. As a result, there is a lack of knowledge of palliative medicine

---

[a]From Gilligan T, Raffin TA. Physician virtues and communicating with patients. *New Horiz* 1997;5:6–14, with permission.
[b]From Nelson J, Meier D. Palliative care in the intensive care unit: part I. *J Intens Care Med* 1999;14:130, with permission.
[c]From Lynn J, Harrell F Jr, Cohn F, et al. Prognoses of seriously ill hospitalized patients on the days before death: implications for patient care and public policy. *New Horiz* 1997;5:56–61, with permission.
[d]From Prendergast TJ. Resolving conflicts surrounding end-of-life care. *New Horiz* 1997;5:62–71, with permission.

ICU may reasonably expect this degree of expertise from their ICU staff, if not now, at least as a goal to be reached in the near future.

First, as mentioned, it is absolutely essential that adequate attention be paid to symptom control. There are very few situations where attention to the physical and psychological needs of patient's conflicts with curative treatment. Palliative care can teach the intensivist about good symptom management.

A second aspect of palliative care applicable to the ICU is to recognize that each individual patient lives within a web of human relationships. To care for a critically ill patient is to have a relationship, not only with the patient but also with all those people to whom the patient is related. Regardless of the caregiver's interest or willingness to explore those relationships, the caregiver cannot escape the complex and frequently difficult communications environment that those relationships create. The ability to communicate effectively with groups of people is absolutely essential to the intensivist. Because of uncertainty about the prognosis is pervasive and colors everything else that occurs in the ICU, a communication strategy that diffuses the power of uncertainty by acknowledging it directly, facilitates good ICU care therefore opening the door to good palliative care.

Third, a fundamental principle of palliative care is acceptance of impending death, by the patient, by loved ones, and by the health care provider. In the ICU, the unexpected nature of illness or injury combined with prognostic uncertainty leads to common self-protective strategies. In their hope of recovery, family members may deny the possibility of death whereas physicians may avoid discussion of death. The approach from palliative care means acknowledging the possibility of death in an ongoing discussion with the family and, when appropriate, moving to limit life-sustaining treatments. It is in the area of withdrawal of life-support that intensivists have most clearly changed their practice and where the most concrete recommendations can be offered.

PAIN AND SYMPTOM CONTROL IN THE INTENSIVE CARE UNIT: GENERAL PRINCIPLES

There are multiple reasons for patients to experience pain, anxiety, dyspnea, and other distressing symptoms during treatment in the ICU. Surgical procedures, bedside instrumentation, placement and maintenance of an endotracheal tube including endotracheal suctioning, and prolonged immobilization, in addition to the trauma or serious illness that warranted hospitalization in the first place, all may cause significant physical and psychological symptoms (36,37). Patients report significant distress associated with pain that may manifest as anxiety or agitation (38). In a recent survey, hunger, thirst, and disruption of sleep were reported as moderate or severe by >50% of ICU patients (39). The act of weaning patients from mechanical ventilation may be associated with significant anxiety even in patients who are clinically improving (40). The overall symptom burden may be particularly high in dying patients (41).

Despite the apparent prevalence of pain and other symptoms, rigorous research into prevalence and control of symptoms has been scarce. Partly, this lack of research reflects the difficulty of symptom assessment in ICU patients. Critically ill patients frequently have altered cognition, they may either be heavily sedated or a significant proportion is endotracheally intubated, which renders them speechless. Although there are symptom assessment tools that can assist providers in obtaining information in many patients (42,43), including intubated and dying patients (39), these tools are time consuming and labor intensive, and have not generally been tested for both reliability and validity (44,45). In the routine practice of critical care medicine, symptom assessment has been subjective and poorly standardized (46).

The most basic principle in the assessment of pain is that pain is irreducibly subjective (42). Therefore, the best indicator of pain is the patient's own report. Patients who can report their pain should be treated accordingly, although their cognition may be altered by illness or medication, and the stress of critical illness may significantly change their ability to cope with or to describe pain. Appropriate treatment always requires a careful pain history, particularly a history of chronic opioid use, to dose analgesics correctly. Instruments available for patients who can communicate range from a simple linear scale to quantify the pain, to more intricate inventories of psychological states such as the McGill pain questionnaire (47). Visual analog scales require less cognitive processing than visual descriptors or numerical rating scales but do require that the patient be able to see (42). None of these scales has been validated in critically ill patients.

Patients who cannot describe pain may manifest it as "agitation." Agitation is not a diagnosis but a description of excessive or inappropriate motor activity. Despite the difficulty of identifying a specific etiology, a diagnostic review of the agitated patient is essential before instituting therapy. Anxiety, fear, frustration with inability to communicate, pain, delirium, dyspnea, and ventilator dyssynchrony all may manifest as agitation. Failure to search for an etiology may lead to inappropriate treatment. To treat pain with sedatives that have no analgesic properties may require excessive sedation to the point of general anesthesia. Delirium may be exacerbated by opioids or benzodiazepines and is best treated with haloperidol.

In >50% of ICU patients who cannot report their subjective experience, assessment is particularly dependent on careful physical examination for potential sources of pain, such as early decubiti, pressure points, intravenous lines, surgical wounds, traumatic fractures, and constricting bandages or restraints. Assessment of the nonverbal patient also depends on the observation of nonspecific physiological data, such as changes in blood pressure and heart rate, tearing or diaphoresis, along with a subjective assessment by the provider of the patient's appearance and how the patient responds to specific treatments such as, turning, positioning, and suctioning (42,48). Observational methods that do not elicit information directly from the patient lack sensitivity and specificity (39,46). Family members may help interpret nonverbal information in such patients, although the validity of such surrogate interpretations is unknown.

Virtually all ICU patients require sedation, analgesia, or both to protect them and facilitate their treatment (49). To administer sedating agents presupposes a therapeutic goal and a way to determine when that goal has been reached. These goals are sometimes poorly defined, the assessments may be made subjective, and documentation of both is frequently poor. A recent systematic review of sedation scoring systems (44) identified 25 sedation instruments, of which only four (one pediatric scale) had been tested for both reliability and validity. The oldest and most widely used scale in adult ICU patients is the Ramsay Scale (50). In many institutions, this has been superseded by instruments that discriminate better among levels of agitation (Table 76.4). A first step in improving sedation practice is to standardize assessment of therapeutic goals and patient assessment using one of these instruments. Systematic assessment can be combined with therapeutic algorithms to perform continuous quality improvement (53). Nonpharmacologic strategies to manage agitation may be underutilized (54,55).

TABLE 76.4

QUANTITATIVE ASSESSMENT OF SEDATION IN CRITICAL CARE

Rating	Ramsay scale[a]	Sedation-agitation scale[b]	Motor-activity assessment[c]
0	N/A	Minimal or no response to noxious stimuli	Unresponsive to noxious stimuli
1	Asleep; no response to light glabellar tap	Arouses to physical stimuli but does not follow commands	Responsive only to noxious stimuli
2	Asleep; sluggish response to light glabellar tap	Difficult to arouse but follows simple commands	Responsive to touch or name
3	Asleep; brisk response to light glabellar tap	Calm, awakens easily, follows commands	Calm and cooperative
4	Awake; responds to commands only	Anxious or mildly agitated, but calms to verbal instructions	Restless and cooperative
5	Awake; cooperative, oriented, and tranquil	Very agitated, does not calm with verbal instructions	Agitated
6	Awake; anxious, agitated, or both	Dangerously agitated, uncooperative	Dangerously agitated, uncooperative

N/A, not applicable.
Numerical coding modified to show parallel elements among the three scales.
[a]From Ramsay MA, Savege TM, Simpson BR, et al. Controlled sedation with alphaxalone-alphadolone. *BMJ* 1974;2:656–659, with permission.
[b]From Riker RR, Picard JT, Fraser GL. Prospective evaluation of the Sedation-Agitation Scale for adult critically ill patients. *Crit Care Med* 1999; 27:1325–1329, (51) with permission.
[c]From Devlin JW, Boleski G, Mlynarek M, et al. Motor Activity Assessment Scale: a valid and reliable sedation scale for use with mechanically ventilated patients in an adult surgical intensive care unit. *Crit Care Med* 1999;27:1271–1275, (52) with permission.

CURRENT PRACTICE

Most of the data regarding symptom control are found in studies of pharmacologic management of pain and agitation. There is a paucity of data on nausea, dyspnea, sleep deprivation, and so on. Studies of pain management in the ICU suggest systematic undertreatment. The SUPPORT study (2) is a major reference point for the management of pain in severely ill, hospitalized patients, half of whom were treated in ICUs during their hospitalizations. Twenty-two percent of patients interviewed in the second week of the SUPPORT study reported that they had "moderate or severe pain almost half the time." Family members of patients who died reported that their loved ones had been in moderate or severe pain half the time. Puntillo reported a series of 24 primarily surgical ICU patients where 63% of patients reported moderate to severe pain (56). Whipple et al. investigated the different perceptions of physicians, nurses, and 17 patients admitted to the ICU after a traumatic injury (57): 95% of house staff and 81% of nurses reported the patients received adequate pain control but 74% of patients reported significant pain (27% moderate and 47% severe). The conclusion seems inescapable: intensivists systematically undertreat pain.

A number of recent papers have raised questions about systematic oversedation. Kress et al. reported the results of a randomized controlled trial in 128 medical ICU patients (58). In the intervention group, sedative infusions were interrupted each morning until the patients were awake or uncomfortable; in the control group, the infusions were not interrupted routinely but at the discretion of the ICU clinicians. The investigators found a shorter duration of mechanical ventilation and shorter ICU length of stay in the intervention group, along with fewer diagnostic studies to assess altered mental status. No measure of patient distress or satisfaction was reported in the original paper. The authors have subsequently published in abstract form a summary of patient interviews that does not reveal any difference in psychological well-being, depression, or post-traumatic stress disorder between intervention and control patients (59). Only 1 patient of 12 recalled awakening

from sedation; the patient was a control subject. These data suggest that, in a medical ICU, the current standard of practice sedates mechanically ventilated patients so heavily that it may prolong their ICU stay.

It is not yet clear how to reconcile these findings with data that pain is undertreated. Sedation may be given excessively whereas analgesics are underdosed. In particular, continuous infusion of sedatives and analgesics may prolong mechanical ventilation but the constant levels so achieved may not suffice for procedural pain from suctioning, turning, and other aspects of ICU care that patients report are uncomfortable (60). Given the paucity of data on patient distress or satisfaction, it may be that adequate symptom control requires medication that itself prolongs ICU treatment (39).

There are even fewer data about the management of pain and sedation in ICU patients at the end of life. This clinical context is very specific: most patients who die in ICUs have life-support withheld or withdrawn. The usual considerations of balancing adequate sedation with hemodynamic stability or avoiding prolongation of mechanical ventilation are no longer issues. There may be new considerations. Some patients may want to remain alert as long as possible to be able to communicate with their families. Some providers may worry about administering large amounts of opioids or sedatives to a patient who will die soon afterwards, for fear that such practice blurs the line between withdrawal of life-support and active euthanasia.

Two studies address to this question. In 1988–89, Wilson et al. retrospectively reviewed over 1 year all patients at the San Francisco General Hospital who had life-support withheld or withdrawn (61). They randomly selected an equivalent number (n = 22) of patients from their affiliated University Hospital. Seventy-five percent (33/44) of the patients who had received either sedation or analgesics or both, at doses that were significantly increased from baseline, once the decision was made to withdraw life-support, died. The rest who did not receive sedation were deeply comatose and died faster than those who received additional medication. The authors concluded that administration of opioids and sedatives was common in the withdrawal of life support from ICU patients and did not appear to hasten death. The latter conclusion was seriously weakened by significant clinical differences between the two patient groups.

Hall and Rocker reviewed charts from 174 consecutive patients who died over a 1-year period in 1996–97 (62). Seventy-nine percent (138/174) had life-support withheld or withdrawn, whereas 21% (36/174) had aggressive therapy continued up to the time of death. Doses of morphine and lorazepam were fivefold higher in patients from whom life-support was withdrawn, and most of this increase occurred in the 4 hours before death. Neuromuscular blocking agents (NMB) were administered to 25 patients, of whom 17 had NMB started in the last 12 hours of life. In 20% (5/25) patients a single dose of NMB was administered to facilitate endotracheal intubation. Nine patients had an NMB infusion at the time of death, five of whom had life-support (but not mechanical ventilation) withdrawn. Sixteen percent (4/25) of patients receiving NMB were also receiving intermittent sedation/analgesia but not continuous infusions.

These and other studies show that the range of opioid doses necessary to control acute pain or dyspnea is very wide; large doses may be necessary. However, the dose in milligrams is much less relevant than careful administration. It is entirely appropriate to give large amounts provided that these doses are carefully titrated to specific effects. In rare cases, it may only be possible to control symptoms with doses that hasten death. Provided that the intended effect is relief of suffering and the doses are carefully titrated to that effect, there is broad consensus in bioethics and the law that ameliorating symptoms is not euthanasia, that is, not the deliberate administration of drugs with the intent to terminate the patient's life (63,64). One of the most egregious failings in end-of-life care is the systematic failure to adequately to treat pain and dyspnea, based on a misunderstanding of this distinction (65).

SPECIFIC RECOMMENDATIONS

There is a modest amount of data describing current practice in pain and symptom management in ICUs. There is much less data to clarify how effective this therapy is to make specific treatment recommendations. A recent, systematic review of randomized controlled trials comparing at least two different agents for the sedation of ICU patients found a discordance between the prevalence of use of sedatives (multiple reviews identified between 11 and 23 different agents used in the United States and United Kingdom) and a paucity of data (66). Of 49 studies identified, only 32 met minimal criteria for adequacy of study design, and of these 32, 20 compared propofol to midazolam. This literature is largely driven by pharmaceutical companies seeking data to support the use of specific medications. If the measure of efficacy is patient/family satisfaction, then there is little information to guide practice. Any recommendations are at the level of consensus guidelines and expert opinion (46).

First, and logically necessary to any improvement in practice, is that intensivists need to place a higher emphasis on specific symptom control. The first step is to incorporate systematic symptom assessment into their routine practice (39).

Second, intensivists must be experts in the use of a fairly small number of analgesic and sedative agents. Expertise includes understanding the pharmacokinetics and metabolism of these agents. With opioids and some benzodiazepines, the plasma elimination half-life is a poor measure of clinical effect because the onset of activity and duration of effect are more closely tied to distribution and redistribution of the drug into and out of the central nervous system (CNS). One must also understand how these properties are altered in the setting of

advanced age (67) and critical illness (68,69). The presence of increased extravascular water increases the volume of distribution of many drugs. Changes in plasma-protein levels will affect protein binding and may increase concentration of free drug. Impairment of hepatic and renal function affects metabolism and clearance. Agents (midazolam) that undergo oxidation-reduction are affected by age, disease states, such as cirrhosis, and competing pharmaceuticals far more than drugs (lorazepam) that undergo glucuronidation (70). Pharmacokinetic data are obtained in studies of healthy volunteers and may not be applicable to critically ill patients (Tables 76.5 and 76.6).

Practically, intravenous administration is preferred in the ICU. Virtually all patients have intravenous access, and many have central venous access that permits administration of agents that are irritating when given by peripheral vein. Intravenous administration reduces the variability in absorption seen in enteral or subcutaneous routes. Enteral administration is complicated in the ICU patient because of impaired gastric emptying, decreased intestinal motility, nasogastric suctioning, diminished intestinal blood flow either due to illness or administration of vasoactive agents, and reduced absorptive surface area (71). Because the exact dose of analgesics or sedatives is less important than titrating the dose to clinical effect, some agents that are well absorbed enterally (lorazepam, diazepam, and haloperidol) can be given through the enteral route. Most medications are dosed by continuous infusion, however. In the case of pain, it is essential to control the pain adequately with bolus dosing before relying on a continuous infusion.

Opioids have a variety of beneficial effects in ICU patients (Table 76.5). Opioids have potent analgesic properties but are only mild sedatives and do not have specific anxiolytic effects apart from those consequent to reduced pain. Opioids may cause euphoria but do not produce amnesia. They are potent antitussives that depress upper airway and tracheal reflexes, facilitating tolerance of an endotracheal tube without coughing or fighting against the ventilator.

Opioids are potent respiratory depressants. They produce dose-dependent inhibition of respiratory rate, tidal volume, minute ventilation, and ventilatory response to CO_2 (73). This effect is potentiated by concomitant administration of benzodiazepines (74). Chronic administration of opioids is associated with tolerance to the respiratory depressant effects of opioids but this process takes many months (75). Therefore, ICU patients typically are sensitive to respiratory depression although it is rarely a pressing concern in patients who are intubated. At equianalgesic doses, no opioid is more or less likely than another to produce respiratory depression. Opioids cause urinary retention, decreased intestinal motility, and delayed gastric emptying. At high doses, they may cause adynamic ileus. Tolerance does not develop to constipation. Opioids may cause nausea through direct stimulation of the chemoreceptor trigger zone.

Benzodiazepines are safe and inexpensive medications that have become the drugs of choice for sedation in intensive care patients (Table 76.6). Benzodiazepines have potent anxiolytic and amnestic properties and are mild hypnotics. At higher doses, they are effective at preventing and treating seizures. They may have some antiemetic effects but this is not a potent property. They have no intrinsic analgesic properties and so are commonly given with an opioid for better control of symptoms at lower doses. Benzodiazepines do not have significant hemodynamic effects at usual doses although midazolam may precipitate hypotension in some patients. They do have mild central respiratory depressant effects that are synergistic with opioids (74). Midazolam has the most effect on the ventilatory response to CO_2 and can cause apnea when given at higher doses (induction of anesthesia) or in susceptible (principally

TABLE 76.5

OPIOID ANALGESICS COMMONLY USED IN INTENSIVE CARE

Drug	Drug interactions	Pharmacokinetics through intravenous route	Metabolism and active metabolites	Specific intensive care unit concerns
Morphine				
Most often given intravenously but may be administered through i.m., s.q., oral, rectal, and inhaled (nebulized) routes. Less potent than fentanyl 1 mg morphine equal to 80–100 µg fentanyl	Nifedipine may increase the analgesic effect, somatostatin may decrease the effect Rifampin and other cytochrome P-450 inducers may decrease plasma concentration	Onset: 5 min Peak effect: 20–30 min Duration of therapeutic effect: 2–7 h Elimination half-life following single dose: 2–3 h in healthy volunteers, 3–6 h in ICU patients	Metabolized mainly in the liver to morphine-3-glucuronide (M3G) and morphine-6-glucuronide (M6G) that are renally excreted. M6G has several times the analgesic potency of morphine and a longer elimination half-life (12 h). M6G accumulates in renal failure and may lead to prolonged sedation in ICU patients M3G is probably inactive, although some data suggest that M3G antagonizes the effect of the parent compound	Opioid most associated with histamine release affecting hemodynamics. May cause hypotension through decreased sympathetic tone in addition to venous and arterial vasodilation ICU states may impair metabolism. Significant liver dysfunction, septic shock, and renal failure all decrease clearance of morphine and its metabolites For patients on chronic opioids, analgesic effect increases linearly with the log of the dose. Therefore, in-patients with uncontrolled pain, large increments may be necessary for amelioration of symptoms
Fentanyl				
Exclusively i.v. administration. High first-pass metabolism in liver makes enteral administration impractical. Available in transcutaneous patch and transmucosal oralet ("lollipop") both rarely used in adult ICU patients More potent than morphine. 80 µg fentanyl equal to 1 mg morphine	Rifampin, human immunodeficiency virus protease inhibitors and other cytochrome P-450 inducers may decrease plasma concentration and analgesic effect	Onset: 30 s–2 min Peak effect: 5–15 min Duration of therapeutic effect: 30–60 min Elimination half-life following single dose: 7–10 h in healthy volunteers, 10–36 h in ICU patients Prolonged in elderly patients	Metabolized through oxidation and hydrolysis in the liver to inactive metabolites that are excreted in bile and urine Hepatic clearance not significantly affected by cirrhosis unless end-stage but very sensitive to hepatic blood flow. Highly protein bound, so free drug increased in hypoproteinemic patients Half-life prolonged in elderly patients because of reduced clearance from decreased hepatic blood flow and decreased plasma protein concentrations Renal failure does not significantly alter pharmacokinetics in most patients	Not associated with histamine release and little effect on cardiac function or vascular tone; therefore, opioid of choice in hemodynamically unstable patients or patients with asthma. May rarely cause bradycardia. May cause muscle rigidity when given in high doses Highly lipid-soluble; therefore, rapid penetration into the CNS and large volume of distribution. Short duration of effect when given as a single bolus reflects redistribution of drug out of the CNS rather than elimination half-life. When given as a continuous infusion, fentanyl may accumulate in fat tissues. Its elimination is then dependent on redistribution out of fat stores rather than half-life

ICU, intensive care unit; CNS, central nervous system, HIV, human immunodeficiency virus.
From multiple sources, including refs. (46,48,67–69,71,72), with permission.

TABLE 76.6

AGENTS COMMONLY USED FOR SEDATION IN INTENSIVE CARE

Drug	Drug interactions	Pharmacokinetics through intravenous route	Metabolism and active metabolites	Specific intensive care unit concerns
Diazepam i.v. formulation common but irritating to veins. Excellent oral absorption but erratic when given i.m. or rectally	Increased clearance with rifampin, phenytoin, phenobarbital Decreased clearance with drugs that compete with cytochrome P-450, e.g. azole antifungals, macrolide antibiotics, calcium channel blockers, HIV protease inhibitors, some antidepressants	Onset: 30–60 s Peak effect: 2–5 min Duration of therapeutic effect dependent on metabolites and, therefore, quite variable: 12–60 h Elimination half-life following single dose: 54–62 h in healthy volunteers, up to 120 h in ICU patients	Hepatic oxidative metabolism to active metabolites oxazepam and desmethyldiazepam. Latter has longer elimination half-life than parent compound, up to 200 h Highly protein bound, so free drug concentrations susceptible to fluctuation in disease states Clearance decreased with liver disease and with increased age	Most lipophilic of benzodiazepines. Rapidly distributes into and out of the CNS Like all the benzodiazepines, has potent amnestic properties
Lorazepam i.v. formulation less irritating to veins than diazepam. Excellent oral and i.m. absorption Five times more potent/mg than diazepam	Valproate sodium increases serum levels through inhibition of glucuronidation	Onset: 5–15 min Peak effect: 30–60 min Duration of therapeutic effect: 4–8 h Elimination half-life following single dose: 13–15 h in healthy volunteers, 10–14 h in ICU patients	Glucuronidation in the liver to inactive metabolites that are renally excreted. Elimination half-life may be prolonged in end-stage cirrhosis and advanced renal failure but least likely of benzodiazepines to be affected by organ dysfunction	Relatively little change in pharmacokinetics with advanced age or in critically ill patients. Time to awakening after prolonged infusion may be shorter than with midazolam
Midazolam Available i.v. only, because first-pass metabolism severely reduces bioavailability when given by oral or rectal route Three times more potent/mg than diazepam	Similar to diazepam: Decreased clearance with drugs that compete with cytochrome P-450, e.g. azole antifungals, macrolide antibiotics, calcium channel blockers, HIV protease inhibitors	Onset: 30–60 s Peak effect: 2–5 min Duration of therapeutic effect: 1–7 h Elimination half-life following single dose: 2–4 h in healthy volunteers, 7–11 h in ICU patients	Oxidation in the liver to hydroxymidazolam, which has activity, although less potent than midazolam Hydroxymidazolam has a larger volume of distribution and a longer elimination half-life than the parent drug Metabolism reported moderately to severely affected by hepatic dysfunction. Free drug increased in renal failure	Very lipid-soluble at physiological pH leading to rapid CNS penetration and equally rapid redistribution. Short duration of effect as bolus because of redistribution. Effects are prolonged when given as a continuous infusion. Elimination half-life prolonged in critically ill patients, especially those with end-organ dysfunction in whom it may be greater than 24 h Time to awakening after prolonged infusion may be longer than with lorazepam

Propofol

i.v. only. Primarily a hypnotic and anesthetic agent but provides effective and titratable sedation at sub-hypnotic doses

May impair the patient's ability to protect the upper airway, so generally reserved for intubated patients but increasingly used in the imminently dying

Propofol is prepared in a lipid emulsion containing 10% soybean oil that contains vitamin K. Therefore, caution is advised when administering propofol to patients receiving warfarin

Onset: <30 s
Peak effect: 90 s
Duration of therapeutic effect: 2–8 min
Elimination half-life after single bolus: 6–8 h
Elimination half-life following continuous infusion in ICU patients: 26–32 h

Hepatic and extrahepatic metabolism. Probably no active metabolites. Mild prolongation of elimination half-life in hepatic disease; clearance unchanged in renal disease
Volume of distribution and elimination half-life increased after prolonged, continuous i.v. administration

Highly lipid-soluble leading to immediate onset and very short distribution half-life (2–8 min)
No intrinsic analgesic properties, so commonly administered with opioids
When given as an i.v. bolus, causes dose-dependent hypotension because of both cardiac depression and peripheral vasodilation. Most commonly given as continuous infusion in ICU patients. Tolerance may develop after continuous infusion for more than 24 h.
Time to awakening shorter than for benzodiazepines, but advantage may be lost with concomitant administration of opioids
Less effective as an amnestic agent than benzodiazepines. Not recommended in pediatric populations because of idiosyncratic metabolic acidosis

Haloperidol

May be given enterally as well as i.v.

Inducers of cytochrome P-450 may reduce plasma concentrations

Onset: 10–30 min
Peak effect: 30–60 min
Duration of therapeutic effect: 4–20 h
Elimination half-life after single bolus: 28–38 h

Hepatic metabolism to multiple metabolites of which only hydroxyhaloperidol has minimal activity. Half-life prolonged in hepatic dysfunction

Relatively nonsedating, especially given potency of antipsychotic effects. Extrapyramidal symptoms rarely seen with i.v. administration
No intrinsic analgesic properties but a potent antiemetic
Minimal cardiovascular or respiratory effects. May cause prolongation of the QT interval and ventricular arrhythmias especially when given at high (>100 mg/d) doses. i.v. infusion not to exceed 5 mg/min

ICU, intensive care unit; CNS, central nervous system; HIV, human immunodeficiency virus.
From multiple sources, including refs. (46,48,67–69,71,72), with permission.

elderly) patients. Lorazepam and, especially, diazepam cause venous irritation when given intravenously. Midazolam is prepared as a water-soluble solution and does not cause phlebitis.

Propofol is a potent intravenous hypnotic and anesthetic that is increasingly used in the ICU for short-term, titratable sedation (Table 76.6). Propofol causes a dose-dependent fall in blood pressure through both direct depression of cardiac output and peripheral vasodilation. This effect is much more pronounced when given as a bolus than when given as a continuous infusion. The hypotensive effect is augmented by concomitant opioid administration. Propofol is a respiratory depressant that causes dose-dependent depression of tidal volumes, minute ventilation, and ventilatory response to carbon dioxide. Apnea is common after induction of anesthesia with propofol. Propofol has demonstrated antiemetic properties during maintenance of anesthesia (76) to reduce postoperative nausea and vomiting after standard anesthesia (77) and to reduce chemotherapy-induced emesis (78,79). Haloperidol is a high-potency, nonspecific dopamine antagonist that is the agent of choice for management of delirium and psychosis in intensive care (Table 76.6) (80).

COMMUNICATIONS: GENERAL PRINCIPLES AND CURRENT PRACTICE

Multiple aspects of critical illness make the ICU a difficult communications environment. Most ICU patients were not terminally ill and many were healthy before an unexpected catastrophic illness or injury. The ability to predict outcome, although excellent across populations, is very limited in individuals (22). The threat of death or significant disability is real but intensivists rarely have an established relationship with their patients. In many cases, they never have the chance to speak to them because most patients are unable to participate in their treatment decisions (24,81,82). Patients admitted to ICUs rarely have completed advance directives (83,84), and the advance directives that are written are frequently too general to be helpful (85) or contain internal inconsistencies (11).

Family members of ICU patients confront difficult choices in a complex and unfamiliar environment. Surrogate decision makers are called on to make decisions about continuing or withdrawing life-support, despite the fact that correlation between the patient preferences and their relatives' predictions of those preferences is poor (86,87). When asked about their needs, family members emphasize communication of information (Table 76.7). Despite the importance to families of clear communication, this does not appear to be strength of critical care practice. Fifty-four percent of families of ICU patients in one study had significant misunderstandings of diagnosis, treatment, or prognosis (91). This lack of comprehension occurred despite the ability of physicians to identify family members who did not understand and despite a positive correlation between understanding and the amount of time physicians spent with the family. Of interest, for the readership of a textbook of supportive oncology, there was a high correlation between family misunderstanding and referral from hematology or oncology.

In addition to the lack of skill or unwillingness to convey medical information to family members, intensivists may not listen carefully to the patient's and family's needs. Twenty-five percent of bereaved families in one study believed that neither the patient nor the family was part of the discussion about end-of-life decisions (92). Only 29% of patients in SUPPORT who preferred palliative care thought that the care they received was consistent with their wishes (93), and they

TABLE 76.7

A DOZEN NEEDS OF THE FAMILY IN THE SETTING OF CRITICAL ILLNESS

To have questions answered honestly
To know specific facts about what is wrong with the patient
To know the prognosis for recovery
To be called at home about changes in the patient's status
To receive information from the physician (at least) once daily
To receive information in understandable language
To believe that hospital personnel care about the patient
To be assured of the patient's comfort
To be comforted
To express emotions
To find meaning in the death of their loved one
To be fed, hydrated, and rested

Adapted from references 33,34,88–90, with permission.

reported low rates of discussions with physicians about their prognoses and preferences. In a survey of American Thoracic Society members, 34% of intensivists reported continuing therapy that the patient/surrogate requested be discontinued, and 82% of physicians made unilateral decisions to withdraw therapy, often without the knowledge or consent of the patient/surrogate and sometimes despite their objections (94).

Prognostic uncertainty and strained communications around unpredictable problems create fertile ground for disagreement. Disputes about management are not the exception in the ICU; they are ubiquitous—an integral part of the critical care environment (95–97). It remains unknown how many physician-family disputes are the result of ineffective communications by physicians. Disputes arise as often among physicians as between physicians and families (24). Despite the common assumption that nurses are more effective communicators than physicians, there is evidence that skills are not different between these groups (98).

RECOMMENDATIONS FOR PRACTICE

Patients and families express needs for better communications with their physicians. In the ICU, this means that intensivists are called to build relationships, facilitate decision making, and negotiate disagreements, in addition to learning how to deliver bad news (99). There are two problems with making concrete recommendations for improved practice in this area (100). First, much of the literature is based on expert opinion and is not grounded in empirical research. Second, the research that exists is written largely from the perspective of the caregiver. Perhaps the most important recent development in this area is the appearance of many attempts to elucidate the patient's and family's perspective (38,88,89,91,101). A first step toward improved ICU communication is to acknowledge this literature and, thereby, the importance of illness (i.e., the patient/family's subjective experience of their biomedical disease) (89). A second step is to eradicate the implicit and false assumption that communication with patients and families is a skill that every nurse and physician possesses. In fact, there are approaches to patients that are demonstrably more and less effective at facilitating communication (102,103). These approaches are skills that can be learned (104–107). Acknowledging the need for training may be difficult because physicians tend to believe that they are communicating effectively despite evidence that they are not (108,109).

A second development that gives hope for improved communications in the ICU is empirical research into the extraordinary complexity of treatment discussions, particularly those surrounding withholding and withdrawal of life-sustaining therapies. Recent work confirms that the act of withdrawing life-sustaining therapy from a patient is not the result of a single decision but emerges from the process of ongoing care (110–112). One implication of this is that intensivists must recognize not only how important family discussions are to families but also how essential they are to the practicing intensivist (113,114).

The astute intensivist sees in the critical care setting opportunities for creating relationships. One rationale for advance directives is an underlying mistrust of physicians (115, 116), and a major hurdle in discussing end-of-life care is to overcome that mistrust. In the outpatient setting, it takes a special effort on the part of physicians to establish a relationship that allows meaningful advance care planning. Insofar as ICU care is an emergent, unexpected event, the lack of previous relationship may open an opportunity to bypass mistrust. The clinician and the patient are brought together under extraordinary circumstances. There is often a sense of shared goals. Family and physician both seek the best possible care for the patient leading to recovery, if possible. Most want to avoid overtreatment if recovery is not possible. These shared goals form the basis of a natural alliance that the skilled intensivist can build upon to facilitate communications (116).

Preferences for end-of-life care are not fixed qualities that a patient discovers upon reflection. A decision to pursue risky therapy or to forego further intensive care is not made in the abstract. Preferences for care emerge from a process of discussion and feedback within the network of the patient's most important relationships (110). Such decisions are inevitably embedded within a social context. The ICU environment can make this communication easier, not harder, because there is a natural iterative pattern in meeting with a family through the course of a critical illness. The ability to meet repetitively over time provides an opportunity to build trust. These meetings also create a new social context where the intensivist plays an important role in the ongoing development of preferences for care. These conversations hold the key to end-of-life decision-making in the ICU (112,115,117).

WITHHOLDING AND WITHDRAWAL OF LIFE SUPPORT: GENERAL PRINCIPLES

Most patients who die in North American ICUs do so following a considered decision to withhold or withdraw some form of life-sustaining therapy (10,62,118). This represents a recent, secular trend in North America toward more active management of dying ICU patients (24,119,120) as well as a dramatic change from earlier practice (Table 76.1). There is a broad ethical and legal consensus that withdrawal of life-sustaining therapy is appropriate in many circumstances (63,64,121–125). Nonetheless, there remains significant variation in practice (Fig. 76.1). The reasons for this variation are not clear, but it does not appear to be associated with size, type of ICU, or the number of admissions (10). The attending physician's status may be a relevant factor (126).

There is a great deal of descriptive research on the process of withdrawal of life-sustaining therapy (61,62,82,85,127–129). Any therapy that sustains life can be withheld or withdrawn. The most common therapies are, in the approximate order of frequency with which they are withdrawn: blood products, hemodialysis, vasopressors, mechanical ventilation, total parenteral nutrition, antibiotics, intravenous fluids, and enteral feedings. Most physicians opt to withdraw therapies in a sequence; the therapies most likely to be withdrawn first are those that are scarce, expensive, or invasive. Many physicians will first withdraw the therapies with which they are most familiar. There are many suggested algorithms for withdrawing different technologies (130–133). These recommendations are based on expert opinion. Few studies report patient comfort, family satisfaction, or the experience of caregivers on which to base a recommendation (134).

Patients and surrogates, or clinicians, or both, may pursue intensive care too long before acknowledging the appropriateness of limiting therapy. Patients and physicians usually move to limit therapy when hope for recovery is outweighed by the burdens of continuing treatment. Most disagreements about continuing therapy are not about the merits of treatment in the face of incontrovertible evidence that it has failed. Physicians and families most often disagree about how to value a small

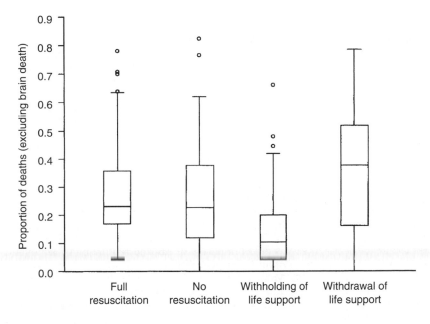

FIGURE 76.1. Variation in the practice of withholding and withdrawal of life-support among 131 American intensive care units. Actual mean percentages (range) are as follows: full support, including cardiopulmonary resuscitation (CPR), 26% (4–79); do not resuscitate (DNR), 24% (0–83); withholding, 11% (0–67); withdrawal, 36% (0–79). (From Prendergast TJ, Claessens MT, Luce JM. A national study of end-of-life care for critically ill patients. *Am J Respir Crit Care Med* 1998;158:1163–1167, with permission.)

chance of improvement, or how to weigh the continuing burdens of treatment, be they physical, emotional, financial, or in loss of dignity. The difficulty in making such judgments in the face of inadequate information naturally leads to disagreements. Most often, these disagreements are handled through an intuitive process of negotiation. The parties agree on a time-limited trial of therapy, followed by review and withdrawal if the patient has not improved. In a small percentage of cases, the perspectives of the patient/surrogate and the treating physicians are difficult to reconcile, and one party may insist on treatment against the strong recommendation of the other. Many physicians attempt to apply the concept of medical futility to such requests to reassert the prerogative to make the decision they favor (135). Because there is no consensus definition of medical futility, this approach should be avoided. The Council on Ethical and Judicial Affairs of the American Medical Association has recently suggested an alternative, procedural approach based upon the experience of researchers in Denver and Houston (136). It is important to recognize that although each side—the medical community and patient advocates—accuses the other of demanding overtreatment, the evidence suggests that physicians and families are about equally responsible (97).

SUGGESTED PROTOCOL FOR WITHDRAWAL OF LIFE SUPPORT

A. *Clarify the decision.* Establish a consensus on withdrawal among the medical team members. Responsibility to proceed with withdrawal remains with the patient/surrogate in consultation with the attending physician, but it is essential to know if there are significant concerns among consulting physicians, nursing, respiratory care, or other members of the critical care team. Members of the team may reach the conclusion that therapy should be discontinued at different times. Unanimity is not to be expected in all cases. Common areas of disagreement include misunderstandings of legal responsibility and liability, disputes over prognosis, and a tendency to focus on survival to ICU discharge that neglects the patient's long-term survival. If disagreements among the critical care team cannot be resolved in advance of the decision, their concerns must be noted as a sign of professional respect.

Identify the appropriate decision maker, patient, or surrogate. Establish consensus on proceeding among patient/family. As with the medical team, unanimity is the goal but is not to be expected in all cases. All critical care providers should hone their skills in understanding the dynamics of family discussions. In particular, speculation as to motivations of family members should be discouraged while encouraging an appreciation for the difficulty of allowing a loved one to die. Providers should be particularly sensitive to framing discussions that suggest that the family's or surrogate's decision is responsible for the patient's death. In almost every case, this is simply inaccurate: the decision is made in accordance with the patient's wishes.

Document the discussion as well as the plan in the medical record.

B. *Identify patient/family goals.* Nearly all patients who have life support withdrawn in a critical care setting die soon thereafter. This is usually not in doubt but should be made clear if it is not already done.

Some patients and most families ask for comfort above all else. Ensuring comfort often comes at the cost of diminished level of consciousness. Occasionally patients will want to visit with loved ones and are prepared to tolerate some physical distress to be present with them. Others simply want to be asleep. To provide excellent care, it is essential to establish with the patient or surrogate the primary treatment goals following the withdrawal of life support.

C. *Review the process with family, and patient, if awake.* Emphasize comfort consistent with patient goals (see preceding text). Describe the plan to deal with any complications of withdrawal. Do not make promises that you cannot keep, for example, adequate analgesia and sedation may not prevent some gasping or gurgling of secretions. Reassure the patient/family that you have a plan to treat these signs should they appear.

Address length of survival. Family members frequently ask how long a patient will live after the withdrawal of life support. They deserve an answer, even if it is only an educated guess. In most cases, it is possible to put a patient's prognosis into categories of minutes to hours, hours to days, days or more. Often, the clinician can be much more specific. Of course, there will always be patients who will surprise their caregivers and prove their predictions wrong. They are few, and it is better to be helpful to the vast majority of families and risk the occasional mistake than to refuse to answer a legitimate question.

D. *Create a calm environment.* To the extent possible, isolate the patient from the noise and activity of the ICU. Provide a private room or draw curtains. Liberalize visiting rules. Allow children at the discretion of the patient/family.

Any technology that is not providing comfort to the patient should be removed. Remove lines and tubes, turn monitors off, disable alarms, and discontinue routine measurement of vital signs. Discretion will be needed with urinary drainage catheters because removal may be uncomfortable and obstruction may ensue. At least one intravenous catheter should remain in place for the administration of sedatives and analgesics.

E. *Principles of symptom management in withdrawal:*
  1. A physician should be at the bedside at the start of a process of withdrawal, regardless of the therapy withdrawn. Most decisions to allow a patient to die are distressing for the family and fraught with second-guessing. The continued presence of the attending physician at the time of withdrawal makes a strong statement to the family of nonabandonment in the face of death, of continued involvement, while dying, to ensure comfort, and of the importance to the medical team and, by inference, to the hospital of the importance of a good death. The absence of the attending physician may send the opposite message. The presence of the attending physician is also valuable to any trainees or students who may have participated in the patient's care. Obviously, a clinician should be available to assess and to respond to significant changes in the patient's status as therapy is withdrawn.
  2. Medications must be immediately available at the bedside.
  3. Administration of medications should be guided by anticipatory dosing, particularly when making changes that are highly likely to cause distress such as discontinuation of assisted ventilation or removal of an endotracheal tube.
  4. Medications should be titrated to effect comfort, not apnea. There is not *a priori* maximal dose. It is difficult to assess discomfort in comatose patients. If

a patient appears uncomfortable, it is an acceptable practice to administer analgesic and/or sedatives under the assumption that the patient may experience something. Family suffering in the presence of an uncomfortable patient may be palpable. It is acceptable practice to administer medication to make the patient appear more comfortable provided that the intent is not to hasten death.

5. Continuous infusion is preferable to bolus dosing although a bolus is often appropriate prior to increasing a continuous infusion dose, particularly for drugs with a longer time to onset (e.g., lorazepam).

6. If a physician is not present, the nurse should be given appropriate latitude to increase dosing to achieve specific goals, such as, to reduce tachypnea to <25 breaths per minute.

F. *Orchestrating withdrawal of therapies.* There is great variation in how clinicians proceed with the withdrawal of life support. There are, however, a few common principles to guide clinicians.

First, any medical treatment that is not essential to the comfort of the dying patient may be withheld or withdrawn. Artificial nutrition and hydration is a medical-treatment like any other but, unlike most, has strong cultural associations with nurturing and caring. It is important to be aware of the strong feelings that nutrition and hydration carry for many people, including caregivers. Although the medical evidence suggests that there is no additional benefit to continuing artificial nutrition and hydration, families may have cultural traditions of caring for the dying that make a decision to forego such therapy very troubling.

Once a decision has been reached to withdraw life-support in a critically ill patient, one must neither prolong dying unnecessarily nor act to hasten it. The former is the more common mistake. A piecemeal withdrawal of therapies that stretches over hours to days is inappropriate (137). In the vast majority of cases, the patient cannot survive without the technology in question, and death is not only expected but also imminent. When a decision is made to withdraw life support, then life support should be withdrawn—all of it. Removal of most therapies does not cause distress. These therapies, therefore, should be stopped rather than gradually reduced. The only therapy where removal commonly results in exacerbation of symptoms is mechanical ventilation (see subsequent text).

One reason for the gradual withdrawal of therapies over days is to create distance between the removal of the medical intervention and the patient's death. Such space is neither legally nor ethically necessary (63,64). However, too close an approximation of death to the withdrawal of therapy is frequently uncomfortable for caregivers and may contribute to a sense of guilt among family members. More important, the time between withdrawal and death is frequently an important vigil for the family: having made the decision to stop therapy may allow them to sit in the presence of the dying.

Withholding and withdrawal are supported by a broad ethical and legal consensus. Euthanasia is universally condemned and it is illegal in Canada and the United States. Medications, such as potassium chloride, that hasten death but have no role in providing comfort, should not be given. Similarly, large bolus doses of sedatives and analgesics should not be given unless and until routine doses have proved ineffective in controlling symptoms. These medications should be titrated up to effect from below, not down from doses that may induce hypotension or apnea. NMB are frequently used in critical care to facilitate mechanical ventilation. Their therapeutic effect makes symptom assessment all but impossible. Their use at the end of life, when symptom control is paramount, is discouraged. There is some evidence that they are used, and sometimes started, in anticipation of withdrawal of life-sustaining therapy (62). Most intensivists recommend stopping any NMB when the decision is made to withdraw life-support and in advance of withdrawing mechanical ventilation (138).

G. *Removal of mechanical ventilation.* Removal of assisted ventilation or an endotracheal tube commonly causes visible signs of distress even in patients comatose from their illness. The goal of ventilator withdrawal is to remove support efficiently over 15 to 30 minutes while maintaining patient comfort. In general, all other life-sustaining therapies should be removed first (Table 76.8). A common concern is whether to leave the endotracheal tube in place (sometimes referred to as *terminal weaning*) or remove it (extubation) (137,139). In patients who can support their own ventilation, even briefly, extubation may improve patient comfort. It allows closer contact between the patient and the loved ones, and may improve communication. It is recommended to leave the endotracheal tube in place in patients on high levels of ventilatory support, who may die immediately if extubated, and in those with difficulty clearing secretions or protecting their airway, who may struggle and gasp when extubated (131).

H. *After-death care.* A physician should acknowledge and confirm to the family when the patient has died. Every intensivist should understand the nature and management of grief and bereavement (140). Recognize that families may second-guess themselves and may need reassurance that their decision was appropriate and correct.

A multidisciplinary team should debrief after every death, to review the technical details of the outcome, to examine the process of decision making among the team members and to allow the team itself to express grief over the death of a patient. This is particularly important in cases where the decision was particularly difficult (young person, tragic circumstances, a person connected to the medical community) or where there was disagreement over the decision.

SUMMARY: IMPLEMENTING PALLIATIVE CARE IN THE INTENSIVE CARE UNIT

Institute mandatory family meetings with the attending physician within 24 hours of admission. Goals of this meeting are as follows:

1. To convey information about the patient, specifically, to review the reason for admission, the treatment plan, and the expected prognosis, along with anticipated decision points

2. To orient the family to the ICU. Clinicians may avail themselves of novel technologies, including written brochures, videotapes, and interactive CDs, to help families understand the people and routines of the ICU (91)

3. To convey a strategy about future communications. The clinicians should identify the responsible physician(s) and nurse(s) and establish a plan for ongoing communications. This plan should offer daily communication between the family and a designated physician, preferably the attending or a critical care fellow and

TABLE 76.8

WITHDRAWAL OF MECHANICAL VENTILATION

1. Establish appropriateness of decision and confirm family's understanding (see text)
2. Optimize existing respiratory function
   Administer breathing treatment, if indicated
   Suction out the mouth and hypopharynx. Endotracheal suctioning prior to withdrawal may or may not be advisable, depending on patient distress and family perception
   Consider administration of scopolamine or glycopyrrolate in patients with excess secretions
   Place the patient at least 30 degrees upright, if possible
   Anticipate distress by assessing respiratory pattern on current level of support. Use opioids to control respiratory distress in dyspneic or tachypneic patients. In the absence of distress, reduce intermittent mandatory ventilation rate below 10, reassess and adjust sedation
3. Recognize that no one sequence applies to all patients because clinical situations are so varied
   For extubation:
   The family should be permitted to observe the extubation, if desired. If so, remove the endotracheal tube into a towel to collect and hide secretions.
   Give appropriate mouth care and humidified air or oxygen by face mask.
   Post-extubation distress is a medical emergency. A physician should be present during and immediately after extubation to assess the patient and to titrate medications. Midazolam (2–5 mg i.v. q7–10 min) or diazepam (5–10 mg i.v. q3–5 min) and/or morphine (5–10 mg i.v. q10min) or fentanyl (100–250 μg i.v. q3–5 min) should be administered.
   For weaning without extubation:
   In general, changes should be made in the following order: eliminate positive end-expiratory pressure (PEEP), reduce fraction of inspired oxygen (FIO_2), reduce mandatory breath rate, reduce pressure support level, eliminate mandatory breaths, place to flow-by or T-piece, extubate to humidified air or oxygen.
   The pace of changes depends on patient comfort and may proceed as quickly as 5–15 min or, in an awake patient you hope to be able to extubate without extreme distress, several hours.
   Patients requiring high levels of ventilatory support may die following reduction or elimination of PEEP, or decrease in FIO_2 to 21%. In such patients, the physician should be present during and immediately after the change in therapy to assess the patient. Distress is a medical emergency and should be treated as described in the preceding text.

Modified from Prendergast TJ. Withholding or withdrawal of life-sustaining therapy. *Hosp Pract (Off Ed)* 2000;35:91–92, 95–100, 102, with permission.

4. To reassure the family of their access to information about sudden changes in the patient's condition. The family should be able to call into the hospital at any time to obtain information about the patient. The hospital must be able to contact the family in the event of a change in status. This may involve loaning a beeper/pager to the family

Highlight the value of good communications skills. Specific areas of need include communicating bad news, group dynamics, how to conduct a family meeting, and how to invite patients into the process of decision making without making them responsible for decisions that may end with the death of the patient (141). Explicit attention needs to be paid to the dynamics of conflict and the importance of negotiating rather than imposing resolution to disagreements.

ICU staff should recognize that the same structural issues that affect communications with families—uncertainty, rapid changes in status, intense personal relationships, exposure to many patient deaths—also affect communication among physicians and between physicians and nurses. A hierarchical model that devalues the input of some members of the multidisciplinary team leads to dissension (3,142). Such dissension may adversely affect patient care (33).

Emphasize the importance of symptom management. One mechanism to accomplish this is to institute regular use of pain and sedation scales. Quantitative attention to symptoms will be especially needed if practice evolves toward reduced sedation to avoid prolonging the length of stay in the ICU. As part of the emphasis on evidence-based symptom management, physicians and nursing staff will need periodic reviews of pharmacology of opioids and sedatives and how their properties are altered in critical illness.

Formalize recognition of the importance of quality of dying and bereavement support through a systematic review of every ICU death. A senior physician and a nurse should institute a quality improvement project based on the review of the first 20 deaths. Bereavement training is essential for ICU staff to help them to recognize and to assist patients/families, as well as attend to the grief reactions that affect professionals who work with many dying patients (143).

References

1. Dougherty CJ. The excesses of individualism. For meaningful healthcare reform, the United States needs a renewed sense of community. *Health Prog* 1992;73:22–28.
2. The SUPPORT Principal Investigators. A controlled trial to improve care for seriously ill hospitalized patients. The study to understand prognoses and preferences for outcomes and risks of treatments (SUPPORT). *JAMA* 1995;274:1591–1598.
3. Asch DA. The role of critical care nurses in euthanasia and assisted suicide. *N Engl J Med* 1996;334:1374–1379.
4. JAMA. A definition of irreversible coma. Report of the Ad Hoc Committee of the Harvard Medical School to Examine the Definition of Brain Death. *JAMA* 1968;205:337–340.
5. *In re Quinlan*, 70 NJ 10, 1976.
6. Lo B. The death of Clarence Herbert: withdrawing care is not murder. *Ann Intern Med* 1984;101:248–251.
7. *Cruzan v Director, Missouri Department of Health*, 497 US 261, 1990.
8. Miles SH. Informed demand for "non-beneficial" medical treatment. *N Engl J Med* 1991;325:512–515.
9. Angell M. The case of Helga Wanglie. A new kind of "right to die" case. *N Engl J Med* 1991;325:511–512.

10. Prendergast TJ, Claessens MT, Luce JM. A national survey of end-of-life care for critically ill patients. *Am J Respir Crit Care Med* 1998;158:1163–1167.

11. Karlawish JH, Hall JB. Managing death and dying in the intensive care unit. *Am J Respir Crit Care Med* 1997;155:1–2.

12. Krakauer EL, Penson RT, Truog RD, et al. Sedation for intractable distress of a dying patient: acute palliative care and the principle of double effect. *Oncologist* 2000;5:53–62.

13. Groeger JS, Lemeshow S, Price K, et al. Multicenter outcome study of cancer patients admitted to the intensive care unit: a probability of mortality model. *J Clin Oncol* 1998;16:761–770.

14. Knaus WA, Wagner DP, Zimmerman JE, et al. Variations in mortality and length of stay in intensive care units. *Ann Intern Med* 1993;118:753–761.

15. Ely EW, Evans GW, Haponik EF. Mechanical ventilation in a cohort of elderly patients admitted to an intensive care unit. *Ann Intern Med* 1999;131:96–104.

16. The Acute Respiratory Distress Syndrome Network. Ventilation with lower tidal volumes as compared with traditional tidal volumes for acute lung injury and the acute respiratory distress syndrome. *N Engl J Med* 2000;342:1301–1308.

17. Rubenfeld GD, Crawford SW. Withdrawing life support from mechanically ventilated recipients of bone marrow transplants: a case for evidence-based guidelines. *Ann Intern Med* 1996;125:625–633.

18. Back A. Cancer. In: Curtis JR, Rubenfeld GD, eds. *Managing death in the intensive care unit.* New York: Oxford University Press, 2001:301–310.

19. Curtis JR, Rubenfeld GD. *Managing death in the intensive care unit: the transition from cure to comfort.* New York: Oxford University Press, 2001.

20. Mularski RA, Bascom P, Osborne ML. Educational agendas for interdisciplinary end-of-life curricula. *Crit Care Med* 2001;29:N16–N23.

21. Lynn J, Harrell F Jr, Cohn F, et al. Prognoses of seriously ill hospitalized patients on the days before death: implications for patient care and public policy. *New Horiz* 1997;5:56–61.

22. Teres D, Lemeshow S. Why severity models should be used with caution. *Crit Care Clin* 1994;10:93–110; discussion 111–115.

23. Kollef MH. Outcome prediction in the ICU. In: Curtis JR, Rubenfeld GD, eds. *Managing death in the intensive care unit.* New York: Oxford University Press, 2001:39–57.

24. Prendergast TJ, Luce JM. Increasing incidence of withholding and withdrawal of life support from the critically ill. *Am J Respir Crit Care Med* 1997;155:15–20.

25. Slomka J. The negotiation of death: clinical decision making at the end of life. *Soc Sci Med* 1992;35:251–259.

26. Block SD. Helping the clinician cope with death in the ICU. In: Curtis JR, Rubenfeld GD, eds. *Managing death in the intensive care unit.* New York: Oxford University Press, 2001:183–191.

27. Danis M, Federman D, Fins JJ, et al. Incorporating palliative care into critical care education: principles, challenges, and opportunities. *Crit Care Med* 1999;27:2005–2013.

28. Chang VT, Thaler HT, Polyak TA, et al. Quality of life and survival: the role of multidimensional symptom assessment. *Cancer* 1998;83:173–179.

29. Lewis KS, Whipple JK, Michael KA, et al. Effect of analgesic treatment on the physiologic consequences of acute pain. *Am J Hosp Pharm* 1994;51:1539–1554.

30. Block SD. Psychological considerations, growth and transcendence at the end of life. *JAMA* 2001;285:2898–2905.

31. Nelson J, Meier D. Palliative care in the intensive care unit: Part I. *J Intensive Care Med* 1999;14:130.

32. Nelson JE. Saving lives and saving deaths. *Ann Intern Med* 1999;130:776–777.

33. Harvey MA, Ninos NP, Adler DC, et al. Results of the consensus conference on fostering more humane critical care: creating a healing environment. Society of Critical Care Medicine. *AACN Clin Issues Crit Care Nurs* 1993;4:484–549.

34. Truog R, Cist AF, Brackett SE, et al. Recommendations for end-of-life care in the ICU. *Crit Care Med* 2001;29:2332–2348.

35. Hoyt JW. Ethics: the new mainstream issue for the ICU and SCCM. *New Horiz* 1997;5:3–5.

36. Desbiens NA, Mueller-Rizner N, Connors AF Jr, et al. The symptom burden of seriously ill hospitalized patients. SUPPORT Investigators. Study to understand prognoses and preferences for outcome and risks of treatment. *J Pain Symptom Manage* 1999;17:248–255.

37. Morrison RS, Ahronheim JC, Morrison GR, et al. Pain and discomfort associated with common hospital procedures and experiences. *J Pain Symptom Manage* 1998;15:91–101.

38. Lynn J, Teno JM, Phillips RS, et al. Perceptions by family members of the dying experience of older and seriously ill patients. SUPPORT Investigators. Study to understand prognoses and preferences for outcomes and risks of treatments. *Ann Intern Med* 1997;126:97–106.

39. Nelson JE, Meier DE, Oei EJ, et al. Self-reported symptom experience of critically ill cancer patients receiving intensive care. *Crit Care Med* 2001;29:277–282.

40. Knebel AR, Janson-Bjerklie SL, Malley JD, et al. Comparison of breathing comfort during weaning with two ventilatory modes. *Am J Respir Crit Care Med* 1994;149:14–18.

41. Somogyi-Zalud E, Zhong Z, Lynn J, et al. Dying with acute respiratory failure or multiple organ system failure with sepsis. *J Am Geriatr Soc* 2000;48:S140–S145.

42. Hamill-Ruth RJ, Marohn ML. Evaluation of pain in the critically ill patient. *Crit Care Clin* 1999;15:35–54.

43. Puntillo KA. The role of critical care nurses in providing and managing end-of-life care. In: Curtis JR, Rubenfeld GD, eds. *Managing death in the intensive care unit: the transition from cure to comfort.* New York: Oxford University Press, 2001:149–164.

44. De Jonghe B, Cook D, Appere-De-Vecchi C, et al. Using and understanding sedation scoring systems: a systematic review. *Intensive Care Med* 2000;26:275–285.

45. Hansen-Flaschen J, Cowen J, Polomano RC. Beyond the Ramsay scale: need for a validated measure of sedating drug efficacy in the intensive care unit. *Crit Care Med* 1994;22:732–733.

46. Shapiro BA, Warren J, Egol AB, et al. Practice parameters for intravenous analgesia and sedation for adult patients in the intensive care unit: an executive summary. Society of Critical Care Medicine. *Crit Care Med* 1995;23:1596–1600.

47. Melzack R, Katz J. Pain measurement in persons in pain. In: Wall PD, Melzack R, eds. *Textbook of pain*, 3rd ed. New York: Churchill Livingstone, 1994:337–351.

48. Foley KM. Pain and symptom control in the dying ICU patient. In: Curtis JR, Rubenfeld GD, eds. *Managing death in the intensive care unit.* New York: Oxford University Press, 2001:103–125.

49. Hansen-Flaschen JH, Brazinsky S, Basile C, et al. Use of sedating drugs and neuromuscular blocking agents in patients requiring mechanical ventilation for respiratory failure. A national survey. *JAMA* 1991;266:2870–2875.

50. Ramsay MA, Savege TM, Simpson BR, et al. Controlled sedation with alphaxalone-alphadolone. *BMJ* 1974;2:656–659.

51. Riker RR, Picard JT, Fraser GL. Prospective evaluation of the sedation-agitation scale for adult critically ill patients. *Crit Care Med* 1999;27:1325–1329.

52. Devlin JW, Boleski G, Mlynarek M, et al. Motor activity assessment scale: a valid and reliable sedation scale for use with mechanically ventilated patients in an adult surgical intensive care unit. *Crit Care Med* 1999;27:1271–1275.

53. American Pain Society Quality of Care Committee. Quality improvement guidelines for the treatment of acute pain and cancer pain. *JAMA* 1995;274:1874–1880.

54. Jastremski CA, Harvey M. Making changes to improve the intensive care unit experience for patients and their families. *New Horiz* 1998;6:99–109.

55. Fontaine DK. Nonpharmacologic management of patient distress during mechanical ventilation. *Crit Care Clin* 1994;10:695–708.

56. Puntillo KA. Pain experiences of intensive care unit patients. *Heart Lung* 1990;19:526–533.

57. Whipple JK, Lewis KS, Quebbeman EJ, et al. Analysis of pain management in critically ill patients. *Pharmacotherapy* 1995;15:592–599.

58. Kress JP, Pohlman AS, O'Connor MF, et al. Daily interruption of sedative infusions in critically ill patients undergoing mechanical ventilation [See comments]. *N Engl J Med* 2000;342:1471–1477.

59. Kress JP, Lacy M, Pliskin N, et al. The long term psychological effects of daily sedative interruption in critically ill patients. *Am J Respir Crit Care Med* 2001;165:A954.

60. de Wit M, Hassoun PM, Epstein SK. Correlation between sedation level and administration of sedative boluses versus continuous infusions. *Am J Respir Crit Care Med* 2001;163:A954.

61. Wilson WC, Smedira NG, Fink C, et al. Ordering and administration of sedatives and analgesics during the withholding and withdrawal of life support from critically ill patients. *JAMA* 1992;267:949–953.

62. Hall RI, Duncan PJ, Rocker G. Death in the ICU—the Halifax experience. *Can J Anaesth* 1999;46:R57–R69.

63. Luce JM, Alpers A. Legal aspects of withholding and withdrawing life support from critically ill patients in the United States and providing palliative care to them. *Am J Respir Crit Care Med* 2000;162:2029–2032.

64. Kapp MB. Legal liability anxieties in the ICU. In: Curtis JR, Rubenfeld GD, eds. *Managing death in the intensive care unit.* New York: Oxford University Press, 2001:231–244.

65. Meier DE, Morrison RS, Cassel CK. Improving palliative care. *Ann Intern Med* 1997;127:225–230.

66. Ostermann ME, Keenan SP, Seiferling RA, et al. Sedation in the intensive care unit: a systematic review. *JAMA* 2000;283:1451–1459.

67. Nielson C. Pharmacologic considerations in critical care of the elderly. *Clin Geriatr Med* 1994;10:71–89.

68. Wagner BK, O'Hara DA. Pharmacokinetics and pharmacodynamics of sedatives and analgesics in the treatment of agitated critically ill patients. *Clin Pharmacokinet* 1997;33:426–453.

69. Park GR. Molecular mechanisms of drug metabolism in the critically ill. *Br J Anaesth* 1996;77:32–49.

70. Bone RC, Hayden WR, Levine RL, et al. Recognition, assessment, and treatment of anxiety in the critical care patient. *Dis Mon* 1995;41:293–359.

71. Volles DF, McGory R. Pharmacokinetic considerations. *Crit Care Clin* 1999;15:55–75.

72. Pohlman AS, Simpson KP, Hall JB. Continuous intravenous infusions of lorazepam versus midazolam for sedation during mechanical ventilatory

support: a prospective, randomized study. *Crit Care Med* 1994;22:1241–1247.

73. Shook JE, Watkins WD, Camporesi EM. Differential roles of opioid receptors in respiration, respiratory disease, and opiate-induced respiratory depression. *Am Rev Respir Dis* 1990;142:895–909.

74. Bailey PL, Pace NL, Ashburn MA, et al. Frequent hypoxemia and apnea after sedation with midazolam and fentanyl. *Anesthesiology* 1990;73:826–830.

75. Santiago TV, Pugliese AC, Edelman NH. Control of breathing during methadone addiction. *Am J Med* 1977;62:347–354.

76. Tramer M, Moore A, McQuay H. Propofol anaesthesia and postoperative nausea and vomiting: quantitative systematic review of randomized controlled studies. *Br J Anaesth* 1997;78:247–255.

77. Gan TJ, El-Molem H, Ray J, et al. Patient-controlled antiemesis: a randomized, double-blind comparison of two doses of propofol versus placebo. *Anesthesiology* 1999;90:1564–1570.

78. Phelps KC, Restino MS. Propofol in chemotherapy-associated nausea and vomiting. *Ann Pharmacother* 1996;30:290–292.

79. Borgeat A, Wilder-Smith O, Forni M, et al. Adjuvant propofol enables better control of nausea and emesis secondary to chemotherapy for breast cancer. *Can J Anaesth* 1994;41:1117–1119.

80. Breitbart W, Marotta R, Platt MM, et al. A double-blind trial of haloperidol, chlorpromazine, and lorazepam in the treatment of delirium in hospitalized AIDS patients. *Am J Psychiatry* 1996;153:231–237.

81. Keenan SP, Busche KD, Chen LM, et al. Withdrawal and withholding of life support in the intensive care unit: a comparison of teaching and community hospitals. The Southwestern Ontario Critical Care Research Network. *Crit Care Med* 1998;26:245–251.

82. Faber-Langendoen K. The clinical management of dying patients receiving mechanical ventilation. A survey of physician practice. *Chest* 1994;106:880–888.

83. Miles SH, Koepp R, Weber EP. Advance end-of-life treatment planning. A research review. *Arch Intern Med* 1996;156:1062–1068.

84. Hanson LC, Danis M, Lazorick S. Emergency triage to intensive care: can we use prognosis and patient preferences? *J Am Geriatr Soc* 1994;42:1277–1281.

85. Faber-Langendoen K. A multi-institutional study of care given to patients dying in hospitals. Ethical and practice implications. *Arch Intern Med* 1996;156:2130–2136.

86. Sulmasy DP, Terry PB, Weisman CS, et al. The accuracy of substituted judgments in patients with terminal diagnoses. *Ann Intern Med* 1998;128:621–629.

87. Covinsky KE, Fuller JD, Yaffe K, et al. Communication and decision-making in seriously ill patients: findings of the SUPPORT project. The Study to Understand Prognoses and Preferences for Outcomes and Risks of Treatments. *J Am Geriatr Soc* 2000;48:S187–S193.

88. Hickey M. What are the needs of families of critically ill patients? A review of the literature since 1976. *Heart Lung* 1990;19:401–415.

89. Kutner JS, Steiner JF, Corbett KK, et al. Information needs in terminal illness. *Soc Sci Med* 1999;48:1341–1352.

90. Furukawa MM. Meeting the needs of the dying patient's family. *Crit Care Nurse* 1996;16:51–57.

91. Azoulay E, Chevret S, Leleu G, et al. Half the families of intensive care unit patients experience inadequate communication with physicians. *Crit Care Med* 2000;28:3044–3049.

92. Hanson LC, Danis M, Garrett J. What is wrong with end-of-life care? Opinions of bereaved family members. *J Am Geriatr Soc* 1997;45:1339–1344.

93. Teno JM, Fisher E, Hamel MB, et al. Decision-making and outcomes of prolonged ICU stays in seriously ill patients. *J Am Geriatr Soc* 2000;48:S70–S74.

94. Asch DA, Hansen-Flaschen J, Lanken PN. Decisions to limit or continue life-sustaining treatment by critical care physicians in the United States: conflicts between physicians' practices and patients' wishes. *Am J Respir Crit Care Med* 1995;151:288–292.

95. Goold SD, Williams BC, Arnold RM. Handling conflict in end-of-life care. *JAMA* 2000;283:3199–3200.

96. Fetters MD, Churchill L, Danis M. Conflict resolution at the end of life. *Crit Care Med* 2001;29:921–925.

97. Prendergast TJ. Resolving conflicts surrounding end-of-life care. *New Horiz* 1997;5:62–71.

98. Maguire P, Faulkner A, Booth K, et al. Helping cancer patients disclose their concerns. *Eur J Cancer* 1996;32A:78–81.

99. von Gunten CF, Ferris FD, Emanuel LL. The patient-physician relationship. Ensuring competency in end-of-life care: communication and relational skills. *JAMA* 2000;284:3051–3057.

100. Ptacek JT, Eberhardt TL. Breaking bad news. A review of the literature. *JAMA* 1996;276:496–502.

101. Singer PA, Martin DK, Kelner M. Quality end-of-life care: patients' perspectives. *JAMA* 1999;281:163–168.

102. Maguire P. Improving communication with cancer patients. *Eur J Cancer* 1999;35:2058–2065.

103. Lo B, Quill T, Tulsky J. Discussing palliative care with patients. ACP-ASIM End-of-Life Care Consensus Panel. American College of Physicians-American Society of Internal Medicine. *Ann Intern Med* 1999;130:744–749.

104. Smith RC, Lyles JS, Mettler J, et al. The effectiveness of intensive training for residents in interviewing. A randomized, controlled study. *Ann Intern Med* 1998;128:118–126.

105. Novack DH, Suchman AL, Clark W, et al. Calibrating the physician. Personal awareness and effective patient care. Working Group on Promoting Physician Personal Awareness, American Academy on Physician and Patient. *JAMA* 1997;278:502–509.

106. Duffy FD. Dialogue: the core clinical skill. *Ann Intern Med* 1998;128:139–141.

107. Hanson LC, Tulsky JA, Danis M. Can clinical interventions change care at the end of life? *Ann Intern Med* 1997;126:381–388.

108. Tulsky JA, Chesney MA, Lo B. See one, do one, teach one? House staff experience discussing do-not-resuscitate orders. *Arch Intern Med* 1996;156:1285–1289.

109. Haidet P, Hamel MB, Davis RB, et al. Outcomes, preferences for resuscitation, and physician-patient communication among patients with metastatic colorectal cancer. SUPPORT Investigators. Study to understand prognoses and preferences for outcomes and risks of treatments. *Am J Med* 1998;105:222–229.

110. Swigart V, Lidz C, Butterworth V, et al. Letting go: family willingness to forgo life support. *Heart Lung* 1996;25:483–494.

111. Miller DK, Coe RM, Hyers TM. Achieving consensus on withdrawing or withholding care for critically ill patients. *J Gen Intern Med* 1992;7:475–480.

112. Cook DJ, Giacomini M, Johnson N, et al. Life support in the intensive care unit: a qualitative investigation of technological purposes. Canadian Critical Care Trials Group. *CMAJ* 1999;161:1109–1113.

113. Tilden VP, Tolle SW, Garland MJ, et al. Decisions about life-sustaining treatment. Impact of physicians' behaviors on the family. *Arch Intern Med* 1995;155:633–638.

114. Gilligan T, Raffin TA. Physician virtues and communicating with patients. *New Horiz* 1997;5:6–14.

115. Drought TS, Koenig BA, Raffin TA. Advance directives. Changing our expectations. *Chest* 1996;110:589–591.

116. Prendergast TJ. Advance care planning: pitfalls, progress, promise. *Crit Care Med* 2001;29:N34–N39.

117. Curtis JR, Patrick DL, Shannon SE, et al. The family conference as a focus to improve communication about end-of-life care in the intensive care unit: opportunities for improvement. *Crit Care Med* 2001;29:N26–N33.

118. Keenan SP, Mawdsley C, Plotkin D, et al. Withdrawal of life support: how the family feels, and why. *J Palliat Care* 2000;16:S40–S44.

119. McLean RF, Tarshis J, Mazer CD, et al. Death in two Canadian intensive care units: institutional difference and changes over time. *Crit Care Med* 2000;28:100–103.

120. Smedira NG, Evans BH, Grais LS, et al. Withholding and withdrawal of life support from the critically ill. *N Engl J Med* 1990;322:309–315.

121. Council on Ethical and Judicial Affairs, American Medical Association. Decisions near the end of life. *JAMA* 1992;267:2229–2233.

122. Withholding and withdrawing life-sustaining therapy. This official statement of the American Thoracic Society was adopted by the ATS Board of Directors, March 1991. *Am Rev Respir Dis* 1991;144:726–731.

123. Task Force on Ethics of the Society of Critical Care Medicine. Consensus report on the ethics of foregoing life-sustaining treatments in the critically ill. *Crit Care Med* 1990;18:1435–1439.

124. *Deciding to forego life-sustaining treatment. President's Commission for the Study of Ethical Problems in Medicine and Biomedical and Behavioral Research*, 1983: www.bioethics.gov/reports/past_commissions/deciding_to_forego_tx.pdf.

125. The Hastings Center. *Guidelines on the termination of life-sustaining treatment and the care of the dying*. The Hastings Center, 1987.

126. Kollef MH, Ward S. The influence of access to a private attending physician on the withdrawal of life-sustaining therapies in the intensive care unit. *Crit Care Med* 1999;27:2125–2132.

127. Asch DA, Faber-Langendoen K, Shea JA, et al. The sequence of withdrawing life-sustaining treatment from patients. *Am J Med* 1999;107:153–156.

128. Christakis NA, Asch DA. Medical specialists prefer to withdraw familiar technologies when discontinuing life support. *J Gen Intern Med* 1995;10:491–494.

129. Cook DJ, Guyatt GH, Jaeschke R, et al. Canadian Critical Care Trials Group. Determinants in Canadian health care workers of the decision to withdraw life support from the critically ill. *JAMA* 1995;273:703–708.

130. Brody H, Campbell ML, Faber-Langendoen K, et al. Withdrawing intensive life-sustaining treatment—recommendations for compassionate clinical management. *N Engl J Med* 1997;336:652–657.

131. Prendergast TJ. Withholding or withdrawal of life-sustaining therapy. *Hosp Pract (Off Ed)* 2000;35:91–92, 95–100, 102.

132. Rubenfeld GD, Crawford SW. Principles and practice of withdrawing life-sustaining treatment in the ICU. In: Curtis JR, Rubenfeld GD, eds. *Managing death in the intensive care unit*. New York: Oxford University Press, 2001:127–148.

133. Faber-Langendoen K, Lanken PN. Dying patients in the intensive care unit: forgoing treatment, maintaining care. *Ann Intern Med* 2000;133:886–893.

134. Campbell ML, Bizek KS, Thill M. Patient responses during rapid terminal weaning from mechanical ventilation: a prospective study. *Crit Care Med* 1999;27:73–77.

135. Prendergast TJ. Futility and the common cold. How requests for antibiotics can illuminate care at the end of life. *Chest* 1995;107:836–844.

136. American Medical Association Council on Ethical and Judicial Affairs. Medical futility in end-of-life care: report of the Council on Ethical and Judicial Affairs. *JAMA* 1999;281:937–941.

137. Gilligan T, Raffin TA. Rapid withdrawal of support. *Chest* 1995;108:1407–1408.

138. Truog RD, Burns JP, Mitchell C, et al. Pharmacologic paralysis and withdrawal of mechanical ventilation at the end of life. *N Engl J Med* 2000;342:508–511.

139. Gianakos D. Terminal weaning. *Chest* 1995;108:1405–1406.

140. Casarett D, Kutner JS, Abrahm J. End-of-life care consensus panel. Life after death: a practical approach to grief and bereavement. *Ann Intern Med* 2001;134:208–215.

141. Cook D. Patient autonomy versus parentalism. *Crit Care Med* 2001;29:N24–N25.

142. Solomon MZ, O'Donnell L, Jennings B, et al. Decisions near the end of life: professional views on life-sustaining treatments. *Am J Public Health* 1993;83:14–23.

143. Cassel CK. *Overview on attitudes of physicians toward caring for the dying patient. Caring for the dying: identification and promotion of physician competency*. Philadelphia, PA: American Board of Internal Medicine, 1996.

RESEARCH ISSUES IN SUPPORTIVE CARE AND PALLIATIVE CARE

CHAPTER 77 ■ OUTCOMES ASSESSMENT IN PALLIATIVE CARE

JOAN M. TENO

Accountability has been called the *third revolution* in medical care (1). Health care providers are now often faced with new questions. For example, what are the outcomes of palliative care that justify its continued institutional support? Or, what is the evidence for the use of a certain medical intervention for a specific patient? Fundamental to answering these questions are defining quality of care for seriously ill patients and determining how care is measured.

Quality care at the end of life is different than during any other period of time. Dying persons, their families, and health care providers are often faced with decisions that involve trade-offs between length of life and quality of life. Reasonable persons may differ in such decisions. Therefore, preferences and values are important to shaping treatment decisions in ways unlike other time periods. Outcomes assessment for the dying must take this into consideration. In this chapter, a practical approach to examining outcomes, whether it is part of an audit prior to quality improvement efforts or for the ongoing assessment of institutional quality of care, will be discussed.

WHY EXAMINE OUTCOMES?

The first response of staff to auditing the quality of care is, "Why?" A typical response is that their work cannot be measured. Yet, audits and ongoing quality monitoring through examining administrative data, reviewing medical records, and/or speaking with dying persons and families, leads to important opportunities to improve quality of care. Simply stated, "If you don't measure it, you won't improve it" (2).

The results of assessing the outcomes of palliative medicine can help create the needed attention to the issue of improving the quality of care. Such tension can create the awareness among health care providers of opportunities to improve and enhance their current practices. Examining the outcomes can be critical to detecting early problems with new medications or other unintended consequences from medical interventions. Examining outcomes can guide organizational efforts to improve the quality of care. For example, knowing that one in four persons now die in a nursing home provides important information for the planning of new programs to meet the needs of the dying (3).

WHAT OUTCOMES TO MEASURE?

Reflecting on the thirtieth anniversary of St. Christopher's Hospice, Dame Cicely Saunders said, "We have never lost sight

of the values that were so important to David: commitment to openness, openness to challenge, and the absolute priority of patients' own views on what they need" (4). Fundamental to palliative care is meeting the needs and expectations of patients and families. Quality in a 42-year-old with an acute myocardial infarction can be measured by whether interventions have been done that minimize infarct size such as the use of aspirin or percutaneous transluminal angioplasty. The vast majority of persons would want efforts to focus on restoring function under these circumstances. On the other hand, the circumstances of a 42-year-old dying of stage IV lung cancer are quite different. Technological interventions require weighting of their impact on both quality and quantity of life—decisions that require the input of an informed patient.

The importance of preferences is reflected in the Institute of Medicine (IOM) definition of quality of care: the "degree to which health services for individuals and populations increased the likelihood of desired health outcomes and are consistent with professional knowledge" (5). This definition implies that conceptual models for quality care (as well as instruments measuring quality) must be based on both professional knowledge *and* informed patient preferences. To date, most conceptual models have been built either around expert opinion *or* qualitative data from patients, families, or health care providers.

Fortunately, both experts and consumers agree in many ways about what is important for end-of-life care—physical comfort, emotional support, and autonomy. However, they have significant areas of disagreement as well, for example, unmet needs (Table 77.1). Family members want more information on what to expect and how they can help their dying loved ones. Patients and families emphasize the importance of closure at the end of life, including issues of personal relationships. Families often speak of frustration with a lack of coordination of medical care. It often is not clear who is in charge; different health care providers provide conflicting information, and transitions can be fraught with confusion (10).

One conceptual model, Patient Focused, Family-Centered Medical Care (Table 77.1) is based on a review of existing professional guidelines *and* results from focus groups conducted with family members (10). According to this model, institutions, and care providers striving to achieve patient-focused, family-centered medical care for the seriously ill patient should:

- Provide the desired level of physical comfort and emotional support
- Promote shared decision making, including care planning in advance

TABLE 77.1

COMPARISON OF DOMAINS OF EXPERT, PATIENTS, FAMILY MEMBERS, HEALTH CARE PROVIDERS, AND PROPOSED COMBINED MODEL IN MEASURING QUALITY OF CARE AT END OF LIFE

	Expert opinion			Consumer opinion			Combined model
Emanuel and Emanuel (6)	Institute of Medicine approaching death: improving care at the end of life (7)	NHO pathway (8)	Patients with human immunodeficiency virus, renal failure on dialysis, and nursing home residents (9)	Patients, families, and health care providers	Bereaved family members	Patient-focused, family-centered medical care (10)
Physical symptoms	Overall quality of life	Safe and comfortable dying	Receiving adequate pain and symptom management	Pain and symptom management	Providing desired physical comfort	Providing desired level of physical comfort and emotional support
Psychological and cognitive symptoms	Physical well-being and functioning	Self-determined life closure	Avoiding inappropriate prolongation of the dying	Clear decision making	Achieving control over health care decisions and everyday decisions	Promote shared decision making
Social relationships and support	Psychosocial well-being and functioning	Effective grieving	Achieving sense of control	Preparation for death	Burden of advocating for quality medical care	Focus on the individual which includes closure, respect, and dignity of the patient
Economic demands and caregiving demands	Family well-being and perceptions		Relieving burden	Completion	Educating on what to expect and increasing confidence in providing care	Attend to the needs of the family for information, increasing their confidence in helping with patient care and providing emotional support prior to and after the patient death.
Hopes and expectations			Strengthening relationship	Contributing to others	Emotional support prior to and after the patient's death	Coordination and continuity of care
Spiritual and existential beliefs				Affirmation of the whole person		Informing and Educating

Nelson EC, Splaine ME, Batalden PB, et al. Building measurement and data collection into medical practice. *Ann Intern Med* 1998;128:460–466 (2).

- Focus on the individual patient by facilitating situations in which patients achieve their desired levels of control, staff members treat patients with respect and dignity, and patients are aided in achieving their desired levels of closure and
- Attend to the needs of caregivers for information and skills in providing care for the patient, and provide emotional support to the family before and after the patient's death

On the basis of this model, a survey intended to be used as part of an initial quality audit of the quality of end-of-life care has been developed and validated. This survey, Brown University Family Evaluation of Hospice Care, has been adopted by National Hospice and Palliative Care Organization with a recent study of "early adopter hospices" showing variation suggesting discriminant validity (11).

WHEN ARE OUTCOMES MEASURED?

The question of when outcomes are measured is an extremely important consideration. Dying is unlike any other period of time. Often, the dying person and her health care providers are balancing the hope for longevity versus the need to make appropriate preparation. Although many outcome measures are not clearly linked to disease trajectory and patient readiness, several outcomes are linked to either. For example, issues around closure are clearly linked to the dying person and family readiness to discuss that the patient is dying. Therefore, the wording of questions and timing of administration of survey must be done in a sensitive manner to reflect where the dying person is in their readiness to discuss existential issues. Other process measures, such as counseling on advance directives or discussion of hospice, should reflect the recommendation of professional guidelines with measures of quality of care to include counterbalancing measures about whether such discussions were done in a sensitive and compassionate manner.

HOW ARE OUTCOMES MEASURED?

Assessment of outcomes refers to measuring the "end results"—the impact or effect of medical care on the dying person and/or the family. Measuring outcomes allows you to judge the effectiveness of medical interventions, innovative programs, and new medications. In addition to examining outcomes, process measures provide important information for quality improvement and examination of the effect of new programs. A *process measure* examines what a service or intervention does for patients and their families. For example, a process measure focuses on whether there is a regular assessment of pain noted in the medical record, while an *outcome measure* examines whether patients report that they received their desired amount of pain relief. Both are important and critical to measure. Ultimately, the quality of medical care is judged by changes in outcome indicators. Yet, an organization will not achieve those outcomes if it does not implement key processes of care that are known to benefit medical care.

Key to choosing an outcome or process measure is the intended use of the quality measures. Table 77.2 notes the four potential uses of measurement tools.

The areas of emphasis and desired characteristics vary for measurement tools intended for different purposes (Table 77.3). For example, the intended audience for quality improvement measures is the institutional and quality

---

TABLE 77.2

PURPOSES OF QUALITY MEASURES

1. Quality improvement—measures to provide information for health care institutions to reform or shape how care is provided
2. Clinical assessment—measures to guide individual patient management
3. Research—measures that assess the phenomenon of interest
4. Accountability—measures that allow comparison of quality of care for the purposes of quality assurance or for consumer choice between health care institutions or practitioners

From Teno JM, Byock I, Field MJ. Research agenda for developing measures to examine quality of care and quality of life of patients diagnosed with life-limiting illness. White paper from the conference on Excellent Care at the End of Life through Fast-Tracking Audit, Standards, and Teamwork (EXCELFAST), September 28–30, 1997. *J Pain Symptom Manage* 1999;17:75–82 (12).

---

improvement team, whereas the intended audience for public accountability is the health care purchaser and consumer.

Measurement tools used for public accountability need further evidence that justifies their use. For example, given the intended audiences and implications of the use of measurement tools for public accountability, more stringent psychometric properties must be used for these measures. In addition, there must be either normative or empirical research that substantiates a claim that the construct being measured for public accountability is under the control of that health care institution.

Typically, measurement tools can review the medical record, examine administrative data (such as death certificate or billing data), or conduct interviews with a patient or a proxy such as a family member. Each potential source of data has strengths and limitations that should be considered when selecting a measurement tool or strategy.

Medical records are legal documents that should reflect the medical care that patients receive. Yet, medical records reflect staff perceptions, and their contents are subject to reporting bias. For example, a nurse may document that a patient understands how to take his/her medications on hospital discharge; this documentation reflects the nurse's perception. Yet, patients and families often report that they did *not* understand that explanation when interviewed after hospital discharge (14). Furthermore, not all discussions are documented in the medical record. Discussions about resuscitation preferences are usually only documented when the patient or family consents to a "do not resuscitate" order. Therefore, a physician and patient may have talked about resuscitation preferences and decided *not* to forgo cardiopulmonary resuscitation, but there is nothing documented in the medical record because cardiopulmonary resuscitation is the default in most of the US hospitals.

Administrative data, such as death certificate data, billing data, or the Minimum Data Set, is readily assessable information that can provide invaluable information. Examining death certificate data that is published on the Internet (see www.cdc.gov) and available in public use files can provide hospice and palliative programs with information about their "market share," that is, what proportion of persons for whom they provide medical care in a certain geographic area. This information can highlight areas that are underserved and opportunities for program expansion. Users of administrative data need to be aware that it can be inaccurate because of

TABLE 77.3

AREAS OF EMPHASIS BASED ON THE PURPOSE OF QUALITY MEASURE

	Purpose of measure			
	Clinical assessment	Research	Improvement	Accountability
Audience	Clinical staff	Science community	Quality improvement team and clinical staff	Payers Public
Focus of measurement	Status of patient	Knowledge	Understand care process	Comparison
Confidentiality	Very high	Very high	Very high	Purpose is to compare groups
Evidence base to justify use of the measure	Important and the measure should have face validity from a clinical standpoint	Builds off existing evidence to generate new knowledge	Important	Extremely important in that proposed domain ought to be under control of that institution
Importance of psychometric properties	Important to the individual provider	Extremely important to that research effort	Important within that setting	Valid and responsive across multiple settings

This table was adapted from an article by Solberg LI, Mosser G, McDonald S. The three faces of performance measurement: improvement, accountability, and research. *Jt Comm J Qual Improv* 1997;23:135–147. (13) on the Three Faces of Performance Measurement: Improvement, Accountability, and Research and reproduced from an article by Teno JM, Byock I, Field MJ. Research agenda for developing measures to examine quality of care and quality of life of patients diagnosed with life-limiting illness. White paper from the conference on Excellent Care at the End of Life through Fast-Tracking Audit, Standards, and Teamwork (EXCELFAST), September 28–30, 1997. *J Pain Symptom Manage* 1999;17:75–82.

coding problems, key punch errors, or economic incentives to upgrade a patient's condition to get more reimbursement.

The Minimum Data Set is used in US nursing homes to systematically collect information on more than 300 items on a quarterly basis. This instrument can provide institution-specific and national estimates of outcomes, such as pain management (15). Yet, these data reflect staff perceptions of patients' levels of pain. Therefore, ascertainment bias is an important concern in the use of these data.

Surveys, either self- or telephone-administered, provide information directly from the patient and family perspective about the quality of care. Typically, satisfaction measures which ask a person to rate the quality of care with response categories that vary from "poor" to "excellent" have not yielded discriminating information about the quality of care. The respondents' task with these rating questions includes several steps: First, determine whether that event occurred; second, formulate their expectations regarding that aspect of care; and third, choose a category from the response categories. Often, persons have lowered expectations regarding their medical care, which, at least in part, explains the finding of high satisfaction in the face of indicators of poor quality of care, for example, severe pain (16,17).

Newer methods have begun using either "patient-centered reports" or "preference-based questions" (i.e., unmet needs) to capture the consumer perspective (Fig.77.1) (18). These methodologies, unlike typical satisfaction questions that rely on ratings questions, provide information that guide improvement of the quality of care. For example, knowing that 85% of patients believe a health care provider is "very good" does not tell that provider in what ways and specific processes of care that he/she can improve. On the other hand, knowing that 20% of patients did not understand a provider's directions for taking pain medications does provide a tangible target for improving and enhancing the quality of care. Moreover, patient-centered reports and preference-based questions have strong face validity with health care providers. In the future, surveys need to rely on all three methodologies—ratings, patient-centered reports, and preference-based questions—to

capture the consumer perspective on the quality of care at the end of life.

WHICH TOOL SHOULD BE USED?

Selecting a measurement tool should be guided by its intended use and the characteristics of the particular tool. The goals of measurement should be clear. As noted in Table 77.3, different psychometric properties (i.e., reliability, validity, and responsiveness of the tool) are needed for different intended uses. In addition, the intended audience is different for each of the four key purposes of measurement listed in Table 77.3. Measurement tools used for accountability, for example, have an intended audience of health insurers, the government, and other such institutions that pay for health care services. The focus of measurement is to compare health care institutions or plans. Given this purpose, it is very important that there is evidence that what is being measured is under the control of that health care institution and that the chosen instrument is reliable, valid, and responsive across the settings.

Reliability is necessary but not sufficient evidence of validity of an instrument or measurement tool. Reliability examines the degree to which the measurement tool is capable of reproducing the same results over time. Therefore, a person should give the same response to a question if asked within a short period of time.

A measurement tool is valid if there is evidence that it measures what it purports to measure. In essence, one is asking whether the measurement tool is reporting the truth. Often, the intent of the measurement tool is to identify a perception or attitude of the respondent. In this case, there is no "gold standard" by which to judge whether the measurement tool is accurately representing the construct that is being measured.

Content validity asks whether the measurement tool examines the correct concepts at face value. Were experts involved as advisors in the creation of the tool? Was the selection of concepts based on a theoretical model? *Construct validity* examines the degree to which the results from that measurement tool are associated with preestablished and

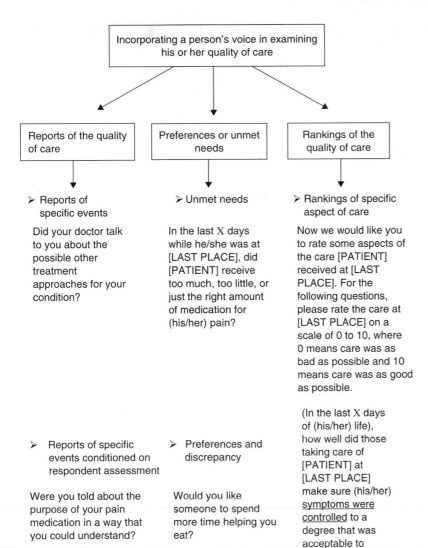

FIGURE 77.1. Proposed classification scheme for measuring a patient and family voice about the quality of medical care. Adapted from **Teno JM. Putting the patient and family voice back into measuring the quality of care for the dying.** *Hosp J* 1999;14: 167–176.

known relationships. For example, a measure of overall satisfaction should be associated with consumer choice of health care plans.

Responsiveness examines the degree to which a measurement tool changes as a result of interventions or historical events. Often, responsiveness is not reported in the initial validation of a measurement tool. Rather, responsiveness is reported at a later date after the measurement tool has been utilized in intervention studies or research that tracks quality over time.

Over the past several decades, an increasing number of measurement tools have been developed for examining the quality of end-of-life care. A web site maintained by the Center for Gerontology and Health Care Research at Brown University offers a structured literature review of existing instruments that focus on examining palliative care outcomes (see www.chcr.brown.edu/pcoc/toolkit.htm). This web site is a good starting point for selecting measurement tools for quality improvement and research purposes. The site provides published instruments in ten domains and selects promising instruments for in-depth review, including psychometric properties and response burden.

For a seriously ill and dying population, the time burden on respondents and staff is an important consideration for selecting an instrument. Limiting the scope of domains covered and the number of individual cases for which data is collected can reduce time burden. For an interview respondent—especially a seriously ill patient—it is particularly important to limit the scope of domains that are covered in the interview. For the purpose of quality improvement, you do not need to collect a large number of cases. A small number of cases collected by a random sample can provide invaluable information to guide a quality improvement effort.

HOW IS THE SAMPLE SELECTED?

A fundamental, yet often perplexing, step is deciding who is to be included in the sample. This relates to the "denominator" for the outcome being measured. Simply stated, a rate is composed of a numerator and a denominator. Determining who is in the denominator can be difficult in palliative medicine. For example, three decades ago, most persons would have considered patients with leukemia in childhood to be among those patients with a terminal illness. However, this no longer is the case due to the tremendous strides made in treating cancers in childhood. Researchers and quality improvement teams, then, must make decisions about which patients to include in the overall group of interest (i.e., the denominator).

The difficulty of accurate prognostication is an additional issue. Physicians are often overly optimistic in their prognoses, resulting in uncertainty about patients' actual time before death. Even the best statistical models are inaccurate because they are applying historical information from a previous cohort of similar patients to predict the future. There is a certain error in those estimates. Moreover, new treatments can invalidate even the best estimates by prediction models.

Although the timing of the interview is not as critical for certain domains, such as pain assessment, other domains are very sensitive to the time from death at which the interview takes place. For example, the timing of a discussion about stopping active treatment depends on the patient's prognosis and condition. The difficulty with prognostication also impacts the ability to compare different health care units or institutions. It is possible that institutions will interview persons at different time periods prior to death. This situation may result in differences in observed quality measures that reflect timing of the interview more than differences in the quality of care provided.

Given these prognostication issues, an institution may do frequent interviews to capture the same time period from death across patients or relies on retrospective interviews with bereaved family members to collect information on a certain time period. Doing a prospective patient data collection has important advantages. First and foremost, the results could improve the quality of care of that individual patient. Second, the information originates from the patient and not a surrogate. Yet, retrospective interviews with bereaved family members remain an important tool to examine the quality of end-of-life care.

If information is desired about the last week of life, often a family member is the only person that is able to provide a consumer perspective on the quality of end-of-life care delivered to the deceased and his/her family. The advantage of this "mortality follow-back" approach is that the denominator can be precisely defined, given that demographic information (including next of kin) is reported on death certificates to state-level departments of vital registries. Therefore, data collection can occur quickly without the costs of case finding for the prospective sample of patients. Because of this, mortality follow-back surveys have been used by both the United Kingdom (19,20) and the United States to collect (21) information on the last year of life of decedents.

WHAT ARE THE NEXT STEPS?

The first step in improving the quality of end-of-life care is taking stock—identifying and understanding the opportunities to improve. Simply stated, if you do not measure it, you will not improve it (2). Measuring or conducting an audit is the first step (Fig. 77.2). The second step is to engage stakeholders and define the goal. Engaging stakeholders means to present the results of the audit in a way that does not assign blame, but rather looks for shared opportunities to improve and enhance the quality of care. Key to the success of this second step is raising awareness and developing a shared goal.

The third step is actually improving the quality of end-of-life care through interventions and measuring whether these interventions succeed in creating change. Often, persons believe that education which provides knowledge and impacts attitudes will achieve change. Many times, even knowledge is not sufficient to change behavior. Instead, changes must be made in the processes of care that provide the cues and default pathways that ensure persons will choose the right behavior. Often, this change can be achieved through a model of rapid improvement that utilizes multiple Plan, Do, Check, and Act cycles (PDCA) (22). PDCA cycles allow testing of interventions first on a small scale (sometimes as small as only one nurse with

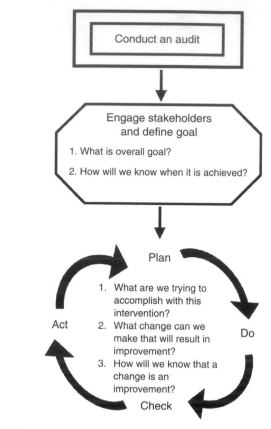

FIGURE 77.2. Quality improvement model.

one patient). From the information learned, the intervention can be refined or a different one can be tested.

Three key questions help to frame the work of the PDCA cycle. First, what is one trying to accomplish with this intervention? Just as an overall goal was identified in Step 2 of the quality improvement model, a goal must be stated for each PDCA cycle. Second, what changes can one make that will result in improvement? This may involve brainstorming with a team of colleagues about what interventions can achieve the goal of the cycle. An effort should be made to be creative, yet one should not be afraid to copy the success of others. Third, how will one know that change is an improvement? It is important to choose either a process or outcome variable that examines whether the goal of that cycle is being met and that data are tracked for the goal of that cycle, as well as the overall goal for the improvement effort. Often, a quality improvement team must test multiple interventions and conduct multiple PDCA cycles to achieve the overall goal. Two recent studies suggest that application of rapid cycle quality improvement can result in substantial gains of the quality of pain management in the nursing homes (23).

CONCLUSIONS

Outcomes assessment is key to improving quality of end-of-life care. At this early stage of development of supportive and palliative care, we urgently need both research and quality improvement efforts that will contribute to the scientific evidence base. Care at the end of life is quite different than care at other time periods. Patients' informed preferences play an even more central role in decision making and outcomes.

Not all persons with stage IV lung cancer, for example, will want experimental chemotherapy, and quality indicators must take into account that reasonable persons have different treatment preferences. Hence, measuring the quality of end-of-life care often requires interviews to examine the consumer perspective.

Even at this early stage, there are several promising measurement tools for quality improvement audits, for research, and for accountability. Selection of these measurement tools must be guided by the intended use of the data. The use of measurement tools for accountability carries two key requirements: an evidence base that suggests that the domain of interest is under the control of health care providers and demonstration of satisfactory psychometric properties of the tool across settings of care.

With an increased focus on accountability, health care providers will need to become familiar with methods to improve the quality of medical care. Measurement plays an important role in quality improvement efforts—from the initial audit that raises awareness of an opportunity to improve, to ongoing assessments of whether interventions are achieving their goals. The ideal quality monitoring system for palliative care should strongly link guidelines and proposed quality indicators. Guidelines should be based on both normative and empirical research. Quality indicators can measure information about the structure of a health care institution (e.g., availability of certain services, existence of policies) about processes of care (i.e., the interactions of health care providers, patients, and family members), and about outcomes of care (i.e., the effectiveness of treatment).

Currently, most quality indicators measure either structure or processes of care. Outcome measures are intuitively more attractive, but they are more difficult to apply because of our limited ability to adjust for differences in patient characteristics and the relatively small numbers of people with a particular condition treated at institutions each year. One argument in favor of collecting process data is that they are a more sensitive measure of quality because adverse outcomes do not occur every time there is an error in the provision of medical care. Furthermore, important outcomes—both positive and negative—often appear months or even years after care has been given. Quality indicators based on measures of structure or process, however, are only as good as their ability to predict outcomes of importance.

ACKNOWLEDGMENTS

This chapter in part is based on a background paper prepared for the National Cancer Policy Board of the Institute of Medicine. The author acknowledges the helpful comments by Ms. Helen Gelband and Cindy Williams for editorial assistance.

References

1. Relman AS. Assessment and accountability: the third revolution in medical care [editorial]. *N Engl J Med* 1988;319:1220–1222.
2. Nelson EC, Splaine ME, Batalden PB, et al. Building measurement and data collection into medical practice. *Ann Intern Med* 1998;128:460–466.
3. Teno JM Facts on dying: brown atlas site of death 1989–1997. accessed February 26, 2004. Web Page. Available at: http://www.chcr.brown.edu/dying/factsondying.htm.
4. Saunders C. Monograph in Commemoration of the 30th Anniversary of St. Christopher's Hospice, 2001.
5. Institute of Medicine. Lohr KN, ed. *Medicare: a strategy for quality assurance.* Washington, DC: National Academy Press, 1990.
6. Emanuel EJ, Emanuel LL. The promise of a good death. *Lancet* 1998;351(Suppl 2):SII21–SII29.
7. Institute of Medicine. Committee on care at the end of life. Field MJ, Cassel CK, eds. *Approaching death: improving care at the end of life.* Washington, DC: National Academy Press, 1997.
8. National Hospice Organization. *A pathway for patients and families facing terminal illness: self-determined life closure, safe comfortable dying and effective grieving.* Alexandria, VA: National Hospice Organization, 1997.
9. Singer PA, Martin DK, Kelner M. Quality end-of-life care: patients' perspectives. *JAMA* 1999;281(2):163–168.
10. Teno JM, Casey VA, Welch L, et al. Patient-focused, family-centered end-of-life medical care: views of the guidelines and bereaved family members. *J Pain Symptom Manage.* 2001;22:738–751.
11. Connor SR, Teno J, Spence C, et al. Family evaluation of hospice care: results from voluntary submission of data via website. *J Pain Symptom Manage* 2005;30:9–17.
12. Teno JM, Byock I, Field MJ. Research agenda for developing measures to examine quality of care and quality of life of patients diagnosed with life-limiting illness. White paper from the conference on Excellent Care at the End of Life through Fast-Tracking Audit, Standards, and Teamwork (EXCELFAST), September 28–30, 1997. *J Pain Symptom Manage* 1999;17:75–82.
13. Solberg LI, Mosser G, McDonald S. The three faces of performance measurement: improvement, accountability, and research. *Jt Comm J Qual Improv* 1997;23:135–147.
14. Cleary PD, Edgman Levitan S, Roberts M, et al. Patients evaluate their hospital care: a national survey. *Health Aff (Millwood)* 1991;10:254–267.
15. Teno JM, Weitzen S, Wetle T, et al. Persistent pain in nursing home residents. *JAMA* 2001;285:2081.
16. Desbiens NA, Wu AW, Broste SK, et al. Pain and satisfaction with pain control in seriously ill hospitalized adults: findings from the SUPPORT research investigations. For the SUPPORT investigators. Study to understand prognoses and preferences for outcomes and risks of treatment. *Crit Care Med* 1996;24:1953–1961.
17. American Pain Society Quality of Care Committee. Quality improvement guidelines for the treatment of acute pain and cancer pain. *JAMA* 1995;274:1874–1880.
18. Teno JM. Putting the patient and family voice back into measuring the quality of care for the dying. *Hosp J* 1999;14:167–176.
19. Cartwright A. Changes in life and care in the year before death 1969–1987. *J Public Health Med* 1991;13:81–87.
20. Addington Hall J, McCarthy M. Regional Study of care for the dying: methods and sample characteristics. *Palliat Med* 1995;9(1):27–35.
21. National Center for Health Statistics. *The national mortality followback survey–provisional data, 1993. Public user data file documentation.* Hyattsville, MD: Centers for Disease Control and Prevention, 1998.
22. Langley G, Nolan K, Nolan T, et al. *The improvement guide: a practical approach to enhancing organizational performance.* San Francisco, CA: Jossey-Bass Publishers, 1996.
23. Baier RR, Gifford DR, Patry G, et al. Ameliorating pain in nursing homes: a collaborative quality-improvement project. *J Am Geriatr Soc* 2004;52:1988–1995.

CHAPTER 78 ■ MEASUREMENT OF QUALITY OF LIFE OUTCOMES

JASON E. OWEN, LAURA BOXLEY, AND JOSHUA C. KLAPOW

INTRODUCTION

For many years, survival was the primary outcome of clinical trials for those diagnosed with cancer. The introduction of formal assessments of health-related quality of life (HRQoL) has changed the way in which clinical trials have been conceptualized, administered, and interpreted. For those providing care for persons at the end of life, quality of life (QOL) concerns assume primary importance, and strong tools for measuring QOL provide both a valid characterization of QOL and an opportunity to detect and manage unaddressed clinical problems. In this chapter we hope to provide a brief conceptualization of HRQoL assessment in oncology populations, discuss the strengths and weaknesses of existing cancer-specific HRQoL assessment instruments and those specific to palliative oncology, and highlight several important methodologic issues of concern to researchers.

OVERVIEW OF HEALTH-RELATED QUALITY OF LIFE ASSESSMENT

A Brief History of Quality of Life Assessment in Palliative Care

The rapid growth of the palliative care movement has paralleled, and perhaps fueled in many respects, the increasing attention that has been given to QOL concerns among those seeking curative cancer treatments. The hospice Medicare benefit was created by the Tax Equity and Fiscal Responsibility Act of 1982 and made permanent by the U.S Congress in 1986. Although preceded by the growth of hospice organizations in Europe, this act made possible the development of community-based hospice services across the United States from the early 1980s to the present time. The rise of modern hospice care represented a paradigm shift for health care in the United States. Survival had been the sole relevant outcome of most clinical trials, and QOL had received only casual treatment in the research literature. By its very definition—"the achievement of the best possible QOL for patients and families (1)"—palliative care challenged dominant ideas about the nature of outcomes assessment in clinical populations.

The field of QOL assessment perhaps owes a great deal to those who fought the political and medical/cultural battles that facilitated the modern hospice movement. Instruments designed to formally measure "QOL" began to appear in the research literature shortly after the Medicare hospice benefit became law. Paralleling the growth of palliative care, the assessment of QOL as an endpoint in cancer clinical trials first emerged in Europe and slowly became integrated into clinical trials protocols in the United States. By 1995, three major clinical trials groups—the U.K. Medical Research Council (MRC), the European Organization for Research and Treatment of Cancer (EORTC), and the National Cancer Institute of Canada (NCIC)-advocated consideration of QOL as an endpoint in all new clinical trials (2). Tracing this development historically, the MRC was among the first clinical trials groups to introduce self-report diaries to track QOL outcomes in 1981 (3). In the early 1980s, the EORTC began to include endpoints related to QOL in its funded clinical trials, and the organization quickly established a study group to develop standardized, psychometrically evaluated tools for measuring QOL within cancer populations (4). A 1986 EORTC protocol titled "Long-term QOL of adult leukemia after BMT versus intensive consolidation in AML" was among the first phase III controlled clinical trials to employ QOL as the primary trial endpoint. In 1993, the EORTC established a separate data-monitoring unit whose sole function was to manage and evaluate QOL data obtained from EORTC clinical trials. The NCIC mandated that all phase III clinical trials consider the use of a QOL endpoint beginning in 1989 (5). Although the U.S. National Cancer Institute was slow to adopt QOL endpoints, Food and Drug Administration guidelines on anticancer drugs specified benefits to QOL as one possible criterion for approval in 1985 (6). QOL is now widely recognized to be the most salient outcome for trials that involve patients with advanced disease or poor prognosis or that involve treatments with little expected difference in survival outcomes (7–9).

Models of Health-Related Quality of Life Assessment

In undertaking efforts to assess HRQoL, it is important to recognize that there are multiple ways in which to conceptualize the construct, and decisions about the choice of assessment instruments to use for any given purpose should be made with these considerations in mind. Wenger and Furberg have defined HRQoL as "those attributes valued by patients, including their resultant comfort or sense of well-being; the extent to which they were able to maintain reasonable physical, emotional, and intellectual function; and the degree to which they retain their ability to participate in valued activities within the family, in the workplace, and in the community (cited in 10)." This definition reflects a growing consensus that HRQoL is a multidimensional construct that involves an individual's perceived health status, life satisfaction, and physical, social, and psychological well-being (10,11). Secondary dimensions of HRQoL are thought to include spirituality, relational intimacy, cognitive function, personal productivity, and symptom burden (12). Despite general agreement about the multidimensional nature of HRQoL, there are a number of ways in which HRQoL assessment has been operationalized. The most commonly employed methods include the assessment of health state utilities, general HRQoL, disease-specific HRQoL, and domain-specific HRQoL.

Health State Utilities

Preference-based HRQoL measures provide health state utilities by asking patients to indicate a preference between two choices under conditions of uncertainty. The most common applications of preference-based HRQoL measures include the time trade-off (TTO) and Standard Gamble techniques. The TTO method addresses an individual's willingness to accept a shorter although healthier life (i.e., how much life expectancy would one trade in exchange for improved QOL). Similarly, the standard gamble assesses the probability that an individual would risk death in order to regain perfect health. Utility-based measures of HRQoL, such as TTO or standard gamble techniques, have not been widely used in cancer populations. However, emerging evidence suggests that patient-based utilities for cancer-related health states are not strongly related to self-report QOL measures (13). Utility scores measured on a 0 to 1.0 scale are typically lower than self-report measures based on the same scale.

One method for measuring patient-based utilities for cancer health states has been proposed by Perez et al. (14). Using a TTO method, Perez et al. (14) asked patients with metastatic disease whether they would be willing to trade days in the upcoming month for a single month of perfect health. Patients who were willing to trade days proceeded through a brief nine-item questionnaire which assessed willingness to trade 3, 5, 10, 15, 20, 25, 27, 29, or 30 days using responses of "Yes," "No," or "Maybe." A "Maybe" response is considered to be an equivalence point at which the patient is indifferent between "Yes" and "No" responses. Utility value for their current health state is then calculated as (30 days traded at equivalence point)/30.

In the standard gamble procedure, an individual is asked whether they would be willing to undergo a treatment with two possible outcomes with varying probabilities: cure or immediate death. The health state utility is identified as the probability at which an individual is indifferent between undergoing and foregoing the hypothetical treatment. For example, an individual nearing the end of life would be likely to agree to undergo a hypothetical treatment with a 90% probability of immediate cure and only a 10% chance of death but might be indifferent at the point at which the probability of immediate cure drops to 50%. This person would have a utility for their current health state of 0.50. Another method for assessing preference-based utilities is through the use of the Health Utilities Index (HUI). The HUI is a 5-item interviewer-administered measure that has been used to estimate patient-derived utilities for their present health state.

Preference-based measures provide a number of benefits over the more traditional questionnaires. Utilities can be used to readily determine quality adjusted survival [e.g., quality adjusted life-years (QALYs)]. Additional benefits include ease of interpretation of a single numerical estimate of HRQoL relative to a profile of subscale scores and, in conjunction with a measure of costs, facilitation of cost-utility analyses (15).

However, these advantages are strongly outweighed by the confusing nature of the assessment techniques and the resulting cognitive burden imposed on patients. Additionally, utility scores are of limited clinical value.

General Health-Related Quality of Life

Unlike utility-based measures, general HRQoL measures are usually derived from self-reports and in most cases do not provide a single point estimate of an individual's overall HRQoL. Rather, such measures typically break HRQoL down into its constituent domains (e.g., physical, social, emotional, and functional well-being) and provide individual scores for each domain. General health status instruments assess the impact of disease and treatment on any medical population, thereby enabling administration to patients with any of a number of different medical conditions. General health status instruments include the Nottingham Health Profile, the Sickness Impact Profile, and the Medical Outcomes Study SF-36. A primary advantage of this approach to QOL assessment is the ease with which resulting QOL scores can be compared with norms derived from populations with other medical conditions. The SF-36 is perhaps the most widely used general measure of HRQoL, but its relevance for patients nearing the end of life is questionable. The instrument contains a number of items that are likely to be inappropriate or result in floor effects for a palliative care population (e.g., "does your health now limit you from engaging in vigorous physical activity," "have you had to cut down on the amount of time you spent on work or other activities as a result of your physical health," and so on. (16)). Although general measures of HRQoL were designed to be broadly applicable across disease conditions, they appear to be of limited value for palliative care patients and have been used only sparingly in end-of-life populations.

Disease-Specific Measures of Quality of Life

Measures of cancer-specific HRQoL sample aspects of QOL which are particularly salient to cancer patients, such as treatment side-effects and pain, in addition to sampling the broader impact of disease on psychological, physical, social, and functional well-being. Cancer-specific measures assess a level of detail that cannot be achieved with generic or preference-based measures. A handful of cancer-specific HRQoL instruments are available to researchers, including the Functional Living Index for Cancer (FLIC), the Cancer Rehabilitation Evaluation System (CARES), the Functional Assessment of Cancer Therapy (FACT), and the EORTC Quality of Life Questionnaire (QLQ-C30) (17–21). The most widely used measures of cancer-specific HRQoL employ a "core-plus" approach, which involves the use of a "core" set of items that can be used with any cancer population "plus" a cancer-specific set of items that evaluate symptoms and experiences that may be unique within a specific type of cancer (e.g., lung or colorectal). In palliative care settings, the QLQ-C30 and FACT (also known as FACIT) have been the most commonly used disease-specific HRQoL instruments, and both employ a "core-plus" assessment methodology.

Utilizing a "core-plus" approach is one way in which researchers and practitioners alike have sought to capture a comprehensive picture of QOL. With the core-plus approach, one uses generalized measures supplemented with disease-specific measures. This enables researchers to compare related groups based on common measures, while addressing the specific characteristics of a target population. For example, the Functional Assessment of Cancer Therapy General Form (FACT G) is a core instrument used in concert with disease specific measures such as the FACT-B to assess QOL in women with breast cancer. Using this approach, one can compare QOL scores across different cancer types as well as have critical information about a specific population. One potential caveat to this approach in palliative care is the increase in response burden for the patient. It is important that the investigator weighs the costs and benefits of increasing the response burden inherent to the assessment procedure. If one's research questions do not include plans for comparative analysis, including a core instrument with potentially irrelevant items may be unnecessarily burdensome.

The European Organization for Research and Treatment of Cancer Quality of Life Questionnaire (EORTC QLQ-C30/Aaronson et al. (17)) is a 30-item HRQoL measure with excellent reliability, and validity has been evaluated favorably in a number of cancer populations. Widely released in 1993, the EORTC QLQ-C30 version 3.0 was designed for international clinical trials and has been translated into many different languages. This instrument provides five subscales of functioning, including physical functioning, role functioning, social functioning, emotional functioning, and cognitive functioning. Symptom-related items, which pertain to dyspnea, fatigue, sleep disturbance, loss of appetite, nausea, vomiting, constipation, and diarrhea, are also assessed. The EORTC Study Group on QOL has developed a number of cancer type–specific modules for use with the QLQ-C30, including lung, breast, head & neck, esophageal, ovarian, gastric, prostate, multiple myeloma, brain, and colorectal cancer-specific items. For example, the "plus" module for colorectal cancer is a 38-item module that covers aspects of QOL that are more specific to patients with colorectal cancer and includes scorable subscales related to body image, sexual function, future perspective, sexual enjoyment, micturition problems, gastrointestinal symptoms, male and female sexual problems, defecation problems, weight loss, and chemotherapy side-effects. The psychometric properties of the EORTC QLQ-C30 have been well studied across a number of patient populations internationally and demonstrate good reliability and validity.

Although used frequently in palliative care, the EORTC QLQ-C30 was not designed for primary use in this field. As a result, the measure has shortcomings when applied to the terminally ill. The EORTC employs a normative approach, basing comparisons to the average ability level of a health individual. This is an unrealistic comparison for terminally ill patients, and may not be optimally informative. A more appropriate comparison for assessment may be to use a model of optimal QOL for an individual's disease stage. One of the unique characteristics of palliative care is the need to address death and end-of-life issues. As such, just meeting the patient's physical needs is not sufficient; an optimal palliative care measure should include a spiritual/existential component to assess patient needs. The QLQ-C30 does not address the specific spiritual needs of palliative care, rendering it ineffective in this domain. The QLQ-C30 questionnaire also includes items that are likely to be inappropriate for many palliative care patients. Examples of these questions include: "Do you have any trouble taking a long walk?" and "Are you limited in any way in doing either your work or doing household jobs?" Fatigue items such as these are likely to produce ceiling affects that will not contribute meaningful information to the QOL assessment. Given the probability of functional and cognitive impairments in study subjects, it is particularly important to avoid including unnecessarily long or insensitive lines of questioning. Some of the QLQ-C30 subscales have performed poorly in studies with patients nearing the end of life. For example, the fatigue subscale of the EORTC QLQ-C30 exhibits clear floor/ceiling effects when used in this population (22). However, a short form of the EORTC QLQ-C30 for use in palliative care is currently in development (see http://www.eortc.be/home/qol/modules.htm).

The FACT-G is a 27-item questionnaire that utilizes 5-point Likert scales to evaluate social well-being, physical well-being, emotional well-being, and functional well-being (18,23). The FACT-G has been widely used in clinical trials in the United States (23). Sixteen cancer-specific modules are available for use with the core FACT-G measure, including breast, bladder, brain, cervical, colorectal, leukemia, lymphoma, and lung cancer–specific items, to name a few. For example, the FACT-C colorectal-specific instrument consists of the 27 items of the FACT-G plus an additional 9 items that pertain to specific symptoms associated with colorectal cancers (e.g., bowel control, ostomy care, and concern about appearance). Importantly, a palliative care specific module (FACIT-PAL) has been developed for use with patients nearing the end of life. This instrument will be discussed in greater detail in the following text.

Domain-Specific Measures of Quality of Life

The term "QOL" has been used broadly in the medical literature, often without formal definition or explication. As a result, a number of clinical trials have reported "QOL" endpoints using measures that are not consistent with multidimensional conceptualizations of HRQoL. Gill and Feinstein (24) report that published studies including QOL analyses have used more than 159 instruments to measure QOL, with little agreement as to which domains, scales, or items actually measure the construct. Accordingly, the reader should be cautious when reviewing studies that use the term "QOL" or purport to have measured QOL. It is not uncommon to see a self-report measure of a single symptom domain referred to as a measure of HRQoL. Instead, we believe this approach can be more accurately conceptualized as assessment of single domains of HRQoL. This approach generally allows researchers to tailor an assessment battery to the population, and study aims, of interest and can be used to bolster a multidimensional measure of HRQoL. Examples of domain-specific constructs (and measures) relevant for palliative care populations include pain (often measured using the Brief Pain Inventory), fatigue (measured using the Multidimensional Fatigue Inventory or the Brief Fatigue Inventory among others), spiritual well-being (assessed with the Spiritual Well-Being scale of the FACIT or the Spiritual Well-Being Scale), and depression (frequently measured using the Center for Epidemiological Studies-Depression Scale, Hospital Anxiety and Depression Scale, or Beck Depression Inventory).

QUALITY OF LIFE ASSESSMENT IN PALLIATIVE CARE

General Considerations

Measurement of QOL in persons at the end of life is quite distinct from the assessment of individuals who are hoping for and perhaps expecting a complete recovery to their pre-diagnosis baseline. In describing the underpinnings of palliative care, Dame Cicely Saunders emphasizes the importance of the following basic principles: symptom control, maximizing the potential of the patient and family's relationships, caring for the family unit, and spiritual needs (25). This concise description highlights potential distinctions between conceptualizations of QOL for those in curative care relative to those nearing the end of life. In the context of palliative care, several domains that are carefully measured in general, health-related, and disease-specific QOL measures are rendered either irrelevant or much less useful than in other settings. For example, a generally outstanding HRQoL measure oft-used in cancer research, the FACT, includes several items that ask patients to rate "worry about [their] condition getting worse" or the extent to which they are "losing hope in the fight against...illness." Similar problems exist for the EORTC QLQ-C30. Other concerns typically measured in QOL instruments that are nonspecific to the end of life are simply decreased in relevance. Functional well-being, for example, is much less important to those who are no longer working or held responsible for instrumental activities of daily living (e.g., balancing checkbooks, doing household grocery shopping, etc.). Other aspects of QOL that are typically minimized in other QOL assessment instruments may be of maximal importance to those at the end of life. Notably, spiritual and existential concerns are among the most strongly endorsed concerns reported by patients in palliative care (26,27). Therefore, an assessment of HRQoL that is based largely on physical symptoms and functional complaints that are quite prevalent in palliative care may *underestimate* actual QOL as perceived by the patient, particularly if there are other salient domains (e.g., spiritual well-being) that may become increasingly salient to the individual.

Search Strategy

A systematic search strategy was employed in order to identify all relevant palliative care-specific measures of HRQoL. The search was conducted in two phases. First, PubMed and PsycInfo were searched using the terms "QOL," "outcomes," "assessment or evaluation or measure or questionnaire," and "hospice or palliat*." Second, previously published reviews of QOL issues in palliative care were collected and reviewed for descriptions of appropriate measures (16,28–30). Given the breadth of the field of QOL assessment and the large number of high-quality reviews of the general HRQoL literature, we chose to limit our discussion to QOL measures that were as follows:

1. Specifically developed for use in persons nearing the end of life
2. Psychometrically evaluated in palliative care populations
3. Based on self-report (rather than clinician) ratings of HRQoL
4. Used in more than one study

These criteria resulted in the identification of nine palliative care QOL measures: the McGill Quality of Life Questionnaire (MQOL), Life Evaluation Questionnaire (LEQ), Palliative Care Outcome Scale (POS), FACIT-PAL, Missoula-VITAS Quality of Life Index (MVQLI), Palliative Care Quality of Life Instrument (PQLI), Hospice Quality of Life Index (HQLI), Assessment of Quality of Life at the End of Life (AQEL), and the Quality of Life at the End-of-Life Instrument (QUAL-E). Once measures of palliative care QOL were identified, systematic searches were repeated in PubMed and PsycInfo to select all published articles in which the measure was administered to patients at the end of life. Each measure will be described, and for each measure we will discuss all available evidence for the instrument's reliability, validity, acceptability, sensitivity to intervention, dissemination/use in clinical trials, and appropriateness for the intended population.

McGill Quality of Life Questionnaire

The MQOL is a 16-item, self-report instrument designed to measure physical symptoms (3 items), physical well-being (1 item) psychological symptoms (4 items), existential well-being (6 items), and social support (2 items). The instrument is scored to generate subscale scores associated with each of these four categories and a total QOL score derived from the average of the five-subscale scores (31). Patients are asked to self-report their QOL concerns using an 11-point Likert-type scale, and

each item is anchored with two verbal descriptors (e.g., 0 = "no problem", 10 = "tremendous problem"). Respondents are asked to describe their QOL only for the previous 2 days. In addition, a single item on the instruction page of the MQOL can be used for those respondents who are unable to complete the questionnaire in its entirety. Item development was based on existing HRQoL and symptom-assessment measures, and item testing and psychometric properties of the MQOL were conducted in samples consisting almost entirely of patients in palliative care or otherwise nearing the end of life (27,31–34). The MQOL was developed in both English and French languages and has been successfully translated into Spanish, Hong Kong Chinese, Taiwan Chinese, and Malaysian (35).

Item characteristics and reliability of the MQOL appear to be acceptable across studies. Two of the five MQOL subscales typically provide negatively skewed distributions (existential well-being and social support), suggesting less than desirable item response characteristics for these items (33). However, it may be possible to transform these skewed distributions in order to more closely approximate normality when the data will be analyzed with parametric statistics whose assumptions involve univariate or multivariate normality. Internal consistency for the entire measure has been shown to be excellent (α's = 0.81 to 0.91 in separate samples (34)). Internal consistency estimates for the subscales are generally in the acceptable range: physical symptoms (α's = 0.65 − 0.88), psychological symptoms (α's = 0.81 − 0.89), existential well-being (α's 0.75 − 0.86), and support (α's = 0.73 − 0.79 (34, 36)). Test-retest reliability for individuals reporting stable QOL over a 2-day period is generally good (α = 0.75 (34)).

With respect to the validity of the instrument, Stromgren et al. (2002) reviewed medical records of newly admitted palliative patients and compared symptoms detailed in the medical record with items on the MQOL. The authors identified 63 distinct symptom domains and problem areas, noting that the content validity of the MQOL was insufficient for many of the symptoms that palliative care patients frequently present on admission. However, the authors appropriately note that the first 3 items of the MQOL allow respondents to identify the symptoms that are most "troublesome," therefore limiting the number of total items to which respondents are exposed by focusing on those that are potentially the most salient. Good convergent validity with other palliative QOL measures has been reported (36,37). Additionally, the MQOL has been shown to be predictive of satisfaction with hospice care received (38).

Like most palliative care–specific quality of life measures, evidence for the acceptability of the MQOL is somewhat mixed. In a study conducted by the lead author of the MQOL, an attempt was made to administer the MQOL to consecutively admitted patients on a palliative care unit. However, among 1131 patients admitted to the palliative care service, only 194 were able to complete the MQOL. One-hundred ninety-four of the 1131 potential participants had sufficient physical and cognitive resources to complete the measure, and only 135 did so- resulting in an overall response rate of 12% (33). To increase response rates and better meet the needs of the target population, the MQOL can be supplemented with a single-item scale. Additionally, the MQOL has been tested with standardized verbal instructions (34). Item non-completion is quite low for the MQOL (0.3% of items left blank (34)). Additional evidence for the acceptability of the instrument is given by the successful use of the MQOL across patient populations, including amyotrophic lateral sclerosis (ALS) (39), HIV/AIDS (32), and cancer (26).

Importantly, the MQOL has been shown to be responsive to change over time. Similar evidence for responsivity is notably lacking in other palliative care–specific quality of life measures. Cohen et al. (33) have shown that the total

MQOL score, 4 of the 5 subscales, and the single-item QOL scale are responsive to change over time. In a study of 88 newly admitted palliative care patients, MQOL scores on all administered subscales (social support was not measured due to poor scale characteristics) increased significantly by 1 week after admission. In a study of 49 patients with ALS, total MQOL and subscale scores were shown to be stable over a 16-month follow-up period (40). In a similar study with those diagnosed with advanced cancers, Lo et al. (35) have shown the MQOL and its subscales to be responsive to change over time. Some studies, however, have failed to show expected changes over time (e.g., (38)). In one of the more sophisticated designs we reviewed, Cohen et al. (34) demonstrated that the total MQOL score and the subscale scores for physical well-being, physical symptoms, psychological symptoms, and existential well-being were responsive to self-reports of "good days," "average days," and "bad days" and transitions over time between "good days" and "bad days." On the basis of these findings, the authors of the MQOL suggest that improving total MQOL scores by 2.6 points is analogous to changing a "bad day" into a "good day," and a score improvement of 1.5 points is analogous to changing a "bad day" into an "average day." Such anchors are easily interpretable, readily understandable to patients, and have clear clinical relevance to those providing palliative care services.

Life Evaluation Questionnaire

The LEQ is a unique QOL measure in that the instrument was designed to reflect the specific concerns and needs voiced by patients themselves. The LEQ is multidimensional and assesses a wide array of concerns related to physical symptoms, psychological symptoms, and existential issues- to name a few. Items were developed on the basis of qualitative interviews conducted with caregivers and patients with incurable cancer (41). The instrument is comprised of 61 statements rated using a 7-point Likert scale. Five factor scores can be derived from the questionnaire: freedom from restriction, life appreciation, contentment, resentment, and social integration. Information on the reliability of the LEQ is sparse. In the initial description of the instrument, the authors report some evidence for construct validity of the LEQ although it is not clear how the five subscales of the LEQ would be expected to correlate with measures of symptom burden and overall QOL (41). In the initial report of the LEQ, it is suggested that participants found the instrument to be highly acceptable, but the length of the instrument is a substantial drawback. Although the instrument has not been widely adopted, researchers with specific interests in the subscales tapped by the LEQ might consider supplementing other measures with items representing the LEQ subscales.

Palliative Care Outcome Scale

The POS is a 10-item self-report scale that purports to measure symptoms, communication with providers, existential concerns, and practical problems common to palliative care settings (42). Eight of the 10 items are rated using a 5-point Likert-type scale, although the remaining 2 items have 3 response categories. Two additional items are used to allow respondents to identify their "main problems" over the past 3 days and to indicate whether they required assistance in completing the questionnaire. As described by the authors, the POS is not designed to generate either an overall estimate of QOL or subscale scores for specific QOL domains. Rather, the instrument was designed as a screen for commonly encountered QOL concerns that could be administered to and completed by patients who would be unable to complete lengthier batteries.

However, a total score consisting of responses to the first 10 items has been used by some researchers (43). A unique feature of the POS is that it includes an analogous measure that can be completed by the respondent's health care providers. Items were chosen from similar QOL instruments by the principle authors.

With respect to item characteristics, reliability, and validity, there are notable limitations of the POS. Internal consistency of the scale is low ($\alpha = 0.64 - 65$ (42,44)). Floor effects have been reported for two items: "how much time do you feel has been wasted on appointments?" and "have any practical matters resulting from your illness, either financial or personal, been addressed (42)?" In a study of the overlap between assessed domains of palliative care QOL measures and issues noted in the medical record, the POS "missed" many of the clinical issues identified in patients' medical charts and fares less favorably than the MQOL (45). However, the instrument appears to be face valid to respondents and has been shown to have significant overlap with the EORTC QLQ-C30 (42).

Despite the attempt to develop an instrument that would be easily completed by those nearing the end of life, completion rates for the POS remain low. In the initial study reporting the development of the instrument and describing its psychometric properties, 37.3% of new referrals to palliative care providers ultimately completed at least one POS (42). Primary reasons for non-completion included physical or mental incapacity (28.7%) and language barriers (3.1%). A subsequent evaluation of the instrument resulted in a response rate of 76.89% (43).

The instrument has been shown to be responsive to changes over time. Stevens et al. (43) have shown that a total POS score declines significantly in the first 4 days after admission to a palliative care unit. Additionally, of the 10 primary issues assessed by the POS, 6 have been shown to be responsive to change upon admission to a palliative care unit: pain, other symptoms, anxiety, family worry/anxiety, information from health care providers, and feeling that life is worthwhile (37,42,43). The POS has been validated in Spanish (44) and used in a variety of clinical populations, including motor neurone disease (46). The instrument has not yet been used in intervention studies.

One indication of the appropriateness of the POS for patients with advanced disease is the time required to complete the instrument. It has been reported that patients complete the POS in an average of 6.9 minutes for the initial administration, and completion times decrease to below 4 minutes on repeat administrations (42). In one study of the POS, 6 of the 10 issues assessed did not appear to be relevant to the population under study: information, sharing feelings with family/friends, feeling that life was worthwhile, feeling good about self as a person, time wasted on appointments, and having practical matters addressed by palliative care team. The median score on these items was 0 or 1, suggesting no concerns or only slight concerns related to that item (43). Participants reported the highest levels of concern for pain, other symptoms (e.g., nausea, coughing, or constipation), anxiety, and perceptions of family anxiety/worries.

FACIT-PAL

The FACIT-PAL is the palliative care version of the widely used FACIT (previously named FACT) system for measuring QOL and uses the core-plus approach to QOL assessment. This approach has clear strengths. Importantly, the core-plus approach allows researchers to compare total QOL and estimates of physical, functional, social, and emotional well-being to norms published for other patient populations (using the FACT-G) and to evaluate clinically meaningful changes in QOL over time. However, this approach also has significant limitations. Notably, the "core" items of the FACIT-PAL are the same items that would be administered to a patient with early stage breast or prostate cancer and may be of substantially less interest or relevance to patients at the end of life. For example, a patient would receive a higher score for the Emotional Well-Being subscale if they indicated less "worry about dying," that they are "losing hope in the fight against [their] illness," or that they are worrying "that [their] condition will get worse." Regardless of their emotional needs, a person nearing the end of life could be understandably confused about how to answer items such as these. More importantly, use of the core-plus approach simply increases the number of items an individual must complete.

There are 27 items on the core FACIT module in addition to 19 items on the palliative care specific portion of the instrument. The palliative care specific items on the FACIT-PAL do provide good representation of the basic QOL concerns identified by Saunders (2000). The instrument assesses six general symptoms common to patients at the end of life (dyspnea, constipation, cachexia, vomiting, swelling, dry mouth) and two items pertaining to cognitive capacity (able to make decisions, thinking clearly (47)). Other symptoms such as pain, nausea, and fatigue are included in the core FACIT questionnaire. Additionally, the FACIT-PAL provides 10 items that measure connections with family and existential concerns. Spiritual well-being is not measured, although an additional 12-item spirituality scale has been developed as part of the FACIT system. The FACIT-PAL has not yet been extensively validated or widely adopted. Although the instrument appears to be promising, particularly when used in conjunction with the core FACIT measure, less information is available about this instrument than for the other HRQoL measures that are described.

Missoula-VITAS Quality of Life Index

The MVQOLI is a 25-item measure using 5-point Likert scales to assess symptom, functional status, interpersonal well-being, emotional well-being, and transcendent subscales (48). Included in this measure is also a single-item global QOL question. This measure is unique for its scoring system that allows subscales to be weighted by the respondent. The response range for this measure is broad, demonstrating a good level of variability in scores obtained. In the initial report of the instrument, total scores spanned 71.5% of the possible range. Internal consistency estimates of the MVQOLI have been shown to be adequate in at least one study ($\alpha = 0.77$ (48)). However, Schwartz et al. (49) report that internal consistencies of the subscales exhibit considerable variation (α's $= 0.23 - 0.70$). Only the symptom subscale seemed to be assessing a single construct. However, test-retest reliabilities appear to be good for the subscales (0.59 $-$.070) and total score (0.77 (49)).

Evidence for the validity of the MVQOLI is mixed. Content and face validity were assessed by providing the measure to hospice professionals for review (48). Fourteen professionals were invited to categorize each of the items into one of five prescribed domains. These items were correctly assigned 77% of the time, indicating that these items could be reliably categorized into the hypothesized dimensions. Convergent validity was assessed by comparing the global QOL item to the remainder of the MVQOLI items. The single QOL item correlated strongly with the complete set of items ($r = 0.43$). Divergent validity was assessed by comparing the MVQOLI items to the Karnofsky Performance Status Scale (KPS), an assessment of functional impairment completed by a qualified observer. Comparison revealed that there was only a small

correlation between the MVQOLI and the KPS ($r = 0.18$). Additional efforts to demonstrate good construct validity of the MVQOLI have produced mixed results (49). However, ecological validity of the instrument is good, with 89% of participants reporting that the MVQLI was strongly or moderately related to their sense of their QOL (49). There is also considerable evidence to suggest that weighting the importance of each QOL domain is unnecessary since nearly all participants rate each domain as being highly important (49). Therefore, the unique use of weighting in this scale is likely an unnecessary complication.

Palliative Care Quality of Life Instrument

The PQLI is a 28-item measure assessing psychological affect, communication, support, health, self-care, activity, and choice of treatment (50). This measure is unique for its inclusion of treatment choice, identified by the authors as an important component to palliative care. The treatment subscale includes two items regarding one's preferences and ability to choose their treatment. Three response choices are provided for these items (i.e., no, sometimes, or yes). The treatment subscale also includes five items to be rated from one to five in the order of perceived importance. The psychological affect, communication, support, health, self-care, and activity subscales of the PQLI are measured in a single metric, where patients may report on a scale from one to three, indicating no, sometimes or yes. The final item on the scale is a single-item measure of QOL, on a scale from 1 to 10. The response complexity of the scale may be cause for hesitation in the implementation of this measure with severely ill patients. More problematic, however, is the wording of the questions themselves. Developed in Greece, this measure was later translated into English, perhaps contributing to the cumbersome question and response format of the PQLI.

The following reliability and validity statistics were calculated using the Hellenistic version of the measure given to 120 Greek cancer patients. Internal consistency of the PQLI is good ($\alpha = 0.79$). Test-retest reliability, after a 7-day interval, is also strong ($r = 0.82$ (Mystakidou et al., 2004)). Interscale correlations were used to assess the validity of the PQLI. Each scale correlated significantly with every other scale included in the measure. The greatest agreement was found between health status, choice of treatment, activity, and self-care. The single-item QOL measure was highly correlated with each of the other subscales (p's < 0.01). Exploratory non-orthogonal factor analysis was also used to assess the validity of the PQLI. The seven factors identified by the analysis corresponded to the seven categories included in the measure. Criterion-related validity was assessed by predicting interview scores on the PQLI from the self-report scores. PQLI constructs were significantly predictive of interview scores. When compared to the EORTC Core QOL Questionnaire (QLQ-C30, version 3.0) and the AQEL, the PQLI demonstrated strong correlational agreement among relevant scales. The strongest agreement was found between items assessing pain and lack of appetite.

As of now, there does not appear to be any evidence supporting the use of the English version of the PQLI in any population. The statistics sited earlier only reflect the validity of the Hellenic version among Greek cancer patients in Athens. Further research is needed to assess the appropriateness and sensitivity of this measure for more generalized use. There is also no evidence to evaluate the ability of the PQLI to assess change over time or to discriminate between patients with differing disease severity.

Hospice Quality of Life Index

The revised HQLI is a 28-item self-report questionnaire, measuring three domains: psychophysiological, functional and social/spiritual well-being (51). Each item is measured on a scale from 1 to 10, with a range of potential scores from 28 to 280. Items were developed using expert opinion, literature review, comparisons to similar measures and qualitative data from patients in hospice care. Reliability of the HQLI was measured by calculating internal consistency, yielding a strong Cronbach's α score of 0.88. Internal consistency estimates for each of the psychophysiological, functional and social/spiritual subscales were also quite good: 0.85, 0.84 and 0.82 respectively.

Several methods were utilized to assess the validity of the latest revised version of the HQLI. Confirmatory factor analysis was used to corroborate the four hypothesized subscales of the 1996 version of the HQLI (51). Analysis revealed, however, a three-factor structure that has been integrated into the revised HQLI. Subscale scores have helped to successfully differentiate healthy individuals from those diagnosed with cancer. Psychophysiological Well-Being subscale scores ranged from zero to 130, with cancer patients averaging 93.2, and healthy adults averaging 105.8. The Functional Well-Being subscale scores ranged from zero to 70, with patients with cancer averaging 35.1 and healthy adults averaging 55.3. Lastly the Social/Spiritual Well-Being subscale scores ranged from zero to 80, with patients with cancer averaging 69.8 and healthy adults averaging 71.7. The highest item scores were in the social/spiritual subscale, and the lowest were found in the functional subscale. The usefulness of these subscales to differentiate healthy individuals from patients with cancer supports the sensitivity of the HQLI. The authors also chose to compare the HQLI to the Eastern Cooperative Oncology Group Performance Status Rating (ECOG-PSR), an assessment of functional status. Total HQLI scores were moderately but significantly correlated to the ECOG-PSR ($r = 0.26$). When compared to the subscales of the HQLI, varying levels of congruence were obtained. Correlations were weak between ECOG-PSR the psychophysiological and social/spiritual subscales, but moderate for the functional subscale.

Assessment of Quality of Life at the End of Life

The AQEL instrument is a 22-item scale, measuring physical, psychological, social, existential and medical care domains. The first 19 items on the questionnaire are measured on a scale from 1 to 10. Depending on the item, reports of high QOL may correspond to high or low values on the scale. The last three items of the questionnaire assess hospital care and any idiographic concerns regarding the experiences of the patient in the last week. The reliability of this questionnaire was assessed using test-retest correlations. Temporal reliabilities of individual items varied from 0.52 to 0.90, with the majority of the items scoring >0.70 indicating good temporal reliability.

The convergent validity of the AQEL was assessed through comparisons with the Cancer Inventory of Problem Situations (CIPS) and the KPS scale. The authors hypothesized that corresponding subscales would be highly correlated (i.e., demonstrating convergent validity), and that dissimilar subscales would not be correlated (i.e., demonstrating divergent validity). Evidence of convergent and divergent validity was mixed. In this analysis, "memory" (AQEL) and "concentration" (CIPS) were significantly associated ($r = 0.49$),

as well as 'physical strength' (AQEL) and "sitting/lying" (CIPS) ($r = -0.62$). Low correlations were observed between "memory" and "eat, dress, wash independently" (CIPS) ($r = 0.11$), and between "physical strength" and "pain" (CIPS) ($r = 0.18$). Subscales assessing physical strength ($r = 0.66$) and global QOL ($r = 0.63$) were strongly correlated with KPS scores. However, items such as "anxiety", "insomnia", "pain", and "sharing worries with any family member" had weak correlations with KPS scores. Additionally, evidence for the ability of the AQEL to detect changes over time has been demonstrated in longitudinal assessments of patients followed from hospice entry until death (29).

These findings suggest that the AQEL may be a sufficiently valid and reliable measure of QOL in a palliative care population. The measure's comprehensiveness and relative brevity make it a practical choice for use among the severely ill. By including a free response item, the AQEL is additionally able to detect factors not described in the scale that may influence a patient's QOL. More research is needed, however, to confirm the psychometric properties of this scale.

Quality of Life at the End-of-Life Instrument

The QUAL-E scale is a 31-item instrument that was developed with particular attention to item phrasing and item response characteristics. In developing the measure, the authors conducted focus groups to identify core attributes associated with a "good death" and validated their focus group findings using national surveys of key stakeholders: palliative care patients, their family members, and health care staff (52). These attributes were then used to develop a potential pool of 54 items, which were administered to 25 participants in order to evaluate item response characteristics. Items exhibiting substantial deviation from normality, poor discrimination, or redundancy with other items were eliminated from the item pool. Remaining items were then administered to 200 terminally ill patients who passed an initial cognitive status screen. Participation in this phase of the study was quite good—85% of all potential participants were eligible and willing to complete the preliminary measure (53).

Although the published instrument consists of 31 interviewer-administered items, only 30 items were factor analyzed. Of these, 24 items loaded strongly on 1 of 5 retained factors: sense of life completion (e.g., being able to say important things to loved ones, being at peace, etc.), relationships with the health care system (e.g., feeling control over treatment decisions, feeling understood by health care providers, etc.), preparation/anticipatory concerns (e.g., worry about becoming a burden to others, fear of dying, etc.), symptom impact (e.g., symptom severity, frequency, and interference with enjoyment of life), and connectedness and affective social support (e.g., having someone to share deepest concerns with, spending time with family). These content domains exhibit good content validity with item domains represented by the MVQOLI, FACT-G and MQOL. The QUAL-E is presented as an interviewer-conducted assessment. The individual is first asked to list the three most troublesome symptoms they have experienced in the last month and to identify the symptom that has been the most bothersome in the past week. Using a 5-point Likert-type scale, the individual is then asked to report the frequency, severity, degree of interference with life enjoyment, worry, and overall importance of the most bothersome symptom. An additional 25 items are provided for the assessment of the five content domains described in the preceding text, and the QUAL-E also provides a single-item assessment of overall QOL that is rated on a scale of 1 to 5 ("very poor,"

"poor," "fair," "good," or "excellent"). Although the published instrument is somewhat lengthy (31 items plus a brief identification of three bothersome symptoms), only 24 items were retained in an item factor analysis, and the response rate among 234 approached participants was quite good. Additional estimates of instrument validity are needed, and the authors have suggested that they are working on a shortened version of this measure.

SUMMARY

In this brief review of existing instruments for measuring palliative care-specific HRQoL, a few tentative conclusions can be made. First, a number of instruments are available to researchers, but validation (particularly by research groups other than the developers of the instrument) studies are incomplete at best. This finding is also true with respect to responsiveness to change over time and acceptability of the instruments to patients nearing the end of life. Second, only two of the reviewed instruments have been extensively employed in palliative care-related studies: the MQOL and the Palliative Care Outcomes Scale. Limitations of each of these measures have been identified, allowing researchers to anticipate the types of problems they are likely to encounter when using these instruments. Given the current state of the literature, the same cannot be said for the other measures reviewed, and these instruments should be employed with some caution or with supplementation from other measures that have been more extensively tested. Third, there is subtle variation across instruments that reflects differences in how HRQoL is conceptualized in palliative care settings. Nearly all of the reviewed instruments provide indices of symptom burden, psychological well-being, interpersonal well-being or social support, and existential/spiritual concerns. Other instruments are unique in their ability to measure certain aspects of HRQoL, including freedom from restriction and resentment (LEQ), communication with providers (POS), cognitive capacity (FACIT-PAL), functional status (MVQLI and HQLI), and self-care abilities (PQLI). Finally, instruments vary substantially in length. The MQOL and POS contained the fewest items (10 and 16 respectively), while the FACIT-PAL and LEQ contained the most (46 and 61 respectively). Given problems associated with poor response rates and missing data in palliative care populations, instrument length should be a primary concern for researchers.

OVERCOMING BARRIERS TO QUALITY OF LIFE ASSESSMENT

Response Rates in Palliative Care

The rate of completion of palliative QOL instruments is poor overall. Most palliative QOL assessment tools are designed to be self-administered and brief enough for patients with dwindling physical and cognitive resources to be able to complete. However, response rates in systematic studies are not infrequently abysmal. In a longitudinal study of 462 patients admitted to a palliative care unit or hospice, fewer than 13% were able to complete the instrument within 2 weeks of death, and most required extensive assistance in completing the measures throughout the study (35). In many studies, overall recruitment/participation rates are unreported. In others, exclusion criteria explicitly exclude those who are unable to complete a verbal interview (37) or fail a brief cognitive

screen (38). Additionally, for studies attempting to follow patient longitudinally, attrition rates are sometimes much higher than would be expected in non-palliative settings. Although Cohen et al. (43) were able to limit attrition from time 1 to time 2 to only 10%, attrition has been much higher in other similar studies (e.g., 38% attrition from time 1 to time 2 (38)).

It is important to recognize two important, but competing issues associated with poor response rates. On the one hand, it is understandable that investigators have great difficulty in recruiting and obtaining consent from study participants who are nearing the end of life. In many ways, it would be quite surprising to have very high response rates for any study, given the responsibilities that investigators have to human-protections research committees (i.e., institutional review boards) and the response burden placed on very ill individuals. However, we must also recognize the potential adverse effects of over-interpretation of studies that have low rates of response. Investigators may be "cream-skimming" when only the healthiest subjects are able to complete the QOL assessments, and these biased samples may have substantial consequences for the interpretation of both longitudinal and intervention studies.

At the very least, investigators must be able to document how those who were able to respond to the QOL assessment differed from those who were unable to respond. Were there differences by disease type? Tumor burden? Cognitive status? By understanding the nature of potential bias, we can begin to better interpret our findings.

The use of emerging technologies may prove to be particularly useful in overcoming some of these barriers to QOL assessment in palliative care. For example, computer adaptive testing (CAT) could be used to greatly reduce the length of current assessment instruments while potentially improving accuracy and clinical utility (54). In CAT, items are presented to patients sequentially such that each item is selected on the basis of the pattern of responses to previous items, such that the assessment is essentially tailored to each individual. In comparison with traditional fixed-length questionnaires, one could expect that fewer items would be administered for domains in which the individual has relatively high QOL, whereas more items might be targeted to those domains in which the individual is exhibiting problems (55). CAT has been successfully implemented in a variety of non-palliative populations (55–59) in one study reducing the number of administered items by 85% and completion time by 80% (60). Other adaptive technologies (e.g., voice recognition, assistive pointing devices, etc.) may also prove to be useful in making QOL assessment easier for patients at the end of life to complete (55).

Response Shift in Self-Report Quality of Life

In the study of QOL, "response shift" refers to the change in self-evaluation based on changes in one's standard of well-being, changes in one's values, or a redefinition of well-being (i.e., a shifting frame of reference). In theory, one's perception of health may remain relatively stable in spite of drastic changes in objective health measures. Alternatively, one's perception of their health may change dramatically without any change in objective health measures. In each scenario, the criterion of health appears to have shifted. To give an example of the response shift phenomenon—consider an individual who has recently been diagnosed with a terminal disease associated with progressive deterioration of functional capacity. When asked to complete a QOL measure shortly after diagnosis, such an individual may complete the measure using an internal, cognitive standard of health that is exemplified by their prior level of functioning. Over time, adjustment to functional impairments (i.e., cognitive reappraisal of the illness experience) may alter the standard of health by which the individual rates their QOL. When the individual completes a follow-up QOL measure, the individual's score on the QOL measure may be relatively preserved despite progressively worsening illness and objective declines in QOL. The idea of response shift has been used to explain the failure of QOL instruments to detect known between-groups differences. For example, in some studies individuals with chronic disease have been observed to rate their QOL similarly to healthy individuals (54). As Rapkin and Schwartz have noted, "QOL can mean different things to different people at different times (61)."

Response shift poses several challenges to QOL assessment. Individuals facing a life-threatening illness may find it adaptive to shift their conception of QOL to accommodate their illness. As such, their perception of well-being could be greatly disparate from their physician's assessment. Alternatively, palliative care patients may also have greater expectations about their functioning than what they are likely to experience. These perceptual differences may obscure measured change in health status. Response shift may play a significant role in treatment evaluation, particularly as it may inflate or underestimate treatment effects. For example, Vielhaber et al. found that individuals with increasing levels of fatigue altered their standards over time, "retrospectively minimiz[ing] their baseline fatigue score, therefore magnifying the degree to which their fatigue has worsened" (62). One popular approach to dealing with response shift includes a retrospective pretest-posttest design to assess subjective change. For example, after completing the MQOL, an individual might be asked to retrospectively rate their QOL at the time of the previous administration. The comparison of one test to the other provides an indication of the extent and direction of response shift. Using the posttest and the retrospective pretest as a comparison, it is hypothesized that each test is completed with the same internal standard of QOL. As such, this contrast could provide an estimation of change not confounded by response shift. Although this method has its drawbacks, it allows researchers to detect and potentially ameliorate response shift confounds. In the translation of QOL data to clinically meaningful applications, one must be cognizant of how response shift may influence research conclusions. By incorporating response shift into one's research design, a better approximation of QOL can be obtained (34).

Ethical Issues in Quality of Life Assessment

When used for clinical purposes, the ethical goal of providing high-quality care to our patients is greatly facilitated when QOL assessment is incorporated into clinical practice. However, when QOL assessment is one of many facets of an ongoing research study, the study objectives and patient care objectives may not always be as obviously aligned. Researchers must be aware of the responsibilities associated with QOL assessment. The MQOL is a particularly useful tool in this regard because it allows patients to self-identify the three physical symptoms that are most burdensome to them, and repeated administration of the MQOL allows us to directly measure success of symptom management efforts. If the assessment results are not part of a feedback mechanism that involves treating clinicians, researchers may identify untreated symptoms, existential crisis, inadequate social support networks, or extreme psychological duress, and may not be aware that they have identified these problems! It is not uncommon in traditional research studies to administer self-report questionnaires, store them in a file cabinet in one of the investigators' offices, and only later have the data screened, entered into a database, and analyzed. Given the sensitive nature of the items typically used to evaluate HRQoL, researchers have an ethical and professional obligation to rapidly discern whether the data that has been obtained from a respondent warrants clinical intervention.

CONCLUSIONS

The assessment of QOL at the end of life is one of the most fundamental tasks facing clinicians and researchers working with these populations. The choice of assessment tools must be made with respect to the research or clinical aims at hand, but we would recommend a standardized approach that minimizes respondent burden. An ideal (and often for this population unrealistic) assessment battery would at minimum include a palliative care specific questionnaire, a disease-specific HRQoL measure, and an assessment of subjective change since the previous assessment (in order to assess and perhaps control response shift). Because patients will vary in their ability and/or willingness to participate in a comprehensive assessment, assessment strategies must to some extent be adaptive. In the absence of validated CAT procedures for palliative care populations, we recommend that all patients receive a single-item QOL measure (e.g., the MQOL single item) that many or most end-of-life patients would be able to answer. Uniform administration of a minimal, single-item measure could reduce problems with attrition and sample bias associated with progressive disease. Interviewers must be mindful of delirium or other cognitive deficits that might impact responses to even a single item. Patients who are able to complete a more thorough assessment could then be asked to respond to a more detailed assessment battery. All measures should be interviewer-administered given the potential for confusion and the eagerness of families to assist (and potentially bias) their loved ones in responding to measures of this type.

It is important to recognize that QOL instruments are not simply measurement tools. The process of asking personal questions about QOL concerns is perceived by many patients as a therapeutic process—giving them the time and attention to reflect on their lives, their relationships with loved ones, and the personal significance of the dying process (63). Supporting this view, Pratheepawanit et al. (36) reported that outpatients in a palliative care clinic preferred completing a multidimensional QOL measure (the MQOL) to being asked to list and rate the severity of their perceived problems, despite the QOL measure taking longer to complete. Additionally, it has been suggested that hospice staff report that QOL assessment is useful for planning clinical care (64). For example, in using QOL instruments to assess existential concerns, some health care workers have noted that the use of a standardized tool serves as a useful bridge for opening dialogues about these particularly difficult issues with their patients (42). An effective QOL assessment not only provides accurate estimates of internal feeling states related to a variety of QOL domains but also both complements and facilitates effective clinical care.

References

1. World Health Organization. *Cancer pain relief and palliative care.* Geneva, Switzerland: WHO, 1990.
2. Fayers PM, de Haes JCJM. Quality of life and clinical trials. *Lancet* 1995; 346:1–2.
3. Fayers PM, Hopwood P, Harvey A, et al. Quality of life assessment in clinical trials- guidelines and a checklist for protocol writers: The U.K. Medical research council experience. *Eur J Cancer* 1997;33:20–28.
4. Kiebert GM, Curran D, Aaronson NK. Quality of life as an endpoint in EORTC clinical trials. *Stat Med* 1998;17:561–569.
5. Sadura A, Pater J, Osoba D, et al. Quality of life assessment: patient compliance with questionnaire completion. *J Natl Cancer Inst* 1992;84: 1023–1026.

6. Beitz J, Gnecoo C, Justice R. Quality of life endpoints in cancer clinical trials: the U.S. Food and drug administration perspective. *Monogr Natl Cancer Inst* 1996;20:7–9.

7. Cook Gotay C, Korn EL, McCabe MS, et al. Quality of life assessment in cancer treatment protocols: research issues in protocol development. *J Natl Cancer Inst* 1992;84:575–579.

8. McMillen Moinpour C, Feigl P, Metch B, et al. Quality of life end points in cancer clinical trials: review and recommendations. *J Natl Cancer Inst* 1997;22:21–25.

9. Italian Psycho-Oncology Society. Consensus development conference: assessment of the quality of life in cancer clinical trials. *Tumori* 1992;78:151–154.

10. Berzon R, Hays RD, Shumaker SA. International use, application and performance of health-related quality of life instruments. *Qual Life Res* 1993;2:367–368.

11. Cella DF, Wiklund I, Shumaker SA, et al. Integrating health-related quality of life into cross-national clinical trials. *Qual Life Res* 1993;2:433–440.

12. Naughton MJ, Shumaker SA. The case for domains of function in quality of life assessment. *Qual Life Res* 2003;12:73–80.

13. Revicki DA, Kaplan RM. Relationship between psychometric and utility-based approaches to the measurement of health related quality of life. *Qual Life Res* 1993;2:477–487.

14. Perez DJ, McGee R, Campbell AV, et al. A comparison of time trade-off and quality of life measures in patients with advanced cancer. *Qual Life Res* 1997;6:133–138.

15. Chapman RH, Berger M, Weinstein MC, et al. When does quality-adjusting life-years matter in cost-effectiveness analysis? *Health Econ* 2004; 13:429–436.

16. Bruley DK. Beyond reliability and validity: analysis of selected quality-of-life instruments for use in palliative care. *J Palliat Med* 1999;2:299–309.

17. Aaronson NK, Ahmedzai S, Bergman B, et al. The European Organization for Research and Treatment of Cancer QLQ-C30: a quality-of-life instrument for use in international clinical trials in oncology. *J Natl Cancer Inst* 1993;85:365–376.

18. Cella DF, Tulsky OS, Gray G, et al. The functional assessment of cancer therapy scale: development and validation of the general measure. *J Clin Oncol* 1993;11:570–579.

19. Padilla GV, Presant C, Grant MM, et al. Quality of life index for patients with cancer. *Res Nurs Health* 1983;6:117–126.

20. Schag CA, Ganz PA, Heinrich RL. CAncer Rehabilitation Evaluation System- Short Form (CARES-SF): a cancer specific rehabilitation and quality of life instrument. *Cancer* 1991;68:1406–1413.

21. Schipper H, Clinch J, McMurray A, et al. Measuring the quality of life of cancer patients: the functional living index-cancer. Development and validation. *J Clin Oncol* 1984;2:472–482.

22. Knobel H, Loge H, Brenne E, et al. The validity of EORTC QLQ-C30 fatigue scale in advanced cancer patients and cancer survivors. *Palliat Med* 2003;17:664–672.

23. Cella D. *FACIT manual*. Evanston, IL: Center on Outcomes, Research, and Education, 1997.

24. Gill TM, Feinstein AR. A critical appraisal of the quality of quality of life measurements. *JAMA* 1994;272:619–626.

25. Saunders C. The evolution of palliative care. *Patient Educ Couns* 2000; 41:7–13.

26. Pelletier G, Verhoef MJ, Khatri N, et al. Quality of life in brain tumor patients: the relative contributions of depression, fatigue, emotional distress, and existential issues. *J Neurooncol* 2002;57:41–49.

27. Cohen SR, Mount BM, Bruera E, et al. Validity of the McGill quality of life questionnaire in the palliative care setting: a multi-centre Canadian study demonstrating the importance of the existential domain. *Palliat Med* 1997;11:3–20.

28. Kaasa S, Loge JH. Quality of life in palliative care: principles and practice. *Palliat Med* 2003;17:11–20.

29. Axelsson B, Sjoden P. Assessment of quality of life in palliative care. *Acta Oncol* 1999;38:229–237.

30. Clinck JJ, Dudgeon D, Schipper H. Quality of life assessment in palliative care. In: Doyle D, Hanks GWC, MacDonald N, eds. *Oxford textbook of palliative medicine*, 2nd ed. New York: Oxford University Press, 2001:83–96.

31. Cohen SR, Mount BM, Strobel MG, et al. The McGill quality of life questionnaire: a measure of quality of life appropriate for people with advanced disease. A preliminary study of validity and acceptability. *Palliat Med* 1995;9:207–219.

32. Cohen SR, Hassan SA, Lapointe BJ, et al. Quality of life in HIV disease as measured by the McGill quality of life questionnaire. *AIDS* 1996; 10:1421–1427.

33. Cohen SR, Boston P, Mount BM, et al. Changes in quality of life following admission to palliative care units. *Palliat Med* 2001;15:363–371.

34. Cohen SR, Mount BM. Living with cancer: "Good" days and "bad" days- what produces them? *Cancer* 2000;89:1854–1865.

35. Lo RSK, Woo J, Zhoc KCH, et al. Cross-cultural validation of the McGill quality of life questionnaire in Hong Kong Chinese. *Palliative Med* 2001;15:387–397.

36. Pratheepawanit N, Salek MS, Finaly IG. The applicability of quality-of-life assessment in palliative care: comparing two quality-of-life measures. *Palliative Med* 1999;13:325–334.

37. Goodwin DM, Higginson IJ, Myers K, et al. Effectiveness of palliative day care in improving pain, symptom control, and quality of life. *J Pain Symptom Manage* 2003;25:202–212.

38. Tierney RM, Horton SM, Hannan TJ, et al. Relationships between symptom relief, quality of life, and satisfaction with hospice care. *Palliative Med* 1998;12:333–344.

39. Robbins RA, Simmons Z, Bremer BA, et al. Quality of life in ALS is maintained as physical function declines. *Neurology* 2001;56:442–444.

40. Bremer BA, Simone A, Walsh S, et al. Factors supporting the quality of life over time for individuals with amyotrophic lateral sclerosis: the role of positive self-perception and religiosity. *Ann Behav Med* 2004;28: 199–125.

41. Salmon P, Manzi F, Valori RM. Measuring the meaning of life for patients with incurable cancer: the Life Evaluation Questionnaire (LEQ). *Eur J Cancer* 1996;32A:755–760.

42. Hearn J, Higginson IJ. Development and validation of a core outcome measure for palliative care: the palliative care outcome scale. *Qual Health Care* 1999;8:219–227.

43. Stevens AM, Gwilliam B, Hern RA, et al. Experience in the use of the palliative care outcome scale. *Support Care Cancer in press*.

44. Serra-Prat M, Nabal M, Santacruz V, et al. Validation of the spanish version of the palliative care outcomes scale. *Med Clin (Barc)* 2004;123: 406–412.

45. Stromgren AS, Groenvold M, Pedersen AK, et al. Symptomatology of cancer patients in palliative care: content validation of self-assessment questionnaires against medical records. *Eur J Cancer* 2002;38: 788–794.

46. Hughes RA, Aspinal F, Higginson IJ. Assessing palliative care outcomes for people with motor neurone disease living at home. *Int J Palliat Nurs* 2004;10:449–453.

47. Greisinger AJ, Lorimor RJ, Aday LA, et al. Terminally ill cancer patients. *Cancer Pract* 1997;5:147–154.

48. Byock IR, Merriman MP. Measuring quality of life for patients with terminal illness: the Missoula-VITAS quality of life index. *Palliat Med* 1998;12:231–244.

49. Schwartz CE, Merriman MP, Reed G, et al. Evaluation of the Missoula-VITAS quality of life index- revised: research tool or clinical tool? *J Palliat Med* 2005;8:121–135.

50. Mystakidou K, Tsilika E, Koulouslias V, et al. The palliative care quality of life instrument in terminal cancer patients. *Health Qual Life Outcomes* 2004;2:8.

51. McMillan SC, Weitzner M. Quality of life in cancer patients. *Cancer Pract* 1998;6:282–288.

52. Steinhauser K, Christakis N, Clipp E, et al. Factors considered important at the end of life by patients, family, physicians and other care providers. *JAMA* 2000;284:2476–2482.

53. Steinhauser KE, Bosworth HB, Clipp EC, et al. Initial assessment of a new instrument to measure quality of life at the end of life. *J Palliat Med* 2002;5:829–841.

54. Norman G. Hi! how are you? Response shift, implicit theories and differing epistemologies. *Qual Life Res* 2003;2:239–249.

55. Andres PL, Black-Schaffer RM, Ni P, et al. Computer adaptive testing: a strategy for monitoring stroke rehabilitation across settings. *Top Stroke Rehabil* 2004;11:33–39.

56. Revicki DA, Cella DF. Health status assessment for the twenty-first century: item response theory, item banking and computer adaptive testing. *Qual Life Res* 1997;6:595–600.

57. Haley SM, Raczek AE, Coster WJ. Assessing mobility in children using a computer adaptive testing version of the pediatric evaluation of disability inventory. *Arch Phys Med Rehabil* 2005;86:932–939.

58. Brodwin MG, Swett EA, Lane FJ, et al. Technology in rehabilitation counseling. In: Parker RM, Szymanski EM, Patterson JB, eds. *Rehabilitation counseling: basics and beyond*, 4th ed. Austin TX: PRO-ED, Inc., 2005: 363–393.

59. Hays RD, Morales LS, Reise SP. Item response theory and health outcomes measurement in the 21st century. *Med Care* 2000;38:28s–42s.

60. Cook KF, Roddey TS, O'Malley KJ, et al. Development of a Flexilevel scale for use with computer-adaptive testing for assessing shoulder function. *J Shoulder Elbow Surg* 2005;14:90s–94s.

61. Rapkin BD, Schwartz CE. Toward a theoretical model of quality-of-life appraisal: Implications of findings from studies of response shift. *Health Qual Life Outcomes* 2004;2:14.

62. Vielhaber A, Homel P, Malamud S, et al. Influence of response shift on the perception of fatigue in patients with advanced cancer. *J Clin Oncol* 2004;22:8116.

63. Annells M, Koch T. 'The real stuff': implications for nursing of assessing and measuring a terminally ill person's quality of life. *J Clin Nurs* 2001;10:806–812.

64. Eischens MJ, Elliott BA, Elliott TE. Two hospice quality of life surveys: a comparison. *Am J Hosp Palliat Care* 1998;15:143–148.

CHAPTER 79 ■ RESEARCH ISSUES: ETHICS AND STUDY DESIGN

JODI LEVINTHAL AND DAVID CASARETT

The goal of good palliative care is to relieve suffering and to improve quality of life. However, it is apparent that access to palliative care is inconsistent, and standards to guide palliative care have not been established clearly. These deficiencies exist, at least in part, because of a lack of solid evidence on which to base clinical decisions (1–3). Therefore, there is an urgent need for research that can provide evidence to define the standard of care and to increase access to quality care.

Recent years have seen a dramatic increase in palliative care research, defined broadly as activities that are designed to contribute to generalizable knowledge (4) about end-of-life care. This growth has created a heterogeneous field that encompasses both qualitative and quantitative techniques, and descriptive as well as interventional study designs (5). Although the past 10 years have seen impressive growth in all of these areas, this rate of growth appears to be particularly rapid for interventional research, including controlled trials of pain medications (6,7), interventional procedures for pain (8), and other nonpharmacologic interventions to improve a variety of aspects of end-of-life care (9–13).

Despite the valuable knowledge that has been produced by this research, and the promise of important advances in future, its progress has been slowed by a persistent uncertainty about the ethics of these studies (14). Indeed, there have been concerns raised from several quarters about whether patients near the end of life should ever be asked to participate in any form of research (15,16). Others have objected to this extreme position (2,17). Nevertheless, many providers, Institutional Review Boards (IRBs), ethics committees, study sections, and even investigators remain uncertain about the ethical limits of research involving dying patients.

These concerns have considerable intuitive appeal, and must be taken seriously. Indeed, it would be unfortunate if the progress of palliative care research were slowed by the sorts of ethical scandals that have threatened other fields of research that involve vulnerable populations, such as those with mental illness (18). However, strict overseeing and tight limits on palliative care research have the potential to do equal damage to the growing field. Therefore, in order to avoid potential scandals, without excessive regulation and overseeing, it will be important that palliative care investigators and clinicians consider these concerns in a fair and balanced way.

This chapter discusses six ethical aspects of palliative care research that investigators and clinicians should consider in designing and conducting palliative care research. These include the following:

1. Whether the study is research or quality improvement
2. The study's potential benefits to future patients
3. The study's potential benefits to subjects
4. The study's risks to subjects
5. Subjects' decision making capacity and
6. The voluntariness of subjects' choices to participate in the research

Each of these is discussed, as well as the opportunities for each to enhance the ethics of palliative care research.

DEFINING RESEARCH

The first, and arguably the most important question that palliative care investigators face in designing an ethical study is whether it is research or quality improvement (QI). This decision is extremely important, and has profound implications for the study's design, and the ethical standards to which it will be held. For instance, federal law requires most research projects to be reviewed by local IRBs to assure that informed consent is obtained from each subject, that research risks are reasonable in relation to expected benefits, and that the subjects are recruited in an equitable fashion (4). In comparison, there are few widely accepted standards that govern QI.

In many situations, it is clear that a planned study is research. For instance, there is likely to be general agreement that randomized clinical trials comparing one or more pain medications, or population-based studies of symptom prevalence are research, and should be held to the ethical standards for research. However, QI activities often share many of the attributes of research. For instance, both QI and research involve systematic data collection methods, such as surveys and chart reviews. Both apply statistical methods to test hypotheses, establish relationships between variables, and to evaluate outcomes. Both QI and research are designed to produce knowledge that could benefit patients other than those directly involved in the activity. In practical terms, therefore, QI and research activities are often difficult to distinguish. This can produce confusion and conflicting opinions from IRBs that review study protocols (19).

Unfortunately, the federal regulations that make the distinction between research and QI so important offer little practical assistance in distinguishing between the two types of activities. In those regulations, research is defined as "a systematic investigation, including research development, testing and evaluation, designed to develop or contribute to generalizable knowledge" (4). Although elegant in its simplicity, this definition may prove prohibitively difficult for palliative care investigators to apply. It is often not clear how systematic an activity needs to be in order to be considered research. Nor is it clear how generalizability should be defined, or how an investigator's intent should be measured.

In an effort to make the distinction between QI and research clearer, additional criteria have been proposed. These include: the degree to which a study deviates from standard care, whether an activity requires identifiable recruitment practices, how individuals are selected to receive a particular intervention, the degree of uncertainty associated with the intervention, and whether the patients involved benefit from the knowledge to be gained (20–22). One of the most recent of these efforts (21) describes a two step algorithm that investigators may find useful when the existing criterion of an intent to produce generalizable knowledge (4) fails to provide adequate guidance. This algorithm is based on the additional risks or burdens that are imposed by a study, and on whether the patients involved in the study will benefit from the knowledge to be gained. Briefly, this algorithm suggests that studies should be considered as research, rather than as QI, if they expose patients to risks in order to generate knowledge that will not benefit them.

This algorithm may prove to be too restrictive, as some have argued (22). In any event, it should not take precedence over existing federal regulations (4). It is at most a guide that palliative care investigators may wish to turn to. When the status of a project is unclear, investigators should also seek guidance from their own IRB.

BENEFITS TO FUTURE PATIENTS: A STUDY'S VALIDITY AND VALUE

Palliative care research is designed to produce knowledge that will advance understanding of end-of-life care. Implicit in this goal is the expectation that this knowledge will eventually improve care for future patients. Therefore, the first ethical aspect of palliative care research that deserves consideration is its potential benefits for future patients. These benefits to others can be described in terms of validity and value.

Validity

First, all studies must be valid. That is, they must use techniques of design and data analysis that peer reviewers can agree as appropriate. In addition, all studies must be designed to produce knowledge that is generalizable. Indeed, generalizability is the cornerstone of the Common Rule's definition of research: "a systematic investigation, including research development, testing, and evaluation, designed to develop or contribute to generalizable knowledge" (4). These requirements collectively describe a study's validity (23). Validity is a threshold requirement for all research, because it is unethical to expose human subjects to risks in studies that peer reviewers agree cannot adequately answer a research question (24). Therefore, at a minimum, investigators must routinely consider a study's validity.

Value

Above this threshold of validity, palliative care studies may offer more or less importance or "value." Broadly, value can be defined as the likelihood that a study's results will improve the health and well-being of future patients (25). Like validity, value is an important measure of a study design's scientific quality, but it is also a measure of its ethical quality. Value is an essential aspect of a study's ethical design because a central goal of research is to produce knowledge that will ultimately be "important" (4,26), "fruitful" (27), or "valuable" (28). In fact, one reason that subjects participate in clinical research is to produce knowledge that will benefit others (29,30). Because subjects are willing to accept risks and burdens of research at least in part in order to benefit others, investigators have accepted an ethical responsibility to maximize the probability that a study will be able to do so. Therefore, in addition to widely accepted scientific arguments for valuable research, there are compelling ethical arguments as well.

Maximizing Validity and Value in Palliative Care Research

Space does not permit a comprehensive overview of ways in which a palliative care study's validity and value can be assessed and improved. Indeed, such a discussion moves quickly beyond ethics and into the technical language of study design and health measurement. Nevertheless, several broad recommendations are possible.

First, a study's sample size should be adequate to answer the research question that is posed. Problems of underpowered studies, and particularly clinical trials, are both widespread and well described (31). But issues of power and sample size are particularly relevant to pain and symptom research, in which random variation can be quite large (32). To minimize these problems, it may be useful to establish consortia or collaborative groups that can participate in multicenter studies. Such arrangements have been highly effective in promoting research on rare disorders, and may be applicable to palliative care research as well, in which investigators are limited and available patients are often sparse.

Second, palliative care investigators can enhance the ethical quality of a study by taking reasonable steps to increase the generalizability of its results. These steps might include sample size calculations that permit subgroup analysis of groups of patients that have typically not been the focus of investigation, such as patients with noncancer diagnoses, or elderly patients. The generalizability of a study's results might also be enhanced by recruiting subjects outside academic medical settings, because preliminary evidence suggests that these patients, and their needs for care, may be different than those who receive care in academic settings (33).

In addition, palliative care investigators can enhance the generalizability, and therefore the value, of their research by making reasonable efforts to include patients who are receiving care at home, and particularly those who are enrolled in a home hospice program. Substantial barriers may make it difficult to include these patients in research. Nevertheless, few data exist to guide the management of home care patients near the end of life, and palliative care investigators can enhance the value of their research by including this population whenever possible (34).

Of course, all of these improvements in generalizability come at a substantial cost. For instance, studies that recruit subjects from several different settings require more elaborate designs for recruitment and follow-up. In addition, investigators who include plans for subgroup analysis in their sample size calculations face rapidly escalating sample size requirements and costs. Nevertheless, steps such as these offer an important way to enhance the value of a palliative care study, and therefore its ethical quality. Therefore, it will also be important that funding agencies understand the ethical importance of generalizability, and that generalizability comes with a financial cost.

BENEFITS TO SUBJECTS

Palliative care investigators can also enhance the ethical rigor of a study by maximizing the benefits that it will offer to subjects. Broadly, these benefits can be considered under two categories: benefits to subjects during the study and benefits to future patients from the data that are collected. Each of these is discussed in the subsequent text.

Benefits to Subjects during the Study

Investigators may have several opportunities to maximize potential benefits of research to the subjects who participate. Perhaps the first, at least in an interventional study, is in their choice of an intervention. Ideally, a new intervention to be studied should have a reasonable chance of success. More important, though, if it is to offer subjects a significant potential benefit, an intervention should offer the possibility of a meaningful improvement over other interventions that are available to subjects outside the study. For instance, a pain management algorithm that is expected to reduce cancer pain (35) would only offer potential benefits if it is qualitatively or quantitatively different than those that constitute the usual standard of care. On the other hand, a comparison of two medications that are commercially available, such as topical fentanyl and sustained release morphine would not offer subjects any potential benefit. This is true even if the study's results offer considerable clinical value (36).

The potential benefits of a study can also be enhanced by choosing an active control design, rather than a placebo (36). If a placebo is used, a study's potential benefits can also be improved by altering the standard 1:1 randomization scheme in a placebo-controlled trial in a way that increases the subjects' chances of receiving an active agent (7). The potential benefits of a placebo-controlled trial can also be enhanced by using a crossover design, so that all subjects are offered potential benefits, if the medication's pharmacokinetic profile makes it possible to avoid carryover effects.

These suggestions should be tempered by two caveats. First, the potential benefits of research are never certain. If they were, a randomized trial would not be ethically acceptable. That is, a legitimate argument for the uncertainty that justifies a clinical trial, or equipoise, could not be made (37). However, investigators generally design studies of interventions for which there is at least some evidence of effectiveness. Therefore, although these potential benefits are not certain, they are more or less likely, and this assessment of likelihood should be considered in the design of pain research.

Second, palliative care studies need not always offer potential benefits. Indeed, many, and perhaps most, will not. Nevertheless, when a study does offer potential benefits, investigators may consider enhancing a study's potential benefits in these ways. The importance of doing so is particularly great if other aspects of a study raise ethical concerns, which might be the case if subjects' decision-making capacity is limited, or if the study's risks are substantial.

Benefits from Data Collected During a Study

Although the opportunities to enhance potential benefits described in the preceding text apply largely to studies involving interventions, another opportunity applies equally well, if not better, to research that is descriptive. A common ethical issue in the design of palliative care research, and particularly descriptive research, is the possibility that data gathered may contribute to a subject's care. For instance, data gathered during a descriptive study may identify pain that is inadequately treated (38–40), dissatisfaction with pain management (41,42), or related clinical problems such as depression (43,44).

In anticipation of instances such as these, investigators can design standard operating procedures that help to ensure that valuable clinical information is made available to the subject and his/her clinicians. At the least, these procedures should include data about the presence of unrecognized and untreated symptoms, and concurrent disorders like depression. This is arguably an ethical obligation of symptom-oriented research (17). Moreover, these procedures offer a significant opportunity for investigators to enhance the potential benefits of pain research.

Benefits to Subjects after a Study Has Ended

Investigators can also enhance the potential benefits for subjects after a study has ended. These sorts of poststudy benefits are not usually included in assessments of a study's balance of risks and benefits. They are also components of a study's value, because these benefits generally come from the knowledge that the study has produced. Nevertheless, subjects may benefit from the knowledge to be gained from a study if the study's results are applied to their care. Investigators have numerous opportunities to ensure that these results are translated into subjects' care and, by doing so, can enhance the study's potential benefits to subjects.

For instance, subjects in palliative care research can benefit after a study if they learn from the study's aggregate results. This might be the case if a study comparing two pain medications found that one resulted in fewer overall side effects (36). Subjects in the study would benefit from these data because this knowledge should allow them to make a more informed choice among available medications. Subjects might also benefit from results that are specific to them. For instance, if a subject receives two medications in a blinded crossover trial, and prefers one to the other, he or she would be better able to choose between these medications in future clinical situations, armed with the results of a blinded comparison of the two.

Finally, investigators can increase the likelihood that subjects have continued access to medications that are studied. If medications are not available, either due to high cost or because the medication has not yet received regulatory approval, subjects will not benefit (immediately) from the study's results. Therefore by arranging reduced rate programs or open label extension phases, investigators can increase a study's potential benefits for subjects by helping to ensure that subjects will benefit from the study's results.

This benefit may be particularly important in palliative care research, because mortality rates in some studies are very high. This means that subjects may not live long enough to see a study medication's approval for clinical use, or to see a study's results published and translated into improved care. For this reason, it is especially important that investigators consider mechanisms by which results can be applied to the care of research subjects in a timely fashion.

MINIMIZING RISKS AND BURDENS

Investigators can also enhance a study's ethical soundness by taking steps to minimize a study's risks and burdens. Although the distinction between risks and burdens is not always clear, a rough heuristic is useful. In general, a risk can be considered as the probability of an adverse medical event or undesirable outcome. Risks might include side effects of a medication, or increased pain during a study. The term *burden* can be used to describe those unpleasant features of participation in a study that are more certain, and which are better thought of as inconveniences. Additional visits to the clinic, time spent filling out questionnaires, or time spent waiting in the clinic might be described as burdens.

Identifying Risks and Burdens

Attention to the ethical design of pain research, and to the minimization of research risks and burdens, requires a clear agreement about how they should be defined. The criteria by which study risks and burdens are identified and evaluated uses the concept of incremental or "demarcated" risks imposed by participation in a study (45). The application of this standard to interventional pain research would mean that investigators designing a trial to compare the effectiveness of two opioids (36) need not go to great lengths to justify the risks of the opioids being evaluated, if subjects in the trial would have received similar medications, with similar risks, off protocol. Of course, the risks of any medication in a clinical trial should be disclosed in the informed consent process (4). Nevertheless, investigators are not under the obligation to minimize or justify these risks as they would be if, for instance, the same medications were being given to patients with mild pain, who would not receive them as part of standard care.

Minimizing Risks: The Choice of Control

Perhaps one of the most contentious and emotional questions in palliative care research (46,47), and indeed in research generally (48–50), is whether a placebo or sham control arm is ethically appropriate. The ongoing debates about the scientific merit of these controls and the competing advantages of active control superiority trials and equivalency trials are beyond the scope of this discussion. However, several general points can be made about the ethics of placebo- and sham-controlled trials. Each of these designs is discussed in the subsequent text.

Broadly, placebos can be defined as interventions that are "ineffective or not specifically effective" for the symptom or disorder in question (51). Increased attention to the ethical issue of placebo controls in recent years has produced a growing consensus that all subjects in a clinical trial should have access to the best available standard of care (52). Therefore in infectious disease research, for instance, all subjects with meningitis would have access to an antimicrobial agent that has proved effective. However, this requirement may be difficult to apply to studies of treatment for pain, other symptoms, or depression, in which the placebo response can be quite substantial. These difficulties are compounded when the symptom being studied is transient, such as incident pain (7).

For these reasons, it may not be practical to prohibit placebos in palliative care research, and a placebo control may be ethically acceptable in several situations. First, placebos are acceptable if subjects receive a placebo in addition to the standard care. For example, subjects might be randomly assigned to receive either an opioid or an opioid plus an adjuvant agent. Second, a placebo arm is justified if the symptom under study has no effective treatment. For example, the transient nature of incident pain often defies adequate treatment on an as-needed basis, and a placebo control might be justified in a randomized controlled trial of a novel agent for the treatment of incident pain. Third, a placebo control is justified if subjects have adequate access to breakthrough, or "rescue" treatment. This may in turn alter a trial's endpoints.

For instance, the free use of breakthrough dosing in a trial suggests the possible inclusion of these doses as a study endpoint either directly (53,54) or as part of a composite endpoint (6,55).

Concrete recommendations about sham procedures are somewhat more elusive, in part because sham procedures themselves are difficult to define. In general, although, sham procedures in palliative care research involve the use of a control procedure such as a nerve block, which is administered in a way that makes it ineffective (8), these procedures create ethical concerns because some subjects, or all subjects, depending on the study's design, are exposed to the risks of the procedure without hope of its benefits (48). Like placebo controls, although shams also have a role in research, because the nonspecific therapeutic effects of surgery may be substantial. For instance, Leonard Cobb's research in the 1950s effectively debunked a widely used cardiac procedure that, if it had been widely disseminated, would eventually have put thousands of patients at risk.

Investigators have an opportunity to reduce these concerns substantially in the design of a sham-controlled study. For instance, investigators might conduct these studies in a setting in which the procedure itself (whether sham or real) poses few if any additional, or "incremental" risks above and beyond the usual care. Investigators might insert a sham epidural catheter that would then be used for postoperative analgesia (56). When this is not possible, investigators can choose a crossover design, in which subjects are assigned to receive either the sham or the real procedure, followed by the other. This design does not decrease the incremental risks of the sham procedure. However, it does ensure that all subjects who bear the risks of the sham procedure also have access to the real procedures potential benefits. This crossover sham design has been used in other settings (57), and might be appropriate for pain research when the risks or discomforts of the sham procedure are substantial.

Minimizing Burdens

For the most part, opportunities to minimize burdens are readily apparent. For instance, it seems reasonable wherever possible to minimize surveys, interviews, and additional study visits (58). These are all burdens that investigators routinely consider carefully in designing studies. However, there may be other needs and concerns that may be unique to, or more common in, patients near the end of life.

Although it is intuitively obvious that all research subjects would like to avoid the added time commitment and inconvenience of travel to and from additional appointment, this concern may be especially important to patients near the end of life, for whom long periods of time spent sitting in a car can exacerbate discomfort. Similarly, patients may view surveys and questionnaires not only as time consuming, but also as a drain on their energy. Therefore, investigators who conduct palliative care research may have an added reason to minimize the burdens of extra visits and data collection procedures, and to rely on telephone data collection strategies whenever possible.

Palliative care investigators may also need to consider the burdens that a study creates for friends and family members who often take on substantial burdens as caregivers (59–62). Although most of the burdens of research participation are borne by the subject, the requirements of time, travel, and perhaps time off from work create burdens for others. Patients may be very sensitive to these burdens and, for some patients with chronic pain, burdens to others can be influential in the decision whether or not to enroll in a study (30). By building flexibility into a study design (e.g., use of brief telephone interviews, multiple options for timing of clinic visits) investigators may be able to reduce the burdens of research participation on others.

ENSURING DECISION-MAKING CAPACITY

Patients who consent to participate in research should have adequate decision-making capacity, which refers to the subjects' ability to understand relevant information, to appreciate the significance of that information, and to reason through to a conclusion that makes sense for them (63). These concerns are parallel concerns in research involving patients with dementia (64), psychiatric illness (65), and patients in the intensive care setting (66) among others. However, deficits in decision-making capacity may create several additional challenges for palliative care investigators.

First, concern about capacity is reasonable given the prevalence of cognitive impairment at the end of life (67,68). Cognitive impairment occurs in 10 to 40% of patients in the final months and in up to 85% of patients in the last days of life (67,68). Cognitive impairment may be difficult to identify in palliative care research because decision-making capacity varies over time (69), and because impairment may result from the experimental or therapeutic medications themselves, such as opioids, benzodiazepines, or corticosteroids (70,71). Investigators who conduct trials of medications will encounter these challenges even more frequently if trials are designed to evaluate treatments for delirium, for which impairment is an inclusion criterion (72).

Second, the effects of cognitive impairment on comprehension may be complicated by clinical depression, which occurs in 5 to 25% of patients near the end of life (43,44,73,74). Clinically significant adjustment disorders may be even more common (43). It is possible that these disorders may impair either comprehension or decision making, or both (65), but studies have not yet supported this conclusion.

Third, even in the absence of overt cognitive impairment or depression, it is possible that severe symptoms or affective disorders may impair subjects' ability to understand the risks and benefits of research participation. For some studies, particularly clinical trials, the presence of one or more of these intractable symptoms is an inclusion criterion (75–77). It is possible that severe symptoms may impair comprehension if patients are unable to concentrate on the information offered in the informed consent process (78).

Finally, these challenges may be compounded in prospective studies that require participation over days or weeks. In these studies, even if patients have the capacity to consent at the time of enrollment, they may not retain that capacity throughout the study. Therefore days or weeks after patients give consent to participate, they may be unable to understand changes in their condition clearly enough to withdraw. The result can be a "Ulysses contract" of sorts, in which research subjects find it easier to enroll than they do to withdraw (79).

None of these challenges is easily remedied. Indeed, it is obstacles such as these that lead some authors to argue that patients near the end of life should not be allowed to enroll in research (15,16). Nevertheless, palliative care investigators have several concrete opportunities to enhance the ethical quality of palliative care research when decision-making capacity is uncertain.

First, at a minimum, investigators whose research involves patients near the end of life who are likely to lack decision-making capacity might institute brief assessments of understanding. Although this strategy cannot assess decision-making capacity, a few simple questions in either open-ended or multiple choice format provide a brief assessment of understanding (80,81). In some situations, investigators may wish to assess decision-making capacity more formally using validated instruments (82).

These sorts of safeguards need not be employed in all studies. Instead, their use should be guided by the prevalence of cognitive impairment in a study population and by the balance of risks and benefits that a study offers (34). For instance, when palliative care research involves only interviews or behavioral interventions that pose minimal risks, informal capacity assessments are generally sufficient. "Minimal risks" are defined as those risks that are encountered during a patient's usual care, or in everyday life (4). When research poses greater than minimal risks, but offers potential benefits, some assessment of understanding may be appropriate. This research includes studies that involve a placebo (7) or invasive interventions such as nerve blocks (83) or epidural catheters (84). When a study that poses greater than minimal risks does not offer potential benefits, or is conducted in a population in which the prevalence of cognitive impairment is high (e.g., an inpatient hospice unit), a formal evaluation of capacity should be considered. This research includes studies that involve a placebo when an effective agent is available (6), and some pharmacokinetic/pharmacodynamic studies that required blood samples and prolonged observation, without potential benefits (85).

If a patient does not have the capacity to give consent, a legally authorized representative may be able to give consent for research. This follows from federal guidelines governing research involving children (4), and is justified by the argument that surrogate decision makers should be allowed to consent to research, just as they are allowed to consent to medical therapy. However, as with other research that involves patients without capacity to consent, investigators should be aware of applicable state laws that may restrict or even prohibit surrogate consent for research. In addition, investigators in this field should be alert to possible future changes in federal regulations that have been discussed (86).

If a patient does not have the capacity to consent, but is still able to participate in decisions, investigators should obtain assent from the patient and informed consent from the patient's surrogate (87,88). This "dual consent" ensures that patients are as involved in the decision as possible, yet provides the additional protection of a surrogate's consent.

If a patient has decision-making capacity intermittently, or is expected to lose capacity, investigators may obtain advance consent. This approach has been used in a study of treatment for delirium, in which informed consent was obtained from patients while they had decision-making capacity (72). Advance consent should be obtained only for specific studies, and should be obtained close to the planned start of research, for instance, at the time of hospitalization or enrollment in a hospice or palliative care program.

PROTECTING VOLUNTARINESS

Another way that investigators can enhance the ethical soundness of a study's design is to examine ways in which the subjects' voluntary participation can be protected (89). In general terms, a choice is voluntary if it is made without significant controlling influences (90,91). At first glance, assurances of voluntariness appear to be an issue of informed consent, and in fact for the most part they are. However, a study's design and plan for subject selection and recruitment may have as great an influence on subjects' freedom to refuse research participation as does the informed consent process. In particular, two features of a study's design are relevant. First, a prospective subject's choice must be made with full knowledge of available alternatives (4). Second, his or her choice must be made with the understanding that he or she can withdraw at any time (4). Each of these creates opportunities in a study's design to ensure voluntariness that are discussed in the subsequent text.

Reasonable Alternatives to Participation

First, investigators can make sure that a study recruits subjects from an environment with excellent standards of palliative care. If patients generally receive excellent care, they will be best able to make a free and uncoerced choice about research participation. If, however, patients do not have access to a bare minimum of treatment options and expertise, they may view research participation more favorably, out of desperation.

One solution, albeit a somewhat draconian one, would be to require that palliative care research be conducted only in settings in which patients have access to a full range of services, treatment, and expertise. Although this requirement would reduce the potential for research participation out of desperation, it would effectively limit research to a small number of academic centers, with a possible loss of generalizability (33). Another more practical option might be to include a lead-in phase when clinical pain research is conducted in settings where the standard of care is poor (17). A lead in phase allows an opportunity to optimize palliative care prior to recruitment. This strategy not only has ethical value but scientific value as well because it provides a uniform baseline prior to randomization.

Opportunities to Withdraw

Investigators can also enhance the ethics of a study's design by ensuring that subjects are able to withdraw at any time. Although a subject's ability to withdraw should be a fundamental aspect of any ethical research (4), there may be unique barriers to withdrawal from palliative care research. For instance, subjects who withdraw from clinical pain research that involves one or more medications will usually need access to a different medication upon withdrawal. This problem may be straightforward in many cases, but can be very challenging if, in an interventional study the investigational medication is an opioid, which requires the subject to get a new prescription and get it filled. Most states have created considerable barriers to opioid prescribing, including triplicate prescriptions, which may make it very difficult for a subject to obtain a new prescription and get it filled in a timely manner. If a subject has his or her medication available, the process may be easier. Nevertheless, considerable challenges of calculating an equianalgesic dose remain. For both of these reasons, investigators can enhance the ethical design of pain research by developing mechanisms to ensure that subjects who drop out continue to receive adequate pain treatment with as little interruption as possible.

CONCLUSION

The field of palliative care, and the standard of care that it represents, depend upon rigorous research to provide data that will guide clinical care. Although this research raises substantial ethical questions, these questions need not curtail what promises to be a valuable, and highly productive area of research. Of course, the concerns discussed in the preceding text should be taken seriously. To do otherwise is to risk the sorts of ethical missteps that have produced scandals in other fields. Nevertheless, these ethical questions can be addressed through careful planning, and with attention to the adequacy of a study's design, and to the informed consent process.

ACKNOWLEDGMENTS

Dr. Casarett is funded by a Health Services Advanced Research Career Development Award from the Department of Veterans Affairs and by a Paul Beeson Physician Faculty Scholars Award.

References

1. Symptoms in Terminal Illness: A Research Workshop. Solar Building, Rockville, Maryland, 2006:http://ninr.nih.gov/ninr/wnew/symptoms_in_terminal_illness.html.
2. Mount B, Cohen R, MacDonald N, et al. Ethical issues in palliative care research revisited. *Palliat Med* 1995;9:165–170.
3. Krouse RS, Easson AM, Angelos P. Ethical considerations and barriers to research in surgical palliative care. *J Am Coll Surg* 2003;196(3):469–474.
4. Department of Health and Human Services. *Protection of human subjects.* Title 45 Part 46: Revised. Code of Federal Regulations. 1991 June 18.
5. Corner J. Is there a research paradigm for palliative care? *Palliat Med* 1996;10:201–208.
6. Dhaliwal HS, Sloan P, Arkinstall WW, et al. Randomized evaluation of controlled-release codeine and placebo in chronic cancer pain. *J Pain Symptom Manage* 1995;10(8):612–623.
7. Farrar JT, Cleary J, Rauck R, et al. Oral transmucosal fentanyl citrate: randomized, double-blinded, placebo-controlled trial for treatment of breakthrough pain in cancer patients. *J Natl Cancer Inst* 1998;90(8):611–616.
8. Polati E, Finco G, Gottin L, et al. Prospective randomized double-blind trial of neurolytic coeliac plexus block in patients with pancreatic cancer. *Br J Surg* 1998;85:199–201.
9. Elliott TE, Murray DM, Oken MM, et al. Improving cancer pain management in communities: main results from a randomized controlled trial. *J Pain Symptom Manage* 1997;13(4):191–203.
10. de Wit R, van Dam F, Zandbelt L, et al. A pain education program for chronic cancer pain patients: follow-up results from a randomized controlled trial. *Pain* 1997;73(1):55–69.
11. Kravitz RL, Delafield JP, Hays RD, et al. Bedside charting of pain levels in hospitalized patients with cancer: a randomized controlled trial. *J Pain Symptom Manage* 1996;11(2):81–87.
12. Teno J, Lynn J, Connors AF Jr, et al. The illusion of end-of-life resource savings with advance directives. *J Am Geriatr Soc* 1997;45(4):513–518.
13. Bredin M, Corner J, Krishnasamy M, et al. Multicentre randomised controlled trial of nursing intervention for breathlessness in patients with lung cancer. *Br Med J* 1999;318(7188):901–904.
14. Casarett D, Knebel A, Helmers K. Ethical challenges of palliative care research. *J Pain Symptom Manage* 2003;25(4):S3–S5.
15. de Raeve L. Ethical issues in palliative care research. *Palliat Med* 1994;8(4):298–305.
16. Annas GJ. *Some choice: law, medicine, and the market.* New York: Oxford University Press, 1998.
17. Casarett D, Karlawish J. Are special ethical guidelines needed for palliative care research? *J Pain Symptom Manage* 2000;20:130–139.
18. Hilts PJ. *VA Hospital is told to halt all research.* New York Times. March 25, 1999.
19. Lynn J, Johnson J, Levine RJ. The ethical conduct of health services research: a case study of 55 institutions' applications to the SUPPORT project. *Clin Res* 1994;42:3–10.
20. Brett A, Grodin M. Ethical aspects of human experimentation in health services research. *JAMA* 1991;265:1854–1857.
21. Casarett D, Karlawish J, Sugarman J. Determining when quality improvement activities should be reviewed as research: proposed criteria and potential implications. *JAMA* 2000;283:2275–2280.
22. Cretin S, Keeler EB, Lynn J, et al. Should patients in quality-improvement activities have the same protections as participants in research studies? *JAMA* 2000;284:1786.
23. Freedman B. Scientific value and validity as ethical requirements for research: a proposed explication. *IRB Rev Hum Subjects Res* 1987;9:7–10.
24. Rutstein DR. The ethical design of human experiments. In: Freund PA, ed. *Experimentation with human subjects.* New York: George Braziller, 1970:383–401.
25. Casarett DJ, Karlawish JH, Moreno JD. A taxonomy of value in clinical research. *IRB Rev Hum Subjects Res* 2002;24(6):1–6.
26. Brody BA. *World Medical Association, declaration of Helsinki. The ethics of biomedical research. An international perspective.* New York: Oxford University Press, 1998.
27. The nuremberg code. Reprinted In: Brody B. *The ethics of biomedical research. An international perspective.* New York: Oxford University Press, 1947:213.
28. Freedman B. Placebo-controlled trials and the logic of clinical purpose. *IRB Rev Hum Subjects Res* 1990;12:1–6.
29. Advisory, Committee, on, Human, Radiation, Experiments. Final Report. Vol 061 00000848-9. Washington, DC: Government Printing Office, 1995.

30. Casarett DJ, Karlawish J, Sankar P, et al. Obtaining informed consent for clinical pain research: patients' concerns and information needs. *Pain* 2001;92:71–79.
31. Meinert CL. *Clinical trials. Design, conduct, and analysis.* Oxford: Oxford University Press, 1986.
32. Moore RA, Gavaghan D, Tramer MR, et al. Size is everything—large amounts of information are needed to overcome random effects in estimating direction and magnitude of treatment effects. *Pain* 1998;78:209–216.
33. Casarett D. How are hospice patients referred from academic medical centers different? *J Pain Symptom Manage* 2001;27:197–203.
34. Casarett D, Kirschling J, Levetown M, et al. NHPCO task force statement on hospice participation in research. *J Palliat Med* 2001;4:441–449.
35. Du Pen SL, Du Pen AR, Polissar N, et al. Implementing guidelines for cancer pain management: results of a randomized controlled clinical trial. *J Clin Oncol* 1999;17(1):361–370.
36. Ahmedzai S, Brooks D. Transdermal fentanyl versus sustained-release oral morphine in cancer pain: preference, efficacy, and quality of life. The TTS-Fentanyl Comparative Trial Group. *J Pain Symptom Manage* 1997; 13(5):254–261.
37. Freedman B. Equipoise and the ethics of clinical research. *N Engl J Med* 1987;317:141–145.
38. Ingham J, Seidman A, Yao TJ, et al. An exploratory study of frequent pain measurement in a cancer clinical trial. *Qual Life Res* 1996;5(5):503–507.
39. Twycross R, Harcourt J, Bergl S. A survey of pain in patients with advanced cancer. *J Pain Symptom Manage* 1996;12(5):273–282.
40. Parmelee PA, Smith B, Katz IR. Pain complaints and cognitive status among elderly institution residents. *J Am Geriatr Soc* 1993;41:517–522.
41. Ward SE, Gordon DB. Patient satisfaction and pain severity as outcomes in pain management: a longitudinal view of one setting's experience. *J Pain Symptom Manage* 1996;11(4):242–251.
42. Desbiens NA, Wu AW, Broste SK, et al. Pain and satisfaction with pain control in seriously ill hospitalized adults: findings from the SUPPORT research investigations. *Crit Care Med* 1996;24(12):1953–1961.
43. Derogatis LR, Morrow GR, Fetting J, et al. The prevalence of psychiatric disorders among cancer patients. *JAMA* 1983;249:751–757.
44. Kathol RG, Mutgi A, Williams J, et al. Diagnosis of depression in cancer patients according to four sets of criteria. *Am J Psychiatry* 1990;147: 1021–1024.
45. Freedman B, Fuks A, Weijer C. Demarcating research and treatment: a systematic approach for the analysis of the ethics of clinical research. *Clin Res* 1992;40:653–660.
46. Kirkham SR, Abel J. Placebo-controlled trials in palliative care: the argument against. *Palliat Med* 1997;11(6):489–492.
47. Hardy JR. Placebo-controlled trials in palliative care: the argument for. *Palliat Med* 1997;11(5):415–418.
48. Macklin R. The ethical problems with sham surgery in clinical research. *N Engl J Med* 1999;341:992–996.
49. Rothman KJ, Michels KB. The continuing unethical use of placebo controls. *N Engl J Med* 1994;331:394–398.
50. Temple RT, Ellenberg SS. Placebo-controlled trials and active control trials in the evaluation of new treatments. Part 1: ethical and scientific issues. *Ann Intern Med* 2000;133:455–463.
51. Shapiro AK, Shapiro E. The placebo: is it much ado about nothing? In: Harrington A, ed. *The placebo effect.* Cambridge: Harvard University Press, 1998.
52. World Medical Association International Code of Medical Ethics; amended by the 35th World Medical Assembly; October, 1983, 2000; Venice, Italy.
53. Broomhead A, Kerr R, Tester W, et al. Comparison of a once-a-day sustained-release morphine formulation with standard oral morphine treatment for cancer pain. *J Pain Symptom Manage* 1997;14(2):63–73.
54. Maxon HRD, Schroder LE, Hertzberg VS, et al. Rhenium-186(Sn)HEDP for treatment of painful osseous metastases: results of a double-blind crossover comparison with placebo. *J Nucl Med* 1991;32(10):1877–1881.
55. Silverman DG, O'Connor TZ, Brull SJ. Integrated assessment of pain scores and rescue morphine use during studies of analgesic efficacy. *Anesth Analg* 1993;77:168–170.
56. Haak van der Lely F, Burm AG, van Kleef JW, et al. The effect of epidural administration of alfentanil on intra-operative intravenous alfentanil requirements during nitrous oxide-oxygen-alfentanil anaesthesia for lower abdominal surgery. *Anaesthesia* 1994;49(12):1034–1038.
57. Hahn AF, Bolton CF, Pillay N, et al. Plasma-exchange therapy in chronic inflammatory demyelinating polyneuropathy. A double-blind, sham-controlled, cross-over study. *Brain* 1996;119(Pt 4):1055–1066.
58. Bruera E. Ethical issues in palliative care research. *J Palliat Care* 1994; 10:7–9.
59. Family Caregiving: Agenda for Action, Improving Services and Support for America's Family Caregivers, National Health Council. Washington, DC: 1999.
60. Steele RG, Fitch MI. Needs of family caregivers of patients receiving home hospice care for cancer. *Oncol Nurs Forum* 1996;23:823–828.
61. Emanuel EJ, Fairclough DL, Slutsman J, et al. Assistance from family members, friends, paid care givers, and volunteers in the care of terminally ill patients. *N Engl J Med* 1999;341:956–963.
62. Takesaka J, Crowley R, Casarett D. What is the risk of distress in palliative care survey research? *J Pain Symptom Manage* 2004;28(6):593–598.
63. Grisso T, Appelbaum PS. *Assessing competence to consent to treatment.* New York: Oxford University Press, 1998.
64. Marson DC, Schmitt FA, Ingram KK, et al. Determining the competency of Alzheimer patients to consent to treatment and research. *Alzheimer Dis Assoc Disord* 1994;8(Suppl 4):5–18.
65. Elliott C. Caring about risks: are severely depressed patients competent to consent to research? *Arch Gen Psychiatry* 1997;54:113–116.
66. Lemaire F, Blanch L, Cohen SL, et al. Working Group on Ethics. Informed consent for research purposes in intensive care patients in Europe—part II. An official statement of the European Society of Intensive Care Medicine. *Intensive Care Med* 1997;23(4):435–439.
67. Breitbart W, Bruera E, Chochinov H, et al. Neuropsychiatric syndromes and psychological symptoms in patients with advanced cancer. *J Pain Symptom Manage* 1995;10(2):131–141.
68. Pereira J, Hanson J, Bruera E. The frequency and clinical course of cognitive impairment in patients with terminal cancer. *Cancer* 1997;79(4):835–842.
69. Bruera E, Franco JJ, Maltoni M, et al. Changing pattern of agitated impaired mental status in patients with advanced cancer: association with cognitive monitoring, hydration, and opioid rotation. *J Pain Symptom Manage* 1995;10(4):287–291.
70. Bruera E, MacMillan K, Kuehn N, et al. The cognitive effects of the administration of narcotics. *Pain* 1989;39:13–16.
71. Stiefel FC, Breitbart W, Holland JC. Corticosteroids in cancer: neuropsychiatric complications. *Cancer Invest* 1989;7:479–491.
72. Breitbart W, Marotta R, Platt MM, et al. A double-blind trial of haloperidol, chlorpromazine, and lorazepam in the treatment of delirium in hospitalized AIDS patients. *Am J Psychiatry* 1996;153(2):231–237.
73. Brown JH, Henteleff P, Barakat S, et al. Is it normal for terminally ill patients to desire death? *Am J Psychiatry* 1986;143:208–211.
74. Massie MJ, Holland JC. Depression and the cancer patient. *J Clin Psychiatry* 1990;51:12–17.
75. Eisenach JC, DuPen S, Dubois M, et al. The Epidural Clonidine Study Group. Epidural clonidine analgesia for intractable cancer pain. *Pain* 1995;61(3):391–399.
76. Pappas GD, Lazorthes Y, Bes JC, et al. Relief of intractable cancer pain by human chromaffin cell transplants: experience at two medical centers. *Neurol Res* 1997;19(1):71–77.
77. Plancarte R, de Leon-Casasola OA, El-Helaly M, et al. Neurolytic superior hypogastric plexus block for chronic pelvic pain associated with cancer. *Reg Anesth* 1997;22(6):562–568.
78. Kristjanson LJ, Hanson EJ, Balneaves L. Research in palliative care populations: ethical issues. *J Palliat Care* 1994;10(3):1010–1015.
79. Dresser R. Bound to treatment: the Ulysses contract. *Hastings Cent Rep* 1984;14:13–16.
80. Miller CK, O'Donnell DC, Searight HR, et al. The deaconess informed consent comprehension test: an assessment tool for clinical research subjects. *Pharmacotherapy* 1996;16(5):872–878.
81. Penman DT, Holland JC, Bahna GF, et al. Informed consent for investigational chemotherapy: patients' and physicians' perceptions. *J Clin Oncol* 1984;2:849–855.
82. Grisso T, Appelbaum PS. The MacArthur treatment competence study III. *Law Hum Behav* 1995;19:149–174.
83. Mercadante S. Celiac plexus block vs. analgesics in pancreatic cancer pain. *Pain* 1993;52:187–192.
84. Boswell G, Bekersky I, Mekki Q, et al. Plasma concentrations and disposition of clonidine following a constant 14-day epidural infusion in cancer patients. *Clin Ther* 1997;19(5):1024–1030.
85. Hoffman M, Xu JC, Smith C, et al. A pharmacodynamic study of morphine and its glucuronide metabolites after single morphine dosing in cancer patients with pain. *Cancer Invest* 1997;15(6):542–547.
86. National Bioethics Advisory Commission. *Research involving persons with mental disorders that may affect decisionmaking capacity.* Rockville, MD: 1998.
87. High DM, Whitehouse PJ, Post SG, et al. Guidelines for addressing ethical and legal issues in Alzheimer disease research: a position paper. *Alzheimer Dis Assoc Disord* 1994;8:66–74.
88. High DM. Advancing research with Alzheimer disease subjects: investigators' perceptions and ethical issues. *Alzheimer Dis Assoc Disord* 1993;7: 165–178.
89. Agrawal M. Voluntariness in clinical research at the end of life. *J Pain Symptom Manage* 2003;25(4):25–32.
90. Beauchamp TL, Childress JF. *Principles of biomedical ethics*, 5th ed. Oxford: Oxford University Press, 2001.
91. Faden RR, Beauchamp TL. *A history and theory of informed consent.* New York: Oxford University Press, 1986.

Note: Page numbers followed by *f* indicate figures; those followed by *t* indicate tables.